D1224210

PATHOLOGIC BASIS *of* VETERINARY DISEASE

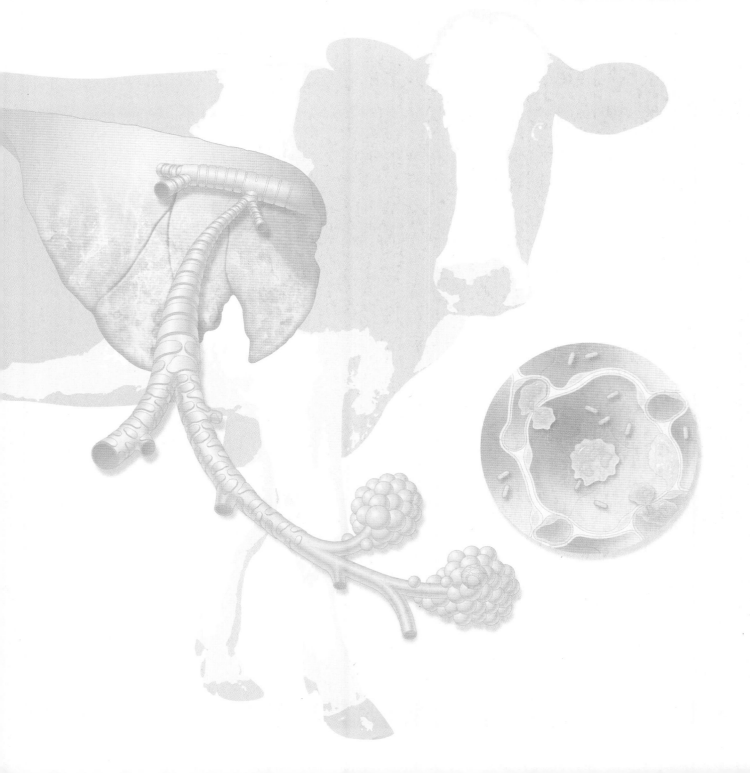

ELSEVIER

evolve

To access your Instructor Resources, visit:

http://evolve.elsevier.com/McGavin/vetdisease

Evolve Student Learning Resources for *McGavin and Zachary: Pathologic Basis of Veterinary Disease,* offers the following features:

Learning Resources

- **WebLinks**
This exciting resource lets you link to hundreds of websites carefully chosen to supplement the content of the textbook. The WebLinks are updated regularly, with new ones added as they develop.

http://evolve.elsevier.com/McGavin/vetdisease

PATHOLOGIC BASIS
of VETERINARY
DISEASE

FOURTH
EDITION

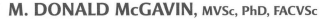

M. DONALD McGAVIN, MVSc, PhD, FACVSc

Diplomate, American College of Veterinary Pathologists
Professor Emeritus of Veterinary Pathology
Department of Pathobiology
College of Veterinary Medicine
University of Tennessee
Knoxville, Tennessee

JAMES F. ZACHARY, DVM, PhD

Diplomate, American College of Veterinary Pathologists
Professor of Experimental Pathology
Department of Pathobiology
College of Veterinary Medicine
University of Illinois
Urbana, Illinois

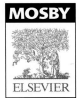

MOSBY

ELSEVIER

With over 2100 illustrations

MOSBY
ELSEVIER

11830 Westline Industrial Drive
St. Louis, Missouri 63146

PATHOLOGIC BASIS OF VETERINARY DISEASE   ISBN-13: 978-0-323-02870-7
Copyright © 2007, 2001, 1995, 1988 by Mosby, Inc.,   ISBN-10: 0-323-02870-5
an affiliate of Elsevier Inc.

All rights reserved. No part of this publication may be reproduced or transmitted in any form or by any means, electronic or mechanical, including photocopy, recording, or any information storage and retrieval system, without permission in writing from the publisher. Permissions may be sought directly from Elsevier's Health Sciences Rights Department in Philadelphia, PA, USA: phone: (+1) 215 239 3804, fax: (+1) 215 239 3805, e-mail: healthpermissions@elsevier.com. You may also complete your request on-line via the Elsevier homepage (http://www.elsevier.com), by selecting 'Customer Support' and then 'Obtaining Permissions'.

Notice

Knowledge and best practice in this field are constantly changing. As new research and experience broaden our knowledge, changes in practice, treatment, and drug therapy may become necessary or appropriate. Readers are advised to check the most current information provided (i) on procedures featured or (ii) by the manufacturer of each product to be administered, to verify the recommended dose or formula, the method and duration of administration, and contraindications. It is the responsibility of the practitioner, relying on his or her own experience and knowledge of the patient, to make diagnoses, to determine dosages and the best treatment for each individual patient, and to take all appropriate safety precautions. To the fullest extent of the law, neither the Publisher nor the Authors assume any liability for any injury and/or damage to persons or property arising out or related to any use of the material contained in this book.

ISBN-13: 978-0-323-02870-7
ISBN-10: 0-323-02870-5

Publishing Director: Linda L. Duncan
Publisher: Penny Rudolph
Managing Editor: Teri Merchant
Publishing Services Manager: Patricia Tannian
Project Manager: Kristine Feeherty
Design Direction: Teresa McBryan

Printed in China

Last digit is the print number: 9   8   7   6   5   4

Working together to grow
libraries in developing countries

www.elsevier.com | www.bookaid.org | www.sabre.org

ELSEVIER   BOOK AID International   Sabre Foundation

To
Beverley Simes Collins McGavin
A true Celtic warrior

Contributors

MARK R. ACKERMANN, DVM, PhD

Diplomate
American College of Veterinary Pathologists;
Professor and JG Salsbury Endowed Chair
Department of Veterinary Pathology
College of Veterinary Medicine
Iowa State University
Ames, Iowa

CHARLES C. CAPEN, DVM, MSc, PhD

Diplomate
American College of Veterinary Pathologists;
Professor and Chairman
Department of Veterinary Biosciences
College of Veterinary Medicine
The Ohio State University
Columbus, Ohio

ANTHONY W. CONFER, DVM, PhD

Diplomate
American College of Veterinary Pathologists;
Regents Professor
Department Head
Sitlington Endowed Chair for Food Animal Research
Department of Veterinary Pathobiology
College of Veterinary Medicine
Oklahoma State University
Stillwater, Oklahoma

JOHN M. CULLEN, VMD, PhD

Diplomate
American College of Veterinary Pathologists;
Professor
Population Health and Pathobiology
College of Veterinary Medicine
North Carolina State University
Raleigh, North Carolina

†VICTOR J. FERRANS, MD, PhD

Senior Research Scientist
Pathology Branch
National Heart, Lung, and Blood Institute
National Institutes of Health
Bethesda, Maryland

ROBERT A. FOSTER, BVSc, PhD, MACVSc

Diplomate
American College of Veterinary Pathologists;
Associate Professor
Department of Pathobiology
Ontario Veterinary College
University of Guelph
Guelph, Ontario

MICHAEL M. FRY, DVM, MS

Diplomate
American College of Veterinary Pathologists;
Assistant Professor
Pathobiology
College of Veterinary Medicine
University of Tennessee
Knoxville, Tennessee

HOWARD B. GELBERG, DVM, PhD

Diplomate
American College of Veterinary Pathologists;
Professor of Pathology
College of Veterinary Medicine
Oregon State University
Corvallis, Oregon

PAMELA E. GINN, DVM

Diplomate
American College of Veterinary Pathologists;
Associate Professor
Infectious Diseases and Pathology
College of Veterinary Medicine
University of Florida
Gainesville, Florida

ANN M. HARGIS, DVM, MS

Diplomate
American College of Veterinary Pathologists;
Affiliate Associate Professor
Department of Comparative Medicine
University of Washington, School of Medicine
Seattle, Washington;
Owner
DermatoDiagnostics
Edmonds, Washington;
Consultant
Phoenix Central Laboratory
Everett, Washington

DONNA F. KUSEWITT, DVM, PhD

Diplomate
American College of Veterinary Pathologists;
Professor
Department of Veterinary Biosciences
College of Veterinary Medicine
The Ohio State University
Columbus, Ohio

†Deceased.

KRISTA M.D. LA PERLE, DVM, PhD

Diplomate
American College of Veterinary Pathologists;
Director
Laboratory of Comparative Pathology and Genetically
Engineered Mouse Phenotyping Core
Assistant Professor of Pathology and Laboratory Medicine
Memorial Sloan-Kettering Cancer Center
Weill Medical College of Cornell University and Rockefeller
University
New York, New York

ALFONSO LÓPEZ, MVZ, MSc, PhD

Professor of Pathology
Department of Pathology and Microbiology
Atlantic Veterinary College
University of Prince Edward Island
Charlottetown, Prince Edward Island

M. DONALD MCGAVIN, MVSc, PhD, FACVSc

Diplomate
American College of Veterinary Pathologists;
Professor Emeritus of Veterinary Pathology
Department of Pathobiology
College of Veterinary Medicine
University of Tennessee
Knoxville, Tennessee

DEREK A. MOSIER, DVM, PhD

Diplomate
American College of Veterinary Pathologists;
Department of Diagnostic Medicine/Pathobiology
College of Veterinary Medicine
Kansas State University
Manhattan, Kansas

RONALD K. MYERS, DVM, PhD

Diplomate
American College of Veterinary Pathologists;
Department of Veterinary Pathology
College of Veterinary Medicine
Iowa State University
Ames, Iowa

SHELLEY J. NEWMAN, DVM, DVSc

Diplomate
American College of Veterinary Pathologists;
Assistant Professor
Anatomic Pathology
Department of Pathology
College of Veterinary Medicine
University of Tennessee
Knoxville, Tennessee

ROGER J. PANCIERA, DVM, MS, PhD

Diplomate
American College of Veterinary Pathologists;
Professor Emeritus
Department of Veterinary Pathobiology
College of Veterinary Medicine
Oklahoma State University
Stillwater, Oklahoma

LAURA J. RUSH, DVM, PhD

Diplomate
American College of Veterinary Pathologists;
Assistant Professor
Department of Veterinary Biosciences
College of Veterinary Medicine
The Ohio State University
Columbus, Ohio

PAUL W. SNYDER, DVM, PhD

Diplomate
American College of Veterinary Pathologists;
Associate Professor of Pathology
Veterinary Pathobiology Department
School of Veterinary Medicine
Purdue University
West Lafayette, Indiana

BETH A. VALENTINE, DVM, PhD

Diplomate
American College of Veterinary Pathologists;
Associate Professor
Department of Biomedical Sciences
College of Veterinary Medicine
Oregon State University
Corvallis, Oregon

JOHN F. VAN VLEET, DVM, PhD

Diplomate
American College of Veterinary Pathologists;
Professor of Veterinary Pathology
Associate Dean for Academic Affairs
School of Veterinary Medicine
Purdue University
West Lafayette, Indiana

STEVEN E. WEISBRODE, VMD, PhD

Diplomate
American College of Veterinary Pathologists;
Professor
Department of Veterinary Biosciences
College of Veterinary Medicine
The Ohio State University
Columbus, Ohio

BRIAN P. WILCOCK, DVM, PhD

Professor Emeritus
Department of Pathobiology
Ontario Veterinary College
University of Guelph;
Chief Pathologist
Histovet Surgical Pathology
Guelph, Ontario

JAMES F. ZACHARY, DVM, PhD

Diplomate
American College of Veterinary Pathologists;
Professor of Experimental Pathology
Department of Pathobiology
College of Veterinary Medicine
University of Illinois
Urbana, Illinois

Preface

Pathologic Basis of Veterinary Disease, the fourth edition in the last two decades in the series previously titled *Thomson's Special Veterinary Pathology*, has been revised and expanded but with the same goal in mind as for the past editions: to provide students of veterinary medicine with a textbook comprehensive enough to meet the needs of the professional curriculum with an emphasis on responses of the cell, tissue, and organ to injury. This book is not meant to be encyclopedic; specific diseases have been selected either because they are of primary importance in veterinary medicine or because they illustrate a basic pathogenetic mechanism. To aid in the understanding of mechanisms, six chapters on basic pathology have been added and pathogenesis and mechanisms of disease have been emphasized by the extensive use of color gross photographs and photomicrographs, schematic diagrams, summary boxes, and tables.

Change not only is a fundamental concept taught in basic cellular pathology but also occurs in the process of writing, editing, and publishing educational textbooks. Advances in technology in publishing during the last decade have provided an opportunity to transform the "traditional" format and content of our textbooks. Thus *Thomson's Special Veterinary Pathology* has become *Pathologic Basis of Veterinary Disease* and was designed to use the expertise of contributors, editors, and the production staff at Elsevier. It should come as no surprise that this book was modeled (unashamedly) on its highly successful counterpart text in human medicine, *Robbins and Cotran Pathologic Basis of Disease*.

The goals of *Pathologic Basis of Veterinary Disease* are to focus the student's attention on how (1) cells and tissues respond to injury in a chronological sequence of events and (2) to understand the interplay of host defense mechanisms with microbes and injurious agents in developing a clear appreciation of the pathogenesis of a disease process. Hence, it is our decision not to cover every disease reported in the veterinary literature or describe and illustrate every nuance of their lesions. Instead, we hope the book will provide a "mechanistic" bridge between the student's understanding of structure, function, microbes, and cell injury learned in the basic sciences and the interpretation of results of physical examination, disease differential diagnoses, imaging modalities, biochemical and molecular diagnostics, and therapeutic strategies presented to the student in the clinical years.

NEW TO THIS EDITION

To accomplish these goals, six new chapters covering basic pathology have been added to the book as Section I: General Pathology, to provide a substantive basis for understanding the materials presented in the chapters within Section II: Pathology of Organ Systems. These latter chapters were revised to incorporate new materials on structure and function of cells and tissues as they relate to disease processes, portals of entry of and defense mechanisms against microbes and injurious agents, and the chronological sequence of events in the mechanism of a disease. The content of most of the chapters was based on materials from the third edition, and these chapters have been extensively updated and revised to fulfill the goal of a mechanistic approach to understanding disease.

Many three-dimensional color diagrams are included to assist students in developing a clearer understanding of the relationships between tissue structure and disease processes. Headings, summary boxes, tables, and glossaries now use color to emphasize the organization and flow of conceptual information. In addition, all diagrams used from the third edition have been either redrawn in color by Elsevier medical artists or replaced by illustrations generously provided by the editors of other Elsevier biomedical textbooks. Although we have used materials from many Elsevier books, we wish to extend our appreciation and special acknowledgment to the editors of the following books for use of some of their illustrative materials:

- Vinay Kumar, Abul K. Abbas, and Nelson Fausto: *Robbins and Cotran Pathologic Basis of Disease*
- Abraham L. Kierszenbaum: *Histology and Cell Biology: An Introduction to Pathology*
- Lee-Ellen C. Copstead and Jacquelyn L. Banasik: *Pathophysiology: Biological and Behavioral Perspectives*
- Kathryn L. McCance and Sue E. Huether: *Pathophysiology: The Biologic Basis for Disease in Adults and Children*
- Sue E. Huether and Kathryn L. McCance: *Understanding Pathophysiology*

EVOLVE SITE

A new Evolve website is a key addition to the fourth edition. The Evolve site provides a variety of resources for both instructors and students. For instructors there is an image collection of all 2100 figures in the book for use in lectures and presentations. For students we have included WebLinks, an exciting resource that links readers to hundreds of websites carefully chosen to supplement the content of the textbook.

ACKNOWLEDGMENTS

We wish to extend our deepest appreciation and thanks to our colleagues throughout the world (truly an international effort), who have so generously provided their illustrative materials for use in this book. Although space limitations preclude listing them here, their names are cited in the figure legend credit for each illustration. We also extend our deepest appreciation to Dr. Barry G. Harmon, Director of Noah's Arkive, and Ms. Lois K. Morrison, Educational Program Specialist, College of Veterinary Medicine, University of Georgia for their patience and assistance in identifying and allowing us to use color illustrations from the Arkive. We have made every attempt to properly credit each illustration to its original source; however, we recognize that inadvertent errors will be made in the long and complicated process of assembling a 1600-page textbook. In addition, veterinary pathologists are a relatively small and tightly integrated community composed of interns, residents, and graduate students as well as faculty members who all share photographs among themselves and with the archives of their institutions. Thus, a contributor of an illustration may not always correctly identify the original source. Please be understanding and address any concerns about credits to mmcgavin@utk.edu or zacharyj@uiuc.edu. We will make every effort to confirm the origin of the photograph and correct the acknowledgement before the book goes into the next printing.

Pathologic Basis of Veterinary Disease was conceived over 3 years ago, and its publication is an acknowledgment of the efforts of the Elsevier staff: Teri Merchant (Managing Editor), Linda McKinley (Book Production Manager), Kristine Feeherty (Project Manager), Don O'Connor (medical artist), Sheryl Krato, Stacy Beane, and John Dedeke. We also appreciate the input of Linda Duncan, Publishing Director. This process has not been without its challenges for them, especially when dealing with two editors, more than 20 chapter contributors, thousands of pages of text and illustrations, and checks and rechecks of edited manuscripts and proofs. Also, the advice of Dr. Robert W. Henry regarding correct anatomic orientation of gross specimens and Dr. David A. Bemis regarding bacteriologic nomenclature, as well as the help of the secretarial staff (Regina Dalton, Diane Dodson, and Colleen Ailor at the University of Tennessee), is gratefully acknowledged.

Finally, we wish to thank our families—Donald McGavin's wife, Beverley, and James Zachary's daughters, Amanda and Briana—for their support and encouragement during this challenging process. They have kindly understood our absences, long spells in the home office, weekends and evenings at work, and trips to St. Louis, Louisville, and Champaign. When we felt ready to give up, they provided the support to sustain the energy required for us to complete this project.

No greater impact can be made on students in their veterinary education than by teachers, including veterinary pathologists, who are willing to share expertise and knowledge with them. We hope that *Pathologic Basis of Veterinary Disease* will aid in this process, foster the student's understanding of mechanistic concepts, and perhaps also alter the way that veterinary pathologists think about teaching pathology.

M. DONALD McGAVIN

JAMES F. ZACHARY

Contents

GENERAL PATHOLOGY

Cellular and Tissue Responses to Injury

RONALD K. MYERS • M. DONALD McGAVIN

INTRODUCTION

The simple definition that pathology is the study of disease understates the wide range and contributions of this discipline to modern medicine. An understanding of pathology is fundamental to understanding how disease works and consequently how it can be diagnosed, treated, and prevented.

To students of medical science, pathology is the course of study that finally connects the study of normal form and function (histology, anatomy, and physiology) to the study of clinical medicine. Pathology is fundamental to making sense of how the various causes of disease (bacteriologic, virologic, and parasitologic causes, for example) interact with the host and result in clinically identifiable conditions.

Pathology is also an important professional practice that directly supports clinical practice. Diagnostic pathologists, for example, perform postmortem examinations (necropsies), which provide clinicians with essential information on how to manage disease outbreaks in herds and how to improve management of individual cases. Surgical pathologists examine tissue removed from live animals (biopsy) and provide diagnoses that help clinicians treat animals under their care. Toxicologic pathologists test and evaluate the effects and safety of drugs and chemicals in laboratory animals. Clinical pathologists perform tests on blood and other body fluids (hematology and serum chemistry, for example) and examine cells (cytology) to provide detailed and essential information for clinicians. Experimental pathologists study the tissue, cellular, and molecular mechanisms of human and animal diseases in the fields of biomedicine and biomedical engineering.

Pathology is also an experimental science that makes essential contributions to further our understanding of disease mechanisms through use of a tremendous variety of techniques. Advanced methods of cell and molecular biology are used to unravel the complexities of how cells and animals respond to injury, so that deeper understanding of diseases can help improve treatment and prevention.

In summary, pathology is according to one dictionary (Stedman's Medical Dictionary) "the medical science, and specialty practice, concerned with all aspects of disease, but with special reference to the essential nature, causes, and development of abnormal conditions, as well as the structural and functional changes that result from the disease processes."

BASIC TERMINOLOGY

If pathology is the study of disease, what is disease? A dictionary definition (Dorland's Medical Dictionary) states that disease is "any deviation from or interruption of the normal structure or function of any part, organ, or system (or combination thereof) of the body that is manifested by a characteristic set of symptoms and signs and whose etiology, pathology, and prognosis may be known or unknown." Disease is not just illness or sickness but includes any departure from normal form (lesions) and function, whether it is clinically apparent or not.

Pathologists study lesions but also the causes (etiologic agents) of the lesions to understand the pathogenesis of a disease. Pathogenesis is the mechanism of how a disease develops from its initiation to its cellular and molecular manifestations. Understanding pathogenesis is essential to understanding how a disease is initiated and progresses, how these changes relate to clinical signs at different stages of the disease, and how appropriate clinical action can be taken.

The relationship of pathology to clinical medicine and the use of some of the basic terms discussed previously along with some additional terms are illustrated in the following clinical scenario.

In a beef feedlot, several steers and heifers are exhibiting difficult breathing, hunched posture, and depression (clinical signs). Physical examination of some of the infected animals reveals elevated temperatures, pulse rates, and respiration rates. Auscultation of the thorax reveals absence of air movement in the cranial region of the thorax along with some crackles and wheezes in other lung fields. A clinical diagnosis of bronchopneumonia is made. Some of the animals die, and a necropsy (postmortem examination) is done. The cranioventral lobes of the lungs are dark red and firm, with fibrin covering the surface (gross lesions). A gross morphologic diagnosis of severe acute fibrinopurulent cranioventral bronchopneumonia is made. Formalin fixed samples are taken for microscopic examination (histopathology), neutrophilic inflammation of airways and alveoli with fibrin are noted (microscopic lesions), and a histologic morphologic diagnosis of severe acute fibrinopurulent bronchopneumonia is made. Fresh samples of lung are taken for bacterial and viral examination, and *Mannheimia haemolytica* and a bovine herpes virus (etiologic agents or causes) are identified. An etiologic diagnosis of *Mannheimia* bronchopneumonia and a disease diagnosis of "shipping fever pneumonia" are made.

The pathogenesis of the above disease might be stated in an abbreviated form like this:

> Various viruses, such as infectious rhinotracheitis virus, and environmental agents, such as dust and noxious gases, disrupt the clearance mechanisms of the airway epithelium allowing opportunistic organisms, such as the bacterium *Mannheimia haemolytica* to colonize and invade the alveoli. Virulence factors of the bacteria, such as endotoxin and various exotoxins, cause necrosis and inflammation, which result in the filling of alveoli and airways with fibrin and neutrophils.

Although the histologic diagnosis of the disease was done by a diagnostic pathologist, the details of this pathogenesis were discovered over time by researchers in many fields, including experimental pathologists.

TYPES OF DIAGNOSIS

Note in the previous scenario that various levels of diagnosis were made. Diagnosis is a concise statement or conclusion concerning the nature, cause, or name of a disease. The accuracy of a diagnosis is limited by the evidence (lesions) available for study. A clinical diagnosis is based on the data obtained from the case history, clinical signs, and physical examination. It often suggests only the system involved, or it provides a list of differential diagnoses. The differential diagnosis (often termed "rule outs" in clinical medicine) is a list of

diseases that could account for the evidence or lesions of the case. A clinical pathologic diagnosis is based on changes observed in the chemistry of fluids and the hematology, structure, and function of cells collected from the living patient. A morphologic diagnosis or lesion diagnosis is based on the predominant lesion(s) in the tissue(s) (see Chapter 3 and Fig. 3-24). It may be macroscopic (gross) or microscopic (histologic) and describes the severity, duration, distribution, location (organ or tissue), and nature (degenerative, inflammatory, neoplastic) of the lesion. An etiologic diagnosis is even more definitive and names the specific cause of the disease. A disease diagnosis is equally specific and states the common name of the disease.

One of the goals in making a diagnosis in a case is to enable a clinician to predict how the disease will progress or resolve. Prognosis is a statement of what the expected outcome of a condition is likely to be. If the lesion is expected to resolve (return to normal) with no expected lasting harm, the prognosis is good or excellent. If the outcome is uncertain—the lesion could resolve or become worse as a result of unforeseen factors— the prognosis is guarded. If the animal is not expected to recover from the lesion or disease, the prognosis is grave. Accurate determination of the prognosis demands a thorough understanding of the disease, especially pathogenesis.

As in this book, the study of pathology is often divided into two basic parts: general pathology and pathology of organ systems. General pathology is the study of basic responses of cells and tissues to insults and injuries, irrespective of the organs, systems, or species of animal involved. This area of pathology is one of the most complex and rapidly growing fields in the natural sciences, largely due to the availability and power of new research techniques. General pathology is studied first, so students will have a thorough understanding of the general principles of disease processes that they will encounter repeatedly in the study of diseases of body systems. Pathology of organ systems (sometimes called systemic or special pathology) involves the study of how each organ system reacts to injury associated with specific diseases.

MORPHOLOGIC CHANGES AND HOW THEY ARE DETECTED AND EVALUATED

The study and practice of pathology historically have been based on the macroscopic and microscopic changes that take place in diseased cells, tissues, and organs, that is to say, the morphology of lesions. Consequently, most pathology texts tend to emphasize anatomic pathology. Morphologic techniques remain the cornerstones of pathology, but progress in our deeper understanding of the mechanisms and in the diagnosis of disease rely more and more on techniques derived from cellular and molecular biology.

The basic tools for the study and practice of pathology begin with an open and inquiring mind, skills in observation, and careful and consistent postmortem techniques. The diagnosis of many diseases can be accurately accomplished with no more than gross examination of a body. Confirmation of gross lesions and discovery and interpretation of microscopic changes typically involves observation of tissue placed on glass microscope slides. Tissues are first fixed (i.e., preserved) usually in 10% formalin, embedded in blocks of paraffin wax, microtome sectioned to about 5 μm thickness, and routinely stained with hematoxylin and eosin (H&E). H&E stained sections are the mainstay of histopathology in both postmortem and surgical pathology, and interpretation of lesions in these specimens can often lead to a final diagnosis. A simplistic explanation of the labeling characteristics of the H&E stain as applied to tissue sections is as follows: Hematoxylin stains nucleic acids (nucleus, ribosomes, mitochondria) blue, whereas eosin stains proteins such as those found intracellularly (e.g., enzymes, actin, and myosin) or those proteins found extracellularly (e.g., collagen and extracellular matrix [ECM]) red or pink.

A variety of ancillary techniques are also used in histopathology. Histochemistry applies a variety of chemical reactions carried out on tissue sections. Glycogen, for example, can be identified in hepatocytes using periodic acid–Schiff (PAS) reaction. Suspected mast cell tumors are routinely stained to demonstrate the metachromatic mast cell granules using toluidine blue or Giemsa stains.

Increasing use in diagnostic laboratories is being made of immunohistochemistry, in which specific antigens are identified in tissue by antibodies linked to a chromogen. Detection of specific intermediate fibers by immunohistochemistry, in tumors for example, can separate malignant striated muscle tumors from other sarcomas. Specific infectious agents, such as the corona virus causing feline infectious peritonitis, can also be identified using immunohistochemistry.

A variety of techniques for identification of molecules or genetic sequences are now in use, with more expected. In situ hybridization, in which labeled nucleic acid probes can identify complementary strands of host or microbe DNA or RNA in intact cells and tissues, is particularly useful in the diagnosis and study of viral disease. These techniques are not as sensitive as PCR (polymerase chain reaction), in which small amounts of target DNA in biologic material are amplified and identified. Small amounts of target DNA of microbes (for example) can be identified in tissues, and RNA sequences can be identified after conversion to DNA and subsequent amplification.

The typical light microscope can magnify to about 1000× and is adequate for routine histopathology. Specialized microscopes such as dark field, phase contrast, and fluorescence microscopes are also used, often for identification of microbes. In both diagnostic and experimental settings, electron microscopy is used to visualize the subcellular structure of cells and microbes. Transmission electron microscopy of ultrathin sections allows resolution of ultrafine structures of less than a nanometer. Scanning electron microscopy allows the ultrafine observation of surfaces. Specialized analytical electron microscopes are also in use. Finally, laser capture microdissection allows pathologists to isolate and capture groups of similar cells from tumors or a diseased tissue Using DNA microarrays, the genes expressed by these cells can be identified and characterized, thus providing a "genetic fingerprint" of the disease process that clinically can be used to develop therapeutic strategies and assess the outcome.

THE NORMAL CELL

COMPONENTS OF NORMAL CELLS AND THEIR VULNERABILITIES

The early pathologists Morgagni and Bichat emphasized the importance of organs and tissues as the seat of disease. Virchow later focused on individual cells as the primary cause of abnormal function and structure associated with diseases. Before we can interpret lesions of sick cells, it is essential that we understand normal cell structure and function. The cell can be visualized simplistically as a membrane-enclosed compartment, subdivided into numerous smaller compartments (organelles) by membranes (Fig. 1-1). This vast interconnecting system of membrane-bound spaces is termed the "cytocavitary network." The function of these organelles is largely determined by the type and quantity of specific enzymes associated with each membrane and in the cytoplasmic matrix.

It is essential to have a clear understanding of the structure and function of the components of normal cells and how they are interrelated in a normally functioning cell. Cell membranes and organelles serve as targets for injury by microbes, harmful environmental agents, and a variety of genetic, metabolic, and toxicologic diseases discussed in greater detail in the Pathology of Organ Systems chapters of this book.

CELL MEMBRANES

Cell membranes are a fluid phospholipid bilayer penetrated by numerous specific proteins (Fig. 1-2). The two main biologic functions of these membranes are (1) to serve as selective barriers and (2) to form a structural base for the enzymes and receptors that

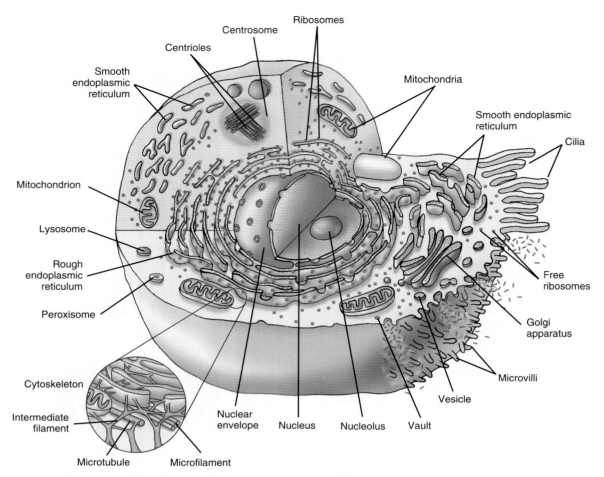

Fig. 1-1 **Cell structure and the organization of organelles, cytoskeleton, and membrane enhancements.** *(From McCance K, Huether S:* Pathophysiology: the biologic basis for disease in adults and children, *ed 4, St Louis, 2002, Mosby.)*

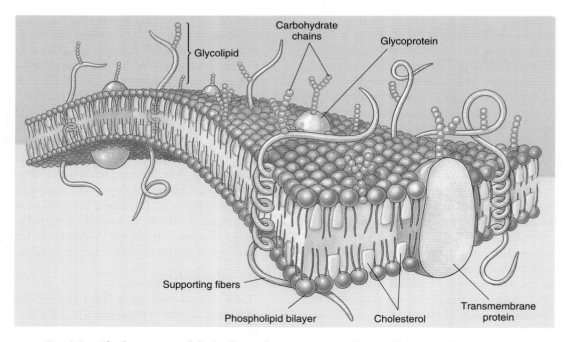

Fig. 1-2 **Fluid mosaic model of cell membrane structure.** The lipid bilayer provides the basic structure and serves as a relatively impermeable barrier to most water-soluble molecules.

(From Thibodeau GA, Patton KT: Structure & function of the human body, *ed 11, St Louis, 2000, Mosby.)*

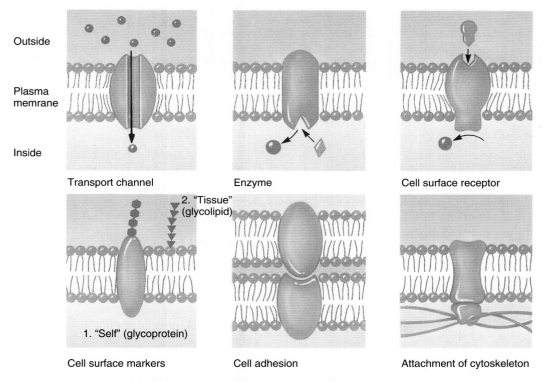

Outside

Plasma memrane

Inside

Transport channel

Enzyme

Cell surface receptor

2. "Tissue" (glycolipid)

1. "Self" (glycoprotein)

Cell surface markers

Cell adhesion

Attachment of cytoskeleton

Fig. 1-3   Functions of transmembrane proteins. A variety of functions are performed by different types of cell membranes as shown. *(From Raven PH, Johnson GB:* Understanding biology, *ed 3, Dubuque, Iowa, 1995, Brown.)*

determine cell function. Cell membranes form the boundaries of many organelles and separate them from the cytosol.

The plasma membrane is the cell's first contact with injurious agents. Microvilli and cilia are specialized areas of the plasma membrane and are often specifically altered in disease (Fig. 1-1). Plasma membranes separate the interior of the cell from external surfaces, neighboring cells, or surrounding matrix. Surface proteins, such as fibronectin, play a role in cell to cell and cell to extracellular matrix interactions. Transmembrane proteins embedded in the phospholipid bilayer serve in variety of structural, transport, and enzymatic functions essential to cell viability (Fig. 1-3). It is these transmembrane proteins that are often used by infectious microbes to enter or use cell systems during their life cycles, thus initiating a process that often results in injury to the host cell.

CYTOSOL

The cytosol is the watery gel in which the cell's organelles and inclusions are dispersed. Many chemical reactions occur in the cytosol mediated by "free" enzymes. The cytosol is a highly organized microtrabecular network.

MITOCHONDRIA

Mitochondria (singular = mitochondrion) are the "powerhouses" of highly specialized eukaryotic cells. They are the site of fatty acid oxidation, the citric acid cycle, and oxidative phosphorylation. Transfer of electrons from reduced cytochrome oxidase to molecular oxygen is the final and critical step culminating in these catabolic pathways. Important structural components of a mitochondrion are the outer membrane, outer compartment, inner membrane, inner compartment (matrix), cristae, and mitochondrial DNA. Damage to mitochondria results in diminished adenosine triphosphate (ATP) production and if damage is unchecked, cell death (Fig. 1-6).

NUCLEUS

The nucleus is that portion of the cell responsible for storage and transmission of genetic information (Fig. 1-1). Chains of DNA, complexed to protein, are chromatin. Areas of uncoiled chromatin (euchromatin) are active in the generation of mRNA for protein synthesis. Highly coiled chromatin (heterochromatin) is inactive in transcription. The outer nuclear membrane is continuous with that of the rough endoplasmic reticulum (RER).

NUCLEOLUS

The nucleolus is a basic organelle of the nucleus and is composed of RNA, nucleolus-associated chromatin, and protein (Fig. 1-1). It functions in the synthesis of rRNA, essential in protein synthesis. The nucleolus can be basophilic or eosinophilic, and its prominence is a subjective measure of the cell's synthetic activity.

ROUGH ENDOPLASMIC RETICULUM

The RER is a network of intracellular membranes studded with ribosomes (Fig. 1-4). RER is prominent in cells producing large amounts of extracellular protein (e.g., reactive fibroblasts, hepatocytes, plasma cells, and pancreatic acinar cells). The RER is responsible for the basophilia of the cytoplasm because of the numerous ribosomes, which contain acid (i.e., RNA).

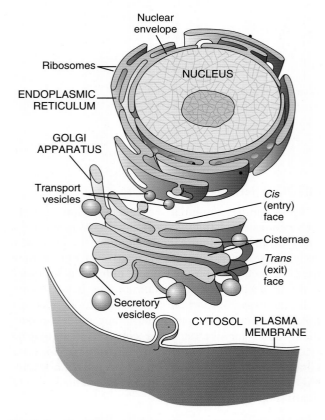

Fig. 1-4 Membrane systems. The rough endoplasmic reticulum and Golgi apparatus are important organelles in cellular biosynthesis of proteins and glycoproteins inserted into cell membranes and used in and secreted from cells. Transcription, translation, assembly, modification, and packaging of these molecules occur in an orderly sequence from the nucleus to the cell membrane as shown. Alterations in one or more of these steps can result in cell injury and serve as the underlying pathogenesis of a disease process.
(From Copstead L, Banasik J: Pathophysiology, ed 3, St Louis, 2005, Mosby.)

SMOOTH ENDOPLASMIC RETICULUM

Smooth endoplasmic reticulum (SER) is a tubular or vesicular form of cell membrane that lacks ribosomes (Fig. 1-1). SER is the locus of enzymes that metabolize steroids, drugs, lipids, and glycogen. It gives the cytoplasm a pale, finely vacuolated appearance as viewed in the light microscope.

GOLGI COMPLEX

The Golgi complex consists of several lamellar stacks or flattened sacs of membranes, vesicles, and vacuoles (Fig. 1-4). It functions in the synthesis of complex proteins by the addition of carbohydrate molecules and in the production of secretory vesicles and lysosomes.

LYSOSOMES

Lysosomes are small membrane-bound vesicles laden with hydrolytic enzymes essential for intracellular digestion (Fig. 1-1). They are discussed more completely as components of phagocytic cells. Peroxisomes are similar to lysosomes but also play a role in energy metabolism.

MICROFILAMENTS, INTERMEDIATE FILAMENTS, AND MICROTUBULES

These structures are composed of protein subunits and function in the cytoskeleton and in cell movement (Fig. 1-5). They have a prominent role in the mitotic spindle, cilia, microvilli, neurons, myocytes, and phagocytic cells. Many cell types besides muscles, for example, contain actin microfilaments.

Intermediate filaments are about 10 nm in diameter and are important in cell shape and movement. Different cell types have different intermediate filaments; for example, cytokeratins are found in epithelial cells, desmin in muscle cells, and vimentin in cells of mesenchymal origin such as fibroblasts. Intermediate filaments can be useful markers for classifyng undifferentiated neoplasms.

CELLULAR INCLUSIONS

Inclusions include glycogen granules, proteinaceous vacuoles, lipid debris, hemosiderin, viral particles, and calcium granules (discussed in greater detail later in this chapter). Some of these are normal, whereas others are the result of cell injury and will be discussed later in this chapter in the section dealing with intracellular and extracellular accumulations.

EXTRACELLULAR MATRIX

Although not part of the cell itself, the ECM and its integrity influences cell health and function (see Chapter 4 and Fig. 4-19). ECM includes basement membranes and interstitial matrices composed of various collagens, proteoglycans, and adhesive glycoproteins

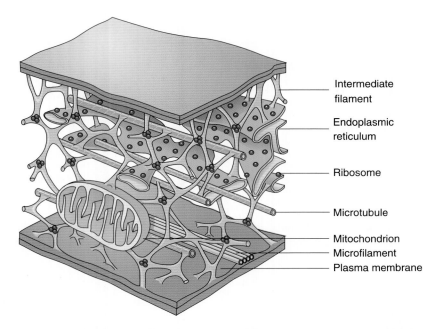

Fig. 1-5   Cytoskeleton. The complexity of and interrelations between intermediate filaments, microtubules, endoplasmic reticulum, and other cytoplasmic organelles that can be involved in the pathogenesis of diseases are shown. *(From McCance KL, Huether SE:* Pathophysiology: the biologic basis for disease in adults and children, *ed 4, St Louis, 2002, Mosby.)*

among a variety of other molecules that interact with cells by means of various integrin molecules. Basement membrane integrity, for example, is essential for the proper structure and functioning of epithelial cells. Other components of the ECM influence how cells grow and differentiate.

CAUSES OF CELL INJURY

Causes of cell injury are numerous and can be classified in a variety of ways. Some causes, such as physical trauma, viruses, and toxins, are clearly extrinsic, whereas others, such as spontaneous genetic mutations, are clearly intrinsic. Others, such as workload imbalance, nutritional abnormalities, and immunologic dysfunctions, can have components of both extrinsic and intrinsic mechanisms. General mechanisms of injury include ATP depletions (often caused by hypoxia), membrane damage (a result of a myriad of causes, including oxygen-derived free radicals), disturbances of cellular metabolism, and genetic damage (Fig. 1-6).

Understanding disease starts with understanding the cell. Until the nineteenth century, the dominant theory of disease in western societies was humoral pathology wherein disease was attributed to a maldistribution of body fluids or "humors." In the mid 1800s, Rudolph Virchow, a German pathologist now considered to be the founder of modern pathology, redefined pathology and medical science by his idea of the body

as an organization of cells, each suited for specific functions. He taught that disease resulted from injury to, or dysfunction of, specific populations of cells. The recent rapid advancement in medical science is owed to a great extent to Virchow's original emphasis on cellular pathology and more recently onmolecular pathology.

Cells can be injured by a large number of causes (etiologic agents). Fortunately the types of responses of the cell to injury are not as large. The responses to injury depend on many factors, including the type of agent, the extent of injury, the duration of injury, and the cell type affected. Renal tubular cells deprived of adequate blood supply, for example, may exhibit only cell swelling, if oxygen is soon restored. Prolonged lack of adequate blood supply (ischemia) can lead to cell death. Diminished but sublethal reduction in blood supply may result in cells adapting by decreasing their metabolic rates, which could lead to recovery or, if adaptation is inadequate, then eventually death.

Cells respond to stimuli and stressors in a variety of ways to maintain homeostasis. Cell injury takes place when a cell can no longer maintain a steady state. Some types of cell injury, such as cell swelling, can be reversible if the extent and duration of injury is not excessive. But if the injury exceeds certain limits, cell death and irreversible change occur. Not all cell injury results in cell death. Cell injury may be sublethal and result in a variety of types of cell degenerations or accumulations and/or adaptations by the cell to the injury.

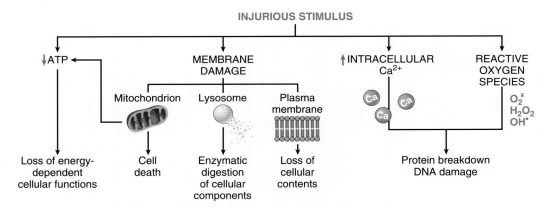

Fig. 1-6   **Cellular and biochemical sites of damage in cell injury.** *ATP,* Adenosine triphosphate.
*(From Kumar V, Abbas A, Fausto N: Robbins & Cotran pathologic basis of disease, ed 7, Philadelphia, 2005,
Saunders.)*

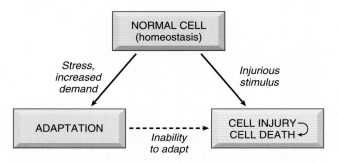

Fig. 1-7   **Stages in the cellular response to stress and injurious
stimuli.** *(From Kumar V, Abbas A, Fausto N: Robbins & Cotran pathologic
basis of disease, ed 7, Philadelphia, 2005, Saunders.)*

In essence, cells or tissues respond to injury (or stress) in
three important ways: (1) adaptation, (2) degeneration or
intracellular or extracellular accumulations, and (3) death
(Fig. 1-7).

Pathologically, reversible cell injury is injury from
which the cell can adapt or recover and thus return to
normal or nearly normal function. Irreversible cell injury
results in a dead cell. This distinction seems clear cut,
but the point at which a cell transitions from reversible
cell injury to irreversible cell injury (i.e., "the point of
no return") has been a major research challenge for the
past few decades and remains so today (Fig. 1-8). The
lesions of reversible and irreversible cell injury will be
discussed in greater detail in subsequent sections; however, in summary, the cytomorphologic changes characteristic of irreversible cell injury include the following:

- Plasma membrane damage
- Calcium entry into the cell
- Mitochondrial swelling and vacuolization
- Amorphous densities (likely calcium) in the
  mitochondria
- Lysosomal swelling

The causes of reversible and irreversible cell injury
resulting in cell death, cell adaptation and degeneration,
and finally cellular accumulations will be now be
discussed.

OXYGEN DEFICIENCY

Hypoxia is one of the most common and important
causes of cell injury and death (Fig. 1-8). Hypoxia is
a partial reduction in the O_2 concentration supplied
to cells or tissue; a complete reduction is referred to
as anoxia. Oxygen is critically important for oxidative
phosphorylation, especially in highly specialized cells
such as neurons, hepatocytes, cardiac myocytes, and
renal tubule cells. Hypoxia can result from inadequate
oxygenation of blood as a result of heart failure or respiratory failure, loss or reduction of blood supply
(ischemia), reduced transport of O_2 in blood (e.g., anemia
or carbon monoxide toxicity), and blockage of cell
respiratory enzymes (cyanide toxicosis).

PHYSICAL AGENTS

Trauma, extremes of heat and cold, radiation, and electrical energy may seriously injure cells. Trauma may cause
direct rupture and death of large numbers of cells, or it
may damage the blood supply to cells. Extreme cold
impairs the blood flow, and intracellular ice crystals
rupture cell membranes. Extreme heat denatures essential cell enzymes and other proteins. Excessive heat can
increase the rate of metabolic reactions so that substrates,
water, and pH changes reach lethal levels. Electricity generates great heat as it passes through tissue. It also alters
conduction of nerves and muscle. Ionizing radiation
causes ionization of cellular water with production of
highly reactive "free radicals" that injure cell components.
Many forms of radiation may damage genetic material

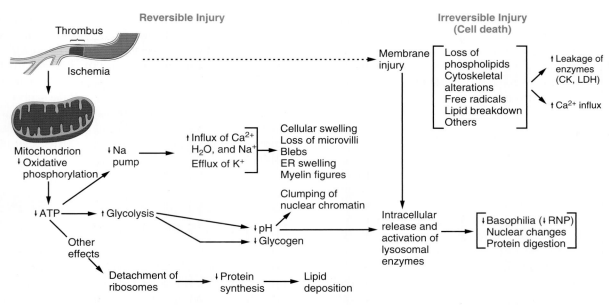

Fig. 1-8   Postulated sequence of events in reversible and irreversible ischemic cell injury. Note that although reduced oxidative phosphorylation and adenosine triphosphate *(ATP)* levels have a central role, ischemia can cause direct membrane damage. *ER,* Endoplasmic reticulum; *CK,* creatine kinase; *LDH,* lactate dehydrogenase; *RNP,* ribonucleoprotein. *(From Kumar V, Abbas A, Fausto N: Robbins & Cotran pathologic basis of disease, ed 7, Philadelphia, 2005, Saunders.)*

resulting in reproductive death of cells, genetic defects, and neoplasia.

INFECTIOUS AGENTS

Viruses are obligate intracellular parasites that redirect host cell enzyme systems toward synthesis of viral proteins and genetic materials, to the detriment of host cells. Cell changes induced by viral agents vary from little effect to cell death or neoplastic transformation.

Injury due to bacterial infection varies and can result from the action of potent toxins on specific host cells (clostridial infections, enterotoxigenic *Escherichia coli* infection) or from an overwhelming or ineffective inflammatory response to uncontrolled bacterial replication in tissue. Some bacteria, such as *Lawsonia intracellularis*, can result in excessive intestinal epithelial cell replication.

Mycotic agents resist destruction by the body that can lead to progressive, chronic inflammatory disease with loss of normal host tissues. Protozoal agents replicate in specific host cells, often resulting in destruction of infected cells. Metazoan parasites cause inflammation, distort tissue, and use host nutrients.

NUTRITIONAL DEFICIENCIES AND IMBALANCES

Dietary protein-calorie deficiencies are seen sporadically in animals and humans (known as kwashiorkor).

These deficiencies require metabolic adaptation by large populations of cells. Lipolysis, catabolism of muscle protein, and glycogenolysis enable short-term survival. Calorie excess, as seen in many pets and people of affluent societies, is implicated in cardiovascular disease and several other diseases. Vitamin and mineral imbalances are common due to errors in formulating rations and hypersupplementation by well-meaning animal owners.

GENETIC DERANGEMENT

A normal genetic apparatus is essential for cell homeostasis. Mutations, whatever their origin, may cause no disease, may deprive a cell of a protein (enzyme) critical for normal function, or may be incompatible with cell survival. A few examples of genetic diseases are defects of clotting factors (hemophilia), lysosomal storage disease (mannosidosis), combined immunodeficiency of Arabian foals, and defects of collagen synthesis (dermatosparaxis). Besides causing overt disease, some genotypes cause the host to be more prone to certain types of extrinsic or intrinsic disease, a condition often termed genetic predisposition.

WORKLOAD IMBALANCE

Cells that are overworked may adapt to the demand or eventually become exhausted and die. Conversely, cells that are no longer stimulated to work may shrink in size and waste away. An example is the way endocrine tissues react to the presence or absence of specific trophic hormones. Muscle fibers, deprived of work or their nerve supply, will atrophy and ultimately disappear, leaving a fibrous stroma.

CHEMICALS, DRUGS, AND TOXINS

Chemicals, drugs, and toxins influence cells by a multitude of mechanisms. Drugs produce their therapeutic effects by modifying the function (and morphology) of specific populations of cells. Most drugs cause these cells to adapt within a tolerable range of homeostasis. Chemicals, including drugs and toxins, can block or stimulate cell membrane receptors, alter specific enzyme systems, produce toxic free radicals, alter cell permeability, damage chromosomes, modify metabolic pathways, and damage structural components of cells.

IMMUNOLOGIC DYSFUNCTION

The immune system may fail to respond to infectious agents and other antigens as a result of congenital or acquired defects of lymphoid tissue or their products. Examples of congenital defects are thymic aplasia of nude mice and combined immunodeficiency of Arabian foals. Affected animals may die at an early age from infection by opportunistic microorganisms. Acquired immunodeficiency disease may be transient and results from damage to lymphoid tissue by viral infection, chemicals, and drugs.

The immune response directed toward foreign antigens (pathogenic organisms) is usually beneficial to the host, but sometimes the response is misdirected against antigens of host cells. This large group of diseases is referred to as autoimmune disease. An inappropriate or exaggerated response to certain antigens results in immunologic disease referred to as hypersensitivity (allergy). Some examples are anaphylaxis, feline asthma, and flea allergy dermatitis. The activity of the immune system is greatly amplified by its effect on serum complement and inflammation. These reactions often lead to serious injury to the kidney, skin, and joints.

AGING

The diminished capacity of aged cells and tissue to carry out their normal functions can hardly be disputed. One can argue that aging is simply the culmination of life's injuries inflicted by chemicals, infectious agents, work imbalances, or poor nutrition. We use the aging category for those lesions commonly found in aged animals; lesions for which we have no other defensible mechanistic explanation. Some of the lesions commonly found

in older animals include: nodular hyperplasia of parenchymal cells in the liver, pancreas, adrenal, spleen, and thyroid. There appear to be defects in growth control of these cell populations, but the cause is unclear. Aged cells may suffer a lifetime of damage to their DNA, or there may be accumulation of cellular debris that interferes with normal cell functions. One could argue that many cancers are caused by old age, rather than by exposure to specific chemicals, foods, viruses, or other insults.

REVERSIBLE CELL INJURY

ACUTE CELL SWELLING

Cell swelling, also called hydropic degeneration, is the most common and fundamental expression of cell injury (Fig. 1-9). It is manifested as increased cell size and volume resulting from an overload of water caused by a failure of the cell to maintain normal homeostasis and regulate the ingress and excretion of water. It is accompanied by modification and degeneration of organelles. Mechanisms responsible for acute cell swelling usually involve damage to cellular membranes, failure of cellular energy production, or injury to enzymes regulating ion channels of membranes. Cell swelling occurs in response to loss of the cell's homeostasis secondary to mechanical, hypoxic, toxic, free radical, viral, bacterial, and immune-mediated injuries.

The functional and morphologic changes begin with increased uptake of water and then to diffuse disintegration of organelles and cytoplasmic proteins. Cell swelling must be distinguished from cell enlargement (hypertrophy) that is caused by an increase of normal organelles. Organs composed of swollen cells are themselves swollen. Affected organs are larger and heavier than normal and pale in color. The parenchyma of swollen organs such as kidney and liver may bulge a little from beneath their capsule when incised. Because of the increase of intracellular water, the specific gravity of affected tissues is slightly less than those of normal tissues.

NORMAL CELL VOLUME CONTROL AND MECHANISMS OF ACUTE CELL SWELLING

In the normal cell, energy derived from ATP drives the Na^+-K^+ ion pumps within cell membranes to continuously drive Na^+ out of the cell in exchange for K^+ moving into the cell. For each molecule of ATP used, the pump moves three Na^+ out of the cell and two K^+ into the cell. By this means the ion pumps maintain the transmembrane ionic gradients required for normal nerve and muscle function. Because water moves passively across cell membranes in response to the osmotic pressure gradient generated by Na^+ and proteins, the

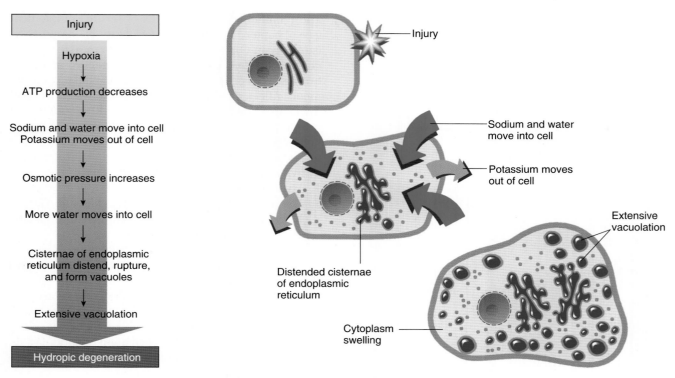

Fig. 1-9   **The process of acute cell swelling (hydropic degeneration).** *ATP,* Adenosine triphosphate. *(From Huether S, McCance K:* Understanding pathophysiology, *ed 3, St Louis, 2004, Mosby.)*

Na^+-K^+ pump is the key to regulation of intracellular water. The best studied laboratory models of cell swelling are: (1) hypoxia induced failure of ATP synthesis and (2) carbon tetrachloride (CCl_4)-induced membrane damage.

HYPOXIC INJURY RESULTING IN ACUTE CELL SWELLING

Hypoxia is probably the most important fundamental cause of acute cell swelling. Hypoxia-induced cell injury results from any defect in the transport of O_2, from inspired air to its role as the final acceptor of electrons from cytochrome oxidase in oxidative phosphorylation. Ischemia is reduced blood flow to a region of the body, usually because of obstruction of the blood supply. Blockage of coronary arteries by atherosclerotic plaque leads to ischemia and hypoxic injury to heart muscle, a common cause of "heart attacks" in humans. Therefore cellular hypoxia occurs with suffocation, anemia, pneumonia, shock or other damage to the circulation, and interference with mitochondrial enzymes.

In acute hypoxic injury, cell O_2 is depleted in moments, aerobic oxidative phosphorylation stops, and ATP levels fall. The drop in cellular ATP stimulates phosphofructokinase, the initial regulator step of anaerobic glycolysis. The metabolic switch to anaerobic metabolism of glucose rapidly depletes the cell's glycogen stores and leads to the accumulation of intracellular lactate and inorganic phosphates. Although the anaerobic generation of ATP is inefficient, it provides for some short-term survival. Some highly specialized cell types such as neurons cannot generate ATP anaerobically and thus are especially prone to hypoxic injury. Ultimately this deficiency of ATP leads to a failure of Na^+-K^+ pumps and loss of cell volume control.

The cardiac glycosides of plant origin, digitalis and ouabain, specifically inhibit the action of the Na^+-K^+ pump. This inhibition modifies the contractility of cardiac myocytes but it may also cause them to swell.

CELL MEMBRANE INJURY IN ACUTE CELL SWELLING

Damage to the cell membranes, both plasma membranes and organelle membranes, destroys the selective permeability barrier that retains proteins and electrolytes within the cytosol and that restricts the entry of Na^+, Ca^{++}, and water from the extracellular space. Failure of the barrier results from chemical modification of phospholipids by free radicals, covalent binding of toxic chemicals to macromolecules, interference with ion channels, and insertion of transmembrane protein complexes (e.g., complement activation).

The hepatotoxicities of CCl_4 and chloroform provide classic examples of cell membrane injury (Fig. 1-10).

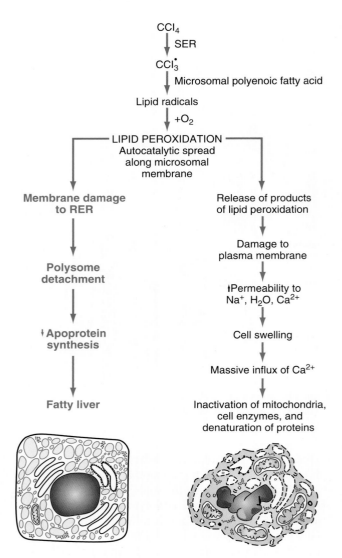

CCl$_4$

↓ SER

CCl$_3^{\bullet}$

↓ Microsomal polyenoic fatty acid

Lipid radicals

↓ +O$_2$

LIPID PEROXIDATION
Autocatalytic spread
along microsomal
membrane

Membrane damage to RER

↓

Polysome detachment

↓

↓ Apoprotein synthesis

↓

Fatty liver

Release of products
of lipid peroxidation

↓

Damage to
plasma membrane

↓

↑Permeability to
Na$^+$, H$_2$O, Ca^{2+}

↓

Cell swelling

↓

Massive influx of Ca^{2+}

↓

Inactivation of mitochondria,
cell enzymes, and
denaturation of proteins

Fig. 1-10 **Sequence of events leading to fatty change and cell necrosis in carbon tetrachloride (CCl$_4$) toxicity.** *RER*, Rough endoplasmic reticulum; *SER*, smooth endoplasmic reticulum. *(From Kumar V, Abbas A, Fausto N:* Robbins & Cotran pathologic basis of disease, *ed 7, Philadelphia, 2005, Saunders.)*

Toxic effects of CCl$_4$ occur when the chemical is converted to the trichloromethyl radical CCl$_3$ by the mixed-function oxidase system of the SER in hepatocytes. The toxic metabolite, CCl$_3$, next causes progressive lipid peroxidation of unsaturated fatty acids of cellular membranes, progressing from the SER to mitochondria and other cell membranes. Chloroform is toxic to hepatocytes when it is metabolized to the electrophilic metabolite, phosgene (CCl$_2$O). The hepatic lesions associated with these two toxins are indistinguishable, and both may result in fatty liver.

Besides toxins, other processes may cause cell membrane injury leading to acute cell swelling.

The membrane-attack complex of serum complement (see Chapter 3) and the hemolysin of streptococci (streptolysin-O) penetrate cell membranes to form a channel for free passage of water, proteins, and electrolytes between intracellular and extracellular compartments. Affected cells are quickly lysed by water overload (hypotonic lysis). Cytotoxic effects of NK (natural killer) cells are mediated in part by the implantation of similar hollow protein-complexes into target cell membranes.

The sequence of events in acute cell swelling caused by hypoxia or ischemia is as follows:
1. Hypoxia—deficiency of O$_2$
2. Decrease of oxidative phosphorylation and ATP
3. Increased glycolysis, increased intracellular lactate, and depletion of glycogen stores
4. Failure of Na$^+$-K$^+$ pump due to ATP deficiency
5. Net influx of Na$^+$, Ca^{++}, and H$_2$O with loss of intracellular K$^+$ and Mg^{++}
6. Swelling of mitochondria and the cytocavitary network (RER, SER, Golgi, and outer nuclear membrane)
7. Detachment of ribosomes, clumping of nuclear chromatin, loss of microvilli, vesiculation of endoplasmic reticulum (ER), formation of membrane whorls ("myelin figures")
8. Severe disruption of cell membranes, influx of Ca^{++} into mitochondria and cytosol, overall cell enlargement, and clearing of the cytosol
9. Irreversible cell injury, cell death (necrosis)

When acute cell swelling results from membrane injury, the sequence of events is similar to those listed previously, except that changes start at about step 5 or 6.

MORPHOLOGY OF ACUTE CELL SWELLING
GROSS APPEARANCE

Acute cell swelling is recognized as pallor, organ swelling, and decreased specific gravity. For example, the liver will be pale and somewhat turgid (Fig. 1-11, *A*). The parenchyma of organs with capsules may bulge, when incised.

MICROSCOPIC APPEARANCE

The influx of water dilutes the cytoplasmic matrix and dilates organelles to give cells a pale, finely vacuolated appearance (cloudy swelling). Renal tubule epithelial cells bulge and impinge on the tubular lumen. Swollen hepatocytes and endothelial cells intrude upon and diminish vascular lumens. Although mechanisms of cell swelling are limited, variations in appearance may occur because of differences in cell type and cause of injury.

Hydropic degeneration (vacuolar degeneration) is a common term used for the microscopic appearance of acute cell swelling (Fig. 1-11, *B*). It occurs in endothelium, epithelium, alveolar pneumocytes, hepatocytes, renal tubular epithelial cells, and neurons and glial cells

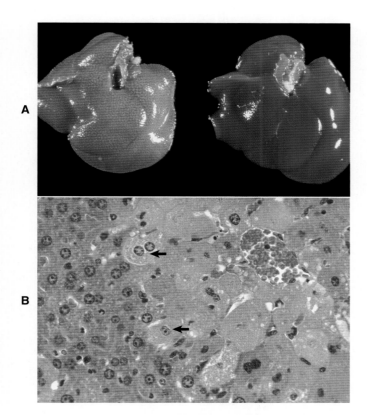

Fig. 1-11   Acute cell swelling, liver, mouse. A, Hepatic swelling in a mouse exposed to chloroform 24 hours previously. The accentuated lobular pattern and slight pallor in the liver on the left are the result of acute cell swelling (hydropic degeneration) and necrosis of centrilobular hepatocytes. The right liver is normal. **B,** Liver from a mouse with chloroform toxicosis. While many hepatocytes in the centrilobular areas (*at right*) are necrotic, several cells at the interface of normal and necrotic (*arrows*) are still undergoing acute cell swelling (hydropic degeneration). H&E stain. (*A* and *B, Courtesy Dr. L.H. Arp.)*

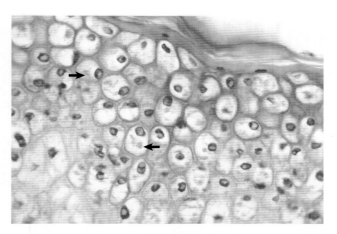

Fig. 1-12   Ballooning degeneration, papular stomatitis, oral mucosa, cow. Cells infected by some types of virus, such as papular stomatitis virus, are unable to regulate their volume and swell at certain stages of the infection. These cells may become very large (ballooning degeneration) and eventually rupture. Some of the cells have viral inclusion bodies (*arrows*). H&E stain. *(Courtesy Dr. M.D. McGavin, College of Veterinary Medicine, University of Tennessee.)*

of the brain. Cytoplasm of affected cells contains translucent vacuoles that fail to stain for fat or glycogen (two other causes of vacuolar degeneration). These vacuoles represent swollen mitochondria and dilated cisternae of the Golgi and ER. Ballooning degeneration is an extreme variant of hydropic degeneration in which cells are greatly enlarged and the cytoplasm is basically a clear space (Fig. 1-12). Ballooning degeneration is typically seen in epidermal cells infected by epitheliotropic viruses (e.g., pox virus). This lesion frequently progresses to the formation of vesicles or bullae (blisters) from lysis of the epidermal cells. These viral infections cause both degradation of cytoplasmic proteins (cytoplasmic proteolysis) and net flux of water into the cytoplasm.

ULTRASTRUCTURAL APPEARANCE

As visualized with the electron microscope, swollen cells have lost and distorted cilia, microvilli, and attachment sites as well as "blebbing" of cytoplasm at the cell surfaces. The cytoplasm is rarefied, and the cisternae of the ER, Golgi, and mitochondria are dilated. The cytocavitary network becomes fragmented into numerous vesicles. Proteins and Ca^{++} precipitate in the cytoplasm and in organelles.

SIGNIFICANCE AND FATE OF ACUTE CELL SWELLING

Injured cells that can no longer regulate water and electrolytes are no better equipped to maintain other cell functions. Significance to the patient depends on the number of cells affected and the immediate importance of the lost cell function. Cells highly vulnerable to hypoxia and cell swelling include cardiac myocytes, proximal renal tubule epithelium, hepatocytes, and endothelium. In the central nervous system (CNS), besides endothelium, also neurons, oligodendrocytes, and astrocytes are swollen, and the process in the CNS is called cytotoxic edema (see Chapter 14). Swollen neurons fail to conduct nervous impulses, resulting in stupor or coma. Swollen myocardial cells contract with less force or with an abnormal rhythm. Swollen renal epithelium may not only fail to absorb and secrete but may also compress delicate interstitial blood vessels, resulting in further injury. Capillaries lined by swollen endothelium are prone to obstruction, exacerbating the lesions by worsening cellular hypoxia. Injured cells with abnormal membrane permeability may be detected by finding their specific cytoplasmic enzymes in serum.

If adequate oxygen is restored to the cells and membrane injury is repaired before a certain point is reached, the "point of no return," most cells can be restored to normal or nearly normal function. What happens when the stage of reversibility is passed is the topic of the subsequent sections beginning with cell death.

In summary, cell swelling is a manifestation of reversible, sublethal cell injury. However, unless the cause of injury to critically important cell types is removed quickly, progressive injury to these dependent cells and tissues may culminate in the death of the animal.

IRREVERSIBLE CELL INJURY AND CELL DEATH

As we have just seen, major mechanisms of acute cell swelling are hypoxia, including ischemia, and membrane injury, often by toxins. Cell swelling can be reversible if the extent and duration of injury is not excessive. But if the injury exceeds certain limits (discussed shortly), cell death occurs (Fig. 1-13). Not all cell injury results in cell death. Cell injury may be sublethal and result in a variety of types of cell degenerations and/or adaptations

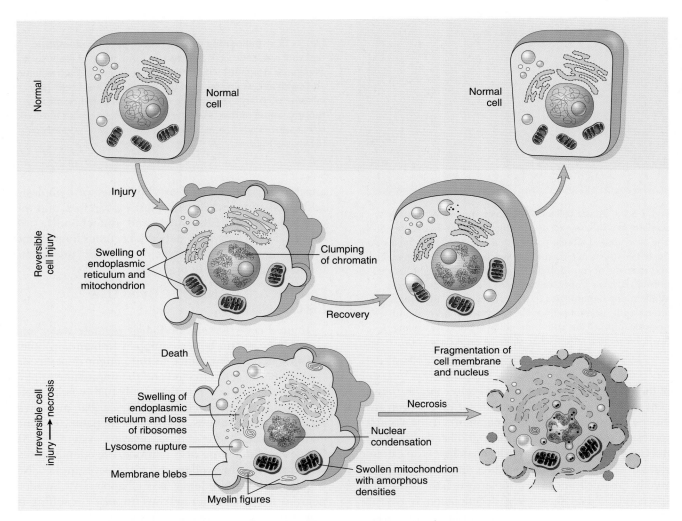

Fig. 1-13   Normal cell and the changes in reversible and irreversible cell injury.
Reversible injury is characterized by generalized swelling of the cell and its organelles, blebbing of the plasma membrane, detachment of ribosomes from the endoplasmic reticulum, and clumping of nuclear chromatin. Transition to irreversible injury is characterized by increasing swelling of the cell, swelling and disruption of lysosomes, presence of large amorphous densities in swollen mitochondria, disruption of cellular membranes, and profound nuclear changes. The latter include nuclear condensation (pyknosis), followed by fragmentation (karyorrhexis) and dissolution of the nucleus (karyolysis). Laminated structures (myelin figures) derived from damaged membranes of organelles and the plasma membrane first appear during the reversible stage and become more pronounced in irreversibly damaged cells. *(From Kumar V, Abbas A, Fausto N: Robbins & Cotran pathologic basis of disease, ed 7, Philadelphia, 2005, Saunders.)*

by the cell to the injury. In essence, cells or tissues respond to injury (or stress) in three important ways: (l) adaptation (with or without accumulations or degenerative changes), (2) reversible injury (again with or without subcellular changes) and (3) death. In this section we will deal with cell death. Various types of cell adaptations, degenerations, and accumulations will be addressed in subsequent sections.

CELL DEATH

Cell death can occur in many ways. For example, extremes of temperature or direct trauma may result in nearly instantaneous destruction or death of cells. On the other hand, death of an animal (somatic death) results in eventual death of all cells that make up the animal (postmortem autolysis). During most of the last century, cell death and necrosis were thought of as being more or less the same and in most pathologic situations, necrosis was usually thought to be preceded by cell swelling as discussed earlier. It is clear that cells die before macroscopic or histologic evidence can be detected. Although necrosis can be defined as the death of cells in a living animal, it should be understood to mean the specific morphologic changes (either macroscopic or microscopic) indicative of cell death in a living animal.

In the last few decades of the twentieth century it became clear that cells die also by shrinkage, both under physiologic and pathologic circumstances, and this complex and now well-studied process has become known as apoptosis. Cell death then began to be classified in two major types: necrosis or apoptosis. Because of the long history of use of necrosis and because apoptosis, cell death with shrinkage, is distinctly different from death following swelling, the term *oncosis* (onco- meaning swelling) has been proposed for what was previously termed necrosis. As in most biologic processes, it is not always possible to make the distinction between these two types of cell death based on histologic examination, and often both swelling and shrinkage are present.

How then are we to use the term *necrosis?* Attempts are being made by toxicologic pathologists to use the term *necrosis* for the histologic changes that occur following cell death by either mechanism, using oncotic cell death or apoptotic cell death when a distinction needs to be made. We will attempt to adhere to this distinction here, but long-used terminology does not easily change. The following sections first will discuss cell death following irreversible cell injury by hypoxia and cell membrane damage (oncotic necrosis), and then apoptosis or apoptotic necrosis (Fig. 1-14).

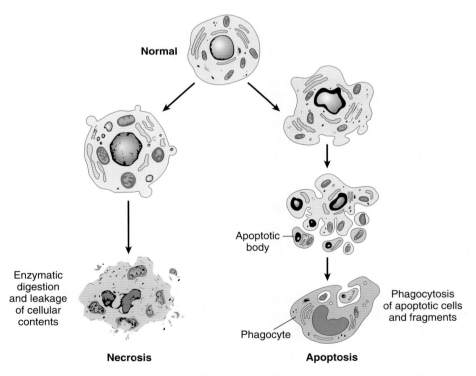

Fig. 1-14   The sequential ultrastructural changes seen in necrosis *(left)* **and apoptosis** *(right).* In apoptosis, the initial changes consist of nuclear chromatin condensation and fragmentation, followed by cytoplasmic budding and phagocytosis of the extruded apoptotic bodies. Signs of cytoplasmic blebs, and digestion and leakage of cellular components characterize necrosis. *(Adapted from Walker NI, Harmon BV, Gobe GC, Kerr JF: Methods Achiev Exp Pathol 13:18-54, 1988.)*

ONCOSIS (ONCOTIC NECROSIS)

Oncosis is cell death following irreversible cell injury by hypoxia, ischemia, and membrane injury. Hypoxic injury, as discussed earlier in Acute Cell Swelling, is a common cause of cell death and oncotic necrosis. It is often due to blockage of or markedly diminished blood supply to an area (ischemia). Ischemic injury is typically more severe than hypoxia alone because not only is the amount of oxygen lowered in the tissue, but the inflow of metabolic substrates and nutrients are also decreased and cell waste and by-products accumulate, some of which are injurious in their own right. Cell membrane damage caused by toxins and other substances and mechanisms can also lead to necrosis, but the resulting morphologic changes are similar.

Acute cell swelling can result in necrosis or can be reversible. There has been much recent interest and research about those circumstances where injury is irreversible and necrosis results, and it is still not clear exactly where the point of no return is. Research has provided convincing evidence for the role of Ca++ in the eventual demise of severely injured cells. Earlier work consistently identified two features of irreversible cell injury: (1) an inability to restore mitochondrial function and (2) evidence of cellular membrane damage.

Research directed at understanding coronary heart disease has led to improved understanding. Heart muscle deprived of its blood supply (ischemia) suffers from hypoxia and substantial loss of cell volume regulation and the influx of Ca++ because of inadequate ATP to run the ion pumps. If the blood supply is resupplied to the ischemic area, often reversal of the injury is not attained, but instead injury is accelerated. It has been shown that restored blood flow results in a tremendous influx of calcium, and added membrane damage occurs shortly after the blood supply is reestablished. This phenomenon is now termed *reperfusion injury*. It has been found that pretreatment with the tranquilizer chlorpromazine prevents much of the Ca++ influx and irreversible cell injury. The reactivity of free Ca++ ion and its role as an intracellular messenger and enzyme activator are better known, and these actions are thought to cause the final demise of the cell in necrosis.

What does Ca++ do to cause the ultimate demise of many severely injured cells as it influxes from the extracellular space (Fig. 1-15)? At least one endogenous, membrane-bound phospholipase (phospholipase A) is activated by free Ca++. Activated phospholipases then break down the normal phospholipids of the inner mitochondrial membrane and other cell membranes. These events then preclude any possibility for cell survival. Activation of phospholipases also generates arachidonic acid, the substrate for many lipid mediators of inflammation (to be discussed later). Therefore it is usual to see some degree of inflammation around foci of necrosis. In addition to phospholipases, Ca++ also

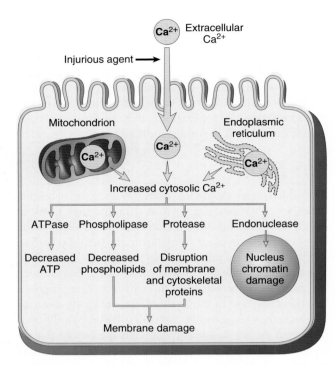

Fig. 1-15 **Sources and consequences of increased cytosolic calcium in cell injury.** *ATP,* Adenosine triphosphate.
(From Kumar V, Abbas A, Fausto N: Robbins & Cotran pathologic basis of disease, ed 7, Philadelphia, 2005, Saunders.)

activates proteases that result in cytoskeleton and membrane damage, adenosinetriphosphatases (ATPases) that accelerate depletion of ATP, and endonucleases that result in chromatin degradation. Irreversible injury to mitochondrial membranes appears to be the death blow to the cell.

There is great interest in control of Ca++ influx into myocardial cells during and following myocardial infarction (heart attack). Drugs that act as Ca++ ion channel-blocking agents are being evaluated and used. Substances—such as antioxidants, including vitamin E—that decrease membrane damage caused by oxygen metabolites (free radicals) that are generated are also important. Decreasing the influx of inflammatory cells and impact of inflammatory mediators is also important in minimizing reperfusion injury.

CELL MEMBRANE INJURY LEADING TO CELL DEATH

Chemical injury to cells in many cases may occur because of membrane damage. Classically studied and referred to in the section on acute cell injury is the toxicity for hepatocytes of CCl_4 (Fig. 1-10). After ingestion and absorption by the gastrointestinal (GI) tract, CCl_4 is transported via the portal vein to the liver where it enters hepatocytes. CCl_4 itself is fairly innocuous, but metabolism by the cytochrome p450 system in the SER results in the formation of a toxic metabolite, CCl_3. This free radical causes lipid peroxidation of organelle membranes starting from the SER and spreading to other organelles and eventually to the limiting cell membrane. This outcome has a variety of consequences. Injury to mitochondria results in decreased oxidative metabolism, decreased ATP production, and consequently an influx of calcium into mitochondria. This outcome results in decreased activity of the sodium-potassium pump and dysregulation of cell volume and massive intracellular increase in calcium with its lethal consequences. Direct damage to the plasma membrane itself by lipid peroxidation can have the same consequences to cell volume control and influx of calcium.

Lysosomal swelling and release of hydrolytic enzymes can result in autodigestion of cell components. Injury to RER of the hepatocyte can result in decreased protein synthesis, and this deficiency then causes insufficient production of lipoproteins required to export lipids and then results in increased fatty acid content in the cell and hepatic lipidosis (see discussion later), if the changes are not lethal.

FREE RADICAL INJURY

Injury to cell and organelle membranes can occur in many ways. One of the most common and important is free radical injury (Fig. 1-16). A free radical is any molecule that has an unpaired electron. These molecules

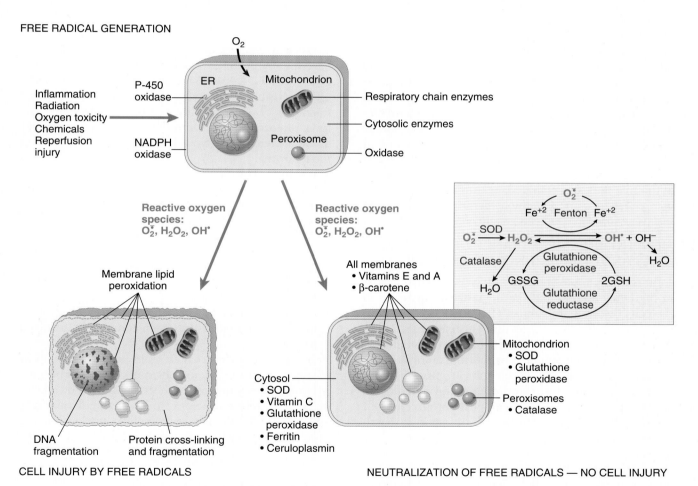

Fig. 1-16   **The role of reactive oxygen species in cell injury.** O_2 is converted to superoxide (O_2^-) by oxidative enzymes in the endoplasmic reticulum *(ER)*, mitochondria, plasma membrane, peroxisomes, and cytosol. O_2^- is converted to H_2O_2 by dismutation and thence to OH by the Cu^{2+}/Fe^{2+}-catalyzed Fenton reaction. H_2O_2 is also derived directly from oxidases in peroxisomes. Not shown is another potentially injurious radical, singlet oxygen. Resultant free radical damage to lipid (peroxidation), proteins, and DNA leads to various forms of cell injury. Note that superoxide catalyzes the reduction of Fe^{3+} to Fe^{2+}, thus enhancing OH generation by the Fenton reaction. The major antioxidant enzymes are superoxide dismutase *(SOD)*, catalase, and glutathione peroxidase. *GSH,* Reduced glutathione; *GSSG,* oxidized glutathione; *NADPH,* reduced form of nicotinamide adenine dinucleotide phosphate. *(From Kumar V, Abbas A, Fausto N: Robbins & Cotran pathologic basis of disease, ed 7, Philadelphia, 2005, Saunders.)*

are highly reactive, transient chemical species, generated as by-products of normal oxidative metabolism or by exposure to radiation, toxic gases, chemicals, and drugs. Most, but not all, are reactive oxygen radicals. Oxygen radicals are also produced by phagocytic cells in inflammatory lesions and account for significant damage to surrounding tissue. Antineoplastic drugs such as doxorubicin generate oxygen radicals that cause significant injury to cardiac myocytes. Cellular components at risk of free radical injury include proteins, membrane lipids, and nucleic acids. Lipid peroxidation of plasma membranes and organelle membranes by free radicals can have similar consequences to those described earlier from CCl_4.

Free radical injury is usually controlled by intracellular antioxidants such as superoxide dismutase (SOD), glutathione peroxidase, and vitamins E and C; however, injury can be catastrophic when these antioxidative systems are defective. In many species of domestic animals, severe cellular damage occurs to heart muscle when there is a deficiency of selenium or vitamin E in the tissues. Vitamin E is one of several cytoprotective molecules that acts as an antioxidant and inhibits production of or quenches free radicals, even in normal cell metabolism. Insufficient antioxidant activity can result in severe cell injury and necrosis as a consequence of the free radicals generated. Selenium is an essential component for some glutathione peroxidases, which also inactivate some free radicals generated within cells.

MORPHOLOGIC APPEARANCE OF NECROTIC CELLS AND TISSUES (ONCOTIC NECROSIS)

In contrast to postmortem autolysis, necrosis occurs in the living animal, but the degradative processes of the cells involved are similar. One challenge to veterinarians and pathologists is to distinguish necrosis, tissues that died before somatic death, from tissues that died with the rest of the animal (postmortem autolysis).

At this point there may be some confusion about the term *autolysis*. Most veterinarians and pathologists use this term synonymously with postmortem changes. Technically, *autolysis* means the self-digestion or degradation of cells and tissues by the hydrolytic enzymes normally present in those tissues. Therefore by the strict definition, autolysis occurs in all tissue that die (and even before they die) regardless of whether cells die before or after the animal dies. Postmortem change includes both autolysis and putrefaction, which is the process by which bacteria break down tissues.

The appearance of necrotic cells varies with the tissue involved, the cause of cell death, and the duration of time. For our immediate purposes, *necrosis* here will for the most part be used to mean oncotic necrosis. Apoptotic necrosis will be discussed later.

ULTRASTRUCTURE OF NECROTIC CELLS (ONCOTIC NECROSIS)

Cells dying after acute cell swelling are obviously swollen. There is tremendous swelling of all mitochondria, ER is dilated and fragmented, chromatin is clumped, the nuclear membrane is folded, the cytoplasm is pale and structureless, and organelles are poorly visualized. As the intracellular and extracellular compartments reach equilibrium across the altered cell membrane, the cell collapses and shrinks like a hot air balloon that has lost its air. The cell is shrunken; cytoplasm and organelles are homogeneous, electron dense, and hard to identify. Specialized areas of the plasma membrane such as desmosomes, microvilli, and cilia are distorted or absent.

HISTOLOGIC CHANGES IN NECROSIS (ONCOTIC NECROSIS)

Nuclear changes of dead cells are variable and are described by the terms pyknosis, karyorrhexis, and karyolysis (Fig. 1-17). All of the following nuclear changes may be visible in the same necrotic lesion. Basophilic fragments of nuclear debris can be confused with bacteria, protozoa, and calcium deposits. Histomorphology of the nucleus of a necrotic cell includes one or more of the following:

- Pyknosis. The nucleus is shrunken, dark, homogeneous, and round. Pyknosis may be a sequel to chromatin clumping of early degeneration.
- Karyorrhexis. The nuclear envelope is ruptured, and dark nuclear fragments are released into the cell cytoplasm.
- Karyolysis. The nucleus is extremely pale due to dissolution of chromatin presumably by action of RNAases and DNAases.
- Absence of nucleus. This is a later stage of karyolysis in which the nucleus has been completely dissolved or lysed.

Some cell lines have a preference for a type of nuclear change in necrosis. Necrotic lymphocytes often become pyknotic, sometimes karyorrhectic, followed by release of nuclear debris. Necrotic renal proximal tubulular epithelial cells often have karyolytic nuclei, but the distal tubules may have predominantly pyknotic nuclei.

Cytoplasmic changes in dead cells

Early in cell necrosis, the cytoplasm becomes homogeneous pink in H&E stained sections (Fig. 1-18). Increased eosinophilia may reflect a loss of ribosomal RNA, which is responsible for cytoplasmic basophilia, or a consolidation of cytoplasmic components as the cell collapses. Degradation of cytoplasmic proteins eventually gives the necrotic cell a pale, ghostlike appearance. Necrotic cells usually lose their adherence to basement membranes and neighboring cells so they are found

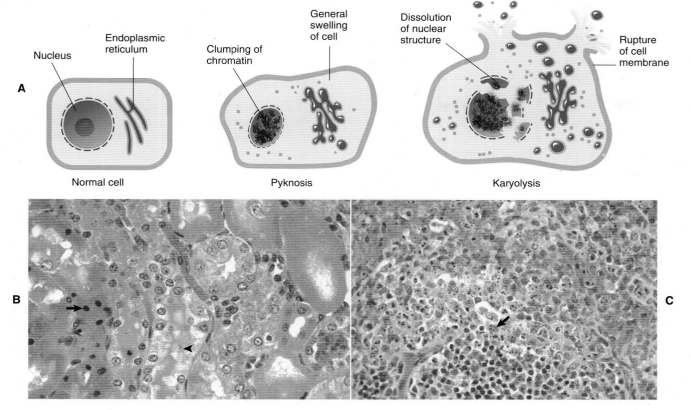

Fig. 1-17 **Cytoarchitecture of cellular necrosis. A,** Schematic representation of nuclear and cytoplasmic changes in the stages of necrosis. **B,** Pyknosis and karyolysis, renal cortex, chloroform toxicosis, mouse. Some epithelial cells exhibit hydropic degeneration, whereas others are necrotic. Some necrotic cells exhibit pyknosis *(arrow)*, whereas others have lost the nucleus or have a very pale nucleus (karyolysis) *(arrowhead)*. H&E stain. **C,** Karyorrhexis, lymphocytes, spleen, dog. Spleen of a dog with parvovirus infection. Lymphocyte nuclei have fragmented because of the infection *(arrow)*. H&E stain. (*A, From Huether S, McCance K: Understanding pathophysiology, ed 3, St Louis, 2004, Mosby. **B** and **C,** Courtesy Dr. L.H. Arp.*)

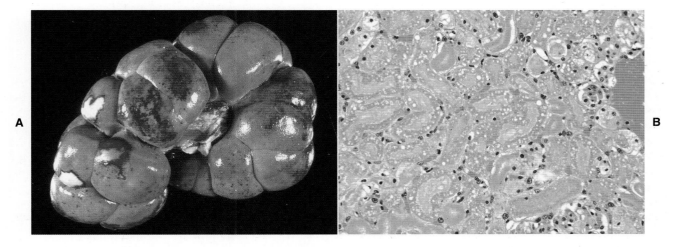

Fig. 1-18 **Coagulation necrosis, infarcts, kidney, cow. A,** Note the pale regions of acute coagulation necrosis surrounded by a red rim of active hyperemia and inflammation *(far left)*. **B,** Acute coagulation necrosis of renal tubular epithelial cells. Necrotic cells have homogeneous eosinophilic cytoplasm, more or less retained cell outlines, and nuclear changes such as pyknosis and nuclear absence. H&E stain. (*A, Courtesy Dr. D.E. Tyler, College of Veterinary Medicine, The University of Georgia; and Noah's Arkive, College of Veterinary Medicine, The University of Georgia. **B,** Courtesy Dr. S. Newman, College of Veterinary Medicine, University of Tennessee.*)

free in tubules, alveoli, follicles, and other lumens or on surfaces. Rupture of cells with loss of cell integrity is the most obvious evidence of cell death.

GROSS APPEARANCE OF NECROTIC TISSUE

Necrotic tissue is usually pale, soft and friable, and sharply demarcated from viable tissue by a zone of inflammation (Fig. 1-18). An exception to the pale color occurs when blood oozes into the necrotic tissue from damaged blood vessels in adjacent viable tissue as happens in renal infarcts which are often surrounded by a narrow (1 to 3 mm) red rim (active hyperemia). A sharp line of demarcation between necrotic and viable tissue is often a reliable means to distinguish necrosis from autolysis. It must be emphasized that necrotic changes are first apparent ultrastructurally (less than 6 hours), then histologically (6 to 12 hours), and finally grossly (24 to 48 hours). Therefore except for vascular changes, morphologic evidence of cell death is often sparse or absent in cases of peracute or acute death.

TYPES OF ONCOTIC NECROSIS

Foci of necrosis in tissue have a limited number of morphologic appearances depending on the tissue involved, the cause of cell injury, and somewhat on the time since injury has occurred. Classification of necrotic lesions enables the pathologist to describe the lesion with a minimum of repetitious detail, but more than one type of necrosis may be seen in an organ or tissue. The following are classically or historically derived and although commonly used do not always accurately describe the complexity of what has happened to the involved cells and tissues.

COAGULATION NECROSIS

Coagulation necrosis (coagulative necrosis) is characterized by preservation of the basic cell outlines of necrotic cells (Fig. 1-18). Cytoplasm is homogeneous and eosinophilic due to coagulation of cell proteins, similar to what happens to heat coagulation of proteins of a cooked egg white. Presumably the injury or subsequent cellular acidosis denatures not only structural proteins but also enzymes. This delays proteolysis of the cell. Nuclei are pyknotic, karyorrhectic, karyolytic, or absent. This form of necrosis may occur in any tissue except brain parenchyma, although it does occur initially in individual neurons. It is classically seen in kidney, liver, and muscle, and the necrotic tissue will eventually lyse within several days and be phagocytosed. Coagulation necrosis suggests hypoxic cell injury as seen in local loss of blood supply or in shock. Bacterial exotoxins and chemical toxins also cause the lesion. Infarction is necrosis due to ischemia. An infarct, for example, occurring in the human heart as a result of the blockage of a coronary artery by an atherosclerotic plaque is an area of coagulation necrosis due to a sudden loss of blood supply to an area.

CASEATION NECROSIS

Caseation necrosis (caseous necrosis) implies conversion of dead cells into a granular friable mass grossly resembling cottage cheese (Fig. 1-19). The necrotic focus is composed of a coagulum of nuclear and cytoplasmic debris. Compared with coagulation necrosis, this is an older (chronic) lesion often associated with poorly degradable lipids of bacterial origin. Any tissue may be affected, and much of the necrotic debris is dead leukocytes. Dystrophic calcification commonly occurs later within the central parts of the lesion. The classic cause of this lesion is tuberculosis. Related bacteria, such as *Corynebacterium*, also cause this lesion in sheep. Delayed degradation of the bacterial cell wall is thought to play a role in the development of a lesion caused by

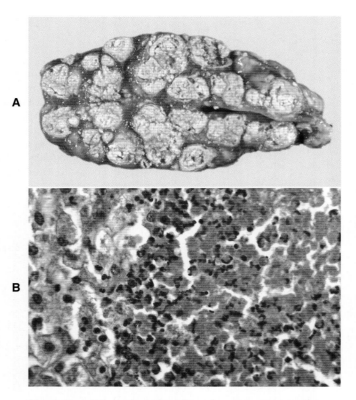

A

B

Fig. 1-19   **Tuberculosis, lymph node, transverse section, ox.** A, The lymph has been replaced by a caseating granuloma. Note the caseous necrosis characterized by a pale yellow, crumbly exudate. B, Granulomatous inflammation in caseous necrosis. Cell walls are disrupted and tissue architecture is lost. Mineralization (not seen here) is common in this type of necrosis. H&E stain. (*A,* Courtesy Dr. M. Domingo, *Autonomous University of Barcelona; and Noah's Arkive, College of Veterinary Medicine, University of Georgia.* *B,* Courtesy Dr. M.D. McGavin, *College of Veterinary Medicine, University of Tennessee.*)

these bacteria and results in a focus of caseous necrosis surrounded by granulomatous inflammatory cells and an outer fibrous connective tissue capsule.

LIQUEFACTIVE NECROSIS

Liquefactive necrosis is the usual type of necrosis in the CNS, although the neuron cell bodies themselves initially show coagulation necrosis, followed by liquefaction (Fig. 1-20). Hypoxic death of cells in the CNS results in rapid enzymatic dissolution of the neuropil (liquefaction), likely due to the large amount of cell membranes present. With loss of astrocytes, and because there is normally very little fibrous connective tissue in the CNS, little remains to support the tissue or fill in dead space. The result is a cavity filled with lipid debris and fluid. These cystic areas are cleared of debris by macrophages that become gitter cells (described further in Chapter 14).

In other tissues, focal infection by pyogenic bacteria leads to release of enzymes from accumulating leukocytes. Early in this process, heterolysis leads to a focal liquid collection of necrotic neutrophils and tissue debris (pus), and the lesion is an abscess that is also a type of liquefactive necrosis. If the abscess persists, loss of fluid or inspissation of the pus results in it becoming more caseous.

GANGRENE

There are three types of gangrene: dry gangrene, moist gangrene, and gas gangrene. They are included here because the initial lesion is coagulation necrosis. Moist gangrene is defined as an area of necrotic tissue (usually coagulation necrosis), which is further degraded by the liquefactive action of saprophytic bacteria

(defined as organisms living in dead organic matter), which usually cause putrefaction (defined as the decomposition of organic matter by microorganisms [i.e., rotten]).

The initial coagulation necrosis can be due to infarction of an extremity (too tight a bandage on a limb, penetrating damage to an artery supplying the leg by a bullet or shrapnel) or of a segment of intestine, or as in the case of the lung, by direct action of aspirated irritants such as medicaments or even ruminal fluid. The saprophytic bacteria contaminate the dead tissue from the local environment (air, skin contaminants, and soil) in the case of a limb, from inhaled air in the lung, and from the adjacent feces in an intestinal infarct.

Grossly, tissues become soft, moist, and reddish-brown to black, and if the saprophytic bacteria produce gas, as they usually do, then gas bubbles and a putrid odor from the hydrogen sulfide, ammonia, and mercaptans may occur (Fig. 1-21, A). With time, if death does not supervene from toxemia, gangrenous tissue of the leg and udder will be separated from the normal tissue by inflammation and may slough.

Microscopically, initially areas of coagulation necrosis contain a few proliferating bacteria. These quickly proliferate and produce liquefaction and, depending on the bacteria, gas bubbles. As the lesion progresses, most of the necrotic tissue will be liquefied by saprophytic bacteria and infiltrating neutrophils.

Dry gangrene is really coagulation necrosis secondary to infarction, which is followed by mummification. It involves the lower portion of an extremity (leg), tail, ears, and udder and can be caused by ingested toxins (ergot and fescue poisoning) or cold (frost bite). Ergot produces

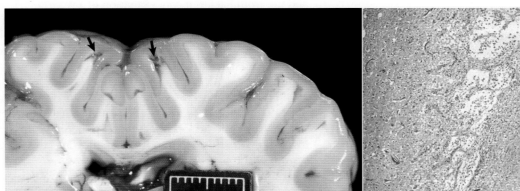
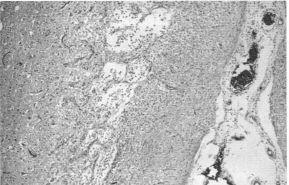

A **B**

Fig. 1-20   Liquefactive necrosis. A, Acute polioencephalomalacia, brain, goat. A thiamine deficiency has resulted in cerebrocortical malacia, which microscopically is liquefaction necrosis and varying degrees of tissue separation *(arrows)*. Scale bar = 2 cm. **B,** Cortical necrosis, cerebrum, dog. The pale vertical band in the cerebral cortex contains areas of near total loss of cells and tissue loss termed liquefactive necrosis. The cells in the spaces are gitter cells. Grossly, this band would have a fluid consistency. H&E stain. (**A,** *Courtesy Dr. R. Storts, College of Veterinary Medicine, Texas A&M University.* **B,** *Courtesy Dr. L.H. Arp.)*

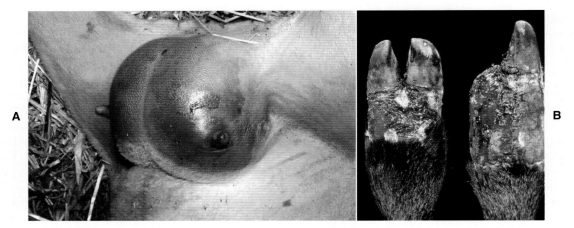

Fig. 1-21   Gangrenous necrosis. A, Moist gangrene, udder, sheep. The surrounding tissue is well vascularized, which contributes to the wet and bloody nature of the lesion. Often saprophytic bacteria and clostridia contaminate areas of necrosis. **B,** Dry gangrene, fescue toxicity, digits, cow. Fescue toxicity is a disease in which the blood supply to the distal extremities is lost because of vasoconstriction from the toxic effect on vessels. The dry leathery appearance adjacent to the hooves is termed dry gangrene. There is still some blood in the skin, indicating that at least a partial blood supply has been retained or restored. Note that one of the claws *(right)* has been lost due to the process. *(**A,** Courtesy Dr. C. Wallace, College of Veterinary Medicine, University of Georgia; and Noah's Arkive, College of Veterinary Medicine, The University of Georgia. **B,** Courtesy Dr. R.K. Myers, College of Veterinary Medicine, Iowa State University.)*

a marked peripheral arteriolar vasoconstriction and damage to capillaries, which leads to thrombosis and infarction. Fescue poisoning in cattle has a similar pathogenesis and lesions. Exposure to very cold temperatures also causes dry gangrene (frostbite). The pathogenesis involves both direct freezing and disruptions of cells by intracellular and extracellular ice crystal formation and vascular damage leading to ischemia and infarction characterized by coagulation necrosis (see Chapter 17).

In dry gangrene, after necrosis, the tissues are depleted of water, for example by low humidity, and this dehydration results in mummification. There is no proliferation of bacteria, as dry tissues do not provide an environment favorable for their proliferation and spread. Grossly, the tissue is shriveled, dry, and brown to black (Fig. 1-21, *B*).

Gas gangrene is also an example of bacteria proliferating and producing toxins in necrotic tissue, but in this case the bacteria are anaerobes, usually microbes such as *Clostridium perfringens* and *Clostridium septicum*. These bacteria are introduced by penetrating wounds into muscle or subcutis. The necrotic tissue then provides an anaerobic medium for growth of the clostridia. Another example, with similar lesions, is caused by *Clostridium chauvoei* (blackleg), which, unlike the bacteria of gas gangrene, is not introduced by a penetrating wound but from spores spread hematogenously from the intestine and lodged in muscle. Here they stay until by some mechanism, such as trauma, necrosis occurs

and thus produces anaerobic conditions in which the spores can germinate and the bacteria proliferate.

Grossly, affected tissues are dark red to black with gas bubbles and a fluid exudate that may contain blood. Microscopically, the lesions are characterized by coagulation necrosis of muscle, a serohemorrhagic exudate, and gas bubble formation (see Chapter 15). Some authors do not classify the lesions of blackleg as gas gangrene, as it is a result of hematogenously disseminated bacterial spores and not from bacterial contamination of a wound.

NECROSIS OF FAT (FAT NECROSIS)

There are three types of fat necrosis: enzymatic necrosis of fat, traumatic necrosis of fat, and necrosis of abdominal fat of cattle. *Enzymatic necrosis of fat*, also called pancreatic necrosis of fat, refers to the destruction of fat in the abdominal cavity and usually adjacent to the pancreas, by the action of activated pancreatic lipases in pancreatic fluid that has escaped from the duct system of the pancreas (Fig. 1-22).

Traumatic necrosis of fat is seen when adipose tissue is crushed. It occurs in fat adjacent to the pelvic canal of heifers following dystocia, and in subcutaneous tissue that has been injured—for example in the subcutaneous and intramuscular fat over the sternum of recumbent cattle.

Fat necrosis of abdominal fat of cattle is characterized by large masses of necrotic fat in the mesentery, omentum, and retroperitoneally. The cause is unknown and it may not be detected until necropsy. In extreme

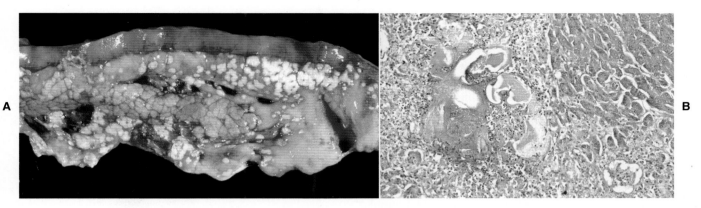

Fig. 1-22   Fat necrosis. A, Enzymatic necrosis of fat (fat necrosis), dog with previous bouts of pancreatitis. Necrotic fat often becomes saponified and so grossly the lesion is chalky to gritty and pale white. **B,** Pancreas, dog. Note the large area (*center*) of fat necrosis and saponification (basophilic). H&E stain. (**A,** *Courtesy Dr. J. Wright, College of Veterinary Medicine, North Carolina State University; and Noah's Arkive, College of Veterinary Medicine, The University of Georgia.* **B,** *Courtesy Dr. J.F. Zachary, College of Veterinary Medicine, University of Illinois.*)

cases, mesenteric fat may surround the intestine and cause stenosis.

Grossly affected fat is white, firm, and chalky. Histologically, necrotic fat is not removed by the fat solvents used in the preparation of the paraffin embedded sections. Necrotic adipocytes are eosinophilic but become basophilic if free fatty acids react with Ca^{++} to form a soap (saponification of fat).

SEQUELAE TO ONCOTIC NECROSIS

In contrast to apoptosis and postmortem autolysis, necrosis incites a notable inflammatory reaction in the surrounding viable tissue. Therefore the necrotic foci are often surrounded by a well-demarcated band of white blood cells and the hyperemia of inflammation. The purpose is to digest (by heterolytic enzymes of leukocytes) and liquefy the necrotic tissue so that it can be removed by macrophages and diffusion into blood and lymph vessels and replaced by normal tissue (regeneration) or fibrous connective tissue (healing). Healing of an abscess occurs after the sequestered pus is phagocytosed and/or carried off by the lymphatics. The process is greatly hastened by drainage, either by rupture to the outside or by surgical drainage of the abscess. Material not liquified is phagocytosed by macrophages and removed via lymphatics or veins. A fragment of necrotic material, especially bone, may resist degradation and form a sequestrum. This may cause chronic irritation and delay repair.

MORPHOLOGIC APPEARANCE OF POSTMORTEM CHANGES

Postmortem autolysis refers to the autolysis of cells occurring after somatic death. These changes are amplified and accelerated by bacterial decomposition from bacteria that have entered the tissue shortly before death or after death (usually by either direct migration from the lumen of the gut of the dead or dying animal, or from the gut into the blood and then disseminated throughout the body by the final beats of the heart). Postmortem bacterial metabolism and dissolution of host tissues (postmortem decomposition) result in the production of color and texture changes, gas production, and odors collectively termed putrefaction.

Somatic death refers to death of the entire body; however, cell types vary greatly in time of viability after cessation of heart beat, respiration, and brain wave activity. In somatic death, many neurons and cardiac myocytes suffer irreversible injury within minutes; kidney and liver cells may survive for an hour; and fibroblasts and bone survive much longer. Interpretation of lesions is usually clouded by changes that occur between the time of death and the time of necropsy (or fixation of tissue). Postmortem autolysis results from total diffuse hypoxia, and cells degenerate as described for hypoxic cell injury. A long death-to-fixation interval can lead to problems in histopathologic diagnosis of necrosis and other lesions; thus keeping postmortem changes to a minimum is important for accurate gross and histopathologic interpretation.

Postmortem changes vary greatly in onset and rate depending on the cause of death, environmental and body temperature, and microbial flora. Cool environmental temperatures and refrigeration (without freezing if possible because freezing induces artefacts such as intracellular and extracellular ice crystals, which disrupt cells and tissues, respectively) inhibit autolysis and delay putrefaction. Animals examined 24 hours after death, after being maintained at 5° C, will have relatively few postmortem changes and artefacts to interpret versus an animal that has been maintained at room temperature for a similar time. An exception is herbivores. In the ruminant forestomach and equine cecum and ascending colon, ingesta will continue to undergo bacterial fermentation after death, with formation of heat and gas. Consequently these animals, even if refrigerated immediately after death, will show considerable intraabdominal postmortem decomposition 24 hours later. High environmental temperatures accelerate autolysis as do fever, high metabolic rate, heat stroke, and exercise before death. Delay in cooling is especially common in fat animals and those with a heavy coat, especially wool. Young and small animals, such as neonates, cool more rapidly than large obese ones. Determining the time since death has occurred can be difficult because of the many factors just listed, influencing the rate of cooling.

In summary, postmortem changes can interfere with accurate interpretation of both gross and histologic changes in tissue. Postmortem changes can be minimized by rapid cooling of the carcass and decreasing the death to tissue fixation time to a minimum. The following are examples of common postmortem changes, with some reference to their sequence of occurrence:

- Rigor mortis is the contraction of muscles occurring after death. It commences 1 to 6 hours after death and persists for 1 to 2 days. When ATP and glycogen (required to relax muscle contraction) are depleted, the contraction is irreversible except by autolysis. Muscular animals often have stronger rigor than those with less muscle mass. High heat and activity before death accelerate the onset of rigor. In animals with cachexia or extreme malnutrition, the energy stores (ATP, glycogen) in the muscles may be so depleted that no contraction of myofibers is possible, and thus these animals do not develop rigor mortis.

- Algor mortis is gradual cooling of the cadaver. Cooling of the carcass depends on temperature of the body at death (e.g., fever, environmental temperature, insulation of the carcass [fat, wool, coverings], body mass, air movement, and other factors) and is difficult to interpret precisely for establishing time of death.

- Livor mortis (hypostatic congestion) (Fig. 1-23) is the gravitational pooling of blood to the down side of the animal. In large vessels, there is clotting followed by separation of blood cells and plasma. This process begins within an hour after death, and the clotted blood can become "fixed" in place (whereby movement of the animal will not influence the distribution of the change) within 12 to 24 hours. It is often not appreciated in animals because of pigmented skin or a thick hair coat and thus is most likely to be evident in white-skinned animals with little hair (e.g., white pigs).

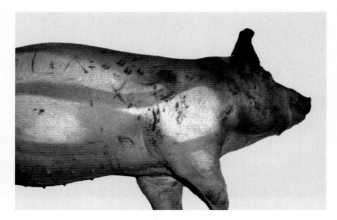

Fig. 1-23   Livor mortis, pig. Note red to purple staining of the skin on the right side, the side on which the pig was lying when it died. This color change is termed livor mortis or hypostatic congestion. The pale white areas are pressure points on the down side into which blood could not flow after death. *(Courtesy Dr. M.D. McGavin, College of Veterinary Medicine, University of Tennessee.)*

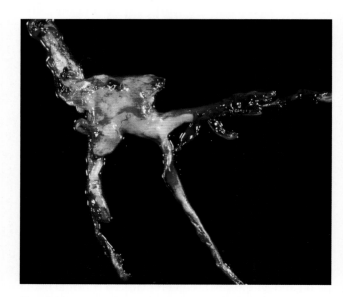

Fig. 1-24   Postmortem clot, dog. The postmortem clot is pale white to yellow (chicken fat clot) in some areas and shiny red (currant jelly clot) in others. Note how it conforms to the shape of the lumen of the vessels from which it was removed. *(Courtesy Dr. R.K. Myers, College of Veterinary Medicine, Iowa State University.)*

- Postmortem clotting (Fig. 1-24) in the heart and vessels occurs within several hours and can be influenced by antemortem changes in blood. Warfarin poisoning and hereditary coagulopathies, for example, will delay or cause failure of blood to clot. Before the blood clots, erythrocytes may settle to the bottom of a large vessel. This results in the clot having two portions: a bottom red mass made up chiefly of

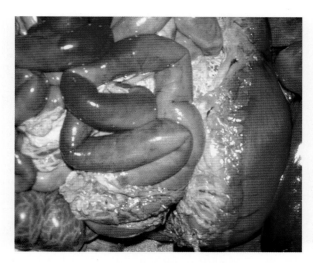

Fig. 1-25   **Imbibition of hemoglobin, viscera, pig that has been dead for several hours before being necropsied.** Note the pink color on the serosal surfaces of the stomach and small intestine. This is termed imbibition of hemoglobin and is due to staining by hemoglobin that has seeped out of autolyzed red blood cells. *(Courtesy Dr. R.K. Myers, College of Veterinary Medicine, Iowa State University.)*

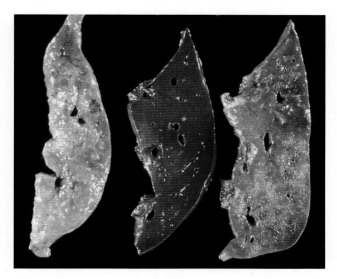

Fig. 1-26   **Postmortem autolysis.** Cross sections of livers from three different pigs at different stages of postmortem autolysis. The section on the right has green staining around the bile ducts due to leakage of bile into the surrounding parenchyma after death (bile imbibition). All of these livers are softer than normal, but the one on the left is notably softer, another characteristic of autolytic tissue. *(Courtesy Dr. R.K. Myers, College of Veterinary Medicine, Iowa State University.)*

erythrocytes and an upper pale yellow mass of clotted serum. The latter type of clot is called a chicken fat clot. This separation depends upon the erythrocyte sedimentation rate (ESR) of the blood. It is high in normal horses and increased in all animals as a systemic inflammatory response. Inflammation results in increased plasma fibrinogen, which causes erythrocytes to form stacks (rouleau formation) that sediment more rapidly. Postmortem clots must be distinguished from antemortem mural thrombi and thromboemboli. Postmortem clots are unattached to vessel walls and tend to be shiny and wet and form a perfect cast of vessel lumens. Antemortem mural arterial thrombi are attached to arterial walls, tend to be dry and duller in color, and are laminated with a tail extending downstream from the point of attachment. Antemortem venous thrombi are also attached, but loosely so, and in many cases may closely resemble postmortem clots.

- Hemoglobin imbibition (Fig. 1-25) is a term applied to the red staining of tissue, especially the heart and arteries (particularly evident in the aorta) and veins beginning some hours after death. Once the integrity of the intima is lost, hemoglobin released by lysed erythrocytes penetrates the vessel wall and extends into the adjacent tissue. Hemoglobin staining of the intima can also occur in acute intravascular hemolysis. It is usually very obvious in aborted fetuses that are retained for hours or days after their in utero deaths.
- Bile imbibition (Fig. 1-26) occurs within hours of death. Bile in the gallbladder starts to penetrate its

wall and stain adjacent tissue yellowish, and later this may become greenish brown. Tissues involved include the adjacent liver and any intestine in contact with the gallbladder. Sometimes similar changes may be seen near the bile ducts.

- Pseudomelanosis. This is the term used for the blue-green discoloration of the tissue by iron sulfide (FeS) formed by the reaction of hydrogen sulfide (H_2S) generated by putrefactive bacteria on iron from hemoglobin released from lysed erythrocytes. Because it depends on bacterial action, it usually takes a day or more to develop.
- Softening (Figs. 1-26 and 1-28) of tissue results from autolysis of cells and connective tissue often aided by putrefactive bacteria.
- Bloating (Fig. 1-27) is the result of postmortem bacterial gas formation in the lumen of the GI tract. Herbivores tend to bloat more rapidly and severely than carnivores. In ruminants the rumen can become markedly distended by gas within hours of death, and this can be so severe as to rupture the diaphragm. The rate of gas formation depends upon the diet, the substrate for the bacteria, and the temperature. Postmortem bloat can sometimes be difficult to distinguish from antemortem bloat (ruminal tympany) in ruminants. Bacteria disseminated hematogenously from the GI tract shortly before death can lodge in a variety of tissues and produce gas (postmortem emphysema).

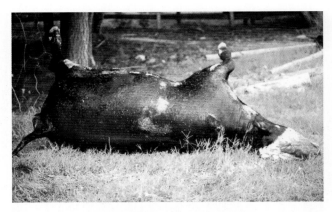

Fig. 1-27   Postmortem bloat or emphysema. Cow killed by lightning several hours earlier. When animals die, especially ruminants, the bacteria in the GI tract continue to grow and produce gas. Rumen microbes may produce very large amounts of gas causing the carcass to swell tremendously. *(Courtesy Dr. W. Crowell, College of Veterinary Medicine, The University of Georgia; and Noah's Arkive, College of Veterinary Medicine, The University of Georgia.)*

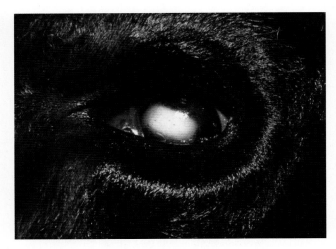

Fig. 1-29   Postmortem autolysis, eye, lens, calf. Note that the cornea is clear. The cloudiness of the lens is due to cooling or freezing and is reversible as the carcass warms up. It should not be confused with cataracts. *(Courtesy Dr. P.N. Nation, University of Alberta; and Noah's Arkive, College of Veterinary Medicine, The University of Georgia.)*

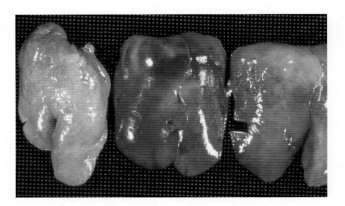

Fig. 1-28   Postmortem autolysis. Pig livers at various intervals after death. Pale foci on the middle liver are due to blood being forced out of the parenchyma by intestinal swelling (intestinal imprints) and from pressure from the overlying ribs (rib imprints). Multiple small pale foci can sometimes be caused by colonies of postmortem bacteria and can be confused with antemortem necrosis. *(Courtesy Dr. R.K. Myers, College of Veterinary Medicine, Iowa State University.)*

- Organ displacement occurs following distention of the viscera; for example, distention of the rumen by gas from fermentation can cause increased intraabdominal pressure, which can result in displacement of abdominal viscera, rectal prolapse, and compression of the diaphragm, which then compresses the thoracic viscera. The latter can result in the expulsion of frothy fluid, originally in the lungs, from the mouth and nose.
- Pale foci subserosally on the liver (Fig. 1-28) can result from two causes: increased intraabdominal pressure, which squeezes blood from these areas (e.g., pressure from the overlying ribs can leave their imprints on the liver), and bacterial action. Under very hot conditions, pale areas can appear on the surface of the bovine liver within hours of death. Histologically these areas resemble coagulation necrosis in which there are extremely numerous bacteria. Presumably these bacteria have been disseminated agonally from the gut into the portal vein.
- Mucosal sloughing occurs rapidly in the rumen, often within a few hours as a result of the enzymes within the ingesta and the low rate of cooling.
- Lens opacity (Fig. 1-29) occurs when the carcass is very cold or frozen. The change will reverse to normal transparency on warming, but it can be confused with cataracts in cold carcasses.

CELL DEATH BY APOPTOSIS

Apoptosis and *programmed cell death* have been used virtually synonymously and refer to individual cell death in a variety of processes. Common to both is the initiation of a self-induced cell death process some refer to as cellular suicide. Although there is much overlap in cellular mechanisms, the term *programmed cell death* should be reserved for physiologic cell death that occurs in developing animals (embryogenesis and normal growth). Production of the keratinized outer layer of skin, for example, involves programmed cell death. For those circumstances in which pathologic cell death occurs with shrinkage first as a feature, *apoptosis* or *apoptotic necrosis* is more appropriately used. Apoptosis occurs

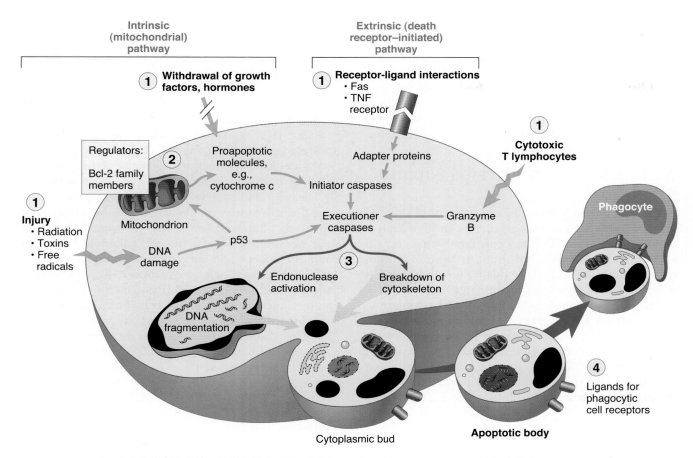

Fig. 1-30   Mechanisms of apoptosis. Labeled *(1)* are some of the major inducers of apoptosis. These include specific death ligands (tumor necrosis factor *[TNF]* and Fas ligand), withdrawal of growth factors or hormones, and injurious agents (e.g., radiation). Some stimuli (such as cytotoxic cells) directly activate execution caspases *(right)*. Others act by way of adapter proteins and initiator caspases, or by mitochondrial events involving cytochrome *c*. *(2)* Control and regulation are influenced by members of the Bcl-2 family of proteins, which can either inhibit or promote the cell's death. *(3)* Executioner caspases activate latent cytoplasmic endonucleases and proteases that degrade nuclear and cytoskeletal proteins. This results in a cascade of intracellular degradation, including fragmentation of nuclear chromatin and breakdown of the cytoskeleton. *(4)* The end result is formation of apoptotic bodies containing intracellular organelles and other cytosolic components; these bodies also express new ligands for binding and uptake by phagocytic cells. *(From Kumar V, Abbas A, Fausto N: Robbins & Cotran pathologic basis of disease, ed 7, Philadelphia, 2005, Saunders.)*

in a variety of pathologic circumstances, including viral diseases such as yellow fever in humans, gland involution following duct blockage, immunologic damage by T lymphocytes, and as a component of injury caused by some chemicals and drugs.

MECHANISMS OF APOPTOSIS*

Mechanisms of programmed cell death and apoptosis have been extensively researched within the last decades.

A variety of stimuli result in a self-programmed, genetically determined, energy-dependent sequence of molecular events involving initiation by cell signaling, control and integration by regulatory molecules, a common execution phase by caspase family genes, and dead cell removal. Some of these mechanisms are initiated by inflammatory mediators such as tumor necrosis factor (TNF) and the Fas ligand (FasL). Others involve deprivation of growth factors, mitochondrial damage, DNA damage, or immune stimulation (Fig. 1-30).

The process of apoptosis may be divided into an initiation phase, during which caspases become catalytically active, and an execution phase, during which these

---

*Portions of this section are from Kumar V, Abbas A, Fausto N: Robbins & Cotran pathologic basis of disease, ed 7, Philadelphia, 2005, Saunders.

enzymes act to cause cell death. Initiation of apoptosis occurs principally by signals from two distinct but convergent pathways: the extrinsic, or receptor-initiated, pathway and the intrinsic, or mitochondrial, pathway. Both pathways converge to activate caspases. We will describe these two pathways separately because they involve largely distinct molecular interactions, but it is important to remember that they may be interconnected at numerous steps.

THE EXTRINSIC (DEATH RECEPTOR–INITIATED) PATHWAY

This pathway is initiated by engagement of cell surface death receptors on a variety of cells. Death receptors are members of the TNF receptor family that contain a cytoplasmic domain involved in protein-protein interactions that is called the death domain because it is essential for delivering apoptotic signals. (Some TNF receptor family members do not contain cytoplasmic death domains; their role in triggering apoptosis is much less established). The best-known death receptors are the type 1 TNF receptor (TNFR1) and a related protein called Fas (CD95), but several others have been described. The mechanism of apoptosis induced by these death receptors is well illustrated by Fas (Fig. 1-31).

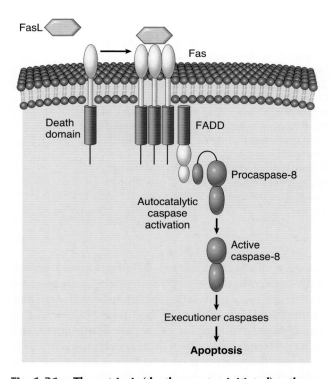

Fig. 1-31   The extrinsic (death receptor–initiated) pathway of apoptosis, illustrated by the events following Fas engagement. *FADD,* Fas-associated death domain; *FasL,* Fas ligand.
(From Kumar V, Abbas A, Fausto N: Robbins & Cotran pathologic basis of disease, ed 7, Philadelphia, 2005, Saunders.)

When Fas is cross-linked by its ligand, membrane-bound FasL, three or more molecules of Fas come together, and their cytoplasmic death domains form a binding site for an adapter protein that also contains a death domain and is called FADD (Fas-associated death domain). FADD is attached to the death receptors, which in turn bind an inactive form of caspase-8 (and, in humans, caspase-10), again via a death domain. Multiple procaspase-8 molecules are thus brought into proximity, and they cleave one another to generate active caspase-8. The enzyme then triggers a cascade of caspase activation by cleaving and thereby activating other procaspases, and the active enzymes mediate the execution phase of apoptosis (discussed later). This pathway of apoptosis can be inhibited by a protein called FLIP, which binds to procaspase-8 but cannot cleave and activate the enzyme because it lacks enzymatic activity. Some viruses and normal cells produce FLIP and use this inhibitor to protect infected and normal cells from Fas-mediated apoptosis. The sphingolipid ceramide has been implicated as an intermediate between death receptors and caspase activation, but the role of this pathway is unclear and remains controversial.

THE INTRINSIC (MITOCHONDRIAL) PATHWAY

This pathway of apoptosis is the result of increased mitochondrial permeability and release of proapoptotic molecules into the cytoplasm, without a role for death receptors. Growth factors and other survival signals stimulate the production of antiapoptotic members of the Bcl-2 family of proteins. This family is named after Bcl-2, which was identified as an oncogene in a B-lymphocyte lymphoma and is homologous to the *Caenorhabditis elegans* protein, Ced-9. There are more than 20 proteins in this family, all of which function to regulate apoptosis; the two main antiapoptotic ones are Bcl-2 and Bcl-x. These antiapoptotic proteins normally reside in mitochondrial membranes and the cytoplasm. When cells are deprived of survival signals or subjected to stress, Bcl-2 and/or Bcl-x are lost from the mitochondrial membrane and are replaced by proapoptotic members of the family, such as Bak, Bax, and Bim. When Bcl-2/Bcl-x levels decrease, the permeability of the mitochondrial membrane increases, and several proteins that can activate the caspase cascade leak out (Fig. 1-32). One of these proteins is cytochrome *c*, well known for its role in mitochondrial respiration. In the cytosol, cytochrome *c* binds to a protein called Apaf-1 (apoptosis activating factor-1, homologous to Ced-4 in *Caenorhabditis elegans*), and the complex activates caspase-9. (Bcl-2 and Bcl-x may also directly inhibit Apaf-1 activation, and their loss from cells may permit activation of Apaf-1.) Other mitochondrial proteins, such as apoptosis inducing factor (AIF), enter the cytoplasm, where they bind to and neutralize various inhibitors of apoptosis, whose

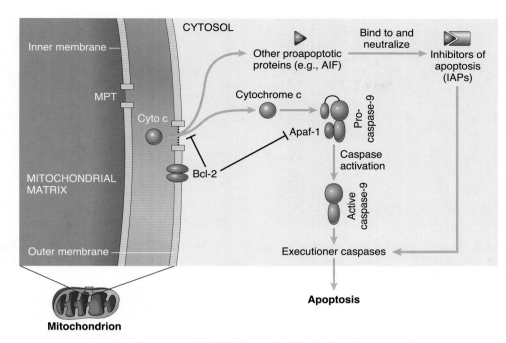

Fig. 1-32   The intrinsic (mitochondrial) pathway of apoptosis. Death agonists cause changes in the inner mitochondrial membrane, resulting in the mitochondrial permeability transition *(MPT)* and release of cytochrome *c* and other proapoptotic proteins into the cytosol, which activate caspases. **AIF,** Apoptosis-inducing factor. *(From Kumar V, Abbas A, Fausto N: Robbins & Cotran pathologic basis of disease, ed 7, Philadelphia, 2005, Saunders.)*

normal function is to block caspase activation. The net result is the initiation of a caspase cascade. Thus the essence of this intrinsic pathway is a balance between proapoptotic and protective molecules that regulate mitochondrial permeability and the release of death inducers that are normally sequestered within the mitochondria. There is quite a lot of evidence that the intrinsic pathway of apoptosis can be triggered without a role for mitochondria. Apoptosis may be initiated by caspase activation upstream of mitochondria, and the subsequent increase in mitochondrial permeability and release of proapoptotic molecules amplify the death signal. However, these pathways of apoptosis involving mitochondria-independent initiation are not well defined. We have described the extrinsic and intrinsic pathways for initiating apoptosis as distinct, but there may be overlaps between them. For instance, in hepatocytes, Fas signaling activates a proapoptotic member of the Bcl family called Bid, which then activates the mitochondrial pathway. It is not known if such cooperative interactions between apoptosis pathways are active in most other cell types.

THE EXECUTION PHASE

This final phase of apoptosis is mediated by a proteolytic cascade, toward which the various initiating mechanisms converge. The proteases that mediate the execution phase are highly conserved across species and belong to the caspase family, as previously mentioned. They are mammalian homologues of the Ced-3 gene in *Caenorhabditis elegans*. The term *caspase* is based on two properties of this family of enzymes: The "c" refers to a cysteine protease (i.e., an enzyme with cysteine in its active site), and "aspase" refers to the unique ability of these enzymes to cleave aspartic acid residues. The caspase family, now including more than 10 members, can be divided functionally into two basic groups: initiator and executioner, depending on the order in which they are activated during apoptosis. Initiator caspases, as we have seen, include caspase-8 and caspase-9. Several caspases, including caspase-3 and caspase-6, serve as executioners. Like many proteases, caspases exist as inactive proenzymes, or zymogens, and must undergo an activating cleavage for apoptosis to be initiated. Caspases have their own cleavage sites that can be hydrolyzed not only by other caspases but also autocatalytically. After an initiator caspase is cleaved to generate its active form, the enzymatic death program is set in motion by rapid and sequential activation of other caspases. Execution caspases act on many cellular components. They cleave cytoskeletal and nuclear matrix proteins and thus

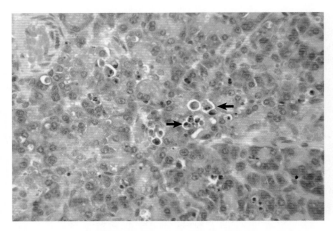

Fig. 1-33   Apoptosis, cytoarchitecture of cells, pancreas, rat. Individual acinar cells are shrunken and their chromatin condensed and fragmented (*arrows*). Cytoplasmic blebs are found in adjacent cells. Inflammation is absent. H&E stain.
(*Courtesy Dr. M.A. Wallig, College of Veterinary Medicine, University of Illinois.*)

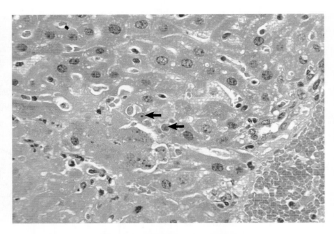

Fig. 1-34   Necrosis and apoptosis, mouse hepatitis virus infection, liver, mouse. This disease causes hepatocyte death, typically by oncotic necrosis but sometimes by apoptosis. Note areas of coagulation necrosis in the lower left and apoptotic bodies in the center, some of which have been taken up by adjacent hepatocytes (*arrows*). H&E stain.
(*Courtesy Dr. R.K. Myers, College of Veterinary Medicine, Iowa State University.*)

disrupt the cytoskeleton and lead to breakdown of the nucleus. In the nucleus, the targets of caspase activation include proteins involved in transcription, DNA replication, and DNA repair. In particular, caspase-3 activation converts a cytoplasmic DNAase into an active form by cleaving an inhibitor of the enzyme; this DNAase induces the characteristic internucleosomal cleavage of DNA, described earlier.

MORPHOLOGIC APPEARANCE OF APOPTOSIS

Morphologically, apoptotic cells have condensed chromatin and cytoplasm, and fragments of them are often found in adjacent or phagocytic cells (Fig. 1-33). Because single cells are dead, gross changes (and even microscopic changes) are usually not obvious. In addition, because the cell fragments into membrane-bound particles, phagocytosis occurs without the inflammation that is so often seen in necrosis.

Although typically discussed separately, necrosis by oncosis and apoptosis can be seen within the same tissue due to the same agent (Fig. 1-34). Cell injury by a chemical, for example, that injures mitochondria may release cytochrome *c* and initiate the apoptosis program. Cells with more severely affected mitochondria may die from swelling or oncosis.

The histopathologic characteristics of apoptosis are listed next:
- Individual cells are shrunken.
- Chromatin is condensed.
- Cytoplasm is fragmented.
- Cytoplasmic buds often containing a fragment of nucleus form on the surface, separate, and are found in adjacent cells and phagocytes as apoptotic bodies.
- Inflammation is absent.

CHRONIC CELL INJURY AND CELL ADAPTATION

As mentioned previously in the discussion of cell swelling and necrosis, cells respond to injury (or stress) in three possible major ways: (1) adaptation, (2) reversible injury with or without degeneration, and (3) death. Sublethal injury to a cell over time can lead to a variety of cell alterations. Cells may adapt by producing more cells (hyperplasia) or by producing more organelles, leading to an increase in size (hypertrophy); in some cases adaptation results in fewer organelles and a decrease in cell and tissue size (atrophy). Cells may degenerate in a variety of ways, some of which involve the accumulation of excess normal or abnormal substances. Impaired function may result, and morphologic changes in the cell and tissue may give a clue as to the cause of the cell injury.

SUBLETHAL INJURY AND SUBCELLULAR CHANGES

AUTOPHAGOCYTOSIS

Autophagocytosis is the uptake and intracellular degradation of damaged or effete organelles. Cells with sublethal injury often have various amounts of damaged organelles. As in organized societies, the cell has a system to clean up after a "storm." In autophagy, portions of the cytoplasmic matrix and its damaged organelles are enveloped by cell membranes to form autophagosomes, which subsequently fuse with lysosomes (Fig. 1-35). When phagocytic white cells ingest dead or dying cells, the process is very similar and termed heterophagy. Autophagy is a common reaction of sublethally injured cells, cells undergoing cyclic physiologic regression (glands), and in atrophy due to many causes. Recent evidence suggests that autophagocytosis pathways may result in a distinct type of cell death.

By light microscopy, autophagic vacuoles may appear as eosinophilic inclusions (see Intracellular Hyaline Proteins) and are common in the liver and kidney. As digestion progresses, electron-dense and lamellar debris is formed. Some vacuoles are evicted from the cell by exocytosis; others remain as residual bodies, and the contents form lipofuscin, the so-called wear-and-tear pigment.

Misfolded proteins or those otherwise altered occur in a variety of circumstances within the cell, both normally and in disease states. These proteins may be repaired by chaperones, or they may be degraded by the ubiquitin-proteasome pathway. The targeted proteins are conjugated to ubiquitin (one of several heat shock proteins) that through a cascade results in polyubiquitination and direction of the protein into a proteasome, a multi-subunit complex with a catalytic core that degrades the protein for removal. Removal of all sorts of proteins, including cell signaling molecules, allows proper control of cell function, growth, and replication. This pathway also plays a role in both activation and inhibition of apoptosis as well as in sublethal injury.

ADAPTIVE CHANGES LEADING TO CHANGE IN CELL SIZE, NUMBER, OR APPEARANCE

Adaptive changes to cell stress or injury can lead to an increase in the size of a tissue or organ (by hyperplasia and/or hypertrophy), a decrease in tissue and cell size (atrophy), or a change to a different cell type (metaplasia) (Fig. 1-36). *Hypertrophy* is an increase in the size of cells or organs. *Hyperplasia* is an increase in the number of cells in a tissue or organ. The two often occur together as an adaptive change and are considered positive responses to injury or stress.

HYPERTROPHY

In simple cellular hypertrophy, the number of cells does not increase. Cells synthesize more organelles, and cell enlargement occurs. The histologic architecture of the organ is normal, but cells are bigger. Hypertrophy can occur in most organs and tissues but tends to occur in cells that undergo little replication (i.e., stable or permanent cells). It is most common in striated muscle. Smooth muscle may have hypertrophy and hyperplasia. Causes of hypertrophy usually involve demands for increased function (e.g., the increased work load on a muscle and resultant hypertrophy of that muscle in weight lifters).

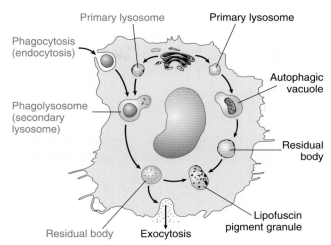

Fig. 1-35   **Autophagy and heterophagy.** Schematic representation of heterophagy (*left*) and autophagy (*right*). The mechanisms are similar for processing cell debris, both from intrinsic sources and extrinsic sources (heterophagy). *(From Kumar V, Abbas A, Fausto N: Robbins & Cotran pathologic basis of disease, ed 7, Philadelphia, 2005, Saunders.)*

The size and configuration of organelles reflect the work requirements of the cell. Chronic exposure to drugs such as phenobarbital, dilantin, and alcohol lead to enlargement of the SER in hepatocytes. SER contains the mixed oxidase enzyme systems that function to catabolize these substances. The increased size of the Golgi complex and RER are a reflection of a need for synthesis of extracellular proteins (e.g., immunoglobulin, collagen, and secretions). These organelles increase in size by duplication of membranes. The number of mitochondria adjusts to the ATP requirements of the cell. The size of nucleoli and proportion of euchromatin also reflect the synthetic activity of the cell.

Physiologic hypertrophy is common and expected following work. Compensatory hypertrophy is a response to the loss of a part of an organ or one of the paired organs or from obstruction of the lumen of a hollow muscular organ. For example, hypertrophy occurs in one kidney after the loss of the opposite kidney. The kidney enlarges due to the increased length of nephrons and not to the increased numbers of nephrons. Functional capacity increases with the increased size. Hypertrophy of the right ventricle of the heart because of stenosis of the pulmonary outflow tract is another example of compensatory hypertrophy (Fig. 1-37).

Hypertrophy is common, protective, limited, and reversible and may rarely cause harm to adjacent structures. Hypertrophy may not always be useful. In myocardial hypertrophy, enlargement of myofibers may occur with a corresponding increase in intercellular

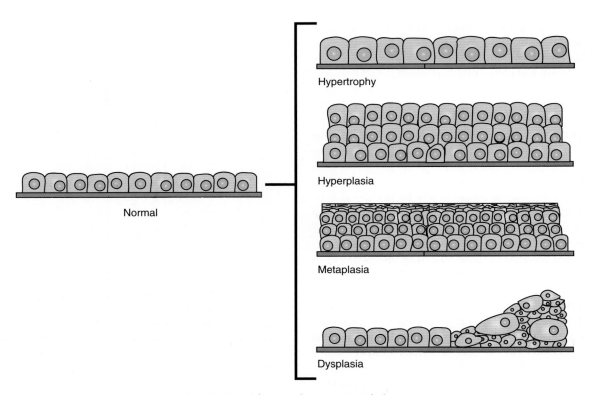

Normal

Hypertrophy

Hyperplasia

Metaplasia

Dysplasia

Fig. 1-36   Adaptive changes in epithelium.

stroma, making the myocardium stiff. In addition, the blood supply may not increase adequately to serve the increased mass of myocytes, and this results in hypoxic injury. The term *hypertrophy* is used in gross pathology to describe lesions that involve gross enlargement of an organ regardless of cause.

Cellular mechanisms leading to hypertrophy vary by tissue and cause, and details are lacking for most entities. Growth factors likely play a role in altering gene expression in many circumstances, whereas in myofiber hypertrophy, the type of mechanical stress can influence the way the muscle enlarges, for example

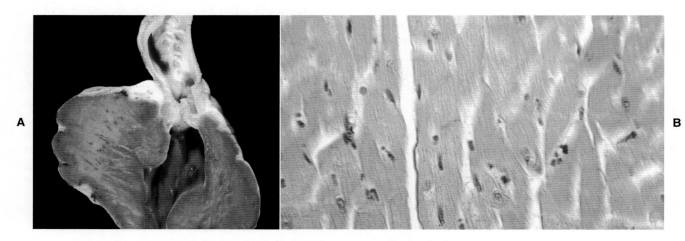

Fig. 1-37   Hypertrophy, heart, dog. A, Narrowing of the pulmonary out flow track caused by pulmonic valve stenosis has forced the right ventricle to contract with much more pressure. This increased workload has caused hypertrophy of the wall of the right ventricle, which is much thicker here than it would normally be. **B,** Note the increased size (hypertrophy) of myocytes in the overworked heart muscle. (**A** and **B,** *Courtesy Dr. L. Miller, Atlantic Veterinary College, University of Prince Edward Island; and Noah's Arkive, College of Veterinary Medicine, The University of Georgia.*)

with increased mitochondria, required for oxidative metabolism in endurance training. Hypertrophy of the uterus results from estrogen binding of cytosolic receptors that in turn lead to activation of genes leading to muscle protein production. These specific changes and others all are likely due to activation of specific genes.

HYPERPLASIA

Because hyperplasia is an increase in the number of cells, increased mitotic division is implied. Hyperplasia increases the size of a tissue, an organ, or part of an organ and may appear grossly as hypertrophy. It is a common change. Microscopically, cells resemble normal cells but are increased in numbers. Hyperplastic cells may also be increased in size (i.e., hypertrophic).

The ability of different adult cell types to undergo hyperplasia varies. Labile cells—those that routinely proliferate in normal circumstances, such as those of the epidermis, intestinal epithelium, and bone marrow cells—readily become hyperplastic. Permanent cells such as neurons and cardiac and skeletal muscle myocytes have very little capacity to regenerate or become hyperplastic in most situations. Stable cells, such as bone, cartilage, and smooth muscle, are intermediate in their ability to become hyperplastic.

Hyperplasia is traditionally divided into physiologic hyperplasia and pathologic hyperplasia. Physiologic hyperplasia is usually either hormonal or compensatory. Hormonal hyperplasia includes conditions such as increased mammary gland epithelial proliferation before lactation and enlargement of the pregnant uterus. Compensatory hyperplasia, or regeneration, occurs after a portion of an organ is lost. For example, if the skin is abraded, the basal layer of the epidermis undergoes mitosis to regenerate superficial layers. Removal of part of the liver can cause mitosis in the remaining hepatocytes resulting in the restoration of the liver to its normal size. This regenerative process takes as little as 2 weeks in rats after partial hepatectomy.

Pathologic hyperplasia is often caused by excessive hormonal stimulation of target cells or chronic irritation. Cystic endometrial hyperplasia of the canine uterus as a result of prolonged progesterone influence is common. Microscopically, there is folding of increased numbers of epithelial cells into glands and onto the lumen surface. The mucosa thickens and may trap or impair secretions, causing dilation of glands and cyst formation within the mucosa. The process is reversible if the stimulus is removed.

Pathologic hyperplasia may cause diffuse enlargement of an organ, such as in benign prostatic hyperplasia in dogs and in goiter (hyperplasia of the thyroid gland) (Fig. 1-38), or be localized as nodular hyperplasia. Nodular hyperplasia may occur without known cause and occurs in the spleen, liver, and pancreas of old dogs. One must differentiate hyperplasia, particularly nodular hyperplasia, from neoplasia.

The significance of hyperplasia usually lies in determining its cause. If it is hormonal in origin, the disturbance in the source organ should be determined.

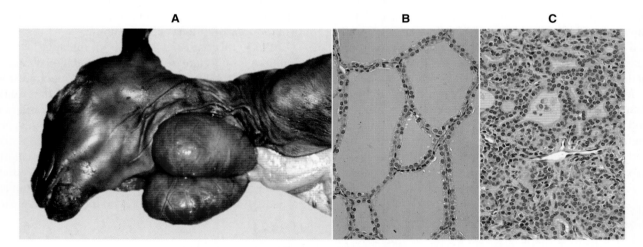

Fig. 1-38   Hyperplasia, thyroid goiter, goat. A, Deficiency of maternal dietary iodine during pregnancy has resulted in hyperplasia (and hypertrophy) of thyroid follicular epithelial cells in this neonatal goat and thus results in a symmetric enlargement of the glands (goiter). **B,** Thyroid follicular epithelial cells from a normal thyroid gland. H&E stain. **C,** Thyroid follicular epithelial cells from a case of thyroid goiter. Note the increased number (and size) of the follicular epithelial cells. H&E stain. (*A, Courtesy Dr. O. Hedstrom, College of Veterinary Medicine, Oregon State University; and Noah's Arkive, College of Veterinary Medicine, The University of Georgia. B and C, Courtesy Dr. B. Harmon, College of Veterinary Medicine, The University of Georgia; and Noah's Arkive, College of Veterinary Medicine, The University of Georgia.*)

If chronic irritation is the cause, determining the agent is often important. Hyperplasia is usually induced by known stimuli. It is a controlled process that stops when the stimulus ceases, can serve a useful purpose (e.g., repair defects, compensate for tissue loss, prepare for increased function, and aid in protection), and is subject to regular growth controls. These features are not part of neoplastic processes, which otherwise may be similar to hyperplastic changes in appearance and behavior.

Cellular mechanisms of hyperplasia vary in details depending on the cell affected and the cause. There are multiple controls as to whether or not a cell enters the replication cycle. In some circumstances hormones trigger cell replication, whereas in others growth factors, increased receptors for growth factors, and activation of cell signaling pathways may all have a role. In some circumstances cytokines are important. Ultimately, transcription factors may influence the expression of a new cadre of genes leading to cell proliferation. In regeneration for restitution of parenchyma to normal amounts (see later discussion), stem cells turn on and lead to appropriate cell replication.

METAPLASIA

Metaplasia is a reversible change in which one adult cell type is replaced by another adult cell type of the same germ line (Fig. 1-39). Usually, specialized epithelium is replaced by less specialized epithelium. One adult cell type does not transform into another type of adult cell. It is the less-differentiated reserve or stem cells that differentiate along a different line. For example, in cigarette smokers, chronic irritation of the normal columnar ciliated epithelium of the trachea and bronchial tree causes it to be replaced by focal or diffuse areas of stratified squamous epithelium. The squamous cells are more resistant to injury but are less protective to the lung, and, as they lack cilia, there is decreased clearance of mucus.

Metaplasia is often but not always an adaptive change to withstand adverse environmental conditions and is reversible if the cause is removed. Epithelial metaplasia is commonly to squamous epithelium and is usually a result of chronic irritation, but it can have other causes (e.g., avitaminosis A). Metaplasia in

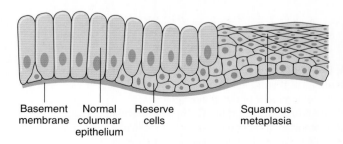

Basement membrane   Normal columnar epithelium   Reserve cells   Squamous metaplasia

Fig. 1-39   Metaplasia. Schematic diagram of columnar to squamous metaplasia. *(From Kumar V, Abbas A, Fausto N: Robbins & Cotran pathologic basis of disease, ed 7, Philadelphia, 2005, Saunders.)*

mesenchymal tissue is less clearly adaptive and is usually a response to change of microenvironment of cells, such as oxygen tension. One type of mesenchymal tissue changes to another; fibrous tissue changes to cartilage or bone, for example.

The following are some examples and causes of metaplasia:

- Chronic irritation from particles and chemicals in the lungs of smokers may cause the normal cuboidal and columnar epithelium of airways to become stratified squamous.
- Vitamin A deficiency causes squamous metaplasia of the transitional epithelium of the urinary tract, cuboidal and columnar epithelial cells lining the ducts within the salivary glands, and the epithelium of the mucous glands of esophageal mucosa in birds (Fig. 1-40).
- Estrogen toxicity, among other things, causes squamous metaplasia of the urinary tract and prostate.
- Healing of glandular epithelium following mastitis may at first be squamous.
- Squamous metaplasia of salivary, biliary, and pancreatic ducts can occur if they are blocked by stones in the lumen.
- Metaplastic bone (osseous metaplasia) occasionally occurs in injured soft tissue.
- Myeloid metaplasia (extramedullary hematopoiesis) in adult spleens and livers occurs commonly after bone marrow injury or insufficiency.
- Metaplasia occurs in some tumors, such as mixed mammary gland tumors of dogs.

Metaplasia is reversible (usually) if the cause is withdrawn. It may, however, be preneoplastic—for example, in the lungs of smokers where it appears before transformation to squamous cell carcinoma.

Cellular mechanisms leading to metaplasia vary. Vitamin A is important in normal differentiation of mucus secreting epithelium by yet unspecified mechanisms. When vitamin A is deficient, these cells differentiate along squamous lines. Estrogen causes differentiation along squamous lines in specific sex hormone responsive epithelia. Growth factors and other trophic substances presumably can influence differentiation along certain pathways from stem cells and ECM (extracelluar matrix) can play an important role. How these metaplastic changes take place in response to injury is less clear.

ATROPHY

Atrophy is the decrease in size or amount of a cell, tissue, or organ after normal growth has been reached (Fig. 1-41). It is due to the decreased number and/or size of cells. It may affect virtually any organ or part of an organ. It is a regressive change usually due to gradual and continuous injury. Some causes and examples of atrophy are:

- Deficient nutritive supply. Starvation and especially a decreased blood supply. For example, liver atrophy

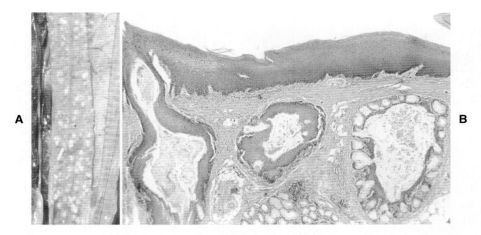

Fig. 1-40   Squamous metaplasia, esophagus, parrot. A, The esophageal mucosa has multiple white raised nodules from squamous metaplasia of mucosal glands. Metaplasia arose from the lack of dietary vitamin A (avitaminosis A). **B,** Note the squamous metaplasia of the esophageal glands. Vitamin A is necessary for maintenance of the normal epithelium. Avitaminosis A results in the replacement of normal mucosal epithelium and goblet cells in the glands by keratinized stratified squamous epithelium. H&E stain. (*A and B, Courtesy Dr. M.D. McGavin, College of Veterinary Medicine, University of Tennessee.*)

results from decreased blood flow through the portal vein (Fig. 1-42).

- Decreased workload. For example, muscle fibers atrophy in sedentary people.
- Disuse. Muscles in a limb that is in a cast atrophy.
- Denervation. Muscle fibers decrease in size if a nerve is severed.
- Pressure. Atrophy, degeneration, and necrosis occur adjacent to tumors because of pressure and compromised blood supply.
- Loss of endocrine stimulation. Atrophy of the zona fasciculata of the adrenal follows prolonged steroid therapy.

Involution is the decrease in size of a tissue caused by reduction in the number of cells (usually by apoptosis) and is usually used to refer to physiologic processes. For example, the thymus involutes with age, and many tissues become smaller because of senile involution. The uterus involutes after parturition, and its smooth muscle cells decrease notably in size and number.

The pathogenesis of atrophy implies an adverse environment. Cells regress to a smaller cell size and survive, but with decreased function. The general cause is inadequate cellular nutrition for any reason. Synthesis of proteins is exceeded by degradation or loss.

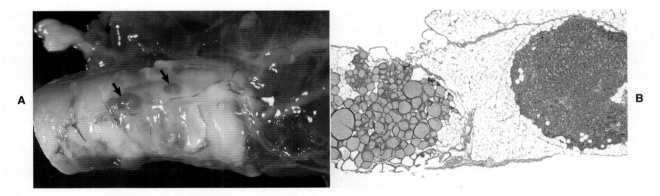

Fig. 1-41   Atrophy, right thyroid gland on trachea, dog. A, The right thyroid gland is extremely small and difficult to discern. Only small pieces of thyroid tissue remain (*arrows*). **B,** The thyroid gland is extremely small, follicles are atrophic and of varied sizes, and colloid has a low concentration of thyroglobulin protein (*pale pink color*). Note that supporting stroma has been replaced by fat cells. The parathyroid gland (*right*) is of normal size. H&E stain. (*A, Courtesy Dr. W. Crowell, College of Veterinary Medicine, The University of Georgia; and Noah's Arkive, College of Veterinary Medicine, The University of Georgia. B, Courtesy College of Veterinary Medicine, University of Illinois.*)

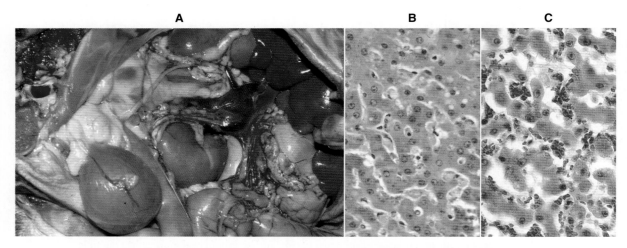

Fig. 1-42   Atrophy, liver, dog. A, Note the small size (up under the rib cage) but normal color of the liver in this dog and the anomalous size of the caudal vena cava in the mesentery (i.e., shunt between the portal vein and the systemic circulation). This shunt caused bypassing of blood from the liver. The reduction in blood flow to the liver causes decreased nutrients (hepatocyte trophic factors) to the hepatocytes and therefore decreased size of hepatocytes. **B,** Normal liver. H&E stain. **C,** Liver, atrophy. Hepatocytes are smaller and narrower than those in the normal liver (**B**). As a consequence, the sinusoids are correspondingly wider. H&E stain. (**A,** *Courtesy Dr. J. Sagartz, College of Veterinary Medicine, The Ohio State University; and Noah's Arkive, College of Veterinary Medicine, The University of Georgia.* **B,** *Courtesy Dr. M.D. McGavin, College of Veterinary Medicine, University of Tennessee.* **C,** *Courtesy Dr. R.K. Myers, College of Veterinary Medicine, Iowa State University.*)

Autophagocytosis, lysosomes, and the ubiquitin proteasome pathway (see earlier discussion under Sublethal Injury and Subcellular Changes) may all play a role in decreasing the organelle and protein content of a cell. The actual triggers and cellular mechanisms are unclear for many circumstances. Atrophy may resolve if the cause is removed. It may persist as is, with or without harm to the organism, or it may progress.

Atrophied organs grossly have a decreased weight and volume, may have a loose covering membrane (e.g., wrinkled skin), have tortuous blood vessels too large for the volume of tissue, and often are firmer due to fibrosis. Microscopically, cells are smaller and/or reduced in number. Ultrastructurally there are fewer mitochondria, less ER, and fewer myofilaments (muscle), and often there is an increase in autophagic vacuoles and maybe lipofuscin.

Serous atrophy of fat is a very important necropsy finding, as it may indicate starvation. Grossly, fat deposits are completely or partially depleted, and a clear or yellowish gelatinous material remains. Histologically, adipocytes are smaller, and interstitial hyaluronic acid mucopolysaccharides are increased. It is most evident in the epidural and perirenal fat, but may affect any fat depot including bone marrow. The cause of starvation may be virtually anything: malnutrition, malabsorption, chronic infection, parasitism, neoplasia, etc. It is common in neonates, often due to mismothering.

INTRACELLULAR ACCUMULATIONS*

One of the manifestations of metabolic derangements in cells is the intracellular accumulation of abnormal amounts of various substances (Fig. 1-43). The stockpiled substances fall into three categories: (1) a normal cellular constituent accumulated in excess, such as water, lipids, proteins, and carbohydrates; (2) an abnormal substance, either exogenous, such as a mineral or products of infectious agents, or endogenous, such as a product of abnormal synthesis or metabolism; or (3) a pigment. These substances may accumulate either transiently or permanently, and they may be harmless to the cells, but on occasion they are severely toxic. The substance may be located in either the cytoplasm (frequently within phagolysosomes) or the nucleus. In some instances, the cell may be producing the abnormal substance, and in other cells they may be merely storing products of pathologic processes occurring elsewhere in the body.

Many processes result in abnormal intracellular accumulations, but most accumulations are attributable to three types of abnormalities.

1. A normal endogenous substance is produced at a normal or increased rate, but the rate of metabolism is inadequate to remove it. An example of this type

---

*Portions of this section are from Kumar V, Abbas A, Fausto N: *Robbins & Cotran pathologic basis of disease,* ed 7, Philadelphia, 2005, Saunders.

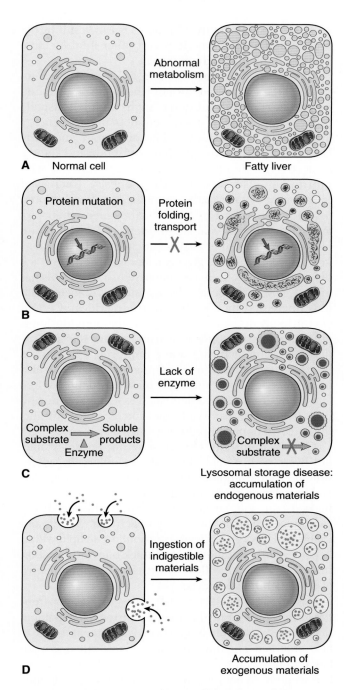

Fig. 1-43   Mechanisms of intracellular accumulations.
A, Abnormal metabolism, as in fatty change in the liver;
B, mutations causing alterations in protein folding and
transport, as in α_1-antitrypsin deficiency; **C,** deficiency
of critical enzymes that prevent breakdown of substrates
that accumulate in lysosomes, as in lysosomal storage
diseases; and **D,** inability to degrade phagocytosed particles,
as in hemosiderosis and carbon pigment accumulation.
(**A** *through* **D,** *From Kumar V, Abbas A, Fausto N: Robbins & Cotran
pathologic basis of disease, ed 7, Philadelphia, 2005, Saunders.*)

of process is fatty change in the liver because of intracellular accumulation of triglycerides (described in a
later section). Another example is the appearance of
reabsorption protein droplets in the epithelial cells of
renal proximal tubules because of increased leakage
of protein from the glomerulus.

2. A normal or abnormal endogenous substance accumulates because of genetic or acquired defects in
the metabolism, packaging, transport, or secretion
of these substances. One example is the group of
conditions caused by genetic defects of specific
enzymes involved in the metabolism of lipid and
carbohydrates resulting in intracellular deposition
of these substances, largely in lysosomes in so-called
storage diseases. Another is α_1-antitrypsin deficiency,
in which a single amino acid substitution in the
enzyme results in defects in protein folding and
accumulation of the enzyme in the ER of the liver in
the form of globular eosinophilic inclusions.

3. An abnormal exogenous substance is deposited and
accumulates because the cell has neither the enzymatic machinery to degrade the substance nor the
ability to transport it to other sites. Accumulations
of carbon particles and nonmetabolizable chemicals
such as silica particles are examples of this type of
alteration.

Whatever the nature and origin of the intracellular
accumulation, it implies the storage of some product by
individual cells. If the overload is due to a systemic
derangement and can be brought under control, the
accumulation is reversible. In genetic storage diseases,
accumulation is progressive, and the cells may become
so overloaded as to cause secondary injury, leading in
some instances to death of the tissue and the patient.

LIPIDS

HEPATIC LIPIDOSIS (FATTY LIVER, FATTY CHANGE, HEPATIC STEATOSIS)

All major classes of lipids can accumulate in
cells: triglycerides, cholesterol/cholesterol esters, and
phospholipids. Phospholipids are components of the
myelin figures found in necrotic cells. In addition,
abnormal complexes of lipids and carbohydrates accumulate in the lysosomal storage diseases.

Lipidosis is the accumulation of triglycerides and
other lipid metabolites (neutral fats and cholesterol)
within parenchymal cells. Although it occurs in heart
muscle, skeletal muscle, and the kidney, clinical manifestations are most commonly detected as alterations in
liver function (elevated liver enzymes, icterus) because
the liver is the organ most central to lipid metabolism.

Hepatic lipidosis, the prototype example of this type
of cellular degeneration, can occur as the result of one
of five mechanisms:

1. Excessive delivery of free fatty acids either from the gut or from adipose tissue
2. Decreased β-oxidation of fatty acids to ketones and other substances because of mitochondrial injury (toxins, hypoxia)
3. Impaired synthesis of apoprotein (CCl₄ toxicity, aflatoxicosis)
4. Impaired combination of triglycerides and protein to form lipoprotein (uncommon)
5. Impaired release (secretion) of lipoproteins from the hepatocyte (uncommon)

The underlying pathogenesis of hepatic lipidosis centers on the biochemical pathways of free fatty acid formation and metabolism. Free fatty acids, derived from triglycerides, provide a large component of the basal energy needs for parenchymal cells. They are obtained directly from the diet through digestive processes, from chylomicrons in the blood, or from adipose cells in body fat stores (adipose tissue). Chylomicrons transport dietary lipids consisting predominately of triglycerides from the alimentary system to the liver, muscle, and adipose tissue. Lipoprotein lipase and other proteins act synergistically within the chylomicron to free fatty acids from triglycerides for their use as an energy source. In the liver, free fatty acids are esterified to triglycerides, converted into cholesterol or phospholipids, or oxidized to ketones. Triglycerides can only be transported out of hepatocytes if apolipoprotein converts them to lipoproteins (Fig. 1-44). Alterations in one or

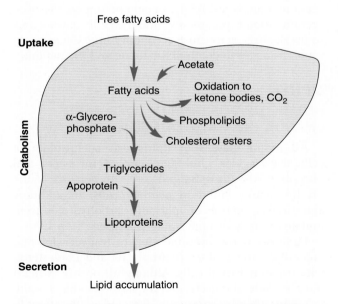

Fig. 1-44   Fatty liver. Schematic diagram of the possible mechanisms leading to the accumulation of triglycerides in a fatty liver. Defects in any of the steps of uptake, catabolism, or secretion can result in lipid accumulation in the cell.
(From Kumar V, Abbas A, Fausto N: Robbins & Cotran pathologic basis of disease, ed 7, Philadelphia, 2005, Saunders.)

more of these biochemical processes can result in the accumulation of triglycerides and other lipid metabolites, resulting in hepatic lipidosis.

In domestic animals, hepatic lipidosis most commonly arises from conditions that cause increased mobilization of body fat stores. Such conditions usually occur when there is increased demand for energy over a short duration, as in late pregnancy and early lactation in dairy cows (pregnancy toxemia and ketosis, respectively). Hepatic lipidosis is also observed with nutritional disorders including obesity (increased transport of dietary lipids or mobilization from adipose tissue), protein-calorie malnutrition (impaired apolipoprotein synthesis), and starvation (increased mobilization of triglycerides), but it also occurs in genetically inherited disorders, such as glycogen storage (Niemann-Pick disease [phospholipid sphingomyelin]) and Wilson's disease, and in endocrine disease, such as diabetes mellitus (increased mobilization of triglycerides). Certain chemical agents, such as CCl₄ (carbon tetrachloride is used in industrial applications) and yellow phosphorus (used in manufacturing other products) for example (rarely seen in clinical medical practice today), can also induce hepatic lipidosis via decreased oxidation of free fatty acids. In some disorders, such as feline hepatic lipidosis (feline fatty liver syndrome) and fat cow syndrome, the cause of hepatic lipidosis is unclear.

Grossly, mild fatty change may not be detectable, but livers with notable lipidosis are enlarged, yellow, soft and friable, and the edges of the lobes are rounded and broad instead of sharp and flat (Fig. 1-45, A). When incised, the cut surface of severely affected livers can bulge and the hepatic parenchyma is soft and friable and has a greasy texture attributable to lipid within hepatocytes. In addition, a 1-cm-thick transverse section from a liver lobe may float in formalin, again indicative of lipid within hepatocytes.

It is important to distinguish these gross lesions from the lesions present in glucocorticoid (steroid) hepatopathy in dogs. The liver in glucocorticoid hepatopathy is also enlarged and has rounded edges, but it is pale beige to tan-white, firm, and nongreasy (Fig. 1-46, A). Cut sections do not float in formalin. These gross lesions are attributable to the accumulation of glycogen and water in the cytoplasm of hepatocytes (see Chapter 8).

Microscopically, hepatocytes with lipidosis are vacuolated, with the extent of the vacuolation depending on the severity of the lipidosis. Initially there are a few small clear vacuoles that increase in size and number and eventually coalesce into larger vacuoles. These vacuoles have sharply delineated borders (Fig. 1-45, B), which are attributed to the hydrophobic interface between water and lipid in the cell's cytoplasm and should be compared with vacuoles that result from glycogen accumulation (Fig. 1-46, B). In hepatocytes

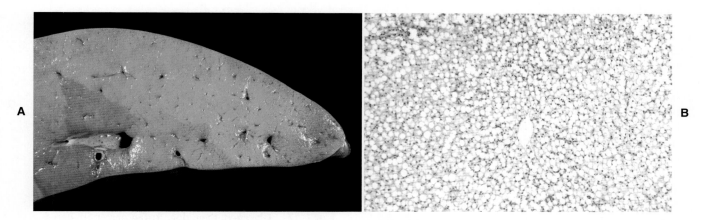

Fig. 1-45   **Steatosis (fatty liver, fatty change, hepatic lipidosis), liver, ox. A,** Note the uniformly pale yellow surface. The liver is usually enlarged and the edges rounded. The cut surface bulges on incision and may feel greasy. **B,** In this severely affected liver, all hepatocytes are vacuolated and their nuclei have been displaced to the side. H&E stain. (**A** *and* **B,** *Courtesy Dr. M.D. McGavin, College of Veterinary Medicine, University of Tennessee.*)

with large amounts of fat, the nucleus can be displaced to the periphery, and the cell can resemble an adipocyte. In extremely affected livers in which all of the hepatocytes are filled with lipid, the liver can resemble fat and can be identifiable only by the presence of portal areas.

Vacuoles in hepatocytes may be due to fat accumulation but can also occur as the result of intracellular accumulation of glycogen or water. Fat is confirmed by special stains, but as alcohol and clearing agents used during the processing of paraffin-embedded sections dissolve fat, formalin-fixed frozen sections—properly stained for fat—must be used to confirm the presence of fat in hepatocytes. Fat stains, which are alcoholic solutions of fat soluble dyes, include Sudan III, Scharlach R, and Oil-Red-O. Glycogen is confirmed by the PAS and PAS-diastase reactions described later (see Glycogen). Vacuoles that do not stain with either fat or PAS are presumed to be a result of the accumulation of water (hydropic degeneration).

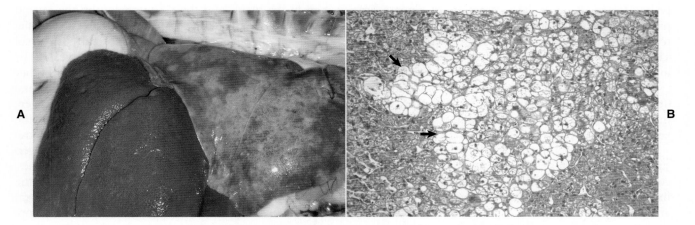

Fig. 1-46   **Glucocorticoid hepatopathy, liver, dog. A,** Extensive accumulation of glycogen in hepatocytes leads to an enlarged and pale brown to beige liver in dogs with glucocorticoid excess from endogenous (Cushing's disease) or exogenous sources. The liver is usually enlarged and the edges rounded. This cut surface would bulge on incision and not be greasy. **B,** Note the swollen hepatocytes (*arrows*) with extensive cytoplasmic vacuolation. H&E stain. (**A,** *Courtesy Dr. K. Bailey, College of Veterinary Medicine, University of Illinois.* **B,** *Courtesy Dr. J. M. Cullen, College of Veterinary Medicine, North Carolina State University.*)

FATTY INFILTRATION

Fatty infiltration should not be confused with fatty change or steatosis, in which the lipid is intracellular (see previous discussion). Adipocytes are normally present in connective tissue and in limited numbers between fasciculi of skeletal muscle and subepicardially between cardiac myocytes. When increased lipid is to be stored, adipocytes increase in number, and the process is called fatty infiltration. It occurs in old age and in obesity in which there is hyperplasia of adipocytes by means of proliferation of preadipocytes. When myocytes of skeletal muscle atrophy and disappear, the lost myocytes may be replaced by adipocytes (see Fig. 15-29).

GLYCOGEN

Variable amounts of glycogen are normally stored in hepatocytes and myocytes (the amount in the liver depends on the interval between sampling and the last meal). Hepatocytes of starved animals are usually devoid of glycogen. Excessive amounts of glycogen are present in animals in which glucose or glycogen metabolism is abnormal, such as diabetes mellitus, or in animals that have received excess amounts of corticosteroids. Large amounts of glycogen can be found in the livers of young growing animals and in animals that are well nourished and on diets of commercially produced feeds.

In diabetes, glycogen is found not only in hepatocytes but also in the epithelial cells of renal proximal tubules and in B cells of the Islets of Langerhans. Hepatocytes are highly permeable to glucose, and hyperglycemia leads to increased glycogen concentration in these cells. Also in diabetes, large amounts of glucose are passed out in the glomerular filtrate and exceed the resorptive capacity of the renal tubule epithelial cells. These cells, when overloaded with glucose, convert it into glycogen, which accumulates intracellularly.

Grossly, physiologic deposits of glycogen cannot be detected, but in steroid-induced hepatopathy, where massive amounts of glycogen are stored, the liver may be enlarged and pale (Fig. 1-46).

Microscopically the amount of glycogen demonstrated in hepatocytes is chiefly a function of the original concentration in the cell, the delay between death and fixation during which time the glycogen is metabolized, and the type of fixation. Despite frequent statements that glycogen is best preserved by fixing tissue in an alcoholic fixative (e.g., absolute alcohol or 10% formalin in absolute alcohol), glycogen can be well preserved by fixation in an ordinary 10% buffered neutral formalin solution at 4° C in a refrigerator during the period of fixation (Fig. 1-47, A). This procedure retains most of the glycogen but avoids the excessive shrinkage and

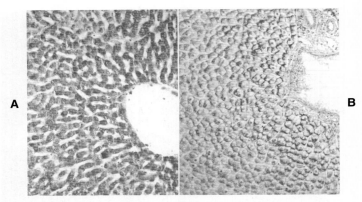

Fig. 1-47   Glycogen, liver, dog. A, Ten-percent buffered neutral formalin fixation at 4° C. Glycogen (purplish-red) is uniformly dispersed throughout the cytoplasm of all hepatocytes. Periodic acid-Schiff technique. **B,** Absolute alcohol (ethanol) fixation at room temperature. The glycogen in each hepatocyte has been pushed to the side of the cell, so-called polarization of glycogen. Periodic acid–Schiff technique. (**A** and **B,** *Courtesy Dr. M.D. McGavin, College of Veterinary Medicine, University of Tennessee.*)

distortion of tissues attributed to fixation in alcoholic fixatives and also avoids "polarization," the phenomenon whereby the glycogen is displaced to the side of the cell away from the surface. Polarization is seen in fixation at room temperature but is worst with alcoholic fixatives (Fig. 1-47, B).

Histologically, glycogen is demonstrated specifically by the PAS reaction using two serial tissue sections mounted on glass slides. The tissue section on the first slide is pretreated with diastase, which digests the glycogen in the tissue, and the tissue section on the second glass slide is untreated. Thus the deposits digested by diastase are glycogen. The PAS reaction breaks 1,2-glycol linkages to form aldehydes, which are revealed by Schiff's reagent. These linkages occur in substances other than glycogen, hence the use of two slides including one pretreated with diastase to specifically identify glycogen. Microscopically, glycogen appears as clear vacuoles in the cytoplasm of the cell. In contrast to intracellular fat whose vacuoles are rounded and sharply delineated, glycogen forms irregular clear spaces with indistinct outlines. Usually the nucleus remains centrally located in the hepatocyte. However, if very large amounts of glycogen are stored in hepatocytes, as in steroid-induced hepatopathy, hepatocyte nuclei may be displaced peripherally.

In glycogen storage diseases (glycogenoses), glycogen accumulates, sometimes in massive amounts in cells as a result of a defective enzyme. Exactly which cells store glycogen depends on the defective enzyme, but skeletal muscle is frequently involved (see Chapters 14 and 15 for more detail).

PROTEINS

In histologic sections, intracellular protein accumulations are of several types and include rounded eosinophilic droplets, vacuoles, and aggregates in cells. The causes of these accumulations vary widely.

HYALINE CHANGE

The adjective "hyaline" is defined by *Dorland's Medical Dictionary* as "glassy and transparent or nearly so," and the noun "hyalin" as a "translucent albuminoid substance." However, histologically the term has come to mean having a homogeneous, eosinophilic, and glassy (translucent) appearance. Some pathologists also add "amorphous," and the lesion has been termed both a change and a degeneration, but the term hyaline is purely descriptive and is rather loosely applied to a variety of changes, none of which is a true cellular degeneration. Hyaline substances may be intracellular or extracellular.

INTRACELLULAR HYALINE PROTEINS

Intracellular hyaline proteins include resorption droplets, Russell bodies in plasma cells, and those caused by defects in protein folding.

Resorption droplets in the epithelial cells of renal proximal tubules

There is normally very little protein in the filtrate from the glomerulus, and what is present is resorbed by the proximal tubule epithelial cells. When the protein concentration of the filtrate is high, as in a proteinuria, for example from glomerular damage, this protein is taken up by the proximal tubule epithelial cells into vesicles where, in H&E stained sections, they appear as hyaline droplets in the cytoplasm (Fig. 1-48, A). The vesicles fuse with the lysosomes to form phagolysosomes, where the protein is metabolized. If the proteinuria ceases, the formation of hyaline droplets also ceases. This condition was once called "hyaline droplet degeneration." It is not a degeneration but an exaggeration of a normal process. Also, similar droplets are seen in the intestinal epithelium of neonatal pigs and calves that have recently ingested colostrum.

Excessive production of normal protein

Hyaline bodies called Russell bodies are seen in the cytoplasm of some plasma cells (Mott cells). These bodies are large, eosinophilic, homogenous, and amorphous and consist of immunoglobulin (γ-globulin). Russell bodies have been described as "manifestations of cellular indigestion" in the ER.

Defects in protein folding

During protein synthesis on ribosomes, proper folding of the protein is essential for its transport in the cell's organelles. Normally, if there is a defect in folding, the protein is eliminated by the proteasome complex. On occasion, these folded proteins accumulate in cells as is seen in some of the human neurodegenerative diseases, including Alzheimer's disease. Sometimes folded proteins may accumulate in tissue, and some types of amyloidosis are examples of this process.

OTHER INTRACELLULAR INCLUSIONS

AUTOPHAGIC VACUOLES

Autophagic vacuoles are large eosinophilic intracytoplasmic inclusions, which ultrastructurally are autophagosomes (Fig. 1-35). They are a common response to injury in cells with sublethal damage, particularly hepatocytes, and are a mechanism by which the cell rids itself of damaged or senescent organelles. A portion of the cell membrane invaginates and envelops the affected organelles to form an autophagosome, which then fuses with a lysosome to cause degradation of the contents. Digestion of the material in autophagic vacuoles may leave some lamellar debris, and this debris may either be exocytosed from the cell or remain intracellularly to form lipofuscin (see later discussion of pigments).

CRYSTALLINE PROTEIN INCLUSION BODIES

Crystalline protein inclusions, sometimes known as crystalloids, occur in normal hepatocytes and renal tubular epithelial cells, particularly in old dogs. They are large, eosinophilic, and rhomboidal and may be so large as to distort the nucleus or the cell (Fig. 1-48, B). Except for being age related, they are of unknown significance. In fact, an increased incidence of these inclusions is the most consistent age-related change in canine hepatocytes.

VIRAL INCLUSION BODIES

Infection of host cells by some types of viruses results in the formation of characteristic inclusion bodies, which may be intranuclear, intracytoplasmic, or both. They are accumulations of viral protein and are useful diagnostically to confirm a specific viral disease.

DNA viruses such as herpesviruses, adenoviruses, and parvoviruses tend to produce only intranuclear inclusions. These inclusions are round to oval and can be eosinophilic (herpesviruses), basophilic, or amphophilic (adenoviruses). Pox viruses are also DNA viruses, but they produce large distinct eosinophilic intracytoplasmic inclusion bodies in infected cells.

A few RNA viruses produce intracytoplasmic inclusions. Examples are the distinctive cytoplasmic neuronal inclusions of rabies (Negri bodies) and the epithelial inclusions of canine distemper. Distemper causes both intranuclear and intracytoplasmic inclusions in nervous tissue (Fig. 1-48, C). Viral inclusions are

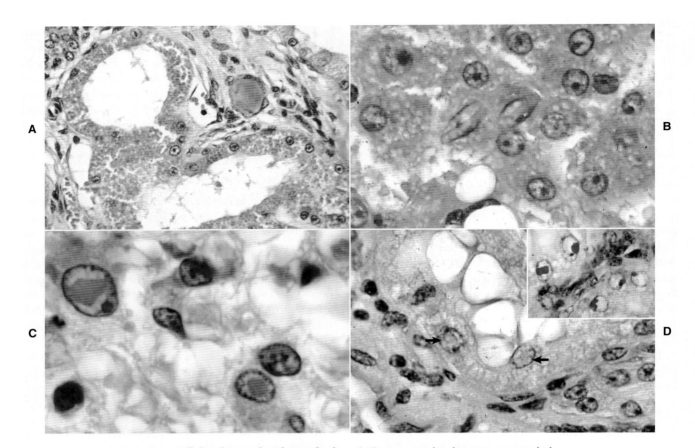

Fig. 1-48 **Cell droplets and inclusion bodies. A,** Resorption droplets, proteinuria, kidney, dog. The cytoplasm of the proximal tubule epithelial cells are filled with eosinophilic homogeneous droplets—protein that has been resorbed by the cells from the glomerular filtrate. H&E stain. **B,** Crystalloids, kidney, dog. Note the elongated crystals in the nuclei of the hepatocytes. **C,** Viral inclusion bodies, brain, dog. Note the intranuclear eosinophilic inclusion bodies in glial cells. H&E stain. **D,** Lead inclusion bodies, kidney, dog. The inclusions in the nuclei of these renal tubular epithelial cells are difficult to see with an H&E stain *(arrows). Inset:* An acid-fast stain is useful in identifying lead inclusions, which stain red. Ziehl Neelsen stain. *(A and C, Courtesy Dr. M.D. McGavin, College of Veterinary Medicine, University of Tennessee. B, Courtesy Dr. D.D. Harrington, College of Veterinary Medicine, Purdue University; and Noah's Arkive, College of Veterinary Medicine, The University of Georgia. D, Courtesy Dr. W. Crowell, College of Veterinary Medicine, The University of Georgia; and Noah's Arkive, College of Veterinary Medicine, The University of Georgia. Inset, Courtesy Dr. W. Crowell, College of Veterinary Medicine, The University of Georgia; and Noah's Arkive, College of Veterinary Medicine, The University of Georgia.)*

usually surrounded by a clear halo, particularly in the nucleus. Cells with inclusion bodies and adjacent cells usually have signs of degeneration or cell death. Many of these viral inclusion bodies will be discussed in the systemic pathology chapters of this book.

LEAD INCLUSION BODIES

In lead poisoning, irregularly shaped intranuclear inclusion bodies that are acid-fast may be present in renal tubular epithelial cells (Fig. 1-48, *D*). They contain both lead and protein. When they are present, they are helpful in the diagnosis of lead poisoning. In dogs, they must be distinguished from the protein crystalline protein inclusions described previously.

EXTRACELLULAR ACCUMULATIONS

HYALINE SUBSTANCES

Extracellular hyaline substances include the following:
1. Hyaline casts in the lumens of renal tubules in a proteinuria
2. Serum or plasma in blood vessels
3. Plasma proteins in vessel walls (e.g., in porcine edema disease). These substances are subendothelial hyaline deposits, primarily seen in arterioles of the brain stem in pigs with porcine edema disease (Fig. 1-51).
4. Old scars. With age, the number of nuclei in collagen deposits decrease as the result of cell senescence,

and the collagen fibers condense and become hyalinized.

5. Thickened basement membranes (e.g., in glomerulonephritis and in the capillaries of the choroid plexus with old age)
6. Hyaline membranes of the alveolar walls (see Chapter 9)
7. Hyaline microthrombi (e.g., platelet microthrombi) in disseminated intravascular coagulation (DIC); often visible in glomerular capillaries and pulmonary alveolar capillaries
8. Amyloid as described next

AMYLOID

The name *amyloid* is given to a chemically diverse group of chiefly extracellular proteinaceous substances that appear histologically and ultrastructurally similar. The name means "starchlike" and was applied to these proteins because when the surface of an affected organ was treated with an iodine solution and then with dilute sulfuric acid, it turned blue, a positive test for starch (Fig. 1-49).

Histologically, amyloid is an eosinophilic amorphous hyaline substance (Fig. 1-50, *A*). It is extracellular and compresses adjacent parenchymal cells, causing atrophy or death from compression and/or ischemia. This outcome is most evident in hepatic amyloidosis, in which the protein is deposited in the space of Disse. Here it compresses the adjacent hepatocytes and interferes with the hepatocytes' access to blood and nutrients in the sinusoids.

The most frequently used special stain for amyloid is Congo red. It stains amyloid orange to orange red (Fig. 1-50, *B*) and under polarized light imparts a light green, so-called apple green fluorescence (see Chapter 11). Congo red staining is not absolutely specific, and

transmission electron microscopy to identify 7.5- to 10-nm filaments may be necessary.

Chemically, amyloid is not one substance. It is a diverse group of glycoproteins whose protein component is configured in a β-pleated sheet pattern, which is responsible for the characteristic staining with Congo red. In human beings, there are three major and several minor forms. In animals, there are two major and two minor forms, which are chemically different but histologically similar.

AL amyloid consists of immunoglobulin light chains, is monoclonal, and is secreted by plasma cells in immunocyte dyscrasias (B-lymphocyte proliferative disorders).

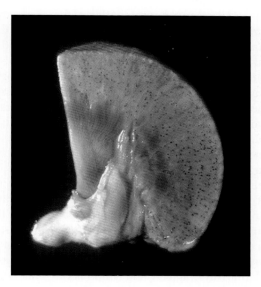

Fig. 1-49   Amyloidosis, kidney, cross section, dog. Note the blue-black foci, which are glomeruli-containing amyloid stained by Lugol's iodine. *(Courtesy Dr. M.D. McGavin, College of Veterinary Medicine, University of Tennessee.)*

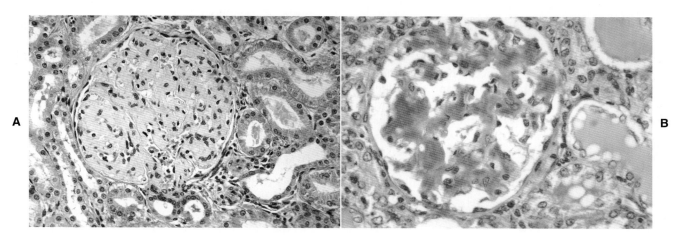

Fig. 1-50   Amyloidosis, kidney, dog. A, The renal glomerulus contains large amounts of pale homogeneous eosinophilic material, which is amyloid. H&E stain. **B,** The amyloid in the glomeruli stains orange. Congo red stain. (**A** and **B,** *Courtesy Dr. M.D. McGavin, College of Veterinary Medicine, University of Tennessee.)*

AA amyloid is not an immunoglobulin but is synthesized from a precursor protein SAA (serum amyloid associated) secreted by the liver. SAA concentration is increased in inflammatory states, but this increase does not necessarily lead to amyloid deposition in all cases in response to IL-1 and IL-6. A minor form of amyloidosis is hereditary amyloidosis found in Shar-Pei dogs and in Abyssinian cats.

β-Amyloid found in Alzheimer's disease in human beings has been detected in the brains of aged dogs.

CLASSIFICATION OF AMYLOIDOSIS

Amyloidosis has been classified in several ways (i.e., primary versus secondary, systemic [generalized] versus localized, and a combination of these categories). Systemic amyloidosis (generalized) is also divided into primary amyloidosis (immunocyte dyscrasia) and secondary amyloidosis (reactive systemic amyloidosis).

- Immunocyte dyscrasia is the most common form of amyloidosis in human beings, but not in animals. The amyloid consists of amyloid light chains and is indicative of a plasma cell dyscrasia. These cells also secrete large amounts of λ- and κ-light chains into blood and urine (Bence Jones proteins), which are diagnostically important.
- Reactive systemic amyloidosis was initially called secondary amyloidosis because it was secondary to chronic inflammatory conditions, particularly those causing a chronic antigenic stimulation with protracted breakdown of cells. It is the most common form of amyloidosis in animals, and the amyloid is deposited in kidney, liver, spleen, and lymph nodes. Functionally, and most often in old dogs, amyloid deposits in the kidney are the most important because they are located in the mesangium and basement membranes of renal glomeruli and cause a proteinuria. The spleen is the most frequent site in reactive systemic amyloidosis, and amyloid is deposited in the periarteriolar lymphoid sheaths and red pulp. The space of Disse of the liver is the usual site for amyloidosis in birds.
- Localized amyloidosis involves a single organ or tissue. Such localized lesions are in the nasal vestibule or rostral portion of the nasal septum and turbinates in horses and in the pancreatic islets in cats.
- β-Amyloidosis. Extracellular accumulation of amyloid-β protein (Aβ) is characteristic of Alzheimer's disease in humans. This type of amyloid has also been identified in the brains of aged dogs, the highest concentration being in the frontal cortex. Dogs older than 13 years had Aβ plaques.

LOCATION OF AMYLOID DEPOSITS IN ANIMALS

The kidney (glomeruli in most animals and medullae in cats), liver (space of Disse in cattle, horses, dogs, and cats), and spleen (germinal centers) are common sites.

Other organs affected include the stomach, intestine (lamina propria), thyroid (C-cell tumor), skin (dermis and subcutis of horses), lymph node (germinal centers), adrenal cortex, pancreas (islets of Langerhans in cats), nasal septum and turbinates (walls of submucosal vessels and basement membranes of mucosal glands of horses), and meningeal and cerebral vessels of older dogs. See the appropriate organ chapters for more detail.

OTHER EXTRACELLULAR ACCUMULATIONS

FIBRINOID CHANGE

Fibrinoid change, also known as the fibrinoid necrosis and fibrinoid degeneration, is a term applied to a pattern of lesions most often observed in the vascular system. The terms *fibrinoid degeneration* and *necrosis* are inappropriate, as the process is not a true regressive alteration of cells. Rather, fibrinoid change is the result of the deposition of immunoglobulin, complement, and/or plasma proteins, including fibrin in the wall of a vessel. This lesion is due to injury to the intima and media such as occurs in the immune-mediated vasculitides.

Grossly, fibrinoid change cannot be observed; however, it is often accompanied by thrombosis and hemorrhage, and when these two lesions are present in a vascular pattern of distribution, fibrinoid change of the vasculature should be considered. Microscopically, direct injury to endothelial cells, basement membrane, or myocytes, such as caused by viruses or toxins, or indirect injury, such as caused by activation complement proteins, can lead to activation of the acute inflammatory cascade and the deposition of plasma proteins in the vessel walls. These proteins, especially fibrin, stain intensely red (eosinophilic) with H&E stains, and involve the vessel wall circumferentially to varying depths of the tunica intima and tunica media (Fig. 1-51). This lesion is also often accompanied by cellular and nuclear debris from injured vascular cells and inflammatory cells. These proteins contribute to the vascular "eosinophilia," which has been described somewhat differently by different pathologists. There is general agreement that the material is eosinophilic, which is sometimes described as "smudgy" or "deeply eosinophilic." Some pathologists add "homogeneous" and others "amorphous" to the descriptive terminology of fibrinoid change.

GOUT

Gout is the deposition of sodium urate crystals or urates in tissue. It occurs in human beings, birds, and reptiles but has not been reported in domestic animals.

In the most common form in human beings, urate crystals are deposited in the articular and periarticular tissues and elicit an acute inflammatory response characterized by the presence of neutrophils and macrophages

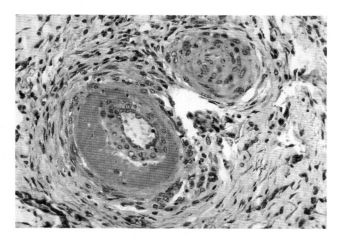

Fig. 1-51   Fibrinoid change, artery. Note the deeply eosinophilic circumferential band in the tunica media. **H&E stain.** *(Courtesy Dr. M.D. McGavin, College of Veterinary Medicine, University of Tennessee.)*

and large aggregations of urate crystals called tophi. These tophi may be visible grossly and are pathognomonic of gout. Later in the course of the disease, the inflammation becomes chronic and a foreign body reaction to the tophi develops. Microscopically, urate crystals are acicular and birefringent and they, or the spaces left after they have been dissolved during the preparation of paraffin-embedded histological sections, are visibly surrounded by numerous neutrophils, macrophages, and giant cells.

In birds and reptiles, there are two forms including: (1) the articular type, which is rare; and (2) a visceral type. The latter characteristically affects the visceral serosae, particularly parietal pericardium, and the kidneys. The serosa is covered with a thin layer of gray granules, and the gross appearance is diagnostic. In the renal form, urate deposits are visible in renal tubules and ureters. Uric acid and urates are the end products of purine metabolism, and in birds and reptiles these products are eliminated as semisolid urates. Visceral gout is usually diagnosed only at necropsy and is seen sporadically due to vitamin A deficiency, high-protein diets, and renal injury.

PSEUDOGOUT

Pseudogout is characterized by deposits of calcium pyrophosphate crystals. It is well recognized in human beings but has been reported in the dog, in which it is rare. The pathogenesis of the canine disease is unknown, but in human beings one form is inherited as an autosomal dominant trait. Grossly, there are chalky white deposits in the joints, which histologically show a chronic reaction with aggregates of crystalline material, macrophages, and fibrosis. The disease may be differentiated from gout by the chemical analysis of the crystalline deposits.

CHOLESTEROL

Cholesterol crystals are the by-products of hemorrhage and necrosis. They are dissolved out of the tissue specimen during the preparation of paraffin-embedded sections, leaving characteristic clefts which, in section, resemble shards of glass. Actually the crystals are thin rhomboidal plates with one corner notched out, their outline resembling that of the state of Utah. Cholesterol crystals in tissue have no significance except that they indicate the site of an old hemorrhage or tissue necrosis, and they may be present in atheromas (i.e., mass of degenerated, thickened arterial intima occurring in atherosclerosis). However, in the choroid plexus of the lateral ventricles of old horses, cholesterol crystals can induce a granulomatous response, and the resultant cholesterol granuloma or cholesteatoma can become so large as to obstruct the outflow of cerebrospinal fluid through the interventricular foramen (foramen of Munro), resulting in obstructive hydrocephalus. It is thought that these granulomas are secondary to cholesterol crystals from hemorrhages into the choroid plexus. Grossly, the cholesterol appears as firm, crumbly gray nodules in the cholesteatomas.

PATHOLOGIC CALCIFICATION*

Calcium salts, usually in the form of phosphates or carbonates, may be deposited in dead, dying, or normal tissue. This process is known as pathologic calcification and occurs in two forms: dystrophic and metastatic. When the deposition occurs locally in dying tissue, it is known as dystrophic calcification; it occurs despite normal serum concentrations of calcium and in the absence of derangements in calcium metabolism. In contrast, the deposition of calcium salts in otherwise normal tissue is known as metastatic calcification, and it almost always results from hypercalcemia secondary to some disturbance in calcium metabolism.

DYSTROPHIC CALCIFICATION

Dystrophic calcification occurs in areas of necrosis, no matter the type of necrosis-coagulative, caseous, liquefactive, or fat necrosis, but is minimal in liquefactive necrosis. Dead and dying cells can no longer regulate the influx of calcium into their cytosol, and calcium accumulates in the mitochondria.

Common sites include necrotic myocardium (Fig. 1-52), necrotic skeletal muscle, granulomas such as tuberculoid granulomas in cattle, and dead parasites, such as hydatid cysts in cattle and trichinae in pigs. Calcium deposits are relatively permanent but harmless

*Portions of this section are from Kumar V, Abbas A, Fausto N: *Robbins & Cotran pathologic basis of disease,* ed 7, Philadelphia, 2005, Saunders.

unless they interfere mechanically (e.g., the movement of a calcified heart valve). Their significance is that they are an indicator of previous injury to a tissue.

Calcification in or under the skin has been designated calcinosis. There are two main forms: (1) calcinosis cutis and (2) calcinosis circumscripta (also see Chapter 17). Calcinosis cutis occurs in dogs with hyperadrenocorticism from either endogenous or exogenous glucocorticoids and has been regarded as idiopathic calcification by some pathologists and dystrophic calcification by others. There is mineralization of the dermal collagen, and epidermal and follicular basement membranes. Calcinosis circumscripta is considered to be dystrophic. It has a preference for German shepherds and Great Danes, in which it is familial. Also, it has been associated with repetitive trauma and at the site of buried sutures of polydioxanone.

Grossly the affected areas of tissue are white and when incised have a gritty feel to them (Fig. 1-52). Microscopically, calcium salts stain blue with hematoxylin and appear as fine amorphous granules or clumps, which can be either intracellular or extracellular. However, the full extent of the calcification may not be evident in H&E stained sections (Fig. 1-53, A) but is revealed more dramatically by special stains, such as von Kossa and Alizarin red S (Fig. 1-53, B). The von Kossa method is not specific for calcium but stains phosphates and carbonates. These substances are almost always complexed with calcium.

METASTATIC CALCIFICATION

Metastatic calcification occurs in normal tissue and is secondary to hypercalcemia. The basic abnormality is the entry of large amounts of calcium ions into cells.

These ions precipitate on organelles, particularly mitochondria.

The four causes of metastatic calcification in order of their importance in veterinary medicine are as follows:
1. Renal failure. Renal failure results in retention of phosphates, which induce a secondary renal hyperparathyroidism and hypercalcemia. Calcium is deposited in the gastric mucosa, kidney, and alveolar septa.

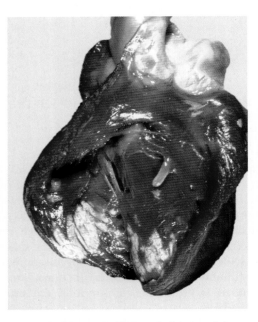

Fig. 1-52 **Calcification, vitamin E/selenium deficiency, myodegeneration, heart, lamb.** The multiple white lesions are areas of necrosis of cardiac myocytes that have been calcified. *(Courtesy Dr. M.D. McGavin, College of Veterinary Medicine, University of Tennessee.)*

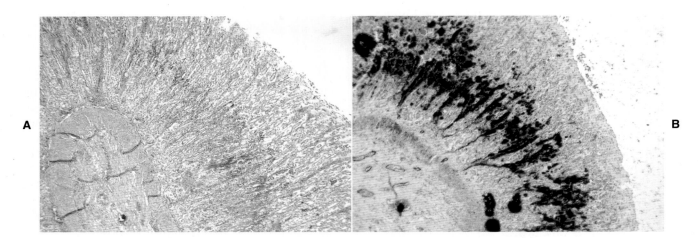

Fig. 1-53 **Uremia, stomach, dog.** A band of calcium has been laid down the middle of the gastric mucosa. **A,** The calcium is stained blue with hematoxylin. H&E stain. **B,** The calcium is stained black. von Kossa stain. (**A** and **B,** *Courtesy Dr. M.D. McGavin, College of Veterinary Medicine, University of Tennessee.*)

2. Vitamin D toxicosis. The ingestion of calcinogenic plants, such as *Cestrum diurnum* by herbivores, results in severe soft tissue mineralization, chiefly involving the aorta, heart, and lungs. In the heart, the endocardium of the right and left atria and left ventricle is often strikingly mineralized. Acute vitamin D toxicosis in dogs and cats is commonly caused by ingestion of rodenticides containing cholecalciferol. Intestinal mucosa, vessel walls, lung, and kidneys are mineralized.

3. Parathormone (PTH) and PTH-related protein. Primary hyperparathyroidism is rare. Hypercalcemia and elevated concentrations of PTH-related protein can be associated with canine malignant lymphomas and canine adenocarcinoma of the apocrine glands of the anal sac. Intestinal mucosa, vessel walls, lung, and kidneys are mineralized.

4. Destruction of bone from primary or metastatic neoplasms.

HETEROTOPIC BONE (ECTOPIC BONE)

Some lesions of dystrophic and metastatic calcification may be confused on gross examination with ectopic ossification, the name given to the process of production of bone at an abnormal site. Ectopic bone is of two types: heterotopic or osseous metaplasia. "Heterotopia" refers to foci of cells or tissues, which are microscopically normal but present at an abnormal location. They are considered to arise from embryonic cell rests. The other type of bone is formed by osseous metaplasia, usually from another type of connective tissue. Fibroblasts differentiate into osteoblasts that form osteoid, which is calcified as in normal bone (Fig. 1-54). This is the more common type.

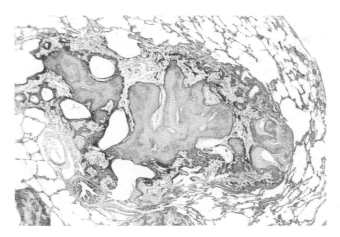

Fig. 1-54   Ectopic bone, lung, dog, A nodule of mature bone in the connective tissue of the lung. H&E stain. *(Courtesy Dr. M.D. McGavin, College of Veterinary Medicine, University of Tennessee.)*

Heterotopic bone is found at many sites, commonly as spicules or nodules of bone in connective tissue of lungs of dogs and cattle, and in the canine dura mater (dural ossification or ossifying pachymeningitis) and at sites of dystrophic and metastatic calcification.

PIGMENTS

It is customary in pathology textbooks to group substances that impart an unusual color to the body (systemic) or its tissues (localized), under the category of pigments. Many of these pigments are unrelated in their origin, but their importance lies in the fact that the clinician and the pathologist need to be able to recognize them grossly, and the pathologist also needs to be able to identify them histologically. Recognition may provide valuable clues in understanding the disease process at hand and its underlying pathogenesis. Because of their diversity, pigments are usually classified broadly into two groups: exogenous (formed outside the body) and endogenous (formed inside the body).

EXOGENOUS PIGMENTS

These pigments include carbon, tattoos, dusts, carotenoids, and tetracycline.

CARBON

Carbon is the most common exogenous pigment. The usual route of entry into the body is via inhalation, and its accumulation in the lung results in a condition called anthracosis (also known as black lung).

Carbon is ubiquitous in the air and all animals are exposed, but those most likely to show gross lesions live in an environment with substantial air pollution, such as adjacent to busy highways (e.g., animals in a zoo near a highway or animals living in a house with a smoker). In the alveoli, the carbon is phagocytosed by macrophages, which transport it via the lymphatics to the regional tracheobronchial lymph nodes. Because elemental carbon is inert and not metabolized by the body, it remains in the tissue for the life of the animal.

Grossly the lungs are usually speckled with fine 1- to 2-mm-diameter subpleural black foci, which are most visible if the lungs are exsanguinated (Fig. 1-55, *A*). In severely affected cases, the medulla of the tracheobronchial lymph nodes may be black. The heavy deposits are in this location because of the concentration of sinus histiocytes (macrophages) in the medulla.

Microscopically, carbon presents as fine black granules and may be extracellular or intracellular (within macrophages). Carbon pigment may be within the alveolar walls or be frequently present as black peribronchiolar or peribronchial foci (Fig. 1-55, *B*). Because of the nonreactiveness of carbon, there are no histochemical

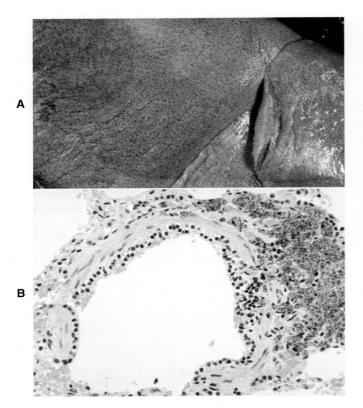

Fig. 1-55   **Anthracosis, lung, aged dog. A,** The fine black foci are peribronchiolar deposits of carbon. The animal was exsanguinated at euthanasia to remove the blood from the lung to render the carbon deposits more visible. **B,** Carbon *(black)* inhaled into the alveoli has been phagocytosed by macrophages and transported to the peribronchial region. H&E stain. *(**A** and **B,** Courtesy Dr. M.D. McGavin, College of Veterinary Medicine, University of Tennessee.)*

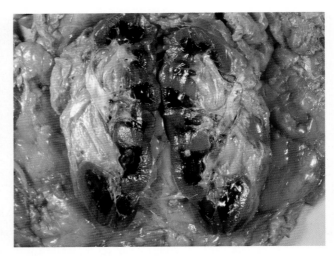

Fig. 1-56   **Carotenosis, kidney and the perirenal fat, Jersey ox.** Accumulation of carotenoids in the adipocytes has colored the fat yellow to dark yellow. *(Courtesy Dr. M.D. McGavin, College of Veterinary Medicine, University of Tennessee.)*

tests for it. Unlike many other pigments, it is resistant to solvents and bleaching agents.

TATTOOS

Animals are frequently tattooed as a method of identification. These pigments, which include carbon, are introduced into the dermis. Some of the pigments are phagocytosed by macrophages, whereas the remainder remains free in the dermis where it can remain indefinitely and does not invoke any inflammatory reaction.

DUSTS

Pneumoconiosis is the general term used for any dust inhaled into and retained in the lung. Anthracosis, from the inhalation of carbon, is a subtype of pneumoconiosis. Inhalation of silicon (e.g., from quarries) is called silicosis. These minute particles enter the lungs by escaping the mucociliary defense mechanisms of the nasal and upper respiratory systems (see Chapter 9) and are deposited in pulmonary alveoli where they may

be phagocytosed and carried to the peribronchial regions. Some types of silica evoke a fibrous reaction, which may ultimately form nodules. Microscopically the mineral is visible as birefringent crystals under polarized light.

CAROTENOID PIGMENTS

These pigments are also called lipochrome pigments, although this term is sometimes confused with lipofuscin (see later discussion). They are fat-soluble pigments of plant origin and include the precursors of vitamin A, namely β-carotene.

Grossly, these pigments normally occur in a wide variety of tissue, such as adrenal cortical cells, corpus luteum-lutein cells, Kupffer cells, and testicular cells, and in the plasma/serum and fat of horses and Jersey and Guernsey cattle and sometimes dogs (Fig. 1-56). Carotenoids discolor fat yellow to orange-yellow. The concentration of carotenoids retained in tissue depends upon the species of animal. Some animals store little or no carotenoids and have white fat and clear serum. These animals include Holstein cattle, sheep, goats, and cats. As fat stores are depleted (e.g., in starvation or cachexia), carotenoids become concentrated in the adipocytes, giving them a dark yellowish-brown color.

Microscopically, carotenoids are not seen in routine formalin-fixed paraffin-embedded sections because the alcohols and clearing agents remove the fat-soluble pigments.

The significance of carotenoids is that they may obscure or confuse the detection of icterus. In those animals whose fat and serum are devoid of carotenoids, a yellow discoloration is easily detected and is most likely to be caused by bilirubin (i.e., icterus).

TETRACYCLINE

Tetracycline-based antibiotics administered during the development of teeth will be deposited in mineralizing dentin, enamel, and cementum, staining the teeth or portions of them yellow or brown (Fig. 1-57). Thus tetracycline administered to a pregnant animal stains the deciduous teeth of the offspring. Tetracycline also stains bone that is being laid down and has been used experimentally as a marker for that bone.

ENDOGENOUS PIGMENTS

MELANIN

Melanin is the pigment normally present in the epidermis and is responsible for the color of the skin and hair. It is also normally present in the retina, iris, and in small amounts in the pia-arachnoid of black animals (e.g., Suffolk sheep [Fig. 1-58]) and in the oral mucous membrane of some breeds (e.g., Jersey cows and Chow dogs).

Melanin is secreted by cells called melanocytes. In the skin of animals, these cells are in the basal layer and transfer their pigment by means of dendritic processes to adjacent keratinocytes, where the melanin is often arranged as a cap over the nucleus to provide some protection from ultraviolet radiation. Melanin is formed by the oxidation of tyrosine, which requires the copper-containing enzyme tyrosinase. Thus in copper deficiency, particularly in cattle and sheep, there is a fading of the coat color, and this is most obvious in black wool. A general lack of melanin can be due to a metabolic defect: a lack of tyrosinase. This condition is called albinism, and the affected animal is called an albino. Histologically the melanocytes appear normal.

Pathologically, melanin is present in hyperpigmentation of the skin associated with many types of chronic injury and endocrinopathies such as hyperadrenalism and in primary neoplasms of melanocytes (melanomas and melanosarcomas), although highly malignant tumors may have little or no pigment.

Microscopically, melanin is stored in melanosomes in the cytoplasm of melanocytes. However, if there is damage to the cells containing melanin (e.g., damage to melanocytes and basal cells of the skin), the free melanin is phagocytosed by macrophages, which are termed melanophages.

Extensive deposits of congenital melanin in tissues is termed congenital melanosis. It occurs in the lungs and aorta (intima) of cattle, sheep, and pigs as brown to black spots up to a couple of centimeters in diameter (Fig. 1-59). Melanosis of the lung is visible both subpleurally and in cross sections of the parenchyma. These deposits of melanin have no adverse effect, but organs with extensive melanosis may be aesthetically unacceptable as food and thus will be condemned at the packing plant.

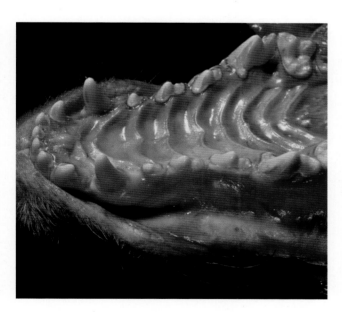

Fig. 1-57   Tetracycline staining, teeth, young dog. The teeth of this dog have been stained yellow by the tetracycline ingested during their development. *(Courtesy Dr. M.D. McGavin, College of Veterinary Medicine, University of Tennessee.)*

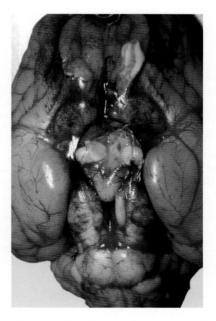

Fig. 1-58   Congenital melanosis, leptomeninges, Suffolk sheep. The leptomeninges have scattered black areas of melanin. This is normal in black-faced sheep. *(Courtesy Dr. M.D. McGavin, College of Veterinary Medicine, University of Tennessee.)*

LIPOFUSCIN-CEROID

Lipofuscin, known as "wear-and-tear" pigment, has in the past been described as accumulating with age and in certain pathologic conditions. However, in recent years, lipofuscin, now referred to as "age pigment," has been differentiated from a pathologically accumulating similar pigment called ceroid, described later.

Lipofuscin accumulates in a time-dependent manner in postmitotic cells (neurons, cardiac myocytes [Fig. 1-60, A], and skeletal muscle myocytes) and in slowly dividing cells, such as hepatocytes and glial cells, and this process is present at a few months of age. Lipofuscin is also found in other cells, but as these replicate, the lipofuscin is divided between the daughter cells and thus does not accumulate to the same extent as it does in postmitotic cells. Lipofuscin is the end result of autophagocytosis of cell constituents, such as organelles, and is the final undegradable remnant of that process. As the pigment cannot be removed by further lysosomal degradation or exocytosis, it accumulates in lysosomes, a form of biologic garbage (Fig. 1-60, B).

Ceroid has many of the same histochemical features as lipofuscin (see later discussion) but is found in response to severe malnutrition, including vitamin E deficiency, cachexia from cancer, irradiation, and in the inherited disease neuronal ceroid-lipofuscinosis. It accumulates in Kupffer cells and to a lesser extent in hepatocytes, skeletal and smooth muscle myocytes, and in inherited neuronal ceroid-lipofuscinosis, where it accumulates in neurons. It can be either intracellular or extracellular. Unlike lipofuscin, it is considered to have a deleterious effect on the cell.

Both lipofuscin and ceroid have many common histologic and histochemical features, such as autofluorescence (golden yellow) and staining with stains for fat such as Sudan black (sudanophilia), although oil-red-O is more sensitive, PAS positiveness, and acid fastness (long Ziehl Neelsen technique). All of these characteristics increase in intensity with age for lipofuscin, but not for ceroid. Lipofuscin consists chiefly of proteins and lipids with very little carbohydrate, but lectin-binding

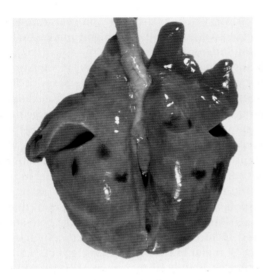

Fig. 1-59   Congenital melanosis, lung, pig. Melanin deposits are subpleural and extend into the substance of a lung. The lesion has no pathological significance. *(Courtesy Dr. M.D. McGavin, College of Veterinary Medicine, University of Tennessee.)*

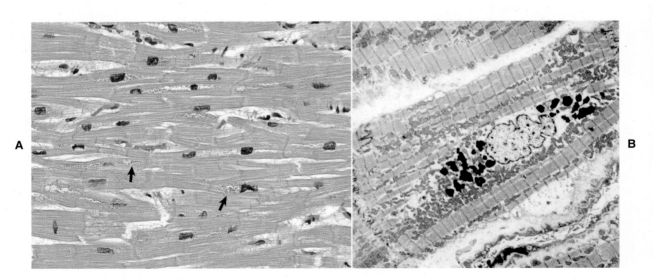

Fig. 1-60   Lipofuscinosis, heart, human. A, Note the brown lipofuscin granules *(arrows)* at the poles of the myocyte nuclei. H&E stain. **B,** Lipofuscin *(black)* is perinuclear and within lysosomes. TEM. Uranyl acetate and lead citrate stain. *(From Kumar V, Abbas A, Fausto N: Robbins & Cotran pathologic basis of disease, ed 7, Philadelphia, 2005, Saunders.)*

histochemistry in human beings and rats has revealed differences in the saccharides of lipofuscin and ceroid.

Grossly, large amounts of lipofuscin in the heart and skeletal muscles impart a brown tinge. It is commonly seen in aged dairy cows sent to slaughter. Ceroid is grossly evident in the small intestine of dogs with so-called intestinal lipofuscinosis (Fig. 1-61) (see Chapter 7) and in nutritional panniculitis in cats, mink, foals, and pigs. Both these conditions are associated with a vitamin E deficiency and the ingestion of unsaturated fatty acids. In the dog the tunica muscularis, usually of the caudal small intestine, is discolored brown because of accumulations of ceroid in myocytes. In the cat with nutritional panniculitis, the subcutaneous fat is discolored lemon yellow to orange. This disease is considered to be the result of the ingestion of fish products with a high concentration of unsaturated fatty acids and a vitamin E deficiency, frequently brought about by the fats becoming rancid and destroying the vitamin E.

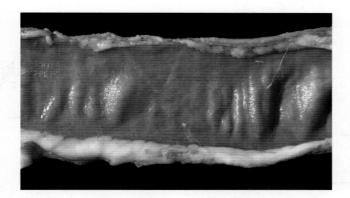

Fig. 1-61   Ceroid, intestine, serosal surface, dog. Note the brown discoloration of the muscular layer. The condition has been called intestinal lipofuscinosis but is not age related. *(Courtesy Dr. M.D. McGavin, College of Veterinary Medicine, University of Tennessee.)*

Microscopically, in routine H&E stained sections or in unstained sections, lipofuscin varies from a light golden brown to dark brown with advancing age. Because it is intralysosomal, it is perinuclear in neurons and in cardiac, skeletal, and smooth muscle myocytes. In feline nutritional panniculitis, globules of ceroid are extracellular in the interstitial tissue or have been ingested by macrophages and giant cells.

The significance of these two pigments is that lipofuscin is a clear indicator of the age of the cell and ceroid is a pathological pigment, often associated with vitamin E deficiency. Lectin binding histochemistry, which has shown differences between lipofuscin and ceroid from rats and human beings, may be applicable to differentiating these pigments in domestic animals, but it is a very laborious research tool and only provides semiquantitative data. Isolation and physicochemical analysis is more precise but even more laborious. Thus, until some other specific test becomes available, differentiation between the two pigments for diagnostic purposes will be based on the features listed in Table 1-1.

HEMATOGENOUS PIGMENTS

This category includes hemoglobin, oxyhemoglobin, unoxygenated hemoglobin, methemoglobin, carboxyhemoglobin, hemosiderin, bilirubin, and hematin. Some are produced normally but can accumulate excessively (unoxygenated hemoglobin, hemosiderin, and bilirubin). Other pigments such as methemoglobin, carboxyhemoglobin, and hematin are pathological.

HEMOGLOBIN

This normal pigment of erythrocytes can be responsible for gross changes in the color of the body. Oxygenated hemoglobin is red and imparts the pink appearance to unpigmented skin and tissues. Normally, arterial blood (oxygenated hemoglobin) is red, and

Table **1-1**   Differences between Lipofuscin and Most Ceroid Pigments in Vivo

	Lipofuscin	Ceroid
Universality (invariably present in humans and all domestic animals)	Yes	No
Intrinsically (intracellularly in lysosomes of postmitotic and stable cells)	Yes	No
Time dependence	Yes	No
Initial occurrence	Infancy	Anytime
Deleteriousness	Never demonstrated	Frequent
Accumulation rate	Very slow	Usually rapid
Tissue distribution	Only intracellular	Intracellular and extracellular
Mode of formation	Mainly autophagy	Mainly heterophagy
Origin of precursors	Mainly intracellular	Mainly extracellular

From Porta EA: *Ann N Y Acad Sci* 959:57-65, 2002.

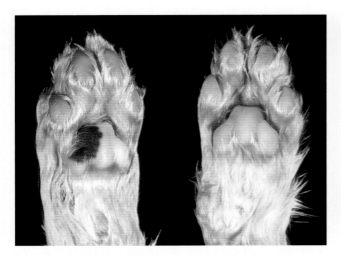

Fig. 1-62 **Cyanosis, feet, cat.** The footpads of the paw on the left are bluish due to unoxygenated hemoglobin, the result of a partial obstruction of the iliac artery at the aortic bifurcation by a saddle thrombus. Normal control paw on the right. *(Courtesy Dr. M.D. McGavin, College of Veterinary Medicine, University of Tennessee.)*

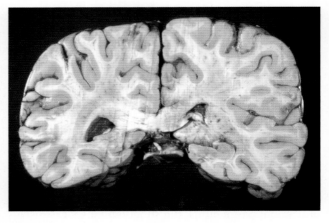

Fig. 1-63 **Carbon monoxide (CO) poisoning, brain, human.** The blood in the brain is cherry red from the carboxyhemoglobin formed by the inhalation of CO in exhaust gases. *(Courtesy Dr. J.C. Parker, School of Medicine, University of Louisville.)*

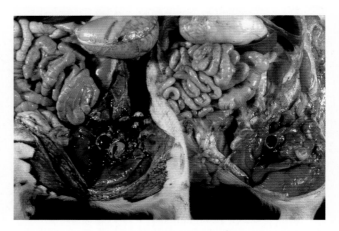

Fig. 1-64 **Methemoglobinemia, experimental nitrite poisoning, hindleg, pig.** *Left,* The methemoglobin in the blood has discolored the blood and muscle chocolate brown. *Right,* Normal control. *(Courtesy Dr. L. Nelson, College of Veterinary Medicine, Michigan State University.)*

venous blood with more unoxygenated blood is bluish. However, if the blood is not sufficiently oxygenated (unoxygenated hemoglobin), the tissues will appear blue, exhibiting so-called cyanosis (Fig. 1-62).

In acute cyanide poisoning, cyanide binds to cytochrome oxidase, the enzyme in the cell responsible for oxidative phosphorylation, and this results in paralysis of cellular respiration. Tissues cannot use the oxygen delivered by the blood. Consequently, in acute cyanide toxicity the oxygen content and color of venous blood may be similar to those of arterial blood, and the venous blood will be bright red.

In carbon monoxide (CO) poisoning, as from exhaust gases from automobiles, the blood is a bright cherry red from the formation of carboxyhemoglobin (Fig. 1-63). Methemoglobin is an oxide of hemoglobin, in which the ferrous ion of hemoglobin is converted to the ferric ion, resulting in a reddish-brown (chocolate brown) color to the blood and tissue (Fig. 1-64). Methemoglobin is seen most often in poisoning by nitrites, especially following ingestion of nitrate-accumulating plants, but has been reported as a result of acetaminophen, naphthalene, local anesthetics (lidocaine, benzocaine, and tetracaine), and chlorates. It may also be congenital due to a genetic condition that occurs in human beings.

In intravascular hemolysis, hemoglobin is released from the lysed erythrocytes and stains the plasma pink. This hemoglobin may be excreted by the kidney, staining it dark red to reddish-black and the urine red (Fig. 1-65). Similar changes can result from myoglobinuria after the destruction of large numbers of myofibers (see Chapter 15).

HEMATINS

This category of pigments includes "formalin pigment" and the excreta of parasites, such as *Fascioloides magna* (liver fluke) and *Pneumonyssus simicola* (lung mite).

FORMALIN PIGMENT

Formalin pigment, also called "acid formalin hematin," is an annoying microscopic artefact that occurs when tissue rich in blood comes in contact with acid solutions of formalin, particularly if there has been a delay between death and fixation, allowing time for the erythrocytes to lyse and release their hemoglobin.

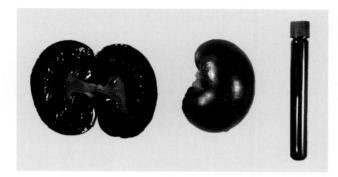

Fig. 1-65   Acute hemolysis from chronic copper poisoning, kidney and urine, sheep. The dark bluish color of the kidney and the dark red of the urine are caused by hemoglobin excreted via the kidney. *(Courtesy Dr. M.D. McGavin, College of Veterinary Medicine, University of Tennessee.)*

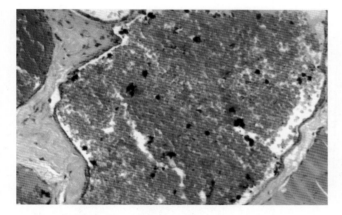

Fig. 1-66   Formalin pigment, blood. Note the black spicules of hematin that lie between and on the erythrocytes, the result of fixation in unbuffered (acid) 10% formalin. H&E stain. *(Courtesy Dr. M.D. McGavin, College of Veterinary Medicine, University of Tennessee.)*

Grossly, formalin pigment is not visible because this change occurs only after fixation. Microscopically the pigment is brown to almost black, fine, and granular (Fig. 1-66), and can have birefringent spicules. It occurs mainly in blood vessels but also in other tissues where there are large accumulations of red blood cells. Pigment can lie between or on top of red blood cells and is negative for iron when stained by the Prussian blue reaction.

Because formalin pigment is formed only during fixation, it has no pathologic significance. Its significance is that it can interfere with the interpretation of histological sections. Fortunately it is easy to prevent its formation. Formalin pigment does not form if the pH of the fixative is above 6. Aqueous solutions of unbuffered

formalin are highly acid. A common fixative is 10% buffered neutral formalin (really buffered neutral 10% formalin), which is buffered with a Sorensen phosphate buffer, and despite the name "neutral" has a pH of 6.8. It does not cause the formation of formalin pigment. Another commonly used and commercially available formalin fixative is Carson's fixative (also called modified Millonig's formalin fixative), with a pH of 7.3 and can be used as a dual-purpose fixative for both routine histopathologic and electron microscopic examinations. If formalin pigment is present in a tissue section, it can be removed by a variety of techniques including soaking the dewaxed tissue section before H&E staining in a saturated alcoholic solution of picric acid.

PARASITE HEMATIN

The two most common causes of parasite hematin in veterinary medicine are *Fascioloides magna* (liver fluke) in ruminants and *Pneumonyssus simicola* in the lungs of macaques.

Parasite hematin from *Fascioloides magna* causes black tracts throughout the liver and is colloquially known as "fluke exhaust" (Fig. 1-67, *A*). This lesion can be so severe as to affect the whole liver. Microscopically the black pigment accumulates adjacent to the migration tracts of the parasite and is phagocytosed by macrophages (Fig. 1-67, *B*). *Pneumonyssus simicola* produces a similar brown to black anisotropic pulmonary pigment presumed to be from the metabolism of hemoglobin by the parasite.

HEMOSIDERIN

Iron is stored in the body in two forms, ferritin and hemosiderin, both of which are protein-iron complexes. Ferritin is in all tissues, but the heaviest concentrations are found in the liver, spleen, bone marrow, and skeletal muscle. Hemosiderin is formed from intracellular aggregates of ferritin (Fig. 1-68). It appears as golden-yellow to golden-brown globules and is the most visible form of storage iron. Normally, most storage iron is found in the spleen.

Excess iron from the breakdown of senescent erythrocytes, or the result of a hemolytic crisis (e.g., because of autoimmune diseases or hemotropic parasites) or reduced erythropoiesis (malnutrition), is stored mainly in the spleen. Rarely in veterinary medicine, excess iron can be present in the body because of excessive absorption from the gut, multiple injections of iron, or from multiple blood transfusions.

Besides splenic storage, there may be local iron storage at sites of erythrocyte breakdown, such as in hemorrhages, and in areas of poor blood flow, as in chronic passive congestion of the lungs. In the latter case, because of the poor blood flow through the lungs, erythrocytes may come to the end of their natural life and be lysed

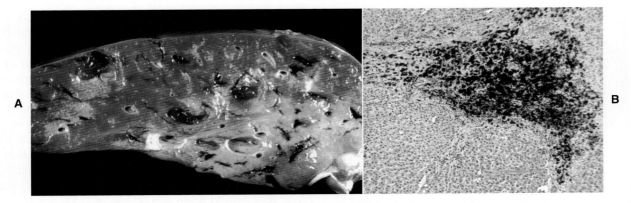

Fig. 1-67 **Hematin pigment from *Fascioloides magna*, liver, ox. A,** Large areas of the liver are black from the pigment excreted by the fluke as it migrated through the liver. **B,** Hematin *(black)* pigment deposited in a fluke migration tract in the liver. H&E stain. *(A, Courtesy Dr. J. Wright, College of Veterinary Medicine, North Carolina State University; and Noah's Arkive, College of Veterinary Medicine, The University of Georgia. B, Courtesy Dr. M.D. McGavin, College of Veterinary Medicine, University of Tennessee.)*

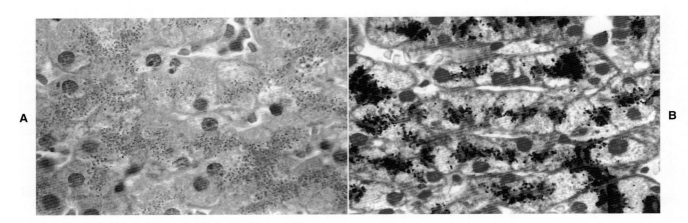

Fig. 1-68 **Hemosiderosis, liver, human being. A,** Hemosiderin is present as fine golden brown granules in hepatocytes H&E stain. **B,** Granules of hemosiderin are stained dark blue by the Prussian blue reaction, which is specific for iron. Prussian blue reaction. *(A and B, From Kumar V, Abbas A, Fausto N: Robbins & Cotran pathologic basis of disease, ed 7, Philadelphia, 2005, Saunders.)*

or enter the alveoli by diapedesis, where they are phagocytosed by alveolar macrophages. These cells are termed "heart failure cells" (Fig. 1-69). Localized deposits of iron may also be present from the intramuscular injection of iron dextran, and this iron may drain to the regional lymph node.

Grossly, no change will be seen in an organ or tissue if there are only small amounts of hemosiderin, but very large amounts will cause a yellow to brown discoloration (Fig. 1-70). This color change can also be seen at sites of old bruises and other hemorrhages or hematomas. The spleen and the liver in hemolytic disease and the lungs in chronic passive congestion will

also appear brown. Microscopically, hemosiderin deposits are golden-yellow to golden-brown globules, which may be intracellular or extracellular (Fig. 1-68, A). It can be confirmed by the Prussian blue reaction (Fig. 1-68, B), which is sometimes incorrectly called a stain but is a chemical reaction, of which the end product is Prussian blue. In the acid solution that liberates ferric iron from the hemosiderin, the ferric iron is reacted with potassium ferrocyanide (colorless) to form ferric ferrocyanide, which is Prussian blue.

The significance of hemosiderin deposits depends on their location and the amount. Normally the spleen contains some hemosiderin, but excess hemosiderin is seen

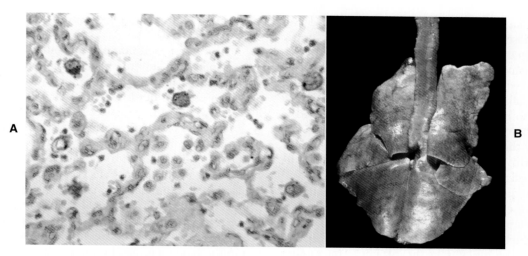

Fig. 1-69   Chronic passive congestion, lung, dog. A, Alveolar macrophages containing hemosiderin *(blue)* are present in the alveoli. Prussian blue reaction. **B,** The lungs have chronic passive congestion attributed to chronic left side heart failure. They are moderately firm and yellow-brown due to alveolar macrophages containing hemosiderin. Inflammatory mediators produced by these macrophages have induced fibroplasia and thus in the long term there has been extensive formation of interstitial collagen. This collagen is the reason the lungs have failed to collapse following incision of the diaphragm, which releases the negative pressure in the pleural cavity (note the rib impressions in the lung). (**A,** *Courtesy Dr. M.D. McGavin, College of Veterinary Medicine, University of Tennessee.* **B,** *Courtesy College of Veterinary Medicine, University of Illinois.*)

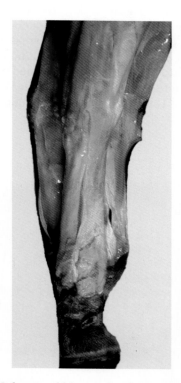

Fig. 1-70   Subcutis, old bruise, leg, horse. The display of colors—red, yellow, and brown—are due to hemoglobin, bilirubin, and hemosiderin, respectively, from the breakdown of the erythrocytes. (*Courtesy Dr. M.D. McGavin, College of Veterinary Medicine, University of Tennessee.*)

in the spleen and liver (Kupffer cells and hepatocytes) from hemolytic diseases, such as in autoimmune hemolytic anemia and hemotropic diseases such as babesiosis, anaplasmosis, or equine infectious anemia. Local tissue aggregations of hemosiderin are usually the result of the breakdown of erythrocytes in an old hemorrhage.

Excess hemosiderin is called hemosiderosis and must be differentiated from hemochromatosis, in which there are extreme accumulations of hemosiderin.

HEMATOIDIN

Grossly, hematoidin is yellow-brown to orange-red pigment derived from hemoglobin but free of iron. Hematoidin closely resembles bilirubin (see next section) but is formed by cells of the macrophage-monocyte system when they phagocytose and digest red blood cells and hemoglobin in areas of hemorrhage. Microscopically, hematoidin is crystalline and polarizes light.

BILIRUBIN

Low concentrations of bilirubin are normally present in the plasma from the breakdown of senescent erythrocytes (see Chapter 13). Briefly, when erythrocytes have come to the end of their natural life span (average 70 days for a cat; average 150 days for cattle and horses), they are phagocytosed by the macrophage-monocyte system, chiefly by macrophages of the spleen and to a lesser extent by those of the bone marrow and liver (Kupffer cells). Within these cells the iron is removed and stored, and the remainder of the porphyrin ring is broken down to bilirubin, which is released into the blood where it attaches to albumin. This bilirubin-albumin complex is too large to be excreted by the kidney. It is carried to the liver, where it enters the space of Disse, where it is taken up by the microvilli of the hepatocytes, is conjugated to form bilirubin glucuronide or diglucuronide, and is then excreted into the bile canaliculus.

Icterus (jaundice), the yellow staining of the tissue by bilirubin, is the result of an imbalance between production and clearance of bilirubin, because there is either excess production or reduced clearance of bilirubin such that it accumulates in the plasma. The mutant Corriedale sheep model is an animal model for Dubin-Johnson syndrome in humans (Fig. 1-71).

Mechanisms leading to icterus can involve one or more of the following:

1. Excess production of bilirubin—as in hemolytic diseases such as babesiosis, anaplasmosis, and equine infectious anemia—or the breakdown of erythrocytes in a large hemorrhage such as a hematoma
2. Reduced uptake of bilirubin from the plasma by hepatocytes
3. Impaired or absent conjugation in hepatocytes, often a congenital or inherited abnormality, as in the Gunn rat
4. Hepatic necrosis. Because the cell membranes of several adjacent hepatocytes form the bile canaliculus, any necrosis of these cells will disrupt the wall of the canaliculus and allow leakage of bilirubin into the circulation. Extensive hepatic necrosis can cause icterus.
5. Decreased excretion of conjugated bilirubin by the hepatocytes into the bile canaliculus
6. Reduced flow of bile from the liver to the intestine caused by either intrahepatic or extrahepatic blockage of the biliary system

Icterus is classified several different ways. A convenient approach uses the classification of prehepatic, hepatic, and posthepatic. The most common cause of prehepatic icterus is a hemolytic crisis, which produces high plasma concentrations of unconjugated bilirubin that exceed the uptake capacity of the hepatocytes. Hepatic icterus is caused by hepatocellular damage, which results in release of bilirubin, both conjugated and unconjugated into the blood and can be the result of one or more of factors 2 to 4. Posthepatic icterus is secondary to obstruction of the biliary system, either intrahepatic or extrahepatic (hepatic bile ducts and the common bile duct), with reflux of the conjugated bilirubin into the blood. In contrast to unconjugated bilirubin, which is carried in the blood attached to albumin and cannot be excreted by the kidney, conjugated bilirubin is excreted.

Grossly, icteric tissues are discolored yellow, and the color change is distributed systemically. Clinically, icterus is most easily recognized in lightly pigmented animals. In living animals, icterus is detected in mucous membranes of the oral cavity, urogenital systems, and alimentary system and in normally white areas, such as the sclera of the eyes. At necropsy, in addition to the sites listed previously, icterus can be identified in the omentum, mesentery, and adipose tissue (Fig. 1-72), except in Jersey and Guernsey cattle, horses, and nonhuman

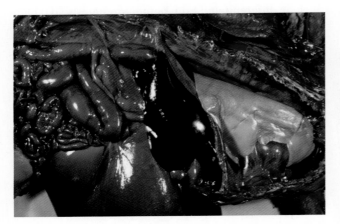

Fig. 1-71   Defective bilirubin excretion, mutant Corriedale sheep, animal model for Dubin-Johnson syndrome. Note the faint yellow discoloration of the lung from bilirubin. The other tissues are discolored dark green from phylloerythrin, which also has a similar defect in excretion from the liver. *(Courtesy Dr. M.D. McGavin, College of Veterinary Medicine, University of Tennessee.)*

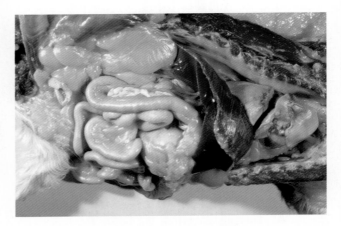

Fig. 1-72   Icterus, hemolytic anemia, abdominal and thoracic viscera, dog. The yellow discoloration from the bilirubin is particularly evident in fat and mesentery. *(Courtesy Dr. M.D. McGavin, College of Veterinary Medicine, University of Tennessee.)*

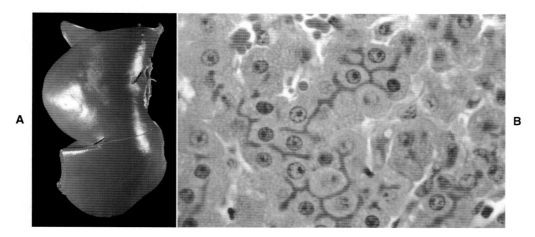

Fig. 1-73   Icterus. A, Icterus, liver, cat. Note the enlarged liver with rounded edges and yellow-orange color caused by retained bilirubin. **B,** Bile casts in bile canaliculi. Acute hemolytic anemia, babesiosis, liver, cow. The bile casts are the result of a high rate of bilirubin excretion by the liver secondary to intravascular hemolysis. H&E stain. (**A,** *Courtesy the College of Veterinary Medicine, University of Illinois.* **B,** *Courtesy Dr. M.D. McGavin, College of Veterinary Medicine, University of Tennessee.*)

primates, whose sera and fat are normally discolored yellow by carotenoids. The intima of the large vessels is also a good site to detect icterus, and unless the plasma concentration is extremely high, the brain is usually unaffected.

Microscopically, icterus is not detected, but excessive quantities of bilirubin can be seen in the bile ducts and bile canaliculi in obstructive jaundice (Fig. 1-73).

Icterus is a very important clinical sign and may be detected by examination of the sclera, and in cases of anemia, in which the mucous membranes are pale, it may be visible there. Laboratory tests to determine the exact plasma or serum concentrations of bilirubin, and preferably whether or not it is conjugated, are essential. It is critical to realize that hyperbilirubinemia is not the same as icterus. Most domestic animals normally have very low serum concentrations of bilirubin, usually less than 1 mg/dl, except for the horse, in which it may range from 1 to 3 mg/dl; however, icterus is not detected until the serum concentration exceeds 1.5 mg/100 ml. Thus hyperbilirubinemia can be present without causing icterus.

PORPHYRIA

Congenital erythropoietic porphyria of calves, cats, and pigs is an inherited metabolic defect in heme synthesis caused by a deficiency of uroporphyrinogen III cosynthetase. The disease is sometimes incorrectly called osteohemachromatosis. It is also known colloquially as "pink tooth" because of the discoloration by the porphyrins accumulating in dentin and bone (Fig. 1-74). The teeth and bones of young animals are

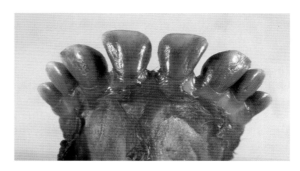

Fig. 1-74   Pink tooth, congenital porphyria teeth, adult ox. The teeth are discolored brown from the accumulation of porphyrins in the dentin. (*Courtesy Dr. M.D. McGavin, College of Veterinary Medicine, University of Tennessee.*)

reddish (pink tooth), and those of adults are dark brown. In these cases both bones and teeth fluoresce red under ultraviolet radiation.

CELLULAR AGING*

The common age-related diseases is animals include renal failure, osteoarthritis, muscle atrophy, cerebral atrophy from loss of cortical neurons, cessation of the growth of the teeth of horses, and loss of elasticity of the skin. The incidence of different causes of mortality in all domestic animals is not available, but data from

---

*Derived and modified slightly from Kumar V, Abbas A, Fausto N: *Robbins & Cotran pathologic basis of disease,* ed 7, Philadelphia, 2005, Saunders.

laboratory beagles maintained for their life span are known. One quarter of these dogs died of neoplastic disease. Of the organ systems involved in the cause of death, the urinary system was responsible for 13%, the respiratory system for 6%, and the CNS for 7%. The leading cause of death from nonneoplastic diseases was renal failure. Death is often the end result of declining cell function, including cellular aging.

Shakespeare probably characterized aging best in his elegant description of the seven ages of man. It begins at the moment of conception, involves the differentiation and maturation of the organism and its cells, at some variable point in time leads to the progressive loss of functional capacity characteristic of senescence, and ends in death.

With age, there are physiologic and structural alterations in almost all organ systems. Aging in individuals is affected to a great extent by genetic factors, diet, social conditions, and occurrence of age-related diseases such as atherosclerosis, diabetes, and osteoarthritis (in human beings). In addition, there is good evidence that aging-induced alterations in cells are an important component of the aging of the organism. Here we discuss cellular aging because it could represent the progressive accumulation over the years of sublethal injury that may lead to cell death or at least to the diminished capacity of the cell to respond to injury.

Cellular aging is the result of a progressive decline in the proliferative capacity and life span of cells and the effects of continuous exposure to exogenous influences that result in the progressive accumulation of cellular and molecular damage (Fig. 1-75). These processes are reviewed next.

STRUCTURAL AND BIOCHEMICAL CHANGES WITH CELLULAR AGING

A number of cell functions decline progressively with age. Oxidative phosphorylation by mitochondria is reduced, as is synthesis of nucleic acids and structural and enzymatic proteins, cell receptors, and transcription factors. Senescent cells have a decreased capacity for uptake of nutrients and for repair of chromosomal damage. The morphologic alterations in aging cells include irregular and abnormally lobed nuclei, pleomorphic vacuolated mitochondria, decreased ER, and distorted Golgi apparatus. Concomitantly, there is a steady accumulation of the pigment lipofuscin, which represents a product of lipid peroxidation and evidence of oxidative damage; advanced glycation end products, which result from nonenzymatic glycosylation and are capable of cross-linking adjacent proteins; and the accumulation of abnormally folded proteins. Advanced glycation end products are important in the pathogenesis of diabetes mellitus, but they may also participate in aging. For example, age-related glycosylation of lens proteins may underlie senile cataracts.

REPLICATIVE SENESCENCE

The concept that cells have a limited capacity for replication was developed from a simple experimental model for aging. Normal human fibroblasts, when placed in tissue culture, have limited division potential. Cells from children undergo more rounds of replication than cells from older people. In contrast, cells from patients with Werner syndrome, a rare disease characterized by premature aging, have a notably reduced in vitro life span. After a fixed number of divisions, all cells become

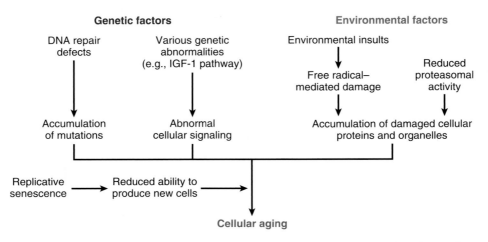

Fig. 1-75 **Mechanisms of cellular aging.** Genetic factors and environmental insults combine to produce the cellular abnormalities characteristic of aging. *IGF-1*, Insulin-like growth factor-1.
(From Kumar V, Abbas A, Fausto N: Robbins & Cotran pathologic basis of disease, ed 7, Philadelphia, 2005, Saunders.)

arrested in a terminally nondividing state, known as cellular senescence. Many changes in gene expression occur during cellular aging, but a key question is which of these are causes and which are effects of cellular senescence.

How dividing cells can count their divisions is under intensive investigation. One likely mechanism is that with each cell division, there is incomplete replication of chromosome ends (telomere shortening), which ultimately results in cell cycle arrest. Telomeres are short repeated sequences of DNA (TTAGGG) present at the linear ends of chromosomes that are important for ensuring the complete replication of chromosome ends and for protecting chromosomal termini from fusion and degradation.

When somatic cells replicate, a small section of the telomere is not duplicated, and telomeres become progressively shortened. As the telomeres become shorter, the ends of chromosomes cannot be protected and are seen as broken DNA, which signals cell cycle arrest. The lengths of the telomeres are normally maintained by nucleotide addition, mediated by an enzyme called telomerase. Telomerase is a specialized RNA-protein complex that uses its own RNA as a template for adding nucleotides to the ends of chromosomes. The activity of telomerase is repressed by regulatory proteins, which restrict telomere elongation, thus providing a length-sensing mechanism. Telomerase activity is expressed in germ cells and is present at low levels in stem cells, but it is usually absent in most somatic tissue. Therefore as cells age, their telomeres become shorter and they exit the cell cycle, resulting in an inability to generate new cells to replace damaged ones. Conversely, in immortal cancer cells, telomerase is reactivated and telomeres are not shortened, suggesting that telomere elongation might be an important—possibly essential—step in tumor formation. Despite such alluring observations, however, the relationship of telomerase activity and telomeric length to aging and cancer still needs to be fully established.

GENES THAT INFLUENCE THE AGING PROCESS

Studies in *Drosophila, Caenorhabditis elegans,* and mice are leading to the discovery of genes that influence the aging process. Analyses of human beings with premature aging are also establishing the fundamental concept that aging is not a random process but is regulated by specific genes, receptors, and signals.

ACCUMULATION OF METABOLIC AND GENETIC DAMAGE

In addition to the importance of timing and a genetic clock, cellular life span may also be determined by the balance between cellular damage resulting from metabolic events occurring within the cell and counteracting molecular responses that can repair the damage. Smaller animals have generally shorter life spans and faster metabolic rates, suggesting that the life span of a species is limited by fixed total metabolic consumption over a lifetime.

One group of products of normal metabolism is reactive oxygen species. These by-products of oxidative phosphorylation cause covalent modifications of proteins, lipids, and nucleic acids. The amount of oxidative damage, which increases as an organism ages, may be an important component of senescence, and the accumulation of lipofuscin in aging cells is seen as the tell-tale sign of such damage. Consistent with this proposal are the following observations: (1) Variation in longevity among different species is inversely correlated with the rates of mitochondrial generation of a superoxide anion radical, and (2) overexpression of the antioxidative enzymes SOD and catalase extends the life span in transgenic forms of *Drosophila*. Thus part of the mechanism that times aging may be the cumulative damage that is generated by toxic by-products of metabolism, such as oxygen radicals. Increased oxidative damage could result from repeated environmental exposure to such influences as ionizing radiation, progressive reduction of antioxidant defense mechanisms (e.g., vitamin E and glutathione peroxidase), or both.

A number of protective responses counterbalance progressive damage in cells, and an important one is the recognition and repair of damaged DNA. Although most DNA damage is repaired by endogenous DNA repair enzymes, some persists and accumulates as cells age. Thus the balance between cumulative metabolic damage and the response to that damage could determine the rate at which we age. In this scenario, aging can be delayed by decreasing the accumulation of damage or by increasing the response to that damage.

Not only damaged DNA but damaged cellular organelles also accumulate as cells age. In part, this may be the result of declining function of the proteasome, the proteolytic machine that serves to eliminate abnormal and unwanted intracellular proteins.

In conclusion, it should be apparent that the various forms of cellular derangements and adaptations described in this chapter cover a wide spectrum, including adaptations in cell size, growth, and function; reversible and irreversible forms of acute cell injury; regulated type of cell death represented by apoptosis; pathologic alterations in cell organelles; and less ominous forms of intracellular accumulations, including pigmentations. Reference is made to all these alterations throughout this book because all organ injury and ultimately all clinical disease arise from derangements in cell structure and function.

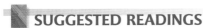

SUGGESTED READINGS

Jubb KVF, Kennedy PC, Palmer N: *Pathology of domestic animals*, vol 1, 2, 3, Boston, 1993, Academic Press, Inc.

Kumar V, Abbas AK, Fausto N: *Robbins & Cotran pathologic basis of disease*, ed 7, Philadelphia, 2005, Saunders.

Levin S, Bucci TJ, Cohen SM et al: The nomenclature of cell death: recommendations of an ad hoc committee of the Society of Toxicologic Pathologists, *Toxicol Pathol* 27:484-490, 1999.

Lockshin RA, Zakeri Z: Review: apoptosis, autophagy, and more, *J Biochem Cell Biol* 36:2405-2419, 2004.

Majno G, Joris I: *Cells, tissues, and disease: principles of general pathology*, ed 2, Oxford, 2004, Oxford University Press.

Merlini G, Bellotti V: Molecular mechanisms of amyloidosis, *N Engl J Med* 349:583-596, 2003.

Mohr U, Carlton WW, Dungworth DL et al, editors: *Pathobiology of the aging dog*, Ames, 2001, Iowa State University Press.

Nezelof C, Seemayer TA: The history of pathology: an overview. In Damjanov I, Linder J, editors: *Anderson's pathology*, ed 10, St Louis, 1996, Mosby.

Pearse AGE: *Histochemistry: theoretical and applied*, Boston, 1961, Little, Brown, and Co.

Porta EA: Pigments in aging: an overview, *Ann N Y Acad Sci* 959: 57-65, 2002.

Riedl SJ, Shi Y: Molecular mechanisms of caspase regulation during apoptosis, *Nat Rev Mol Cell Biol* 5(11):897-907, 2004.

Trump BF, Berensky IK: The reaction of cells to lethal injury: oncosis and necrosis—the role of calcium. In Lockshin RA, Zakeri Z, Tilly J, editors: *When cells die*, New York, 1998, Wiley-Liss.

2

Vascular Disorders and Thrombosis

DEREK A. MOSIER

INTRODUCTION

Free-living unicellular organisms, such as amoebas, obtain nutrients and eliminate metabolic waste products directly into the external environment. In multicellular organisms, most cells do not have direct access to the external environment, and they require a circulatory system to deliver nutrients and remove their waste products. The movement of fluid and cells through the circulatory system links the external and local cell environments, and provides a means of communication between cells in complex, multicellular organisms. In this chapter, the basic abnormalities that affect fluid circulation and balance within an animal are described.

CIRCULATORY SYSTEM

The circulatory system consists of blood, a central pump (heart), blood distribution (arterial) and collection (venous) networks, and a system for exchange of nutrients and waste products between blood and extravascular tissue (microcirculation) (Fig. 2-1). A network of vessels (lymphatics) that parallel the veins also contribute to circulation by draining fluid from extravascular spaces into the blood vascular system.

The heart provides the driving force for blood distribution. Equal volumes of blood are normally distributed to the pulmonary circulation by the right side of the heart and the systemic circulation by the left side of the heart. The volume of blood pumped by each half of the heart per minute (cardiac output) is determined by the beats per minute (heart rate) and the volume of blood pumped per beat by the ventricle (stroke volume). Typically, each half of the heart pumps the equivalent of the entire blood volume of the animal per minute.

Arteries have relatively large diameter lumens to facilitate rapid blood flow with minimal resistance.

The walls of arteries are thick and consist predominantly of smooth muscle fibers for tensile strength and elastic fibers for elasticity (Fig. 2-2). These fibers allow arteries to act as pressure reservoirs, expanding to hold blood ejected from the heart during contraction and passively recoiling to provide continuous flow and pressure to arterioles between heart contractions.

Arterioles are the major resistance vessels within the circulatory system; intravascular pressure can fall by nearly half after blood passes through the arterioles. Arterioles have relatively narrow lumens, the diameter of which is controlled by the smooth muscle cells that are the major component of their walls. Extrinsic sympathetic innervation and local intrinsic stimuli regulate the degree of arteriolar smooth muscle contraction, causing arterioles to dilate or constrict to selectively distribute blood to the areas of greatest need.

Capillaries are the site of nutrient and waste product exchange between the blood and tissue. Capillaries are the most numerous vessel in the circulatory system, with a total cross-sectional area nearly 1300 times that of the aorta. However, they normally contain only about 5% of the total blood volume. The velocity of blood flow through the capillaries is very slow, and red blood cells generally move through a capillary in single file to further facilitate the diffusion of nutrients and wastes. Capillaries have narrow lumens (approximately 8 μm) and thin walls (approximately 1 μm) consisting of a single epithelial cell layer (endothelium). At the junctions between capillary endothelia are interendothelial pores, which make the capillary semipermeable to facilitate diffusion of nutrients and waste products between the blood and tissues. There are three types of capillaries: continuous, fenestrated, and discontinuous. The basic functions and tissue locations of these types of capillaries are illustrated in Fig. 2-3. These types of capillaries are central to disease processes in most organs, and they will be discussed in greater detail in the chapters covering the diseases of organ systems.

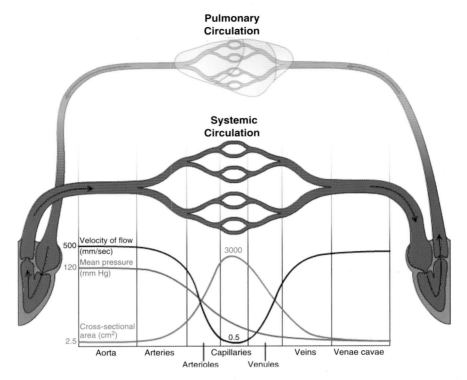

Fig. 2-1   **The vascular system.** Blood travels from the left side of the heart to the right side of the heart via the systemic circulation, and from the right side of the heart to the left side via the pulmonary circulation. Blood flow rate and pressure in the systemic arterial circulation decrease in conjunction with increased total arterial cross-sectional area. In the venous systemic circulation, blood flow rate, but not pressure, increases in conjunction with decreased total venous cross-sectional area. The flow, pressure, and cross-sectional area relationships are similar but reversed (i.e., veins deliver blood and arteries collect blood) in the pulmonary circulation. *(Courtesy Dr. D.A. Mosier and L. Schooley, College of Veterinary Medicine, Kansas State University.)*

The return trip of blood to the heart begins in the postcapillary venules. Venules have a composition similar to capillaries but may have thin layers of muscle as they become more distant from the capillary bed. Arterioles, metarterioles, capillaries, and postcapillary venules are only visible microscopically, and they are collectively referred to as the microcirculation (Fig. 2-4).

Veins are composed mainly of collagen with smaller amounts of elastin and smooth muscle (Fig. 2-5). Venules and veins provide a low resistance pathway for the return of blood to the heart. Because of their distensibility, they can store large amounts of blood; nearly 65% of total blood volume is normally present within the systemic veins. Pressure and velocity of flow are low within venules and veins. Therefore other factors are necessary to help move venous blood toward the heart, such as venous valves to prevent backflow of blood, skeletal muscle contraction, venous vasoconstriction, an increased pressure gradient due to decreased pressure in the heart during filling (cardiac-suction effect), and decreased pressure in the thoracic veins due to negative pressure within the thoracic cavity (respiratory pump).

The lymphatic system originates as blind-ended lymphatic capillaries, which permeate the tissue surrounding the microcirculation (Fig. 2-4). Lymphatic capillaries have overlapping endothelial cells and large interendothelial gaps so that external pressure allows movement of fluid and molecules into the vessel. However, intravascular lymphatic pressure forces these overlapping edges together to prevent the flow of lymph back out of the vessel. Lymphatic capillary gaps are much larger than those between blood capillary endothelium, so they can accommodate movement of larger particles and substances. Lymphatic capillaries converge into progressively larger lymph vessels that drain into lymph nodes and then ultimately empty into the venous system. Similar to the venous vessels, lymphatics are low pressure, distensible vessels that require lymphatic valves and contraction of surrounding muscles to facilitate return of fluid to the blood.

All components of the circulatory system are lined by a single layer of endothelium. Endothelium forms a dynamic and heterogenous interface between blood and tissue, and is also a critical participant in events

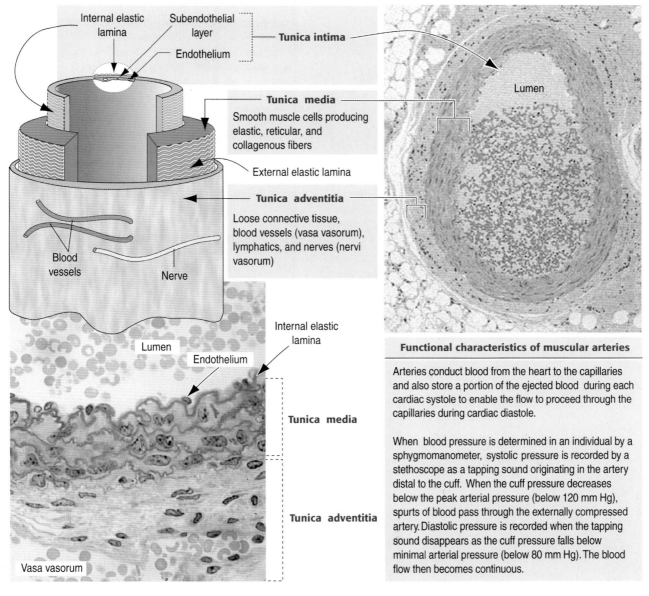

Functional characteristics of muscular arteries

Arteries conduct blood from the heart to the capillaries and also store a portion of the ejected blood during each cardiac systole to enable the flow to proceed through the capillaries during cardiac diastole.

When blood pressure is determined in an individual by a sphygmomanometer, systolic pressure is recorded by a stethoscope as a tapping sound originating in the artery distal to the cuff. When the cuff pressure decreases below the peak arterial pressure (below 120 mm Hg), spurts of blood pass through the externally compressed artery. Diastolic pressure is recorded when the tapping sound disappears as the cuff pressure falls below minimal arterial pressure (below 80 mm Hg). The blood flow then becomes continuous.

Fig. 2-2   **Structure of a muscular artery.** (*From Kierszenbaum AL: Histology and cell biology: an introduction to pathology, St Louis, 2002, Mosby.*)

such as fluid distribution, inflammation, immunity, angiogenesis, and hemostasis (Fig. 2-6). Normal endothelium has antithrombotic and profibrinolytic properties that maintain blood in a fluid state, but upon injury endothelium becomes prothrombotic and antifibrinolytic. This allows endothelium to respond locally to promote or restrict a host response to a specific area, while not affecting the normal function of endothelium and flow of blood in nonstimulated areas. Endothelial activation by oxidative stress, hypoxia, inflammation, infectious agents, tissue injury, or similar events results in the production and release of numerous substances with wide-ranging roles in physiology and pathology (Fig. 2-7, Box 2-1).

MICROCIRCULATION, INTERSTITIUM, AND CELLS

The exchange of fluid, nutrients, and waste products between blood and cells takes place through the interstitium, the space between cells and the microcirculation. The interstitium is composed of an extracellular matrix (ECM), which has structural, adhesive, and absorptive components. Type I collagen is the major structural

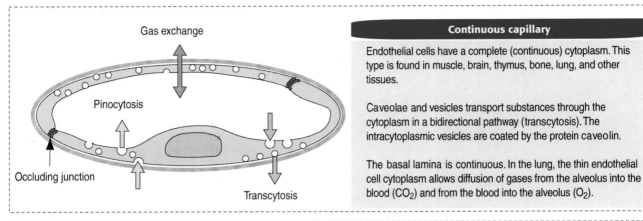

Continuous capillary

Endothelial cells have a complete (continuous) cytoplasm. This type is found in muscle, brain, thymus, bone, lung, and other tissues.

Caveolae and vesicles transport substances through the cytoplasm in a bidirectional pathway (transcytosis). The intracytoplasmic vesicles are coated by the protein caveolin.

The basal lamina is continuous. In the lung, the thin endothelial cell cytoplasm allows diffusion of gases from the alveolus into the blood (CO_2) and from the blood into the alveolus (O_2).

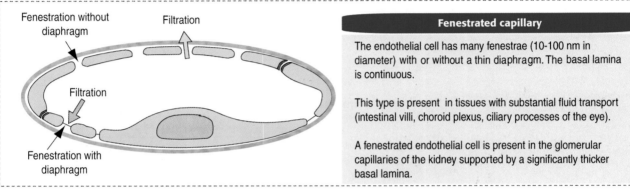

Fenestrated capillary

The endothelial cell has many fenestrae (10-100 nm in diameter) with or without a thin diaphragm. The basal lamina is continuous.

This type is present in tissues with substantial fluid transport (intestinal villi, choroid plexus, ciliary processes of the eye).

A fenestrated endothelial cell is present in the glomerular capillaries of the kidney supported by a significantly thicker basal lamina.

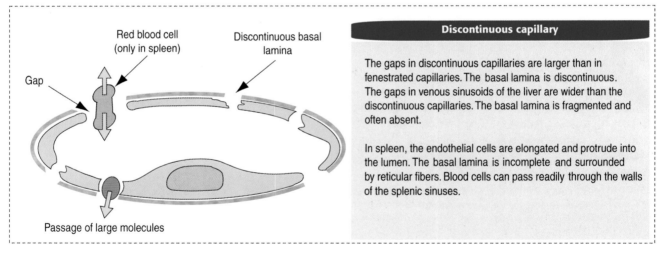

Discontinuous capillary

The gaps in discontinuous capillaries are larger than in fenestrated capillaries. The basal lamina is discontinuous. The gaps in venous sinusoids of the liver are wider than the discontinuous capillaries. The basal lamina is fragmented and often absent.

In spleen, the endothelial cells are elongated and protrude into the lumen. The basal lamina is incomplete and surrounded by reticular fibers. Blood cells can pass readily through the walls of the splenic sinuses.

Fig. 2-3 **Types of endothelium lining capillaries.** *(From Kierszenbaum AL:* Histology and cell biology: an introduction to pathology, *St Louis, 2002, Mosby.)*

component of the ECM and forms the framework in which cells reside. This is intimately associated with type IV collagen of cell basement membranes. Adhesive glycoproteins provide sites of attachment for structural components and also serve as receptors for cells, such as phagocytes and lymphocytes, which move through the interstitium. Absorptive disaccharide complexes (glycosaminoglycans) and protein-disaccharide polymer complexes (proteoglycans) are hydrophilic and can bind large amounts of water and other soluble molecules. In most cases, no more than 1.0 mm of interstitial space separates a cell from a capillary.

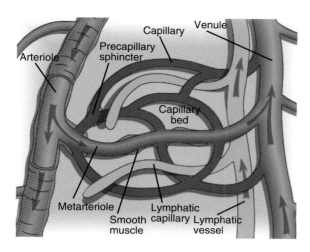

Fig. 2-4   The microcirculation. The microcirculation consists of arterioles (small arteries proximal to a capillary bed), metarterioles (arterial capillaries), capillaries (thin, semipermeable vessels that connect arterioles and venules), and postcapillary venules (small vessels that merge to form veins after collecting blood from a capillary network). Smooth muscle of the arterioles and metarterioles regulates flow of blood into the capillary bed. There is a dramatic drop in pressure and blood flow rate from the arterial to the venous side of the microcirculation, facilitating interactions between capillary blood and interstitial fluid. Blind-ended lymphatic vessels that originate near capillary beds interact intimately with the microcirculation. *(Courtesy Dr. D.A. Mosier and L. Schooley, College of Veterinary Medicine, Kansas State University.)*

FLUID DISTRIBUTION AND HOMEOSTASIS

The distribution of fluid, nutrients, and waste products between the blood, interstitium, and cells is controlled by physical barriers as well as pressure and concentration differences between each compartment. The cell's plasma membrane is a selective barrier that separates interstitial and intracellular compartments. Nonpolar (uncharged) lipid soluble substances such as O_2, CO_2, and fatty acids move relatively freely across the plasma membrane based on concentration gradients. Polar (charged) lipid insoluble particles and molecules such as electrolytes, calcium, glucose, and amino acids enter the cell by carrier-mediated transport. Water readily moves across the plasma membrane down its concentration gradient. Although approximately 100 times the volume of water in a cell crosses the plasma membrane in 1 second, cell fluid content remains relatively stable because of the activity of energy-dependent membrane pumps (e.g., Na^+/K^+ adenosine triphosphatase [ATPase] pump) and the balance between osmotic pressures exerted by interstitial and intracellular solutes.

The capillary wall is a semipermeable barrier that influences the movement of fluid, nutrients, and waste products between the blood and interstitium. Lipid soluble substances can pass through capillary endothelium by dissolving in the membrane lipid bilayer, and large proteins can move through the cell by transport within vesicles. Most importantly, water and polar molecules move through interendothelial pores. Normally, these pores are large enough to allow the passage of water, small nutrients (ions, glucose, amino acids), and waste products, yet small enough to prevent the movement of cells and large proteins (albumin and other plasma proteins such as complement, kinin, and coagulation proteins). Local stimuli, such as inflammation, can cause endothelial cells to contract to widen interendothelial pores and allow the passage of larger molecules. Under normal conditions, the composition of plasma and interstitial fluid is very similar, with the exception of the large plasma proteins.

Movement of substances through interendothelial pores and cell membranes is generally passive in response to concentration and pressure gradients. Nutrient-rich arterial blood contains O_2, glucose, and amino acids that move down their concentration gradients into the interstitium, where they are available for use by cells. CO_2 and waste products generated by cells accumulate in the interstitium and move down their gradient into the venous blood. These gradients become larger in areas where cells are metabolically active.

Water distribution between the plasma and interstitium is determined mainly by osmotic and hydrostatic pressure differentials between the compartments and is described by the following formula (Fig. 2-8):

$$\text{Net filtration across the endothelium} = K[(P_{cap} - P_{int}) - \sigma(\pi_{cap} - \pi_{int})]$$

K = Capillary endothelial permeability constant
P = Hydrostatic pressure
σ = Reflection coefficient
π = Colloid osmotic pressure
cap = capillary
int = interstitium

Although sodium and chloride account for approximately 84% of the total osmolality of plasma, free movement of these electrolytes through interendothelial pores balances their concentrations in the plasma and interstitium, so their contribution to differences in osmotic pressure between these compartments is minimal. In contrast, nonpermeable, suspended plasma proteins comprise less than 1% of the total osmolality of plasma. However, because these proteins (particularly albumin) do not readily move through interendothelial pores, they exert a colloidal osmotic pressure that is responsible for the majority of the difference in osmotic pressure between the plasma and interstitium.

In the microcirculation, intravascular and interstitial osmotic pressures and interstitial hydrostatic forces

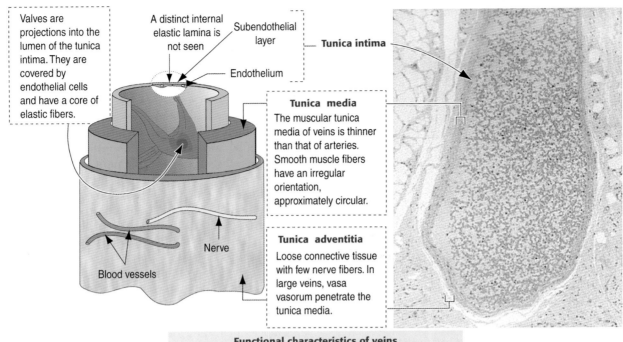

Valves are projections into the lumen of the tunica intima. They are covered by endothelial cells and have a core of elastic fibers.

A distinct internal elastic lamina is not seen

Subendothelial layer

Endothelium

Tunica intima

Tunica media
The muscular tunica media of veins is thinner than that of arteries. Smooth muscle fibers have an irregular orientation, approximately circular.

Tunica adventitia
Loose connective tissue with few nerve fibers. In large veins, vasa vasorum penetrate the tunica media.

Nerve

Blood vessels

Functional characteristics of veins

Veins are high-capacitance vessels containing about 70% of the total blood volume.

In contrast to arteries, the tunica media contains fewer smooth muscle cell bundles associated with reticular and elastic fibers.

Although veins of the extremities have intrinsic vasomotor activity, the transport of blood back to the heart depends on external forces provided by the contraction of surrounding skeletal muscles and on valves that ensure one-way blood flow.

Fig. 2-5 **The structure of a vein.** *(From Kierszenbaum AL: Histology and cell biology: an introduction to pathology, St Louis, 2002, Mosby.)*

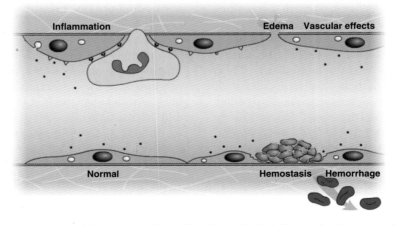

Fig. 2-6 **Structure and function of the endothelium.** Endothelium is both a physical barrier between intravascular and extravascular spaces, and it is an important mediator of fluid distribution, hemostasis, inflammation, and healing. *(Courtesy Dr. D.A. Mosier and L. Schooley, College of Veterinary Medicine, Kansas State University.)*

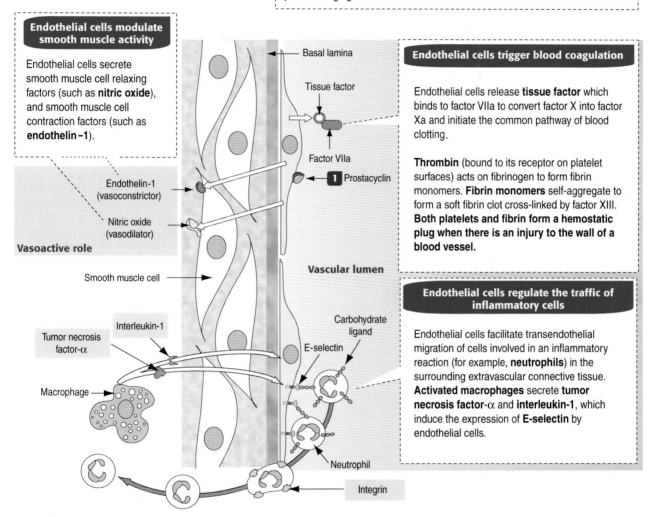

Endothelial cells produce prostacyclin

1 Prostacyclin is formed by endothelial cells from arachidonic acid by a process catalyzed by prostacyclin synthase. Prostacyclin prevents the adhesion of platelets to the endothelium, and prevents intravascular clot formation.

Endothelial cells control vascular cell growth

Angiogenesis occurs during normal wound healing and vascularization of tumors. Endothelial cells secrete factors that stimulate angiogenesis.

Some of these factors induce endothelial cell proliferation and migration; others activate endothelial cell differentiation or induce a secondary cell type to produce angiogenic factors.

Endothelial cells modulate smooth muscle activity

Endothelial cells secrete smooth muscle cell relaxing factors (such as **nitric oxide**), and smooth muscle cell contraction factors (such as **endothelin-1**).

Basal lamina

Tissue factor

Endothelin-1 (vasoconstrictor)

Nitric oxide (vasodilator)

Vasoactive role

Factor VIIa

1 Prostacyclin

Smooth muscle cell

Vascular lumen

Endothelial cells trigger blood coagulation

Endothelial cells release **tissue factor** which binds to factor VIIa to convert factor X into factor Xa and initiate the common pathway of blood clotting.

Thrombin (bound to its receptor on platelet surfaces) acts on fibrinogen to form fibrin monomers. **Fibrin monomers** self-aggregate to form a soft fibrin clot cross-linked by factor XIII. **Both platelets and fibrin form a hemostatic plug when there is an injury to the wall of a blood vessel.**

Tumor necrosis factor-α

Interleukin-1

Macrophage

Carbohydrate ligand

E-selectin

Neutrophil

Integrin

Endothelial cells regulate the traffic of inflammatory cells

Endothelial cells facilitate transendothelial migration of cells involved in an inflammatory reaction (for example, **neutrophils**) in the surrounding extravascular connective tissue. **Activated macrophages** secrete **tumor necrosis factor-α** and **interleukin-1**, which induce the expression of **E-selectin** by endothelial cells.

Fig. 2-7   **Bioactive mediators from endothelial cells.** *(From Kierszenbaum AL: Histology and cell biology: an introduction to pathology, St Louis, 2002, Mosby.)*

remain relatively constant and favor intravascular retention of fluid. However, high hydrostatic pressures within the arteriolar end of the capillary bed result in a net filtration of fluid into the interstitium. Lower hydrostatic pressures in the venular end of the capillary bed result in a net absorption pressure and reentry of fluid into the microvasculature. Alternatively, filtration and absorption may not occur because of a drop in

hydrostatic pressure across individual capillary beds. Instead, filtration may occur across the entire length of capillary beds with open precapillary sphincters and high rates of blood flow, whereas absorption may occur across the entire length of capillary beds with closed precapillary sphincters and low blood flow rates. The slight excess of fluid that is retained in the interstitium and any plasma proteins that have escaped

Box **2-1**

Endothelial Properties in Health and Disease: Endothelial Products

FLUID DISTRIBUTION AND BLOOD FLOW

Semipermeable membrane for fluid distribution
• Interendothelial junctions
Vasodilation
• Nitric oxide
• Prostacyclin (PGI$_2$)
Vasoconstriction
• Endothelin

HEMOSTASIS

Antihemostatic substances
• PGI$_2$
• Endothelial cell protein C receptor
• Tissue factor pathway inhibitor (TFPI)
• Tissue plasminogen activator
• Heparan sulfate
• Adenosine diphosphatase (ADPase) and adenosine triphosphatase (ATPase)
• Protein S
Prohemostatic substances
• von Willebrand's factor
• Tissue factor (TF) (factor III)
• Plasminogen activator inhibitor-1 (PAI-1)

INFLAMMATORY MEDIATORS

Cytokines
• Interleukin (IL)-1, IL-6, IL-8
Enhanced expression of TF
Expression of leukocyte adhesion molecules:
• Cell adhesion molecule family
  • Mucosal addressin cell adhesion molecule 1 (MAdCAM-1)
  • Intercellular adhesion molecule 1 (ICAM-1),
  • Vascular cell adhesion molecule 1 (VCAM-1)
  • Platelet/endothelial cell adhesion molecule 1 (PECAM-1)
• Selectin family
  • P-selectin
  • E-selectin

GROWTH FACTORS

Platelet-derived growth factor (PDGF)
Colony-stimulating factor (CSF)
Fibroblast growth factor (FGF)
Transforming growth factor-β (TGF-β)
Heparin

FIBRINOLYSIS

Synthesis and secretion of fibrinolytic components under certain circumstances
Regulation of formation of plasmin
Tissue plasminogen activator (tPA)
Urokinase plasminogen activator receptor
Plasminogen activator inhibitor-1 (PAI-1)
Annexin II

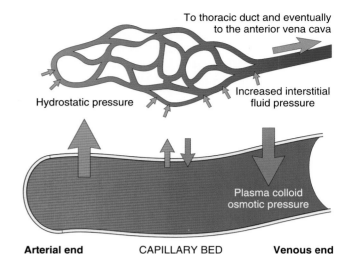

Fig. 2-8 **Factors affecting fluid balance in the microcirculation.** Intravascular and interstitial hydrostatic and osmotic forces and lymphatic drainage are normally balanced so that there is no net loss or gain of fluid across the capillary bed. However, increased intravascular hydrostatic pressure or diminished plasma osmotic pressure leads to a net accumulation of extravascular fluid (edema). As the interstitial fluid pressure increases, tissue lymphatics remove much of the excess volume, eventually returning it to the circulation via the thoracic duct (except lymph from the head and neck, which is returned through the tracheal trunks and right lymphatic duct to empty into the cranial vena cava). If the ability of the lymphatics to drain tissue is exceeded, persistent tissue edema results. *(From Kumar V, Abbas AK, Fausto N: Robbins & Cotran pathologic basis of disease, ed 7, Philadelphia, 2005, Saunders.)*

the vasculature enter lymphatic capillaries to be drained from the area.

The constant flow of fluid between the microcirculation and interstitium allows exchange of nutrients and waste products between these two fluid compartments to support cell functions. Additionally, the interstitium provides a fluid buffer to either increase or decrease the plasma volume to assure effective circulatory function. Excessive fluid intake will expand plasma volume and increase hydrostatic pressure, resulting in greater filtration into the interstitium to maintain a relatively constant plasma volume. Reduced fluid intake will decrease plasma volume, shifting the movement of water from the interstitium into the plasma to increase circulating fluid volume.

EDEMA (ABNORMAL FLUID DISTRIBUTION)

Alteration in any of the factors that regulate normal fluid distribution between the plasma, interstitium, and cells can lead to pathologic imbalances between these compartments.

IMBALANCE BETWEEN INTRACELLULAR AND INTERSTITIAL COMPARTMENTS

Distribution of fluid between the interstitium and cells is generally dynamic but stable. This stability is necessary to maintain a relatively constant intracellular environment for cell function. Generalized conditions (such as alterations in plasma volume) and local stimuli (such as inflammation) can result in slight and usually transient shifts in fluid distribution between the interstitium and cells. Excess plasma volume (hypervolemia) results in movement of additional water into the interstitium and ultimately into the cell along both osmotic and hydrostatic gradients to result in cell swelling. In contrast, reduced plasma volume (hypovolemia) can result in a flow of water in the opposite direction resulting in cell shrinkage and decreased interstitial volume. Increased interstitial volume will also cause a slight flow of fluid into cells in the affected region.

Disruption of any of the mechanisms that maintain proper fluid distribution between the cell and interstitium can have serious consequences for the cell. Failure to maintain proper osmotic balance as a result of cell membrane damage or failure of the energy-dependent plasma membrane pumps result in cell swelling, which if not quickly corrected can lead to cell death caused by osmotic lysis.

IMBALANCE BETWEEN INTRAVASCULAR AND INTERSTITIAL COMPARTMENTS

Changes in distribution of fluid between the plasma and interstitium are most commonly manifested as edema, an accumulation of excess interstitial fluid. Edema occurs by four major mechanisms: (1) increased microvascular permeability, (2) increased intravascular hydrostatic pressure, (3) decreased intravascular osmotic pressure, and (4) decreased lymphatic drainage (Box 2-2).

Box 2-2

Causes of Edema

INCREASED VASCULAR PERMEABILITY

Vascular leakage associated with inflammation
  Infectious agents
  - Viruses (e.g., influenza and other respiratory viruses, canine adenovirus 1, equine and porcine arteriviruses, morbilliviruses)
  - Bacteria (e.g., *Clostridium* sp., Shiga-like toxin–producing *Escherichia coli*, *Erysipelothrix rhusiopathiae*)
  - Rickettsia (e.g., *Cowdria ruminantium*, *Ehrlichia risticii*, *Ehrlichia equi*, *Rickettsia rickettsii*)
  Immune-mediated
  - Type III hypersensitivity (e.g., feline infectious peritonitis, purpura hemorrhagica)
Neovascularization
Anaphylaxis (e.g., type I hypersensitivity to vaccines, venoms, and other allergens)
Toxins (e.g., endotoxin, paraquat, noxious gases, zootoxins)
Clotting abnormalities (e.g., pulmonary embolism, disseminated intravascular coagulation)
Metabolic abnormalities (e.g., microangiopathy due to diabetes mellitus, encephalomalacia due to thiamine deficiency)

INCREASED INTRAVASCULAR HYDROSTATIC PRESSURE

Portal hypertension (e.g., right-side heart failure, hepatic fibrosis)
Pulmonary hypertension (e.g., left-side heart failure, high altitude disease)
Localized venous obstruction (e.g., gastric dilation and volvulus, intestinal volvulus and torsion, uterine torsion or prolapse)
Iatrogenic fluid overload

DECREASED INTRAVASCULAR OSMOTIC PRESSURE

Decreased albumin production (e.g., malnutrition/starvation, debilitating diseases, severe hepatic disease)
Excessive albumin loss (e.g., gastrointestinal disease [protein-losing enteropathies] or parasitism [haemonchosis or trichostrongylosis in sheep], renal disease [protein-losing nephropathies], severe burns)
Water intoxication

DECREASED LYMPHATIC DRAINAGE

Lymphatic obstruction or compression (e.g., inflammatory or neoplastic masses)
Congenital lymphatic aplasia or hypoplasia
Intestinal lymphangiectasia
Lymphangitis (e.g., paratuberculosis, sporotrichosis, epizootic lymphangitis of horses)

MECHANISMS OF EDEMA FORMATION
INCREASED MICROVASCULAR PERMEABILITY

Increased microvascular permeability is most commonly associated with the initial microvascular reaction to inflammatory or immunologic stimuli. These stimuli induce localized release of mediators that cause vasodilation and increased microvascular permeability. Immediate increases in permeability are induced by mediators such as histamine, bradykinin, leukotrienes, and substance P, which cause endothelial cell contraction and widening of interendothelial gaps. Subsequent release of cytokines such as interleukin-1 (IL-1), tumor necrosis factor (TNF), and γ-interferon induces cytoskeletal rearrangements within endothelial cells that result in endothelial cell retraction and more persistent widening of interendothelial gaps. Movement of intravascular fluid through these gaps into the interstitium results in localized edema that can dilute an acute inflammatory agent. The reaction terminates as localized edema and regresses when the stimulus is mild. However, most cases progress to the leakage of plasma proteins and emigration of leukocytes as early events in the formation of an acute inflammatory exudate.

INCREASED INTRAVASCULAR HYDROSTATIC PRESSURE

Increased intravascular hydrostatic pressure is most often due to increased blood volume in the microvasculature. This can be due to an active increased flow of blood into the microvasculature (hyperemia), such as occurs with acute inflammation. But more commonly it results from passive accumulation of blood (congestion), often caused by heart failure or localized venous compression or obstruction. Increased microvascular volume and pressure cause increased filtration and reduced or even reversed fluid absorption back into the vessel. When increased hydrostatic pressure affects a localized portion of microvasculature, the edema is localized. In the case of heart failure, congestion and increased hydrostatic pressure can occur in the portal venous system (right heart failure) causing ascites; in the pulmonary venous system (left heart failure) causing pulmonary edema; or in both venous systems (generalized heart failure) causing generalized edema. Generalized edema can result in a reduction of circulating plasma volume, which activates a variety of volume-regulating compensatory responses. Plasma volume is increased through sodium retention induced by activation of the renin-angiotensin-aldosterone pathways, and water retention mediated by antidiuretic hormone (ADH) release following activation of intravascular volume and pressure receptors. The resulting intravascular volume overload further complicates the dynamics of fluid distribution that accompany heart failure.

DECREASED INTRAVASCULAR OSMOTIC PRESSURE

Decreased intravascular osmotic pressure most commonly results from decreased concentrations of plasma proteins, particularly albumin. Hypoalbuminemia reduces the intravascular colloidal osmotic pressure resulting in increased fluid filtration and decreased absorption, culminating in edema. Hypoalbuminemia can result from either decreased production of albumin by the liver or excessive loss from the plasma. Decreased hepatic production most commonly occurs because of a lack of adequate protein for the synthetic pathway as a result of malnutrition or intestinal malabsorption of protein. Less often, severe liver disease with decreased hepatocyte mass or impaired hepatocyte function can result in inadequate albumin production. Loss of albumin from the plasma can occur in gastrointestinal diseases characterized by severe blood loss, such as that caused by parasitism. Renal disease in which glomerular and/or tubular function is impaired can result in loss of albumin into the urine. Plasma exudation accompanying severe burns is a less frequent cause of albumin loss. Due to the systemic nature of hypoalbuminemia, edema caused by decreased intravascular osmotic pressure tends to be generalized.

DECREASED LYMPHATIC DRAINAGE

Decreased lymphatic drainage reduces the ability of the lymphatic system to remove the slight excess of fluid that normally accumulates in the interstitium during fluid exchange between the plasma and interstitium. This can occur because of lymph vessel compression by a neoplastic or inflammatory swelling, lymph vessel constriction caused by fibrosis, or internal blockage of a lymph vessel by a thrombus. Edema occurs once the capacity of the damaged lymphatics is exceeded and is localized to the area served by the affected lymphatic vessels.

MORPHOLOGIC CHARACTERISTICS OF EDEMA

Edema is morphologically characterized by clear to slightly yellow fluid that generally contains a small amount of protein (transudate), which thickens and expands affected interstitium (Fig. 2-9). When edema occurs in tissues adjacent to body cavities or open spaces, such as alveolar lumens, the increased interstitial pressure often forces fluid into these cavities and spaces. The result can be fluid within alveolar lumens (pulmonary edema) (Fig. 2-10), the thoracic cavity (hydrothorax), the pericardial sac (hydropericardium), or the abdominal cavity (ascites or hydroperitoneum) (Fig. 2-11). Histologically, edema is an amorphous,

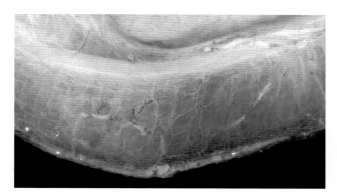

Fig. 2-9   Edema, intestine, submucosa, horse. Note the clear to slightly yellow fluid (that generally contains a small amount of protein [transudate]), which thickens and expands the affected submucosa. *(Courtesy Department of Veterinary Biosciences, The Ohio State University; and Noah's Arkive, College of Veterinary Medicine, The University of Georgia.)*

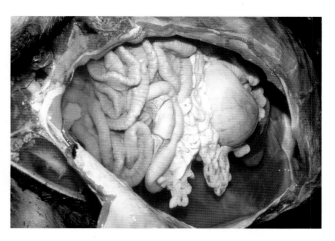

Fig. 2-11   Ascites (hydroperitoneum), peritoneal cavity, dog. Slightly yellow fluid is present in the peritoneal cavity. When edema occurs in tissue adjacent to body cavities, the increased interstitial pressure forces the edema fluid, which is usually clear to slightly yellow (transudate), into these cavities. *(Courtesy Dr. D.A. Mosier, College of Veterinary Medicine, Kansas State University.)*

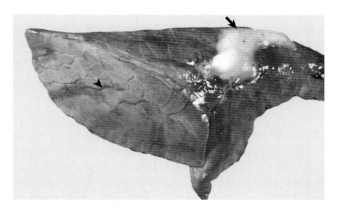

Fig. 2-10   Pulmonary edema, lung, pig. The lung failed to collapse and has a firm rubbery texture attributable to edema fluid in alveoli and the interstitium. Note the prominent interlobular septa caused by edema *(arrowhead)* and the frothy edema fluid exuding from the bronchus *(arrow)*. *(Courtesy Dr. M.D. McGavin, College of Veterinary Medicine, University of Tennessee.)*

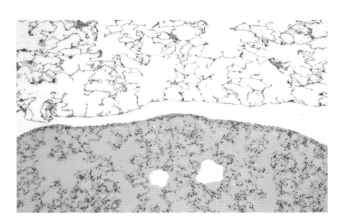

Fig. 2-12   Pulmonary edema, lung, rat. There is eosinophilic (pink staining) fluid distending the alveoli in the lower specimen. Histologically, edema is an amorphous, pale eosinophilic fluid, and the depth of the eosinophilia is proportional to its protein content. The fluid in this specimen has a high protein content. The upper specimen is normal rat lung. H&E stain. *(Courtesy Dr. A. López, Atlantic Veterinary College; and Noah's Arkive, College of Veterinary Medicine, The University of Georgia.)*

pale eosinophilic fluid (hematoxylin and eosin [H&E] stain) because of its protein content (Fig. 2-12). The clinical significance of edema is variable, depending mainly on its location. Subcutaneous edema results in doughy to fluctuant skin and subcutis that is often cooler than adjacent nonaffected tissue, but alone has minimal clinical impact (Fig. 2-13). Likewise, ascites does not generally have an impact on the function of abdominal organs. In contrast, edema of a tissue within a confined space, such as the brain in the cranial vault, can result in pressure within the organ that results in serious organ dysfunction. Similarly, filling a confined space with fluid, such as in hydrothorax or hydropericardium, can have a substantial impact on the function of the lungs and heart, respectively. In these situations edema can have immediate and life-threatening implications.

HEMOSTASIS

Hemostasis is the arrest of bleeding. It is a physiologic response to vascular damage and provides a mechanism to seal an injured vessel to prevent blood loss

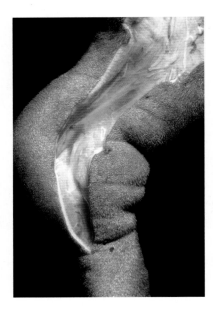

Fig. 2-13 **Subcutaneous edema, congenital lymphedema, skin, dog.** This form of edema results in doughy to fluctuant skin and subcutis. Edematous skin is often cooler than adjacent nonaffected skin. In congenital lymphedema the lymph vessels are hypoplastic or aplastic. *(Courtesy Dr. H. Liepold, College of Veterinary Medicine, Kansas State University.)*

(hemo = blood, stasis = halt, slow). Hemostasis is a finely regulated process that predominantly involves interactions between endothelium, platelets, and coagulation factors. It normally occurs only at the site of vascular injury, without affecting fluidity and flow of blood in normal undamaged vasculature. Disruption of the delicate balance of hemostasis can result in the pathologic states of blood loss (hemorrhage) or inappropriate thrombus formation (thrombosis).

Normal endothelium provides a surface that promotes the smooth, nonturbulent flow of blood. It produces and responds to mediators that enhance vasodilation and inhibit platelet adhesion, aggregation, and coagulation. In contrast, following injury or activation, endothelium produces or responds to mediators that induce vasoconstriction, enhance platelet adhesion and aggregation, and stimulate coagulation (Box 2-3).

Platelets are anucleate cell fragments derived from megakaryocytes. Their major role in hemostasis is to form the initial plug that covers and seals a small area of vascular damage. Following vascular damage, platelets adhere to subendothelial collagen and other ECM components (e.g., fibronectin, adhesive glycoproteins, and proteoglycans). Adhered platelets express receptors that promote aggregation of additional platelets and become activated to release the products of their cytoplasmic granules and produce other mediators of coagulation (e.g., thromboxane) (Box 2-4). The phospholipid

surfaces of aggregated platelet membranes also serve to promote coagulation.

Coagulation factors are plasma proteins produced mainly by the liver. Their purpose in hemostasis is to form fibrin. Coagulation factors are divided into: (1) a structurally related and functionally interdependent contact group (prekallikrein, high molecular weight kininogen [HMWK], and factors XII and XI); (2) a vitamin K–dependent group (factors II, VII, IX, and X); and (3) a highly labile fibrinogen group (factors I, V, VIII, and XIII). Circulating coagulation factors are activated in a cascade fashion by hydrolysis of arginine- or lysine-containing peptides to convert them to enzymatically active serine proteases (except for factor XIII, which has cysteine-rich active sites). The contact group factors are activated by contact with collagen or subendothelial components to initiate coagulation by the intrinsic pathway. The extrinsic pathway of coagulation is activated by release of tissue factor (TF, factor III) from damaged cells. The vitamin K–dependent coagulation factors play an important role in localizing coagulation by γ-carboxylating glutamic acid residues of N-terminal ends of precursor factors so that they can bind calcium to form calcium bridges with platelet phospholipids.

HEMOSTATIC PROCESS

The sequence of events that contribute to hemostasis are: (1) transient vasoconstriction and platelet aggregation to form a platelet plug at the site of damage (primary hemostasis), (2) coagulation to form a meshwork of fibrin (secondary hemostasis), (3) fibrinolysis to remove the platelet/fibrin plug (thrombus retraction), and (4) tissue repair at the damaged site (Fig. 2-14).

PRIMARY HEMOSTASIS

Primary hemostasis includes the initial vascular and platelet response to injury. Neurogenic stimuli and mediators released locally by endothelium and platelets causes vasoconstriction immediately following damage (Fig. 2-14, A). The nature and effectiveness of vasoconstriction is partially determined by the size of the affected vessel, the amount of smooth muscle it contains, and endothelial integrity. Narrowing of the vessel lumen allows opposing endothelial surfaces to come into contact with and sometimes adhere to each other to reduce the volume of blood flowing through the damaged area. Platelets can directly adhere to the exposed subendothelial matrix of collagen, fibronectin, and other glycoproteins and proteoglycans (Fig. 2-14, B). However, more efficient adhesion occurs when von Willebrand's factor released by local activated endothelium coats subendothelial collagen to form a specific bridge between collagen and platelet receptor GpIb. At this stage and without further stimulation, adhered and aggregated

Box **2-3**

Endothelial Mediators of Hemostasis

ANTICOAGULANT
Prostacyclin (PGI$_2$)

Maintains vascular relaxation and inhibits platelet adhesion and activation

Nitric Oxide (NO)

Maintains vascular relaxation and inhibits platelet aggregation. Acts synergistically with the protein C pathway and antithrombin III (ATIII) to suppress thrombin production.

Thrombomodulin

Membrane protein that binds thrombin to initiate activation of protein C

Protein S

Cofactor in protein C pathway; independently inhibits activation of factors VIII and X

Heparin-Like Molecules

Heparan sulfate proteoglycans bind and concentrate ATIII on the endothelial surface

Tissue Plasminogen Activator (tPA)

Activates fibrinolysis by stimulating plasminogen conversion to plasmin

Ectoenzyme Adenosine-Diphosphatase

Degradation of adenosine diphosphate (ADP) to inhibit its procoagulant effects

Annexin V

Binds negatively charged phospholipids and calcium to displace phospholipid-dependent coagulation factors

on the endothelial surface to inhibit formation of thrombin and factor Xa

Tissue Factor Pathway Inhibitor-1 (TFPI-1)

A direct inhibitor of the TF:VIIa complex

PROCOAGULANT
Tissue Factor

Produced following endothelial activation by substances such as cytokines, endotoxin, thrombin, immune complexes, and mitogens

von Willebrand's Factor

Released following endothelial exposure to substances such as thrombin, histamine, and fibrin

Plasminogen Activator Inhibitor-1 (PAI-1)

Reduces fibrinolysis by inhibiting tissue plasminogen activator (tPA) and urokinase-like plasminogen activator (uPA)

VASCULAR REPAIR
Platelet-Derived Growth Factor (PDGF)

Stimulates mitogenesis of smooth muscle and fibroblasts

Fibroblast Growth Factor (FGF)

Stimulates fibroblast proliferation

Transforming Growth Factor-β (TGF-β)

Modulates vascular repair by inhibition of proliferation of various cell types, including endothelium

---

platelets may disaggregate. Otherwise, platelets within the aggregate secrete the contents of their dense bodies and α-granules and produce substances such as thromboxane to accelerate hemostasis. Adenosine diphosphate (ADP) released from dense granules triggers the binding of fibrinogen to platelet receptor GpIIb-IIIa, resulting in the formation of bridges that link platelets into a loose aggregate. Platelet contraction consolidates this loose aggregate into a dense plug, which covers the damaged area. When vascular injury is minimal, platelet plugs alone may resolve the damage. If not, the exposed collagen and aggregated platelet phospholipids promote secondary hemostasis at the site.

SECONDARY HEMOSTASIS

In most cases of vascular damage, the formation of fibrin is important for the prevention of blood loss.

Fibrin is the end-product of a series of enzymatic reactions involving coagulation factors, nonenzymatic cofactors, calcium, and phospholipid membranes derived mainly from platelets (Fig. 2-14, C). Three integrated pathways have been classically used to describe the coagulation process and formation of fibrin. The cascade model of coagulation provides a useful starting point for understanding coagulation (Figs. 2-15 and 2-16). However, more recent concepts of coagulation emphasize the interrelatedness of these pathways, the multiple positive and negative control loops within the system, and amplification of the process on affected cell surfaces.

INTRINSIC PATHWAY

Intrinsic coagulation is a complex and highly interrelated process that is initiated by the contact group of

Box 2-4

Platelet Mediators in Hemostasis

PROCOAGULANT
Thromboxane A$_2$ (TXA$_2$)
Induces vasoconstriction and enhances platelet
   aggregation

Phospholipids (i.e., Phosphatidyl Serine)
Provides sites for coagulation reactions

Adenosine Diphosphate (ADP)
Mediates platelet aggregation and activation

Calcium
Cofactor in many coagulation reactions and promotes
   platelet aggregation

Platelet Factor 4
Promotes platelet aggregation and inhibits heparin
   action

Thrombospondin
Promotes platelet aggregation and inhibits heparin
   action

Fibrinogen
Fibrin precursor, concentrated by binding to platelet
   receptor GpIIb-IIIa

Factors V, XI, and XIII
Factors involved in coagulation reactions

von Willebrand's Factor
Promotes platelet adhesion to subendothelial collagen
   via platelet receptor GpIb

α$_2$-Antiplasmin and α$_2$-Macroglobulin
Inhibition of plasmin

Plasminogen Activator Inhibitor-1 (PAI-1)
Inhibits tissue plasminogen activator (tPA) and
   activated protein C to promote clot stabilization

Serotonin
Promotes vasoconstriction

ANTICOAGULANT
Adenosine Triphosphate (ATP)
Inhibits platelet aggregation

Protease Nexin II
Inhibits factor XIa

Tissue Factor Pathway Inhibitor (TFPI)
Inhibits TF:factor VIIa of the extrinsic pathway

Protein S
Cofactor in the protein C pathway for inhibition
   of factors Va and VIIIa

VASCULAR REPAIR
Platelet-Derived Growth Factor (PDGF)
Stimulates mitogenesis of smooth muscle and
   fibroblasts for vessel repair

β-Thromboglobulin
Promotes fibroblast chemotaxis for vessel repair

Vascular Endothelial Growth Factor (VEGF)
Stimulates endothelial cell proliferation

Transforming Growth Factor-β (TGF-β)
Modulates vascular repair by inhibition of proliferation
   of various cell types, including endothelium

Epidermal Growth Factor (EGF)
Promotes fibroblast proliferation

coagulation factors (Figs. 2-15 and 2-16). Prekallikrein and factor XI normally circulate bound to HMWK, which acts as a catalytic factor for their activation. Following vascular injury, circulating prekallikrein-HMWK and factor XII form a complex on negatively charged endothelial or subendothelial surfaces, which results in activation of factor XII (factor XIIa). Factor XIIa initiates a complex series of reactions that affect coagulation as well as kinin formation, complement activation, and fibrinolysis. Factor XIIa activates factor XI (XIa) and interacts with prekallikrein to form kallikrein, and interacts with HMWK to form kinins. Cleavage of factor XIIa by kallikrein, plasmin, and other proteolytic enzymes forms fragments (factor XIIf), which have activity that is similar to, but much weaker than, factor XIIa. Both kallikrein and factor XIa with Ca^{2+} can activate factor IX (factor IXa). Factor IXa then binds to platelet phospholipids in a complex with Ca^{2+} and factor VIII. Following modification of factor VIII by thrombin into factor VIIIa, this complex of factor VIIIa-factor IXa/Ca^{2+}-phospholipid (tenase) activates factor X to initiate the common coagulation pathway.

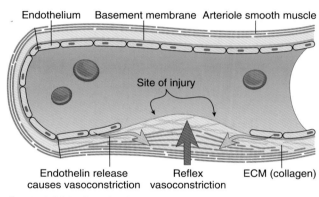

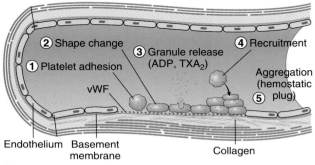

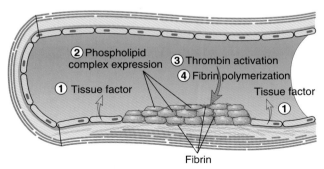

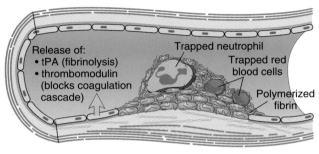

D   THROMBUS AND ANTITHROMBOTIC EVENTS

EXTRINSIC PATHWAY

Release of factor III (TF) from cells underlying damaged endothelium, or from activated endothelium, initiates the extrinsic pathway (Figs. 2-15 and 2-16). TF is a high molecular weight phospholipid-containing glycoprotein found in the plasma membrane of many cells, including activated, but not resting, endothelium. Endothelial cell production of TF is stimulated by substances such as endotoxin, TNF, IL-1, transforming growth factor-β (TGF-β), and thrombin. When circulating factor VII comes into contact with TF, it forms a Ca^{2+}-dependent TF:VII complex on the TF-expressing surface. Although this complex may have some enzymatic activity, activation of factor VII by substances such as factors XIIa, XIIf, IXa, Xa, IIa, and kallikrein results in the much more active TF:VIIa complex. This complex along with Ca^{2+} activates factor X to initiate the common pathway.

COMMON PATHWAY

The intrinsic and extrinsic pathways merge with the activation of factor X (Figs. 2-15 and 2-16). Factor Xa is bound to endothelial or platelet membrane phospholipids where it can directly convert factor II into factor IIa (thrombin). However, when factor Xa is combined with factor Va and Ca^{2+} (prothrombinase complex), this reaction occurs much more rapidly. Thrombin is a multifunctional mediator whose major function is to cleave fibrinopeptides A and B from factor I (fibrinogen) to form fibrin monomers (Fig. 2-17). Removal of these fibrinopeptides reduces intermolecular repulsive forces so that fibrin monomers spontaneously form weak H^+ bonds and self-polymerize into soluble fibrin polymers.

Fig. 2-14   Diagrammatic representation of the normal hemostatic process. A, After vascular injury, local neurohumoral factors induce a transient vasoconstriction. **B,** After endothelial injury and disruption that exposes the subendothelial extracellular matrix *(ECM)*, platelets adhere to the ECM via von Willebrand's factor *(vWF)* and are activated, undergoing a shape change and granule release; released adenosine diphosphate *(ADP)* and thromboxane A₂ *(TXA₂)* lead to further platelet aggregation to form the primary hemostatic plug. **C,** Local activation of the coagulation cascade (involving tissue factor and platelet phospholipids) results in fibrin polymerization, "cementing" the platelets into a definitive secondary hemostatic plug. **D,** Counter-regulatory mechanisms, such as release of tissue plasminogen activator *(tPA)* (fibrinolytic) and thrombomodulin (interfering with the coagulation cascade), limit the hemostatic process to the site of injury. (**A** *through* **D,** *From Kumar V, Abbas AK, Fausto N: Robbins & Cotran pathologic basis of disease, ed 7, Philadelphia, 2005, Saunders.*)

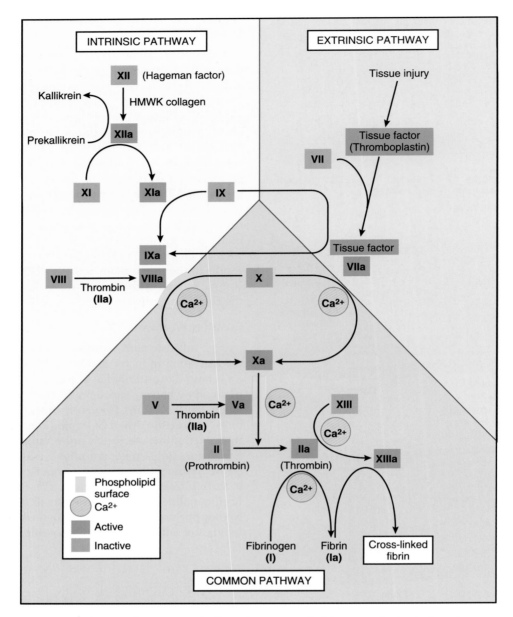

Fig. 2-15   The coagulation cascade. Note the common link between the intrinsic and extrinsic pathways at the level of factor IX activation. Factors in red boxes represent inactive molecules; activated factors are indicated with a lower case "a" and a green box. *PL*, Phospholipid surface; *HMWK*, high molecular weight kininogen. Not shown are the anticoagulant inhibitory pathways. *(From Kumar V, Abbas AK, Fausto N: Robbins & Cotran pathologic basis of disease, ed 7, Philadelphia, 2005, Saunders.)*

Factor XIIIa, formed by the action of factors Xa and IIa on factor XIII, along with Ca²⁺, catalyzes the formation of covalent bonds that cross-link adjacent fibrin molecules to make the polymer insoluble. Cross-linking of the fibrin network, along with concurrent platelet contraction and the presence of abundant calcium, thrombin, and adenosine triphosphate (ATP), causes retraction of the fibrin-platelet thrombus. Retraction reduces the size of the thrombus to allow blood flow to continue and to pull damaged vessel edges closer together for efficient healing.

INTEGRATED MODEL OF COAGULATION

In vivo coagulation is more like an integrated web rather than a series of independent cascades. The major stimulus for coagulation in vivo is exposure of

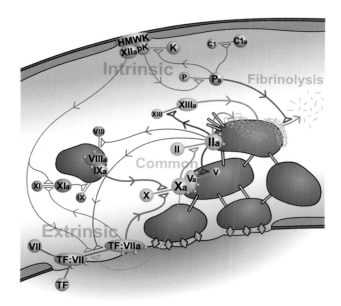

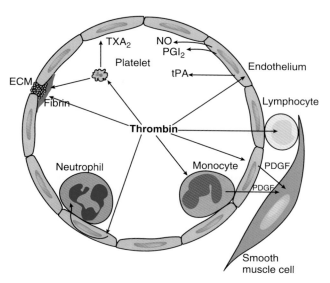

Fig. 2-16   Coagulation, fibrinolysis, and other pathways are highly integrated to balance the host response to injury. Intrinsic coagulation is initiated by binding of high molecular weight kininogen (*HMWK*), factor XII, and prekallikrein (*pK*) to altered endothelial surfaces. Activated products of this reaction (factor XIIa and kallikrein [*K*]) directly or indirectly result in the formation of factor XIa (intrinsic coagulation pathway), factor VIIa (extrinsic coagulation pathway), plasmin (*Pa*) (fibrinolysis), and complement fragments C3a, C3b, C5a (complement cascade). Extrinsic coagulation is initiated by release of tissue factor (*TF*) from areas of damaged endothelium, with subsequent binding of TF to factor VII. The TF:VII complex can be activated by a wide variety of agents. Activation of factor X initiates the common cascade to ultimately result in cleavage of fibrinogen into fibrin. In addition to its role in the common pathway, factor IIa (thrombin) also influences both the intrinsic (factors XI and VIII) and extrinsic (*TF:VII*) coagulation pathways. Additional interactions between these factors, which are not shown in the figure, are described in the text. Specific effects of kallikrein include cleavage and activation of factors XII, IX, and VII, plasminogen, HMWK, and complement fragment C5. *(Courtesy Dr. D.A. Mosier and L. Schooley, College of Veterinary Medicine, Kansas State University.)*

Fig. 2-17   The central roles of thrombin in hemostasis and cellular activation. In addition to a critical function in generating cross-linked fibrin (via cleavage of fibrinogen to fibrin and activation of factor XIII), thrombin also directly induces platelet aggregation and secretion (e.g., TXA_2). Thrombin also activates endothelium to generate leukocyte adhesion molecules and a variety of fibrinolytic (*tPA*), vasoactive (*NO*, PGI_2), or cytokine (*PDGF*) mediators. Likewise, mononuclear inflammatory cells may be activated by the direct actions of thrombin. *ECM*, Extracellular matrix; *NO*, nitric oxide; *PDGF*, platelet-derived growth factor; PGI_2, prostacyclin; TXA_2, thromboxane A_2; *tPA*, tissue plasminogen activator. *(From Kumar V, Abbas AK, Fausto N:* Robbins & Cotran pathologic basis of disease, *ed 7, Philadelphia, 2005, Saunders.)*

plasma to TF and subsequent extrinsic coagulation. Two important events occur following the formation of the TF/factor VIIa complex on damaged, TF-expressing surfaces. Factor X is activated as described for the common pathway, and factor IX is activated to allow a bypass of the contact phase of classical intrinsic coagulation. Factor Xa remains localized upon the damaged cell surface to initiate the formation of a small amount of thrombin. Although the amount of thrombin generated is insufficient to convert significant amounts of fibrinogen into fibrin, it does activate platelets and

factors V, VIII, XI, and XIII on TF-expressing surfaces. Factor IXa can bind to the surface of activated platelets in the area to initiate the formation of tenase complexes, which activates additional factor X of the common pathway. Thrombin-activated or intrinsically activated factor XIa can also participate by activating additional factor XI upon platelet surfaces. The thrombin-initiated activation of these different factors provides an amplification of the critical reactions necessary to generate large amounts of thrombin for the subsequent conversion of fibrinogen into fibrin. Other, probably less important links between the pathways also exist. For example, intrinsic factors XIIa, XIIf, and IXa, and kallikrein can activate extrinsic factor VII to provide additional amplification of this pathway.

The interrelatedness of coagulation pathways also extends to anticoagulant reactions. When excessive levels of thrombin are generated, thrombin destroys rather than activates factors V and VIII. When thrombin binds to thrombomodulin on endothelial surfaces, it activates protein C, a potent anticoagulant (see Coagulation Inhibitors). Intrinsic pathway factors XIIa,

XIIf, and XIa, and kallikrein not only participate in fibrin formation but also initiate fibrinolysis by cleaving plasminogen into plasmin (see Thrombus Dissolution, next).

THROMBUS DISSOLUTION

The purpose of a fibrin-platelet thrombus is to form a temporary patch that is dissolved following healing of the vessel (thrombolysis). The rate of dissolution must be balanced so that it does not occur so quickly that bleeding returns but is not prolonged so that vessel occlusion may occur (Fig. 2-18). Fibrin dissolution (fibrinolysis) is initiated immediately upon vessel injury by the cleavage of the plasma protein plasminogen into plasmin (Fig. 2-19). Plasminogen is activated by a wide variety of proteases, including activated contact group coagulation factors, plasminogen activators present within endothelium and other tissues (tissue plasminogen activator, tPA), and activators present in secretions and fluids. Plasminogen adsorbs to fibrin within a thrombus, so that upon activation the plasmin is localized to the site of the thrombus. The presence of fibrin increases the efficiency of tPA-dependent plasmin generation by nearly twofold. Additionally, by binding to fibrin, plasmin is protected from its major inhibitor (α_2-antiplasmin). The bound plasmin restricts thrombus size by degrading both cross-linked (insoluble) fibrin within the thrombus and fibrinogen, so that additional fibrin formation is inhibited. Dissolution of insoluble, but not soluble, fibrin by plasmin results in the formation of fibrin degradation products (FDPs). FDPs are various-sized fragments of fibrin and fibrinogen that can impair hemostasis. Collectively, FDPs inhibit thrombin, interfere with fibrin polymerization, and can coat platelet membranes to inhibit platelet aggregation.

REGULATION OF HEMOSTASIS

The potent biologic effects of hemostatic products must be finely regulated to achieve appropriate hemostasis, without creating detrimental effects associated with too little or too much activity. Coagulation factors are continuously activated at a low, basal level to keep the system primed for a rapid response to an injurious stimulus. Proteins that inhibit or degrade activated hemostatic products are present in the plasma or are locally produced at the site of hemostasis (Fig. 2-19). These products help confine hemostasis to a site of

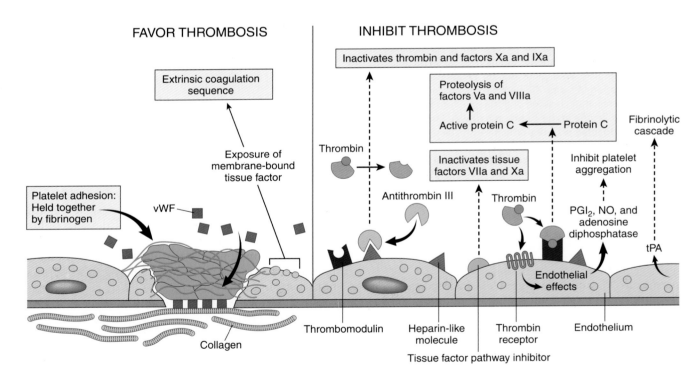

Fig. 2-18   **Schematic illustration of some of the procoagulant and anticoagulant activities of endothelial cells.** Not shown are the profibrinolytic and antifibrinolytic properties. *vWF*, von Willebrand's factor; *PGI₂*, prostacyclin; *NO*, nitric oxide; *tPA*, tissue plasminogen activator. **Thrombin receptor is referred to as protease activated receptor (PAR).** *(From Kumar V, Abbas AK, Fausto N: Robbins & Cotran pathologic basis of disease, ed 7, Philadelphia, 2005, Saunders.)*

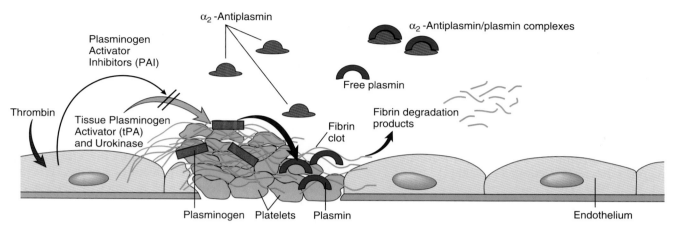

Fig. 2-19   The fibrinolytic system, illustrating the plasminogen activators and inhibitors. *(From Kumar V, Abbas AK, Fausto N: Robbins & Cotran pathologic basis of disease, ed 7, Philadelphia, 2005, Saunders.)*

vascular damage and inhibit hemostatic reactions in normal vasculature. Regulation is also achieved by simple dilution of activated agents as blood removes them from the area, and the factors are removed from the circulation by the liver and spleen.

COAGULATION INHIBITORS

The major anticoagulant-antithrombotic systems upon endothelial cells are the protein C-protein S-thrombomodulin system and endothelial heparan sulfate to which antithrombin III (ATIII) and tissue factor pathway inhibitor (TFPI) are bound. ATIII is the most potent and clinically significant of the coagulation inhibitors, accounting for nearly 80% of the thrombin-inhibitory activity of plasma. ATIII is a circulating serine protease produced by endothelium and hepatocytes that will degrade all activated coagulation factors except for factor VIIa. However, its most important action is the neutralization of thrombin and factor Xa. ATIII can bind heparan sulfate present on the surface of normal endothelium and platelets to localize it to the site where it is most needed to inactivate thrombin and factor Xa. Through this binding, heparin accelerates the rate of ATIII-induced serine protease inactivation by 2000- to 10,000-fold. ATIII also inhibits fibrinolysis (by inhibiting plasmin and kallikrein), kinin formation, and complement activation. Although the major role of heparin is to bind and enhance the activity of ATIII, it also inhibits coagulation by enhancing the release of TFPI from endothelial cells and interfering with binding of platelet receptors to von Willebrand's factor.

The protein C pathway also plays a critical role in preventing thrombosis. Proteins C and S are vitamin K–dependent glycoproteins that, when complexed together on phospholipid surfaces, potently inhibit coagulation by destroying factors Va and VIIIa. An important step in this process is the activation of protein C by thrombin, a reaction that normally occurs at low levels but that increases nearly 20,000-fold following the binding of thrombin to the endothelial receptor thrombomodulin. This reaction is further enhanced by the presence of a protein C receptor on the surface of endothelial cells. Protein S, in addition to serving as a nonenzymatic cofactor with protein C, can independently inhibit factors VIIIa, Xa, and Va. Binding of thrombin to thrombomodulin also results in the loss of the procoagulant functions of thrombin. The protein C-S complex may also enhance fibrinolysis by neutralizing plasminogen activator inhibitors.

TFPI is a significant inhibitor of extrinsic coagulation, which functions synergistically with protein C and ATIII to suppress thrombin formation. TFPI is a plasma protein derived mainly from endothelium and smooth muscle cells that forms a complex with factor Xa on the endothelial-bound TF:VIIa molecule to inhibit subsequent factor X activation. TFPI can interact with VIIa without Xa, but at a slow rate. Therefore TFPI does not substantially inhibit extrinsic coagulation until factor Xa levels increase, after which TFPI provides negative feedback for further generation of Xa by the TF:VIIa complex.

FIBRINOLYTIC INHIBITORS

Major inhibitors of fibrinolytic agents include plasminogen activator inhibitor-1 (PAI-1) and antiplasmins, which include α_2-antiplasmin, α_2-macroglobulin, α_1-antitrypsin, antithrombin III, and C-1 inactivator. PAI-1 inhibits tPA and urokinase, therefore inhibiting fibrinolysis and promoting fibrin stabilization. PAI-1 also inactivates activated protein C, plasmin, and thrombin. The antiplasmins function in a cooperative fashion to prevent excessive plasmin activity so that a thrombus can dissolve at a slow and appropriate rate. α_2-Antiplasmin is the first to bind and neutralize plasmin. When its binding capacity is saturated, excess plasmin is taken up by α_2-macroglobulin. α_2-Macroglobulin also binds to certain activated factors, such as thrombin, and physically entraps but does not degrade their active sites. When α_2-macroglobulin is saturated, plasmin binds to α_1-antitrypsin. α_1-Antitrypsin is a weak inhibitor of fibrinolysis, but a potent inhibitor of factor XIa. In addition to their fibrinolytic roles, α_1-antitrypsin and α_2-macroglobulin are the major plasma inhibitors of activated protein C.

HEMOSTATIC INTEGRATION WITH OTHER HOST RESPONSES

Hemostatic pathways are highly integrated, and many factors within the pathways have multiple roles. Thrombin has a major procoagulant role to cleave factor I to yield fibrin monomers. Thrombin also activates factors V, VIII, XI, and XIII, and is a potent activator of platelets. In contrast, high concentrations of thrombin destroy, rather than activate, factors V and VIII. When thrombin binds to thrombomodulin on endothelial surfaces, it activates protein C, a potent anticoagulant.

A prothrombotic environment is also proinflammatory. Inflammatory stimuli, such as IL-1 and TNF, activate endothelium to produce TF and to increase their expression of leukocyte adhesion molecules. Thrombin and histamine released by degranulating mast cells also stimulate the expression of the adhesin P-selectin. In early stages of inflammation, leukocytes can loosely attach and roll along endothelium or adhered platelets by interacting with endothelial or platelet P-selectin. During this interaction the neutrophil $\alpha_M\beta_2$ integrin may bind to fibrinogen bound to GPIIb/IIIa on the surface of activated platelets to promote the conversion of fibrinogen into fibrin. An enhanced prothrombotic environment during inflammation also occurs because of decreased thrombomodulin function in response to inflammatory products such as endotoxin, IL-1, TNF, and TGF-β. Additionally, adhered or migrating neutrophils and platelets can release lysosomal proteases (e.g., elastase, collagenase, and acid hydrolases), which cleave many products upon the endothelial or platelet surfaces. The conversion of prekallikrein to kallikrein during the contact phase of intrinsic coagulation is another source of integration between hemostatic, fibrinolytic, and inflammatory pathways. Kallikrein is chemotactic, can directly cleave C5 to C5a and C5b, and can cleave HMWK to form bradykinin. The major fibrinolytic protein plasmin also influences other host responses by cleaving C3 to generate C3a and C3b. Mitogenic factors produced by activated endothelium and platelets (e.g., platelet-derived growth factor [PDGF], TGF-β, and vascular endothelial growth factor [VEGF]) contribute to the healing of the damaged tissue. These are just a few of the many relationships between these different host responses.

An important link between intrinsic and extrinsic pathways is the TF/factor VIIa complex. This complex is the major component of extrinsic coagulation, but it can also activate factor IX to allow a bypass of the contact phase of intrinsic coagulation. In turn, intrinsic factors XIIa, XIIf, and IXa, and kallikrein can activate factor VII, which greatly increases the efficiency of extrinsic coagulation. These features give the TF/factor VIIa complex a central role in efficient hemostasis. Extrinsic coagulation and the TF/factor VIIa complex are probably the most important mechanism for in vivo coagulation because bleeding tendencies are not usually associated with factor XII, prekallikrein, and HMWK deficiencies and some factor XI deficiencies in humans and animals.

Some hemostatic reactions initiate pathways that have multiple and sometimes opposite outcomes. Intrinsic pathway factors XIIa, XIIf, and XIa, and kallikrein not only initiate the formation of fibrin but also initiate fibrinolysis by cleaving plasminogen into plasmin. Factor XIIa not only participates directly in intrinsic coagulation and fibrinolysis but indirectly initiates kinin formation and complement activation by converting prekallikrein to kallikrein. Kallikrein is chemotactic, can directly cleave C5 to C5a, can cleave HMWK to form bradykinin, and can convert plasminogen to plasmin. Plasmin also influences complement activation by cleaving C3 to generate C3a and C3b. Additionally, both kallikrein and plasmin can directly activate factor XII to result in autoamplification of all factor XIIa pathways. Other hemostatic products that influence other host systems include factor Xa, thrombin, and fibrinopeptides, all of which have inflammatory and coagulation functions. These interactions indicate the fine balance within the hemostatic system and the interrelatedness between hemostasis and other host response mechanisms.

DISORDERS OF HEMOSTASIS: HEMORRHAGE AND THROMBOSIS

The purpose of hemostasis is to prevent blood loss following vascular damage, while at the same time maintaining blood in a fluid state so that it flows freely through a normal vasculature. Failure of hemostasis can result in the extravascular loss of blood (hemorrhage) or the inappropriate formation of intravascular thrombus (thrombosis).

HEMORRHAGE

Hemorrhage occurs because of abnormal function or integrity of one or more of the major factors that influence hemostasis—the endothelium and blood vessel, platelets, or coagulation factors.

Abnormalities in blood vessels can result from various inherited or acquired problems. Trauma can physically disrupt a vessel and cause hemorrhage by rhexis (rhexis = breaking forth, bursting). Hemorrhage by rhexis can also occur following vascular erosion by inflammatory reactions or invasive neoplasms. Certain fungi commonly invade and damage blood vessels to cause extensive local hemorrhage (e.g., internal carotid artery erosion secondary to guttural pouch mycosis in horses). More commonly, small defects in otherwise intact blood vessels allow small numbers of erythrocytes to escape by diapedesis (dia = through, pedian = leap). Endotoxemia is a common cause of endothelial injury that results in small widespread hemorrhages (Fig. 2-20). Infectious agents, such as canine adenovirus-1, or chemicals, such as uremic toxins, can also damage endothelium. Similarly, immune complexes can become entrapped between endothelial cells and activate complement and neutrophil influx to result in damage to the endothelium and vessel wall (type III hypersensitivity reaction). Developmental collagen disorders, such as the Ehlers-Danlos syndrome, are sometimes accompanied by hemorrhage. Affected blood vessels contain abnormal collagen in their basement membranes and surrounding supportive tissue, resulting in vascular fragility and predisposition to leakage or damage. Similar hemorrhages occur because of the collagen defects in guinea pigs or primates with vitamin C deficiency.

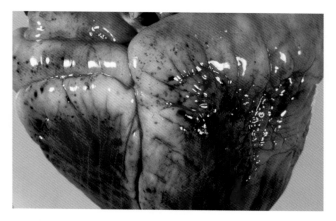

Fig. 2-20   Hemorrhage, endotoxemia, heart, cow. Note the epicardial and subepicardial hemorrhages in the fat of the coronary groove (a common site), from injury to the endothelium from endotoxin (component of the cell wall of gram-negative bacteria). The smaller, pinpoint hemorrhages (1 to 2 mm) are petechiae. The larger, blotchy hemorrhages (3 to 5 mm) are ecchymoses. *(Courtesy Dr. M. D. McGavin, College of Veterinary Medicine, University of Tennessee.)*

Decreased platelet numbers (thrombocytopenia) or abnormal platelet function can cause hemorrhage. Thrombocytopenia can result from decreased production, increased destruction, or increased use of platelets. Decreased production generally occurs following megakaryocyte damage or destruction as a result of causes such as radiation injury, estrogen toxicity, cytotoxic drugs, and viral or other infectious diseases (e.g., feline and canine parvoviruses). Increased platelet destruction is often immune-mediated. Autoimmune destruction due to antibody production against platelet membrane components, such as GPIIb and GPIIIa, can occur following immune dysregulation (e.g., systemic lupus erythematosus). Alteration of platelet membranes by drugs or infectious agents may also stimulate immune-mediated destruction or removal of platelets from the circulation. Isoimmune destruction of platelets in neonatal pigs has occurred following ingestion of colostrum-containing antiplatelet antibodies. Viral diseases (e.g., equine infectious anemia and feline immunodeficiency syndrome) and arthropod-borne agents are often associated with platelet destruction and their removal by the spleen. The most common cause of increased platelet use is diffuse endothelial damage or generalized platelet activation, which initiates disseminated intravascular coagulation (DIC). With DIC there is widespread intravascular coagulation and platelet activation, which rapidly results in consumption of platelets and coagulation factors (see thrombosis section). This results in progressive thrombocytopenia and hemorrhage as the syndrome escalates. Another platelet consumption disease that is not accompanied by coagulation is thrombotic thrombocytopenic purpura. In this condition, platelet aggregates form in the microvasculature, possibly due to increased release of proagglutinating substances by normal or damaged endothelium.

Decreased platelet function is usually associated with an inability to adhere or aggregate at a site of vascular injury. Inherited problems of platelet function in humans include deficiency of GPIb on the platelet surface (Bernard-Soulier syndrome), deficient or defective GPIIb and GPIIIa on the platelet surface (Glanzmann's thrombasthenia), and deficient release of platelet granule content ("storage pool disease"). Glanzmann's thrombasthenia is a rare disease that has been reported in Otterhound and Great Pyrenees dogs. In these dogs there is prolonged bleeding and hematoma formation from minor injury and spontaneous epistaxis because of a mutation affecting a Ca^{+2}-binding domain of the extracellular portion of GPIIb. Abnormal synthesis or release of platelet granule content has been reported in Simmental cattle, dogs (Spitz, Basset hound, American foxhounds), cats, and fawn-hooded rats. Defective platelet storage of ADP occurs in the Chédiak-Higashi syndrome (Aleutian mink, cattle, Persian cats, killer whales).

Acquired platelet inhibition and dysfunction is most often associated with administration of nonsteroidal antiinflammatory drugs, such as aspirin. Aspirin inhibits the cyclooxygenase pathway of arachidonic acid metabolism, thus decreasing thromboxane production to result in reduced platelet aggregation. Platelet function is also inhibited by uremia because of renal failure. Secondary platelet dysfunction can also occur because of deficiencies of factors necessary for normal platelet function. In von Willebrand's disease, or in autoimmune or myeloproliferative disorders in which autoantibodies against von Willebrand's factor are produced, the amount of functional von Willebrand's factor is decreased. This results in decreased platelet adhesion following vascular damage with either subclinical or severe hemorrhage.

Decreased concentrations or function of coagulation factors can also result in hemorrhage. Inherited deficiencies in coagulation factors have been recognized in many different breeds of dogs and less often other species (Box 2-5). These conditions are characterized by hemorrhage that can range from subclinical to severe. In many cases, the coagulation factor deficiency is recognized because of prolonged bleeding following venipuncture or surgery, but otherwise has minimal significance to the animal. Other inherited deficiencies are characterized by severe episodes of hemorrhage that begin soon after birth.

Acquired defects in coagulation can be caused by decreased production or increased use of coagulation factors. Severe liver disease results in decreased synthesis of most coagulation factors. Production of coagulation factors II, VII, IX, X and proteins C and S is reduced by vitamin K deficiency. Decreased vitamin K production, absorption, or function will reduce conversion of glutamic acid residues into γ-carboxyglutamic acid on these factors. Common substances that competitively inhibit this conversion include dicumarol in moldy sweet clover (*Melilotus alba*), warfarin-containing rodenticides, and sulfaquinoxaline (Fig. 2-21). An inherited deficiency of binding of γ-glutamyl-carboxylase with vitamin K has been reported in British Devon Rex cats. The most common cause of decreased coagulation factors is increased consumption associated with DIC.

The appearance of hemorrhage depends on cause, location, and severity. Hemorrhage within tissue is often characterized based on size. A petechia (pl. petechiae) is a pinpoint (1 to 2 mm) hemorrhage that occurs mainly because of diapedesis associated with minor vascular damage (Fig. 2-20). An ecchymosis (pl. ecchymoses) is a larger (up to 2 to 3 cm in diameter) hemorrhage that occurs with more extensive vascular damage (Fig. 2-22), whereas suffusive hemorrhage affects larger contiguous areas of tissue then the

---

Box **2-5**

Examples of Inherited Coagulation Deficiency Disorders

FACTOR I
Rare, goats and dogs (Bernese mountain dogs, borzoi, Lhasa apso, vizsla, collie). Mild bleeding tendencies in dogs, more severe in goats.

FACTOR II
Rare, dogs (boxer, Otterhound, English cocker spaniel). Mild bleeding in adults; epistaxis and umbilical cord bleeding in puppies.

FACTOR VII
Rare, dogs (beagles, also Alaskan malamutes, boxer, bulldog, miniature schnauzer, mix breeds). Mild, more easily bruised.

FACTOR X
Rare, dogs (cocker spaniels, mix breeds, Jack Russell terrier). Fatal in severely affected dogs, mild to moderate hemorrhage in less severe cases.

FACTOR XII
Cats and rarely dogs (miniature poodle, standard poodle, German shorthair pointer, Shar-Pei). No bleeding.

FACTOR XI
Cattle (Holstein and Japanese black) and dogs (Great Pyrenees, English springer spaniel, Kerry blue terrier). Spontaneous hemorrhage is insignificant but can be severe after surgery. Most common hereditary coagulation problem in cattle.

FACTOR IX (HEMOPHILIA B)
Dogs and cats. Variable bleeding depending on the molecular damage; generally mild in cats and small dogs, more severe in large dogs.

FACTOR VIII (HEMOPHILIA A)
Dogs, horses, cattle, sheep, and cats. Bleeding can be severe in large dogs and horses; mildly affected animals do not spontaneously bleed.

VON WILLEBRAND'S DISEASE
Dogs, cats, horses, and pigs. Mild to severe hemorrhage depending on form of molecular damage; epistaxis, mucosal hemorrhage, postsurgical bleeding. Most common inherited canine bleeding disorder.

VITAMIN K-DEPENDENT FACTORS (II, VII, IX, X)
Rare, Devon Rex cats. Severe, sometimes fatal hemorrhages.

PREKALLIKREIN
Some dogs and Belgian horses and miniature horses. Mucosal or postsurgical bleeding.

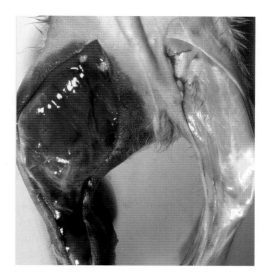

Fig. 2-21   Hemorrhage, anticoagulant (warfarin-containing) rodenticide toxicosis, skin and subcutis, medial aspect of the right hindleg, dog. There is a large area of extensive hemorrhage in the subcutis. This lesion was attributed to decreased production of coagulation factors II, VII, IX, and X and proteins C and S resulting from a deficiency of vitamin K induced by warfarin. *(Courtesy Dr. D.A. Mosier, College of Veterinary Medicine, Kansas State University.)*

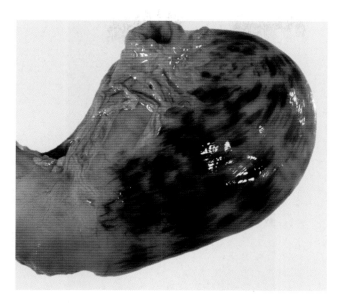

Fig. 2-23   Suffusive hemorrhage, serosa, stomach, dog. Suffusive hemorrhage results from severe injury to endothelial cells in the capillary beds. *(Courtesy Dr. D.A. Mosier, College of Veterinary Medicine, Kansas State University.)*

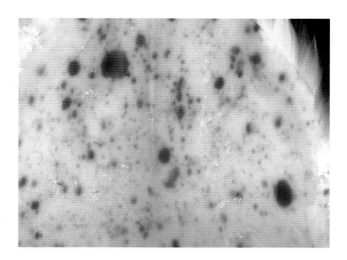

Fig. 2-22   Ecchymotic hemorrhages (ecchymoses), subcutis, rabbit. Ecchymoses result from moderate injury to endothelial cells in the capillary beds. *(Courtesy Dr. D.A. Mosier, College of Veterinary Medicine, Kansas State University.)*

other two types (Fig. 2-23). Hemorrhage that occurs into a focal, confined space forms a hematoma. Hematomas are most common in the ears of long-eared dogs or pigs and in the spleen following trauma to the vasculature (Fig. 2-24). The hematoma grows in size until the pressure exerted by the extravascular blood matches that within the injured vessel or the vessel seals internally by hemostasis. Hemorrhage into body cavities results in pooling of coagulated or noncoagulated blood within the cavity and is classified by terms such as hemoperitoneum (blood in the peritoneal cavity), hemothorax (blood in the thoracic cavity), and hemopericardium (blood in the pericardial sac) (Fig. 2-25).

The significance of hemorrhage depends mainly on the amount, rate, and location of the blood loss. In most cases, blood loss occurs locally and is quickly stopped by hemostatic processes that seal the damaged vessel. In more severe cases, blood loss continues until local tissue pressure matches intravascular pressure and ends the hemorrhage (such as occurs with hematoma formation). When these mechanisms fail to stop blood loss, significant hemorrhage can occur externally or internally into body cavities. Rapid loss of substantial amounts of blood, such as occurs because of traumatic injury of a large vessel, can lead to hypovolemia, decreased tissue perfusion, and hypovolemic shock (see later discussion in this chapter). In contrast, slow rates of blood loss can be totally or partially compensated for by increased hematopoiesis. Many cases of gastric ulceration and hemorrhage are characterized by persistent but slow rates of blood loss. Some hemorrhages can create pressure that interferes with tissue function. This is most significant in vital organs or in tissue with little room to expand in response to the pressure, such as the brain and heart.

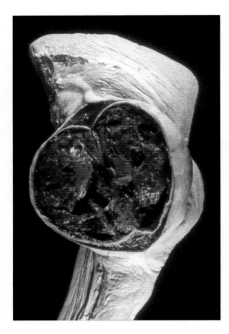

Fig. 2-24   Organizing hematoma, spleen, horse. Trauma to the spleen has caused damage to the splenic red pulp and its vessels, resulting in bleeding into the splenic parenchyma, forming a hematoma. Note that this hematoma is not acute but is several days old, because the blood clot is being degraded. The hematoma is contained by the splenic capsule. *(Courtesy Dr. H.B. Gelberg, College of Veterinary Medicine, Oregon State University.)*

THROMBOSIS

Thrombosis is characterized by the formation of an inappropriate thrombus of fibrin and/or platelets along with other blood elements (thrombus; pl. thrombi) on the wall of a blood or lymphatic vessel or heart (mural thrombus), or free in their lumens (thromboembolus). Major determinants of thrombosis are historically referred to as Virchow's triad and include the endothelium and blood vessels (vascular injury), coagulation factor and platelet activity (coagulability), and the dynamics of blood flow (stasis or turbulence) (Fig. 2-26, Box 2-6).

Changes in the endothelium are the most important factor in thrombosis. Endothelial injury and exposure of tissue factor (TF) and subendothelial components, such as collagen and fibronectin, are potent stimuli for platelet aggregation and coagulation. Causes of injury are widely varied in their severity and cause, and include trauma, vasculitis caused by infection or immunologic reactions, metabolic disorders, neoplasia, and toxins. Additionally, loss of anticoagulant properties of normal endothelium combined with local release of procoagulant substances can result in fibrin formation. Platelets may also adhere to intact endothelium by interacting with altered proteoglycans in the endothelial glycocalyx. Reduced prostacyclin synthesis may also increase platelet adhesion to endothelium.

Abnormal blood flow increases the risk of thrombosis. Reduced blood flow may occur systemically with heart failure or in a local region of congestion caused by vascular obstruction or vascular dilation. Reduced blood

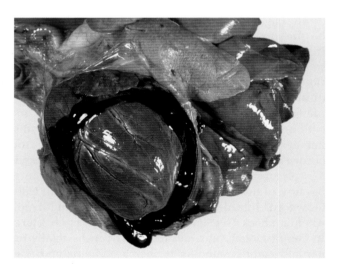

Fig. 2-25   Hemopericardium, pericardial sac, dog. Hemorrhage into the pericardial sac has caused its distention. Extensive hemopericardium can interfere with the dilatation and contraction of the ventricles, causing cardiac tamponade. Both coagulated and noncoagulated blood are present in the **pericardial sac.** *(Courtesy Dr. D.A. Mosier, College of Veterinary Medicine, Kansas State University.)*

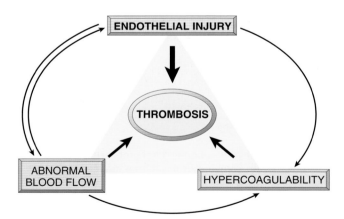

Fig. 2-26   Virchow triad in thrombosis. Endothelial integrity is the single most important factor. Note that injury to endothelial cells can affect local blood flow and/or coagulability; abnormal blood flow (stasis or turbulence) can, in turn, cause endothelial injury. The elements of the triad may act independently or may combine to cause thrombus formation. *(From Kumar V, Abbas AK, Fausto N: Robbins & Cotran pathologic basis of disease, ed 7, Philadelphia, 2005, Saunders.)*

Box **2-6**

Causes of Thrombosis

ENDOTHELIAL INJURY

Viruses (e.g., canine adenovirus 1, equine morbillivirus, herpesvirus and arterivirus, ovine orbivirus, bovine and porcine pestivirus)

Bacteria (e.g., *Salmonella typhimurium, Mannheimia hemolytica, Erysipelothrix rhusiopathiae, Hemophilus somnus*)

Fungi (e.g., *Aspergillus, Mucor, Absidia, Rhizopus*)

Nematode parasites (e.g., *Strongylus vulgaris* larvae, *Dirofilaria, Spirocerca, Aelurostrongylus,* angiostrongylosis)

Immune-mediated vasculitis (e.g., purpura hemorrhagica, feline infectious peritonitis)

Toxins (e.g., endotoxin, *Claviceps*)

Vitamin E/Selenium deficiency (microangiopathy)

Local extension of infection (e.g., hepatic abscesses, metritis)

Disseminated intravascular coagulation (DIC)

Faulty intravenous injections

Renal glomerular and cutaneous vasculopathy of greyhounds

ALTERATIONS IN BLOOD FLOW

Local stasis or reduced flow (e.g., gastric dilation and volvulus, intestinal torsion and volvulus, varicocele, external compression of vessel)

Cardiac disease (e.g., cardiomyopathy, cardiac hypertrophy)

Aneurysm (e.g., copper deficiency in pigs, *Strongylus vulgaris, Spirocerca lupi*)

Hypovolemia (e.g., shock, diarrhea, and burns)

HYPERCOAGULABILITY

Enhanced platelet activity (e.g., diabetes mellitus, nephrotic syndrome, malignant neoplasia, heartworm disease, uremia)

Increased clotting factor activation (e.g., nephrotic syndrome, DIC, neoplasia)

Antithrombin III deficiency (e.g., DIC, hepatic disease, glomerular amyloidosis)

Metabolic abnormalities (e.g., hyperadrenocorticism, hypothyroidism)

Glomerulopathies

---

flow is most important in veins, where the slow flow rate favors accumulation of activated coagulation factors and contact of platelets with the endothelium. Venous thrombosis is common in horses with occlusion of intestinal veins secondary to intestinal torsion. Inactivity can also lead to venous stasis and thrombosis in the limbs, a common problem in humans but not in animals. Dilated heart chambers (e.g., dilatative cardiomyopathy) or dilated vessels (e.g., aneurysms) are also areas where reduced blood flow predisposes to thrombosis.

Turbulent blood flow also enhances the potential for thrombosis. Turbulence disrupts laminar blood flow so the thin layer of plasma that normally separates the endothelium from cellular elements, particularly platelets, is disrupted, and platelets interact more readily with the endothelium. Similarly, turbulence results in mixing of the blood, which provides greater opportunity for interactions between coagulation factors. Turbulence can also physically damage endothelium, creating a strong stimulus for platelet adhesion and coagulation. Turbulence, along with increased risk of thrombosis, is usually greatest in areas where vessels branch, where there is narrowing of the vessel lumen, or at sites of venous or lymphatic valves.

Increased coagulability of blood (hypercoagulability) is another factor that predisposes patients to thrombosis. Hypercoagulability usually reflects an increase or decrease in the concentration of activated hemostatic proteins (e.g., coagulation factors and coagulation or fibrinolytic inhibitors) caused by enhanced activation or decreased degradation of these proteins. Less often, an alteration in hemostatic protein function may influence coagulability. Activity of coagulation and fibrinolytic proteins can increase in certain conditions such as inflammation, stress, surgery, neoplasia, pregnancy, and renal disease (e.g., the nephrotic syndrome). Transient increases in factor I occur with inflammation, stress, and tissue necrosis. Factor I and factor VIII are elevated by trauma, acute illness, surgery, and increased metabolism that accompanies hyperthyroidism. Deficiency of antithrombin III, a major inhibitor of thrombin, occurs relatively often in dogs with the nephrotic syndrome. In this syndrome, ATIII is depleted because of loss through damaged glomeruli. In affected dogs, there is an increased incidence of venous thrombosis and pulmonary embolism. Increased platelet activation (e.g., heartworm disease, nephrotic syndrome, and neoplasia) can also contribute to hypercoagulability of blood.

The appearance of a thrombus depends on its underlying cause, location, and composition (relative proportions of platelets, fibrin, and erythrocytes). Thrombi composed predominantly of platelets and fibrin tend to be pale, whereas those containing many erythrocytes are red. Cardiac and arterial thrombi are usually initiated by endothelial damage. This damage provides a site for firm platelet attachment and subsequent incorporation of fibrin. Rapid blood flow in these arteries and arterioles inhibits passive incorporation of erythrocytes into the thrombus (Fig. 2-27). Cardiac and arterial thrombi are dull, usually firmly attached to the vessel, wall and red-gray (pale thrombi) (Fig. 2-28). The thrombus may or may not occlude the vessel lumen, and large thrombi tend to have tails that extend downstream from the point of endothelial attachment.

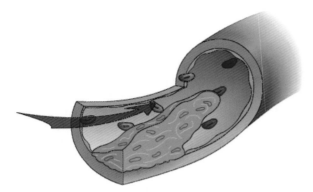

Fig. 2-27   Thrombus (mural), artery. Thrombus formation is usually initiated by endothelial damage, forming a site of attachment for the thrombus. Growth of the thrombus is downstream, resulting in a tail that is not attached to the vessel wall. Portions of the tail can break off to form thromboemboli. *(Courtesy Dr. D.A. Mosier and L. Schooley, College of Veterinary Medicine, Kansas State University.)*

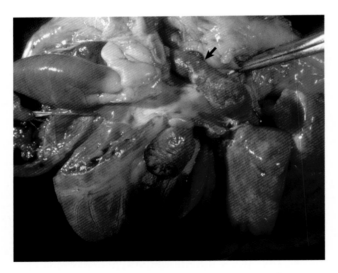

Fig. 2-28   Arterial thrombus, pulmonary artery, dog. Arterial thrombi are composed primarily of platelets and fibrin because of the rapid flow of blood, which tends to exclude erythrocytes from the thrombus; thus they are usually pale beige to gray *(arrow)*. *(Courtesy Dr. D.A. Mosier, College of Veterinary Medicine, Kansas State University.)*

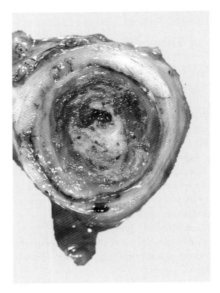

Fig. 2-29   Arterial thrombus, lines of Zahn, cranial mesenteric artery, horse. Cardiac and larger arterial thrombi often have a laminated appearance characterized by alternating layers of platelets *(dark)* and fibrin *(pale)* intermixed with erythrocytes and leukocytes (lines of Zahn). These lines are the result of rapid blood flow in the heart and arteries/arterioles that favors the deposition of fibrin and platelets and the exclusion of erythrocytes from the thrombus. This horse had verminous arteritis (*Strongylus vulgaris* fourth stage larvae) in the affected artery. *(Courtesy Dr. P.N. Nation, University of Alberta; and Noah's Arkive, College of Veterinary Medicine, The University of Georgia.)*

Cardiac and larger arterial thrombi often have a laminated appearance created by rapid blood flow and characterized by alternating layers of platelets, interspersed by fibrin intermixed with erythrocytes and leukocytes (lines of Zahn) (Fig. 2-29).

Venous thrombi often occur in areas of stasis. Because of the slow blood flow and reduced clearance rate of activated clotting factors in these areas, erythrocytes are commonly incorporated into a loose meshwork of fibrin and platelets (Fig. 2-30). Venous thrombi are typically gelatinous, soft, glistening, and dark red (red thrombi) (Fig. 2-31). They are almost always occlusive and molded to the vessel lumen, and often extend for a considerable distance upstream from their point of origin. They commonly have points of attachment to the vessel wall, but these are often very loose and difficult to discern. Venous thrombi are morphologically similar to postmortem clots (see Chapter 1, Fig. 1-24). Compared with venous thrombi, postmortem clots are softer and do not have a point of vascular attachment. In larger vessels or the heart, erythrocytes may settle to the bottom of the clot, leaving a yellow upper layer (chicken fat clot) indicative of postmortem formation. The presence or absence of associated lesions is often a major factor in distinguishing between an antemortem venous thrombus and a postmortem clot.

The significance of a thrombus is determined by its location and its ability to disrupt perfusion in a dependent tissue. Disruption of tissue perfusion is influenced mainly by the size of the thrombus, its rate of formation, and its method of resolution or repair. In general,

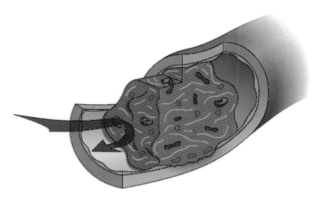

Fig. 2-30   Venous thrombus. Thrombus formation often occurs in areas of slow blood flow or stasis. Venous thrombi are dark red and gelatinous due to large numbers of erythrocytes that are loosely incorporated into the thrombus due to the slow blood flow. Most venous thrombi are occlusive. *(Courtesy Dr. D.A. Mosier and L. Schooley, College of Veterinary Medicine, Kansas State University.)*

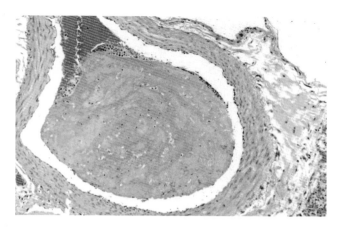

Fig. 2-32   Large thrombus, pulmonary artery, cow. Large thrombi are less readily dissolved by thrombolysis and therefore heal by other methods. This thrombus consists of a large coagulum of fibrin that has undergone little to no resolution. **H&E stain.** *(Courtesy Dr. M.A. Miller, College of Veterinary Medicine, University of Missouri; and Noah's Arkive, College of Veterinary Medicine, The University of Georgia.)*

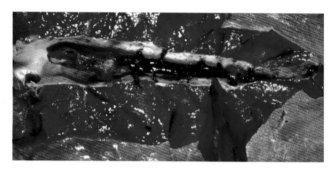

Fig. 2-31   Venous thrombi, pulmonary vein, lung, horse. Venous thrombi become molded to the shape of the lumen of the vein and grow upstream from the site of initiation. *(Courtesy Dr. J. King, College of Veterinary Medicine, Cornell University; and Noah's Arkive, College of Veterinary Medicine, The University of Georgia.)*

thrombi that rapidly develop are more detrimental than those that slowly develop. A slowly developing thrombus will create progressive narrowing of the vessel lumen, but the slow rate of development provides opportunity for collateral blood flow to increase into the affected area. Small thrombi are usually less damaging than large thrombi. Small thrombi are more easily removed by thrombolysis with little residual vessel damage or tissue compromise. In contrast, large thrombi substantially narrow the vessel lumen to restrict blood flow, are often occlusive, and are less readily dissolved by thrombolysis (Fig. 2-32). Occlusive thrombi block blood flow either into (occlusive arterial thrombus) or out of (occlusive venous thrombus) an area and often result in ischemia (decreased oxygenation of tissue) or infarction (necrosis of tissue caused by lack of oxygen).

Under most circumstances and following removal of the injurious stimulus, the well-regulated cascade of events in thrombosis results in the return to normal function of the endothelium and subendothelial collagen (Fig. 2-33, A). However, blood flow through a vessel containing a chronic large or occlusive thrombus can change over time. The thrombus provides an ongoing stimulus for platelet adhesion and coagulation, so thrombus propagation can occur to result in progressive narrowing and possible occlusion of the vessel lumen. A thrombus can also be incorporated into the wall of the vessel by a process similar to that used to replace irreversibly damaged tissue. Products of the aggregated platelets stimulate permanent healing of the damaged area by recruiting fibroblasts to the damaged area. Thrombotic debris is removed by macrophages, and granulation tissue and subsequent fibrosis (organization) occur at the site of the thrombus. Concurrently, there is regrowth of endothelium over the surface of the scar. Although there is a permanent narrowing of the vessel lumen, the regrowth of endothelium over the healed thrombus decreases the stimulus for continued thrombosis (Fig. 2-33, B). In occlusive and some large thrombi, this healing process may be accompanied by invasion and growth of endothelial-lined blood channels through the fibrosed area (recanalization) (Figs. 2-33, C and 2-34). This provides alternate routes for blood flow to reestablish through or around the original thrombus. Although reestablishment of blood flow increases tissue perfusion, the permanent vascular narrowing and altered, more turbulent blood flow at the site of a healed thrombus result in an increased risk for subsequent thrombosis at the site.

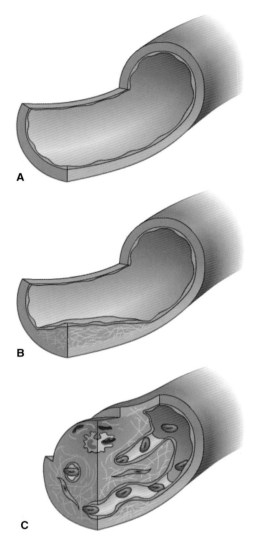

Fig. 2-33   Thrombus resolution. A, Small thrombi are removed by thrombolysis, and the blood vessel returns to normal structure and function. **B,** Larger, more persistent thrombi are resolved by removal of thrombotic debris by phagocytes with subsequent granulation tissue formation and fibrosis with regrowth of endothelium over the surface to incorporate the affected area into the vessel wall. **C,** In large mural or occlusive thrombi that are not removed by thrombolysis or phagocytosis of the thrombotic debris, the thrombus is organized by the invasion of fibroblasts and later by the formation of new vascular channels (recanalization), which provides alternate routes for blood flow through and around the site of the original thrombus. (*A, B,* and *C, Courtesy Dr. D. A. Mosier and L. Schooley, College of Veterinary Medicine, Kansas State University.*)

In some cases, a thrombus or portions of a thrombus can break loose and enter the circulation as an embolus (pl. emboli), a piece of free-floating foreign material within the blood. Thromboemboli (emboli derived from fragments of a thrombus) eventually become lodged in

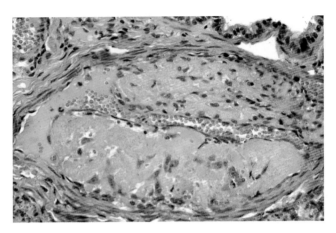

Fig. 2-34   Occlusive mural thrombus, recanalization, cat. In occlusive and large thrombi, the healing process may occur by fibrosis and the invasion and growth of endothelial-lined vascular channels through the fibrosed area (recanalization). Note the vascular channel, horizontally in the middle of the thrombus. This provides alternate routes for blood flow to reestablish through or around the original thrombus. The permanent vascular narrowing and altered, more turbulent blood flow at the site of a healed thrombus result in an increased risk for subsequent thrombosis at the site. H&E stain. (*Courtesy Dr. B.C. Ward, College of Veterinary Medicine, University of Mississippi; and Noah's Arkive, College of Veterinary Medicine, The University of Georgia.*)

a smaller-sized vessel as the vessel diameter reaches a size that prevents the passage of the embolus, a process called embolization. Venous thromboemboli typically lodge in the pulmonary circulation where they can cause pulmonary infarcts or right-side heart failure. Arterial thromboemboli typically lodge within a smaller artery downstream from the site of the thrombus, often near sites of vascular bifurcation. Arterial emboli frequently result in infarction of dependent tissue, depending on the tissue and nature of its vascular supply. Cardiac thromboemboli usually lodge at the bifurcation of the external iliac arteries with a portion of the thromboembolus entering each iliac vessel to form a saddle thrombus (Fig. 2-35).

Emboli can also originate from substances other than thrombi. Fat from the bone marrow can be released into the circulation following a fracture of a long bone. Most fat emboli lodge in the pulmonary circulation. Fibrocartilaginous emboli consist of portions of an intervertebral disk, which are released following rupture of a degenerative disk. These can result in occlusion of local vessels and sometimes cause localized spinal cord infarction. Bacteria from inflammatory lesions such as vegetative valvular endocarditis or abscesses can enter the blood to form bacterial emboli. When these lodge within vessels, they may cause infarction and secondary sites of infection. Intravascular parasites,

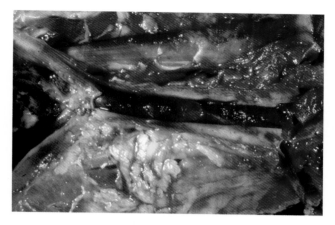

Fig. 2-35 **Saddle thrombus, iliac-aortic bifurcation, cat.** Cardiac thromboemboli usually lodge at the bifurcation of the aorta into the external iliac arteries with a portion of the thromboembolus entering each iliac vessel to form a saddle thrombus. A saddle thrombus is not attached to the wall of the aorta or iliac arteries and is easily removed at necropsy. The thromboembolus is composed of layers of platelets and fibrin in which there are enmeshed erythrocytes. *(Courtesy Dr. M.D. McGavin, College of Veterinary Medicine, University of Tennessee.)*

such as heartworms (e.g., *Dirofilaria*), or flukes (e.g., schistosomes) can form parasitic emboli. Malignant neoplasms that invade a vessel result in the formation of neoplastic emboli composed of neoplastic cells. Less common sources of emboli include hematopoietic cells from the bone marrow, amniotic fluid, aggluti-nated erythrocytes, or clumps of other cells, such as hepatocytes, released following tissue trauma. In any case, the significance of these emboli is their potential to occlude a vessel and inhibit blood flow to dependent tissue.

A serious manifestation of abnormal coagulation is DIC. This is a severe dyshomeostasis caused by the generation of excess thrombin. There are many causes, including diffuse vascular damage (e.g., trauma, vas-culitis, and burns), which results in exposure of blood to TF. Intravascular generation of TF by endothelial cells and monocytes can also occur in response to bac-teremia, other systemic infections, or any other stimuli that activate the release of inflammatory mediators. The result is TF-induced activation of extrinsic coagula-tion to produce thrombin. Thrombin causes platelet aggregation and activation of coagulation factors V, VIII, and I to form fibrin, resulting in widespread microvascular clots. Concurrently the high levels of thrombin stimulate clot dissolution by binding to thrombomodulin to activate protein C, by converting plasminogen into plasmin, and by binding to ATIII to become inactivated. The widespread nature of the coag-ulation response results in the consumption of these

and other factors, resulting in widespread hemorrhages. This combination of microthrombosis with concurrent or rapidly sequential hemorrhage represents one of the most profound and dramatic examples of dyshome-ostasis in animals.

NORMAL BLOOD FLOW, DISTRIBUTION, AND PERFUSION

The heart provides the driving pressure for blood distribution. Baroreceptors in the carotid sinus and aortic arch signal the cardiovascular control center in the medulla to balance sympathetic and parasympa-thetic output to maintain appropriate blood pressure. Left atrial volume receptors and hypothalamic osmore-ceptors also help regulate pressure by altering water volume and sodium balance. Sodium concentration is an important contributor to blood volume, osmolal-ity, and pressure, and is controlled by the renin-angiotensin-aldosterone system. Secretion of ADH by the hypothalamus in response to a water deficit increases renal tubular reabsorption of water to help maintain blood volume.

Distribution of blood within the circulatory system is highly variable. Organs that alter or recondition blood (e.g., lungs, gastrointestinal tract, kidney, and liver) receive substantially greater blood flow than is required for their metabolic needs. Oxygen and CO_2 are exchanged in the lungs, nutrients are obtained from the gastrointestinal tract and processed by the liver, wastes are removed and electrolytes are balanced by the kidneys, heat is dissipated in the skin, and regula-tory hormones enter from endocrine tissues. Systemic neural and hormonal influences can cause general changes in blood distribution. Blood vessel B_2 recep-tors, most abundant in cardiac and skeletal muscle, cause vasodilation and increased flow when stimulated by epinephrine. In contrast, vessel α-receptors, notably absent in the brain, induce vasoconstriction and reduced flow in most organs upon stimulation with norepinephrine. Local intrinsic controls alter arteriolar radius to adjust the blood flow to a tissue based on that tissue's metabolic needs. These local controls generally override any central controls to maintain adequate blood flow to support normal cell function. At rest, more than 60% of the circulating blood volume is in the veins, pro-viding a storage pool that can be quickly returned to the heart during periods of increased tissue need. In contrast, most capillary beds are closed at any given time; blood flows through only about 10% of the total capillaries of resting skeletal muscle. The orchestration of central pressure, blood composition, and blood distribution is critical to meet the varying perfusion needs of all the cells in the body despite constantly changing conditions.

ALTERATIONS IN BLOOD FLOW AND PERFUSION

INCREASED BLOOD FLOW

Hyperemia is an active engorgement of vascular beds with a normal or decreased outflow of blood. It occurs because of increased metabolic activity of tissue that results in localized increased concentrations of CO_2, acid, and other metabolites. These cause a local stimulus for vasodilation and increased flow (hyperemia). Hyperemia can occur as a physiological mechanism within the skin to dissipate heat. It also occurs because of increased need, such as increased blood flow to the gastrointestinal tract after a meal. Hyperemia is also one of the first vascular changes that occur in response to an inflammatory stimulus (Fig. 2-36). Neurogenic reflexes and release of vasoactive substances, such as

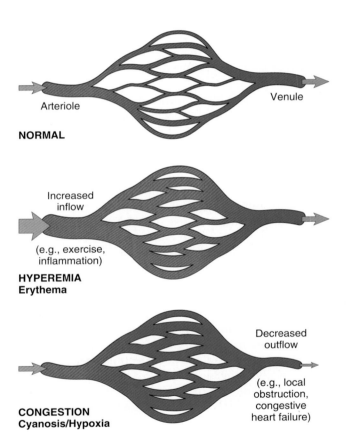

NORMAL

Arteriole   Venule

Increased inflow

(e.g., exercise, inflammation)

**HYPEREMIA
Erythema**

Decreased outflow

(e.g., local obstruction, congestive heart failure)

**CONGESTION
Cyanosis/Hypoxia**

Fig. 2-36   Hyperemia versus congestion. In both cases, there is an increased volume and pressure of blood in a given tissue with associated capillary dilation and a potential for fluid extravasation. In hyperemia there is increased inflow leading to engorgement with oxygenated blood. In congestion, diminished outflow leads to a capillary bed swollen with deoxygenated venous blood resulting in cyanosis. *(From Kumar V, Abbas AK, Fausto N: Robbins & Cotran pathologic basis of disease, ed 7, Philadelphia, 2005, Saunders.)*

histamine and prostaglandins, mediate the change to promote delivery of inflammatory mediators to the site. Tissues with hyperemic vessels are bright red and warm, and there is engorgement of the arterioles and capillaries.

DECREASED BLOOD FLOW

Congestion is the passive engorgement of a vascular bed generally caused by a decreased outflow with a normal or increased inflow of blood (Fig. 2-36). Passive congestion can occur acutely (acute passive congestion) or chronically (chronic passive congestion). Acute passive congestion occurs following euthanasia or in acute heart failure (cardiac arrhythmias) in dependent organs, such as the lung and liver (Fig. 2-37), or in organs in which relaxation of smooth muscle from barbiturate euthanasia results in dilation of the vasculature and vascular sinusoids, such as in the spleen. Most passive congestion occurs and is recognized clinically as chronic passive congestion. It can occur locally because of the obstruction of venous outflow caused by a neoplastic or inflammatory mass, displacement of an organ, or fibrosis resulting from healed injury. Generalized passive congestion occurs because of decreased passage of blood either through the heart or the lungs. This is most often caused by heart failure or conditions (e.g., pulmonary fibrosis) that inhibit the flow of blood through the lungs. Right sided heart failure causes portal vein and hepatic congestion (Fig. 2-38). Left sided heart failure results in pulmonary congestion (Fig. 2-39). Chronically, there may be fibrosis caused by the hypoxia and cell injury

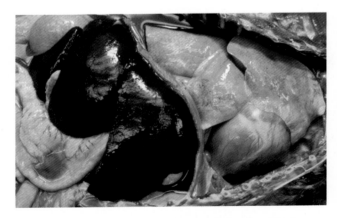

Fig. 2-37   Acute passive congestion, liver, dog. The liver is enlarged and dark red. Acute passive congestion occurs in the vascular system and dependent organs (heart, lungs, portal system) when there is a sudden interruption of the return of blood to the heart as occurs in heart failure resulting from arrhythmias and following euthanasia. *(Courtesy Dr. D.A. Mosier, College of Veterinary Medicine, Kansas State University.)*

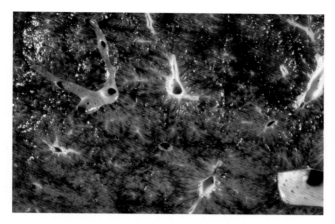

Fig. 2-38   Chronic passive congestion (nutmeg liver), liver, cut surface, dog. The cut surface has a repeating pattern of red and tan mottling (an accentuated lobular pattern). Chronic passive congestion leads to persistent hypoxia in centrilobular areas and atrophy, degeneration, and/or eventually necrosis of centrilobular hepatocytes. The red areas are dilated central veins and adjacent areas of sinusoidal dilation and congestion due to centrilobular hepatic necrosis. The tan areas are normal, uncongested parenchyma. *(Courtesy Dr. D.A. Mosier, College of Veterinary Medicine, Kansas State University.)*

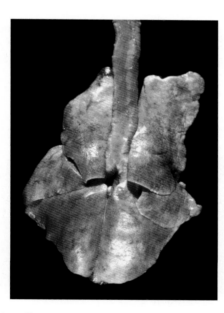

Fig. 2-39   Chronic passive congestion, lung, dog. The lungs are moderately firm and yellow-brown because of alveolar macrophages containing hemosiderin. Inflammatory mediators produced by these macrophages also induce fibroplasia, and thus long-term there is extensive formation of interstitial collagen. This collagen is the reason the lungs fail to collapse following loss of negative pressure in the pleural cavity when the diaphragm is incised at necropsy. *(Courtesy College of Veterinary Medicine, University of Illinois.)*

that accompanies congestion (e.g., chronic hepatic congestion). Congested tissues are dark red, swollen (edema), and cooler than normal. The microvasculature is engorged with blood, and there is often surrounding edema and sometimes hemorrhage caused by diapedesis.

DECREASED TISSUE PERFUSION

Reduced blood flow to an area is usually caused by a local obstruction of a vessel, local congestion, or decreased cardiac output. Local obstruction results in either reduced blood flow into an area or inadequate blood flow out of an area. Ischemia occurs when the perfusion of tissue in the affected area becomes inadequate to meet the metabolic needs of the tissue. Ischemia caused by arterial disease is most commonly due to incomplete luminal blockage by a thrombus or embolus. The result is a decreased flow of oxygenated blood into the area. Arteriolar vasoconstriction, if prolonged, can also result in ischemia. Ischemia due to venous lesions can be caused by intraluminal obstruction, such as a venous thrombus. However, external pressure that occludes the vein, such as inflammatory or neoplastic masses, is a common cause. Venous obstruction leads to congestion characterized by slowing and stagnation of blood flow, with loss of tissue oxygenation, local increased hydrostatic pressure, and leakage of fluid into the interstitium (edema). Increased interstitial pressure may partially inhibit arterial inflow into the area to compound the problem. Capillaries can also become occluded by thrombi or external pressure. The severity of ischemia is determined by the local vascular anatomy and degree of anastomoses and collateral circulation, the number of microcirculatory vessels and degree of resistance of the arteriole supplying the capillaries, the extent of the decreased perfusion, the rate at which the occlusion occurred, and the metabolic needs of the tissue. Ischemia can be tolerated to different levels by different tissue. The brain and heart are most susceptible because of a high need for O_2 and nutrients combined with poor collateral circulation. In contrast, organs that recondition blood (e.g., lungs, gastrointestinal tract, kidneys, and skin) can tolerate substantial reductions in flow because they already receive more blood than necessary for their metabolic needs. Other tissues receive blood based on their immediate needs (e.g., skeletal muscle during physical activity). Rapid and complete occlusion that affects large areas of tissue is generally more severe because collateral circulation may not be able to reestablish flow to certain areas quickly enough to prevent tissue necrosis.

In tissue in which there has been a return of blood flow after brief ischemia, the tissue often returns to normal. The ATP of ischemic tissue is degraded to adenosine, a potent vasodilator, which relieves the ischemia and allows ATP production to resume. However, after prolonged ischemia, the return of blood flow can result in a variety of detrimental effects. Reflow results in fluid loss to the interstitium, resulting in high tissue pressure, which compresses veins and inhibits local venous return. The congested capillaries hemorrhage, TF is released, and vessels are occluded by thrombi. In ischemic cells, a breakdown product of ATP is hypoxanthine. In the absence of oxygen, this is nonreactive. However, upon the return of oxygen, xanthine oxidase converts hypoxanthine into urates, hydrogen peroxide, and superoxide anions. Subsequent reaction of superoxide results in the formation of additional reactive oxygen species, such as hydroxyl radicals. Collectively, these oxygen free radicals formed during reperfusion can create damage in addition to that caused by ischemia and energy depletion of the cell.

An infarct is a local area of peracute ischemia that undergoes coagulative necrosis. Infarction is caused by the same events that result in ischemia and is most commonly secondary to thrombosis or thromboembolism. The characteristics of an infarct are variable based on the type and size of vessel that was occluded (artery or vein), the duration of the occlusion, the tissue in which it occurs, and the prior perfusion and vitality of the tissue. Complete arterial blockage usually results in immediate infarction (Fig. 2-40). In contrast, when venous obstruction occurs, such as due to torsions or displacements of the bowel, there is extensive congestion and edema of the affected bowel that precedes and promotes infarction. Concurrent disease, decreased cardiovascular function, anemia, or decreased tissue vitality will increase the likelihood of localized areas of ischemia progressing to infarction. In tissue with a single blood supply and minimal anastomoses (e.g., brain, heart, kidney, and spleen), occlusion of nearly any sized vessel typically results in infarction of the dependent tissue (Fig. 2-41). In tissue with parallel blood supplies that have numerous anastomoses (e.g., skeletal muscle and gastrointestinal tract), occlusion is less serious unless it occurs in a large vessel. Tissues with dual blood supplies (e.g., liver and lung) are not commonly susceptible to infarction unless concurrent underlying disease is present that compromises the overall blood supply.

Most infarcts are dark red soon after their occurrence because of hemorrhage from damaged vessels in the infarcted area, and backflow of blood into the area from surrounding vessels (Fig. 2-41). As cells undergo necrosis, there is swelling of the affected area, which can force blood out of the infarcted region, giving it a pale appearance (Fig. 2-42). Additionally, hemolysis of erythrocytes and degradation and diffusion of hemoglobin give the infarct a progressively paler appearance. This change in color can occur within 1 to 5 days depending on the tissue and extent of the infarction. Certain types of tissue that have a loose (spongy) consistency, such as the lungs and storage-type spleens (e.g., dogs and pigs), usually remain red because the

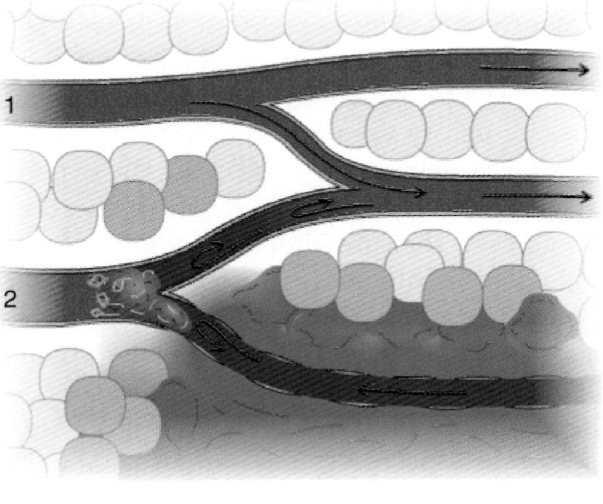

Fig. 2-40   Infarction due to arterial obstruction. Arterial obstruction results in loss of blood flow to downstream tissue, resulting in abrupt coagulative necrosis. The amount of necrosis is dependent on factors such as the type and prior health of the tissue affected, its metabolic rate (neurons versus myocytes and fibroblasts), and amount of collateral circulation or alternative blood supply. *1,* Normal arterial flow; *2,* arterial flow obstructed by an arterial thrombus. *(Courtesy Dr. D.A. Mosier and L. Schooley, College of Veterinary Medicine, Kansas State University.)*

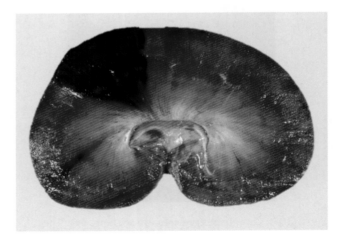

Fig. 2-41   Acute hemorrhagic infarct, kidney, dog. There is a focal wedge-shaped hemorrhagic area of cortical necrosis. The capsular surface of the infarct bulges above that of the adjacent normal kidney, indicating acute cell swelling and hemorrhage. *(Courtesy Dr. W. Crowell, College of Veterinary Medicine, The University of Georgia; and Noah's Arkive, College of Veterinary Medicine, The University of Georgia.)*

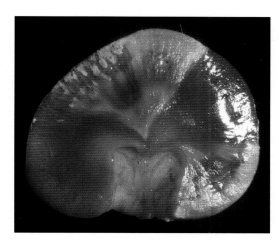

Fig. 2-42   **Acute pale infarcts, kidney, rabbit.** Multiple, pale white to tan pyramidal-shaped infarcts extend from the renal cortex to the medulla. The infarcts bulge above the capsular surface *(center top)*, indicative of acute cell swelling. The glistening areas on the right are highlights from the photographic lamps. *(Courtesy Dr. M.D. McGavin, College of Veterinary Medicine, University of Tennessee.)*

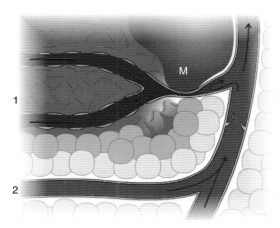

Fig. 2-43   **Infarction due to venous obstruction.** Venous obstruction results in stagnation of blood flow and reduction or loss of venous return. There is progressive ischemia and ultimately coagulative necrosis of the tissue upstream of the site of vessel obstruction. The amount of necrosis is dependent on factors such as the type and prior health of the tissue affected, metabolic rate, and amount of collateral circulation or alternative blood supply. *1,* Venous return to a larger vein (note the valve) obstructed by a mass *(M)*; *2,* normal venous return to a larger vein. *(Courtesy Dr. D.A. Mosier and L. Schooley, College of Veterinary Medicine, Kansas State University.)*

interstitial areas are expandable and necrosis-induced pressure does not build up to force blood out of the infarcted region (Figs. 2-43 and 2-44). Parenchymal tissues with a less expansible interstitium (e.g., kidney) generally become pale over time because of the pressure that forces blood from the necrotic area. Inflammation occurs at the periphery of the dead tissue so that leukocytes, then macrophages, enter the area to clear the necrotic debris, and subsequently neovascularization and granulation occur to replace the necrotic region with fibrous tissue. This process can occur over a period of weeks or months depending on the extent of the damage. In contrast to the coagulative necrosis caused by infarction in most tissue, infarction in the brain and nervous tissue is characterized by liquefactive necrosis. Subsequently there is glial cell removal of damaged tissue and astrocytic production of glial fibers (astrogliosis) to replace the affected area.

SHOCK

Shock (cardiovascular collapse) is a circulatory dyshomeostasis associated with loss of circulating blood volume, reduced cardiac output, and/or inappropriate peripheral vascular resistance. Although causes can be diverse (e.g., severe hemorrhage or diarrhea, burns, tissue trauma, endotoxemia), the underlying events of shock are relatively stereotyped. Hypotension results in impaired tissue perfusion and cellular hypoxia and a shift to anaerobic metabolism by cells, cellular degeneration, and death (Fig. 2-45). Although the cellular

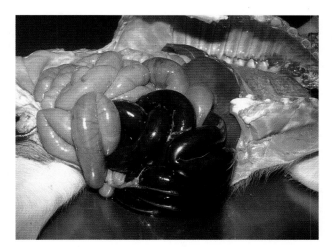

Fig. 2-44   **Venous infarction, small intestinal volvulus, pig.** Note the intensely congested loops of small intestine undergoing early venous infarction. The veins have been compressed by a volvulus that has compressed the veins but not the arteries, thus preventing the venous return. If the volvulus had rotated further, it would also have compressed the arteries. *(Courtesy Dr. D.A. Mosier, College of Veterinary Medicine, Kansas State University.)*

effects of hypoperfusion are initially reversible, persistence of shock results in irreversible cell and tissue injury. Shock is rapidly progressive and life threatening when compensatory responses are inadequate. Shock can be classified into three different types based on

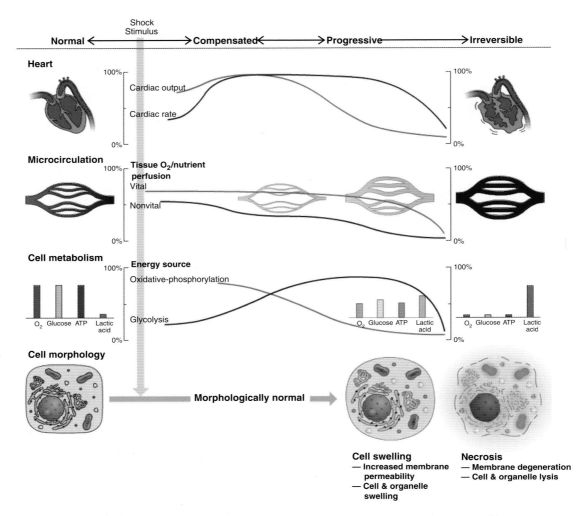

Fig. 2-45   **Shock.** In hypovolemic shock, there is initially compensation characterized by increased cardiac rate and output, vasoconstriction of nonessential vascular beds, and predominantly oxidative metabolism by morphologically normal cells. With progression, cardiac output falls as peripheral vasodilation occurs and cell metabolism shifts to glycolysis with progressive morphological changes in cells. *(Courtesy Dr. D. A. Mosier and L. Schooley, College of Veterinary Medicine, Kansas State University.)*

the fundamental underlying problem: (1) cardiogenic, (2) hypovolemic, and (3) blood maldistribution. Shock attributed to blood maldistribution can be further divided into septic shock, anaphylactic shock, and neurogenic shock.

CARDIOGENIC SHOCK

Cardiogenic shock results from failure of the heart to adequately pump blood. Cardiac failure can occur due to myocardial infarction, ventricular tachycardia, fibrillation or other arrhythmias, dilatative or hypertrophic cardiomyopathy, obstruction of blood flow from the heart (e.g., pulmonary embolism and pulmonary or aortic stenosis), or other cardiac dysfunctions. In all cases, there is a decrease in both stroke volume and cardiac output. Major compensatory mechanisms (e.g., sympathetic stimulation of the heart), which increase heart contractility, stroke volume, total cardiac output, and heart rate, are only variably successful depending on the nature of the cardiac damage and the ability of the damaged heart to respond. Unsuccessful compensation leads to stagnation of blood and progressive tissue hypoperfusion.

HYPOVOLEMIC SHOCK

Hypovolemic shock arises from reduced circulating blood volume due to blood loss caused by hemorrhage, or due to fluid loss secondary to vomiting, diarrhea, or burns. Reduced circulating blood volume leads to decreased vascular pressure and tissue hypoperfusion. Immediate compensatory mechanisms (e.g., peripheral vasoconstriction and fluid movement into the plasma) act to increase vascular pressure and maintain blood flow to critical tissues, such as the heart, brain, and kidney. Increased pressure provides an adequate driving force upon which local mechanisms can draw on to increase blood flow based on their needs. When the insult is mild, compensation is generally successful and the animal returns to homeostasis. Loss of about 10% of blood volume can occur without a decrease in blood pressure or cardiac output. However, if greater volumes are lost, adequate pressure and perfusion can not be maintained and there is insufficient blood flow to meet the needs of the tissues. When blood loss approaches 35% to 45%, blood pressure and cardiac output can fall dramatically.

BLOOD MALDISTRIBUTION

Blood maldistribution is characterized by decreased peripheral vascular resistance and pooling of blood in peripheral tissues. This is caused by neural or cytokine-induced vasodilation that can result from situations such as trauma, emotional stress, systemic hypersensitivity to allergens, or endotoxemia. Systemic vasodilation results in a dramatically increased microvascular area, and although the blood volume is normal, the effective circulating blood volume is decreased. Unless compensatory mechanisms can override the stimulus for vasodilation, there is pooling and stagnation of blood with subsequent tissue hypoperfusion. The three major types of shock due to blood maldistribution are anaphylactic, neurogenic, and septic shock.

Anaphylactic shock is a generalized type I hypersensitivity. Common causes include exposure to insect or plant allergens, drugs, or vaccines. The interaction of the inciting substance with immunoglobulin E bound to mast cells results in widespread mast cell degranulation and the release of histamine and other vasoactive mediators. Subsequently, there is systemic vasodilation and increased vascular permeability, causing hypotension and tissue hypoperfusion.

Neurogenic shock may be induced by trauma, particularly trauma to the nervous system; electrocution such as by lightning strike; fear; or emotional stress. In contrast to anaphylactic and endotoxic shock, cytokine release is not a major factor in the initial peripheral vasodilation. Instead, there are autonomic discharges that result in peripheral vasodilation, followed by venous pooling of blood and tissue hypoperfusion.

Septic shock is the most common type of shock associated with blood maldistribution. In septic shock, peripheral vasodilation is caused by components of bacteria or fungi that induce the release of excessive amounts of vascular and inflammatory mediators. The most common cause of septic shock is endotoxin, a lipopolysaccharide (LPS) complex within the cell wall of gram-negative bacteria. Less often, peptidoglycans and lipoteichoic acids of gram-positive organisms initiate shock. Local release of LPS from degenerating bacteria is a potent stimulus for many of the host responses that are necessary to respond to the infectious agent. LPS often gains entry from microflora of the bowel, entering the circulation into the reticuloendothelial system, then accumulating in the liver, spleen, alveoli, and leukocytes. LPS activates cells (mainly endothelium and leukocytes) through a series of reactions involving LPS-binding protein (an acute phase protein), CD14 (a cell membrane protein and soluble plasma protein) and Toll-like receptor 4 (TLR4, a signal-transducing protein). Endothelial activation by LPS inhibits production of anticoagulant substances (e.g., TFPI and thrombomodulin). Activation of monocytes and macrophages by LPS induces the direct or indirect release of TNF and IL-1 and other cytokines (e.g., IL-6, IL-8, chemokines). LPS directly activates factor XII to initiate intrinsic coagulation and other factor XIIa–related pathways (kinins, fibrinolysis, complement). LPS can also directly activate the complement cascade pathway to generate the anaphylatoxins C3a and C5a. Although these events are important for enhancing the inflammatory response to control localized infections associated with relatively low concentrations of LPS, they can be detrimental if the response becomes more pronounced. This may occur with overwhelming infections by bacteria (generating large concentrations of LPS), or when prolonged intestinal ischemia due to other types of shock results in breakdown of the mucosal integrity and leakage of bacteria and toxins into the blood. These higher concentrations of LPS induce even more production of TNF, IL-1, and other cytokines, and the secondary effects of these cytokines become more prominent. TNF and IL-1 induce TF expression and endothelial activation of extrinsic coagulation and enhance the expression of endothelial leukocyte adhesion molecules. IL-1 also stimulates the release of platelet activating factor (PAF) and tissue plasminogen activator inhibitor (TPAI) to enhance platelet aggregation and coagulation. PAF released from leukocytes, platelets, and endothelium can cause platelet aggregation and thrombosis, increased vascular permeability, and, similar to

TNF and IL-1, stimulation of arachidonic acid metabolite production (particularly PGI_2 and thromboxane). TNF and IL-1 induce nitric oxide production, which also contributes to vasodilation and hypotension. Neutrophils become activated by TNF and IL-1 to enhance their adhesion to endothelium, which further interferes with blood flow through the microvasculature. The end result of the activation of these myriad vascular, proinflammatory, and procoagulant alterations is the profound systemic vasodilation, hypotension, and tissue hypoperfusion characteristic of septic shock.

STAGES AND PROGRESSION OF SHOCK

Regardless of the underlying cause, shock generally progresses through three different stages: (1) a nonprogressive stage, (2) a progressive stage, and (3) an irreversible stage.

Nonprogressive shock is characterized by compensatory mechanisms that counteract reduced functional circulating blood volume and decreased vascular pressure. Baroreceptors respond to decreased pressure by increasing medullary sympathetic nervous output and epinephrine/norepinephrine release, which increases cardiac output and causes arteriolar vasoconstriction (increased peripheral resistance) in most tissues in an attempt to raise vascular pressure. Notable exceptions are critical tissues, such as the heart, brain, and kidney, to which the blood flow is preserved. Left atrial volume receptors and hypothalamic osmoreceptors help regulate pressure by altering water and sodium balance. Reduced plasma volume stimulates ADH release and water retention, and activates angiotensin II production by the renin-angiotensin system to result in aldosterone release and sodium retention. ADH and angiotensin II are also vasoconstrictors and help contribute to increased peripheral resistance. Vasoconstriction also results from endothelial release of endothelin, cold, increased O_2, or decreased CO_2. Decreased microvascular pressure results in a shift in fluid movement from the interstitium into the plasma to also help increase blood volume. The results of these and other responses are increased heart rate and cardiac output, and increased vascular pressure. This provides an adequate driving force upon which local mechanisms can draw on to increase blood flow based on their needs. When the insult is mild, compensation is generally successful and the animal returns to homeostasis.

In the case of severe or prolonged hypovolemia or cardiac damage that inhibits the ability of the heart to increase output, compensatory mechanisms are inadequate and shock enters the progressive stage. In this stage there is blood pooling, tissue hypoperfusion, and progressive cell injury. Cellular metabolism becomes less efficient and shifts from aerobic to anaerobic with pyruvate converted to lactate without entering the Krebs cycle. The deficient production of ATP and overproduction of lactic acid inhibits normal cell functions and results in cellular and systemic acidosis. Metabolic products (e.g., adenosine and potassium), increased local osmolarity, local hypoxia, and increased CO_2 eventually result in arteriolar relaxation and dilation. In the case of septic shock, these events exacerbate preexisting cytokine- and mediator-induced vasodilation of the microvasculature. In hypovolemic and cardiogenic shock, the decreased vascular resistance initiates pooling and stagnation of blood within previously closed vascular beds. Widespread arteriolar dilation due to local influences overrides systemic controls and dramatically contributes to further decreases in vascular plasma volume and pressure. When oxygen and energy stores of the cell are depleted, membrane transport mechanisms are impaired, lysosomal enzymes are released, structural integrity is lost, and cell necrosis occurs. In addition to the detrimental metabolic effects of deficient oxygenation, cell and tissue injury occur in response to the dramatic accumulation of mediators that is characteristic of progressive shock regardless of its underlying cause. These include histamine, kinins, PAF, complement fragments, and a wide variety of cytokines (e.g., TNF, IL-1, IL-8). These mediators are associated with inappropriate systemic inflammation and systemic activation of complement, coagulation, fibrinolysis, and kinin pathways.

The exact point where shock enters the irreversible stage is not clear. At the cellular level, metabolic acidosis that results from anaerobic metabolism inhibits enzyme systems needed for energy production. Decreased metabolic efficiency allows vasodilatory substances to accumulate in the ischemic cells and tissues. Once these local products and reflexes override centrally mediated vasoconstriction to produce vasodilation, it is unlikely that shock will be reversed. The fall in peripheral resistance due to widespread peripheral vasodilation decreases vascular pressure even more. Irreversibility is generally assured when shock progresses into the syndrome of multiple organ dysfunction. As each organ system fails, particularly the lung, liver, intestine, kidney, and heart, there is a reduction in the metabolic support each system provides to the others. Vicious cycles occur in which the failing function of one organ or tissue contributes to the failure of another (e.g., decreased cardiac output causes renal and pancreatic ischemia; electrolyte imbalances caused by renal ischemia then result in cardiac arrhythmias and myocardial depressant factor released by the ischemic pancreas contribute to even greater reductions in cardiac output). The end point of irreversible shock is often manifested as DIC, the profound and paradoxical dysfunction of hemostasis.

CLINICAL AND MORPHOLOGICAL FEATURES OF SHOCK

Clinical features of shock are rapidly progressive and include hypotension, weak pulse, tachycardia, hyperventilation with pulmonary rales, reduced urine output, and hypothermia. Organ and system failure occur in later stages, each manifesting with signs specific to that organ or tissue.

The lesions of shock are variable and depend on the nature and severity of the initiating stimulus, and the stage of progression of shock. Characteristically there are vascular changes accompanied by cell degeneration and necrosis. Generalized congestion and pooling of blood are present in most cases, unless there has been substantial blood loss. Edema, hemorrhage (petechial and ecchymotic), and thrombosis may be present as reflections of the vascular deterioration that accompanies shock. Thrombosis and platelet plugging of capillaries can be prominent in septic shock. Vascular abnormalities are most obvious in those cases that progress to DIC. Cell degeneration and necrosis is most prominent in those cells that are most susceptible to hypoxia, such as neurons and cardiac myocytes, and cells that do not obtain adequate preferential blood flow during shock. Hepatocytes, renal tubular epithelium, adrenal cortical epithelium, and gastrointestinal epithelium are often affected. With the exception of neuronal and myocyte loss, virtually all of these tissue changes can revert to normal if the animal survives. Specific changes may include severe pulmonary congestion, edema, and hemorrhage with alveolar epithelial necrosis, fibrin exudation, and hyaline membrane formation. Passive congestion and centrilobular hepatic necrosis, as well as renal tubular necrosis, are often present in these metabolically important organs. Intestinal congestion, edema, and hemorrhage with mucosal necrosis may occur. In the heart there is myofibril coagulation due to hypercontraction of sarcomeres. This is most likely a response to high sarcoplasmic calcium levels due to lack of energy and membrane damage. Cerebral edema, and in some cases cerebrocortical laminar necrosis, as a result of cerebral ischemia may be present.

SUGGESTED READINGS

Darien BJ: Fibrinolytic system. In Feldman BF, Zinkl JG, Jain NC, editors: *Schalm's veterinary hematology*, ed 5, Baltimore, 2000, Lippincott Williams & Wilkins.

de Gopegui RR, Navarro T: Vascular wall: endothelial cell. In Feldman BF, Zinkl JG, Jain NC, editors: *Schalm's veterinary hematology*, ed 5, Baltimore, 2000, Lippincott Williams & Wilkins.

Eto M, Luscher TF: Modulation of coagulation and fibrinolytic pathways by statins, *Endothelium* 10(1):35-41, 2003.

Gentry PA: Platelet biology. In Feldman BF, Zinkl JG, Jain NC, editors: *Schalm's veterinary hematology*, ed 5, Baltimore, 2000, Lippincott Williams & Wilkins.

Giallourakis CC, Rosenberg PM, Friedman LS: The liver in heart failure, *Clin Liver Dis* 6(4):947-967, 2002.

Hajjar KA: Molecular mechanisms of fibrinolysis. In Beutler E, Lichtman MA, Coller BS, editors: *Williams hematology*, ed 6, New York, 2001, McGraw-Hill.

Hajjar KA, Esmon NL, Marcus AJ: Vascular function in hemostasis. In Beutler E, Lichtman MA, Coller BS, editors: *Williams hematology*, ed 6, New York, 2001, McGraw-Hill.

Kierszenbaum AL: Cardiovascular system. In Kierszenbaum AL: *Histology and cell biology: an introduction to pathology*, St Louis, 2002, Mosby.

Lee KW, Lip GY: Acute coronary syndromes: Virchow's triad revisited, *Blood Coagul Fibrinolysis* 14(7):605-625, 2003.

Lip GY, Blann AD: Thrombogenesis, atherogenesis and angiogenesis in vascular disease: a new "vascular triad," *Ann Med* 36(2):119-125, 2004.

Loscalzo J, Schafer AI: *Thrombosis and hemorrhage*, ed 3, Philadelphia, 2003, Lippincott Williams & Wilkins.

Majno G, Joris I: *Cells, tissues, and disease: principles of general pathology*, ed 2, New York, 2004, Oxford University Press.

Majno G, Joris I: Vascular disturbances. In Majno G, Joris I, editors: *Cells, tissues, and disease: principles of general pathology*, ed 2, New York, 2004, Oxford University Press.

Michiels C: Endothelial cell functions, *J Cell Physiol* 196(3):430-443, 2003.

Mitchell RN: Hemodynamic disorders, thromboembolic disease, and shock. In Kumar V, Abbas AK, Fausto N, editors: *Robbins & Cotran pathologic basis of disease*, ed 7, Philadelphia, 2005, Saunders.

Parise LV, Smyth SS, Coller BS: Platelet morphology, biochemistry and function. In Beutler E, Lichtman MA, Coller BS, editors: *Williams hematology*, ed 6, New York, 2001, McGraw-Hill.

Roberts HR, Monroe DM, Hoffman M: Molecular biology and biochemistry of the coagulation factors and pathways of hemostasis. In Beutler E, Lichtman MA, Coller BS, editors: *Williams hematology*, ed 6, New York, 2001, McGraw-Hill.

Rubin E: *Rubin's pathology: clinicopathologic foundations of medicine*, ed 4, Philadelphia, 2004, Lippincott Williams & Wilkins.

Seligsohn U: Disseminated intravascular coagulation. In Beutler E, Lichtman MA, Coller BS, editors: *Williams hematology*, ed 6, New York, 2001, McGraw-Hill.

Shebuski RJ, Kilgore KS: Role of inflammatory mediators in thrombogenesis, *J Pharmacol Exp Ther* 300(3):729-735, 2002.

Shen GX: Impact and mechanism for oxidized and glycated lipoproteins on generation of fibrinolytic regulators from vascular endothelial cells, *Mol Cell Biochem* 246(1-2):69-74, 2003.

Slauson DO: Disturbances of blood flow and circulation. In Slauson DO, Cooper BJ, editors: *Mechanisms of disease: a textbook of comparative general pathology*, ed 3, St Louis, 2002, Mosby.

Stockham SL, Scott MA: Hemostasis. In Stockham SL, Scott MA, editors: *Fundamentals of veterinary clinical pathology*, Ames, 2002, Iowa State Press.

Stokhof AA: The extracardiac peripheral circulation and shock. In Dunlop RH, Malbert CH, editors: *Veterinary pathophysiology*, Ames, Iowa, 2004, Blackwell Publishing.

Tablin F: Platelet structure and function. In Feldman BF, Zinkl JG, Jain NC, editors: *Schalm's veterinary hematology*, ed 5, Baltimore, 2000, Lippincott Williams & Wilkins.

3

Acute Inflammation

MARK R. ACKERMANN

INTRODUCTION

When cells are injured by stimuli such as mechanical trauma, tissue necrosis, cancerous cells, or infectious microbes, as discussed in Chapter 1, these stimuli can trigger a well-organized cascade of fluidic and cellular changes within living vascularized tissue called acute inflammation (Fig. 3-1). These changes result in the accumulation of fluid, electrolytes, and plasma proteins as well as leukocytes in extravascular tissue and are recognized clinically by redness, heat, swelling, pain, and loss of function of the affected tissue. Inflammation is often a protective mechanism whose biologic purpose is to dilute, isolate, and eliminate the cause of injury and to repair tissue damage resulting from the injury. Without inflammation, animals would not survive their daily interactions with environmental microbes, foreign materials, and trauma, and with some degenerate, senescent, and neoplastic cells.

Our understanding of inflammation has evolved over the last 5000 years of recorded history (Table 3-1). Clinical signs attributable to inflammation were first described in Egypt in 3000 BC. Celcus, a Roman writer (de Medicina Celcus, 25 BC to 50 AD), was the first individual to describe the four cardinal signs of inflammation (redness, heat, swelling, and pain) that are commonly used today to diagnose inflammation in medicine. In the mid 1800s, Rudolf Virchow, the founder of modern pathology, added the fifth cardinal sign of inflammation, loss of function. In addition to his numerous contributions to cellular pathology, Dr. Virchow, by the age of 25, had discovered fibrinogen, described the processes of leukocytosis, and later characterized pus and necrosis. In 1859, his book titled *Cell Pathology* became the basis for all microscopic study of disease. Phagocytosis by macrophages, an important component of inflammation and immunologic responses, was first described by Elie Metchnikoff in 1883. In 1908 he was awarded the Nobel Prize in Medicine for these studies. Finally, the first experiment to demonstrate the role of a chemical mediator (histamine) in inducing vascular changes (flare and wheal reactions) was conducted by Sir Thomas Lewis in 1927. Work of these pioneers, as well as additional experimental studies conducted during the past century, has provided: (1) an in-depth and clearer understanding of inflammation and (2) the foundation for development of therapeutic compounds to treat undesirable effects of inflammatory responses. In fact, such treatments are so widely used and commonplace in veterinary medicine today, that the contributions and discoveries of these scientists are often taken for granted.

Acute inflammation, a provoked response, is the progressive reaction of vascularized living tissue to injury over time. This process is usually a well-ordered cascade mediated by chemoattractants, vasoactive molecules, proinflammatory and inflammatory cytokines and their receptors, and antimicrobial or cytotoxic molecules. Acute inflammation has a short duration ranging from a few hours to a few days and its principal characteristics are microvascular exudation of electrolytes, fluid, and plasma proteins and leukocytic emigration, principally neutrophils, followed by rapid repair and healing. For convenience in this chapter, the acute inflammatory response will be divided into three sequential phases: fluidic, cellular, and reparative.

Chronic inflammation is considered to be inflammation of prolonged duration, usually weeks to months, in which active inflammation is characterized predominately by lymphocytes and macrophages, tissue necrosis, and accompanied by tissue repair, such as healing, fibrosis, and granulation tissue formation, all of which may all occur simultaneously. Chronic inflammation can be a sequela to the failure to eliminate an inciting stimulus that caused the initial acute inflammation or it can occur as a direct result of an inciting stimulus. Examples of the latter include infections by *Mycobacterium* spp.; prolonged exposure to foreign materials such as plant material and grass awns; and autoimmune diseases,

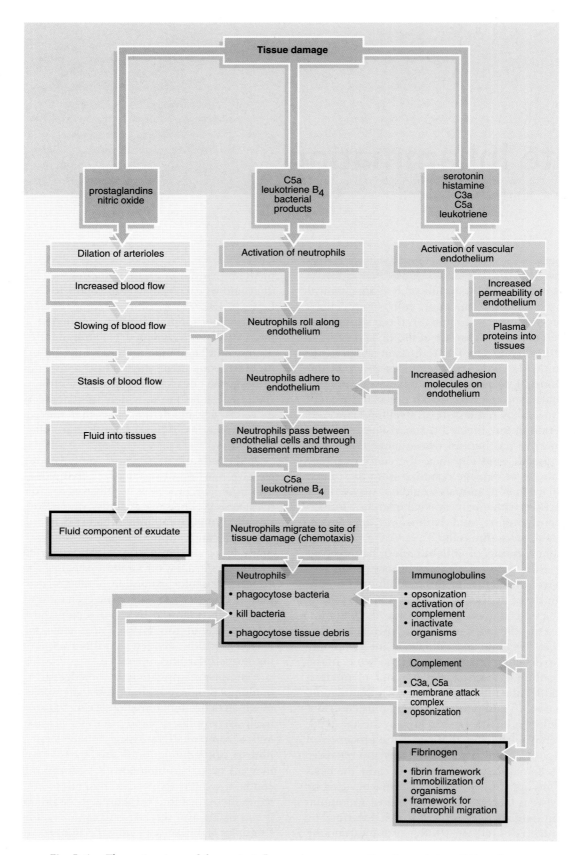

Fig. 3-1   The major steps of the acute inflammatory process. *(From Stevens A, Lowe JS, Young B: Wheater's basic histopathology: a colour atlas and text, ed 4, New York, 2002, Churchill Livingstone.)*

Table **3-1**   Highlights of the Historical Contributions to the Understanding and Characterization of Inflammation

Contributor	Time	Contribution
Egyptians	3000 BC	Descriptions of inflammation
Celsus (Italy)	25 BC–50 AD	Four cardinal signs of inflammation: rubor (redness), tumor (swelling), calor (heat), dolor (pain)
John Hunter (Scotland)	1793	Inflammation is a *salutary* (favorable to health) effect, not a disease per se
Julius Cohnheim (Germany)	1839-1884	Observed inflamed vessels microscopically
Elie Metchnikoff (Russia)	1882	Observed and described phagocytosis
Rudolf Virchow (Germany)	1821-1902	Fifth cardinal sign of inflammation: functio laesa (loss of function); cellular injury
Sir Thomas Lewis (England)	1927	Determined that chemicals (histamine) induce vascular changes

such as arthritis. Although there are some clear biologic, pathologic, and mechanistic differences and similarities between acute and chronic inflammation, discussion of acute inflammation is separated from chronic inflammation (covered in Chapter 4) as a matter of convenience.

BENEFICIAL AND HARMFUL ASPECTS OF INFLAMMATION

As a general rule, inflammatory responses are beneficial in the following:

- Diluting and/or inactivating biologic and chemical toxins
- Killing or sequestering microbes and neoplastic cells
- Providing wound healing factors to ulcerated surfaces and traumatized tissue
- Degrading foreign materials
- Restricting movement of appendages and joints to allow time for healing and repair

However, in some instances, excessive and/or prolonged inflammatory responses can be detrimental and are often more harmful than the inciting stimulus. In several disorders of human beings, such as myocardial infarction, cerebral thrombosis, and atherosclerosis, excessive and prolonged inflammatory responses can exacerbate the severity of the disease process. In veterinary medicine, exuberant or uncontrolled inflammatory responses occurring in certain diseases listed in Table 3-2 can also result in increased severity of disease. Fortunately, basic research has resulted in a clearer understanding of the fundamental biologic interactions in the fluidic, cellular, and reparative phases of the acute inflammatory response and of the stimuli and mediators playing key roles in the chronic inflammatory response. As a result, antiinflammatory drugs—such as corticosteroids, aspirin, and nonsteroidal antiinflammatory drugs (NSAIDs)—have been developed and used to reduce the severity of the inflammatory response by modulating defined biologic pathways in the inflammatory cascade.

The disciplines of pharmacology, physiology, and molecular pathology are providing information that is leading to the evolution of more targeted, potent, and clinically efficacious antiinflammatory drugs. In the future, as veterinarians use new antimicrobials, chemotherapeutic agents, and therapies that regulate gene expression to treat disease, it may become important to precisely modify the inflammatory response with antiinflammatory drugs and continually monitor this therapy. For example, in *Mannheima haemolytica* pneumonia of cattle, the use of targeted antiinflammatory drugs that modulate leukocyte infiltration and vascular leakage may reduce exudate in alveoli and alveolar walls and provide improved gaseous exchange and a reduction in the extent of pulmonary damage and fibrosis. At the same time, potent antibiotics or other drugs can be used to reduce bacterial proliferation.

OVERVIEW OF THE ACUTE INFLAMMATORY RESPONSE

The acute inflammatory response, as diagrammed in Fig. 3-2, can be initiated by a variety of exogenous and endogenous stimuli that result in injury to vascularized tissue. The response to injury begins as active hyperemia, with an increased flow of blood to injured tissue secondary to dilation of arterioles and capillaries (redness and heat) facilitated by chemical mediators, such as prostaglandins, leukotrienes, and nitric oxide (Table 3-3). Active hyperemia is rapidly followed by changes in junctional complexes of endothelial cells induced by vasoactive amines, complement components C3a and C5a, bradykinin, leukotrienes, and platelet-activating factor (PAF), resulting in leakage of plasma and plasma proteins into the extracellular space (swelling and pain [stretching of pain receptors])

Table **3-2**   **Selected Disorders That Are Induced or Exacerbated by Inflammatory Responses**

DISORDERS IN WHICH THE MECHANISM OF INJURY IS INFLAMMATION

Human beings: Alzheimer's disease, atherosclerosis, atopic dermatitis, chronic obstructive pulmonary disease, Crohn's disease, gout, graft rejection, Hashimoto's thyroiditis, multiple sclerosis, pemphigus psoriasis, rheumatoid arthritis, sarcoidosis, systemic lupus erythematosus (SLE), type I diabetes mellitus, ulcerative colitis, vasculitis (Wegner's, polyarteritis nodosa, Goodpasture's disease)

Cats: eosinophilic stomatitis, lymphoplasmacytic syndrome, pemphigus

Dogs: granulomatous meningoencephalitis, pemphigus, systemic and discoid lupus erythematosus

Common to many species: anaphylaxis, spondylitis, asthma, reperfusion injury, osteoarthritis, glomerulonephritis

INFECTIOUS DISEASE EXACERBATED BY INFLAMMATION

Human beings: dysentery, Chagas' disease, cystic fibrosis pneumonia, filariasis, *Helicobacter* gastritis, hepatitis C, Influenza virus pneumonia, leprosy, Neisseria/pneumococcal meningitis, poststreptococcal glomerulonephritis, schistosomiasis, sepsis, tuberculosis

Dogs: *Helicobacter* gastritis

Cattle: *Mannheimia haemolytica* pneumonia, mastitis, *Mycobacterium bovis, Mycobacterium avium-intracellularis-paratuberculosis*

Pigs: circovirus

Ferrets/mink: Aleutian mink disease

Common to many species: vegetative valvular endocarditis

CONDITIONS IN WHICH POSTINFLAMMATORY FIBROSIS OCCURS

Human beings: bleomycin pulmonary fibrosis, allograft rejection, idiopathic pulmonary fibrosis, hepatic cirrhosis (postviral, alcohol, or toxin), radiation-induced pulmonary fibrosis

Dogs: idiopathic pulmonary fibrosis (West Highland white dogs)

Cattle/sheep/horses: plant toxins (hepatic fibrosis)

Modified from Nathan C: *Nature* 420:846-851, 2002.

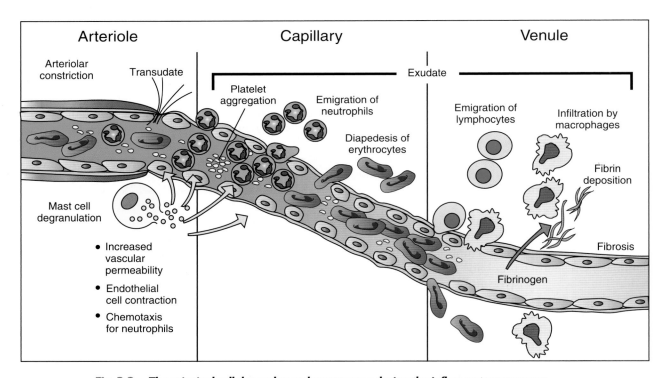

Fig. 3-2   **The principal cellular and vascular responses during the inflammatory response.** **The majority of leukocyte transmigration and hemorrhage occurs in the capillaries and postcapillary venules.** *(Modified from McCance KL, Huether SE: Pathophysiology: the biologic basis for diseases in adults and children, ed 3, St Louis, 1998, Mosby.)*

Table **3-3**   **Key Responses of Acute Inflammation and the Principal Inflammatory Mediators That Mediate These Processes**

VASODILATION

Nitric oxide
Prostaglandins: PGD_2
Leukotrienes: LTB_4

INCREASED VASCULAR PERMEABILITY

Vasoactive amines: histamine, substance P
Complement factors: C5a, C3a
Prostaglandins: PGE_2
Leukotrienes: LTC_4, LTD_4, LTE_4
Platelet-activating factor, substance P

CHEMOTAXIS, LEUKOCYTE ACTIVATION

Complement factors: C5a
Leukotrienes: LTB_4
Chemokines: IL-8
Defensins: α- and β-defensins
Bacterial products: lipopolysaccharide, peptidoglycan,
   teichoic acid
Surfactant proteins A and D

FEVER

Cytokines: IL-1, TNF, IL-6
Prostaglandins: PGE_2

NAUSEA

Cytokines: IL-1, TNF, high mobility group factors

PAIN

Bradykinin
Prostaglandins: PGE_2

TISSUE DAMAGE

Neutrophil and macrophage lysosomal/granule contents:
   matrix metalloproteinases
Reactive oxygen species: superoxide anion,
   hydroxyl radical, nitric oxide

C3a, Complement factor C3a; *C5a*, complement factor C5a; *IL-1, IL-6, IL-8*, interleukins 1, 6, and 8, respectively; *LTB_4, LTC_4, LTD_4, LTE_4*, leukotrienes B_4, C_4, D_4, and E_4, respectively; *PGD_2, PGE_2*, prostaglandins D_2 and E_2, respectively; *TNF*, tumor necrosis factor.

mainly from the postcapillary venules. The volume and protein concentration of leakage through gaps between the endothelial cells is related to the size of the gaps and the molecular weight of electrolytes and plasma proteins, such as albumin and fibrinogen. With more severe injury resulting in destruction of individual endothelial cells, hemorrhage occurs and plasma and plasma proteins can leak directly through a breach in the wall of the capillary or venule. Once activated,

endothelial and perivascular cells such as mast cells, dendritic cells, fibroblasts, and pericytes can produce cytokines and chemokines that regulate the expression of receptors for inflammatory mediators and adhesion molecules.

The plasma proteins and fluid that initially accumulate in the extracellular space in response to injury form a transudate. A transudate is a fluid that lacks protein (specific gravity <1.012 [<3 g of protein/dL]) and cellular elements (<1500 leukocytes/μL), and is essentially a balanced electrolyte solution—an ultrafiltrate of plasma. Most commonly the formation of a transudate is due to hypertension in veins and capillaries or hypoproteinemia resulting in edema; however, transudates occur in the early stages of the acute inflammatory response when intercellular gaps that open between endothelial cells are so small that only water and electrolytes can pass through them. In time, neutrophils and additional protein can enter injured areas resulting in the formation of an exudate. An exudate is an opaque and often viscous fluid (specific gravity >1.020) that contains more than 3 g of protein/dL and more than 1500 leukocytes/μL. As will be discussed in a later section, the morphologic classification of inflammatory responses into categories such as serous, fibrinous, and/or suppurative is based on the character of the fluid that leaks and of the leukocytes that migrate from vessels into the extracellular space.

Fibrinogen is an important plasma protein in exudates that polymerizes in extravascular tissues to form fibrin. Plasma dilutes the effects of the inciting stimulus, whereas polymerized fibrin confines the stimulus to an isolated area, thus preventing its movement into adjacent tissue. This confinement provides leukocytes with a well-defined target for migration during the cellular phase of the acute inflammatory response. Neutrophils are the first leukocytes to enter the exudate, and their accumulation in the exudate after they liquify is termed "pus." Neutrophils have a variety of cytoplasmic granules, such as lysosomes, containing antimicrobial peptides and proteins as well as matrix metalloproteinases, elastases, and myeloperoxidases that kill pathogens and degrade foreign material by two mechanisms: (1) phagocytosis and fusion with primary and secondary lysosomes and (2) secretion of the contents of granules into the exudate. This latter mechanism can often result in severe tissue injury. Fibrin and its products have additional activities, including chemotactic properties and blood clotting. It is also forms a framework during the initial stages of wound healing (see Chapter 4).

Neutrophils and other leukocytes do not migrate randomly to find areas of tissue injury. Fortunately, microbes, foreign materials, and some neoplastic cells release chemoattractant molecules into the exudate that diffuse through the exudate to encounter capillaries and venules. As would be expected, the greatest concentration of chemoattractant would exist nearest the microbes or foreign material, with the concentration decreasing in a gradient-like manner at distances away from the source. This process forms a "chemotactic gradient" that essentially creates a pathway for leukocytes to follow to reach the site of tissue injury. Chemoattractants activate receptors and molecules on neutrophils that result in neutrophil (1) movement and attachment to the luminal surface of capillaries and venules, (2) migration through the intercellular junctions formed by gaps between endothelial cells, and (3) migration within the exudate up the concentration gradient to the source of injury. This transmigration process is called the leukocyte adhesion cascade. This cascade has a well-characterized sequence of events occurring on the luminal surface of endothelial cells. These events, discussed in detail in a later section, include capture, rolling, slow rolling, firm adhesion, and transmigration of leukocytes into the exudate.

The reparative phase of the acute inflammatory response begins early and is only completed after the stimulus-causing injury is removed. This matter is not of minor consequence because failure to remove the stimulus can result in exuberant proliferation of granulation tissue in response to chronic unresolved injury. In the reparative phase, necrotic cells and tissue are replaced by differentiation and regeneration of epithelial and mesenchymal stem cells, by filling the defect with connective tissue and covering the denuded surface by reepithelialization (see Chapter 4). When the acute inflammatory response is completed in the proper sequence and the stimulus of injury is removed, the injured tissue returns to normal structure and function, and the inflammatory process is terminated.

STIMULI INDUCING THE ACUTE INFLAMMATORY RESPONSE

There are two classes of stimuli, endogenous and exogenous, capable of causing injury to cells and tissue and inducing the acute inflammatory response. Endogenous stimuli include those that primarily cause autoreactive inflammatory responses, such as newly developed antigens from degenerate, dysplastic, or neoplastic cells and hypersensitivity reactions. Exogenous stimuli include microbes such as viruses, bacteria, protozoa, and metazoan parasites; foreign bodies such as plant fibers and suture material; mechanical stimuli such as traumatic injury; physical stimuli such as thermal or freezing injury, ionizing radiation, and microwaves; chemical stimuli such as caustic agents, poisons, and venoms; and nutritive stimuli such as ischemia and vitamin deficiencies.

The acute inflammatory response to endogenous and exogenous stimuli occurs simultaneously with activation of the innate immune system. Innate immunity is a nonspecific defense against potentially harmful environmental stimuli and consists of the following:

- Physical barriers and microenvironments provided by the lining epithelia of the skin (low pH, lactic and fatty acids) and mucosal surfaces such as the respiratory and reproductive tracts (mucociliary activity) and alimentary system (saliva, mucous secretions, and peristalsis)
- Molecular products released by mucosal epithelia, such as lactoferrin, antimicrobial peptides (alpha [α] and beta [β] defensins, anionic peptide), and surfactant proteins
- Preformed (in cytoplasmic granules) and synthesized (released from cell immediately after synthesis) chemical mediators from effector cells distributed in the connective tissue of these barriers, such as mast cells (histamine and tumor necrosis factor [TNF]-α), leukocytes (cytokines, degradative enzymes), and macrophages (cytokines)
- Effector molecules in the blood, such as plasma proteases (complement, kinin, and clotting systems) and in certain nerve fibers (sensory fibers, C-reactive fibers) that release substance P

The physical and biologic stimuli that activate the acute inflammatory and innate immune responses can exert their actions directly on effector cells in mucosal surfaces and vascularized connective tissue, on effector molecules in the blood, on endothelial cells, or on a combination of these components. The location, severity, and clinical signs of the acute inflammatory response depend on the route of exposure, such as dermal, alimentary, respiratory, urinary, or hematogenous, and the physical or biologic characteristics of the stimulus. More specifically, stimuli of the acute inflammatory response include but are not limited to visible and ultraviolet light spectra (sunburn and photosensitization), γ-radiation, blunt force trauma (abrasion, bruising, incision, and laceration), thermal injury (hot and cold), chemotherapeutics, environmental chemicals, microbial molecules (lipids and proteins), venom (insect, snake, and reptile), and responses of the adaptive immune system (type I to IV hypersensitivities) to microbial and environmental antigens. Stimuli must either penetrate (light spectra) or break/penetrate (microbes and foreign bodies) epithelial barriers of the skin and alimentary, urinary, and respiratory systems to irritate the tissue and incite an acute inflammatory response. When microbes cross these barriers, they immediately encounter tissue macrophages and other leukocytes that express membrane pattern-recognition receptors (Toll-like receptors [TLRs]). There are currently 23 known TLRs that recognize a few highly conserved

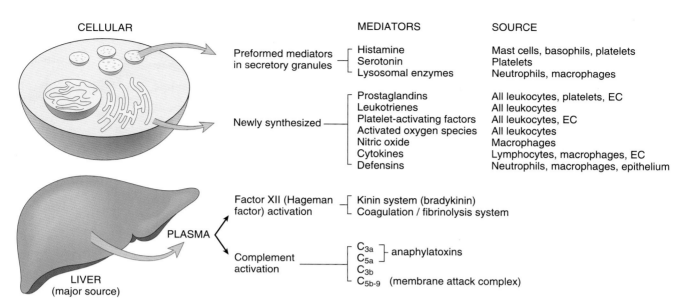

Fig. 3-3   Chemical mediators of inflammation. EC, Endothelial cells. *(From Kumar V, Abbas A, Fausto N: Robbins & Cotran pathologic basis of disease, ed 7, Philadelphia, 2005, Saunders.)*

ligands in microbes called pathogen-associated molecular patterns. Of the 23 TLRs, binding ligands have been characterized for only TLRs 1 through 11 to date. These patterns include the expression of lipopolysaccharide (LPS) (gram-negative bacterial cell wall), lipoteichoic acids (gram-positive bacterial cell wall), mannose, peptidoglycan, bacterial DNA, N-formylmethionine (in bacterial proteins), double-stranded RNA (viruses), and glucans (fungal cell walls). When these molecular patterns are recognized by receptors, such as TLRs, on macrophages, leukocytes, and mucosal epithelia, they trigger the release of chemokines and cytokines, and cellular activation, all of which initiate and/or participate in the acute inflammatory response.

In contrast to the innate immune system, adaptive immunity results in an antigen-specific immune response, the production of protective antibodies, and effector leukocytes that attempt to eliminate the inciting stimulus of injury, and the generation of memory cells that make subsequent adaptive immune responses against a specific microbial antigen more efficient. Because acute inflammation is a vasocentric provoked response, it would be reasonable to assume that just about any exogenous or endogenous stimulus could induce inflammation. In reality, this assumption is true, but because the inflammatory response has numerous redundant checks and balances that regulate the occurrence and severity of expression of the response, harmful effects of inflammation are minimized.

The effects of inflammatory stimuli are manifested through a group of biologic molecules called the chemical mediators of inflammation, which include vasoactive amines, such as histamine and serotonin; plasma proteases, such as complement, kinin, and clotting system proteins; lipid mediators, such as arachidonic acid metabolites; PAF; cytokines; chemokines; and nitric oxide (Fig. 3-3). Mast cells are rich in histamine and many of the chemical mediators listed previously. Mast cells are widely distributed in connective tissue adjacent to blood vessels, and alterations in the permeability of these vessels in the fluidic phase of the acute inflammatory response often occur as the result of mast cell activation. Histamine, preformed in mast cell granules, is released through a process called degranulation. Bradykinin, another vasoactive amine, is produced during vascular and/or endothelial cell injury. Both histamine and bradykinin cause changes in the caliber of arterioles, capillaries, and postcapillary venules and permeability changes in capillaries and postcapillary venules. These changes occur early in the fluidic phase of the acute inflammatory response and are quickly followed by the cellular phase.

FLUIDIC (EXUDATIVE) PHASE OF THE ACUTE INFLAMMATORY RESPONSE

In general, normal vascular capillaries limit the exchange of molecules to those less than 69,000 MW, the size of albumin. The exchange of small molecules and water between the vessel lumen and the interstitial space is extremely rapid. For example, the water of plasma is exchanged with the water of the interstitial space 80 times before the plasma can move the entire length of the capillary. Physiologically, increased amounts of fluid can pass across the vascular wall when there is: (1) excessive hydrostatic pressure caused by hypertension and/or sodium retention, (2) decreased plasma proteins (colloid), or (3) lymphatic and/or venous obstruction. If fluid leakage is excessive, edema (transudate) develops. If the leakage is not excessive and postcapillary venules and lymphatic vessels are functioning normally, all of the fluid released from arterioles and small capillaries is returned to the circulation via paracellular gaps of postcapillary venular and lymphatic vessels. During acute inflammatory responses, there is a net outflow of fluid from arterioles, capillaries, and venules into extracellular tissue (Fig. 3-4).

The principal function of the fluidic phase of the acute inflammatory response is to dilute and localize the stimulus. The sequence of vascular events in the acute inflammatory response includes the following:

- Increased blood flow to the site of injury
- Increased permeability of capillaries and postcapillary venules to plasma proteins and leukocytes (chemical mediators of inflammation)
- Emigration of leukocytes (inflammatory mediators and the leukocyte adhesion cascade) into the exudate

In this phase there is an immediate vasocentric reaction (arterioles, capillaries, and postcapillary venules) to the stimulus.

Initially, arterioles dilate and capillary beds in the affected area expand in volume to accommodate an increased blood flow (heat and redness) in response to the stimulus (Fig. 3-5). Secondly, vascular flow through the capillary beds is then slowed as a result of permeability changes induced by chemical mediators. Reduced vascular flow results from plasma that becomes more viscous following leakage of water from capillary beds into extracellular space. Microscopically, capillaries are often packed with erythrocytes as a result of hemoconcentration and viscosity changes caused by leakage of fluid from the capillaries and postcapillary venules into the extravascular space. This process results in stasis of blood flow and provides a microenvironment that facilitates leukocytic margination along the luminal surface of endothelial cells before their emigration through intercellular junctions of endothelial cells into the inflammatory exudate in the extravascular space. Changes in capillary flow and permeability serve to dilute, isolate, and confine the stimulus within extravasated transudates and exudates.

ENDOTHELIAL CELL DYNAMICS DURING THE ACUTE INFLAMMATORY RESPONSE

Endothelial cells are the interface between plasma in the lumen and the perivascular connective tissue. Endothelial cells are polarized cells (luminal versus

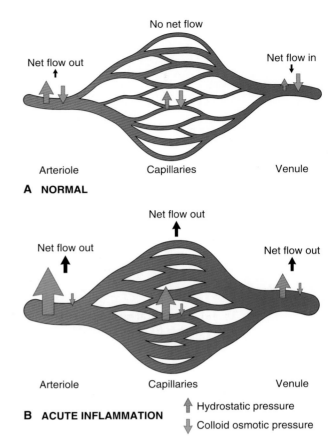

Fig. 3-4 **Blood pressure and plasma colloid osmotic forces in normal and inflamed microcirculation. A,** Normal hydrostatic pressure (*red arrows*) is about 32 mm Hg at the arterial end of a capillary bed and 12 mm Hg at the venous end; the mean colloid osmotic pressure of tissue is approximately 25 mm Hg (*green arrows*), which is equal to the mean capillary pressure. Although fluid tends to leave the precapillary arteriole, it is returned in equal amounts via the postcapillary venule, so that the net flow (*black arrows*) in or out is zero. **B,** Acute inflammation. Arteriole pressure is increased to 50 mm Hg; the mean capillary pressure is increased because of arteriolar dilation, and the venous pressure increases to approximately 30 mm Hg. At the same time, osmotic pressure is reduced (averaging 20 mm Hg) because of protein leakage across the venule. The net result is an excess of extravasated fluid. (*A* and *B, From Kumar V, Abbas A, Fausto N: Robbins & Cotran pathologic basis of disease, ed 7, Philadelphia, 2005, Saunders.*)

abluminal surfaces) that are adapted to fit the physiologic needs of the vascular bed of the organ in which they reside. Transport across the endothelial cell layer occurs by: (1) transcytosis (transcellular passage) via small vesicles and caveolae or (2) paracellular passage. Transcytosis, the process of transporting substances across the endothelium by uptake into and release from coated vesicles, facilitates the transport of albumin, low-density lipoproteins (LDLs), metalloproteinases, and insulin.

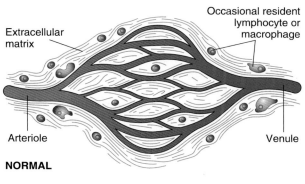

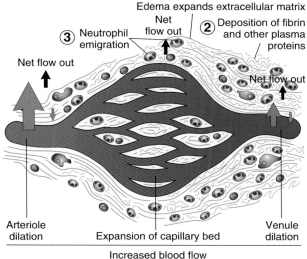

Fig. 3-5 **The major local manifestations of acute inflammation compared with normal.** (*1*) Vascular dilation (causing erythema and warmth), (*2*) extravasation of plasma fluid and proteins (edema), and (*3*) leukocyte emigration and accumulation in the site of injury. (*From Kumar V, Abbas A, Fausto N: Robbins & Cotran pathologic basis of disease, ed 7, Philadelphia, 2005, Saunders.*)

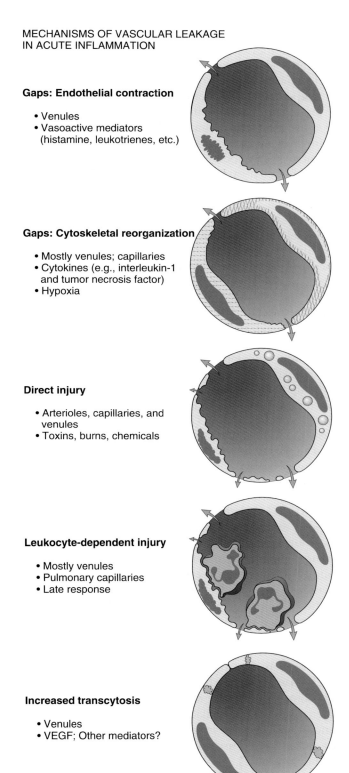

Fig. 3-6 **Diagrammatic representation of five mechanisms of increased vascular permeability in inflammation.** *VEGF*, Vascular endothelial growth factor. (*From Cotran RS, Kumar V, Collins T, Robbins SL: Robbins pathologic basis of disease, ed 6, Philadelphia, 1999, Saunders.*)

Paracellular passage allows transport of water and ions between cells (cell junctions). Paracellular passage is especially active in postcapillary venules. Roughly 30% of endothelial cell junctions in postcapillary venules can open to a width of 6 μm, roughly the width of a red blood cell.

Leakage of fluid from the vasculature can occur within seconds after a stimulus induces the acute inflammatory response. The mechanisms by which this leakage occurs depend on the biologic and physical characteristics of the inciting stimulus. Mechanisms of vascular extravasation in the acute inflammatory response are illustrated in Fig. 3-6 and can include the following:

• Opening of junctional complexes (endothelial gaps) between endothelial cells

- Direct injury that results in necrosis and detachment of endothelial cells, as occurs with certain viral and protozoal infections
- Leukocyte-dependent injury that results in necrosis and detachment of endothelial cells and is induced by enzymes and mediators released from leukocytes during the transmigration phase of the acute inflammatory response
- Increased endothelial cell transcytosis

Endothelial gaps, resulting in vascular leakage, can occur by (1) contraction (actin/myosin) of apposing endothelial cells, the most common mechanism of extravasation, and through (2) the reorganization of the cytoskeletal microtubule and microfilament proteins within the endothelial cell, resulting in the formation of gaps between endothelial cells. In either of these two types of endothelial cell gap formation, the gaps result from the opening of junctional complexes between endothelial cells. The formation of gaps due to endothelial cell contraction occurs in postcapillary venules where there is a high density of receptors for histamine, serotonin, bradykinin, and angiotensin II. Gaps formed by cytoskeletal reorganization occur most commonly in postcapillary venules and, to a lesser extent, in capillaries in response to cytokines, such as interleukin (IL)-1 and TNF and hypoxia. Gap formation is transient and lasts 15 to 30 minutes after the stimulus occurs. Vascular leakage resulting from direct injury of endothelial cells is caused by endothelial cell necrosis and detachment of the cell from the underlying basement membrane and establishes conditions favorable for the activation of the platelet, clotting, and complement cascades. This type of extravasation usually occurs immediately after necrotizing injury induced by, for example, thermal injury, chemotherapeutics, and bacterial cytotoxins, and it affects arterioles, capillaries, and postcapillary venules. Vascular leakage resulting from leukocyte-induced injury results from neutrophils and other leukocytes interacting with endothelial cells during the leukocyte adhesion cascade. Activated leukocytes release reactive oxygen species, such as singlet oxygen and oxygen free radicals, and proteolytic enzymes, such as matrix metalloproteinases and elastase from lysosomes during degranulation of the cells, which then result in endothelial cell necrosis and detachment and thus an increase in vascular permeability. This type of extravasation usually affects capillaries and postcapillary venules.

CELLULAR PHASE OF THE ACUTE INFLAMMATORY RESPONSE

The principal function of the cellular phase of the acute inflammatory response is to deliver leukocytes into the exudate that has sequestered the site of injury so they can internalize stimuli through phagocytosis and, as required, kill and/or digest the stimulus. Neutrophils, eosinophils, basophils, monocytes, and lymphocytes play an integral role in protecting the mucosas, skin, and other surfaces of the body, such as the pleura, pericardium, and peritoneum, from infection by microbes through phagocytosis or release of proteolytic degradative enzymes, chemical mediators, and reactive oxygen species. Neutrophils also have an important role in responding to foreign materials and toxins and in responding to neoplastic cells.

The movement of leukocytes from the lumina of capillaries and postcapillary venules into the interstitial connective tissue occurs through a process called the leukocyte adhesion cascade (Fig. 3-7). This process is actually initiated during the fluidic phase of the acute inflammatory response and is driven by chemokines, cytokines, and chemoattractant substances such as complement. Vasodilation and permeability changes result in the slowing of blood flow and lead to changes in hemodynamic forces and the movement of leukocytes to the periphery of the vascular lumen in apposition to the surface of endothelial cells. This process is called margination. When the surface of the endothelium becomes lined by leukocytes, this outcome, when observed microscopically, is called pavementing (Fig. 3-8). Finally, leukocytes migrate between endothelial cells to enter the exudate through a process called emigration or transmigration. The leukocyte adhesion cascade has a well-characterized sequence of events including: tethering (capture), rolling, slow rolling, activation and firm adhesion, and transmigration of leukocytes toward a chemotactic stimulus. Each of these steps is important in the process of eliminating the stimulus because blocking any of these steps results in fewer numbers of leukocytes in the exudate. Temporally, tethering, rolling, slow rolling, activation and firm adhesion, and transmigration all occur concurrently, involving different leukocytes in the same capillaries and postcapillary venules. This process is mediated by the interaction of ligands expressed on the surface of neutrophils, lymphocytes, and macrophages and their receptors expressed on luminal surfaces of activated endothelial cells (Table 3-4). Chemokines and cytokines influence this process by modulating the surface expression and/or avidity of these adhesion molecules. Adhesion molecules are divided into: (1) selectins (E-, L-, and P-selectin), (2) integrins (very late antigen [VLA] family of β_1 integrins; β_2 integrins [Mac-1, LFA-1, p150,95, $\alpha d\beta_2$]), (3) cytoadhesion family (vitronectin, β_3 integrins, and β_7 integrins used predominately by lymphocytes), (4) the immunoglobulin superfamily (intercellular adhesion molecule [ICAM-1 to ICAM-3], vascular cell adhesion molecule [VCAM-1], platelet-endothelial cell adhesion molecule [PECAM-1], and mucosal

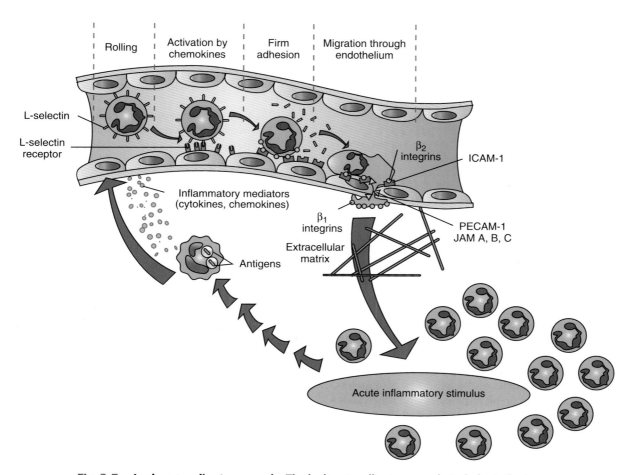

Fig. 3-7   Leukocyte adhesion cascade. The leukocyte adhesion cascade includes tethering (capture) and rolling, which are largely mediated by L- and P-selectins and their receptors. Upon activation of leukocytes and endothelial cells, there is proteolytic cleavage of L-selectin molecules and enhanced expression of β_2 integrins (Mac-1; CD11a/CD18) by leukocytes and intercellular adhesion molecule-1 *(ICAM-1)* by endothelial cells. Once leukocytes are attached to the vascular endothelium, they adhere to platelet-endothelial cell adhesion *(PECAM-1)* molecules present at the endothelial cell junction and transmigrate through the junction into the perivascular tissue, where they express β_1 integrins that adhere to extracellular matrix proteins such as laminin, fibronectin, vitronectin, and collagen. The process is mediated by chemokines (CXCL8; interleukin-8), complement fragments, vasoactive amines, cytokines, and membrane-derived mediators such as platelet-activating factor and leukotrienes. Inhibition of this process is increasingly becoming possible with specific "molecular" agonists that inhibit selectin, ICAM-1, and integrin binding. *JAM A, B, C,* Junction adhesion molecules A, B, and C. *(Redrawn with permission from Dr. M.R. Ackermann, College of Veterinary Medicine, Iowa State University.)*

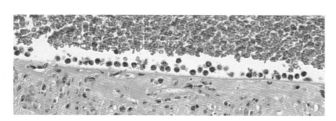

Fig. 3-8   Pavementing of neutrophils, acute inflammation, arteriole. H&E stain. *(Courtesy Dr. J.F. Zachary, College of Veterinary Medicine, University of Illinois.)*

addressin adhesion molecule-1 (MAdCAM-1)), and (5) other molecules such as CD44 (Table 3-5).

Tethering (capture) (Fig. 3-7) occurs after margination and represents the first contact leukocytes have with the luminal surfaces of endothelial cells. Tethering occurs by transient, weak binding interactions between the selectin family of adhesion molecules and their receptors. During tethering, leukocytes temporarily bind to endothelia and then release, resulting in a closer association between the leukocyte and endothelial

Table **3-4** **Endothelial Cell/Neutrophil Adhesion Molecules**

Endothelial Molecule	Leukocyte Receptor	Major Role
P-selectin	Sialyl-Lewis X PSGL-1	Rolling (neutrophils, monocytes, lymphocytes)
E-selectin	Sialyl-Lewis X ESL-1, PSGL-1	Rolling, adhesion to activated endothelium (neutrophils, monocytes, T lymphocytes)
ICAM-1	CD11/CD18 (integrins) (LFA-1, Mac-1)	Adhesion, arrest, transmigration (all leukocytes)
PECAM-1	PECAM-1	Transendothelial cell migration
JAM A	JAM A, LFA-1	Transendothelial cell migration
JAM C	JAM B, Mac-1	Transendothelial cell migration

From Cotran RS, Kumar V, Collins T, Robbins SL: *Robbins pathologic basis of disease*, ed 6, Philadelphia, 1999, Saunders.
ESL-1, E-selectin ligand-1; *ICAM-1*, intercellular adhesion molecule-1; *JAM*, junctional adhesion molecule; *LFA-1*, lymphocyte function antigen-1; *Mac-1*, macrophage antigen-1; *PECAM-1*, platelet endothelial cell adhesion molecule-1; *PSGL-1*, P-selectin glycoprotein ligand-1; *VCAM-1*, vascular cell adhesion molecule-1; *VLA*, very late antigen.

cell membranes and reduced speed of the traveling leukocyte. This process is mediated by selectins, including L-selectin expressed by neutrophils and P-selectin, a carbohydrate binding molecule stored in Weibel-Palade bodies of endothelial cells and α-granules of platelets. L-selectin is expressed on all leukocytes and binds sialyl Lewis X receptor (and other receptors) on endothelial cells. P-selectin molecules expressed on endothelial cell surfaces bind to P-selectin glycoprotein ligand-1 (PSGL-1) present on neutrophils, eosinophils, monocytes, and lymphocytes. E-selectin also mediates leukocyte-endothelial cell adherence and is expressed on endothelial cell surfaces for binding glycoprotein receptors expressed on leukocytes.

Rolling, the next step after tethering, is the process in which L-selectin and also P-selectin mediated attachments result in continued contact between the leukocyte and endothelium (Fig. 3-7). During rolling, bonds are formed at the leading edge of the rolling leukocyte and broken at the trailing edge. Leukocytes begin to roll along the surface of the endothelium under the pressure of blood flow hemodynamics. Even slight disturbances such as surgical manipulation, heat, temporary ischemia, and mast cell products induce rolling of neutrophils along the surface of vascular endothelial cells. Rolling then progresses to the slow rolling stage. Slow rolling occurs following interaction of endothelial cells with proinflammatory cytokines, such as TNF-α and the expression of E-selectin by endothelia and β_2 integrins (CD11a [LFA-1] and CD11b [Mac-1]) by neutrophils. By slowing leukocyte transit time through capillaries and postcapillary venules, combined with the continual close proximity of slow rolling leukocytes to the endothelium, and the expression of chemokines on the surface of endothelial cells, these events contribute to the proper microenvironment for slow rolling to occur and for progression to the "firm adhesion" stage.

Firm adhesion (Fig. 3-7) occurs after leukocytes have progressed through the rolling and slow rolling stages. For firm adhesion to occur, neutrophils and endothelial cells become activated by a variety of cytokines (such as interleukin-1 [IL-1], interleukin-6 [IL-6], tumor necrosis factor [TNF]), complement factors (C5a), platelet activating factor (PAF), platelet-derived growth factor (PDGF), chemokines, and other inflammatory mediators. Once neutrophils are activated, L-selectin molecules are proteolytically cleaved from the neutrophil surface, and the neutrophils express a new set of membrane proteins (integrins) by rapid exocytosis of cytoplasmic vesicles. Firm adhesion to endothelial cells is mediated by binding of β_2 integrin molecules, such as Mac-1 (CD11a/CD18) expressed on neutrophils to ICAM-1 and other ICAM molecules on endothelial cells. E-selectin adherence also contributes to the process of firm adhesion. There are four β_2 integrins (LFA-1, Mac-1, p150, 95, and $\alpha d\beta_2$), each of which are heterodimers that differ only in their subunit CD11 a, b, c, and d for LFA-1, Mac-1, p150,95, and $\alpha d\beta_2$, respectively. CD18 (the β-subunit) is identical in all four β_2 integrins. Three β_2 integrins (LFA-1, Mac-1, and p150,95) are involved with leukocyte adherence; however, the β_2 integrin $\alpha d\beta_2$, which was first identified in dogs and subsequently in human beings, is apparently not meaningfully involved with the adherence of neutrophils or other leukocytes to endothelium.

In postcapillary venules, neutrophil movement decreases from 10 μm/sec to a complete stop after margination. Firmly adhered leukocytes emigrate (transmigrate) through the endothelial layer between endothelial cells if an exogenous chemoattractant is present in the exudate. A number of leukocyte adhesion molecules are involved in this process. Neutrophils and other leukocytes

Table **3-5** Summary of Various Leukocyte Adhesion Molecules

Common Name	CD	Expressed on	Binds	Expressed on
INTEGRINS				
β_1 integrins	CD29			
VLA-1	CD49a/CD29	EC	Collagen	ECM
VLA-2	CD49b/CD29	EC	Collagen	ECM
VLA-3	CD49c/CD29	EC	Fibronectin	ECM
VLA-4	CD49d/CD29	L (except PMNs)	VCAM-1	EC
VLA-5	CD49e/CD29	EC	Fibronectin	ECM
VLA-6	CD49f/CD29	EC	Laminin	ECM
β_2 integrins	CD18			
LFA-1	CD11a/CD18	L	ICAM-1	EC
Mac-1	CD11b/CD18	L	ICAM-1	EC, L
gp150,95	CD11c/CD18	L	ICAM-1	EC
$\alpha_d\beta_2$	CD11d/CD18	Mac, CD8$^+$ T lymphocytes	ICAM-3	L, EC
β_3 integrins	CD61			
$\alpha_{IIb}\beta_3$	CD41/CD61	Platelets	Fibrinogen	EC
$\alpha_v\beta_3$	CD41/CD61	EC, Mac, M	Fibronectin	ECM
β_4 integrins				
$\alpha_6\beta_4$		EC, SC	Laminin	ECM
β_5 integrins				
$\alpha_v\beta_5$		EC, epithelia	Vitronectin	ECM
β_6 integrins				
$\alpha_v\beta_6$		Epithelia	Fibronectin	ECM
β_7 integrins				
α_4		EC, lympho	MAdCAM-1, VCAM-1	EC
α_e		Intraepithelia, lympho	E-cadherin	EC
β_8 integrins				
$\alpha_v\beta_8$			Laminin	ECM
IMMUNOGLOBULIN SUPERFAMILY				
ICAM-1	CD54	EC, epithelia, SC, PMN, MQ	β_2 integrins	L
ICAM-2	CD102	EC, lympho	β_2 integrins	L
ICAM-3		EC, lympho, PMN, M	β_2 integrins	L
ICAM-4		Red blood cells	β_2 integrins	L
ICAM-5		Subset of neurons	β_2 integrins	L
VCAM-1	CD106	EC	VLA-4	L (except PMNs)
PECAM-1	CD31	EC, L	PECAM-1	EC, L
MAdCAM-1		EC (mucosal)	L-selectin	PMN, lympho, $\alpha_4\beta_7$ integrin
Selectins				
L-selectin	CD62L	L, trophoblasts, blastula	GlyCAM-1, CD34, MAdCAM-1	EC, uterus
E-selectin	CD62E	EC	ESL-1, sLe^x	L
P-selectin	CD62P	EC, platelets	PSGL-1, GlyCAM-1, sLe^x	EC, P
OTHER				
Hyaluronic acid receptor	CD44	L	Hyaluronic acid	ECM
JAM A	CD321	EC junction, L, platelets	JAM A, LFA-1	L
JAM B	CD322	HEV	JAM B, JAM C, VLA-4	L, DC
JAM C		EC junction, L, platelets	JAM B, Mac-1	
CD99	CD99	L, M, EC		EC

This table is not comprehensive for cellular expression and binding activity.

DC, Dendritic cells; *EC,* endothelial cells; *ECM,* extracellular matrix; *ESL-1,* E-selectin ligand; *GlyCAM-1,* glycoprotein cell adhesion molecule-1; *HEV,* high endothelial cell venule; *L,* leukocytes; *lympho,* lymphocytes; *M,* monocytes; *Mac,* macrophages; *MAdCAM-1,* mucosal addressin cell adhesion molecule-1; *PMN,* polymorphonuclear cells (neutrophils); *PSGL-1,* P-selectin glycoprotein ligand-1; *SC,* Schwann cells; *sLe^x,* Sialyl-Lewis X. See text for definition of adhesion molecule abbreviations.

transmigrate between endothelial cells at the intercellalular junctions. PECAM-1, a molecule that is present on endothelial cell membranes and junctional adhesion molecules (JAMs) A, B, and C mediate adherence activities and the adherence process. Contributions to this process also include β_2 integrin binding of ICAM-1 and E-selectin binding. Pseudopodia from neutrophils and other leukocytes extend between endothelial cells and come into contact with and bind to the basement membrane (composed of laminin and collagens) and subjacent extracellular matrix proteins (proteoglycans, fibronectin, vitronectin). This binding interaction is mediated, at least in part, by the β_1 integrins. Transendothelial migration of neutrophils across the vascular wall leads to accumulation of neutrophils in the perivascular connective tissue stroma within the inflammatory exudate and can be accompanied by vascular leakage and injury. Neutrophils, drawn out of the blood vessels by chemoattractants, now migrate to the stimulus along the established chemotactic gradient.

LEUKOCYTE ADHESION DEFICIENCIES

Leukocyte adhesion deficiencies (LADs) type I, type I variant, and type II and E-selectin deficiency occur due to one or more defects in the sequence of steps leading to migration of leukocytes into the site of inflammation. These deficiencies occur in human beings and recently have been recognized and characterized in cattle and dogs (Table 3-6). The debilitation that often occurs in human beings and animals with severe forms of leukocyte adhesion deficiencies underscores the importance of leukocytes in host defense and the vital nature of the adhesion molecules integral to the transmigration process.

Cattle, dogs (Irish setters), and human beings with LAD type I lack functional expression of the β_2 integrins. They often have high numbers of neutrophils in the blood, which can exceed 125,000/µL in cattle; however, these neutrophils have impaired passage across vascular walls (Fig. 3-9) and numerous other functional abnormalities related to inadequate membrane adherence activity.

Cattle with bovine leukocyte adhesion deficiency (BLAD) develop severe gingivitis, tooth loss, oral ulcers, enteric ulcers, cutaneous ulcers, abscesses that lack pus formation, and pneumonia (Fig. 3-10). Most affected cattle die within few days or weeks after birth due to diarrhea and/or pneumonia. The hallmark lesion histologically is a sparse infiltration of neutrophils into

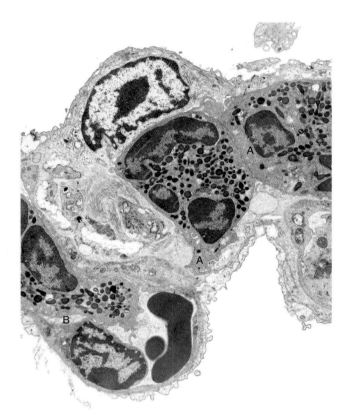

Fig. 3-9 **Bovine leukocyte adhesion deficiency, intravascular neutrophils partially adhered (rolling) on endothelial cells, capillary, alveolar septum, lung.** The septum is thickened because of two neutrophils (A) within the septal wall and a neutrophil (B) within the lumen of a vascular capillary (adherence). TEM. Uranyl acetate and lead citrate stain. (*Courtesy Dr. M.R. Ackermann, College of Veterinary Medicine, Iowa State University.*)

Table **3-6** **Molecular Defects of Various Leukocyte Adhesion Molecule Deficiencies Identified in Animals and Humans**

Name	Species	Molecular Defect	Severity
LAD, type I	Human beings	Mutations in CD18, CD11	Mild to severe
	Bovine	Mutation in CD18	Severe
	Canine	Mutation in CD18	Severe
LAD, type II	Human beings	Impaired selectin fucosylation	Severe
LAD variant	Human beings	Proteolysis of E-selectin	Severe

LAD, Leukocyte adhesion deficiency.

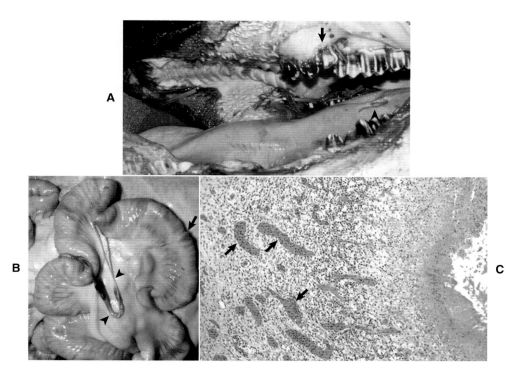

Fig. 3-10   Bovine leukocyte adhesion deficiency (BLAD), gross and microscopic characteristics. A, The oral cavity has irregularly arranged molar teeth *(arrow)*, oral ulcers *(arrowhead)*, and grass material within the oral cavity secondary to impaired mastication. **B,** The serosa of the small intestine is thickened *(arrow)*, and there are fibrous tags between serosal surfaces *(arrowheads)*. **C,** Microscopically the mucosa underlying the areas of thickened serosa is ulcerated and covered by cell debris. Vascular lumina contain elevated numbers of neutrophils, which do not adhere to the vascular endothelium *(arrows)* despite the ulcerated and "inflamed" mucosa. Lymphocytes, macrophages, and plasma cells are present perivascularly in Peyer's patches, but the lymphoid tissue virtually lacks neutrophils. The lack of neutrophil adherence to the vascular endothelium and of infiltration into the perivascular areas is caused by the lack of expression of β_2 integrins in BLAD. H&E stain. (**A, B,** and **C,** *Courtesy Dr. M.R. Ackermann, College of Veterinary Medicine, Iowa State University.*)

ulcerated mucosal surfaces or pulmonary alveoli, despite high numbers of neutrophils within lumina of submucosal and pulmonary septal blood vessels. There are no effective treatments for calves and Irish setters with LADs, although cattle with BLAD can survive into adulthood with intensive medical care.

The deficiency in β_2-integrin expression in Holstein calves is due to a single point mutation (adenine → guanine) at position 128 resulting in a single amino acid change (aspartic acid → glycine) in the β-subunit (CD18) of the β_2 integrins. This defect occurs in a highly conserved extracellular region (amino acids 96 through 389) of the protein. A second, silent mutation has also been detected in cattle with BLAD and does not alter the amino acid sequence. In Irish setters with canine leukocyte adhesion deficiency (CLAD), there is a single missense mutation resulting in a G to C transversion at nucleotide 107 of the cDNA sequence, resulting in a serine that replaces a highly conserved cysteine.

A variant form of LAD type I has been described in human beings in which β_2 integrins are expressed but do not undergo conformational change upon leukocyte stimulation. In 1992 a second form of LAD was discovered: LAD type II. In LAD type II, patients lack sialoglycoproteins that are utilized for selectin-mediated adherence. Their CD18 binding remains intact. Interestingly, these patients suffer from the same types of lesions and infections as do patients with CD18 deficiency. Therefore these observations demonstrate the importance of CD18-independent adherence. Finally, as indicated earlier, individuals with clinical disease similar to LAD type I and II (recurrent mucosal infections) had expression of adhesion molecules but enhanced proteolytic cleavage of E-selectin.

CADHERINS

Cadherins are a group of functionally related glyco-proteins expressed in epithelial cells of skin and mucosal epithelium that mediate calcium-dependent, cell-to-cell adhesion. There are three cadherin subtypes: epithelial (E) cadherin or uvomorulin, placental (P) cadherin, and neural (N) cadherin. E- and P-cadherin are present in intercellular junctions (adherens). Intraepithelial lymphocytes that express $\alpha_4\beta_7$ integrin bind to E-cadherin expressed by epithelial cells. E-cadherin is present in most epithelial cells and P-cadherin is present in the placenta and in epithelium in conjunction with E-cadherin. N-cadherin is present in neural tissue, muscle, kidney, and lens of the eye. Autoantibodies to cadherins are the basis for the skin disease pemphigus vulgaris (see Chapter 17). Cadherins are vital to innate immune activity and tissue repair.

THERAPEUTIC STRATEGIES: INHIBITION OF LEUKOCYTE ADHESION MOLECULES

Inhibition of leukocyte infiltration may be useful to treat diseases such as stroke, myocardial infarction, asthma, and autoimmune diseases in human beings and laminitis, reperfusion injury postcolic, gastric dilation/volvulus, mastitis, enteritis, allergic lung disease, pneumonia, and autoimmune diseases in domestic animals. For example, studies have shown that initial neutrophil infiltration into bronchi and bronchioles of cattle with *Mannheima haemolytica* pneumonia require functional β_2 integrins; however, β_2 integrins are not vital for neutrophil infiltration into alveoli. In addition, infiltration into alveoli can be inhibited by the selectin inhibitor TBC1269 (Bimosiamose, Encysive Pharmaceuticals, Bellaire, Tex). Inhibition of leukocyte infiltration during infectious diseases such as *Mannheima haemolytica* pneumonia may prevent excessive leukocyte infiltration and leukocyte-mediated damage if combined with appropriate antibiotic therapy. Also manipulation of leukocyte infiltration into precise regions of the lung or other tissue may make it possible to "site-direct" infiltration into a location of interest. For example, it may be possible to develop inhibitors that allow leukocyte infiltration into bronchi of animals with a bronchus-specific pathogen, such as *Bordetella bronchiseptica* in dogs and pigs, but prevent infiltration into alveoli (the site of gaseous exchange). Inhibitors may also allow infiltration into the renal pelvis and cortical tubular area during ascending bacterial infections (pyelonephritis), but not glomeruli, for example.

Nonspecific types of inhibition of leukocyte adhesion molecules include NSAIDs, corticosteroids, and drugs that inhibit the production or release of inflammatory cytokines. Specific inhibitors to adhesion molecules include selectin antagonists (TBC1269 [Encysive Pharmaceuticals], Efomycine [Bayer Pharmaceutical Group, Leverkusen, Germany], Cylexin [Epimmune Inc., San Diego, Calif]), β_1 integrin antagonists (TBC4746 [Encysive Pharmaceuticals], BIO1211 [Biogen Inc., Cambridge, Mass]), and antagonists to β_2 integrins (A304470 [Abbott Laboratories, Abbott Park, Ill] and BIRT377 [Boehringer Ingelheim Pharmaceuticals, Ingelheim, Germany]). Other inhibitors include peptides derived from fibronectin fragments, monoclonal antibodies, and small inhibitory RNA (siRNA). These drugs are being tested in animal models of myocardial infarction, stroke, multiple sclerosis, graft-versus-host disease, psoriasis, rheumatoid arthritis, inflammatory bowel disease, asthma, and colitis. Some of these drugs are available commercially or are being used in human clinical trials.

REPARATIVE PHASE OF THE ACUTE INFLAMMATORY RESPONSE

OUTCOMES OF THE ACUTE INFLAMMATORY RESPONSE

There are four main outcomes of acute inflammation:
- Resolution (the return to normal structure and function)
- Healing by fibrosis
- Abscess formation
- Progression to chronic inflammation

These outcomes are determined by the severity of tissue damage, the ability of cells to regenerate, and the biologic characteristics of the stimulus that caused the injury. In the acute inflammatory response, the desired outcome is resolution; that is, the complete return of normal structure and function. Resolution occurs if:
- The acute inflammatory response is completed in the correct sequence
- Macrophages and lymphatic vessels remove the exudate
- The inciting stimulus is eliminated
- The stroma (connective tissue) of the affected tissue is intact and can provide support for regeneration of epithelial cells
- Denuded or necrotic epithelial cells are replaced by regeneration of adjacent epithelial cells on an intact basement membrane

Mechanistically, the critical first stage of resolution involves the killing and/or removal of the inciting stimulus, neutralization or decay of chemical mediators, return to normal of vascular flow and capillary permeability, cessation of leukocyte emigration, apoptotic cell death of remaining neutrophils in the exudate, and the removal of the exudate via phagocytosis by cells of the monocyte-macrophage system and drainage to regional

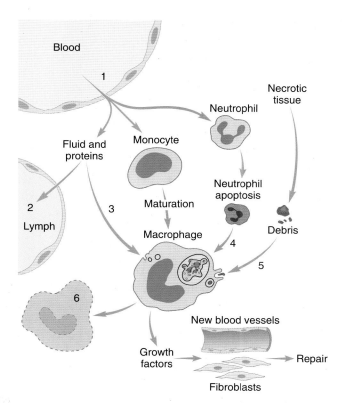

Fig. 3-11   Events in the resolution of inflammation.
(1) Return to normal vascular permeability; *(2)* drainage of
edema fluid and proteins into lymphatics or *(3)* by pinocytosis
into macrophages; *(4)* phagocytosis of apoptotic neutrophils
and *(5)* phagocytosis of necrotic debris; and *(6)* disposal of
macrophages. Macrophages also produce growth factors that
initiate the subsequent process of repair. Note the central role
of macrophages in resolution. *(Modified from Haslett C, Henson PM:*
Resolution of inflammation. In Clark R, Henson PM, editors: The molecular
and cellular biology of wound repair, New York, 1996, Plenum Press.)

lymph nodes (Fig. 3-11). Regeneration is the second
stage of resolution and is dependent on the availability
of progenitor epithelial cells to replace lost cells and the
presence of a supportive stroma and intact basement
membrane for cellular migration. As an example, acute
renal tubular necrosis can be caused by aminoglycoside antibiotics and results in detachment and necrosis
of tubular epithelial cells from the tubular basement
membrane. If the supporting stroma and basement
membrane remain intact, progenitor epithelial cells
can divide and migrate to replace lost cells and thus
return the tubule to normal function. If the basement
membrane is not intact to guide the proliferating cells,
functional tubules will not form. Instead, regenerative
tubular epithelial cells will atrophy or form into small
aggregates with syncytial giant cells. Simultaneously,
the microvascular supply to the region must be restored
and this occurs mechanistically by the proliferation of

endothelial cells in response to molecules, such as vascular endothelial growth factor (VEGF), as discussed
with wound healing in Chapter 4.

EFFECTOR CELLS OF THE ACUTE INFLAMMATORY RESPONSE

VASCULAR ENDOTHELIAL CELLS

Central to the integrity of the vasculature and any type
of acute inflammatory response is the endothelial cell.
Once considered simply a cell that, in the most simplistic view, offered physical separation between the
blood and the surrounding tissue, endothelial cells are
now known to have an extremely sophisticated role in
regulating: (1) hemostasis/coagulation, (2) vascular pressure, (3) angiogenesis during wound healing, (4) carcinogenesis, (5) leukocyte homing, and (6) inflammation.
During inflammation, endothelial cells have a major
role through contraction, release of chemical mediators,
and expression of adhesion molecules and receptors
that include E-selectin, P-selectin, L-selectin ligand,
PECAM-1, JAM A, B, and C, and the immunoglobulin
superfamily, such as ICAM-1, which serves as ligands
for leukocyte β_2 integrins.

MAST CELLS AND BASOPHILS

The origin and relationship between mast cells and
basophils has been a traditional point of debate and
confusion. Current research clearly indicates that mast
cells and basophils represent distinct cell types even
though they share several morphologic and functional
characteristics. Mast cells and basophils originate and
differentiate in bone marrow from a common CD34+
precursor cell along with other granulocytes and
monocytes. Differentiation of CD34+ precursor cells
into mast cells or basophils is dependent on stem cell
factor, a glycoprotein that acts with other cytokines and
is produced in the bone marrow by fibroblasts and vascular endothelial cells. There is no evidence to suggest
that basophils differentiate into tissue mast cells.

Mammalian mast cells are normally distributed
throughout connective tissue adjacent to small blood
and lymphatic vessels of skin and mucous membranes,
which allows them to interact with resident dendritic
cells (macrophages) and respond to foreign proteins
and microbes in the perivascular spaces. Experimental
studies suggest that cutaneous mast cells in tissue have
a life span of 4 to 12 weeks depending on their location.
Mast cells represent an extremely heterogeneous
population of cells. In the 1960s Enerback identified
two separate types of mast cells: "mucosal" and "connective tissue." The mucosal mast cells, typically located
in the respiratory and intestinal mucosa, can increase

in numbers during some types of T_H2 cell–dependent immune responses. In contrast, the connective tissue mast cells show little or no T-cell dependence. Mast cells express high affinity receptors for immunoglobulin E (IgE) (Fc ε-RI) on their surface and the release of mast cell granules is stimulated by cross-linking of IgE receptors by antigens such as pollens, allergens, and parasites. Substance P released from sensory (C-reactive) nerve fibers and macrophages also causes degranulation of mast cells. Degranulation results in the release of preformed TNF-α histamine, neutral proteases, proteoglycans (chondroitin sulfates and heparin), serotonin (in rodent species but not human beings), tryptase, chymase, and stem cell factor into tissue. Histamine and substance P activity appears interrelated because histamine released by mast cells can downregulate release of substance P by nerve fibers, thereby reducing excessive amounts of the two proinflammatory molecules. The mast cell–substance P fiber interrelationship is an often cited example of the neuroinflammatory-neuroimmune pathways.

Mast cells also synthesize leukotriene C_4 (LTC$_4$), PAF, prostaglandin D_2, numerous cytokines, and C-C chemokines (macrophage inflammatory protein [MIP]-1-α and macrophage chemotactic protein [MCP]-1). The release of these mediators contributes significantly to the initiation of the acute inflammatory response. In addition, at physiologic concentrations these products likely counteract the effects of dense populations of mast cells in tissue and thus assist in regulating vascular permeability. Mast cells also release proteolytic enzymes, such as tryptase and chymase, which are involved with remodeling of the extracellular matrix. Tryptase is mitogenic to epithelial cells and likely contributes to proliferation of epithelial cells during wound repair.

Basophils are similar to neutrophils and eosinophils in that they mature in the bone marrow, circulate in the peripheral blood, are recruited into the tissue, and have a life span of several days in tissue. Basophils express high affinity IgE receptors similar to mast cells and release granules and inflammatory mediators. Basophils appear to lack heparin, have a more limited cytokine repertoire than mast cells, and release mainly IL-4 and IL-13. Basophils express CD40L and CCR3 (eotaxin receptor), both of which point to a role as a cell that can enter sites of inflammation and release regulatory cytokines where they upregulate VCAM-1 expression by endothelial cells and switch B lymphocytes to produce IgE, further contributing to the IgE type of response. Basophils can be prominent in IgE-mediated leukocyte infiltration into the mucosa of the nose, sinuses, respiratory tract, and skin, and all of these sites are particularly predisposed to allergic conditions.

The role of mast cells and basophils in IgE-mediated hypersensitivity reactions has been known for decades.

These cells appear to represent critical effector cells in disorders of IgE-dependent immediate type I hypersensitivities (see Chapter 5). The release of their granules and mediators at inflammatory concentrations results in mucus secretion, accumulation of seroproteinaceous fluid in airways, bronchoconstriction, and vasodilation. The excessive release of tryptase and chymase by mast cells may enhance degradation of the extracellular matrix and contribute to fibrosis and tissue remodeling. Chemokines and cytokines from mast cells and basophils contribute to innate immune defenses and enhanced adhesion molecule expression with subsequent leukocyte infiltration.

NEUTROPHILS

Neutrophils are often the first type of leukocyte recruited into the inflammatory exudate. Their purpose is to: (1) kill microbes, such as bacteria, fungi, protozoa, and viruses; (2) kill tumor cells; or (3) to eliminate foreign materials. The biologic activities of neutrophils are primarily designed to kill microbes, but if killing does not occur they can limit the growth of microbes, allowing time for adaptive immunologic responses to develop.

Neutrophils perform two important functions to accomplish their effects: (1) phagocytosis of microbes or foreign material and then fusion of the phagosome with the neutrophil's lysosomes to form a phagolysosome in which the microbes or foreign material are killed or degraded, respectively, and (2) secretion and/or release of the contents of their granules into the inflammatory exudate to enhance the acute inflammatory response. They also infiltrate areas of acute tissue necrosis, such as those that occur with ischemia in infarcts and in necrotic areas of tumors.

Neutrophils are produced in the bone marrow, circulate in the blood stream, and if not recruited into tissue by an acute inflammatory response, can enter tissue where they eventually are destroyed by macrophages via apoptosis and phagocytosis or are lost from the body by migration across mucosal surfaces, such as the alimentary and respiratory tracts. The average transit time in the blood is 10 hours, and the half-life varies between species but ranges from 5 to 10 hours; neutrophils within tissue survive from 1 to 4 days. Cytokines, such as IL-1 and TNF, and growth factors, such as granulocyte-macrophage colony-stimulating factor (GM-CSF), granulocyte colony-stimulating factor (G-CSF), and IL-3 can increase release of neutrophils from the bone marrow and induce granulopoiesis in 2 to 4 days. GM-CSF and G-CSF are also present in tissue during acute inflammatory response and prevent apoptosis of tissue neutrophils. Growth factor withdrawal, which occurs during resolution of acute inflammation, induces

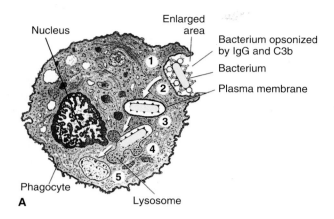

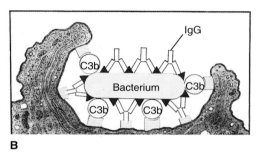

Fig. 3-12   Phases of phagocytosis. A, Opsonized microbes (*1*) bind to the surface of a phagocyte and (*2*) are ingested into a phagocytic vacuole or phagosome (*3*). Lysosomes fuse with the phagosome (*4*), releasing their digestive enzymes into the vacuole. This process results in the formation of a phagolysosome (*5*), within which the microbe is killed and digested. **B,** Enlargement showing microbe opsonization. *IgG,* Immunoglobulin G; *C3b,* complement component. (***A*** *and **B,** From McCance K, Huether S: Understanding pathophysiology, St Louis, 1996, Mosby.*)

apoptosis and this outcome can be accelerated by TNF. During apoptosis, neutrophils lose the capacity to degranulate and become activated, which prevents excessive tissue damage from their lysosomal enzymes and allows for their phagocytosis by macrophages.

Neutrophils entering tissue become activated (phagocytosis, killing, and locomotion) through stimulation by inflammatory mediators and adherence to ligands by surface adhesion molecules (Fig. 3-12). Inflammatory mediators bind receptors on neutrophils, such as: (1) G protein-linked seven membrane domain receptors for PAF, C5a, IL-8 and substance P (the neurokinin-1 receptor) and (2) single-transmembrane-domain receptors for growth factors such as GM-CSF and cytokines such as TNF. Many of these mediators induce chemotaxis; when leukocyte adhesion molecules— such as the selectins and integrins—bind their respective ligands, they induce mitogen-activated protein kinase (MAPK) and G proteins (ρ-A) resulting in locomotion of neutrophils usually toward a chemotactic gradient and activation.

Neutrophils can internalize by phagocytosis large particles up to 0.5 μm in diameter, such as microbes, foreign bodies, senescent cells, and debris. Neutrophils can internalize nonopsonized particles; however, opsonization greatly facilitates phagocytosis. The principal opsonin receptors are Fc receptors (Fc γ-receptor I, IIA, IIIB), which bind the Fc portion of immunoglobulins. Such binding initiates activity of the GTPase Rac-1 and the β_2 integrin Mac-1 (CD11b/CD18), which also binds complement fragment C3bi and initiates GTPase-ρ. Such binding-inducing proteins and lipid kinases (e.g., protein kinase C and phosphatidylinositol 3-kinase) mediate actin assembly for formation of filopodia or lamellipodia, which surround and then internalize particles via phagocytosis by activated neutrophils. The activation process also leads to the release of calcium stored in the endoplasmic reticulum, which can induce a respiratory (oxidative) burst. Oxidative burst is the process by which nicotinamide adenine dinucleotide phosphate (NADPH) oxidase in phagosomes catalyzes the formation of free radicals that are used to kill microbes or degrade internalized material.

Once a particle is internalized, phagosomes can "mature" by fusing with lysosomes and endosomes or remove parts of internalized particles. The fusion process is likely mediated by calmodulin, a calcium-binding protein, and soluble NSF (N-ethylmaleimide-sensitive factor) attachment protein receptors (SNARE; a fusion protein) that bind ligands on another vesicle to bring the membranes together for fusion. The maturation process results in lowering of the pH within the phagosome and the activation of microbicidal enzymes; NADPH oxidase, which forms oxidative radicals; and myeloperoxidase complexes. Smaller particles are taken up by receptor-mediator or nonspecific endocytosis, a process that is similar to phagocytosis.

The ability of neutrophils to kill microbes or to degrade foreign material depends largely on the contents of the neutrophil granules, which store degradative enzymes, peroxidative enzymes, adhesion molecules, and antimicrobial peptides and/or proteins. Myeloperoxidase is an enzyme used to convert hydrogen peroxide to hypochlorous acid. Hypochlorous acid, hydrogen peroxide, and a halide cofactor form the myeloperoxidase system, which is an effective microbicidal mechanism used by neutrophils to kill internalized microbes and degrade internalized substances. Defensins, cathelicidins, and antimicrobial proteins contribute to the degradation of microbes through the formation of pores in microbial membranes. They also have an effect on chemotaxis and activation of the adaptive immune response. Lactoferrin inhibits the growth of phagocytosed bacteria by sequestering free iron, and elastase hydrolyzes bacterial cell wall proteins and tissue elastin. The enzymatic contents of granules—such as gelatinase (matrix metalloproteinase 9 [MMP 9]) and myeloperoxidase—and nonenzymatic substances—such as antimicrobial peptides and lactoferrin—are also commonly released by the cell into the extracellular space and play a role in the extracellular killing of microbial pathogens and degradation of the extracellular matrix. The effects of neutrophil proteases, if not inactivated, can cause serious injury to tissue; therefore protease inhibitors are present in plasma and are present in inflammatory lesions following vascular leakage.

Neutrophil granule formation begins during myeloid cell differentiation in the bone marrow (Box 3-1). Granules are observed initially in myeloblasts and promyelocytes when immature transport vesicles bud from Golgi and fuse to form primary granules. Primary granules are also called azurophilic granules because of their affinity for the dye azure A. These granules contain myeloperoxidase, elastase, defensins, and small amounts of lysozyme. Myelocytes and metamyelocytes form secondary (specific) granules that contain defensins, lactoferrin, lysozyme, and lesser amounts of myeloperoxidase, CD11b/CD18, and elastase. Band cells, the penultimate stage of neutrophil development, form tertiary (gelatinase) granules that contain lysozyme, gelatinase (MMP 9), cysteine-rich secretory protein-3 (CRISP-3), and adhesion molecules CD11b/CD18

(Mac-1), but have smaller amounts of myeloperoxidase, lactoferrin, proteinase 3, elastase, and defensins. Band and mature neutrophils also have secretory vesicles that contain plasma proteins, alkaline phosphatase, and numerous CD antigens, including CD11b/CD18 adhesion molecules. The secretory vesicles are mobilized quickly after neutrophil activation, allowing leukocyte infiltration.

Neutrophil granules have evolved phylogenetically and are specially adapted for each species. In most mammals, enzymes released into an exudate from neutrophil granules cause liquefaction of the exudate and the process results in the formation and accumulation of pus. Reptiles and birds that either lack or have reduced concentrations of these enzymes cannot liquefy the exudate, and a caseous material forms to be degraded by the next available line of inflammatory cells, macrophages. Granules in chicken heterophils (the avian, rabbit, and guinea pig neutrophil equivalent is termed heterophils) have little myeloperoxidase, but concentrations are also reduced in neutrophils of cattle and pigs. Cattle and sheep neutrophils have limited lysozyme levels. α-Defensins are present in rabbits, guinea pigs, hamsters, rats, and cattle neutrophils, but have not been identified in those of dogs, cats, mice, pigs, and horses. The effect of these granule differences in various animal species on host defense and neutrophil function is not fully understood.

Box 3-1

Enzymes and Molecules Present in Neurophil Granules

SPECIFIC GRANULES

Lactoferrin
Lysozyme
Alkaline phosphates
Type IV collagenase
Leukocyte adhesion molecules
Plasminogen activation
Phospholipase A_2

AZUROPHIL GRANULES

Myeloperoxidase
Lysozyme—bactericidal factors
Cationic proteins
Acid hydrolases
Elastase
Nonspecific collagenase
BPI
Defensins
Cathepsin G
Phospholipase A_2

From Cotran RS, Kumar V, Collins T, Robbins SL: *Robbins pathologic basis of disease,* ed 6, Philadelphia, 1999, Saunders.
BPI, Bactericidal/permeability-increasing protein.

EOSINOPHILS

Eosinophils are recruited from the blood stream into vascularized connective tissue of most organs in response to eosinophil chemoattractants present in allergic and parasitic diseases. As examples, the skin, the respiratory and alimentary systems, and the liver are common organ systems in which eosinophils are present in certain inflammatory responses. Eosinophils have prominent granules that release basic proteins and when activated produce cytokines, chemokines, proteases, and oxidative radicals. This array of mediators is often released in response to helminthic infections, and eosinophilic infiltration has been more recently implicated in resistance to the development of some cancers. On the other hand, eosinophil products contribute to tissue damage in several organs, including the lungs (asthma), heart, skin, and gastrointestinal tract.

Eosinophils were first recognized as blood cells (leukocytes) having numerous cytoplasmic granules with affinity for acidic dyes such as eosin. Therefore, the name "eosinophil" ("eosin-loving") was proposed by Ehrlich in the late 1800s for these unique cells. By 1939, eosinophils were postulated to have a role in the immune response to helminths, and by the 1970s eosinophils were well known to increase in the

Table **3-7**   **Morphologic Features and Function of Eosinophilic Granules**

Granule Type	Morphology	Content	Function
Small granules	Few, small, homogeneous	Acid phosphatase, arylsulfatase	Inactivate leukotrienes
Primary granules	Few, round, electron-dense		
Secondary granules (specific granules)	Electron-dense, crystalline core	Major basic protein	Toxic to parasites, tumor cells, host tissue; causes histamine release; inhibits heparin activity
	Electron-lucent matrix	Eosinophil cationic protein	Toxic to parasites, causes histamine release, antiparasitic
		Eosinophil-derived neurotoxin	Neurotoxic with H_2O_2/halide, microbicidal
		Eosinophil peroxidase	Microbicidal
		Catalase	Inactivates leukotrienes

blood (eosinophilia) in parasitic and allergic diseases. Eosinophils are slightly larger than neutrophils. The nucleus is lobulated (bilobed) and composed primarily of heterochromatin (condensed). Eosinophil granules are known for their large size, especially in horses; are rich in arginine; and have reddish brown tinctorial properties.

Eosinophils have several types of granules listed in Table 3-7, including large specific granules, small granules, primary granules, and secondary granules. Large specific granules contain four distinct basic proteins: (1) major basic protein, (2) eosinophil cationic protein, (3) eosinophil-derived neurotoxin, and (4) eosinophil peroxidase. These proteins exert biologic effects on microbes and on the tissue in which the microbes replicate by damaging lipid membranes. In addition, histaminase and a variety of hydrolytic lysosomal enzymes, such as collagenase and gelatinase, are also present in the large specific granules. Small granules contain enzymes, such as arylsulphatases, acid phosphatases, metalloproteinases, and gelatinases. Eosinophils also elaborate cytokines, such as ILs 1, 2, 3, 4, 5, 6, 8, 10, 12, 16, GM-CSF, transforming growth factor (TGF)-α and TGF-β and chemokines. The contents of eosinophil granules are released in response to inflammatory stimuli in a manner similar to those used to activate neutrophils. However, products of eosinophil granules can result in extensive tissue degradation, including the degradation of collagen, which is commonly seen in eosinophilic granulomas of cats, horses, and dogs. Nearly all mast cell tumors in dogs and some mast cell tumors in cats contain eosinophils.

Major chemoattractants for eosinophils include histamine and eosinophilic chemotactic factor A (from mast cells), neutrophil peptides, C5a, cytokines (IL-4, IL-5, and IL-13) and chemokines (CCL-5, known as RANTES [regulated on activation, normal T lymphocytes expressed and secreted], and CCL-11, known as eotaxin) released from epithelial cells, eosinophils, mast cells, and helminths. 5-Oxo-6,8,11,14-eicosatetraenoic acid (5-oxo-ETE) is a strong activator of human eosinophils with a chemotactic potency comparable with those of eotaxin and RANTES, both of which enhance 5-Oxo-ETE–induced chemotaxis. 5-Oxo-ETE and these chemokines contribute to the accumulation of eosinophils in the respiratory system in diseases such as asthma.

MONOCYTES AND MACROPHAGES

Monocytes and macrophages are components of the monocyte-macrophage system. The number of macrophages in tissue is maintained by: (1) influx of monocytes from the blood, (2) proliferation of recruited monocytes locally in tissue, and (3) biologic turnover of macrophages via apoptotic cell death (life span in tissue of less than 3 weeks). During inflammatory responses, monocytes that have receptors (IgG Fc-domains, C3b) for chemical mediators of inflammation exert migratory, chemotactic, pinocytic, and phagocytic activities in response to inflammatory stimuli. When monocytes emigrate into tissue, they undergo additional differentiation to become tissue macrophages. There are two types of tissue macrophages: macrophages that reside within specific organs/tissue (free macrophages and fixed macrophages) and macrophages derived from monocytes in response to inflammatory stimuli. Macrophages residing in organs/ connective tissue first enter these sites as blood monocytes under physiologic (rather than inflammatory) conditions. These macrophages include macrophages in connective tissue (histiocytes [free macrophages]), liver (Kupffer cells [fixed macrophages]), lung (alveolar macrophages [free macrophages] and intravascular macrophages [fixed macrophages]), lymph nodes (free and fixed macrophages), spleen (free and fixed macrophages), bone marrow (fixed macrophages), serous fluids (pleural and peritoneal macrophages [free macrophages]), and skin (histiocytes [fixed macrophages]). As indicated, during inflammatory conditions monocytes are recruited by inflammatory mediators, such as chemokines, to leave the circulatory system, enter sites of inflammation, and become activated macrophages. This process can occur virtually anywhere in the body and often sets the stage for the development of chronic inflammation.

Functionally, macrophages are a component of the innate immune system in terms of their role in phagocytosis and cytokine release during the acute inflammatory response. However, macrophages are one of the main triggers of the adaptive immune response because of their ability to process and present antigen and regulate T-cell activity. Monocytes, macrophages, dendritic cells, and other cell types of the chronic inflammatory response will be discussed in greater detail in Chapter 4.

CHEMICAL MEDIATORS OF THE ACUTE INFLAMMATORY RESPONSE

Chemical mediators of the acute inflammatory response (Fig. 3-3, Table 3-3, Appendix 3-1) are often produced as preformed or synthesized molecules in the liver and in neutrophils, basophils, macrophages/monocytes, platelets, mast cells, endothelial cells, smooth muscle cells, fibroblasts, and most epithelial cells. Preformed molecules, such as histamine are transcribed, translated, processed, and stored, often in granules or vacuoles within inflammatory cells. They can be released immediately upon cellular activation and are therefore active in seconds. Other molecules, such as most cytokines, adhesion molecules, and prostaglandins, are largely synthesized after an inflammatory cell becomes activated. Endothelial cells, for example, often express low, basal levels of the adhesion molecule ICAM-1, but after the cell becomes activated (by cytokines such as IL-1), they rapidly transcribe the ICAM-1 gene generating ICAM-1 mRNA that is translated into ICAM-1 protein, which is processed, transported, and expressed on the cell surface. This process is somewhat rapid, resulting in ICAM-1 expression within hours; however, it is not nearly as rapid as the release of histamine. Inflammatory mediators originating from plasma proteins, such as kinin, and the coagulation and complement system proteins are constantly secreted by the liver in precursor forms that must be activated via proteolytic cleavage in the circulatory system to their active forms; however, once the proteolytic cleavage is initiated, kinin and complement activity is immediate, similar to histamine.

Inflammatory mediators, whether preformed, synthesized, or derived from plasma, generally bind to receptors on target cells and often activate target cells or cause the target cell to secrete additional inflammatory mediators. In the latter case, the mediators may amplify or suppress secretion by target cells of additional mediators. Once activated and released or secreted, most inflammatory mediators:

- Have short half-lives and quickly decay
- Are enzymatically destroyed by kinases
- Are scavenged by protective mechanisms, such as antioxidants
- Are blocked by endogenous inhibitors such as complement inhibitors

This arrangement provides a check and balance system on the severity of the acute inflammatory response and also can be exploited in the development of drugs to inhibit excessive inflammatory responses. Inflammatory mediators, if excessively unregulated, have the potential to cause severe injury to tissue in and surrounding the acute inflammatory response.

Preformed inflammatory proteins include histamine, serotonin, bradykinin, and tachykinins (substance P and neurokinins). These substances are released during the initial phases of the acute inflammatory response. Mast cells and basophils are the principal sources of histamine and serotonin. Bradykinin is released by leukocytes and vascular endothelial cells, and substance P is released by mast cells, basophils, and C-reactive (sensory) nerve fibers. As indicated, the mediators are rapidly active (in seconds to minutes) and contribute to increased vascular permeability that lasts from minutes to hours.

Histamine rapidly enhances vascular permeability and is one of the earliest recognized mediators of inflammation. Experiments by Sir Thomas Lewis in 1927 and Dale and Laidlaw in 1911 indicated the potential role of histamine and other local mediators in acute inflammation. Histamine is derived from the amino acid histidine through the action of histidine decarboxylase. This enzyme catalyzes the decarboxylation of histidine to histamine and carbon dioxide. Histamine is stored (preformed) in granules of mast cells, basophils, and platelets.

As a mediator of inflammation, major effects of histamine are: (1) vasodilation (active hyperemia) via both H_1 and H_2 receptors, (2) increased microvascular permeability via predominantly the H_1 receptor, (3) neural reflexes, vagal reflexes, bronchial constriction, (4) release of $PGF_{2\alpha}$, (5) pain and itching, (6) tachycardia, and (7) eosinophil chemotaxis. The acute vascular effects of histamine are immediate (within minutes) and transient (last about 30 to 90 minutes). Whether histamine has a role in chronic inflammation is speculative, but it may act to modulate the inflammatory response and the reactivity of various leukocytes, including lymphocytes.

Antihistamines inhibit binding of histamine to H_1 receptors located on target cells (leukocytes, endothelial cells, and smooth muscle). In addition, eosinophils release histaminases that degrade histamine.

The release of histamine from mast cells is in response to a variety of stimuli including IgE, C3a, C5a, heat, cold, substance P, adenosine triphosphate (ATP), and products from leukocytes, endothelial cells, and platelets. Three histamine receptors of the 7TM receptor family have been described: H_1, H_2, and H_3. Free histamine reacts within minutes with H_1 receptors on venular endothelium to cause contraction and gap formation (cytoskeletal reorganization [actinomycin filaments]), resulting in increased vascular permeability. Histamine H_1 receptor activation may lead to the production of cytokines and antibodies by T lymphocytes and B lymphocytes, respectively. In addition, H_1 receptors are also found on a variety of blood leukocytes, such as T lymphocytes, B lymphocytes, and monocytes.

Histamine also acts through H_2 receptors found on many cells, such as endothelial cells, gastric epithelial cells, and neurons. The action of histamine on leukocytes is also mediated through histamine H_1 and H_2 receptors. H_3 receptors serve as inhibitory autoreceptors on histamine-containing nerve terminals and regulate the release of neurotransmitters in the central nervous system (CNS) and peripheral nervous system (PNS).

There is substantial overlap of activities by these receptors on many types of cells. Many of the actions of histamine can be mimicked by H_1 and H_2 receptor agonists (a molecule or drug that binds to a receptor and triggers a response by the cell), whereas these actions can be blocked by H_1 and H_2 antagonists, molecules or drugs that block a receptor and prevent a response by the cell. This latter effect is the basis for therapies used in veterinary medicine today. Histamine receptors, for example, are involved in the pathogenesis of allergies, and H_1 receptor antagonists reduce symptoms associated with allergic rhinitis such as sneezing, pruritus, and rhinorrhea (runny nose). In allergic bronchiolitis of cats and horses, H_1 receptor activation results in increased vascular permeability leading to serous inflammation in the bronchi and bronchioles. If this response can be blocked, the effects of allergens can be minimized in affected patients.

Serotonin (5-hydroxytryptamine) is an important preformed vasoactive amine with actions similar to those described previously for histamine. Serotonin is also an important neurotransmitter. Serotonin is found in mast cell granules of rodents and platelets of mammals. Serotonin and histamine are released from platelets after they are activated by the following:

- Aggregation and following contact with collagen in an exposed basement membrane from areas of endothelial necrosis and detached cells
- Thrombin from activation of the coagulation cascade
- Adenosine diphosphate released from injured endothelial cells
- Immune complex activation of the complement cascade (C3a, C5a)

Kinins, such as the tachykinins and bradykinin, are chemical mediators of the acute inflammatory response and also act by modulating the responses of the clotting and complement cascades. Kinin system activation leads ultimately to the formation of bradykinin. Bradykinin, a prototype kinin and a vasoactive peptide, has proinflammatory (makes the disease worse) properties that result in the following:

- Increased vascular permeability
- Vasodilation (venules)
- Increased sensitivity to pain
- Smooth muscle contraction
- Increased arachidonic acid metabolism (stimulation of phospholipase A_2)
- Hypotension
- Bronchoconstriction

Kinins are formed by two distinct pathways: the plasma kinin pathway and the tissue kinin pathway. The plasma kinin pathway is activated by the contact of a protein complex formed by high molecular weight kininogen (HMWK), factor XI, and prekallikrein with negatively charged surfaces, such as exposed basement membrane. When Hageman factor (factor XII, HF) binds to this surface and interacts with the bound protein complex, there is reciprocal activation/generation of activated Hageman factor (Hfa) and kallikrein (contact activation system). Kallikrein then acts on HMWK to yield bradykinin, an oligopeptide containing nine amino acid residues.

The tissue kinin pathway is generated by the action of tissue kallikrein on a low molecular weight kininogen (LMWK) to produce lysyl bradykinin and finally bradykinin. Tissue kallikrein is chemically and antigenically distinct from plasma kallikrein, although it is capable of acting on either HMWK or LMWK to generate bradykinin. Control of the proinflammatory effects of kinins is through rapid inactivation of bradykinin and kallikrein. Bradykinin is broken down by kininase. Plasma kallikrein is inhibited by C1-INH esterase (serum α_2-macroglobulin), a member of the serpin family of proteases. This family of proteases forms approximately 20% of the proteins in blood plasma and includes α_1-antichymotrypsin, α_1-antitrypsin, and antithrombin III. They act to block proteolytic activity in the clotting and complement systems and thus serve as a regulatory check on these systems.

Tachykinins are a family of vasoactive neuropeptides that includes substance P and neurokinin A and B, which are synthesized by sensory afferent nerve fibers of the lungs and alimentary system. These substances are involved in allergic reactions and asthma. Substance P can induce vasoconstriction, vasodilation, increased permeability changes leading to edema, leukocyte activation, and chemotaxis. Substance P also induces activation and degranulation of mast cells, basophils, and eosinophils and their release of histamine and other inflammatory mediators. The released histamine, in a feedback mechanism, binds the H_3 receptors of nerve fibers and partially inhibits the production of substance P, thus regulating the level of activity. One of the main receptors for substance P, neurokinin-1 receptor (NK-1R), is expressed on a variety of cells including mast cells, epithelial cells, endothelial cells, and macrophages. NK-1R is regulated by substance P expression. Often, increased levels of substance P result in decreased NK-1R expression. The release of substance P from afferent sensory nerve fibers in skin and mucous membranes can also be induced by capsaicinoids such as capsaicin and dihydrocapsaicin. Capsaicinoids are natural compounds present in chile peppers of the genus *Capsicum*, which cause the burning sensation in commercial pepper sprays (less-than-lethal, self-defense weapons). Capsaicin binds the vanilloid receptor-1 of afferent sensory fibers, leading to release of substance P from these fibers. Thus the tachykinins induce inflammatory responses when released by activated and degranulated mast cells, basophils, and eosinophils, and also from stimulated nerve fibers.

COMPLEMENT CASCADE

The complement cascade is a unique sequence of molecular events occurring within the vascular system in which inactive plasma proteins synthesized by the liver are activated following tissue injury (Fig. 3-13). This cascade results in the generation of numerous biologically active molecules that have proinflammatory, chemotactic, opsonizing, antigen solubilization, antibody formation, permeability, and microbicidal (cell lysis) effects that are usually beneficial to the animal. A large number of plasma proteins (20 including their cleavage products) make up the complement system and nearly 10% of serum proteins are complement factors. Traditionally divided into the "classical" and "alternative" pathways, activation or "fixation" of complement proteins eventually results in formation of a membrane attack complex (MAC) that perforates the cell membranes of foreign invaders and naïve host cells alike. In the generation of MAC, a variety of complement components are elaborated that have important inflammatory and immune effects.

Complement proteins C1 through C9 are inactive components of plasma that are activated by substances including microbial molecules such as endotoxins, aggregated immunoglobulin, complex polysaccharides,

and venoms. The critical step in unleashing the biological functions of the complement cascade is activation of C3 through either the classical or alternative complement activation pathways. The classical pathway of the complement cascade can be activated by antibody complexes. Activation occurs when IgG and/or IgM are cross-linked with C1. C1 has three components: C1q, r, and s. C1q binds the Fc regions of IgG and/or IgM and brings C1r, which is proteolytic, into proximity to C1s, which is cleaved; through interactions with C4 and C2, and leads to the formation of classical pathway C3 convertase (C4b2a) and the eventual formation of classical pathway C5 convertase (C4b2a3b). Classical pathway C3 convertase converts C3 to C3a, and classical pathway C5 convertase converts C5 to C5a.

The alternative pathway is initiated by products from microorganisms including LPS (lipopolysaccharide) from gram-negative bacteria and polysaccharides from fungal cell walls. In addition, other activated plasma proteins, including kallikrein, plasmin, and activated factor XII, can cleave C3 resulting in its activation to C3b. C3b combines with factor B and, coupled with factor D activity, forms the alternative pathway C3 convertase (C3bBb). Alternative pathway C3 convertase converts C3 to C3b. C3b combines with alternative pathway C3 convertase to form alternative pathway C5 convertase (C3bB3b), which converts C5 to C5a. Because the alternative pathway can be activated by clotting and kinin factors, once the clotting or the kinin systems are activated, complement activity follows and vice versa. Therefore the clotting, kinin, and complement systems are closely interactive, and often activation of one system leads to activation of others (Fig. 3-14).

C3a increases vascular permeability by inducing histamine release from mast cells. C5a, once formed, is released into the inflammatory exudate and behaves as an anaphylatoxin (a molecule that causes the release of histamine and other chemical mediators from mast cells or basophils), a chemoattractant for leukocytes, and an inducer of adhesion molecule expression by endothelial cells. C3b is an important opsonin and enhances neutrophil phagocytosis. The plasma enzyme carboxypeptidase can degrade both C3a and C5b.

A MAC results from the cleavage of C5 by C5 convertase, leading to the formation of C5a and C5b. C5b serves as the anchor for the assembly of a single molecule composed of C6, C7, and C8. This MAC (C5b with C6, C7, C8) facilitates polymerization of C9 (up to 18 molecules of C9) into a tube that is inserted into the lipid bilayer of the plasma membrane of, for example, a bacterium. A channel is formed through the cell membrane allowing the passage of ions, small molecules, and water into the bacterium by osmosis. Bacterial lysis ensues. This process can also injure naïve host cells, such as occurs in hemolytic anemias.

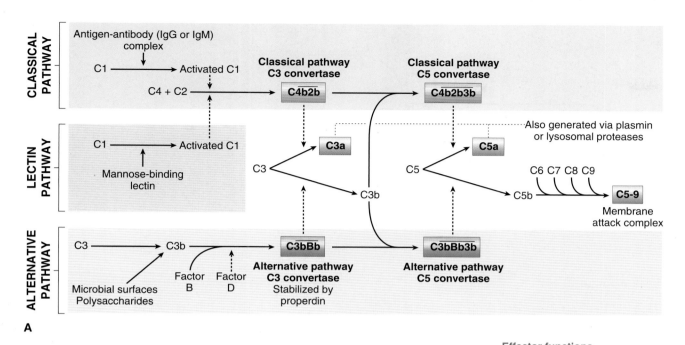

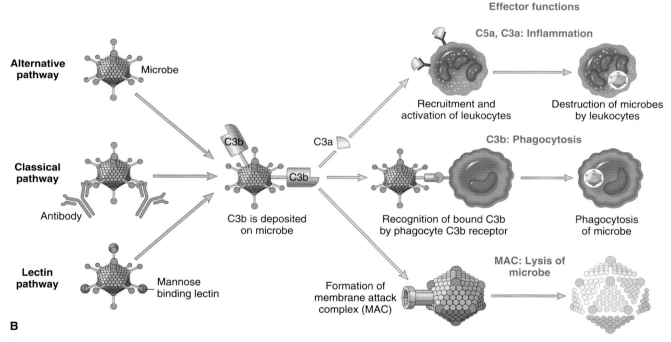

Fig. 3-13   A, Components and pathways of the complement cascade. **B,** Effector functions of the complement system. *IgG,* Immunoglobulin G; *IgM,* immunoglobulin M. *(A and B, From Kumar V, Abbas A, Fausto N: Robbins & Cotran pathologic basis of disease, ed 7, Philadelphia, 2005, Saunders.)*

ARACHIDONIC ACID METABOLITES

When cells are injured by inflammatory stimuli or other chemical mediators of inflammation, their cell membrane lipids are rapidly rearranged to create a variety of biologically active lipid mediators derived from arachidonic acid. Arachidonic acid metabolites are lipid-derived autocoid (acting as a local hormone) mediators of inflammation that serve as intracellular and extracellular signals influencing the coagulation cascade and mediating nearly every step of the acute inflammatory response (Fig. 3-15). Effects are short-lived because these lipid metabolites decay rapidly or

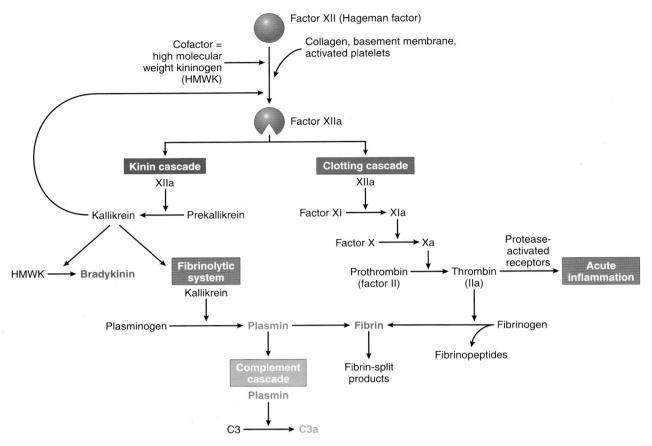

Fig. 3-14 **Interrelationships between the four plasma mediator systems triggered by activation of factor XII (Hageman factor).** Note that thrombin induces inflammation by binding to protease-activated receptors (PARs) (principally PAR-1) on platelets, endothelium, smooth muscle cells, and other cells. *(From Kumar V, Abbas A, Fausto N: Robbins & Cotran pathologic basis of disease, ed 7, Philadelphia, 2005, Saunders.)*

are destroyed by enzymes. Arachidonic acid metabolites include prostaglandins, leukotrienes, and lipoxins and encompass the cyclooxygenase (COX) and lipoxygenase pathways.

Arachidonic acid (eicosatetraenoic acid) is an essential 20-carbon fatty acid derived from linoleic acid, which is present in plasma membranes of dietary red meats. It is an integral component of esterified membrane phospholipids and serves as the major precursor for eicosanoids. Eicosanoids are synthesized by two important classes of enzymes: (1) cyclooxygenases and (2) lipoxygenases, and their respective products (eicosanoids) are: (1) prostaglandins and thromboxanes and (2) leukotrienes and lipoxins. These molecules are synthesized in endothelial cells, leukocytes, and platelets and principally exert their biologic effects on vascular and airway smooth muscle cells, endothelial cells, and platelets during the acute inflammatory response.

Arachidonic acid is released from membrane phospholipids of many cell types, but particularly endothelial cells and leukocytes, through the action of cytoplasmic phospholipase A_2 (cPLA$_2$) and to a lesser degree, soluble (extracellular) phospholipase A_2 (sPLA$_2$). This outcome occurs in response to physical and chemical stimuli including C5a. cPLA$_2$ is translocated from the endoplasmic reticulum to plasma membrane when intracellular calcium concentrations increase. The activity of sPLA$_2$ also requires the participation of calcium; however, its contribution to the formation of intracellular arachidonic acid varies among the different cell types when compared with that of cPLA$_2$. Membrane phospholipids contain a glycerol backbone attached to which is often a saturated fatty acid at the sn-1 position, an unsaturated fatty acid at the sn-2 position, and a base at the sn-3 position. Arachidonic acid is often in the sn-2 position and released by cPLA$_2$ or sPLA$_2$ to become free arachidonic acid.

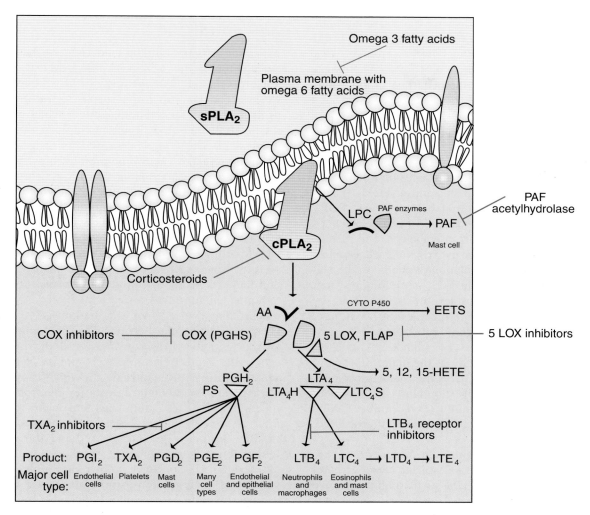

Fig. 3-15   Key inflammatory mediators derived from the plasma membrane.
Cytoplasmic phospholipase A_2 *(cPLA$_2$)* activity on the plasma membrane leads to free arachidonic acid *(AA)* and lysophosphatidylcholine *(LPC)*. Arachidonic acid metabolites include prostaglandins and leukotrienes, and LPC is a substrate for platelet-activating factor *(PAF)*. The type of prostaglandin formed by a cell is dependent on the cell type. Platelets, for example, form thromboxane, whereas endothelial cells form prostacyclin. Leukotrienes are formed by leukocytes. Inhibitors specific to the various enzymes or products are listed in red. *COX*, Cyclooxygenase; *EETs*, epoxyeicosatrienoics; *FLAP*, 5-lipoxygenase-activating protein; *HETE*, hydroxyeicosatetraenoic acid; *LOX*, lipoxygenase; *LTA$_4$, LTB$_4$, LTC$_4$, LTE$_4$*, leukotrienes A$_4$, B$_4$, C$_4$, and E$_4$, respectively; *LTA$_4$H*, leukotriene A$_4$ hydrolase; *LTC$_4$S*, leukotriene C$_4$ synthase; *PGD$_2$, PGE$_2$, PGF$_2$, PGH$_2$, PGI$_2$*, prostaglandins D$_2$, E$_2$, F$_2$, H$_2$, and I$_2$, respectively; *PGHS*, prostaglandin H synthase; *PS*, polysaccharides; *sPLA$_2$*, soluble phospholipase A$_2$; *TXA$_2$*, thromboxane A$_2$.
(Redrawn with permission from Dr. M.R. Ackermann, College of Veterinary Medicine, Iowa State University.)

Free arachidonic acid is metabolized in one of three pathways: (1) the COX pathway for the formation of prostaglandins and thromboxanes; (2) the lipoxygenase pathway for the formation of leukotrienes and lipoxins; and (3) the cytochrome p450 pathway for the formation of epoxyeicosatrienoic acids (HPETE and HETE). There are three COX isoenzymes—COX-1, COX-2, and COX-3—that are actually components of prostaglandin H

synthase and work in concert with a peroxidase heme group. The COX-1 isoenzyme is constitutively expressed, is present in almost all tissues, and is considered a housekeeping enzyme with physiologic roles in hemostasis and gastroprotection. COX-2 isoenzyme expression is induced by exogenous and endogenous stimuli and occurs locally in sites of inflammation. It is present in leukocytes, endothelial cells of blood vessels, and synovial fibroblasts. COX-3 isoenzyme is a splice variant of COX-1 (and also termed COX-1b or COX-1v). It is present in greatest abundance in the cerebral cortex of dogs and human beings and is also detected in human aortas and rodent cerebral endothelia, heart, kidney, and neuronal tissues.

PROSTAGLANDIN FORMATION AND INHIBITION

Arachidonic acid metabolites from COX isoenzymes induce an intermediate prostaglandin, PGH_2 that is converted into at least five metabolites (PGD_2, PGF_2, PGE_2, PGI_2, and TXA_2) by prostanoid synthase enzymes unique for each of these five metabolites. The relative concentration of each of these five types of prostaglandins synthesized following stimulation depends on the cell type stimulated. For example, PGI_2–a thromboresistant prostaglandin termed prostacyclin–is produced by endothelial cells via PGI_2 (prostacyclin) synthase, whereas TXA_2–a thrombogenic prostaglandin termed thromboxane–is produced by platelets via TXA_2 (thromboxane) synthase. PGD_2 is the major prostanoid produced by mast cells; PGE_2 is the major prostanoid produced by epithelial cells, fibroblasts, and smooth muscle cells. These factors inhibit (PGI_2), induce (TXA_2) coagulation/thrombosis, or affect vascular permeability (PGD and PGE).

Aspirin, indomethacin, ibuprofen, and naproxen are COX-1 inhibitors (Fig. 3-15). Aspirin, naproxen, and ibuprofen also inhibit COX-2, as do the highly selective COX-2 inhibitor drugs celecoxib, rofecoxib, valdecoxib, lumiracoxib, and etoricoxib. Acetaminophen inhibits COX-3 in dogs; however, acetaminophen's activity in human beings and rodents is less clear. Because COX-3 is present in greatest abundance in the cerebral cortex and acetaminophen crosses the blood-brain barrier (unlike other NSAIDs), these observations were initially thought to explain why acetaminophen was sometimes more effective for treating headaches and pain relief and less effective in inhibiting inflammation in the body. Although this may be the case in dogs, the mechanistic basis of acetaminophen's activity in human beings is not fully understood at this time. Acetaminophen may inhibit COX-2 to a minor degree and also slightly inhibit COX-3 (COX-1b), and yet have other activity/activities. Much of the antiinflammatory effect of corticosteroids is due to their inhibition of phospholipase A_2, the enzyme that releases arachidonic acid from membrane phospholipids. Corticosteroids signal the cell to synthesize a polypeptide known as lipocortin (lipomodulin), which then acts to inhibit phospholipase A_2. Therefore the antiinflammatory effect of corticosteroids is delayed. A variety of other natural and synthetic compounds can inhibit phospholipase A_2.

LEUKOTRIENE FORMATION AND INHIBITION

In leukocytes, arachidonic acid can also be metabolized through the 5-lipoxygenase pathway to form leukotrienes and lipoxins (Fig. 3-15). 5-Lipoxygenase works in concert with 5-lipoxygenase activating protein as an arachidonic acid binding protein, which optimizes the proximity of 5-lipoxygenase to interact with arachidonic acid. The complex formed by 5-lipoxygenase and 5-lipoxygenase activating protein called 5-HPETE (hydroperoxyeicosatetraenoic acid) is converted to an intermediate complex, leukotriene A_4, which is subsequently converted to either leukotriene B_4 or leukotriene C_4, via leukotriene A_4 hydrolase or leukotriene C_4 synthetase, respectively. Leukotriene C_4 synthetase is a glutathione transferase, and once leukotriene C_4 is secreted from a cell, it is metabolized to leukotriene D_4 and leukotriene E_4 by sequential removal of the glutathione, glutamic acid, and glycine moieties.

The major effects of the leukotrienes include: (1) increased vascular permeability, (2) chemotaxis for leukocytes, and (3) vasoconstriction, all of which exacerbate the acute inflammatory response. Neutrophils produce primarily leukotriene B_4, which is one of the most potent chemotactic factors for neutrophils and macrophages. It also stimulates leukocytes to release their lysosomal contents. Mast cells and eosinophils produce primarily leukotriene C_4, and the group of leukotrienes–leukotriene C_4, leukotriene D_4, and leukotriene E_4, formerly known as "slow reacting substance"–causes intense vascular leakage from the venules. Macrophages produce both leukotriene B_4 and leukotriene C_4. In addition to the leukotrienes, 5-HPETE and its end product 5-HETE (hydroxyeicosatetraenoic acid) are highly chemotactic for neutrophils and macrophages.

Lipoxins, secreted primarily by platelets, are also produced from arachidonic acid via the lipoxygenase pathway. Platelets cannot form lipoxins directly, but through cell-to-cell interactions with leukocytes and the transfer of arachidonic acid metabolites to platelets, cooperation between different cells types can result in the formation of eicosanoids via transcellular biosynthesis. Neutrophils can transfer their leukotriene A_4 to platelets. Platelets contain 12-lipooxygenase, which converts the neutrophil derived and transferred leukotriene A_4 to lipoxin A_4 and lipoxin B_4. Lipoxins have proinflammatory and antiinflammatory effects and appear to counteract the effects of leukotrienes. They stimulate macrophage adhesion to endothelial cells in blood vessels, but inhibit neutrophil adhesion and chemotaxis. Lipoxin A_4 causes vasodilation and dampens the actions of leukotriene C_4-induced vasoconstriction.

The 5-lipoxygenase pathway can be inhibited by a variety of new chemical agents (5-lipoxygenase inhibitors and leukotriene receptor antagonists) (Fig. 3-15). In addition, eosinophils release arylsulfatase from granules, which inactivates leukotrienes.

OMEGA 3 FATTY ACIDS (FISH OILS) AND INHIBITION OF EICOSANOID ACTIVITY

Many studies have demonstrated that omega 3 fatty polyunsaturated fatty acids, which are in high concentrations in certain fish, can reduce inflammatory responses, particularly prostaglandin and leukotriene activity (Fig. 3-15). This effect occurs because omega 3 fatty acids, when acted upon by phospholipase A and subsequent enzymes, form the "3" series of prostaglandins (thromboxane A_3) and the "5" series of leukotrienes (LTB_5) instead of the "2" series of prostaglandins (thromboxane A_2) and the "4" series of leukotrienes (LTB_4), which occur with omega 6 fatty acids. The "3" and "5" series of prostaglandins and leukotrienes derived from omega 3 fatty acids are less biologically active than their omega 6 series counterparts. Roughly two thirds of the polyunsaturated fatty acids in the body have an omega 6 structure; the remaining have an omega 3 structure. This two-thirds to one-third ratio can be altered by consumption of diets high in fish oils and thereby result in more omega 3 in the tissue and less active prostaglandin and leukotriene products.

PLATELET-ACTIVATING FACTOR

PAF is another potent molecule of phospholipid origin derived from cell membranes of platelets, basophils, mast cells, neutrophils, macrophages, and endothelial cells. PAF has potent pathophysiologic effects and contributes to inflammation, endotoxic shock, and allergic reactions (asthma) through vasoconstriction, bronchoconstriction, platelet aggregation, and leukocyte adhesion, chemotaxis, and degranulation. However, at low concentrations (experimentally induced), PAF can cause vasodilation and increased vascular permeability. PAF also contributes to the inflammatory response by increasing the oxidative burst in neutrophils following phagocytosis of bacteria and enhances the synthesis of eicosanoids by leukocytes. PAF can also cause platelet aggregation followed by release of serotonin and histamine when mast cells are degranulated in response to PAF released during IgE-mediated hypersensitivities in the lung. Thus platelet aggregation can increase vascular permeability in acquired immunologic responses and result in inflammation.

LysoPAF acetyltransferase (lysoPAF-AT) and PAF-synthesizing phosphocholinetransferase (PAF-PCT) are two enzymes that control the final synthesis of PAF from lipid membranes and thus promote PAF production. PAF mediates its effects on target cells through a single G protein–coupled receptor. These receptors have been identified on endothelium, neutrophils, eosinophils, macrophages, smooth muscle, and glial cells in the brain, and thus to a certain extent an autocoid regulatory system exists. PAF activity is reduced/regulated by PAF acetylhydrolase, which is expressed in the previously listed target cells. PAF acetylhydrolase degrades PAF through hydrolysis of its acetate moiety in the *sn-2* position of glycerol and thus inhibits the proinflammatory activity of PAF. PAF acetylhydrolase is thus potentially an enzyme that could be used for the development of drugs to reduce inflammatory responses.

CYTOKINE FAMILY
OVERVIEW

Cytokines are a group of proteins produced by many cell types including lymphocytes (lymphokines), macrophages (monokines), endothelial cells, neutrophils, basophils, mast cells, eosinophils, epithelial cells, and connective tissue cells (Appendix 3-1). Their primary purpose is to modulate, via enhancement or suppression, the functional expression of other cell types during the inflammatory response. Chemokines are produced from almost all cell types and are cytokines that promote leukocyte chemotaxis and migration across capillaries and postcapillary venules. Cytokines also play major roles in: (1) hematopoiesis, including granulopoiesis by cytokines, such as IL-3 and G-CSF; and (2) adaptive immunity, such as the proliferation of lymphocytes by cytokines, including IL-2, and activation of T_H1 or T_H2 responses by IL-10 and IL-12, respectively. More than 29 major cytokines are now recognized, which have been organized into the following categories according to their principal functional activities:

- Hematopoietic growth factors, including IL-3, GM-CSF, possibly IL-9, IL-11, and stem cell factor
- Inflammatory mediators, which induce acute phase reactants and natural immunity (IL-1, IL-6, TNF)
- Chemotactic cytokines (IL-8)
- T-cell proliferation, activation, and differentiation cytokines (ILs 2, 4, 5, 7, 9, 10, 12 on up to IL-29)

Concerning T-lymphocyte activity, there are cytokines and proteins that exert lymphocyte regulatory activity (interferon [IFN]-γ, TGF-β). Of particular importance in allergic disease is the recognition of the control of dendritic cells by T-lymphocyte regulatory cells that release IL-4 and IL-10, and two lineages of T-lymphocyte helper cells (T_H1 and T_H2). Dendritic cells (part of the monocyte-macrophage system) are cells of the adaptive immune system. They are present in tissue in contact with the environment and include Langerhans' cells of the skin and dendritic cells of the mucosal surfaces of the respiratory and alimentary systems. They are sentinel cells constantly monitoring for and phagocytosing microbes and foreign materials. In cooperation with lymphocytes and macrophages in lymphoid tissue, they act as antigen presenting cells to activate T helper cells and cytotoxic T cells and B cells. The T_H1 lineage, normally driven by IL-12 and IFN-γ, induces cell-mediated immune responses within specific diseases, such as the granulomatous inflammatory response to mycobacterial infections, whereas the T_H2 cells induce humoral responses and humoral-related diseases, such as asthma and atopy.

Biochemically, cytokines can be divided into type I and type II cytokines. Type I cytokines have four α helix units. Type II cytokines have six α helix units and are likely derived from a single ancestral gene. Type I and II cytokines bind receptors specific for the I and II ligand structures. Despite the similarities within type I and type II cytokines and their receptors, there is still much diversity in structure and function of cytokines within each type.

CYTOKINE RECEPTORS AND SIGNALING

Cytokine activity can be altered in several ways, usually via binding to and activating cytokine receptors. Briefly, there are class I cytokine receptors (receptors for IL-2 through IL-9, IL-11 through ILs 13, 15, 21, 23, 27, erythropoietin (EPO), G-CSF, GM-CSF, leptin, and others) and class II cytokine receptors (receptors for IFN-α, IFN-β, IFN-γ, and ILs 10, 19, 20, 22, 24, 26, 28, and 29). EPO agonists are commonly used for patients with anemia and are drugs abused by endurance athletes, such as marathoners, cross-country skiers, and cyclists. Other G-CSF agonists, such as Neupogen (Amgen Inc., Thousand Oaks, Calif), increase granulopoiesis and are commonly used for cancer patients with decreased blood neutrophil levels (neutropenia) secondary to chemotherapy. Agonists have also been developed for IFN-β.

Many cytokine receptors, including those for the interferons IL-2 through IL-7, IL-11, IL-13, erythropoietin, and GM-CSF, activate the JAK/STAT signaling pathway (Fig. 3-16). JAK stands for Janus kinase, and STAT is an abbreviation for signal transducer and activator of transcription. Members of the JAK family are cytoplasmic protein tyrosine kinases physically associated with ligand-bound receptors. JAK phosphorylates amino acids in a protein on STAT, and STAT dimers (a molecule consisting of two identical simpler molecules) enter the nucleus to bind DNA and induce transcription and the expression of specific gene products and cellular responses to activation. There are three isoforms of JAK (JAK1 to JAK3) and a fourth JAK family member TYK2. All of these have slightly different activities depending on the stimulus. JAK1, for example, is integral to lymphocyte development,

whereas JAK2 mediates erythropoiesis. There are several isoforms in the STAT family including STAT 1 to 6, which also have subtle signaling differences. STAT 1 and 2 are especially involved with interferon signaling, STAT 3 mediates responses to pathogens, STAT 4 is involved with T_H1/IL-12 activity, STAT 5 mediates cell growth and natural killer (NK) growth, and STAT 6 mediates T_H2 responses. Suppressors of cytokine signaling (SOCS) are signaling proteins that inhibit activity of some cytokines whose receptors induce the JAK/STAT pathway of signaling through the inhibition of JAK. Protein tyrosine phosphatases (PTPs) such as SHP2 (SH2-domain–containing PTP) can inhibit JAK and STAT. Phosphorylated STAT proteins in the nucleus can be inhibited by PIAS (protein inhibitor of activated signal transducer and activator of transcription) proteins as well. These proteins regulate the activity of cytokine activity on cells, and as discussed later, these pathways may be potentially useful as a mechanism to target and inhibit specific components of the acute inflammatory response with existing or newly developed antiinflammatory drugs.

TNF-α receptors are trimers of three identical cell surface transmembrane proteins. Binding of the receptor triggers phosphorylation of I kappa B (IKB) and thereby allows release of IKB from nuclear factor (NF) kappa B in the cytosol. IKB becomes ubiquinated and degraded, and NF kappa B moves to the nucleus, where it binds promoter and enhancer regions of DNA of more than 60 genes, including genes for IL-1 and other cytokines, and genes for cell proliferation, cell adhesion, and angiogenesis. TNF can also bind receptors that lead to apoptosis.

Cytokine activity can also be inhibited. Nonspecific inhibitors include corticosteroids, aspirin, and ibuprofen. More precisely, "molecular" inhibitors can inhibit cytokine activity through anticytokine antibodies, such as anti-TNF MAb (Remicade, Centocor Inc., Horsham, Penn), or the blockage of receptors, such as soluble TNF-R (Embrel, Wyeth Pharmaceuticals, Madison, NJ). Specific inhibitors are also under development for cytokine receptors including SOCS and PTP.

CYTOKINES THAT REGULATE NATURAL KILLER CELL FORMATION AND ACTIVITY

IL-21 has been recently described and appears to regulate differentiation and apoptotic death induced by NK cells. NK cells are specialized to kill certain types of target cells, such as tumor cells or cells infected with viruses that may be the underlying cause of inflammation. NK cells are considered lymphocytes but do not express T-cell receptors or CD3, an antigen expressed on the surface of T lymphocytes; however, they do have an intrinsic ability to engage in perforin-mediated killing. NK cells secrete specialized granules

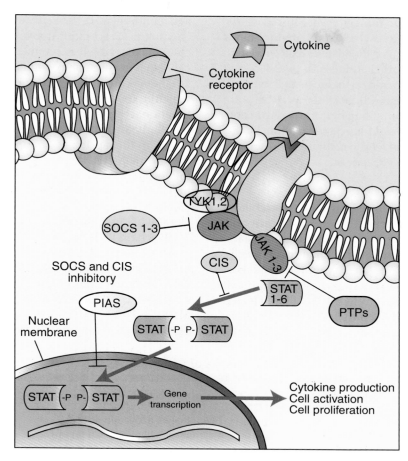

Fig. 3-16   **Several families of cytokines activate the JAK/STAT (Janus kinase/signal transducer and activator of transcription) pathway.** The STAT class of proteins function both as a signal transducer and transcription activator. Activation of STAT involves dimerization and phosphorylation by JAK, a tyrosine kinase. Signaling by JAK/STAT proteins is regulated by proteins such as the SOCS (suppressor of cytokine signaling). JAK/STAT signaling leads to transcription of genes that drive inflammatory responses, including cell activation, immune regulation, and cell proliferation. *CIS,* Cytokine-inducible SH2 domain-containing protein; *PIAS,* protein inhibitor of activated signal; *PTPs,* protein tyrosine phosphatases; *TYK,* tyrosine kinase (of the JAK family). *(Modified from Leonard W: Nat Rev Immunol 1:200-208, 2001.)*

that contain potent cytotoxic molecules, such as perforin, which cause lysis of target cells on contact. Inactive NK cells can be stimulated by Flt-3 ligand, a hematopoietic cytokine that stimulates proliferation of dendritic cells and antitumor immune responses, and also by IL-4, IL-12, IL-15, and IL-21. Once activated, IL-21 induces NK cell differentiation and upregulation of CD16, the low affinity IgG receptor necessary for antibody-dependent cellular cytotoxicity, and also NK release of IFN-γ required for macrophage and dendritic cell activation. Finally, IL-21 initiates a delayed apoptotic program for death of the differentiated NK cell and prevents recruitment of uninvolved NK cells.

PROTEINS WITH CYTOKINE-LIKE FUNCTIONS
HIGH MOBILITY GROUP BOX PROTEIN-1

High mobility group box protein-1 (HMGB-1) is a nonhistone nuclear protein that has cytokine-like functions. It was first described as a nonhistone chromosome protein transcription and replication regulator, a nucleosome stabilizer, a mediator of cell differentiation, a regulator of metastasis by neoplastic cells, and a mediator of neurite outgrowth. Now HMGB-1 is recognized as a mediator of endotoxemia, sepsis, inflammation, and sickness behavior (nausea and the feeling of being ill or sick). IL-1, TNF, and interferons induce macrophages to secrete HMGB-1 and lysophosphatidylcholine; the latter molecule plays a key role in the response of monocytes to LPS released from gram-negative bacteria. HMGB-1, an advanced glycosylation end product, binds macrophage RAGE (receptor for advanced glycosylation end products), which further induces IL-1, TNF-α, and IFN-γ release. HMGB-1 and cytokines—such as IL-1, TNF, IL-6—and prostaglandins such as PGE$_2$ are involved with hypothalamic function in food aversion, hypophagia, anorexia, weight loss, and sickness behavior (see later discussion of febrile response) and serve to amplify the inflammatory response.

CHEMOKINES

Chemokines, released in response to inflammatory stimuli, are secreted proteins that induce neutrophil, macrophage, and lymphocyte chemotaxis into inflammatory exudates. They also activate inflammatory cells, induce antiviral activity, regulate immune responses, and induce hematopoiesis, angiogenesis, and cell growth. Chemokines are produced by all nucleated cells in the body, including epithelial cells, fibroblasts, macrophages, mast cells, keratinocytes, dendritic cells,

and endothelial cells. Leukocytes secrete all types of chemokines, except for fractalkine (used for monocyte chemotaxis), which is produced by nonhematopoietic cells such as vascular endothelial cells.

Chemokines can be classified based on biochemical structure (position of their cysteine residues) or by the functional behavior they induce (inflammatory or homing). Structural classification of chemokines is based on their primary amino acid structure depending on their cysteine residues that induce secondary folding (Table 3-8). Most numerous are the chemokines in: (1) the CC family, which bind the CCR (receptor); (2) the CXC family, which bind the CXCR, (3) the XC chemokine lymphotactin, which binds CR, and (4) the CX3C chemokine fractalkine, which binds CX3CR.

The functional classification of chemokines includes inflammatory chemokines or homing chemokines. Inflammatory chemokines (IL-8, GCP-2, ENA-78, Gro, NAP-2, IP-10, Mig, I-Tac, RANTES, MIP-1-α and MIP-1-β, HCC-1, MCP 1 to 5, and eotaxins 1 to 3) are expressed by resident cells and infiltrating leukocytes

Table **3-8** **Name, Abbreviation, and Common Name of Chemokines**

Name	Abbreviation	Common Name
CCL1	TCA	T-lymphocyte activation (I-309)
CCL2	MCP-1	Macrophage chemotactic protein-1
CCL3	MIP-1-α	Macrophage inflammatory protein-1-α
CCL4	MIP-1-β	Macrophage inflammatory protein-1-β
CCL5	RANTES	Regulated on activation, normal T lymphocytes expressed and secreted
CCL7	MCP-3	Macrophage chemotactic protein-3
CCL8	MCP-2	Macrophage chemotactic protein-2
CCL11		Eotaxin-1
CCL12	MCP-5	Macrophage chemotactic protein-5
CCL13	MCP-4	Macrophage chemotactic protein-4
CCL17	TARC	Thymus and activation-regulated cytokine
CCL19	MIP-3-β	Macrophage inflammatory protein-3-β
CCL20	LARC/MIP-3-α	Liver and activation-regulated chemokine/Macrophage inflammatory protein-3-α
CCL21	SLC	Secondary lymphoid organ chemokine
CCL22	MDC	Macrophage-derived chemoattractant
CCL24		Eotaxin-2
CCL26		Eotaxin-3
CXCL1	Gro-α	Growth-related oncogene-α
CXCL2	Gro-β	Growth-related oncogene-β
CXCL3	Gro-γ	Growth-related oncogene-γ
CXCL5	ENA-78	Epithelial neutrophil-activating peptide-78
CXCL6	GCP-2	Granulocyte chemotactic protein-2
CXCL8	IL-8 (NAP-1)	Interleukin-8
CXCL9	MIG	Monokine induced by γ-interferon
CXCL10	IP-10	Interferon-inducible protein
CXCL11	ITAC	Interferon-inducible T lymphocyte α chemoattractant
CXCL12	SDF-1	Stromal derived factor-1
CXCL13	BCA-1/BLC	B lymphocyte attracting chemokine
CXCL14	BRAK	Breast and kidney expressed chemokine
CXCL16		

Table **3-9**   **Chemokine Ligands of the C-C and C-X-C Families and Their Receptors**

Family	Ligand	Receptor
C-C	CCL 3, 7, 9, 15, 16, 23	CCR1
	CCL 2, 7, 8, 12, 13	CCR2
	CCL 5, 7, 8, 11, 13, 24, 26	CCR3
	CCL 17, 22	CCR4
	CCL 3, 4, 5	CCR5
	CCL 20	CCR6
	CCL 19, 21	CCR7
	CCL 1, 16, 17	CCR8
	CCL 25	CCR9
	CCL 27, 28	CCR10
	CCL 2, 7, 8, 11, 12, 13	CCR11
C-X-C	CXCL 1, 6, 7, 8	CXCR1
	CXCL 1, 2, 3, 5, 6, 7, 8	CXCR2
	CXCL 9, 10, 11	CXCR3
	CXCL 12	CXCR4
	CXCL 13	CXCR5
	CXCL 14	Unknown
	CXCL 16	CXCR6

in response to cytokines, bacterial toxins, and other agents during the acute inflammatory response. Receptors for these chemokines include CXCR1, 2, 3 and CCR1, 2, 3, and 5; these receptors often bind several different chemokines (Table 3-9). Chemokines for leukocyte homing are generally produced constitutively in lymphoid tissue. Receptors for these chemokines are usually present on lymphocytes and dendritic cells, and they typically bind only one or maybe two chemokines. The expression of receptors by these cells varies with the state of cellular differentiation, thereby preventing immature cells from entering the wrong location. For example, naïve cells express CCR1-10 and CXCR1-3,5 as well as CR1 and CX3CR1; memory T lymphocytes express CCR 8-10, CXCR1,2,4,5, and CR1 but do not express CCR1-7, CXR3, and CXCR31. Commonly studied chemokines include IL-8, MCP-1 (macrophage chemotactic protein), RANTES, IP-10, SDF-1, and eotaxin.

CHEMOKINE RECEPTORS AND SIGNALING

Chemokines are the only cytokines that bind G protein–coupled seven transmembrane (7TM) spanning receptors, and although chemokines are relatively small (8 to 10 kDa), they are somewhat large for the 7TM receptor family, which also binds larger proteins such as histamine, dopamine, and serotonin. Once bound, the 7TM receptor activates a G protein, which initiates production of second messengers, most commonly cyclic adenosine monophosphate (cAMP) and inositol 1,4,5-triphosphate IP_3. cAMP and IP_3, in turn, phosphorylate enzymes and stimulate the release of calcium. Enzymatic activity induced by cAMP activates the transcription factor CREB (cAMP response element binding protein). Chemokine receptors bound by ligand are endocytosed and either recycled or degraded by the cell.

Experimentally, chemokines can be inhibited at several stages: (1) inhibition of interaction between the ligand and the glycosylated molecules on the cell surface, (2) inhibition of ligand/receptor binding, (3) inhibition of receptor activity, and (4) inhibition of cell signaling. The development of new drugs to treat specific aspects of inflammatory diseases will likely target one or all of these pathways in the chemokine cascade.

OXYGEN-DERIVED FREE RADICALS AND NITRIC OXIDE

Free radicals such as superoxide anion, hydroxy radical, and nitric oxide derivatives result in lipoperoxidation of phospholipid membranes, damage to DNA molecules resulting in strand breaks and adduct formation, and oxidization of signaling molecules—thus affecting (increasing or decreasing) cytokine and other signaling pathways. The oxidative radicals can: (1) injure vascular endothelial cells, leading to increased vascular permeability: (2) inactivate antiproteases, such as α_1-antitrypsin, resulting in damage to extracellular matrix proteins; (3) enhance cytokine expression secondary to signaling changes and cell damage; (4) activate endothelial cells and increase adhesion molecule expression; and (5) increase the formation of chemotactic factors (LTB_4). They can also inactivate neurotransmitters (adrenaline and noradrenaline), leading to hypotension.

Oxygen-derived free radicals are released from neutrophils and macrophages following exposure to chemokines and immune complexes, and after phagocytosis by the leukocyte. They damage cells through peroxidation of cell membrane lipids, cross-linking of proteins, cleaving glycoconjugates, directly damaging DNA phosphate backbone and bases, and inducing the formation of DNA adducts. Fortunately, the body has antioxidants that are: (1) enzymatic, such as superoxide dismutase (SOD isoforms 1, 2, and 3), catalase, and glutathione peroxidase; (2) nonenzymatic, such as ceruloplasmin, transferrin, and melatonin; and (3) nonenzymatic dietary substances, such as vitamins A, C, and E and lycopenes, flavonoids, genistein, and reserpines. All of these minimize the damage to tissue caused by free radicals.

Nitric oxide is a chemical mediator of inflammation that causes vasodilation by relaxing vascular smooth muscle cells. In response to injury and inflammatory stimuli, nitric oxide derivatives are synthesized by endothelial cells, macrophages, and specific populations of neurons in the brain from L-arginine, molecular oxygen, NADPH, other cofactors, and the enzyme nitric oxide synthase (NOS). There are three forms of nitric oxide synthase that mediate nitric oxide formation: neuronal (nNOS), inducible (iNOS), and endothelial (eNOS). In addition to its vasodilatory activities, nitric oxide inhibits platelet aggregation and adhesion, inhibits mast cell-induced inflammation, oxidizes lipids and other molecules, and regulates leukocyte chemotaxis.

RECEPTORS FOR EXOGENOUS AND ENDOGENOUS INFLAMMATORY STIMULI AND TOLL-LIKE RECEPTORS

TLRs are a family of pattern-recognition receptors (PRRs) in mammals that can distinguish between chemically diverse classes of genetically conserved microbial products (Table 3-10). These receptors play a central role in the release of inflammatory cytokines from the innate immune system in response to microbial structures, such as exogenous microbial substances and endogenous products. In addition, TLRs likely play a role in the adaptive immune response, which develops during the acute inflammatory response.

Exogenous microbial products, often with redundant molecular structure, are termed pathogen associated molecular patterns (PAMPs) and include substances such as LPS, peptidoglycan, and lipoteichoic acid.

PAMPs can bind several types of receptors (PRRs). These receptors include secreted receptors that circulate in the blood (LPS binding protein), surface receptors (macrophage mannose receptors), nucleotide-binding oligomerization domain (NOD) receptors, and surface receptors (TLRs) of the TLR family (Fig. 3-17, Table 3-10). These receptors have different mechanisms by which they activate the cell and some work together. LPS, for example, is bound by LPS binding protein which, in turn, binds CD14 and TLR4. The formation of a PRR-PAMP complex initiates transmembrane signaling that often involves a MyD88 protein event leading to NF kappa B activation and MAPK (p38) signaling. The NF kappa B family of transcription factors initiates gene transcription and translation, resulting in the expression of proteins involved in many cellular processes such as cell proliferation, differentiation, apoptosis, and cell responses to injury, stress, and external pathogens (Fig. 3-18). NF kappa B and p38 then can induce phagocytosis by leukocytes, dendritic cell activation, release of inflammatory cytokines and chemokines, and the activation of the innate (defensin and antimicrobial peptide release) and adaptive (T_H1 and T_H2 activity) immune systems. On some occasions,

Table 3-10   Types of Pathogen Associated Molecular Pattern (PAMP) Exogenous Ligands, Their Pattern Recognition Receptors (PRRs), and the Subsequent Action Related to Acute Inflammation

Exogenous PAMP Ligands	Secreted PRRs	Action
Mannose	Mannan-binding lectin (MBP)	Complement activation
Microbial membranes	C-reactive protein (CRP) and serum amyloid protein (SAP)	Opsin, complement activation
Lipopolysaccharide (LPS)	LPS-binding protein (LBP)	LPS binding
	Cell Surface PRRs	
LPS, peptidoglycan	CD14	Co-receptor for TLR
Mannose	Macrophage mannose receptor	Phagocytosis
Bacterial cell walls	MARCO	Phagocytosis
	Intracellular PRRs	
dsRNA	dsRNA activated protein kinase	NF kappa B and MAPK signaling
Peptidoglycans	Nucleotide-binding oligomerization domain (NOD)	NF kappa B and MAPK signaling
Numerous ligands (Table 3-12)	Toll-like receptors (TLR)	NF kappa B and MAPK signaling
Endogenous PAMP ligands	**Endogenous PRPs**	**Action**
Heparan sulfate, hyaluronic acid, heat shock protein 60 and 70, endoplasmic reticulum glycoprotein 96, fibronectin, fibrinogen, surfactant protein A	Growth factor receptors, CD44, Toll-like receptors, TGF-βR, gp IIb/IIIa, surfactant protein receptor 210 (myosin XVIIIA)	Numerous cellular responses including cellular activation, proliferation, and/or apoptosis

Data from Medzhitov R: *Nat Rev Immunol* 1:135-142, 2001.
Endogenous inflammatory stimuli are those produced by host cells.
gp, Glycoprotein; *MAPK*, mitogen-activated protein kinase; *MARCO*, class A scavenger receptor macrophage receptor with collagenous structure; *NF*, nuclear factor; *TGF-βR*, transforming growth factor-β receptor.

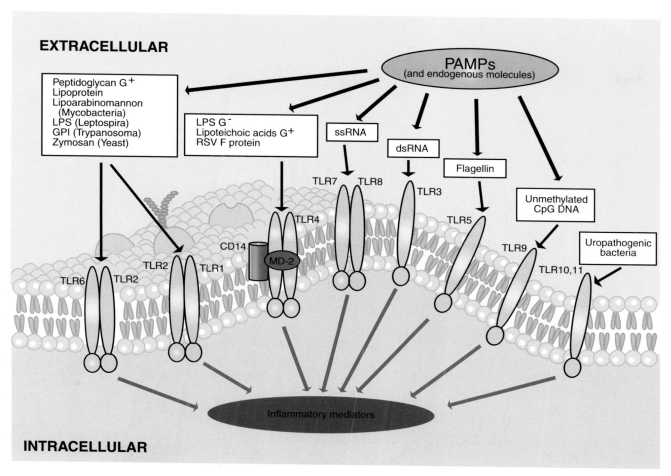

Fig. 3-17 **Pathogen associated molecular patterns (*PAMPs*).** PAMPs such as lipopolysaccharide (*LPS*), teichoic acid, and CpG, as well as other endogenous substances, have affinities to certain Toll-like receptors (*TLRs*) and result in activation of TLR signaling as well as inflammatory and other responses. Endogenous molecules can also activate TLRs and include: heparan sulfate, hyaluronan, heat shock protein 60 (mitochondria), heat shock protein 70 (cytoplasm), fibronectin, fibrinogen, and surfactant protein A. Ligands for TLR10 are not known; TLR11 ligands include uropathogenic bacteria. *CD14*, LPS binding protein receptor; *CpG*, bacterial cytosine-phosphate-guanine motifs; *GPI*, glycosylphosphatidylinositol; *MD-2*, accessory extracellular adaptor protein that binds TLR4; *RSV*, respiratory syncytial virus. (*Modified from Medzhitov R: Nat Rev Immunol 1:135-142, 2001.*)

TLR4 signaling does not engage MyD88 (MyD88-independent signaling) and results in the formation of interferon-β (IFN-β) and IFN-inducible gene products. Intracellular receptors, such as the NOD receptors, bind peptidoglycan. NOD1 binds to peptidoglycan-derived tripeptide structures, whereas NOD2 binds peptidoglycan-derived muramyl dipeptides. Bound NOD 1 and 2 activate the protein kinase RICK, which then induces NF kappa B activity and eventual secretion of proinflammatory cytokines, such as IL-1 and TNF.

Endogenous molecules (not produced by microbes) such as exudate sulfate, hyaluronan, HSP 60 (mitochondria), HSP 70 (cytoplasm), Gp 96 (endoplasmic reticulum), fibronectin, fibrinogen, and surfactant protein A can also bind PRRs such as TLR4 and initiate cell signaling, inflammation, and activation of the innate immune system (Table 3-10). These molecules are often overlooked when considering acute inflammation in the context of microbial infections, because microbial products, such as teichoic acid and LPS are very potent activators of acute inflammation. However, endogenous molecules likely have a significant role in inflammation generated against neoplastic cells, toxins, and mechanical injury.

ANTIMICROBIAL PEPTIDES AND COLLECTINS

Antimicrobial peptides, such as the α- and β-defensins, cathelicidins, and others—such as anionic peptides,

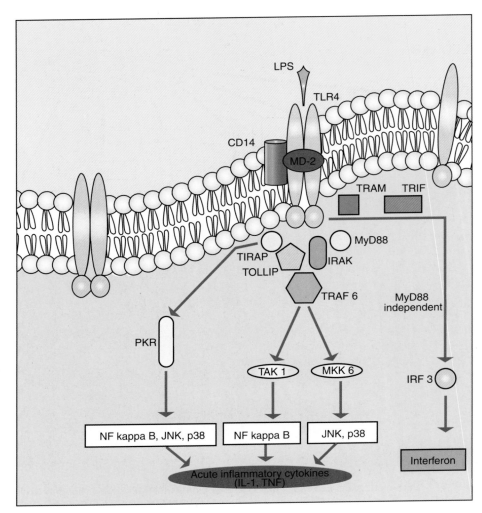

Fig. 3-18 **Toll-like receptor 4** *(TLR4)*. TLR4, when bound by certain microbial or endogenous products, initiates signaling that leads to release of inflammatory cytokines, such as interleukin *(IL-1)* and tumor necrosis factor *(TNF)*, antimicrobial peptides, and molecules that initiate adaptive immunity. Ligand: Lipopolysaccharide *(LPS)*. Selected signaling molecules: Toll/IL-1 receptor (TIR) cytoplasmic domain, cytoplasmic protein adaptors to TIR *(TIRAP, MyD88, TRAF)*, IL-1 receptor-associated kinases *(IRAK)*, dsRNA-responsive protein kinase *(PKR)*, TNF receptor-associated factor 6 *(TRAF 6)*, protein kinase *(TAK 1)*, map-kinase kinase *(MKK)*, interferon regulatory factor 3 *(IRF 3)*. Transcription factors: Nuclear factor kappa B *(NF kappa B)*, c-Jun N-terminal kinase *(JNK)*, p38. *MD-2*, accessory protein; *TRAM*, TRIF-related adaptor molecule; *TRIF*, TIR-containing adaptor inducing interferon-β. *(Modified from Medzhitov R: Nat Rev Immunol 1:135, 2001.)*

histatins, and dermacidins—are small peptides with microbicidal activity against gram-negative and gram-positive bacteria, fungi, mycobacteria, and some enveloped viruses such as human immunodeficiency virus (HIV) (Table 3-11). They are encoded by genes of the cells involved in the inflammatory response, especially neutrophils, and by epithelial cells forming the skin and the mucosal barriers of the respiratory and alimentary systems. The microbicidal activity likely occurs through the formation of pores within bacterial membranes and viral envelopes. In addition to the microbicidal activity, antimicrobial peptides are increasingly becoming appreciated for their role in other nonmicrobial activities related to inflammation and wound repair. These activities include chemotaxis of leukocytes and dendritic cells, cell proliferation, wound repair, cytokine release, and the protease-antiprotease balance. There is also much evidence that antimicrobial peptides link the innate and adaptive immune responses.

There are a wide variety of antimicrobial peptides; however, the defensins have received the most attention for activities other than microbial killing. There are three types of defensins: the α-, β- and θ-defensins.

Table **3-11**   **Inflammatory and Other Activities of Antimicrobial Peptides and Surfactant Proteins**

Antimicrobial Peptide/Protein	Major Cell of Production	Activity
α-Defensins	Enterocytes, leukocytes	Microbicidal activity, induce interleukin-8 production (cryptidins), inhibit angiogenesis (neutrophil α-defensins)
β-Defensins	Epithelia, leukocytes	Microbicidal activity, chemotactic for neutrophils, dendritic cells, other leukocytes, induce cell proliferation
Cathelicidins	Leukocytes, epithelia	Microbicidal activity, induce cytokine and histamine release, regulate cell proliferation, angiogenesis, wound healing, prevent apoptosis (PR-39)
Surfactant proteins A and D	Epithelia	Opsonization of pathogens, macrophage activation

Cryptidins = a type of α-defensin produced by Paneth cells; neutrophil α-defensins = α-defensins produced by human neutrophils; PR-39 = a cathelicidin molecule produced by porcine neutrophils.

α-Defensins are produced by neutrophils and Paneth cells. β-Defensins are produced by neutrophils and epithelial cells. θ-Defensins are produced in neutrophils of primates. The defensins are cationic proteins with three pairs of intramolecular disulfide bonds. α-Defensins and β-defensins can stimulate mast cell degranulation, induce IL-8 synthesis, induce T lymphocyte chemotaxis, and activate T lymphocytes, macrophages, and dendritic cells, thus interconnecting innate and adaptive immunity. The importance of defensins in immunity is underscored by the fact that HIV-1 infected individuals that are healthy and in "remission" have high concentrations of α-defensins, which are thought to enhance T-lymphocyte activity and may also have direct anti–HIV-1 activity.

Collectins are molecules with a collagen-like domain and lectin binding-portion that also activate and regulate inflammatory responses. Surfactant proteins (SPs) are collectins that mediate inflammatory responses in the lung, other areas of the respiratory tract mucosa, and other organs such as the ear canal. There are four surfactant proteins (A, B, C, and D) involved with surfactant production, processing, and regulation in the lung. Two of these, A and D, also regulate inflammatory responses. SP-AD can opsonize and aggregate viral and bacterial pathogens and also activate macrophages, induce uptake of apoptotic cells, and increase or decrease production of TNF and reactive oxygen species in response to infectious agents. SP-AD bind several different receptors that include SIRP (signal inhibitory regulatory protein) and SHP1 (SRC homology SH2 domain containing protein tyrosine phosphatase 1); SP-R210 (surfactant protein receptor 210); TLR2; TLR4; CD91; AND C1qr (complement 1 receptor). Once triggered, these receptors alter NF kappa B activity and inflammatory cell activation. Mannose-binding protein is a collectin produced by hepatocytes (acute phase protein) and is present in the serum. Mannose-binding protein can opsonize pathogens and activate complement. Impaired expression of SP-A, SP-D, and mannose-binding protein is associated with increased susceptibility to infection.

ACUTE PHASE PROTEINS

Acute phase proteins are plasma proteins synthesized in the liver whose concentrations increase (or decrease) by 25% or more during inflammation. These proteins serve as inhibitors or mediators of the inflammatory processes and include C-reactive protein, α_1-acid glycoprotein, haptoglobin, mannose-binding protein, fibrinogen, α_1-antitrypsin, and complement components C3 and C4. The concentration of these acute phase proteins usually increases during inflammation, whereas the concentration of prealbumin and albumin (also acute phase proteins) decreases in inflammation. Acute inflammatory conditions that are severe enough to raise blood plasma concentrations of cytokines, such as IL-1 and TNF, increase the blood concentrations of acute phase proteins. C-reactive protein has recently received attention as a marker of inflammatory conditions, especially atherosclerosis in human beings. In addition to its role diagnostically, C-reactive protein binds to bacteria and fungi and also activates complement. Once acute phase proteins and systemic levels of inflammatory cytokines are elevated, they affect the heart rate, blood pressure, and the hypothalamic regulation of temperature by directly or indirectly stimulating neurons within specific hypothalamic nuclei. The previously described changes also affect respiratory rates and gaseous exchange.

SUMMARY OF THE CHEMICAL MEDIATORS OF ACUTE INFLAMMATION

Various exogenous and endogenous stimuli can activate TLRs, Fc receptors for IgE, or simply cause mechanical or other damage to invoke an acute inflammatory response (Table 3-3). This response can occur very rapidly as the result of the release of preformed or rapidly activated inflammatory mediators such as histamine, kinins, complement factors like C3a and C5a, and tachykinins (substance P). These molecules generally affect vascular caliber and permeability and activate leukocytes and endothelial cells. Concurrently, lipid-based products such as prostaglandins, leukotrienes, and PAF contribute to chemotaxis, vascular tone, and leukocyte activity, all of which work in concert with chemokines and cytokines to activate endothelial cells and leukocytes and enhance neutrophil infiltration. Nitric oxide released by macrophages and endothelia induce vasodilation and also contribute to tissue damage caused by other reactive oxygen species. Inflammatory mediators bind receptors that subsequently induce cytoplasmic signaling and cellular activation, resulting in the production of additional cytokines, adhesion molecules, and other inflammatory mediators that may either exacerbate or inhibit the inflammatory process. Activated neutrophils expressing leukocyte adhesion molecules, such as the integrins, enter inflamed tissue and can release hydrolytic enzymes and other granule contents that further damage tissue. Systemically, increases in acute phase proteins and cytokines can affect body temperature, cardiovascular function, locomotion, sleep, appetite, and other activities.

As the previously described process has been studied over the years, therapeutic intervention to regulate the inflammatory process has become more precise. Early on, some home remedies, such as the use of the bark of the willow tree (*Salix* sp.) by Greeks, Chinese, Europeans, and Native Americans to alleviate pain, seemed far from scientific until it was discovered that the bark of these trees contained salicin, a component of acetylsalicylic acid (aspirin). Now, drugs that inhibit receptors, receptor signaling, and gene expression can prevent very specific pathways of the inflammatory process. It is up to the veterinary clinician to remain current in her or his knowledge of the steps of the inflammatory response to gain optimal benefit from newly developed therapies.

INFLAMMATION AND THE SENSATION OF PAIN

Several features of inflammatory response activate sensory nerve fibers. Mechanoreceptors can sense changes in tissue swelling secondary to the accumulation of edema fluid and/or exudates. Thermoreceptors can sense changes in localized or systemic temperatures. Pain receptors can also become activated. Concerning pain, release of prostaglandin E_2 is a crucial mediator of the inflammatory pain sensation. PGE_2 mediates this activity through a specific glycine receptor subtype (GlyR α-3) of the dorsal gray horn of the spinal cord. Inhibition of PGE_2 expression through inhibition of COX enzymes reduces pain and future therapies may target GlyR α-3 receptors.

THE EFFECT OF INFLAMMATION ON THE FEBRILE RESPONSE AND OTHER ACTIVITIES

Cytokines such as IL-1, TNF, and IL-6, as well as high mobility group protein box-1 (HMGB-1) molecules are often produced during acute inflammatory responses. These inflammatory mediators, along with LPS (microbial factor) and other potentially toxic microbial or chemical molecules, are important regulators of body temperature (fever), malaise, headache, confusion, anorexia, locomotion, and unconsciousness. Many of these actions occur through: (1) the effects of these cytokines on sensory fibers in the vagus nerve, which extends to the brain stem, and (2) their effects on cerebral endothelial cells, perivascular microglia, and meningeal macrophages and the ability of the cells to induce COX-1, COX-2, and COX-3 activity for the formation and release of prostaglandins such as PGE_2. PGE_2 then activates various hypothalamic nuclei, including the ventromedial preoptic nucleus, paraventricular nucleus, solitary tract nucleus, ventrolateral medulla, and parabrachial nucleus, which regulate fever and the other clinical responses listed previously.

UNIQUE TYPES OF INFLAMMATION

SEPTICEMIA AND ENDOTOXIC SHOCK

SEPTICEMIA

Septicemia is a clinically significant form of bacteremia complicated by toxemia, fever, malaise, and often shock (Table 3-12). Septicemia is characterized by the multiplication of microorganisms within the bloodstream and "seeding" into blood from fixed microcolonies present in one or more tissues. In septicemia, inflammation is not a well-controlled local reaction to injury, but instead mediators of inflammation are generated systemically leading to diffuse "leakage" of plasma into the interstitium and sequestration of leukocytes in the microvasculature. Generation of cytokines, kinins, vasoactive amines, and lipid mediators of inflammation, combined with widespread endothelial damage, leads to profound circulatory disturbances. Because of the systemic nature of this host-microbial interaction, quantities of phagocytic cells, antibody, complement components, and coagulation proteins may become depleted unless septicemia is controlled in the early stages. Septic shock and disseminated intravascular

Table **3-12**   **Examples of Differing Types of Inflammatory and Clinical Responses to Stimuli**

| | TYPE OF INFLAMMATORY STIMULI | | |
	Skin Allergen	Gram-Negative Bacterial Infection in Dermis	Gram-Negative Septicemia
Stimulus	Allergen	LPS, toxins	LPS, toxins
Site	Epidermis/dermis	Dermis	Blood
Molecular trigger	Immunoglobulin E-cross-linking, dendritic cell binding	TLR4, CD14	Hageman factor, complement, TLR4
Major response	Histamine, leukotrienes	IL-1, TNF, prostaglandins, PAF, neutrophil products	Kinins, bradykinin, PAF, prostaglandins, IL-1, TNF
Extent of response	Local	Local	Systemic
Clinical finding	Swelling, pruritus (bronchoconstriction)	Swelling, exudate (pus)	Fever, nausea, malaise
Desired resolution	Limited, resolves in hours/days	Limited, resolves in days	Transient, resolves
Possible sequelae	Severe wheal and flare, anaphylaxis	Cellulitis leading to ulceration, eventual fibrosis/granuloma	Septic shock

CD14 = receptor for LPS-binding protein.
Hageman factor = clotting factor.
IL-1, Interleukin-1; *LPS*, lipopolysaccharide (endotoxin); *PAF*, platelet-activating factor; *TLR4*, Toll-like receptor 4; *TNF*, tumor necrosis factor.

coagulation (DIC) are the usual sequelae of advanced bacterial septicemia.

Septicemia should be differentiated from a bacterial embolism. For example, some strains of *Streptococcus* spp. may break free from vegetative lesions (valvular endocarditis), as large colonies are protected by cell debris and fibrin. The bacterial emboli may then mechanically lodge in the lung, liver, kidney, or brain to produce a secondary focus of infection (abscess), but the whole process remains subclinical. In such a case, the blood sample taken for culture often lacks viable bacteria.

ENDOTOXIC SHOCK

The systemic interaction of microorganisms and their products (toxins) with a spectrum of host cells and chemical mediators results in a clinical syndrome recognized as sepsis or septic shock (Table 3-12). The host mediators and amplification systems initiating the syndrome vary with the type of organism and the nature of the infectious process (local or systemic). Regardless of the specific cause, the major elements of septic shock form a continuum including: (1) hemodynamic derangements, (2) abnormal body temperature, (3) progressive hypoperfusion of the microvasculature, (4) hypoxic injury to susceptible cells, (5) quantitative adjustments in blood leukocytes and platelets, (6) DIC, (7) multiple organ failure, and (8) death.

Bacterial endotoxin, the LPS from the outer membrane of gram-negative bacteria, has been studied extensively as an initiator of septic shock. The peptidoglycan layer of gram-positive bacteria and bacterial exotoxins can initiate many of the same host responses.

Other important initiators are products of the interaction of neutrophils, macrophages, and platelets with microorganisms in the tissue. Endotoxin is bound in the serum by lipopolysaccharide binding protein (LPB) that binds CD14. Endotoxin has numerous ways to induce systemic activation of inflammatory mediators. Three direct effects of endotoxin are the activation of Hageman factor (a clotting factor), the complement cascade, and induction of the TLR4 pathway. These pathways can ultimately activate bradykinin, PAF, arachidonic acid metabolites, and cytokines (IL-1 and TNF), all of which have a role in many of the coagulation, hemodynamic, thermoregulatory, and leukocyte derangements observed in septic shock. TNF is capable of producing most clinical and pathologic features of septic shock, including: hypotension, metabolic acidosis, hemoconcentration, intestinal hemorrhage, fever, neutrophil and endothelial activation, and predisposition to thrombosis. IL-1 shares many of the biologic activities of TNF in the mediation of septic shock. Secretion of TNF by activated macrophages can be partially inhibited by pretreatment with glucocorticoids such as dexamethasone, which have been used therapeutically, often with limited success. In addition, lethal shock is prevented with anti-TNF antibody or TNF receptor inhibitors.

In severe septicemia, a systemic inflammatory response syndrome (SIRS) can develop in which there is extensive accumulation of cytokines, activated neutrophils, and platelets in the ciriculatory system. This result leads to multiple organ failure (MOF) and shock. Most patients survive initial SIRS insults, but these individuals are at increased risk of secondary or opportunistic infections termed compensatory antiinflammatory response syndrome (CARS). The initial activation of innate immunity can lead to decreased macrophage activity, T-cell anergy, and apoptosis of lymphocytes contributing to CARS.

Multiple organ failure (MOF) represents a late stage in septic shock and accounts for much of the irreversibility of organ failure. Systemic tissue ischemia and hypoxia, associated with progressive cardiovascular derangements, increased vascular leakage, and DIC, lead to generalized organ failure. Organs that are particularly sensitive to these effects include: heart, brain, kidney, lung, liver, and intestinal mucosa. Cells injured by ischemia revert to anaerobic energy production (glycolysis), resulting in rapid depletion of substrates (glycogen, glucose), accumulation of lactate, and a deficiency of ATP. Without sufficient ATP, cell membrane ion pumps fail to maintain electrolyte balances, membrane integrity, and protein synthesis. The influx of sodium into cells with water causes cells to swell with further loss of function. Influx of calcium ions activates many intracellular enzymes, including phospholipase, which breaks down cellular membranes and generates arachidonic acid products. Loss of the proton gradient of the inner mitochondrial membrane makes oxidative phosphorylation impossible. Irreversible cell injury is believed to be closely related to generalized failure of mitochondria and loss of selective permeability of cell membranes.

Animals dying of septic shock typically have evidence of fluid in the body cavities, pulmonary edema, petechial hemorrhages, congestion of the liver and intestines, and dehydration. Common microscopic lesions include acute necrosis of renal tubules, centrolobular hepatocytes, cardiac myocytes, adrenals, and tips of intestinal villi.

MORPHOLOGIC CLASSIFICATION OF EXUDATES IN ACUTE INFLAMMATORY LESIONS

The gross and microscopic appearance of different types of acute inflammatory reactions in tissue can often be classified according to the vascular and cellular components of the response, thus providing a mechanistic basis for understanding the pathogenesis. Histopathologic lesions of acute inflammation are most commonly grouped into five categories: serous, catarrhal, fibrinous, suppurative or purulent, and hemorrhagic, or a combination of these lesions, such as fibrinosuppurative. Similar histopathologic patterns of lesions also occur in chronic inflammation (lymphomonocytic/ lymphohistiocytic or granulomatous [macrophages, multinucleate giant cells, lymphocytes, plasma cells, fibrosis]) and will be discussed in Chapter 4.

It should be recognized that the histopathologic lesions of acute inflammation often represent: (1) a continuum of progressive changes of the same type of inflammation occurring over time or (2) different types of inflammatory responses occurring concurrently in the same or different areas of an affected tissue. Therefore as an example, rhinitis could progress in a sequence from serous to catarrhal to mucopurulent to purulent. If the inciting stimulus is severe, changes could progress rapidly from serous to fibrinous to hemorrhagic.

SEROUS INFLAMMATION

Serous inflammation is the term used to describe a pattern of acute inflammation in which the tissue response consists of the leakage or accumulation of fluid with a low concentration of plasma protein and no to low numbers of leukocytes. This watery material is released from small gaps between endothelial cells and from hypersecretion of inflamed serous glands. This response is essentially a transudate (specific gravity <1.012) and is seen with: (1) thermal injury to skin, such as burns and photosensitization, in which the lesion can appear as a fluid-filled blisters or (2) acute allergic responses characterized by watery eyes and a runny nose with a clear, colorless transudate.

Grossly, lesions, for example, with serous inflammation consist of tissue that: (1) contains excessive clear to slightly yellow, watery fluid that leaks from the tissue on cut section or (2) forms raised fluid-filled vesicles protruding above the surface of the mucous membrane of the nasal cavity (serous rhinitis) or of the skin (Fig. 3-19). Microscopically, connective tissue fibers are separated, often widely, and capillaries and postcapillary venules are dilated with erythrocytes (active hyperemia). Endothelial cells lining these vessels can vary from flattened to hypertrophied.

CATARRHAL INFLAMMATION

Catarrhal inflammation or mucoid inflammation is the term used to describe a pattern of acute inflammation in which the tissue response consists of the secretion or accumulation of a thick gelatinous fluid containing abundant mucus and mucins from a mucous membrane. This response occurs most commonly in tissue with abundant goblet cells and mucus glands, such as in certain types of chronic allergic and autoimmune gastrointestinal diseases and with chronic inflammation of the airways of the respiratory system (chronic asthma). Grossly the surface or cut surface of affected tissue may be covered with or contain, a clear to slightly opaque, thick fluid (Fig. 3-20). Microscopically the lesion can include hyperplastic epithelial cells of mucus

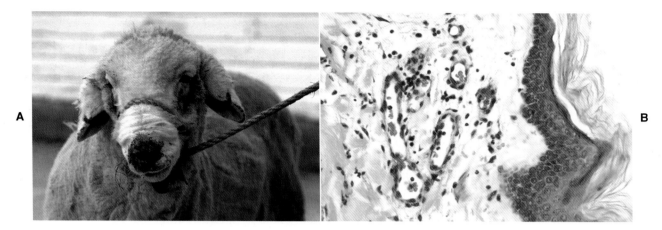

Fig. 3-19   Serous exudate/subcutaneous edema, photosensitiaization, skin of the nose and ears, ewe. A, The nonhaired skin of the nose is covered by a crust resulting from dehydration of the serous exudate released from injured blood vessels following a short exposure to the sun. The ears are edematous and droopy. **B,** Microscopically, there is moderate expansion of the superficial dermis with edema secondary to vascular leakage (serous inflammation). The post-capillary venules are dilated (active hyperemia), and leukocytes can be observed marginating on endothelia. H&E stain. (*A and B,* Courtesy Dr. M.D. McGavin, College of Veterinary Medicine, University of Tennessee.)

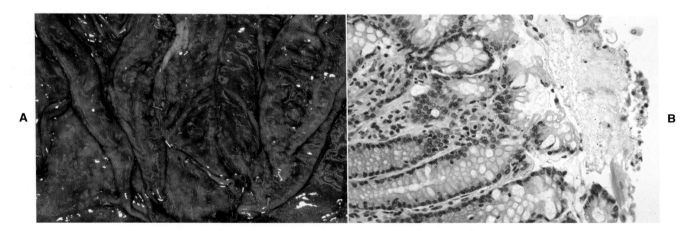

Fig. 3-20   Catarrhal inflammation. A, Abomasum, cow. The mucosal epithelium is moderately thickened, covered by a glistening layer of clear mucus, and has a subtle nodular appearance caused by accumulation of mucinous secretory products (catarrhal exudate) in the gastric pits. **B,** Colon, cow. Microscopically, there is a catarrhal colitis with hyperplasia of mucosal epithelial cells and increased accumulation of mucus on the mucosal surface. H&E stain. (*A and B,* Courtesy Dr. M.D. McGavin, College of Veterinary Medicine, University of Tennessee.)

glands and goblet cells, as well as connective tissue fibers separated by mucins.

FIBRINOUS INFLAMMATION

Fibrinous inflammation is the term used to describe a pattern of acute inflammation in which the tissue response consists of the accumulation of fluid with a high concentration of plasma protein (specific gravity >1.02) and no to low numbers of leukocytes. This response is an exudate. Fibrinous inflammation occurs with more severe endothelial cell injury that allows leakage of large molecular weight proteins, such as fibrinogen. Fibrinogen leaks from capillaries and post-capillary venules during the fluidic phase of the acute inflammatory response and polymerizes outside of the vessels to fibrin, a homogenous and vividly pink (eosinophilic) protein when stained with hematoxylin and eosin (H&E). This lesion is most commonly caused by infectious microbes and is seen in the serous membranes of the body cavities, such as those lined by pleura (fibrinous pleuritis), pericardium (fibrinous pericarditis), peritoneum (fibrinous peritonitis), and in the synovial membranes of joints (fibrinous synovitis or polyserositis) and the meninges (fibrinous leptomeningitis). Common examples include the lesions in pulmonary alveoli in fibrinous pneumonia (*Mannheima haemolytica*), atypical interstitial pneumonia (3-methylindol), and respiratory viral infections (infectious bovine rhinotracheitis [IBR] in cows). When fibrin forms a distinct layer covering an ulcer, it is referred to as a fibrinous pseudomembrane, whereas when it lines the pneumonocyte surface of lung alveoli and is mixed with necrotic cell debris such as occurs with bovine respiratory syncytial virus (BRSV) infection, it is called a hyaline membrane.

Grossly the surfaces of affected tissue are red (active hyperemia) and covered with a thick, stringy, elastic, white-gray to yellow exudate that can be removed from the surface of the tissue (in contrast to a fibrous response) (Fig. 3-21). A classic example of fibrinous inflammation occurs in fibrinous pneumonia caused by acute *Mannheima haemolytica* infection, where both alveoli and stromal connective tissue (interlobular septa) contain notable fibrinous exudate that rapidly becomes infiltrated by neutrophils, resulting in a fibrinosuppurative exudate. Another example of fibrinous inflammation occurs in IBR, caused by a herpesvirus that injures epithelial cells of the respiratory tract, resulting in an acute fibrinous inflammatory response. Noninfectious causes, such as heat and smoke inhalation, can cause fibrinous exudate in the trachea. Microscopically, capillaries and postcapillary venules are dilated with erythrocytes (active hyperemia), and endothelial cells are reactive (hypertrophied). The stromal connective tissue or the mesothelial surfaces of the affected organ contains or is covered by red to vividly red layers of coagulated and/or polymerized fibrin, albumin, and other plasma proteins. The fibrinous exudate is often rapidly infiltrated by neutrophils resulting in fibrinosuppurative inflammation.

SUPPURATIVE INFLAMMATION

Suppurative inflammation is the term used to describe a pattern of acute inflammation in which the tissue response consists of the accumulation of fluid with a high concentration of plasma protein (specific gravity >1.02) and high numbers of leukocytes, predominately neutrophils. This material is an exudate commonly known as pus. Pus can be a creamy liquid, but if dehydrated it can be more caseous and firm in consistency and occasionally laminated in diseases such as ovine caseous lymphadenitis. A circumscribed collection of pus visible grossly is called an abscess, whereas, if visible only microscopically, it is called a microabscess.

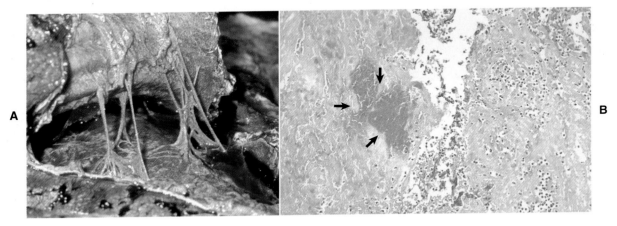

Fig. 3-21 **Fibrinous inflammation, pleural cavity, visceral and parietal pleurae, horse.**
A, The pleural surfaces are covered by a yellow-gray, thick, friable exudate consisting of fibrin mixed with other plasma proteins. This exudate can be easily pulled apart and should not be confused with fibrous adhesions. The latter response occurs over time and consists of a similar appearing material that contains collagen fibers. These fibers provide tensile strength to the material and form adhesions between opposing surfaces that can only be broken with some difficulty. **B,** Microscopically, there are layers of homogenous red material (fibrin-fibrinous exudate) that contain occasional neutrophils and a focus of bacteria (*arrows*). H&E stain.
(*A* and *B*, *Courtesy Dr. J.F. Zachary, College of Veterinary Medicine, University of Illinois.*)

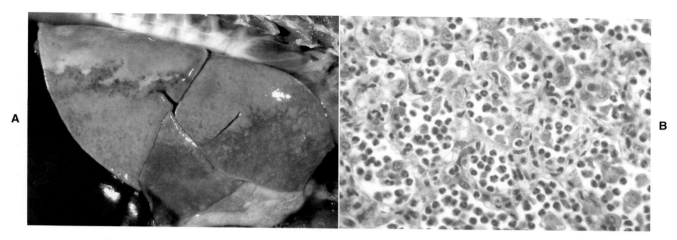

Fig. 3-22   **Suppurative (purulent) inflammation, secondary bacterial bronchopneumonia, infectious canine distemper, puppy. A,** The cranioventral areas of the lung are firm and beige to brown. This lesion is caused by neutrophils transmigrating into alveoli in an acute inflammatory response secondary to bacterial infection of the lung. **B,** Microscopically, alveoli contain numerous neutrophils (suppurative exudate) and sloughed pneumocytes. H&E stain. (**A** *and* **B,** *Courtesy Dr. M.D. McGavin, College of Veterinary Medicine, University of Tennessee.*)

Dense neutrophil accumulation (pus) can also be distributed in tissue layers such as fascial planes and subcutaneous connective tissue and is referred to as cellulitis or phlegmonous inflammation. Instead of producing a focal abscess, the neutrophils evoke a watery suppurative exudate distributed along fascial planes and tissue spaces, as in some cases of blackleg or extensive gram-positive (staphylococcal) infection. Suppurative inflammation, microabscesses, abscesses, and exudates are most commonly caused by bacteria, including *Staphylococcus* spp., *Streptococcus* spp., and *Escherichia coli,* and can occur in many organs. These genera can also cause suppurative bacterial meningitides in the CNS. Abscesses in the brains of horses caused by *Streptococcus equi* and microabscesses in the brains of cows caused by *Listeria monocytogenes* are good examples of suppurative inflammation. Bacteria-induced suppurative inflammation also occurs commonly in: (1) the pelvis and tubules (pyelonephritis) of the kidney, (2) the bronchi of the lungs (bronchopneumonia), (3) the nasal and sinus cavities (rhinitis and sinusitis), (4) the glandular epithelium of the prostate (prostatitis), (5) the lumina of the gall bladder (cholecystis) and urinary bladder (urocystitis), and (6) the acini and ducts of the mammary gland (mastitis). Unresolved suppurative inflammation can progress to chronic inflammation.

Grossly the surfaces and/or connective tissues of affected organs are hyperemic and covered by or contain, respectively, a thick white-gray to yellow pus (Fig. 3-22). In some cases, pus will be mixed with fibrin, forming a fibrinosuppurative exudate. Microscopically, affected tissues have large numbers of neutrophils; many degenerate and often are mixed with necrotic cellular debris, bacteria, plasma proteins, and fibrin.

NOMENCLATURE OF THE INFLAMMATORY RESPONSE (MORPHOLOGIC DIAGNOSES)

Nomenclature, a system of names assigned to structures and processes in a scientific discipline, used in veterinary pathology provides clinicians with a morphologic diagnosis, a precise description of the process, type of inflammation, and disease. A morphologic diagnosis has six components listed in the following sequence: degree of severity, duration, distribution, exudate, modifier, and tissue (Table 3-13). Based the results of a postmortem examination and/or histologic evaluation of tissue specimens, a pathologist will construct a morphologic diagnosis by including, in sequential order, the components of the nomenclature that best describe the specimens. For example, using the kidney as the injured tissue, the central component of a morphologic diagnosis is the name of the tissue derived from its Latin term, "nephro-." If the kidney is inflamed, the prefix "nephro-" is combined with the suffix "itis" (inflammation or disease of) to form the word "nephritis," meaning inflammation of the kidney. The other components of the morphologic diagnosis, such as degree, duration, distribution, exudate, and modifier, precede nephritis and are used to describe the characteristics of the inflammatory process. The pattern of distribution of the inflammatory lesion not only provides location but in many instances implies a mechanism of injury.

Table **3-13**   The Nomenclature of a Morphologic Diagnosis

Degree	Duration	Distribution	Exudate	Modifier	Tissue
Minimal	Acute	Focal	Serous	Necrotizing	Nephritis
	Subacute	Multifocal	Catarrhal	Bronchointerstitial	Cystitis
Mild	Chronic	Locally	Fibrinous	Hemorrhagic	Enteritis
Moderate	Chronic-active	extensive	Suppurative	Embolic	Pneumonia*
Marked		Diffuse	Granulomatous		Hepatitis
(severe)		(interstitial)			
		Cranioventral†			

This table provides an example of how nomenclature can be used to construct a morphologic diagnosis. It is not intended to be all inclusive and may vary from schemes used in other veterinary colleges.

*In the lung, it is customary to use the term *pneumonia* to indicate inflammation of the lung.

†Used only for diseases of the lungs.

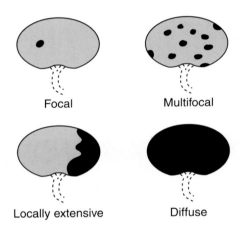

Fig. 3-23 Patterns of lesion distribution used to construct morphologic diagnosis, as an example, in the kidney.
(From Slauson DO, Cooper BJ: Mechanisms of disease: a textbook of comparative general pathology, ed 3, St Louis, 2002, Mosby.)

These patterns of distribution are shown in Fig. 3-23 and include focal, multifocal, locally extensive, and diffuse. They will be covered in greater detail in each organ system. The subtleties of this process are learned through advanced training in the discipline of pathology, and terms describing the degree and duration evolve from professional experience and are not likely to be mastered by veterinary students during their professional training.

For completeness in this discussion, morphologic diagnoses can also use the suffixes "osis" (diseased or abnormal condition) or "opathy" (disease). In this context, such diseases or conditions refer to those caused by degenerative or aging processes without inflammation. Therefore the same nomenclature can be used to diagnose a degenerative condition in the kidney by using the term "nephrosis or nephropathy." The other components are then added to nephrosis or nephropathy to describe the characteristics of the degenerative process. Finally, some metabolic and neoplastic diseases do not fit into this nomenclature, but equally valid morphologic diagnoses can be constructed. An enlarged, soft and friable, yellow, and greasy liver can be morphologically diagnosed as "fatty liver" (hepatic lipidosis), whereas a solid, firm, white expansile mass in the liver could be morphologically diagnosed as "hepatic malignant lymphoma."

SUGGESTED READINGS

Aderem A, Ulevitch RJ: Toll-like receptors in the induction of the innate immune response. *Nature* 406:782-787, 2000.

Alexander WS: Suppressors of cytokine signaling (SOCS) in the immune system, *Nat Rev Immunol* 2:1-7, 2002.

Calder PC, Grimble RF: Polyunsaturated fatty acids, inflammation, and immunity, *Eur J Clin Nut* 56(S3):S14-S19, 2002.

Elmquist JK, Scammell TE, Saper CB: Mechanisms of CNS response to systemic immune challenge: the febrile response, *Trends Neurosci* 20(12):565-570, 1997.

Faurschou M, Borregaard N: Neutrophil granules and secretory vesicles in inflammation, *Microbes Infect* 5:1317-1327, 2003.

Foster D, Parrish-Novak J, Fox B et al: Cytokine-receptor pairing: accelerating discovery of cytokine function, *Nat Rev Drug Discov* 3:160-170, 2003.

Gangur V, Birmingham NP, Thanesvorakul S: Chemokines in health and disease, *Vet Immunol Immunopathol* 86:127-136, 2002.

Giger U, Boxer LA, Simpson PJ et al: Deficiency of leukocyte surface glycoproteins Mo1, LFA-1, and Leu M5 in a dog with recurrent bacterial infections: an animal model, *Blood* 69:1622-1630, 1984.

Kehrli ME Jr., Ackermann MR, Shuster DE et al: Animal model of human disease: bovine leukocyte adhesion deficiency: beta-2 integrin deficiency in young Holstein cattle, *Am J Pathol* 140:1489-1492, 1992.

Mayadas T, Cullere X: Neutrophil β_2 integrins: moderators of life or death decisions, *Trends Immunol* 26(7):388-395, 2005.

Ramierez-Romero R, Brogden KA, Gallup JM et al: Mast cell density and substance P–like immunoreactivity during initiation and progression of lung lesions in ovine *Mannheimia haemolytica* pneumonia, *Microb Pathog* 30:325-335, 2001.

Rottman JB: Key role of chemokines and chemokine receptors in inflammation, immunity, neoplasia, and infectious disease, *Vet Pathol* 36:357-367, 1999.

Simionescu M, Gafencu A, Antohe F: Transcytosis of plasma macromolecules in endothelial cells: a cell biological survey, *Microsc Res Tech* 57:269-288, 2002.

Ulbrich H, Eriksson EE, Lindobom L: Leukocyte and endothelial cell adhesion molecules as targets for therapeutic interventions in inflammatory disease, *Trends Pharm Sci* 24:640-647, 2003.

Wedemeyer J, Tsai M, Galli SJ: Roles of mast cells and basophils in innate and acquired immunity, *Current Opin Immunol* 12: 624-631, 2000.

Yang D, Biragyn A, Hoover DM et al: Multiple roles of antimicrobial defensins, cathelicidins, and eosinophil-derived neurotoxin in host defense, *Ann Rev Immunol* 22:181-215, 2004.

APPENDIX 3-1

Mediators of Inflammation

Mediator	Source	Structure	Stimulus	A*	B*	C*	Activity	Receptor/ Signaling	Inhibitors
VASOACTIVE AMINES									
Histamine	Mast cells, basophils, platelets	Decarboxylated histidine	Trauma, cold, cross-linking of IgE, C3a, C5a	+	++	+/−	Endothelial cell retraction, smooth muscle cell contraction	Histamine binds H_1 and H_2 receptors	H_1 and H_2 inhibitors, enzymatic degradation
Serotonin	Rodent mast cells and basophils	5-hydroxy-tryptamine	Trauma, cold, cross-linking of IgE, C3a, C5a	+	++	+/−	Endothelial cell retraction, smooth muscle contraction		
TACHYKININS									
Substance P Neurotachykinin A Neurotachykinin B	Nerve fibers, macrophages		Neuronal activation, histamine	+	++	+	Endothelial cell retraction, smooth muscle contraction, leukocyte activation	Neurokinin receptors	
PLASMA PROTEASES									
Bradykinin Lysylbradykinin	Plasma proteins	9 amino acid peptide	Negative surfaces, collagen, endotoxin, immune complexes	+	+	−	Endothelial cell retraction, smooth muscle cell relaxation, contraction	Plasma and tissue kallikrein with XII, prekallikrein, HMWK, and XI	Kininase I, angiotensin-converting enzyme (kininase II)
Kallikrein	Plasma factor (Fletcher)	80 kD protein	Contact activation	−	−	+	Cleaves XII, HMWK, activates collagenase	Activated by XIIa	
COAGULATION AND FIBRINOLYTIC SYSTEMS									
Clotting cascade and fibrinolysis enzymes	Plasma	60-450 kD proteins	Plasma contact with collagen, basement membranes, endotoxin, immune complexes	−	+/−	+/−	Thrombosis and fibrinolysis; activation of kallikrein, bradykinin, complement	Enzymatic cleavage of nonactivate factors results in activity	PGI_2, heparin, antithrombin III, proteins C and S, II, and X inhibitors; plasminogen activators

COX, Cyclooxygenase; *CRF 2*, cytokine receptor family 2; *DD*, death domain; *FADD*, Fas-associated death domain; *G-CSF*, granulocyte colony-stimulating factor; *GM-CSF*, granulocyte-macrophage colony-stimulating factor; *HMGB-1*, high-mobility group box protein-1; *HMWK*, high molecular weight kininogen; *IFN*, interferon; *IgE*, immunoglobulin E; *IL-1 through IL-29*, interleukin-1 through interleukin-29; *JAK/STAT*, Janus kinase/signal transducer and activator of transcription; *LTB₄, LTC₄, LTD₄, and LTE₄*, leukotrienes B₄, C₄, D₄, and E₄, respectively; *LOX*, lipoxygenase; *M-CSF*, macrophage colony-stimulating factor; *MHC*, major histocompatibility complex; *MORT*, mediator of receptor-induced toxicity; *N/A*, not applicable; *NK*, natural killer; *NOD*, nucleotide-binding oligomerization domain; *PAF*, platelet-activating factor; *PGE₂, PGF₂, and PGI₂*, prostaglandins E₂, F₂, and I₂, respectively; *PLA₂*, phospholipase A₂; *RNA*, ribonucleic acid; *TGF-β*, transforming growth factor-β; *TNF*, tumor necrosis factor; *TXA₂*, thromboxane A₂.

	Source	Stimulus				Function	Mechanism/Effects	Inhibitors
CELLULAR PROTEASES								
Tryptase/chymase	Mast cells	Histamine, substance P	–	–	–	Cleaves extracellular matrix, activates receptors	Protease activation of receptors: cleavage of certain receptors results in activation; degrades matrix proteins	
COMPLEMENT								
C3a	Plasma proteins	Immune complexes, endotoxin, plasmin, proteases	–	+	+/–	Chemotaxis, leukocyte activation	C3a binds C3a receptor and induces histamine release from mast cells	
C5a		Complement fragments range in size of 75-410 kD	–	+	++	Chemotaxis, leukocyte activation	C5a binds C5a receptor and induces histamine release from mast cells	
C5, C6, C7		Complement fragments range in size from 75-410 kD	–	–	–	Membrane attack complex that forms pores	Forms pores in microbial and other membranes	
C3b		Complement fragments range in size from 75-410 kD	–	–	–	Opsonin	Opsonizes microbes and binds leukocyte receptor	
EICOSANOIDS PROSTAGLANDINS								
Prostacyclin (PGI_2)	Endothelial cells	Arachidonic acid metabolite via COX	Cell injury, intracellular calcium release, with PLA_2 activity	+	–	–	Inhibits platelet aggregation on endothelial cells, reduces thrombosis, vasodilation	G protein-coupled receptor	Aspirin, COX 1-3 inhibitors, corticosteroid

Continued

APPENDIX **3-1**

Mediators of Inflammation—Cont'd

Mediator	Source	Structure	Stimulus	A*	B*	C*	Activity	Receptor/ Signaling	Inhibitors
Thromboxane (TXA$_2$)	Platelets	Arachidonic acid metabolite via COX	Platelet activation, with PLA$_2$ activity	+	–	–	Platelet activation and thrombosis, vasoconstriction	G protein-coupled receptor	Aspirin, COX 1-3 inhibitors, corticosteroid
PGE$_2$	Variety of cells	Arachidonic acid metabolite via COX		+	+	–	Mediators of sensation to pain, can reduce inflammatory responses, vasodilation	G protein-coupled receptor	Aspirin, COX 1-3 inhibitors, corticosteroid
PGF$_2$	Endothelial and epithelial cells	Arachidonic acid metabolite via cells		+	–	–	Smooth muscle contraction, vasoconstriction	G protein-coupled receptor	Aspirin, COX 1-3 inhibitors, corticosteroid
LEUKOTRIENES									
LTB$_4$	Leukocytes	Arachidonic acid metabolite via LOX	Membrane injury, with PLA$_2$ activity	–	+/–	++ +	Chemotaxis, leukocyte and endothelial cell activation	G protein-coupled receptor	Aspirin, LOX inhibitors, corticosteroid
LTC$_4$, LTD$_4$, LTE$_4$	Mast cells, basophils	Arachidonic acid metabolite via LOX	Membrane injury with PLA$_2$ activity	+	++ +	–	Slow-reacting substance of inflammation, vasoconstriction	G protein-coupled receptor	Aspirin, LOX inhibitors, corticosteroid
PAF	Platelets, endothelial cells, leukocytes	Glycerol-based lipid mediator	PAF	+	++	++ +	Chemotaxis, leukocyte, and endothelial cell activation, vasoconstriction	G protein-coupled receptor	PAF acetylhydrox-ylase
INTERLEUKINS/CYTOKINES									
IL-1	Macrophages, endothelial cells, leukocytes	17 kD protein	Activated leukocytes and endothelial cells	+	+	+	Chemotaxis, leukocyte activation, acute phase protein release, fever, hemodynamics	IL-1 R 1-9, JAK/STAT signaling	IL-1 receptor inhibitors, IL-1 mimetics, COX inhibitors, corticosteroid

Cytokine	Cellular source	Structure	Stimulus for production				Principal actions	Receptor	Therapeutic potential
IL-2	T-helper lymphocytes	15 kD protein	Antigenic stimulation, IL-1	–	–	–	Proliferation of lymphocytes	IL-2 receptor, JAK/STAT signaling	IL-2 receptor inhibitors, IL-1 mimetics, cell-cycle inhibitors
IL-3	T lymphocytes	20 kD protein	Antigenic stimulation, mitogens	–	–	–	Growth of bone marrow stem cells, hematopoietic cells, mast cells	CD23	IL-3 receptor inhibitors, mimetics, cell cycle inhibitors
IL-4	T_H2 lymphocytes	14 kD protein		–	–	–	T_H2 response; NK cell activation	CD124, CD132	IL-4 receptor inhibitors, mimetics
IL-5	T_H2 lymphocytes	13 kD protein repeated α helix		–	–	–	T_H2 response, eosinophil proliferation	IL-5 R, CD125	IL-5 receptor inhibitors, mimetics
IL-6	T lymphocytes, macrophages, fibroblast, other cells	26 kD protein	IL-1 and TNF	–	–	–	Acute phase protein synthesis, antiviral activity, B-lymphocyte differentiation, lung mucus production (with IL-17)	CD126, CD130	IL-6 receptor inhibitors, mimetics
IL-7	Bone marrow stromal cells	25 kD protein		–	–	–	B- and T-lymphocyte proliferation in bone marrow	CD127, CD132	IL-7 receptor inhibitors, mimetics
IL-8	Endothelial cells, leukocytes		Cellular activation	–	++	+	Leukocyte, especially neutrophils, chemotaxis	IL-8 R	IL-8 receptor inhibitors, mimetics, COX inhibitors, corticosteroid
IL-9				–	–	–	T_H2 response, hematopoiesis	IL-9 R	
IL-10	T regulatory lymphocytes, T_H2 lymphocytes, dendritic cells	α Helix		–	–	–	Decreases dendritic cell activity and T_H2 response; in family with IL-19, 20, 22, 24, 26, 28, 29	CRF 2	
IL-11				–	–	–	Megakaryocyte hematopoiesis	IL-9 R	
IL-12	Dendritic cells and macrophages			–	–	–	T_H1 response, growth, and differentiation of T lymphocytes, NK cell activation	IL-12 R B1, 2	
IL-13				–	–	–	T_H2 response, growth, and differentiation	IL-13 R	

Continued

APPENDIX 3-1

Mediators of Inflammation—Cont'd

Mediator	Source	Structure	Stimulus	A*	B*	C*	Activity	Receptor/ Signaling	Inhibitors
IL-14				—	—	—			
IL-15	T lymphocytes			—	—	—	IL-2-like activity (lymphocyte proliferation) and NK cell activation	IL-15 R, CD122	
IL-16	Memory T lymphocytes, mast cells, eosinophils			—	—	—		CD4	
IL-17	CD4 memory cells			—	—	+	Chemoattractant for CD4 T-helper lymphocytes	IL-17 R	
IL-18	Macrophages, Kupffer cells			—	—	—	Synergistic with IL-12 for Th-1 induced activity and IFN-γ release	IL-1 R-related protein	
IL-19		α Helix		—	—	—	In family with IL-10, 20, 22, 24, and 26	CRF 2	
IL-20		α Helix		—	—	—	In family with IL-10, 19, 22, 24, and 26, implicated in psoriasis	CRF 2	
IL-21	CD4 T lymphocytes			—	—	—	Induces differentiation of NK cells previously activated by IL-4, IL-12, and IL-15; inhibits recruitment of nonactivated NK cells	IL-2-like R	
IL-22		α Helix		—	—	—	Induces acute phase protein release; in IL-10 family	CRF 2	
IL-23				—	—	—	T_H1 response similar to IL-12, acts on CD4 lymphocytes		
IL-24		α Helix		—	—	—	IL-10 family with IL-19, 20, 22, and 26	CRF 2	
IL-25	Mast cells			—	—	—	T_H2 response, induces production of IL-4, 5, and 13		

Cytokine	Structure	Cell source	Stimulus / target				Actions	Receptor	Therapeutic agents
IL-26	α Helix			—	—	—	IL-10 family with IL-19, 20, 22, and 24	IL-26 R (IL-20 & IL-10 components)	
IL-27				—	—	—	T$_H$1 response, stimulates naïve CD4 T lymphocytes; synergistic with IL-12	IL-27 R	
IL-28				—	—	—	Possibly antiviral like IFN and IL-10	CRF 2	
IL-29				—	—	—	Similar to IL-28; possibly antiviral	CRF 2	
Il-31		T$_H$2 lymphocytes	Macrophage activation, epithelial cells	—	—	—	Induces dermatitis in mice	Gp130-like receptor	Receptor inhibitors, JAK/STAT inhibitors
IL-32		Lymphocytes and epithelia	Monocytes	—	—	—		Synergistic with NOD 1 and 2 ligands	
IL-33		Lymphocytes	T helper type 2 lymphocytes	—	—	—		IL-1 receptor induces T$_H$2 responses	
TNF-α	17 kD protein	Macrophages	Macrophage activation, endotoxin, phagocytosis	+	+	+	Activation of endothelial cells, leukocytes, acute phase protein synthesis, apoptosis	TNF receptor, FADD, MORT, DD	TNF receptor inhibitors, TNF mimetics, COX inhibitors, corticosteroid
TNF-α	17 kD protein	T lymphocytes	Antigenic stimulation, mitogen	+	+	+	Activation of endothelial cells, leukocytes, acute phase protein synthesis, apoptosis	TNF receptor, FADD, MORT, DD	TNF receptor inhibitors, TNF mimetics, COX inhibitors, corticosteroid
TGF-β	Cystine knot	Fibroblasts, endothelial cells, macrophages, T regulatory lymphocytes		—	—	—	Fibrosis, decreased dendritic cell activity, relative decrease in T$_H$1 and T$_H$2 responses, decreased epithelial cell proliferation	TGF-β receptor	
IFN-γ		T lymphocytes, NK cells	Antigenic stimulation or mitogen	—	—	—	T$_H$1 response, antiviral activity, phagocytosis, induction of MHC I and II expression, MHC	IFN receptor, JAK/STAT signaling	
IFN-α	16-20 kD glycoprotein	Many cell types	Virus, double-stranded RNA	—	—	—	Antiviral activity through MHC I expression oligoadenylate synthetase, Mx proteins	IFN receptor, JAK/STAT signaling	

Continued

APPENDIX 3-1

Mediators of Inflammation—Cont'd

Mediator	Source	Structure	Stimulus	A*	B*	C*	Activity	Receptor/Signaling	Inhibitors
IFN-β	Many cell types	20 kD glycoprotein	Virus, double-stranded RNA	–	–	–	Antiviral activity through MHC I expression oligoadenylate synthetase, Mx proteins	IFN receptor, JAK/STAT signaling	
GM-CSF	T lymphocytes, endothelial cells, fibroblasts	22 kD glycoprotein	Antigen stimulation, IL-1-activated endothelial cells and fibroblasts	–	–	–	Proliferation and maturation of precursors to neutrophils, eosinophils, and monocytes		
G-CSF	Many cell types	20 kD glycoprotein	Infection	–	–	–	Proliferation of neutrophil precursors		
M-CSF	Many cell types	70-90 kD glycoprotein (dimmer)	Infection	–	–	–	Proliferation, maturation of monocytes/macrophages		
Stem cell factor	Mast cells		Mast cell activation	–	–	+?	Proliferation of mast cells	c-Kit ligand	
Nitric oxide	Endothelial cells, macrophages, neurons	N/A	Cellular activation, calcium release	+	+	–	Vascular dilation, macrophage endosomal killing, lipoperoxidation of membranes	Nitric oxide synthase conversion of L-arginine to	
HMGB-1	Many cell types		IL-1, TNF-α, IFN-γ, lysophosph-atidylcholine	–	–	–	Activates macrophages to release IL-1, TNF, and IFN-γ and induces food aversion and weight loss during sickness	Macrophage RAGE	

4

Chronic Inflammation and Wound Healing*

MARK R. ACKERMANN

INTRODUCTION

Chronic inflammation is inflammation of prolonged duration (weeks to months to years) in which acute inflammation, tissue destruction, and tissue repair occur simultaneously. Chronic inflammation arises: (1) when the acute inflammatory response fails to eliminate the inciting stimulus, (2) after repeated episodes of acute inflammation, or (3) in response to unique biochemical characteristics and/or virulence factors in the inciting stimulus or microbe. Table 4-1 lists some of the most common causes of chronic inflammation in domestic animals. The underlying biologic mechanisms that result in chronic inflammation include: persistence/resistance, isolation in tissue, unresponsiveness, autoimmunity, and unidentified mechanisms.

- Persistence/resistance: Persistent infections, such as those caused by *Mycobacterium* spp.; *Nocardia* spp.; deep-seated mycoses, such as *Blastomyces dermatitidis* and *Histoplasma capsulatum*; and parasites, such as *Toxocara canis* larvae, can avoid and/or resist phagocytosis by neutrophils and macrophages—or once internalized in these cells, can prevent fusion with lysosomes or killing by lysosomes. Such microbes also usually do not produce biologic molecules that cause severe tissue injury, but their presence continually incites chronic inflammatory and immune responses. Tissue destruction, granulomatous inflammation, and fibrosis are common sequelae.
- Isolation: Some microbes, such as *Streptococcus* and *Staphylococus* spp., are not naturally resistant to phagocytosis and/or destruction but are able to isolate themselves from effective innate and adaptive immune responses and from antimicrobial drugs by "hiding" themselves in pus.
- Unresponsiveness: Certain foreign materials are virtually indestructible and therefore are unresponsive to phagocytosis and/or enzymic breakdown. They include plant material, grass awns, silica dust, asbestos fibers, some suture materials, and surgical prostheses.
- Autoimmunity and leukocyte defects: Alterations in the regulation of adaptive immune responses to self-antigens result in autoimmune diseases, such as polyarteritis nodosa, with a chronic inflammatory response. Defects in leukocyte function, as occurs in humans with Wegener's granulomatosis, also result in chronic inflammation.
- Unidentified mechanisms: In some diseases, such as canine granulomatous meningoencephalitis, the cause of chronic inflammation remains unknown.

As the chronic inflammatory response develops, cytokines, chemokines, and other inflammatory mediators are released and incite: (1) active inflammation (chronic to granulomatous with lymphocytes, macrophages, plasma cells, and multinucleated giant cells [MGCs]); (2) tissue destruction (necrosis); (3) proliferation of fibroblasts and deposition of collagen (desmoplasia and/or fibroplasia); (4) angiogenesis and neovascularization (granulation tissue formation); and (5) initiation of wound healing (reepithelialization and tissue repair).

BENEFICIAL AND HARMFUL ASPECTS OF CHRONIC INFLAMMATION

The body initially responds to injury through acute inflammation. Once the acute inflammatory response fails, chronic inflammation ensues as the body attempts

---

*See Appendix 4-1 for a listing of the acronyms, terms, and functions of the chemical mediators of inflammation.

Table **4-1**   Selected Examples of Conditions That Can Cause or Lead to Chronic Inflammation in Domestic Animals

Microbial Agents	Toxins	Autoimmune Diseases	Foreign Bodies	Other

Bacteria:
    Brucella spp.
    Mycobacteria spp.:
        canine/feline leprosy
        M. avium-intracellulare
        M. bovis tuberculosis
        atypical (e.g., *M. marinum*)
    Rhodococcus equi
Virus:
    Porcine circovirus
Fungi:
    Trichophyton spp.
    Microsporum spp.
    Aspergillus spp.
Protozoa/Parasites:
    Leishmania spp.
    Trypanosoma spp.
    Draschia spp.
    Habronema spp.
	Vicia villosa
	    (Hairy vetch)
		Lupus erythematosus
		Allergic contact dermatitis
		Irritant contact dermatitis
		Rheumatoid arthritis
		Polyarteritis nodosa
			Retained suture
			Plant fibers
			Silica
			Asbestos
			Beryllium
			Inhaled smoke
			Inhaled dust
				Canine granulomatous
				    meningoencephalitis
				Lick granuloma
				Sterile nodular granuloma
				Sperm granuloma
				Chalazion
				Eosinophilic granulomas
				    of dogs, cats, horses
				    (see Table 4-2)

to overcome the inciting stimulus via macrophages and the adaptive immune response. If these responses fail, the stimulus is then "walled-off" with collagen produced by fibroblasts, encapsulating the stimulus and functionally placing it "outside" of the body. Often this response can be beneficial and in time can lead to a return to normal activity. Small granulomas or abscesses in the lung, liver, or even in some areas of the skin, with time, eventually go unnoticed by the innate and adaptive immune systems and do not stimulate pain or mechanical interference to movement or function.

On the other hand, chronic inflammation can be detrimental. The mononuclear leukocyte infiltrates (macrophages, lymphocytes, natural killer [NK] cells) within areas of chronic inflammation take up space and often displace, replace, and sometimes obliterate the structure of the original tissue. At the same time, new blood vessels form, fibroblasts proliferate and deposit collagen, and if the lesion expands, the inflammatory response can affect function of adjacent tissues and/or cells and ultimately the function of the entire organ. For example, chronic inflammatory lesions in the skin can result in ulcerations and obliterate adjacent hair follicles. In the lung, they can destroy alveoli, and the lesion can become so severe or extensive that it can impair gaseous exchange. In the brain, chronic inflammation can destroy neurons and glia, elevate the intracranial pressure, and obstruct the flow of cerebrospinal fluid (CSF) within the ventricular system and thus contribute to elevated intracranial pressure.

The extent of debilitation in animals with chronic inflammatory lesions depends on the location of the lesion and extent of tissue involvement. Even very small chronic lesions in the brain can rapidly incite clinical signs through either the destruction of neuroparenchyma or, perhaps, by impairing flow or resorption of CSF. In contrast, some widespread chronic inflammatory lesions—such as those in inflammatory bowel disease of dogs and cats, and Johne's disease of cattle—can involve extensive areas of the intestine and often precede clinical signs (diarrhea) by months or even years. Yet other diseases, such as embolic hepatic or lung abscesses or disseminated tuberculoid granulomas, can be debilitating over time through the loss of parenchymal function and the continual release of inflammatory mediators, such as tumor necrosis factor (TNF) and interleukin (IL)-1, both of which affect temperature and appetite (see Chapter 3).

In chronic inflammation, the first clinical intervention is to remove the inciting factor, if possible. Thus antibiotics and antifungal drugs are used against bacterial and mycotic infections. Some foreign bodies can be removed surgically, and it may be possible to identify, opsonize, chelate, or sequester immunologic allergens/antigens. Unfortunately, few medical therapies completely resolve certain types of chronic inflammation, especially if granulomas and/or extensive scar tissue has developed. In the future, perhaps surgical debulking of large lesions may be followed by gene or stem cell therapy to effectively eliminate specific types of granulomas, such as those caused by mycobacterial infection.

PROGRESSION OF THE ACUTE INFLAMMATORY RESPONSE TO CHRONIC INFLAMMATION, FIBROSIS, AND ABSCESS FORMATION

Acute inflammatory responses can either fully resolve with return of the tissue to normal structure and function, or repair by healing. If conditions do not allow for complete resolution of the acute inflammatory response, three outcomes can result: (1) progression to chronic/granulomatous inflammation, (2) healing by fibrosis, or (3) abscess formation (Fig. 4-1). These outcomes are determined by the severity of tissue damage, the ability of cells to regenerate, and the biologic characteristics of the stimulus that caused the injury.

PROGRESSION TO CHRONIC/GRANULOMATOUS INFLAMMATION

Progression to chronic/granulomatous inflammation occurs when the acute inflammatory response fails (Fig. 4-9). Failure is characterized by: (1) the inciting stimulus persisting for a long period of time (weeks to months); (2) extensive tissue injury and necrosis (third-degree burn); (3) a shift of the cellular elements

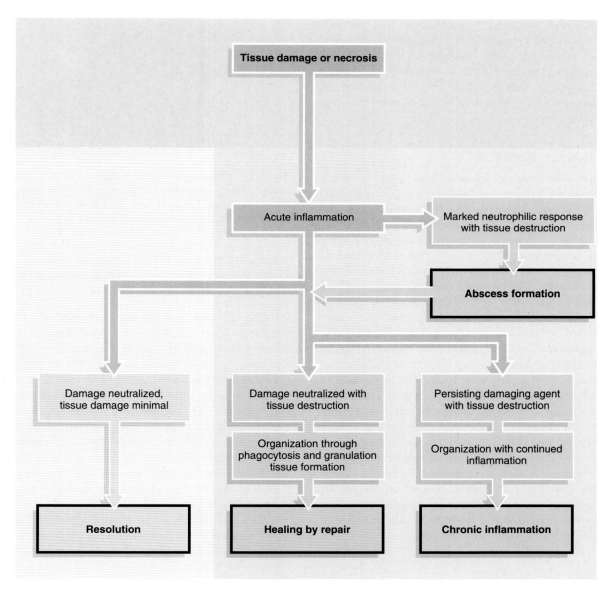

Fig. 4-1   The outcomes of tissue injury and unresolved acute inflammation. *(From Stevens A, Lowe JS, Young B: Wheater's basic histopathology: a colour atlas and text, ed 4, New York, 2002, Churchill Livingstone.)*

of the inflammatory response from neutrophils to lymphocytes, macrophages, and sometimes multinucleate giant cells; and/or (4) extensive connective tissue reorganization followed by fibrosis (fibroplasia).

Deep-seated mycoses, such as *Blastomyces dermatitidis* and *Histoplasma capsulatum*; bacteria, such as *Nocardia, Brucella, Mycobacterium,* or *Salmonella* spp.; protozoa, such as *Leishmania* or *Trypanosoma* spp.; parasites, such as *Toxocara* larva or *Habronema*; autoantigens, such as those occurring in sperm granulomas or in autoimmune diseases like lupus erythematosus; and foreign bodies (plant awns, sticks, metals, asbestos, and suture material) are examples of stimuli that often result in chronic inflammatory responses. Such agents continually induce the release of inflammatory mediators from indigenous parenchymal cells and leukocytes, leading to macrophage infiltration and activation; T lymphocyte, NK cell, and perhaps mast cell or eosinophil infiltration; and fibroblast and endothelial cell proliferation. Some of the inflammatory cytokines, such as transforming growth factor-β (TGF-β), may interfere with regeneration of epithelial and parenchymal cells (see Wound Healing and Angiogenesis).

HEALING BY FIBROSIS

Healing by fibrosis occurs following tissue injury in which there is necrosis of the tissue framework provided by stromal elements (connective tissue) and of the epithelial cells required to regenerate and successfully reconstitute the parenchymatous elements of the tissue (Fig. 4-27). With necrosis, dead tissue and the acute inflammatory exudate are removed by macrophages (phagocytosis by cells of the monocyte-macrophage system), and the space is filled with fibrovascular tissue (granulation tissue) commonly seen in the healing process. Granulation tissue is eventually replaced by immature fibrous connective tissue that is poorly collagenized and then by mature connective tissue that is well collagenized, healing the wound and forming a scar (cicatrix). Structural integrity may be reestablished, but functional integrity is dependent on the extent of the loss of epithelial cells. For example, with severe skin burns or extensive lacerations, dermal scarring eventually replaces lost tissue and to a limited extent restores structural integrity; however, its functional integrity is extremely limited if the scar reduces the range of motion of the limbs and digits. The degree and extent of fibroblast and myofibroblast proliferation in such wounds is largely dependent upon mediators such as TGF-β and interleukin-13 (IL-13). (see Wound Healing and Angiogenesis).

ABSCESS FORMATION

Abscess formation (Fig. 4-2) occurs when the acute inflammatory response fails to rapidly eliminate the

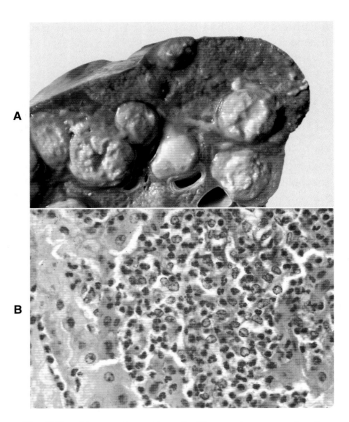

Fig. 4-2   Abscess formation. A, Abscess, lung, cow. A cut section of lung has numerous abscesses. Note the white-to-gray exudate and how it bulges from the cut surface. **B,** In Fig. 4-2, **A,** the exudate consists of cell debris and a large number of neutrophils admixed with lesser numbers of degenerating macrophages and lymphocytes, and bacteria (the latter not visible with H&E stain). H&E stain. (*A and B, Courtesy Dr. M.D. McGavin, College of Veterinary Medicine, University of Tennessee.*)

inciting stimulus and the enzymes and inflammatory mediators from neutrophils in the exudate liquefy the affected tissue and neutrophils to form "pus." Abscesses can have a septic or sterile origin. Septic abscesses most commonly originate from bacterial infection, whereas sterile abscesses arise from incompletely degraded foreign bodies or from the failure of injected medications to be completely absorbed. Pyogenic bacteria, such as *Staphylococcus* and *Streptococcus* spp., commonly cause septic abscesses. They enter tissue hematogenously or by direct extension from the skin following trauma. The pus within an abscess can range in consistency from serous to purulent to caseous and in color from white, to yellow, to green, depending on the inciting stimulus. The color of the exudate often depends on the pigment produced by the inciting bacterium; for example, yellow exudates caused by abscesses formed by *Staphylococcus* and *Streptococcus* spp., green exudate caused by abscesses formed by *Pseudomonas aeruginosa*, and red exudate caused by abscesses formed by *Serratia marcescens*.

Initially, after an acute inflammatory response has been established, a newly formed septic abscess site consists of a collection of neutrophils that may not be encapsulated or is surrounded by a "thin" vascularized connective tissue wall. At this point, antibiotics can penetrate the capsule and enter the exudates. If the septic abscess persists, the initial "thin" connective tissue wall surrounding the exudates can mature into a fibrous capsule, which is thick and largely impermeable, in an attempt to "wall-off" the exudates from normal tissue. Abscesses with this response can present serious problems in systemic (hematogenous) or local (topical diffusion) antibiotic treatments. In large abscesses with abundant pus, the pus itself may dilute the antibiotic and further prevent the drug from reaching the optimal concentration required to kill the bacteria. It is for these reasons that larger abscesses are often lanced to drain the pus. Sterile abscesses do not require antibiotics or other drugs to kill the inciting stimulus, but they do require breakdown of the capsule by lancing or some other means.

MECHANISMS OF CHRONIC INFLAMMATORY RESPONSES

T_H1 AND T_H2 IMMUNOLOGIC RESPONSES AND T REGULATORY CELLS

T lymphocytes expressing $CD4^+$ (T helper cells) and $CD8^+$ T lymphocytes (T suppressor or cytotoxic cells) play important roles in the adaptive immune response. Immunologists use the terms T_H1 and T_H2 as immunological response categories useful in understanding the inflammatory process. T_H1 immunologic responses are generally cell mediated, whereas T_H2 immunologic responses are generally humoral. When $CD4^+$ T lymphocytes bind foreign antigens presented by macrophages and dendritic cells, they release lymphokines that attract leukocytes into the lesion site; some of these cells are directed toward a T_H1 response, whereas others are directed toward a T_H2 response. In addition to macrophages and dendritic cells, B lymphocytes can also present antigens to $CD4^+$ T lymphocytes.

In contrast to $CD4^+$ cells, $CD8^+$ T lymphocytes secrete molecules that kill cells to which they bind. This is a particularly effective defense mechanism if the cell is infected with a virus. The cell will be destroyed before it releases new virions able to infect additional cells. In general, $CD8^+$ T lymphocytes monitor all the cells of the body and will kill any cells that express foreign antigen fragments.

Many chronic inflammatory conditions and their lesions are exacerbated by the presence of poorly degradable exogenous or endogenous antigens. These lesions are usually of long duration, smolder, and often develop insidiously. Initially, lesions are small and undetectable,

but they eventually evolve and expand to a size that results in clinical signs and/or makes them detectable via palpation or diagnostic modalities. It is during this insidious phase that dendritic cells, macrophages, and B lymphocytes present antigen to $CD4^+$ T lymphocytes to initiate an adaptive immune response. Dendritic cells are the predominant cell type that presents antigens to naïve $CD4^+$ T lymphocytes, whereas macrophages are the predominant cell type that presents antigens to memory $CD4^+$ T lymphocytes. The biologic characteristics of antigens, including the amount and structure of protein, polysaccharide, and lipid, contribute to whether the resulting T-lymphocyte response will be balanced between a cell-mediated response (T_H1) and humoral response (T_H2) (Fig. 4-3). However, in many chronic inflammatory conditions, there is often a predominance of either T_H1 type cells (cell-mediated responses) over T_H2 type cells (humoral responses) or vice versa. T regulatory lymphocytes (T reg) and regulatory dendritic cells can affect the strength and the balance of T_H1 and/or T_H2 responses through inhibition of either or both responses (see Effector Cells of the Chronic Inflammatory Response, Lymphocytes).

T_H1 IMMUNOLOGIC RESPONSES

T_H1 immunologic responses often occur in response to: (1) foreign bodies; (2) endogenous antigens, such as those in myelin basic protein (which can occur in murine experimental allergic encephalomyelitis [EAE] and is an experimental model of multiple sclerosis); and (3) endogenous antigens, such as those in intracellular microbes like *Mycobacteria* spp., *Listeria monocytogenes*, *Histoplasma capsulatum*, and *Leishmania* spp. In fact, some immunologists believe that the persistence of many intracellular microbes is caused by an inadequate or suboptimal T_H1 immunologic response or an inappropriately strong T_H2 immunologic response.

T_H1 chronic inflammatory responses are composed, histologically, of T and B lymphocytes, macrophages, dendritic cells, and occasionally fibroblasts. They are induced by: IL-12, interferon (IFN)-γ, and ILs 18, 23, and 27 (Fig. 4-3). Briefly, antigen presenting dendritic cells release IL-12 (also ILs 18, 23, and 27) that induces pre-T_H/$CD4^+$ cells to commit to the T_H1 pathway. The T_H1-committed $CD4^+$ cells then release IL-2 for proliferation of T lymphocytes that produce IFN-γ and TNF-β which activates macrophages. In addition, IFN-γ can inhibit the commitment of pre-Th_H/$CD4^+$ cells to the T_H2 pathway.

T_H2 IMMUNOLOGIC RESPONSES

T_H2-predominant responses are often seen in chronic inflammatory conditions with an allergic basis, such as asthma, chronic allergic inhalant, or food allergic dermatitis, or inflammatory bowel disease. In addition

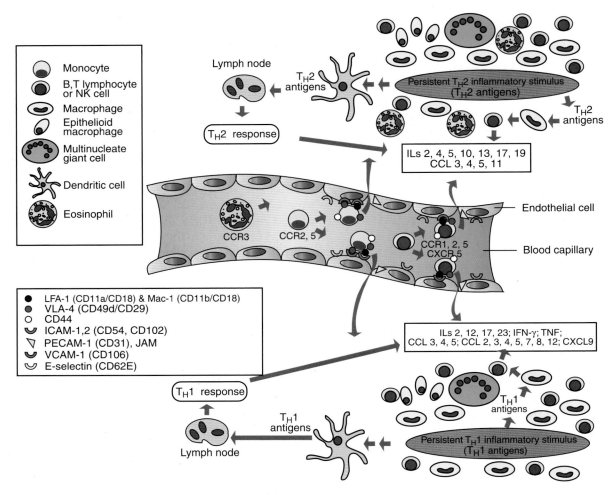

Fig. 4-3   Schematic illustration of the T$_H$1- and T$_H$2-mediated chronic inflammation.
T$_H$1-(below the blood vessel) and T$_H$2-(above the blood vessel) mediated types of chronic
inflammation and some of the key inflammatory mediators, chemokines, and adhesion molecules that mediate the process. *CCL, CXCL,* Chemokine ligand; *ICAM-1,2,* intercellular adhesion
molecule-1,2; *IL,* interleukin; *INF-γ,* interferon-γ; *JAM,* junctional adhesion molecule; *LFA-1,* lymphocyte function antigen-1; *Mac-1,* macrophage-1 antigen; *NK,* natural killer; *PECAM-1,* platelet
endothelial cell adhesion mlecule-1; *TNF,* tumor necrosis factor; *VCAM-1,* vascular cell adhesion
molecule-1; *VLA-4* very late antigen-4. *(Redrawn with permission from Dr. M.R. Ackermann, College of
Veterinary Medicine, Iowa State University.)*

to increasing the number of T and B lymphocytes,
macrophages, dendritic cells, and fibroblasts in the
inflammatory milieu, T$_H$2 responses can also lead to
increased numbers of mast cells and eosinophils associated with IgE and other humoral responses. T$_H$2
responses are induced by high concentrations of IL-4,
IL-10, also ILs 5, 9, 13, 17, and, to some degree,
perhaps ILs 19, 20, 22, 24, 26, 28, and 29 (Fig. 4-3).
Briefly, T$_H$2 dendritic cells present antigen to pre-
T$_H$/CD4$^+$ cells committing them to the T$_H$2 pathway.
T$_H$2-committed CD4$^+$ cells release IL-4 and ILs 5, 10,
13, 17 and 19 (also ILs 19, 20, 22, 24, 26, 28, and 29)
to act on B lymphocytes thus resulting in antibody
production and, in some cases, increased activity of
eosinophils and mast cells. In addition, ILs 4, 5, 10, and

13 can also inhibit pre-Th/CD4$^+$ cells from committing
to the T$_H$1 pathway.

GRANULOMATOUS INFLAMMATION AND GRANULOMA FORMATION

Granulomatous inflammation is a distinct type of chronic
inflammation in which cells of the monocyte-
macrophage system are predominant and take the form
of macrophages, epithelioid macrophages (activated
macrophages), and MGCs. Granulomatous inflammation
occurs secondarily in response to endogenous or exogenous antigens or idiopathically as in granulomatous
meningoencephalitis of dogs. Development and regulation of granulomatous inflammation requires multiple

factors: (1) an inciting agent, usually with indigestible, poorly degradable, and persistent antigens (e.g., *Mycobacteria* spp.): (2) a host immune response, usually an intense T lymphocyte–mediated response; and (3) the interplay of various cytokines produced by cells within the chronic inflammatory lesion.

Classification of granulomatous inflammation by pathologists has evolved over the years because of the increased understanding of disease pathogenesis and advances in molecular biology. For simplicity, this chapter will discuss two morphologic forms of granulomatous inflammation: diffuse (lepromatous) granulomas, which are currently thought to be consistent with a T_H2-biased immunologic response, and nodular (tuberculoid) granulomas, which are currently thought to be consistent with a T_H1-biased immunologic response. Both of these types are derived from granulomatous lesions in humans and are increasingly becoming defined and seen as distinct, both immunologically and molecularly.

DIFFUSE (LEPROMATOUS) GRANULOMAS (T_H2-BIASED GRANULOMAS)

Mycobacterium leprae, the cause of human leprosy, produces noncaseating aggregates of macrophages and chronic inflammatory cells often around nerve fibres in the distal extremities and upper respiratory tract mucosa (sites in the body with temperatures lower than core body temperature) of infected humans. This type of granulomatous inflammation appears to form with a T_H2-type bias.

These lesions can be poorly delineated (e.g., poorly defined borders) and have a widespread distribution, a heavy bacterial burden, relatively few lymphocytes, and variable fibrosis. Similar granulomatous lesions are seen in animals. Feline leprosy and canine lepromatous-like granulomas are somewhat similar to human leprosy in lesion formation. *Mycobacterium avium-intracellulare* paratuberculosis—the cause of Johne's disease in cattle, sheep, and goats—also induces a diffuse (lepromatous) type of granulomatous inflammation consisting of diffuse sheets of macrophages with few lymphocytes and plasma cells. This lesion most commonly occurs in the lamina propria of the ileum and colon (Fig. 4-4) and in mesenteric lymph nodes. Special stains, such as an acid-fast histochemical stain and immunohistochemical stains to specific bacterial antigens, can be used to identify these bacteria within the cytoplasm of macrophages (Fig. 4-5). Because bacteria are present in large numbers in these lesions, they are commonly identified by these techniques. Nodular (tuberculoid) granulomas, defined later, are not seen in Johne's disease lesions. Finally, *Mycobacterium avium-intracellulare* infection also occurs in the lung and other organs of birds and other species and induces lesions with similar sheets of macrophages containing abundant bacteria detectable with special stains.

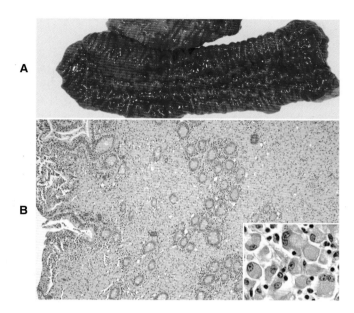

Fig. 4-4 **Diffuse (lepromatous) type of granulomatous inflammation, Johne's disease (*Mycobacterium avium-intracellulare* paratuberculosis), ileum, cow. A,** The mucosa is thickened because of a dense infiltrate of granulomatous inflammatory cells in the lamina propria. **B,** The lamina propria contains numerous macrophages arranged in sheets. The ileal lumen is to the left; scattered crypts still remain in the central area of the specimen. H&E stain. *Inset:* Higher magnification of macrophages and lymphocytes within the granulomatous inflammation present in the granulomatous inflammatory exudate. H&E stain. (**A,** *Courtesy Dr. J. Andrews, College of Veterinary Medicine, University of Illinois.* **B,** *Courtesy Dr. J. Hostetter, College of Veterinary Medicine, Iowa State University.* **Inset,** *Courtesy College of Veterinary Medicine, University of Illinois.*)

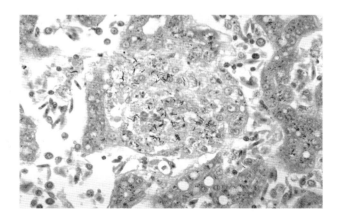

Fig. 4-5 ***Mycobacterium avium-intracellulare* bacilli.** Diffuse (lepromatous) type of granulomatous inflammation with numerous macrophages and multinucleate giant cells that contain abundant bacilli stained red. Acid-fast stain. (*Courtesy Dr. M.D. McGavin, College of Veterinary Medicine, University of Tennessee.*)

NODULAR (TUBERCULOID) GRANULOMAS (T$_H$1-BIASED GRANULOMAS)

Examples of nodular (tuberculoid) granulomas are those that have been classically caused by *Mycobacterium bovis* or *Mycobacterium tuberculosis* and by some deep fungal infections, such as coccidioidomycosis (Fig. 4-6). Tuberculoid granulomas develop with a T$_H$1-type bias and occur in many species but have been described extensively from lesions of infected human beings, cattle, and rhesus monkeys. Because the portal of entry is often the respiratory tract, these lesions often involve the lung and other parenchymal organs and induce the formation of granulomas with three distinctive morphologic areas. The innermost area is often, but not always, a centrally located region of cellular necrosis (cell debris and caseation) surrounded by a middle area containing macrophages, epithelioid macrophages, and multinucleate giant cells. The outermost area surrounding the entire lesion consists of T and B lymphocytes, plasma cells, macrophages, and a fibrous capsule.

Mycobacterial organisms and their antigens are very sparse in these granulomas and not commonly detected with acid-fast stains and immunohistochemical stains for mycobacterial antigens. Mineralization can occur in tuberculoid granulomas, but this outcome depends on the species of animal affected. It is common in cattle, present to a lesser degree in pigs, and uncommon in sheep. "Atypical" mycobacteria, such as *Mycobacterium marinum*, can also cause nodular (tuberculoid) granulomas in the subcutaneous tissues of dogs, cats, and other species, and very few organisms are detected with stains.

Microscopically, nodular (tuberculoid) granulomas may or may not have a central core of necrotic cell debris (caseating and noncaseating granulomas) (Fig. 4-6).

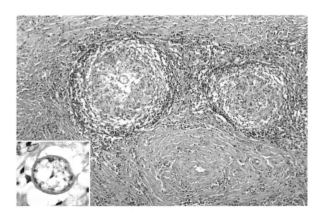

Fig. 4-6   Nodular (tuberculoid) type of granulomatous inflammation, coccidioidomycosis. Granulomas are round to oval with a central core of numerous macrophages surrounded by lymphocytes, plasma cells, macrophages, and a peripheral zone of fibroblasts, which produce a fibrous capsule. The granuloma on the left contains a single central fungal element (*inset*). H&E stain. (*Figure* and *Inset*, *Courtesy Dr. M.D. McGavin, College of Veterinary Medicine, University of Tennessee.*)

Those granulomas lacking caseation (noncaseating) often have multinucleate giant cells in the central area in lesions from human beings; however, in granulomatous inflammation of most animals, multinucleate giant cells are often located in the outer area of the inflammation. Still, other granulomas develop this classic morphologic arrangement but do not contain significant infiltrates of macrophages.

CONTENT AND FORMATION OF T$_H$1 AND T$_H$2 GRANULOMAS

T$_H$1 or T$_H$2 chronic inflammatory responses (Fig. 4-7) and granulomas often can differ somewhat in cellular content (number of T$_H$1 and T$_H$2 cells) and the degree of fibrosis. However, for both T$_H$1 or T$_H$2 granulomas, roughly 30% to 60% of the T lymphocytes in a granuloma are specific for antigens inducing the granuloma, whether the antigens are from an endogenous or exogenous source, foreign body, or microbe. Co-stimulatory molecules are important for T lymphocyte activation, and the co-stimulatory molecule CD40 ligand is required for recruitment of CD4$^+$ cells into the granuloma and for IFN-γ production, whereas granuloma formation is unaffected in mice lacking another co-stimulatory molecule, CD28. CD8$^+$ T lymphocytes can lyse bacteria-infected macrophages containing microbial antigens, thus releasing the organisms and further allowing them to participate in T$_H$1 or T$_H$2 responses. The role of γ/δ-T lymphocytes and NK cells is less clear, but they may have a role in the formation and clearing of either T$_H$1 or T$_H$2 granulomas.

Experimentally, schistosome eggs induce T$_H$2 granulomas in a mouse model, which results in severe fibrosis and eosinophil accumulation (Fig. 4-7). Cytokines of T$_H$2 bias that are present in the schistosome granulomas include ILs 4, 5, 10, and 13 along with TGF-β, resulting in granulomatous lesions with eosinophils. T$_H$2 cytokines induce Arg-1 activity (metabolism of arginine) in macrophages. The Arg-1 activity results in the production of polyamines, which induce cell proliferation, and proline, which induces collagen production. The presence of fibrosis in this model fits well with parasite-induced granulomas seen in animals and humans; however, it is not a consistent feature of many lepromatous granulomas in animals, such as those in Johne's disease and infections with *Mycobacterium avium-intracellulare*.

Mycobacterium bovis antigens induce tuberculoid T$_H$1 granulomas. T$_H$1 cytokines include IFN-γ, IL-12, TNF-α, nitric oxide (NO and its intermediates, NO$_2$-, NO$_3$-, N$_2$O$_2$, and ONOO–), and TGF-β. In contrast to the Arg-1 pathway used in T$_H$2 granulomas, macrophages in T$_H$1 granulomas use the nitric oxide synthetase 2 (NOS$_2$) pathway to produce nitric oxide and citrulline, which reduces the degree of fibrosis. In granulomas with a T$_H$1 bias, the regulation of fibrosis and collagen deposition occurs largely by the influence of IL-13 and TGF-β.

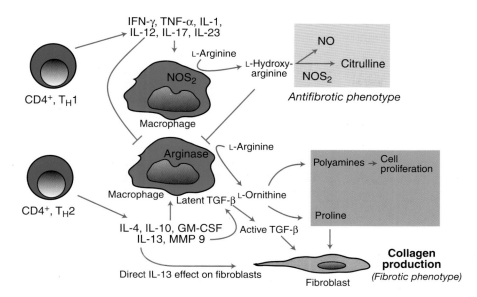

Fig. 4-7   Mechanistic basis for fibrosis in experimentally induced T$_H$1- and T$_H$2-mediated responses by macrophages. In T$_H$1-mediated responses, nitric oxide synthetase 2 (*NOS$_2$*) enzyme is activated by interferon-γ (*IFN-γ*), tumor necrosis factor-α (*TNF-α*), and interleukin-1 (*IL-1*) produced by T lymphocytes. The *NOS$_2$* enzyme converts L-hydroxy-arginine to citrulline, which is antifibrotic. With the T$_H$2 pathway, *NOS$_2$* is not activated in the presence of the T$_H$2 cytokines (*ILs 4, 10, and 13*) and granulocyte-macrophage colony-stimulating factor (*GM-CSF*), and ornithine is converted to polyamines and praline, which induce cell proliferation of fibroblasts and collagen production, respectively, thereby contributing to fibrosis. *TGF-β*, Transforming growth factor-β. (*Redrawn with permission from Dr. M.R. Ackermann, College of Veterinary Medicine, Iowa State University.*)

SARCOIDOSIS OF HUMAN BEINGS

Sarcoidosis is a disease of human beings characterized by the spontaneous formation of granulomas. To date, no counterpart in domestic animals has been found. However, studies of sarcoid granulomas have led to an improved understanding of granuloma formation that may apply generally to other animal species. Individuals with sarcoidosis develop granulomatous reactions in the lung hilus, lung parenchyma, eye, and skin. The disease appears to be caused by a persistent, ineffective reaction to an unknown antigen in individuals who may have a predisposition to the disease. It begins with an accumulation of antigen-presenting cells, which trigger T lymphocytes to release cytokines important for granuloma formation.

Sarcoid patients have an accumulation of CD4+ T lymphocytes with receptors for CXC3 chemokines and IL-12, and they release IFN-γ and IL-2. There is an expansion of T lymphocytes with TNF receptors, B lymphocyte proliferation with immunoglobulin synthesis, and the accumulation of activated macrophages expressing major histocompatibility complex (MHC) II antigens and adhesion molecules. Macrophages and T lymphocytes have an increased propensity for proliferation in situ. The macrophages release IL-1, IL-6, IL-8, IL-15, TNF-α, granulocyte-macrophage colony-stimulating factor (GM-CSF), regulated on activation, normal T lymphocytes expressed and secreted (RANTES), IP-10, monocyte chemotactic protein-1 (MCP-1), and macrophage inflammatory protein-α (MIP-1-α), which contribute to macrophage infiltration and activation. In some patients, the macrophages also release fibrogenetic cytokines, such as TGF-β, platelet-derived growth factor (PDGF), and insulin-like growth factor, thus inducing fibrosis.

SARCOIDS OF HORSES

Sarcoids of horses are not a correlate to sarcoids in human beings. Sarcoids that occur in the skin of horses are not granulomas but are locally aggressive skin tumors, and the most common dermatologic neoplasm reported in horses. They are composed of proliferating fibroblasts and do not contain the numerous macrophages, lymphocytes, and plasma cells seen in human sarcoids. There is no consistently effective therapy for equine sarcoid. Bovine papillomavirus (BPV) types 1 and 2 are associated with the development of equine sarcoid. Most sarcoid tumors express the BPV types 1 and 2 major transforming protein, E5, but appear not to produce infectious virions. E5 may contribute to virus persistence and disease pathogenesis by down-regulating MHC class I expression and thereby reducing immunosurveillance. The mode of transmission of BPV infection has not been determined.

EOSINOPHILIC GRANULOMAS

Certain types of chronic inflammation have dense infiltrates of eosinophils and many of these form eosinophilic granulomas (Table 4-2; also see Chapter 17). Some eosinophilic granulomas develop in response to migrating parasites, such as *Toxocara canis* (larval migrans). In certain other conditions of cats, dogs, and horses, it is suspected that some of these conditions form in response to antigen in a T_H2-directed manner; however, no specific antigen has been identified for many of these conditions.

Grossly, eosinophilic granulomas in cats appear as papules, nodules, plaques (sometimes linear), and ulcers in the skin. They also occur as nodular or ulcerated lesions in the oral mucosas and footpads. Microscopically, the inflammatory response consists of eosinophils, macrophages, and areas of dense eosinophilia around collagen (Fig. 4-8). For many years, the densely eosinophilic, collagen-rich areas were considered regions of collagen degradation; however, the eosinophilic material is composed largely of major basic protein (MBP), a protein present in large amounts in the granules of eosinophils (see Chapter 3). Apparently eosinophils degranulate in these regions, releasing MBP, which accumulates over time.

OTHER CHRONIC INFLAMMATORY/ GRANULOMATOUS CONDITIONS

Several conditions of human beings and animals are characterized by chronic inflammatory and/or granulomatous lesions. One such condition, polyarteritis nodosa, is seen in human beings and rats and only rarely in other species. It is characterized by perivascular infiltrates of lymphocytes, plasma cells, and macrophages. Dogs can develop idiopathic canine polyarteritis, a condition in which arterial lesions not only involve coronary arteries, but also medium to small arteries of other organs. As indicated earlier, eosinophilic granulomas occur in cats, dogs, and horses, and the causes of

Table **4-2**   **Eosinophilic Granulomas of Domestic Animals**

Species	Type of Eosinophilic Granuloma
Feline	Eosinophilic plaque, granuloma, and dermatitis
Canine	Eosinophilic granuloma of the oral cavity of huskies and other dogs
Equine	Equine collagenolytic granuloma, axillary nodular necrosis, unilateral papular dermatosis
All species	Eosinophilic (T_H2) granulomas secondary to parasitic infections

these granulomas have not been determined but are thought to occur secondary to parasitic larval migration, microbial infections, or foreign material. Finally, a variety of other human diseases are characterized by varying degrees of perivascular granulomatous inflammation, but to date have no or very rarely seen veterinary correlates. These diseases occur around blood vessels, may be secondary to immunologic mechanisms, and include: large-vessel vasculitis (giant cell [temporal] arteritis, Takayasu arteritis), medium-sized vessel arteritis (Kawasaki disease, [and polyarteritis nodosa]), and small-vessel vasculitis (Wegener's granulomatosis, Churg-Strauss syndrome, microscopic polyangiitis, Henoch-Schönlein purpura, essential cryoglobulinemia vasculitis, and cutaneous leukocytoclastic angiitis).

INHIBITION OF MACROPHAGES IN THE CHRONIC INFLAMMATORY RESPONSE

Although macrophage activation is most commonly discussed and studied, macrophages can also be inhibited For example, macrophage activity is inhibited/reduced after phagocytosis of apoptotic bodies and low-density lipoproteins (LDLs) in some inflammatory foci. In addition, macrophages can be inhibited by several chemical mediators, including IL-10, TGF-β, IFN-γ, monocyte colony-stimulating factor, CD47, CD200R, CD36, $\alpha_5\beta_3$-integrins, and glucocorticoid receptor activation (Table 4-3). These mediators are often present in inflamed areas and thus can regulate

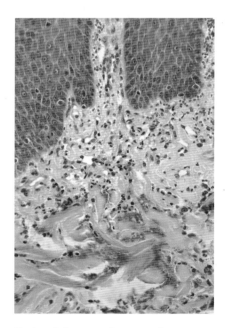

Fig. 4-8   Eosinophilic granuloma, oral mucosa, cat. Note the mixture of eosinophils, macrophages, and lymphocytes in the superficial dermis accompanied by collagenolysis *(bottom half of illustration)*. H&E stain. *(Courtesy Dr. M.D. McGavin, College of Veterinary Medicine, University of Tennessee.)*

Table **4-3**   **Stimuli that Affect the Activation Status of Macrophages**

Type of Activation	Activating Factor	Macrophage Response	Macrophage Activity
Innate activation to microbes	Toll-like receptor CD14 (LPS binding) β-Glucan receptor TREM	Co-stimulatory expression ROS, NO expression Cytokine release	Inflammation, antigen presentation to memory T lymphocytes
Humoral activation	Fc receptor Complement receptors	Ig/Fc internalization Cytolytic activity Cytokine release	Inflammation, antigen presentation to memory T lymphocytes
Classical activation T_H1	IFN-γ	MHC II expression Cytokine release (IL-1, IL-6, TNF) Respiratory burst NO release	Cell-mediated immunity Microbial killing DTH
Alternative activation T_H2	IL-4 IL-13	MHC II expression Mannose receptor expression	Humoral immunity Allergic response Response to parasites Arginase repair
Deactivation by innate/ adaptive stimuli	IL-10 TGF-β IFN-α, IFN-β GM-CSF CD47 CD200R CD36 (scavenger receptor) $\alpha_5\beta_3$-Integrin Glucocorticoid receptor Internalized ox LDL	MHC II down-regulation PGE_2 release IL-10 release TGF-β release PPAR inhibition of NF kappa B	Immunosuppression

DTH, Delayed type hypersensitivity; *IFN*, interferon; *Ig*, immunoglobulin; *IL*, interleukin; *MHC*, major histocompatibility complex; *NF*, nuclear factor; *NO*, nitric oxide; *ox LDL*, oxidized low-density lipoprotein; *PGE_2*, prostaglandin type E_2; *PPAR*, peroxisome proliferator-activated receptor; *ROS*, reactive oxygen species; *TGF*, transforming growth factor; *T_H1*, T helper cell type 1 lymphocyte response; *T_H2*, T helper cell type 2 lymphocyte response; *TREM*, triggering receptor expressed on myeloid cells.

macrophage activity. Recent work has also shown that macrophage activity can also be reduced by acetylcholine (Ach) and peroxisome proliferator-activated receptor (PPAR). Macrophages express Ach receptors, which are ligand-gated ion channels. They are most often associated with the neuromuscular junction and the peripheral and central nervous systems. Vagal release of Ach modulates macrophage activity and TNF-α release. It is termed the "cholinergic antiinflammatory pathway." Inhibition of macrophage activity can be beneficial in preventing overexuberant activity of the chronic inflammatory response. On the other hand, research may find that inhibition may be detrimental in certain conditions.

PEROXISOME PROLIFERATOR-ACTIVATED RECEPTORS: TRANSCRIPTION FACTORS THAT REDUCE CHRONIC INFLAMMATORY RESPONSES

Activated PPARs are nuclear transcription factors that can alter and often reduce inflammatory responses by macrophages, dendritic cells, endothelial cells, and T lymphocytes. The PPARs affect inflammatory responses through transrepression of signal transduction pathways by binding to peroxisome proliferator binding elements (PPBEs) and enhancing transcription or inhibiting transcription factors. PPARs can inhibit NF kappa B, STATs and AP-1, and the T-lymphocyte activator NFAT. Through inhibition of NF kappa B and AP-1 signaling in macrophages, PPAR activity decreases iNOS expression, reduces macrophage survival, and inhibits cytokine (IL-6 and IL-12) and vascular cell adhesion molecule-1 (VCAM-1) expression. Thus PPARs generally inhibit inflammatory activity of chronic inflammatory cells, such as macrophages and T lymphocytes, and thereby prevent overzealous reactions. Agonists to PPARs have promise as therapeutic agents that may reduce the inflammatory response in atherosclerosis and other chronic inflammatory or granulomatous lesions.

GROSS AND MICROSCOPIC LESIONS AND NOMENCLATURE OF THE CHRONIC INFLAMMATORY RESPONSE

The term *chronic inflammation* implies two underlying and often concurrently occurring processes: fibroplasia and cellular infiltration. Fibroplasia, the formation of fibrous connective tissue, includes any stage of the process from the formation of fibrous connective tissue that includes newly formed "immature" connective tissue with newly formed blood vessels to "mature" connective tissue that contains well-collagenized and remodeled granulation tissue. Cellular infiltrates are composed of predominantly macrophages, lymphocytes, and plasma cells, depending on the inciting stimulus and the duration of the inflammatory process. It is important to understand the meaning of these terms mechanistically and in the context of developing morphologic diagnoses for gross and histopathologic lesions. To clinicians, these terms imply duration of illness, whereas to pathologists, they imply the characteristics of the tissue's response to injury.

Grossly, chronic inflammatory lesions are often gray to white, firm, and have either a nodular surface in the case of granulomas or an indented or pitted surface in the case of fibrosis. The gray-to-white color is largely a result of the infiltrates of macrophages and lymphocytes, proliferation of fibroblasts, and deposition of fibrous connective tissue. The firm texture is attributable to fibrous connective tissue (fibroblasts and endothelial cells) and the consolidation (i.e., solidification) of the leukocytes in the exudate. The irregular shape occurs because of the haphazard accumulation of leukocytes and the fibrosis/scarring and contraction of the lesion by myofibroblasts within the fibrous connective tissue (see Wound Healing and Angiogenesis).

The lungs of dogs with *Blastomyces dermatitidis* infection often have a nodular appearance because of the formation of numerous granulomas and/or pyogranulomas (Fig. 4-9). The use of and distinction between terms such as granuloma and pyogranuloma are dependent on the number of neutrophils in the overall inflammatory exudate or in the center of the granuloma and often reflects the interpretation of the examining pathologist.

The kidneys of dogs, cats, or other species with chronic interstitial nephritis or chronic pyelonephritis, for example, frequently have pitted surfaces that correspond to areas where fibrous tissue formed within renal parenchyma during the chronic inflammatory response that pulls the renal capsule into the parenchyma as part of the healing process. In chronic pyelonephritis, the inflammatory bands often radiate from the renal medulla into the cortex and to the renal capsule, and obliterate or surround and separate cortical tubules and glomeruli. Fibrous adhesions between the renal cortex and the capsule can occur. This fibrous connective tissue may also contain lymphocytes, plasma cells, and macrophages.

Grossly, scars, abscesses, and granulomas that occur with the persistence of chronic inflammation are often easily seen. Severe scarring results in an area that is generally gray to white with extensive contraction,

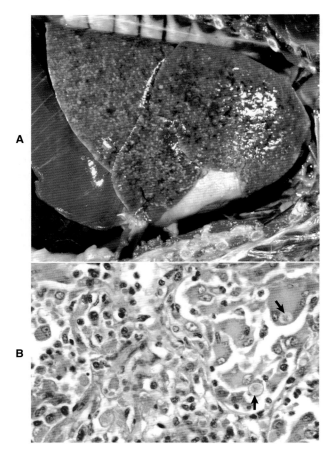

Fig. 4-9   **Granulomas and pyogranulomas, blastomycosis, lung, dog. A,** Numerous multifocal discrete and coalescing variably sized gray-white nodules are scattered at random (embolic pattern) in the lung parenchyma. They are composed of granulomatous inflammatory cells. Note that the lung lobes fail to collapse. **B,** The granulomatous inflammatory exudate contains activated and multinucleate giant cells with intracellular *Blastomyces dermatitidis* organisms *(arrows)*. Lymphocytes and plasma cells are also present in the exudate. H&E stain. (**A,** *Courtesy Dr. M.D. McGavin, College of Veterinary Medicine, University of Tennessee.* **B,** *Courtesy Dr. J.F. Zachary, College of Veterinary Medicine, University of Illinois.*)

whereas abscesses are often round with a fibrous capsule and a central area of pus. Granulomas are often gray to white, round to oval, and firm to hard, whereas diffuse granulomatous inflammation is often gray to white; expansile, but poorly demarcated from adjacent tissue; and firm. Grossly the three main differential diagnoses for a white, firm, oval to irregular nodular mass are abscess, granuloma, and neoplasm. Most commonly, histopathology is required to differentiate the three as they can appear very similar grossly.

Microscopically, chronic inflammatory responses are classified into categories based on the types and distribution of the inflammatory cells in the exudate. These categories include: (1) chronic inflammation,

(2) chronic-active inflammation, (3) granulomatous inflammation, (4) pyogranulomatous inflammation, (5) granulomas, and (6) pyogranulomas.

- The simplest type of chronic inflammation has a basic cellular exudate consisting predominantly of lymphocytes with lesser numbers of macrophages and plasma cells (Fig. 4-10). Sometimes lymphocytes and macrophages predominante over plasma cells, and such lesions can be called lymphohistiocytic. "Histiocytic" is a term used for macrophage infiltration; however, a few pathologists use the term "macrophagic." This type of inflammatory response is characteristically seen in the early stages of the chronic inflammatory response and in response to specific microbes, such as viruses.
- Chronic-active inflammation has the same cellular components as chronic inflammation, but also contains neutrophils, fibrin, and plasma proteins that are constituents of the acute inflammatory response. Chronic-active inflammation occurs when the inciting stimulus has not been removed from the exudate in the chronic inflammatory response, and it continues to elicit an acute inflammatory response. One should be careful not to confuse the morphologic diagnosis of chronic-active inflammation with the hepatic disease entity of dogs termed chronic-active hepatitis.

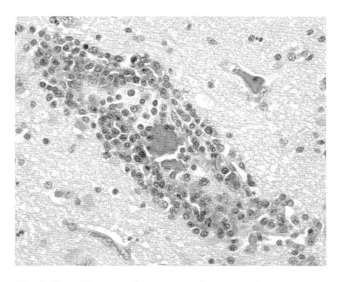

Fig. 4-10   Chronic inflammation, distemper, brain, raccoon. In its simplest form, chronic inflammation, as seen with some viral infections, consists of an exudate of lymphocytes with occasional macrophages and plasma cells. In many tissues, especially in the central nervous system, these cells can have a perivascular pattern of distribution. In certain animal species (exotic wildlife species, horses) and specific disease categories (parasitic, protozoal, viral), perivascular chronic inflammatory exudates may also contain variable numbers of eosinophils. H&E stain. *(Courtesy Dr. J. F. Zachary, College of Veterinary Medicine, University of Illinois.)*

- Granulomatous inflammation has a basic cellular exudate consisting predominantly of activated macrophages and perhaps also epithelioid macrophages, multinucleate giant cells, and lesser numbers of lymphocytes and plasma cells. Granulomatous inflammation can be arranged in a diffuse or haphazard manner as seen in the thickened intestinal mucosa (i.e., lamina propria) of cattle with Johne's disease (Fig. 4-4). If the macrophages are arranged in solid, nodular-like masses, they are termed granulomas (see later). Granulomatous inflammation is characteristically seen in deep-seated mycoses; infections with more evolved bacteria, such as *Nocardia*, *Brucella*, and *Mycobacteria* spp., and protozoal infections.
- Pyogranulomatous inflammation has the same cellular exudate as granulomatous inflammation but also contains multifocal/random infiltrates of neutrophils, fibrin, and plasma proteins, which are constituents of the acute inflammatory response. Pyogranulomatous inflammation occurs when the inciting stimulus has not been removed from the exudate in the granulomatous inflammatory response, and it continues to elicit an acute inflammatory response. A nodular-like granulomatous area with neutrophils is termed a pyogranuloma (see later). Pyogranulomatous inflammation is often seen with infections caused by *Blastomyces dermatitidis* (Fig. 4-9).
- Granulomas are a distinct type of granulomatous inflammatory response that occurs when macrophage infiltration is present in a well-defined area and thus forms a distinct mass on gross observation. Granulomas can occur as noncaseating and caseating types. Noncaseating granulomas are often round to oval and composed of numerous macrophages with variable numbers of epithelioid macrophages, perhaps multinucleate giant cells, with a peripheral zone of fibroblasts, lymphocytes, and plasma cells (Fig. 4-6). Caseating granulomas have the same morphologic features as noncaseating granulomas; however, the center is formed by a core of gray-white-yellow pasty (thick-dehydrated) necrotic debris resembling cheese (Latin caseus = cheese). Caseating granulomas most commonly occur in tuberculosis.
- A pyogranuloma is a granuloma with a central area of neutrophils.

EFFECTOR CELLS OF THE CHRONIC INFLAMMATORY RESPONSE

The primary effector cells of the chronic inflammatory response are fibroblasts, macrophages, dendritic cells, α-β and γ-δ lymphocytes, NK cells, plasma cells, mast cells, eosinophils, and endothelial cells. These cells comprise chronic inflammatory lesions and also mediate adaptive immune responses and tissue repair.

FIBROBLASTS

Fibroblasts are multipurpose cells whose function is often overlooked in tissue responses to injury (Figs. 4-11 and 4-12). Fibroblasts are elongated cells that contribute to the structural integrity of tissue and have abundant rough endoplasmic reticulum, which is used for the synthesis of collagen. In addition, they also produce other extracellular matrix (ECM) proteins, cytokines, matrix metalloproteinases, and chemokines that regulate the composition of the extracellular microenvironment in physiologic and pathologic conditions.

With tissue injury or certain hypoxic conditions, fibroblasts undergo proliferation in response to the release of fibroblast growth factors (FGFs), TGF-β, IL-13, PDGF, vascular endothelial growth factor (VEGF), and other mediators/molecules. Continued release of these substances in response to chronic inflammatory stimuli leads to the extensive fibrosis and collagen deposition characteristic of chronic inflammation. The mechanistic basis for fibrosis in experimentally induced T_H1 and T_H2 mediated responses by macrophages is illustrated in Fig. 4-7 (also see Fibroblasts and the Mechanistic Basis of Fibrosis).

MONOCYTES/MACROPHAGES

Along with fibroblasts, monocytes/macrophages are one of the hallmark cell types of chronic inflammation. They produce a wide variety of inflammatory mediators, including chemokines, cytokines, nitric oxide, and are often situated at strategic locations within tissues of the body to: (1) quickly sense the initial activity of acute inflammation, (2) migrate in response to chemotaxins, (3) internalize agents and particulate matter for sequestration/removal, and (4) process antigens for presentation to effector cells of the adaptive immune response.

Macrophages arise from bone marrow-derived monocytes, which circulate hematogenously with some monocytes localizing in tissues physiologically. The differentiation of monocyte stem cells into blood monocytes proceeds rapidly in the bone marrow (i.e., $1^{1}/_{2}$ to 3 days) and is regulated by growth and differentiating factors, cytokines, and adhesion molecules, such as IL-3, colony-stimulating factors, and TNF. Under physiologic conditions, monocytes in the blood localize throughout the body and differentiate into tissue macrophages. Several organs have specialized tissue macrophages, including bone (osteoclasts), liver

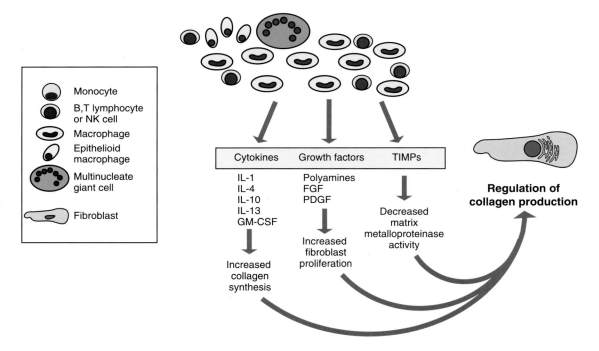

Fig. 4-11   Development of fibrosis in chronic inflammation. In most chronic inflammatory lesions, activated macrophages, lymphocytes and other cells secrete cytokines, growth factors, and tissue inhibitors of matrix metalloproteinases (*TIMPs*) that lead to fibroblast proliferation and collagen synthesis. *FGF*, Fibroblast growth factor; *GM-CSF*, granulocyte-macrophage colony-stimulating factor; *IL*, interleukin; *NK*, natural killer; *PDGF*, platelet-derived growth factor.
(Redrawn with permission from Dr. M.R. Ackermann, College of Veterinary Medicine, Iowa State University.)

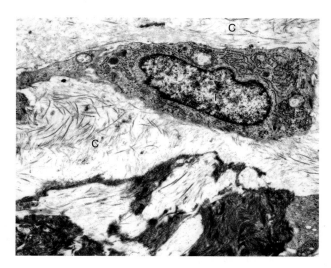

Fig. 4-12   Fibroblast, fibrosis in chronic inflammation.
A fibroblast (*F*) is surrounded by collagen fibrils (*C*), many of
which extend from the fibroblast plasma membrane. Edema
fluid also separates many of the fibrils. The fibroblast has a
large amount of rough endoplasmic reticulum because of the
high level of collagen protein synthesis. Adjacent to the collagen fibers is a modest amount of polymerized fibrin (*dark
area, bottom of illustration*). TEM. Uranyl acetate and lead
citrate stain. (*Courtesy Dr. M.R. Ackermann, College of Veterinary
Medicine, Iowa State University.*)

(Kupffer cells), lung (pulmonary alveolar macrophages
and pulmonary intravascular macrophages [in rumi-
nants]), brain (microglial cells), testis (interstitial
macrophages), and spleen and lymph node (sinus
histiocytes). With acute inflammatory stimuli, mono-
cytes/macrophages typically enter affected tissue
within 24 to 48 hours. Certain mediators, such as the
chemokine, monocyte/macrophage chemotactic factor
(MCP), monocytes recruit from the blood into areas of
inflammation. Once present, monocytes rapidly
become activated by cytokines, antigens, and other
stimuli. In chronic inflammatory lesions, macrophages
are the cell of last resort and accumulate in sites of persistent antigen, persistent microbes, foreign material,
or repeated injury.

MONONUCLEAR CELL MATURATION AND TRAFFICKING IN THE CHRONIC INFLAMMATORY RESPONSE

The macrophage is a key part of the development
and persistence of chronic inflammation. Monocytes,
derived from the bone marrow, enter tissues to form
the macrophage-monocyte system (e.g., Kupffer cells,
alveolar macrophages, and microglial cells) and thus
are part of the innate and adaptive immune systems.
Monocytes can also be recruited from the blood stream
to enter tissue and differentiate into macrophages that
can also respond to tissue injury. The population of

macrophages in a tissue is maintained by three mechanisms: (1) entry of monocytes from blood, (2) local proliferation, and (3) loss of macrophages when they reach
their tissue life span. Under noninflammatory conditions, the replenishment of tissue macrophages occurs
through local proliferation and not via monocyte influx.
However, with inflammatory stimuli, monocytes are
recruited from the blood into tissue in response to the
stimulus.

In noninflamed tissue, monocytes expressing
CX3CR1 and CCR5 chemokine receptors are attracted
to tissues releasing their respective ligands (i.e.,
fractalkine (CX3CL) and MIP-1-α [CCL3]). In areas of
inflammation, monocytes expressing CCR2 chemokine
receptors are attracted by MCP-1 (CCL2) (Table 4-4).
Attracted monocytes enter these areas in a manner
similar to that described for the leukocyte adhesion
cascade outlined for neutrophils in Chapter 3. Slow
rolling is mediated by L-selectin adherence to L-selectin
receptors expressed by endothelial cells. However, firm
adherence by monocytes to endothelial cells is largely
mediated by LFA-1 (CD11a/CD18), very late antigen-4
(VLA-4) ($\alpha_4\beta_1$-integrin), and also Mac-1 (CD11a/CD18)
molecules that adhere to the respective endothelial cell
ligands: intercellular adhesion molecule (ICAM)-1/2,
VCAM-1, and ICAM-1/2, respectively. Transmigration
of monocytes between endothelial cells is mediated by
leukocyte adhesion molecules expressed on the monocyte such as LFA-1, VLA-4, Mac-1, platelet endothelial
cell adhesion molecule-1 (PECAM-1), and junctional
adhesion molecule JAM A, JAM B, and JAM C. These
molecules bind to adhesion molecules such as
PECAM-1 and the JAM molecules expressed by
endothelial cells at the intracellular junction. As monocytes and other leukocytes pass between endothelial
cells, they separate the tight junctions and VE-cadherins
to allow intercellular migration.

ACTIVATION OF MONOCYTES/MACROPHAGES

Activation of monocytes/macrophages occurs in
response to various stimuli (Fig. 4-13), each of which
incites a slightly different response by the macrophage
(Table 4-3). Monocytes/macrophages are activated by
stimuli that include the following:
- Innate immune activation during microbial infections through the binding of microbial products (e.g.,
  LPS and teichoic acid) or endogenous molecules
  (e.g., heat shock proteins and oxidized LDLs) to Toll-
  like receptors
- Classic activation mediated by IFN-γ, IL-12, and
  T helper lymphocyte type 1 responses (T_H1
  responses)
- Alternative activation mediated by IL-4 and IL-13
  during T helper lymphocyte type 2 responses (T_H2
  responses)

Table **4-4**   **Key Adhesion Molecules and Chemokines Involved with Homing of Naïve Lymphocytes, Adherence/Transmigration of Monocytes, and Activated T Lymphocytes in Sites of Chronic Inflammation**

Cell Type	Endothelial Cell Type	Slow Rolling by the Leukocyte-Endothelial Cell	Chemokine Receptor-Ligand	Firm Adhesion (Leukocyte-Endothelial Cell)	Transmigration
PERIPHERAL LYMPH NODE HOMING					
Naïve T lymphocyte	HEV	L-selectin-PNAD	CCR7-CCL19/21	LFA-1–ICAM-1,2	LFA-1–ICAM-1,2 LFA-1–JAM A
Naïve B lymphocyte	HEV	L-selectin-PNAD	CXCR4-CXCL12	LFA-1–ICAM-1,2	LFA-1–ICAM-1,2 LFA-1–JAM A
PEYER'S PATCH HOMING					
Naïve T lymphocyte	HEV	L-selectin-L-selectin R $\alpha_4\beta_7$-MAdCAM-1	CXCR7-CCL19/21 CXCR4-CXCL12	$\alpha_4\beta_7$-MAdCAM-1 LFA-1–ICAM-1,2	LFA-1–ICAM-1,2 LFA-1–JAM A
Naïve B lymphocyte	HEV	L-selectin-L-selectin R $\alpha_4\beta_7$-MAdCAM-1	CXCR4-CCL12 CXCR5-CXCL13	$\alpha_4\beta_7$-MAdCAM-1 LFA-1–ICAM-1,2	LFA-1–ICAM-1,2 LFA-1–JAM A
ACTIVATED T LYMPHOCYTES IN SITES OF INFLAMMATION					
T lymphocyte*	Non-HEV	E-, P-selectin R-E-, P-selectin R	CCR7-CCL19/21	E-, P-selectin LFA-1–ICAM-1,2	LFA-1–ICAM-1,2 LFA-1–JAM A PECAM-1–PECAM-1
MONOCYTES					
Monocyte	Non-HEV	L-selectin-L-selectin R E-selectin R-E-selectin P-selectin R-P-selectin	CX3CR-CX3CL CCR5-CCL3 CCR2-CCL2	LFA-1–ICAM-1,2 VLA-4–VCAM-1 Mac-1–ICAM-1,2	LFA-1–JAM A VLA-4–JAM A Mac-1–JAM C PECAM-1–PECAM-1

Slow rolling is the process of decreased vascular transit of leukocytes within the blood by selectin-mediated adherence/tethering; Firm adhesion is the stable binding of leukocytes to endothelial cells (see Chapter 3). L-selectin-PNAD denotes the leukocyte adherence molecule (L-selectin) and the endothelial cell molecule (PNAD) as does LFA-1 (leukocyte adherence molecule) and ICAM-1 (endothelial cell molecule).
E- and P-selectin R are expressed on monocytes at low levels and increase with activation; E- and P-selectin are expressed at increased levels on endothelial cells in areas of chronic inflammation.
$\alpha_4\beta_7$, α_4 β_7 Integrin; *CCL*, CC-type chemokine ligand; *CCR*, CC-type chemokine receptor; *HEV*, high endothelial venule; *ICAM*, intercellular adhesion molecule; *JAM*, junctional adhesion molecule; *LFA*, lymphocyte function antigen; *MAdCAM*, mucosal addressin cellular adhesion molecule; *PECAM*, platelet endothelial cell adhesion molecule; *PNAD*, peripheral lymph node addressin; *R*, receptor; *VCAM*, vascular cell adhesion molecule.
*Activated T lymphocyte in this case is a generic term for $T_H 1$, $T_H 0$, $T_H 2$ effector memory and central memory cells, and T-lymphocyte clones.
Note that effector memory cells have only minimal to no CCR7 expression. Activated B lymphocytes likely migrate similarly.

- Humoral activation by the attachment of immunoglobulins to Fc receptors and complement factors to complement receptors

The outcome of these different types of activation leads to specific responses:

- Innate activation can lead to release of reactive oxygen species (ROS), nitric oxide (NO), and IFN-α and IFN-β.
- Classic activation with IFN-γ leads to expression of MHC II antigen, respiratory burst, release of IL-1 and TNF for microbial killing, cellular immunity, and delayed type hypersensitivity.
- Alternative activation enhances MHC class II expression and mannose receptor expression for humoral immunity and allergic responses.
- Innate deactivation and reduced inflammatory responses can occur with the uptake of apoptotic cells or storage of oxidized LDLs in lysosomes.

FORMATION OF EPITHELIOID MACROPHAGES AND MULTINUCLEATE GIANT CELLS

Both epithelioid macrophages and multinucleate giant cells often form in response to foreign bodies or persistent intracellular pathogens. The molecular mechanisms by which epithelioid macrophages and multinucleate giant cells form are poorly understood. It is a fascinating biologic phenomena requiring membrane fusion and integration of the cytoplasm and nuclei of multiple cells. Studies in human patients with sarcoidosis, a special type of granulomatous inflammation in humans (see Sarcoidosis) have elucidated some of the important factors and conditions that contribute to MGC formation. This process involves cytokines, such as IFN-γ, IL-3, 4, 13, and GM-CSF; pathogen factors, such as muramyl dipeptide,

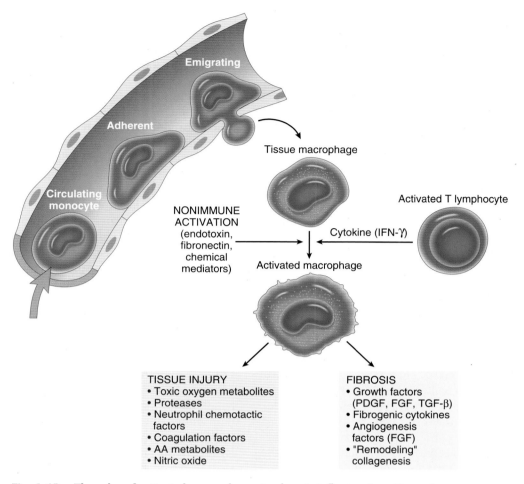

Fig. 4-13   **The roles of activated macrophages in chronic inflammation.** Macrophages are activated by cytokines from immune-activated T lymphocytes (particularly interferon-γ *[IFN-γ]*) or by nonimmunologic stimuli, such as endotoxin. The products made by activated macrophages that cause tissue injury and fibrosis are indicated. *AA,* Arachidonic acid; *FGF,* fibroblast growth factor; *PDGF,* platelet-derived growth factor; *TGF-β,* transforming growth factor-β. Also see Table 4-3. *(From Kumar V, Abbas A, Fausto N: Robbins & Cotran pathologic basis of disease, ed 7, Philadelphia, 2005, Saunders.)*

a peptidoglycan portion of bacterial cells walls; macrophage receptors, such as P2X$_7$ (a ligand-gated ion channel activated by adenosine triphosphate); integrins (LFA-1 and ICAM-1); CD98 (ligand for the cell-surface lectin galectin-3 and may function with β$_1$-integrins); macrophage fusion protein receptor (MFPR; CD47 is a ligand); CD44 (binds hyaluronic acid and works in concert with MFPR); and ADAM9 (a disintegrin and metalloproteinase).

HISTOLOGIC CHARACTERISTICS OF MACROPHAGES

Activated macrophages within tissues are relatively large cells histologically (20 to 25 μm in diameter) with abundant, often clear cytoplasm and a single, oval to polygonal, often slightly eccentric, reniform nucleus (Fig. 4-14). With time, activated macrophages can

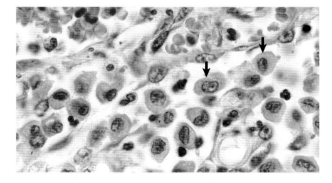

Fig. 4-14   **Macrophages, lung, dog.** Cells have abundant cytoplasm and slightly eccentric, often reniform nuclei *(arrows).* Note the small vacuoles in the cytoplasm, probably phagocytosed material. H&E stain. *(Courtesy Dr. N. Cheville, College of Veterinary Medicine, Iowa State University.)*

sometimes further differentiate into epithelioid macrophages and MGCs (see Multinucleate Giant Cells).

EPITHELIOID MACROPHAGES

Epithelioid macrophages are larger than activated macrophages. They have abundant cytoplasm, and the cell membrane occasionally assumes a polygonal to elongated shape forming sheets and thus can resemble to a limited degree squamous epithelium (Fig. 4-14). These cells have diminished phagocytic capacity, but they contain large amounts of RER, Golgi, vesicles, and vacuoles. These latter structures suggest that the main function of epithelioid macrophages involves extracellular secretion; however, the physiologic activity of epithelioid macrophages is poorly understood and requires additional investigation.

MULTINUCLEATE GIANT CELLS

MGCs are common elements of granulomatous inflammation. MGCs are syncytial cells formed by the fusion of two or more activated macrophages into one large cell having two or more nuclei (Fig. 4-15). These nuclei can be distributed in the cell in a haphazard manner or aggregated in the center of the cytoplasm. This form is called a foreign body type of MGC (Fig. 4-15). The nuclei can also be arranged in a horseshoelike semicircle at the periphery of the cell. This form is called a Langhans'-type cell (Fig. 4-15). The Langhans'-type giant cell should not be confused with Langerhans' cells, which are dendritic cells (see next discussion) of the skin.

DENDRITIC CELLS

Dendritic cells are central to antigen processing, presentation, and the stimulation of adaptive immunity. Functionally, they serve as sentinel cells of the adaptive immune response. Nearly all tissues and organs contain dendritic cells; however, they are most plentiful in tissues that cover the body, such as the skin and the mucous membranes that line the respiratory and alimentary systems. In skin, for example, specialized dendritic cells, termed Langerhans' cells, are present in the epithelium and function to present antigen taken up in the epidermis to inflammatory cells. Langerhans' cells commonly become neoplastic in dogs and form cutaneous histiocytomas, which are benign tumors of the skin that usually have a good long-term prognosis.

Although dendritic cells have some resemblance to macrophages, they have numerous distinct filopodia, which extend from their surface (Fig. 4-16). Increasingly, several subtypes of dendritic cells are being identified (Table 4-5). In general, immature dendritic cells (CD34+) migrate to sites of antigen exposure, take up antigen, migrate to and mature in a lymphoid organ where they present antigen to T and B lymphocytes (Fig. 4-17). This migration process is mediated by chemokines and adhesion molecules, and most dendritic cells enter lymph nodes via the afferent lymphatic vessels in lymph fluid under the influence of chemokines, particularly CCL21. Once in the lymph node, dendritic cells often localize in the parafollicular (T lymphocytes) area in the vicinity of high endothelial venules (HEVs), a site where naïve T lymphocytes enter the node. In this location, dendritic cells activate naïve T lymphocytes. In addition

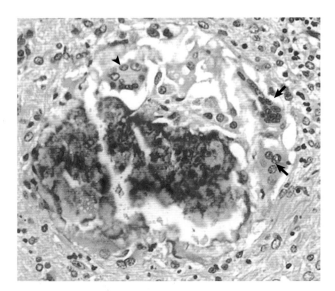

Fig. 4-15   Multinucleate giant cells, chronic granulomatous inflammation, central nervous system, rabbit. This focus contains both foreign body-type (*arrows*) and Langhans'-type (*arrowhead*) multinucleate giant cells. H&E stain. (*Courtesy Dr. A. Loretti, Ontario Veterinary College, University of Guelph.*)

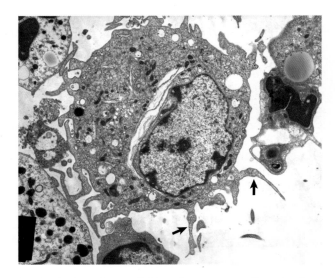

Fig. 4-16   Dendritic cell. Note the numerous filopodia that extend from the cell surface (*arrows*). TEM. Uranyl acetate and lead citrate stain. (*Courtesy Dr. S. Sacco and S. Fach, USDA/ARS-National Animal Disease Center.*)

Table **4-5**   **Subpopulations of Dendritic Cells (DCs) and Activities**

DC Subpopulation	Location	Activity	Other
CD8⁻DCs	T, S, LN, PP, L	$\downarrow T_H1, \uparrow T_H2, \downarrow$ IL-12	Present antigen
CD8⁺DCs	T, S, LN, PP, L	$\uparrow T_H1, \downarrow T_H2, \uparrow$ IL-12	Present antigen
CD8ⁱⁿᵗDCs	LN	Enter LN via lymphatics	
Langerhans cells	Skin epidermis	Antigen capture	Migrate to LN
Dermal DCs	Skin dermis	Antigen capture	Migrate to LN
Plasmacytoid DCs	T, S, LN, PP	Viruses induce type I IFN	Antiviral activity

IFN, interferon; IL-12, interleukin-12; L, liver; LN, lymph node; PP, Peyer's patch; S, spleen; T, thymus; T$_H$1 and T$_H$2, T helper cell type 1 and 2 lymphocyte response, respectively.

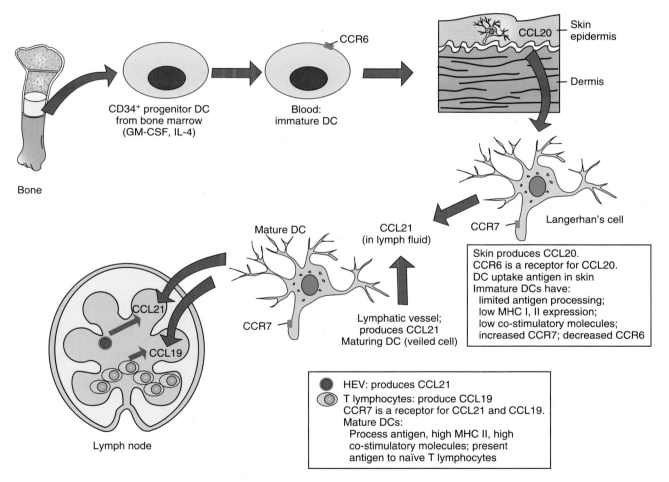

Fig. 4-17   Dendritic cell *(DC)* precursor migration. In this example, migration to the skin is mediated by chemokine receptors located on the dendritic cell and by chemokine ligands *(CCL)* in the skin. Eventually, the dendritic cell takes up antigen and migrates to the lymph node under chemokine influence to present the antigen. In the lymph node, the dendritic cell localizes to the parafollicular area and presents antigen to lymphocytes. *CCR,* Chemokine receptor; *GM-CSF,* granulocyte-macrophage colony-stimulating factor; *HEV,* high endothelial venule; *IL-4,* interleukin-4; *MHC,* major histocompatibility complex. *(Redrawn with permission from Dr. M.R. Ackermann, College of Veterinary Medicine, Iowa State University.)*

to their activity as antigen presenting cells, dendritic cells also contribute to the inflammatory process through release of chemokines and cytokines; however, there are fewer dendritic cells than macrophages in the body and within inflammatory lesions. Although macrophages also present antigen to naïve T lymphocytes, macrophage antigen presentation is more efficient for memory T lymphocytes than for naïve T lymphocytes, the forte of dendritic cells. Through recruitment of naïve T lymphocytes, dendritic cells contribute to the ongoing persistence of a stimulus in certain chronic inflammatory lesions.

Tolerogenic dendritic cells

Tolerogenic dendritic cells can suppress immune responses. They accomplish this activity through the sampling of small amounts of self-antigens, harmless environmental antigens, and inciting the deletion of self-reactive T lymphocytes.

Dendritic cell trafficking

Trafficking immature monocytic dendritic cells express chemokine receptors CCR1 and CCR5 and are recruited by chemokine ligands CCL3 and CCL4 released from lymphocytes and macrophages in tissue. There are several subtypes of dendritic cells, and those dendritic cells that express CD11c antigen express CCR2, which responds to CCLs 2, 7, 8, 12 and 13. After dendritic cells take up antigen and become exposed to an endogenous (e.g., TNF-α) or exogenous (a ligand for a Toll-like receptor) mediator, the dendritic cell matures and expresses CCR7 (Fig. 4-17). Mature dendritic cells expressing CCR7 migrate from the site of the inflammatory lesion into the vasculature and then spread hematogenously throughout the body until they are recruited by high endothelial venules in the paracortical areas of lymph nodes in which lymphocytes express CCL19 and CCL21. In this location, dendritic cells present antigen and thus contribute to the amplification of the adaptive immune response.

LYMPHOCYTES

Lymphocytes play a key role in most chronic inflammatory lesions, especially in autoimmune diseases and in diseases with persistent antigen. As with macrophages, lymphocytes enter unresolved areas of acute inflammation within 24 to 48 hours, being attracted by chemokines, cytokines, and other stimuli. Histologically, they are often aggregated around blood vessels and surround granulomas or are distributed haphazardly within injured tissue (Fig. 4-10). In viral encephalitides, lymphocytes are commonly distributed in a perivascular pattern, primarily in the gray matter. In other types of conditions, such as lymphoplasmacytic

stomatitis and pododermatitis of cats, lymphocytes and plasma cells are the predominant cell types in the lesions.

γ/δ-T LYMPHOCYTES

γ/δ-T lymphocytes are often the first type of T lymphocyte to arrive in the lesion of chronic inflammation and can contribute to the formation of granulomas. This mechanism is supported by the fact that mice lacking γ/δ-T lymphocytes have defects in granuloma formation. However, the role of γ/δ-T lymphocytes in the establishment and persistence of granulomas has not been fully determined. Cattle have high numbers of circulating γ/δ-T lymphocytes, relative to other T lymphocytes, and are a useful model for assessing the role of γ/δ-T lymphocytes, in the formation of classic granulomas in *Mycobacterium tuberculosis* and *Mycobacterium bovis* infections and in the formation of diffuse granulomatous lesions in *Mycobacterium avium-paratuberculosis* infections.

α/β-T LYMPHOCYTES (CD4/CD8)

α/β-T lymphocytes (CD4 and CD8 lymphocytes) enter areas of chronic inflammation and are key to the regulation of the type of adaptive immune response that ensues, albeit a T_H1, T_H2, or T_H0 response of chronic inflammation and/or granuloma formation. Under the influence of cytokines, these lymphocytes can further differentiate into: (1) effector memory lymphocytes, which enter extralymphoid sites; and (2) central memory lymphocytes, which settle into the blood and lymphoid organs. Memory lymphocytes contribute to the persistence of the chronic inflammatory response and granuloma formation.

B LYMPHOCYTES

B lymphocytes contribute to chronic inflammation in at least two major ways. B lymphocytes can: (1) take up and present antigen and (2) differentiate into immunoglobulin producing cells (plasma cells or immunocytes) that secrete immunoglobulins that can bind to and opsonize antigens facilitating phagocytosis. Certain persistent, poorly degradable antigens, such as those in foreign bodies and in microbes such as *Nocardia* spp., can have eosinophilic proteinaceous aggregates of immunoglobulin on their outer surfaces, which can be seen histologically and are termed Splendore-Hoeppli proteins.

T REGULATORY LYMPHOCYTES

T regulatory (T reg) lymphocytes can influence the strength and the balance of T_H1 and/or T_H2 responses through inhibition of dendritic cells. T regulatory lymphocytes are thought to release IL-10 and TGF-β and small amounts of IL-4. This T reg activity appears to inhibit dendritic cells and both T_H1 and T_H2 immunologic responses. If T reg lymphocytes are not activated, then dendritic and antigen presenting cells are free to be activated and initiate T_H1 or T_H2 immunologic responses.

TRAFFICKING OF NAÏVE AND ACTIVATED T AND B LYMPHOCYTES

HOMING OF NAÏVE LYMPHOCYTES VIA HIGH ENDOTHELIAL VENULES

After formation, naïve T and B lymphocytes traffic (home) to various locations, such as peripheral lymph nodes, lymphoid follicles in the mucosal surfaces of the colon and cecum, Peyer's patches in the mucosal surfaces of the small intestine, and organs such as the spleen. These cells express L-selectin and migrate in the blood and often enter these areas through specialized vessels termed high endothelial venules (HEVs), which are postcapillary venules that have a thick basal lamina, endothelial cells with a plump morphology due to a cuboidal appearance, and abundant cytoplasm. HEVs produce certain chemokines constitutively (CCL19, CCL21, CXCL12, and CXCL13) to attract naïve T and B lymphocytes expressing the corresponding chemokine receptors CCR7 (receptor for CCL19, CCL21) and/or CXCR4 (receptor for CXCL12) and/or CXCR5 (receptor for CXCL12) (Table 4-4). HEVs are located principally in T-lymphocyte zones (paracortical areas of lymph nodes, interfollicular areas of Peyer's patches, and lymph nodes), but some are located in the B-lymphocyte zones, especially the periphery of B-lymphocyte follicles. Both peripheral lymph nodes and Peyer's patch HEVs express the adhesion molecules that mediate T-lymphocyte and B-lymphocyte adherence, including peripheral node addressin ligand for L-selectin, ICAM 1, ICAM-2, VE-cadherin; however, only Peyer's patch HEVs express MAdCAM-1, a receptor for the α-4/β-7 adhesion molecule expressed by T and B lymphocytes destined for Peyer's patches and enteric lymph nodes, which are key components of the gut-associated lymphoid tissue (GALT).

ADHERENCE AND TRANSENDOTHELIAL MIGRATION OF ACTIVATED T LYMPHOCYTES

Lesions transitioning into sites of chronic inflammation release chemokines, sphingosine 1-phosphate, and other chemoattractive stimuli that attract and activate T lymphocytes. Although naïve T lymphocytes express high concentrations of L-selectin and the antigen CD45RB, in acutely activated T lymphocytes and in effector/memory T lymphocytes and T lymphocyte clones, L-selectin expression decreases along with expression of the CD45RB antigen. Instead of L-selectin, acutely activated T_H1 and T_H2 cells, effector and central memory lymphocytes, and T lymphocyte clones begin to express high to low levels of E- and P-selectin ligands, which bind to E- and P-selectin receptors, which are expressed by endothelial cells activated in sites of chronic inflammation.

Lymphocytes adhere to these areas by eventually binding firmly to the vascular wall via adhesions between LFA-1 adhesion molecule expressed on lymphocytes, which binds to ICAM-1 and ICAM-2 expressed on endothelial cells. Lymphocytes transmigrate across the vascular wall by adherence between LFA-1 integrins and the ICAM-1 molecules, JAM molecules, and also contributions from PECAM-1.

NATURAL KILLER CELLS

Natural killer (NK) cells elaborate cytokines and have cytolytic activity. They are present in chronic inflammatory lesions, but their role varies based on the characteristics of the inflammatory stimulus. NK cells can kill cells recognized as foreign without previous antigen specificity as is required by T lymphocytes. NK cells are activated by type I interferons and IL-12. Similar to T lymphocytes, NK cells can kill cells with perforin and/or granzyme and TNF-related apoptosis-inducing ligand (TRAIL). They also release IFN-γ, TNF-β, and TNF-α. Because NK cells lack some of the antigenic specificity required for T lymphocytes, they may contribute to autoimmune disease.

Two subsets of human NK cells have been identified according to surface CD56 expression. One type, CD56dim NK cells, are the majority of NK cells and function as effector cells of natural cytotoxicity and antibody-dependent cellular cytotoxicity. In contrast, CD56bright NK cells secrete cytokines that modulate the immune response.

PLASMA CELLS

Under appropriate stimuli, such as intense antigenic stimulation and B lymphocyte presentation of antigens, B lymphocytes differentiate into plasma cells, which can secrete immunoglobulins that bind to and opsonize antigens and facilitate phagocytosis. Plasma cells form within lymph nodes, mucosal surfaces, and wound sites. The bone marrow also contains a resident population of plasma cells, which can increase in certain disease conditions and must be differentiated from neoplastic accumulations as can occur with multiple myelomas. Bone marrow plasma cells have immediate access to the vasculature. Similarly, plasma cells within the medullary sinus of lymph nodes can enter lymphatic vessels and eventually the blood; however, peripheral blood often contains few plasma cells. In the chronic inflammatory exudate, plasma cells are usually found mixed, although in lesser numbers, with lymphocytes and macrophages. Plasma cells predominate in certain chronic inflammatory conditions, such as inflammatory bowel disease of dogs and cats, lymphoplasmacytic stomatitis and pododermatitis of cats, chronic dermatitis of any domestic animal species, and interstitial nephritis of dogs and cats.

EOSINOPHILS

Different types of chronic inflammatory conditions and granulomas contain a low to high number of eosinophils. Eosinophils are recruited into and stimulated to proliferate within chronic inflammatory exudates by several mediators, most notably IL-5 and eotaxin. In some chronic inflammatory conditions that contain eosinophils, such as human asthma, there is thought to be a T_H2 shift, resulting in increased concentrations of chemokines such as eotaxin in the tissue. The same result is likely true for other as yet poorly characterized conditions, such as the eosinophilic complex of cats, eosinophilic infiltrates in the base of the tongue of Siberian huskies and other dogs, eosinophilic enteritis in boxer dogs, and eosinophilic inflammatory lesions in the skin of horses. For these conditions, it may be that some type of persistent yet unidentified T_H2-inducing antigen is present locally.

MAST CELLS

Mast cells tend to look similar to macrophages in hematoxylin and eosin (H&E) stained tissue sections and therefore are often not considered to be a part of the chronic inflammatory lesion. However, when special stains, such as a Giemsa stain, are applied to foci of chronic or granulomatous inflammation, these lesions frequently contain a surprisingly large number of mast cells identified by their characteristic metachromatic granules. For example, chronic lung lesions (e.g., fibrosis and alveolar epithelial hyperplasia) that develop following severe *Mannheimia haemolytica* pneumonia often contain increased numbers of mast cells and reduced levels of substance P fibers (see Chapter 3).

The reason for the presence of mast cells in chronic inflammatory conditions likely relates to their production of proteolytic enzymes, such as chymase and tryptase. Such enzymes likely help physiologically in remodeling and fine-tuning components of the ECM. With persistent inflammation and fibrosis, there can be increased proliferation of mast cells. In addition to the increased mast cell numbers present in the subacute and chronic phases of *Mannheimia haemolytica* pneumonia, mast cells are also increased in areas of fibrosis. Increased mast cell numbers in these lesions occur by increased infiltration and also by increased proliferation of mast cells in situ. With severe inflammation, there can be loss of substance P fibers, and mast cells can respond to this loss by increasing their expression of c-kit, an important regulator of mast cell proliferation.

ENDOTHELIAL CELLS

Endothelial cells are required for neovascularization of chronic inflammatory lesions. The process of angiogenesis (neovascularization) in chronic lesions is similar to that which occurs during wound healing (see Wound Healing and Angiogenesis) and is induced by hypoxia and release of endothelial cell growth factors, such as FGF, VEGF, and PDGF.

Endothelial cells are interconnected by tight junctions composed of occludins, claudin, and JAMs along with adherens junctions composed of vascular endothelial cadherin (VE-cadherin). As leukocytes migrate between endothelial cells, leukocyte adhesion molecules bind some of these intercellular molecules. For example, LFA-1 molecule (CD11-α/CD18) binds JAM-A, VLA-4 molecule (α-4/β-1) binds VCAM-1 and JAM-B, and Mac-1 (CD11b/CD18) binds JAM-C to mediate leukocyte passage between endothelial cells. These molecules are especially important for the transmigration of monocytes and lymphocytes through endothelial cell junctions into sites of chronic inflammation by providing a stable yet temporary site of attachment of leukocyte filopodia and lamellipodia.

WOUND HEALING AND ANGIOGENESIS

Almost immediately after a wound develops, the process of healing begins. Injured tissue goes through four temporal phases to repair the wound: hemostasis, acute inflammation, proliferation (granulation), and remodeling (maturation, contraction) (Fig. 4-18). These phases occur in this sequence but may progress at different rates. Even in one lesion site, different areas may be in different phases of repair.

Hemostasis occurs immediately after injury unless there is a clotting disorder. Initially following injury,

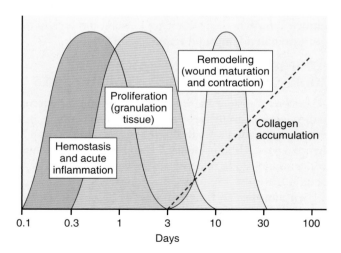

Fig. 4-18   Temporal phases of wound healing (see text for more detail). *(Modified from Clark RAF: Wound repair. In Clark RAF, editor: The molecular and cellular biology of wound repair, ed 2, New York, 1996, Plenum Press.)*

hemostasis is controlled via vasospasm, a process in which blood vessels constrict in response to injury. But this spasm subsides rapidly, and the injured (transected) blood vessels will subsequently relax, allowing additional bleeding if platelets do not become involved. During the initial period of vasoconstriction, platelets aggregate and adhere to exposed collagen, especially collagen in the basement membrane underlying injured endothelial cells. Once adhered, platelets secrete vasoconstrictive substances to: (1) maintain constriction of the transected vessels, (2) initiate the process of thrombogenesis to "plug" the leak in the vessel and prevent additional bleeding, and (3) initiate blood vessel healing (angiogenesis). This process also occurs with large blood vessels, but additional physiologic factors are involved, such as blood shunting and decreased blood pressure.

By 24 hours after vascular injury, the inflammation phase (acute inflammation) of wound healing is fully established and can last up to 96 hours or longer if the healing process is disrupted by infection, trauma, or some other perturbation. It is in this phase that the "cardinal signs of inflammation—redness, swelling, heart pain, and loss of function" are observed (see Chapter 3). Neutrophils and macrophages, through phagocytosis and their degradative enzymes, breakdown and remove ("clean up") the cell debris resulting from tissue injury. Macrophages secrete a variety of chemotactic and growth factors that establish the microenvironment for the proliferation (granulation) phase. See Chapters 2 and 3 for greater detail about hemostasis and acute inflammation, respectively.

The proliferation phase begins approximately 4 days after injury and can last up to 3 to 4 weeks or longer depending on the size of the wound. This phase is characterized by the generation of new endothelium (angiogenesis), epithelium (epithelialization), and connective tissue stroma (fibroplasia/desmoplasia) to restore normal structure and function to the injured tissue. The healing of skin following third-degree burns or severe ulcerations is an excellent example of this process. The return to normal structure and function is dependent on: (1) the retention of normal stromal elements of the ECM to provide the structural framework for repair, and (2) normally functioning fibroblasts, myofibroblasts (contractile fibroblasts), endothelial cells, pericytes (nonendothelial components of blood vessels), and epithelial cells.

The remodeling (maturation, contraction) phase begins approximately 3 to 4 weeks following injury, but only after the inflammation and proliferation phases have been successfully completed. This phase includes remodeling of granulation tissue by immature connective tissue and the conversion of immature connective tissue to mature connective tissue through extracellular

collagen formation. Remodeling can last for 2 or more years. It essentially provides the time some tissues and organs, such as bone, need to return to the near normal tensile strength as required for normal axial and appendicular skeletal function.

A key component of wound repair is the ECM and stromal stem cells (fibroblasts, myofibroblasts) (Fig. 4-19). In mild or moderate injury, partially degraded collagen, proteoglycans, and elastin are completely degraded by matrix metalloproteinases and other enzymes removed by macrophages and then resynthesized by surviving fibroblasts. Simultaneously, fibroblasts and endothelial cells proliferate to fill tissue defects (granulation tissue) and epithelial cells, endothelial cells, and some parenchymal cells proliferate along basement membranes to restore the normal structure of the tissue. If basement membranes are degraded in the injury and the healing process disrupted, then complete healing is delayed because of a requirement for a new basement membrane to be deposited by endothelial cells that attach to and line the contiguous remaining basement membrane. Should healing be continually delayed (infection) or prevented (large tissue defect with loss of stroma and basement membrane), then dysregulated healing can occur in the form of extensive fibrosis (scars and hypertrophic scars) with haphazard arrangement and/or metaplasia of the overlying epithelial cells.

The four phases of wound healing described are applicable to all tissues and organ systems, but each system has its unique mesenchymal and parenchymal cell types that influence the process of healing. Bone healing with callus formation and skin healing with reepithelization are good examples of healing and the specialization of cell types involved (see Chapters 16 and 17). Overall the success of wound healing, especially in the skin, is often determined by whether the process occurs via first or second intention healing. Healing in other tissue is similar. In bone, for example, optimal healing occurs in bone fragments that are stabilized and in direct apposition.

FIRST AND SECOND INTENTION HEALING

First intention healing in skin occurs when the edges of a wound site are directly apposed and reattach and heal to each other rapidly. Wounds lacking such close, intimate apposition are termed second intention healing. In the simplest type of wound, such as a cut or incision in the skin by a surgeon, there is initial hemorrhage from the damaged vasculature and retraction and constriction of blood vessels. In the wound area, there is deposition of fibrin, leakage of plasma proteins, clot formation, platelet aggregation, and neutrophil infiltration. The nature of repair is dependent

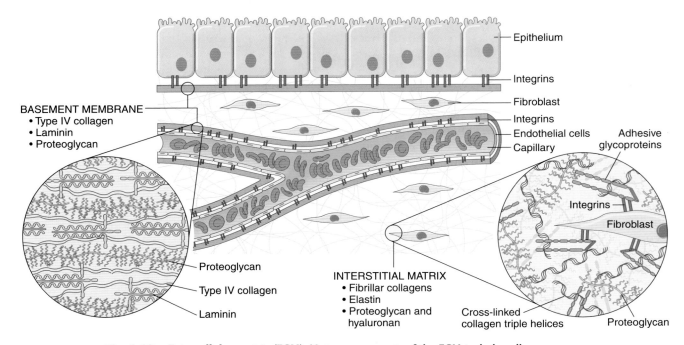

Fig. 4-19 **Extracellular matrix (ECM).** Major components of the ECM include collagens, proteoglycans, and adhesive glycoproteins. Both epithelial and mesenchymal cells (e.g., fibroblasts) interact with ECM via integrins. To simplify the diagram, many ECM components (e.g., elastin, fibrillin, hyaluronan, and syndecan) are not included. *(From Kumar V, Abbas A, Fausto N: Robbins & Cotran pathologic basis of disease, ed 7, Philadelphia, 2005, Saunders.)*

upon several factors, including the proximity of the cut edges to each other, the presence or absence of foreign bodies or infectious microbes, and the general health capacity of the animal to repair wounds. Under ideal conditions, such as in surgery, first intention healing is desired (Fig. 4-20). First intention healing occurs in nonseptic wounds, whereas second intention healing occurs in septic wounds, with foreign bodies, or gaping wounds with nonopposed edges. If the wound healing process is disrupted or delayed, the process is shifted to second intention healing.

FIRST INTENTION HEALING

First intention healing occurs in 2 to 3 days in the skin, if the cut edges of a nonseptic wound are positioned in close proximity to each other by sutures or bandages. During this time, the hemorrhage, plasma proteins, and cell debris within the wound are phagocytosed and removed by macrophages, new blood vessels sprout and grow into the lesion, and the ECM is synthesized to fill the gap between the apposed tissue edges. With time (weeks), this stable interconnection in the dermis will be replaced by collagen fibers that undergo continual maturation, thus providing the skin with near normal tensile strength after wound healing. Concurrently, basal cells of the squamous epithelium will undergo hyperplasia and cover the defect in 3 to 5 days. This type of repair leaves little trace of the

wound, except for perhaps mild fibrosis in the superficial dermis and loss of adnexa (e.g., hair follicles, sebaceous glands, and sweat glands) at the site of the wound. The tensile strength is nearly the same as that of adjacent tissue. First intention healing is the goal of the surgeon for repair of incision sites made during surgery.

SECOND INTENTION HEALING

Second intention healing occurs when the cut edges of the skin, for example, are not brought into appropriate apposition for healing (Fig. 4-20). In such wounds, connective tissue is haphazardly synthesized and arranged and there is little or no organization in the healing process; however, fibrous connective tissue fills the defect in the superficial and deep dermis. This disorganization can also delay or prevent the migration of epithelial cells that attempt to cover the surface of the wound and disrupt the orderly deposition of ECM in the wound. In addition, new fibrous connective tissue will lack adnexa (hair follicles, sebaceous and sweat glands). In some cases, fibrous connective tissue can form into granulation tissue (see later section) in which histologically, proliferating fibroblasts are arranged perpendicular to new capillaries, and the long axes of the new capillaries are arranged perpendicular to the surface of the skin (Fig. 4-28, B). Tensile strength of granulation tissue is diminished and the lesions can

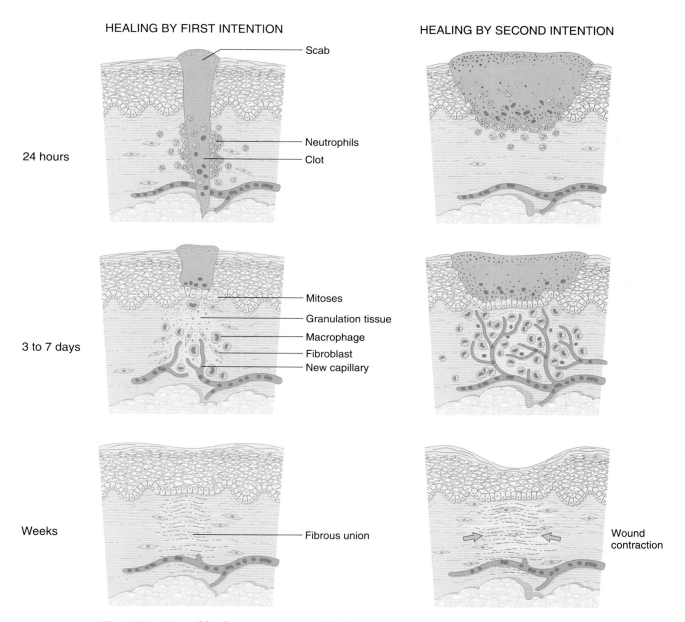

HEALING BY FIRST INTENTION

HEALING BY SECOND INTENTION

24 hours — Scab / Neutrophils / Clot

3 to 7 days — Mitoses / Granulation tissue / Macrophage / Fibroblast / New capillary

Weeks — Fibrous union / Wound contraction

Fig. 4-20   Wound healing. Steps in wound healing by first intention (*left*) and second intention (*right*). Note large amounts of granulation tissue and wound contraction in healing by second intention. (*From Kumar V, Abbas A, Fausto N: Robbins & Cotran pathologic basis of disease, ed 7, Philadelphia, 2005, Saunders.*)

tear or split. Thus with second intention healing, the site can remain ulcerated, lack hair, and in some cases, the fibrous connective tissue can undergo continuous proliferation and protrude from the skin surface as a hyperplastic scar.

IMPAIRED WOUND HEALING

In addition to spontaneously occurring impairments of wound healing, such as foreign bodies, infection, and neoplasms, certain other conditions can prevent or impair wound healing, even first intention healing. For example, altered deposition of collagen and ECM proteins can occur with osteogenesis imperfecta because of impaired production of type I collagen. Similarly, impaired synthesis, cross-linking, hydroxylation, or posttranslational processing of collagen can delay wound healing in individuals with Ehlers-Danlos syndrome. Hyperglycosylation of proteins, which can occur with prolonged diabetes mellitus, can alter the vasculature, lead to diabetic ulcers, and inhibit wound healing.

Chemotherapeutic drugs can also prevent cellular proliferation and may reduce healing. Several new chemotherapeutic drugs specifically target endothelial cell proliferation, which may greatly influence the process of neovascularization so vital to efficient wound repair. In human beings, guinea pigs, and other species that require dietary vitamin C, deficiencies in intake can lead to scurvy, a disease in which there is decreased collagen hydroxyproline synthesis and poor wound healing. Extreme starvation, malnutrition, and cachexia from cancer or severe weight loss from chemotherapy can impair the synthesis and deposition of ECM proteins as a result of negative energy balance and a lack of amino acid substrates, normally synthesized in the liver. Additionally, such individuals and severe burn victims often lack adequate levels of serum proteins such as albumin, which results in lowered osmotic plasma pressure, impaired fluid resorption from the wound site, and enhanced edema fluid accumulation.

EXPRESSION OF GENES RESPONSIBLE FOR WOUND REPAIR

Wound repair requires activation of genes of the viable cells, such as macrophages, fibroblasts, and endothelial cells adjacent to the sites of tissue injury. As indicated, macrophages internalize through phagocytosis cell debris to "clear up" an area and degrade the ECM. In concert with fibroblasts, macrophages release growth factors that enhance the proliferation of: (1) endothelial cells for neovascularization, (2) fibroblasts for deposition of a new ECM, (3) myofibroblasts for wound contraction, and (4) parenchymal cells for return to normal structure and function of the affected tissue.

Gene expression by cells in a wound is regulated to a large degree by oxygen levels. In the milieu of a wound, there is generally a reduced oxygen tension caused by vascular damage. Normal tissues have oxygen levels >90% oxygen saturation, and there is increased activity of prolyl hydroxylase, an enzyme that places a hydroxyl group on hypoxia-inducing factor-α (HIF-α) (Fig. 4-21).

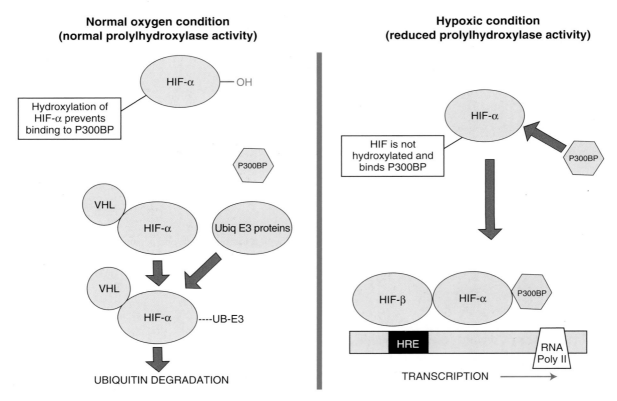

Fig. 4-21   Hypoxia-inducing factor (*HIF*). Initiation of wound healing and regulation of gene expression by HIF. When oxygen levels are normal, HIF is not active, and hypoxia responsive genes are not activated. With hypoxia, however, HIF activates transcription of genes of the hypoxia response elements (*HRE*). *UB, Ubiq,* Ubiquitin; *VHL,* von Hippel-Lindau disease. These genes increase blood vessel formation, iron sequestration, and hypoxia metabolism.

(Redrawn with permission from Dr. M.R. Ackermann, College of Veterinary Medicine, Iowa State University.)

Hydroxylated HIF-α is degraded by the ubiquitin pathway. In hypoxic tissue, however, as occurs in wounds or within neoplastic masses, there is reduced prolyl-hydroxylase activity and thereby less hydroxylation of HIF-α. Nonhydroxylated HIF-α aggregates with HIF-β and induces transcription of hypoxia responsive elements (HREs) in the genome. The HREs include genes for glycolytic enzymes, growth factors, and iron binding proteins. Early growth response gene 1 (EGR-1) is another transcription factor activated in wounds that leads to expression of growth factors and cytokines. Therefore both HIF-α and EGR-1 activity in hypoxic conditions lead to increased cellular transcription that up-regulates genes for glycolysis (glucose transporters, hexokinase 1 and 2, lactate dehydrogenase, phosphofructokinase), endothelial and fibroblast proliferation (TGF-β, VEGF), and iron sequestration (ceruloplasmin, transferring receptor). These genes promote cell survival in hypoxic conditions, enhance cell proliferation, especially of cells vital to repair (endothelial cells, fibroblasts), and delay or alter differentiation of other cells (epithelia or parenchymal cells) until endothelial and fibroblast proliferation is well established.

DEGRADATION OF CELLS AND TISSUE COMPONENTS IN WOUNDS

Wounds generally have a central core that is composed of: (1) degenerate and/or necrotic cells, such as parenchymal cells, fibroblasts, and endothelial cells as well as infiltrating leukocytes, such as neutrophils, platelets, lymphocytes, mast cells, and macrophages; (2) inflammatory products (cytokines, eicosanoids, chemokines, and their respective receptors); (3) serum proteins (albumin, acute phase proteins, complement); (4) clotting proteins (fibrin); and (5) ECM. Many of these cells and mediators need to be removed before optimal healing will take place. Phagocytic cells, such as neutrophils and macrophages, are very important in the clean-up process through phagocytosis of particulate matter and subsequent lysosomal degradation and the release of digestive enzymes into the tissue. In addition, macrophages have a major role in the uptake of apoptotic cells that form in response to TNF-α or other proapoptotic inflammatory stimuli. The ECM can be especially difficult to degrade. However, macrophages and fibroblasts are key to this process through the release of matrix metalloproteinases that degrade the ECM.

DEGRADATION OF THE EXTRACELLULAR MATRIX IN WOUNDS

The ECM is composed of: (1) proteins and (2) the hydrated gel of proteoglycans in which they lie. It surrounds and interconnects cells in connective tissue, such

as fibroblasts, blood vessels, lymphatic vessels, resident mast cells, macrophages, dendritic cells, and nearby parenchymal cells and/or epithelia (Fig. 4-19). The ECM influences cellular development, polarity (organization), and function of epithelial cells (Fig. 4-22).

With tissue injury, there is often destruction and degradation of the ECM. This process occurs through physical separation or tearing, dilution from plasma proteins, infiltration by inflammatory cells, and degradation by enzymes, largely the matrix metalloproteinases (MMPs) (Fig. 4-23). Macrophages, fibroblasts, mast cells, and most leukocytes produce MMPs (Table 4-6). Many MMPs were initially named after the type of ECM protein that they were found to degrade (e.g., collagenase), but because the MMPs are now known not to be uniquely specific for a particular ECM substrate, they have been reclassified in a numerical manner, matrix metalloproteinases 1 through 20.

For example, collagenase is now termed MMP-1, gelatinase is MMP-2, stromelysin is MMP-3, and matrilysin is MMP-7. Matrix metalloproteinases degrade collagen, gelatin, elastin, aggrecan, versican, proteoglycan, tenascin, laminin, fibronectin, and other ECM components. The MMP enzymatic domain contains three histidine residues that form a complex with zinc. A regulatory domain is responsible for latency and allows activation in the presence of zinc. MMP activity is also regulated by tissue inhibitors of MMP (TIMP). In addition to MMP, serine proteases, such as tissue plasminogen-activator (tPA) and urokinase plasminogen activator (uPA) degrade and remodel ECM components (Box 4-1). Fragments of proteins degraded by MMP, tPA, uPA, and other degradative processes are removed from wounds by lymphatic drainage and phagocytosis by macrophages and neutrophils. Proteoglycans are largely degraded by lysosomal enzymes of macrophages and neutrophils (Box 4-1).

RESYNTHESIS OF THE EXTRACELLULAR MATRIX WITH WOUND HEALING

SYNTHESIS OF COLLAGEN AND MATRIX PROTEINS

As wounds repair, the body attempts to reestablish the ECM. The structural proteins of the ECM include several types of collagens, elastin, and adhesive types proteins including fibronectin, laminin, tenascin, and vitronectin (Fig. 4-19). The fibrillar collagens (types I, II, III, V, and XI) are triple-stranded helical structures aggregated into fibrils in the extracellular space and surrounded by collagens IX and XII, which interconnect the collagen fibrils with one another and the ECM. Most tissues have a predominance of one collagen type. For example, collagen type I is present in

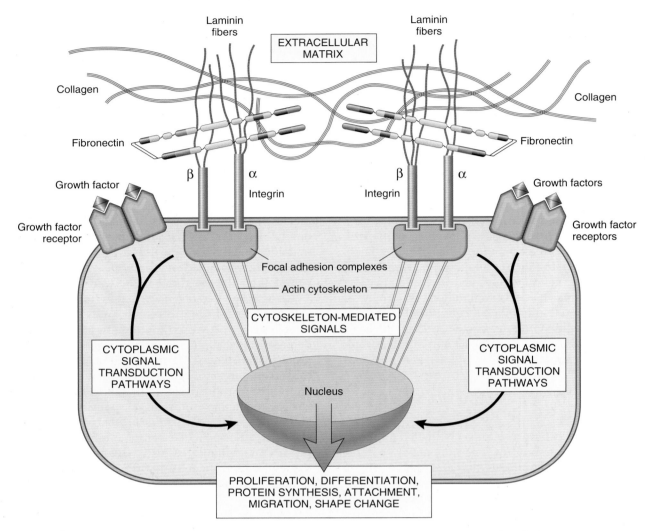

Fig. 4-22 **Extracellular matrix (ECM) regulation of cell functions.** Mechanisms by which ECM (e.g., fibronectin and laminin) and growth factors can influence cell growth, motility, differentiation, and protein synthesis. Integrins bind ECM components and interact with the cytoskeleton at focal adhesion complexes (protein aggregates that include vinculin, α-actin, and talin). This can initiate the production of intracellular messengers or can directly mediate nuclear signals. Cell-surface receptors for growth factors may activate signal transduction pathways that overlap with those activated by integrins. Collectively, these are integrated by the cell to yield various responses, including changes in cell growth, locomotion, and differentiation. (From Kumar V, Abbas A, Fausto N: Robbins & Cotran pathologic basis of disease, ed 7, Philadelphia, 2005, Saunders.)

bone, skin, and tendon; collagen type II is present in cartilage and vitreous humor; collagen type III is present in skin and muscle; collagens type V and VI are present in interstitial tissues; collagen type VI is present near epithelia; collagen type VIII is present near endothelial cells; and collagens type X and XI are present in cartilage.

Collagen type IV is largely present in basal lamina along with laminin, entactin, a heparin sulfate proteoglycan, and perlecan. Throughout the ECM are molecules of elastin, which stretch, recoil, and allow flexibility in the tissue. Collagen fibers, laminin, fibronectin, tenascin and other ECM proteins bind to cells in the connective tissue via extracellular domain of integrin molecules of cells by means of a specific amino acid sequence, the RGDS sequence. For example, laminin binds $\alpha_2\beta_1$-integrins of endothelial cells, some collagens bind $\alpha_6\beta_1$-integrins of epithelial cells, and fibronectin and vitronectin bind $\alpha_5\beta_3$-integrins. The intracellular portion of integrin molecules interact with the cellular cytoskeleton (i.e., actin assembly) and thereby link the extracellular milieu with cellular

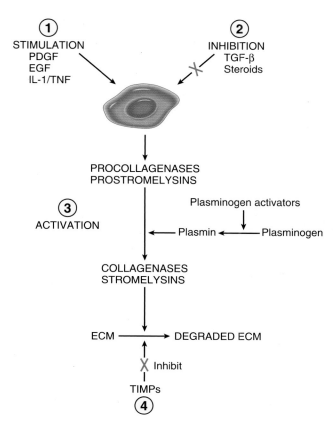

Fig. 4-23   Matrix metalloproteinase activities. Four mechanisms are shown: *1*, regulation of synthesis by growth factors or cytokines; *2*, inhibition of synthesis by corticosteroids or transforming growth factor-β *(TGF-β)*; *3*, regulation of the activation of the secreted but inactive precursors; and *4*, blockage of the enzymes by specific tissue inhibitors of metalloproteinase *(TIMPs)*. *ECM,* Extracellular matrix; *EGF,* epidermal growth factor; *IL-1,* interleukin-1; *PDGF,* platelet-derived growth factor. *(Modified from Matrisian LM:* Trends Genet *6:122, 1990.)*

Table **4-6**   **Matrix Metalloproteinase (MMP) Activity, Regulation, and Cellular Production**

Function: Degrade basement membrane and extracellular matrix proteins
Co-factors necessary: Zinc (Zn^{2+})
Regulation: Cellular synthesis, lysosomal degradation and release, and tissue inhibitors of metalloproteinases

Type of MMP	Cell Type
MMP 1, 2, 3, 11, 14	Fibroblasts
MMP 9, 12	Macrophages
MMP 9	Neutrophils
MMP 2, 3, 9	Endothelial cells
MMP 9	Pericytes
MMP 1, 3, 7, 9, 13	Some cancer cells

Box **4-1**

Enzymes Responsible for Degradation of the Extracellular Matrix (ECM) Proteins and Proteoglycans

PROTEINASES THAT DEGRADE ECM PROTEINS:

Matrix metalloproteinases
Cathepsin G
Cysteine protease
Urokinase-PA
Serine protease

PROTEOGLYCANS ARE DEGRADED BY:

Lysosomal uptake
  Heparinases—an endoglucuronidase that degrades
    hyaluronates, chondroitins, heparans, and heparins
  Galactosidases—degrades dermatans and keratans

activities, such as cell growth, differentiation, proliferation, and senescence (Fig. 4-22).

COLLAGEN PRODUCTION BY FIBROBLASTS

Fibroblasts are induced by TGF-β and other cytokines to synthesize collagen (see later). Ribosomes in fibroblasts produce approximately 30 types of collagen α-chains that are composed of repetitive glycine-x-y segments. Although within the rough endoplasmic reticulum, praline and lysine residues in these chains are hydroxylated, and this hydroxylation process requires vitamin C (Fig. 4-24). The chains are then glycosylated, arranged in a triple helix, and eventually released into the extracellular space as procollagen. The ends of procollagen are cleaved enzymatically resulting in the formation of fibrils termed tropocollagen. Cross-linkages between collagen fibrils occur at lysine and hydroxylysine residues through the activities of the enzyme lysyl oxidase, and this cross-linking process provides the tensile strength of collagen.

SYNTHESIS OF PROTEOGLYCANS

Proteoglycans are produced by fibroblasts. They retain water and are vital to the hydration of the ECM. Proteoglycans have a protein backbone surrounded by a network of glycosaminoglycan (GAG) chains. The GAGs are negatively charged, often highly sulfated, polysaccharide chains covalently linked to the serine residues on a protein backbone (Fig. 4-25). Most GAGs contain high concentrations of N-acetylglucosamine. Hyaluronic acid lacks sulfation and is not connected to the protein backbone (Table 4-7). GAGs are key to the water retention properties of proteoglycans. Proteoglycan hydration of the ECM allows tissue to be pliable and have elasticity.

Heparan sulfate proteoglycans such as syndecan, decorin, and perlecan encircle and surround cells and

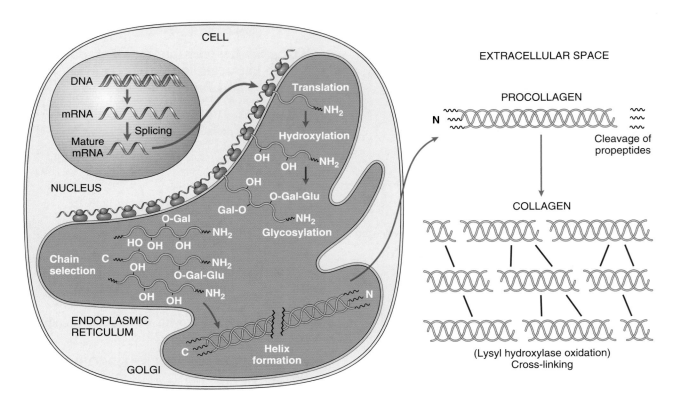

Fig. 4-24 **Steps in collagen synthesis.** *(From Kumar V, Abbas A, Fausto N: Robbins & Cotran pathologic basis of disease, ed 7, Philadelphia, 2005, Saunders.)*

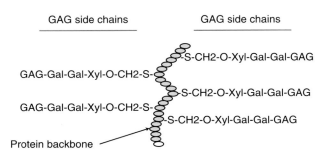

Fig. 4-25 **Proteoglycan molecule.** Proteoglycans have a central protein backbone that supports glycosaminoglycan (GAG) side chains. The GAGs retain water and contribute to the hydration of tissue. *(Redrawn with permission from Dr. M.R. Ackermann, College of Veterinary Medicine, Iowa State University.)*

basal laminae. Syndecan is an integral transmembrane protein that can bind chemokines. With inflammation, syndecan can release the chemokine, which then induces leukocyte infiltration.

FIBROBLASTS AND THE MECHANISTIC BASIS OF FIBROSIS

Fibroblasts align along planes of tissue stress during development (Langer's lines or tension lines). In quadrupeds, these lines are generally dorsoventral over the thorax and abdomen (axial body plane) and parallel to the long axis of the limbs (appendicular body plane). Surgical incisions along Langer's lines extend between, rather than transect, bands of fibrous connective tissue and tend to pull the margins of surgical skin incisions together. Such incisions reduce the degree of postsurgical scar formation.

Fibroblasts of cats appear to be especially responsive to injury and inflammation. In fact, injury of fibroblasts has been associated with their neoplastic transformation in cats. For example, traumatic lens rupture can lead to intraocular inflammation and fibroblast proliferation, and in some cases, fibrosarcomas. In addition, fibroblast proliferation and fibrosarcomas are common in cats at vaccination sites.

Initially during the hemostasis and inflammation phases of wound repair, fibrin and serum proteins form a loose gel-like framework for the migration of fibroblasts and endothelial cells into the wound to form granulation tissue. Simultaneously, leukocytes and other cells, such as fibroblasts and endothelial cells, are stimulated by HIF-α and epidermal growth factor (EGF) (see Expression of Genes Responsible for Wound Repair) to synthesize and release a variety of growth factors that result in fibroblast proliferation and migration. These factors include FGF-1 and FGF-2, PDGF, EGF, and TGF-β-1, 2, and 3. FGF, PDGF, IL-13, and

Table **4-7**   Composition and Tissue Specificity of Selected Glycosaminoglycans (GAGs)

GAG	Carbohydrate Components	Localization
Hyaluronate	Hyaluronic acid	Synovial fluid, vitreous humor, extracellular matrix of connective tissue
Chondroitin sulfate	D-glucuronate + N-acetylgalactosamine	Cartilage, bone, heart valves
Heparan sulfate	Glucuronate + glucosamine	Basement membranes, cell surfaces, intracellular granules of mast cells
Heparin	Glucuronate + glucosamine	Lines arteries of lungs, liver, skin
Dermatan sulfate	L-idurante + N-acetylgalactosamine	Skin, blood vessels, heart valves
Keratan sulfate	Galactose + N-acetylglucosamine	Cartilage, aggregated with chondroitin sulfate

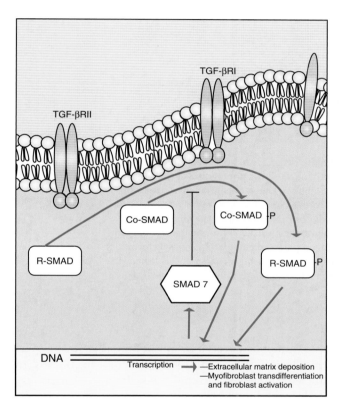

Fig. 4-26   Transforming growth factor-β (TGF-β) signaling. This process results in fibroblast and myofibroblast activation and collagen deposition R, Receptor. *(Redrawn with permission from Dr. M.R. Ackermann, College of Veterinary Medicine, Iowa State University.)*

TGF-β induce fibroblasts to produce collagen, whereas FGF, VEGF, TGF-β, angiopoietin, and mast cell tryptase induce endothelial cells to proliferate and migrate and produce basement membrane for formation of new capillaries.

With time the newly formed, provisional, connective tissue is remodeled into a more mature matrix. In the entire process, TGF-β has a central role in fibroblast activity and collagen deposition, because it is produced by platelets and macrophages and induces macrophage chemotaxis, fibroblast migration and proliferation, and synthesis of collagen and ECM proteins. TGF-β binds TGF-β receptor II, which dimerizes with TGF-βRI.

The TGF receptor then phosphorylates R-SMAD and Co-SMAD to overcome inhibition of SMAD 7 (Fig. 4-26). This signaling process induces fibroblast activity, and regulation of the signaling may be useful in therapeutic strategies to control scarring and/or fibrosis.

In addition to collagen production, fibroblasts can migrate to a certain degree, and this process is mediated by adhesion molecules that bind to the ECM. This binding is a complicated event in which the adherence process is essential for migration of the cell and also its anchoring to extracellular proteins. During wound repair, proliferating fibroblasts will often align themselves parallel with lines of tension stress.

MORPHOLOGY OF GRANULATION TISSUE AND FIBROUS CONNECTIVE TISSUE

GRANULATION TISSUE

Some lesions develop a distinctive type of arrangement of connective tissue fibers, fibroblasts, and blood vessels termed granulation tissue. Granulation tissue is the exposed connective tissue that forms within a healing wound. It is often red, is hemorrhagic, and bleeds easily when bumped or traumatized because of the fragility of the newly formed capillaries (Fig. 4-27). It is especially common in horses. When viewed with a magnifying glass, the surface of granulation tissue has a granular appearance and thus the term *granulation tissue* arose. In granulation tissue, fibroblasts and connective tissue fibers grow parallel to the wound surface and are arranged perpendicularly to the proliferating capillaries. Often the penetrating blood vessels are evenly spaced. Excessive granulation can lead to a type of hypertrophic scar called proud flesh.

HYPERTROPHIC SCARS

Hypertrophic scars occur as a result of exuberant proliferation of fibroblasts and collagen in wounds that fail to heal properly. The best example of this condition occurs in skin wounds of the distal limbs of horses and is known as "proud flesh," as indicated proliferating connective tissue forms a large cauliflower-like mass

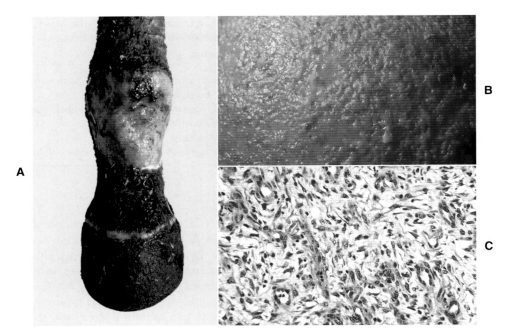

Fig. 4-27   Granulation tissue, nonhealing ulcer, skin, distal limb, horse. A, In the bed of the ulcer, there is extensive fibrosis and granulation tissue. **B,** Gross photograph of the surface of granulation tissue. Note the fine nodules or "granulations" on the surface that gave rise to the term *granulation tissue*. They are a mixture of newly formed blood vessels, extracellular matrix (ECM), and fibroblasts, with no to minimal collagen deposition. It provides the support for wound repair and remodeling via fibroplasia and reepithelization. **C,** Photomicrograph of granulation tissue. Note how the new fibroblasts are arranged perpendicularly to the newly formed blood vessels in a rich bed of ECM *(clear spaces)*. Collagen deposition is sparse at this time. H&E stain. (**A, B,** *and* **C,** *Courtesy Dr. M.D. McGavin, College of Veterinary Medicine, University of Tennessee.*)

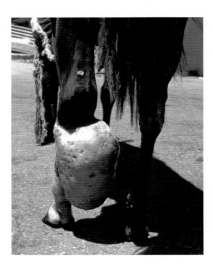

Fig. 4-28   Exuberant granulation tissue (proud flesh), chronic ulcer, skin, distal hindlimb, horse. Note the large proliferating mass of fibrous tissue on the lower portion of the left hindlimb. It often lacks superficial epithelium. *(Courtesy Dr. M.D. McGavin, College of Veterinary Medicine, University of Tennessee.)*

that cannot be covered by epithelium (Fig. 4-28). Why this lesion most commonly occurs in horses in unclear; however, the epidermis of horses is often very "tight" with limited elasticity.

Keloid is a special type of excessive connective tissue deposit that occurs in human beings. It has an incidence of 5% to 16% following skin trauma in high-risk populations, such as blacks, Hispanics, and Asians. Clinical management of hypertrophic scars, proud flesh, and keloids can be difficult but includes intralesional corticosteroids, compression, occlusive dressings, pulsed-dye laser therapy, cryosurgery, surgical excision, radiation, fluorouracil chemotherapy, topical silicone, interferons, and drugs, such as imiquimod, that induce IFN-γ.

FIBROUS CONNECTIVE TISSUE

Fibrous connective tissue is the dense accumulation of fibroblasts and collagen formed within a wound site. Histological characteristics depend on wound severity and duration. Fibrous connective tissue contains variable numbers of fibroblasts and collagen along with inflammatory cells (Fig. 4-29). In recently formed wounds, the collagen can be very immature and edematous with a variety of inflammatory cells, perhaps neutrophils. With time, the fibrous connective tissue progresses into mature, densely packed collagen with few inflammatory cells. Once formed and matured, fibrous connective tissue often persists for years, perhaps life.

WOUND CONTRACTION

THE SCIRRHOUS REACTION

With severe thermal/chemical burns or extensive abrasions of a large surface area of the skin, the healing process and the formation of connective tissue becomes extensive. In time, these areas of connective tissue contract and place tension on the surrounding normal skin, resulting in a scirrhous reaction that can cause immobility of the surrounding skin and perhaps limbs along with pain and deformation. Contraction of such wounds is mediated largely by myofibroblasts.

Similarly, within areas of necrosis and/or inflammation in the liver, lung, spleen, and kidney, excessive fibrosis in parenchymal areas can result in the formation of connective tissue tracts between the healing area and capsular and interstitial connective tissue. When this new connective tissue contracts during the healing process, it grossly results in local indentation or pitting on the organ surface, such as occurs with chronic renal cortical infarcts. If there are multiple such areas, the organ surface develops an undulating and/or nodular appearance, such as occurs in a cirrhotic liver. Contraction of such wounds is again mediated largely by myofibroblasts.

MYOFIBROBLASTS

Myofibroblasts are specialized fibroblasts with contractile activity. They form within wounds in response to tissue plane stress and the secretion of TGF-β by platelets and macrophages as wounds develop, and they increase in number with time and severity. Their function is to contract the wound and thus bring together injured tissue separated by edema and inflammation. Physiologically, myofibroblasts also occur in tissues with contractility, such as uterine submucosa, intestinal villi, testicular stroma, the ovary, periodontal ligament, bone stroma, capillaries, and pericytes.

Myofibroblasts have stress fibers, actin and myosin fibers, gap junctions, and a fibronexus. The fibronexus is a mechanotransduction region of the plasma membrane, which is rich in integrin molecules. The fibronexus interconnects intracellular actin fibers with extracellular proteins, such as fibronectin. This provides an anchor point during myofibroblast contraction. In contrast, fibroblasts lack contractile myofilaments and a fibronexus. Actin polymerization and contractility in myofibroblasts is stimulated by Rho GTPases. The Rho signaling that induces contractility in myofibroblasts results in

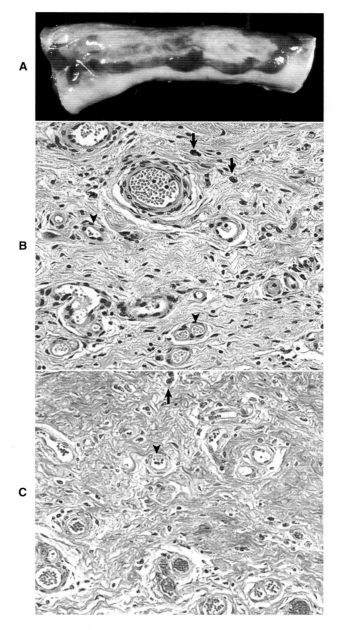

Fig. 4-29 **Fibrous connective tissue. A,** Hemomelasma ilei, ileum, antimesenteric serosal surface, horse. This lesion is approximately 1 to 2 weeks old. *Strongylus edentatus*-induced injury to the serosal vasculature results in hemorrhage followed by wound healing. Note the raised areas of fibrosis (raised gray-white areas), hemosiderosis (yellow-brown areas), and hemorrhage (red-brown areas). **B,** Healing response in hemomelasma ilei. Note the abundant newly formed capillaries (*arrowheads*) and intervening fibrous connective tissue (bands of red fibers). This healing response is the next step following the granulation tissue phase demonstrated in Fig. 4-27. Hemosiderin (*arrows*) is present in the connective tissue and is indicative of hemorrhage having occurred in the injury at an earlier time (weeks). H&E stain. **C,** Fibrous connective tissue in the healing response. Collagen is readily demonstrated in fibrous connective tissue by a Trichrome stain (*blue stained fibers*). Masson trichrome stain. (*A, B,* and *C, Courtesy Dr. J.F. Zachary, College of Veterinary Medicine, University of Illinois.*)

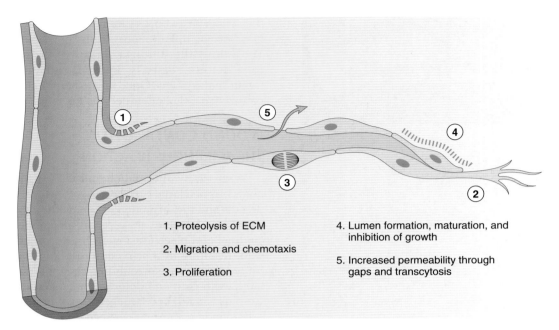

Fig. 4-30   Steps in the process of angiogenesis. *ECM,* Extracellular matrix. *(Modified from Motamed K, Sage EH: Kidney Int 51:1383, 1997.)*

1. Proteolysis of ECM

2. Migration and chemotaxis

3. Proliferation

4. Lumen formation, maturation, and inhibition of growth

5. Increased permeability through gaps and transcytosis

continual contraction of filaments in myofibroblasts. Such contractions condense wound sites. This type of contraction by myofibroblasts differs from the periodic contractility that occurs in smooth muscle cells.

ANGIOGENESIS IN WOUND REPAIR

Angiogenesis in simple terms is the formation of new blood vessels. It is a process essential for all living organisms with a cardiovascular system and involves a series of steps, as illustrated in Fig. 4-30, for the formation of new capillaries, including the following:

- Proteolysis of the ECM and basement membrane of parental vessels at the margins of the wound so a new capillary "bud" can form and initiate cellular migration
- Migration of immature endothelial cells into the wound
- Proliferation of endothelial cells to form solid "endothelial tubes"
- Maturation of endothelial tubes into new capillaries with the formation of lumina
- Establishment of inter-endothelial gap junctions and the receptors/ligands responsible for the leukocyte adhesion cascade along the luminal surface of the endothelial cells
- Recruitment of pericytes and smooth muscle cells to support the final differentiation stage of the newly formed vessel

This process occurs because as wounds heal, new vessels are necessary to supply the injured site with oxygen, remove carbon dioxide and other waste products, drain excess fluid, and provide a vascular pathway for cells and stem cells into the wound. This same beneficial process has also been adapted by primary and metastatic neoplastic cells to grow and spread throughout tissues of the body.

INITIATION OF ENDOTHELIAL CELL PROLIFERATION
ENDOTHELIAL CELL GROWTH FACTORS

The formation of new blood vessels in wounds begins from the proliferation of endothelial cell buds from blood vessels in viable tissue adjacent to the wound or can be derived from bone marrow endothelial precursor cells (EPCs) (Fig. 4-31). These buds grow into the "healing" wound, form elongated vascular tubular structures within the wound, interconnect and revascularize the wound, and then eventually differentiate into mature vessels. Initially, endothelial cell buds form, and cells migrate into wounds under the autocrine (see Fig. 12-1) influence of HIF-α and EGF (see Expression of Genes Responsible for Wound Repair), which enhance expression of genes that improve cell survival in hypoxic conditions.

Concurrently, growth factors such as FGF, VEGF A, angiogenins, and ephrins released from macrophages, endothelial cells, and fibroblasts bind receptors on endothelial cells and induce their proliferation (Fig. 4-32). VEGF A stimulates the initial stages of endothelial cell proliferation through binding the VEGF R2 receptor on endothelial cells. The secondary stages of endothelial cell proliferation appear to involve angiopoietin 1 and its receptor, Tie2.

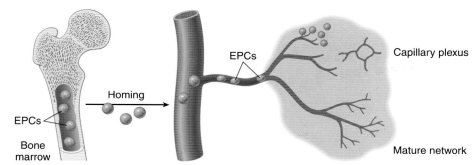

A Angiogenesis by Mobilization of EPCs from the Bone Marrow

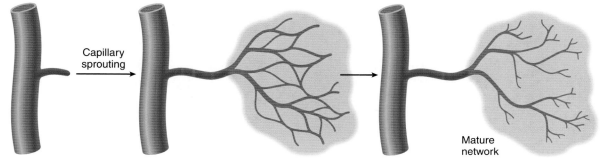

B Angiogenesis from Preexisting Vessels

Fig. 4-31   **Angiogenesis by mobilization of endothelial precursor cells (*EPCs*). A,** Bone marrow. EPCs are mobilized from the bone marrow and may migrate to a site of injury. The homing mechanisms have not yet been defined. At these sites, EPCs differentiate and form a mature network by linking with existing vessels. **B,** Preexisting vessels (capillary growth). In angiogenesis from preexisting vessels, endothelial cells from these vessels become motile and proliferate to form capillary sprouts. Regardless of the initiating mechanism, vessel maturation (stabilization) involves the recruitment of pericytes and smooth muscle cells to form the periendothelial layer. (**A** and **B,** *Modified from Conway EM, Collen D, Carmeliet P: Cardiovasc Res 49:507, 2001.*)

ENDOTHELIAL CELL MIGRATION IS MEDIATED BY INTEGRINS

Newly formed endothelial cells and fibroblasts migrate into wound sites and bind to fibrinogen and plasma proteins as well as newly deposited ECM substances, such as heparan sulfate, chondroitin sulfate, type III collagen, laminin, vitronectin, and fibronectin. This adherence is mediated by adhesion molecules expressed by new endothelial cells and fibroblasts. These adhesion molecules include α_5- and β_3-integrins, which bind fibrin and fibronectin (Fig. 4-32). It is interesting that for wound repair, enhancement of angiogenesis is beneficial and vital; however, in neoplasia, inhibition of angiogenesis and thus the growth of the tumor has potential therapeutic benefits.

VASCULAR REMODELING

Once blood vessels are initially formed, they are loosely arranged and require remodeling to become mature. With remodeling, endothelial cells produce a mature basement membrane. In addition, smooth muscle cells and pericytes can form within the wall, and fibroblasts can form adventitial fibers, depending on whether the vessel is a capillary, artery, vein, or lymphatic vessel. Other endothelial cell growth factors and receptors involved with vascular remodeling include angiopoietin 2, which also binds Tie2 and ephrin B2 and its receptor, EphB4. Proliferation of lymphatic endothelial cells is mediated largely by VEGF C and its receptor, VEGF R3, as well as prox 1 gene expression.

REGULATORS/INHIBITORS OF ENDOTHELIAL CELL GROWTH

Inhibitors of angiogenesis are produced by endothelial cells, macrophages, and fibroblasts. These inhibitors balance the proliferative healing responses of angiogenesis and to prevent overexuberant proliferation of endothelial cells. These inhibitors include angiostatin, endostatin, thrombospondin, and specialized CXC chemokines (lacking ELR motif). Such inhibitors of

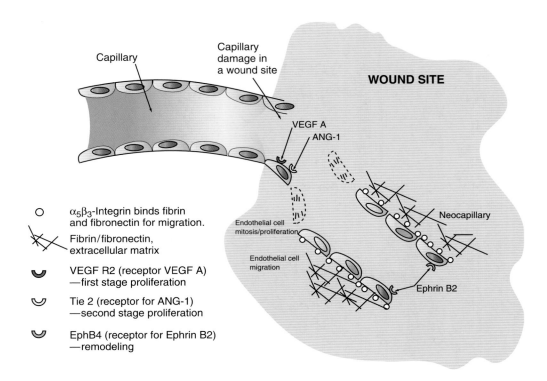

Angiogenesis inhibitors (not shown): angiostatin, endostatin,
special CXC chemokines, PEDF

Fig. 4-32   **Molecular mediators of angiogenesis.** Growth factors, such as vascular endothelial growth factor A *(VEGF A)* and angiopoetin-1 *(ANG-1)*, bind receptors on endothelial cells that induce proliferation and migration. The migration is mediated by $\alpha_5\beta_3$-integrins expressed by endothelial cells that bind molecules, such as fibrin and fibronectin. Factors such as Ephrin B2 bind endothelial receptors Ephrin B4 and mediate vascular remodeling. *(Redrawn with permission from Dr. M.R. Ackermann, College of Veterinary Medicine, Iowa State University.)*

angiogenesis are being studied intensely for their potential chemotherapeutic role against certain types of cancer.

EPITHELIALIZATION IN WOUND REPAIR

Epithelialization (reepithelialization) is the process by which the skin and mucous membranes replace superficial epithelial cells damaged or lost in a wound. Epithelial cells at the edge of a wound proliferate almost immediately following injury to cover the denuded area. Under normal conditions, this process is rapid, and first intention healing occurs in 3 to 5 days to repair the wound. During wound repair, keratinocytes and mucosal epithelial cells must move laterally across the wound surface to fill the void. Before this lateral movement can occur, epithelial cells must disassemble their connections to the underlying basement membrane and their junctional complexes with neighboring cells. They must also express surface receptors that permit movement over the ECM of the wound surface.

INTACT BASEMENT MEMBRANES ENHANCE REEPITHELIZATION

The presence or rapid deposition of basement membrane into the wound greatly facilitates proliferation of viable epithelial cells at the margins of the wound. For example, with initial loss of enterocytes that cover the surface of intestinal villi or renal tubular cells that line proximal convoluted tubules, the immediate response is for the adjacent normal epithelial cells to extend over the denuded basement membrane and to cover the area, if it is larger, by becoming thin, elongated cells. At the same time, there is proliferation (mitosis) of viable adjacent epithelial cells, and these cells migrate along the basement membrane to cover the denuded surface and replace lost cells. Without a basement membrane, proliferative cells lack a clear path of migration. The immature cells may loiter at the site of proliferation and fuse, thus forming syncytial cells, as can be seen with renal tubular injury and the failure of the tubular epithelium to migrate.

Similarly, regenerating skeletal muscle cells and transected axons will regenerate inside a tube surrounded by basal lamina and endoneurium. Components of the basement membrane, including laminin, type III collagen, and the associated proteoglycans, provide a substratum for epithelial and other cells to bind the basement membrane via integrins, proliferate, and migrate along the basement membrane surface.

INITIATION OF CELL PROLIFERATION IN EPITHELIA

Growth factors are vital for the proliferation of keratinocytes, mucosal epithelia, renal tubular cells, and other parenchymal epithelial cells. In skin and other surface epithelia, for example, keratinocyte growth factor (KGF) and EGF bind receptors on epithelial cells and induce signal transduction, which activates mitogen-activated protein kinases (MAPKs) that induce cells in the nonproliferating G_o phase of the cell cycle to enter the cycle and proliferate (see Chapter 6). Hepatocyte growth factor (HGF) induces proliferation of hepatocytes, and nerve growth factor (NGF) enhances growth of nerve fibers. Cell proliferation is regulated by: (1) the amount of growth factor produced, (2) the level of expression of the growth factor receptor, (3) inhibitory signals from other growth factors, (4) the microenvironment including the availability of oxygen and nutrients, and (5) integrin attachment to an established basement membrane. Although TGF-β induces fibroblast proliferation and collagen deposition, TGF-β inhibits proliferation of epithelial cells in many parenchymal organs.

DIFFERENTIATION OF EPITHELIA

Once epithelial cells have filled in a gap in the epithelium of a tissue or an organ, cellular differentiation is required for return of the tissue or organ to normal function. FGF 10 is a key initiator of wound repair in skin and lung epithelia (Fig. 4-33). FGF 10 binds FGF R III, which through bone morphogenic protein 4 and sonic hedgehog (a signaling protein for developmental patterning) enhances expression of several transcription factors, including GATA-6, thyroid transcription factor-1 (TTF-1), hepatocyte nuclear factor-β (HNF-β), and hepatocyte factor homolog-4 (HFH-4). Each of these transcription factors enhance expression of genes, which regulate a specific function for a particular cell. In the lung, for example, TTF-1 induces production of surfactant proteins A, B, and C, and HFH-4 stimulates cilia formation. Activity of these transcription factors is reduced in the presence of NF kappa B, an important mediator of inflammation. Therefore concurrent inflammation can impair differentiation of epithelial and parenchymal cells and thus inhibit or delay reepithelization.

METAPLASIA IN WOUND REPAIR

Some wounds do not heal properly and can turn into hypertrophic scars that impair epithelial and parenchymal cell growth. Such wounds may remain ulcerated or in parenchymal organs; the injured site may be replaced by fibroblasts and inflammatory cells rather than parenchymal cells. In either case, epithelial and parenchymal stem cells may continually attempt to cover or fill wound defects. With time, these cells may convert to another cell or tissue type. For example, regions of the lung constantly exposed to smoke can change from pseudostratified epithelium to stratified squamous epithelium, or regions of lower esophagus continually exposed to gastric acidity

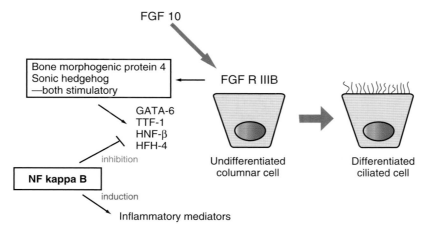

Fig. 4-33 **Epithelial cell differentiation, growth, and transcription factors.** Fibroblast growth factor 10 *(FGF-10)* binds epithelial receptor fibroblast growth factor receptor IIIB *(FGF R IIIB)*, which activates bone morphogenic protein and sonic hedgehog that induce activity of transcription factors for epithelial cell differentiation. This process is inhibited with inflammatory conditions that have increased levels of nuclear factor *(NF)* kappa B. *HFH-4,* Hepatocyte factor homolog-4; *HNF-β,* hepatocyte nuclear factor-β; *TTF-1,* thyroid transcription factor-1. *(Redrawn with permission from Dr. M.R. Ackermann, College of Veterinary Medicine, Iowa State University.)*

can undergo metaplasia into squamous cells. Osseous and chondroid metaplasia can occur in persistent wounds. In general, cells that undergo metaplasia have either: (1) enhanced expression of an altered set of transcription factors and/or (2) decreased expression of transcription factors generally active for the affected tissue. The result is conversion of the cell's phenotype into a new phenotype. Often, if the initiating stimulus is removed, cells can revert to the original phenotype.

SUGGESTED READINGS

Alter TS, Tanzi EL: Hypertrophic scars and keloids: etiology and management, *Am J Clin Dermatol* 4(4):235-243, 2003.

Boros DL: The cellular immunological aspects of the granulomatous response. In: *Granulomatous infections and inflammations: cellular and molecular mechanisms*, Washington, DC, 2003, ASM Press.

Borovikova LV, Ivanoa S, Zhang M et al: Vagus nerve stimulation attenuates systemic inflammatory response to endotoxin, *Nature* 405:458-462, 2000.

Braddock M: Wound repair in skin and bone, *Sci Med* July/August:218-229, 2002.

Hostetter J, Huffman E, Byl K, Steadham E: Inducible nitric oxide synthase immunoreactivity in the granulomatous intestinal lesions of naturally occurring bovine Johne's disease, *Vet Pathol* 42:241-249, 2005.

Imhof BA, Aurrand-Lions M: Adhesion mechanisms regulating the migration of monocytes, *Nat Rev Immunol* 4:432-444, 2004.

Ley K, Kansas GS: Selectins in T-cell recruitment to non-lymphoid tissues and sites of inflammation, *Nat Rev Immunol* 4:1-11, 2004.

Lingen MW: Role of leukocytes and endothelial cells in the development of angiogenesis in inflammation and wound healing, *Arch Pathol Lab Med* 125:67-71, 2001.

Majno G: Chronic inflammation. Links with angiogenesis and wound healing, *Am J Pathol* 153:1035-1039, 1998.

Miyasaka M, Tanaka T: Lymphocyte trafficking across high endothelial venules: dogmas and enigmas, *Nat Rev Immunol* 4:360-371, 2003.

Nissen NN, Polverini PJ, Koch AE et al: Vascular endothelial growth factor mediates angiogenic activity during the proliferative phase of wound healing, *Am J Pathol* 152:1445-1452, 1998.

Okamoto H, Mizuno K, Horio T: Monocyte-derived multinucleate giant cells and sarcoidosis, *J Dermatol Sci* 31:119-128, 2003.

APPENDIX 4-1

Acronym	Term	Function
Ach	Acetylcholine	Parasympathetic and antiinflammatory responses
ADAM9	Disintegrin and metalloproteinase	Cell fusion
Arg-1	Argininase-1	T_H2 fibrotic response
BPV	Bovine papillomavirus	Papilloma in cattle, sarcoid in horses
CD4	Cluster determinant 4 lymphocyte	Lymphocyte responses
CD8	Cluster determinant 8 lymphocyte	Lymphocyte killing
CD36	Cluster determinant 36	Monocyte scavenger receptor
CCL, CX3CL (see Chapter 3, Table 3-8)	Chemokine ligand	Chemotaxis
CCR, CX3CR (see Chapter 3, Table 3-8)	Chemokine receptor	Chemotaxis
CSF	Cerebrospinal fluid	Central nervous system function
ECM	Extracellular matrix	Proteinaceous matrix between cells
EPC	Endothelial precursor cell	Endothelial precursor cell
FGF	Fibroblast growth factor	Promotes proliferation of many cell types
GAG	Glycosaminoglycan	Extracellular glycoconjugates
GATA-6	Transcription factor	Transcription factor for differentiation
GM-CSF (see Chapter 3, Table 3-8)	Granulocyte-macrophage colony-stimulating factor	Cell proliferation
HEV	High endothelial venule	Lymphocyte trafficking
HFH-4	Hepatocyte factor homolog-4	Growth factor
HGF	Hepatocyte growth factor	Transcription factor for cell differentiation
HIF	Hypoxia-inducing factor	Regulator of cell activity in hypoxic conditions
HNF	Hepatocyte nuclear factor	Transcription factor for cell differentiation
HRE	Hypoxia response elements	Response elements to HIF
ICAM-1	Intercellular adhesion molecule-1	Leukocyte adhesion
IFN (see Chapter 3, Table 3-8)	Interferon	Antiviral and T_H1 responses
IL (see Chapter 3, Table 3-8)	Interleukin	Cytokine

Acronym	Term	Function
JAM	Junctional adhesion molecule	Cell/leukocyte adhesion
LDL	Low-density lipoprotein	Vascular lipid transport
LFA-1	Lymphocyte function antigen-1	Leukocyte adhesion
Mac-1	Macrophage-1 antigen	Leukocyte adhesion
MAPK	Mitogen-activated protein kinase	Cell signaling
MBP	Major basic protein	Eosinophil granule product
MCP (see Chapter 3, Table 3-8)	Macrophage chemotactic protein	Macrophage chemotaxis
MFPR	Macrophage fusion protein receptor	Receptor for CD47 ligand
MGC	Multinucleate giant cell	Sequester persistent antigen
MHC	Major histocompatibility complex	Immunity
MIP (see Chapter 3, Table 3-8)	Macrophage inflammatory protein	Macrophage chemotaxis
MMP	Matrix metalloproteinase	Degradation of ECM
NF kappa B	Nuclear factor kappa B	Inflammation transcription factor
NGF	Nerve growth factor	Growth factor
NK	Natural killer	Specialized lymphocyte-like cell
NOS	Nitric oxide synthase	Nitric oxide and T_H1 response
PDGF	Platelet-derived growth factor	Growth factor
PECAM-1	Platelet endothelial cell adhesion molecule-1	Leukocyte adhesion
PPAR	Peroxisome proliferators activated receptor	Transcription factor that reduces inflammatory response by cells
STAT	STAT kinase receptor	Cytokine receptor signaling
T reg	Regulatory T lymphocyte	Regulated dendritic cell activity
TGF-α	Transforming growth factor-α	Stimulates the growth of parenchymal cells
TGF-β	Transforming growth factor-β	Stimulates the growth of fibroblasts
T_H1	T helper lymphocyte type 1	Cell-mediated lymphocyte responses
T_H2	T helper lymphocyte type 2	Humoral lymphocyte responses
TIMP	Tissue inhibitor of matrix metalloproteinase	Reduction of ECM degradation
TNF (see Chapter 3, Table 3-8)	Tumor necrosis factor	Inflammation
TTF	Thyroid transcription factor	Transcription factor for cell differentiation
VCAM-1	Vascular cell adhesion molecule-1	Adhesion molecule for monocytes
VEGF	Vascular endothelial cell growth factor	Angiogenesis
VLA-4	Very late antigen-4	Leukocyte adhesion

5

Diseases of Immunity

PAUL W. SNYDER

GENERAL FEATURES OF THE IMMUNE SYSTEM

The immune system is a defensive system whose primary functions are to protect against infectious organisms such as bacteria, viruses, fungi, and parasites and the development of cancer. The complexity by which these functions occur is evidenced not only by the cell types, recognition molecules, and soluble factors involved and interactions with other systems (e.g., endocrine, nervous), but also by the ability to recognize virtually any foreign antigen. Immunologic responses result in pathologic processes, primarily inflammatory responses, as a result of either normal immune responses to foreign antigens (e.g., microbial pathogens) or from aberrations of the immune system as in the case of hypersensitivity reactions and autoimmune diseases. Finally, the importance of a normal functional immune system cannot be more evident than in instances when it is deficient as the result of a genetic defect or as the result of an acquired immunodeficiency disease.

Immunity is the result of nonspecific (innate) and specific (adaptive) responses that together provide effective protection. The immune system's recognition and response functional capabilities are key components of both innate and adaptive immune responses. The recognition capabilities are highly specific and allow immune responses to develop against a diverse group of foreign (nonself) antigens and prevent the development of immune responses to self-antigens. Innate and adaptive immune responses feature effector mechanisms for eliminating or neutralizing the antigen, whereas adaptive immunity has the additional feature of memory. The emphasis of this chapter is on diseases that are the result of inadequate or inappropriate immune responses. Before one can understand the pathogenic mechanisms of these diseases, one must first have an understanding of the basic elements of the immune system. The chapter begins with an overview of our current understanding of

innate and adaptive immunity, cells of the immune system, cytokines, and major histocompatibility complex (MHC) molecules. This overview will facilitate our discussion of disorders of the immune system that will include hypersensitivity reactions, autoimmunity, and immunodeficiency. This chapter concludes with a discussion of amyloidosis, a diverse group of conditions characterized by the deposition of a pathologic extracellular protein. One of the conditions is associated with the deposition of immunoglobulin components. Although the focus of this text is on the pathologic basis of veterinary diseases, with an emphasis on domestic species, in this chapter we use the vast knowledge base regarding human and rodent immunology (applicable to most mammalian species studied to date) as our basis and interject major known relevant species differences as appropriate.

INNATE IMMUNITY (NONSPECIFIC IMMUNITY)

As stated previously, the function of the immune system is to protect against infectious pathogens and the development of cancer. There are two categories of immune responses that are based in part on their specificity for the antigen: (1) innate immunity and (2) adaptive immunity (Fig. 5-1). Innate immune responses are considered the first-line defense mechanisms, are not specific to the antigen, and lack memory. These defense mechanisms are the result of anatomic (e.g., skin, mucosal epithelia, cilia) and physiologic (stomach pH, body temperature, etc.) properties, and phagocytic and inflammatory responses. Major components of innate immunity are intact epithelial barriers, phagocytic cells, natural killer (NK) cells, and a number of plasma proteins, the most important of which are the proteins of the complement system. Phagocytic cells are recruited to sites of infection during an inflammatory

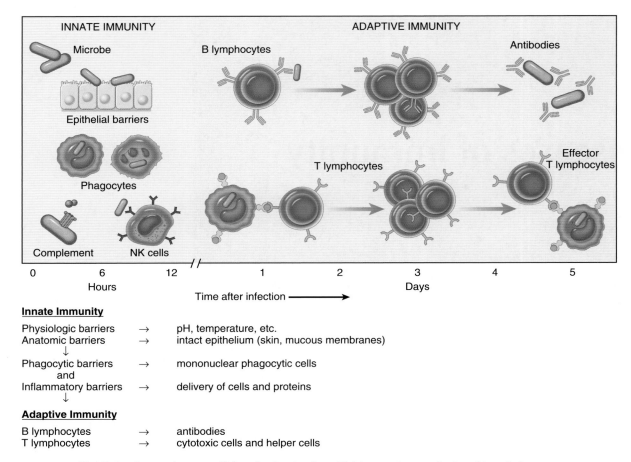

Fig. 5-1 **Innate (nonspecific) and adaptive (specific) immunity are depicted in relation to the time course of an infection.** *NK,* **Natural killer.** *(From Kumar V, Abbas AK, Fausto N:* Robbins & Cotran pathologic basis of disease, *ed 7, Philadelphia, 2005, Saunders.)*

response where they have a number of functions, two of which are to ingest and destroy pathogenic organisms and neutralize toxins. Neutrophils, monocytes, and tissue macrophages are the major cells involved in phagocytosis. These cells recognize components of microbial pathogens through the expression of several membrane receptors, including receptors for mannose residues and N-formyl-methionine containing peptides and a newly discovered family of Toll-like receptors (TLRs) that are homologues of the Toll receptor. TLRs are a family of pattern recognition receptors that, when activated by microbial components, signal the activation of transcription factors that facilitate the microbicidal mechanisms of the phagocytic cell. NK cells are the cytotoxic cells of innate immunity and are discussed later. The complement system, discussed in Chapter 3, is a complex cascade of proteins that has a number of biologic functions, including the formation of the membrane attack complex that efficiently lyses plasma membranes of microbial pathogens. The complement system can be activated by either the innate immune system (alternative and mannose/lectin pathways) or the adaptive immune system (classical pathway). Other important plasma proteins of the innate immune system include mannose-binding protein and C-reactive protein; two of the functions of these proteins are to facilitate phagocytosis through opsonization of pathogens and complement activation. Inflammatory responses comprise vascular, permeability, and cellular phases that act in response to damage to vascularized tissue. The features of the inflammatory response are also presented in Chapter 3.

TOLL-LIKE RECEPTORS

TLRs are the mammalian homologue of the Toll receptor originally identified in *Drosophila*. It has not only an embryologic function but also an immunologic function. In mammals, TLRs are membrane molecules that function in cellular activation by a wide range of microbial pathogens. TLRs are classified as pattern recognition receptors (PRRs) because they recognize pathogen associated molecular patterns (PAMPs) and signal to the host the presence of an infection. Pathogen associated

Table **5-1** **Toll-like Receptors (TLRs) and TLR Ligands and Their Microbial Source**

TLR	Ligand	Microbial Source
TLR2	Lipoproteins	Bacteria
	Peptidoglycan	Gram-positive bacteria
	Zymosan	Fungi
	LPS	*Leptospira*
	GPI anchor	Trypanosomes
	Lipoarabinomannan	Mycobacteria
	Phosphatidylinositol dimannoside	Mycobacteria
TLR3	Double-stranded RNA	Viruses
TLR4	LPS	Gram-negative bacteria
	HSP60	Chlamydia
TLR5	Flagellin	Various bacteria
TLR6	CpG DNA	Bacteria, protozoans
TLR7	Single-stranded RNA	Viruses
TLR8	Single-stranded RNA	Viruses
TLR9	CpG DNA	Bacteria, viruses

Modified from Kumar V, Abbas AK, Fausto N: *Robbins & Cotran pathologic basis of disease*, ed 7, Philadelphia, 2005, Saunders.
CpG, Cytosine and guanine linked oligonucleotide; *GPI*, glycosyl phosphatidyl inositol; *HSP60*, heat shock protein 60; *LPS*, lipopolysaccharide.

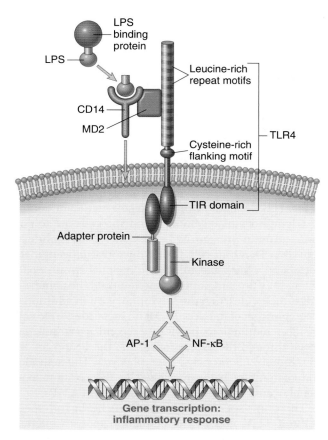

Fig. 5-2 **Signaling pathway for Toll-like receptor 4 (*TLR4*) in response to bacterial lipopolysaccharide (*LPS*).** The binding of LPS to TLR4 results in activation of a signal transduction pathway, leading to gene transcription and the elicitation of an inflammatory response. *AP-1*, Activating protein 1; *NF-κB*, nuclear factor kappa B; *TIR*, Toll/interleukin-1 receptor.
(From Kumar V, Abbas AK, Fausto N: Robbins & Cotran pathologic basis of disease, ed 7, Philadelphia, 2005, Saunders.)

molecules include lipopolysaccharide (LPS) from gram-negative bacteria, peptidoglycan from gram-positive bacteria, double-stranded RNA from viruses, or α-glucans from fungi (Table 5-1). In general, TLRs 1, 2, 4, and 6 recognize unique bacterial products that are found on the cell surface, and TLRs 3, 7, 8, and 9 are involved in viral detection and nucleic acid recognition within endosomes. The specificity of TLRs for microbial products is dependent on interactions between TLRs and non-TLR adapter molecules. All TLRs contain an extracellular domain characterized by a leucine-rich repeat motif flanked by a cysteine-rich motif (Fig. 5-2). They also contain a conserved intracellular signaling domain, Toll/interleukin (IL)-1 receptor (TIR), that is identical to the cytoplasmic domain of the IL-1 and IL-18 receptors. Fig. 5-2 illustrates how TLRs function in the recognition of LPS. In the blood or extracellular fluid, the binding of LPS to LPS binding protein (LBP) facilitates the binding of LPS to CD14, a plasma protein and glycophosphatidylinositol-linked membrane protein present on most cells. The binding of LPS to CD14 results in the dissociation of LBP and the association of the LPS-CD14 complex with TLR4. An accessory protein, MD2, complexes with the LPS-CD14-TLR4 molecule and results in LPS-induced cell signaling.

Briefly, TLR signaling through the binding of PAMP to a TLR leads to the activation of TIR, which forms a complex with the cytoplasmic adapter protein MyD88, an IL-1 receptor associated kinase (IRAK), and tumor necrosis factor receptor–associated factor 6 (TRAF6).

Activated TRAF then activates the mitogen-activated protein kinase (MAPK) cascade leading to the activation of nuclear factor (NF) kappa B, a transcription factor. MyD88 is a universal signaling molecule for NF kappa B activation, and MyD88 deficient mice are incapable of activation by TLR, IL-1 and IL-18. Recent information suggests that there are also signaling mechanisms unique to individual TLRs.

TLRs and their pathogen-associated ligands are important recognition molecules for the innate immune system and trigger a number of antimicrobial and inflammatory responses. Up to 15 different TLR genes have been identified. The importance of these receptors in immunity is further supported by the observation of polymorphisms in the genes encoding them.

Although the individual TLRs exhibit ligand specificity, they differ in their cellular expression patterns and the signal pathways they activate, similar to that described for cytokines, which exhibit pleiotropy, redundancy, synergy, and antagonism. There are constitutively and inducibly expressed TLRs in different tissues. TLRs regulate cell recruitment to sites of infection through the up-regulation of the expression of adhesion molecules, chemokines, and chemokine receptors during an inflammatory response. TLRs activate leukocytes (primarily neutrophils and NK cells of the innate immune system) and epithelial, endothelial, and hematopoietic cells. TLRs are also hypothesized to be essential for linking the innate immune response to the adaptive immune responses. Central to this hypothesis is the TLR-dependent dendritic cell-mediated control of T lymphocyte activation. Dendritic cells are important antigen-presenting cells for T lymphocyte activation. Dendritic cells uptake microbial antigens in the peripheral tissues and migrate to regional lymph nodes where they present peptide fragments, in the context of MHC molecules, to naïve T lymphocytes. In addition to the expression of the peptide-MHC signal, dendritic cells are also required to provide a second, co-stimulatory signal through the expression of B7, the ligand for the CD28 molecule on naïve T lymphocytes. The activation and maturation pathway related to the co-stimulatory signal occurs through TLR recognition of PAMPs.

There are species differences in the ligand specificity of TLRs and in the cellular responses elicited. Although sequences for canine, feline, and chicken TLR4 have been identified, no functional data have been published. With regard to domestic animals, a significant body of literature exists on TLRs of cattle.

Finally, TLRs have been implicated in "innate autoimmunity," with several reports of TLRs recognizing fibrinogen, heat-shock proteins, or DNA. There are also reports of TLR binding of DNA as a factor in directing antibody production by autoreactive B lymphocytes contributing to the pathogenesis of rheumatoid arthritis and systemic lupus erythematosus. Further studies are necessary to more fully understand these observations and the underlying immunopathogenesis.

ADAPTIVE IMMUNITY (SPECIFIC IMMUNITY)

Adaptive immunity in general consists of cell-mediated immunity, mediated by T lymphocytes against intracellular pathogens, and humoral immunity, mediated by B lymphocytes against extracellular pathogens and toxins (Fig. 5-3). The adaptive immune response is the second-line defense mechanism and is characterized by antigen specificity, diversity, memory, and self/nonself recognition. Antigen specificity and self/nonself recognition are the result of distinct membrane molecules. Mature B lymphocytes are activated by a specific antigen-binding molecule on its membrane. The antigen receptor is membrane-bound immunoglobulin. Mature T lymphocytes express a specific antigen-binding molecule, the T-cell receptor (TCR), on their membrane. Unlike membrane-bound immunoglobulin on the B lymphocyte, which can recognize antigen alone, TCRs can recognize only antigens that are associated with cell membrane proteins called major histocompatibility complex (MHC) molecules. Self/nonself recognition is the result of MHC molecules. There are two major classes of MHC molecules. Class I molecules are present on all nucleated cells, and class II molecules are present primarily on antigen-presenting cells. T lymphocytes and B lymphocytes are the major cells of adaptive immunity.

CELLS AND TISSUES OF THE IMMUNE SYSTEM

T LYMPHOCYTES

T lymphocytes are small nongranular cells that constitute 50% to 70% of the peripheral blood mononuclear cells. They originate in the bone marrow and migrate to the thymus (thus the "T" designation), where they undergo differentiation, selection, and maturation processes before exiting to the periphery as effector cells. In secondary lymphoid tissues, they are located primarily in the paracortical regions of lymph nodes and the periarteriolar sheaths (PALS) of the spleen. These specific anatomic sites elaborate chemoattractant cytokines (chemokines), for which the T lymphocytes express receptors. The definitive marker for T lymphocytes is the TCR, the polymorphic antigen-binding molecule. The antigen specificity of individual lymphocytes is attributed to their respective TCR, which is genetically determined. TCRs are classified as either αβ-TCR or γδ-TCR based on the composition of their disulfide-linked heterodimers. The individual polypeptide chains of the heterodimers contain variable (antigen-binding) and constant regions. In mammals, most peripheral blood T lymphocytes express αβ-TCR; however, in ruminants and swine these cells make up only 10% to 50%, and 10% of peripheral blood T lymphocytes, respectively. Both TCRs are associated with CD3, and together they form the TCR-CD3 complex. There are significant activation and functional differences between αβ-TCR- and γδ-TCR-expressing lymphocytes. Unlike membrane bound immunoglobulin on B lymphocytes that can recognize soluble antigen, the αβ-TCR can only recognize antigen after it has been processed into peptide fragments and associated with MHC molecules (the MHC is discussed later). In most instances the antigen is associated with the MHC on the surface of an antigen-presenting cell, a virally infected cell, a neoplastic cell, or a cell of a foreign tissue graft. Individual αβ-TCRs are covalently linked

Antigens

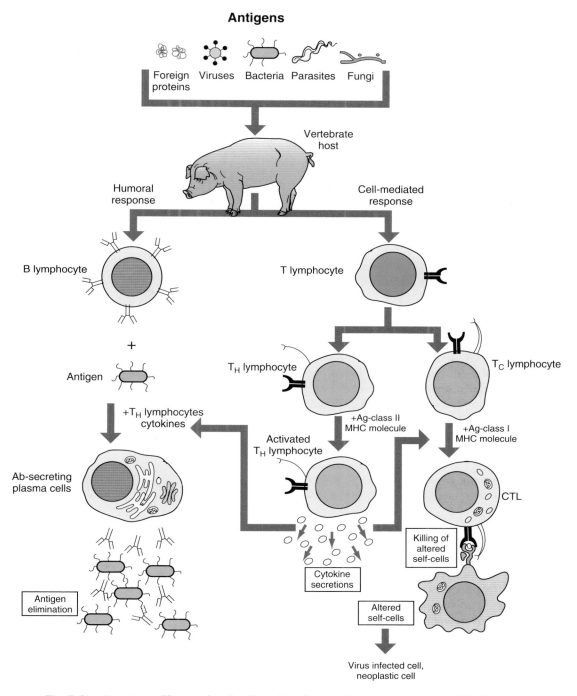

Fig. 5-3 **Overview of humoral and cell-mediated arms of adaptive immunity.** *CTL,* Cytotoxic T lymphocyte. *(Adapted from Goldsby RA, Kindt TJ, Osborne BA: Kuby immunology, ed 4, New York, 2000, WH Freeman.)*

to a cluster of five polypeptide chains, three comprising the CD3 molecule and two comprising the β-chain. The CD3 molecule and the β-chain are invariant, and although they do not bind antigen, they do function in the signal transduction following antigen binding by the TCR. Each T lymphocyte expresses a unique TCR

with regard to structure and antigen specificity. The genes that encode α-, β-, γ-, and δ-chains of the TCR can undergo somatic rearrangements during their development in the thymus, resulting in tremendous diversity for antigen recognition. Not only are these rearrangements important for diversity, they can also be used to molecularly phenotype proliferating populations of T lympho-cytes as a diagnostic tool for the identification of clonal populations (neoplastic) and polyclonal populations (nonneoplastic) (see Chapter 6).

In most species a minority of T lymphocytes express γδ-TCR. The γδ-TCR lymphocytes develop in the thymus and migrate to the epithelium of the skin and intestine, mammary gland, and reproductive organs. Although these cells can be found with in regional lymph nodes and the lamina propria, in these organs they primarily reside as intraepithelial lymphocytes (IELS). As stated already, in some species, notably ruminants, γδ-TCR lymphocytes are the predominant circulating popula-tion of T lymphocytes. In contrast to the αβ-TCR lym-phocytes, γδ-TCR lymphocytes can recognize native antigen in the absence of MHC binding and they do not rely exclusively on the δ-chain as a signal trans-ducer. Most γδ-TCR lymphocytes use the γ-chain for signal transduction following activation. The diversity of antigens recognized by γδ-TCR is limited in most species except ruminants and swine, indicating their importance in these species. Some have suggested that they may provide early cell-mediated immune responses in neonates. The precise function of γδ-TCR lympho-cytes remains unknown. Another small subset of T lym-phocytes, called NK-T lymphocytes, expresses molecules found on NK cells in addition to a limited diversity of TCRs. NK-T lymphocytes primarily recognize glycolipids that are associated with an MHC-like molecule, CD1. The function of NK-T lymphocytes remains unknown.

Although all T lymphocytes express the TCR-CD3 complex, they are further classified according to acces-sory CD4 and CD8 molecules. These nonpolymorphic accessory molecules include CD4, CD8, CD2, integrins, and CD28. CD4 and CD8 functionally subdivide T lymphocytes into CD8+ cytotoxic T lymphocytes (T_C) and CD4+ helper T lymphocytes (T_H). During antigen presentation, CD4+ lymphocytes only recognize antigen bound to MHC class II molecules (Fig. 5-4), whereas CD8+ lymphocytes only recognize antigen bound to MHC class I molecules. This co-receptor requirement is commonly referred to as MHC class I and MHC class II restriction, the basis for positive selection in the thymus. Although there have been reports in some species of CD4 cells that are functionally cytotoxic and CD8 cells that are functionally "helper"-like, these appear to be anomalies and for the purposes of this text are excluded. In most species, peripheral blood T lymphocytes express either CD4 or CD8. Except for ruminants and swine, cells negative for both CD4 and CD8–"double nega-tive" lymphocytes–are rare in the peripheral blood. So-called double lymphocytes cells positive for both CD4 and CD8, positive are rare except in swine, where they can approach 25% of the T lymphocytes in the

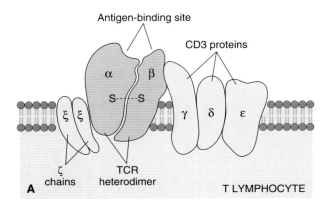

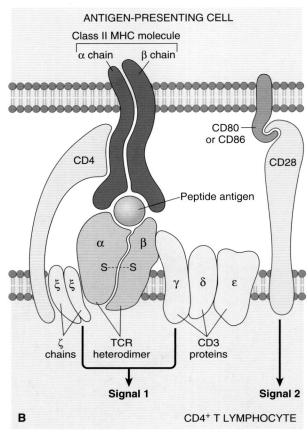

Fig. 5-4   **The T-lymphocyte receptor complex (T-cell recep-tor [TCR]). A,** TCR-α and TCR-β chains complexed with CD3 γ-, δ-, and ε-chains and the invariant, ζ-chains. **B,** Illustrating how the TCR recognizes antigen in the context of major histocompatibility complex on the antigen-presenting cell *(top)* and how the ζ-chains and CD3 γ-, δ-, and ε-chains deliver one of the two required signals for activation of the T lymphocyte. The second required signal is delivered by the co-stimulator molecules CD28 on the T lymphocyte and B₇ on the antigen-presenting cell. *MHC,* Major histocompatibility complex. *(A and B, From Kumar V, Abbas AK, Fausto N: Robbins & Cotran pathologic basis of disease, ed 7, Philadelphia, 2005, Saunders.)*

peripheral circulation. T lymphocytes require two sig-nals for activation. Signal 1 is provided by the TCR and the MHC-antigen complex, and the CD4 or CD8 MHC complex. Signal 2 is provided by another accessory mol-ecule expressed by T lymphocytes, the CD28 molecule. The ligands for CD28 are B7-1 (CD80) and B7-2 (CD86) expressed on activated dendritic cells, B lym-phocytes and macrophages (Fig. 5-4). An inability to deliver the second signal results in an unresponsive T lymphocyte that either undergoes apoptosis or remains anergic. These molecules provide an impor-tant co-stimulatory signal for T lymphocyte activation, and are discussed in more detail later in the chapter regarding anergy and the development of tolerance with regard to autoimmunity. When T lymphocytes are activated by antigen and receive the appropriate co-stimulatory signals, they clonally expand as a result of their secretion of IL-2. This clonally expanded popu-lation of T lymphocytes, of the same antigen specificity, differentiates into populations of effector cells and memory cells.

T_H lymphocytes can be classified based on their functional capacity and ability to elicit primarily an antibody response or a cell-mediated immune response. Following activation of T_H lymphocytes, by recognition of antigen bound to MHC class II molecules on the sur-face of an antigen-presenting cell, there is clonal expan-sion of T_H lymphocytes of the same antigen specificity. These clonally expanded cells are important in directing the immune response as either primarily an antibody response or a cellular response. The type of response is dictated by a restricted cytokine profile that primarily activates B lymphocytes in the case of an antibody response or activates T_C lymphocytes and macrophages in a cellular response. The restricted cytokine profile for T_H lymphocytes allows for their classification as either T_H1 or T_H2 lymphocytes (Table 5-2). T_H1 lym-phocytes synthesize and secrete IL-2 and interferon-γ (IFN-γ), stimulating T_C lymphocytes and macrophages, and induce a cell-mediated immune response. T_H2 lymphocytes synthesize and secrete IL-4, IL-5, IL-6, and IL-13 that stimulate B lymphocytes to develop into antibody-secreting plasma cells and inhibit macrophage functions, and induce an antibody response. The type of immune response (antibody versus cell-mediated) can have a profound influence on the outcome of a disease. In the instance of an intracellular protozoal infection, a T_H2 type response results in rapid proliferation of the organism and death of the host, whereas a T_H1 type response results in elimination of the organism and survival of the host. Similarly, a T_H2 response to an allergen results in the elaboration of immunoglobulin (Ig)E, through IL-4 production, stim-ulation of eosinophils, through IL-5 production, and

Table 5-2 Basic Cytokine and Functional Profiles of T_H1 and T_H2 Lymphocytes

Cytokine	T_H1	T_H2
IL-2	+	
IFN-γ	++	
TNF-β	++	
GM-CSF	++	+
IL-3	++	++
IL-4		++
IL-5		++
IL-13		++
Function		
Antibody*	+	++
IgE		++
Eosinophils, mast cells		++
Macrophages	++	
Type IV hypersensitivity	++	
Cytotoxic T lymphocytes	++	

GM-CSF, Granulocyte-macrophage colony-stimulating factor; *IFN-γ*, inter-feron-γ; *IgE*, immunoglobulin E; *IL*, interleukin; *TNF-β*, tumor necrosis factor-β.
*Opsonizing and complement fixing antibodies.

the development of an allergic reaction. The exact reg-ulation of the T_H1 versus the T_H2 lymphocyte response is unknown, but studies suggest that IL-12 produced by activated macrophages stimulates the T_H1 response, whereas IL-4 inhibits the T_H1 response, allowing the T_H2 response to dominate. Again, one must recognize that this is an oversimplification of a complex regula-tory mechanism, and that as additional knowledge is gained about T_H1 and T_H2 responses, we will be able to understand pathogenic mechanisms of diseases, which will lead to the development of more specific therapeu-tic targets.

B LYMPHOCYTES

B lymphocytes constitute 5% to 20% of the peripheral blood mononuclear cells. B-lymphocyte development occurs in two phases, an antigen-independent phase in the primary lymphoid tissues, followed by an anti-gen-dependent phase in secondary lymphoid tissues. B lymphocytes can be found in primary lymphoid tissues like the bone marrow and ileal Peyer's patches (a primary lymphoid tissue in some species because it is the site of B-lymphocyte development, rather than the bone marrow), and in secondary lymphoid tissues like the spleen, lymph nodes, tonsils, and Peyer's patches. Within secondary lymphoid tissues B lympho-cytes are aggregated in the form of distinct lymphoid follicles, which upon activation expand to form promi-nent pale regions called germinal centers (Fig. 5-5).

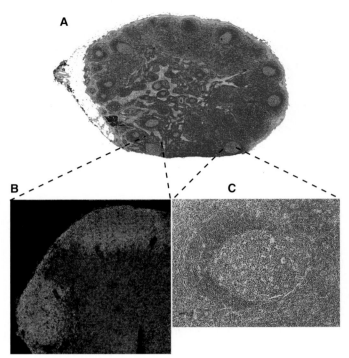

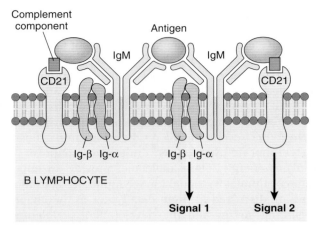

Fig. 5-6   **The B-lymphocyte antigen receptor complex.** Membrane IgM (or IgD, not shown) and the signaling molecules Ig-α and Ig-β. CD21, also known as complement receptor-2, binds complement components and activate B lymphocytes. *Ig,* Immunoglobulin. *(Courtesy Dr. Alex McPherson, University of California, Irvine.)*

Fig. 5-5   **Histology of a hyperplastic lymph node. A,** Outer cortex, containing numerous secondary lymphoid follicles with characteristic pale centers, and inner medulla are easily identifiable. **B,** Localization of B lymphocytes (labeled with a B-lymphocyte marker conjugated with a green fluorochrome) and T lymphocytes (labeled with a T-lymphocyte marker conjugated with a red fluorochrome). Immunoflourescence photomicrograph. **C,** Higher magnification of a secondary lymphoid follicle illustrating the central pale, germinal center, which contains primarily proliferating B lymphocytes, CD4+ lymphocytes and dendritic cells, surrounded by densely packed small B lymphocytes. H&E stain. (**A, B,** and **C,** *From Kumar V, Abbas AK, Fausto N: Robbins & Cotran pathologic basis of disease, ed 7, Philadelphia, 2005, Saunders.)*

This anatomic localization, similar to T lymphocytes in the PALS and paracortex, is the result of elaboration of chemokines for which the B lymphocyte has receptors. The antigen receptor of the B lymphocyte is the membrane bound immunoglobulin. Following the antigen-independent phase of development B lymphocytes express IgM and IgD on their surface that signifies a mature B lymphocyte. In the antigen-dependent phase, antigen-activated mature B lymphocytes differentiate into IgM-secreting plasma cells or switch to another antibody isotype. Immunoglobulins can be generated against an almost unlimited number of antigenic determinants through the rearrangement of genes encoding the light chain and heavy chain components. As in the case of the TCR, an evaluation of the rearranged genes of a B lymphocyte can be used to molecularly phenotype B lymphocyte neoplasms (see Chapter 6).

Like the T lymphocyte, the B lymphocyte also has accessory molecules that function to form the antigen receptor complex (Fig. 5-6). These nonpolymorphic molecules are heterodimers composed of Ig-α (CD79a) and Ig-β (CD79b) that do not bind antigen but do interact with the transmembrane portion of surface immunoglobulin involved in cell activation. B lymphocytes, unlike T lymphocytes, can recognize soluble antigens. Additional nonpolymorphic molecules that are important to B-lymphocyte functions are CD21 and CD40. The CD21 molecule is the complement receptor-2 molecule whose ligands are C3b and C3d. B lymphocyte responses to protein antigens are dependent on cytokines produced by activated T lymphocytes (CD4+). The CD40 molecule interacts with CD40 ligand on the surface of T_H lymphocytes and functions to allow B-lymphocyte development into antibody-secreting plasma cells. A failure to express CD40 ligand has been associated with an inability to isotype switch, resulting in a hyper-IgM syndrome. B lymphocytes activated by antigen develop into antibody secreting plasma cells and memory cells of the same antigenic specificity.

MACROPHAGES

Mononuclear phagocytic cells include circulating monocytes and tissue-based macrophages. In the spleen, macrophages are located in the marginal zone, white pulp, and red pulp, where they function primarily as phagocytic cells. In the lymph node, macrophages are located in the subcapsular sinus, which is analogous to the marginal zone of the spleen, and the medulla. These physical locations, the subcapsular sinus of lymph nodes and marginal zone of the spleen, facilitate their exposure to potential antigens. Nonlymphoid tissue-based macrophages have different functions and are named according to the tissue in which they reside (Table 5-3).

Table **5-3**   **Nomenclature and Location of Nonlymphoid Monocyte-Macrophage Cell Types**

Organ/Tissue	Name	Location
Lung	Alveolar macrophages	Alveolar spaces
	Pulmonary intravascular macrophages	Capillaries of the lung
Connective tissues	Histiocytes	Interstitium
Kidney	Mesangial cells	Glomerular tuft
Brain	Microglial cells	Neuroparenchyma and perivascular areas
Bone	Osteoclasts	Bone marrow
Blood	Monocytes	Circulation
Liver	Kupffer cells	Hepatic sinusoids

One primary function of these cells is phagocytosis, as discussed in Chapter 3 regarding inflammation. Macrophages express Fc receptors for antibody and can phagocytose antigens opsonized by antibody or complement components. Another primary function is their involvement in the immune response as antigen-presenting cells. In this instance they phagocytose antigen, process it into peptide fragments which are then presented to T lymphocytes and the induction of cell-mediated immune responses. Although all nucleated cells express MHC class I molecules and could be considered antigen-presenting cells, only three cell types normally express MHC class II molecules and are regarded as the major antigen-presenting cells. They are the macrophage, dendritic cell, and B lymphocyte. Whereas B lymphocytes and dendritic cells constitutively express MHC class II molecules, macrophages express MHC class molecules upon activation.

Macrophages also have an important role in generation of a cell-mediated immune response, and are essential to type IV hypersensitivity reactions. Activated T_H1 lymphocytes synthesize IFN-γ, a potent activator of macrophages. Under the influence of IFN-γ, macrophages have increased phagocytic activity and are more efficient at killing.

DENDRITIC CELLS

Dendritic cells comprise a distinct population of cells that are characterized by elongate cell processes. Most dendritic cells are antigen-presenting cells, which process antigens and present fragments to T lymphocytes. They are more efficient than macrophages and B lymphocytes at antigen presentation. Antigen-presenting dendritic cells are nonphagocytic, bone marrow–derived cells. They are the most important antigen-presenting cell for initiating primary immune responses to protein antigens (Fig. 5-7).

Antigen-presenting dendritic cells express a number of molecules, such as TLRs and mannose receptors, that make them efficient at capturing and responding to antigens. They also express high concentrations of MHC class II molecules and B7 co-stimulatory molecules. By expressing chemokine receptors similar to T lymphocytes, they have the ability to localize in T lymphocyte regions of lymphoid tissue. By colocalizing to these areas, they are uniquely positioned to present antigens to recirculating T lymphocytes. Antigen-presenting dendritic cells function to capture antigen and then migrate to T lymphocyte areas of secondary lymphoid organs where they present fragments of the antigen on their surface and increase their expression of co-stimulatory molecules that activate T lymphocytes. Specifically, migrating dendritic cells, derived from Langerhans' cells that have captured antigen, enter the lymph node through efferent lymphatics and localize in lymphoid organs where they present antigenic peptides to T lymphocytes that facilitate B lymphocyte activation and the production of antibody-secreting plasma cells. In addition to their function as antigen-presenting cells, they are also important in the process of negative selection in the thymus and in the maintenance of peripheral tolerance. The four types of antigen-presenting dendritic cells and their locations are listed in Table 5-4. Circulating dendritic cells, also known as "veiled cells," make up less than 1% of peripheral blood mononuclear cells. The second type of dendritic cell, the follicular dendritic cell, is primarily located in lymphoid follicles. These cells are not bone marrow derived, do not express MHC class II molecules, and do not function as an antigen-presenting cell. Follicular dendritic cells have Fc receptors and receptors for C3b. They store antigen-antibody and antigen-C3b complexes and are thought to be involved in the development and maintenance of memory B lymphocytes.

NATURAL KILLER CELLS

NK cells are nonspecific cytotoxic cells that are important in early responses to tumor cells and viral infections. NK cells are bone marrow–derived, large granular lymphocytes that make up 5% to 15% of the peripheral blood mononuclear cells. Their size, slightly larger than that of a small lymphocyte, and the presence of abundant granular cytoplasm distinguish them from T lymphocytes (Fig. 5-8). They are commonly referred to as large granular lymphocytes. The cytoplasm of NK cells and cytotoxic T lymphocytes is characterized by cytotoxic granules that contain perforin and granzymes, two potent pathways mediating lysis of the target cell. NK cells and T lymphocytes express numerous similar surface molecules and kill virus infected cells and tumor cells by similar mechanisms. Two membrane molecules, CD16 and CD56, are commonly used to identify NK cells. NK cells express Fc-γ-receptors

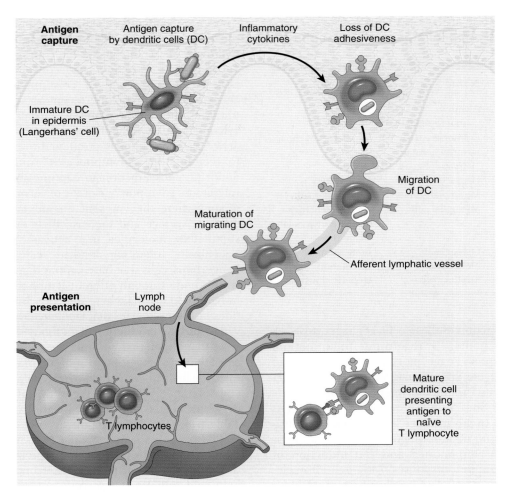

Fig. 5-7 **Dendritic cell functions.** Specialized dendritic cells in the epidermis (Langerhans' dendritic cells) capture antigen via phagocytosis or endocytosis and migrate to regional lymph nodes, where they present peptide fragments of the antigen to naïve T lymphocytes. *(From Kumar V, Abbas AK, Fausto N: Robbins & Cotran pathologic basis of disease, ed 7, Philadelphia, 2005, Saunders.)*

Table **5-4** **Antigen-Presenting Dendritic Cells and Their Primary Location**

Dendritic Cells	Location
Langerhans' cells	Skin, mucous membranes, iris, ciliary body
Interstitial dendritic cells	Most major organs
Interdigitating dendritic cells	T-lymphocyte area of secondary lymphoid tissue and thymic medulla
Circulating dendritic cells	Peripheral blood

(CD16) and the β-subunit of the IL-2 receptor (CD2). They do not express antigen-specific TCR or CD3 molecules. In contrast to cytotoxic lymphocytes, NK cells are not MHC restricted, are constitutively cytolytic, and do not develop memory cells. Because NK cells are activated early in an immune response and do not require a previous sensitization phase to develop memory cells following activation, they are the cytotoxic cell of innate immunity, the counterpart to the adaptive immune response's cytotoxic T lymphocyte.

Although NK cells do not express any antigen-specific molecules, they are very efficient at recognizing and killing altered or virally infected cells. NK cell activity is regulated through activating and inhibitory receptor molecules expressed on their cell surface (Fig. 5-9). These NK cell receptor molecules fall into two distinct categories: the immunoglobulin-like NK receptors and the C-type lectinlike NK receptors. Ligands for these receptors are cell surface molecules whose expression has been altered as a result of infection or damage. Ligands for activating receptors that stimulate NK cell activity commonly include viral and stress-induced proteins. Ligands for inhibitory receptors that block NK cell activity, most commonly involve class I MHC molecules. A decreased expression of class I MHC molecules makes

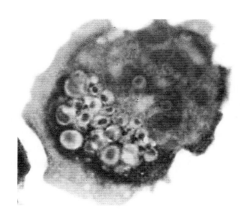

Fig. 5-8   Activated natural killer cell with numerous cytoplasmic granules that are characteristic of these large granular lymphocytes. *(Courtesy Dr. Noelle Williams, Department of Pathology, University of Texas Southwestern Medical School, Dallas.)*

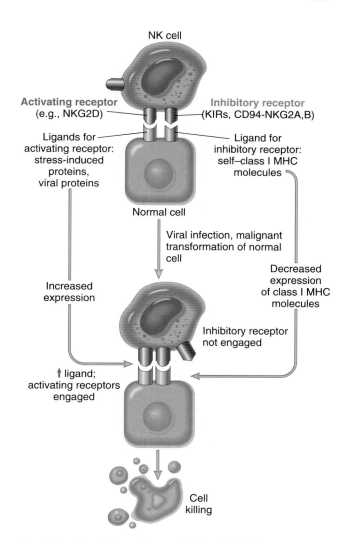

Fig. 5-9   **Regulation of natural killer** *(NK)* **cell activity through activating and inhibitory receptors.** *MHC,* Major histocompatibility complex. *(From Kumar V, Abbas AK, Fausto N: Robbins & Cotran pathologic basis of disease, ed 7, Philadelphia, 2005, Saunders.)*

cells susceptible to NK cell–mediated lysis. A decrease in MHC class I expression often occurs in virus-infected cells and in neoplastic cells, making them susceptible to attack by NK cells. Normal cells are protected from NK cell killing because all nucleated cells express class I MHC molecules. This is an oversimplification of the "opposing-signals" model of NK cell regulation of how cytotoxic activity is limited to altered self-cells. Recent studies on the molecular mechanisms of NK cell regulation indicate that the absence of an inhibitory stimulus by itself is insufficient for triggering NK cell killing. NK cells also require triggering of activating receptors. Several activating receptors have been identified. One is the NKG2D receptor, a C-type lectin-like molecule that recognizes a number of stress-induced proteins. These stress-induced proteins are normally only constitutively expressed in the intestinal epithelium or as a result of cellular distress caused by infection or neoplastic transformation. There are a number of additional activating receptors, some of which recognized viral proteins, that are structurally similar to class I MHC molecules.

Because NK cells express Fc-γ-receptors (CD16), they can also function in antibody-dependent cellular cytotoxicity (ADCC). In the case of NK cells, ADCC allows for antibody-bound targets to be identified and targeted for NK cell–induced lysis.

NK cells also facilitate the early response to viral infections not only by responding to cytokines produced early in a viral infection, but also by producing cytokines that help direct the immune response. NK cells are activated by IFN-α and IFN-β, released by virus-infected cells, and by IL-12, released by macrophages. Following activation NK cells have the ability to produce IFN-γ, a major cytokine directing the development of T_H1-type immune response early in the infection. IL-2 and IL-15 stimulate NK cell proliferation, and IL-12 enhances NK cell killing.

CYTOKINES: MESSENGER MOLECULES OF THE IMMUNE SYSTEM

GENERAL PROPERTIES OF CYTOKINES

Cytokines make up a vast group of low molecular weight soluble glycoprotein proteins that are produced by immune and nonimmune cells, are largely produced locally, and act locally to direct the immune response. The expression of cytokine receptors and their respective ligands is highly regulated and contributes to the complexity of the systemic organization of the immune response. Cytokines are involved in every aspect of leukocyte biology and the immune response and are essential to leukocyte development, recirculation, differentiation, and activation and in maintaining self-tolerance. Cytokines can influence the cytokine-producing cell itself (autocrine), other cells present locally (paracrine), or distant cells (endocrine) (see Fig. 12-1). Cytokines use common signal transducing pathways, converting an extracellular signal through a cell surface receptor to activate or inhibit the target cell.

The nomenclature of cytokines has evolved from a system that originally named them according to their cellular source (e.g., lymphokine from lymphocytes and monokines from monocytes) to one that named them according to not only the cellular source but also the target cell (e.g., interleukin, a cytokine produce by a leukocyte that influences another leukocyte) or to the primary function (e.g., chemokine, a cytokine that affects chemotaxis). As cytokines were characterized, it became apparent that they have pleiotropic, redundant, synergistic, and antagonistic features that do not allow for such a simplistic classification scheme. More recently, cytokines and their receptors have been classified based on their molecular structure and common signaling pathways. Many cytokines share a similar, α-helix structure that is also shared by their respective receptors and are classified as type I cytokines and receptors. As will be discussed later, the classification of cytokines and cytokine receptors according to their structural similarities allowed for the identification of the cause of the profound cytokine defects associated with x-linked severe combined immunodeficiency disease in humans and dogs. Unfortunately, type I cytokines also have now been found to include other regulatory proteins, such as growth hormone, prolactin, erythropoietin, thrombopoietin, and leptin. Type II cytokines include type I interferons (IFN-α and IFN-β), type II interferon (IFN-γ), and the IL-10 family of cytokines.

The breadth and depth of knowledge regarding the function, regulation, and control of cytokines is overwhelming; however, an overview of the major cytokines and their primary functions is important for understanding the pathogenic mechanism of many disease processes. Some of the major cytokines and their primary biologic activities are presented here and in Chapters 3 and 4 as they pertain to acute and chronic inflammatory responses.

Cytokines that broadly influence innate and adaptive immune responses include IL-1, interferons (type 1), IL-6, and TNF-α. These cytokines are produced and influence a wide array of cell types. Cytokines that are involved in hematopoiesis and lymphocyte development include IL-2, IL-3, IL-4, IL-5, IL-12, IL-15, TGB-β, and granulocyte-macrophage colony-stimulating factor (GM-CSF) to mention a few. Chemokines are a large group of cytokines that influence leukocyte development, trafficking, and function. They are organized into subfamilies, with distinct functions, based on the position of cysteine residues. The C-X-C subfamily of chemokines is primarily produced by activated macrophages and tissue cells (e.g., endothelium), and the C-C subfamily

is largely produced by activated T lymphocytes. Chemokines are responsible for the anatomic localization ("homing") of lymphocytes within lymphoid and nonlymphoid tissue. Chemokines and the other proinflammatory cytokines are more thoroughly covered in Chapter 3. The most important functional group of cytokines related to the pathogenesis of a number of diseases of immunity are those involved in the regulation of T_H lymphocytes. As discussed previously, T_H lymphocytes are classified based on their functional capacity and ability to elicit primarily an antibody response or a cell-mediated immune response rather than on their expression of specific cell markers (Fig. 5-10). T_H1 lymphocytes are activated by IL-12 and IL-18 and produce primarily IL-2, IFN-γ, and TNF-β to direct a cell-mediated immune response. T_H2 lymphocytes are activated by IL-4 and produce primarily IL-3, IL-4, IL-5 IL-6, IL-10, and IL-13 to direct a humoral immune response. As discussed later in the chapter, the type of response (T_H1 versus T_H2 type) may determine if a diseased state will occur. IL-15 regulates the growth and activity of NK cells. As indicated in Fig. 5-10, some cytokines, such as IL-10 and TGF-β, down-regulate immune responses. In summary, cytokines produced by the T_H1 or T_H2 subset of lymphocytes not only promote the activation and functional capacities of the subset that produces them (autocrine effect), they also inhibit the development and activity of the other subset. This is known as cross-regulation and has important implications with regard to protective immune responses and adverse immune responses, as will be discussed later.

Finally, a number of cytokine inhibitors identified and one of the more studied ones include a factor called IL-1 receptor antagonist, which is produced by macrophages, hepatocytes, and keratinocytes. This factor inhibits the local and systemic effects of IL-1 by blocking the IL-1 receptor. Another group of inhibitors are the soluble cytokine receptors, which are the enzymatic product of cleavage of the extracellular domain of cytokine receptors that bind their respective cytokines, preventing interaction with the membrane-bound receptor form. The best characterized soluble cytokine receptor is the soluble IL-2 receptor. A number of pathogenic organisms have adapted this as an evasion strategy by producing cytokine-binding proteins or mimics to influence the development of the immune response. Although soluble receptors have been identified in a number of human diseases, their exact role remains to be determined.

STRUCTURE AND FUNCTION OF HISTOCOMPATIBILITY ANTIGENS

The MHC represents a complex of genes that encode specialized molecules involved in intercellular recognition

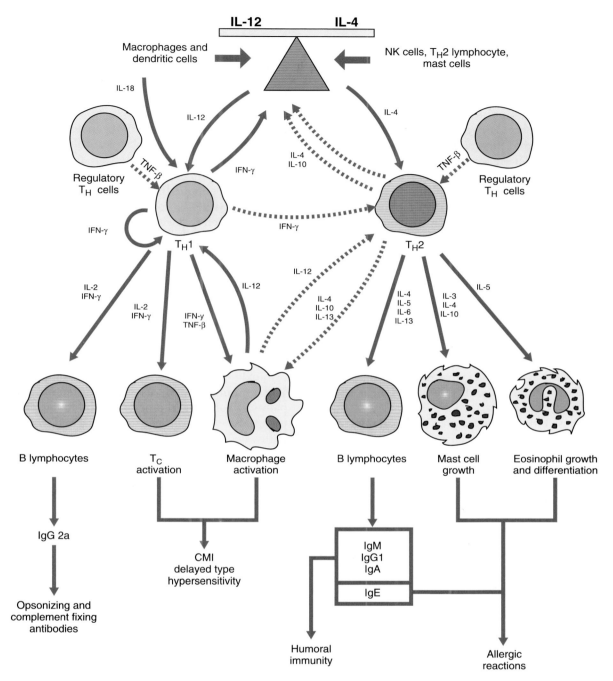

Fig. 5-10   **Cross-regulation of immunity.** Cross-regulation of T_H1 and T_H2 lymphocytes in part determines if an immunity is primarily a cell-mediated response or a humoral response. T_H1 lymphocytes, activated primarily by interleukin *(IL)*-12 and IL-18, promote cell-mediated immunity *(CMI)* by activating macrophages and cytotoxic T lymphocytes. T_H2 lymphocytes, activated primarily by IL-4, promote humoral immunity by producing cytokines that activate B lymphocytes to develop into antibody-secreting plasma cells. T_H2 lymphocytes also produce cytokines that activate mast cells and eosinophils in the pathogenesis of allergic diseases. The cross-regulation of T_H1 and T_H2 lymphocytes provides an inverse relationship between cell-mediated and humoral immunity. *IFN-γ,* Interferon-γ; *Ig,* immunoglobulin; *NK,* natural killer; *TNF-β,* tumor necrosis factor-β. *(Adapted from Goldsby RA, Kindt TJ, Osborne BA: Kuby immunology, ed 4, New York, 2000, WH Freeman.)*

and the distinguishing of self from nonself. These cell surface molecules have immunologic and nonimmunologic functions. The histocompatibility designation originated from the identification of these molecules in determining the compatibility of transplanted tissues. The MHC is an essential component in humoral and cell-mediated immunity. Most T lymphocytes only recognize fragments of antigen when they are bound to MHC molecules, and this requirement is the basis for MHC restriction. The repertoire of MHC molecules is genetically controlled and determines an individual's ability or inability to respond to specific antigens. MHC molecules are present throughout vertebrates and are maintained in gene clusters, each of which encodes different MHC products, which are linked. The primary function of cell surface MHC molecules is to bind peptide fragments of foreign proteins for presentation to antigen-specific T lymphocytes. There are three major classes of genes, and these encode for MHC molecules that are grouped according to their structure, tissue distribution, and function. Class I and class II genes encode cell surface molecules. Class III genes encode components of the complement system, enzymes 21-hydroxylase A and B, cytochrome p450, tumor necrosis factor (TNF)-α and TNF-β, and heat shock protein 70.

MHC class I molecules are present on all nucleated cells (and platelets in some species). Their major function is presentation of peptide fragments of antigens to cytotoxic T lymphocytes (CD8+). This requirement results in CD8+ lymphocytes being MHC class I restricted. MHC class I molecules are further subdivided into highly polymorphic loci, referred to as Ia, and relatively nonpolymorphic loci, referred to as Ib, Ic, and Id. Each class I molecule is composed of a heterodimer consisting of a polymorphic α-chain that is linked to a nonpolymorphic β_2-microglobulin. The extracellular region of the α-chain consists of three domains (α_1, α_2, and α_3). The α_1 and α_2 domains form a groove where the peptide fragments bind the MHC molecule (Fig. 5-11). Although MHC class I molecules differ in their ability to bind peptide fragments, they are not as restrictive as antibodies and TCRs. The intracellular processing of antigen into peptide fragments, the association of those fragments with MHC class I molecules, and their transport to the cell surface is a complex process.

Antigen uptake by antigen-presenting cells is by phagocytosis or endocytosis. Antigen processing is the degradation of an antigen into peptide fragments, which are complexed with MHC molecules. Antigen presentation is the transport of the peptide-MHC complex to the membrane, where they are displayed. Antigens can arise intracellularly (endogenous) and extracellularly (exogenous) and the immune system most effectively eliminates these antigens through the elaboration of cytotoxic T lymphocytes or secretion of antibody. The immune system uses two different processing pathways for antigen processing and antigen presentation. Intracellular antigens are processed in a cytosolic pathway and presented in association with MHC class I molecules (Fig. 5-12). Extracellular antigens are processed in an endocytic pathway and presented in association with MHC class II molecules. Endogenous antigens are degraded into small peptide fragments

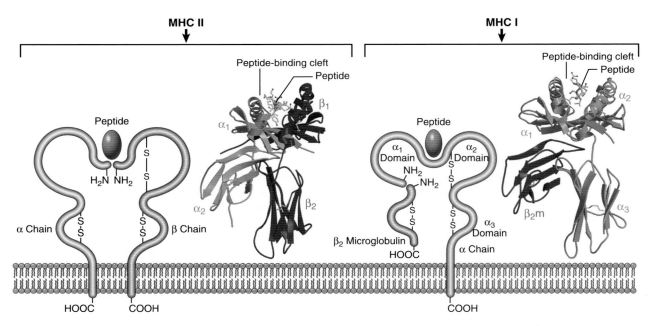

Fig. 5-11 Schematic diagram and crystal structures of class I and II major histocompatibility complex **(MHC)** molecules. *(Courtesy Dr. P. Bjorkman, California Institute of Technology, Pasadena.)*

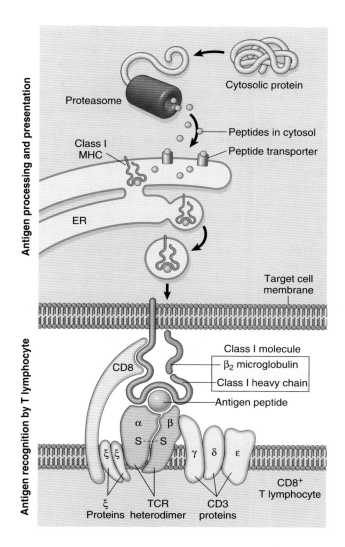

Antigen processing and presentation

Cytosolic protein

Proteasome

Class I MHC

Peptides in cytosol

Peptide transporter

ER

Target cell membrane

Antigen recognition by T lymphocyte

CD8

Class I molecule

β₂ microglobulin

Class I heavy chain

Antigen peptide

α β

S—S

ξ ξ   γ δ ε

CD8⁺ T lymphocyte

ξ   TCR   CD3
Proteins   heterodimer   proteins

Fig. 5-12   Antigen processing and presentation by an antigen-presenting cell, and antigen recognition by T lymphocytes. (A class I major histocompatibility complex [MHC]-restricted CD8⁺ lymphocyte is depicted.) *ER,* Endoplasmic reticulum; *TCR,* T-cell receptor. *(From Kumar V, Abbas AK, Fausto N: Robbins & Cotran pathologic basis of disease, ed 7, Philadelphia, 2005, Saunders.)*

heavy chain. Because cytotoxic T lymphocytes only recognize peptides when they are presented as a complex with MHC class I molecules, they are referred to as being MHC class I restricted. MHC restriction is the result of positive selection of lymphocytes during T-lymphocyte development in the thymus. Portions of some antigens, those portions not processed for presentation, and in some cases entire antigens are completely degraded by exopeptidases of the antigen-presenting cell into amino acids and do not initiate an immune response. Endogenous antigens are most frequently encountered during viral infections and thus cytotoxic T lymphocytes are an important defense mechanism for eliminating virally infected cells.

Class II molecules have a variable tissue distribution depending on the species of domestic animal, but in general they are present on antigen-presenting cells (B lymphocytes, dendritic cells, and macrophages) and can be induced on T lymphocytes, keratinocytes, and endothelial cells by IFN-γ. There are significant species differences with regard to the constitutive expression of MHC molecules. The major function of MHC class II molecules is the induction of helper T lymphocytes. Class II MHC molecules are heterodimers consisting of an α-chain and a β-chain. The antigen binding site of the class II molecule, unlike that of the class I molecule, is formed by portions of both the α₁ and β₁ domain. Additionally, as with the class I MHC molecules, polymorphism of the class II MHC molecules is associated with determining an individual's response to antigens of infectious organisms (see next section). Peptides that bind to class II MHC molecules are in general derived from exogenous antigens, which have been internalized and processed within endosomes and lysosomes of antigen-presenting cells. Antigen-presenting cells can internalize antigen by phagocytosis or endocytosis (receptor mediated or pinocytosis). Macrophages are the only cell type capable of both, as other antigen-presenting cells are poorly phagocytic. Extracellular antigens are processed into peptide fragments in an endocytic pathway and presented in association with MHC class II molecules on the cell membrane. During the synthesis of a class II molecule within the ER, it associates with another protein called the invariant chain, which prevents the molecule from binding endogenously derived peptides. The complex is then transported from the ER to the Golgi complex and into an endocytic compartment (vesicles) that contains the antigenic peptide fragments derived from exogenous antigens. Proteolytic cleavage of the invariant chain allows for the association of the peptide fragment with the class II MHC molecule. The peptide–class II MHC complex is then transported to the cell surface for presentation to CD4⁺ T helper lymphocytes. The CD4 molecule acts as a co-receptor for induction of T$_H$ cell activation. Because T-helper

within the cytoplasm by the proteasome complex. Peptide fragments are transported to the endoplasmic reticulum (ER) by an adenosine triphosphate–binding peptide transporter, TAP. Within the ER, the newly synthesized MHC class I α-chain and associated β₂-microglobulin bind the antigenic peptide and form a complex that is transported from the ER to the Golgi and then to the plasma membrane for presentation to CD8⁺ cytotoxic T lymphocytes. The antigen recognition molecule of the cytotoxic T lymphocyte (T$_C$) recognizes the MHC-peptide complex by means of its CD8 molecule, which functions as a co-receptor, binding to the nonpolymorphic α₃ domain of the MHC class I lymphocytes only recognize peptides when they are presented as a complex with class II MHC molecules, they are referred to as being class II MHC restricted. It is worth mentioning that of the two scientists, Peter Doherty and Rolf Zinkernagel, who received the Nobel Prize in Medicine in 1996 for discovering MHC restriction, Dr. Doherty is an Australian veterinarian.

MHC molecules are important in regulating T-lymphocyte development in the thymus and in the peripheral lymphoid tissues determining specific responses to different forms of antigens. During the development and maturation process in the thymus, only T lymphocytes capable of recognizing self-MHC molecules are selected (positive selection) for export to the peripheral lymphoid tissues. These developmental processes influence an individual's T-lymphocyte repertoire, which is the functional population that influences immunity. An individual's ability to mount an effective immune response is determined in part by his or her ability to recognize endogenous and exogenous antigens and their MHC haplotype. Thus in one case, the association of an antigenic peptide fragment with a specific MHC molecule may result in a protective antibody response with elimination of an infectious agent, whereas in another case, the association of an antigenic peptide fragment with a specific MHC molecule may result in an inappropriate immune response to an innocuous antigen, producing an allergic reaction.

The organization (chromosomal location) and characterization (number of loci, etc.) of the MHC of each species of domestic animals appears to be fairly conserved and present in higher vertebrates and mammals. Most mammalian species studied have class I, II, and III genes, with differences between species being the arrangement and number of genetic loci comprising the MHC. In general, class I genes are more closely related within a species than between species, and the avian MHC is smaller and less complex, with many genes found in the mammalian MHC being absent. Although it is beyond the scope of this chapter to discuss the details regarding the differences between domestic species, the preceding overview is relevant to most domestic species.

MAJOR HISTOCOMPATIBILITY COMPLEX AND DISEASE ASSOCIATION

The MHC influences transplant acceptance or rejection, immune responsiveness, and the pathogenesis of a number of diseases. The MHC represents a complex of genes that encode specialized molecules involved in antigen presentation and thus regulate immune responses. The ability of the immune system to respond to an antigen is determined in part by the binding of peptide fragments to MHC molecules, which are then presented on the surface of antigen-presenting cells.

There is a growing body of information associating certain MHC alleles with increased or decreased susceptibility to certain diseases (Table 5-5). Because the MHC genes of most domestic species are not well characterized, it is difficult to distinguish if the observed effects are due to the MHC itself or to other tightly linked genes. These conclusions are generally the result of an observation that some MHC alleles occur at a higher frequency among individuals affected with the disease, as compared with the general population. The association of an increased risk with certain MHC alleles is never the sole basis for determining if an individual will develop the disease, as often other hereditary and environmental factors also play an important role. The diseases most often associated with certain MHC alleles have a pathogenesis that incorporates a significant immunologic component. The types of diseases identified are diverse; however, they frequently include autoimmune, infectious, and allergic diseases. Additionally, MHC diversity may increase or decrease the susceptibility to infectious diseases. There is evidence that MHC polymorphisms may significantly impact disease resistance and is best illustrated in species in which there is a loss of MHC diversity attributed to a limited breeding pool of animals. In the case of the cheetah and Florida panther, the current breeding stocks of both species are derived from a limited genetic pool thus resulting in reduced MHC diversity. In both species, there is an increased susceptibility to infectious agents that is not seen in other species of big cats.

Although there are a number of hypotheses to account for the role of MHC molecules in disease susceptibility, the actual mechanisms remain elusive. The most often hypothesized mechanism is attributed to the role of MHC alleles in determining responsiveness or nonresponsiveness to a particular pathogen. On the one hand, through antigen presentation and activation of cytotoxic or helper T lymphocytes, it determines whether or not a protective immune response is generated to a particular pathogen. On the other hand, certain MHC alleles may encode molecules that are used by infectious agents, as in the case of receptors for viruses or bacterial toxins, and facilitate their infectivity or pathogenicity.

DISORDERS OF THE IMMUNE SYSTEM

As has been discussed, immunity is a complex defensive system of recognition and effector mechanisms for protecting the host from infectious pathogens and cancer. During the normal immune response, there are mechanisms for eliminating the inciting foreign antigen, and associated with this is some degree of tissue damage that elicits an inflammatory response of appropriate duration and severity for the antigen. However, there

Table **5-5**   **Major Histocompatibility Complex (MHC) Polymorphisms Related to Resistance or Susceptibility to Diseases**

Major Histocompatibility Complex	Alleles	Polymorphisms Related to Resistance or Susceptibility to:
BOVINE LEUKOCYTE ANTIGEN (BoLA)		
Class I	Aw-7, Aw-12, Aw-8	Bovine leukosis virus infection
	A*6	Development of mastitis
Class II	DRB3	Bovine leukosis virus infection
	DRB*3.2*23	Coliform mastitis
	DR	*Dermatophilus*
OVINE LEUKOCYTE ANTIGEN (OvLA)		
Class I	SY1	*Trichostrongylus*
		Scrapie
		Caseous lymphadenitis
CAPRINE LEUKOCYTE ANTIGENS (CLA)		
Class I	Be7, Be1, and Be14	Caprine arthritis-encephalitis virus
EQUINE LEUKOCYTE ANTIGENS (ELA)		
Class I	Aw-7	*Culicoides* hypersensitivity
	A3, A15	Sarcoids
	A9	Recurrent uveitis
Class II	Dw13	Sarcoids
SWINE LEUKOCYTE ANTIGENS (SLA)		
Class I	Various	*Trichinella spiralis*
DOG LEUKOCYTE ANTIGENS (DLA)		
Class I	A3, A7	Diabetes mellitus
	A10, B4	Atopy
	A1, A7, B5	Systemic lupus erythematosus
Class II	DRB1	Visceral leishmaniasis

are a number of instances in which the immune response elicits an inflammatory response that is not appropriate to the inciting antigen and these fall into three general categories. The largest category is the hypersensitivity reactions, which are associated with a large number of diseases covered throughout this text. The second category is the autoimmune diseases, in which the immune response is inappropriately directed at a self-antigen, resulting in damage to normal organs or tissue. The third category is the immunodeficiency diseases, in which a genetic or acquired defect results in an inability to mount an immune response and thus control infections, resulting in severe systemic inflammation. The chapter will now focus on general features of immunologic tissue injury, with discussion of some specific immunologic diseases that are attributable to disorders of the immune system. Finally, we will conclude with a discussion of amyloidosis, a condition that is the result of a number of mechanisms, some of which have an immunologic basis.

MECHANISMS OF IMMUNOLOGIC TISSUE INJURY: HYPERSENSITIVITY REACTIONS

A hypersensitivity reaction is defined as the altered reactivity to a specific antigen that results in pathologic reactions upon the exposure of a sensitized host to that specific antigen. The designation of these immune responses as "hyper" is somewhat of a misnomer because the reactions elicited are better characterized as inappropriate or misdirected responses. An immune response can be either beneficial or harmful. By characterizing hypersensitivity responses as inappropriate or misdirected, we are not implying that these responses are any different from those that occur as a normal "beneficial" defense mechanism. To state it more clearly: If the immune response is beneficial it is immunity, and if it is harmful it is hypersensitivity. All hypersensitivity reactions are characterized by sensitization and effector phases. The sensitization phase requires that the host must have had either a previous exposure or a prolonged exposure to the antigen such that he or she can develop an immune response to the inciting antigen. The pathology associated with hypersensitivity reactions occurs in the effector phase and is most commonly manifested as an inflammatory reaction or as cell lysis.

Hypersensitivity reactions have historically been classified on the basis of the immunologic mechanism that mediates the disease, as type I, type II, type III, or type IV. Type I, II, and III are mediated by antibody, and type IV is mediated by macrophages and T lymphocytes. Type I is also known as immediate type hypersensitivity and most often is the result of an IgE response that is directed against an environmental or exogenous antigen (also known as an allergen). The result is the release of vasoactive mediators from IgE sensitized mast cells, and these mediators produce an acute inflammatory response. Type II is also known as cytotoxic hypersensitivity and most often occurs when IgG or IgM is directed against either an altered self-protein or a foreign antigen bound to a tissue or cell.

The result can lead to either destruction of the tissue or cell by antibody-dependent phagocytosis (ADCC), complement-mediated lysis, or altered cellular function without evidence of tissue or cell damage. Type III is also known as immune complex hypersensitivity and is due to the formation of insoluble antibody-antigen complexes (also known as immune complexes). The result is activation of the complement system and the development of an inflammatory reaction at the sites of immune complex deposition. Type IV is also known as delayed-type hypersensitivity (DTH) and is the result of activation of sensitized T lymphocytes to a specific antigen. The resulting immune response is either mediated by direct cytotoxicity or by the release of cytokines that act primarily through macrophages. This original classification, as proposed by Gell and Coombs, was based largely on the primary initiating event involved in the individual reactions and not on the actual pathogenesis as it relates to what is seen clinically or pathologically. Although the original classification of hypersensitivity

Table **5-6** **Mechanisms of Hypersensitivity Diseases**

Type	Immunologic Component	Antigen	Prototype Disorder	Immune Mechanisms	Pathologic Lesions
Immediate (type I) hypersensitivity	IgE mediated	Allergens	Anaphylaxis; allergies (atopic forms)	Production of IgE antibody → immediate release of vasoactive amines and other mediators from mast cells; recruitment of inflammatory cells (late-phase reaction)	Vascular dilation, edema, smooth muscle contraction, mucus production, inflammation
Antibody-mediated (type II) hypersensitivity	IgG and IgM mediated	Cell- or matrix-associated antigens Cell surface receptor	Autoimmune hemolytic anemia; neonatal isoerythrolysis; transfusion reactions; drug reactions; Pemphigus	Production of IgG, IgM → binds to antigen on target cell or tissue → phagocytosis or lysis of target cell by activated complement or Fc receptors; recruitment of leukocytes	Cell lysis; inflammation
Immune complex-mediated (type III) hypersensitivity	IgG and IgM mediated	Soluble antigen (e.g., bacterial and viral antigens)	Systemic lupus erythematosus; some forms of glomerulonephritis; serum sickness; Arthus reaction	Deposition of antigen-antibody complexes → complement activation → recruitment of leukocytes by complement products and Fc receptors → release of enzymes and other toxic molecules	Necrotizing vasculitis (fibrinoid necrosis); inflammation

Ig, Immunoglobulin.

Table **5-6**   Mechanisms of Hypersensitivity Diseases—Cont'd

Type	Immunologic Component	Antigen	Prototype Disorder	Immune Mechanisms	Pathologic Lesions
Cell-mediated (type IV) hypersensitivity	T-lymphocyte mediated	Soluble antigen (e.g., bacterial and viral antigens) Contact antigens Cell-associated antigen	Contact dermatitis; transplant rejection; tuberculosis; chronic allergic diseases	Activated T lymphocytes → (i) release of cytokines and macrophage activation; (ii) T-lymphocyte mediated cytotoxicity	Perivascular cellular infiltrates; edema; cell destruction; granuloma formation

reactions is still valid, "newer" versions that are based on the pathogenesis better illustrate the complexity of these reactions and the specific pathology (lesions) associated with them. For the purposes of our discussion, we will use the original version of the Gell and Coombs classification presented in Table 5-6, understanding that many of the diseases associated with hypersensitivity reactions are actually complex and may involve more than one type. In humans, genetic mapping studies of most diseases characterized by a hypersensitivity reaction suggest that there are disease-associated susceptibility genes, further supporting the complex pathogenesis of these diseases. Finally the pathogenesis of many diseases rarely involves a single hypersensitivity reaction, and in fact some diseases may begin as an immediate hypersensitivity but progress to be predominantly DTH. For clarity, the hypersensitivity diseases are discussed in the context of their predominant mechanism except when it is appropriate to elaborate on the progression of a disease.

TYPE I HYPERSENSITIVITY (IMMEDIATE HYPERSENSITIVITY)

Type I hypersensitivity reactions are most commonly the result of an IgE-mediated immune response directed against environmental antigens (i.e., allergens) and parasite antigens. Harmful IgE-mediated responses to innocuous environmental antigens resulting in allergic reactions are termed hypersensitivity, whereas similar IgE-mediated protective responses to parasite antigens are considered immunity. This distinction emphasizes the fact that these are not unique immunologic reactions but rather misdirected or inappropriate "normal" immune responses. Type I hypersensitivity occurs in a previously sensitized host and is initially manifested as acute inflammatory process that occurs within minutes ("immediate hypersensitivity") of exposure to the

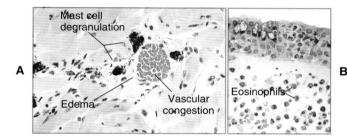

Fig. 5-13   **Immediate hypersensitivity reaction. A,** Early reaction (minutes) is characterized by mast cell degranulation and release of preformed vasoactive substances that cause vasodilation and increased vascular permeability, resulting in edema of interstitial tissue. **B,** As the lesion progresses to the late phase (hours), the inflammatory infiltrate is primarily composed of eosinophils and fewer lymphocytes and neutrophils. (**A** and **B,** Courtesy Dr. Daniel Friend, Department of Pathology, Brigham and Women's Hospital, Boston.)

specific antigen. In many instances the reaction progresses from an early acute inflammatory response to a late phase response and/or chronic inflammatory lesion that persists (Figs. 5-13 and 5-14). The basic pathogenesis involves a sensitization phase and an effector phase. The sensitization phase occurs during the initial exposure to an antigen when the host develops an antigen-specific IgE response, which results in sensitization of the host by the binding of the antigen-specific IgE to Fcε receptors on the surface of mast cells (Fig. 5-15). The host is now sensitized, and either through a second exposure or prolonged initial exposure to the IgE-specific antigen, there is cross-linking of two or more IgE molecules on the surface of the mast cell. This results in its activation and release of preformed and newly synthesized mediators, resulting in the effector phase. The effector phase can be limited to an acute inflammatory

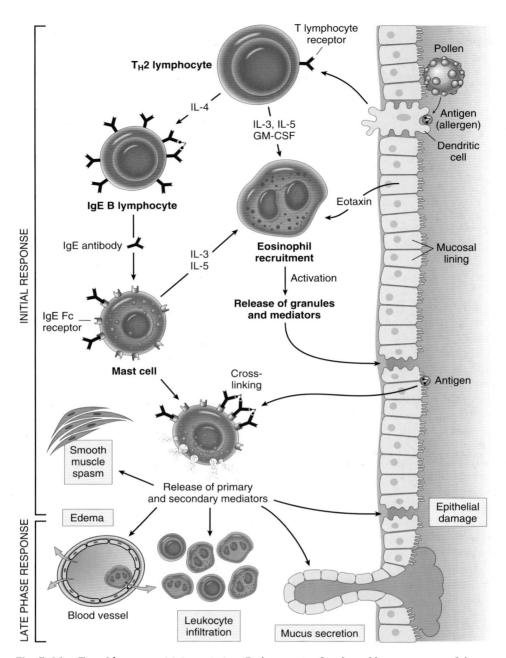

Fig. 5-14 **Type I hypersensitivity reaction.** Pathogenesis of early and late responses of the type I hypersensitivity reaction. *GM-CSF,* Granulocyte-macrophage colony-stimulating factor; *IgE,* immunoglobulin E; *IL,* interleukin. *(From Kumar V, Abbas AK, Fausto N: Robbins & Cotran pathologic basis of disease, ed 7, Philadelphia, 2005, Saunders.)*

reaction (occurring within minutes), resulting primarily from the release of mast cell mediators, or can progress to a late-phase reaction (over a period of hours), or to a chronic reaction (persisting for days to years). The acute reaction is characterized by responses associated with release of preformed vasoactive amines from the mast cell and includes increased vascular permeability, smooth muscle contraction, and influx of inflammatory cells. The late phase and chronic reactions, often associated with repeated or prolonged antigen exposures, are largely the result of a more intense inflammatory cell infiltration (primarily eosinophils, neutrophils, macrophages, and T lymphocytes) and tissue damage. Because the mast cell is central to the pathogenesis of a type I hypersensitivity reaction, we will review their biologic features and primary functions.

Mast cells are a heterogeneous population of bone marrow–derived cells that reside in vascularized tissue.

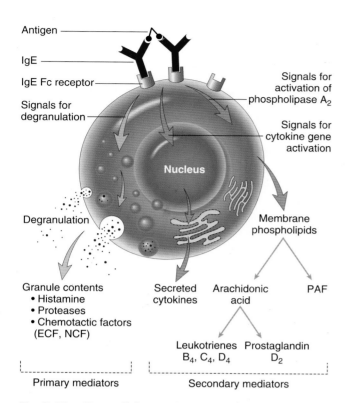

Antigen

IgE

IgE Fc receptor

Signals for degranulation

Signals for activation of phospholipase A$_2$

Signals for cytokine gene activation

Nucleus

Degranulation

Membrane phospholipids

Granule contents
• Histamine
• Proteases
• Chemotactic factors (ECF, NCF)

Secreted cytokines

Arachidonic acid

PAF

Leukotrienes B$_4$, C$_4$, D$_4$

Prostaglandin D$_2$

Primary mediators

Secondary mediators

Fig. 5-15   Mast cell degranulation and activation. Cross-linking of a sensitized (immunoglobulin E *[IgE]* bound to membrane FcE receptors) mast cell by antigen results in mast cell activation and degranulation. Degranulation results in release of preformed mediators (histamine, proteases, and chemotactic substances). Activation results in synthesis of arachidonic acid from the plasma membrane and the production of prostaglandins and leukotrienes. *ECF,* Eosinophil chemotactic factor; *NCF,* neutrophil chemotactic factor; *PAF,* platelet-activating factor. *(From Kumar V, Abbas AK, Fausto N: Robbins & Cotran pathologic basis of disease, ed 7, Philadelphia, 2005, Saunders.)*

Mast cells are easily identified by their abundant metachromatic cytoplasmic granules. Metachromasia is defined as the staining of a tissue component so that the color (absorption spectrum) of the tissue-dye complex differs from the color of the original dye and of the other stained tissue. In other words, the metachromatic substance is a different color from those of the dye and the other stained tissue. For example, toluidine blue is a metachromatic dye, and it stains most tissues blue, but mast cell granules are purple. Other commonly used metachromatic dyes include methylene blue and thionine. Wright's and Giemsa stains are dye mixtures that include a metachromatic dye. Mast cells can be divided into mucosal and connective tissue subpopulations, not only based on their location but also on their phenotypic, morphologic, histochemical, and functional characteristics. This suggests that individual subpopulations of mast cells may have specific functions in normal and pathologic responses that are a result of their activation.

The tyrosine kinase receptor, c-kit, expressed on mast cells, their precursors, and its ligand–stem cell factor (SCF)–is essential to mast cell development and function. Alterations in c-kit have been used to molecularly identify poorly differentiated mast cell tumors.

Mast cell activation can occur through a number of immunologic and nonimmunologic mechanisms. In addition to the activation of mast cells through cross-linking of membrane-bound IgE by antigen, other substances and stimuli can also activate mast cells. Mast cells can be activated by FcE receptor-independent mechanisms, including cytokines (IL-8), complement products (the anaphylatoxins C3a and C5a), drugs (nonsteroidal antiinflammatory drugs, codeine, and morphine) and physical stimuli (heat, cold, and trauma). Non-IgE-mediated activation of mast cells is referred to as an anaphylactoid reaction, whereas the IgE-mediated activation is referred to as type I hypersensitivity. There are species and tissue differences in the how type I reactions are manifested, and these are attributable to the types and proportions of mediators produced by the mast cell. Mast cells are a heterogeneous population of cells with regard to their structure and function. Although they are generally divided into mucosal-based and connective tissue–based populations, in either case they are primarily found adjacent to blood vessels and nerves where their mediators have their greatest influence. Mediators released by mast cells are broadly classified as preformed (primary) or newly synthesized (secondary), and as presented in Table 5-7 and Fig. 5-15, they influence local tissues and other cell types. Primary mediators are stored in cytoplasmic

Table **5-7**   **Summary of Mast Cell Mediators and Their Actions**

Action	Mediator
Vasodilation, increased	Histamine
Vascular permeability	PAF
	Leukotrienes C$_4$, D$_4$, E$_4$
	Neutral proteases that activate complement and kinins
	Prostaglandin D$_2$
Smooth muscle spasm	Leukotrienes C$_4$, D$_4$, E$_4$
	Histamine
	Prostaglandins
	PAF
Cellular infiltration	Cytokines (e.g., TNF)
	Leukotriene B$_4$
	Eosinophil and neutrophil chemotactic factors (not defined biochemically)
	PAF

PAF, Platelet-activating factor; *TNF,* tumor necrosis factor.

granules and include the vasoactive amines histamine, serotonin, and adenosine; chemotactic factors for eosinophils and neutrophils; enzymes including neutral proteases and acid hydrolases; and proteoglycans, such as heparin and the chondroitin sulfates. Newly synthesized mediators consist largely of the lipid mediator products of cyclooxygenase and lipoxygenase metabolism of arachidonic acid (see Chapter 3), a number of cytokines and platelet-activating factor (PAF). The major products of arachidonic metabolism are the prostaglandins and leukotrienes, of which prostaglandin D_2 and leukotrienes C_4, D_4, and E_4 are most important. The major cytokines released from mast cells during a type I reaction include IL-4, IL-5, IL-6, and TNF-α. IL-4 and IL-5 contribute to B-lymphocyte activation and IgE synthesis. IL-5 is chemotactic for eosinophils. IL-6 and TNF-α are involved in the pathogenesis of shock during a systemic type I (anaphylactic) reaction. The biochemical events involved in IgE-mediated activation and mediator release by mast cells are similar to those described for leukocyte activation in Chapter 3. The primary actions of preformed and newly synthesized mediators are attributable to cellular infiltration, vasoactive responses, and smooth muscle contraction. PAF, first identified as an initiator of platelet aggregation and degranulation, functions not only in the acute phase by increasing vasodilation and vascular permeability, but is also important early in the late phase by recruiting and activating inflammatory cells. Finally, it is of note that recent studies have identified TLR pathways that mediate interactions between dendritic cells, T lymphocytes, and mast cells, thus modulating type I responses.

A type I reaction begins as an acute inflammatory reaction mediated largely by the vasoactive amines released by degranulation of mast cells. It is during this early stage that mast cells also release large quantities of chemotactic factors and cytokines. These mediators recruit and activate the inflammatory cells that will not only sustain the inflammatory response in the absence of antigen, but also cause tissue damage. The immediate response is characterized by increased blood flow, increased vascular permeability (edema), and smooth muscle spasm. As the reaction progresses, additional leukocytes are recruited, and they release biologically active substances that cause cell damage. Of these leukocytes, eosinophils are particularly important.

Eosinophils are recruited to the sites of type I hypersensitivity reactions by chemokines, such as eotaxin, and their survival is influenced by IL-3, IL-5, and GM-CSF, which are largely derived from T_H2 lymphocytes. Eosinophils recruited during the early response play an active role in the late phase response by releasing components of their granules, synthesizing lipid mediators, and producing cytokines. The basic proteins released by eosinophils are toxic to parasites and host tissue. In particular, eosinophil major basic protein is toxic not only to parasites but also to tumor cells and normal cells. These proteins contribute to the epithelial cell damage associated with chronic type I reactions. Lipid mediators synthesized by activated eosinophils include PAF, leukotrienes, and lipoxins. Cytokines produced and released by eosinophils include growth factors, chemokines, cytokines involved in inflammation and repair, and regulatory cytokines. Macrophages and lymphocytes also participate in the late phase response to varying degrees.

Epithelial cells further contribute to the inflammation by becoming activated and producing factors that recruit and activate additional inflammatory cells. It is this complex series of cell activation, recruitment, and mediator release that amplifies the immune response and sustains the inflammatory reaction long after the antigen has gone.

The factors that determine whether a host will develop a type I hypersensitivity reaction are complex. The genetic makeup of the host and the dose and route of antigen exposure are most important. These factors influence whether the individual will have a T_H1 or T_H2 response. The development of an IgE-secreting B lymphocyte from an immature (naïve) B lymphocyte is dependent on activated CD4+ lymphocytes of the T_H2 type. The cytokines that define a T_H2-lymphocyte response have important roles in regulating the cells involved in a type I hypersensitivity reaction. IL-3, IL-4, and IL-10 influence mast cell production; IL-4 is involved in isotype switching to IgE; and IL-3 and IL-5 influence eosinophil maturation and activation. IL-13 promotes the production of IgE. The major cytokine that defines a T_H1 response, IFN-γ, inhibits the T_H2 response. Thus an animal that develops predominantly a T_H2 response to a particular antigen would be more likely to develop a type I hypersensitivity reaction as compared with one that develops predominantly a T_H1 response. The CD4+ T lymphocyte plays a central role in the pathogenesis of a type I hypersensitivity. In humans, additional genetic influences can be linked to the human leukocyte antigen (HLA)-linked immune response genes. These genes appear to control allergen-specific IgE responses. As mentioned previously, the association of specific class I MHC molecules with an increased susceptibility to atopy in the dog have been proposed. As with the mast cell and the eosinophil, a role for the CD4+ T lymphocyte in the late phase response has also been described. Studies suggest that the continued production of T_H2 cytokines contributes to the chronic inflammation associated with some chronic type I hypersensitivity reactions.

In summary, type I hypersensitivity is a complex disease process that occurs in sensitized hosts, which can result in three types of responses: (1) an acute inflammatory response, (2) a late phase response, and (3) a chronic inflammatory response. In sensitized hosts, the cross-linking of IgE on the surface of mast cells results in the immediate release of mediators that influence local tissue and recruit additional inflammatory cells. The acute response is dependent on resident mast cells, whereas the late phase and chronic responses are dependent on recruited cells, especially the eosinophil. Central to the pathogenesis of a type I hypersensitivity reaction are the T_H2 lymphocytes and the cytokines they produce, which influence IgE production and the recruitment and activation of leukocytes.

Systemic and localized type I hypersensitivity reactions occur in animals. The pathogenesis of many infectious and noninfectious diseases involves the production of IgE and the development of a type I hypersensitivity reaction. Type I hypersensitivity is an allergic reaction that occurs within minutes of exposure to an antigen to which the host has been previously sensitized. Allergy has become synonymous with type I hypersensitivity. By definition, type I hypersensitivity reactions are mediated by IgE. Systemic type I hypersensitivity reactions are called anaphylaxis. Atopy is the genetic predisposition to develop localized type I hypersensitivity reactions to innocuous antigens. Atopy is often limited to an organ or tissue, such as in allergic dermatitis and rhinitis, food allergies, and asthma. Non–IgE-mediated allergic-like reactions are referred to as anaphylactoid reactions.

SYSTEMIC TYPE I HYPERSENSITIVITY (ANAPHYLAXIS)

Anaphylaxis refers to an acute systemic hypersensitivity reaction to an antigen that is mediated by IgE and involves mast cell activation, resulting in a shocklike state often involving multiple organ systems. The clinical signs and pathology attributable to a systemic anaphylactic reaction vary by species and often correlate to the primary shock organ in its most severe manifestation–death. This variation reflects differences in the distribution of the mast cells, the mediator content of their granules that are unique to individual species, and the primary target tissue. The primary target tissues are blood vessels and smooth muscle. Blood vessel beds and smooth muscles vary in their histamine receptor content, and as such some are more susceptible than others to the influences of histamine. Because of the aforementioned, the early signs of anaphylaxis can be varied. Cutaneous signs include pruritus, hyperemia, and angioedema. Cardiovascular signs include hypotension and an accompanying sinus tachycardia (characteristic of a vasovagal response). Respiratory signs include bronchospasms, laryngeal edema, and dyspnea. As the anaphylactic reaction progresses, hypotension or hypoxia may lead to unconsciousness. Fatal anaphylaxis may occur as the result of asphyxiation secondary to edema of the upper airway, circulatory failure as a result of dilation of the splanchnic vascular bed, or hypoxemia as a result of severe bronchospasms. In humans, a body of evidence also implicates human heart mast cells (HHMCs) in myocardial anaphylaxis as a primary mechanism. Other than in cases with upper airway edema or pulmonary hyperinflation (emphysema), there are no pathognomonic lesions of anaphylaxis. The species most sensitive to the development of anaphylaxis is the guinea pig. The most common pathologic findings in most species are pulmonary edema and emphysema, except for dogs, for which the major shock organ is the liver, and severe hepatic congestion and visceral hemorrhage are the most common findings.

The types of antigens that can elicit a systemic anaphylactic reaction are diverse, but most commonly include drugs (especially penicillin-based antibiotics), vaccines, venom of stinging insects, and heterologous sera. Although the greatest risk for the development of an anaphylactic reaction occurs during parenteral administration, it must be noted that in some cases even a small quantity of antigen in a highly sensitized host can elicit a systemic response.

LOCALIZED TYPE I HYPERSENSITIVITY

In a localized type I hypersensitivity reaction, the clinical signs and pathologic findings are restricted to a specific tissue or organ. Localized reactions most commonly occur at epithelial surfaces, such as the surfaces of the skin and mucosa of the respiratory and gastrointestinal tract. As discussed previously, species differences on the location of mast cells, the mediators contained within them, and the histamine receptor distribution on target tissue may explain the different spectra of diseases seen among individual species.

Allergic dermatitis is a cutaneous manifestation of a type I hypersensitivity reaction that results in inflammation of the skin. The route of exposure to the antigen may be by inhalation, ingestion, or percutaneous absorption. If the allergic dermatitis is thought to have a genetic predisposition, then the disease is referred to as atopic dermatitis. Dietary type I hypersensitivity reactions in the dog and cat more commonly present as a cutaneous disease rather than a gastrointestinal disease. Other common cutaneous manifestations of type I hypersensitivity are flea and other arthropod bites and urticaria and angioedema (hives). All of these diseases are characterized by an acute inflammatory reaction, often perivascular, caused by mediators released from sensitized mast cells. In some instances, as in atopic dermatitis, the lesion may progress to a late phase response or chronic inflammation characterized by more intense inflammatory infiltrates (e.g., atopic dermatitis) or to a type IV hypersensitivity reaction (arthropod bites).

Other secondary changes, such as acanthosis, hyperpigmentation, sebaceous gland metaplasia, and pyoderma, occur in long-standing cases or in animals that have significant trauma related to pruritus.

Allergic rhinitis is a respiratory manifestation of a type I hypersensitivity reaction that most commonly develops in ruminants. The most common antigens are grass and weed pollens and mold spores (*Micropolyspora faeni*). This disease also frequently progresses from an acute inflammatory disease to a late phase response and chronic inflammation. In cattle, long-standing allergic rhinitis may progress to a type IV hypersensitivity reaction with the formation of nasal granulomas. Mold spores (*Micropolyspora faeni*) are more frequently associated with a type III hypersensitivity reaction, resulting in an allergic pneumonitis (extrinsic allergic alveolitis).

Although an inherited predisposition has been implicated in some species, the exact mode of inheritance remains to be determined. In humans, a link to genes encoding IL-4 and certain MHC antigens, important components of allergic diseases, has been made.

TYPE II HYPERSENSITIVITY (CYTOTOXIC HYPERSENSITIVITY)

In the original Gell and Coombs classification, the type II hypersensitivity reaction was designated as antibody-mediated cytotoxic hypersensitivity. This type of hypersensitivity most often occurs as the result of the development of antibodies directed against antigens on the surface of a cell or in a tissue, with the result that the cell or tissue is destroyed. Antigens may be either endogenous (normal cellular or tissue protein) or exogenous (e.g., a drug or microbial protein adsorbed to the cell). In some instances, the antigen may be a cell surface receptor and the antibody may activate or block the activation of the cell rather cause cytotoxicity. The pathogenesis of many immune-mediated and autoimmune diseases is centered on the development of antireceptor or antisurface antigen antibodies and a type II hypersensitivity reaction. The largest group of "cytotoxic" hypersensitivity reactions involves the hematologic diseases, with antibodies directed against antigens present on the surface of red blood cells and platelets. Type II hypersensitivity reactions are mediated by antibodies directed against antigens on the surface of tissue or cells, such that the tissue or cell is destroyed or the function of the cell is altered. Type II hypersensitivity reactions most frequently involve IgM and IgG and occur within hours after exposure in a sensitized host.

There are three basic antibody-mediated mechanisms that result in type II hypersensitivity (Fig. 5-16). Complement-dependent reactions occur as a result of the complement activating capability of IgG and IgM. Complement activation can mediate cytotoxicity by either the formation of the membrane attack complex, resulting in cell lysis, or the fixation of C3b fragments (opsonization) to the surface facilitating phagocytosis (see Chapter 3). Antibody-dependent reactions can similarly opsonize cells, facilitating phagocytosis, or result in cell lysis by antibody-dependent cellular cytotoxicity. Opsonization of cells by antibody makes them susceptible to destruction by macrophages, neutrophils, NK cells, and eosinophils, all of which bear Fc receptors. This is commonly referred to as antibody-dependent cellular cytotoxicity (ADCC). Finally, antibodies directed against surface receptors may result in altered cell or tissue function. The antireceptor antibodies can function as agonists, stimulating cell function or as antagonists, blocking receptor function.

Diseases with a type II hypersensitivity pathogenesis are presented in Table 5-8. The physical and biochemical properties of red blood cells, platelets, and leukocytes make them susceptible to cytotoxic reactions. Two properties of red blood cells make them uniquely susceptible to being involved in type II reactions. First, their surface contains a complex array of blood group antigens that can become targets of antibody responses as is commonly the case in transfusion reactions or immune-mediated hemolytic disease of the newborn. Second, the biochemical properties of red blood cells make them prone to adsorb substances, such as drugs or antigenic components of infectious agents or tumors. In these instances, the red blood cell may be either directly targeted because the substance alters a surface protein to an extent that it is now recognized as foreign, or indirectly targeted if there is an antibody response to the substance itself. Finally, in autoimmune forms of hemolytic anemia, agranulocytosis, and thrombocytopenia, there is a breakdown of tolerance and the subsequent development of antibodies to normal cells, and as a result they are destroyed.

The majority of cytotoxic type II diseases result in a decrease or loss of a population of cells (e.g., anemia, thrombocytopenia). Noncytotoxic type II diseases are initially characterized by activation or inhibition of cell or tissue function followed by inflammation, which may cause inflammatory damage to the targeted organ. In a type II reaction, the pathogenesis commonly begins with cell surface antigens eliciting an antibody response, whereby the antibodies bind to the cell and the cell is either lysed or complement components attract phagocytic cells that damage tissues by releasing proteolytic enzymes.

TYPE III HYPERSENSITIVITY (IMMUNE COMPLEX HYPERSENSITIVITY)

Type III hypersensitivity is designated as immune complex hypersensitivity. This reaction occurs through the formation of antigen-antibody complexes that activate

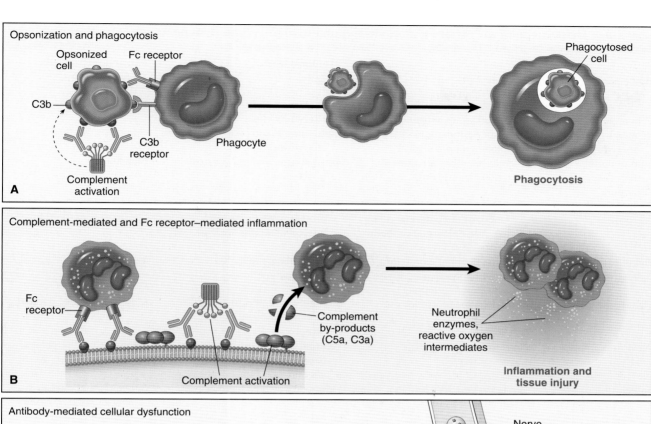

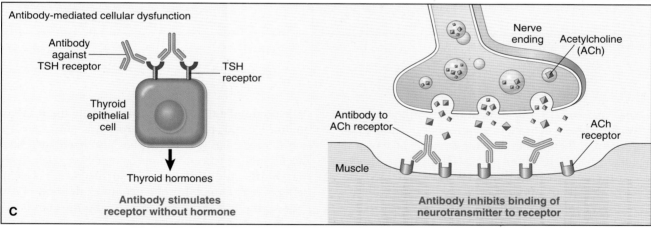

Fig. 5-16 **Schematic depiction of the three major mechanisms of an antibody mediated injury. A,** Opsonization by antibodies (or complement) enhances phagocytosis of antigen by monocyte-macrophage cells. **B,** Antibody can activate the complement system, via the classical pathway, resulting in the elaboration of inflammatory mediators, such as C5a and C3a. **C,** Antibodies against cell receptors can activate (depicted) or inhibit (not depicted) cell functions. *TSH,* Thyroid-stimulating hormone. (**A, B,** *and* **C,** *From Kumar V, Abbas AK, Fausto N: Robbins & Cotran pathologic basis of disease, ed 7, Philadelphia, 2005, Saunders.)*

complement and result in tissue damage (Fig. 5-17). The cell or tissue injury is similar to a type II hypersensitivity reaction, although the underlying pathogenesis is different. With a type III reaction, the cell or tissue is being destroyed not because the antibody is being directed against that cell or tissue, but rather because immune complexes either become "stuck" to that cell or are deposited in that tissue. Think of it as an "innocent bystander" reaction: The targeted tissue is not a direct target of the immune response. The pathogenesis begins with the formation of immune complexes that become lodged or are formed in or deposited in tissue and are capable of activating the complement system. Products of complement activation, anaphylatoxins, chemotactic

Table **5-8**   Diseases with a Primary Cytotoxic Hypersensitivity (Type II Hypersensitivity) Pathogenesis

Disease	Target Antigen	Mechanisms of Disease	Clinicopathologic Manifestations
Autoimmune hemolytic anemia	Erythrocyte membrane proteins (blood group antigens)	Opsonization and phagocytosis of erythrocytes	Hemolysis, anemia
Neonatal isoerythrolysis	Erythrocyte membrane proteins (blood group antigens)	Opsonization and phagocytosis of erythrocytes	Hemolysis, anemia
Autoimmune thrombocytopenic purpura	Platelet membrane proteins (gpIIb:IIIa integrin)	Opsonization and phagocytosis of platelets	Bleeding
Pemphigus diseases	Proteins in intercellular junctions of epidermal cells (e.g., the epidermal cadherin desmoglein 1)	Antibody-mediated activation of proteases, disruption of intercellular adhesions	Vesiculobullous (diseases of the skin)
Vasculitis caused by ANCA	Neutrophil granule proteins, presumably released from activated neutrophils	Neutrophil degranulation and inflammation	Vasculitis
Myasthenia gravis	Acetylcholine receptor	Antibody inhibits acetylcholine binding, down-modulates receptors	Muscle weakness, paralysis
Pernicious anemia	Intrinsic factor of gastric parietal cells	Neutralization of intrinsic factor, decreased absorption of vitamin B_{12}	Abnormal erythropoiesis, anemia
Bullous pemphigoid	Collagen type XVII within hemidesmosomes	Antibodies against basal cells	Subepidermal vesicles characterized by basement membrane clefts

ANCA, Antineutrophil cytoplasmic antibody.

factors, and so on result in neutrophil infiltration and activation. Upon activation, neutrophils release their enzymes and these result in tissue damage. Like type II hypersensitivity reactions, type III hypersensitivity reactions most frequently involve IgM and IgG and occur within hours after exposure in a sensitized host.

Antigen-antibody complexes form as a part of a normal immune response and usually facilitate the clearance of antigen by the phagocytic system without resulting in a type III hypersensitivity reaction. Although a number of factors determine whether a type III reaction will occur, the most important is the relationship of the antibody response to the quantity of antigen. When antibody is in great excess of antigen, the antigen-antibody complexes formed are large and insoluble, and easily removed by the phagocytic system. When antigen is in great excess of the quantity of antibody, the antigen-antibody complexes formed are too small to be capable of becoming lodged in tissues or of activating the complement system. However, when antigen is in slight excess of antibody, these small soluble complexes can become lodged in tissue and activate the complement system. When this type of small soluble antigen-antibody complex is formed in the circulation,

their accumulation in tissue is essentially the result of anatomic and physiologic processes and has no immunologic basis. Finally, it has also been suggested that in some instances immune complex hypersensitivity may be the result of the normal phagocytic system being overwhelmed. Immune complex deposition can be localized to a tissue or generalized if the complexes are formed in circulation. Blood vessels, synovial membranes, glomeruli, and the choroid plexus are particularly vulnerable to deposition of immune complexes. The concentration and size of the complexes determine the sites of deposition.

Type III reactions can develop from antibody responses to endogenous or exogenous antigens and immune complexes can be deposited in a number of tissues (Table 5-9). Although a number of diseases of domestic species involve a type III hypersensitivity pathogenesis, a majority of diseases are the result of persistent infections, autoimmune disease, or inhalation of foreign antigen. Organisms that result in persistent infections are often characterized by a weak antibody response and the development of immune complex formation. A number of autoimmune and immune-mediated diseases result in the development of antibody

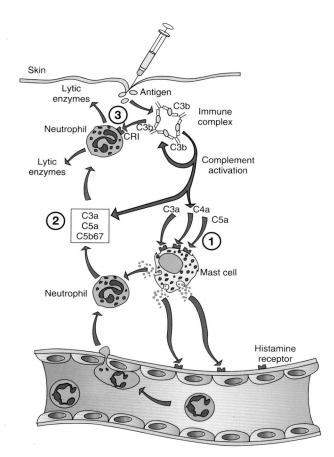

Fig. 5-17 **A localized type III hypersensitivity reaction (Arthus reaction) in the dermis.** Antigen-antibody complexes, formed at the site of injection, activate the complement system to elaborate components that activate resident mast cells *(1)* and attract circulating neutrophils *(2)*. Inflammation is the result of tissue damage caused by mediators and enzymes released from both cell types *(3)*. *CRI,* complement receptor 1. *(Adapted from Goldsby RA, Kindt TJ, Osborne BA: Kuby immunology, ed 4, New York, 2000, WH Freeman.)*

responses to self-antigens or antigens complexed to self-proteins, and these are capable of generating complement activating immune complexes. Immune complexes formed against commonly inhaled environmental antigens can lead to the development of an allergic alveolitis. Type III hypersensitivity reactions are mediated by the formation of antigen-antibody complexes, which results in complement activation leading to an influx of neutrophils and subsequent cell or tissue destruction. Antigen-antibody complexes may be formed in the circulation and lodge in tissue, or may be formed in the tissue directly. The cell or tissue injury is largely determined by physiologic or anatomic properties rather an immunologic basis. The pathogenesis of a number of diseases of domestic animals have a type III hypersensitivity basis.

LOCALIZED TYPE III HYPERSENSITIVITY

Localized type III hypersensitivity reactions are best exemplified by the Arthus reaction (Fig. 5-17). The parenteral administration of an antigen to an animal that has a circulating antibody specific for that antigen results in a localized acute inflammatory response. The complexes are formed either within the tissue at the site of antigen deposition or localized within blood vessels, as the antigen and antibody diffuse into the vascular wall. Early, within hours, the reaction is characterized by margination and emigration of neutrophils to and from the blood vessels and progressively results in tissue and vascular damage. The quantity of antigen-antibody complexes formed in the wall of the vessel determines the extent of the tissue damage. Small quantities of complexes may result in only mild hyperemia and edema. Large quantities of complexes may result in tissue and vascular necrosis as a result of neutrophils releasing the contents of their granules. In some cases, the damage to the wall may be so severe as to cause thrombosis and localized ischemic injury. The Arthus reaction is still used today as an experimental model of a localized type III reaction. Recent studies, using the cutaneous Arthus reaction in complement-deficient mice, document the requirement of Fc receptor (FcR) activation for eliciting an inflammatory response and a revision of the hypothesis of the mechanism of immune complex-mediated inflammation. Complement components, such as C5a, are generated as a result of FcR activation. Conversely, the use of FcR-deficient mice and the Arthus reaction establish the requirement of this receptor, because immune complexes and C3 alone are not sufficient to trigger an inflammatory response and tissue damage.

Many diseases have a progressive clinical course, and immune complex reactions often play a role, even though they may not be involved in the initial immunologic response. There are limited clinical examples of diseases characterized primarily by a localized immune complex reaction. One dramatic example is blue eye in the dog, which is an anterior uveitis that develops in a small percentage of dogs naturally infected with or vaccinated against canine adenovirus type I. Other organs commonly affected by localized immune complex disease include the lung and skin. In the lung, chronic exposure of the lower airways to inhaled antigens can lead to the development of antigen-specific antibodies that form complexes within alveolar walls. This form of allergic lung disease is commonly referred to as allergic pneumonitis (extrinsic allergic alveolitis). Common antigens include spore-forming organisms (e.g., some actinomycetes and fungi). Allergic diseases of the lower airways frequently lead to type II pneumocyte hyperplasia, emphysema, and fibrosis, which are all secondary to inflammation and tissue damage mediated by

Table **5-9**   **Diseases with a Primary Type III Hypersensitivity (Immune Complex Hypersensitivity) Pathogenesis**

Disease	Antigen Involved	Clinicopathologic Manifestations
Systemic lupus erythematosus	DNA, nucleoproteins, others	Glomerulonephritis, arthritis, vasculitis
Blue eye	Canine adenovirus 1 antigen	Anterior uveitis
Equine infectious anemia	Viral antigens	Anemia, thrombocytopenia
Poststaphylococcal hypersensitivity	Staphylococcal cell wall antigens	Dermatitis
Cutaneous vasculitis	Bacterial antigens, viral antigens, drugs	Vasculitis
Poststreptococcal (*Streptococcus equi* ssp. *equi*) hypersensitivity	M protein	Purpura hemorrhagica, glomerulonephritis
Acute glomerulonephritis	Bacterial antigens; parasite antigens; viral antigens; tumor antigens	Nephritis
Reactive arthritis	Bacterial antigens	Acute arthritis
Arthus reaction	Various foreign proteins	Cutaneous vasculitis
Serum sickness	Various proteins (e.g., foreign serum)	Arthritis, vasculitis, nephritis
Hypersensitivity pneumonitis	Fungal spores, dust	Alveolitis, vasculitis
COPD	Fungal spores, dust	Bronchiolitis
Aleutian mink disease	Viral antigens	Glomerulonephritis, vasculitis
Rheumatoid arthritis	IgG	Erosive polyarthritis

COPD, Chronic obstructive pulmonary disease; *IgG*, Immunoglobulin G.

type III hypersensitivity. Chronic obstructive pulmonary disease (COPD) in horses may be caused in part by a localized type III reaction to spore-forming organisms or dust that results in bronchiolitis (see Chapter 9). In dogs, staphylococcal infections of the skin may develop a type I, III, or IV reaction. In the case of a type III reaction, a neutrophilic dermal vasculitis is often evident (see Chapter 17).

GENERALIZED TYPE III HYPERSENSITIVITY

When antigen is present in the circulation at appropriate concentrations relative to circulating antibody concentrations (as discussed previously), the result is the formation of immune complexes capable of generating a type III hypersensitivity reaction. Serum sickness is the prototypical disease with a type III hypersensitivity pathogenesis. Early examples of this disease were the result of the administration of heterologous serum, which led to the formation of circulating immune complexes that became lodged primarily in blood vessels, glomeruli, and joints. The blood vessel, glomerulus, or joint was not a target of the immune response but rather an "innocent bystander," because the resulting inflammation occurred as a result of the complement activating capacity of the immune complexes that lodged there.

The pathogenesis of a systemic immune complex disease is best illustrated in three phases as depicted in Fig. 5-18. The first phase, as discussed previously, occurs when the host develops an antibody response to an antigen such that the ratio of antigen to antibody is

appropriate for the formation of small, soluble, circulating complexes that are not adequately cleared by the monocyte-macrophage system. Because the formation of antigen-antibody complexes can be a normal component of an immune response, the presence of immune complexes in circulation by itself is not sufficient to diagnose an immune complex disease. In the second phase, the complexes adhere to cells or lodge in tissues that are uniquely susceptible to circulating immune complexes. The biochemical properties of the antigen-antibody complexes (overall quantity and size, charge, etc.), and the physiologic and anatomic characteristics of some cells and tissues account for their unique susceptibility to immune complex deposition. Other factors may also contribute to the formation or deposition of immune complexes in certain tissues. As an example, in rheumatoid arthritis it has been proposed that lymphocytes within the joint may produce an altered IgG molecule that stimulates the production of rheumatoid factor (anti-IgG). Complexes become lodged within blood vessel walls and extravascular tissues as a result of the increased vascular permeability caused by the anaphylatoxins and vasoactive amines released from neutrophils, activated through the binding of antigen-antibody complexes to complement and Fc receptors on their surface. The result is phase three: the activation of the complement system and the development of an acute inflammatory reaction centered on the vasculature. Neutrophils and macrophages are activated similarly through Fc receptors and produce a number of inflammatory cytokines that attract and

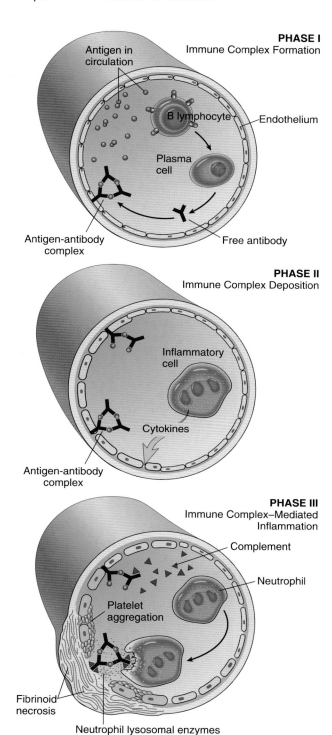

PHASE I
Immune Complex Formation

Antigen in circulation

B lymphocyte

Endothelium

Plasma cell

Antigen-antibody complex

Free antibody

PHASE II
Immune Complex Deposition

Inflammatory cell

Cytokines

Antigen-antibody complex

PHASE III
Immune Complex–Mediated Inflammation

Complement

Neutrophil

Platelet aggregation

Fibrinoid necrosis

Neutrophil lysosomal enzymes

Fig. 5-18   Schematic depiction of the three phases of a systemic type III hypersensitivity reaction. The first phase results in immune complex formation. In the second phase, the antigen-antibody complexes become lodged in the vessel wall and activate inflammatory cells. The end result, the third phase, is the elicitation of tissue damage and an inflammatory response.

(From Kumar V, Abbas AK, Fausto N: Robbins & Cotran pathologic basis of disease, ed 7, Philadelphia, 2005, Saunders.)

activate additional inflammatory cells. The inflammatory cells and mediators have been thoroughly discussed in Chapter 3. Immune complexes that lodge in blood vessels, glomeruli, or joints result in vasculitis, glomerulonephritis, and arthritis, respectively. The damage to the vessels also results in damage to the intima and exposure of collagen, which initiates the formation of microthrombi by the activation of the coagulation cascade and platelets.

The two primary cell types involved in a type III hypersensitivity reaction are Fc receptor–bearing neutrophils and macrophages (Fig. 5-19). Complement activation leads to the elaboration of factors (primarily C5a) that are chemotactic and attract neutrophils and macrophages to the site. These cells are activated and produce a number of proinflammatory cytokines. Early in the response, these cells release vasoactive amines that cause increased vascular permeability, allowing the immune complexes to lodge within the vessel wall. Many of these phagocytic cells are also stimulated to release their proteolytic enzymes and toxic free radicals, and these processes result in tissue and vascular damage. Platelets also contribute to the developing inflammatory reaction by releasing vasoactive amines and other proinflammatory constituents.

Diseases associated with type III hypersensitivity reactions are most commonly associated with a single exposure to a large quantity of antigen (e.g., administration of heterologous serum or from an immune response to systemic infections) or from continuous exposures to small quantities of antigen as in the case of autoimmune diseases (e.g., rheumatoid arthritis and systemic lupus erythematous). In either of these instances, the development of type III hypersensitivity is dependent on antigen being in excess of antibody.

TYPE IV HYPERSENSITIVITY (DELAYED-TYPE HYPERSENSITIVITY)

Type IV hypersensitivity is also known as cell-mediated hypersensitivity because it is the result of the interaction of T lymphocytes and the specific antigen to which they have been sensitized. The resulting immune response is mediated either by direct cytotoxicity by CD 8+ T lymphocytes or by the release of soluble cytokines from CD 4+ lymphocytes, which act through mediator cells (primarily macrophages) to produce chronic inflammatory reactions (Fig. 5-20). Because these responses are dependent on sensitized T lymphocytes and require 24 to 48 hours to develop, they are also referred to as delayed-type hypersensitivity (DTH). Unlike type I, II, and III hypersensitivity reactions, type IV hypersensitivity is not dependent on an antibody. We will first discuss the response mediated primarily by activated CD4+ lymphocytes. The prototypical DTH

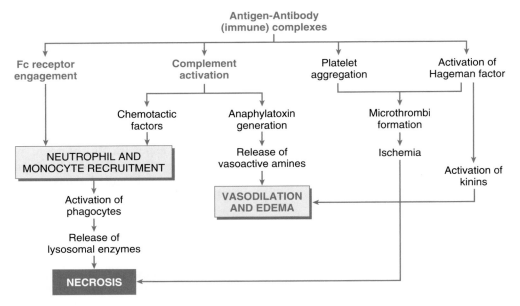

Fig. 5-19 **Pathogenesis of type III hypersensitivity reactions and the morphologic consequences.** Locally or systemically deposited immune complexes result in tissue damage and inflammation by activation of the complement system and through activation of neutrophils and macrophages through their Fc receptors. Activation of a component of the coagulation system also contributes to the tissue damage. *(From Kumar V, Abbas AK, Fausto N: Robbins & Cotran pathologic basis of disease, ed 7, Philadelphia, 2005, Saunders.)*

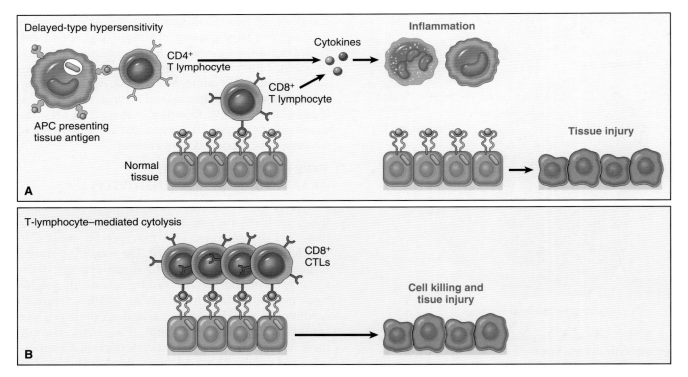

Fig. 5-20 **The two primary mechanisms of T lymphocytes that cause type IV hypersensitivity reaction. A,** CD4+ T lymphocytes (and occasionally CD8+ lymphocytes) are activated by antigen and produce cytokines that attract other cell types and promote an inflammatory response. **B,** CD8+ T lymphocytes (cytotoxic T lymphocytes [CTLs]) are also activated by antigen and can cause inflammation by killing targeted cells and tissue. *APC,* Antigen-presenting cell. (**A** *and* **B,** *From Kumar V, Abbas AK, Fausto N: Robbins & Cotran pathologic basis of disease, ed 7, Philadelphia, 2005, Saunders.)*

reaction is the localized tuberculin response. Following an intradermal exposure of tuberculin, a purified protein derivative (PPD) of the tubercle bacillus, a previously sensitized host will develop a localized type IV reaction at the site of inoculation at 24 to 72 hours. The intradermal antigens are taken up and processed by dendritic Langerhans' cells, which present antigenic peptides to antigen-specific CD4+ lymphocytes that are activated to produce and secrete cytokines that attract and activate other inflammatory cells. Grossly the site appears as a swollen, firm nodule. Microscopically the nodule is composed of interstitial edema and a mononuclear infiltrate that is primarily centered around blood vessels. Early (<12 hours), the infiltrate is primarily neutrophilic, which is replaced largely by macrophages and lymphocyte (>12 hours). The DTH response is generally minimal and short lived, as the concentration of PPD injected is small and rapidly degraded. A similar DTH reaction can be used to test for previous exposures to a number of intracellular organisms.

In addition to the tuberculin response, type IV hypersensitivity is the underlying pathogenesis for allergic contact hypersensitivity and granulomatous inflammatory responses. As mentioned with the other hypersensitivity reactions, the components of a type IV hypersensitivity reaction can be considered beneficial (protective immunity) when they occur as an appropriate response to intracellular organisms, or they can be considered harmful (hypersensitivity), for example, when they occur as an inappropriate response to exogenous chemicals or substances that are complexed with proteins, as in the case of allergic contact hypersensitivity. Type IV hypersensitivity, also known as delayed-type hypersensitivity or cell-mediated hypersensitivity, occurs when sensitized T lymphocytes encounter antigens and are activated to produce cytokines that induce a cell-mediated immune response, which develops over a 24- to 72-hour period. The classic type IV reaction is the tuberculin response.

In the tuberculin reaction, the quantity of antigen limits the extent of the inflammatory response, and resolution of the inflammation generally occurs in 5 to 7 days. This is in contrast to chronic infections with persistent intracellular organisms or poorly degradable intracellular antigens (Table 5-10) that develop into a specific type of chronic inflammatory response called granulomatous inflammation. DTH reactions frequently occur in response to intracellular organisms and cause extensive tissue damage. These diseases are characterized by granulomatous inflammation. In this type of response, the host is unable to destroy or eliminate the organism, resulting in antigen persistence. Compared with the tuberculin reaction, the type of inflammatory infiltrate is different. As discussed in Chapter 4, granulomatous inflammation designates that the inflammatory infiltrate has specific attributes, notably the presence of morphologically transformed macrophages into epithelial-like cells commonly called epithelioid macrophages (Figs. 5-21 and 5-22). Concurrently, there may be many multinucleated giant cells that represent fused macrophages. A number of fusion-related monocyte-macrophage surface proteins have been identified and include receptors for mannose and β_1 integrin, SHPS-1, and the chemoattractant chemokine ligand 2. Lymphocytes can also represent a significant component of the inflammatory infiltrate. Generally, CD4+ lymphocytes are interspersed with the macrophages, and CD8+ lymphocytes are localized to the periphery. As these lesions progress, they may become organized into nodules commonly called granulomas (Fig. 5-22). Depending on the inciting antigen, there may also be varying proportions of necrosis (often as a necrotic center), calcification of the necrotic tissue, and peripheral fibrous encapsulation. These features are largely the result of lytic enzymes released from activated macrophages. Nonimmunologic granulomas can occur in cases of foreign-body type granulomas, which typically have fewer lymphocytes. In either case, the body is trying to limit the spread or wall off the inciting antigen.

Table **5-10**   **Diseases with a Primary Type IV Hypersensitivity (Delayed-Type Hypersensitivity) Pathogenesis**

Disease	Specificity of Pathogenic T Lymphocytes	Clinicopathologic Manifestations
Tuberculosis	*Mycobacteria* spp. antigens	Granuloma formation
Allergic contact dermatitis	Haptens	Perivascular dermatitis
Rheumatoid arthritis	Unknown antigen in joint synovium (type II collagen?); role of antibodies and type III hypersensitivity?	Chronic arthritis with inflammation, destruction of articular cartilage and bone
Johne's disease	*Mycobacterium paratuberculosis* antigens	Granulomatous enteritis
Allograft rejection	MHC molecules	Inflammation of graft tissue
Equine recurrent uveitis	Unknown	Uveitis

MHC, Major histocompatibility complex.

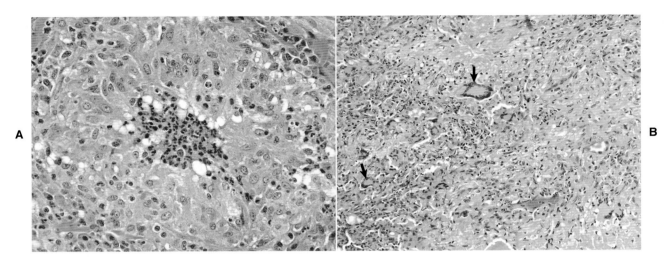

Fig. 5-21   Granulomatous inflammation associated with chronic infections.
A, Blastomycosis, skin, dog. Note the partially encapsulated nodule composed of sheets of epithelioid macrophages and the central area of neutrophils. H&E stain. **B,** Mycobacteriosis, lung, gazelle. Numerous epithelioid macrophages and multinucleated giant cells *(arrows)* constitute the granulomatous tissue that has replaced normal lung parenchyma. H&E stain.
(**A** and **B,** Courtesy Dr. P.W. Snyder, School of Veterinary Medicine, Purdue University.)

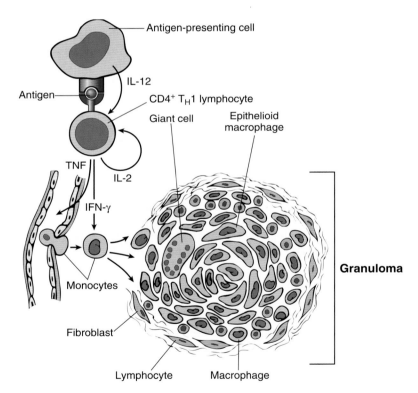

Fig. 5-22   Schematic depiction of granuloma formation in a type IV hypersensitivity reaction. A T_H1 lymphocyte synthesizes cytokines in response to interleukin *(IL)*-12 production and antigen presentation by an antigen-presenting cell. The cytokines activate additional T_H1 lymphocytes *(IL-2)* and monocyte-macrophage cells (interferon-γ *[IFN-γ]*), and promote localized and systemic inflammatory responses (tumor necrosis factor *[TNF]*-α). As the response develops, macrophages fuse to form multinucleated giant cells, and fibroblasts are stimulated to synthesize collagen, resulting in the formation of a granuloma. *(From Kumar V, Abbas AK, Fausto N: Robbins & Cotran pathologic basis of disease, ed 7, Philadelphia, 2005, Saunders.)*

The type IV hypersensitivity reaction is immunologically specific and like all the hypersensitivity reactions involves a sensitization phase and an effector phase. The sensitization phase occurs with the initial exposure to the antigen and results in the development of antigen-specific memory T lymphocytes. These CD4+ lymphocytes recognize peptides presented in the context of class II molecules on the surface of antigen-presenting cells. In this context, the naïve CD4+ T lymphocytes develop into functional T_H1 lymphocytes. These activated T_H1 lymphocytes are sometimes designated as T_{DTH} lymphocytes. Once the host is sensitized, a prolonged exposure or repeat exposure to the antigen results in the development of an effector phase. The effector phase can occur as a cytotoxic response mediated by CD8+ lymphocytes or more commonly as a T_H1 response through the elaboration of cytokines by CD4+ lymphocytes (Fig. 5-22). T_H1 cytokines (most importantly, IL-2, IL-3, IFN-γ and TNF-β) and chemokines (IL-8, macrophage chemotactic and activating factor, and macrophage-inhibition factor) enhance the function of cytokine-producing T lymphocytes (autocrine and paracrine fashion) and attract and activate macrophages. IL-2 induces the proliferation and long-term survival of T lymphocytes. IL-3 supports the growth and differentiation of T_H1 lymphocytes and NK cells. IFN-γ, the key mediator of type IV hypersensitivity, activates macrophages not only to enhance their phagocytic and killing mechanisms but also to enhance their ability to present antigen by inducing increased expression of class II MHC molecules. Activated macrophages and dendritic cells produce IL-12, which also facilitates the development of T_H1 lymphocytes. Activated macrophages also produce IL-1 and TNF-α, both of which act locally to increase the expression of adhesion molecules on endothelial cells, which further facilitates the extravasation of additional inflammatory cells. The production of cytokines and chemokines by the CD4+ T_H1 lymphocytes influences macrophage function and mediates the production of cytokines that influence CD4+ lymphocytes, resulting in a response that potentially goes from a beneficial protective response (immunity) to a harmful response that results in tissue damage (hypersensitivity).

The beneficial protective response of T lymphocyte–mediated hypersensitivity is not limited to intracellular organisms. It also can be a primary component of transplant rejection and immunity to cancer. There are other harmful T lymphocyte–mediated responses that result in disease. One example is allergic contact hypersensitivity. In allergic contact hypersensitivity, the antigen is often too small to elicit an immune response by itself. These antigens must be complexed with other, larger proteins to become antigenic and are specifically referred to as haptens or generally called contact antigens (Box 5-1). Allergic contact hypersensitivity is also dependent on processing and presentation

of the antigen by dendritic Langerhans' cells to CD4+ lymphocytes in regional lymph nodes. In the case of allergic contact dermatitis, the keratinocyte may also participate by producing a number of cytokines that activate Langerhans' cells, mast cells, and other inflammatory cells. In the sensitization phase, the protein-hapten complex is taken up and processed by Langerhans' cells that migrate to regional lymph nodes.

Box 5-1

Pathogens and Contact Antigens Commonly Associated with Type IV Hypersensitivity Reactions in Domestic Animals

SOURCES OF ANTIGEN

Infectious Agents

Bacteria

Mycobacterium tuberculosis
Mycobacterium bovis
Mycobacterium avium ssp. *paratuberculosis*
Mycobacterium avium spp.
Listeria
Yersinia

Viruses

Lymphocytic choriomeningitis virus

Fungi

Blastomyces dermatitidis
Histoplasma capsulatum
Cryptococcus neoformans

Protozoa

Toxoplasma gondii
Leishmania

Contact Antigens (haptens)

Components of insecticides in:

Flea collars
Sprays
Dips

Chemical Components of Plastics, Leather, Metals, and Dyes
Components of shampoos
Topically applied drugs
Pollens
House Plants

Allograft Tissues and Cells
MHC molecules

Neoplastic Cells
Tumor-associated antigens
Tumor-specific antigens

MHC, Major histocompatibility complex.

In the paracortex region of the lymph node (T-lymphocyte area), they present antigenic components to CD4+ lymphocytes. The host develops a population of memory cells and is now sensitized to the antigen. In a sensitized host, continuous exposure to the antigen, or more commonly repeat exposure to the antigen, results in an effector phase response seen as epidermal vesicle formation with dermal and epidermal infiltrates of mononuclear inflammatory cells. The result is tissue damage that is disproportionate to any beneficial effects of the immune response.

Finally, as mentioned earlier, another form of DTH can occur that is mediated by direct cytotoxicity by CD 8+ T lymphocytes. This response is most commonly associated with viral infections. CD 8+ T lymphocytes, bearing viral antigen-specific TCRs, kill antigen-expressing target cells. These cells are commonly referred to as cytotoxic T lymphocytes (CTLs). The expression of viral proteins on the surface of an infected cell in association of class I MHC molecules serves as the recognition signal for the TCR-CD3 membrane complex. Following recognition of antigen by the CTL, there is up-regulation of adhesion molecules on the CTL and the target cell, resulting in a CTL-target cell conjugate. This stimulates an activating signal pathway that results in death of the target cell by apoptosis. The two principal mechanisms of CTL-mediated apoptosis are: (1) the directional delivery of cytotoxic proteins, and (2) the interaction of membrane-bound Fas ligand on the CTL, with the Fas receptor on the target cell. Both are dependent on the activation of caspases. Perforins and granzymes are preformed cytotoxic proteins contained in the cytoplasmic granules of CTLs. Perforin, released between the conjugated CTL and the target cell, is polymerized in the presence of Ca^{2+} and forms pores in the plasma membrane of the target cell, not only causing lysis but also permitting the delivery of granzymes. Granzymes activate caspases, normally present in an inactive proenzyme form, that ultimately result in apoptotic death of the cell. The cross-linking of Fas by its ligand, membrane-bound Fas ligand, results in the activation of the extrinsic (death-receptor–initiated) pathway of apoptosis covered in greater detail in Chapter 1.

CYTOKINE-RELATED DISEASES

A number of diseases are characterized by severe disruptions, either overproduction or underproduction, of cytokines or cytokine receptors. One of the most profound examples is the excessive elaboration of cytokines during bacterial septicemia and shock. The basic pathogenesis involves an infection with a gram-negative, endotoxin producing bacterium that stimulates macrophages to overproduce IL-1 and TNF-α. High concentrations of these two cytokines in circulation cause septic shock (see Chapter 2). A number of microbial

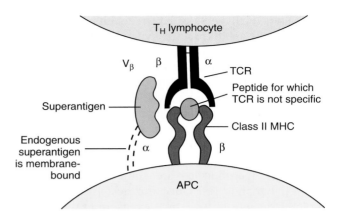

Fig. 5-23 **Superantigens.** Schematic depiction of superantigens that bind to the V_β domain of the T-lymphocyte receptor *(TCR)* and the α-chain of a class II major histocompatibility complex *(MHC)* molecule and activate large numbers of T lymphocytes irrespective of their antigen specificity. *APC,* Antigen-presenting cell. *(Adapted from Goldsby RA, Kindt TJ, Osborne BA: Kuby immunology, ed 4, New York, 2000, WH Freeman.)*

pathogens also produce toxins or other antigenic molecules that are referred to as superantigens. Superantigens bind to class I MHC molecules and V_β domains of the T-lymphocyte antigen receptor (TCR). This binding is outside the normal antigen binding site and activates all T lymphocytes expressing the same V_β domains, irrespective of their antigen specificity (Fig. 5-23). The result is the activation of numerous T lymphocytes (between 5% and 20% versus a normal response of <0.01%) and the elaboration of cytokines. Superantigens are subclassified as exogenous or endogenous. Exogenous superanti-gens are produced by bacteria and include some enterotoxins, exfoliating toxin, and toxic shock syndrome toxin (TSST1). Endogenous superantigens are specific cell-membrane molecules produced during viral infections of cells. The best characterized is minor lymphocyte stimulating (Mls) determinants associated with mouse mammary tumor virus infections. Similar to bacterial septic shock, increased serum concentrations of IL-1 and TNF-α, cause systemic responses like fever, disseminated intravascular coagulation (DIC), and shock.

TRANSPLANT REJECTION

Immunologic responses are responsible for transplant rejection, and some of the basic features of those responses are discussed here. Although the frequency and success of transplantation of tissues in humans is increasing, the frequency and success in domestic species remains very low. Most of the literature on domestic species is related to the development and characterization of animal models rather than as a form of medical treatment. The most common tissue transplants in veterinary medicine are kidney grafts in dogs and cats with end-stage renal disease. The most common graft is an allograft, defined as a graft between two individuals of the same species. Graft rejection largely occurs as a result of the recipient recognizing the grafted tissue as foreign. The antigens responsible are the MHC molecules and blood group antigens of the graft. As discussed previously, MHC molecules are widely distributed and function as specialized molecules involved in intercellular recognition and the differentiation of self and nonself. Blood group antigens in domestic species are far more complex than those in humans. Transplant rejection is a complex process that involves both cell-mediated immunity and humoral immunity.

As we have discussed throughout this chapter, the cell-mediated immune response is primarily composed of two mechanisms that are mediated by T lymphocytes. Both mechanisms are involved in graft rejection (Fig. 5-24). The first mechanism, referred to as the direct pathway of graft rejection, is mediated by CD8+ cytotoxic T lymphocytes (CTLs). In this instance

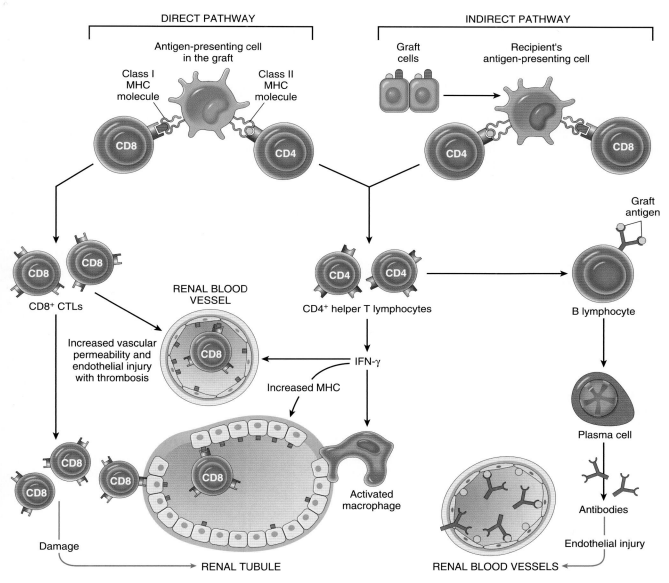

Fig. 5-24   Schematic depiction of the two primary pathways of graft rejection. The direct pathway is mediated by antigen-presenting cells within the graft recognizing major histocompatibility complex (MHC) molecules of the recipient and are recognized by CD4+ and CD8+ T lymphocytes. The indirect pathway is mediated by graft antigens presented by antigen-presenting cells of the recipient that activate CD4+ and CD8+ T lymphocytes, resulting in a type IV hypersensitivity reaction, CTLs, Cytotoxic T lymphocytes; IFN-γ, interferon-γ. (From Kumar V, Abbas AK, Fausto N: Robbins & Cotran pathologic basis of disease, ed 7, Philadelphia, 2005, Saunders.)

the recipient's CTLs recognize allogenic MHC molecules expressed by antigen-presenting cells within the graft (donor origin). The molecular basis for the recognition signals are complex and poorly understood. The second mechanism, referred to as the indirect pathway of graft rejection, is mediated by the recipient's T lymphocytes that recognize antigens of the graft presented by the antigen-presenting cells of the recipient. In this mechanism the uptake of antigen (recipient MHC molecules), processing, and presentation to CD4[+] cells is identical as for any other foreign peptide, as we have discussed previously. However, in this instance the CTLs generated cannot directly kill graft cells because they are only recognizing graft antigens presented by the recipient's antigen-presenting cells. The indirect pathway is dependent on the activation of CD4[+] lymphocytes and the elaboration of cytokines and development of a DTH reaction. These activated CD4[+] cells also function to facilitate the development of an antibody (humoral) response against alloantigens in the graft. Generally graft rejection reactions are classified based on the pathologic findings within the rejected tissue as hyperacute, acute, and chronic. The human classification scheme for grading rejected renal transplants has been applied to feline renal transplant rejection reactions and was found to be less reliable in accurately characterizing the severity of the rejection reaction.

AUTOIMMUNE DISEASE

Autoimmunity is by definition a specific immune response to self-antigens. Autoimmunity reflects a loss of immunologic tolerance to self-tissue or cellular antigens and is characterized by abnormal or excessive activity of self-reactive immune effector cells. Autoimmunity can be organ specific, localized, or systemic. Autoimmunity can be mediated by both autoantibodies and by self-reactive T lymphocytes. The etiology of most autoimmune diseases remains elusive, as they are often multifactorial and have a genetic and an environmental component. Criteria for diagnosing an autoimmune disease may include: (1) direct proof such as the fact that the disease can be transferred through cells or autoantibodies; (2) indirect proof as in identifying the antigen, then isolating the homologous antigen in an animal model, and reproducing the disease through administration of the antigen; (3) isolating self-reactive antibodies or T lymphocytes; and (4) circumstantial evidence such as familial occurrence, lymphocyte infiltrate, MHC associations, and clinical improvement with immunosuppressive therapy. The complexity of autoimmune diseases is also supported by the fact that nonpathologic autoreactive T lymphocytes and antibodies can be found in normal individuals. Most autoimmune

diseases have a tendency to be characterized by cyclical periods of alternating clinical disease and convalescence, an increased susceptibility of the female sex, and a predisposition to multiple autoimmune phenomena as in the case of the mixed connective tissue disorders.

How does a loss of self-tolerance occur? In order to understand the mechanisms related to a loss of self-tolerance, one must first understand the basic concepts of maintaining immunologic tolerance to self-antigens.

IMMUNOLOGIC TOLERANCE

When exposed to an antigen, the immune system can be responsive and develop an immune response or it can be nonresponsive and develop a state of tolerance. In either case, responsive or nonresponsive, the reaction is immunologically specific and has to be carefully regulated, as a response to a self-antigen or a nonresponse to a pathogen could be equally detrimental. Immunologic tolerance is an active physiologic process and is not simply the lack of an immune response. Immunologic tolerance is defined as a failure of the immune system to respond to a specific antigen after previous exposure to that antigen. It is an absence of a functional response rather than a lack of any response at all. The development of autoimmunity can be simply described as an escape from the mechanism by which self-tolerance is maintained.

Tolerance is maintained by a number of mechanisms including deletion, anergy, and suppression. Deletion, also referred to as self-tolerance, is the process of clonally eliminating self-reactive lymphocytes. For T lymphocytes, self-tolerance occurs as a developmental process of immature lymphocytes in the thymus, termed central tolerance, and as a component of mature effector cells upon exposure to antigens in the peripheral tissues, known as peripheral tolerance (Fig. 5-25). Although immature B lymphocytes undergo selection processes in the bone marrow, independent of antigen, these are not referred to as central tolerance. Not all self-reactive B and T lymphocytes are deleted during their development. However, there are mechanisms of anergy and suppression that prevent the activation of self-reactive T or B lymphocytes outside the thymus and bone marrow.

CENTRAL TOLERANCE

Central tolerance occurs during T lymphocyte development in the thymus, where self-reactive T lymphocytes are clonally eliminated. Central tolerance has been most extensively studied in the thymus (Fig. 5-25), where developing T lymphocytes undergo two selection processes that are essential for their development into mature effector cells and are based on the ability of developing lymphocytes to recognize self-peptides in association with MHC molecules. Positive selection is

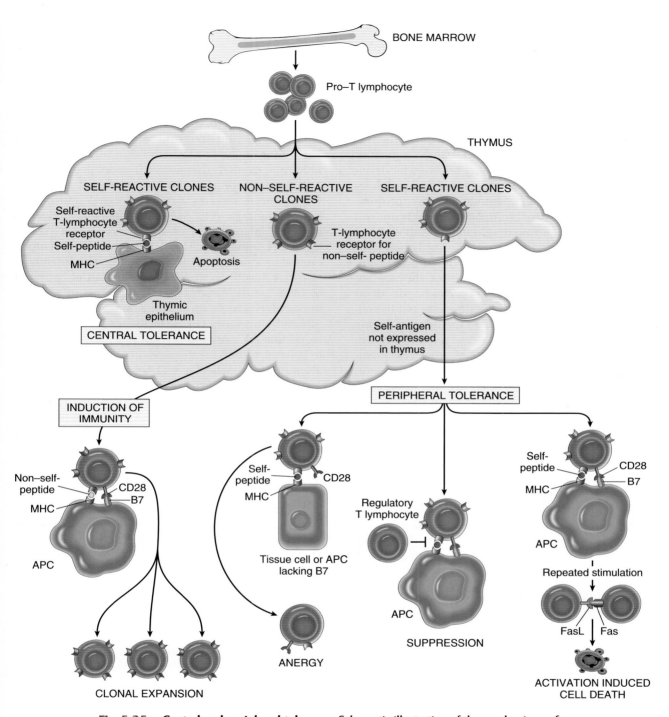

Fig. 5-25 **Central and peripheral tolerance.** Schematic illustration of the mechanisms of central and peripheral tolerance of T lymphocytes. *APC,* Antigen-presenting cell, *FasL,* Fas ligand; *MHC,* major histocompatibility complex. *(From Kumar V, Abbas AK, Fausto N:* Robbins & Cotran pathologic basis of disease, *ed 7, Philadelphia, 2005, Saunders.)*

the clonal expansion of those cells capable of self-MHC restriction. Negative selection is the clonal deletion of those cells expressing TCRs capable of recognizing self-antigens in association with MHC molecules. Developing T and B lymphocytes expressing high avidity

receptors for self-antigens are deleted from further development, resulting in a peripheral effector cell population lacking self-reactive cells. Self-reactive lymphocytes are eliminated by an apoptotic mechanism. For T lymphocytes, it is the interaction of an immature lymphocyte and an antigen-presenting cell that triggers the process of clonal deletion of self-reactive T lymphocytes. This process of clonal deletion involves an apoptotic pathway mediated by the Fas-Fas ligand. The exact molecular signals that trigger this apoptotic pathway remain elusive. The expression of peripheral antigens in the thymus is thought to be partially mediated by a protein called AIRE (autoimmune regulator), which is thought to be essential for the deletion of immature self-reactive T lymphocytes. Negative selection for developing B lymphocytes also occurs through a clonal deletion process involving an apoptotic pathway for those cells that have "excessive" stimulation of their antigen receptor molecules during development. Although the mechanisms regulating tolerance during lymphocyte development are very effective at identifying and eliminating self-reactive T and B lymphocytes, they are not perfect, as self-reactive lymphocytes can be identified in normal individuals. Lastly, the development of central tolerance requires exposure to the antigen during lymphocyte development, and many self-antigens are not present in the thymus or bone marrow. These self-antigens are commonly referred to as sequestered antigens because they are not seen by the developing lymphocytes. Some of the tissue antigens that fall into this class of antigens include: myelin basic protein, lens proteins, and sperm, to mention a few. These antigens can be released as a result of infection or trauma and result in an immunologic response by self-reactive lymphocytes against myelin, lens, and sperm, respectively.

Because the development of self-reactive lymphocytes may escape the mechanisms of central tolerance, the immune system has developed peripheral tolerance mechanisms to prevent these cells from becoming activated and developing into effector cells capable of causing autoimmunity.

PERIPHERAL TOLERANCE

In peripheral tolerance, self-reactive T lymphocytes that are not eliminated as a result of negative selection processes in the thymus have the potential to cause tissue injury when they exit the thymus and enter the peripheral tissues. Within the peripheral tissues there are mechanisms to prevent the activation of these self-reactive lymphocytes, and these occur as a consequence of the normal immune response to antigen and involve the same signals required for activation of lymphocytes during an immune response. Regulation of cellular activation occurs primarily by three mechanisms, which are briefly discussed next.

Anergy

Anergy is the functional inactivation of lymphocytes that encounter antigen. As previously discussed, two signals are required for the activation of naïve T lymphocytes by antigen-presenting cells. The first is generated by interaction of peptide antigen in association with MHC molecules on the surface of antigen-presenting cells within the TCR-CD3 complex, and the second is generated by the presence of co-stimulatory molecules. Co-stimulatory molecules are essential for the activation of naïve T lymphocytes and involve the interaction between T lymphocyte molecules (CD28) and their ligands (B7-1 and B7-2) on antigen-presenting cells. The interaction of CD28 with B7 results in T-cell activation and its survival. However, if an antigen-presenting cell does not provide the co-stimulatory signal, the T lymphocyte receives a negative signal, and the cell becomes anergic (Fig. 5-25). Another mechanism for inducing anergy involves the delivery of a specific inhibitory signal by CTLA-4 molecules on T lymphocytes that also bind to B7 molecules. The interaction of CTLA-4 with B7 results in inhibition of activation by blocking IL-2 production. The process of anergy is irreversible. The limited expression of co-stimulatory molecules by normal tissue facilitates the maintenance of peripheral tolerance to self-reactive lymphocytes. In general, CD 28 is expressed on resting and activated T lymphocytes, whereas CTLA-4 is only expressed on activated T lymphocytes. What drives a T lymphocyte, expressing CD 28 molecules, to recognize B7 molecules that lead to activation or to express CTLA-4 molecules that recognize the same B7 molecules that leads to anergy is unknown. Anergy of B lymphocytes occurs largely through the absence of specific T-helper cell activation, although negative selection of mature self-reactive B lymphocytes is known to occur. An inability of B lymphocytes to receive appropriate signals from T-helper lymphocytes, subsequent to antigen exposure, results in their deletion from lymphoid tissues.

Suppression by regulatory T lymphocytes

This mechanism of peripheral tolerance occurs through the activation of regulatory cells that prevent immune reactions to self-antigens. Suppression can occur as a result of cross-regulation of CD4$^+$ T$_H$1 cells by a specific population of CD4$^+$ T$_H$2 cells. Specifically, CD25$^+$ and CD4$^+$ T$_H$2 cells producing IL-4, IL-10, and TGF-β down- regulate T$_H$1 responses, effectively inhibiting lymphocyte activation and its effector function.

Clonal deletion by activation-induced cell death

As discussed previously, one of the possible outcomes following lymphocyte activation as a result of antigen recognition during an immune response is lymphocyte proliferation. A second possible out come following antigen exposure is cell death. For CD4$^+$ T lymphocytes, both outcomes—proliferation and death—are largely regulated by the expression of accessory co-stimulatory molecules. Activation-induced cell death (AICD) of T lymphocytes occurs by Fas-Fas ligand signaling following persistent stimulation by antigen-presenting cells expressing antigen. During the normal immune response, AICD functions to down-regulate immune responses and results in the return to immune home-ostasis. Lymphocytes can be induced to express Fas (CD95), a member of the TNF-receptor family. The ligand for Fas, Fas ligand (FasL), is expressed primarily on activated T lymphocytes. The binding of Fas to FasL results in apoptosis of activated T lymphocytes. Antigens that are expressed to a high level in normal tissue would result in persistent stimulation of self-reactive T lymphocytes, thus resulting in deletion through Fas-FasL–mediated apoptosis. In the case of an auto-reactive B lymphocyte exposed to soluble antigen in the periphery, the cell becomes anergic. If the anergic autoreactive B lymphocyte is recognized by a T lym-phocyte specific for the autoantigen, the interaction of the Fas ligand on the T lymphocyte binding to the Fas molecule on the B lymphocyte results in activation-induced cell death of the B lymphocyte. Two strains of mice have been identified with a mutation in either the Fas molecule (lpr mice) or the FasL (gld mice). The lpr and gld strains have severe autoimmune disease develop with a phenotype similar to that of humans with sys-temic lupus erythematosus (SLE).

Antigen sequestration

Antigens that are not expressed in the thymus or are "cryptic" in nature have the potential to induce a self-reactive immune response. Certain physiologic charac-teristics of some tissue (e.g., testis, eye, and brain) are considered to render them as "immunologically privi-leged sites" because of the difficulty in eliciting an immune response to antigens in these tissue. Antigens in these sites cannot be seen by the immune system because they are sequestered. The sequestering of anti-gens may occur through the blood-brain barrier, an absence of lymphatic drainage, or the limited ability to express MHC molecules. A mechanism for the eye is referred to as the anterior chamber–associated immune deviation (ACAID), thought, in part, to be the result of inhibitory cytokines, such as TGF-β, produced by the cells of the iris and ciliary body. However, if the antigens in these tissues are released as the result of trauma or infec-tion, they have the potential to cause a severe immune response as a consequence of activating self-reactive lym-phocytes. Posttraumatic uveitis and orchitis are thought to be the result of the release of sequestered antigens.

MECHANISMS OF AUTOIMMUNITY

Although central tolerance is important in lymphocyte development, it is the mechanisms of peripheral toler-ance that have a greater influence on the development of autoimmunity. We have described the complexities of central and peripheral tolerance, and thus it is understandable that the mechanisms responsible for allowing autoreactive lymphocytes to become activated and develop into self-reactive T lymphocytes or autoan-tibody-producing plasma cells are equally diverse and complex (Fig. 5-26). Although autoantigens have been described for a number of autoimmune diseases, it is the identification of the initiating antigen that remains elusive. The cause of most autoimmune diseases remains unknown, as they often are multifactorial and have genetic and environmental components (Fig. 5-27).

FAILURE OF PERIPHERAL TOLERANCE

Previously we discussed the mechanisms self-tolerance, which will now serve as a basis for present-ing how a failure to maintain those mechanisms can contribute to the pathogenesis of autoimmunity.

GENETIC FACTORS IN AUTOIMMUNITY

The majority of autoimmune diseases in humans have a strong genetic predisposition. The most well-studied genetic component centers around the MHC molecules. As previously discussed, MHC molecules are important in the development of lymphocytes and in the regulation of peripheral effector lymphocytes. Just as autoreactive lymphocytes have been identified in normal individuals without autoimmune disease, the presence of certain MHC molecules themselves is not sufficient to result in autoimmune disease. These observations would suggest that the expression of an autoimmune phenotype is not likely to be the result of a single-gene defect. Other genes that regulate proteins involved in other aspects of the immune response, or that are involved in the inflammatory or healing response, may also be involved. Additionally, experi-mental variations in the expression and activity of tran-scription factors can influence the expression of certain autoimmune diseases.

Several strains of mice with specific genetic muta-tions of factors involved in the maintenance of central and peripheral tolerance that results in autoimmune disease have been identified. Mice with defects of Fas or FasL have disruption of the activation-induced cell death signal in lymphocytes, resulting in autoimmune disease. Mice lacking the transcriptional factor AIRE, which is responsible for thymic expression of self-antigens, and mice defective in the expression of CTLA-4, the inhibitory receptor involved in T-lymphocyte anergy, also develop autoimmunity. An important regulatory cytokine—IL-2, the major growth factor for lymphocytes—is also required for the development and function of regulatory T lymphocytes. Mice lacking either IL-2 or the IL-2 receptor develop autoimmune disease charac-terized by inflammatory bowel disease, anti-DNA antibod-ies, and autoimmune hemolytic anemia. The proposed mechanism of autoimmunity in these mice is thought to involve T lymphocytes and be a result of a failure

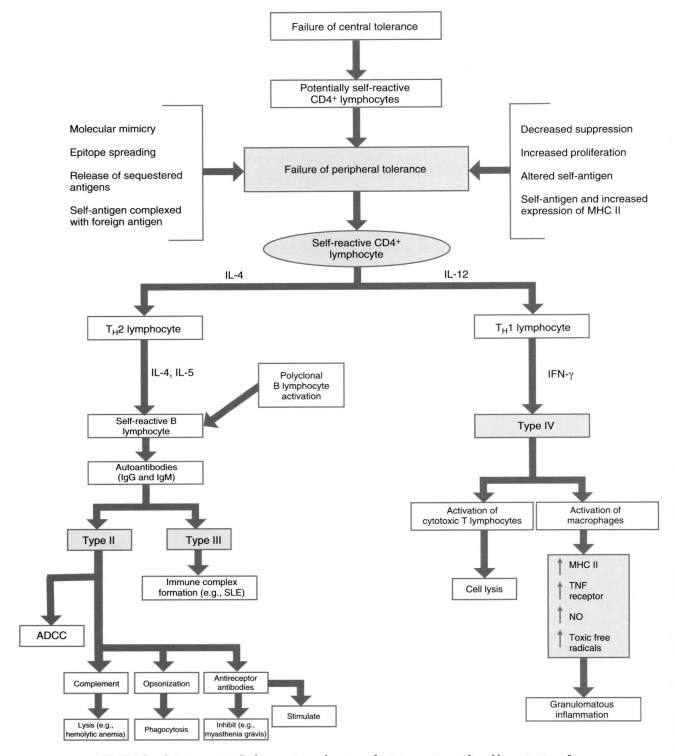

Fig. 5-26 **Autoimmunity.** Pathogenetic mechanisms of autoimmunity mediated by activation of T lymphocytes (CD4+). *ADCC,* Antibody-dependent cellular cytotoxicity; *IFN-γ* interferon-γ; *Ig,* immunoglobulin; *IL,* interleukin; *MHC,* major histocompatibility complex; *NO,* nitric oxide; *SLE,* systemic lupus erythematosus; *TNF,* tumor necrosis factor.

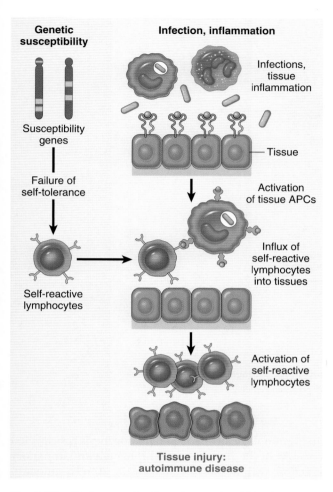

Fig. 5-27   Pathogenesis of autoimmunity. *APCs,* Antigen-presenting cells. *(From Kumar V, Abbas AK, Fausto N: Robbins & Cotran pathologic basis of disease, ed 7, Philadelphia, 2005, Saunders.)*

of suppression by regulatory T lymphocytes and a failure of activation induced cell death, two mechanisms of peripheral tolerance. These mouse models of autoimmune disease have facilitated the identification of pathogenic mechanisms of autoimmunity. Although all of these mechanisms have now been identified in human autoimmune diseases, it is likely only a matter of time before they are identified in other species.

Of the domestic species, there have been a number of autoimmune diseases in dogs documented to have a familial tendency, and the mechanism is in part attributed to certain MHC alleles. These recognized associations of specific autoimmune diseases and MHC molecules have been limited to a few specific breeds. It should also be noted that other diseases of immunity, for example, immunodeficiency and atopy, also have a higher incidence in some breeds.

MICROBIAL AGENTS IN AUTOIMMUNITY

The recognition that certain infections may result in the development of an autoimmune disease is the result of two observations. First, experimentally, one can induce autoimmunity in specific strains of mice by infection with certain strains of virus. Second, many spontaneous autoimmune diseases occur following viral infections, although attempts to isolate and identify viral agents in patients with autoimmune diseases have been equivocal. Again, these observations would suggest that these diseases have a complex pathogenesis with a genetic and an environmental component.

The role of infections as environmental factors in the pathogenesis of autoimmune diseases may be explained by understanding how infectious agents may cause a break down of anergy to self-molecules (loss of self-tolerance). As discussed earlier, not all self-reacting B and T lymphocytes are eliminated during the differentiation and development process. These potentially self-reacting lymphocytes are regulated in the periphery by clonal anergy. Therefore a loss of this regulation could explain how autoimmune diseases develop. Plausible mechanisms of why infectious agents cause aberrations of peripheral clonal anergy are twofold (Fig. 5-28). One mechanism may be the result of nonspecific disruption of the regulatory cells, which results in the induction of co-stimulatory molecules on antigen-presenting cells that are expressing self-molecules. This mechanism is not specific to the antigens of the infectious agent and is likely the result of the overall inflammatory response to the pathogen. Additionally, during an inflammatory response, some cells are induced by the inflammatory cytokine IFN-γ to increase their expression of MHC molecules. This can result in the expression of MHC molecules by cells that normally do not express them. Although the expression of MHC molecules in the absence of co-stimulatory molecules will not activate T lymphocytes, it does increase the potential to do so if co-stimulatory molecules are inappropriately expressed. The second mechanism is specific to the antigens of the infectious agent and is the result of cross-reactivity of T lymphocytes with an infectious agent's antigen and a self-antigen. Many infectious agents express antigens that have similar peptide sequences to those of normal peptides as a part of their immune evasion mechanism. Therefore the potential exists for any immune response to an infectious agent to cross-react with a normal peptide, resulting in an immune response directed against self-cells or self-tissues. This mechanism is called molecular mimicry. The result is the activation of T lymphocytes that recognize the infectious agent peptide–MHC complex. These T lymphocytes can potentially attack self-peptide–MHC complexes that are cross-reactive.

Once an autoimmune disease is initiated, the clinical course is generally progressive and characterized by cyclical periods of exacerbation and remission. As with any immune-mediated disease, antigen persistence is required to maintain the functional immune response. In autoimmune diseases, antigen persistence is thought

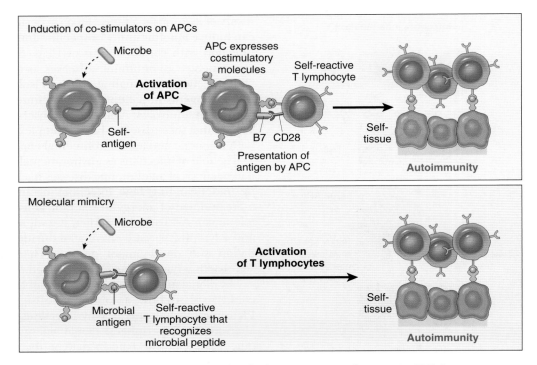

Fig. 5-28   **Autoimmunity and the role of infections in its pathogenesis.** *APC,* Antigen-presenting cell. *(From Kumar V, Abbas AK, Fausto N: Robbins & Cotran pathologic basis of disease, ed 7, Philadelphia, 2005, Saunders.)*

in part to occur through epitope spreading. Epitope spreading is the process by which the immune response spreads from one epitope of an antigenic molecule to another, non–cross-reacting, epitope of the same antigenic molecule, or from one epitope of different peptides that are a part of a large complex. The epitopes involved are frequently ones that the immune response has not developed tolerance against because they are not normally presented by MHC molecules in sufficient concentrations. These so-called cryptic epitopes are normally not expressed at sufficient concentrations or are "hidden" during differentiation and development of lymphocytes. However, during an infection or inflammatory response, there may be tissue or cell damage that results in the release or expression of cryptic or hidden epitopes of self-antigens, and these become targets for the immune response. Because these epitopes were hidden, the immune system has not developed tolerance to them. Epitope spreading is thought to maintain the initiated immune response by means of the continued recruitment of autoreactive T lymphocytes specific for normal "cryptic" self-peptides.

With this basic understanding of self-tolerance, and the possible molecular mechanisms involved in the pathogenesis of autoimmunity, we can present some of the more common autoimmune diseases of domestic species. Autoimmune diseases can be organ specific or systemic. With many of the organ-specific diseases,

an immunologically mediated pathogenesis is suspected because of the finding of a lymphocytic inflammatory reaction within the affected tissue. Rarely, autoantibodies may be identified in the circulation. The organ-specific autoimmune diseases are discussed in the appropriate chapters covering individual organ systems. This chapter will focus on some of the systemic autoimmune diseases of domestic species, beginning with the multisystemic disease systemic lupus erythematosus.

SYSTEMIC LUPUS ERYTHEMATOSUS

SLE is one of the most well-studied systemic autoimmune diseases in humans and is characterized by the production of autoantibodies directed against a wide array of normal tissue and cellular components. The predominant autoantibody, commonly known as antinuclear antibody (ANA), is directed against nuclear antigens. The disease has been described in humans, nonhuman primates, mice, horses, dogs, cats, snakes, and iguanas. As with many autoimmune diseases, SLE has a highly variable and often progressive clinical course characterized by a variety of clinical and immunologic abnormalities. Unlike humans, in whom the disease predominantly affects women, there is no clear sex predilection in domestic species. There are certain breeds of dogs that have a higher incidence. The average age of diagnosis is approximately 5 years. Epidemiologic data on other species is limited.

ETIOLOGY AND PATHOGENESIS

The cause of SLE remains undetermined, although the presence of autoantibodies directed against a number of tissues and cellular components suggests that the underlying immunologic abnormality is a failure to maintain self-tolerance. Antibodies against nuclear and cytoplasmic components, which are neither organ specific or species specific, and those directed against cell surface antigens, particularly red blood cell antigens, are central to the pathogenesis of the disease. Detection of autoantibodies also facilitates the diagnosis and monitoring of human patients with SLE. The autoantibodies and self-antigens form immune complexes, which can be deposited in glomeruli (glomerulonephritis), blood vessels (vasculitis), skin (dermatitis), and joints (arthritis), resulting in the major clinical signs associated with the disease.

Antinuclear antibodies are found in a high percentage of patients with SLE. In humans, antinuclear antibodies are grouped into four categories: (1) antibodies against DNA, (2) antibodies against histones, (3) antibodies to nonhistone proteins bound to RNA, and (4) antibodies against nucleolar antigens. The most common method of measuring antinuclear antibodies is indirect immunofluorescence. The pattern of immunofluorescence is used to help identify the type of autoantibody present. Other methods can be used to more specifically identify the target of ANA. In human beings, the majority of ANAs are directed against nucleic acids in native double-stranded DNA, in contrast to the dog, in which the majority of ANAs are directed against nuclear proteins such as histones and extractable nuclear antigens (ENAs). ANAs are also found in normal patients and in patients with other diseases; however, their frequency is much lower. In the dog, the incidence of ANA in normal dogs and dogs with other canine diseases is 16% and 20%, respectively, compared with 97% to 100% in dogs with SLE. The indirect immunofluorescence test for ANA is sensitive but not specific because of the relatively high incidence in normal dogs and those with non-SLE diseases. Two anti-ENA antibodies appear to be specific for canine SLE. These are the anti-Sm and the anti-T1 antibodies.

Patients with SLE frequently have autoantibodies in an array of tissue and cells. Many patients have rheumatoid factors and thus have a positive Coombs' test for anti-IgG antibodies. Antibodies directed against cellular antigens on red blood cells, platelets, and lymphocytes are frequently noted. In these instances they may lead to clinical signs of hemolytic anemia (anti-RBC antibodies), thrombocytopenia (anti-platelet antibodies), and immune system abnormalities (anti-lymphocyte antibodies). Other autoantibodies to components of muscle (myositis) and skin (dermatitis) are also frequently detected. While there can be an extensive number of autoantibodies identified in patients with SLE, the major clinical signs are attributed to the deposition of immune complexes in the joint, skin, and kidney and the elaboration of a type III hypersensitivity reaction. The tissues most frequently involved are in the joint, skin, and kidney.

Canine lupus primarily affects middle-aged dogs and in some studies has been reported to occur more frequently in males than females. Breeds overrepresented are the Shetland sheepdog, German shepherd, Old English sheepdog, Afghan hound, beagle, Irish setter, and poodle. Affected dogs usually present with a spectrum of clinical signs and the disease has a progressive clinical course. Common clinical findings include fever, nonerosive polyarthritis, glomerulonephritis, mucocutaneous lesions, lymph node and splenic enlargement, and hematologic abnormalities (e.g., anemia, thrombocytopenia, and leukopenia). ANAs are the most common immunologic finding. In some reports, up to 100% of affected animals have been positive for ANAs. Dogs can also have antierythrocyte antibodies (Coombs' positive), anti-IgG antibodies (rheumatoid factor positive), circulating immune complexes and deposits of these in the skin. Only the direct Coombs' test is valid in the dog. In the dog, as in other species, the immunologic abnormalities involve both humoral and cellular immunity. The abnormalities in humoral immunity are largely attributed to the already discussed presence of autoantibodies and are centered on the activation of self-reactive B lymphocytes. The abnormalities in cellular immunity include a lymphopenia that is characterized by a decrease in the percentage and absolute number of CD8+ lymphocytes and a concurrent increase in the percentage and a decrease in the absolute number of CD4+ lymphocytes. This translates into a high CD4+:CD8+ ratio (as high as 6 in dogs with SLE versus <2 in normal dogs).

LESIONS OF SYSTEMIC LUPUS ERYTHEMATOSUS

A wide spectrum of morphologic lesions is associated with canine SLE. The most common finding, polyarthritis, is characterized as a nonerosive lesion that commonly affects the intervertebral, carpal, tarsal, and temporomandibular joints. The acute arthritis is characterized by exudation of neutrophils and fibrin into the synovial membrane and concurrent perivascular cuffing by mononuclear cells. The primary differential diagnosis for the arthritis is rheumatoid arthritis, which is an erosive lesion. The renal lesion, the result of immune complex deposition, involves the glomerulus, blood vessels, and the basement membranes of renal tubules (Fig. 5-29). The resulting glomerulonephritis is variable in appearance and ranges from slight mesangial alterations to diffuse proliferative lesions. The renal lesions have a common pathogenic mechanism that is a result of the deposition of immune complexes and the activation of complement (type III hypersensitivity).

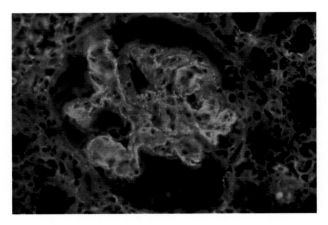

Fig. 5-29 **Immune-complex glomerulonephritis, Aleutian mink disease, kidney, glomerulus, mink.** Intraglomerular immunoglobulin deposits demonstrated by immunofluorescence. Note the granular ("lumpy-bumpy") pattern of fluorescence in this case of Aleutian mink disease. **Immunoflourescence microscopy.** *(Courtesy Dr. S.J. Newman, College of Veterinary Medicine, University of Tennessee.)*

Glomerular lesions are often indicated by a persistent proteinuria (>0.5 g/dL).

Skin lesions are highly variable and nonspecific in canine SLE. The face, ears, and digital extremities are frequently involved and characterized by erythema, ulceration, and exfoliative dermatitis. The distribution of the lesions suggests that photosensitization may play a role. Histologically, the epidermis is characterized by basal cell vacuolation and necrosis, and the dermis is variably edematous with a superficial infiltration of mononuclear inflammatory cells at the dermal-epidermal junction (interface dermatitis). Additionally, there may be a panniculitis, composed primarily of lymphocytes and plasma cells, and vasculitis, with fibrinoid necrosis of the vessel wall. By indirect immunofluorescence, there are deposits of immunoglobulin and complement components at the dermal-epidermal junction. Other dermatologic variants of lupus are covered in Chapter 17. The definitive diagnosis of SLE is based on accepted criteria rather than pathognomonic findings. Using 11 established criteria for the dog, modified from the American Rheumatism Association criteria for humans, a definitive diagnosis requires the presence of four or more criteria. A "probable" diagnosis is based on the presence of three criteria or the presence of polyarthritis with the identification ANAs. Other diagnostic schemes, using "major" and "minor" signs along with a positive ANA or SLE prep test, are also used to make definitive and probable diagnoses.

In the cat, SLE is less well recognized and manifests with fever, glomerulonephritis, dermatitis, and hemolytic anemia. The ANA test in cats is less reliable because many normal cats can have positive tests results. Horses with SLE similarly present with generalized skin disease and may also have glomerulonephritis, arthritis, and hemolytic anemia.

GENETIC FACTORS

SLE in humans is characterized as a disease with a complex genetic component with MHC and multiple non-MHC genes involved. Extensive genetic studies in domestic animals are lacking, yet it is reasonable to suggest that the disease in other species will also be characterized by involvement of multiple genes. The association of SLE with certain MHC alleles in human beings indicates that the MHC genes that regulate the production of specific antibodies are involved—specifically, MHC alleles that are linked to the production of anti–double-stranded DNA, anti-Sm, and antiphospholipid antibodies. Other than the observation of breed predilections for the dog and cat and the report of an association with the canine MHC allele DLA-A7, there are no definitive genetic studies similar to those reported in humans. Interestingly a low percentage of humans with SLE also have inherited deficiencies of complement components, such as C2, C4, or C1q. Because complement components are important in the removal of circulating immune complexes by the monocyte-macrophage system, such a deficiency may contribute to the deposition of circulating complexes into tissue rather than to their removal. There is an increase in lupuslike autoimmunity in mice lacking certain complement components. Finally a well-described animal model of SLE is the NZB × NZW mouse strain, in which a number of genetic loci have been identified as being associated with the development of the disease.

ENVIRONMENTAL FACTORS

In addition to the genetic factors, SLE in humans has also been associated with a number of environmental factors. Specifically, drugs such as hydralazine, procainamide, and D-penicillamine can induce an SLE-like disease. In domestic animals, exposure to specific drugs and viral infections are suspected. Exposure to ultraviolet light is known to exacerbate the disease in the dog. These patients present with dermatologic manifestations localized to areas exposed to sunlight (e.g., face and dorsal regions) or areas lacking adequate hair coat (e.g., axillary region). A similar association has been noted in humans with SLE. The influence of UV radiation may be attributed to tissue damage and inflammation that result in activation of keratinocytes and the elaboration of IL-1, or the modification of DNA through the induction of apoptosis that renders the DNA immunogenic. The influence of sex hormones on the occurrence and manifestations of SLE in humans has not been documented in domestic species.

IMMUNOLOGIC FACTORS

As discussed previously, SLE is characterized by a number of immunologic abnormalities and is clinically noted to have manifestations attributable to specific immune components. It is therefore reasonable to suggest that the pathogenesis of SLE involves aberrations of humoral and/or cell-mediated immunity. Previously, as a result of the documentation of autoantibodies in patients with SLE, it was hypothesized that the pathogenesis centered on an intrinsic B lymphocyte defect. Additionally, polyclonal B lymphocyte activation is a common immunologic abnormality seen in patients with SLE and in animals that are models for the disease. Recent studies, however, indicate that the autoantibodies associated with the development of clinical SLE are not the result of polyclonal B-lymphocyte activation, but rather the result of antigen-specific helper T-lymphocyte–dependent B-lymphocyte responses. This observation is consistent with our overall understanding of autoimmunity, and the current hypothesis is that these diseases are more likely to be the result of an immunologic dysregulation centered on helper T lymphocytes. The currently proposed model for the pathogenesis of SLE is presented in Fig. 5-30. This model is an oversimplification of a complex disease with genetic and nongenetic factors that contribute to the development of a complex multisystemic disease with numerous clinical presentations, a progressive disease course, and an absence of specific cause.

Although the underlying cause of autoantibody production in SLE remains unknown, the elaboration of antibody-peptide complexes are central to the mechanism of tissue damage. The majority of lesions in SLE are the result of immune complex disease (type III hypersensitivity). Antibodies directed against cell surface antigens also lead to the destruction of leukocytes, red blood cells, and platelets through direct cell lysis and enhanced removal by opsonization and phagocytosis. ANAs bind to cell-free nuclei to produce characteristic hematoxylin bodies or lupus erythematosus (LE) bodies. These bodies are frequently found in the skin, kidney, lung, lymph node, spleen, and heart of patients with SLE. These ANAs can also lead to the formation of LE cells, which are typically present in the bone marrow and are a phagocytic cell (macrophage or neutrophil) that has engulfed an opsonized nucleus. This phenomenon is also used as an in vitro diagnostic test to demonstrate the presence of ANA (LE test or LE prep).

In summary, SLE represents the prototypical multiorgan autoimmune disease with a highly variable clinical presentation, a complex cause, and pathogenesis involving multiple genetic and environmental factors and a multitude of immunologic abnormalities. The current pathogenesis suggests that these factors contribute to the activation of T and B lymphocytes, resulting in the production of autoantibodies directed against a number of self-constituents, namely molecules within the nucleus, in the cytoplasm, or on the cell surface.

RHEUMATOID ARTHRITIS

Rheumatoid arthritis is an autoimmune disease characterized by the presence of rheumatoid factors (anti-IgG antibodies) and is recognized in most species. The disease is discussed in Chapter 16.

SJÖGREN-LIKE SYNDROME

Sjögren-like syndrome is a systemic autoimmune disease characterized by keratoconjunctivitis sicca, xerostomia, and lymphoplasmacytic adenitis. In humans, Sjögren syndrome can manifest itself alone or in association with other autoimmune or immune-mediated diseases, such as rheumatoid arthritis, pemphigus, SLE, polymyositis, and immune-mediated thyroiditis. A Sjögren-like syndrome has been described in the dog and cat.

ETIOLOGY AND PATHOGENESIS

The keratoconjunctivitis sicca (dry eyes) and xerostomia (dry mouth) result from the lymphocytic infiltration and fibrosis of lacrimal and salivary glands (lymphoplasmacytic sialoadenitis). In humans the infiltrate is primarily composed of activated CD4+ lymphocytes and fewer B lymphocytes and plasma cells. Affected dogs are frequently hypergammaglobulinemic and less frequently have identifiable ANAs and rheumatoid factors. Many human patients have ANAs, rheumatoid factors, and nonorgan specific autoantibodies.

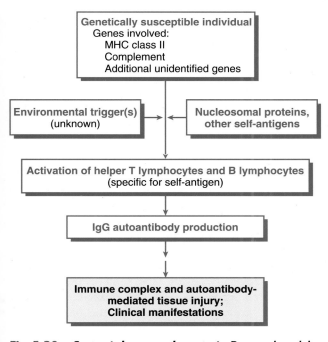

Fig. 5-30   **Systemic lupus ergthematosis.** Proposed model for the pathogenesis of systemic lupus erythematosus. *IgG,* Immunoglobulin G; *MHC,* major histocompatibility complex. *(Modified from Kotzin BL: Cell 65:303-306, 1996.)*

Two autoantibodies specific to Sjögren syndrome in humans are directed against ribonucleoproteins: SS-A (Ro) and SS-B (La), which are considered serologic markers of the disease. Although autoantibodies can be identified, there is no direct evidence that they are the primary cause of tissue injury in any species evaluated to date. With the identification of autoantibodies and the presence of T lymphocytes within affected tissues, it is likely that the disease is the result of immunologic dysregulation centered on helper T lymphocytes. Sjögren syndrome in humans also is weakly correlated with certain MHC alleles, suggesting that as in SLE, the presence of certain MHC alleles may predispose the development of the disease.

As with many autoimmune diseases, viruses are suspected as potential causal agents. In most species in which viruses have been implicated, the evidence is largely circumstantial and Koch's postulates have rarely been satisfied. The mechanisms by which infectious agents can induce autoimmunity were discussed earlier.

CLINICAL SIGNS AND LESIONS

Dogs with Sjögren-like syndrome have an adult onset of conjunctivitis and keratitis. Other findings include gingivitis and stomatitis. A case reported in the cat was characterized by dry eyes and enlarged salivary glands. The keratoconjunctivitis frequently leads to blepharospasm and conjunctival hyperemia. The xerostomia leads to dysphagia. Involvement of tissues other than salivary and lacrimal glands, as is reported in about one third of human cases, has not been documented in the dog and cat. Human patients have lymph node involvement that is characterized as a pleomorphic infiltrate with increased mitoses, and are at a fortyfold increased risk for developing lymphoid malignancies. Microscopically the salivary and lacrimal glands are infiltrated predominately by lymphocytes (Fig. 5-31). In the cat, immunohistochemical analysis of lesions in these glands indicated that the predominant cell type was positive for CD79 (B lymphocyte marker) with fewer, scattered CD3+ cells (T-lymphocyte marker) and plasma cells. A mild interstitial fibrosis was also noted.

INFLAMMATORY MYOPATHIES

Inflammatory myopathies in domestic species comprise an uncommon, heterogeneous group of disorders that are characterized by skeletal muscle damage and inflammation. An immune-mediated pathogen is suspected. Four distinct disorders—masticatory muscle myositis, generalized inflammatory myositis, dermatomyositis, and extraocular myositis—are included in this category. They may occur alone or in association with other immune-mediated or autoimmune diseases.

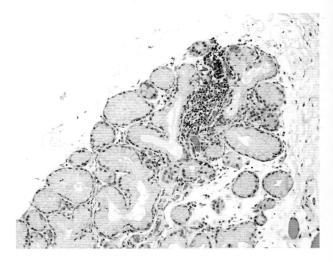

Fig. 5-31   Lymphoplasmacytic sialoadenitis, Sjögren syndrome, salivary gland, cat. Note the accumulation of lymphocytes and macrophages around salivary acini. H&E stain. *(Courtesy Dr. P.W. Snyder, School of Veterinary Medicine, Purdue University.)*

Of these diseases, only dermatomyositis is covered here; the remaining diseases are covered in Chapter 15.

DERMATOMYOSITIS

Dermatomyositis is an inflammatory disease of the skin, muscles, and vasculature affecting primarily young dogs. The cause and pathogenesis are unknown. The disease has a higher incidence in the collie and Shetland sheepdog breeds, and in these breeds, it is often referred to as canine familial dermatomyositis, an inheritable inflammatory disease of the skin and muscle. The disease has also been diagnosed in a number of other breeds. A sex predilection has not been reported. The clinical and pathologic findings suggest that an immune-mediated or an autoimmune mechanism is involved in the pathogenesis.

LESIONS

The dermatologic manifestations of the disease are variable but generally begin at an early age (between 2 and 6 months) and are characterized by alopecia and erythematous dermatitis that involve the face, ears, and bony prominences of the distal extremities. Erosions and ulcers are common early in the disease and scarring and pigmentary changes are seen in chronic cases. Histopathologically, degeneration and necrosis of basal cells of the epidermis and follicular epithelium are characteristic. Frequently, vacuolation of the basal epithelium leads to subepidermal cleft formation. Infiltration of the superficial dermis is often composed of lymphocytes, plasma cells, and macrophages with fewer mast cells and neutrophils. Follicular atrophy and secondary ulceration and fibrosis can also be noted. The skeletal muscle manifestations of the disease are a myositis composed of a variable infiltrate of primarily mononuclear inflammatory cells and occasional neutrophils. There are varying degrees of myofiber degeneration characterized by myofiber fragmentation, vacuolation, and hyalinization. In chronic cases, there may be fibrosis and evidence of myofiber regeneration. The temporal and masseter muscles are commonly involved, although in severe cases there may be generalized muscle involvement. Involvement of the esophageal muscles can lead to the development of megaesophagus.

VASCULITIS

Vasculitis is inflammation of the walls of blood vessels. It is most often seen as a component of an underlying systemic disease process (e.g., infectious or neoplastic) or as an adverse reaction to drug or vaccine administration. In these instances, the pathogenesis involves a type III hypersensitivity reaction with the formation of immune complexes that are either formed in the vessel wall or formed in the circulation and lodge in the vessel wall. The inflammation of the blood vessel is not the result of an immunologic response to components of the blood vessel but rather an "innocent bystander" phenomenon with the formation or deposition of complexes in the wall and then activation of the complement system. The pathogenesis of a type III reaction was covered earlier in the chapter. An idiopathic febrile disease characterized by a systemic necrotizing vasculitis that occurs primarily in young (4 to 10 months of age) beagle dogs is suspected to be immune-mediated, based on clinical signs, immunologic abnormalities, and pathologic findings. The syndrome has been designated as juvenile polyarteritis or beagle pain syndrome, and there appears to be a familial predisposition in some colonies. A similar syndrome has been reported in other breeds. Males and females are equally affected.

CLINICAL SIGNS AND IMMUNOLOGIC ABNORMALITIES

The classic presentation is a febrile (104° F to 107° F) young dog with anorexia, hunched stance, cervical pain, and an unwillingness to move the head and neck. The disease has a cyclic course, with two to seven periods of signs that resolve. They have a moderate to notable leukocytosis, with neutrophilia, nonregenerative anemia, and hypoalbuminemia. Cerebral spinal fluid analysis indicates a neutrophilic pleocytosis with mild to moderate increases in microprotein. On serum protein electrophoresis, they have a high α_2-globulin fraction. ANA tests, LE preparations, and rheumatoid factor tests are generally negative. Immunologic abnormalities include an increase in serum IgA concentration, an increase in the percentage of peripheral B lymphocytes, and a decrease in the percentage of total peripheral T lymphocytes, a marked suppression of the blastogenic response to mitogenic stimulation, an inability to generate immunoglobulin-secreting plasma cells following polyclonal activation, and evidence of monocyte-macrophage activation. There are increased concentrations of IL-6 in the serum of acutely affected dogs, and these return to base-line concentrations during periods of remission or following corticosteroid therapy.

LESIONS

Severe necrotizing vasculitis and perivasculitis with thrombosis of small- to medium-sized blood vessels in the leptomeninges of the cervical spinal cord, cranial mediastinum, and heart are commonly seen (Fig. 5-32). In severe cases, a more widespread distribution of vascular lesions occur and commonly involves the thyroid gland, small intestine, testes, diaphragm, esophagus, and urinary bladder. Most patients experience multiple episodes, but some may have only one to two episodes before becoming normal, and clinical signs appear to resolve in all but the most severely affected patients by 12 to 18 months of age. Some dogs that experience repeated acute episodes develop splenic, hepatic, and renal amyloidosis. The pathogenesis of amyloidosis is attributed to serum amyloidal A production and the development of reactive systemic amyloidosis secondary to the vascular inflammation.

IMMUNODEFICIENCY SYNDROMES

Immunodeficiency diseases occur when there is a failure of the immune system to protect the host from infectious organisms or the development of cancer. An immunodeficiency syndrome that is the result of a

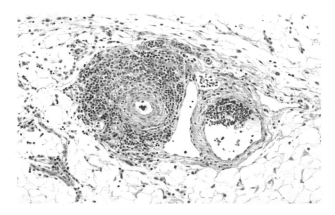

Fig. 5-32   Perivasculitis and vasculitis, polyarteritis, beagle dog. Note the accumulation of lymphocytes and macrophages around the arteriole. H&E stain.
(Courtesy Dr. P.W. Snyder, School of Veterinary Medicine, Purdue University.)

congenital or genetic defect in a component of the immune system is called a primary immunodeficiency. Although the defect may be present at birth, the disease may not be manifested until later in life. An immunodeficiency syndrome that is an acquired loss of immune function as a complication of infections, malnutrition, or aging or a side effect of immunosuppression, irradiation, or chemotherapy for cancer or autoimmune disease is called a secondary immunodeficiency. It is important to differentiate between a primary and secondary state of immunodeficiency with respect to treatment and prognosis. In some instances, it is useful to subclassify immunodeficiency diseases into those that affect adaptive (specific) or noninnate (nonspecific) immune responses. The study of immunodeficiency diseases has provided valuable insights and has enhanced our understanding of the complexities of the immune system. The ability to specifically identify the defective component provides great potential for the development of screening tests and of effective therapies. Naturally occurring and experimentally induced defects have made significant contributions to the field of immunology. There are a greater number of well-characterized immunodeficiency diseases in humans that likely have a domestic animal counterpart that have not yet been recognized. With the advent of new reagents and methodologies for characterizing cells and components of the immune system of domestic species, there should be a better chance in identifying immunodeficiency syndromes. Most primary immunodeficiency diseases are inherited, and the gene defect has been identified. There are additional forms of immunodeficiency that are the result of developmental defects that impair the function of an organ of the immune system. Finally, secondary immunodeficiency is a component of a large number of diseases of domestic species (ranging from malnutrition to viral infections that target lymphoid cells) and is beyond the scope of this chapter. This portion of the chapter will cover some of the better characterized primary immunodeficiency diseases of domestic animals.

PRIMARY IMMUNODEFICIENCIES

Most primary immunodeficiency diseases are the result of a genetic defect (inherited or congenital) and affect specific (i.e., humoral and cell-mediated arms of the adaptive immune response) or nonspecific immunity (i.e., components of innate immune responses, such as complement, phagocytosis, NK cells, etc.). Specific defects in adaptive immune responses can be divided into those affecting T lymphocytes or B lymphocytes or both (Fig. 5-33). As already discussed, interactions between B and T lymphocytes are necessary for the development of many immune responses. In some instances, the clinical distinction between a primary

B-lymphocyte defect and a T-lymphocyte defect may not be obvious with respect to humoral immunity. For example, T-lymphocyte defects almost always result in impaired antibody synthesis and as such are indistinguishable from B-lymphocyte defects or combined B-lymphocyte and T-lymphocyte defects. In general, most primary deficiencies manifest themselves early in life and affected patients clinically have a failure to thrive and a susceptibility to recurrent infections. In many instances, the type of infection suggests to some extent the likely component of the immune system that is defective (Table 5-11). It is beyond the scope of this chapter to present all of the forms of human and rodent immunodeficiency, and thus only a few are referenced for clarity to facilitate understanding diseases that have been characterized in domestic species.

PRIMARY IMMUNODEFICIENCIES OF SPECIFIC IMMUNITY
SEVERE COMBINED IMMUNODEFICIENCY DISEASE

Severe combined immunodeficiency disease (SCID) is a family of genetic defects that have in common deficiencies in both humoral and cell-mediated immunity. In its extreme form, SCID results from a defect in the common lymphoid stem cell that results in defective cell-mediated and humoral immune responses. More commonly, SCID defects affect either T lymphocytes or B and T lymphocytes and are best characterized in humans, mice, dogs, and horses. T-lymphocyte defects often clinically have a combined immunodeficiency because there is a secondary impairment of humoral immunity that is the result of an inability of the T lymphocyte to provide the necessary signals for B-lymphocyte activation. These defects result in an inability to generate a specific immune response and can have an autosomal recessive, X-linked, or sporadic inheritance pattern. The types of underlying defects are diverse and may involve enzyme systems or proteins necessary for lymphocyte development and differentiation, or signal transduction pathways involved in lymphocyte activation. Often the most common infectious manifestation of SCID is a viral or fungal infection. Immunity to viral and fungal infections is largely dependent on cell-mediated immunity. Immunity to most bacterial infections (especially extracellular bacteria) are largely dependent on humoral immunity, and neonates have adequate humoral immunity from the passive transfer of maternal antibodies that protect them.

SCID in horses is an autosomal recessive disorder described in the Arabian or Arabian-cross breed. The defect results in a severe lymphopenia (less than 1000/mm³) attributed to an inability to produce functional T and B lymphocytes. At birth, before they acquire maternal antibodies via colostrums, affected animals are deficient in serum IgM, and following

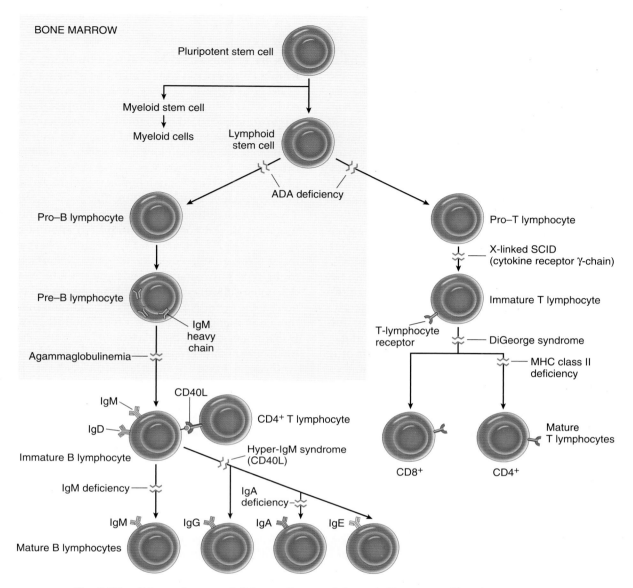

Fig. 5-33   Primary immunodeficiency diseases. Schematic illustration of lymphocyte development and differentiation with known sites of disruption that cause primary immunodeficiency diseases. *ADA,* Adenosine deaminase; *Ig,* immunoglobulin; *MHC,* major histocompatibility complex; *SCID,* severe combined immunodeficiency disease. *(From Kumar V, Abbas AK, Fausto N: Robbins & Cotran pathologic basis of disease, ed 7, Philadelphia, 2005, Saunders.)*

Table **5-11   Examples of Infections in Immunodeficiencies**

Pathogen Type	T-Lymphocyte Defect	B-Lymphocyte Defect	Granulocyte Defect	Complement Defect
Bacteria	Bacterial sepsis	Streptococci, staphylococci	Staphylococci, *Pseudomonas*	Pyogenic bacterial infections
Viruses	Cytomegalovirus, chronic infections with respiratory and intestinal viruses	Enteroviral encephalitis		
Fungi and parasites	*Candida, Pneumocystis carinii*	Intestinal giardiasis, aspergillosis	*Candida, Nocardia, Aspergillus*	
Special features	Aggressive disease with opportunistic pathogens, failure to clear infections, adverse reactions to attenuated vaccines	Chronic recurrent gastrointestinal infections, sepsis, meningitis	Neutrophilia	

catabolism of passively transferred antibodies, they have agammaglobinemia develop. Recurrent infections are typical and death is commonly the result of infection with equine adenovirus, *Pneumocystis carinii*, *Cryptosporidium parvum*, or a variety of common equine bacterial pathogens. Grossly the thymus is small and maybe undetectable. Microscopically, there is profound lymphoid hypoplasia of primary and secondary lymphoid tissue. Thymuses contain small lobules with no corticomedullary differentiation, few lymphocytes, Hassall's corpuscles, and occasional cysts. Spleens are characterized as having no lymphoid follicles, periarteriolar lymphoid sheaths, or plasma cells. Additionally, it has been noted that the lymphoid follicle sites in the spleen lack connective tissue stroma, and this characteristic can be used to differentiate hypoplasia from atrophy. Lymph nodes lack lymphoid follicles, plasma cells, and corticomedullary differentiation. The molecular basis for the defect has been identified as a spontaneous mutation in the gene encoding, the catalytic subunit of a DNA-dependent protein kinase (DNA-PKcs) that is located on chromosome 9. Affected foals have a complete absence of functional DNA-PKcs. DNA-PK is required for the recombination of immunoglobulin heavy chain and TCR genes during development, which when defective results in an inability to form functional V regions. Interestingly, as a result of the DNA-PKcs mutation, affected horses also are defective in their DNA repair mechanisms. The importance of DNA repair mechanisms in preventing the development of cancer (see Chapter 6) would suggest that affected foals and heterozygous carriers would be at an increased risk for cancer. Although affected foals rarely live beyond 5 months of age, heterozygous carriers do, and they have been observed to be at a greater risk for developing sarcoids, a locally aggressive fibroblastic cutaneous neoplasm.

SCID in dogs was first described in Basset hounds as an X-linked defect (XSCID) characterized by lymphopenia, with increased numbers of B lymphocytes and few to no T lymphocytes. The lymphopenia is not as profound as it is in foals with SCID. At approximately 6 to 8 weeks of age, as maternally derived antibody concentrations decline, they develop recurrent infections of the skin, respiratory, or gastrointestinal system. Phenotypically, there is a decrease in the number of circulating CD8+ lymphocytes resulting in a CD4+:CD8+ ratio of approximately 15:1 (compared with 2:1 in normal dogs) and normal percentages of B lymphocytes. Dogs with XCSID are hypogammaglobulinemic with normal serum IgM concentrations and decreased concentrations of IgG and IgA. Affected dogs rarely live past 4 months of age, and death is frequently attributed to septicemia or systemic viral infections. At necropsy, lymph nodes, tonsils, Peyer's patches, and the thymus are extremely small and

may be undetectable. Microscopically, there is severe lymphoid hypoplasia with similar characteristic features as described previously for lymphoid tissues of the foal with SCID. Thymuses of affected puppies are small (approximately 10% the weight of age-matched controls) and are characterized by a lack of corticomedullary demarcation and small lobules with few to no lymphocytes (Fig. 5-34). Thymuses have markedly increased percentages of CD8/CD4 lymphocytes (46% versus 16% in age-matched controls) compatible with a block in T lymphocyte differentiation. Canine XSCID is due to a mutation in the common gamma (γ_c) subunit of the IL-2, IL-4, IL-7, IL-9, and IL-15 receptors. These receptors, for five immunologically different cytokines, belong to the type I cytokine receptor family. A four base pair deletion results in a stop codon that prevents full translation of the γ_c mRNA. T lymphocytes are nonfunctional due to an inability to express a functional IL-2 receptor. B lymphocytes are only activated by T-lymphocyte-independent antigens, and although they are capable of synthesizing IgM, they are incapable of class-switching to IgG. A similar molecular form of XSCID has also been described in the Cardigan Welsh Corgi breed. An insertional mutation, due to the insertion of a cytosine in exon 4, also results in a stop codon preventing complete translation of γ_c mRNA. In human SCID, mutations of the γ_c are the most common molecular mechanism with numerous distinct point, insertion, and deletion mutations identified. An autosomal recessive form of SCID has been described in Jack Russell terriers that is the result of a mutation in DNA-PKcs similar to that described previously in the Arabian horse and the CB-17 mouse.

SCID in mice occurs in the CB-17 strain and is an autosomal recessive trait characterized by an absence of mature B and T lymphocytes. The molecular basis for the SCID phenotype is attributed to a defect resulting in decreased DNA-PK enzyme activity. Although mice are highly susceptible to opportunistic infections, they can be maintained in environments that minimize their exposure to pathogenic agents and kept alive for more than a year of age. An interesting, although poorly understood, immunologic finding in older (greater than 6 months of age) mice with SCID is the ability to produce small quantities of immunoglobulin and low numbers of mature T lymphocytes. This phenotype is referred to as "leaky SCID." This leaky phenotype has not been described in other forms of SCID. As in other species with defective DNA repair mechanisms, there is an increased sensitivity to ionizing radiation damage.

COMMON VARIABLE IMMUNODEFICIENCY

Common variable immunodeficiency is a primary immunodeficiency disease characterized by an adult onset of hypogammaglobulinemia attributed to an intrinsic B-lymphocyte defect, which results in an inability to produce much of the antibody. The disease has been

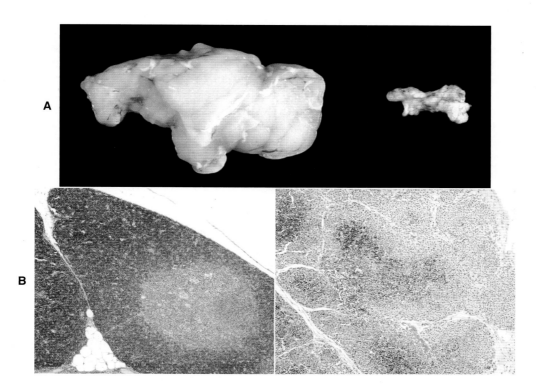

Fig. 5-34   X-linked severe combined immunodeficiency disease (XSCID) thymuses, normal puppy and littermate. A, The gland from the normal puppy *(left)* weighed 7.4 g, and the gland from the XSCID puppy *(right)* weighed 0.2 g. **B,** Thymus from a normal neonatal dog *(left)* and from a neonatal dog with XSCID *(right).* The normal thymic lobule has a pale medullary region and a dark cortical region that is densely packed with small lymphocytes. The XSCID thymus has small lobules with no corticomedullary distinction and a paucity of small lymphocytes. H&E stain. (**A** *and* **B,** *Courtesy Dr. P.W. Snyder, School of Veterinary Medicine, Purdue University.*)

described in a litter of miniature Dachshund dogs. The dogs were characterized as having an absence of B lymphocytes in lymphoid tissues and little to no serum immunoglobulins. At necropsy, the affected animals had lesions characterized as atrophy of lymphoid tissue and pneumonia. Lymph nodes were further characterized as lacking lymphoid follicles. The pneumonia was caused by *Pneumocystis carinii*, a common opportunistic pathogen in immunocompromised animals and humans. In humans there have been a number of identified defects intrinsic to B lymphocytes that prevents their terminal differentiation and affects their ability to produce immunoglobulin, thus the designation as variable immunodeficiency. A similar disease has also been described in a 12-year-old Quarter Horse, which was characterized by hypogammaglobulinemia and an absence of B lymphocytes in circulation, bone marrow, and spleen.

AGAMMAGLOBULINEMIA

Agammaglobulinemia is a primary immunodeficiency characterized by an inability to produce immunoglobulins and an absence of mature B lymphocytes and plasma cells. The disease has been described in Thoroughbred,

Quarter Horse, and Standardbred breeds of horses. To date, all cases have been males, suggesting that, as in the human disease, it is an X-linked trait. Microscopically, there was an absence of plasma cells, primary follicles, and germinal centers in lymph nodes. Affected horses commonly have extracellular bacterial infections of the joints and respiratory system. In humans there is a mutation of the BTK gene located on the X chromosome that encodes a tyrosine kinase that results in an arrest of B-lymphocyte development at the pre-B stage. The disease in humans is referred to as X-linked agammaglobulinemia (XLA).

SELECTIVE IMMUNOGLOBULIN DEFICIENCIES

Selective deficiencies are represented by a number of diseases characterized by a deficiency of an individual class of immunoglobulin. Forms of these diseases have been identified and described in horses and dogs. The most common forms are selective IgM deficiency and selective IgA deficiency, characterized by a serum level of IgM or IgA, respectively, that is at least 2 standard deviations below normal. Serum concentrations of other classes of immunoglobulin are normal, and B lymphocyte numbers are normal. These deficiencies may not result in clinical signs until there is degradation of passively transferred maternal antibody. In horses, there are distinct forms of selective IgM deficiency with most affected animals succumbing to septicemia or pneumonia by 10 months of age. A few affected foals live beyond 10 months and commonly die of recurrent respiratory infections before reaching adulthood. Some horses reach adulthood before they show clinical signs of selective IgM deficiency. Selective IgA deficiency has been described in a number of breeds of dogs, including the German shepherd, Shar-Pei, Irish setter, and beagle. Because of the importance of IgA in mucosal immunity, many affected animals have respiratory, gastrointestinal, and skin infections. Some affected dogs, like human patients with IgA deficiency, have a predisposition to developing atopic disease. In most instances there are normal numbers of IgA-producing plasma cells, suggesting an inability to synthesize or secrete IgA. Although the molecular basis for selective immunoglobulin deficiencies is unknown, they are thought to relate to the differentiation of naïve B lymphocytes into immunoglobulin-secreting plasma cells.

THYMIC HYPOPLASIA

Thymic hypoplasia represents a number of immunodeficiency diseases characterized by a failure to develop a functional thymus, resulting in a T-lymphocyte deficiency. Mice homozygous for the genetic trait nu (nu/nu) are hairless, and this athymic strain is commonly referred to as the nude mouse. Affected mice have a developmental arrest of the thymus, which occurs around day 12 of gestation and results in an absence of a functional thymus. Nude mice have defective cell-mediated immune responses and are unable to develop antibody responses. The immunologic abnormalities are attributed to a deficiency of T-lymphocyte responses. Heterozygous (nu/+) animals are normal. The few circulating T lymphocytes in affected mice have TCRs of the γ/δ-type rather than the α/β-type. Under conventional housing conditions, mortality is high during the first 2 weeks of life; however, when maintained in germfree environments, they can survive longer. This strain of mice is an important animal model, as they can tolerate allografts and xenografts. Similar, although less well-characterized, hairless and athymic conditions have been described in other species. A condition in humans characterized by thymic hypoplasia is referred to as DiGeorge syndrome. DiGeorge syndrome is a T lymphocyte deficiency resulting from an embryologic defect affecting the development of the third and fourth pharyngeal pouches. Affected humans have thymic (fourth pharyngeal pouch) and parathyroid (third pharyngeal pouch) defects. They have decreased circulating T lymphocytes, and T-lymphocyte areas of lymphoid tissues (paracortical areas of lymph nodes and periarteriolar

sheaths of the spleen) are depleted of lymphocytes. There is an absence of cell-mediated immune responses. DiGeorge syndrome is not familial, but rather the result of the deletion of a specific gene that is a member of the T-box family of transcription factors. Specifically, how or why this transcription factor influences the development of the thymus and parathyroid is unknown.

PRIMARY IMMUNODEFICIENCIES OF NONSPECIFIC IMMUNITY
DEFICIENCIES OF THE COMPLEMENT SYSTEM

The complement system contains more than 30 soluble and cell-bound proteins that influence immune and inflammatory responses. The pathways of complement activation, regulation of the complement system, and biologic consequences of complement activation have been previously covered in Chapter 3. In humans, inherited deficiencies have been described for nearly all components and two of the inhibitors. Although a deficiency of C2 is the most common, humans with deficiencies in components of the classical pathway have little to no increased risk for infections, suggesting that the alternative and lectin pathways of activation are sufficient for controlling infections. Deficiencies of the classical pathway components are associated with an increased incidence of SLE-like autoimmune disease, which has been attributed to impaired clearance of immune complexes by the monocyte-macrophage system. Although deficiencies of components of the alternative pathway (properdin and factors D and H) are rare, when they do occur they are associated with recurrent pyogenic infections. A deficiency of C3, which is required for all three pathways of complement, is the most serious deficiency and results in serious recurrent infections. An autosomal recessive trait resulting in a genetically determined deficiency of C3 has been described in the Brittany spaniel dog. Homozygous dogs have serum concentrations of C3 and also opsonic and chemotactic activities that are severely decreased compared with normal dogs. Affected dogs are predisposed to recurrent infections and type 1 membranoproliferative glomerulonephritis. Bacterial infections with *Clostridium* spp., *Escherichia coli*, and *Klebsiella* spp. resulting in pneumonia, septicemia, and pyometra, respectively, are the most common clinical manifestations.

The molecular basis for the deficiency has been identified as a deletion mutation that results in a premature stop codon, preventing adequate translation and resulting in decreased concentrations of mRNA. Heterozygous dogs have serum concentrations of C3 that are approximately 50% of normal, but these dogs are clinically normal. C3 deficiency has also been described in guinea pigs and rabbits.

An autosomal recessive trait resulting in a deficiency of factor H, a component of the alternative pathway of complement, has been described in the Norwegian Yokshire breed of pig. Factor H is a regulator of complement activation that blocks the formation of C3 convertase and is a cofactor for cleavage of C3b by factor I. Deficiencies of factor H result in unregulated elaboration of C3b upon activation of the alternative pathway. The most common clinical manifestation is renal disease. Affected pigs develop a type II membranoproliferative glomerulonephritis characterized by glomerular changes consisting of thickened capillary walls, proliferation of mesangial cells, dense intramembranous deposits, and glomerular deposits of C3 components. The disease is commonly referred to as porcine dense deposit disease.

The molecular basis for the decreased serum concentrations of factor H has been reported to be the result of nucleotide sequence alterations in the factor H gene that cause a block in protein secretion. Hepatocytes of affected animals have increased intracellular concentrations of factor H. Hereditary factor H deficiency in humans can be characterized by a variety of clinical manifestations ranging from recurrent bacterial infections to glomerular disease to hemolytic uremic syndrome. Deficiencies of the terminal components (C5, C6, C7, C8, and C9), which are required for the formation of the membrane attack complex and the lysis of cell membranes, do occur and generally result in increased bacterial infections.

Deficiencies of C1 inhibitor and other complement regulatory proteins, although described in humans, have yet to be described in domestic animals. C1 inhibitor deficiency is an autosomal dominant trait that causes hereditary angioedema. C1 inhibitor is a protease inhibitor that targets C1r and C1s enzymes of the classical pathway of complement, Hageman factor (factor XII) of the coagulation pathway, and the kallikrein system. As indicated in Chapter 4, these three pathways are closely linked and result in the elaboration of vasoactive amines, notably bradykinin. Affected human patients develop episodes of edema involving the skin and mucosal membranes, such as those of the larynx and gastrointestinal system. Deficiencies of membrane-bound regulator proteins, such as decay-accelerating factor and homologous restriction factor, result in paroxysmal nocturnal hemoglobinuria. In the absence of these regulatory factors, red blood cells can be more easily lysed by concentrations of complement that are much lower than normally required. The increased lysis of red blood cells causes chronic hemolytic anemia and hemoglobinuria.

CHÉDIAK-HIGASHI SYNDROME

Chédiak-Higashi syndrome is an inherited disease caused by defective lysosomes, melanosomes, platelet-dense granules, and cytolytic granules. The disease has been described in cats, cattle, killer whales, beige mice, rats, Aleutian mink, and humans. Common clinical manifestations of the disease may include hypopigmentation, a bleeding tendency, ocular abnormalities, and recurrent infections. Some species are more susceptible to recurrent infections than others. The hallmark of the disease is the presence of enlarged granules within melanocytes, neutrophils, eosinophils, and monocytes. The enlarged granules are melanosomes (melanocytes), lysosomes (many cell types), or cytoplasmic granules (e.g., fused primary and secondary granules of neutrophils). Neutrophils containing giant granules have impaired functions, such as defective chemotaxis and intracellular killing. NK cells are also defective and may also contribute to the increased susceptibility to infections reported in some species. Mink with Chédiak-Higashi syndrome have an increased susceptibility to Aleutian mink disease virus. The hypopigmentation is the result of an inability of melanocytes, containing abnormally large melanosomes, to migrate and release their contents, resulting in a deficiency of pigment most commonly evident in the skin, hair, and eye. The bleeding tendency is a coagulopathy resulting from defective platelets. Platelet counts are generally normal. In most species studied, most recently cattle, there is insufficient platelet aggregation because of a decreased response to collagen. Research suggests that the GPIa/IIa ($\alpha_2\beta_1$-integrin) glycoprotein or rhodocytin pathway of platelet activation may be defective. Ocular abnormalities identified in cattle, cats, mink, mice, and humans are similar and are characterized by abnormal ocular pigmentation and an associated photophobia. Cats with Chédiak-Higashi syndrome frequently develop cataracts. The molecular basis for Chédiak-Higashi syndrome has been identified in some human forms and in beige mice and cattle to be a result of a mutation of the Lyst gene. The Lyst gene encodes a membrane-associated protein, which is thought to regulate intracellular protein trafficking. Exactly how the protein regulates intracellular trafficking remains unknown.

LEUKOCYTE ADHESION DEFICIENCY

Leukocyte adhesion deficiency (LAD) is a primary immunodeficiency disease characterized by the inability of leukocytes to migrate from circulation into sites of inflammation, resulting in recurrent bacterial infections (see Chapter 3). The disease is best characterized in humans and in bovine (BLAD) and canine (CLAD) species, in which the defect is inherited as an autosomal recessive trait. The Irish setter breed of dogs and Holstein breed of cattle are commonly affected domestic species. The hallmark of the disease is a profound leukocytosis characterized by a marked neutrophilia, and the disease was initially referred to in these species as canine granulocytopathy syndrome and bovine granulocytopathy syndrome, respectively. In Irish setters, CLAD-affected puppies often initially have omphalophlebitis just after birth and by 4 months of age commonly have episodes of gingivitis, osteomyelitis, or lymphadenopathy. An inability to form pus and delayed wound healing may also be observed. Dogs rarely survive beyond 6 months of age as a result of the recurrent infections. In affected calves, BLAD causes a similar spectrum of recurrent infections and leads to death by 7 months of age. The molecular basis for the disease is a defective expression of the β_2-integrin subunit of a large group of heterodimeric (α- and β-subunits) leukocyte adhesion molecules. The β_2-integrins are a family of adhesion molecules that all share the same β-subunit (CD18), but have unique α-subunits (CD11a, b, c). Members of the β_2-integrin family include: leukocyte function–associated antigen, LFA-1 (CD11a/CD18); Mac-1 or complement receptor 3 (CD11b/CD18); and p150,95 or CR4 (CD11c/CD18). As discussed in Chapter 3, these surface molecules are in part required for neutrophil adhesion to the endothelium and extravasation into the tissue, migration to sites of inflamma-tion or infection (chemotaxis), and phagocytosis of C3b-opsonized bacteria. The binding of neutrophils to cytokine-activated endothelial cells at sites of inflammation is also mediated in part by selectins, which are not affected in LAD. Therefore in LAD, neutrophils marginate, but fail to migrate from the endothelium. Human, bovine, and canine LAD are caused by missense mutations in the β_2-integrin subunit gene, resulting in a functionally defective β_2-integrin protein.

AMYLOIDOSIS

Although there is no evidence to suggest that amyloidosis is always the result of a primary immunologic

abnormality, the pathogenesis of amyloidosis may involve components of the immune system and as such is discussed here. Amyloidosis represents a broad spectrum of clinical and pathologic conditions that all have in common the deposition of amyloid material. Amyloid is a pathologic proteinaceous substance of different chemical entities with an identical conformational property of forming β-pleated sheets of non-branching fibrils as identified by x-ray crystallography and infrared spectroscopy (Fig. 5-35). By light microscopy, and standard hematoxylin and eosin staining, amyloid appears as an amorphous, eosinophilic, hyaline, extracellular substance that with progressive accumulation results in pressure atrophy of adjacent cells and tissue (Fig. 5-36). Although amyloid can be derived from

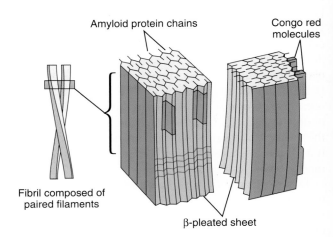

Fig. 5-35 Schematic depiction of amyloid fibrils, β-pleated sheets, and binding sites for Congo red dye. *(Modified from Glenner GG: N Engl J Med 52:148, 1980.)*

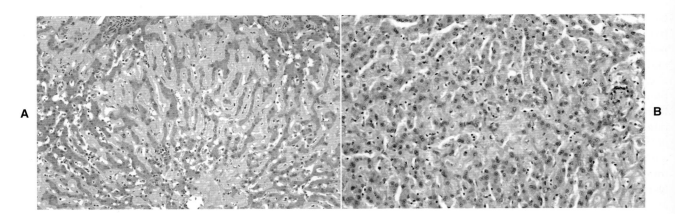

Fig. 5-36 **Amyloidosis, liver, dog.** This dog had repeated episodes of vasculitis. The amyloid was attributed to systemic reactive amyloidosis (AA amyloid) caused by increased concentrations of serum amyloid A (SAA). **A,** Liver. The spaces of Disse are expanded by eosinophilic proteinaceous material (amyloid) that had caused atrophy of the hepatic cords. H&E stain. **B,** The deposits of amyloid are stained orange by the Congo red stain. (*A and B, Courtesy Dr. P.W. Snyder, School of Veterinary Medicine, Purdue University.*)

different chemical entities, all deposits have the same appearance and tinctorial characteristics. In humans, there are three major and several minor biochemical forms. Amyloidosis is a feature of several different pathologic mechanisms and as such should not be considered a single disease, but rather a group of diseases having in common the deposition of similar-appearing proteins. It is often necessary to differentiate amyloid from other similar-appearing extracellular deposits, such as collagen and fibrin. Differentiating these proteins is readily accomplished using histochemical techniques. The most common technique for identifying amyloid is the Congo red stain, which does not have chemical specificity for amyloid but is dependent on the conformational property of being arranged in β-pleated sheets. Congo red stains amyloid an orange to red color, and when viewed by polarized light reveals a characteristic green birefringent material (see Chapter 11). A loss of Congo red staining by pretreating sections with potassium permanganate may suggest that the amyloidogenic protein is of amyloid-associated origin (see next section).

CHEMICAL NATURE OF AMYLOID

Amyloid contains approximately 95% fibrillar proteins and 5% P component and other glycoproteins. Of the 15 biochemically distinct forms of amyloid recognized in humans, 3 are most common: (1) amyloid light chain (AL), derived from immunoglobulin light chains of plasma cells; (2) amyloid associated (AA), derived from the acute phase protein serum amyloid A (SAA); and (3) Aβ amyloid, derived from amyloid precursor protein (APP). These forms of amyloid are also recognized in domestic species.

The AL form of amyloid can contain complete immunoglobulin light chains, the NH_2-terminus portion of immunoglobulin light chains, or both. Of the two immunoglobulin light chains, λ and κ, most AL forms consist of λ-light chains or their fragments. Immunoglobulin-secreting cells, B lymphocytes, and plasma cells are associated with deposition of AL amyloid.

The AA form of amyloid consists of a proteolytic fragment of a larger acute phase protein called SAA, which is found in the plasma and is synthesized in the liver and released during systemic inflammatory reactions.

The Aβ form of amyloid contains a proteolytic fragment of the APP and is associated with the cerebral amyloid angiopathy of Alzheimer's disease in humans and with some forms of neurodegeneration in the canine brain. This form of amyloid will be discussed more extensively in Chapter 14.

Of the large number of other biochemically distinct proteins that have been associated with the formation of amyloid in a number of human clinical diseases, only a few are relevant to domestic species. One of these is islet amyloidosis, affecting the feline pancreas.

Islet amyloid is derived from islet amyloid polypeptide (IAPP), which is a hormone synthesized by the β cells of the pancreatic islets. All forms of amyloid contain other minor components, including serum amyloid P protein, proteoglycans, and glycosaminoglycans. Serum amyloid P may function to stabilize the fibrils and decrease their susceptibility to proteolysis.

CLASSIFICATION OF AMYLOIDOSIS

In addition to the classification based on the primary biochemical constituent as discussed previously, it is also useful from a pathologist's perspective to categorize these conditions according to their clinical disease and pathogenesis (Table 5-12). Amyloid can be systemic (generalized), with deposits in many organ systems, or it can be localized, with deposits limited to a single organ. The systemic or generalized category can be further subclassified into primary amyloidosis (AL), when associated with immunocyte dyscrasia, or secondary amyloidosis (SAA), when associated with a chronic inflammatory or destructive tissue process. Hereditary or familial amyloidosis comprises a separate heterogeneous category with several distinctive patterns of organ involvement that are primarily recognized in humans.

PRIMARY AMYLOIDOSIS

Primary amyloidosis is the most common systemic form of amyloidosis and is of the AL type. Many cases of AL amyloidosis are attributable to the presence of some type of immunocyte dyscrasias. The most common immunocyte dyscrasias associated with AL amyloidosis in domestic species is a neoplasm of plasma cells. Plasma cell-derived neoplasms include the extramedullary plasmacytoma and the myeloma or more common multiple myeloma that are most often limited to the bone marrow. Although neoplastic plasma cells often synthesize abnormal amounts of complete immunoglobulin or components of immunoglobulins (light or heavy chain only), only a small percentage of patients with these neoplasms develop amyloidosis. On serum protein electrophoresis, there may be a monoclonal gammopathy that is compatible with the presence of a single specific immunoglobulin. Additionally, in some cases the serum may contain only the light chain component (referred to as Bence Jones protein). Because an individual plasma cell can only synthesize either the λ- or κ-type of light chain and because plasma cell-derived neoplasms are of clonal origin, only one light chain type will be present. The λ-light chain is most often identified in AL-type amyloidosis. Because light chains are small proteins (approximately 50 kD), they are frequently detected in the urine of affected patients. The mere presence of Bence Jones proteins itself is not sufficient to produce AL amyloidosis, as many cases of plasma cell neoplasms with identifiable Bence Jones proteins occur in most domestic species without the

Table **5-12** **Classification of Amyloidosis**

Clinicopathologic Category	Associated Diseases	Major Fibril Protein	Chemically Related Precursor Protein
SYSTEMIC (GENERALIZED) AMYLOIDOSIS			
Immunocyte dyscrasias with amyloidosis (primary amyloidosis)	Multiple myeloma and other monoclonal B-cell proliferations	AL	Immunoglobulin light chains, chiefly λ-type
Reactive systemic amyloidosis (secondary amyloidosis)	Chronic inflammatory conditions	AA	SAA
Familial amyloidosis	Some animals have systemic deposition of amyloid in addition to renal deposits	AA	
LOCALIZED AMYLOIDOSIS			
Amyloid of aging	Neurodegenerative disease, senile plaques, cerebral amyloid angiopathy	Aβ	APP
Endocrine tumors		A Cal	Calcitonin, polypeptide hormones or prohormones
Nonendocrine tumors	Amyloid-producing odontogenic tumor, ameloblastomas		
Islets of Langerhans	Diabetes mellitus	IAPP	Islet amyloid polypeptide
Isolated amyloid of pulmonary vasculature	–	Apolipoprotein A-1	Apolipoprotein A-1
Prion diseases	Various prion diseases of the CNS, spongiform encephalopathy	Misfolded prion protein (PrPsc)	Normal prion protein PrP
Familial amyloidosis of the dog	Renal disease	AA	Likely SAA
Familial amyloidosis of the cat	Renal disease	AA	Likely SAA
Gastrointestinal amyloidosis	Age-related finding		Unknown (not AA)

A Cal, Amyloid of hormone origin; *AA,* amyloid associated; *AL,* amyloid light chain; *APP,* amyloid precursor protein; *CNS,* central nervous system; *IAPP,* islet amyloid polypeptide; *SAA,* serum amyloid A.

development of amyloidosis. In contrast to amyloidosis in humans, in which the majority of patients with AL amyloid do not have any overt B lymphocyte or plasma cell neoplasm but do have monoclonal antibodies or light chains in their serum or urine, domestic species rarely have AL-type amyloid without evidence of an immunocyte dyscrasias. A more complete discussion of these neoplasms may be found in Chapter 13.

REACTIVE SYSTEMIC AMYLOIDOSIS

This form of amyloidosis has a systemic distribution and is also referred to as secondary amyloidosis because it is often secondary to a chronic inflammation of the destructive tissue process. Reactive systemic amyloidosis in domestic animals is a form of AA amyloid, which is most often either secondary to chronic inflammatory or neoplastic (nonimmunocyte dyscrasias) conditions or idiopathic, where no underlying disease is found. A prolonged increased serum concentration of SAA protein is necessary but by itself insufficient for the development of AA amyloid. This form of amyloidosis

is recognized in most species. A form of the disease is also recognized in captive cheetahs and closely related Siberian tigers. In the cheetahs, in which renal deposits were primarily in the medullary interstitium, inflammatory conditions, most often gastritis, were found in all affected cats.

FAMILIAL AMYLOIDOSIS

This is a systemic form of AA amyloidosis that is hereditary in some breeds of cats and dogs. Familial AA amyloid has been described in the Abyssinian and Siamese breeds of cat and the Shar-Pei breed of dog. The organ systems affected are varied, but deposits most commonly occur in the kidney (primarily a glomerular deposition in the Abyssinian cat and medullary interstitium deposition in the Shar-Pei dog) and liver (Siamese cat). The amyloid fibrils consist of AA proteins, suggesting that this form may be related to chronic inflammatory conditions. Preliminary analysis of the different isoforms of SAA in the cat suggests that certain SAA genes may contribute to the development of this form of amyloid. Most domestic species have at least three isoforms of SAA.

LOCALIZED AMYLOIDOSIS

Occasionally, amyloid deposits are limited to a single organ or tissue. In many instances, the localized deposits are grossly visible as masses. Localized amyloidosis is present in calcifying epithelial odontogenic tumors (amyloid-producing odontogenic tumor) of the cat and dog. Of the prominent features of these rare neoplasms, one is the presence of amyloid, which often calcifies. Some forms of naturally occurring transmissible spongiform encephalopathies, such as chronic wasting disease (CWD), are characterized by amyloid plaques in the brain in addition to the intraneuronal vacuolation. The lesions of CWD and other prion diseases are discussed in Chapter 14.

ENDOCRINE AMYLOIDOSIS

Deposition of amyloid in the pancreas of cats, nonhuman primates (macaques and baboons), and humans can lead to the development of type 2 diabetes mellitus. The amyloid is deposited in the pancreatic islets and is derived from islet amyloid polypeptide (IAPP), a normal protein secreted by the β cell of the pancreas. How a normal protein product becomes amyloidgenic in some instances remains unknown. It is not known if the deposition of amyloid and the development of clinical diabetes mellitus is the result of progressive loss of β cells from the amyloid or if the deposition of amyloid occurs as a result of prolonged stimulation of the β cells as a consequence of insulin resistance. The disease in cats is discussed in Chapter 11. Amyloid deposition can also occur in the cortex of the adrenal gland; however, it is not associated with any functional deficiencies.

AMYLOID OF AGING

Amyloid deposition can occur as an age-related change in a number of organ systems. Similar to senile systemic amyloidosis in humans, old dogs can develop neurodegenerative changes that may include cerebrovascular amyloidosis or the formation of senile plaques. These deposits can consist of a number of extracellular proteins, but most commonly contain Aβ type amyloid. Other organ systems rarely containing amyloid deposits in the aged dog are heart, gastrointestinal tract, and lungs. The deposition of amyloid in the pulmonary vasculature of aged dogs was reported to be derived from apolipoprotein AI (Apo AI). These forms of amyloidosis are discussed in the appropriate chapters covering these respective organ systems.

PATHOGENESIS OF AMYLOIDOSIS

Amyloid deposition is the result of abnormal folding of pathogenic proteins, deposited extracellularly as fibrils organized into β-pleated sheets. Although there are many diverse proteins associated with the formation of amyloid, they are all characterized by misfolded proteins leading to the formation of fibrils that are unstable and self-associated. Equally diverse are the number of conditions that can be associated with the formation of amyloid, and each of these conditions are characterized by excessive production of amyloidgenic proteins that are prone to misfolding. The two general categories of amyloidgenic proteins are: (1) those that are normal proteins that have an inherent tendency to misfold and form fibrils when produced in excess quantities, and (2) those that are abnormal protein products as a result of genetic mutations that are structurally unstable and form fibrils that self-associate. Misfolded proteins are normally degraded intracellularly within proteasomes or extracellularly by macrophages. In amyloidosis, these degradative processes are inadequate and may be responsible for the accumulation of misfolded proteins extracellularly. A simplified pathogenic scheme for the major forms of amyloidosis is presented in Fig. 5-37. As discussed previously, the overproduction of a precursor protein, although necessary, by itself is not sufficient to result in the formation of amyloid. In secondary reactive systemic amyloidosis, a component of a systemic inflammatory reaction results in the activation of macrophages that elaborate endogenous pyrogens IL-1 and IL-6, which stimulate hepatocytes to synthesize and secrete SAA.

During an inflammatory reaction, the quantity of SAA in the serum may increase several 100 times normal concentrations; however, not all systemic inflammatory reactions result in the formation of AA amyloid. Why is it that only some inflammatory reactions lead to amyloidosis? Two theories, one based on a defective degradation system for SAA and one based an abnormal SAA protein that is resistant to degradation, have been proposed. SAA is normally degraded to soluble protein products by enzymatic components of the monocyte-macrophage system. An enzymatic defect in this system may result in incomplete degradation and the production of insoluble AA molecules that form fibrils. Alternatively, a mutation of an SAA gene may result in the synthesis of an abnormal SAA protein that is resistant to degradation and prone to producing insoluble AA molecules that form fibrils. Finally, in the AL form of amyloidosis plasma cells synthesize excessive quantities of immunoglobulin light chains that are resistant to complete degradation and susceptible to forming insoluble fibrils. Although there have been numerous attempts to identify specific sequence motifs unique to AA and AL forms of amyloid, to date none has been identified. Another research interest has focused on the existence the diversity of SAA isoforms and their relationship to the formation of AA amyloid.

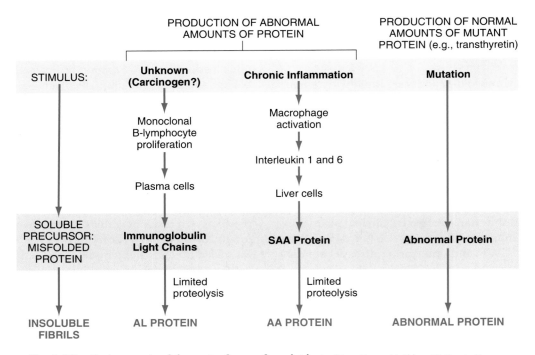

Fig. 5-37   **Pathogenesis of the major forms of amyloidosis.** *(From Kumar V, Abbas AK, Fausto N: Robbins & Cotran pathologic basis of disease, ed 7, Philadelphia, 2005, Saunders.)*

MORPHOLOGY OF AMYLOIDOSIS

Although there are no consistent or characteristic patterns for the distribution of amyloid deposition in any of the categories discussed, a few generalizations can be made. Reactive systemic amyloidosis, secondary to chronic inflammatory conditions, is often the most severe of the systemic forms. Liver, kidney, spleen, lymph nodes, and adrenal glands are most commonly affected. Animals with renal amyloidosis frequently die from renal failure.

Grossly affected organs are often enlarged, moderately firm, and abnormally discolored. In some instances, the application of an iodine solution (e.g., Lugol's iodine) to an affected tissue may stain the deposits brown, which develops into a blue-violet color when exposed to dilute sulfuric acid solution.

Microscopically the diagnosis of amyloid is based on its extracellular location and staining characteristics. As discussed previously, Congo red is the most commonly used stain for the identification of amyloid. Congo red stains amyloid orange to red under light microscopy, which is seen under polarized light as an apple-green birefringent material. All forms of amyloid stain with Congo red, as the reaction is based on the presence of fibril organized into β-pleated sheets. Immunohistochemistry can also be used not only to identify amyloid deposits but also to identify the specific constituents composing the deposits (e.g., anti-β-light chain antibodies). By electron microscopy, amyloid fibrils are characterized as nonbranching, 7.5- to 10-nm

diameter tubules. Descriptions of individual organ system involvement are covered in their respective chapters.

SUGGESTED READINGS

Abbas AK: Diseases of immunity. In Kumar V, Abbas AK, Fausto N, editors: *Robbins & Cotran pathologic basis of disease*, ed 7, Philadelphia, 2005, Saunders.

Akira S, Takeda K: Toll-like receptor signaling, *Nat Rev Immunol* 4:499-511, 2004.

Bauer TR Jr, Gu YC, Creevy KE et al: Leukocyte adhesion deficiency in children and Irish setter dogs, *Pediatr Res* 55:363-367, 2004.

Buckley RH: Primary immunodeficiency diseases: dissectors of the immune system, *Immunol Rev* 185:206-219, 2002.

Chabanne L, Fournel C, Rigal D et al: Canine systemic lupus erythematosus. Part I. Clinical and biological aspects, *Comp Cont Ed* 21:135-141, 1999.

Goldsby RA, Kindt TJ, Osborne BA, Kuby J: *Immunology*, ed 5, New York, 2003, WH Freeman.

Janeway CA, Jr, Medzhitov R: Innate immune recognition, *Annu Rev Immunol* 20:197-216, 2002.

Kyewski B, Derbinski J: Self-representation in the thymus: an extended view, *Nat Rev Immunol* 4:688-698, 2004.

Leonard WJ: Type I cytokines and interferons and their receptors. In Paul WE, editor: *Fundamental immunology*, New York, 2004, Lippincott Williams & Wilkins.

Merlini G, Bellotti V: Molecular mechanisms of amyloidosis, *N Engl J Med* 349:583-596, 2003.

Mok CC, Lau CS: Pathogenesis of systemic lupus erythematosus, *J Clin Pathol* 56:481-490, 2003.

O'Garra A, Vieira P: Regulatory T cells and mechanisms of immune system control, *Nat Med* 10:801-805, 2004.

Pedersen NC: A review of immunologic diseases of the dog, *Vet Immunol Immunopathol* 69:251-342, 1999.

Perryman LE: Primary immunodeficiencies of horses, *Vet Clin North Am Equine Pract* 16:105-116, 2000.

Perryman LE: Molecular pathology of severe combined immunodeficiency in mice, horses, and dogs, *Vet Pathol* 41:95-100, 2004.

Schwartz RH: T cell anergy, *Annu Rev Immunol* 21:305-334, 2003.

Sharpe AH, Freeman GJ: The B7-CD28 superfamily, *Nat Rev Immunol* 2:116-126, 2002.

Simonte SJ, Cunningham-Rundles C: Update on primary immunodeficiency: defects of lymphocytes, *Clin Immunol* 109:109-118, 2003.

Takeda K, Kaisho T, Akira S: Toll-like receptors, *Annu Rev Immunol* 21:335-376, 2003.

Tizard IR: *Veterinary immunology: an introduction*, Philadelphia, 2000, Saunders.

Ward DM, Shiflett SL, Kaplan J: Chédiak-Higashi syndrome: a clinical and molecular view of a rare lysosomal storage disorder, *Curr Mol Med* 5:469-477, 2002.

Werling D, Jungi TW: Toll-like receptors linking innate and adaptive immune response, *Vet Immunol Immunopathol* 91:1-12, 2003.

Wills-Karp M, Hershey GKK: Immunologic mechanisms of allergic disorders. In Paul WE, editor: *Fundamental immunology*, New York, 2004, Lippincott Williams & Wilkins.

6

Neoplasia and Tumor Biology

DONNA F. KUSEWITT • LAURA J. RUSH

Despite the relatively short life span of most animals, neoplasia is an important concern for veterinary practitioners, diagnosticians, and researchers. Tumor diagnosis and treatment for individual animals is becoming an increasingly prominent part of small animal practice. In food animals, infectious and environmental causes of cancer can have a major impact on herd or flock health. Furthermore, animal models provide important insights into the cause and treatment of human cancer.

DEFINITIONS

A neoplasm is a "new growth" composed of cells, originally derived from normal tissues, that have undergone heritable genetic changes allowing them to become relatively unresponsive to normal growth controls and to expand beyond their normal anatomic boundaries. Other common terms for neoplasms describe their clinical appearance or behavior: tumor ("swelling") and cancer ("crab"). Although the terms *neoplasm* and *tumor* may refer to benign or malignant growths, the term *cancer* always denotes a malignant growth. Oncology is the study of neoplasia; the term is derived from the Greek word *oncos* ("tumor").

Benign tumors do not invade surrounding tissue or spread to new anatomic locations within the body; thus these tumors are usually curable and are rarely responsible for the death of the host. Malignant tumors, if left untreated, will invade locally, may spread by metastasis ("change of place"), and will ultimately kill the host. Interestingly, tumors of the nervous system very rarely metastasize; however, many of these tumors are notably invasive and kill their hosts, thus the tumors are malignant.

With the recognition that tumor development is a stepwise process, potentially preneoplastic changes have assumed new diagnostic and clinical significance. These changes include hyperplasia (increased cell number in a tissue), metaplasia (transformation of one differentiated cell type into another), and dysplasia (abnormal pattern of tissue growth) (Fig. 6-1). Hyperplasia, which is an increase in the number of cells in a tissue, should be distinguished from hypertrophy, which is an increase in individual cell size rather than number. Metaplasia is seen most commonly in epithelial tissue. In several species of animals, vitamin A deficiency is characterized by squamous metaplasia of respiratory and digestive epithelium. Dysplasia usually refers to disorderly arrangement of cells within epithelium. In general, preneoplastic changes are reversible. They arise in response to physiologic demands, injury, or irritation and resolve with the removal of the inciting factor. For example, epidermal hyperplasia is a normal part of wound repair, and skeletal muscle hypertrophy is an adaptive response to increased workload. Preneoplastic changes often indicate an increased risk for neoplasia in the affected tissue, and preneoplastic lesions may themselves progress to neoplasia. The terms *dysplasia* and *metaplasia* can be applied to tumors to describe changes that persist during the transition from preneoplasia to neoplasia; however, the terms *hyperplasia* and *hypertrophy* are not appropriate in descriptions of true neoplasms.

NOMENCLATURE

Most tumors appear to consist of a single cell type, and the name of the neoplasm reflects the cell type (mesenchymal or epithelial) from which the tumor is presumed to arise.

MESENCHYMAL TUMORS

Mesenchymal tumors arise in cells of embryonic mesodermal origin. Benign tumors originating from mesenchymal cells are usually named by adding the suffix *-oma* to the name of the cell of origin. Thus a lipoma is a benign tumor derived from a lipocyte ("fat cell") (Fig. 6-2, *A*), and a fibroma is a benign tumor

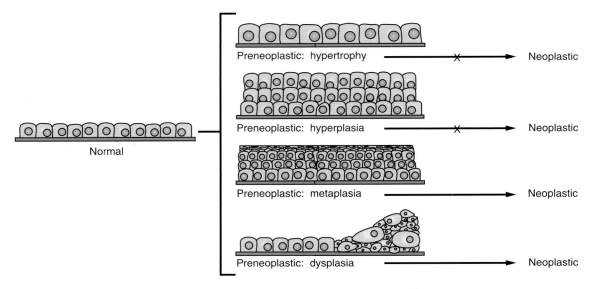

Fig. 6-1   **Preneoplastic changes that may precede tumor emergence.** Preneoplastic changes in tissues include alterations in cell number, size, and organization. Some of these terms can also be applied to neoplastic tissues, as indicated. In this example, preneoplastic changes are illustrated in simple cuboidal epithelium, although such changes may also occur in other epithelial and mesenchymal cell types. *(Redrawn with permission from Dr. D.F. Kusewitt, College of Veterinary Medicine, The Ohio State University.)*

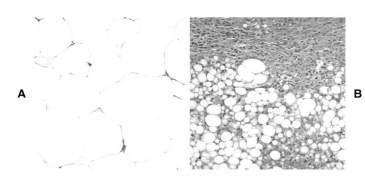

Fig. 6-2   Comparison of benign and malignant tumors of lipocyte origin, dog. A, The benign lipoma is composed of mature fat cells indistinguishable from normal cells. H&E stain. **B,** The liposarcoma consists of poorly differentiated cells, many of which do not have the morphologic features characteristic of lipocytes H&E stain. (**A** and **B,** *Courtesy College of Veterinary Medicine, The Ohio State University.*)

of fibroblast origin. A malignant tumor of mesenchymal origin is a sarcoma ("fleshy growth"). A prefix or modifier indicates the tissue of origin. For instance, a liposarcoma is a malignant tumor of lipocyte origin (Fig. 6-2, *B*), and a fibrosarcoma is a tumor composed of malignant fibroblasts. The cells comprising the hematopoietic system are mesenchymal. Tumors arising from circulating blood cells or their precursors are termed leukemias ("white blood"); neoplastic hematopoietic cells are

usually found in large numbers in the blood stream (Fig. 6-3), although they may also form solid tumor masses.

EPITHELIAL TUMORS

All of the three embryonic cell layers—endoderm, mesoderm, and ectoderm—can give rise to epithelial tissue and to tumors derived from this tissue. Terms for both benign and malignant epithelial tumors are frequently modified by prefixes or adjectives describing their appearance or the response they elicit in surrounding tissue. For instance, the adjective "squamous" is applied to an epithelial neoplasm that demonstrates squamous differentiation.

Benign tumors that arise from glandular epithelium are called adenomas, whatever their microscopic appearance. However, the term is also applied to many tumors that are derived from nonglandular epithelial tissues but that have a tubular appearance, such as renal adenomas. The term *papilloma* refers to a benign exophytic growth arising from an epithelial surface, whereas a polyp is a grossly visible, benign epithelial tumor projecting from a mucosal surface (Fig. 6-4).

All malignant tumors of epithelial origin are termed carcinomas ("cancers"). The general term *carcinoma* may be further modified to indicate the organ of origin, as in hepatocellular carcinoma. The prefix *adeno-* indicates

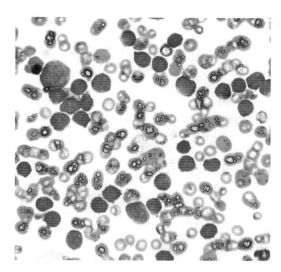

Fig. 6-3   Acute lymphoid leukemia, peripheral blood, dog. The peripheral blood smear contains numerous neoplastic large lymphocytes. Flow cytometry identified these cells as B lymphocytes. The white blood cell count of this animal was 293,000 leukocytes per μL. **Wright's stain.** *(Courtesy Dr. M.L. Wellman, College of Veterinary Medicine, The Ohio State University.)*

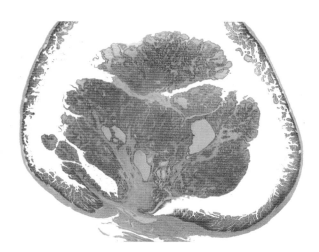

Fig. 6-4   Polyp, small intestine, mouse. The neoplastic growth arises from the mucosa and extends into the lumen of the intestine. There is no invasion of the intestinal wall. **H&E stain.** *(Courtesy College of Veterinary Medicine, The Ohio State University.)*

a glandular pattern of tumor growth. Adenocarcinomas may be described as papillary, tubular, or cystic. Carcinomas and adenocarcinomas that stimulate the formation of abundant collagen in surrounding connective tissue (desmoplasia) may be termed scirrhous. The neoplastic epithelial cells of mucinous carcinomas and adenocarcinomas produce abundant mucin. Carcinoma in situ is a preinvasive form of carcinoma

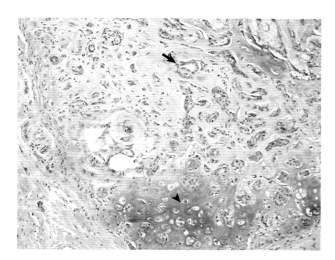

Fig. 6-5   Mixed mammary tumor, mammary gland, dog. Mixed mammary tumors of dogs contain both epithelial structures (*arrow*) and mesenchymal elements, such as cartilage and bone (*arrowhead*). **H&E stain.** *(Courtesy College of Veterinary Medicine, The Ohio State University.)*

that remains within the epithelial structure from which it arises and does not penetrate the basement membrane to enter the stroma.

UNDIFFERENTIATED TUMORS

The appearance of some malignant tumors gives no clue to their cell of origin; thus they are termed undifferentiated neoplasms.

MIXED TUMORS

Mixed tumors contain multiple cell types derived from a single or multiple germ layers. Mixed tumors are believed to arise from a single pluripotential or totipotential cell capable of differentiating into a variety of more mature cell types. Teratomas and teratocarcinomas arise from totipotential germ cells; thus they contain tissue derived from all embryonic cell layers and consist of a bizarre mixture of adult and embryonic tissue types. The mixed mammary gland tumor of dogs is generally considered a mixed tumor. A mixed mammary tumor is composed of a variable admixture of neoplastic epithelial elements (luminal epithelium and myoepithelium) and mesenchymal elements (fibrous connective tissue, fat, cartilage, and bone) (Fig. 6-5).

TUMORLIKE LESIONS

Hamartomas are disorganized but mature mesenchymal or epithelial tissues found in their normal anatomic location. Many of the hamartomas identified in animals consist of abnormal proliferations of blood vessels.

Hamartomas apparently represent the result of aberrant differentiation rather than true neoplasia, and their behavior is completely benign. Choristomas are composed of normal mature tissue located at an ectopic site. An example is the dermoid, a mass consisting of mature skin and its appendages, which may be found in a variety of unusual sites, including the cornea.

VETERINARY NOMENCLATURE

In Table 6-1, the names of common benign neoplasms in animals and their malignant counterparts are shown. The names given are those commonly employed in veterinary medicine. The terms used by veterinary pathologists to describe tumors in animals may differ from the terms used by medical pathologists to describe human tumors. This is partly because conventional usage plays an important role in tumor nomenclature; thus tumor nomenclature may be dictated by historical precedent rather than by logic. Moreover, attempts to standardize diagnostic terms for tumors in veterinary medicine have lagged far behind such efforts in the medical arena. A significant difference between veterinary and human nomenclature is that a benign tumor arising from melanocytes is termed a "benign melanoma" or "melanocytoma" by veterinary pathologists and a "nevus" by medical pathologists. Medical pathologists reserve the term *melanoma* for a malignant tumor of melanocyte origin, whereas veterinary pathologists term such tumors "malignant melanomas."

Table **6-1**   **Tumor Nomenclature**

	ORIGIN	Tissue of Origin	Cell of Origin	Benign	Malignant
MESENCHYMAL	Connective tissue and related tissue	Fibrous connective tissue	Fibroblast	Fibroma	Fibrosarcoma
		Fat	Adipocyte	Lipoma	Liposarcoma
		Cartilage	Chondrocyte	Chondroma	Chondrosarcoma
		Bone	Osteoblast	Osteoma	Osteosarcoma
	Endothelium and related tissue	Blood vessel	Vascular endothelium	Hemangioma	Hemangiosarcoma
		Lymphatic vessel	Lymphatic endothelium	Lymphangioma	Lymphangiosarcoma
		Synovium	Synovial lining cell	Synovioma	Synovial sarcoma
		Mesothelium	Mesothelial cell		Mesothelioma
		Meninges	Meningeal connective tissue cell	Meningioma	Malignant meningioma
		Ovary	Modified mesothelium	Adenoma	Adenocarcinoma
	Hematopoietic and lymphoid tissue	Lymphoid tissue	Lymphocytes	*	Lymphoma
		Bone marrow	Leukocytes and erythrocytes	*	Leukemia
		Connective tissue	Mast cell	Mast cell tumor	Malignant mast cell tumor
			Histiocytes	Histiocytoma	Malignant histiocytosis
	Muscle	Smooth muscle	Smooth muscle cell	Leiomyoma	Leiomyosarcoma
		Skeletal muscle	Skeletal muscle cell	Rhabdomyoma	Rhabdomyosarcoma
EPITHELIAL	Lining or covering epithelia	Skin	Squamous epithelial cell	Papilloma	Squamous cell carcinoma
			Adnexal cells	Adenoma	Adenocarcinoma Carcinoma
			Melanocyte	Benign melanoma	Malignant melanoma
		Upper alimentary tract	Squamous epithelial cell	Papilloma	Carcinoma
		Lower alimentary tract	Columnar epithelium	Adenoma	Adenocarcinoma Carcinoma
		Upper respiratory tract	Columnar epithelium	Adenoma	Adenocarcinoma Carcinoma
		Lung	Columnar epithelium of bronchi and bronchioles	Adenoma	Adenocarcinoma Carcinoma

*Not generally recognized.

Table **6-1**   **Tumor Nomenclature—Cont'd**

	ORIGIN	Tissue of Origin	Cell of Origin	Benign	Malignant
EPITHELIAL—Cont'd			Alveolar epithelium	Adenoma	Adenocarcinoma
		Urinary tract	Transitional epithelium	Papilloma	Transitional cell carcinoma
		Uterus	Columnar epithelium	Uterine polyp	Endometrial carcinoma Endometrial adenocarcinoma
	Solid epithelial organs	Lining of glands or ducts	Prostate, thyroid, bile ducts of liver, etc.	Adenoma	Adenocarcinoma Carcinoma
		Glands	Pancreas, salivary gland, etc.	Adenoma	Adenocarcinoma
		Liver	Hepatocyte	Hepatoma	Hepatocellular carcinoma
		Kidney	Renal tubular cell	Renal tubular adenoma	Renal cell carcinoma
		Testicle	Sertoli cell Interstitial cell	Sertoli cell tumor Interstitial cell tumor	Sertoli cell tumor
			Germ cell	Seminoma Teratoma	Seminoma Teratocarcinoma
		Ovary	Stromal cell	Granulosa cell tumor	*
				Luteoma	*
				Thecoma	*
			Germ cell	Dysgerminoma Teratoma	Dysgerminoma Teratocarcinoma
NERVOUS TISSUE	Glial cells	Central nervous system	Astrocyte	*	Astrocytoma Glioblastoma
			Oligodendrocyte	*	Oligodendroglioma
			Microglial cell	*	Microgliomatosis
		Peripheral nervous system	Schwann cell	Schwannoma	Malignant schwannoma
	Neural cells	Central nervous system	Neuron	*	Primitive neuroecto-dermal tumor
		Peripheral nervous system	Neuron	Ganglioneuroma	
MIXED TUMORS	Various	Mammary gland	Epithelium and myoepithelium	Benign mixed mammary tumor (dog) Adenoma	Malignant mixed mammary tumor (dog) Adenocarcinoma
		Testicle	Germ cell	Teratoma	Teratocarcinoma
		Ovary	Germ cell	Teratoma	Teratocarcinoma

TUMOR CHARACTERISTICS

BENIGN VERSUS MALIGNANT TUMORS

The most important distinction between benign and malignant tumors is that malignant tumors are able to invade locally and metastasize systemically, but benign tumors are not. The invasive capabilities of malignant tumors are associated with enhanced tumor cell motility, increased production of proteases, and altered tumor cell adhesion characteristics. Although benign tumors are ultimately distinguished from their malignant counterparts based on invasiveness, a variety of morphologic and behavioral features are generally considered to predict the potential for malignant behavior (Table 6-2). Although both benign and malignant tumors are composed of proliferating cells, malignant tumors have essentially unlimited replicative potential. The tumors are relatively independent of exogenous growth stimulatory molecules and are insensitive to growth inhibitory signals from their environment.

Table **6-2**   **Comparisons between Benign and Malignant Tumors**

Characteristic	Benign	Malignant
Differentiation	Well-differentiated appearance	Usually some lack of differentiation
	Structure similar to tissue of origin	Structure often atypical
	Little or no anaplasia	Variable degree of anaplasia
Growth rate	Slow, progressive expansion	Slow to rapid growth; erratic growth rate
	Rare mitotic figures	Mitotic figures often numerous
	Normal-appearing mitotic figures	Mitotic figures sometimes abnormal
Local invasion	No invasion	Local invasion
	Cohesive and expansile growth	Infiltrative growth
	Capsule often present	Usually no capsule
Metastasis	No metastasis	Frequent metastasis (definitive criterion for malignancy)

Moreover, malignant cells are better able than benign cells to evade programmed cell death (apoptosis) and to escape the host's cytotoxic immune response. Compared with benign tumors, malignant tumors stimulate marked angiogenesis (the formation of new blood vessels), thus assuring adequate tumor nutrition.

Because some benign tumors evolve into malignant neoplasms and some malignant tumors develop increasingly aggressive behavior over time (a process termed malignant progression), tumors may be graded to reflect where they lie on the continuum from benign to highly malignant and/or staged to indicate the extent of tumor spread. Together the grade and stage of the tumor indicate the risk the tumor poses to the host and help determine therapeutic strategy. It should be noted, however, that many benign tumors, such as equine sarcoids, have little or no malignant potential and rarely if ever evolve into malignant tumors.

DIFFERENTIATION

HALLMARKS OF DIFFERENTIATION
MORPHOLOGY

Each normal, fully differentiated, mature tissue type has a characteristic gross and microscopic appearance that varies little from individual to individual of a species. Neoplastic tissues lose these differentiated features of cellular morphology and organization to a variable extent. In general, malignant tumors appear less differentiated than benign tumors. Loss of morphologic hallmarks of tissue maturity is often accompanied by loss of functional capacity and development of aggressive behavior.

Neoplastic cells often show considerable morphologic variability compared with the normal tissue from which they are derived. Tumor cells, especially malignant tumor cells, may exhibit anaplasia (cellular atypia). Anaplastic cells are poorly differentiated cells that exhibit notable cellular and nuclear pleomorphism (variation in size and shape). In some tumors, bizarre tumor giant cells are seen (Fig. 6-6). Nuclei may exhibit

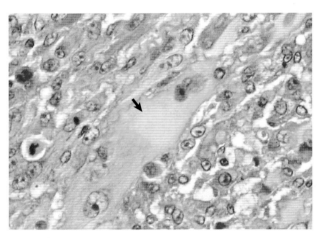

Fig. 6-6   Rhabdomyosarcoma, skeletal muscle, chicken. Rhabdomyosarcomas often contain bizarre tumor giant cells such as the cell indicated by the arrow. H&E stain. (*Courtesy College of Veterinary Medicine, The Ohio State University.*)

extreme variability in number, size, shape, chromatin distribution, and nucleolar size and number (Fig. 6-7). Anaplastic nuclei are often hyperchromatic (darkly staining) because of increased DNA content; are disproportionately large relative to cell size, resulting in an increased nuclear:cytoplasmic ratio; and have prominent nucleoli. Mitotic figures in tumor cells may be numerous. Many of the nuclear changes seen in neoplastic cells reflect the frequent cell division, chromosomal abnormalities, and active metabolic state that characterize these cells.

Neoplastic cells often exhibit loss of characteristic cytoplasmic as well as nuclear features. For instance, poorly differentiated mast cell tumors often lack the prominent cytoplasmic granules that are a hallmark of normal mast cells (Fig. 6-8). Special stains or immunohistochemistry may be able to highlight some characteristic morphologic feature retained in at least a subpopulation of tumor cells. As an example, characteristic granules may be revealed in some cells of feline and canine mast

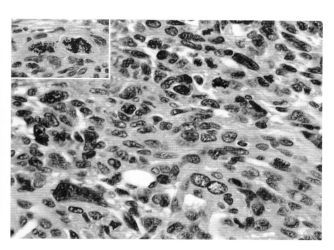

Fig. 6-7   Anaplastic sarcoma, heart, mouse. This tumor exhibits marked nuclear pleomorphism and has a fairly high mitotic index. The inset shows a notably abnormal mitotic figure. H&E stain. (***Figure** and **Inset,** Courtesy College of Veterinary Medicine, The Ohio State University.*)

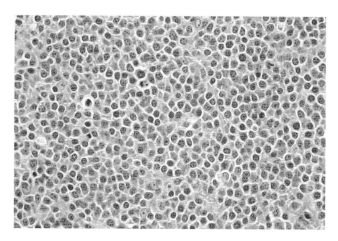

Fig. 6-9   Lymphoma (lymphosarcoma), lymph node, dog. The normal lymph node architecture has been completely effaced by solid sheets of neoplastic lymphocytes. H&E stain. (*Courtesy College of Veterinary Medicine, The Ohio State University.*)

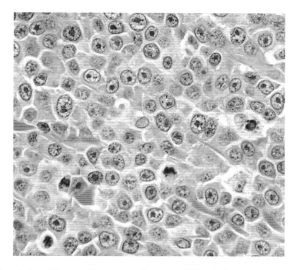

Fig. 6-8   Mast cell tumor, skin, cat. With H&E staining, hallmark mast cell granules are not visible. To see these granules, the section must be stained with a metachromatic stain such as toluidine blue or giemsa. Note the very large single nucleolus and marginated chromatin in the neoplastic cells. H&E stain. (*Courtesy College of Veterinary Medicine, The Ohio State University.*)

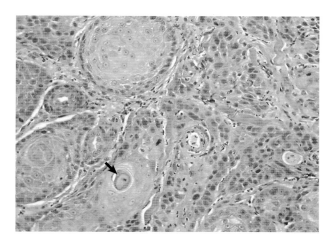

Fig. 6-10   Squamous cell carcinoma, tongue, cat. The orderly pattern of epidermal maturation seen in normal oral mucosa is absent from this squamous cell carcinoma. An occasional "keratin pearl" (*arrow*) reveals the tissue of origin for this tumor. H&E stain. (*Courtesy College of Veterinary Medicine, The Ohio State University.*)

cell tumors by staining with toluidine blue or Giemsa. Many tumor cells have noticeably basophilic cytoplasm as a result of the presence of large numbers of ribosomes required for rapid cell growth and frequent cell division.

In tumors, normal tissue organization is usually lost to some extent. Increasing loss of normal architecture in tumors correlates with increasing independence of tumor cells from their surrounding tissue. As an example, lymphomas arising in lymph nodes often consist of solid sheets of neoplastic cells that partially or completely efface normal lymph node architecture (Fig. 6-9). In tissue that normally undergoes continual renewal, such as the skin and oral mucosa, the normal maturation sequence may be altered. Thus in squamous cell carcinomas, the orderly morphologic progression from basal cell layer to fully keratinized stratum corneum may not be seen (Fig. 6-10).

FUNCTION

Loss of differentiated function frequently accompanies loss of differentiated morphology in tumors.

Thus neoplastic cells arising from alveolar lining cells of the lung generally fail to perform normal respiratory functions and tumors of primitive germ cell origin do not form normal sperm or ova. Some aspects of normal function may be retained. Thyroid adenomas may continue to produce thyroid hormones and plasma cell tumors may secrete immunoglobulins. However, in the majority of cases, these functions are no longer regulated appropriately because the neoplastic cells have lost responsiveness to and dependence upon normal regulatory pathways. Thus thyroid adenomas may produce clinical hyperthyroidism, and plasma cell tumors may cause hypergammaglobulinemia.

BEHAVIOR

Benign tumors are generally expansile and may compress adjacent tissue, whereas malignant tumors have invasive and in many instances metastatic capabilities. In malignant tumors, alterations in adhesion, motility, and protease production allow tumor cells to leave the tumor mass and penetrate surrounding tissue. Moreover, for malignant cells to invade and ultimately metastasize, they must become completely independent of local growth regulatory controls and acquire an independent blood supply. Acquisition of these features allows tumors to spread well beyond their ordinary anatomic niches.

STEM CELLS AND DIFFERENTIATION

Most tumors are composed of cells that lack fully differentiated morphologic, functional, and behavioral characteristics. Furthermore, many neoplastic cells share some features with the embryonic cells that gave rise to the mature tissue in which the tumor originated. This similarity between embryonic and neoplastic cells may be accounted for in two different ways. First, normal mature cells may undergo dedifferentiation as they evolve into tumor cells, leading to the reemergence of more primitive characteristics. Second, tumors may arise from the small population of stem cells found in all adult tissue; such stem cells are required for normal tissue renewal. The appearance and behavior of the tumor that develops from a neoplastic stem cell is determined by the stage of differentiation at which the malignant phenotype is manifested; the neoplastic stem cell is said to have undergone maturation arrest at that stage of its development. The diversity of cell types that can arise from a single progenitor stem cell is limited by the differentiation potential of that cell.

Totipotent stem cells, such as embryonic stem cells, can give rise to all tissues of the body, whereas multipotent or pluripotent stem cells can give rise to a smaller variety of tissue types. The plasticity of most adult stem cells is generally considered to be relatively restricted. Leukemias provide excellent examples of neoplasms arising from stem cells. A leukemia almost always arises

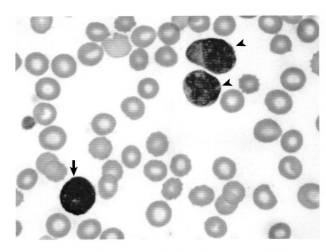

Fig. 6-11 **Myelomonocytic leukemia, peripheral blood, dog.** In this unusual case, leukemic cells of both monocytic (*arrowheads*) and granulocytic (basophil) (*arrow*) origin were present in peripheral blood. The animal had a marked leukocytosis (103,000 white blood cells per μL) and thrombocytopenia. Wright's stain. *(Courtesy Dr. M.J. Burkhard, College of Veterinary Medicine, The Ohio State University.)*

from a single hematopoietic stem cell that has undergone heritable genetic change. The progeny of this stem cell all exhibit the same genetic change, although the cell type and degree of differentiation of the progeny may vary. Thus in myelogenous leukemia, a neoplastic multipotential stem cell may give rise to a combination of leukemic cells of the granulocytic, monocytic, and erythroid series (Fig. 6-11). The concept of a stem cell origin for cancer explains not only the embryonic characteristics of neoplastic cells, but also the success of treatment strategies that use differentiating agents, such as retinoids (vitamin A derivatives used to induce maturation of some human leukemia cells).

PROLIFERATION

THE CELL CYCLE

The cell cycle consists of G_1 (presynthetic), S (DNA synthesis), G_2 (premitotic), and M (mitotic) phases (Fig. 6-12). Quiescent cells are in a physiologic state called G_0. In adult tissue, many cells reside in G_0 and are unable to enter the cell cycle at all or do so only when stimulated by extrinsic factors.

CONTROL OF NORMAL CELL PROLIFERATION AND TISSUE GROWTH*

In adult tissues, the size of a cell population is determined by the relative rates of cell proliferation, differentiation, and death by apoptosis. Fig. 6-13 depicts these relationships and shows that increased cell

---

*Portions of this section are from Kumar V, Abbas A, Fausto N: *Robbins & Cotran pathologic basis of disease*, ed 7, Philadelphia, 2005, Saunders.

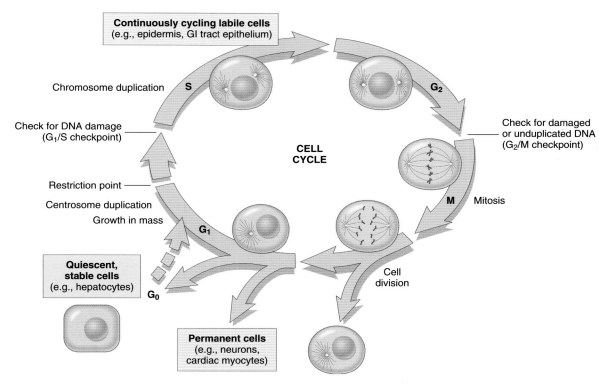

Fig. 6-12   Cell-cycle landmarks. The figure shows the cell-cycle phases (G_0, G_1, G_2, S, and M), the location of the G_1 restriction point, and the G_1/S and G_2/M cell-cycle checkpoints. Cells from labile tissues, such as the epidermis and the gastrointestinal (*GI*) tract, may cycle continuously; stable cells, such as hepatocytes, are quiescent but can enter the cell cycle; permanent cells, such as neurons and cardiac myocytes, have lost the capacity to proliferate. *(Modified from Pollard TD, Earnshaw WC: Cell biology, Philadelphia, 2002, Saunders.)*

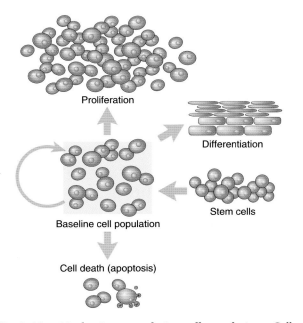

Fig. 6-13   Mechanisms regulating cell populations. Cell numbers can be altered by increased or decreased rates of stem cell input, by cell death due to apoptosis, or by changes in the rates of proliferation or differentiation. *(Modified from McCarthy NJ, Smith CA, Williams GT: Cancer Metastasis Rev 11:157-178, 1992.)*

numbers may result from either increased proliferation or decreased cell death.

PROLIFERATION

Cell proliferation is largely controlled by signals (soluble or contact-dependent) from the microenvironment that either stimulate or inhibit cell proliferation. An excess of stimulators or a deficiency of inhibitors leads to net growth and, in the case of cancer, uncontrolled growth. Although accelerated growth can be accomplished by shortening the cell cycle, the most important mechanism of growth is the conversion of resting or quiescent cells into proliferating cells by making the cells enter the cell cycle. Both the recruitment of quiescent cells into the cycle and cell-cycle progression require stimulatory signals to overcome normal physiologic blocks to cell proliferation. Cell proliferation can be stimulated under both physiologic and pathologic conditions. The proliferation of mammary epithelium under hormonal stimulation during lactation is an example of physiologic proliferation. Pathologic conditions, such as tissue injury, cell death, and mechanical alterations, also stimulate cell proliferation. Excessive physiologic stimulation may create pathologic conditions, such as enlargement of the thyroid as a consequence of increased serum levels of thyroid-stimulating hormone.

DIFFERENTIATION

Differentiation also impacts the size of a cell population and its proliferative potential. For example, myocytes and neurons are terminally differentiated cells (i.e., they are at an end stage of differentiation and are not capable of replicating). In some adult tissues, such as liver and kidney, differentiated cells are normally quiescent but are able to proliferate when necessary. In proliferative tissue, such as bone marrow and the epithelia of the skin and gut, the mature cells are terminally differentiated, short-lived, and incapable of replication, but they may be replaced by new cells arising from stem cells. Thus in such tissues there is a homeostatic equilibrium between the proliferation of stem cells, their differentiation, and the death of fully differentiated cells.

APOPTOSIS

Apoptosis, sometimes called "programmed cell death," is a physiologic process required for tissue homeostasis. In proliferative tissue, such as gut epithelium, terminally differentiated and functionally effete cells undergo apoptosis and are thus removed from the cell population. Apoptosis can also be induced by a variety of pathologic stimuli. Apoptosis may occur in response to withdrawal of survival factors from the cell environment or by binding of death factors, such as Fas ligand and tumor necrosis factor (TNF)-α, to cell surface receptors. Hypoxia and lack of essential nutrients may end in apoptosis. DNA damage may also induce apoptosis; in this case, apoptosis is triggered by p53. Apoptosis may be stimulated by the activity of cytotoxic immune cells, including T lymphocytes and natural killer (NK) cells. Signals for apoptosis activate a variety of signaling pathways, many of which ultimately result in the release of cytochrome C from mitochondria. The final effectors of apoptosis are the caspases, intracellular proteases that selectively destroy cellular organelles and degrade genomic DNA into nucleosome-sized fragments. The morphologic hallmarks of apoptosis include margination of chromatin, condensation and fragmentation of the nucleus, and condensation of the cell with preservation of organelles. Ultimately the cell breaks into membrane-bound apoptotic bodies that are engulfed by surrounding cells without stimulating an inflammatory response (Fig. 6-14).

TISSUE PROLIFERATIVE ACTIVITY

Tissue may be composed primarily of quiescent cells in G_0, but most mature tissue contains some combination of continuously dividing cells, terminally differentiated cells, stem cells, and quiescent cells that enter

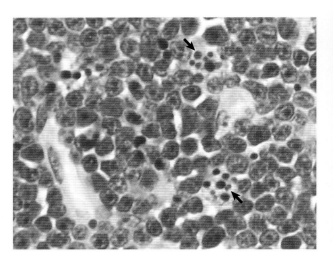

Fig. 6-14   Lymphoma, apoptotic lymphoma cells, spleen, mouse. The light microscopic appearance of apoptosis is characterized by condensation and fragmentation of nuclei (*arrows*), cell shrinkage, engulfment of apoptotic bodies by surrounding cells, and lack of inflammation. H&E stain. (*Courtesy College of Veterinary Medicine, The Ohio State University.*)

the cell cycle. Stem cells have special properties, which were described previously. The tissues of the body may be divided into three groups on the basis of their proliferative activity.

CONTINUOUSLY DIVIDING TISSUES (LABILE TISSUES)

In continuously dividing tissues (also called labile tissues), cells proliferate throughout life, replacing those that are lost. These tissues include surface epithelia, such as stratified squamous surfaces of the skin, oral cavity, vagina, and cervix; the lining mucosa of all the excretory ducts of the glands of the body (e.g., salivary glands, pancreas, and biliary tract); the columnar epithelium of the gastrointestinal tract and uterus; the transitional epithelium of the urinary tract; and cells of the bone marrow and hematopoietic tissue. In most of these tissues, mature cells are derived from stem cells, which have an unlimited capacity to proliferate and whose progeny may differentiate into a variety of mature cell types.

QUIESCENT TISSUES (STABLE TISSUES)

Quiescent (or stable) tissues normally have a low level of replication; however, cells from these tissues can undergo rapid division in response to stimuli and are thus capable of reconstituting the tissue of origin. They are considered to be in the G_0 stage of the cell cycle but can be stimulated to enter G_1. In this category are the parenchymal cells of the liver, kidneys, and pancreas; mesenchymal cells, such as fibroblasts and smooth muscle; vascular endothelial cells; and resting lymphocytes and other leukocytes. The regenerative capacity of stable cells is best exemplified by the ability of the liver to regenerate after partial hepatectomy and after acute chemical injury. Fibroblasts, endothelial cells, smooth muscle cells, chondrocytes, and osteocytes are quiescent in adult mammals but proliferate in response to injury. Fibroblasts in particular may proliferate extensively.

NONDIVIDING TISSUES (PERMANENT TISSUES)

Nondividing (permanent) tissues contain cells that have left the cell cycle and cannot undergo mitotic division in postnatal life. To this group belong neurons, and skeletal and cardiac muscle cells. If neurons in the central nervous system are destroyed, the tissue is generally replaced by the proliferation of the central nervous system supportive elements—the glial cells. However, recent results demonstrate that limited neurogenesis from stem cells may occur in adult brains.

Although mature skeletal muscle cells do not divide, skeletal muscle does have some regenerative capacity, through the differentiation of the satellite cells that are attached to the endomysial sheaths. If the ends of severed muscle fibers are closely juxtaposed, muscle regeneration in mammals can be excellent, but this is a condition that can rarely be attained under practical conditions. Cardiac muscle has very limited, if any, regenerative capacity, and extensive injury to the heart muscle, as may occur in myocardial infarction, is followed by scar formation.

TUMOR GROWTH

As illustrated in Fig. 6-15, the latent period for a tumor is the time before a tumor becomes clinically detectable. The smallest clinically detectable mass is about 1 cm in diameter and contains about 10^9 cells.

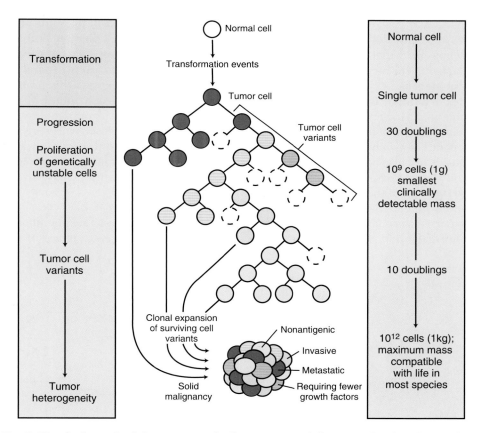

Fig. 6-15   Biology of solid tumor growth. The center panel illustrates clonal evolution of a tumor and generation of tumor-cell heterogeneity. New subclones arise from descendents of the original transformed cell. With progressive growth, the tumor mass becomes enriched for those variants that are more adept at evading host defenses and are likely to be more aggressive. The left panel shows the corresponding stages of tumor progression, and the right panel depicts minimal estimates of tumor-cell doublings that precede the formation of a clinically detectable tumor mass. It is evident that by the time a solid tumor is detected, it has already completed a major portion of its life cycle, as measured by population doublings. The maximum tumor size compatible with life depends to some extent on the species affected. *(Modified from Kumar V, Abbas A, Fausto N: Robbins & Cotran pathologic basis of disease, ed 7, Philadelphia, 2005, Saunders.)*

To form a tumor that size, a single transformed cell must undergo about 30 rounds of cell division, if all the progeny remain viable and capable of replication. Thus, by the time most tumors become clinically evident, they have probably been developing in the host for many years. However, once tumors reach a clinically detectable size, their growth may appear to be very rapid, because only 10 doubling cycles are required to convert a 1-g tumor into a 1-kg tumor. In fact, volume doubling times for tumors vary considerably, depending upon the rate at which tumor cells divide, the fraction of tumor cells that are replicatively competent, and the rate at which tumor cells die. In general, benign neoplasms grow more slowly than malignant tumors, although there is considerable variation among tumors. Moreover, tumors may grow erratically depending on their blood supply, the effect of extrinsic growth-regulating factors such as hormones, the efficacy of the host immune response, and the emergence of subpopulations of particularly aggressive tumor cells.

The mitotic index is usually defined as the number of cells in a microscopic field that contain condensed chromosomes and lack nuclear membranes (Fig. 6-16). Such cells are interpreted as being actively dividing, and the mitotic index of a tumor is considered to indicate its malignant potential. However, the mitotic index can be misleading. The fraction of tumor cells observed to be in mitosis depends not only on the number of cells undergoing mitosis but also on the length of time required to complete the process. In tumor cells, the time required for completion of the cell cycle is generally as long as or even longer than for normal cells. Mitotic figures may persist in cells unable to complete cell division and abnormal mitotic figures may be seen.

PROLIFERATIVE POTENTIAL

Essentially unlimited proliferative potential is a hallmark of neoplasia, especially of malignant neoplasms. Unlike normal cells, many tumor cells are immortal. This immortality is due to a combination of the alterations discussed later. In general, neoplastic cells escape normal limits on cell division, become independent of external growth stimulatory and inhibitory factors, and lose their susceptibility to apoptotic signals. This results in an imbalance between cell production and cell loss and a net increase in tumor size. However, it should be noted that the growth of a tumor is not completely exponential. A proportion of tumor cells is continually lost from the replicative pool because of irreversible cell-cycle arrest, differentiation, and death (Fig. 6-17).

TELOMERASE

Because the DNA replication machinery is unable to duplicate the extreme ends of DNA templates, the telomeres that form the ends of chromosomes are shortened at each cell division. Embryonic cells express telomerase, a riboprotein enzyme that allows telomeres to be replicated and even expanded; however, most adult cells do not express this protein and their telomeres shrink with each round of cell division. Very short telomeres are incompatible with continued cell division. Many neoplastic cells regain the ability to produce telomerase and thus to replicate their telomeres. Reexpression of telomerase appears to play an important role in tumor cell immortality.

CELL CYCLE

Many adult cell types are not mitotically active. These cells have exited the G_1 phase of the cell cycle and

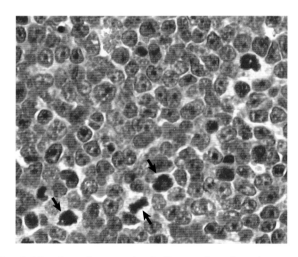

Fig. 6-16   Lymphoma, mitotic figures, lymph node, mouse. The arrows indicate mitotic figures. This tumor has a high mitotic index. H&E stain. *(Courtesy College of Veterinary Medicine, The Ohio State University.)*

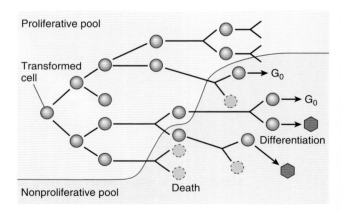

Fig. 6-17   Schematic representation of tumor growth. As the cell population expands, a progressively higher percentage of tumor cells leave the replicative pool by reversion to G_0, differentiation, and death. *(From Kumar V, Abbas A, Fausto N: Robbins & Cotran pathologic basis of disease, ed 7, Philadelphia, 2005, Saunders.)*

reside in G_0. Moreover, in response to DNA damage, even actively dividing normal cells undergo cell-cycle arrest, usually at one of several cell-cycle checkpoints. Cell-cycle arrest is initiated by the multifunctional tumor suppressor gene product p53 and gives the cell time to repair DNA damage. Many neoplastic cells no longer respond to extrinsic or intrinsic signals directing them into G_0 and no longer express functional p53. Thus the cells move continuously through the cell cycle. Moreover, because the tumor cells do not undergo cell-cycle arrest following DNA damage, they progressively accumulate potentially mutagenic DNA damage (Fig. 6-18).

GROWTH MODULATION

For homeostasis to be maintained, normal cells must engage in a continual dialogue with their environment. There is a constant exchange of information among cells via soluble mediators, including growth stimulatory factors, growth inhibitory factors, and hormones. These soluble mediators tightly control the growth of nonneoplastic cells. Neoplastic cells, on the other hand, often lose both their dependence upon extrinsic growth stimulatory substances and their susceptibility to growth inhibitory signals from their environment. The mechanisms by which this occurs are discussed later. The end result is that tumor cells are no longer responsive to the needs of the organism as a whole and develop the capacity to drive their own replication.

APOPTOSIS

Although virtually all normal cells in the body can undergo apoptosis (programmed cell death) in response to appropriate physiologic signals, many cancer cells acquire resistance to apoptosis. This blocks a major route of tumor cell loss and enhances the overall growth rate of the tumor. Many tumor cells circumvent apoptosis by functional inactivation of the p53 gene, thus removing a key proapoptotic molecule. Additionally, tumor cells may constitutively activate survival signaling pathways, rendering the cells independent of exogenous survival factors. Finally, tumor cells may develop mechanisms for inactivating death factor signaling pathways, thus evading apoptosis in response to homeostatic signals from the cellular environment.

GENOMIC INSTABILITY

Evolving genomic instability is a hallmark of cancer. Many tumor cells fail to undergo cell-cycle arrest or apoptosis in response to DNA damage. They produce long and unstable telomeres subject to breakage, they lose the ability to carry out effective DNA repair, they demonstrate aberrant DNA methylation, and they exhibit increased rates of gene amplification, recombination, conversion, and transposition. These factors contribute to an increased rate of mutation and chromosomal aberration in neoplastic cells. Ultimately, this genomic instability results in aneuploidy, a chromosome complement that is not a simple multiple of the haploid chromosome content, or polyploidy, a chromosome complement more than twice the haploid chromosome number. The karyotypes of cancer cells may thus be notably abnormal and unstable. As a rule, increasing aneuploidy is correlated with increasingly malignant behavior. Genomic instability will be discussed in more detail later in the chapter.

TUMOR EVOLUTION

STEPWISE TUMOR DEVELOPMENT

Neoplasms develop as the result of multiple genetic and epigenetic changes that occur over a relatively long time course. It is the cumulative effect of these alterations that create a tumor. The stepwise evolution of tumors has been studied most thoroughly in carcinomas. There are several types of carcinoma that develop in an orderly and predictable fashion. For instance, squamous cell carcinoma arises from the epithelium of the eyelid in many species of animals, including cattle, horses, cats, and dogs. In all species, these tumors develop through the same sequence of steps: epidermal hyperplasia, carcinoma in situ, and invasive carcinoma. Extensive studies of experimentally induced squamous cell carcinomas in the skin of mice have revealed a similar morphologic pattern of tumor evolution (Fig. 6-19) and have led to a detailed model of stepwise carcinoma development as described in the following section (Fig. 6-20).

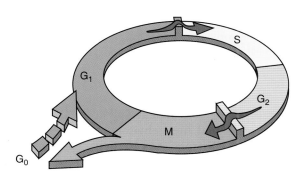

Fig. 6-18   **Schematic representation of the cell cycle.** Many normal cells reside in G_0, a nonreplicative state. When they do enter the proliferative cycle, they can arrest at cell-cycle checkpoints at the G_1-S and G_2-M boundaries in response to a variety of stimuli, including DNA damage. In contrast, tumor cells spend little time in G_0 and often do not undergo cell-cycle arrest in response to DNA damage or lack of extrinsic growth stimuli. *(Modified from Kumar V, Abbas A, Fausto N:* Robbins & Cotran pathologic basis of disease, *ed 7, Philadelphia, 2005, Saunders.)*

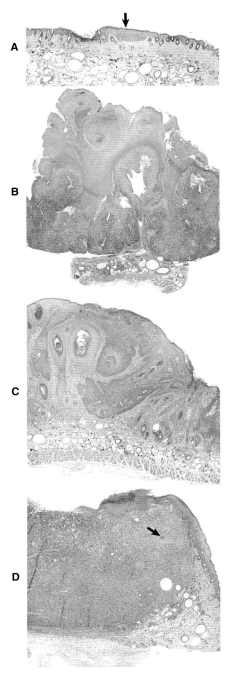

Fig. 6-19   **Development of squamous cell carcinoma in the skin of a hairless mouse exposed to ultraviolet radiation.** **A,** A focus of epidermal hyperplasia *(arrow)* is the earliest lesion seen. **B,** This develops into a papilloma, a benign exophytic papillary growth that is highly keratinized and does not penetrate into the dermis. **C,** As the papilloma undergoes conversion into a malignant squamous cell carcinoma, it begins to invade the dermis and to lose the regular pattern of epithelial differentiation. **D,** A fully developed squamous cell carcinoma has lost most differentiated characteristics and extends deep into the dermis. Only a few keratin "pearls" *(arrow)* indicate the origin of this tumor from the epidermis of the skin. All figures were taken at the same magnification. H&E stain. (*A* through *D,* Courtesy Dr. T.M. Oberyszyn, The Ohio State University.)

INITIATION

The first step is initiation, the introduction of irreversible genetic change into basal cells of the skin by the action of a mutagenic initiating agent or initiator. Initiators are chemical or physical carcinogens that damage DNA. Mutation induction requires not only the introduction of a DNA lesion, but also mispairing of the DNA lesion during subsequent DNA replication to produce an altered complementary DNA strand. Thus at least a single round of DNA replication is necessary for fixation of the genetic change to occur. Initiated cells appear morphologically normal and may remain quiescent for many years. However, these cells harbor mutations that provide them with a growth advantage under special conditions. For instance, the initiated cells may respond more vigorously to mitogenic signals or be more resistant to apoptosis-inducing stimuli than their neighbors.

PROMOTION

The second stage of tumor development is promotion. Promotion refers to the outgrowth of initiated cells in response to selective stimuli. Most of these selective stimuli, termed promoting agents or promoters, drive proliferation. For example, the skin irritant croton oil is an effective skin tumor promoter. In general, promoters are not mutagenic; instead, they alter gene expression in initiated and uninitiated cells to create an environment in which initiated cells have a growth advantage. Because promoters are nonmutagenic, their effects are usually reversible, and some papillomas can actually undergo regression. What emerges at the end of the promotion phase of tumor development is a papilloma, a benign tumor.

PROGRESSION

The final stage of tumor development, progression, includes the conversion of a benign tumor to an increasingly malignant tumor and, ultimately, to a metastatic tumor. Malignant conversion represents an irreversible change in the nature of the developing tumor. Progression is a complex and poorly understood process involving both genetic and epigenetic changes in tumor cells and their environment that select for increasingly malignant clones of tumor cells. Karyotypic instability in tumor cells and increasing tumor cell heterogeneity are hallmarks of progression.

TUMOR HETEROGENEITY AND CLONAL SELECTION

Most tumors are believed to be of clonal origin (i.e., they are ultimately derived from a single transformed cell). Tumor cell heterogeneity is generated during the course of tumor growth by the progressive accumulation of heritable changes in tumor cells (Fig. 6-15). With each

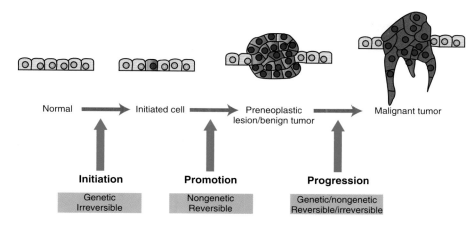

Fig. 6-20   **Illustration of stepwise tumor development.** Initiated cells have irreversible genetic damage. In the presence of a promoter, these initiated cells expand to form a preneoplastic lesion or benign tumor. With further genetic and epigenetic alterations, a malignant tumor emerges from a subclone of cells within the benign precursor lesion. *(Redrawn with permission from Dr. D.F. Kusewitt, College of Veterinary Medicine, The Ohio State University.)*

new genetic alteration, the progeny of the genetically altered tumor cell constitute a subclone of tumor cells. The generation of subclones is fostered by the marked genetic instability of tumor cells compared with normal cells. Successful subclones are those that have a high proliferative rate, are able to evade the host immune response, can stimulate the development of an independent blood supply, are independent of exogenous growth factors, and are able to escape from the primary tumor and spread to distant sites. These characteristics give successful subclones a selective advantage over other subclones of cells within the tumor. A tumor subclone with a selective advantage will eventually predominate.

MOLECULAR CHANGES UNDERLYING TUMOR PROGRESSION

In a few well-studied tumor types, such as chemically induced skin tumors in mice and colonic carcinomas in humans, the stepwise molecular changes that underlie morphologic changes in the tumors have been determined. Many of these genetic changes are associated with proliferation, DNA repair, angiogenesis, and invasiveness, as detailed later.

TUMOR SPREAD

FEATURES OF TUMOR SPREAD

Malignant tumors are often highly invasive. They do not respect anatomic boundaries, and they infiltrate adjacent normal tissue. Benign tumors, on the other hand, are generally expansile rather than infiltrative. The border between a benign tumor and adjacent tissue is usually distinct, and benign tumors of epithelial origin are often encapsulated (surrounded by a connective

tissue capsule). Metastasis occurs when colonies of tumor cells take up residence at some distance from the parent tumor. Metastasis is the single most reliable hallmark of malignancy. Benign tumors do not metastasize. However, some malignant tumors, notably those of the central nervous system, are also nonmetastatic. Metastatic disease is believed to be responsible for 90% of human cancer deaths. Moreover, it is estimated that approximately 30% of solid cancers in humans have already metastasized by the time of initial diagnosis, greatly reducing the possibility of successful therapy. Cancer may metastasize by seeding of the body cavities and surfaces (transcoelomic spread), by lymphatic spread, or by hematogenous spread.

PATHWAYS OF TUMOR METASTASIS

TRANSCOELOMIC

When cancers arise on the surface of an abdominal or thoracic structure, they encounter few anatomic barriers to spread. Thus mesotheliomas may be confined to the abdominal or pleural cavities, but the tumor cells within these cavities readily spread to cover all visceral and parietal surfaces (Fig. 6-21). In both humans and dogs, ovarian adenocarcinomas preferentially spread transcoelomically. Although such tumors are rare in dogs, they are commonly encountered in women. Even in the absence of invasion into the underlying organs, tumors such as mesotheliomas and ovarian adenocarcinomas are extremely difficult to treat and are generally fatal.

LYMPHATIC

In general, most carcinomas metastasize via the lymphatic system, although sarcomas may also employ this route of spread. The pattern of lymph node

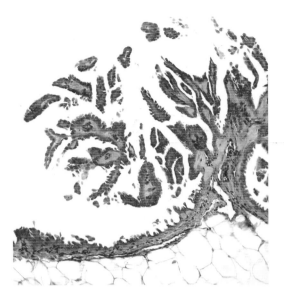

Fig. 6-21 **Mesothelioma, peritoneum of the abdominal cavity, dog.** Mesotheliomas spread extensively within body cavities, but rarely metastasize by lymphatic or hematogenous routes. Note in the figure that neoplastic mesothelial cells cover the serosal surfaces and form papillary fronds, but they do not infiltrate underlying tissue. H&E stain. (*Courtesy College of Veterinary Medicine, The Ohio State University.*)

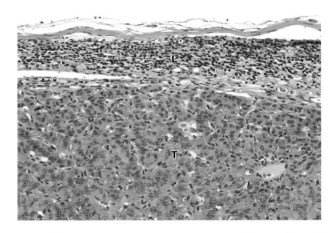

Fig. 6-22 **Pancreatic carcinoma, metastatic, hepatic (portal) lymph node, dog.** Tumor cells (*T*) have almost completely replaced the normal architecture of the lymph node, except for a thin subcapsular rim of lymphocytes (*L*). The tumor was confirmed by immunohistochemistry to be a functional pancreatic islet β-cell carcinoma. H&E stain. (*Courtesy College of Veterinary Medicine, The Ohio State University.*)

involvement is usually dictated by preexisting routes of regional lymphatic drainage. The lymph nodes closest to the tumor are usually colonized earliest and develop the largest metastatic tumor masses (Fig. 6-22). Thus adenocarcinomas of the intestine in all species usually metastasize first to the mesenteric lymph nodes and

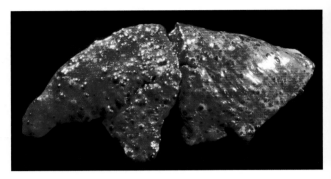

Fig. 6-23 **Hemangiosarcoma, metastatic, lung, dog.** The multifocal (embolic) distribution of tumor nodules of relatively uniform size throughout the lung is characteristic of hematogenous metastasis. (*Courtesy College of Veterinary Medicine, The Ohio State University.*)

later to other lymph nodes within and outside the abdominal cavity. For many years, it was assumed that cancers spread in a stepwise manner from the primary site to regional lymph nodes, then to distant sites, such as the lung, and that regional lymph nodes actually represented a mechanical barrier to the spread of cancer. Thus removal of regional lymph nodes containing tumor tissue was believed to protect the patient from further spread of the tumor. However, regional lymph nodes may be bypassed as a result of natural, tumor-related, or treatment-induced anomalies in lymphatic drainage. More recent studies suggest that lymphatic spread does not occur in an orderly fashion and that metastasis to regional lymph nodes indicates that neoplastic disease has become widely systemic.

HEMATOGENOUS

Because lymphatic vessels connect with the vascular system, the distinction between lymphatic and hematogenous spread is somewhat artificial. However, sarcomas do tend to use the hematogenous route of spread more frequently than carcinomas. Tumors generally invade veins rather than do arteries because arterial walls are much thicker and more difficult to penetrate. Tumors that enter veins ultimately enter the vena cava and lodge in the lungs (Fig. 6-23) or enter the portal system and lodge in the liver. Neoplasms metastatic to the lungs may secondarily enter the arterial circulation. Some tumors have a notable predilection for veins. Pheochromocytomas of many species frequently enter the adrenal veins, where they may form large tumor masses extending into the vena cava.

MECHANISMS OF INVASION AND METASTASIS

Metastasis is a complex process requiring invasion of the extracellular matrix (ECM), entry into blood vascular

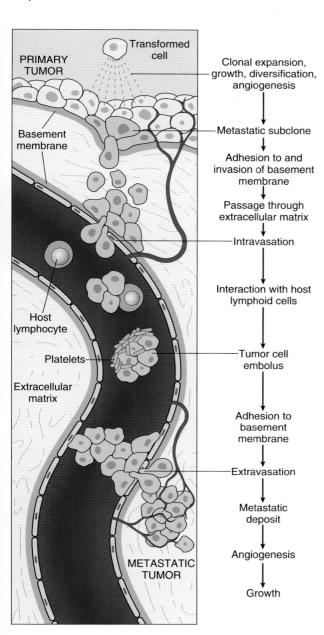

Fig. 6-24   The metastatic cascade. This figure illustrates the sequential steps involved in the hematogenous spread of a tumor. Similar events occur during lymphatic spread. *(From Kumar V, Abbas A, Fausto N: Robbins & Cotran pathologic basis of disease, ed 7, Philadelphia, 2005, Saunders.)*

or lymphatic vessels, extravasation of tumor cells, and colonization of the metastatic site (Fig. 6-24). These activities require many coordinated alterations in cell-cell and cell-matrix adhesion, motility, and invasiveness. Due to the complexity of the metastatic process and the heterogeneity of tumor cells, metastasis is inefficient. Of the many tumor cells that enter the circulation, only a few are able to produce metastases. Local invasion is a prerequisite for metastasis; thus the two processes share many features.

ADHESION

As a first event in invasion and metastasis, tumor cells must detach from the main tumor mass, penetrate the basement membrane, and enter the ECM. For cells to separate from each other, intercellular adhesion structures, including desmosomes and adherens junctions, must be dismantled. In many tumor cells of epithelial origin, this occurs because of the loss of cadherin or catenin function. These molecules are essential structural elements of intercellular junctions. At the same time that tumor cells detach from each other, they must also establish contacts with ECM components. Integrins and other specific receptors on the tumor cell membrane recognize and bind to a variety of ECM components, such as fibronectin, laminin, collagen, and vitronectin. During invasion and metastasis, carcinoma cells often express increased numbers of these receptors. Moreover, instead of being localized to the basal surface of the tumor cell, the receptors are redistributed to cover the entire cell membrane. Tumor cells also appear to be able to modulate the types of ECM receptors that they express, allowing the cells to adapt to different microenvironments.

INVASION

Nonneoplastic epithelial cells generally rest on a specialized extracellular structure called the basement membrane to which they are firmly attached by hemidesmosomes. In benign epithelial tumors the basement membrane usually remains intact, whereas in malignant tumors the neoplastic epithelial cells penetrate the basement membrane to invade surrounding tissue. Tumor cells actively degrade basement membrane and ECM components by increasing the net protease activity in their vicinity (Fig. 6-25). Net protease activity is determined by a variety of interacting factors, including the rate of protease synthesis, the rate at which proteases are activated, and the rate at which protease inhibitors are produced. Proteases and antiproteases may be produced and activated by the tumor cells themselves, or tumor cells may induce nonneoplastic stromal cells to produce these enzymes. Proteases that appear to play an important role in tumor metastasis include matrix metalloproteinases, such as type IV collagenase, and urokinase, a serine protease.

MIGRATION

At many points during invasion and metastasis, tumor cells migrate actively. This migration appears to be mediated by coordinated alterations in the cytoskeleton and the cellular adhesion structures with which they are intimately associated. Tumor cell migration is stimulated by autocrine growth factors, such as hepatocyte growth factor, also called "scatter factor," and by

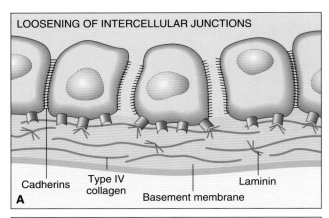

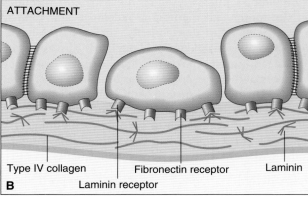

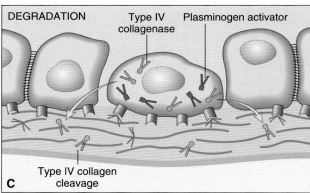

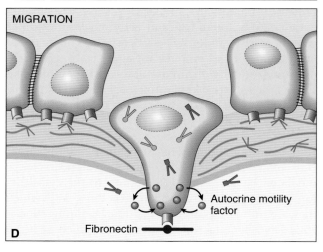

cleavage products of ECM components, including fragments of collagen.

TUMOR EMBOLI

The processes by which tumor cells invade blood and lymphatic vessels, extravasate from these vessels, and invade the ECM at a metastatic site are variations on those discussed earlier. Once inside a lymphatic or blood vessel, tumor cells tend to associate to form small emboli. In vessels, tumor cells may be recognized and attacked by host lymphocytes or may be surrounded by platelets. Interestingly, platelets may actually protect the tumor embolus and enhance tumor metastasis. The site at which tumor cells exit the blood vascular or lymphatic system is determined both by the pattern of lymphatic or vascular drainage of the primary tumor and by the ability of tumor cells to interact with adhesion molecules on endothelial cells. In addition, metastatic sites must provide a suitable microenvironment for tumor cell growth. Some tumors preferentially metastasize to specific sites. For example, prostate carcinomas in both humans and dogs frequently spread to bone (Fig. 6-26).

METASTASIS SUPPRESSION

A wide variety of genetic and epigenetic changes affect tumor cell adhesion, motility, and protease production. Thus metastatic potential is probably the cumulative effect of many different genetic alterations, and it seems unlikely that any individual genetic change single-handedly makes a tumor metastatic. On the other hand, a small number of genes have been identified that seem to function to suppress metastasis effectively. A good example of a candidate metastasis suppressor gene is the gene encoding E-cadherin, a component of adherens junctions, because loss of intercellular junctions appears to be essential for tumor metastasis.

TUMOR STROMA

COMPOSITION OF THE STROMA

A tumor consists of tumor cells proper, the tumor parenchyma, and nonneoplastic supporting structures, the stroma (Fig. 6-27). The stroma is composed largely of

Fig. 6-25 **Schematic illustration of the sequence of events in the invasion of epithelial basement membranes by tumor cells.** Tumor cells detach from each other because of reduced adhesiveness (**A**). Cells then attach to the basement membrane via laminin receptors (**B**) and secrete proteolytic enzymes, including type IV collagenase and plasminogen activator. Degradation of the basement membrane (**C**) and tumor cell migration (**D**) follow. *(From Kumar V, Abbas A, Fausto N: Robbins & Cotran pathologic basis of disease, ed 7, Philadelphia, 2005, Saunders.)*

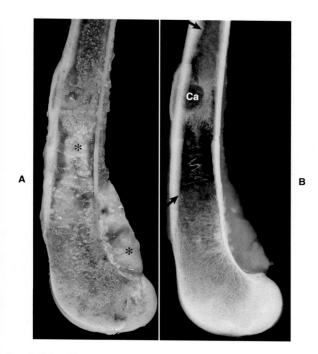

Fig. 6-26   Prostate carcinoma, metastasis, femur, dog.
A, The gross photograph of a sectioned femur reveals metastatic prostate carcinoma (*). **B,** The radiograph illustrates an osteolytic bone metastasis (*Ca*). In the regions between the arrows, extensive proliferation of new bone has occurred in response to the tumor. (*A and* **B,** *Modified from Rosol TJ, Tannehill-Gregg SH, LeRoy BE et al: Animal models of bone metastasis. In Keller ET, Chung LWK, editors:* Cancer treatment and research, *Boston, 2004, Kluwer Academic Publishers.*)

extracellular connective tissue and consists of proteins and glycoproteins, such as collagen, embedded in a complex matrix of proteoglycans. The stroma contains the blood vessels that supply nutrients to the tumor, fibroblasts, and a variety of inflammatory and immune cells. The amount of stroma associated with tumors can vary considerably. The extracellular material in the stroma of epithelial tumors is produced primarily by surrounding nonneoplastic mesenchymal cells, whereas many mesenchymal tumors can produce the ECM in their stroma. For instance, many osteosarcomas produce bone, a specialized form of connective tissue stroma. Stromal tissue may form a connective tissue capsule around epithelial tumors that limit neoplastic spread. In general, encapsulated epithelial tumors are considered to have a better prognosis than unencapsulated tumors (Fig. 6-28).

In the stroma of rare tumors, both mesenchymal and epithelial, there is an amorphous eosinophilic substance termed amyloid. Amyloid consists of one of a variety of abnormal proteins arranged in β-pleated fibrils. The proteins that form amyloid are usually secreted by the tumor cells themselves; for instance, λ-light chain protein secreted by neoplastic plasma cells forms the amyloid sometimes seen in the extramedullary plasmacytomas of various species.

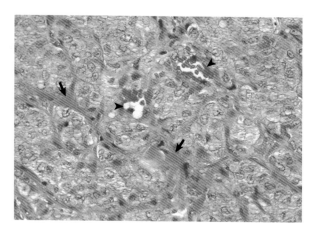

Fig. 6-27   Pancreatic adenocarcinoma, pancreas, dog. The tumor parenchyma is divided into incomplete lobules by the tumor stroma (*arrows*) composed of collagen and extracellular matrix components in which blood vessels (*arrowheads*), fibroblasts, and inflammatory and immune cells are embedded. H&E stain. (*Courtesy College of Veterinary Medicine, The Ohio State University.*)

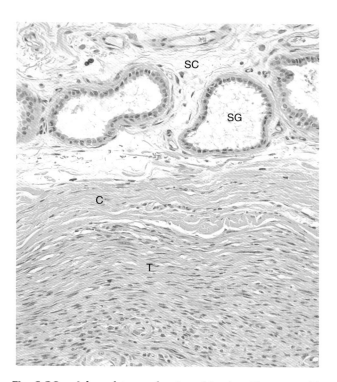

Fig. 6-28   Adnexal tumor, benign, skin, dog. This tumor (*T*) lies within the subcutis (*SC*) and is surrounded by a thick connective tissue capsule (*C*), which is more frequently associated with benign than with malignant tumors. *SG,* Normal apocrine sweat glands of the subcutis. H&E stain. (*Courtesy College of Veterinary Medicine, The Ohio State University.*)

TUMOR-STROMAL INTERACTIONS

Tumor cells interact with their stroma in a complex fashion, exchanging a wide variety of signaling molecules,

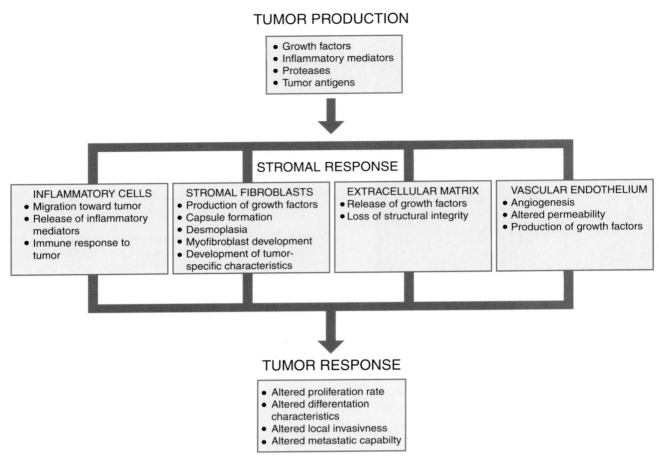

Fig. 6-29   Tumor-stromal interactions. Tumor cells and the stroma in which they are embedded interact in a variety of ways that serve to modify the growth and behavior of both elements. Tumor stroma may both enhance and limit tumor development and spread. *(Redrawn with permission from Dr. D.F. Kusewitt, College of Veterinary Medicine, The Ohio State University.)*

including growth factors, cytokines, hormones, and inflammatory mediators (Fig. 6-29). These exchanges modulate the growth rate, differentiation state, and behavior of both stromal and tumor cells. Platelet-derived growth factor released by tumor cells stimulates tumor-associated fibroblasts to increase the production of collagen. In some cases, this process leads to an extensive fibrous reaction, termed a scirrhous or desmoplastic response, in the stroma. Transforming growth factor-α of tumor origin can stimulate tumor-associated fibroblasts to differentiate into myofibroblasts, which are fibroblasts with contractile capabilities. Tumor-associated fibroblasts may acquire special characteristics that distinguish them from normal fibroblasts. Such fibroblasts may secrete a fetal type of ECM. In some tumors, tumor-associated fibroblasts acquire heritable genetic and epigenetic changes that allow them to co-evolve with adjacent tumor cells. Tumor cells may induce surrounding stromal cells to produce cytokines that promote tumor cell proliferation and motility.

Furthermore, growth factors are sequestered in the ECM of the stroma, where they bind to proteoglycans. This interaction controls the bioavailability of these factors, which can be released from the ECM by the activity of proteases secreted by tumor cells, stromal fibroblasts, or inflammatory cells.

ANGIOGENESIS

Continued growth of solid tumors is absolutely dependent upon an adequate blood supply to provide oxygen and nutrients to tumor cells. Without the development of new blood vessels, a process termed angiogenesis, tumors are limited to a maximum diameter of 1 to 2 mm. At some point during tumor development, an angiogenic switch occurs that confers on tumor cells the ability to induce and sustain new tumor vasculature. Angiogenesis is a complex process involving recruitment of endothelial cells from preexisting blood vessels, endothelial cell proliferation, directed migration of endothelial cells through the ECM, and maturation and differentiation of the capillary sprout. Angiogenesis is controlled by the balance between a plethora of angiogenesis-stimulating and angiogenesis-inhibiting factors. Tumors induce angiogenesis by the production and release of angiogenic factors, such as vascular endothelial growth factor, or by down-regulating production of antiangiogenic factors, such as thrombospondin. In addition, angiogenic and antiangiogenic factors bound to ECM components can be released and activated by tumor protease activity. Vascular endothelial growth factor and acidic and basic fibroblast growth factors are among the most potent angiogenic factors produced by tumors. The tumor blood vessels that develop in response to angiogenic signals are usually more dilated, more tortuous, and more permeable than normal blood vessels (Fig. 6-30).

In addition to supplying nutrients, tumor vasculature plays other roles in tumor development. Vessel leakiness allows perivascular deposition of a fibrin network that promotes formation of collagenous tumor stroma. The endothelial cells of tumor blood vessels produce growth factors, such as platelet-derived growth factor and interleukin (IL)-1, that can stimulate the growth of tumor cells. Moreover, without access to the circulatory system, tumors cannot metastasize. Because solid tumor growth is absolutely dependent on an adequate blood supply, therapeutic strategies to inhibit angiogenesis are being developed.

Investigation of the development of lymphatic vasculature of tumors has demonstrated that tumor lymphangiogenesis shares many features with tumor angiogenesis. Tumor-associated lymphatic vessels

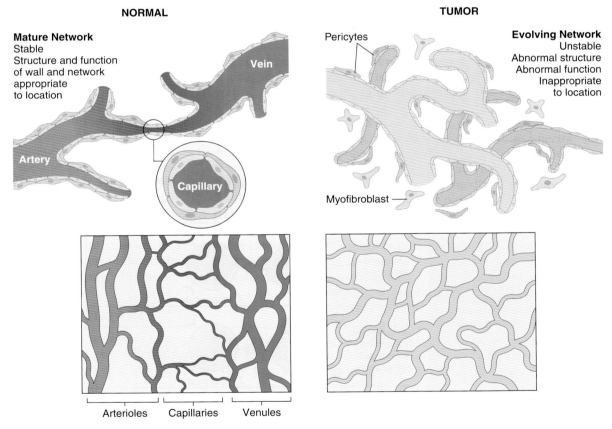

NORMAL   **TUMOR**

Fig. 6-30   Tumor angiogenesis. Compared with normal vessels *(left panels)*, tumor vessels are tortuous and irregularly shaped *(right panels)*. The tumor vasculature is formed from circulating endothelial precursor cells and existing host vessels; myofibroblasts give rise to pericytes that surround vessels. In contrast to the stable vessel network of normal tissue, the networks formed by tumor vessels are unstable and leaky. Arterioles, capillaries, and venules are clearly distinguishable in normal vasculature; in the tumor, vessels are disorganized and specific vessel types cannot be identified. *(From Kumar V, Abbas A, Fausto N: Robbins & Cotran pathologic basis of disease, ed 7, Philadelphia, 2005, Saunders.)*

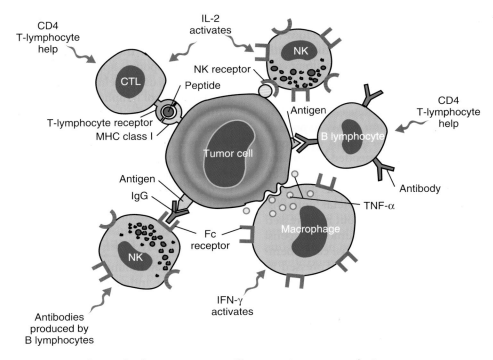

Fig. 6-32   **Cells involved in immunosurveillance against tumors.** Antitumor responses involve cytotoxic CD8+ and helper CD4+ lymphocytes, natural killer (*NK*) cells, macrophages, B lymphocytes, and a variety of immunomodulatory cytokines. *CTL*, Cytotoxic T lymphocyte; *IFN-γ*, interferon-γ; *IgG*, immunoglobulin G; *IL-2*, interleukin-2; *MHC*, major histocompatibility complex; *TNF-α*, tumor necrosis factor-α. (*Modified from Kumar V, Abbas A, Fausto N: Robbins & Cotran pathologic basis of disease, ed 7, Philadelphia, 2005, Saunders.*)

of receptors, both inhibitory and activating, that recognize MHC molecules and stress-induced ligands on tumor cells. NK cells can kill a wide variety of neoplastic and virally infected cells. Cells that express MHC class I molecules are preferentially spared by NK cells, whereas cells lacking MHC molecules are specifically targeted. After binding to a tumor cell, the NK cell releases lytic granules that activate apoptosis in the target cell. This mechanism of cell killing or cytolysis is shared with T lymphocytes and is discussed in more detail next.

MACROPHAGES

Macrophages are migratory phagocytic cells capable of killing tumor cells by releasing reactive oxygen intermediates, lysosomal enzymes, nitric oxide, and tumor necrosis factor. Their antitumor activity is stimulated by interferon (IFN)-γ, which is produced by both T lymphocytes and NK cells. Macrophage-mediated tumor cell killing is independent of MHC antigens, tumor-specific antigens, and the type of transformed cell being targeted, but direct contact between the macrophage and tumor cell is required.

T LYMPHOCYTES

Cytotoxic T lymphocytes (CTLs) are the primary effector cells of the adaptive antitumor immune response.

Most CTLs are CD8+ T lymphocytes that have been primed by dendritic cells to recognize and engage tumor antigens on the surface of tumor cells. When a CTL attaches to its target cell, a well-organized immunologic synapse is rapidly formed at the site of cell-to-cell contact and persists for more than an hour. Into this synapse, the CTL releases lytic granules containing perforin, a pore-forming protein, and granzymes, which are serine proteases. Perforin mediates the entry of granzymes into the target cell. Once inside the target cell, granzymes initiate both caspase-dependent and caspase-independent apoptosis. CD4+ T lymphocytes do not appear to be essential for the generation or maintenance of a CTL response; instead, CD4+ lymphocytes are generally considered to function as helper T lymphocytes that enhance the function of CD8+ CTLs and antigen-producing B lymphocytes. CD4+ T lymphocyte helper activities are largely mediated through secretion of cytokines such as IL-2, which drives CD8+ cell proliferation, and IFN-γ, which stimulates CD8+ T-lymphocyte differentiation.

B LYMPHOCYTES

Many tumor antigens can incite both cell-mediated and humoral immune responses. Antibody-producing B lymphocytes mediate the humoral immune response to tumors. Antibodies that recognize tumor antigens kill tumor cells by binding to the cells and activating a local complement cascade. Activation of the complement cascade generates a membrane attack complex that induces loss of tumor cell membrane integrity and rapid cell death with the morphologic hallmarks of necrosis. In addition, antitumor antibodies may be bound by their constant regions to NK cells or macrophages, leaving the variable regions of the immunoglobulins available for specific recognition of tumor antigens. This allows the effector cells to recognize, attach to, and kill tumor cells by the mechanism of antibody-dependent cell-mediated cytotoxicity (ADCC).

EVASION OF THE IMMUNE RESPONSE

Many tumors are able successfully to evade immuno-surveillance, using a variety of mechanisms (Fig. 6-33).

ALTERED MAJOR HISTOCOMPATIBILITY COMPLEX EXPRESSION

CTLs recognize tumor antigens only on tumor cells that display the antigens in the context of MHC class I molecules. Thus tumor cells that lose or down-regulate expression of class I MHC antigens may have a distinct selective advantage. However, tumors that fail to express class I antigens are more susceptible to NK cell killing. Tumors may also down-regulate expression of class II MHC antigens. Class II antigens are required for activation of the helper T lymphocytes that stimulate CTL differentiation, and loss of these antigens prevents the generation of an optimal antitumor CTL response.

ANTIGEN MASKING

Tumors may become invisible to the immune system by losing or masking tumor antigens. The outgrowth of

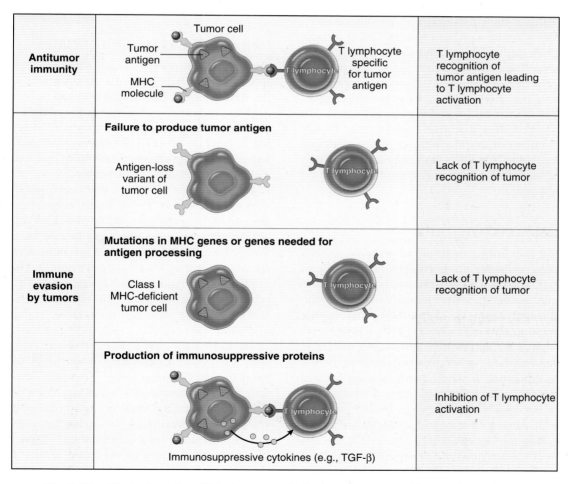

Fig. 6-33   Mechanisms by which tumors evade the immune system. Tumor cells employ a variety of mechanisms to avoid attack by cytolytic T lymphocytes. *MHC*, Major histocompatibility complex; *TGF-β*, transforming growth factor-β. (*From Kumar V, Abbas A, Fausto N: Robbins & Cotran pathologic basis of disease, ed 7, Philadelphia, 2005, Saunders.*)

clonal tumor variants that do not express tumor antigens will be favored during tumor evolution. Tumor antigens on the cell surface may be hidden from the immune system if they are complexed with glycocalyx molecules, fibrin, or even antibodies. Some humoral responses to tumor antigens may therefore promote tumor survival by protecting tumor antigens from recognition by CTLs.

TOLERANCE

Although the immune system responds vigorously to non–self-antigens, it is tolerant to self-antigens. Thus tumor antigens shared with normal tissue usually are not able to evoke an immune response because the body has already been "tolerized" to the antigen. Tolerance can also result from presentation of non-self-antigens in a "tolerogenic" context (i.e., in the absence of co-stimulatory molecules required for effective T-lymphocyte activation).

IMMUNOSUPPRESSION

Tumor cells or their products may be immunosuppressive. Many tumors produce transforming growth factor-α, which inhibits the proliferation and function of lymphocytes and macrophages. Tumors may also produce Fas ligand. Fas ligand expressed by tumor cells binds to Fas receptors on nearby T lymphocytes and triggers their apoptosis. By this mechanism, T-lymphocyte clones that recognize a tumor may be specifically deleted. Finally, tumor cells release tumor antigens into the circulation that form immune complexes with antibodies, and these immune complexes may be immunosuppressive.

TUMOR IMMUNOTHERAPY

The fact that the antitumor immune response attacks only the tumor cells and not normal tissue makes it an attractive candidate as a therapeutic modality. Moreover, effective immunotherapy would reduce or eliminate the need to use highly cytotoxic chemotherapeutic agents that indiscriminately target dividing cells. These drugs can cause significant morbidity and mortality in cancer patients. To date, immunotherapy results have been variable and disappointing; however, many new approaches are presently under investigation, some of which show promise.

In general, immunotherapeutic strategies are aimed at (1) providing the patient with mature effector cells or antibodies that recognize and destroy tumors (passive immunotherapy) or (2) stimulating the immune response of the host against the tumor (active immunotherapy).

Administration of monoclonal antibodies raised against tumor antigens or tumor-specific effector lymphocytes generated in vitro generates rapid but short-lived passive tumor immunity. Monoclonal antibodies raised in other species have a limited usefulness because the tumor host may develop an immune response to these antibodies that abrogates their effectiveness. However, coupling toxins to monoclonal antibodies may allow targeted delivery of therapeutic agents to tumor cells. Antitumor lymphocytes are generated by removing lymphocytes from the host or tumor and expanding them in vitro by incubation with IL-2; these autologous immune cells are then readministered to the patient. Many approaches to stimulate the activity immunity of patients against their tumors have been attempted. These include vaccination with tumor cells or tumor antigens to generate antitumor CTLs, administration of cytokines to increase effector cell number and function, and nonspecific stimulation of the immune system by treatment with proinflammatory substances, such as bacterial products.

SYSTEMIC EFFECTS ON THE HOST

DIRECT EFFECTS VERSUS PARANEOPLASTIC SYNDROMES

Tumors directly compromise the function of the organs in which they arise by replacing normal tissue and by disrupting normal anatomic relationships of affected organs. Both in the tissue of origin and in metastatic sites, expanding tumor tissue may compress surrounding normal tissue or the blood vessels that supply this tissue, resulting in pressure atrophy or frank necrosis. This is a particularly severe problem in organs encased in bone, such as the brain, that can expand to only a very limited extent. In the brain, even benign tumors that are not surgically accessible may prove fatal. Seizure activity is a common manifestation of brain tumors. Tumor invasion into the wall of a hollow organ such as the stomach may lead to organ rupture. Tumors may erode blood vessel walls, causing acute hemorrhage, whereas tumor extension into blood vessels may lead to the formation of tumor emboli that produce infarcts at distant sites.

In addition to direct effects, tumors may cause a variety of systemic clinical signs termed paraneoplastic syndromes. Paraneoplastic disorders are indirect and usually remote effects that are caused by tumor cell products rather than by the primary tumor or its metastases. Approximately 75% of human cancer patients develop paraneoplastic syndromes, but the incidence in veterinary cancer patients is not known. These syndromes are best described for the dog, although some affecting the cat and the horse have been reported (Table 6-3). Recognition of paraneoplastic syndromes is important for the following reasons: (1) Paraneoplastic syndromes may appear early in the course of tumor

Table **6-3**   **Paraneoplastic Syndromes in Animals**

System	Syndrome
Systemic	Anorexia/cachexia
	Fever
Endocrine	Hypercalcemia
	Hypoglycemia
	Hyperestrogenism
	Hypergastrinemia
	Thyrotoxicosis
	Hyperhistaminosis
	Hypercatecholaminemia
	Cushing's disease
Skeletal	Hypertrophic osteoarthropathy
	Myelofibrosis
Vascular/hematopoietic	Leukocytosis
	Leukopenia
	Thrombocytosis
	Thrombocytopenia
	Erythrocytosis
	Anemia
	Eosinophilia
	Disseminated intravascular coagulation
	Hyperviscosity syndrome
Neurologic	Peripheral neuropathy
	Myasthenia gravis
Cutaneous	Alopecia
	Nodular dermatofibrosis

Modified from McCullen JM, Page R, Misdorp W: An overview of cancer pathogenesis, diagnosis, and management. In Meuten DJ, editor: *Tumors in domestic animals*, Ames, 2002, Iowa State Press.

development and may be associated with specific tumor types, thus recognition of these syndromes can facilitate early tumor diagnosis; (2) treatment of the metabolic abnormalities associated with paraneoplastic syndromes and antitumor therapy may be required to assure effective cancer management; and (3) the severity of paraneoplastic abnormalities reflects the tumor burden; thus monitoring such abnormalities may be useful in determining tumor response to therapy and identifying tumor recurrence or spread.

CACHEXIA

Many animals with cancer show notable weight loss and debility. In cancer cachexia, both muscle and fat are lost, whereas in simple starvation fat is lost preferentially. Also, in starvation, there is a compensatory decrease in basal metabolic rate not seen in cancer cachexia. The etiology of cancer cachexia is complex. Contributing factors include anorexia, impaired digestion, nutritional demands of tumor tissue, nutrient loss in cancer-related effusions or exudates, and a variety of metabolic and endocrine derangements. Extra calories do not reverse the catabolic state of cancer cachexia. Many humoral factors, including cytokines and hormones, contribute to the development of cachexia. Among the best characterized of these factors are TNF-α, IL-1, IL-6, and prostaglandins.

ENDOCRINOPATHIES

A functioning neoplasm of an endocrine tissue produces the normal hormonal products of the tissue of origin, but the host is usually able to regulate this hormone production only to a very limited extent. Frequently, the result is an overproduction of hormone due to increased numbers of hormone-producing tumor cells, increased production of hormone by individual neoplastic cells, or both. In endocrine glands with more than one cell type, such as the pancreatic islet, the anterior pituitary, the thyroid, and the adrenal, generally only a single cell type becomes neoplastic. Thus a pancreatic islet cell adenoma will probably produce only a single hormone such as insulin, glucagon, gastrin, or somatostatin, and not a combination of hormones. Several clinically significant endocrinopathies are seen fairly commonly in veterinary medicine. These include hyperthyroidism due to thyroid neoplasia in the cat, and Cushing's disease (hyperadrenocorticism) due to pituitary tumors in several species. A variety of nonendocrine neoplasms may also produce hormonally active substances not normally found in the tissue of tumor origin. This is termed ectopic hormone production. The hormone produced may be identical to the normally produced hormone, may be a modified form of the normal hormone, or may be the product of a gene that encodes a protein related to but not identical with the true hormone.

Probably the two most frequently observed metabolic derangements resulting from cancer-associated endocrine abnormalities in animals are hypercalcemia of malignancy and hypoglycemia. Hypercalcemia is seen with functional tumors of the parathyroid gland that produce excess parathyroid hormone, the major regulator of calcium levels in the body. In the great majority of cases, however, hypercalcemia of malignancy is due to ectopic production of parathyroid hormone and parathyroid hormone-related protein by neoplastic tissue, including a wide variety of carcinomas and sarcomas. In dogs, hypercalcemia is seen most frequently with adenocarcinoma of the anal sac (~90% of cases) (Fig. 6-34), lymphoma (~20% of cases), and multiple myeloma (~15% of cases). Hypercalcemia of malignancy in cats appears to be relatively rare. Parathyroid hormone and parathyroid-related hormone are encoded by two separate genes. The genes are regulated independently and produce proteins of somewhat

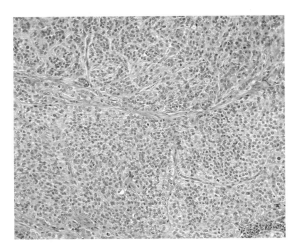

Fig. 6-34 Apocrine gland carcinoma, anal sac, dog. This tumor is composed of the typical solid lobules of malignant epithelial cells that characterize apocrine gland adenocarcinomas. Apocrine gland carcinoma, lymphoma, and multiple myeloma may be associated with hypercalcemia of malignancy. H&E stain. *(Courtesy College of Veterinary Medicine, The Ohio State University.)*

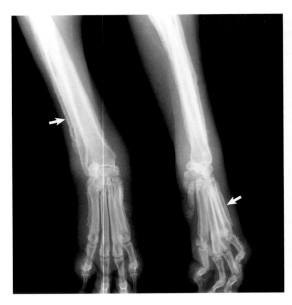

Fig. 6-35 Hypertrophic osteopathy, forelimbs, dog with a pulmonary tumor. On this radiograph, the arrows indicate newly deposited bone that is less dense than normal cortical bone. Note that multiple bones on both limbs are affected and that new bone deposits are located primarily in the diaphyseal region of the long bones. *(Courtesy Dr. J. Mattoon, College of Veterinary Medicine, The Ohio State University.)*

different size and sequence. However, the amino terminal 34 amino acids of the two proteins are functionally equivalent. The hormones increase serum calcium by increasing calcium release from bones, enhancing reabsorption of calcium in the kidneys, and stimulating absorption of calcium in the intestine. Clinical signs of hypercalcemia include muscle weakness, cardiac arrhythmia, anorexia, vomiting, and renal failure. Hypercalcemia may also occur as a result of tumor metastasis to bone and resultant bone resorption; however, this is not a true paraneoplastic disorder because it is a direct effect of the tumor.

Hypoglycemia is seen primarily with insulinomas, functioning tumors of the pancreatic islet β cells. However, profound hypoglycemia of unknown origin may also occur with other tumor types. Due to the absolute dependence of the nervous system on glucose for energy, clinical signs of hypoglycemia are mostly neurologic and may include lethargy, incoordination, muscle weakness, and seizures.

SKELETAL SYNDROMES

Hypertrophic osteopathy occurs in both cats and dogs. It usually presents clinically as a symmetric lameness. Radiographically, there is evidence of extensive periosteal new bone growth (Fig. 6-35). Hypertrophic osteopathy occurs with a variety of tumor types, although there is a strong association with space-occupying thoracic lesions, both neoplastic and nonneoplastic. The cause of this condition is not known, although abnormalities of growth hormone production are suspected. Myelofibrosis results from overgrowth of nonneoplastic fibroblasts in the bone marrow. It may be associated with myeloproliferative disease or with distant tumors. The cause is unknown.

VASCULAR AND HEMATOLOGIC SYNDROMES

Nonhematopoietic cancer in animals may result in a variety of vascular and hematologic syndromes, including eosinophilia and neutrophilic leukocytosis. The etiology of these conditions is unclear, but circulating cytokines are likely to be involved. Anemia is commonly seen in veterinary cancer patients. There are numerous potential causes for anemia in these animals, including anemia of chronic disease, bone marrow invasion, blood loss, and hemolysis. Polycythemia associated with ectopic production of erythropoietin has been reported. Thrombocytopenia is seen in approximately one third of all dogs with cancer. Disseminated intravascular coagulation (DIC) may be secondary to any large tumor. Anemia and DIC are frequently seen in dogs with hemangiosarcoma, a tumor that accounts for 7% of canine malignancies. Excessive immunoglobulin production by tumors, particularly monoclonal gammopathies due to multiple myeloma, can result in hyperviscosity syndrome, manifested as altered neurologic function, congestive heart failure, or bleeding disorders.

NEUROLOGIC SYNDROMES

Paraneoplastic neurologic disease in veterinary cancer patients is usually related to hypercalcemia, hypoglycemia, or hyperviscosity and is often manifested as seizure activity. Primary peripheral nervous system disease has also been reported. In many dogs with cancer, there is microscopic evidence of peripheral neuropathy; however, clinical signs of disease, such as areflexia, muscle weakness, reduced muscle tone, or paralysis, are much less common. Myasthenia gravis is occasionally seen in veterinary cancer patients, usually in association with a mediastinal tumor such as thymoma. The underlying defect in myasthenia gravis is a failure of nerve impulse transmission at neuromuscular junctions. Clinical signs include muscle weakness, reduced exercise tolerance, and dysphagia. Many neurologic paraneoplastic syndromes in humans are immune mediated, and this is likely to be the case in animals as well.

CUTANEOUS SYNDROMES

There are only a few reports of cutaneous manifestations of paraneoplastic disease in dogs and cats. Clinical signs of flushing, alopecia, or necrolytic dermatitis have been associated with a variety of tumor types. The syndrome of nodular dermatofibrosis in German shepherd dogs is a heritable disorder characterized by multiple benign-appearing fibrous nodules in the skin in conjunction with bilateral renal cystadenocarcinomas.

MISCELLANEOUS SYNDROMES

Gastrin-secreting tumors have been reported in dogs and cats. These tumors can cause gastroduodenal ulceration, abdominal pain, vomiting, and blood loss. Mast cell tumors are very common in dogs. Neoplastic mast cells produce a wide variety of biologic mediators, including histamine, heparin, platelet-activating factor, TNF-α, prostaglandins, and proteases. Release of these compounds, particularly histamine, is responsible for such paraneoplastic disorders as gastrointestinal ulceration and hemorrhage. Although widespread mastocytosis is frequently associated with clinical signs, cutaneous mast cell tumors rarely produce systemic signs.

GENETICS AND CANCER

Cancer is ultimately due to heritable changes in the DNA of the tumor cells. These changes are manifested in enhanced expression of normal proteins, decreased or absent expression of normal proteins, and expression of abnormal proteins. For instance, tumor suppressor proteins such as that encoded by p53 may fail to be expressed or may be expressed in an inactive form.

Oncogene-encoded proteins may be overexpressed or expressed in constitutively active form. The altered protein repertoire of the tumor cell determines its *phenotype*. Such changes create cells with the features of neoplasia, including unlimited proliferative potential, growth factor independence, resistance to apoptosis, and invasive capabilities.

Genetic alterations in the coding region of a gene clearly may result in the production of an altered protein as a result of an altered coding sequence or premature protein termination. However, changes in other regions of the genome may also affect the sequence of the encoded protein and the level at which it is expressed. An alteration in splice site sequence can yield incorrectly spliced mRNA that is translated into an aberrant protein. Because the 5′ untranslated region of a gene generally contains its promoter and the 3′ untranslated region often contains mRNA stabilization motifs, sequence alterations in these regions of the genome may also have profound effects on gene expression level.

STEPWISE ACCUMULATION OF CHANGES

Cancer is associated with a progressive accumulation of genetic and epigenetic abnormalities. These defects lead to disruption of cell growth, cell death, apoptosis, differentiation, DNA repair, and other critical pathways. Some model systems demonstrate an orderly morphologic progression through premalignant to malignant to invasive and metastatic disease, and molecular genetic investigations of these various stages have made important contributions to our understanding of cancer biology. The molecular events that occur in the development of familial adenomatous polyposis, a form of human colorectal cancer, provide an excellent example of the genetic evolution that underlies progressive morphologic changes in cancer (Fig. 6-36). The initiating event is loss or mutation of the APC (adenomatous polyposis coli) tumor suppressor gene, leading to adenoma formation. This is followed by an activating mutation of a RAS oncogene and loss of genetic material harboring additional tumor suppressor genes. Ultimately a malignant carcinoma emerges.

As illustrated in Fig. 6-37, DNA is susceptible to many types of chemical and physical alterations. Some of these changes are due to injurious endogenous and exogenous agents. In addition, DNA alterations occur as part of normal processes of genome replication, repair, and rearrangement. Under some circumstances, these normal processes can lead to changes in DNA structure that contribute to the neoplastic phenotype. Furthermore, as tumors evolve, they often demonstrate reduced DNA repair capabilities and increased genomic instability. These developments accelerate the accumulation of genetic alterations in tumor cells.

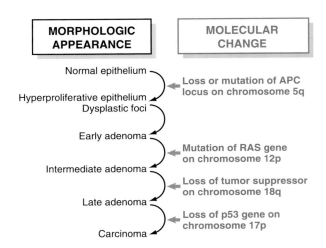

Fig. 6-36   **Molecular model for the evolution of human colorectal cancers through the adenoma-carcinoma sequence.** Although adenomatous polyposis coli (APC) mutation is an early event and loss of p53 occurs late in the process of tumorigenesis, the timing for the other changes may show variations. Note also that individual tumors may not have all of the changes listed. *(Adapted from Vogelstein B, Kinzler KW: Colorectal tumors. In Vogelstein B, Kinzler KW, editors: The genetic basis of human cancer, New York, 2002, McGraw-Hill.)*

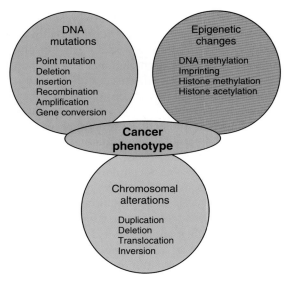

Fig. 6-37   **Heritable alterations contributing to carcinogenesis.** Many genetic changes caused by extrinsic and intrinsic DNA-damaging agents, normal physiologic processes, and aging alter the amino acid sequences of encoded proteins and the levels at which these proteins are expressed. These changes in turn are responsible for the neoplastic phenotype. *(Redrawn with permission from Dr. D.F. Kusewitt, College of Veterinary Medicine, The Ohio State University.)*

Why do we study the molecular basis of cancer? Cancer is often treated using cytotoxic drugs and/or radiation therapy, neither of which discriminates between normal and tumor cells. Nonselective cell killing is responsible for many of the deleterious side effects of cancer treatment. More rational therapies would specifically target molecularly altered tumor cells, leaving nontumor cells lacking the molecular defect(s) relatively unharmed. Examples of molecularly targeted therapies used in humans include Gleevec, which is active against the BCR/ABL chromosomal translocation in chronic myeloid leukemia, and Iressa, which targets the epidermal growth factor receptor (EGF-R) in lung cancer. Specific molecular defects can also be exploited for early detection and/or early intervention at a stage when the tumor may be more responsive to treatment. Mutations in the BRCA1 gene are associated with a high risk for development of breast and/or ovarian cancer in women. Identification of the carrier status gives women the option of prophylactic mastectomy and/or oophorectomy. Mutations and other molecular defects can also be used to stratify patients for treatment and/or prognostic purposes.

GENETIC CHANGES IN CANCER
DNA DAMAGE AND MUTATION

DNA damage, per se, does not constitute mutation. Mutation occurs during DNA replication, when the DNA strand containing unrepaired or misrepaired DNA damage is used as a template for the synthesis of a complementary DNA strand (see later discussion). At this time, unrepaired DNA lesions are misread by DNA polymerases, which insert incorrect bases in the newly synthesized DNA strand, and incorrectly repaired DNA lesions are reproduced in the daughter DNA strand. This process is known as mutation fixation; at least one and sometimes two rounds of replication are required for mutations to become fully fixed in the genome.

A chemical or physical change in an individual base may lead to the substitution of one base for another. The point mutation thus created can lead to altered protein sequence, if it is located in an exon or at a splice site, and to altered levels of expression, if it is located in the promoter or in the mRNA stabilization motif of a gene. Single- and double-strand breaks in DNA are caused by physical and chemical agents and viruses; they may also occur during normal physiologic processes, such as recombination of immunoglobulin genes and T-lymphocyte receptor genes. Although single-strand breaks are usually readily repaired, they can in some circumstances lead to gene conversion, the replacement of a gene or part of a gene by DNA derived from a closely related gene. Gene conversion is one mechanism by which organisms routinely generate diversity in large families of related genes, for example, major histocompatibility antigen genes. Double-strand breaks produce unprotected, recombinogenic DNA ends and often lead to major chromosomal anomalies, including deletions and translocations. Clearly, such large-scale chromosomal changes have the potential to alter the gene expression repertoire of a cell in a dramatic fashion. Insertions of DNA bases into the genome may be as small as a single base or larger than a viral genome. Insertion of individual bases by the enzyme terminal deoxynucleotide transferase is part of the system by which antibody diversity is normally generated. Retroviral genomes replicate only after insertion into the host genome, and these large insertions can interrupt the coding sequence of host genes, abrogating their expression. On the other hand, juxtaposition of viral promoter elements adjacent to cellular coding sequences can lead to dysregulated, often markedly increased, host gene expression. Unscheduled amplification of DNA segments is a poorly understood process by which multiple rounds of localized DNA replication produce hundreds or thousands of copies of DNA segments up to several megabases in length. Such amplified DNA segments may be visible in cytogenetic preparations as homogeneously staining regions in chromosomes or as episomal double minutes. Amplification of oncogenes or drug resistance genes may have significant effects on the life history of a tumor. Expansion or contraction of a small region of tandemly repeated DNA sequences can occur as the result of DNA polymerase slippage during replication. This process can introduce sequence alterations into protein encoding genes.

CHROMOSOMAL INSTABILITY

The karyotypes of many tumor cells are extremely abnormal because of changes in chromosome number and configuration. These alterations are the result of chromosomal instability. In tumors with notable chromosomal instability, each cell in a tumor may have a different karyotype and exhibit a remarkable array of duplications, deletions, and reciprocal and nonreciprocal translocations. Such abnormalities can dramatically affect the levels of gene expression by altering the numbers of gene copies present and by juxtaposing regulatory and structural elements of unrelated genes. In some cases, specific chromosomal abnormalities are associated with specific disease entities. Probably the best studied example of such an association is the relationship between chronic myeloid leukemia in humans and a reciprocal translocation between chromosomes 9 and 22 that yields an abnormal chromosome called the Philadelphia chromosome. This translocation fuses portions of the BCR and ABL genes; the fusion gene thus produced encodes an abnormal protein that appears to be responsible for neoplastic transformation of myeloid cells.

TYPES OF GENETIC ALTERATIONS IN CANCER CELLS
ANEUPLOIDY

The numerical aberrations in cancer can involve many different chromosomes or can be limited to a single chromosome. Cytogenetic analysis can determine the copy number of each chromosome. Monosomy is the term used when only one copy of a chromosome exists. Trisomy is the term used when three copies of a chromosome exist. For example, one quarter of canine lymphomas show trisomy of chromosome 13. In mice, trisomy of chromosome 15 occurs in almost all T-lymphocyte lymphomas and leukemias, suggesting that overexpression of a gene or genes on this chromosome plays an important role in tumor causation. Alterations in chromosome number (aneuploidy) are largely the result of mistakes in chromosome segregation due to multipolar spindles, centrosome amplification, kinetochore malfunction, or abnormal cytokinesis.

TRANSLOCATION

Translocations often occur when the cell response to DNA damage is dysregulated. When cells respond appropriately to DNA damage, multiple signaling cascades, such as the p53 pathway, are activated, leading to cell-cycle arrest, enhanced DNA repair, and, in the face of excessive DNA damage, apoptosis. However, if these pathways are no longer functional, chromosomal instability results. Dysfunctional telomeres also contribute to chromosomal instability (Fig. 6-38). The precise mechanisms by which an intact DNA damage response and normal telomerase activity maintain chromosomal integrity are not known.

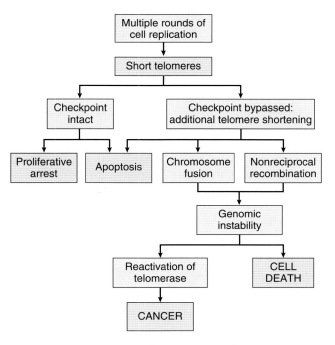

Fig. 6-38   Cellular responses to telomere shortening. The figure shows the response of cells with intact cell-cycle checkpoints and of cells with checkpoint defects. *(From Kumar V, Abbas A, Fausto N: Robbins & Cotran pathologic basis of disease, ed 7, Philadelphia, 2005, Saunders.)*

MUTATION

In addition to abnormal numbers of chromosomes, mutations (heritable change in the DNA sequence) are also present in most tumors. Mutations can result in a lack of or inactivation of a protein. On the other hand, some mutations cause uncontrolled activation of a protein. One example is a point mutation of the RAS oncogene. This mutation causes constitutive and unregulated activation of the protein and gives the affected cell a growth advantage over surrounding normal cells. Another type of mutation is a dominant-negative mutation, in which the mutant gene product causes inactivation of the wild-type product, effectively eliminating the cellular contribution of the normal gene. A missense mutation that changes a codon for one amino acid into a codon for a different amino acid has been identified in the Birt-Hogg-Dubé (BDH) gene in German shepherd dogs with hereditary multifocal renal cystadenocarcinoma and nodular dermatofibrosis (see later discussion).

DELETION

Deletions involve loss of DNA from a chromosome and can be as small as one base pair or as large as an entire arm of a chromosome. Heterozygous deletions occur on only one chromosome, whereas homozygous deletions occur on both chromosomes. Small deletions of one or two base pair cause a shift in the reading frame during protein synthesis (frameshift mutation). One possible consequence is that the mutated sequence codes for a premature stop codon, resulting in a truncated protein. Large deletions often encompass chromosome regions that harbor tumor suppressor genes.

AMPLIFICATION

Genomic amplifications result in the presence of more than one diploid copy of a DNA sequence. The amplified region can involve large segments of a chromosome and encompass millions of base pairs. Alternatively the amplified region may be very small and contained within a portion of a single gene, such as the internal tandem duplication (ITD) of the c-kit gene in canine mast cell tumors. Regions of genomic amplification are useful for identifying potential oncogenes.

EPIGENETIC MECHANISMS OF ALTERED GENE EXPRESSION
DEFINITION OF "EPIGENETIC"

Epigenetic alterations have recently come to light as being major players in tumor biology. The term *epigenetic* refers to a heritable change in gene expression in somatic cells resulting from something other than a change in the DNA sequence. The most frequently studied epigenetic changes are DNA cytosine methylation and histone modifications. These epigenetic modifications can enhance or suppress gene expression and can be transmitted to daughter cells during cell division. Although DNA methylation and histone modifications are carried out by normal cellular enzymes, the activity and specificity of these enzymes can be altered by exogenous agents acting through a variety of oncogenic pathways. And although epigenetic changes are stable for the most part, they can be modulated with various pharmacologic agents. This quality makes them attractive targets for therapeutic intervention designed to restore gene expression to its normal state.

TYPES OF EPIGENETIC CHANGES IN CANCER CELLS
DNA methylation

DNA methylation involves the addition of a methyl group to the No. 5 carbon of cytosine, in cytosines located immediately 5′ to guanine (CpG dinucleotide). The methylation process is carried out by various methyltransferase enzymes. Methylation is essential for regulating gene expression in normal cells. Cancer cells, however, are characterized by an overall decrease in 5-methylcytosine in the bulk of the genome (global hypomethylation) with a paradoxical increase in gene-specific methylation of clusters of CpG sites located in the promoter and/or exon 1 of genes (CpG islands). In general, hypomethylation of genes, particularly of promoter regions, leads to gene activation, whereas hypermethylation results in gene silencing. Promoter methylation has been found in every type of human cancer studied (Fig. 6-39).

Imprinting

Another situation in which methylation plays a role is in imprinting. Genomic imprinting refers to the parent-of-origin, allele-specific expression of certain genes whereby only the maternal or paternal allele is expressed. This monoallelic expression is controlled in part by DNA methylation, but this regulation is sometimes lost in cancer. The loss of imprinting can allow a double dose of a growth-promoting gene product. For example, insulin-like growth factor-2 (IGF-2) is an imprinted gene that is expressed from only the paternal allele in most normal tissue. If a cancer cell undergoes relaxation of imprinting, the methylation-mediated silencing of one allele is lost, enabling biallelic expression and higher than normal levels of this growth-promoting gene product.

Histone modification

In addition to DNA methylation, a second type of epigenetic regulation involves histone modification. DNA is wound around histones to form chromatin. Chromatin can exist in an open configuration in which DNA is accessible to transcription factors (euchromatin) or in a closed, compact configuration in which DNA is

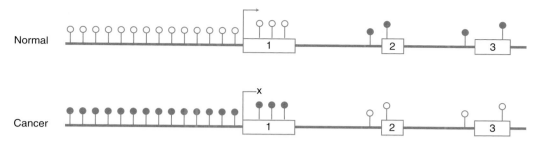

Fig. 6-39   CpG island methylation. In most normal tissues, the dense clusters of CpG sites in the 5′ regions of genes (CpG islands) are unmethylated (*open lollipops*), whereas those in the body of the gene are methylated (*filled lollipops*). The reverse is often seen in cancer where 5′ CpG islands become hypermethylated, and there is concurrent hypomethylation of CpG sites in the body of the gene. Unmethylated 5′ CpG islands are associated with active transcription (*arrow*), whereas methylated 5′ CpG islands are associated with transcriptional repression (*x*). (*Redrawn with permission from Dr. L.J. Rush, College of Veterinary Medicine, The Ohio State University.*)

inaccessible to transcription factors (heterochromatin). Posttranslational modifications, such as acetylation, methylation, and phosphorylation, take place on the histone tails. In the aggregate, these modifications form the "histone code," which plays an important role in determining gene expression. For example, the addition of a negatively charged acetyl group (CH_3CO^-) to certain lysine residues in a histone tail results in a weaker bond between the DNA and the histone. This allows a relaxed chromatin configuration and increases transcription of the associated gene. (Fig. 6-40).

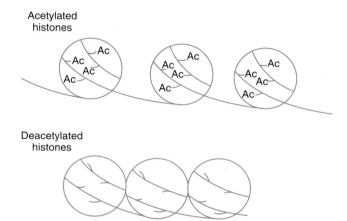

Fig. 6-40   Histone acetylation. DNA is wound around histones. The presence of acetyl groups (*Ac*) on histone tails is associated with relaxed chromatin, which is permissive to gene transcription. Removal of acetyl groups by histone deacetylases results in a closed chromatin configuration that is less permissive to the transcription machinery. (*Redrawn with permission from Dr. L.J. Rush, College of Veterinary Medicine, The Ohio State University.*)

CANCER ETIOLOGY

The genetic alterations that contribute to cancer development include both heritable changes in germline sequences present in all cells within an organism, and somatic changes that accumulate in individual cells and tissues of the body over time. Human families and genetically related animals that exhibit distinct mendelian inheritance of specific types of cancer are said to have cancer syndromes. In these cases, a single germline mutation is generally responsible for tumor development. In contrast, sporadic tumors occur randomly in the population and are not associated with specific germline characteristics.

GERMLINE MUTATIONS AND CANCER SYNDROMES

Heritable genetic lesions undergo germline transmission from one generation to the next, and the affected individual is born with one defective copy of a gene in each cell. Heritable mutations may be linked to familial cancer syndromes. Characteristics of heritable familial cancers include an early age of onset compared with sporadic cases, the formation of bilateral tumors in

paired organs, the occurrence of multiple primary tumors in nonpaired organs, and a family history of cancer. Although many of the familial cancer syndromes are due to mutations in recessive tumor suppressor genes, the syndromes generally show a predominantly autosomal dominant pattern of inheritance. This apparent paradox is explained later in the discussion of hereditary retinoblastoma. Some cancer syndromes show a recessive mode of inheritance. In such syndromes, the affected individual must inherit the genetic defect from both parents. For instance, the mutant *ter* gene carried by strain 129/Sv-ter mice confers high susceptibility to testicular teratoma when present in the homozygous state, but not when carried in the heterozygous condition. Interestingly, the role of germline mutations in oncogenes in hereditary cancer syndromes remains unclear.

The seminal work that identified the retinoblastoma (RB) tumor suppressor gene came about through the study of such inherited cancer syndromes (see later discussion). Other well-known inherited cancer syndromes in humans include germline mutations of p53 in Li-Fraumeni syndrome, mutations of NF1 and NF2 that lead to neurofibromatosis, mutations of BRCA1 and BRCA2 associated with breast and ovarian cancers, and mutations in MEN1 and RET, which are associated with multiple endocrine neoplasia. A well-documented veterinary cancer syndrome is the disease with the unwieldy name "hereditary multifocal renal cystadenocarcinoma and nodular dermatofibrosis" that occurs in the German shepherd dog. This disease is characterized by bilateral and multifocal renal tumors, uterine leiomyomas, and nodules in the skin (dermatofibrosis). The gene responsible has been mapped to a locus homologous to the human Birt-Hogg-Dubé locus, mutations which cause a phenotypically similar human disease.

Although the inherited cancer syndromes account for less than 10% of all human cancers, they have led to the identification of a number of important tumor suppressor genes that also play a significant role in sporadic tumors. In dominant cancer syndromes, tumor risk is very markedly increased because of changes in a single gene; however, there are also a variety of tumor susceptibility genes that alter cancer incidence to a considerably lesser extent. A variety of cancer susceptibility patterns have been identified in the dog as shown in Table 6-4. The tumor susceptibility genes identified to date generally encode proteins involved in carcinogen metabolism or DNA repair. Their effects are substantially modified by interactions with each other and with the environment. For instance, the lack of pigmentation in white cats contributes to their susceptibility to squamous cell carcinoma of the ears; however, sun exposure makes a major contribution to tumor incidence in these animals.

ACQUIRED SOMATIC MUTATIONS

In contrast to germline mutations, acquired mutations occur in somatic cells and are restricted to individual cells and their progeny. These mutations are not passed through the germline. Whatever the germline genetic background upon which a tumor develops, additional genetic changes are required in the specific cells that give rise to the tumor. Somatic genetic alterations are caused both by intrinsic and extrinsic agents. These changes accumulate randomly over time, thus aging dramatically increases the risk of cancer. The graph shown in Fig. 6-41 illustrates the increased risk of cancer with age in the human population, for which

Table **6-4**   **Cancer Susceptibility in Dogs**

Tumor Site	Tumor Type	Susceptible Breeds	Resistant Breeds
Hematopoietic system	Lymphoma	Boxer	Crossbreeds
	Malignant histiocytosis	Bernese mountain dog	
Brain	Various	Boston terrier, boxer, bulldog	
Skin	Mast cell tumor	Boxer, bulldog, retriever	
	Vascular tumor		
	Hemangiosarcoma	German shepherd	
Mammary gland	Various	Boxer,* Brittany spaniel, dachshund, English setter, Labrador retriever, pointer, Springer spaniel	Boxer,* German shepherd, crossbreeds
Nose and sinuses	Various	Airedale, collie, Scottish terrier	
Oropharynx	Various	Boxer, cocker spaniel, golden retriever	Beagle, dachshund
Ovary	Carcinoma	Pointer	
Pancreas	Carcinoma, insulinoma	Airedale terrier, poodle	
Thyroid	Carcinoma	Beagle, boxer, retriever	Poodle
Skeleton	Osteosarcoma	Giant breeds, boxer, Danish dog, German shepherd, rottweiler	Crossbreeds
Testis		Boxer, collie, German shepherd	
Urinary bladder	Carcinoma	Beagle, collie, Scottish terrier	

Modified from McCullen JM, Page R, Misdorp W: An overview of cancer pathogenesis, diagnosis, and management. In Meuten DJ, editor: *Tumors in domestic animals*, Ames, 2002, Iowa State Press.
*Information obtained from two independent studies.

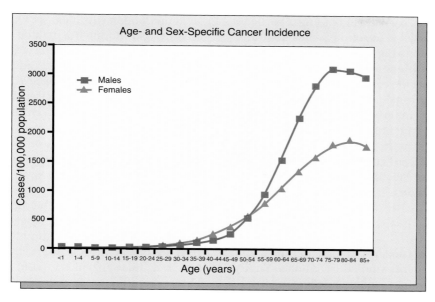

Fig. 6-41   **Cancer incidence by age in the human population of the United States for the year 2001.** Cancer incidence is shown as the number of cases of invasive cancer per 100,000 persons. Data for all races and all cancer sites are combined. Basal and squamous cell carcinomas of sun-exposed skin and all in situ cancers except urinary bladder cancers are excluded. Data are from selected state and metropolitan area cancer registries and cover approximately 92% of the U.S. population. *(Compiled by Dr. D.F. Kusewitt from data released by the Centers for Disease Control and Prevention.)*

solid epidemiologic data are available. Somatic mutations are responsible for the majority of cancers in humans and probably in animals.

INTRINSIC FACTORS

As a byproduct of ordinary metabolism, a variety of DNA damaging agents are produced, including reactive oxygen species. Moreover, DNA is susceptible to ordinary hydrolytic attack. These processes induce a variety of DNA lesions that can result in mutation. Moreover, in the course of many rounds of replication, DNA changes are introduced as a result of DNA polymerase errors. Illegitimate recombination, inappropriate nucleotide addition, and altered DNA methylation, activities carried out by normal cellular enzymes, can lead to the accumulation of DNA alterations. Chromosomal abnormalities also arise as a result of decreased telomere length, altered telomerase activity, and mistakes in chromosome segregation.

EXTRINSIC FACTORS

Extrinsic factors that interact with DNA to cause cancer include chemical, physical, and infectious agents. Mutagens are agents that create DNA damage that gives rise to mutations, whereas carcinogens are agents that cause cancer. Many mutagens are also carcinogens. However, there are carcinogens with

unknown mechanisms of action; such carcinogens may or may not be mutagens.

CHEMICALS

Chemical carcinogens are widespread in the environment. All animals are exposed to low levels of carcinogens in air, water, food, and medications; accidental exposure to very high levels of carcinogens occasionally occurs. One notable chemical cause of cancer in animals is the bracken fern plant, the toxin of which causes urinary bladder cancer in cattle grazing pastures containing the plant. Unlike humans, however, animals do not voluntarily expose themselves to potent carcinogens, such as tobacco smoke.

RADIATION

Natural sources of radiation include the sunlight and cosmic rays that bombard the earth and naturally occurring radioisotopes, such as radon, in the soil. Medical procedures, including diagnostic radiographs and radiation therapy, can provide substantial radiation exposure. Radiant energy with wavelengths greater than 5×10^{-5} cm (visible light, infrared radiation, microwaves, radio waves, and electrical waves) is generally considered to be noncarcinogenic. However, shorter wavelength γ-rays, x-rays, and ultraviolet radiation can cause notable DNA damage and resultant mutation.

In addition, high-energy particles, including α-particles (helium nuclei), β-particles (electrons), and neutrons, can be carcinogenic. Ionizing radiation includes those forms of radiation with enough energy to eject electrons from target molecules (γ-rays, x-rays, α-particles, β-particles, and neutrons). Because most animals have hair, ultraviolet radiation is generally not an important veterinary carcinogen. There are, however, two instances in which the ultraviolet radiation in sunlight poses a significant risk to animals: squamous cell carcinoma of the ears in white cats and ocular squamous cell carcinoma in Hereford cattle with nonpigmented eyelids.

INFECTIOUS AGENTS

Viruses as a cause of cancer were first identified and have been most thoroughly studied in animals. Virally induced tumors in animals often affect a relatively large number of animals in a flock or herd, frequently arise in relatively young animals, and generally show a pattern of occurrence consistent with an infectious cause. There are many types of oncogenic viruses that induce cancer by a large variety of mechanisms. Table 6-5 summarizes those viruses of significance to veterinary medicine. Oncogenic retroviruses are small RNA viruses that cause many neoplastic diseases of importance in animals, including avian leukosis, feline leukemia, and bovine leukosis. Oncogenic DNA viruses include papillomaviruses that cause skin cancer, hepadnaviruses associated with liver cancer, and herpesviruses that induce adenocarcinomas, lymphomas, and leukemias. Species of *Helicobacter* bacteria have been recently demonstrated to play a role in gastric carcinoma and gastric lymphoma in ferrets and mice and in hepatocellular carcinoma in mice.

MECHANISMS OF CARCINOGENESIS

CHEMICAL

A very wide variety of chemicals can cause cancer. Direct-acting chemical carcinogens are effective in the form in which they enter the body, but most carcinogens are procarcinogens that require metabolic activation by cellular enzymes to form ultimate carcinogens. These are thus termed indirect-acting carcinogens. Despite their varied composition, the effective form of most carcinogens is an electrophilic compound that binds covalently to DNA to form DNA adducts. Fig. 6-42 illustrates the general mechanism of chemical carcinogenesis.

As discussed previously, experimental carcinogenesis studies have been critical in elucidating the stepwise development of cancer. Moreover, these studies have clearly defined the contribution of initiating versus

Table **6-5**   **Oncogenic Viruses of Animals**

Classification	Virus	Species Affected	Associated Tumors
Retrovirus	Mouse mammary tumor virus	Mouse	Mammary adenocarcinomas
	Avian sarcoma-leukosis virus complex	Fowl	Various sarcomas, carcinomas, lymphomas, leukemias
	Avian reticuloendotheliosis virus complex	Fowl	Lymphomas, leukemias
	Mouse leukemia and sarcoma viruses	Mouse	Various sarcomas, carcinomas, lymphomas, leukemias
	Feline leukemia virus	Cat	Leukemias, lymphomas
	Bovine leukosis virus	Cattle	Leukemias, lymphomas
	Primate leukemia and sarcoma viruses	Primate	Fibrosarcomas, leukemias
	Mason-Pfizer monkey virus	Primate	Fibrosarcomas
	Feline immunodeficiency viruses	Cat	Lymphomas
	Jaagsiekte sheep retrovirus	Sheep	Pulmonary carcinomas
Hepadnavirus	Hepatitis B group	Primate, rodent, duck	Hepatocellular carcinomas
Papovavirus	Polyoma	Mouse	Various carcinomas, sarcomas
	SV40	Primate	Sarcomas (in rodents)
	Papilloma	Many species	Papillomas, carcinomas
Adenovirus	Types 2, 5, 12	Human	Sarcomas (in hamsters)
Herpesvirus	Frog herpesvirus	Frog	Adenocarcinomas
	Marek's disease	Fowl	Lymphoproliferative disease
	Herpesvirus ateles	Primate	Lymphomas, leukemias
	Herpesvirus saimiri		
Poxvirus	Various	Various	Fibromas, papillomas

Modified from Wyke J: Viruses and cancer. In Franks LM, Reich NM, editors: *Cellular and molecular biology of cancer*, New York, 2003, Oxford University Press.

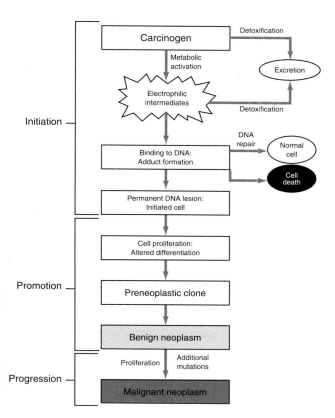

Fig. 6-42   General schema of events in chemical carcinogenesis. Note that promoters cause clonal expansion of the initiated cell, thus producing a preneoplastic clone. Further proliferation induced by the promoter leads to formation of a benign neoplasm. Accumulation of additional mutations during the phase of tumor progression results in emergence of a malignant tumor. *(Modified from Kumar V, Abbas A, Fausto N: Robbins & Cotran pathologic basis of disease, ed 7, Philadelphia, 2005, Saunders.)*

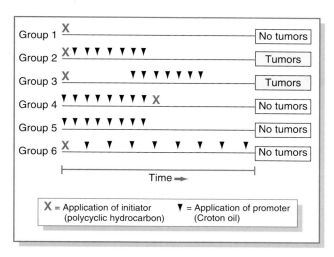

Fig. 6-43   Experiments demonstrating the initiation and promotion phases of chemical skin carcinogenesis in mice. Tumors arose only if application of an initiator was followed by multiple applications of a promoter. For group 2, application of the promoter was repeated at twice-weekly intervals for several months. For group 3, application of the promoter was delayed for several months and the promoter was then applied twice weekly. When the promoter was applied at monthly rather than twice-weekly intervals (group 6), it did not effectively promote tumor emergence. *(From Kumar V, Abbas A, Fausto N: Robbins & Cotran pathologic basis of disease, ed 7, Philadelphia, 2005, Saunders.)*

promoting agents to cancer development (Fig. 6-43). In multistage tumorigenesis models, such as the skin carcinogenesis model in mice, the initiator must be administered before the promoting agent. The initiator is ineffective without subsequent application of a promoter. Moreover, multiple closely spaced promoter treatments are required to drive tumor emergence.

RADIATION

Unlike chemicals, all forms of radiation are complete carcinogens (i.e., they are able both to initiate and, with continued exposure, to promote tumorigenesis). Direct DNA damage due to ionizing radiation consists primarily of single- and double-strand breaks and base elimination. However, ionizing radiation also generates free radicals from many cellular molecules. The interactions of these highly reactive molecules result in many forms of indirect DNA damage, including altered bases and DNA-protein cross-links. Absorption of ultraviolet radiation by DNA results in the formation of hallmark

DNA adducts, pyrimidine dimers, which are potentially mutagenic. To a lesser extent, ultraviolet radiation generates reactive oxygen species, leading to indirect DNA damage like strand breaks and DNA-protein cross-links.

VIRAL

Although a common feature of most oncogenic viruses is the requirement for a DNA stage during viral replication, they employ a remarkable array of direct and indirect mechanisms to induce cancer.

DOMINANT ONCOGENE

The genomes of many rapidly transforming viruses include a dominant oncogene that drives tumor development. Oncogenes may be of ancient or more recent host cell origin, such as the *fes, fgr, abl, fms*, and *kit* genes transduced by oncogenic retroviruses of cats. Viruses may also contain oncogenes not of host cell origin. For example, papillomavirus genomes include the E6 and E7 genes that encode inhibitors of the p53 and pRb tumor suppressor proteins, respectively; some viruses contain genes that encode growth stimulatory molecules, such as the small T antigen of SV40.

INSERTIONAL MUTAGENESIS

Viruses that do not possess their own oncogenes can instead activate expression of cellular oncogenes by a process of insertional mutagenesis. For example, most tumors caused by the avian leukosis virus exhibit a similar site of viral insertion, suggesting that virally induced alterations in genes at that site in the host genome are essential for tumorigenesis.

HIT AND RUN MECHANISM

In the two mechanisms discussed previously, the viral genome or portions of the genome persist in the host cell. However, some viruses also cause tumors merely by transient residence in target cells. The precise mechanism by which this might occur has not been elucidated. Bovine papillomavirus uses such a *hit and run* mechanism of cell transformation.

INDIRECT MECHANISMS

Viruses may also stimulate tumorigenesis by suppression of the host immune system or stimulation of target cell proliferation. The herpesvirus that causes Marek's disease is an example of a virus that suppresses the ability of the host to eliminate transformed cells, whereas hepatitis viruses exemplify viruses that stimulate cell proliferation.

MOLECULAR DETERMINANTS OF CANCER

TUMOR SUPPRESSOR GENES

Cells receive signals for both growth stimulation and inhibition, and must maintain the proper balance between these stimuli. The designation of tumor suppressor gene was originally given to genes that inhibited cell growth. Over time, the class of tumor suppressor genes has expanded to include many different types of cancer-related genes that, when inactivated through genetic and/or epigenetic means, lead to uncontrolled proliferation or tumor growth. This includes genes that control cell cycle, apoptosis, DNA repair, and other fundamental pathways.

The pivotal concept of tumor suppressor genes was posited by Alfred Knudson in 1971, based on his observations of children with familial and sporadic retinoblastoma, an uncommon tumor arising in retinoblasts. Knudson's two-hit hypothesis states that both alleles of a tumor suppressor gene must undergo mutation (i.e., a genetic "hit") for cancer to develop. In inherited cancer syndromes, the person is born with a mutation in one allele of all cells in the body (Fig. 6-44). The second hit is acquired as a somatic mutation of the tumor suppressor gene in one cell and leads to cancer development at a much earlier age than in a person who was not born with the germline mutation. The development of a sporadic tumor requires that a person sustain two hits, one on each allele of the same gene

in the same cell, which has a much lower probability of occurrence.

Loss of both alleles in a single cell is a rare event; however, loss of only one allele occurs much more frequently. If this takes place in a cell that already lacks a functional copy of the gene, expression of the tumor suppressor gene is completely abrogated and cancer is likely to result. It has subsequently been shown that loss of the second allele can occur by a variety of mechanisms, including point mutation in the allele, deletion of the allele or the chromosomal segment where it resides, deletion of the entire chromosome containing the allele, or mitotic recombination resulting in replacement of the normal allele by the mutant allele. When the normal allele has been completely lost, the cell and its progeny contain only the single abnormal allele. This is called loss of heterozygosity.

Tumor suppressor genes are frequently located in areas of the genome that are deleted in cancer. The areas of chromosomal loss can be limited to small deletions of a few hundred base pairs or encompass a whole chromosome arm or even an entire chromosome. By examining a large number of tumors, the minimal region of loss can be defined as the common region, which is deleted in all tumors of the type under investigation. Candidate tumor suppressor genes within the boundaries of this area can then be further interrogated for the presence of inactivating mutations in the remaining allele. Confirmation of the candidate gene as a *bona fide* tumor suppressor gene involves complex *in vitro* and *in vivo* experiments, such as demonstrating that (1) loss of the gene product leads to increased ability to form colonies in soft agar, (2) the presence of mutation, deletion, or hypermethylation along with the absence of the gene product in primary tumors, and (3) loss of the gene correlates with increased tumorigenicity in mouse models. In addition to loss of genetic material and inactivating mutations, it is now widely recognized that DNA methylation, discussed earlier, is an alternative method of silencing tumor suppressor genes.

Many tumor suppressor genes are key components of the cell cycle. One of the most widely studied tumor suppressor genes is p53, and it is inactivated most commonly by mutation in more than half of human cancers. It is a DNA-binding protein that regulates transcription of numerous genes and plays a critical role in cell-cycle arrest and induction of apoptosis following DNA damage. For these reasons, it has been entitled the guardian of the genome. Levels of p53 are rapidly elevated in response to DNA damage. This leads to increased transcription of p53 target genes, such as p21 and GADD45, which function in cell-cycle arrest and DNA repair, respectively. The half-life of p53 is short (about 20 minutes) and is rapidly degraded following completion of DNA repair. If the DNA repair

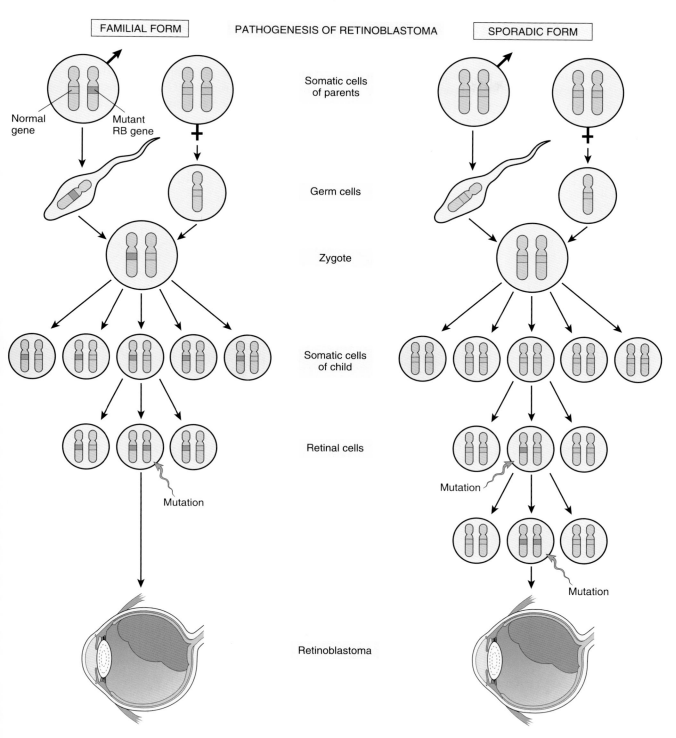

FAMILIAL FORM   PATHOGENESIS OF RETINOBLASTOMA   SPORADIC FORM

Normal gene   Mutant RB gene

Somatic cells of parents

Germ cells

Zygote

Somatic cells of child

Retinal cells

Mutation

Mutation

Mutation

Retinoblastoma

Fig. 6-44   Schematic illustration of the pathogenesis of retinoblastomas (*RBs*) and the "two hit" hypothesis. Two mutations of the RB gene lead to neoplastic proliferation of the retinal cells. In the familial form (*left*), all somatic cells have one mutant copy of the RB gene inherited from a carrier parent. The second mutation affects the RB locus in one of the retinal cells after birth. In the sporadic form (*right*), both RB mutations are acquired by the retinal cells after birth. (*From Kumar V, Abbas A, Fausto N:* Robbins & Cotran pathologic basis of disease, *ed 7, Philadelphia, 2005, Saunders.*)

is unsuccessful, p53 directs cell death by activating BCL2-associated X protein (BAX), a key component of the apoptotic cascade (Fig. 6-45). It is clear then that loss of functional p53 can have devastating consequences for maintaining integrity of the genome. Without p53, mutagenic DNA damage goes unchecked, the cell proceeds through division, and the mutation becomes fixed in the genome.

Another widely studied tumor suppressor gene is the retinoblastoma gene. As described earlier, RB is a target for inactivation both in germline and somatic cells and, like p53, plays an important role in cell-cycle control. In quiescent cells, RB is hypophosphorylated and active. When RB is hyperphosphorylated and inactive, the cell can proceed through the G_1/S transition. Control of proper RB function and phosphorylation status involves a host of other genes, including p16INK4a, cyclin D, and CDK4. Therefore a defect in any one of these gene products disrupts the RB pathway and leads to unregulated progression through the cell cycle.

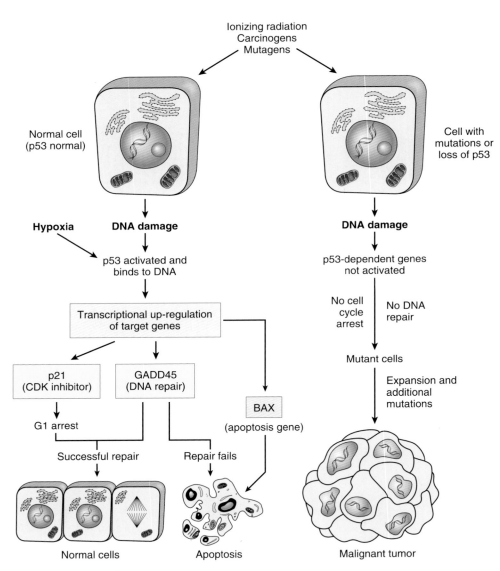

Fig. 6-45   The role of p53 in maintaining integrity of the genome. DNA damage or hypoxia activate normal p53, leading to G_1 arrest and induction of DNA repair by upregulation of p21 and GADD45, respectively. Successful DNA repair allows cells to proceed through the cell cycle. If DNA repair fails, BCL2-associated X protein (*BAX*) promotes apoptosis. In cells with loss or mutation of p53, DNA damage does not induce cell-cycle arrest or DNA repair. The genetically damaged cells proliferate and may eventually give rise to malignant neoplasms.
(From Kumar V, Abbas A, Fausto N: Robbins & Cotran pathologic basis of disease, ed 7, Philadelphia, 2005, Saunders.)

Although the classic definition of a tumor suppressor gene dictates that both alleles must be inactivated (through loss, mutation, or promoter methylation), recent evidence suggests that for certain genes inactivation of only one copy is sufficient for tumor growth (haploinsufficiency). Haploinsufficiency can contribute to tumor development by a number of mechanisms. One mechanism is a simple gene-dosage effect in which half the normal amount of a protein is insufficient to maintain the normal homeostatic balance in the cell. Alternatively, a mutation in one allele can give rise to a dominant-negative protein whereby the abnormal protein blocks the function of the normal protein produced by the remaining wild-type allele. A third mechanism occurs when a mutation in one allele of a tumor suppressor gene decreases the amount of normal protein in a cell, which may in turn influence other pathways that may have concurrent abnormalities.

ONCOGENES

Oncogenes are derived from proto-oncogenes—normal cellular genes that regulate cell growth and differentiation. Proto-oncogenes encode products involved in diverse pathways and include molecules such as growth factors and their receptors, cell-cycle regulators, DNA-binding proteins, transcription factors, protein kinases, and others. Oncogenes were first identified as RNA tumor virus proteins. Later it was discovered that normal cells have the equivalent gene products.

There are a number of ways in which oncogenes can be abnormally activated to promote tumor growth. The genomic region containing the gene can be amplified, resulting in dramatically increased copy number. For example, the N-MYC oncogene can be amplified up to 100 times in human neuroblastomas. Oncogenes can undergo mutations that cause constitutive activation of the gene. In these cases, the gene is always "turned on" and is unresponsive to inhibitory signals. This scenario is often the case for cell surface receptors, such as the epidermal growth factor receptor (EGF-R) in carcinomas. Many tyrosine kinase receptors have activating mutations that result in constitutive activation even in the absence of ligands. Tumor cells can also produce large amounts of stimulatory molecules along with their cognate receptors, forming a growth-promoting autocrine loop. All of these mechanisms serve to drive proliferation and render the cell unresponsive to normal inhibitory signals.

The prototype of signal transduction oncogenes is the RAS family of guanine triphosphate binding proteins (G proteins). There are several members of this family, including HRAS, KRAS, and NRAS. In normal cells, RAS transmits growth stimulatory signals from outside the cell to the nucleus, ultimately activating transcription of genes for cell-cycle progression. RAS alternates between an active and inactive state in its normal location on the cytoplasmic side of the cell membrane where it is closely associated with farnesyl transferase. Inactive RAS binds guanine diphosphate (GDP). Upon receiving a stimulatory signal from a growth factor, RAS exchanges GDP for guanine triphosphate (GTP). RAS bound to GTP is the active form, which triggers the RAS–RAF–mitogen-activated protein kinase (MAPK) pathway and results in transcription of genes that promote cell division (Fig. 6-46). The activation of RAS is normally short lived, as RAS has an intrinsic GTPase that hydrolyzes GTP to GDP and converts RAS to its inactive state. In many cancers, RAS is constitutively activated either by mutations in RAS itself or by failure of the GTPase to inactivate RAS. RAS family members, the farnesyl transferase anchor to the plasma membrane, and other components of the signal transduction pathway are all attractive molecular targets for therapeutic intervention in cancer patients.

DEFECTS IN DNA REPAIR

Defects in DNA repair enzymes are one cause of mutations and genomic instability. If mutations inactivate tumor suppressor genes and activate oncogenes, the cell has a selective growth advantage. Specific types of DNA repair mechanisms have evolved to repair specific DNA lesions. Mismatch repair enzymes, such as MLH1 and MSH2 proofread DNA, much like the "spell check" function on a computer, to locate and fix single nucleotide mismatches that occur on a regular basis. For example, if an adenine is mistakenly paired with a guanine during DNA replication, this error will be recognized and corrected.

It is well recognized that exposure to ultraviolet light leads to cross-linking of pyrimidine residues and formation of pyrimidine dimers. These lesions require a large cohort of DNA repair proteins to perform a nucleotide excision repair procedure. This process is similar to the "cut and paste" function of a computer in which the dimer is excised and the correct nucleotides are replaced and ligated in its stead. As discussed earlier, p53 levels rise in response to DNA damage from any number of agents and give the cell time to carry out the repair processes.

Additional DNA repair genes include ATM, BRCA1, and BRCA2 in humans. Failure of DNA repair of any type can lead to the mutation becoming fixed in the genome and passed on with subsequent rounds of cell division. When the DNA repair gene itself is defective, either through mutation, promoter methylation, or genomic loss, the result is a myriad of mutations throughout the genome with widespread genomic instability and increased cancer susceptibility.

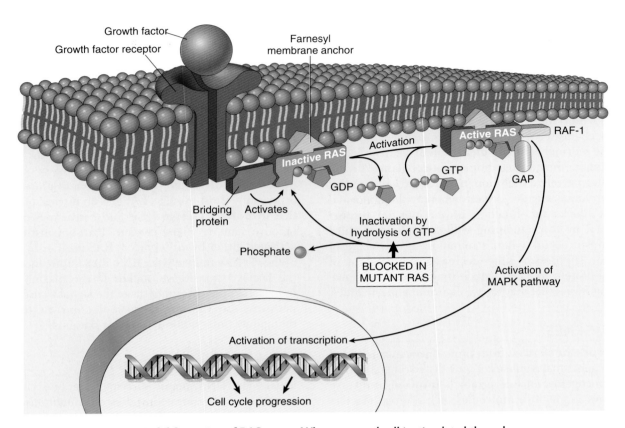

Fig. 6-46   Model for action of RAS genes. When a normal cell is stimulated through a growth factor receptor, inactive (guanine diphosphate [*GDP*]-bound) RAS is activated to a guanine triphosphate (*GTP*)-bound state. Activated RAS recruits RAF and stimulates the mitogen-activated protein kinase (*MAPK*) pathway to transmit growth-promoting signals to the nucleus. In cancer, mutated RAS is permanently activated because of the inability to hydrolyze GTP, leading to continuous stimulation of cells in the absence of an external trigger. The anchoring of RAS to the cell membrane by the farnesyl moiety is essential for its action. *GAP*, GTPase-activating protein. (*From Kumar V, Abbas A, Fausto N: Robbins & Cotran pathologic basis of disease, ed 7, Philadelphia, 2005, Saunders.*)

ANIMALS AND CANCER

ANIMAL MODELS OF CANCER

Animal models have been and remain critically important tools for understanding the cause of human cancer and for testing cancer therapeutic agents. Animal models of cancer include both experimentally induced and naturally occurring. In experimentally induced cancer models, administration of carcinogenic substances or transplantation of human cancer cells results in *de novo* development of cancer in test animals. Naturally occurring models of cancer rely on the spontaneous development of tumors in the test animal.

EXPERIMENTALLY INDUCED TUMORS

A major advantage of experimental model systems is the rapid and reproducible induction of cancer in a very large proportion of experimental animals. Rodents, mice in particular, are often used for such studies. Mice are small and relatively inexpensive

to maintain. Moreover, mice reproduce rapidly and their genetics are highly defined and readily manipulated. The mouse genome has recently been sequenced, essentially in its entirety, and detailed comparative maps of the human and mouse genomes have been developed. Many inbred mouse strains, each consisting of genetically identical or syngeneic individuals, are available. Syngeneic mice readily accept tissue grafts from each other. Genetic homogeneity of syngeneic mice tends to standardize responses and thus reduce the numbers of animals required for studies. A number of inbred mouse strains have been developed that are particularly suited to specific needs in cancer research. For instance, Sencar mice are highly susceptible to tumors of keratinocyte origin and are thus employed for many skin carcinogenesis studies. Nude mice, which are profoundly immunodeficient, accept tumor or normal tissue grafts from other species and provide an environment in which these xenografts can be maintained, manipulated, and studied. Differences in strain susceptibility to different experimentally induced cancers have been exploited to identify modifier genes that dramatically affect tumor incidence. With the advent of effective means for creating genetically engineered mice, specific genes of interest can be introduced into or inactivated in the mouse genome. A gene introduced into the mouse genome is generally termed a transgene. A mouse lacking a functional normal gene is a knockout for that gene. Moreover, the timing, location, and level of gene expression in genetically engineered mice can now be precisely controlled, thus allowing gene expression to be turned on or off in particular tissues as required for specific studies. Gene expression modulated in this fashion is termed conditional gene expression.

Conventional inbred mice have been used extensively to determine the carcinogenicity of chemical and physical agents and to test the safety and efficacy of anticancer therapeutics. Studies in mice, particularly studies of chemically induced skin cancer, have been critical in defining the stages of carcinoma progression. Genetically engineered mice have been essential for identifying the mechanisms by which specific genes act to retard or enhance tumor development, growth, and spread. However, mice have several inherent shortcomings as models of human cancer. The genetic homogeneity of inbred mice does not reflect the high degree of genetic diversity within the general human population. The spectrum of experimentally induced tumors in mice differs from the spectrum of naturally occurring tumors in humans. Moreover, experimentally induced tumors in mice rarely metastasize; in humans, on the other hand, tumor metastasis is of overwhelming importance. Finally, the short life span and small size of mice make them less than ideal for long-term testing of tumor therapies.

NATURALLY OCCURRING TUMORS

Several naturally occurring cancers in animals, including avian leukosis, bovine lymphoma, and feline leukemia, have provided invaluable information about the cause, transmission, and prevention of virally induced cancers. However, virally induced cancers do not appear to account for a large proportion of human cancers. Recently the dog has become the focus of increasing attention as a useful animal model of nonviral human cancers. The recent sequencing of the canine genome and comparative alignment with human and murine genomes enhance the usefulness of dogs as a naturally occurring cancer model.

The age-adjusted cancer incidence in dogs is 381 per 100,000; this is comparable with the cancer incidence in humans. With the large number of pet dogs in this country, many cancer cases are thus available for entry into clinical trials. Like humans, dogs are outbred.

Moreover, dogs share a common environment with humans and are exposed to many of the same carcinogens. As in humans, many canine tumors metastasize widely. Because tumors in dogs progress more rapidly than human tumors, studies can be completed within a reasonable time frame. On the other hand, the time course of tumor development is sufficiently long to allow meaningful comparison of response times in different treatment groups. Because dogs are relatively large, they provide abundant tumor tissue for diagnostic and experimental purposes. In addition, many therapeutic approaches that are difficult to test in small rodents can readily be examined using larger dogs. Clinical trials in dogs are much easier to instigate and much cheaper to carry out than comparable studies in humans. Many dog owners are enthusiastic participants in clinical trials that may benefit their pets. Tumor types for which dogs are particularly good models of human cancer include osteosarcoma and lymphoma.

CLINICAL ONCOLOGY

HISTOPATHOLOGIC DIAGNOSIS

A definitive diagnosis of cancer is frequently obtained by standard histopathology and/or cytology from incisional or excisional biopsies or aspirates. Biopsy specimens are analyzed by routine hematoxylin and eosin (H&E) staining for histopathologic evaluation, and by Wright's stain or Diff-Quik for aspirates. Cells are scrutinized for features of malignancy, including abnormal morphology, evidence of invasion and/or metastasis, high mitotic index, presence of abnormal mitoses, high nuclear:cytoplasmic ratio, and absence of encapsulation. The degree of differentiation is evaluated. Malignant neoplasms are frequently poorly to moderately differentiated, and some may be so anaplastic that the cell of origin cannot be determined. Abnormal structures or cellular products may also provide clues to the presence of malignancy.

Special staining techniques may be used to aid in the diagnosis of some tumors. For example, immunohistochemistry can establish if a lymphoma originates from B lymphocytes or T lymphocytes (Fig. 6-47). This knowledge may be useful to the clinician in designing treatment or delivering a prognosis. The type of intermediate filaments present in an undifferentiated malignancy can indicate if the tumor is of epithelial (positive for cytokeratin staining) or mesenchymal (positive for vimentin staining) origin. Some neoplasms, such as mesotheliomas and synovial cell sarcomas, are often positive for both cytokeratin and vimentin. Squamous cell carcinomas that have undergone epithelial-to-mesenchymal transformation will have areas positive for one stain or the other, and the transition areas may be positive for both. An exhaustive list

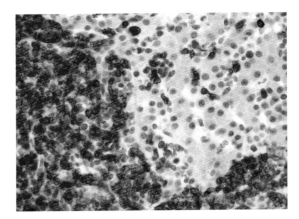

Fig. 6-47   Lymphoma, liver, dog. Note the neoplastic lymphocytes invading the liver. The malignant cells are immunohistochemically positive for CD3 *(brown color),* indicating a T-lymphocyte neoplasm. The surrounding hepatocytes are not labeled. Immunohistochemistry. *(Courtesy Dr. D.F. Kusewitt, College of Veterinary Medicine, The Ohio State University.)*

of antibodies is beyond the scope of this chapter, but immunohistochemical staining is becoming a widely used tool that assists the pathologist in providing a more complete diagnosis in cases in which routine H&E evaluation is limited.

Histochemical stains can also aid in diagnosis. Poorly differentiated canine mast cells may have granules that are not clearly visible by H&E staining. Staining with toluidine blue often highlights the granules and confirms the diagnosis in otherwise challenging cases.

CLONALITY ASSAYS

Although cells can exhibit some degree of heterogeneity within a tumor as a result of clonal selection (see previous discussion), all of the neoplastic cells originated from expansion of a single transformed cell. *Clonality* can be assessed using the HUMARA (human androgen receptor assay) method in females who are polymorphic at the X-linked androgen receptor locus (Fig. 6-48). Other X-linked genes that can be interrogated include G6PD or PGK. Because females have random inactivation of one X chromosome in each cell, clonality can be demonstrated by showing that each cell within a tumor population has the same X chromosome inactivated (thus the need to use polymorphic markers). If the tumor population has equal distribution of inactivated X chromosomes, it is not monoclonal. These assays have not been well established in companion animals.

Clonality can be determined by a different method in lymphoid malignancies. Sometimes it is difficult to distinguish benign lymphoid hyperplasia from lymphoma by morphology alone. Establishing that the lymphocyte population is clonal gives more weight to the diagnosis of a malignancy. This can be done by

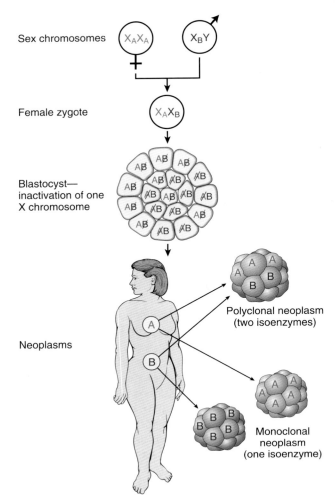

Fig. 6-48   Diagram depicting the use of X-linked isoenzyme markers to assess monoclonality of tumors. Because of random X-inactivation, all females are mosaics with two cell populations (G6PD isoenzyme A or B in this case). Monoclonal neoplasms are composed of cells that contain the active maternal (X_A) or the paternal (X_B) X chromosome, but not both. These assays can only be used in females who are heterozygous at the X-linked marker being tested. *(From Kumar V, Abbas A, Fausto N:* Robbins & Cotran pathologic basis of disease, *ed 7, Philadelphia, 2005, Saunders.)*

analyzing the lymphocytes for T- or B-lymphocyte receptor rearrangement using the polymerase chain reaction (PCR). If the entire lymphocyte population has a single rearrangement, this is indicative of a clonal population. Conversely, if each lymphocyte has a different receptor rearrangement, this indicates a nonclonal population, which is more consistent with a reactive specimen. It must be remembered that the presence of a clonal population does not, by itself, mean that the specimen is a malignancy. Some nonneoplastic conditions, such as canine ehrlichiosis, can give rise to clonal lymphocyte populations. Therefore results need to be interpreted in conjunction with clinical signs and other clinicopathologic data.

OTHER MOLECULAR DIAGNOSTIC TECHNIQUES

A full description of molecular techniques used in cancer diagnosis is beyond the scope of this chapter. However, it is certain that their use will be become more widespread and commonplace in veterinary medicine. Cytogenetic analysis can be a useful tool for diagnosis, determining the presence of residual disease after treatment, stratification of high- and low-risk patients. The discovery of recurrent chromosomal abnormalities and translocations, particularly in leukemias and lymphomas, will aid in diagnosis and understanding the pathogenesis of these diseases.

The increasing use of microarrays for global gene expression analysis in the research setting will undoubtedly lead to identification of panels of specific biomarkers that can be used for diagnosis in the future. Microarrays, which allow the measurement of thousands of genes simultaneously in a single sample, are already available for dogs and horses, and it is anticipated that other species will be added to the list. Large-scale studies using carefully selected tumor samples will be necessary to identify significant diagnostic and prognostic changes in gene expression patterns, which can be applied to individual tumors to provide important information to the clinician. Likewise, the advancement of proteomics for the large-scale interrogation of protein expression in tumors will add to our diagnostic armamentarium.

Finally, identification of genes involved in inherited cancers can be accomplished through the detailed analysis of well-described pedigrees, particularly in certain cancer-prone breeds. As is the case in humans, the elucidation of these genes is important not only in the diagnosis and screening of high-risk animals but also in providing insight into the pathogenesis of sporadic tumors.

GRADING

A tumor grade is assigned by the pathologist to provide some indication of how similar or dissimilar the neoplastic cells are to their normal counterparts. The underlying assumption is that this provides some indication about biologic behavior. This is not universally true, however, and experience has demonstrated that tumor stage (see next section) is sometimes a more useful parameter. Grading schemes vary depending on the tumor type. The ideal scheme incorporates criteria that are easily identified on an H&E stained section, and the grade is strongly linked to prognosis or response to therapy.

All grading schemes evaluate the degree of differentiation of tumor cells. The tumor grade classifications usually include well-differentiated (cells appear very similar to normal cells), moderately differentiated (somewhat similar to normal cells), and poorly differentiated (anaplastic) cells. These categories translate to low, medium, and high grade, or grades I, II, and III, respectively. Other criteria that may be included in grading schemes include the mitotic rate (i.e., the number of mitotic figures in ten $40\times$ fields), the degree of necrosis, location and invasiveness of the tumor, and overall cellularity. To be biologically relevant, the grading system for a particular tumor type should be based on objective criteria that can be assessed on routine sections with high concordance between different evaluators and provide the clinician with useful information. As such, criteria need to be periodically reevaluated in light of new discoveries and diagnostic capabilities.

STAGING

Tumor stage gives an indication of the extent of tumor growth and spread. In general, staging guides the clinician in developing a therapeutic plan and offering an estimate of prognosis to the client. One of the most widely used schemes is the TNM system, which is based on the size of the primary tumor (T), degree of lymph node involvement (N), and extent of metastasis (M). Within each category, a number is assigned based on clinical, diagnostic, and histopathologic evaluation. A designation of T_0 is given to carcinoma in situ, whereas T_1 to T_4 indicate increasing size of the primary tumor. N_0 indicates the absence of detectable lymph node involvement, whereas N_1 to N_3 indicate progressive involvement. Similarly, M_0 signifies no detectable metastasis, whereas M_1 and M_2 indicate metastasis to one and two organs, respectively.

Overall, TNM staging provides a standard measurement by which the natural course of disease and impact of treatment modalities can be compared. Increased availability of more sophisticated diagnostic testing, such as computerized tomography (CT) and magnetic resonance imaging (MRI), as well as more sensitive histologic detection, such as the use of immunohistochemistry for cytokeratin to detect micrometastases in lymph nodes of patients with carcinoma, may influence comparisons of studies among investigators.

SURGICAL MARGINS

Typically, excisional biopsies are performed with the intent of complete removal of the tumor mass to effect a cure or greatly reduce tumor burden. Histologic evaluation of surgical margins has long been a valuable service provided by the diagnostic pathologist. Margins of the tumor are evaluated microscopically for the presence or absence of tumor cells to confirm that the tumor was completely excised. Residual malignant cells at the surgical site may warrant a second surgical procedure.

Evaluation of margins is not always straightforward. Sometimes it is difficult for the pathologist to properly orient the gross specimen with respect to lateral, deep, and superficial margins. At other times it may be difficult to distinguish true surgical margins from those produced at trimming. This uncertainty can be diminished if the surgeon marks the tumor with ink (preferable) or sutures upon removal of the tumor from the body, and indicates in the pathology request which margins (lateral, deep) are so marked. In select circumstances, evaluation of surgical margins on frozen tissue sections while the patient remains under anesthesia may be beneficial. If residual tumor cells are present at the margins, the surgeon then has the opportunity to immediately make a wider excision without subjecting the patient to a second operative procedure. It is important to realize that having clean surgical margins on a histologic slide does not guarantee that the patient is free of tumor. Neoplasms are three-dimensional lesions that often have irregular growth patterns. Only a portion of the mass is examined in any one section, and although that particular section may have clean margins, other portions of the mass may not. In addition, multifocal or multicentric lesions may not be submitted to the pathologist. Lastly, lymphatic or hematogenous spread may not be evident on the section or sections examined.

The American College of Veterinary Pathologists has formed an Ad Hoc Committee on Oncology to provide guidance on new diagnostic techniques in oncology and develop written guidelines to promote more consistent methods for tumor grading and reporting of margins.

Taken together, the tumor type, grade, stage, and completeness of excision are used by the clinician to develop the most appropriate treatment plan for the patient. As we learn more about the molecular pathogenesis of certain tumors, the need for specialized diagnostic tests will certainly increase. Targeted molecular therapies will be effective only if the target is present in the patient's tumor. For example, a compound that is designed to be active against the internal tandem duplication (ITD) of c-kit in canine mast cell tumors will probably not be very effective if administered to patients without the ITD. Open lines of communication between clinicians and pathologists are vital to the integration and use of such knowledge.

SUGGESTED READINGS

Franks LM, Teich NM: *Introduction to the cellular and molecular biology of cancer*, ed 3, Oxford, 2001, Oxford University Press.

Hanahan D, Weinberg RA: The hallmarks of cancer, *Cell* 100(1): 57-70, 2000.

Herman JG, Baylin SB: Gene silencing in cancer in association with promoter hypermethylation, *N Engl J Med* 349(21): 2042-2054, 2003.

Kufe DW, Bast RC Jr, Hait W et al: *Holland Frei cancer medicine*, ed 7, Hamilton, Ontario, Canada, BC Decker (in press).

Meuten DJ, editor: *Tumors in domestic animals*, ed 4, Ames, 2002, Iowa State Press.

Payne SR, Kemp CJ: Tumor suppressor genetics, *Carcinogenesis* 26(12):2031-2045, 2005.

Pitot HC: *Fundamentals of oncology*, ed 4, New York, Marcel Dekker, 2002.

Sell S: Stem cell origin of cancer and differentiation therapy, *Crit Rev Oncol Hematol* 51(1):1-28, 2004.

Vail DM, MacEwen EG: Spontaneously occurring tumors of companion animals as models for human cancer, *Cancer Invest* 18(8):781-792, 2000.

PATHOLOGY OF ORGAN SYSTEMS

7

Alimentary System*

HOWARD B. GELBERG

INTRODUCTION

The alimentary system is a long and complex tube that varies in its construction and function among animal species. For example, herbivores need fermentation chambers (either a rumen or expanded cecum) for the digestion of cellulose, a feature not present in carnivores. Although a large variety of gastrointestinal disturbances are clinically important in all species of animals, the predominant form of disease varies by species. Pet carnivores, partly because of their long life span, effective vaccines, and a lifestyle and diet similar to that of human beings, have alimentary neoplasia develop far more often than herbivores. Meat, milk, and fiber-producing animals (ruminants and pigs) are host to a variety of infectious diseases that are largely resistant to vaccines. These pathogens may have evolved as a result of the herding instinct of these animals and the opportunity for pathogens to mutate within a large socially structured host population. Equids are most prone to displacements of alimentary viscera.

A large part of the practice of veterinary medicine is devoted to the diagnosis and treatment of alimentary disorders. Many of the newer molecular and imaging tools have been designed specifically to increase the clinician's ability to make accurate diagnoses of the varied conditions of the alimentary system. Additionally, every physical examination includes the opportunity for a fecal analysis that allows the clinician a window into the functioning of the alimentary system as a whole.

Tools such as the polymerase chain reaction (PCR) allow the clinician to rapidly diagnose an infectious cause of enteritis without having to culture the organism in the traditional manner. Diagnosis of the cause of an infectious disease of the alimentary system can also be made after biopsy from paraffin-embedded tissue by immunohistochemical staining or by in situ hybridization that allows demonstration of the pathogen within target cells.

With the advent of fiberoptic endoscopes combined with laparoscopy, a thorough knowledge of normal and abnormal anatomy of the entire alimentary system is of clinical importance in disease diagnosis. This knowledge is now a necessity in clinical practice because gastrointestinal lumens, from the oral mucosa through the esophagus, stomach, duodenum, and the large colon, can be directly viewed in the live animal. With a small abdominal incision and insertion of a fiberoptic laparoscope, the entire serosal surface of the abdominal viscera can be viewed and sampled.

STRUCTURE AND FUNCTION

The most important point to keep in mind when examining the alimentary system is that normal mucosal and serosal surfaces should be smooth and shiny. The exception to this rule is the rumen, in which the papillae may normally have a roughened, towel-like surface appearance. When they do not, animals should be examined thoroughly to determine why they deviate from normal. The function of the alimentary system in its entirety is to take ingested feedstuffs, grind them and mix them with a variety of secretions from the oral cavity, stomach, and intestines (digestion) and absorb the constituent nutrients into the blood stream and lacteals. Undigested ingesta, effete neutrophils, fresh (hematochezia) or digested (melena) blood, and excess secretions are passed from the body into the alimentary lumen and thus become a component of the feces. The quality and quantity of the feces is often an early indicator of alimentary dysfunction, as is regurgitation and vomiting.

*Previous chapters on this subject in earlier editions were written or partially written by Dr. H. Van Kruningen of the Department of Pathobiology, University of Connecticut.

PORTALS OF ENTRY

There are limited numbers of ways that pathogenic agents gain entry into the alimentary system (Box 7-1). The most common, of course, is through ingestion. However, under certain circumstances pathogens may be coughed up by the lungs and swallowed. Systemic blood-borne infections of viruses (viremia), bacteria (bacteremia), and systemic toxins (septicemia and toxemia) may make their way through the blood stream and attach to specific receptors on the epithelial lining cells of the alimentary system. Parasites may migrate through various regions of the body to find a home within the mucosa or free in the lumen of the alimentary tract.

DEFENSE MECHANISMS

Considering the types of materials that are ingested by domestic animals, it is significant to note that they are not constantly ill. This resistance to disease occurs because the alimentary system is well suited to protect itself against most potentially pathogenic insults (Box 7-2). These protective mechanisms include oral secretions such as saliva; "normal" resident flora and fauna; the gastric pH; opening of tight junctions between cells to allow macromolecules such as immunoglobulins into the lumen; vomiting; extraintestinal secretions from the liver and pancreas; intestinal proteolytic enzymes, phagocytes, and other effector cells within the submucosa, which are exuded into the alimentary lumen; the high rate of epithelial turnover; increased peristalsis resulting in diarrhea; Paneth cells; and the immune system. Paneth cells produce antimicrobial peptides and proteins, including lysozyme and secretory phospholipase A_2. They also produce α-defensins (cryptdins).

Box 7-1
Portals of Entry in the Alimentary System
• Ingestion • Coughed up by the lungs and swallowed • Systemic blood-borne infections • Parasite migration

Box 7-2
Defense Mechanisms in the Alimentary System
• Saliva • Resident flora and fauna • Gastric pH • Secreted immunoglobulins • Vomiting • Extraintestinal secretions from the liver and pancreas • Intestinal proteolytic enzymes • Phagocytes and other effector cells within the submucosa • High rate of epithelial turnover • Increased peristalsis resulting in diarrhea • Paneth cells • Adaptive immune system

DISEASES

ORAL CAVITY

INTRODUCTION

Examination and evaluation of the oral cavity is one of the many places where the practice of pathology and clinical medicine merge. This result is because the oral cavity can be examined by the clinician or pathologist using the same criteria for abnormality. The same can be said of the rectal mucosa.

STRUCTURE AND FUNCTION

The physiologically normal oral mucosa is smooth, shiny, and pink. In animals in which the oral mucosa is heavily pigmented (melanosis), assessment of circulatory function (capillary refill time) and color as an indicator of red blood cell concentration (packed cell volume) can be difficult. In these cases, examination of conjunctiva, rectal, and urogenital mucosa can be substituted. The oral cavity is where ingested materials are masticated; mixed with digestive enzymes, such as saliva; and passed on through the oropharynx to the esophagus.

DEFENSE MECHANISMS

Defense mechanisms of the oral cavity include the taste buds, which reject potentially toxic materials based on taste and tongue feel, an indigenous bacterial flora that occupy attachment sites of pathogens, and saliva (Box 7-3). Saliva provides a flushing action so potential pathogens are cleared from the oropharynx. Saliva also forms a protective coating of the mucosa and contains antimicrobial lysozyme and immunoglobulins. Neutrophils at the end of their life span are eliminated by migrating through the alimentary tract. This includes the oral cavity. In their absence, stomatitis results.

DEVELOPMENTAL ANOMALIES

A variety of developmental abnormalities occur in the oral cavity. Some are incompatible with life unless surgically corrected. Of these congenital lesions, only a few have a proven hereditary component. Most are idiopathic. Thorough physical examination of neonates must include examination of the oral cavity for these defects.

Box **7-3**

Defense Mechanisms in the Oral Cavity

- Taste buds that reject potentially toxic materials based on taste and tongue feel
- Indigenous bacterial flora that occupy attachment sites of pathogens
- Saliva
  - Flushing action so potential pathogens are cleared from the oropharynx
  - Protective coating of the mucosa
  - Contains antimicrobial lysozyme and immuno-globulins

Palatoschisis or cleft palate and cheiloschisis or cleft lip are among the most common developmental abnormalities of the oral cavity. Cheiloschisis is sometimes referred to as "hare lip," because this is a normal feature of the rabbit. It is a failure of fusion of the upper lip along the midline or philtrum. Palatoschisis can be genetic or toxic in origin. It results from a failure of fusion of the lateral palatine processes. It can be caused by steroid administration during pregnancy in primates, including human beings. Depending on the size of the defect, which may involve only the soft palate or both the soft and hard palates (Fig. 7-1), the lesion may be surgically correctable. It is a matter of some ethical concern whether to correct such defects without also sterilizing the patient, because the potential for cleft palate to have a genetic cause is present. Important sequelae to the host from cleft palate are starvation due to an inability to create a negative pressure in the mouth and resultant failure to suckle and aspiration pneumonia, because no effective separation is present between the oral and nasal cavities.

STOMATITIS AND GINGIVITIS

Stomatitis and gingivitis refer to inflammation of the mucous membranes of the oral cavity and gingiva, respectively. Because the oral cavity is constantly bombarded with ingested substances that are moved around by the tongue, the final result of a variety of insults to the lining of the oral cavity is a loss of mucosa—erosions, ulcerations, and necrosis. Thus, although inflammation is apparent, clues as to the initiating process may be absent. Lesions are classified as macules, papules, vesicles, erosions, and ulcers. These lesions can be caused by infectious agents, particularly viruses, chemical injury, trauma, intoxicants, autoimmune disease, and by systemic diseases. They often result in anorexia due to painful mastication. Hypersalivation (ptyalism) is also apparent, whether from overproduction or lack of swallowing. In the cat, gingivitis is the first and most consistent sign of feline immunodeficiency virus infection associated

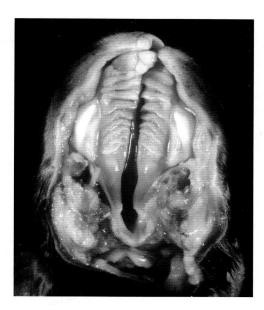

Fig. 7-1   Palatoschisis and cheiloschisis, hard and soft palate, puppy. The lateral palatine processes have failed to fuse during the first trimester of gestation (palatoschisis). In dogs, palatoschisis has been attributed to genetic abnormalities, excessive intake of vitamin A during gestation, and the administration of cortisone during gestation. The upper lip is also cleft (cheiloschisis). *(Courtesy Dr. H. Gelberg, College of Veterinary Medicine, Oregon State University.)*

with a reduction in CD4 lymphocytes, thymic atrophy, and lymph node atrophy.

VESICULAR STOMATITIDES

The vesicular stomatitides are listed in Table 7-1. Blistering or vesiculation of the oral epithelium is present early in the course of these diseases. They are all virus-induced, and all have identical appearances at gross and histopathologic examination. None of these conditions is fatal. They produce great economic loss in the affected animals because of poor weight gain and sometimes abortions in gravid females. The exact cause of the abortions is unknown, but it is probably related to the stress induced by the painful oral, cutaneous, and pedal (hoof or foot) lesions. Secondary bacterial invaders, both gram-negative and gram-positive, of these lesions can result in endotoxemia. Several diseases, such as foot-and-mouth disease and vesicular exanthema, affect the coronary bands of the digits and interdigital clefts, resulting in lameness. Some of these diseases (foot-and-mouth disease, vesicular exanthema, swine vesicular disease) are exotic to the United States and thus are reportable to state or federal authorities, or both, if suspected by the examining clinician or pathologist. This requirement is due to the great expense involved in eradicating these diseases from the United States and their

Table 7-1   Vesicular Stomatitides

Disease	Cause	Ruminant	Pigs	Horses
Foot-and-mouth disease	Picornavirus	+	+	−
Vesicular stomatitis	Rhabdovirus	++	+	+
Vesicular exanthema of swine	Calicivirus	−	++	−
Swine vesicular disease	Enterovirus	−	++	−

+ = Species in which disease occurs; − = species in which disease does not occur.

potential use as agents of agroterrorism. Nontariff export barriers often arise from the presence of infectious agents in livestock that are foreign to countries with which we trade. These restrictions are designed to prevent introduction of highly contagious agents, such as foot-and-mouth disease, into resident animal populations.

The gross lesions of the vesicular stomatitides are epitheliotropic. Fluid-filled vesicles are present in the oral cavity, lips, rostral plate, and tongue (Fig. 7-2, A). Entry of virus in these cases is most likely oral into areas of temporary loss of mucosa due to normal mastication and trauma. The viruses are cytolytic, and the resultant release of virus from cells infects neighboring cells. The lesions enlarge centripetally, forming vesicles. Bullae result from vesicle coalescence. The epithelium covering large bullae easily ruptures with handling. Subsequently, ulcers are created. These ulcers are typically hyperemic (Fig. 7-2, B). Viremia, often transient, sometimes occurs.

Similar vesicular lesions occur in the nasal mucosa, particularly in pigs with vesicular exanthema and in the proximal epithelium of the alimentary system (esophagus and rumen) of cattle with foot-and-mouth disease. Some animals have conjunctivitis and vesicular dermatitis of the teats and vulva. Microscopically, the lesions of these four diseases (foot-and-mouth disease, vesicular stomatitis, vesicular exanthema, and swine vesicular disease) are similar. Virus-induced, intracellular edema progresses to cell swelling of the stratum spinosum. Cell lysis and intercellular edema and vesicles result. The epithelium overlying the virus-rich vesicular fluid contains large amounts of intracellular virus. Even slight friction can rupture vesicles and bullae, creating an ulcer. Healing progresses from the normal fibrin and/or neutrophil rich acute stages to the more chronic stages of granulation.

Lesions and signs of the vesicular stomatitides include vesicles, bullae, oral epithelium that detaches to leave a raw, ulcerated surface, ptyalism, lameness, fever, and anorexia. The lesions develop as a result of rupture of initially infected cells and centripetal spread of virus to adjacent susceptible epithelium and multiple repeats of this infectious, lytic cycle. The vesicular

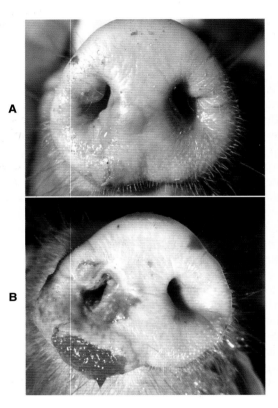

Fig. 7-2   Cutaneous vesicles, vesicular exanthema, snout, pig. A, Vesicles, both intact (upper vesicle) and ruptured (lower vesicle), are present on the planum rostrale and are caused by the infection of injured mucosal epithelial cells with vesicular exanthema of swine virus, a calicivirus. **B,** Ruptured vesicles with cutaneous ulceration, vesicular exanthema (later stage of the disease). Note the ruptured vesicles which can cause pain resulting in inappetence. (**A,** From Gelberg H, Lewis RM: Vet Pathol 19:424-443, 1982. **B,** Courtesy Dr. H. Gelberg, College of Veterinary Medicine, Oregon State University.)

stomatitides are tentatively diagnosed based on the clinical signs and lesions resulting from oral and nasal ulceration, conjunctivitis, and ulceration of the genitalia and mammary gland. Lameness is secondary to hoof involvement that is focused at the coronary band.

Definitive diagnosis is important and is performed at federal laboratories equipped to rapidly respond to putative outbreaks. Federal quarantine of infected herds is an important control mechanism, followed by eradication, slaughter, and carcass disposal.

SPECIFIC VESICULAR DISEASES

Foot-and-mouth disease is an extremely important disease worldwide but has not appeared in U.S. livestock since 1929, when it was eradicated after an outbreak in California. It is characterized in its early stages by vesicles in the planum nasale, in the oral cavity, and tongue. Fluid from ruptured vesicles spreads to areas of abraded skin; for example, that of mammary gland. The coronary bands of the hooves can also be affected. Coronary band vesiculation may eventually lead to sloughing of the hoof. Although this disease is not fatal, the pain and accompanying inappetence lead to weight loss. If allowed to heal, the hoof will regrow into a ball-like structure. Young animals with foot-and-mouth disease frequently have a viral myocarditis.

Vesicular stomatitis is common in calves, but does not occur in sheep or goats. In northern latitudes, it is generally a warm weather disease, suggesting that insects act as vectors. As the name implies, vesicles in the oral cavity characterize the disease. Clinically the disease is often recognized by inappetence in the affected animal, accompanied by ptyalism.

Vesicular exanthema is a specific disease of pigs that is indistinguishable clinically and pathologically from foot-and-mouth disease. This disease is uniquely American and was believed eradicated from pigs in 1956 through enactment of federal laws requiring the cooking of garbage fed to pigs. The evidence indicates that vesicular exanthema of swine serovars are variants of San Miguel sea lion virus. This latter marine calicivirus occurs in coastal sea lion and fur seal populations from California to Alaska (Fig. 7-3).

Swine vesicular disease is indistinguishable from the other vesicular diseases and is exotic to the United States.

EROSIVE AND ULCERATIVE STOMATITIDES

Erosions are defined by a loss of part of the surface epithelium, whereas ulcers are full-thickness epithelial losses exposing the basement membrane. Thus erosions may progress to ulcers that may become perforating ulcers. Erosive and ulcerative stomatitis can have a variety of causes. Agents responsible include the viruses of bovine viral diarrhea (BVD) (Fig. 7-4), rinderpest, malignant catarrhal fever (Fig. 7-5), feline calicivirus, and bluetongue. Other causes include uremia (Fig. 7-6); foreign bodies, such as foxtail awns; the feline eosinophilic granuloma complex; and vitamin C deficiency in primates and guinea pigs (Fig. 7-7). Often the

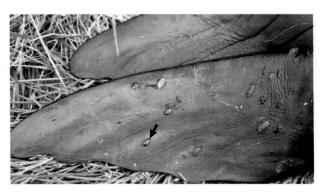

Fig. 7-3   Cutaneous vesicles, San Miguel sea lion virus infection, foreflippers, northern fur seal. On the nonhaired portion of the foreflipper are vesicles both intact *(arrow)* and ruptured, caused by the infection of injured mucosal epithelial cells with San Miguel sea lion virus, a calicivirus. These vesicles will rupture with trauma, resulting in cutaneous erosion and ulceration. *(Courtesy Dr. H. Gelberg, College of Veterinary Medicine, Oregon State University.)*

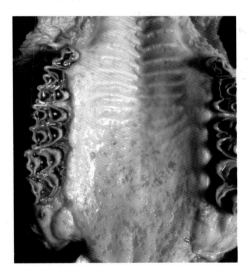

Fig. 7-4   Erosions and ulcers, bovine viral diarrhea virus infection, hard palate, cow. Erosions and ulcers caused by this pestivirus are particularly evident here on the mucosal epithelial surface of the caudal hard palate. These lesions are characteristic of the ulcerative stomatitides, which, unlike the pox and parapox viruses, do not form vesicles. *(Courtesy Dr. M.D. McGavin, College of Veterinary Medicine, University of Tennessee.)*

oral lesions must be evaluated in the context of the clinical signs, together with histopathologic findings and ancillary testing, to arrive at a definitive diagnosis. Additionally, the vesicular stomatitides can progress, secondary to abrasion, to the point that they cannot be distinguished from the ulcerative stomatitides.

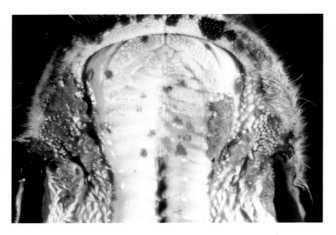

Fig. 7-5 **Erosions and ulcers, malignant catarrhal fever (MCF), hard palate, dental pad and buccal papillae, cow.** The erosions and ulcers *(red areas on mucosal surface)* are due to MCF virus, a herpes virus, but are characteristic of many ulcerative stomatitides. *(Courtesy Dr. H. Gelberg, College of Veterinary Medicine, Oregon State University.)*

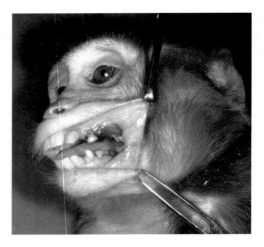

Fig. 7-7 **Ulcerative gingivitis secondary to scurvy (vitamin C deficiency), gingiva, monkey.** There is a deep ulcer at the commissure of the mouth and smaller ulcers periodontally. Vitamin C deficiency in primates and guinea pigs can result in gingival erosions and ulcers, and even tooth loss. *(Courtesy College of Veterinary Medicine, University of Illinois.)*

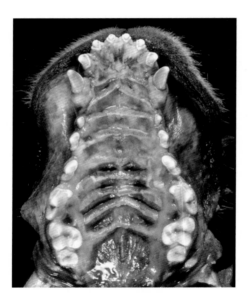

Fig. 7-6 **Uremic ulcers, hard palate, dog.** Ulcers present on the transverse palatine ridges and periodontal gingiva are secondary to vascular damage associated with increased concentrations of serum blood urea nitrogen and creatinine from kidney failure. Affected animals often have an ammoniacal or uremic odor to the breath. *(Courtesy Dr. H. Gelberg, College of Veterinary Medicine, Oregon State University.)*

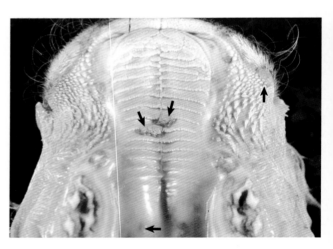

Fig. 7-8 **Epithelial plaques, papular stomatitis, hard palate mucosa, calf.** Virus-induced (parapoxvirus) epithelial plaques and papules are present on the mucosal epithelium of the hard palate and adjacent gingiva *(arrows)*. *(Courtesy Dr. H. Gelberg, College of Veterinary Medicine, Oregon State University.)*

PAPULAR STOMATITIDES

Parapoxviruses cause the papular stomatitides. The two major diseases in this category, bovine papular stomatitis and contagious ecthyma, are zoonotic. Bovine papular stomatitis is recognized by papules on the nares, muzzle, gingiva, buccal cavity, palate, and tongue (Fig. 7-8). Lesions also occur in the esophagus, rumen,

and omasum. Microscopically, there is ballooning degeneration of the epithelial cells of the stratum spinosum. At a later stage, these cells may contain intracytoplasmic eosinophilic parapoxvirus inclusions (Fig. 7-9). Disease is more common in immunosuppressed animals, such as those persistently infected with bovine viral diarrheal virus. In human beings, the disease is called milker's nodules and is characterized by papules of the hands and arms.

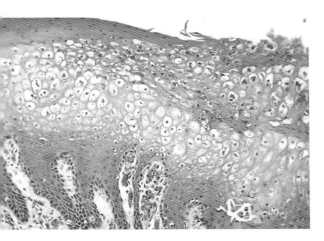

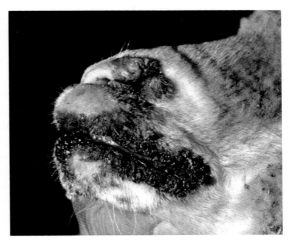

Fig. 7-9   Ballooning degeneration, papular stomatitis, hard palate mucosa, cow. There is ballooning degeneration of the epithelial cells of the stratum spinosum. At a later stage, these cells may contain intracytoplasmic eosinophilic parapoxvirus inclusions (not visible here). H&E stain. *(Courtesy Dr. M.D. McGavin, College of Veterinary Medicine, University of Tennessee.)*

Fig. 7-10   Contagious ecthyma, oral mucous membranes, lamb. Note crusts around nose and lips. Multiple pustules and coalescing ruptured pustules covered by scabs are present on the skin. The parapoxvirus induces epithelial proliferation (acanthosis), followed by vesicle formation. These vesicles rupture and are quickly covered by scabs. Lesions develop at the sites of trauma, such as occur with a nursing kid, where damage to the superficial oral epithelium allows entry of the virus into skin. *(Courtesy Dr. M.D. McGavin, College of Veterinary Medicine, University of Tennessee.)*

Contagious ecthyma, or sore mouth, is a condition of sheep and goats characterized by macules, papules, vesicles, pustules, scabs, and scars in areas of skin abrasions, including the corners of the mouth (Fig. 7-10), mouth, udder, teats, coronary bands, and anus. Occasionally the mucosa of the esophagus and rumen also can be affected. Eosinophilic cytoplasmic inclusion bodies are visible at microscopic examination of lesions early in the course of disease. The condition in human beings is called orf.

NECROTIZING STOMATITIDES

Necrotizing stomatitis occurs in cattle, sheep, and pigs. In cattle, it is sometimes referred to as calf diphtheria (Fig. 7-11). Necrotizing stomatitis is characterized by yellow-gray, round foci surrounded by a rim of hyperemic tissue in the oral cavity, larynx, pharynx, or tongue. Necrotizing stomatitis is the end stage of all other forms of stomatitis when they are complicated by infection with *Fusobacterium necrophorum*, a filamentous to rodlike to coccoid, gram-negative anaerobe. Bacterial toxins are responsible for the extensive lesions. Clinical signs include swollen cheeks, inappetence, pyrexia, and halitosis. Infection may become systemic if severe, resulting in lesions throughout the alimentary system and associated lymphoid tissue. Well-demarcated foci of coagulation necrosis typify the histologic appearance of necrotizing stomatitis. As might be expected in foci of inflammation, there is a circumferential rim of leukocytes and increased vascularity. Noma is a severe form of oral avascular necrosis associated with the presence of spirochetes and fusiform bacteria. Although rare, it is

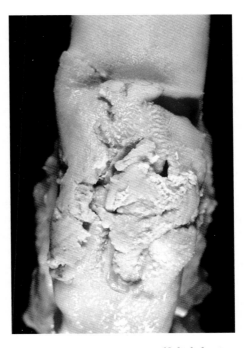

Fig. 7-11   Necrotizing stomatitis, calf diphtheria, tongue, calf. The dorsal surface of the tongue is ulcerated, and the ulcers are covered by a diphtheric membrane. Calf diphtheria is caused by infection with the bacterium *Fusobacterium necrophorum* secondary to abrasion and/or trauma to the mucosal epithelium of the oral cavity or larynx. *(Courtesy Dr. M.D. McGavin, College of Veterinary Medicine, University of Tennessee.)*

seen most commonly in primates, including humans, and dogs. It is characterized by severe necrotizing gingivitis, osteolysis, and sometimes death.

Ulcerative gingivitis (trench mouth), caused by anaerobic spirochetes, affects humans, some nonhuman primates, and rarely puppies. Similar to necrotizing stomatitis, ulcerative gingivitis is characterized by acute inflammation and necrosis, oral ulceration and pain, halitosis, a fragile oral mucosa, and ptyalism. In addition to *Fusobacterium* spp., *Borrelia vincentii* is causative. Debilitated animals and those with intercurrent infections are at increased risk for these secondary invaders. The morphologic diagnosis is an acute, necrotizing gingivitis. Unlike the case in necrotizing stomatitis, the causative agents are readily identified by tissue smears or by culture.

EOSINOPHILIC STOMATITIDES

Oral granulomas or ulcers ("rodent ulcers") occur frequently in cats. Similar lesions occur sporadically in a variety of canine breeds. In cats, they are termed oral eosinophilic granulomas. Although the etiology of this condition is unknown, the histologic appearance of lesions suggests an immune-mediated mechanism, possibly a hypersensitivity reaction to an unknown antigen. Antibodies to intercellular material can often be demonstrated in affected cats. In the majority of cases of both dogs and cats, an increase in circulating eosinophils is present.

In cats, lip lesions are commonly visible near the philtrum and may extend through the adjacent haired skin. Oral lesions may occur anywhere in the mouth including the gingiva, hard and soft palates, oral and nasal pharynx, tongue, and occasionally draining lymphoid tissues (Fig. 7-12). In dogs, eosinophilic granulomas typically are raised, fungating masses on the ventral and lateral lingual epithelium and palate. Collagenolysis (because collagen is acellular, it cannot undergo necrosis) is characteristically central in the lesion. The surrounding inflammatory tissue contains mixed inflammatory cells with increased numbers of eosinophils, mast cells, and multinucleated giant cells. Lesions grouped as the eosinophilic granuloma complex of cats include eosinophilic ulcers, linear granulomas, and eosinophilic plaques. The latter two lesions are strictly dermatologic and do not affect the oral cavity. No proven etiologic link has been established between these cutaneous conditions and oral eosinophilic granulomas. The cause of the canine lesions is unknown.

LYMPHOPLASMACYTIC STOMATITIS

Lymphoplasmacytic stomatitis is an idiopathic condition of the cat named on the basis of the histologic appearance of the lesions (Fig. 7-13). It is a chronic condition characterized by red, inflamed gums, fetid breath,

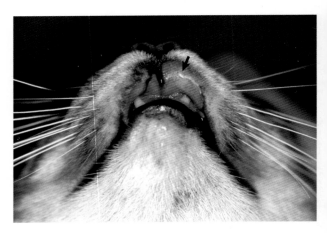

Fig. 7-12 **Eosinophilic granuloma, skin, upper lip, cat.** Bilateral ulceration of the upper lip is present. The upper left lip is more extensively affected (**arrow**). (*Courtesy Dr. Ann M. Hargis, DermatoDiagnostics.*)

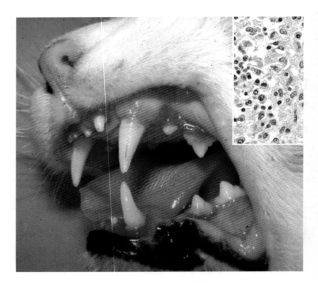

Fig. 7-13 **Lymphoplasmacytic stomatitis, gingiva, cat.** This chronic condition of cats is characterized by red, inflamed gums, fetid breath, and inappetence. The oral mucosa can also be hyperplastic and ulcerated. *Inset:* There is a florid infiltrate of mixed inflammatory cells, including many lymphocytes and plasma cells in the lamina propria beneath the epithelium. H&E stain. (**Figure,** *Courtesy Dr. C. Patrick Ryan, Veterinary Public Health, Los Angeles Department of Health Services; and Noah's Arkive, College of Veterinary Medicine, University of Georgia.* **Inset,** *Courtesy Dr. J.F. Zachary, College of Veterinary Medicine, University of Illinois.*)

and inappetence. The oral mucosa can be hyperplastic and ulcerated. Associations have been hypothesized between this condition and the presence of bacteria or calicivirus associated with feline leukemia virus (FeLV) and/or feline immunodeficiency virus infection.

CHRONIC ULCERATIVE PARADENTAL STOMATITIS

This condition of dogs, also known as ulcerative stomatitis and lymphocytic-plasmacytic stomatitis, is caused by apposition of "kissing ulcers" to dental plaque. The condition is painful with resultant inappetence and anorexia. Affected dogs drool and have halitosis. This condition occurs in older dogs of any breed, but Malteses and cavalier King Charles spaniels are particularly susceptible. The lymphocytic-plasmacytic lesions noted on histologic examination are suggestive of an inflammatory rather than infectious etiology. If untreated, bone resorption may occur.

HYPERPLASIA AND NEOPLASIA

In the dog, 70% of tumors of the alimentary system are in the oral cavity. These tumors run the gamut of biologic behavior from simple epithelial hyperplasia to malignant neoplasms with metastases to distant sites.

HYPERPLASTIC DISEASES

Gingival hyperplasia is a simple overgrowth of gum tissue. The hyperplasia can become so severe as to bury incisor teeth (Fig. 7-14). Gingival hyperplasia is most common in brachycephalic dog breeds and is present in 30% of boxer dogs older than 5 years.

Grossly, gingival hyperplasia can be indistinguishable from an epulis (Fig. 7-15). Epulis is a nonspecific term that designates a growth of the gingiva. The several kinds of epulides can only be distinguished by histopathologic examination. This distinction is not just an academic exercise because, although all epulides are considered benign, one form—acanthomatous epulis—invades bone and can be quite destructive. Fortunately, this type of

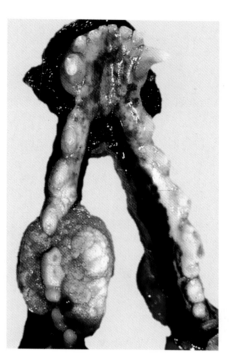

Fig. 7-15   Fibromatous epulis, left mandible, molar teeth, dog. This growth is an epulis (fibromatous type); however, epulides are often indistinguishable from gingival hyperplasia. Epulis is a term used to designate a growth of the gingiva that is firm, periodontal, and usually solitary, in contrast to gingival hyperplasia. This distinction is not just an academic exercise because, although all epulides are considered benign, one form, acanthomatous epulis, is locally invasive. It invades bone and can be quite destructive. *(Courtesy Dr. J. King, College of Veterinary Medicine, Cornell University.)*

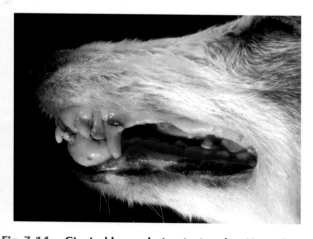

Fig. 7-14   Gingival hyperplasia, gingiva, dog. Hyperplastic gingiva has enveloped the lower incisor teeth. Dental calculus (*tartar, brown*) is also present on both upper and lower incisor and molar teeth. *(Courtesy Dr. H. Gelberg, College of Veterinary Medicine, Oregon State University.)*

epulis can be managed therapeutically. Whether the epulides represent fibrous and epithelial hyperplasia or benign neoplasms of tooth germ is controversial.

NEOPLASIA

Squamous cell carcinomas occur in the oral cavity, particularly in old cats, in which they account for 60% of oral neoplasms. They generally occur on the ventrolateral surface of the tongue and tonsils. Lingual squamous cell carcinomas occur more commonly in felids, and tonsillar squamous cell carcinomas are more common in canids. Although often appearing histologically aggressive, only a small percentage of lingual neoplasms metastasize, most commonly to draining lymph nodes: the mandibular and medial retropharyngeal. Unfortunately, most tonsillar carcinomas do metastasize, often to distant sites.

Squamous cell carcinomas vary both in size and in gross appearance—from flat to proliferative (Fig. 7-16). These tumors are often quite aggressive locally, invading subjacent tissues. Some tumors contain more differentiated cells, keratin, often in whorls (keratin pearls) and

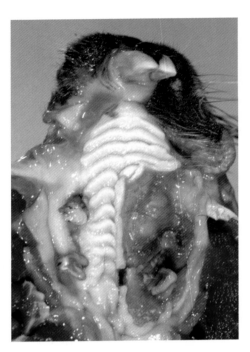

Fig. 7-16 **Squamous cell carcinoma, palate, woodchuck.** A mass of proliferating neoplastic squamous epithelial cells has displaced and replaced the mucosa and underlying tissue of the left hard palate and gingiva. *(Courtesy Dr. H. Gelberg, College of Veterinary Medicine, Oregon State University.)*

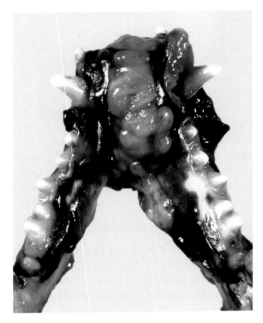

Fig. 7-17 **Amelanotic melanoma, mandibular symphysis, dog.** A proliferative, ulcerated nonpigmented mass is present on the oral mucosa at the mandibular symphysis and protrudes into the oral cavity, likely resulting in malocclusion. Incisor teeth have been lost. Note the absence of pigmentation (melanin) in this tumor. *(Courtesy Dr. M.D. McGavin, College of Veterinary Medicine, University of Tennessee.)*

visible desmosomes (intracellular bridges), whereas others are less well differentiated, with significant mitotic activity. In these latter cases, intracellular immunohistochemical markers for cytokeratin are useful in determining a definitive diagnosis. The amount of fibrous tissue within an individual tumor is variable. Some carcinomas induce a scirrhous response, whereas others have areas of necrosis caused by rapid tumor growth, "collision necrosis" of the tightly packed proliferating cells, and loss of contiguity with the blood supply.

Ninety percent of melanomas of the oral cavity of dogs are malignant. A breed predilection exists for Scottish terriers, Airedales, cocker spaniels, golden retrievers, Bedlington terriers, Duroc pigs, and others. Most melanomas contain copious intracellular pigment and are visibly black. Some melanomas without pigment, termed amelanotic melanomas, present a greater diagnostic challenge to both the clinician and pathologist (Fig. 7-17). Immunohistochemical staining for tyrosinase-related protein-2 is useful for identifying amelanotic tumors. Melanomas are composed of melanocytes and are of neural crest origin. Cellular morphology within melanomas varies from spindloid to epithelioid. Thus some neoplasms are histologically difficult to differentiate from squamous cell carcinomas, and others from fibrosarcomas.

Canine oral papillomatosis is a papovavirus-induced transmissible condition that usually occurs in animals younger than 1 year. The lesions usually regress spontaneously. Immunity is long-lasting. The lesions are papilliform or cauliflower-like and can become quite florid. They are generally white and friable and occur on the mouth, tongue, palate, larynx, and epiglottis. These oral tumors are usually multiple, white to gray, raised, and pedunculated with a keratinized surface and a stromal core. The epithelial cells comprising the lesion can be acanthotic, hyperplastic, and rest on a hyperplastic folded connective tissue stroma. The stratum spinosum is also hyperplastic and ballooned. Cytoplasmic inclusion bodies are sometimes present.

Fibrosarcomas arise from the collagen-producing cells (fibroblasts) of the oral cavity. Fibrosarcomas are most common in the cat, accounting for 20% of oral neoplasia in that species.

TEETH*

INTRODUCTION

Teeth provide mechanical advantage for prehension, tearing and/or mastication of food. Among domestic

---

*Previous contributions to this section were authored by Dr. Richard Dubielzeg of the School of Veterinary Medicine, University of Wisconsin-Madison.

animals, there are differences in the growth pattern and numbers of teeth. Hypsodont teeth, such as in the horse, continue to grow throughout life, and appropriate leveling of the occlusive surfaces (floating) may be necessary as the horse ages. Brachydont teeth, such as in carnivores, do not continue to grow after they are fully erupted. Most species of mammals have deciduous teeth that are replaced near maturity by permanent teeth. In many species, the approximate age of the animal may be obtained by eruption dates and examination of wear patterns and shape of the teeth.

STRUCTURE AND FUNCTION

Molar teeth in general are designed for grinding feedstuffs, whereas incisors in ruminants (mandibular only) are for cropping forage. Canine teeth are designed for tearing flesh. Brachydont teeth consist of a crown, which is the portion above the gingiva (the neck that is slightly constricted), and just below the gingiva are the roots, which are embedded in the bony socket (alveolus) of the jaw. Enamel covers the crown, cementum covers the roots, and both cover the dentin. Besides carnivores, the incisor (lower) teeth of ruminants and porcine teeth, except the canines of the boar, are brachydont.

Hypsodont teeth have an elongated body, but the neck and roots may form later in life. Cementum covers the tooth, and enamel is beneath the cementum. Beneath the enamel is the dentin. The cementum and enamel invaginate into the dentin, forming the infundibula. Enamel crests result from normal wear, with enamel being the hardest of the layers. The cheek teeth of ruminants and tusks of boars and the teeth of horses are hypsodont.

In simple-toothed animals, such as carnivores, the tooth root is not covered by enamel. Receding gum lines therefore expose the dentin, resulting in pain and invasion by bacteria. Domestic animal species seldom get caries, although buildup of plaque can result in gingival infections and tooth loss.

MALOCCLUSIONS

Abnormal development and positioning of the teeth may affect dental function. Malocclusion refers to a failure of the upper and lower incisors to interdigitate properly. This feature is "normal" for some dogs, particularly the brachycephalic breeds. In the extreme, malocclusions can lead to difficulty in the prehension and mastication of food. Malocclusions are named according to the position of the mandible. Protrusion of the lower jaw is termed prognathia, whereas a short lower jaw with resultant protrusion of the upper jaw is termed brachygnathia and sometimes hypognathia (Fig. 7-18). Sometimes these terms are incorrectly used, referring to brachygnathia as superior prognathia and prognathia as superior brachygnathia.

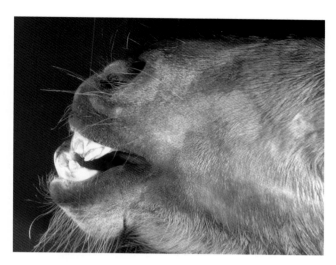

Fig. 7-18   **Prognathia, head, horse.** The mandible is elongated compared with the maxilla. *(Courtesy Dr. H. Gelberg, College of Veterinary Medicine, Oregon State University.)*

Malocclusions result from abnormal jaw conformation or rarely from abnormal tooth eruption patterns. In some animals, such as rodents and rabbits, the teeth continue to grow throughout the animal's lifetime. If these animals are not provided with sufficient roughage in their diets, the teeth (both incisors and cheek teeth) overgrow and either "lock" the jaw or, because of a lack of occlusal grinding surfaces, prevent the animal from receiving proper nutrition (Fig. 7-19).

ANOMALIES OF TOOTH DEVELOPMENT

In simple-toothed animals, agenesis of a tooth or teeth occurs and is generally of no clinical significance. Supernumerary tooth development is less common than tooth agenesis and is similarly of little clinical significance. Some animals, such as elasmobranchs (sharks), continue to produce row upon row of teeth as the outer most rows are lost. Dental dysgenesis may be primarily due to dysplasias of the enamel-forming organ or secondary to trauma, infection and hyperthermia, toxicosis, or other metabolic irregularities.

Dentigerous cysts result from dental dysgenesis. Epithelial-lined, cystic structures in tissue, including the bone of the jaw, results. Dentigerous cysts develop from abnormal proliferation of the cell rests of Malassez. Although rare, dentigerous cysts are often painful, and although not usually neoplastic, they can destroy the jaw. Dentigerous cysts are epithelial-lined and may become impacted with keratin. Rudimentary, malformed teeth may be found within these cysts, and painful fistulas may develop, especially in horses. These draining tracts are seen most often rostral and ventral to the ear (ear tooth). Dentigerous cysts occur less frequently in otherwise normal, mature animals.

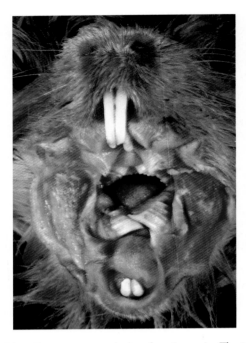

Fig. 7-19 **Overgrown teeth, head, guinea pig.** The incisors and molars are longer than normal and the tongue is entrapped by the lower molar teeth, which will lead to starvation unless properly corrected. *(Courtesy Dr. H. Gelberg, College of Veterinary Medicine, Oregon State University.)*

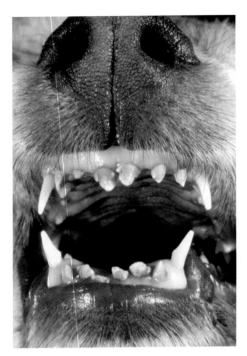

Fig. 7-20 **Enamel hypoplasia, permanent incisor teeth, dog.** There is a lack of enamel formation with resultant discrete deep pits and exposure of the dentin *(light yellow to beige areas of the teeth)*, the result of infection with canine distemper virus and necrosis of the ameloblasts during enamel formation. Permanent adult teeth (shown in illustration) are infected with virus before their eruption and while they are still within their sockets (dental alveoli). *(Courtesy Dr. H. Gelberg, College of Veterinary Medicine, Oregon State University.)*

Segmental enamel hypoplasia occurs before eruption of the permanent teeth of dogs as a result of hyperthermia and viral infection. Most often, this is due to canine distemper virus infection. Enamel is fully formed when the teeth are erupted; therefore virus infection of ameloblasts must occur during enamel formation, before 6 months of age, if enamel hypoplasia is to occur. The epithelium of the enamel organ during virus infection is necrotic and disorganized. After clearing the virus infection, there is a return to normal structure and function of the enamel organ. Segmental enamel hypoplasia results because of the temporal lack of enamel formation (Fig. 7-20).

Chemicals, most notably tetracycline antibiotics, can cause permanent discoloration of otherwise normal teeth if such agents are present during the process of mineralization. Congenital porphyria, a defect in red blood cell production, may result in incorporation of porphyrins into dentin, resulting in pink discoloration of the teeth (pink tooth) (Fig. 7-21). Both tetracycline and porphyrins fluoresce under ultraviolet light, dramatically demonstrating these lesions.

Fluoride incorporation into the enamel and dentin occurs in fluoride toxicosis, particularly in cattle and sheep. A relationship exists in beef cattle between fluorosis and selenium supplementation, with supplementation

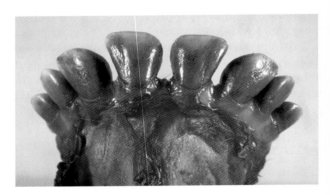

Fig. 7-21 **Pink tooth, congenital porphyria teeth, adult ox.** The teeth are discolored brown from the accumulation of porphyrins in the dentin. *(Courtesy Dr. M.D. McGavin, College of Veterinary Medicine, University of Tennessee.)*

being protective in high fluoride areas. Excessive dietary concentrations of fluorine during odontogenesis (from 6 to 36 months of age) may result in incorporation of the fluoride in the enamel and dentin of the permanent teeth. The result is soft, chalky, discolored enamel, usually

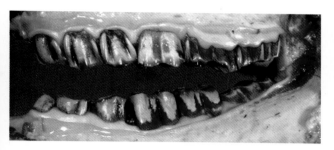

Fig. 7-22 **Fluorosis, cheek teeth, cow.** The enamel is chalky and weak, and the teeth are usually rapidly worn down. *(Courtesy Dr. L. Krook, College of Veterinary Medicine, Cornell University.)*

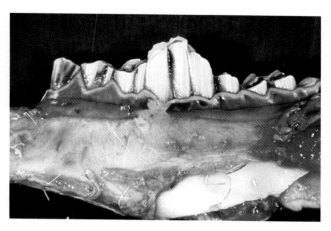

Fig. 7-23 **Dental attrition, molar teeth, antelope.** Age-associated dental wear results in improper mastication of feedstuffs and malnutrition. This condition occurs most commonly in horses and is referred to as "step-mouth." *(Courtesy College of Veterinary Medicine, University of Tennessee.)*

yellow, dark brown, or black (Fig. 7-22). Occlusal grinding of affected soft teeth against more normal enamel results in rapid dental wear. One wonders therefore about the cumulative effect of fluoride supplementation in municipal drinking water, vitamins with added fluoride, fluoride-supplemented toothpaste, fluoride treatment of teeth, reconstituted and bottled soft drinks made with fluoridated water, and so forth. It is difficult to calculate the total fluoride load ingested by individuals or what the effects of that fluoride supplementation may be.

LESIONS CAUSED BY ATTRITION AND ABNORMAL WEAR

Loss of normal dental structure and function often results from rapid and irregular and/or abnormal wear of occlusal surfaces in many species of domestic animals. In those species with hypsodont teeth, attention to the dentition as the animal ages is often a major factor in overall body conditioning and health (Fig. 7-23). Aggressive treatment of occlusal surface irregularity by filing of high points in the dental arcade (floating) can notably prolong an animal's life. Rock chewing or other compulsive oral behaviors in dogs may result in accelerated dental wear. In all species, exposure of dentin or the pulp canal may lead to dental infection with serious consequences.

FELINE EXTERNAL RESORPTIVE NECK LESIONS

Cats suffering from feline external resorptive neck lesions often have pain upon chewing that may be reflected by inappetence and/or abnormal masticatory movements. External neck resorption of the teeth of otherwise dentally normal cats is caused by odontoclastic resorption of dental tissue, particularly in the neck area or root of the tooth. Cementum or osteoid ingrowths partially or completely line the resorptive cavity. The resultant cavity may attract bacterial plaque, resulting in intense inflammation and osteoclastic resorption of dental tissue. The primary cause of this condition is not known.

INFUNDIBULAR IMPACTION

Impaction of the infundibulum, infundibular necrosis or infundibular caries, may cause serious dental disease in ruminants and more rarely in horses. Incomplete infundibular cementum formation before tooth eruption likely predisposes to infundibular impaction. The pathogenic mechanism is comparable to dental caries in simple-toothed animals. Feed material is ground into the infundibulum, where bacteria metabolize it to form acid, which causes demineralization. Bacterial enzymes digest the organic matrix of enamel and dentin. As a result of this destruction, the pulp cavity becomes infected, resulting in pulpitis and endodontitis. Dental abscesses and fistulous tracks may develop. The inflamed infundibular cavities often continue to become impacted with feed, creating a vicious cycle.

PERIODONTAL DISEASE

Bacterial films resident on the tooth surface and the acids and enzymes they produce may damage their enamel substrate (cavities) and also destroy the subjacent gingival tissue and periodontal ligament (periodontal disease). More than 200 species of bacteria and fungi have been associated with dental plaque (a film of an organic matrix, food particles and bacteria on the tooth surface). This plaque often becomes mineralized (tartar or dental calculus). The mineralized material contributes to atrophy and inflammation of the gingival epithelium and supporting stroma by acting as a nidus for additional plaque accumulation.

The initial site for destructive inflammation is in the gingival crevice-forming pockets. With time, this inflammation spreads distally along the tooth, resulting in gingival-epithelial attachment only on the root of the tooth, deep in the alveolar socket. Progression of inflammation destroys the connective tissue of the periodontal ligament, resulting in loosening of the tooth. Alveolar osteomyelitis and pulpitis can form apical abscesses, bacteremic spread of inflammation, significant oral pain, reluctance to masticate, and halitosis. Periodontal disease is common in carnivores and humans. Mildly abrasive diets and brushing of the teeth of pet carnivores, combined with regular dental examination, is preventative in carnivores as it is in human beings.

DENTAL NEOPLASIA

Proliferative, cystic or neoplastic diseases of the dental arcade can originate from cell rests that form from the dental lamina or the enamel organ (the cell rests of Malassez). Dental neoplasms usually arise in proximity to the teeth, either deeply in the jaw or from the surface epithelium. There is a relatively precise method of naming dental neoplasms based on the tissue or cell of origin and the extent of differentiation and odontogenesis present within the neoplastic tissue. The histologic appearance of these neoplasms is complex; pathologists with considerable experience in differentiating these uncommon neoplasms should be consulted when a precise diagnosis is indicated.

Odontomas are hamartomas originating in the enamel organ, usually of puppies and foals (Fig. 7-24). They usually contain well-recognizable dentin and enamel as well as ameloblasts, odontoblasts, and dental pulp.

Ameloblastoma is a term applied to epithelial neoplasms of enamel organ origin. Several subtypes can be

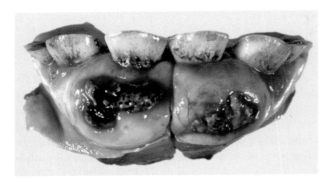

Fig. 7-24   **Odontoma, incisor teeth, cow.** This is a hamartoma (a benign tumorlike nodule) of the enamel organ and in this case has expanded bilaterally on the rostral mandibles. There is extensive hemorrhagic ulceration over the tumor. Diagnosis can be confirmed by radiographic and histopathologic examination. *(Courtesy Dr. M.D. McGavin, College of Veterinary Medicine, University of Tennessee.)*

distinguished histologically. They are ameloblastic fibroma, ameloblastic odontoma, calcifying epithelial odontogenic tumor, peripheral odontogenic fibroma, and other rare tooth neoplasms.

Ameloblastoma appears randomly in the dental arcade, usually in adult dogs. They are often osteolytic and thus are locally invasive. Histologic examination by an expert is often necessary to distinguish ameloblastoma from acanthomatous epulis and squamous cell carcinoma.

TONSILS

STRUCTURE AND FUNCTION

The palatine tonsils are pharyngeal lymphoid structures covered by stratified squamous epithelium. Their function is uncertain, although it is likely they serve in lymphocyte production and antibody formation. In carnivores, they are found in crypts or recesses at the dorsolateral aspect of the caudal oropharynx. In pigs, they are flat and recognized by tiny pores in the surface epithelium of the caudal soft palate. Equids, ruminants, and pigs have lingual tonsils in addition to palatine tonsils.

PORTALS OF ENTRY

Tonsils do not possess afferent lymphatics and do not serve as lymph filters. Therefore only primary (or direct) or hematogenous infections occur (tonsillitis) (Fig. 7-25), and primary neoplasms of either the lymphoid (lymphosarcoma) (Fig. 7-26) or epithelial (squamous cell carcinoma) (Fig. 7-27) components. In many viremias of mammals, such as pseudorabies of pigs, virus may be isolated from the tonsils.

SALIVARY GLANDS

INTRODUCTION

Salivary glands are found in a variety of locations in the head and neck regions. They arise from oral ectoderm. In all species the major salivary glands include the parotid, mandibular, and sublingual. Carnivores have a zygomatic gland as well. Minor salivary glands include buccal, labial, lingual, palatine, and others similarly named by location.

STRUCTURE AND FUNCTION

Most salivary glands are discrete aggregates of compound tubuloalveolar tissue. Saliva is a mixture of serous and mucoid secretions. Saliva lubricates the mouth and esophagus and moistens ingesta. Saliva also dissolves water-soluble components of food so the taste buds can function. The mucus in saliva binds to masticated food and creates a bolus that is more easily swallowed. Salivary mucus also coats the epithelium of the

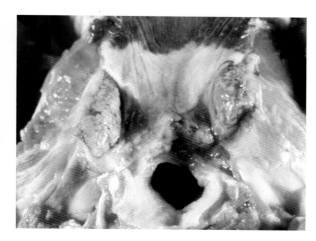

Fig. 7-25   Necrotizing tonsillitis, tonsils, dog. The palatine tonsils are enlarged and discolored. The left tonsil is covered by a diphtheritic membrane, and the right tonsil is extensively ulcerated. Because there are no afferent lymphatics to the tonsils, infection is either primary (by direct spread) or hematogenous. *(Courtesy Dr. M.D. McGavin, College of Veterinary Medicine, University of Tennessee.)*

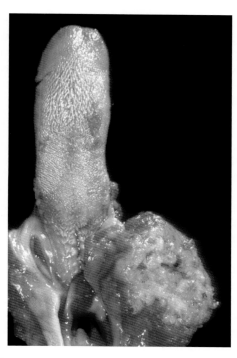

Fig. 7-27   Squamous cell carcinoma, tonsil, cat. The right tonsil has been replaced by a large expansile neoplasm. The left tonsil is normal and remains in its crypt. *(Courtesy Dr. R. Storts, College of Veterinary Medicine, Texas A&M University.)*

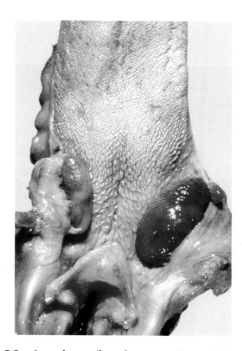

Fig. 7-26   Lymphoma (lymphosarcoma), tonsil, dog. Proliferation of malignant lymphocytes has expanded the tonsils so that they now protrude beyond their crypts. *(Courtesy Dr. M.D. McGavin, College of Veterinary Medicine, University of Tennessee.)*

mouth, preventing mechanical damage to the tissue. Saliva, through its flushing action, reduces bacterial populations. Saliva contains a lysozyme that lyses bacteria. Carbohydrate digestion begins in the oral cavity as a result of the presence of α-amylase, which changes starch into maltose. There are very small quantities of this enzyme in carnivores and cattle. Saliva also is an effective buffer, especially in ruminants, whose forestomach have no glands. In carnivores, evaporation of saliva is a major mechanism of thermoregulation.

PORTAL OF ENTRY

Salivary glands are generally affected by blood-borne pathogens, direct penetration by foreign objects, obstruction of the excretory ducts, or bite wounds. In humans, ascending infections from the salivary ducts occur. There is no reason to suspect that ascending infections do not occur in other mammals as well. The serous portions of the salivary gland are radiosensitive.

INFLAMMATORY DISEASES

Sialoadenitis or inflammation of a salivary gland is relatively rare in veterinary medicine. Although diagnosis of systemic diseases is not made by examining the salivary gland, rabies and canine distemper are two very important diseases that cause inflammation of the salivary glands. Saliva is a particularly important medium of spread, in bite wounds, of the rhabdovirus that causes rabies. In the rat, a coronavirus termed sialodacryoadenitis virus is responsible for inflammation of the salivary gland and some adnexal ocular glands. *Salmonella typhisuis* has caused parotid sialoadenitis in pigs.

Gross lesions of sialoadenitis are subtle and include swelling and edema. Sialoadenitis can be accompanied by pain on palpation. Abscesses occasionally occur and are especially noticeable when they occur in the retrobulbar zygomatic gland where they may cause ocular protrusion (proptosis).

MISCELLANEOUS DISEASES OR CONDITIONS

Changes in the salivary glands are uncommon in domestic animal species. A ranula is a cystic saliva-filled distention of the duct of the sublingual or submaxillary salivary gland that occurs on the floor of the mouth alongside the tongue (Fig. 7-28). It is thus epithelial lined. The cause is generally unknown, although some cases are due to sialoliths. A salivary mucocele, in contrast, is a pseudocyst not lined by epithelium but filled with saliva. The cause of this lesion is also unknown, but it may occur secondary to traumatic rupture of the duct of a sublingual salivary gland with resultant leakage and encapsulation of saliva by reactive connective tissue.

Sialoliths are rare in domestic animal species. When they do occur, they are considered to be caused by inflammation of the salivary gland with sloughed cells or inflammatory exudate forming a nidus for mineral accretion (Fig. 7-29). Thus they are one cause of ranula formation.

NEOPLASIA

Salivary gland neoplasms, both benign and malignant, are uncommon but occur in all species (Fig. 7-30). They are composed of glandular or ductular elements or a combination of epithelial and mesenchymal components similar to those in mixed mammary neoplasms. A grossly appearing similar condition, salivary gland infarction, occurs infrequently in cats and rarely

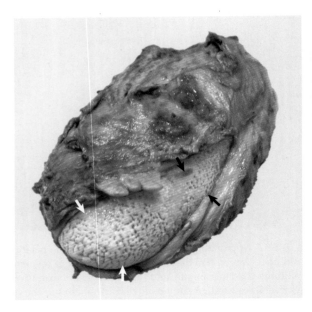

Fig. 7-29   Sialolith, horse. Pressure necrosis from this large stonelike mass (*arrows*) has destroyed the gland in which it formed. (*Courtesy Dr. B. Cooper, College of Veterinary Medicine, Oregon State University.*)

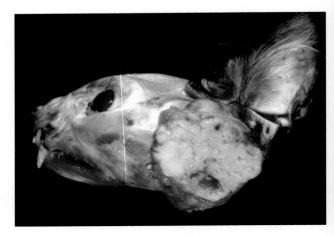

Fig. 7-30   Salivary gland carcinoma, left parotid salivary gland, cat. A large proliferative carcinoma of the salivary gland has replaced the normal gland. (*Courtesy Dr. H. Gelberg, College of Veterinary Medicine, Oregon State University.*)

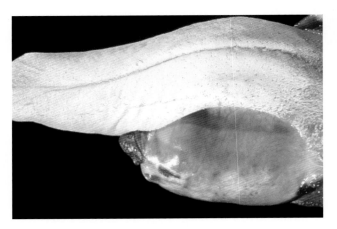

Fig. 7-28   Ranula, mandibular salivary duct, dog. This is a cystic distention of the left mandibular salivary duct along the ventral-lateral aspect of the tongue. (*Courtesy Dr. P. Stromberg, College of Veterinary Medicine, The Ohio State University.*)

in dogs. The cause of the infarction is unknown. The gross appearance of firmness and swelling of an infarcted gland must be distinguished microscopically from neoplasia (Fig. 7-31). In salivary gland infarction, there are discrete foci of parenchymal necrosis with peripheral hemorrhage and inflammatory cells. Regeneration of the gland can be mistaken for neoplasia unless one is familiar with the former condition.

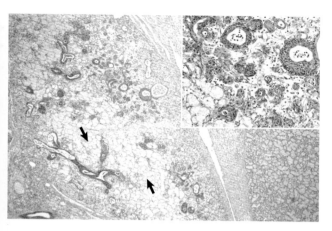

Fig. 7-31 Salivary gland infarction, salivary gland, cat.
Note the areas that lack cell definition (necrosis) secondary to infarction (*arrows*). Normal salivary gland is present in the right third of this illustration. *Inset:* Abortive regeneration as evidenced by hyperplasia of surviving salivary duct epithelial cells. H&E stain. (***Figure*** *and* ***Inset,*** *Courtesy Dr. J.F. Zachary, College of Veterinary Medicine, University of Illinois.*)

TONGUE

INTRODUCTION

The tongue is a muscular organ covered by stratified epithelium and is functionally connected to the esophagus via the epiglottis.

STRUCTURE AND FUNCTION

The tongue is necessary for prehension, mastication, and swallowing of feedstuffs and water. The epithelial covering of the tongue is stratified squamous dorsally with various degrees of keratinization, but ventrally the epithelium is not keratinized and attaches the tongue to the floor of the oral cavity by a frenulum. Keratinized papillae are most prominent in ruminants and cats. There are various types of papillae, some with secondary lamellas. Vallate papillae, for example, are on the dorsal surface of the tongue near its root and are flat structures completely surrounded by a cleft. Some surface macroscopic papillae contain taste buds. The tongue is a highly vascular (functioning in heat loss in many animals, especially carnivores that have no sweat glands) and sensitive organ containing a variety of serous and mucus glands and sensory cells (taste buds). The muscular part of the tongue is striated in randomly arranged bundles. A cordlike structure enclosed in dense collagen extending lengthwise near the ventral central surface of the tongue of carnivores is called the lyssa. Porcine and equid tongues have a similar structure. The lyssa appears to be a structure without a function. Historically the lyssa was removed as "prevention" for rabies. Lyssa bodies are synonymous with Negri bodies, and rabies used to be called lyssa. Adipose tissue becomes more abundant in the caudal part of the tongue in most species.

DEVELOPMENTAL ANOMALIES

Congenital diseases of the tongue include epithelial defects such as fissures, epitheliogenesis imperfecta, macroglossia and microglossia, bifid tongue, and hair growing from the tongue (Fig. 7-32). Lethal glossopharyngeal defect, or bird tongue of dogs, is characterized by a pointed tongue that cannot wrap around a nipple and create the negative pressure required for nursing. Without intervention, starvation results. Ventral ankyloglossia, fusion of the tongue to the floor of the oral cavity, has been reported in related Anatolian shepherd dogs. The cause of these congenital lesions is not known, but they sometimes occur in association with other defects. As in the case of other congenital defects, ingestion of teratogenic substances by the dam during gestation is an etiologic possibility, as is mutation of T-box genes.

SYSTEMIC DISEASE: PRIMARY INVOLVEMENT OF THE TONGUE

Disease agents that principally target the tongue are relatively rare. The exception to this rule is *Actinobacillus lignieresii*, a gram-negative bacillus that is a normal inhabitant of the oral cavity. *Actinobacillus lignieresii* is an opportunistic invader of damaged lingual tissue, principally in bovids and occasionally in equids and small ruminants. The granulomas resulting from infection contain centrally located actinobacilli rimmed by radiating

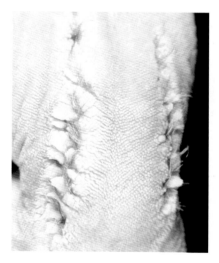

Fig. 7-32 Hamartoma ("hair tongue"), tongue, dog.
Dysplastic hair is growing from the hamartoma in the tongue.
(Courtesy Dr. H. Gelberg, College of Veterinary Medicine, Oregon State University.)

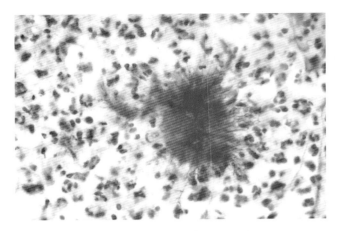

Fig. 7-33 Actinobacillosis (wooden tongue), tongue, cow. Splendore-Hoeppli reaction (colony of bacteria with surrounding radiating "clubs") is surrounded by suppurative inflammation. H&E stain. *(Courtesy Dr. M.D. McGavin, College of Veterinary Medicine, University of Tennessee.)*

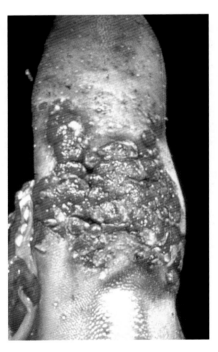

Fig. 7-34 Actinobacillosis, tongue (dorsal surface), cow. Proliferative and ulcerative chronic-active inflammatory lesions containing neutrophils mixed with mononuclear inflammatory cells (lymphocytes, macrophages, plasma cells) and fibrous tissue are present on the tongue. *(Courtesy Dr. M.D. McGavin, College of Veterinary Medicine, University of Tennessee.)*

amorphic eosinophilic, clublike structures composed of immunoglobulin molecules from lesion plasmacytes (Fig. 7-33). Mixed mononuclear inflammatory cells, including multinucleated Langhans' giant cells, often surround these foci (Splendore-Hoeppli phenomenon)

and may be present in regional lymph nodes. The amount of fibrous tissue present is dependent on the duration of the inflammation. The resulting lingual disease is called wooden tongue; the name is derived from the swelling, inflammation, and fibrosis that causes increased firmness of the tongue and linguomegaly (Fig. 7-34). Horses are rarely affected by *Actinobacillus lignieresii* infections, but they are manifested as cutaneous or lymph node abscesses, mastitis, and occasional glossitis.

SYSTEMIC DISEASE: SECONDARY INVOLVEMENT OF THE TONGUE

Thrush is a *Candida albicans* (yeast) infection of intact mucous membranes of the tongue and esophagus (Fig. 7-35). It occurs principally in ungulates but has also been seen in carnivores. Thrush is not a primary disease but often indicates an underlying debility, particularly in young animals. This infection presents as a gray-green pseudomembrane that is easily scraped off the intact underlying mucosal surface (Fig. 7-36). It occurs as a result of antibiotic treatment that kills

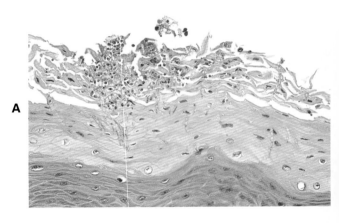

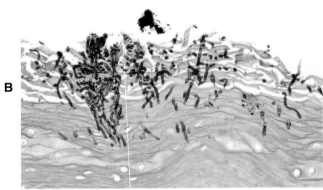

Fig. 7-35 Thrush (oral candidiasis), tongue, foal. **A,** Hyphae of *Candida albicans* are growing in the superficial epithelium of the tongue. H&E stain. **B,** Same specimen as **A.** Gomori's methenamine silver stain. *(A and B, Courtesy Dr. J.F. Zachary, College of Veterinary Medicine, University of Illinois.)*

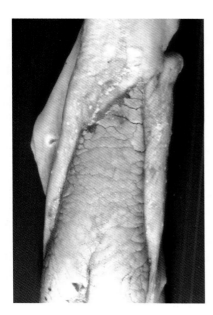

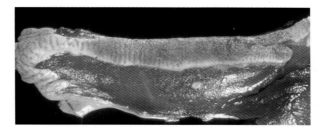

Fig. 7-37   Ulcerative glossitis, uremia (uremic glossitis), tongue, horse. There is extensive ulceration of the mucosal epithelium of the tongue associated with increased concentrations of serum blood urea nitrogen and creatine from kidney failure. *(Courtesy Dr. H. Gelberg, College of Veterinary Medicine, Oregon State University.)*

Fig. 7-36   Thrush, tongue, foal. A pseudomembrane of hyphae of *Candida* is present on the dorsal surface. It has been scraped off the rostral end of the tongue *(top)* to reveal normal mucosa beneath the fungal mat. *(Courtesy Dr. H. Gelberg, College of Veterinary Medicine, Oregon State University.)*

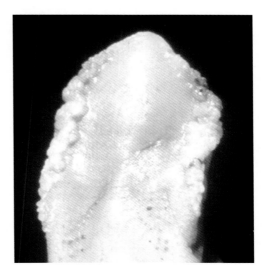

normal flora, increased serum glucose concentrations as a result of diabetes mellitus, a high-sugar diet, or intravenous glucose therapy. The availability of iron is a limiting factor for the indigenous bacteria, which compete with yeast for mucosal colonization. Immunodeficiency states also contribute to the development of thrush. All of these scenarios provide tissue conditions suitable for the proliferation of yeast forms. Rarely, systemic infection may result. Factors predisposing to systemic infections include multiple antibiotic usage, indwelling catheters, and endotracheal tubes.

Often, lingual lesions are manifestations of systemic diseases, such as BVD, foot-and-mouth disease, multisystemic amyloidosis, and uremia (Fig. 7-37). Some of these diseases are discussed in more detail elsewhere in other chapters of this book.

HYPERPLASTIC AND NEOPLASTIC CONDITIONS

Epithelial hyperplasia of the lateral edges of the tongue is common in piglets before nursing, when the fringelike epithelium is rubbed off (Fig. 7-38).

Lingual (glossal) neoplasms are rare but, when they occur, are generally of epithelial origin. Squamous cell carcinomas are most common (Fig. 7-39), but papillomas (Fig. 7-40), rhabdomyomas, rhabdomyosarcomas, fibrosarcomas, melanomas, and granular cell tumors have all been reported in domestic animals.

Fig. 7-38   Lingual epithelial hyperplasia, tongue, neonatal pig. The lateral surfaces of the tongue are covered by a hyperplastic epithelial fringe. This fringe is normal at birth and will be lost through mechanical trauma to the fringe during nursing. *(Courtesy Dr. H. Gelberg, College of Veterinary Medicine, Oregon State University.)*

PARASITES

Parasites of the tongue are uncommon, with the exception of those that reside in muscles, such as *Sarcocystis* spp. and *Trichinella spiralis* in pigs and occasionally in carnivorous wildlife such as polar bears. *Gongylonema* spp. can be present in the mucosa of pigs and ruminants and are of no clinical significance.

ESOPHAGUS
INTRODUCTION

Under normal circumstances, the esophageal lumen is a potential space. The wall collapses when the esophagus is not transporting ingesta.

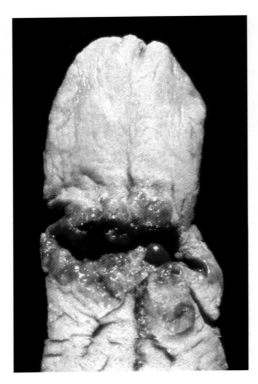

Fig. 7-39   Squamous cell carcinoma, tongue (dorsal surface), dog. Note the proliferative, ulcerated, and hemorrhagic neoplasm growing transversely across the surface of the tongue. *(Courtesy Dr. H. Gelberg, College of Veterinary Medicine, Oregon State University.)*

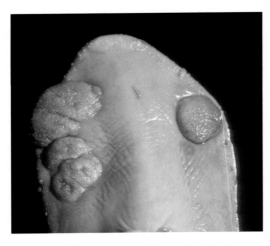

Fig. 7-40   Papillomas, tongue (ventral surface), cow. Papillomas, often caused by bovine papillomavirus, are present on the ventral surface of the tongue. The virus infects traumatized mucosal epithelial cells and induces epithelial cell proliferation. *(Courtesy Dr. M.D. McGavin, College of Veterinary Medicine, University of Tennessee.)*

STRUCTURE AND FUNCTION

The esophagus extends from the distal end of the oropharynx, passes through the mediastinum, and ends at the cardia of the stomach at the diaphragmatic hiatus. Protrusion of the stomach through the diaphragm into the thoracic cavity at this location is termed a hiatal hernia. The esophagus is lined by nonkeratinizing stratified squamous epithelium in carnivores and is keratinized in pigs, horses, and ruminants. Keratinization is greatest in ruminants, less in horses, and least in pigs. Longitudinal and oblique mucosal folds are present to varying degrees.

The tunica muscularis is completely striated in ruminants and dogs. In the horse, the distal third of the esophagus contains smooth muscle. The pig is similar to the horse, except that the middle third of the esophagus contains a mixture of smooth and striated muscle. In the cat, opossum, and primates, the distal two thirds of the esophagus is composed of smooth muscle. The smooth muscle is arranged as an inner circular layer and an outer longitudinal layer.

Mixed mucinous glands are present in the tunica submucosa of pigs and dogs. In pigs the glands are most abundant in the cranial half of the esophagus, and in dogs they are present throughout. Glands are present in cats, horses, and ruminants only at the junction of the esophagus and pharynx.

It is important to remember that unlike the rest of the tubular digestive tract, the esophagus is unique in that it lacks a serosa in all but the abdominal portion. This means that sutures are not likely to seal an incision. Combine this with the strong muscular contractions that characterize this organ and it is easy to understand why esophageal surgery is not often performed and is even less often successful. For the same anatomic reason, perforating foreign bodies of the esophagus do not seal themselves off.

PORTALS OF ENTRY

All materials passed from the oral cavity traverse through the esophagus to the stomach or rumen, including caustic chemicals. Penetration or obstruction by foreign objects is the most common portal of entry (Fig. 7-41). Some parasites spend part or all of their life cycles in the esophagus. Iatrogenic puncture of the esophagus is a not uncommon sequela to passage of stomach tubes. Gastric reflux is an additional portal of entry into the esophagus.

DEVELOPMENTAL ANOMALIES

Esophageal motility disorders are termed achalasia. In this condition, the sequential contractility of the esophagus is defective and the lower sphincter fails to function properly. Achalasia results in difficulty in swallowing and may be associated with regurgitation and weight loss.

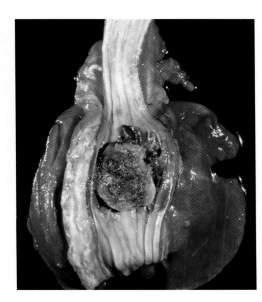

Fig. 7-41   Foreign body with necrosis, esophagus, dog.
A ham bone lodged in this dog's esophagus dorsal to the base
of the heart has caused esophageal dilation and pressure
necrosis of the esophageal mucosa. *(Courtesy Dr. C.S. Patton,
College of Veterinary Medicine, University of Tennessee.)*

Cricopharyngeal achalasia is a congenital, possibly
neurogenic, disorder of the upper esophageal (cricopharyngeal) sphincter. It occurs in young, small breed dogs,
particularly terriers, cocker spaniels, and miniature
poodles. Postweaning dysphagia and regurgitation
after a meal of solid food is characteristic of this
functional disorder. Liquids are generally swallowed
without incidence. Gagging or choking behavior of the
patient after swallowing is a good indicator, in the
appropriately aged dog, of this condition.

Acquired canine achalasia is extremely uncommon.
In this condition, there is often a visible abnormality of
the musculature of deglutition (cricopharyngeus). There
does not appear to be a characteristic change in the
affected musculature. Esophageal myotomy is therapeutic for this idiopathic condition.

MEGAESOPHAGUS

Megaesophagus or esophageal ectasia is dilation of
the esophagus because of insufficient or uncoordinated
peristalsis in the mid and cervical esophagus. It has been
described in dogs, cats, cows, ferrets, horses, and new
world camelids. Causes include motility problems related
to innervation or denervation disorders and to partial
physical obstructions and stenosis, secondary to inflammatory diseases of esophageal musculature or persistence of the right aortic arch. Many cases are idiopathic.

Congenital megaesophagus is due to partial blockage of the lumen of the esophagus by a persistent right
fourth aortic arch. Because of the persistence of the
arch, a vascular ring forms around the esophagus and
trachea, preventing full dilation of the esophagus. The
ring is formed by the aorta, pulmonary artery, and
ductus arteriosus. This form of megaesophagus is
unique in that the esophageal obstruction, and thus
dilation, occurs cranial to the heart because of the location of the obstructing vascular ring (Fig. 7-42; also see
Fig. 10-23). Persistent right aortic arch is likely hereditary in German shepherds, Irish setters, and greyhounds. All other forms of megaesophagus result in
dilation cranial to the stomach.

Congenital megaesophagus also occurs as an idiopathic denervation of the esophagus, most notably in
Great Danes, Irish setters, miniature schnauzers,
Labrador retrievers, wire hair fox terriers, Shar-Peis,
Newfoundlands, and Siamese cats. Myasthenia gravis
(see later discussion) may be of genetic origin in a small
number of cases.

Acquired megaesophagus or esophageal achalasia is
the result of failure of relaxation of the distal esophageal
or cardiac sphincter of the stomach in human beings.
The obstruction, and thus dilation, occurs cranial to the
stomach (Fig. 7-43). Although the gross appearance of
acquired megaesophagus in animals is similar to that of
human beings, the cause of the condition in animals
does not involve the cardiac sphincter. Causes are idiopathic or secondary to polymyositis (inflammation of
the esophageal muscle), myasthenia gravis (an autoimmune disease directed against acetylcholine receptors
of the neuromuscular junction), hypothyroidism (which
can result in muscle atrophy and denervation disease),
congenital myopathy, lead and thallium poisoning
(via effect on innervation), peripheral neuropathies,
esophagitis, and recurrent gastric dilation. Increased
risk is seen in German shepherds, golden retrievers,
and Irish setters.

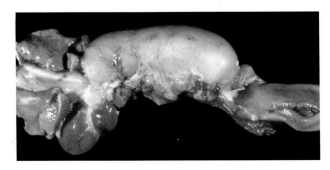

**Fig. 7-42   Megaesophagus from a persistent right aortic
arch, esophagus, dog.** Dilation of the esophagus cranial to
the heart is the result of failure of the right fourth aortic arch
to regress during embryonic life (vascular ring abnormality).
*(Courtesy Dr. C.S. Patton, College of Veterinary Medicine, University of
Tennessee.)*

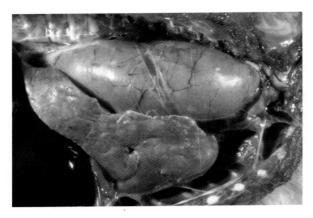

Fig. 7-43   **Megaesophagus, thoracic esophagus, dog.** A notably dilated thoracic esophagus cranial to the diaphragm has displaced the right lung caudally and ventrally. This form of megaesophagus is often attributable to an abnormality (mass, foreign body, innervation disorder) affecting the cardiac sphincter. *(Courtesy Dr. H. Gelberg, College of Veterinary Medicine, Oregon State University.)*

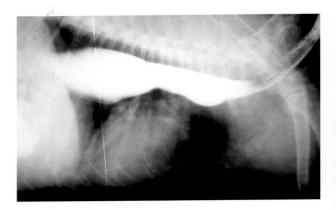

Fig. 7-44   **Megaesophagus, thoracic radiograph, dog.** Swallowed radiopaque imaging agent (barium sulfate) demonstrates dilation of the esophagus cranial to the diaphragm. *(Courtesy Dr. H. Gelberg, College of Veterinary Medicine, Oregon State University.)*

Megaesophagus is recognized clinically by regurgitation after ingestion of solid food. Thus congenital megaesophagus is often recognized at weaning. Often animals are thin and may have aspiration pneumonia. Radiographically, in megaesophagus, the esophagus is dilated and retains radiopaque dyes (Fig. 7-44). Dilation may vary from diffuse to locally extensive depending on its cause. Putrid ingesta are sometimes found in the dilated, atonic portions of the esophagus. Although degenerated nerve fibers are occasionally found within vagus nerves, megaesophagus can occur without histologic lesions.

ESOPHAGEAL PARASITES

With notable exceptions, parasitic diseases of the esophagus are generally of no clinical importance. The more common parasites of the esophagus are *Gongylonema* spp., which affect ruminants, pigs, horses, primates, and occasionally rodents. These nematodes reside in the mucosa, and are characteristically thin, red, and serpentine. They can be 10 to 15 cm in length and are easily visible (Fig. 7-45). The intermediate hosts are cockroaches and dung beetles.

Gasterophilus spp. occur in equids. These fly larvae have interesting life cycles because their eggs are laid on the skin in varying locations. The warmth and moisture from licking activates them. The larvae burrow into the oral mucosa, molt, and then migrate down the esophagus. They occur both in the distal esophagus and stomach where they attach to the mucosa via oral hooks. They eventually detach, leaving craters at the site of attachment, and pass in the feces.

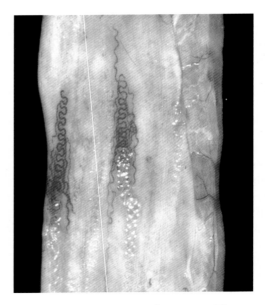

Fig. 7-45   **Gongylonemiasis, esophagus, cow.** The serpentine intramucosal nematodes are characteristic of *Gongylonema*, a nematode of the superfamily Spiruroidea. *(Courtesy Dr. M.D. McGavin, College of Veterinary Medicine, University of Tennessee.)*

Hypoderma lineatum is the larvae of the warble fly of ruminants. These parasites eventually migrate to the esophageal adventitia and then to the subcutaneous tissue of the back.

Probably the most pathogenic of the esophageal parasites is *Spirocerca lupi* of canids. These nematodes reach the esophageal submucosa after migrating from the stomach through the aortic wall. A passage forms between the esophageal lumen and the granuloma containing the parasite, allowing discharge of ova into the lumen of the alimentary system and eventually into inflammation spreads distally along the tooth, resulting in gingival-epithelial attachment only on the root of the tooth, deep in the alveolar socket. Progression of inflammation destroys the connective tissue of the periodontal ligament, resulting in loosening of the tooth. Alveolar osteomyelitis and pulpitis can form apical abscesses, bacteremic spread of inflammation, significant oral pain, reluctance to masticate, and halitosis. Periodontal disease is common in carnivores and humans. Mildly abrasive diets and brushing of the teeth of pet carnivores, combined with regular dental examination, is preventative in carnivores as it is in human beings.

DENTAL NEOPLASIA

Proliferative, cystic or neoplastic diseases of the dental arcade can originate from cell rests that form from the dental lamina or the enamel organ (the cell rests of Malassez). Dental neoplasms usually arise in proximity to the teeth, either deeply in the jaw or from the surface epithelium. There is a relatively precise method of naming dental neoplasms based on the tissue or cell of origin and the extent of differentiation and odontogenesis present within the neoplastic tissue. The histologic appearance of these neoplasms is complex; pathologists with considerable experience in differentiating these uncommon neoplasms should be consulted when a precise diagnosis is indicated.

Odontomas are hamartomas originating in the enamel organ, usually of puppies and foals (Fig. 7-24). They usually contain well-recognizable dentin and enamel as well as ameloblasts, odontoblasts, and dental pulp.

Ameloblastoma is a term applied to epithelial neoplasms of enamel organ origin. Several subtypes can be distinguished histologically. They are ameloblastic fibroma, ameloblastic odontoma, calcifying epithelial odontogenic tumor, peripheral odontogenic fibroma, and other rare tooth neoplasms.

Ameloblastoma appears randomly in the dental arcade, usually in adult dogs. They are often osteolytic and thus are locally invasive. Histologic examination by an expert is often necessary to distinguish ameloblastoma from acanthomatous epulis and squamous cell carcinoma.

TONSILS
STRUCTURE AND FUNCTION

The palatine tonsils are pharyngeal lymphoid structures covered by stratified squamous epithelium. Their function is uncertain, although it is likely they serve in lymphocyte production and antibody formation. In carnivores, they are found in crypts or recesses at the dorsolateral aspect of the caudal oropharynx. In pigs, they are flat and recognized by tiny pores in the surface epithelium of the caudal soft palate. Equids, ruminants, and pigs have lingual tonsils in addition to palatine tonsils.

PORTALS OF ENTRY

Tonsils do not possess afferent lymphatics and do not serve as lymph filters. Therefore only primary (or direct) or hematogenous infections occur (tonsillitis) (Fig. 7-25), and primary neoplasms of either the lymphoid (lymphosarcoma) (Fig. 7-26) or epithelial (squamous cell carcinoma) (Fig. 7-27) components. In many viremias of mammals, such as pseudorabies of pigs, virus may be isolated from the tonsils.

SALIVARY GLANDS
INTRODUCTION

Salivary glands are found in a variety of locations in the head and neck regions. They arise from oral ectoderm. In all species the major salivary glands include the parotid, mandibular, and sublingual. Carnivores have a zygomatic gland as well. Minor salivary glands include buccal, labial, lingual, palatine, and others similarly named by location.

STRUCTURE AND FUNCTION

Most salivary glands are discrete aggregates of compound tubuloalveolar tissue. Saliva is a mixture of serous and mucoid secretions. Saliva lubricates the mouth and esophagus and moistens ingesta. Saliva also dissolves water-soluble components of food so the taste buds can function. The mucus in saliva binds to masticated food and creates a bolus that is more easily swallowed. Salivary mucus also coats the epithelium of the

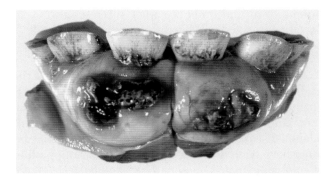

Fig. 7-24   **Odontoma, incisor teeth, cow.** This is a hamartoma (a benign tumorlike nodule) of the enamel organ and in this case has expanded bilaterally on the rostral mandibles. There is extensive hemorrhagic ulceration over the tumor. Diagnosis can be confirmed by radiographic and histopathologic examination. *(Courtesy Dr. M.D. McGavin, College of Veterinary Medicine, University of Tennessee.)*

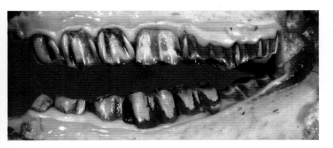

Fig. 7-22   Fluorosis, cheek teeth, cow. The enamel is chalky and weak, and the teeth are usually rapidly worn down. *(Courtesy Dr. L. Krook, College of Veterinary Medicine, Cornell University.)*

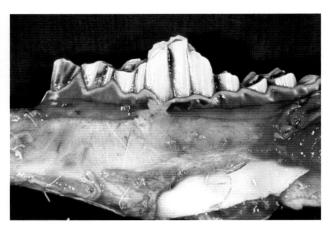

Fig. 7-23   Dental attrition, molar teeth, antelope. Age-associated dental wear results in improper mastication of feedstuffs and malnutrition. This condition occurs most commonly in horses and is referred to as "step-mouth." *(Courtesy College of Veterinary Medicine, University of Tennessee.)*

yellow, dark brown, or black (Fig. 7-22). Occlusal grinding of affected soft teeth against more normal enamel results in rapid dental wear. One wonders therefore about the cumulative effect of fluoride supplementation in municipal drinking water, vitamins with added fluoride, fluoride-supplemented toothpaste, fluoride treatment of teeth, reconstituted and bottled soft drinks made with fluoridated water, and so forth. It is difficult to calculate the total fluoride load ingested by individuals or what the effects of that fluoride supplementation may be.

LESIONS CAUSED BY ATTRITION AND ABNORMAL WEAR

Loss of normal dental structure and function often results from rapid and irregular and/or abnormal wear of occlusal surfaces in many species of domestic animals. In those species with hypsodont teeth, attention to the dentition as the animal ages is often a major factor in overall body conditioning and health (Fig. 7-23). Aggressive treatment of occlusal surface irregularity by filing of high points in the dental arcade (floating) can notably prolong an animal's life. Rock chewing or other compulsive oral behaviors in dogs may result in accelerated dental wear. In all species, exposure of dentin or the pulp canal may lead to dental infection with serious consequences.

FELINE EXTERNAL RESORPTIVE NECK LESIONS

Cats suffering from feline external resorptive neck lesions often have pain upon chewing that may be reflected by inappetence and/or abnormal masticatory movements. External neck resorption of the teeth of otherwise dentally normal cats is caused by odontoclastic resorption of dental tissue, particularly in the neck area or root of the tooth. Cementum or osteoid ingrowths partially or completely line the resorptive cavity. The resultant cavity may attract bacterial plaque, resulting in intense inflammation and osteoclastic resorption of dental tissue. The primary cause of this condition is not known.

INFUNDIBULAR IMPACTION

Impaction of the infundibulum, infundibular necrosis or infundibular caries, may cause serious dental disease in ruminants and more rarely in horses. Incomplete infundibular cementum formation before tooth eruption likely predisposes to infundibular impaction. The pathogenic mechanism is comparable to dental caries in simple-toothed animals. Feed material is ground into the infundibulum, where bacteria metabolize it to form acid, which causes demineralization. Bacterial enzymes digest the organic matrix of enamel and dentin. As a result of this destruction, the pulp cavity becomes infected, resulting in pulpitis and endodontitis. Dental abscesses and fistulous tracks may develop. The inflamed infundibular cavities often continue to become impacted with feed, creating a vicious cycle.

PERIODONTAL DISEASE

Bacterial films resident on the tooth surface and the acids and enzymes they produce may damage their enamel substrate (cavities) and also destroy the subjacent gingival tissue and periodontal ligament (periodontal disease). More than 200 species of bacteria and fungi have been associated with dental plaque (a film of an organic matrix, food particles and bacteria on the tooth surface). This plaque often becomes mineralized (tartar or dental calculus). The mineralized material contributes to atrophy and inflammation of the gingival epithelium and supporting stroma by acting as a nidus for additional plaque accumulation.

The initial site for destructive inflammation is in the gingival crevice-forming pockets. With time, this

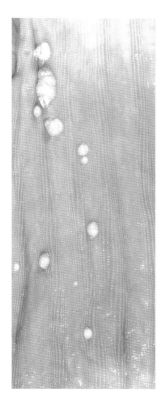

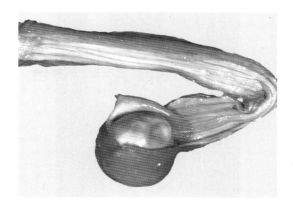

Fig. 7-56 **Leiomyoma, esophagus, dog.** A mass consisting of submucosal proliferation of smooth muscle cells bulges into the distal esophageal lumen causing obstruction. *(Courtesy Dr. H. Gelberg, College of Veterinary Medicine, Oregon State University.)*

Fig. 7-55 **Papillomatosis, bovine papilloma virus, esophagus, bull.** Multiple papillomas, characteristic of this viral-induced disease, occur following trauma to the esophageal mucosa and infection of mucosal epithelial cells. Oral papillomas may be present concurrently. *(Courtesy Dr. H. Gelberg, College of Veterinary Medicine, Oregon State University.)*

occasionally palpable, but are most often intraluminal rather than mural. Epithelial tumors include papillomas (Fig. 7-55) and squamous cell carcinomas. The later have wide metastatic potential. Smooth muscle tumors of the esophagus are also rare, but may result in similar clinical signs whether benign or malignant (Fig. 7-56). Esophageal fibrosarcomas of dogs are often associated with *Spirocerca lupi* infestation. Esophageal lymphosarcoma occurs sporadically in most species (Fig. 7-57).

RUMEN, RETICULUM, AND OMASUM

INTRODUCTION

The three compartments of the ruminant forestomach are the reticulum, rumen, and omasum. The forestomach is subdivided by folds and compartments. Normal forestomach motility, and thus innervation, is critical in maintaining digestive homeostasis. The forestomach is aglandular. The resident flora and fauna are responsible for digestion and fermentation. In general, the rumen is a large fermentation vat where microorganisms break down ingesta by mechanical and chemical action into

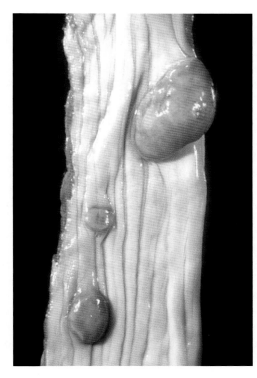

Fig. 7-57 **Lymphoma (lymphosarcoma), esophagus, dog.** Masses of submucosal proliferating malignant lymphocytes bulge into the esophageal lumen, causing partial obstruction. Note that the mucosal epithelium is intact (smooth and shiny). *(Courtesy Dr. M.D. McGavin, College of Veterinary Medicine, University of Tennessee.)*

short chain fatty acids, which are directly absorbed across the epithelial lining into the blood and constitute more than half of the absorbable energy. The reticulum and omasum act mechanically to further reduce the ingesta to fine particles.

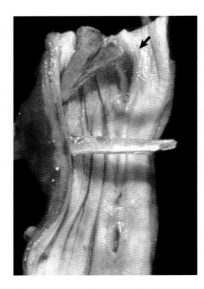

Fig. 7-52 **Ulcers and perforation, foreign body, esophagus, dog.** The esophagus has been perforated by an ingested chicken bone. Note that the end of the bone opposite the perforation site has caused a deep ulcer *(arrow)*. There are also several chronic ulcers caudal to the perforation, presumably from abrasion by other bones as they moved down the esophagus. *(Courtesy Dr. C.S. Patton, College of Veterinary Medicine, University of Tennessee.)*

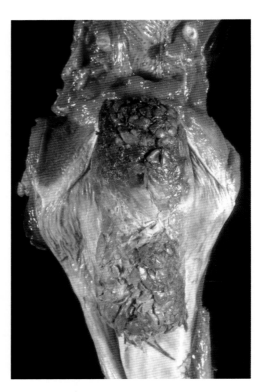

Fig. 7-53 **Foreign body (choke), esophagus, cow.** A corn cob has lodged in the esophagus subjacent to the larynx. *(Courtesy Dr. H. Gelberg, College of Veterinary Medicine, Oregon State University.)*

most frequently as a result of ingestion of large foreign bodies such as potatoes, apples, bones (Fig. 7-52), corn cobbs (Fig. 7-53), or medicaments such as large gelatin-filled capsules or tablets (dry boluses). If these bodies are lodged against the epithelium for longer than 2 days, the interaction often results in circumferential pressure necrosis of the esophageal mucosa (Fig. 7-54), which forms strictures during healing. These strictures then can cause reflex regurgitation after ingestion of food.

In older horses, poor dentition causes feed to be incompletely masticated, resulting in impaction in the esophagus. Neoplastic or inflammatory lesions of the esophagus or periesophageal tissues also cause obstruction. Persistence of the right aortic arch has already been discussed as a cause of esophageal stenosis and megaesophagus.

NEOPLASIA

Neoplasms of the esophagus are rare. Bracken fern (*Pteridium aquilinum*) consumption has been associated with squamous cell carcinomas in felids and equids. The clinical signs are similar to those of other causes of esophageal blockage and include dysphagia, regurgitation, weight loss, and dilation of the esophagus proximal to the mass. Tumors of the esophagus are

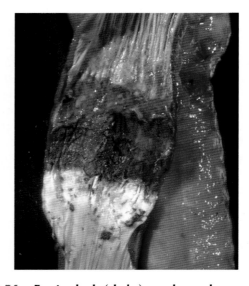

Fig. 7-54 **Foreign body (choke), esophagus, horse.** Pressure necrosis of the proximal esophageal mucosa, adjacent to the larynx has occurred secondary to lodgment of a foreign body (compacted chaff). As a general rule, pressure necrosis usually occurs if the foreign body remains in place against the mucosal epithelium for longer than 2 days. *(Courtesy Dr. M.D. McGavin, College of Veterinary Medicine, University of Tennessee.)*

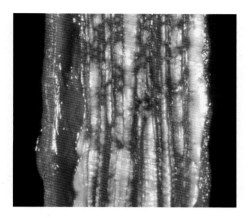

Fig. 7-49 **Acid reflux esophagitis, esophagus, horse.** The dark red streaks on the surface of the esophagus are areas of epithelial loss secondary to gastric acid reflux. The white streaks and vertically linear areas on the surface of the esophagus are areas of unaffected and likely hyperplastic mucosal epithelium. As would be expected, erosions are most severe on the esophageal mucosa adjacent to the cardia and extend rostrally. This distribution is diagnostic of acid reflux esophagitis. (*Courtesy Dr. H. Gelberg, College of Veterinary Medicine, Oregon State University.*)

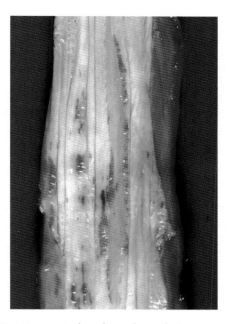

Fig. 7-50 **Trauma-induced esophageal ulceration, esophagus, horse.** These red linear ulcers are the result of abrasion from improper stomach tubing, either from an overly large diameter tube, from a too-vigorous insertion, or from a tube with a roughened edge. (*Courtesy Dr. H. Gelberg, College of Veterinary Medicine, Oregon State University.*)

heartburn in human beings. Other causes of esophageal ulcers include improper use of stomach tubes, which cause linear scraping on the crests of the longitudinal folds of the esophageal mucosa (Fig. 7-50), and infectious diseases, such as BVD (Fig. 7-51), which cause mucosal injury in other locations as well.

Leukoplakia of the esophagus and stomach is characterized by discrete, flat, white mucosal elevations (epithelial plaques) of no clinical significance and of unknown cause. They are sometimes mistaken for thrush lesions or neoplasia. Unlike thrush lesions, they do not scrape off easily, and their regularity, number, and location distinguish them from neoplasms. Histologically the stratum germinativum and prickly cell layers are notably thickened, and the surface cells have pyknotic nuclei and some parakeratosis. In human beings, about 5% of these lesions become cancerous. They are present in the oral cavity and esophagus and are believed related to chronic irritation most often associated with smoking or chewing tobacco. Alcohol consumption and restorative dental amalgams may also predispose to leukoplakia.

CHOKE

Choke is a clinical term referring to esophageal obstruction subsequent to stenoses or blockage. Choke most often occurs in those anatomic locations where the esophagus cannot fully expand. These locations are dorsal to the larynx and at the thoracic inlet, base of the heart, and the diaphragmatic hiatus. Choke occurs

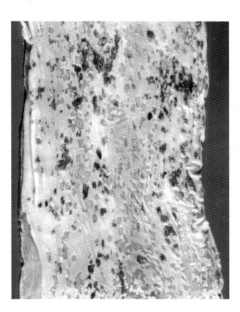

Fig. 7-51 **Ulcerative esophagitis, bovine viral diarrhea, esophagus, cow.** Note the multiple variably sized (millimeter range) and variably shaped esophageal mucosal ulcers caused by the pestivirus of bovine viral diarrhea. (*Courtesy Dr. H. Gelberg, College of Veterinary Medicine, Oregon State University.*)

the feces. Clinical sequelae of infestation include dysphagia, aortic aneurysms, hemothorax, and rarely esophageal fibrosarcomas or osteosarcomas (Fig. 7-46). Spondylosis deformans develops occasionally in the vertebral bodies of chronically affected canids adjacent to the aortic granulomas. *Spirocerca lupi* infestations occur in warmer climates. The intermediate hosts are dung beetles, and the paratenic hosts are chickens, reptiles, and rodents.

MISCELLANEOUS ESOPHAGEAL LESIONS AND CONDITIONS

Idiopathic muscular hypertrophy of the distal esophagus is a peculiar lesion in horses and pigs that can be quite spectacular at necropsy (Fig. 7-47), but usually it is of no clinical significance. The esophageal musculature can be several centimeters thick, and the lesion can extend along the distal quarter of the esophagus. Rarely this condition plays a role in esophageal impaction. Similarly, dilation of the esophageal glands of aged dogs can be a spectacular gross lesion of no clinical consequence. It is therefore important to carefully evaluate these lesions either at necropsy or during fiberoptic viewing in the live animal to determine whether what appear to be erosions and ulcers are rather mucosal elevations filled with mucus. Because the lesions are subepithelial, the overlying mucosa is smooth and shiny. Dilated esophageal glands vary in number and location but are generally only a few millimeters in diameter (Fig. 7-48). They are most numerous in the distal esophagus.

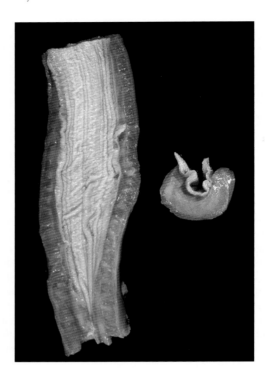

Fig. 7-47   Muscular hypertrophy, distal esophagus, horse. Longitudinal (*left*) and transverse (*right*) sections of the esophagus demonstrate the marked increase in the thickness of the smooth muscle in the tunica muscularis of the distal esophagus. *(Courtesy Dr. C.S. Patton, College of Veterinary Medicine, University of Tennessee.)*

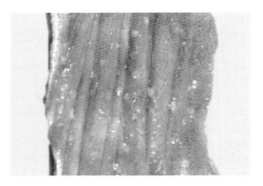

Fig. 7-48   Cystic esophageal glands, distal esophagus, dog. Multiple white mucosal cysts are present in the esophageal glands of the mucosa and submucosa. These cysts are common and insignificant findings in aged dogs. *(Courtesy Dr. H. Gelberg, College of Veterinary Medicine, Oregon State University.)*

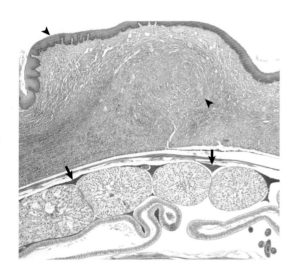

Fig. 7-46   Fibrosarcoma, esophagus, dog. *Spirocerca lupi* (longitudinal section) *(arrows)* is present in the esophageal submucosa deep to the fibrosarcoma, which it has induced *(arrowheads).* H&E stain. *(Courtesy Dr. H. Gelberg, College of Veterinary Medicine, Oregon State University.)*

Esophageal erosions and ulcers are relatively common and have a variety of causes. One of the more common causes of esophageal erosions and ulcers is reflux of stomach acid. This reflux of gastric acids causes chemical burning of the lower esophagus and is commonly called acid reflux esophagitis (Fig. 7-49) or

STRUCTURE AND FUNCTION

The rumen has small papillae that vary by diet up to 1.5 cm in length. Papillae are longer with high roughage diets and shorter when more concentrates are in the ration. There is a dorsal and ventral compartment. The reticulum has a honeycomb appearance, and the omasum consists of a series of about 100 longitudinal folds similar to the pages of a book. The nonglandular stratified squamous mucosa of the reticulum, rumen, and omasum can be acutely inflamed when the contents have an acid pH and the abnormal milieu permits bacterial and mycotic overgrowth.

The epithelial lining of the forestomach functions as a protective barrier for the forestomach and for the metabolism of ingesta and the absorption of volatile fatty acids. Because the reticulo-omasal orifice is more dorsal than the floor of the compartments, the reticulum can trap foreign bodies, especially dense metallic ones. These can irritate or penetrate the mucosa ("hardware disease"). Problems with motility and imbalances of rumen flora and fauna are the most frequent abnormalities of forestomach function. Often the changes in flora and fauna are precipitated by a change in ingested substrate promoting the growth of particular organisms. These changes alter ruminal pH and thus affect the integrity of the mucosal lining of the compartments of the forestomach or cause the production of excessive gas, resulting in distention.

Parts of compartment one (C1) (and of C2 and C3) of the camelid forestomach are lined by mucinous glandular epithelium. Concretions of ingesta are sometimes found within the saccules that contain the glands. The saccules are also the sites of water and other solutes. The nonglandular portions of C1 and C2 are lined by nonkeratinized stratified squamous epithelium. The forestomach of new world camelids contracts at two to three times the rate of other ruminants (and in reverse order), and with each cycle the saccules empty and refill. This results in high digestive efficiency across the saccules.

BLOAT (RUMINAL TYMPANY)

Ruminal tympany or bloat is, by definition, an overdistention of the rumen and reticulum by gases produced during fermentation. Mortality of affected animals is approximately 50%. A hereditary predisposition to bloat might exist in cattle because cases are on record of bloat in monozygotic twins. Bloat can be divided into primary tympany and secondary tympany.

Primary tympany is also known as legume bloat, dietary bloat, or frothy bloat. It generally occurs up to 3 days after animals begin a new diet. Certain legumes, such as alfalfa, ladino clover, and grain concentrates, promote the formation of stable foam. The nonvolatile acids of legume and ruminal fermentation lower the rumen pH to between 5 and 6, which is optimal for formation of bloat. Foam mixed with rumen contents physically blocks the cardia, preventing eructation and causing the rumen to distend with the gases of fermentation. Clinical signs include a distended left paralumbar fossa, a distended abdomen, increased respiratory and heart rates, and late in the disease, decreased ruminal movements. Death, when it occurs, is attributable to distention of the abdomen and compression of the diaphragm with resultant decreased pleural cavity size, respiratory embarrassment, and increased intraabdominal and intrathoracic pressure, resulting in decreased venous return to the heart, which becomes generalized congestion cranial to the thoracic inlet.

The lesions of primary tympany are often difficult to detect if there is an interval between death and postmortem examination, because the foam can collapse. Conversely, fermentation can occur after death in a nonbloated animal, resulting in the production of abundant gas. The most reliable postmortem indicator of antemortem bloat is the sharp line of demarcation between the pale, bloodless distal esophagus and the congested proximal esophagus at the thoracic inlet. This line may sometimes form even after death before the blood clots. This division is known as a bloat line (Fig. 7-58).

Secondary tympany is caused by a physical or functional obstruction or stenosis of the esophagus resulting in failure to eructate. Vagus indigestion or other innervation disorders, esophageal papilloma, lymphosarcoma, and esophageal foreign bodies are examples of causes of secondary tympany.

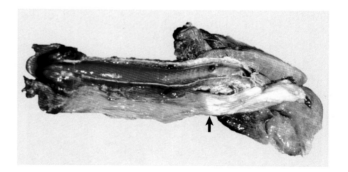

Fig. 7-58   **Bloat line, esophagus and trachea at the thoracic inlet, cow.** There is a sharp demarcation between the caudal (blanched) and the cranial (congested) mucosa of the esophagus *(arrow).* This demarcation is caused by compromised venous return, the result of a grossly distended rumen displacing the diaphragm cranially and causing increased intrathoracic pressure, thus preventing the flow of venous blood into the thorax. In this illustration, a similar demarcation can be seen on the mucosa of the trachea. The subcutaneous tissues of the neck and head are also congested. *(Courtesy Department of Veterinary Pathology, Cornell University.)*

FOREIGN BODIES

Foreign bodies can collect or lodge in the rumen. These include trichobezoars (hair balls) and phytobezoars (plant balls). Trichobezoars are sometimes a sequelae to a habit of bucket-fed calves sucking on each other to satisfy their nursing instincts. Trichobezoars can form in utero because of hair circulating in the amniotic fluid and being swallowed by the fetus. Phytobezoars result from an excess of indigestible roughage.

Ingestion of nails and wire, common where straw and hay bales are bound by wire, can result in perforation of the wall of the reticulum with resultant reticulitis, peritonitis, or pericarditis (hardware disease) (Fig. 7-59). Often, in areas in the United States where ruminants are at high risk of hardware disease because of farming practices, magnets are placed in rumens to prevent the ingested wires and nails from penetrating the reticular mucosa. Occasionally, ruminants ingest plates from storage batteries and suffer lead poisoning.

INFLAMMATORY DISEASES

Inflammation of the rumen, rumenitis, is generally considered synonymous with lactic acidosis. Lactic acidosis is synonymous with grain overload, rumen overload, carbohydrate engorgement, and chemical rumenitis. All ruminants are susceptible. The pathophysiology of lactic acidosis usually involves a sudden dietary change to an easily fermentable feed or a change in the feed volume consumed. The latter scenario is most likely to occur during weather changes, especially among feedlot cattle when a sudden cooling rainstorm will stimulate food intake of cattle that had previously lost appetite due to high environmental temperatures and humidity.

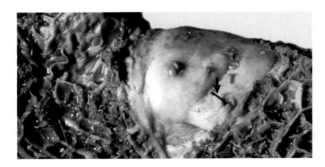

Fig. 7-59   Traumatic reticulitis, reticulum, cow. Several ingested wires have perforated the wall of the reticulum *(arrow)* and lodged in the tunica muscularis. Each wire is surrounded by a sinus tract draining to the surface of the reticulum. A chronic ulcer has formed around each area penetrated by the wires. *(Courtesy Dr. M.D. McGavin, College of Veterinary Medicine, University of Tennessee.)*

Ruminal microflora is generally rich in cellulolytic gram-negative bacteria necessary for the digestion of hay. A sudden change to a highly fermentable, carbohydrate-rich feed promotes the growth of gram-positive bacteria, *Streptococcus bovis*, and *Lactobacillus* spp. The lactic acid produced by the fermentation of ingested carbohydrates decreases the ruminal pH below 5 (normal = 5.5 to 7.5). This acidic pH eliminates normal ruminal flora and fauna and damages ruminal mucosa. Increased concentrations of dissociated fatty acids lead to ruminal atony. Death, when it occurs, is due to dehydration secondary to the increased osmotic effect of ruminal solutes (organic acids) causing movement of fluids across the damaged ruminal mucosa into the rumen, acidosis (from absorption of lactate from the rumen), and circulatory collapse. Mortality among animals with lactic acidosis ranges from 25% to 90% and usually occurs within 24 hours.

At necropsy, the ruminal and intestinal contents are watery and acidic. Often abundant grain is found in the rumen. The mucosa of the ruminal papillae is brown and friable and detaches easily, especially from the ventral ruminal sac. Caution must be exercised in interpreting this latter finding as a lesion because the ruminal mucosa often detaches easily in animals that have been dead for even a few hours at high environmental temperatures. Hydropic change and coagulative necrosis of the ruminal epithelium followed by an influx of neutrophils are common microscopic lesions. Animals surviving lactic acidosis have stellate scars develop, visible because of their color difference from the unaffected surrounding mucosa. Scars are pale; unaffected mucosa is dark brown to black.

Bacterial rumenitis generally occurs because of lactic acidosis or mechanical rumen injury. Bacteria that colonize the damaged rumen can be transported into the portal circulation and to the liver, resulting in multiple abscesses. *Arcanobacterium (Actinomyces) pyogenes* is a common cause of bacterial abscesses in the liver. *Fusobacterium necrophorum*, also transported from the rumen to the liver, results in necrobacillosis, which has distinctive liver lesions.

Mycotic infections of the rumen also occur because of damage to the ruminal mucosa caused by lactic acidosis and mechanical rumen injury. Mycotic rumenitis also results from the administration of antibiotics, usually in calves but also in adult cattle. The antibiotics reduce the number of normal flora and allow fungi to proliferate. In cases of mycotic rumenitis, lesions are generally circular and well delineated and are caused principally by infarction from thrombosis secondary to fungal vasculitis (Fig. 7-60). Offending fungi include *Aspergillus, Mucor, Rhizopus, Absidia*, and *Mortierella* spp. These fungi can spread to the placenta hematogenously and cause mycotic placentitis, which leads to abortions.

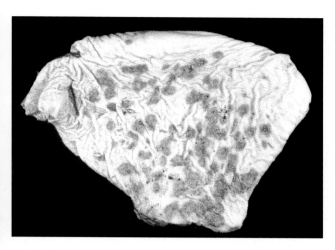

Fig. 7-60   **Mycotic rumenitis, rumen, calf.** Note the numerous well-demarcated foci of necrosis and hemorrhage (infarcts) in the ruminal mucosa that can be caused by angioinvasive fungi such as *Aspergillus, Mucor, Rhizopus, Absidia,* and *Mortierella* spp. This type of mycotic infection is usually preceded by a chemical (lactic acid) rumenitis (overeating). *(Courtesy Dr. H. Gelberg, College of Veterinary Medicine, Oregon State University.)*

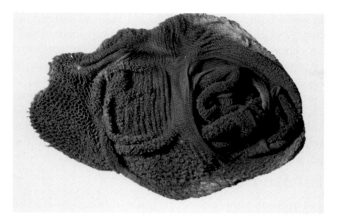

Fig. 7-61   **Parakeratosis, reticulo-rumen, calf.** A diet that was almost devoid of roughage has resulted in atrophy and parakeratosis of ruminal papillae. Normal papillae are leaf shaped, but some of these papillae have become finger shaped, cauliflower shaped, or clumped. The parakeratotic epithelium has been stained brown to black by components of the feed because of the lack of abrasion by the ground feed. These lesions are most marked on the ventral floor of the ventral sac of the rumen. *(Courtesy Dr. M.D. McGavin, College of Veterinary Medicine, University of Tennessee.)*

Ruminal candidiasis occurs as an incidental finding at necropsy. There is usually an underlying debilitating condition, glucose therapy, or an antibiotic-induced kill-off of resident flora and fauna. Ruminal candidiasis is seldom diagnosed in a live animal.

MISCELLANEOUS DISEASES OR CONDITIONS

Ruminal papillae vary in length, becoming longer with high-roughage diets (Fig. 7-61). Such diets also can cause the papilla to become tongue- or leaf-shaped. Animals consuming diets with less than 10% roughage can develop ruminal parakeratosis. These rumens have hard, brown, often clumped, papillae. This lesion has little to no clinical consequence.

Ruminal papillomas are viral-induced in some cases, but in certain countries, bracken fern has been implicated as a cause of these rumen neoplasms (Fig. 7-62).

Vagal indigestion results in a functional outflow problem from the forestomach. Damage to the vagus nerve can occur anywhere along its length and can result in functional pyloric stenosis. Causes of vagal indigestion include inflammation of the vagus nerve due to traumatic reticuloperitonitis, liver abscesses, volvulus of the abomasum, and bronchopneumonia. Mechanical obstruction of the forestomach or abomasal outflow can be due to lymphosarcoma or papillomas or to blockage following ingestion of indigestible or foreign materials. Diet and dwarfism are sometimes associated with vagus indigestion. Many cases are idiopathic. Clinical signs

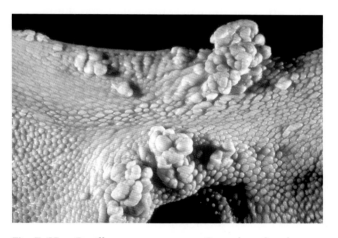

Fig. 7-62   **Papillomas, rumen, cow.** Smooth-surfaced, squamous papillomas are present on the dorsal wall. *(Courtesy Dr. H. Gelberg, College of Veterinary Medicine, Oregon State University.)*

include ruminoreticular distention. The presence of abomasal distention is dependent on the precise location of the damage to the vagus nerve. Vagal indigestion is divided into four types, based on the anatomic location of the functional obstruction. Type I is usually due to inflammatory lesions around the vagal nerve and is a failure of eructation resulting in bloat. Type II is a functional or anatomic condition that results in failure of omasal transport into the abomasum. Usual causes are adhesions and abscesses on the medial wall of the reticulum associated with or secondary to traumatic reticuloperitonitis. Abomasal lymphosarcoma and physical obstruction of the omasal canal (e.g., neoplasia or ingested placenta) may also be causative. Type III is caused by physical impaction by roughage and thus is dietary in origin. Abomasum displacements and volvulus are also potential causes. Type IV is pregnancy related, perhaps as a result of shifting of position of the abomasum secondary to the expanding uterus.

RUMINAL PARASITISM

Paramphistomiasis is a fluke infestation of the ruminant forestomach in warmer latitudes around the world. These trematodes are found in the genera *Paramphistomum*, *Calicophoron*, and *Cotylophoron*. They are similar in size and appearance to ruminal papillae (Fig. 7-63). Although the presence of adult organisms in the forestomach is usually of no clinical significance, heavy infestations of larvae in the proximal small intestine, before migration to the rumen and reticulum, can cause hypoproteinemia, anemia, and death. Larvae burrow deeply into, and sometimes through, the wall of the small intestine and can be found in the peritoneal cavity. The intermediate host is a snail. Cercariae encyst on aquatic vegetation and are eaten by the ruminant.

STOMACH AND ABOMASUM

INTRODUCTION

Although some differences exist, the stomachs of the simple-stomached animals and the abomasum of ruminants (third compartment of new world camelids)

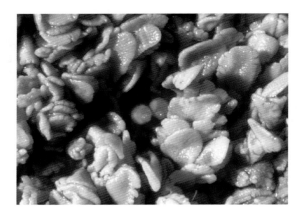

Fig. 7-63 Paramphistomiasis, rumen, cow. The pink conical structures located in the center of the illustration are paramphistomes (ruminal flukes). They are considered to be innocuous, but massive numbers of immature flukes in the duodenum may cause a severe catarrhal duodenitis. Note the normal leaf-shaped ruminal papillae, indicative of a high-roughage diet. *(Courtesy Dr. M.D. McGavin, College of Veterinary Medicine, University of Tennessee.)*

are very similar in structure and function. A fundus and body make up the cranial portion lined by numerous spiral folds and produces acid and pepsin. The aboral portion, the pyloric part, is lined by epithelium with mucous-secreting glands and G cells that produce gastrin. Stomachs have an indigenous flora. Most of these organisms cannot be cultured by traditional methods.

STRUCTURE AND FUNCTION

The gastric mucosa of simple-stomached animals contains numerous folds or rugae that can be flattened when the stomach is distended. Foveolas or gastric pits communicate with the lumen of the stomach and they transport gastric cell secretions. The glandular stomach functions in the enzymatic and hydrolytic digestion of ingested food substances. Epithelial cell types include columnar mucus and bicarbonate-secreting surface epithelial cells, mucous neck cells arranged in tubuloalveolar glands, acid-secreting parietal cells, pepsinogen-secreting chief cells, and neuroendocrine (enterochromaffin, argentaffin) cells.

Multiple submucosal lymphoid patches are present in monogastric animals. In ruminants a single lymphoid patch is present at the fold separating the omasum and abomasum.

In some species, such as the horse and rat, the cranial stomach (nonglandular part or pars nonglandularis) is lined by stratified squamous epithelium, whereas the distal portion (pars glandularis) is lined by glandular epithelium. In the horse, the dividing line between the two is called the margo plicatus. The pars nonglandularis in the pig is a small square to rectangular area of stratified squamous epithelium surrounding the esophageal entrance to the stomach.

DEFENSE MECHANISMS

The gastric mucosal barrier is of significant importance in preventing autodigestion and bacterial overgrowth. There is, however, a resident flora that is difficult to grow on artificial media. Microorganismal overgrowth is prevented under normal physiologic conditions by abomasal or gastric motility, prostaglandin E_2, a protective layer of mucus and bicarbonate, secretory immunoglobulin A (IgA), transforming growth factor-α, epidermal growth factor, an extremely acid luminal pH, and an effective pyloric sphincter that prevents regurgitation into the stomach or abomasum of duodenal, hepatic, and pancreatic secretions. An intact epithelial layer and adequate blood flow also prevent acid-induced damage.

GASTRIC DILATION AND VOLVULUS

Simple gastric dilation occurs in a variety of animals and in human beings (Fig. 7-64). In dogs, particularly in the large, deep-chested breeds, the acute gastric

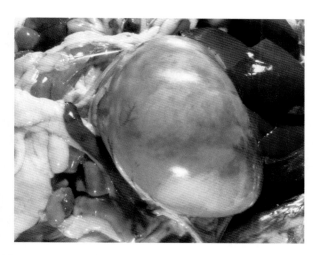

Fig. 7-64   **Simple gastric dilation, stomach, rabbit.** The stomach is markedly dilated and filled with gas, occurs most commonly following aerophagia or overeating, and is relieved by eructation or vomiting. *(Courtesy Dr. H. Gelberg, College of Veterinary Medicine, Oregon State University.)*

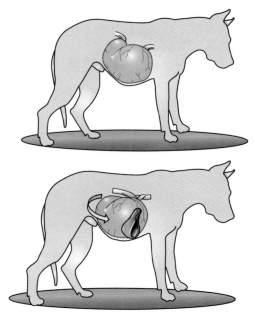

Fig. 7-65   **Schematic illustration, gastric dilation and volvulus, stomach, dog.** The stomach is distended with food and gas (*top example*). It rotates (*arrow*) on the mesenteric axis (*bottom example*) clockwise (180, 270, or 360 degrees on a ventrodorsal axis when the abdomen is viewed from the ventral surface), resulting in a gastric volvulus with an obstructed esophagus that prevents eructation and thus further contributes to gastric dilation. The spleen, attached to the stomach by the gastrosplenic ligament, rotates with the stomach and is thus folded back upon itself and located in the right cranial abdomen against the diaphragm (*bottom example*). The splenic vein is compressed, resulting in a congested spleen, because the arterial blood supply remains patent longer than venous drainage. *(Modified from Van Kruiningen HJ, Gregoire K, Meuten DJ: J Am Anim Hosp Assoc 10:294-324, 1974.)*

dilation and volvulus syndrome occurs. This lesion is life threatening and should not be confused with simple gastric dilation that is common in young puppies after overeating. Predisposing factors to acute gastric dilation include a source of distending gas, fluid, or feed, obstruction of the cardia that prevents eructation, and emesis and obstruction of the pylorus that prevents passage of gastric contents into the small intestine. The source of gas is not well understood. Theories include gas production by *Clostridium perfringens*, spores of which are present in the feed, CO_2 from physiologic mechanisms of digestion, or simple aerophagia.

The result of repeated episodes of gastric dilation is stretching and relaxation of the gastrohepatic ligament. Recurrent dilation combined with overfeeding, postprandial exercise, and perhaps a hereditary predisposition results in gastric rotation. Gastric rotation is recognized by splenic displacement and a twisted esophagus and results in vascular compression and decreased venous drainage and hypoxemia (Figs. 7-65 and 7-66). The stomach generally is rotated clockwise on the ventrodorsal axis when the abdomen is viewed from the ventral surface. Rotation is 180 to 360 degrees. The combination of gastric hypoxemia, acid-base imbalance, obstruction of the pylorus and cardia, and increased intragastric pressure leads to antiperistaltic waves followed by atony, cardiovascular ischemia, arrhythmias, and shock. Decreased portal venous return leads to pancreatic ischemia and release of myocardial depressant factor, cardiac collapse, and death.

Epidemiologic evidence suggests that dry dog foods that list oils or fats among the first four ingredients increase the risk of gastric dilation and volvulus syndrome. Gastric dilation and volvulus is sometimes associated with gastric eversion or intussusception into the distal esophagus. This latter condition can also occur independently of gastric dilation and volvulus.

ABOMASAL DISPLACEMENT

Normally the abomasum lies over the xiphoid process at the abdominal ventral midline. Abomasal displacement is usually to the left side, although right-sided displacements also occur (Fig. 7-67). Left-sided displacement of the abomasum is a generally nonfatal entity of high-producing dairy cattle during the 6 weeks following parturition. Strenuous activity can predispose nonpregnant cows to displacement. In the post-calving period, abomasal atony can occur as a result of heavy grain feeding (volatile fatty acids decrease motility) and hypocalcemia. Meanwhile, the gravid uterus may have displaced the rumen and abomasum cranially

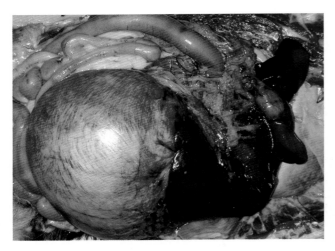

Fig. 7-66   Gastric dilation and volvulus, abdomen, dog.
The stomach is filled with gas and its serosa is congested.
The duodenum and engorged spleen have been displaced to
the right. *(Courtesy Dr. A. Paulman, College of Veterinary Medicine, University of Illinois.)*

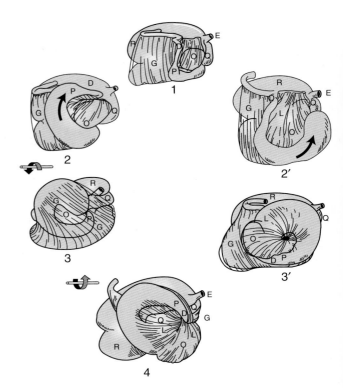

**Fig. 7-67   Schematic diagrams illustrating two possible
modes of rotation of the omasum, abomasum, and cranial
part of the duodenum in volvulus.** *1,* Normal relations; *2,*
simple dilation and displacement on the right; *3,* 180-degree
volvulus around the longitudinal axis of the lesser omentum,
counterclockwise as seen from the rear; *2′,* 90-degree rotation
of the abomasum in a sagittal plane, counterclockwise as seen
from the right; *3′,* 180-degree rotation of the abomasum and
omasum around the transverse axis of the lesser omentum,
drawing the duodenum cranially, medial to the omasum;
4, 360-degree counterclockwise volvulus, final stage resulting
from either mode of rotation. *D,* Duodenum; *E,* esophagus;
G, greater omentum; *L,* lesser omentum; *O,* omasum;
P, pylorus; *Q,* reticulum; *R,* rumen. *(Modified from Habel RE,
Smith DF: J Am Vet Med Assoc 179:447-455, 1981.)*

and to the left, rupturing the attachment of the greater
omentum to the abomasum. The abomasum then occupies the cranial left quadrant of the abdomen and dis-
places the rumen medially. This change leads to partial
obstruction of abomasal outflow. Metabolic acidosis
contributes to rumen atony and impaired movement of
ingesta. The associated hypochloremia is a result of HCl
secretion and is common along with hypokalemia.
Abomasal ulcers and peritoneal adhesions can result in
chronic displacement.

Fifteen percent of abomasal displacements are right
sided. The abomasum can be overdistended, displaced
dorsally, and rotated on its mesenteric axis. Twenty percent of such cases lead to abomasal volvulus. Right-
sided displacements occur in postparturient dairy
cows and in calves.

Clinical features of displaced abomasums, whether
right sided or left sided, include anorexia, cachexia,
dehydration, lack of feces, ketonuria, and a characteristic high-pitched ping subsequent to percussion, over
the abomasum. Idiopathic abomasal volvulus occurs
occasionally in ruminants and calves (Fig. 7-68).

GASTRIC DILATION AND RUPTURE

Gastric dilation occurs in horses as a result of the
ingestion of fermentable feeds or grain, a situation analogous to grain overload with lactic acidosis in cattle.
Acute gastric dilation and rupture in equids occurs most
frequently as a terminal event in intestinal obstruction
and displacement. Because gastric dilation and rupture
can occur after death, the diagnostic challenge is to

determine if the rupture occurred antemortem or
postmortem. The only reliable indicator of the time of
rupture, in relation to the death of the animal, is the
presence of hemorrhage and evidence of inflammation, such as fibrin strands, along the margins of the
rupture (usually the greater curvature), because such
inflammatory responses occur only in live animals
(Figs. 7-69 and 7-70).

In Northern Europe, acute gastric dilation occurs in
horses on pasture as part of the syndrome called grass
sickness or dysautonomia. The esophagus and stomach
are often dilated and atonic. Although serologic evidence suggests an association of grass sickness with
Clostridium perfringens type A enterotoxin, noninflammatory degeneration of associated autonomic ganglia

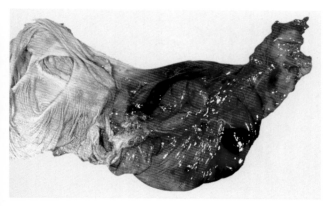

Fig. 7-68 **Volvulus, abomasum, calf.** The volvulus took place at the omasal-abomasal junction, compromising the abomasum's venous return and resulting in severe passive congestion of the abomasal mucosa. *(Courtesy Dr. J. King, College of Veterinary Medicine, Cornell University.)*

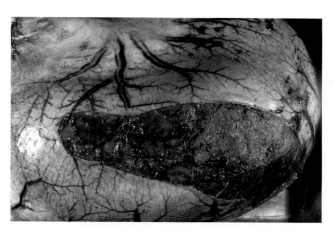

Fig. 7-70 **Rupture, stomach, horse.** The hemorrhage visible on the right margin of the rupture indicates that the rupture occurred antemortem. Note also that the rent through the tunica muscularis is longer than that through the mucosa, which still covers the ingesta on the left and right sides. The mucosal and serosal surfaces are congested. *(Courtesy Dr. H. Gelberg, College of Veterinary Medicine, Oregon State University.)*

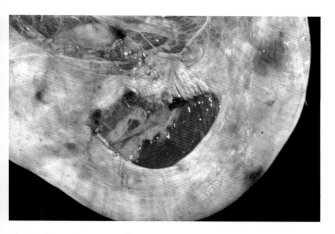

Fig. 7-69 **Rupture, abomasum, calf.** Multifocal hemorrhages along the upper margin of the tear and subserosally adjacent to the greater curvature indicate that the rupture occurred antemortem. *(Courtesy Dr. M.D. McGavin, College of Veterinary Medicine, University of Tennessee.)*

have also been described. This condition can be experimentally produced in the horse with whole blood from affected animals, suggesting that a soluble toxin may be causative.

Chronic gastric dilation is also associated with ingestion of poorly digestible substances. The habits of cribbing and aerophagia may also be contributory.

Dysautonomia also occurs in pet carnivores secondary to ganglionic death in cranial nerves, spinal nerves, and autonomic nerves. Associated ganglionic peptides are reduced in an amount consistent with the functional aberrations. Ganglioneuritis creates a similar syndrome to dysautonomia in a variety of species and is

infrequently diagnosed. Gastrointestinal signs of dysautonomia include xerostomia, decreased anal tone, vomiting, and regurgitation.

Chronic abomasal and/or rumen dilation may occur in cows with overeating disease, dystocia, exhaustion, poor-quality or frozen feedstuffs, abomasal ulcers with or without abomasal lymphoma, and vagal indigestion. A sequela of abomasitis may be a mycotic infection similar to that which occurs in the rumen (Fig. 7-71).

In monkeys, an increased frequency of acute gastric dilation often occurs during weekends, when there may be changes in feeding behavior secondary to nonfamiliar keepers. Studies have implicated *Clostridium perfringens* overgrowth secondary to an increase in fermentable feed consumption in the pathogenesis of gastric dilation in primates.

Chronic gastric dilation in canids is usually secondary to gastric ulcer, mural gastric lymphomas, uremia affecting gastric structure and function, pyloric stenosis or obstruction, acute gastric dilation, intervertebral disc disease, or vagotomy. Chronic gastric dilation is characterized by reduced feed intake, diminished gastric motility, and increased gastric gas accumulation sometimes resulting in abdominal distention similar to that of bloat.

IMPACTION

Impaction of the monogastric stomach and abomasum has a variety of causes. Lesions of the thorax such as pneumonia, pleuritis, lymphadenopathy, and lymphosarcoma can infiltrate and damage the vagal nerves. Roughage, hairballs, and other foreign materials also cause impaction. Gastric trichobezoars and phytobezoars

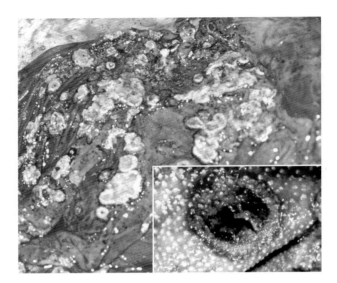

Fig. 7-71 **Mycotic abomasitis and omasitis, calf.** The mucosal surface of the abomasum has discrete and coalescing ulcers covered by yellow-white diphtheritic membranes and a red outer margin of active hyperemia and inflammation. These lesions are indicative of infarcts and are likely secondary to vasculitis and thrombosis by angioinvasive fungi such as *Aspergillus, Mucor, Rhizopus, Absidia,* and *Mortierella* spp. The diphtheritic membranes are a mixture of necrotic cellular debris from the infarct, inflammatory cells, and hyphae from the inciting fungus. *Inset:* Mycotic omasitis. The lesion is similar to the one in the abomasum. The diphtheritic membrane has been lost due to omasal peristalsis, but the necrotic center (infarct) and red outer margin of active hyperemia and inflammation are prominent. *(Figure, Courtesy College of Veterinary Medicine, University of Illinois. Inset, Courtesy Dr. H. Gelberg, College of Veterinary Medicine, Oregon State University.)*

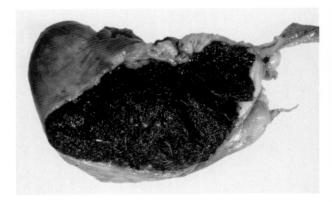

Fig. 7-72 **Trichobezoar, stomach, rabbit.** The stomach is impacted with ingested hair. *(Courtesy Dr. H. Gelberg, College of Veterinary Medicine, Oregon State University.)*

of monogastric animals are similar to those that occur in the rumen (Fig. 7-72).

Abomasal emptying defect is principally a condition of Suffolk sheep 2 to 6 years of age. It is characterized by an impacted, dilated abomasum. Clinical signs include anorexia, weight loss, and increased ruminal chloride levels. The latter feature is believed to be secondary to abomasal reflux. Scattered chromatolysis and neuronal necrosis in the celiac and mesenteric ganglia are consistent with neurotoxicosis. The process is likely mediated by excitotoxins, although viruses have not been ruled out. Clusters of affected animals in a single flock are suggestive of an environmental causality. Inflammation is minimal. Abomasal emptying defect may be a form of acquired dysautonomia.

INFLAMMATORY DISEASES

Inflammation of the simple stomach or abomasum, gastritis and abomasitis, respectively, must be distinguished from simple hyperemia and petechiae, which are often nonspecific agonal lesions. Gastritis is often associated clinically with vomiting, dehydration, and metabolic acidosis. Hemorrhage, edema, increased amounts of mucus, abscesses, granulomas, foreign body penetration, parasites, inflammatory cells of various types, erosions, ulcerations, and necrosis characterize the changes in the mucosal surface and subsequent inflammatory reaction.

Clostridium septicum is a cause of hemorrhagic abomasitis with submucosal emphysema of sheep and cattle, a disease known as braxy. Although this disease is most common in the United Kingdom and Europe, it occurs in North America as well. Generally the disease follows ingestion of frozen feeds contaminated with the causative *Clostridium* spp. The lesions are produced by the exotoxin of the bacteria, and death therefore is due to an exotoxemia.

Sarcina-like organisms have been reported in association with abomasal bloat in several calves. Sarcinas are anaerobic, gram-positive, nonmotile cocci found in rafts or pockets. They are suspected gastric pathogens in a variety of animal species. The lesions are similar to braxy.

In many septicemias of pigs, bacterial emboli lodge in the vessels of the gastric submucosa and cause thrombosis resulting in hyperemia, hemorrhage, infarction, and ulceration. This occurs in salmonellosis, swine dysentery, Glasser's disease, and colibacillosis. Certain intoxicants such as vomitoxin produced by *Fusarium* spp. can cause similar lesions (Fig. 7-73).

A deep mycosis that causes a granulomatous gastritis is due to *Histoplasma capsulatum* (see Intestinal Diseases of Carnivores). Very rarely, *Mycobacterium tuberculosis* causes granulomatous gastritis in a variety of species. In granulomatous gastritis there is epigastric discomfort after eating (postprandial), emesis, progressive cachexia, weakness, vomiting of blood (hematemesis), and pyloric obstruction due to the space-occupying

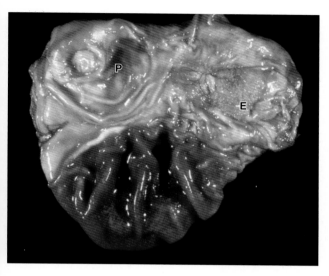

Fig. 7-73 **Acute "hemorrhagic gastritis," stomach, pig.** The fundus of the stomach is hemorrhagic. This type of gastric change is often seen in the pig in acute septicemia, for example, from salmonella, and the severe congestion is attributed to venous infarction from endotoxemia. *E*, Esophageal os; *P*, pylorus. *(Courtesy Dr. H. Gelberg, College of Veterinary Medicine, Oregon State University.)*

inflammatory reaction. In both histoplasmosis and tuberculosis, regional (gastric, splenic, and hepatic) lymph nodes may be affected. Nodular or diffusely thickened gastric and lymphoid lesions contain predominately macrophages. Mononuclear inflammatory cells, fibroblasts, granulocytes (including eosinophils), and multinucleate giant cells are also present. Often the causative organisms can be demonstrated within the granulomatous inflammation, but special stains such as acid-fast for mycobacteria and periodic acid–Schiff (PAS) reaction or Gomori's methenamine silver stain may be necessary to demonstrate fungi.

Eosinophilic gastritis is uncommon in all species of domestic animals, but has been reported in pet carnivores and humans. The etiologic basis for this condition is in general poorly understood. There are three types of gastritis characterized by an influx of eosinophils.

A characteristic focal eosinophilic infiltrate is sometimes associated with trapped nematode larvae, especially *Toxocara canis*. Larvae of *Toxocara canis* pass to puppies through nursing, through fecal soiling of bedding, or from dirt or other fomites harboring eggs or larvae. It is the parasite's larval sheath, feces, and saliva that are antigenic. In dogs and cats, tissue reaction to these larvae results in epithelial cell hyperplasia, resulting in a polyplike proliferation of the antral mucosa. Pyloric obstruction sometimes results.

In other cases of eosinophilic gastritis, the infiltration of eosinophils is more diffuse and is believed to be a hypersensitivity reaction. The offending antigen is not known. In many of these cases, there is a peripheral eosinophilia, especially when associated with eosinophilic infiltration of the small intestine (eosinophilic gastroenteritis). This form of eosinophilic gastritis may become transmural, with necrosis and scarring.

The third type, scirrhous eosinophilic gastritis of dogs and cats, for the most part has unknown causes. The fibrosis associated with scirrhous changes in the stomach and lymph nodes result in persistent emesis, weight loss, and malnutrition.

The gross lesions of eosinophilic gastritis are rather nonspecific and consist of diffuse or nodular mural thickenings. Microscopic lesions are characterized by infiltrates of eosinophils in the mucosa and the submucosa and are seen extensively through the muscle layers of the stomach and sometimes in segments of the small intestine and colon. In the dog, there is sometimes necroproliferative eosinophilic perivasculitis and eosinophilic lymphadenopathy. In the scirrhous form, the eosinophilic infiltrate is followed by transmural fibroplasia and scarring.

HYPERTROPHIC OR HYPERPLASTIC DISEASES

Hypertrophic gastritis, characterized by thickened rugae, is the result of hyperplasia of the gastric glands. This effect is believed to be a response to chronic retention of gastric fluid and reflux of intestinal bile. Similar mucosal glandular changes are seen in immune-mediated lymphoplasmacytic gastritis of dogs. Hypertrophic gastritis has also been described in primates, horses, pigs, and rodents. The nematode *Nochtia nocti* causes this lesion in the stomachs of monkeys. Equine hypertrophic gastritis is a focal or more diffuse lesion associated with the nematodes *Habronema* spp. and *Trichostrongylus axei*, respectively.

Chronic giant hypertrophic gastropathy of dogs affects the basenji, beagle, boxer, and bull terrier breeds, among others. The disease is similar to Ménétrier's disease in human beings. Clinical signs include weight loss, diarrhea, vomiting, and hypoproteinemia. The chronic gastritis results in increased mucosal permeability to serum proteins with subsequent protein-losing gastropathy. Unlike normal gastric mucosal folds, in giant hypertrophic gastropathy the mucosa does not flatten with distention of the organ (Fig. 7-74). Microscopically the mucosa is hypertrophic and hyperplastic. The incorporation of folds of submucosa and muscularis mucosa is variable, as is the presence of inflammatory cells. The cause of this condition is unknown.

ULCERS AND EROSIONS

An ulcer is a mucosal defect in which the entire epithelial thickness, down to or through the basement membrane, has been lost. Penetration through the

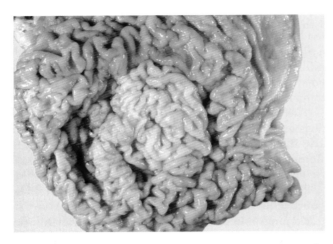

Fig. 7-74   Chronic giant hypertrophic gastropathy, stomach, dog. A cerebriform mass of redundant mucosa is present in the center of the gastric mucosa. Chronic inflammation in the mass results in increased mucosal permeability to serum proteins and a subsequent protein-losing gastropathy. *(Courtesy College of Veterinary Medicine, Cornell University.)*

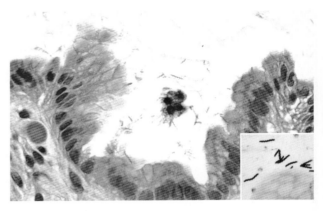

Fig. 7-75   *Helicobacter* spp. infection, stomach, cat. Numerous spiral bacteria are present in the superficial mucous layer. There is no inflammation in the adjacent mucosa; however, in some areas the epithelium is hyperplastic. H&E stain. *Inset:* The helical shape of the *Helicobacter* organisms is demonstrated with a Steiner's silver stain. *(**Figure,** Courtesy Dr. H. Gelberg, College of Veterinary Medicine, Oregon State University. **Inset,** Courtesy Dr. C.S. Patton, College of Veterinary Medicine, University of Tennessee.)*

remaining tissue layers to the peritoneal cavity is termed a perforating ulcer. Partial-thickness epithelial loss is termed an erosion. Chronic ulcers differ from acute ulcers by the presence of an indurated rim caused by fibrosis and attempts at epithelial regeneration. The identification of gastric ulcers is not challenging, both at necropsy and by endoscopy. They are sharply bordered cavities often coated with exudate. Thrombosis of blood vessels is sometimes associated with some ulcers in ruminants with mycotic vasculitis secondary to lactic acidosis. Thus, it is an infarct. The pathogenesis of most gastric and duodenal ulcers in human beings has been demonstrated to be a result of a helical bacterium. Although similar gastric *Helicobacter*-like organisms (GHLOs) are readily demonstrated in dogs and cats, their association with ulcer formation is not established. It appears that as many animals without gastritis or ulcers are as heavily colonized by these bacteria as are those animals with ulcers (Fig. 7-75). More than 90% of cats are infected with *Helicobacter* spp. *Helicobacter felis* can be cultured in vitro, but the noncultivatable *Helicobacter heilmannii* is present most often. Pathologic and clinical outcomes depend on a number of bacterial virulence factors as well as on the host response to these agents. Investigations suggest there may be a link to *Helicobacter* presence and other disease entities, including coronary and neurologic disease.

Theories abound as to the causes of most gastric ulcers in animals. None have been proven. There may be a heritable component to ulcer susceptibility.

The conditions necessary for ulcer development boil down to an imbalance between acid secretion and mucosal protection. This imbalance occurs as a result of the following:

- Local disturbances or trauma to the mucosal epithelial barrier; this injury can be due to back flush of bile salts from the duodenum or ingestion of lipid solvents, such as alcohol.
- Normal or high gastric acidity
- Local disturbances in blood flow (stress-induced and sympathetic nervous system–mediated arteriovenous shunts) resulting in ischemia
- Steroids and nonsteroidal antiinflammatory drugs (NSAIDs) that depress prostaglandin formation (PGE_2, PGI_1) or concentration, thus decreasing phospholipid secretions, which are protective

All of the above mechanisms allow pepsin and hydrochloric acid into the submucosa.

Severe gastric hyperacidity and gastric ulcers is sometimes associated with islet cell tumors producing gastrin. Some of these gastrin-producing tumors arise in the duodenum, but the majority are endocrine or pancreatic in origin. These neoplasms release histamine into the blood stream, which binds to receptors on parietal cells of the stomach, increasing HCl secretion. The gastric ulceration produced associated with these tumors is known as Zollinger-Ellison syndrome.

In dogs, gastric ulceration causes vomiting, inappetence, abdominal pain, and anemia secondary to gastric bleeding (Fig. 7-76). Melena may also occur if the ulceration persists, and significant amounts of blood are lost

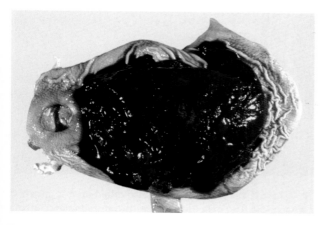

Fig. 7-76   **Ulcer, stomach, dog.** The stomach contains a large volume of clotted and unclotted blood from a gastric ulcer (idiopathic). The hemorrhage was so severe that the dog died from exsanguination. *(Courtesy Dr. H. Gelberg, College of Veterinary Medicine, Oregon State University.)*

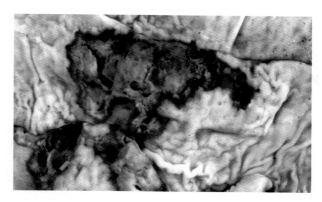

Fig. 7-78   **Ulcers, abomasum, cow.** The ulcers consist of a central area of necrosis surrounded by an outer red margin characteristic of active hyperemia and inflammation. The discrete rounded outline of these ulcers suggests that they are infarcts, possibly from vasculitis and thrombosis caused by angioinvasive fungi. *(Courtesy Dr. H. Gelberg, College of Veterinary Medicine, Oregon State University.)*

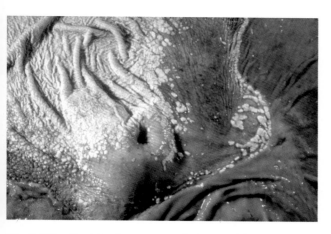

Fig. 7-77   **Gastric ulcers, stomach, horse.** Administration of nonsteroidal antiinflammatory drugs (NSAIDs) has caused extensive ulceration of the stratified squamous epithelium of the nonglandular mucosa. The ulceration extends from the cardia (*center*) to the margo plicatus (*right*). *(Courtesy College of Veterinary Medicine, Cornell University.)*

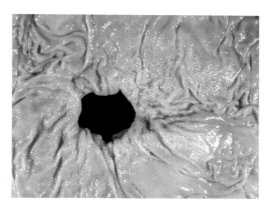

Fig. 7-79   **Perforating ulcer, abomasum, cow.** The rounded borders of the ulcer indicate an attempt at repair and therefore chronicity. Death was due to peritonitis. *(Courtesy Dr. H. Gelberg, College of Veterinary Medicine, Oregon State University.)*

to the gastrointestinal system. Gastric ulcers in dogs and cats are generally idiopathic but can occur in these animals with mast cell or other tumors.

Ulcers are idiopathic in foals. Foals with gastric ulcers may have abdominal pain, bruxism (grinding of the teeth), ptyalism, and gastric reflux and may lie in dorsal recumbency. Gastric ulcers associated with administration of NSAIDs are common in horses but are also described in other species given these drugs (Fig. 7-77). Equine gastric ulcer syndrome occurs in 40% to 90% of competitive and performance horses, with the most severe ulcers occurring in those animals that are worked

the hardest. More than a third of horses used less strenuously develop mild ulcers.

Cattle with abomasal ulcers have partial or complete anorexia, decreased milk production, palpable discomfort to pressure applied to the right xiphoid area, and melena. In any species, the vomiting of coffee grounds–like material (hematemesis) or melena is highly suggestive of gastric ulcer disease. Abomasal ulcers of ruminants vary from subclinical to fatal (Figs. 7-78 and 7-79). In calves, ulcers are associated with dietary changes or mechanical irritation of the abomasum by roughage. Dietary changes involve substitution of roughage for milk or milk replacer, together with the associated stress. In dairy cattle, ulcers are associated with heavy

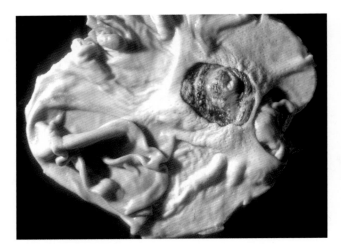

Fig. 7-80   Gastric ulcer (pars esophagea), stomach, pig.
This type of gastric ulcer occurs exclusively in pigs and most commonly in confined growing pigs. The lesion is limited to the stratified squamous epithelium surrounding the cardia (pars esophagea). Ulcers in this location characteristically have a multifactorial cause, including the ingestion of finely ground grain or pelleted feed (possibly deficient in vitamin E), fermentation of sugars in the feed, and stress of confinement rearing. These ulcers frequently bleed and can cause exsanguination.
(Courtesy Dr. M.D. McGavin, College of Veterinary Medicine, University of Tennessee.)

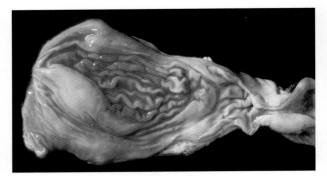

Fig. 7-81   Uremic gastropathy (also called uremic gastritis), stomach, cat. The major lesion here is congestion and edema of the gastric mucosa caused by injury to capillaries within the lamina propria associated with elevated concentrations of nitrogen-derived metabolic waste products in the systemic circulation from kidney failure. With chronicity, there is calcification of the gastric mucosa, visible as fine white stippling and lines in the mucosa (not shown here). *(Courtesy Dr. C.S. Patton, College of Veterinary Medicine, University of Tennessee.)*

grain feeding (lactic acidosis) at the time of parturition, displacement of the abomasum, BVD, impaction, torsion, and gastric lymphosarcoma.

In pigs, gastric ulcers are common and occur in penned pigs fed finely ground grain. These ulcers always are limited to the stratified squamous epithelium of the esophageal portion of the gastric mucosa that surrounds the cardia (Fig. 7-80). Death can result from exsanguination into the gastric lumen. Evidence suggests that a high-carbohydrate diet is not sufficient alone to produce erosions and ulcers, but rather that the appropriate diet in combination with fermentative commensal bacteria, such as *Lactobacillus* and *Bacillus* spp., produce lesions.

MISCELLANEOUS DISEASES AND CONDITIONS

Uremic gastritis occurs most frequently in carnivores as a result of chronic renal disease (Fig. 7-81). In ungulates, it is a rare event and is usually secondary to obstructive kidney disease (postrenal uremia). Uremic gastritis is characterized by mineralization of the glands, vessels, and interstitium of the gastric mucosa and sometimes results in ulcer formation.

Amyloidosis occasionally is present in the stomach in association with systemic amyloid infiltrates. Generalized AA amyloidosis with gastric deposits of amyloid has been reported in bats, Siamese and Abyssinian cats, goats, rhesus monkeys, sheep, and Siberian tigers.

Pyloric stenosis can be due to an anatomic problem or an inability of the pyloric sphincter to function properly. This condition may be congenital or acquired. This lesion occurs most often in dogs (particularly brachycephalic breeds), Siamese cats, horses, and human beings. Congenital pyloric stenoses may be hereditary, at least in human beings. Pyloric stenosis is often first recognized in recently weaned animals by projectile vomiting, retention of gastric contents, gastromegaly, and the presence of strong peristaltic waves (Fig. 7-82).

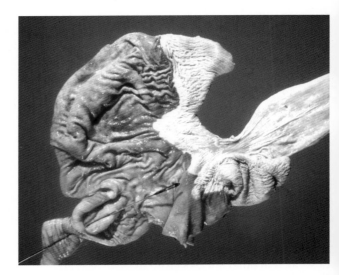

Fig. 7-82   Pyloric stenosis, stomach, horse. The probe passes through the narrowed pyloric canal. *(Courtesy Dr. H. Gelberg, College of Veterinary Medicine, Oregon State University.)*

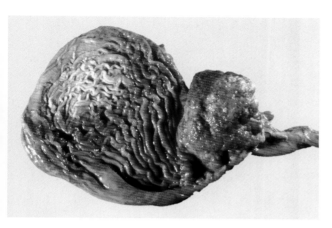

Fig. 7-83 **Giant hypertrophic pyloric gastropathy, stomach, dog.** The mass of hyperplastic glandular tissue at the pylorus could be mistaken for a neoplasm. *(Courtesy Dr. H. Gelberg, College of Veterinary Medicine, Oregon State University.)*

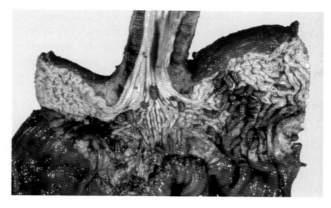

Fig. 7-84 **Gasterophiliasis, stomach, horse.** Fly larvae (bots) of *Gasterophilus intestinalis* are attached to the epithelium of the nonglandular portion of the stomach. Note the muscular hypertrophy of the distal esophagus. Although not shown in this illustration, *Gasterophilus nasalis*, another similar equine gastric parasite, attaches to the epithelium of the glandular portion of the stomach. *(Courtesy Dr. H. Gelberg, College of Veterinary Medicine, Oregon State University.)*

Pyloric muscular hypertrophy, variable submucosal edema, vascular ectasia, and degeneration of myenteric ganglion cells may be identified histologically. Functional pyloric stenosis can be a feature of vagus indigestion of ruminants. In general, the cause of pyloric stenosis is not well understood.

Giant hypertrophic pyloric gastropathy, not to be confused with giant hypertrophic gastropathy of basenjis and other dogs, is a lesion seen most often in older small breed dogs. To the uninitiated, the gross and microscopic features of this pyloric lesion strongly imitate carcinoma (Fig. 7-83). Microscopically, there is notable foveolar and glandular hyperplasia with variable hypertrophy of smooth muscle, small mucosal erosions, and ulcerations. There is usually a lymphoplasmacytic infiltrate of variable degree. The cause of this condition is unknown.

PARASITES
HORSES

Many parasites cause disease of the stomach, especially in ungulates. Modern anthelmintics have made these diseases relatively easy to prevent and control both in individual animals and in herds.

Equine bots, *Gasterophilus intestinalis* and *Gasterophilus nasalis*, are commonly seen in animals on inadequate deworming regimens (Fig. 7-84). *Gasterophilus intestinalis* colonizes the stratified portion of the stomach. The adult fly lays eggs on the hairs of the distal limbs of the horse. *Gasterophilus nasalis* lays its eggs around the nose of the horse. The larvae hatch after being moistened and warmed by licking. They are swallowed and live in the duodenum. Both species attach to the mucosa via their anterior pincers. The larvae pass in the feces, pupate, and develop into flies.

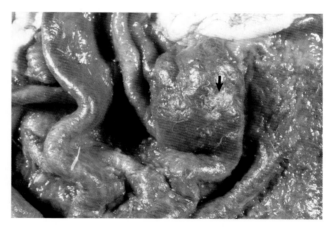

Fig. 7-85 **Focal granulomatous gastritis, *Draschia* brood pouch, stomach, horse.** A large parasitic brood pouch is present in the glandular mucosa adjacent to the margo plicatus *(right center of illustration)*. Nematodes have been squeezed from the pouch and are visible on the surface *(arrow)*. Histologically, the mucosa is expanded by focal granulomatous inflammation containing clusters of adult *Draschia megastoma*. *(Courtesy Dr. H. Gelberg, College of Veterinary Medicine, Oregon State University.)*

Draschia megastoma is found in brood pouches in the glandular mucosa adjacent to the margo plicatus (Fig. 7-85). Infection is sometimes referred to as habronemiasis, based on antiquated taxonomic nomenclature in which the nematodes were classified as *Habronema* spp. Eggs produced in the cysts are extruded through a pore in the brood pouch to the gastric lumen. The eggs pass out with the feces and are consumed by fly larvae that are intermediate hosts. Both *Draschia* spp. and *Gasterophilus* spp. can cause gastric ulcers. Considering their location and means of survival in the stomach, it is remarkable that they do not cause serious damage more often.

RUMINANTS

Haemonchus contortus, the barber pole worm, is relatively common in ruminant abomasums. The common name of this parasite is related to the macroscopically visible entwining of the blood-filled intestine and white uterus in the female worm (Fig. 7-86). Hyperinfested pastures containing numerous third-stage larvae are the source of infection. Lambs are particularly at risk. Larvae on grasses are ingested by the host and enter the abomasum, where they may lie dormant within the gastric glands. After development to adults they enter the abomasal surface. Eggs pass in the feces, completing the life cycle. *Haemonchus* are blood feeders and can cause severe anemia, hypoproteinemia, and resultant edema. This edema is characteristically present in the intermandibular space resulting in a physical resemblance to a bottle ("bottle jaw"). As with any process resulting in anemia and hypoproteinemia, there are pale mucus membranes, stunting, and diarrhea. Diagnosis is by fecal egg counts and, at necropsy, by semiquantification of abomasal parasite load along with the attendant lesions of anemia and hypoproteinemia.

In temperate climates, ostertagiosis is considered the most important parasitic disease in cattle (*Ostertagia ostertagia*) and small ruminants (*Ostertagia circumcincta*). Affected animals are unthrifty. *Ostertagia* spp. have a direct life cycle similar to that of *Haemonchus* spp. The nematodes are smaller than those of *Haemonchus* and are uniformly brown. Third-, fourth-, and fifth-stage larvae reside in the abomasal gastric glands. *Ostertagia* spp. are often present along with *Trichostrongylus* spp. in other gastrointestinal locations. Intercurrent gastrointestinal parasitism with other trichostrongyles has an additive effect on clinical symptomatology. Unthriftiness, lack of proper mentation, diarrhea, hypoproteinemia, and

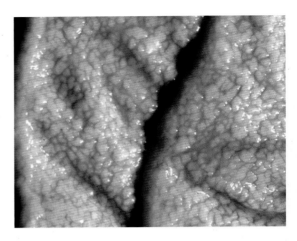

Fig. 7-87   Ostertagiosis, abomasum, cow. The granular Moroccan leather appearance of the abomasal mucosa is characteristic of chronic ostertagiosis and is due to epithelial hyperplasia of the gastric glands, which may also contain *Ostertagia* larvae. *(Courtesy Dr. M.D. McGavin, College of Veterinary Medicine, University of Tennessee.)*

ventral edema may result. The multinodular appearance of the abomasum of heavily infested animals resembles Morocco leather (Fig. 7-87). This cobblestone appearance is due to mucous cell hyperplasia and lymphoid nodules in the abomasal submucosa elevating the overlying epithelium. Differential diagnoses include lymphosarcoma.

Abomasitis produced by *Ostertagia* spp. is characterized by an infiltration of mononuclear inflammatory cells and eosinophils. There are also increased numbers of globule leukocytes, a decrease in the number of parietal and chief cells, and hyperplasia of abomasal mucous cells. *Ostertagia* spp. are visible macroscopically. The nematodes are brown, are smaller than those of *Haemonchus contortus*, and are present within the gastric glands and mucosal nodules formed as a result of the host's response to the parasite's presence.

PIGS

Hyostrongylus rubidus of pigs is a gastric parasite that causes a thickening of the mucosa, with mucus accumulation and submucosal pockets. The parasite is threadlike and red. Clinically, hyostrongylosis is associated with the "thin sow syndrome." Grossly the gastric mucosa is thickened, catarrhal, and somewhat cobblestone. Microscopically, there is mucus metaplasia of parasitized and adjacent gastric glands. Submucosal lymphoid follicles develop in chronic infections.

CARNIVORES (DOGS AND CATS)

Several genera of nematodes, principally *Ollulanus*, *Gnathostoma*, and *Cylicospirura*, rarely cause gastritis in dogs and cats.

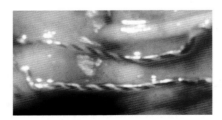

Fig. 7-86   *Haemonchus contortus*, abomasum, sheep. The white spiral reproductive tract wrapped around the blood filled intestine is responsible for the striped appearance, hence the common name "barber's pole worm." *(Courtesy Dr. H. Gelberg, College of Veterinary Medicine, Oregon State University.)*

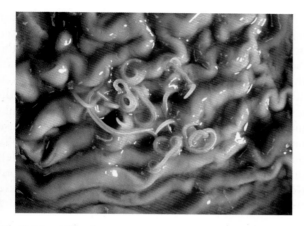

Fig. 7-88   **Physalopteriasis, stomach, dog.** Stout coiled nematodes, *Physaloptera canis* are firmly attached to the gastric mucosa by dentate pseudolabia. *(Courtesy Dr. M.D. McGavin, College of Veterinary Medicine, University of Tennessee.)*

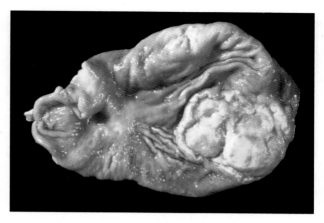

Fig. 7-90   **Lymphoma (lymphosarcoma), stomach, cat.** A large expansile mass is present in the submucosa of the stomach *(top edge)* and is covered by an intact mucosal epithelium. Note the other lymphomatous mass, which is ulcerated *(lower right)*. This latter lesion is somewhat atypical of this disease, because ulceration is uncommon and occurs in late-stage disease when the mass is quite large and protrudes into the gastric lumen. In most cases of gastric lymphoma, the mucosal epithelium is intact and not ulcerated. *(Courtesy Dr. C.S. Patton, College of Veterinary Medicine, University of Tennessee.)*

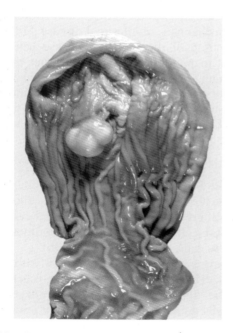

Fig. 7-89   **Leiomyoma, stomach, dog.** This tumor arose from smooth muscle in the tunica muscularis and is covered by intact mucosa. *(Courtesy Dr. H. Gelberg, College of Veterinary Medicine, Oregon State University.)*

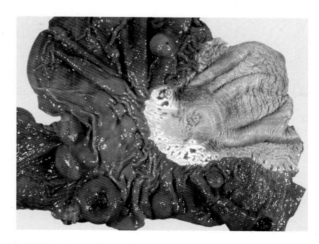

Fig. 7-91   **Lymphoma (lymphosarcoma), stomach, horse.** Large smooth-surfaced submucosal nodules, two of which have a central hemorrhagic ulcer, are present in the glandular portion of the stomach. Ulcers in the stratified squamous portion of the stomach are sites of *Gastrophilus intestinalis* attachment. *(Courtesy Dr. H. Gelberg, College of Veterinary Medicine, Oregon State University.)*

Physaloptera spp. are often thought of as gastric parasites of carnivores because they are sometimes found in the stomach on endoscopic examination or at necropsy. They are occasionally responsible for vomiting. They appear similar to ascarids but generally attach by anterior hooks to the proximal duodenal mucosa at the gastric valve (Fig. 7-88). Intermediate hosts are coprophagous beetles.

NEOPLASIA

Gastric neoplasia, although uncommon, manifests in different ways in domestic animals. Leiomyoma and more rarely leiomyosarcoma arise from the tunica muscularis (Fig. 7-89). Lymphosarcoma can be primary, metastatic, or multicentric in origin (Figs. 7-90 and 7-91). In cattle, lymphosarcoma is often caused by the bovine leukemia

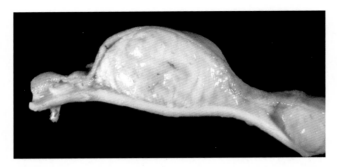

Fig. 7-92   Lymphoma (lymphosarcoma), transverse section of the abomasum, cow. This cross section demonstrates a white, space-occupying submucosal mass. The intact mucosa is located at the top of the specimen. *(Courtesy Dr. H. Gelberg, College of Veterinary Medicine, Oregon State University.)*

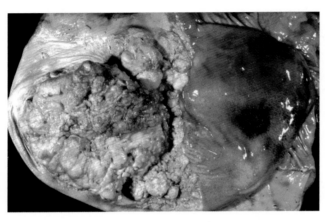

Fig. 7-93   Squamous cell carcinoma, stomach, horse. A large proliferative, ulcerative mass has arisen from the epithelium of the nonglandular (squamous) mucosa of the stomach. *(Courtesy Dr. A. Paulman, College of Veterinary Medicine, University of Illinois.)*

virus and has a predilection for the abomasum and the right atrium and uterus (Fig. 7-92). Squamous cell carcinoma of the stratified squamous (esophageal) portion of the stomach is relatively common in the horse (Fig. 7-93). Glandular neoplasms, adenomas, and adenocarcinomas occur in all species but are seen most often in dogs and cats.

INTESTINE

INTRODUCTION

The intestines might be thought of as a tube within the body cavity that carries material (ingesta) through the body. The overall anatomic and histologic organization of this digestive tube is demonstrated in Fig. 7-94. By the action of enzymes, resident flora, and added secretions, ingesta are broken down, useful substances are absorbed into the body, and waste products are

excreted. To perform these functions, the intestine needs a very large surface area. Creation of this surface area is accomplished by coiling the intestine in the abdomen. Herbivores have longer intestines than carnivores or omnivores and need a fermentation vat, either the rumen or cecum, to digest cellulose. In addition to its length, the intestinal mucosa is thrown into numerous folds that contain villi that notably increase the number of cells contacting the ingesta (Fig. 7-95). Finally, each enterocyte has a microvillous border, further increasing the surface area available for digestive and absorptive processes. Damage to any of these structures can result in intestinal dysfunction and resultant diarrhea.

STRUCTURE AND FUNCTION

The intestinal mucosa is composed of epithelial cells lining the intestinal lumen and mesenchymal cells of the lamina propria and muscularis mucosa. An understanding of these cell types and their functional roles in digestion and absorption is important in understanding the mechanisms of intestinal disease. Similarly, an understanding of the biology of these cell types is important in predicting clinical outcomes and therapeutic strategies for intestinal disease. The structure and function of the intestine and categorization of veterinary pathogens by cell-type tropism was admirably described by Dr. H.W. Moon in both editions of *Cell Pathology*, by Dr. N. Cheville.

EPITHELIAL CELLS

There are six types of epithelial cells lining the intestine. These absorptive epithelial cells are called enterocytes, undifferentiated or crypt epithelial cells, goblet cells, Paneth cells, enterochromaffin (neuroendocrine, argentaffin) cells, and M cells (Fig. 7-96).

Enterocytes are tall and columnar with luminal microvilli. They contain a surface glycocalyx that houses the digestive and absorptive enzymes. The mature cells do not proliferate, but they provide feedback inhibition of mitosis of the crypt cells by chalones. Many nutrients are absorbed through the lateral intercellular spaces between cells. Enterocytes move up the crypt and intestinal villus to the extrusion zone at the villus tip, where effete enterocytes are discarded into the fecal mass. The turnover rate for enterocytes is the most rapid of any fixed-cell population in the body. In neonatal pigs, for instance, the turnover rate is 7 to 10 days. In 3-week-old pigs that have achieved climax flora, that rate accelerates to 2 to 3 days.

Undifferentiated crypt epithelial cells have little or no digestive capability. They are the progenitor cells that replace all of the other epithelial cell types. They have short, sparse microvilli. Crypt cells are considered the source of secretory component that acts as a receptor for IgA and immunoglobulin M (IgM) produced by

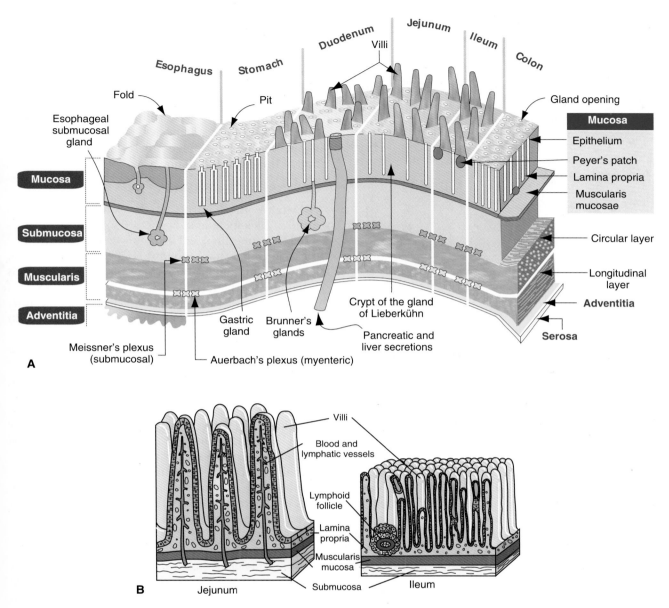

Fig. 7-94   **Schematic diagram of the anatomic and histologic organization of the digestive tube. A,** Entire digestive tube. **B,** Higher magnification of the jejunum and ileum. (**A,** *From Kierzenbaum AL: Histology and cell biology: an introduction to pathology, St Louis, 2002, Mosby.*)

plasmacytes in the intestinal lamina propria. The migration rate of crypt cells up the villus is dependent on several factors, one of which is an adaptation to gut microflora. In germ-free or gnotobiotic animals, the enterocyte replacement rate is similar to that of the neonate. Crypt cells are considered a source of chloride ion secretion into the intestinal lumen.

Goblet cells function in mucus secretion. They occur in both villous and crypt regions. Their numbers tend to increase caudally through the intestine.

Paneth cells are located near the crypt base in some species, notably primates, horses, and rodents. Paneth cells are considered to have both secretory and phagocytic functions. They produce cryptdin and lysins. These substances are toxic to bacteria and probably protect the proliferating crypt cells from infection. Collectively, Paneth cells consist of a cellular mass similar to that of the pancreas. It has been suggested that Paneth cells play a role in elimination of heavy metals because they are selectively damaged by methylmercury.

Enterochromaffin cells, also known as argentaffin cells because of their affinity for silver, are enteroendocrine cells. They occur primarily in the crypts and produce serotonin, catecholamines, gastrin, somatostatin, serotonin, cholecystokinin, secretin, bombesin, enteroglucagon, and likely others. They secrete these

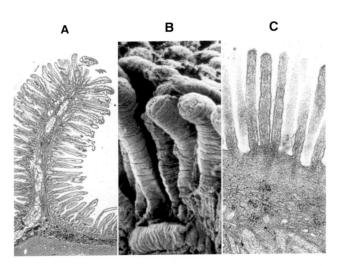

Fig. 7-95 **Organization of the intestine.** The digestive and absorptive surfaces of the intestine are markedly increased by the presence of villi and microvilli on the enterocytes. **A,** Intestinal villus. Villus epithelial cells are present on a basement membrane (not seen) on a core of lamina propria. H&E stain. **B,** Small intestine, intestinal villi, scanning electron microscopy. Carbon sputter coat. **C,** Enterocyte microvilli. TEM. Uranyl acetate and lead citrate stain. (*A, B,* and *C, From Damjanov I, Linder J:* Anderson's pathology, *ed 10, St Louis, 1996, Mosby.*)

products into the tissue rather than the gut lumen and thus are truly endocrine. Occasionally, they form neoplasms called carcinoids.

M cells are so named because they have a microfolded or membranous surface. They form the dome epithelium that covers the gut-associated lymphoid tissue (GALT). They serve important functions in the uptake of antigens from the intestinal lumen and in the transport of these antigens to the GALT. M cells also serve as a portal of entry for some pathogens, including bacteria such as *Salmonella, Yersinia,* and *Rhodococcus* spp. and some viruses, such as BVD virus.

MESENCHYMAL CELLS

Mesenchymal cells reside in the lamina propria. Their numbers increase with exposure to antigen, although there is a resident population of these cells in normal animals. The intestinal lymphoid tissue is 25% of the body's lymphoid mass (Fig. 7-97) and consists of those in the lamina propria and the GALT. This volume is larger than that of the spleen. In spite of the fact that the average person ingests 700 tons of antigens in a lifetime, the gut is adept at not responding to these food antigens. Data are beginning to accumulate identifying the different T-lymphocyte types in the lamina propria.

Neutrophils are transient within the lamina propria of the intestine. Neutrophils are short-lived in the blood and tissues; their normal route of removal from the body is to migrate through the wall of the alimentary tract to the lumen and be digested or excreted from the body via feces.

Eosinophils, when present in the intestinal lamina propria and submucosa, indicate a hypersensitivity reaction, often to food antigens or parasites.

Globule leukocytes are large granular lymphocytes that are interepithelial or within the lamina propria. They are found in all species and occasionally form neoplasms, most notably in the cat. The normal function of these cells is unknown.

DEFENSE MECHANISMS

Defense mechanisms of the intestinal tract are diverse. They include indigenous (nonpathogenic) bacterial flora, intestinal and extraintestinal secretions, gastric acidity, intestinal motility, epithelial cell turnover, bile salts, immunologic mechanisms, and, although a secondary mechanism, the Kupffer cells of the liver.

Secretions of the oral cavity, saliva, and intestine, called mucins, inhibit the adherence of organisms to the mucosa of the alimentary system.

Normal gastric acidity kills many organisms before they have the chance to interact with enterocytes. Very young animals are achlorhydric; thus they may be more susceptible to some organisms, such as pathogenic *Escherichia coli.*

Helical bacteria in the stomach are the single greatest cause of gastric ulcers in human beings. Although similar organisms occur in the stomachs of domestic animals, particularly carnivores, their role in gastritis of animals is less certain. Normal gastric acidity apparently does not kill all potentially pathogenic bacteria (helical bacteria) in the stomach and proximal small intestine of domestic animals.

Indigenous (nonpathogenic) bacterial flora competitively bind to putative attachment sites on the enterocytes thus preempting pathogen attachment. They also compete for substrate with pathogens and alter the microenvironmental pH, making competitive growth difficult. In addition, they produce inhibitory growth substances that are toxic to other bacteria called bacteriocins. Colicins are bacteriocins produced by *Escherichia coli.*

Intestinal peristalsis is protective in that loss of motility may lead to bacterial overgrowth in the intestine and increased susceptibility to toxins that are not moved out of the gut. Diarrhea can be in part a defense mechanism that rids the body of bacteria and toxins.

Epithelial cells of the intestine have the greatest turnover rate of any cell population in the body. In effect this means that pathogens with a life cycle that exceeds that of the enterocytes will likely not be successful because their host cell will slough before the pathogen can reproduce.

Bile salts inhibit the growth of many organisms, and the Kupffer cells of the liver act as a secondary line of

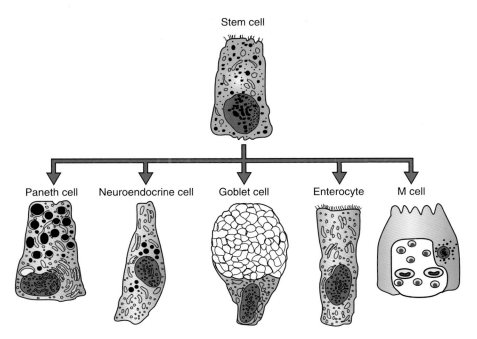

Fig. 7-96   **Schematic illustration of the epithelial cell types of the small intestine.** Progenitor cells, located in the intestinal crypts, give rise to all other epithelial cell types lining the crypt and covering the villi. *(From Damjanov I, Linder J: Anderson's pathology, ed 10, St Louis, 1996, Mosby.)*

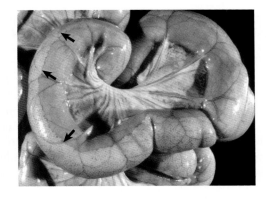

Fig. 7-97   Normal gut-associated lymphoid tissue, intestine, pig. The lymphoid tissue on the antimesenteric surface of the intestine is outlined by arrows and makes up one quarter of the animal's total lymphoid mass. *(Courtesy Dr. H. Gelberg, College of Veterinary Medicine, Oregon State University.)*

defense. Because all the blood from the intestine percolates through the hepatic sinusoids, the Kupffer cells are perfectly positioned to phagocytose bacteria and endotoxins with which they come in contact. In pigs, goats, and cattle (artiodactyls), these functions are performed by intravascular pulmonary macrophages.

Secretory IgA and IgM constitute very important mechanisms of humoral immunity and function largely to prevent attachment of pathogens to intestinal epithelium. Crypt epithelial cells produce the secretory component of IgA.

Bacterial growth is inhibited by lactoferrin and peroxidase from the pancreas and lysozyme from Paneth cells.

DIARRHEA
PATHOGENESIS

Diarrhea is defined as secretion of abnormally fluid feces accompanied by an increased volume of feces and an increased frequency of defecation. There are four major mechanisms by which diarrhea may occur:
- Malabsorption with or without bacterial fermentation leading to osmotic diarrhea. Generally, this is a problem of the small intestine, but secondary colonic malfunctions can occur because of malabsorption of bile salts and fatty acids that stimulate fluid secretion in the large intestine.
- Hypersecretion by a structurally intact mucosa. This activity results in a net efflux of fluid and electrolytes independent of permeability changes, absorptive capacity, or exogenously generated osmotic gradients.
- Exudation caused by increased capillary or epithelial permeability (protein-losing enteropathy).
- Hypermotility generally is involved in diarrhea, but usually not as a primary mechanism in domestic animals. Hypermotility is defined as an increased rate, intensity, or frequency of peristalsis. Theoretically, with decreased mucosal contact time, digestion and absorption of nutrients should be less efficient. It is suspected that

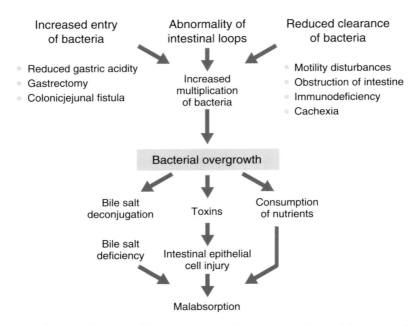

Fig. 7-98   Schematic diagram of the mechanism of how intestinal bacterial overgrowth causes malabsorption and diarrhea. *(From Damjanov I, Linder J: Anderson's pathology, ed 10, St Louis, 1996, Mosby.)*

decreased motility in some diseases allows for increased bacterial proliferation (Fig. 7-98). Conversely, some enterotoxins can stimulate intestinal motility.

As might be expected, the pathogenesis of diarrhea is much more complicated than as just explained. Involved are a complex interplay of cells and factors that are currently being elucidated by a variety of molecular techniques. For example, when a pathogen invades an enterocyte, the pathogen can release an enterotoxin. This toxin causes the enterocyte to release cytokines, particularly interleukin-8 (IL-8). These cytokines activate resident macrophages and recruit new macrophages into the lamina propria from the blood. The activated leukocytes release soluble factors (histamine, serotonin, adenosine) that increase intestinal secretion of chloride ions and water and inhibit absorption.

Other factors (prostaglandins, leukotrienes, platelet-activating factor) act on enteric nerves to induce neurotransmitter-mediated intestinal secretion. Cell damage is possibly a consequence of inflammation mediated by T lymphocytes or proteases and oxidants secreted by mast cells. T lymphocytes also may affect epithelial cell maturation, causing villous atrophy and crypt hyperplasia. Cell death can result from pathogen invasion into enterocytes, multiplication of the pathogen, and extrusion of the affected enterocytes. These changes lead to notable distortion of villous architecture with a lack of absorptive mature enterocytes accompanied by nutrient malabsorption and osmotic diarrhea.

Additionally, there are nonintestinal causes of diarrhea that must be considered in addition to diseases of

the intestine. Among this group are hyperthyroidism, Addison's disease, pancreatic insufficiency, pancreatitis, chronic renal failure, and others. These diseases are discussed in their respective chapters of this book.

CONSEQUENCES

The consequence of excess fluid loss in the feces through diarrhea is dehydration. Dehydration results in hypovolemia. Hypovolemia results in hemoconcentration that results in inadequate tissue perfusion. Energy therefore is generated in tissue by anaerobic glycolysis. The resultant hypoglycemia leads to ketoacidosis. Acidosis is, by definition, a reduction in blood and tissue pH. Acidosis causes a reduction in pH-dependent enzyme system functions. Acidosis is compounded by fecal bicarbonate loss in diarrhea and the results of inadequate renal excretion of hydrogen ions and inadequate absorption of bicarbonate, which is a late effect of inadequate renal perfusion. The resultant electrolyte imbalance results in an increase in intracellular hydrogen ion concentration and a decrease in intracellular potassium ion concentration. The imbalances decrease neuromuscular control of myocardial contraction, leading to a further decrease in tissue perfusion. A vicious cycle results, culminating in hypovolemic shock.

DEVELOPMENTAL ANOMALIES

Occlusion of the intestinal lumen due to anomalous development of the intestinal wall is called atresia (Fig. 7-99). Atresia is generally named for the part of the bowel that is occluded, such as atresia ani or atresia coli.

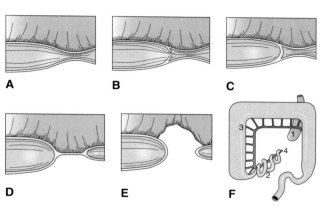

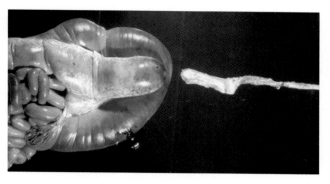

Fig. 7-99 **Schematic illustration of the types of stenosis and atresia. A,** Stenosis. **B,** Stenosis with partial membrane. **C,** Membrane atresia. **D,** Cord atresia. **E,** Blind end atresia. **F,** Christmas tree atresia (*1,* jejunum; *2,* ileum; *3,* colon; *4,* ileocolic artery). (**A** through **F,** *From van der Gaag I, Tibboel D: Vet Pathol 17(5):565-574, 1980.*)

Fig. 7-101 *Atresia coli,* **colon, cow.** There is a blind-ended atretic segment of the spiral colon. The smaller segment at the right of the photograph is distal, the terminal part of the colon. (*Courtesy Dr. H. Gelberg, College of Veterinary Medicine, Oregon State University.*)

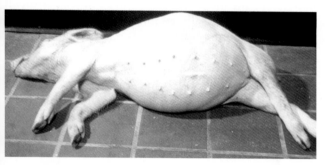

Fig. 7-100 **Abdominal distention, atresia coli, feeder pig.** This pig has been unable to defecate since birth because of an atretic developmental malformation of the distal colon. Note the greatly distended abdomen. (*Courtesy Dr. J. King, College of Veterinary Medicine, Cornell University.*)

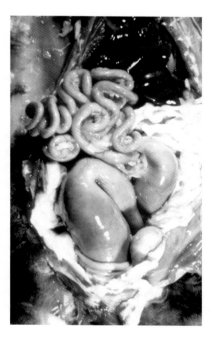

Fig. 7-102 **Megacolon, colon, cat.** This disease may be congenital due to a lack of intestinal innervation or atresia of the distal colon or anus. It can also be acquired secondary to nerve injury. (*Courtesy Dr. H. Gelberg, College of Veterinary Medicine, Oregon State University.*)

The causes of atresia in domestic animals are not completely understood, but it can be a result of mechanical lesions to blood vessels in a portion of the gut, such as caused by malpositioning, that compromises circulation and results in vascular accidents and ischemia. Release of meconium into the abdominal cavity of the fetus may result in sterile peritonitis and may be responsible for some cases of atresia, such as in cystic fibrosis of human beings. In still other cases, the embryonic cells that occlude the lumen fail to break down, resulting in atresia. The end result is segmental atresia in which a segment of the bowel is either entirely missing or completely occluded because of a lack of epithelial development and confluence between two contiguous portions (Figs. 7-100 and 7-101).

Meckel's diverticulum is a remnant of the omphalomesenteric duct. It is near the termination of the ileum and represents the stalk of the yolk sac. Generally, it disappears after the first trimester of gestation. It can persist in all mammalian species and although blind-ended, should not be confused with the cecum.

Megacolon, as its name implies, is a large, usually fecal-filled colon (Figs. 7-102 and 7-103). It occurs in pigs, dogs, cats, overo foals, and human beings. It may be caused by a congenital lack of myenteric plexuses (Hirschsprung's disease) secondary to the failure of

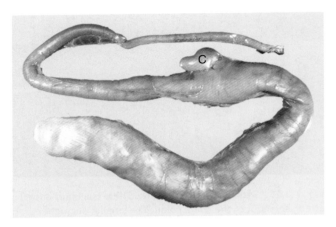

Fig. 7-103 **Megacolon, colon, dog.** The large colon from the cecum (*C*) to the anus is dilated with feces. In dogs, this disease has pathogeneses similar to those described in cats (Fig. 7-102). (*Courtesy Dr. H. Gelberg, College of Veterinary Medicine, Oregon State University.*)

migration of neuroblasts from the neural crest to the colorectal myenteric plexuses.

The equine overo pattern of spotting is defined by white patches of epidermis on the ventral or lateral abdomen that extend dorsally up to, but do not include, the dorsal midline. The epidermis is also nonpigmented on the lateral neck and flank. The overo pattern typically includes at least one pigmented leg. Affected foals are white and appear normal at birth. They do not pass meconium; subsequently they have colic develop and die. These white foals are nonperistaltic because of absence of the myenteric (Auerbach's) plexus or submucosal (Meissner's) plexus particularly in the colon and rectum. Thus these anomalies can be termed aganglionosis. A congenital aganglionic megacolon is contracted and nonperistaltic. Dilation or megacolon occurs proximal to the aganglionic section of the gut.

Acquired megacolon is secondary to damage to the colonic innervation. Such events are usually traumatic and most common in carnivores struck by automobiles. Atresia ani can also result in megacolon.

INTESTINAL OBSTRUCTION

Mechanical obstruction of the intestinal tract occurs in all species of domestic and wild animals. Although foreign bodies of all types have been removed from animals at surgery, the long-term systemic effects of some foreign bodies are also important. These include copper and zinc toxicosis from ingestion of coins in dogs, seals, ruminants, and horses, and lead poisoning in cattle from ingestion of old batteries. Primates caged in outdated facilities with lead paint or lead bars can also succumb to lead poisoning. *Pythium insidiosum* infection has caused intestinal obstruction in a puppy.

ENTEROLITHS AND IMPACTION

Enteroliths are rare in species other than the horse, with an increased incidence in the Arabian breed. Generally, affected animals are more than 4 years old. The stones are usually formed by ammonium magnesium phosphate (struvite) and collect around a small central nidus, often a metallic foreign body (Fig. 7-104). Enteroliths vary greatly in size from several centimeters in diameter to greater than 20 cm, and they can weigh several kilograms. They generally lodge at the pelvic flexure or transverse colon. Diets high in magnesium and phosphorus predispose to enterolith formation. In the past, millers' horses (grain and feed mills) had access to large amounts of inexpensive bran, and thus their horses were more prone to enteroliths. In California, the feeding of high-protein, magnesium-rich alfalfa hay may partially explain the higher incidence of enteroliths in California equids.

The presence of aggregated ingesta that cannot move along the intestinal tract (impaction) occurs in all species. It is especially common in horses following anthelmintic administration and is the result of the rapid

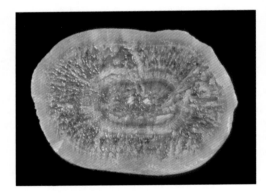

Fig. 7-104 **Enterolith, horse.** This cross section demonstrates concentric laminations. A metallic nidus was present in the center of the enterolith. (*Courtesy Dr. H. Gelberg, College of Veterinary Medicine, Oregon State University.*)

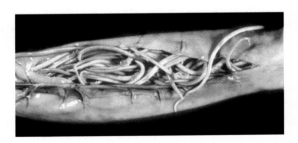

Fig. 7-105 **Ascarid impaction, jejunum, horse.** Impaction was the result of a rapid "die off" of the ascarids as the result of administration of an anthelmintic. (*Courtesy Dr. H. Gelberg, College of Veterinary Medicine, Oregon State University.*)

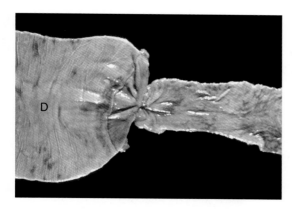

Fig. 7-106 **Stricture, intestine, horse.** The dilated intestine (*D*) is proximal to the stricture. Such strictures can be caused by penetrating or nonpenetrating wounds of all kinds from the luminal side or to vascular injury. *(Courtesy Dr. H. Gelberg, College of Veterinary Medicine, Oregon State University.)*

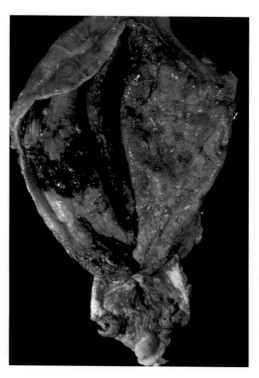

Fig. 7-107 **Stricture, colon, pig.** This lesion in pigs has been attributed to thrombosis of the cranial hemorrhoidal artery from vasculitis and thrombosis caused by *Salmonella*. *(Courtesy Dr. C.S. Patton, College of Veterinary Medicine, University of Tennessee.)*

die-off of large numbers of nematodes, particularly ascarids (Fig. 7-105). Cecal impaction occurs in old horses because of a high-roughage (indigestible) diet, debility, or poor dentition caused by a lack of mechanical leveling of the teeth (floating). Fibrous ingesta can also result in ileal impaction. Large amounts of ingested sand can accumulate anywhere in the equine colon, resulting in impaction.

STRICTURES WITH OBSTRUCTION

Strictures (luminal narrowing) due to penetrating or nonpenetrating wounds of all kinds or to vascular injury can obstruct the intestine (Fig. 7-106). For example, rectal stricture is a sequela of salmonellosis in pigs and is due in part to thrombosis of the cranial hemorrhoidal artery and lack of collateral circulation (Fig. 7-107) that could otherwise allow the intestinal segment to remain viable.

INTUSSUSCEPTION

When one segment of intestine becomes telescoped into the immediately distal segment of intestine, the lesion is called an intussusception (Figs. 7-108 and 7-109). The intussusceptum is the trapped segment and the intussuscipiens is the enveloping portion of the intestine. The cause is generally unknown but is thought to be associated with intestinal irritability and hypermotility. Irritability and hypermotility can occur secondary to enteritis, irritation that is caused by parasites of all sorts, and general debility. Foreign bodies, neoplasms, and some parasites, such as the nodular worm of sheep (*Oesophagostomum* spp.), by means of the subserosal nodules it produces, can provide a toehold for the intestine to telescope into itself. In the dog, intussusception of the intestine has been related to, or caused by, handling of the small intestine during surgery,

hypertrophied lymphoid nodules, and granulomas secondary to inflammatory and parasitic diseases, linear foreign bodies (string) (Fig. 7-110, *A*), and ascarids.

In bovids and equids, tumors, abscesses and granulomas may be causes of intussusceptions. In equids, verminous arteritis may uniquely cause intussusceptions. Ileoileal, ileocecal, cecocecal, and cecocolic intussusceptions are sometimes associated with *Anoplocephala perfoliata*. Rarely, duodenogastric and gastroesophageal intussusceptions occur.

Clinical features of intussusception are similar to those of intestinal obstruction. In small animals with thin abdominal walls, they can sometimes be palpated. Intussusceptions are enlarged, thickened segments of intestine that vary in length. Intussusceptions are grossly swollen, doughy-feeling segments of the intestine. They resemble the folds of an accordion (Fig. 7-110, *B*). Red to black discoloration depends on the degree of vascular compromise, ranging from congestion to hemorrhage and necrosis. The mesenteric attachment of the intussusceptum may be seen extending from the lesion. Ischemic necrosis, congestion, and edema may occur in both the intussusceptum and intussuscipiens.

Because peristalsis continues after death, intestinal invaginations can occur after death. Before attributing

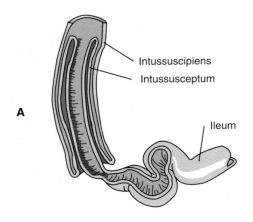

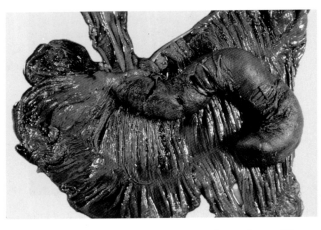

Fig. 7-109   Ileocecal intussusception, ileum, horse. The necrotic intussuscipiens is present in the lumen of the opened cecum. *(Courtesy Dr. M.D. McGavin, College of Veterinary Medicine, University of Tennessee.)*

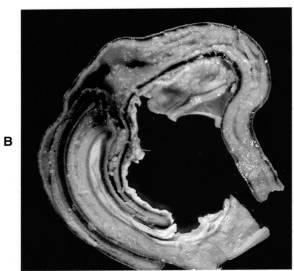

Fig. 7-108   Intussusception. A, Schematic diagram showing the anatomic positioning of small intestinal segments in an intussusception. **B,** Longitudinal section of small intestinal intussusception demonstrating the position of the intussusceptum (trapped segment) and the intussuscipiens (the enveloping portion) of the small intestine. (**A,** *Redrawn with permission from Dr. T. Boosinger;* **B,** *Courtesy Dr. T. Boosinger, College of Veterinary Medicine, Auburn University; and Noah's Arkive, College of Veterinary Medicine, The University of Georgia.)*

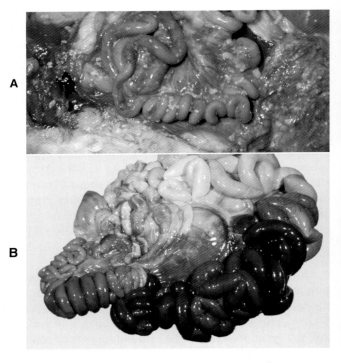

Fig. 7-110   Accordion-folded intestines. A, Small intestine, cat. A linear foreign body (roast beef string) has caused the accordion-folded appearance of the small intestine *(lower).* Peristalsis of the intestine over the string, which is taut, in the intestinal lumen causes a sawing, abrasive effect and perforation of the intestine resulting in peritonitis, the white exudate seen on the serosal surfaces. **B,** Intussusception, intestine, pig. The accordion-folded intussusception *(left)* is contiguous with infarcted bowel, the result of vascular strangulation. (**A,** *Courtesy College of Veterinary Medicine, University of Illinois.* **B,** *Courtesy Dr. H. Gelberg, College of Veterinary Medicine, Oregon State University.)*

death to intestinal obstruction caused by intussusception, there is a need to determine if the intussusception took place before or after death. Because inflammation only occurs in the living organism, postmortem invaginations are easily reduced because there are no adhesions and they are not accompanied by hyperemia or fibrin on the peritoneal surfaces, which remain smooth and glistening. On rare occasions, antemortem intussusceptions spontaneously reduce by sloughing of the infarcted intussusceptum, which then passes in the feces. Often the site of sloughing is replaced with fibrous tissue, and a circumferential scar or stricture forms.

ILEUS

Paralytic ileus (adynamic ileus) is a nonmechanical hypomotility resulting in a functional obstruction of the bowel (pseudoobstruction). It can be due to paralysis of the bowel wall (generally the result of bowel manipulation at surgery), peritonitis from any cause, shock, severe pain, abnormal stimulation of splanchnic nerves, toxemia, electrolyte imbalances (especially hypokalemia), vitamin B-complex deficiency, uremia, tetanus, diabetes mellitus, or heavy-metal poisoning.

The gut is not paralyzed but because of continuous nerve discharge it becomes refractory, resulting in lack of tonic stimulation of the bowel musculature. In most cases of paralytic ileus, there are no gross lesions. It occurs in most animal species.

Grass sickness of equids in Europe is associated with gastrointestinal hypomotility and subsequent colic. Degenerative lesions of this idiopathic condition are present in the autonomic ganglia, suggesting it is an acquired dysautonomia. An occasional outbreak in equids is associated with the temporospatial occurrence of similar lesions in rabbits.

INTESTINAL DISPLACEMENTS

Intestinal displacements include herniations that lead to incarcerations (fixation) of the displaced bowel and finally strangulations (interference with blood flow) of the incarcerated segment of intestine. Herniations are characterized as internal or external.

Internal herniations are displacements of intestine through a normal or pathologic foramen in the abdominal cavity. The most common of these displacements occurs in horses. They include herniation through the epiploic foramen and through mesenteric tears. The dorsal border of the epiploic foramen is formed by the caudate lobe of the liver and the caudal vena cava. The ventral boundary is the right lobe of the pancreas, the gastropancreatic ligament, and the portal vein. The cranial boundary is the hepatoduodenal ligament, and the caudal boundary is the junction of the pancreas and mesoduodenum. The epiploic cavity is only a potential space. It is proposed that the caudate lobe of the liver atrophies in older animals, enlarging the foramen and allowing loops of intestine to slip through and become incarcerated and strangulated (Fig. 7-111).

External hernias are formed when a hernial sac, formed by a pouch of parietal peritoneum, penetrates outside the abdominal cavity. Types of external herniation include umbilical, ventral, diaphragmatic (Fig. 7-112), hiatal, inguinal, scrotal (Fig. 7-113), and perineal. Perineal hernias are seen in old male dogs with prostate gland enlargement and obstipation. Some of these herniations (diaphragmatic, perineal) are more correctly termed eventrations (protrusion of the intestine through the abdominal wall or diaphragm) because they are not

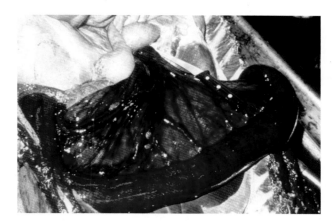

Fig. 7-111   Herniation of small intestine through the epiploic foramen, abdomen, horse. An enlarged epiploic foramen has allowed the small intestine to herniate through the foramen, become incarcerated, and then strangulated. *(Courtesy Dr. J. King, College of Veterinary Medicine, Cornell University.)*

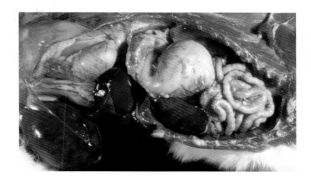

Fig. 7-112   Diaphragmatic hernia, abdomen, cat. Traumatic rupture of the diaphragm has allowed intestines, stomach, and liver into the thoracic cavity, resulting in displacement and compression of the thoracic viscera and consequently compromise of cardiopulmonary function. *(Courtesy Dr. H. Gelberg, College of Veterinary Medicine, Oregon State University.)*

accompanied by a peritoneal pouch. Postoperative wound dehiscence of a ventral abdominal incision also causes eventration.

It should be noted that umbilical hernias are generally caused by a defect in the abdominal wall and not by the chewing on the umbilical cord by the dam. Umbilical hernias may have a genetic basis, so it may be a matter of some ethical concern whether to surgically repair these hernias in show and breeding animals. In calves, umbilical infections are also associated with an increased risk for hernia development.

Rectal prolapse may occur secondary to tenesmus or excessive postpartum straining (Fig. 7-114).

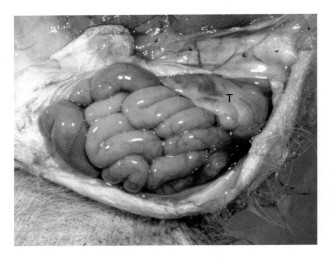

Fig. 7-113   Scrotal hernia, scrotum, pig. Loops of intestine within the scrotum entered through the inguinal canal to lie in the scrotal cavity and have displaced the testis (*T*) caudally. (*Courtesy Dr. H. Gelberg, College of Veterinary Medicine, Oregon State University.*)

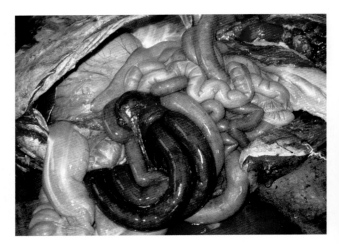

Fig. 7-115   Infarction, small intestine, horse. Volvulus of the intestine has resulted in vascular compromise and infarction of several loops of bowel. (*Courtesy Dr. M.D. McGavin, College of Veterinary Medicine, University of Tennessee.*)

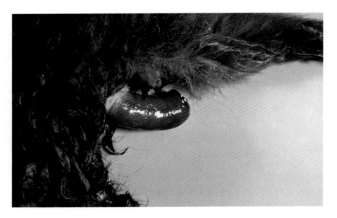

Fig. 7-114   Prolapsed rectum, anus, cat. Tenesmus caused the rectum to prolapse. (*Courtesy Dr. M.D. McGavin, College of Veterinary Medicine, University of Tennessee.*)

VOLVULUS AND TORSION

A volvulus is a twisting of the intestine on its mesenteric axis. A torsion is a rotation of a tubular organ along its long axis. The latter is most common in the cecum of cattle and horses and occasionally of the abomasum of calves. Both volvulus and torsion result in vascular obstruction and ischemic injury. Infarction is a result of occlusion of the thin-walled mesenteric veins. Because the mesenteric arterial supply is anatomically more resistant to occlusion, blood is pumped into the twisted segment but cannot drain. Edema, congestion, hemorrhage, and eventual necrosis result (Figs. 7-115 and 7-116). It is probable that the mechanism of intestinal twisting is secondary to movement of the abdominal cavity (i.e., the intestine stays still and the horse rolls or otherwise moves around the static intestine).

At surgery or necropsy, the twisted segment of intestine is distended with gas and fluid and is discolored either dark red or black. There is usually a sharp line of demarcation between the affected and normal intestine. This line marks the site for surgical resection. A volvulus may result in a rotation of the intestine up to 720 degrees, either clockwise or counterclockwise on its mesenteric axis. Therefore surgical correction of a volvulus may be difficult and complex. It is very important to determine the viability of the bowel after reduction of a volvulus. The affected segment of intestine is often necrotic, congested, and hemorrhagic. Intestinal stasis and toxemia and/or bacteremia may result from bacterial overgrowth and anoxic bowel necrosis. Reperfusion injury may also occur. Toxemia and intestinal rupture may result in death.

Volvulus of the equine large intestine occurs most commonly in the left colon. In equids, the left ventral colon is an extension of the right ventral colon beginning at the sternal flexure. The left ventral colon doubles back on itself in the pelvic inlet to form the left dorsal colon. This pelvic flexure can be palpated rectally. The left dorsal colon becomes the right dorsal colon at the diaphragmatic flexure. The diaphragmatic flexure lies cranial to the sternal flexure and usually contacts the ventral body wall. The left dorsal colon is sacculated with one taenia; the left ventral colon is sacculated with four taeniae. When twisting occurs, it is usually clockwise around the mesocolon and is thus a volvulus. Torsion of the large colon of mares accounts for half of their intestinal displacements in the peripartum period.

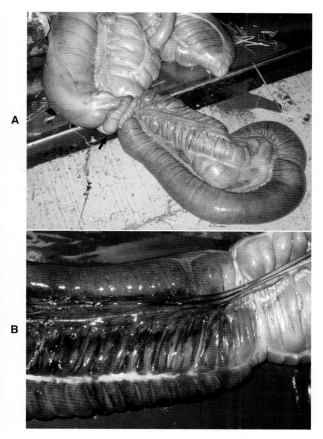

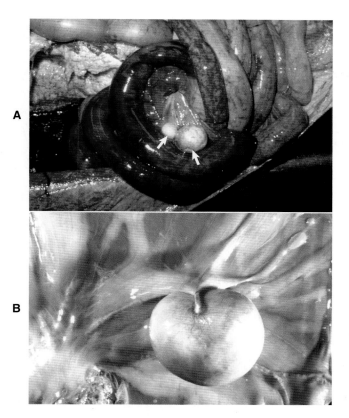

Fig. 7-116 **Torsion, large colon, horse. A,** Rotation of the colon on its long axis has resulted in severe colic with strangulation (*arrow*). Note the red to blue discoloration of the colon distal to the torsion caused by obstruction of venous blood flow. **B,** Note the sharp line of demarcation (point where the torsion occurred) between viable colon (to the right) and nonviable colon (to the left) caused by obstruction of venous blood flow. In this case, the torsion was not found at the time of necropsy; however, a torsion will commonly untwist itself (reduce itself) during transport of the dead animal to the postmortem room. The lesion is characteristic of a torsion. (**A,** *Courtesy Dr. H. Gelberg, College of Veterinary Medicine, Oregon State University.* **B,** *Courtesy Dr. M.D. McCracken, College of Veterinary Medicine, University of Tennessee.*)

Fig. 7-117 **Pedunculated lipomas. A,** Intestinal strangulation by pedunculated lipomas, small intestine, horse. Two lipomas (*arrows*) have wrapped around the mesentery and strangled the bowel resulting in infarction. **B,** Mesentery, horse. Closer view of a pedunculated lipoma. (**A,** *Courtesy College of Veterinary Medicine, Cornell University.* **B,** *Courtesy College of Veterinary Medicine, University of Illinois.*)

A peculiar type of intestinal strangulation occurs in horses in which lipomas, which are pedunculated, wrap around the intestinal mesentery or the bowel itself, causing ischemia, colic, and death (Fig. 7-117). However, most mesenteric lipomas are of no clinical consequence. Although rare, intestinal strangulation by pedunculated lipomas has been reported in the dog.

RENOSPLENIC ENTRAPMENT

Renosplenic entrapment of the large colon in horses is due to left dorsal displacement of the left dorsal colon or left ventral colon between the spleen and left body wall. Entrapment occurs over the renosplenic ligament that runs between the left kidney and the spleen. The cause of the displacement is unknown but could occur secondary to rolling behavior in horses or gaseous distention of the large colon. If not corrected either by rolling the horse or by surgery, intestinal rupture and death may result.

MISCELLANEOUS DISEASES AND CONDITIONS

Cecal or large intestinal rupture occurs most commonly in postparturient mares (Fig. 7-118), but can also result from impaction and as a complication of anesthesia. The sites of rupture vary, and the mechanisms are unknown. Iatrogenic rectal tearing may occur secondary to rectal palpation (Fig. 7-119). The presence of blood on a rectal sleeve after palpation is cause for concern because peritonitis may be the result of penetration of the abdominal cavity.

Diverticula (singular, diverticulum) are epithelium-lined cavities that are derived from mucosal epithelium

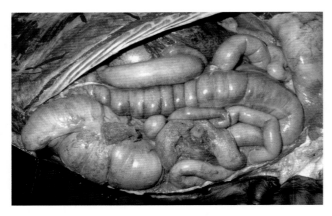

Fig. 7-118   Fibrinous peritonitis, abdomen, horse. The presence of fibrin and ingesta adherent to serosal surfaces indicates antemortem perforation or rupture of the intestine. *(Courtesy Dr. M.D. McGavin, College of Veterinary Medicine, University of Tennessee.)*

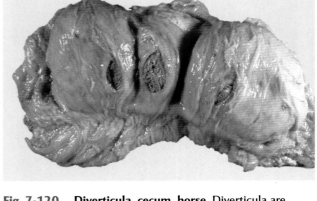

Fig. 7-120   Diverticula, cecum, horse. Diverticula are mucosal outpouchings into the subjacent smooth muscle layers of the colon. They are filled with ingesta and lined by intact mucosa. *(Courtesy Dr. H. Gelberg, College of Veterinary Medicine, Oregon State University.)*

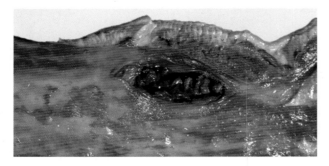

Fig. 7-119   Ulceration, rectum, horse. Hemorrhage, ulcers, and tears in the rectum are often caused by inexperienced persons or overvigorous rectal palpation. *(Courtesy Dr. M.D. McGavin, College of Veterinary Medicine, University of Tennessee.)*

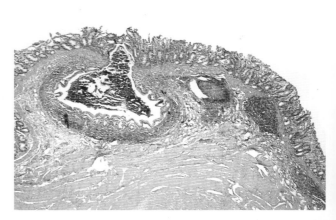

Fig. 7-121   Diverticulum, colon, cow. A diverticulum lined by superficial mucosa has penetrated through the submucosa to lie next to the muscularis. H&E stain. *(Courtesy Dr. M.D. McGavin, College of Veterinary Medicine, University of Tennessee.)*

that extend through the muscularis mucosa, submucosa, and muscularis and often reach the serosa, where they sometimes rupture, causing peritonitis (Figs. 7-120 through 7-122). Muscular hypertrophy of the tunica muscularis associated with diverticulosis has been recorded in young Yorkshire pigs and in Romney Marsh and Hampshire sheep.

Muscular hypertrophy of the distal ileum is an idiopathic condition of horses and pigs. Although generally an incidental finding, hypertrophy of the tunica muscularis can lead to impaction and rupture of the ileum. The lesion in horses is sometimes segmental, affecting the ileum and variably the jejunum. Often the lesion is a sequela of muscular hypertrophy caused by a damaged or stenotic ileocecal valve. Muscular hypertrophy of equids may also affect the duodenum and jejunum in association with diverticula. Horses with muscular

hypertrophy of the distal ileum may have mild colic, occasional diarrhea, and weight loss. Often muscular hypertrophy is asymptomatic. Muscular hypertrophy of the ileum in pigs generally occurs as an idiopathic, asymptomatic lesion. The lesion is suspected to be secondary to a functional obstruction of the ileocecal valve. Diverticulosis and/or intestinal rupture may result.

Cats can have a severe hypertrophy of the inner, circular layer of the tunica muscularis of the ileum and sometimes the jejunum. In cats with hypereosinophilic syndrome, a disease characterized by intramural eosinophil infiltrates, hypertrophy of the gastric antrum

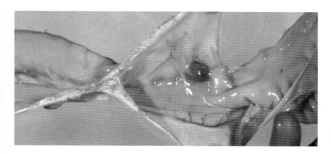

Fig. 7-122   Mesodiverticulum, ileum, horse. An intestinal mucosal outpouch has penetrated the wall of the intestine and extended into the mesentery (*red nodule*). *(Courtesy Dr. J. King, College of Veterinary Medicine, Cornell University.)*

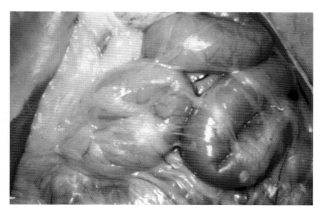

Fig. 7-124   Leiomyometaplasia, intestine, dog. "Brown dog gut" is a rare condition caused by the accumulation of a brown pigment now known to be ceroid (formerly called lipofuscin) in the lysosomes of smooth muscle cells of the tunica muscularis. It is a dietary condition due to vitamin E deficiency. *(Courtesy Dr. C.S. Patton, College of Veterinary Medicine, University of Tennessee.)*

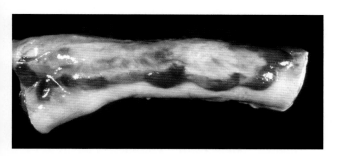

Fig. 7-123   Hemomelasma ilei, ileum, horse. Hemorrhagic and siderotic fibrovascular plaques on the antimesenteric serosa are attributed to strongyle larval migration (*Strongylus edentatus*). *(Courtesy Dr. H. Gelberg, College of Veterinary Medicine, Oregon State University.)*

and small intestinal musculature can occur. Muscular hypertrophy of the intestine and medial hyperplasia of the pulmonary arteries occur in cats given large oral doses of *Toxocara cati* larvae. These conditions are often accompanied by diarrhea and eosinophilic enteritis. Fibrosis of the lamina propria and hypertrophy of the inner layer of the tunica muscularis may result.

Another unique lesion in the horse is hemomelasma ilei. These lesions are pink to black plaques that vary in length from several millimeters to many centimeters and can occur anywhere in the intestine but are generally limited to the ileum (Fig. 7-123). They are attributed to larval migrations of strongyles (usually *Strongylus edentatus*) and are located on the antimesenteric serosal surface. These fibrovascular serosal plaques are putatively formed in response to tissue damage caused by the migrating parasites. However, parasites have never been reported in the lesions and therefore the cause of hemomelasma ilei is unknown. They are generally of no clinical consequence, but can on occasion lead to intestinal strictures and intermittent colic.

Intestinal lipofuscinosis or leiomyometaplasia is also called "brown dog gut." The discolored intestinal smooth

muscle may occur in association with chronic enteritis and pancreatitis. Experimentally, leiomyometaplasia can be produced in dogs by vitamin E deficiency, in association with excess dietary lipids. The canine and human intestinal pigmentation is the result of vitamin E deficiency. The dietary requirement for vitamin E is proportional to the concentration of polyunsaturated fatty acids in the diet. Intestinal lipofuscinosis probably does not cause clinical signs but may be an indicator of a metabolic or nutritional disorder. In this condition, the intestinal serosa varies from tan to dark brown (Fig. 7-124). The stomach and large bowel are variously affected, as is the small intestine. Accumulation of brown, granular, acid-fast–staining lipofuscin in the perinuclear lysosomes of the leiomyocytes is characteristic of this condition.

Amyloidosis occasionally is present in the intestines in association with systemic amyloid AA infiltrations in a variety of animal species.

Tiger striping is a nonspecific congestion of colonic ridges secondary to diarrhea and/or tenesmus (Fig. 7-125).

SMALL INTESTINAL INTOXICANTS

Because most toxins enter the body through ingestion, those that are irritants can cause contact lesions in the oral cavity, esophagus, stomach, and intestine. The lesions that result are generally those of hemorrhage and inflammation. In many cases of intoxication, induction of vomiting is contraindicated because what burns going down will also burn coming up. The numbers and types of chemicals and intoxicants animals are exposed to makes a listing of them a monumental undertaking.

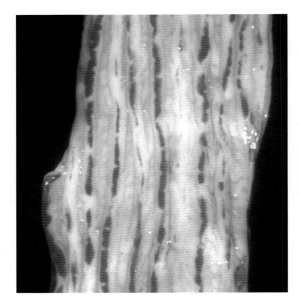

Fig. 7-125   Tiger striping, colon, dog. Nonspecific congestion and hemorrhage of the colonic ridges is due to tenesmus and/or diarrhea. *(Courtesy Dr. H. Gelberg, College of Veterinary Medicine, Oregon State University.)*

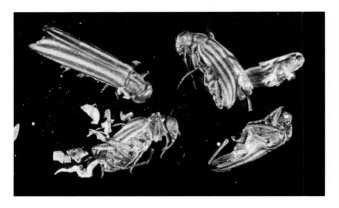

Fig. 7-126   Striped blister beetles. Numerous species of blister beetles (*Epicauta* spp.) such as gray, black, and striped can be found throughout the United States. They contain a vesicant (blister-causing substance) that causes inflammation and blistering of mucosal surfaces when they are ingested. Usually, these beetles are trapped and crushed in crimped hay. *(Courtesy Dr. W. Crowell, College of Veterinary Medicine, University of Georgia; and Noah's Arkive, College of Veterinary Medicine, University of Georgia.)*

A few examples are phosphorus, arsenic, bracken fern (cattle), mercury, oak, copper, nitrate, thallium, and blister beetles. Blister beetles, a specific toxicity, are sometimes incorporated into crimped hay (Fig. 7-126). They contain a topical irritant called cantharidin. Lesions include sloughing of the epithelium of the stomach and enterocytes of the proximal small intestine (Fig. 7-127).

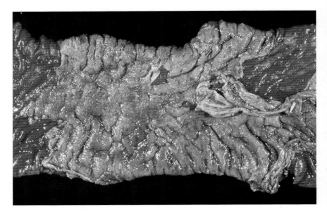

Fig. 7-127   Acute necrohemorrhagic enteritis, small intestine, horse. The severe necrosis with sloughing of intestinal mucosa is the result of cantharidin, a toxin contained in ingested blister beetles. *(Courtesy Dr. R. Panciera, School of Veterinary Medicine, Oklahoma State University; and Noah's Arkive, College of Veterinary Medicine, The University of Georgia.)*

In addition, cantharidin can cause hemorrhagic ulcers of the urinary bladder and myocardial necrosis.

Although not generally considered an intoxicant, corticosteroids cause colonic perforation in some treated dogs and can delay gastrointestinal healing. They do this by decreasing cell turnover, decreasing mucus production, and stimulating gastrin secretion, leading to increased acid production. NSAIDs can cause right dorsal colitis in equids. This colitis is characterized by necrosis, resulting in erosions and ulcers. Epithelial loss may be severe, with only regenerating, rounded islands of normal mucosa remaining. The massive edema of the denuded intestine causes rupture of the submucosa in an elongated diamondlike pattern. The mechanism of injury is direct by topical application (oral administration) and through inhibition of prostaglandin synthesis. Neutrophils play a role by increasing synthesis of tumor necrosis factor-α, leukotriene B_4, and up-regulation of leukocyte adhesion molecules.

VASCULAR DISEASES OF THE INTESTINE
PARASITES

In horses, *Strongylus vulgaris* fourth-stage larvae are present in the wall of the cranial mesenteric artery, resulting in arteritis. So-called aneurysms (some with osseous metaplasia and bone marrow) and mural thromboses develop (Fig. 7-128). In many cases, even complete occlusion of the anterior mesenteric artery does not result in bowel infarction because collateral circulation will develop if the vascular occlusion develops slowly (Fig. 7-129). Therefore it is important to ascertain if the colonic arteries are thrombosed before assigning the cause of bowel death to *Strongylus vulgaris*. Severe colic

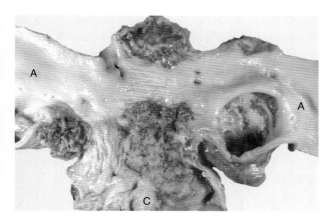

Fig. 7-128   Verminous arteritis, cranial mesenteric artery (C), horse. Chronic proliferative arteritis and mural thrombosis have resulted from the migration of *Strongylus vulgaris* fourth-stage larvae through and within the vessel wall at or near its origin from the aorta *(A)*. The arteritis can lead to mural thrombosis, formation of aneurysms *(lower right)*, arterial mineralization, and infarction of the bowel. *(Courtesy Dr. H. Gelberg, College of Veterinary Medicine, Oregon State University.)*

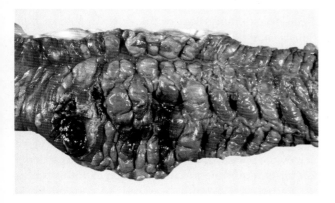

Fig. 7-129   Infarcts, small intestine, horse. Thromboemboli from sites of verminous arteritis in the cranial mesenteric artery will often lodge in end arteries of segments of the small intestine, resulting in sudden vascular occlusion and bowel infarction. *(Courtesy Dr. H. Gelberg, College of Veterinary Medicine, Oregon State University.)*

and death often results from bowel infarction secondary to verminous arteritis and thrombosis.

Third-stage larvae are ingested and molt to fourth-stage larvae in the small intestine. They then invade small arterioles on their way to the anterior mesenteric artery. It takes 3 to 4 months in this location until fifth-stage larvae are produced and migrate through the blood vessels to the cecocolonic subserosa. They may be walled off similarly to *Oesophagostomum* spp. in ruminants and pigs. In the lumen of the large intestine, adults develop. The entire cycle takes up to 6 months or more. Thus the

prepatent period in foals is considerable, and by the time ova appear in the feces, significant vascular damage may have occurred. Modern and effective deworming regimens are quite effective and will hopefully succeed in making this disease of historic significance only.

LYMPHANGIECTASIA

Lymphangiectasia, or lacteal dilation, is the most commonly reported cause of protein-losing enteropathy in dogs. Clinical signs include diarrhea, steatorrhea, hypoproteinemia, and ascites (Fig. 7-130). Lymphangiectasia can be due to a congenital developmental disorder of the lymphatic vessels, or it can be acquired secondary to lymph vessel obstruction caused by granulomatous or neoplastic diseases. An inherited cause is suspected in some canine breeds. A special case is lipogranulomatous lymphangiectasia of the dog, the name of which is descriptive of the lesions present. Most cases of acquired lymphangiectasia are idiopathic. Gross and microscopic lesions are those of lymphangiectasia and include a thickened intestinal mucosa with dilated lymphatics and lacteals (Figs. 7-131 and 7-132). There are variable increases in lymphocyte and plasma cell numbers in affected tissue.

DISEASES OF THE INTESTINAL EPITHELIUM

A number of diseases are characterized by colonization or destruction of the epithelial components of the intestinal mucosa. Although the disease-producing effects of pathogens are complex and multifactorial, a simplified understanding of the principal cell under attack is

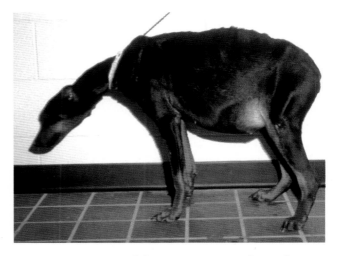

Fig. 7-130   Ascites, abdomen, emaciation, dog, Doberman pinscher. Protein-losing enteropathy, secondary to idiopathic intestinal lymphangiectasia resulted in hypoproteinemia and then ascites. *(Courtesy Dr. H. Gelberg, College of Veterinary Medicine, Oregon State University.)*

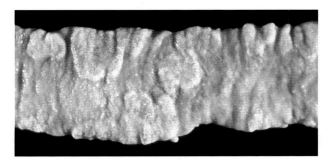

Fig. 7-131   Lymphangiectasia, jejunum, dog. Intestinal villi are expanded by ectasia of the lymphatics *(raised white areas)*. Lymphangiectasia can be a congenital developmental disorder of the lymphatic vessels, or it can be acquired secondary to lymph vessel obstruction caused by granulomatous or neoplastic diseases. *(Courtesy College of Veterinary Medicine, University of Illinois.)*

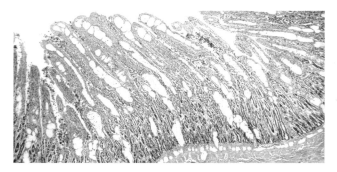

Fig. 7-132   Lymphangiectasia, jejunum, dog. Lacteals are dilated, thus resulting in diminished lymph absorption by lacteals in the lamina propria and subsequent loss of protein (hypoproteinemia) and other nutrients into the intestinal lumen. H&E stain. *(Courtesy Dr. H. Gelberg, College of Veterinary Medicine, Oregon State University.)*

helpful in predicting disease outcome and managing treatment.

DISEASES OF THE ABSORPTIVE ENTEROCYTES

A number of agents have a tropism for the absorptive cells lining the intestinal villi. These agents include viruses such as rotavirus, enteric coronavirus, and the coronavirus of transmissible gastroenteritis of pigs. Intracellular bacteria and parasites can likewise invade and multiply in absorptive epithelial cells. Examples include the agent of swine dysentery (*Brachyspira hyodysenteriae*), coccidia, and cryptosporidia.

Some pathogens with a tropism for absorptive lining cells of the intestine cause destruction of these cells. This results in loss of enterocytes and at least temporary villous atrophy. The loss of the absorptive-digestive villous enterocytes causes maldigestion, and malabsorption results.

Furthermore, because ingesta and normal alimentary secretions are unabsorbed, they are degraded further and fermented in the intestine by bacteria, increasing the osmolality of intestinal contents, with a subsequent increase in the fluid content of the bowel.

Because the regenerative crypt cells are not attacked by pathogens with tropism for villous enterocytes, diseases with villous enterocyte damage are not necessarily fatal. The lost cells are replaced by the maturing cells migrating along the basement membrane from the crypt to the villus. The naked basement membrane contracts, causing villous atrophy. This contraction may be a function of the smooth muscle in the lamina propria. The functionally immature migrating crypt cells cover the villi. Often these immature cells become squamoid in an effort to cover the maximum area of basement membrane. However, if naked basement membranes contact each other, they will adhere, resulting not only in villous blunting but also villous fusion, preventing the reformation of normal villi.

DISEASES OF UNDIFFERENTIATED CRYPT CELLS

Loss of the undifferentiated epithelial cells in the base of the crypts means loss of the cells capable of rapid mitosis, and thus regeneration of the epithelium is impaired. Therefore the clinical effect of crypt cell loss can be delayed for several days because the villi are initially still covered by enterocytes. This type of loss is more severe, and often fatal, compared with villous enterocyte loss. Agents that target the crypt cells are called radiomimetic because they mimic the effects of radiation on the rapidly dividing enterocytes. Examples of these agents include the parvoviruses of carnivores, BVD virus, rinderpest virus, and some mycotoxins such as vomitoxin.

ABNORMALITIES OF THE MICROVILLI AND GLYCOCALYX

Because the microvilli and glycocalyx on the villous enterocytes are largely responsible for the immense surface area and enzymes responsible for nutrient digestion and absorption, it follows that damage to either of these structures can result in intestinal malfunction and resultant diarrhea. A prime example of this is human lactose intolerance. Such persons lack lactase in the glycocalyx. Because of this lack, they are unable to digest lactose from dairy products. The lack of lactase results in failure of uptake, and the lactose is fermented by bacteria in the colon. This results in an osmotic drain of fluid into the gut with resultant diarrhea. Thus the malabsorption in this case is limited to a single substrate. Histologically the intestine is normal.

Some bacteria, such as attaching and effacing *Escherichia coli*, damage the microvilli by their attachment. This attachment disrupts enzyme systems housed in the microvilli and glycocalyx and causes diarrhea. The antibiotic neomycin can similarly cause fragmentation of microvilli and destruction of the glycocalyx with resultant diarrhea. Cessation of neomycin therapy results in a return to normal structure and function.

DISEASES IN WHICH THE EPITHELIAL TARGETS ARE UNKNOWN OR NONSPECIFIC

In a number of enteric diseases, the targeted epithelial cell is unknown or nonspecific. Many of the pathogens causing these diseases are of importance in the young of food-producing animals. Enterotoxic *Escherichia coli* infection of neonatal pigs, calves, lambs, and human beings causes what is known as a secretory diarrhea. These bacteria are able to colonize the small intestinal enterocytes by way of their surface or pili antigens, which anchor them to the enterocytes. Different pili antigens adhere to glycoconjugate receptors on enterocytes in different regions of the small intestine. Thus these bacteria are not washed out by peristalsis. Because the enterocytes are not damaged, no lesions are observed, although microscopically the bacteria can be seen attached to the epithelial surface. The bacteria produce a toxin that causes enterocytes to secrete water and electrolytes. Although cAMP (cyclic adenosine monophosphate) and cGMP (cyclic guanosine monophosphate) mediate this process, the exact mechanism by which this secretion occurs is unknown. Some secretions, especially those of chloride ions, occur via the crypt cells. Intestinal secretion exceeds the ability of the colon to absorb the surplus fluid. The net result is diarrhea.

Clostridium perfringens type C is a pathogen of neonatal pigs, lambs, calves, and foals. Unlike the enterotoxic *Escherichia coli*, which produces a toxin affecting enterocytes, *Clostridium perfringens* produces a nonspecific cytotoxin. This toxin causes necrosis of villous absorptive cells, which then extends to the lamina propria and blood vessels. The result is massive and acute necrohemorrhagic enteritis.

SEPARATION OF APICAL JUNCTIONAL COMPLEXES

Apical junctional complexes, also called tight junctions or zona occludens, join enterocytes to each other. Normally, these junctions are a barrier to macromolecular transepithelial transport. In certain parasitic diseases, such as ostertagiosis, these tight junctions are pathologically opened, allowing transport of macromolecules into the intestinal (abomasal) lumen. This opening of tight junctions is also important in allowing macromolecules, such as immunoglobulin, into the lumen where the parasites can be attacked.

DISEASE OF THE LAMINA PROPRIA

Lesions within the lamina propria can be infiltrative, necrotizing, or vascular, all of which can cause diarrhea even though the epithelium is not the primary cell type injured.

INFLAMMATION

Chronic injury of the lamina propria that results in dense cellular infiltration can cause diarrhea in a variety of ways, none of which are completely understood. These mechanisms include simple physical impairment of mucosal diffusion by space-occupying cells with resultant disruption of the overlying epithelium causing increased permeability. Examples of these diseases in domestic animals are canine histiocytic ulcerative colitis (boxer colitis), Johne's disease (paratuberculosis) of cattle, amyloidosis, and lymphoma.

NECROTIZING PROCESSES

Primary necrotizing processes of the lamina propria generally involve necrosis of the GALT with extension to the overlying epithelium. Examples of diseases with these lesions include BVD of bovids and *Rhodococcus equi* infection of equids.

VASCULAR CHANGES AND LYMPHANGIECTASIA

Vascular changes and dilation of lacteals are idiopathic or secondary to obstruction of flow. These lesions are seen most commonly as part of the syndrome resulting from space-occupying lesions of the lamina propria, such as occurs in Johne's disease and lymphoma. Endotoxemia that results in vascular damage and disseminated intravascular coagulopathy can cause thrombi in small vessels, and hemorrhage, necrosis, and ulceration of the intestine.

DISEASES DUE TO SPECIFIC PATHOGENS

A number of pathogens affect different animal species in similar ways. The mechanism of damage is similar among these animal species and pathogens. Therefore it is useful to discuss the diseases caused by these organisms across species. Specific diseases that do not have analogs in other species are described later in this chapter.

VIRAL DISEASES
Group A rotavirus enteritis

Rotaviruses are ubiquitous pathogens present everywhere in the environment, including air and water. Each species of animal has its specific rotavirus, and although broad similarities exist in pathogenesis among viral infection of individual species, in general the viruses are not cross infective among species. These viruses are important pathogens. Human group A rotavirus, for example, kills a million children a year in the developing countries of the world. In all species, these viruses cause disease in association with other enteropathogens of neonates.

In calves, the disease is most important during the first week of life and in piglets in the first 7 weeks of life. These ages correspond to the reduction of colostral and milk-associated antirotavirus antibody titers that occur after weaning. Specific diagnosis of these diseases is difficult for a variety of reasons. The virus is ubiquitous and therefore can be isolated or detected in many animals, most of whom do not have clinical disease. Additionally, because the viruses are cytolytic, some animals with viral diarrhea can be negative for viruses because the cells harboring the virus have been shed previously in the feces.

Rotaviruses are about 70 nm in diameter and are tri-layered. Only the complete triple-layered virion is infectious. Rotaviruses have double-stranded RNA at their core, and protein spikes project from the surface. The complete particle looks like a wheel, thus the appellation rotavirus. Piglets and calves with rotavirus disease have dehydration and yellow, watery diarrhea and are weak and depressed. Production of clinical disease is dependent on the amount of villous epithelium that is lost. This varies by host species. The epithelial cells over the upper two thirds of the affected villi of the proximal small intestine are infected first in those species that suffer with severe diarrhea from rotavirus infection (Fig. 7-133). Sloughing of villous cells results in shortening and sometimes fusion of villi, if basement membranes are exposed (Fig. 7-134). Depending on the degree of enterocyte loss, recovery may be delayed or incomplete depending on the amount of absorptive surface that is permanently lost. Death, when it occurs, is generally associated with intercurrent infections with

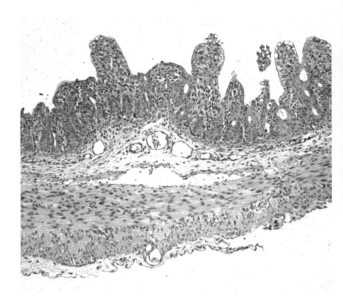

Fig. 7-134   Rotavirus enteritis, jejunum, piglet. There is notable blunting and fusion of intestinal villi secondary to virus-induced cytolysis of enterocytes covering the tips and sides of intestinal villi. H&E stain. *(Courtesy Dr. H. Gelberg, College of Veterinary Medicine, Oregon State University.)*

those organisms that also target villous epithelial cells, such as coronavirus, cryptosporidia, *Escherichia coli*, coccidia, and others.

Coronavirus enteritis

Coronaviruses responsible for calfhood enteritis (at 100 to 120 nm) are larger than a rotavirus. Their genetic core is single-stranded RNA. Peplomers project from the surface, resulting in the appearance of a corona, such as created by the sun; hence the appellation coronavirus. The clinical course of the disease, histologic lesions, mechanism of diarrhea production, and age of affected calves is very similar to that of rotavirus enteritis although somewhat prolonged. Virus infection is more virulent than in rotavirus enteritis and death more common. Colitis occurs in addition to small intestinal involvement, but the principal disease signs and pathogenicity are related to the small intestinal lesions. In the colon, similar to the small intestine, enterocytes when lost are initially replaced by less mature and often squamoid cells. Unlike in rotavirus enteritis, crypt lumens contain cell debris and crypt cells may be focally hyperplastic. The lamina propria and draining lymph nodes often contain increased numbers of inflammatory cells. A hemorrhagic form of the disease with extensive colitis has been reported.

Although generally a mild and self-limiting disease of neonates, feline enteric coronavirus has been associated with fatal enteritis in a series of cats.

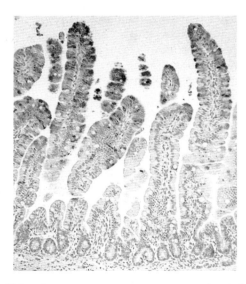

Fig. 7-133   Rotavirus enteritis, jejunum, piglet. Infected enterocytes contain large amounts of viral antigen *(brown)*. Note that infected enterocytes are those that cover the tips and upper sides of intestinal villi. Antirotavirus immunoperoxidase stain. *(Courtesy Dr. H. Gelberg, College of Veterinary Medicine, Oregon State University.)*

Lesions consist of degeneration and loss of enterocytes from jejunal villous tips. Cats 2 months to 7 years old are affected.

Adenovirus enteritis

Adenoviral infection occurs in cattle, sheep, pigs, goats, Spanish ibex, cervids, horses, and inland bearded dragons. Each species-specific virus causes inapparent respiratory disease and under some circumstances clinical enteric disease. Other organs may also be affected, such as liver and kidneys. Endothelial cells are often affected. In Arabian horses and Arabian crossbreeds, adenovirus enteritis occurs in horses with combined immunodeficiency (CID). Adenovirus is transmitted by aerosols, feces, and fomites. When enteritis is produced, characteristic basophilic to amphophilic intranuclear inclusion bodies are present in villous enterocytes, usually in young animals that are immunosuppressed. Endothelial cells also are affected and have similar inclusions. Loss of enterocytes results in villous blunting and fusion. In general, adenovirus infection is subclinical.

BACTERIAL DISEASES
Escherichia coli diseases (colibacillosis)

Coliform bacteria arrive early among the normal flora that colonizes the intestinal tract of virtually all animals. Young animals are at highest risk for coliform diarrhea, especially pigs and calves. There is interplay of many intrinsic and extrinsic factors that act together to determine if disease will be produced by infection. Some of the factors are the genetic make-up of the host animals, the passive transfer of specific antibodies in the colostrums, the constant bathing of the intestine with milk-associated antibodies from nursing, environmental contamination, and the nutritional plane of the host. Environmental stressors predisposing to disease production include temperature extremes, crowding, and intercurrent infections with rotavirus, coronavirus, cryptosporidia, coccidia, and others. The development of unique serotypes of *Escherichia coli* may cause problems in individual environments. In the past, autogenous vaccines, made to order for these environments, have been reasonably effective in controlling some disease outbreaks. Probiotics containing several *Escherichia coli* types and/or *Lactobacillus* spp. have shown promise as a preventative in calves. Lytic phages have also been promising in eliminating infection.

There are a variety of classification schemes for the *Escherichia coli* enteritides. They include enterotoxic, septicemic, edema disease, postweaning, enteroinvasive, and attaching and effacing.

Escherichia coli attach to cells by a variety of pili or fimbriae (Fig. 7-135). Enterotoxigenic *Escherichia coli* may have fimbrial antigens F4 (K88), 5 (K99), 6 (987P), 18,

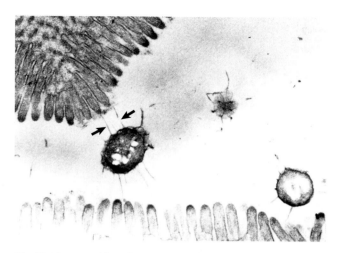

Fig. 7-135 **Colibacillosis, intestine, piglet.** *Escherichia coli* pili *(arrows)* are attached to enterocytes. TEM. Uranyl acetate and lead citrate stain. *(Courtesy Dr. R. Isaacson, College of Veterinary Medicine, University of Minnesota.)*

or 41 and may also produce up to three enterotoxins (STa, STb, LT) and shigatoxins. Fimbrial and nonfimbrial adhesins such as AIDA-1 may also be present. *Escherichia coli*–induced diseases are grouped into several clinical syndromes.

Many *Escherichia coli* produce verotoxins (VTEC) important in disease pathogenesis. More than 200 serotypes of VTEC have been isolated from cattle alone. Diagnosis of toxin-producing *Escherichia coli* is by selective culture properties of the bacteria, immunomagnetic separation, and other monoclonal-based immunoassays for the Vero-Shiga toxins. More recent developments are the use of real-time polymerase chain reaction (PCR) to detect pathogenic gene sequences.

Enterotoxic colibacillosis. *Enterotoxic colibacillosis* occurs most often in animals 2 days to 3 weeks of age. Calves and piglets are most often affected. Why enterotoxic colibacillosis is a disease of neonates is not well understood. Some speculation is that enteric bacterial colonization is a function of gastric acidity and that the low pH of the stomach of postneonatal animals kills the bacteria.

The diarrhea that occurs is a function of bacterial endotoxin-induced sodium and chloride secretion into the intestinal lumen. Water is drawn into the intestine to normalize the resultant NaCl. Thus the diarrhea is termed secretory. Diarrhea is voluminous, yellow to white, and watery to pasty. Affected animals are dehydrated, with a "tucked up" abdomen. Subsequent to dehydration, the eyes of affected animals may be recessed deeply into their sockets (sunken eyeballs). Animals that die of enterotoxic *Escherichia coli* infection are often emaciated and have diarrheic feces pasted around their perineum. At necropsy, the small intestine is

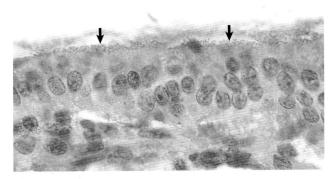

Fig. 7-136 Enterotoxic colibacillosis, jejunum, piglet. Mats *(arrows)* of *Escherichia coli* are attached to the microvillous surface of the enterocytes. H&E stain. *(Courtesy Dr. H. Gelberg, College of Veterinary Medicine, Oregon State University.)*

dilated, flaccid, and filled with translucent, yellow fluid and sometimes gas. Chyle is present in the mesenteric lymphatic vessels similar to animals without enteric disease, indicating that unlike the malabsorptive diseases of the small intestine, absorption proceeds normally in cases of enterotoxic colibacillosis. Microscopically the intestine is also normal. Diagnosis can be made by light microscopic examination in freshly dead animals by noting the presence of bacteria lining the luminal surface of the enterocytes (Fig. 7-136).

Septicemic colibacillosis. Septicemic colibacillosis is a disease of newborn calves, lambs, and occasionally foals that have not received sufficient colostrum to develop immunity. Although the lesions produced are generally those of septicemia, similar to those caused by other organisms, infection can localize in the intestine, causing enteritis. Diagnosis is generally made by finding fibrin in any location in the body, such as the eye, joints, abdomen, heart sac, or chest. The bacteria gain entry to the body through the respiratory system, oral cavity, or umbilicus. Fibrinous arthritis, ophthalmitis, serositis, meningitis, (polyserositis) and white-spotted kidneys (cortical abscesses) characterize the septicemia. Mixed bacterial infections often occur with enterotoxic *Escherichia coli*.

Edema disease. Edema disease, also known as enterotoxemic colibacillosis, is an *Escherichia coli* infection that is specific for pigs. Edema disease is caused by a bacterial enterotoxin (verotoxin) produced in the small intestine and spread hematogenously via induction of IL-8. This interleukin attracts neutrophils that carry the toxin throughout the body. It is generally a disease of pigs 6 to 14 weeks of age and is usually associated with dietary changes at weaning. It is often noted that the best pigs in a group are the ones affected. Edema disease is characterized by neurologic signs

including incoordination, poor balance, weakness, tremors, and convulsions.

Hemolytic *Escherichia coli* proliferates in the small intestine subsequent to dietary changes and produces a heat-labile exotoxin called the edema disease principle. This systemic toxin (angiotoxin) causes generalized vascular endothelial injury of arterioles and arteries, resulting in fluid loss and edema. The edema can be found anywhere but is most characteristic in the gastric submucosa, eyelids (Fig. 7-137), forehead, gallbladder, and mesentery of the spiral colon (Fig. 7-138). In the brain, arterial damage causes focal malacia in the medulla, thalamus, and basal ganglia. These nervous tissue lesions are collectively known as focal symmetric

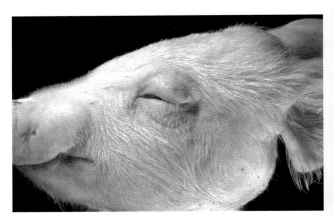

Fig. 7-137 Edema disease, head, pig. The skin of the eyelids, snout, and submandibular area are edematous due to production of angiotoxin by *Escherichia coli*, which increases the permeability of capillaries. *(Courtesy Dr. H. Gelberg, College of Veterinary Medicine, Oregon State University.)*

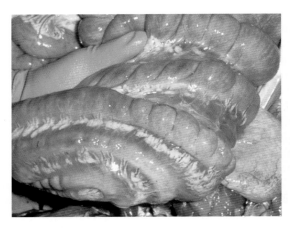

Fig. 7-138 Edema disease, spiral colon, pig. Edema of the mesentery is a result of an angiotoxin produced by *Escherichia coli*. *(Courtesy Dr. M.D. McGavin, College of Veterinary Medicine, University of Tennessee.)*

encephalomalacia or swine cerebral angiopathy and are responsible for the variety of clinical signs. Death is due to an endotoxic shocklike syndrome. Some animals suffer from a Shwartzman-like bilateral renal cortical necrosis. Morbidity within a herd is approximately 35% and all affected animals die.

Postweaning colibacillosis.   Postweaning colibacillosis is another specific disease of pigs caused by a hemolytic *Escherichia coli*. The disease appears identical to enterotoxic colibacillosis of the neonate in that it produces a secretory diarrhea and therefore no lesions. It is a distinct strain of *Escherichia coli*, however, and is associated with feed and management changes at weaning.

Enteroinvasive colibacillosis.   This disease is described in human beings, laboratory animals, and occasionally cattle and pigs. It has not been reported as a field problem in livestock. The pathogenesis of the disease is similar to that of other invasive bacteria such as *Salmonella* spp. In human beings, the colon is affected. A Shiga toxin gene, a locus for enterocyte effacement, and a plasmid encoding for hemolysin are produced by *Escherichia coli*, which results in hemorrhagic colitis and sometimes the hemolytic-uremic syndrome. These strains are also called VTEC or verotoxin *Escherichia coli* strains based on the Vero (African green monkey kidney) cell line on which the bacteria are sometimes grown. Outbreaks of enteroinvasive colibacillosis in human beings are often food-borne illnesses. These organisms are pathogenic because of their acid resistance and ability to survive the acid environment of the stomach. Shiga toxin–producing enterohemorrhagic *Escherichia coli* O157:H7 rarely causes naturally occurring disease in domestic livestock but often contaminates ground beef. Surveys have indicated that O157:H7 *Escherichia coli's* seroprevalence in dairy herds is 38.5%, with an individual cow prevalence of 6.5%, and is most often isolated from the skin surface. This finding is an important reason not to eat undercooked ground beef. Steaks are a different matter because bacterial contamination is only a surface phenomenon and bacteria are killed by surface searing of meat. Experimentally, calves may have necrohemorrhagic or mucohemorrhagic diarrhea develop. Human disease can be serious, resulting in hemorrhagic colitis, thrombocytopenic purpura, and the hemolytic uremic syndrome. Deer, sheep, cattle, horses, dogs, and rabbits, including laboratory rabbits, may be carriers. Stable flies and fecal contamination of a variety of substances may create fomites.

Attaching and effacing *Escherichia coli*.   This disease has been infrequently reported in rabbits, calves, pigs, lambs, dogs, and human beings. The actual incidence of this disease in domestic animals is unknown. Lesions are characterized by *Escherichia coli* attachment to the microvillous border of enterocytes and gallbladder

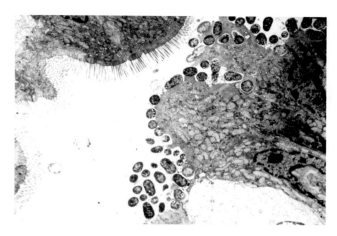

Fig. 7-139   **Attaching and effacing *Escherichia coli*, intestine, rabbit.** Bacterial rods have attached to and effaced the microvillous border of enterocytes. TEM. Uranyl acetate and lead citrate stain. *(From Thulin, J, Kuhlenschmidt M, Gelberg H: Lab Invest 54:719-731, 1991.)*

epithelium via cups and pedestals (Fig. 7-139). Intimin, a bacterial outer membrane protein, facilitates bacterial attachment to the host cell's membrane, resulting in attachment and effacement. Gross lesions are not present except that the intestine is dilated and fluid-filled. Colonization of the epithelium by attaching and effacing *Escherichia coli* is relatively common; disease occurs most often in association with other enteropathogens of calves of this age, namely rotavirus, *Cryptosporidium parvum*, enterotoxigenic *Escherichia coli*, coronavirus, BVD, and coccidia. In contrast to enterotoxic *Escherichia coli* infection, in attaching and effacing *Escherichia coli* infection the brush border of the enterocytes is disrupted and can be seen on select enterocytes in hematoxylin and eosin (H&E) stained tissue sections. Microvillous disruption results in loss of the glycocalyx digestive enzymes, resulting in maldigestion, malabsorption, and diarrhea.

Mucoid enteropathy.   This subacute and fatal disease of young rabbits is characterized by copious quantities of mucus in the feces concurrent with impaction of the cecum and sometimes the sacculated colon. Although the cause is unknown, coliform bacteria are suspect.

Salmonellosis

Salmonella spp. are enteroinvasive bacteria. All known species of *Salmonella* are pathogenic, and it is an important zoonosis and nosocomial infection. Salmonellosis is a significant cause of acute and chronic diarrhea and death in numerous animal species and in human beings. *Salmonella typhimurium* is the second most common food-borne pathogen in human beings. In veterinary medicine, salmonellosis can occur epizootically, enzootically, or sporadically. The species most often isolated from diseased animals include *Salmonella typhimurium*, *Salmonella enteritidis*, *Salmonella dublin*, *Salmonella choleraesuis*, and *Salmonella typhosa*.

The salmonellas are gram-negative, aerobic to facultatively anaerobic and motile. They survive and multiply within phagocytic cells, resulting in granulomatous inflammation. The form of salmonellosis that occurs—septicemic, acute enteric, or chronic enteric—depends on the challenge dosage of the bacterium, previous exposure to the bacterium, and stress factors, such as overcrowding, transport, cold temperatures, feed changes, pregnancy, parturition, surgery, anesthesia, and antibiotic administration. Some recovered animals become carriers and shed the organism in their feces, particularly after stress. This may make diagnosis by culture difficult because carriers may not be ill. Conversely, antibiotic treatment of ill animals may create false-negative bacterial cultures. Although dogs and cats rarely get clinical salmonellosis, 10% are carriers and can infect their human companions. Recently, it has been documented that fatal salmonellosis may occur in cats in association with homemade, raw-meat diets.

The most common route of bacterial entry is fecaloral. Effective hand washing is thus of paramount importance for food handlers. Besides being present in contaminated feed, water, and aerosols, flies and fomites can transmit salmonella. Transplacental infection may also occur. After ingestion, salmonella may colonize regional lymphoid tissue in the oral cavity and gut. Some species are enteroinvasive.

Salmonella enterica serovars choleraesuis and *typhimurium* in pigs have been shown to adhere to apical membranes of M cells, enterocytes, goblet cells, and sites of cellular extrusion. Salmonellas produce disease via enterotoxins, cytotoxins (verotoxins), and endotoxins. Experimental infections of calves with *Salmonella typhimurium* demonstrate up-regulation of CXC chemokines (IL-8, GRO-α, and GCP2), IL-1-β, IL-1R-α, and IL-4 associated with a neutrophilic influx. Once in contact with macrophages of the lamina propria or Peyer's patches, the organisms are phagocytosed and transported to regional lymph nodes or by way of the portal circulation to the liver. The organisms colonize the small intestine, colon, mesenteric lymph nodes, and gallbladder, which may serve as reservoirs in carrier animals. Salmonellosis infects the young more frequently; the young are more severely affected than are adults; and the young are more likely to succumb to septicemia.

Peracute *Salmonella* septicemia. Peracute *Salmonella* septicemia is a disease of calves, foals, and pigs. Young animals are generally at greater risk than older animals, although the reasons for this difference are not understood. In foals, the feces of affected animals are typically green. The species of *Salmonella* most often involved in septicemic salmonellosis is *Salmonella choleraesuis*. Gross lesions of animals dying of peracute *Salmonella* septicemia are minimal and are due to fibrinoid necrosis of blood vessels. Necrosis of blood vessels causes a widespread petechiation and a blue discoloration (cyanosis) of the extremities and ventrum of white pigs. Fibrinous polyserositis may be present. Peracute *Salmonella* septicemia is usually fatal in animals 1 to 6 months of age. Death is usually attributable to disseminated intravascular coagulopathy secondary to the generalized Shwartzman reaction.

Acute enteric salmonellosis. This disease is caused most frequently by *Salmonella typhimurium* and occurs in cattle, pigs, and horses. Carnivores are rarely affected. Characteristic of the disease is diffuse catarrhal enteritis with diffuse fibrinonecrotic ileotyphlocolitis. Intestinal contents are malodorous and contain mucus, fibrin, and occasionally blood. The feces have a septic tank odor. Multiple foci of hepatocellular necrosis and hyperplasia of Kupffer cells (paratyphoid nodules), when present, are characteristic of acute enteric salmonellosis. Lymphadenopathy is usually present. Fibrinous cholecystitis at necropsy is pathognomonic for acute enteric salmonellosis in calves.

Chronic enteric salmonellosis. This disease occurs in pigs, cattle, and horses. Lesions are seen principally in pigs that have discrete foci of necrosis and ulceration, principally in the cecum and colon. These are termed button ulcers (Figs. 7-140 and 7-141).

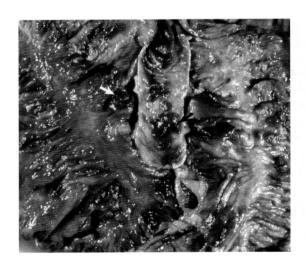

Fig. 7-140 **Button ulcers (*arrows*), colon, pig.** Multiple foci of necrosis (infarcts) due to chronic enteric salmonellas are termed "button ulcers" and are pathognomonic for this disease in North America and in other areas where hog cholera has been eradicated. The morphology of this lesion is attributable to bacterial toxin-induced vasculitis and thrombosis of blood vessels in the lamina propria and submucosa resulting in focal intestinal infarcts. *(Courtesy Dr. H. Gelberg, College of Veterinary Medicine, Oregon State University.)*

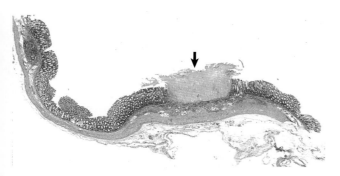

Fig. 7-141 **Chronic enteric salmonellosis, colon, pig.** Multiple foci of mucosal necrosis *(arrow)* are termed "button ulcers" and are pathognomonic for chronic enteric salmonellosis in hog cholera–free areas. H&E stain. *(Courtesy Dr. M.D. McGavin, College of Veterinary Medicine, University of Tennessee.)*

Additionally, because salmonellosis causes vascular thrombosis and pigs have poor or no collateral blood supply to the rectum (cranial hemorrhoidal artery), in affected animals rectal strictures develop, with resultant abdominal distention secondary to fecal retention.

Clostridial enteritis

Many diseases that affect animals and human beings are caused by clostridial organisms. This discussion is limited to those clostridia that produce diarrheal disease. All clostridial enteritides produce enterotoxemias.

Clostridium perfringens is a gram-positive, anaerobic bacillus that normally inhabits the gastrointestinal tract and is ubiquitously present in the environment. It is the most important cause of clostridial enteritis in domestic animals. At least 17 exotoxins have been described, but only 4 are believed to be involved in the pathogenesis of disease. These spore-forming bacilli produce their toxins when circumstances provide them with an excess of growth that requires nutrients in an anaerobic environment. The four major toxins—α,β,ε, and ι—are used to classify the toxigenic types of *Clostridium perfringens* into five major groupings: A through E. The toxins are protein exotoxins, some of which are proenzymes. Some of the toxins have enzymatic activity. *Clostridium perfringens* type A produces the α-toxin responsible for necrotic enteritis of birds, enterotoxemia of calves and lambs, necrotizing enterocolitis of piglets, canine hemorrhagic enteritis, and possibly equine colitis. Type B produces α-,β-, and ε-toxins and the diseases lamb dysentery, hemorrhagic enteritis of neonatal calves and foals, and hemorrhagic enterotoxemia of sheep. Type C produces α- and β-toxins and necrotic enteritis of birds, hemorrhagic enterotoxemia of neonatal farm animal

species, and struck of sheep. Type D produces α- and ε-toxins and pulpy kidney disease of lambs and enterocolitis of goats of all ages. Type E produces α- and ι-toxins and enteritis of lagomorphs and possibly enterotoxemia in calves and lambs.

Enterotoxigenic strains of *Clostridium perfringens*, particularly type A, are responsible for clostridial food poisoning. This generally occurs when cooked foods are improperly stored, and spores that survive the cooking environment germinate and produce enterotoxin.

Enterotoxemia. Enterotoxemia is produced by one of the five *Clostridium perfringens* types described previously. Type D occurs most often. Clostridial enterotoxemia most often affects the better-fleshed animals within a group. Outbreaks often follow an abrupt change in the amount or quality of feed such as occurs in an animal being "finished" for sale or slaughter. In foals, enterotoxemia has been associated with feeding materials rich in carbohydrates and proteins. This diet leads to a change in the intestinal microbial balance. *Clostridium perfringens* proliferates and produces abundant toxin. Clinical signs may be absent before death or may include diarrhea, sometimes with blood. Glycosuria occurs only in lambs with enterotoxemia and is a helpful feature in preliminary necropsy diagnosis.

The small intestine, the target organ of clostridial enterotoxemia, typically has serosal and mucosal petechiae, ecchymoses, and paintbrush or diffuse hemorrhage similar in appearance to those of intestinal strangulation. The intestines are atonic and dilated. Emphysematous enteritis is variably present, as is coagulative necrosis of skeletal musculature. Congestive splenomegaly is present. Upon exposure to enterotoxin, villous tip enterocytes and midvillous enterocytes degenerate and are sloughed into the intestinal lumen, leaving denuded basement membranes. The exposed basement membranes allow fluid leakage and attract leukocytes into the lamina propria. Death is usually rapid.

***Clostridium perfringens* type A.** *Clostridium perfringens* type A is the most frequently occurring clostridium in mammals and birds. It is also the most common clostridium found in the environment. *Clostridium perfringens* type A produces enteric disease in a great variety of animals. These diarrheal diseases are generally mild with minimal damage noted in the intestinal mucosa. In addition to enteritis, infection produces gas gangrene and other anaerobic wound infections. In the western United States, it causes hemorrhagic abomasitis in young ruminants, often accompanied by severe diarrhea. In the Pacific Northwest, principally in Washington and Oregon, a condition called yellow lamb disease is associated with *Clostridium perfringens* type A. Death is rapid and accompanied by clinical and pathologic signs of red cell lysis, hence the yellow discoloration of the carcass.

Clostridium perfringens type B. *Clostridium perfringens* type B is the cause of lamb dysentery. This is generally a disease of very young lambs, although older animals may be affected in prolonged disease outbreaks. Unexpected death is usual, but occasionally there is an antecedent anorexia and abdominal pain with or without severe bloody diarrhea. Other young ruminants and foals may also be affected. This disease occurs sporadically in the United States but is more common in Europe, South Africa, and the Middle East.

Clostridium perfringens type C. Enterotoxic hemorrhagic enteritis affects calves, lambs, and foals during the first few days of life and piglets during the first 8 hours of life. Clinical signs vary from none to bloody diarrhea. When piglets are affected, the whole litter dies. Lesions at necropsy include hemorrhagic or necrotizing enteritis of the small intestines, sometimes with gas in the lumen and within the walls of the intestine (Figs. 7-142 and 7-143). Struck is a disease affecting adult sheep, goats, and feedlot cattle in winter and early spring. Also caused by *Clostridium perfringens* type C, it is characterized by hemorrhagic enteritis with ulceration, ascites, and peritonitis.

Clostridium perfringens type D. This bacterium affects fattening sheep, goats, and calves. The disease is diet-related and associated with grain overload or "overeating disease." The sudden change in diet promotes growth of organisms in the small intestine. The disease is often characterized by unexpected death sometimes preceded by central nervous system signs or "blind staggers." Endothelial cell damage is produced by a bacterial toxin (angiotoxin). This lesion can result in

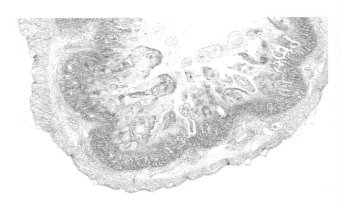

Fig. 7-143   Clostridial enteritis, small intestine, pig. Nonspecific necrotizing enteritis results from the toxins produced by *Clostridium perfringens* type C. H&E stain. *(Courtesy Dr. H. Gelberg, College of Veterinary Medicine, Oregon State University.)*

bilateral symmetric encephalomalacia, which is similar in its regional distribution to edema disease of pigs (swine cerebral angiopathy). Lesions of *Clostridium perfringens* type D infection are multisystem hemorrhages, particularly of serosal surfaces. Pericardial effusion is present along with mild gastroenteritis. The angiotoxin produces "pulpy kidney disease" of sheep.

Clostridium perfringens type E. Case reports of necrohemorrhagic diarrhea associated with *Clostridium perfringens* type E infection are poorly documented. It is safest to state that *Clostridium perfringens* type E may rarely cause enterotoxemia of lambs, calves, and rabbits.

Peracute hemorrhagic gastroenteritis of dogs. Known as canine hemorrhagic gastroenteritis, the cause of this disease is undiscovered, but is considered likely a result of infection with *Clostridium perfringens* type E. The disease most often occurs in dogs of toy and miniature breeds younger than 2 years. Blood is observed at the anus before death. As the name of the disease denotes, there is hemorrhagic necrosis of the gastrointestinal mucosa anywhere from the stomach caudally. Numerous clostridial organisms are present in the intestinal debris but are not attached to intact mucosa. Unlike parvoviral enteritis in which crypts are preferentially destroyed, in hemorrhagic gastroenteritis the crypts are spared.

Lincomycin or antibiotic enteritis. This enteritis is associated with antibiotic administration and is seen most commonly in rabbits and horses; both are cecal fermenters. It has been suggested, but not proven, that antibiotic administration causes death of normal enteric flora, which allows overgrowth of *Clostridium perfringens* type A. Clinical signs and gross and microscopic lesions are similar to those observed in animals with

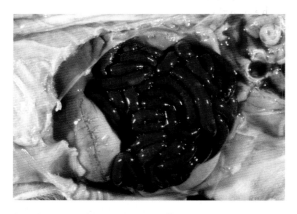

Fig. 7-142   Enterotoxemia, small intestine, pig. The entire small intestinal mucosa is hemorrhagic. Necrosis can extend through the muscularis mucosa and is caused by toxins of the *Clostridium perfringens* type C group acting directly on the intestinal mucosa in the intestinal lumen. The entire litter of piglets was affected. *(Courtesy Dr. H. Gelberg, College of Veterinary Medicine, Oregon State University.)*

Clostridium spp. enteritis, but bacterial organisms are often lacking.

Clostridium piliformis.   Commonly called Tyzzer's disease, *Clostridium piliformis* infects multiple mammalian species. Although pathogen entry is usually via the intestine, the principal target is the liver, but lesions also occur in the intestine and heart. Intestinal involvement is variable and most common in rodents and rabbits. Colitis occurs in some cats. The enteric manifestations of Tyzzer's disease are generally in the distal small intestine, particularly the ileum. Mucosal necrosis and edema extend into the muscularis. Definitive diagnosis is made by finding the causative bacillus (best done with silver stains, such as Dieterle's or Steiner's) in the characteristic hepatic or intestinal lesions (Fig. 7-144). The target organs of *Clostridium piliformis* vary among affected animals.

Clostridium difficile.   *Clostridium difficile* spores are common in the environment and in the intestinal tract of many mammals. They cause pseudomembranous colitis in primates including human beings, hemorrhagic necrotizing enterocolitis in foals, necrotizing typhlocolitis in horses (colitis X) and possibly cats, and enteritis in a variety of laboratory animals. *Clostridium difficile* also affects suckling pigs in outbreaks characterized by mesocolonic edema and typhlocolitis. Dogs, especially those hospitalized, may also shed the organism. *Clostridium difficile's* disease producing ability in the dog is not understood, but its zoonotic potential may be important. The induction of disease by *Clostridium difficile* is likely dose-related, but the reasons for bacterial overgrowth, apart from those caused by oral antibiotic administration, are not understood. The lesions are similar to those produced by *Clostridium perfringens* infection.

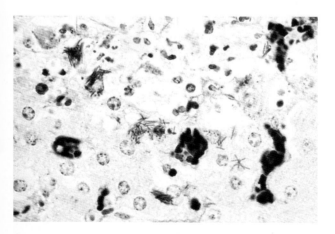

Fig. 7-144   Tyzzer's disease, intestine, foal. Criss-crossed bacilli resembling Chinese characters or pickup sticks are diagnostic of infection with *Clostridium piliformis*. Warthin-Starry stain. *(Courtesy Dr. H. Gelberg, College of Veterinary Medicine, Oregon State University.)*

Clostridium spiroforme.   *Clostridium spiroforme* causes enterotoxemia in lagomorphs and rodents. The bacterium is semicircular in vivo and has a coiled appearance in vitro when bacteria are joined end to end. In the rabbit, weaning and/or antibiotic treatment with a concomitant change in cecal flora precede diarrhea and death. Lesions include a dilated cecum with liquid contents. As is the case with other clostridia, the cause is confirmed by mouse lethality studies or Vero cell cytotoxicity studies; the appropriate toxin is isolated from intestinal contents soon after death of the animal.

Clostridium colinum.   Also known as quail disease, this ulcerative colitis is restricted to gallinaceous birds. The disease occurs in birds secondary to stress that is often a result of intercurrent infections. Classically, there is hemorrhagic enteritis of the small intestine often accompanied by necroulcerative enterotyphlitis. Necrohemorrhagic hepatosplenitis is often present. Death is rapid and losses are high, especially in quail.

Campylobacteriosis (*Lawsonia*)

Campylobacter spp. are the cause of a proliferative segmental enteropathy in a variety of species, including human beings. *Campylobacter* are curved, gram-negative, motile, obligate intracellular bacteria that cannot be grown on artificial media. 16S ribosomal DNA of organisms from lesions shows a close resemblance to that of *Lawsonia intracellularis* of pigs, and isolates can cross-infect among species. Lesions of proliferative enteropathy have been reported in pigs, dogs, horses, sheep, rabbits, guinea pigs, hamsters, rats, ferrets, foxes, cervids, monkeys, ostriches, and emus. In the dog, the majority of cases occur in puppies younger than 3 months. Clinically, diarrhea is of 5 to 15 days' duration. The diarrhea is mucoid or watery, with or without blood, and accompanied by partial anorexia, vomiting, and a slight fever. Lesions consist of surface erosions and proliferation of cryptal enterocytes with the presence of bacteria in the apical cytoplasm of affected cells. Diagnosis depends on characteristic histopathologic findings of crypt cell proliferation and by the presence of comma-shaped bacteria in the intestinal crypt epithelial cytoplasm. *Campylobacter* infections from poultry are an important issue in food safety and thus an important emerging zoonotic disease.

Mycobacterial enteritis

Intestinal mycobacteriosis.   Intestinal tuberculosis, caused by *Mycobacterium tuberculosis* and *Mycobacterium bovis*, is an uncommon disease in cattle, nursing calves, nonhuman primates, and human beings. Although historically associated with drinking unpasteurized milk, more recently intestinal tuberculosis is an important AIDS-associated disease in human beings.

The bacteria are ingested and then taken up by the M cells of the GALT, particularly in the distal ileum. Like Johne's disease of cattle, intestinal tuberculosis is a chronic wasting disease characterized by a roughened, rugaelike appearance to the intestine.

In small animals, it is sometimes clinically possible to palpate the thickened intestine. A thickened colon is sometimes palpable rectally in large animals. Granulomatous lymphadenopathy is often present, sometimes with mineralization and necrosis. The intestinal lamina propria and submucosa, as in Johne's disease, are enlarged and the architecture distorted by epithelioid macrophages and giant cells. Fewer acid-fast organisms are seen as compared with Johne's disease. In most cases of *Mycobacterium avium-intracellulare*-induced intestinal tuberculosis, lepromatous (noncaseating) granulomatous inflammation occurs similar to that of Johne's disease of small ruminants and dogs.

Pigs often contract intestinal tuberculosis as a result of the husbandry practice of feeding them avian litter as an inexpensive protein source. As might be expected, early lesions develop in the retropharyngeal lymph nodes.

DISEASES IN ANIMAL SPECIES
INTESTINAL DISEASES OF HORSES

Bacterial

***Rhodococcus equi* enteritis.**   *Rhodococcus equi* is a soil saprophyte and a normal inhabitant of the equine intestine. The disease caused by this large, potentially zoonotic, gram-positive, facultatively anaerobic rod is often characterized by pulmonary pyogranulomas in foals under 6 months and in immunocompromised adult horses and human beings, or those with intercurrent disease (AIDS patients). The bacterium is not resistant to neutrophil-mediated destruction but can resist the intracellular environment of macrophages. All pathogenic *Rhodococcus equi* isolated from horses but not human beings have a large plasmid and the encoded surface-expressed lipoprotein VapA, which is associated with virulence. The frequent intercurrence of helminths and *Rhodococcus equi* infection suggests that migrating larvae aid in distributing the bacterium through the body of the foal. Stringent control of helminth infections may therefore help to reduce or eliminate *Rhodococcus equi* infection.

Equine abortion, pneumonia, and placentitis have been associated with infection, as have sporadic infections, sometimes fatal, of a wide variety of mammalian species. *Rhodococcus equi* can be isolated from a large number of otherwise healthy mammals of different species.

When coughed up and swallowed in large numbers, the bacteria enter the intestinal M cells overlying the GALT, resulting in pyogranulomatous lymphadenitis of GALT and lymph nodes and pyogranulomatous ulcerative enterotyphlocolitis.

Intestinal infection commences in Peyer's patches, which are ultimately replaced by granulomatous inflammation, abscess formation, and necrotic tissue, and the patches are ulcerated. Infection then spreads to mesenteric lymph nodes with a similar result. Macrophages, often laden with intact bacteria, fill the intestinal lamina propria and submucosa, resulting in a markedly thickened, corrugated intestine. The grossly observable abscesses and foci of necrosis and ulceration often correspond to the distribution of GALT (Fig. 7-145). Mesenteric, cecal, and colonic lymph nodes are enlarged, firm, and gray (Fig. 7-146). They may contain granulomas

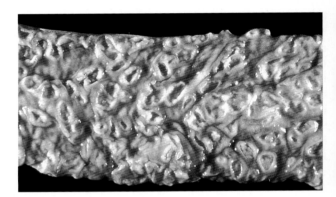

Fig. 7-145   Multifocal ulcerative colitis, colon, horse.
Rhodococcus equi infection causes multiple mucosal ulcers centered over gut-associated lymphoid tissue. *(Courtesy Dr. H. Gelberg, College of Veterinary Medicine, Oregon State University.)*

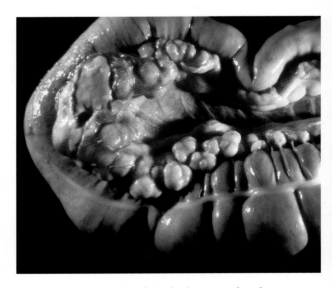

Fig. 7-146   Mesenteric lymphadenitis, colon, horse.
Infection of colic lymph nodes with *Rhodococcus equi* causes pyogranulomatous lymphadenomegaly. *(Courtesy Dr. H. Gelberg, College of Veterinary Medicine, Oregon State University.)*

and abscesses. The large number of macrophages and multinucleated giant cells within the lamina propria and lymphoid tissue is characteristic of this infection. Bacteria may be seen within these cells with Giemsa and tissue Gram stains. The florid inflammatory infiltrate expands the intestinal villi and may distort the crypts of the entire intestinal tract.

Contamination of cutaneous wounds by *Rhodococcus equi* may result in cutaneous ulcerative lymphangitis in horses. Swine cervical lymphadenopathy may also be a result of infection.

Rickettsial

Equine monocytic ehrlichiosis. Equine monocytic ehrlichiosis, also known as Potomac horse fever, was first reported in 1983. It appears that the disease was present for at least the previous 5 years. First described in the Potomac River valley of Maryland, Virginia, and Pennsylvania, it is now found throughout the United States and elsewhere. The common denominator is a proximity of horses to slow-moving bodies of water. Fever, depression, severe diarrhea, dehydration, and laminitis characterize the disease. Equine monocytic ehrlichiosis is apparently the same disease known as churrido equino (equine scours), which has been present for more than a century in Uruguay and Brazil.

The causative agent, *Neorickettsia risticii* (formally called *Ehrlichia risticii*)–an intracytoplasmic rickettsial pathogen of epithelial cells, macrophages, and monocytes–is found in trematodes in freshwater snails. A reduction in pollution levels of the Potomac River basin is believed to have resulted in an increase in the number of freshwater snails. Mayflies and caddis flies have been implicated in transmission. Horses are believed to become infected by eating the dead flies that may accumulate in water buckets and feed troughs. Rickettsia are often transmitted by arthropods, and this disease is seasonal in northern latitudes (May through September). Without treatment, one third of cases with diarrhea die as a result of dehydration.

Clinical signs associated with equine monocytic ehrlichiosis include fever, watery diarrhea, depression, dehydration, variable colic, and subcutaneous edema of the thorax, abdomen, and hind legs. Experimental evidence indicates that *Neorickettsia risticii* may be abortigenic. The gross lesions of Potomac horse fever are subtle, consisting of congestion, petechiae, and edema, primarily in the cecum and colon. There is a variable superficial necrotizing enterocolitis. Sometimes the small intestine is affected. Intestinal contents are tan, watery, and malodorous.

Because the experimental reproduction of clinical disease in germ-free animals has not been done, the microscopic appearance of lesions is not certain. Intercurrent bacteria may be responsible for some of the reported lesions. Interestingly, horses with Potomac horse fever have a mild necrotizing typhlocolitis similar in distribution to colitis X and enteric salmonellosis. The nature of the gross lesions is somewhat controversial because experimental infections produce variable results. Like hog cholera, Potomac horse fever is sometimes associated with concurrent *Salmonella* infection, perhaps accounting for the *Salmonella*-like lesions.

Monocytes and macrophages in all layers of the intestine can be demonstrated with stains such as Giemsa to contain *Ehrlichia* organisms.

Idiopathic

Equine granulomatous enteritis. This sporadic disease, characterized by wasting and hypoalbuminemia, has been reported most often in thoroughbred and standardbred horses younger than 5 years old. The pathogenesis of the disease is unknown. In a few cases, *Mycobacterium avium* was isolated from lesions. The disease is characterized by diffuse or segmental transmural noncaseating granulomatous inflammation of the small and occasionally large intestines. Giant cells are present in about half the cases. The result is a notably thickened bowel (Figs. 7-147 and 7-148).

Clostridial enteritis (colitis X). The severe diarrhea seen in cases of colitis X contains no blood and is rapidly fatal. The cause is unknown. However, the disease is associated with certain environmental and clinical variables. These include exhaustion; shock or other stressors; enterotoxemia, perhaps associated

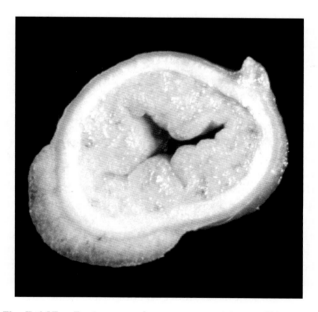

Fig. 7-147 **Equine granulomatous enteritis, small intestine (formalin fixed), horse.** The lamina propria is greatly thickened by granulomatous inflammatory cells. *(Courtesy Dr. H. Gelberg, College of Veterinary Medicine, Oregon State University.)*

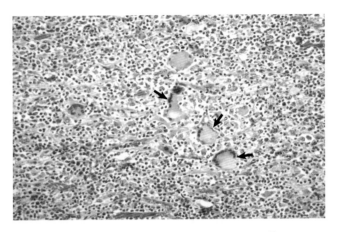

Fig. 7-148   Equine granulomatous enteritis, small intestine, horse. Mononuclear inflammatory cells (macrophages, lymphocytes, plasma cells) and multinucleate giant cells (*arrows*) are present in the lamina propria and submucosa. H&E stain. *(Courtesy Dr. H. Gelberg, College of Veterinary Medicine, Oregon State University.)*

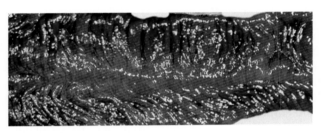

Fig. 7-149   Clostridial enteritis, colon, horse. Commonly called "colitis X," this disease is characterized by mucosal edema, congestion, and hemorrhage. The lesions are attributed to endotoxemia caused by *Clostridium perfringens* type A or *Clostridium difficile.* *(Courtesy Dr. H. Gelberg, College of Veterinary Medicine, Oregon State University.)*

with overgrowth of *Clostridium perfringens* type A (antibiotic enteritis); *Clostridium difficile;* or anaphylaxis. Lesions are limited to the mucosa of the cecum and colon and consist of edema, congestion, and hemorrhage (Fig. 7-149). The location and nature of these lesions overlap with those of acute enteric salmonellosis and equine monocytic ehrlichiosis. Therefore elimination of *Salmonella* spp. and *Ehrlichia risticii* as causes is necessary before a diagnosis of colitis X can be made. Thus colitis X is a diagnosis made by exclusion of other causes. At necropsy, in addition to the intestinal lesions, evidence of endotoxic shock, such as disseminated intravascular coagulopathy, thrombosis, and hemorrhage of the adrenal cortices (Waterhouse-Friderichsen syndrome) can be present, as in salmonellosis and other septicemic diseases.

Hemorrhagic fibrinonecrotic duodenitis-proximal jejunitis.   Also known as anterior enteritis and gastroduodenojejunitis, the morphologic description of the lesions is the same as the name of this idiopathic disease. The disease is characterized microscopically by submucosal edema and a neutrophilic infiltrate of the submucosa and lamina propria. *Salmonella* and clostridial infections are suspected as the cause. This disease occurs in horses older than 9 years of age, and the definitive diagnosis is made at necropsy by the characteristic hemorrhagic necrotizing lesions in the small intestine. The duodenum is always involved; jejunal involvement is variable.

Chronic eosinophilic gastroenteritis and multisystemic eosinophilic epitheliotropic disease. Soft stools accompanied by weight loss characterize this uncommon condition. The inflammatory reaction consists of eosinophils among other inflammatory cells in both nodular and diffuse accumulations within all portions and layers of the gastrointestinal system, salivary glands, and mesenteric lymph nodes. A circulating eosinophilia may be present. Clinical signs relating to the gastrointestinal system may include watery diarrhea and hypoproteinemia secondary to protein-losing enteropathy. The histology of the condition, especially the presence of eosinophils, suggests a hypersensitivity reaction that in at least one instance was associated with *Pythium* spp. infection. With the exception of the rare cases with a specific etiologic agent, affected horses die. The disease is associated with an up-regulated T_H2 response and increased IL-5 production. In humans and occasionally in horses, the lymphoplasmacytic infiltrates in this condition are precursors to lymphosarcoma.

Anaphylactoid purpura.   Leukocytoclastic vasculitis associated with numerous discrete foci of necrosis and hemorrhage throughout the intestine and in the mucosa of the larynx and skeletal muscles, is termed anaphylactoid purpura in the horse, and Henoch-Schöenlein disease in human beings. Anecdotal evidence suggests that an Arthus-like hypersensitivity reaction to a streptococcal respiratory infection is the mechanism of lesion production.

INTESTINAL DISEASES OF RUMINANTS
Viral
Bovine viral diarrhea.   Also known as mucosal disease, bovine viral diarrhea (BVD) affects cattle of all ages but is most common in animals 8 months to 2 years of age. In this respect, clinical cases are typically younger than in animals susceptible to Johne's disease. Animals infected early in life with noncytopathic BVD virus develop a persistent infection. Later in life, if exposed to cytopathic virus, they may have disease develop. Clinical signs may include anorexia, depression, profuse watery diarrhea with staining of the perineum and tail, agalactia,

pyrexia, rumen atony, ptyalism, lacrimation, and a mucopurulent nasal discharge. Multifocal, sharply demarcated erosions and ulcers in the tongue, gingiva, palate, esophagus, rumen, abomasum (Fig. 7-150), and coronary bands of the hooves characterize BVD. In the

intestine, the characteristic lesion is sharply demarcated foci of necrosis in the epithelium over the GALT (Figs. 7-151 and 7-152). Calves infected in utero may have cerebellar hypoplasia, cataracts, microphthalmia, renal dysplasia, and other congenital defects develop. Abortions, stillbirths, and mummified fetuses can also result from in utero infection. Aborted calves often have enlarged hemal lymph nodes. BVD is caused by a pestivirus. Morbidity in a herd varies from 2% to 50%. All affected animals die.

Lesions in the stratified squamous epithelium begin in the stratum spinosum. Necrosis of the epithelium is soon followed by the formation of erosions and ulcerations. Villous and crypt enterocytes become necrotic. There is lympholysis in the GALT. Follicular medullary regions of intestinal lymphoid tissue may be filled with cell debris and dead enterocytes. There is commonly a fibrinonecrotic pseudomembrane over the damaged GALT. Ulcerative lesions have already been described in the oral cavity, tongue, esophagus, and rumen.

A more common outcome from BVD infection occurs in immunocompetent animals that are seronegative at the time of exposure to either the cytopathic or noncytopathic virus. Variable signs develop, but they are mostly mild or subclinical. Most cattle in the United States have serologic evidence of exposure to nonvaccine BVD. Exotic ruminants may also become infected. Under certain circumstances pigs may become subclinically infected. This is of interest because the viruses of BVD and hog cholera are antigenically closely related. This may cause confusing serologic results when testing hogs for cholera. New World camelids may also succumb to BVD infection, although infections are often subclinical. The diagnosis of persistent infection is by immunohistochemistry of skin biopsies because calves shed large amounts of virus through the skin.

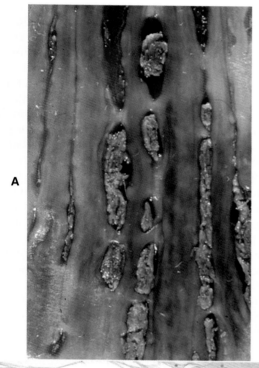

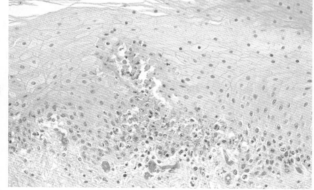

Fig. 7-150   Acute multifocal esophageal ulcers, esophagus, cow. A, Grossly, there are multiple sharply demarcated ulcers *(vertically linear red streaks)* and similar areas covered by diphtheritic membranes *(vertically linear yellow-brown streaks).* The cause is the pestivirus of bovine viral diarrhea. **B,** Microscopically, there is a focus of necrosis of cells of the stratum basale and stratum spinosum caused by the pestivirus of bovine viral diarrhea. **H&E stain.** *(A, Courtesy Department of Veterinary Biosciences, College of Veterinary Medicine, The Ohio State University; and Noah's Arkive, College of Veterinary Medicine, The University of Georgia. B, Courtesy Dr. J.S. Haynes, College of Veterinary Medicine, Iowa State University; and Noah's Arkive, College of Veterinary Medicine, The University of Georgia.)*

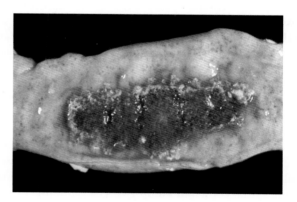

Fig. 7-151   Bovine viral diarrhea, ileum, mucosa, cow. Peyer's patches and the overlying epithelium are necrotic and covered with suppurative exudate. *(Courtesy Dr. H. Gelberg, College of Veterinary Medicine, Oregon State University.)*

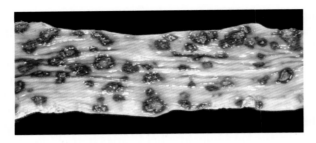

Fig. 7-152   Multifocal ulcerative colitis, bison, colon. Multiple mucosal ulcers were caused by bovine viral diarrhea virus. *(Courtesy Dr. H. Gelberg, College of Veterinary Medicine, Oregon State University.)*

Feedlot cattle that are persistently infected are believed to be more susceptible to mannheimiosis, chronic pneumonia and polyarthritis syndrome, salmonellosis, infectious bovine rhinotracheitis, bovine respiratory syncytial virus, and mycoses. Other diagnostic means are virus isolation, reverse transcription (RT)-PCR, and antigen capture enzyme-linked immunosorbent assay (ELISA).

Rinderpest.   Lesions similar to those of BVD occur in cattle with rinderpest. This morbillivirus disease of cattle, however, has characteristic multinucleate enterocytes in the intestinal lesions that do not occur in BVD. Rinderpest does not occur in the United States or Europe, but it is a significant disease in Africa and Asia. In immunologically naïve populations of animals, morbidity and mortality may be high. Recovered animals have solid immunity. Vaccines are efficacious.

Malignant catarrhal fever.   Caused by closely related rhadinoviruses (γ-herpesviruses), malignant catarrhal fever occurs in a variety of species of ruminants, including cervids and bison. The African form of the disease, caused by alcelaphine herpesvirus-1 (AHV-1) is common in wildebeests and other ruminants. In the United States and worldwide, ovine herpesvirus-2 (OHV-2), caprine herpesvirus-2 (CpHV-2), and white-tailed deer herpesvirus (MCF-WTD) are most often reported in ruminants. The respiratory form of the disease, associated with keratoconjunctivitis, is most commonly seen in cattle in the United States.

Lesions include widespread lymphoplasmacytic necrotizing arteritis and phlebitis of the subcutis and especially in the rete mirabile surrounding the base of the pituitary gland. Hoof walls may be shed. Coagulation necrosis is found in lymph nodes, and lymphoplasmacytic infiltrates are present in the retina, myocardium, brain, spinal cord, and meninges. The alimentary form of the disease is characterized as multifocal ulcerative stomatitis, glossitis, esophagitis, abomasitis, and enterotyphlocolitis associated with vasculitis. Hemorrhagic cystitis may also be present.

Winter dysentery.   Winter dysentery is a somewhat enigmatic, acute, generally nonfatal disease of adult cattle. As the disease progresses in a herd, virtually all members become ill. As the name implies, it is a seasonal disease and additionally occurs only in northern latitudes. Catarrhal ileitis and jejunitis characterize this highly contagious disease.

Although its cause is unknown, a coronavirus has been implicated as causative and can sometimes be demonstrated immunohistochemically in colonic basal enterocytes of affected animals. Acute onset of profuse diarrhea, decreased milk production in dairy cattle, variable depression, and anorexia are characteristic. Malodorous green to black (melena) diarrhea lasts for up to 4 days and may contain fresh blood and mucus. Immunity in dairy herds is protective for years. Older animals are more severely affected than are younger ones. Calves appear to be refractory to disease development.

Mild lesions are noted in the rare animal that dies of winter dysentery. The intestinal mucosa is intact, but there is variable congestion and petechiae of the abomasum and small intestine. The intestine may be atonic. The colon may have congestion and hemorrhage of the colonic mucosal folds, a nonspecific lesion associated with tenesmus (tiger striping).

Diagnosis is generally made by epizootic information, clinical signs, its seasonal occurrence, and lack of significant mortality.

Bovine torovirus diarrhea.   The shedding of bovine torovirus (Breda virus, BoTV) has been associated with diarrhea of neonatal veal calves. BoTV is a single-stranded, enveloped RNA virus, which currently cannot be grown in cell culture. BoTV is associated with the presence of other enteropathogens of neonates, including rotavirus, coronavirus, *Cryptosporidium*, *Salmonella*, and *Giardia*. Although it is not uncommon to have intercurrent infections producing diarrhea in calves, especially in the presence of immunosuppression, malnutrition, and other stressors, BoTV may cause disease independently. Necrosis and sloughing of enterocytes on the middle and lower villi, extending into the crypts, are noted on histologic examination. Diagnosis is confirmed by antigen-capture ELISA or RT-PCR in feces in the absence of evidence of other enteric pathogens. Death, when it occurs, is due to dehydration.

Bacterial

Paratuberculosis.   Paratuberculosis or Johne's disease has been described in numerous ruminant species. In cattle, the disease is characterized by intractable diarrhea, emaciation, and hypoproteinemia in animals older than 19 months. In the average infected herd, 32% to 42% of animals are infected. In small ruminants (sheep and goats), the clinical disease is similar to that observed in cattle except that diarrhea does not occur. The pygmy goat is an exception to the course of disease in small ruminants in that some pygmy goats have explosive diarrhea develop and die unexpectedly. In other ruminants, the disease has a protracted course and is considered a wasting disease because of the loss of body mass (Fig. 7-153). Ruminants are infected from feces-contaminated soil. Newer methods of bacterial classification suggest that the causative bacterium *Mycobacterium paratuberculosis* should be reclassified as *Mycobacterium avium* ssp. *paratuberculosis*.

The causative organisms are very resistant to environmental stressors, particularly in regions with acid soils. After ingestion, the bacilli penetrate the gastrointestinal mucosa and are taken up by macrophages. Lesions in the lamina propria of the intestines, particularly in the ileum, include the accumulation of macrophages. There is little correlation between the severity of the gross lesions and the severity of clinical disease. An age-related immune resistance to infection and disease develops in animals older than 2 months. Fetuses can be infected, but disease is delayed until the animals are much older. Isolation of newborns from fecal contamination is a useful measure to reduce the incidence of infection in a particular herd.

Diagnosis is made by observing clinical signs together with the signalment. The gross lesion in Johne's disease is a chronic, segmental thickening of the ileum, cecum, and proximal colon (Fig. 7-154). The ileocecal valve region is usually affected. Affected segments have a variably thickened, rough, rugose mucosa, often with multiple foci of ulceration. There is mesenteric lymphadenopathy.

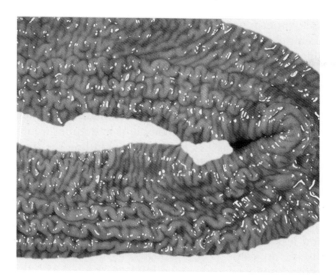

Fig. 7-154   Granulomatous enteritis, Johne's disease (*Mycobacterium avium* ssp. *paratuberculosis*), ileum, sheep. There is notable thickening of the mucosa, which is smooth and shiny (intact) and not ulcerated. *(Courtesy Dr. M.D. McCracken, College of Veterinary Medicine, University of Tennessee; and Noah's Arkive, College of Veterinary Medicine, The University of Georgia.)*

Noncaseating granulomas contain numerous foamy macrophages with large numbers of acid-fast organisms (Fig. 7-155). In contrast, sheep, goats, and deer may have tuberculoid (caseating) granulomas in the intestines, lymphatics, and lymph nodes. These granulomas

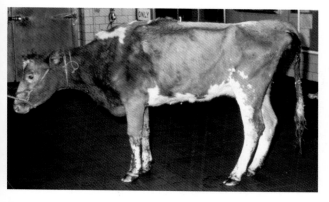

Fig. 7-153   Granulomatous enteritis, Johne's disease (*Mycobacterium avium* ssp. *paratuberculosis*), cow. There is chronic wasting and diarrhea in this 18-month-old heifer. The age at which this cow showed clinical signs is not typical of the disease. Signs usually occur two or more years after initial infection. *(Courtesy College of Veterinary Medicine, Cornell University.)*

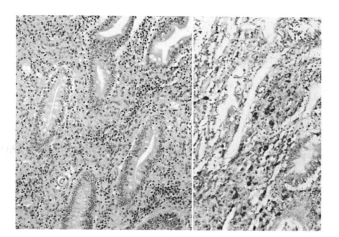

Fig. 7-155   Granulomatous enteritis, Johne's disease (*Mycobacterium avium* ssp. *paratuberculosis*), small intestine, cow. A, The lamina propria of the intestine is markedly expanded by granulomatous inflammatory cells, which compress the crypts and eventually result in their loss (atrophy). H&E stain. **B,** *Mycobacterium*-containing macrophages distend the lamina propria. Ziehl-Neelsen stain. (**A** and **B,** *Courtesy Dr. P.N. Nation, Animal Pathology Services; and Noah's Arkive, College of Veterinary Medicine, The University of Georgia.)*

are sometimes mineralized and contain whorled accumulations of epithelioid macrophages with variable numbers of Langhans'-type giant cells. It is more difficult to find acid-fast mycobacteria in these mature granulomas.

Mycobacterium avium ssp. *paratuberculosis* can be isolated from feces of affected animals, from diseased intestines and regional lymph nodes, and sometimes from a variety of other tissues and fluids, including the liver, uterus, fetus, milk, urine, and semen. Acid-fast bacteria in rectal mucosal scrapings are found in 60% of the cases. Hepatic microgranulomas occur in about 25% of affected animals. Aortic mineralization (arteriosclerosis), when it occurs in association with the clinical signs and lesions of paratuberculosis, is specific for Johne's disease in cattle. The pathogenesis of this vascular lesion is not well understood but is associated with the severe cachexia associated with the disease. The epizootiology of Johne's disease leads many to believe it is one of the most important diseases facing the dairy industry. Speculation has existed for many years that Johne's disease is zoonotic and somehow causative of Crohn's disease in human beings.

Hemorrhagic bowel syndrome of dairy cattle. Also known as fatal jejunal hemorrhage syndrome and intraluminal-intramural hemorrhage of the small intestine, this condition of dairy cattle is characterized by intraluminal hemorrhage resulting in blood clots that lead to intestinal obstruction. It is characterized by dark, clotted blood in the feces; variable and multifocal distention of the small intestine; small intestinal ileus; and necrohemorrhagic jejunitis or enteritis (Fig. 7-156). The cause is unknown, but *Clostridium perfringens* type A is suspected. The mortality rate is high.

Miscellaneous

Chlamydiosis. Bovine chlamydia (strains of *Chlamydophila psittaci*—formerly *Chlamydia psittaci*) has been recovered from spontaneous enteritis of young calves. Affected calves have diarrhea, fever, anorexia, and depression. Following experimental inoculation, newborn calves have fever and diarrhea develop within 24 hours and become moribund within 4 to 5 days. Grossly the ileum is most severely affected, but the jejunum and large intestine also have lesions. In diseased segments, the mucosa is congested and marked with petechiae. The intestinal wall and mesentery are edematous. The lumen contains watery, yellow fluid mixed with a yellow, tenacious, fibrin-rich material attached to the surface. Colonic ridges are hyperemic and have small erosions. Bleeding from petechiae and ecchymoses of the colonic or rectal ridges occurs infrequently. Regional lymph nodes are enlarged.

Microscopically, villous epithelial cells, enterochromaffin cells, goblet cells, macrophages, fibroblasts of

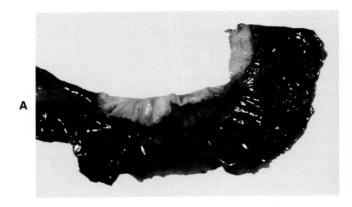

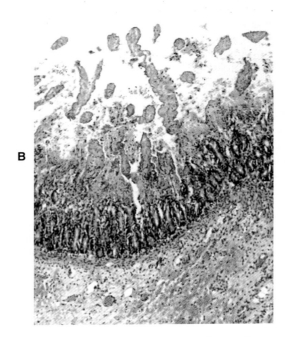

Fig. 7-156 **Necrohemorrhagic enteritis, hemorrhagic bowel syndrome, small intestine, cow. A,** The massive small intestinal hemorrhage and necrosis is characteristic of clostridial infections of the intestine. **B,** Note the horizontal linear "band" of acute coagulative necrosis affecting the superficial half of the mucosa *(light pink zone)* of the intestine caused by clostridial toxins. H&E stain. (**A,** *Courtesy Dr. M.D. McGavin, College of Veterinary Medicine, University of Tennessee.* **B,** *Courtesy Dr. C.W. Qualls, College of Veterinary Medicine, Oklahoma State University; and Noah's Arkive, College of Veterinary Medicine, The University of Georgia.*)

the lamina propria, and endothelial cells of lacteals are parasitized by the chlamydia. In the epithelial cells, the chlamydia are located in the apical cytoplasm. The chlamydia are endocytosed and multiply in epithelial cell apices. They subsequently are liberated into the lamina propria. Villi are enlarged by dilated lacteals and infiltrates of mononuclear cells and neutrophils. Crypts of both small and large intestines are dilated and have sloughed epithelial cells and inflammatory exudate (colitis cystica superficialis). The centers of lymphoid follicles of Peyer's patches are necrotic. The mucosa and submucosa of the intestines are thickened by a diffuse granulomatous reaction. The abomasum also has lesions, and, in some calves, foci of inflammation extend transmurally, thereby causing focal peritonitis.

INTESTINAL DISEASES OF PIGS

Enteric diseases of pigs are an important cause of economic loss. Rapid and accurate on-farm diagnosis is critical in controlling disease outbreaks. If one takes into account the epidemiology of the outbreak and the age of the affected animals and the location and nature of lesions, one can generally be fairly accurate in rendering an on-farm diagnosis, pending laboratory confirmation. This listing of specific infectious causes of enteritis in pigs is exclusive of those agents already discussed. When formulating a differential diagnosis, all causes of enteritis must be considered, including intestinal displacements, colibacillosis, rotavirus, *Salmonella*, parasites, toxins, and so on.

Viral

Transmissible gastroenteritis.   Transmissible gastroenteritis (TGE) is an important disease in pigs younger than 10 days. The coronavirus that causes this disease cross-reacts with, but is distinct from, the coronavirus that causes feline infectious peritonitis. The virus is inactivated by sunlight; therefore TGE disease occurs mostly in winter. Piglets suffer from acute diarrhea, weight loss, vomiting, and dehydration. Morbidity and mortality, especially in neonates, approach 100% in susceptible herds. Death occurs within 48 hours to 5 days after the commencement of clinical signs. Target cells for the virus are villous enterocytes, and therefore lesions consist of notable atrophy of villi of the small intestine (Fig. 7-157). Sows are susceptible to the virus, and morbidity among the sows is 100%, but the clinical signs are mild and transient (fever, vomiting, inappetence, agalactia), and none die. Immunity is complete. Diagnosis is by positive immunostaining of intestinal sections in piglets acutely ill with the disease.

Similar to rotavirus or non-TGE coronavirus infections, the virus is lytic and sloughed enterocytes carry virus into the feces. The difference in pathogenicity between rotavirus and non-TGE coronavirus infections and TGE is the number of villous enterocytes destroyed by a virus. In TGE, most of the villous enterocytes are destroyed and therefore the clinical disease is more severe.

The diarrhea contains odoriferous undigested milk. The loss of the majority of villous enterocytes results in continued significant intestinal malabsorption. Because of fusion of adjacent villi, the enterocyte mass may never fully be restored. Affected surviving animals remain chronic "poor doers." In feeder pigs, transmissible

gastroenteritis virus infection causes transient clinical signs with eventual recovery.

Piglets dead from TGE are dehydrated and their perineum is stained with liquid, yellow, fecal material. The small intestine is dilated and thin walled because of the loss of enterocytes, and contains yellow fluid and gas (Fig. 7-158). Mesenteric lymph vessels are devoid of chyle as a result of malabsorption. The diagnosis is partially based on the presence of villous atrophy. The decrease in villous height: crypt depth ratio is marked and may be appreciated subgrossly (Fig. 7-159). Colibacillosis, coccidiosis, cryptosporidiosis, rotavirus infection, and non-TGE coronavirus infection are among the differential diagnoses.

Bacterial

Swine dysentery.   Unlike most of the other diseases of the porcine gut, swine dysentery is generally confined to the large intestine. The gross lesions of

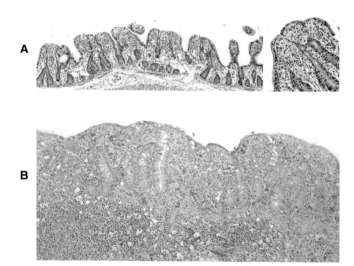

Fig. 7-157   Transmissible gastroenteritis, small intestine, piglet. A, Early stage of the disease. Transmissible gastroenteritis virus targets epithelial cells of the tips and upper sides of intestinal villi causing necrosis of the enterocytes and atrophy of the villi. These cells are sloughed and replaced by flattened epithelial cells migrating up the basement membrane from progenitor cells in the crypts. *Inset:* Note the flattened epithelial cells covering the tips and sides of the atrophic villi and the fusion of the adjacent villi. Inflammation is minimal. H&E stain. **B,** Later stage of the disease. There is severe blunting (marked villus atrophy) of intestinal villi with fusion of their basement membranes. Chronic inflammation is prominent in the lamina propria and submucosa. H&E stain. (**A,** *Courtesy Dr. B.G. Harmon, College of Veterinary Medicine, The University of Georgia; and Noah's Arkive, College of Veterinary Medicine, The University of Georgia.* **B,** *Courtesy Dr. H. Gelberg, College of Veterinary Medicine, Oregon State University.*)

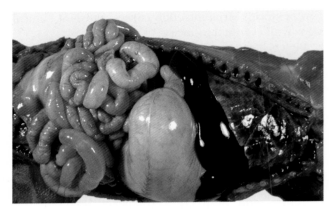

Fig. 7-158   Transmissible gastroenteritis, small intestine, piglet. The small intestine is dilated by gas, is thin walled, and contains undigested milk. *(Courtesy Dr. M.D. McGavin, College of Veterinary Medicine, University of Tennessee.)*

the disease closely approximate those of acute enteric salmonellosis except that bloody feces are more usual in dysentery. Weanling pigs 8 to 14 weeks old are usually affected, and the disease spreads rapidly through a herd. Morbidity approaches 90%, and mortality is around 30%. Lesions of mucohemorrhagic enteritis are present in the spiral colon, colon, cecum, and rectum. The intestine often has a fibrinonecrotic pseudomembrane that correlates with the severe diarrheic feces that contains blood, mucus, and fibrin (Fig. 7-160). The diarrhea and electrolyte loss that occur are caused by colonic absorptive failure.

The causative bacterium, *Brachyspira hyodysenteriae*, previously known as *Treponema* and *Serpulina*, acts synergistically with anaerobic colonic flora, such as *Fusobacterium necrophorum* or *Bacteroides vulgatus* to produce disease. This synergism is believed to be partially responsible for the age restriction (8 to 14 weeks old) of the disease because neonatal animals have not yet developed the appropriate anaerobic gut flora. *Brachyspira hyodysenteriae* produces a cytotoxic hemolysin, which is a virulence determinant. *Brachyspira hyodysenteriae* is identified by impression smear (Fig. 7-161), dark-field microscopy, immunolabeling techniques, and by newer methods, such as PCR.

***Lawsonia* enteritis.**   This disease manifests in a variety of ways as indicated by the number of names applied to it: proliferative enteropathy, proliferative ileitis, intestinal adenomatosis, distal ileal hypertrophy, terminal ileitis, and proliferative hemorrhagic enteropathy. The genus of the causative agent has undergone several recent changes in nomenclature. For many years, this disease was believed to be caused by *Campylobacter* spp. (*Campylobacter sputorum mucosalis*, *Campylobacter jejuni*, *Campylobacter hyointestinalis*). Newer methods of bacterial classification caused the name to be changed first to *Ileobacter* and now *Lawsonia*. Pigs older than 4 weeks of age are susceptible; thus this condition is a postweaning disease. The nature of the lesions is a function of the extent of intestinal mucosal necrosis. The disease begins as a bacteria-induced stimulation of intestinal crypt epithelial cells of the small intestine, particularly in the ileum (Figs. 7-162 and 7-163). Lesions are generally most severe in the ileum. With time, the

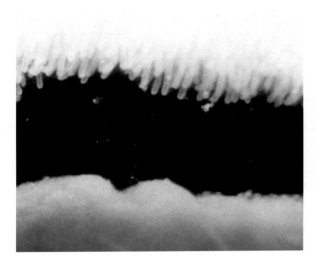

Fig. 7-159   Wet mount, intestinal villi, transmissible gastroenteritis, small intestine, piglet. There is notable villous atrophy *(bottom)* compared with normal intestine *(top)*. *(Courtesy Dr. H. Gelberg, College of Veterinary Medicine, Oregon State University.)*

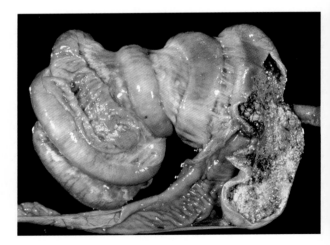

Fig. 7-160   Necrohemorrhagic enterocolitis, swine dysentery, spiral colon, pig. There is marked necrosis and hemorrhage of the intestinal mucosa caused by the bacterium *Brachyspira hyodysenteriae*. *(Courtesy Department of Veterinary Biosciences, College of Veterinary Medicine, The Ohio State University; and Noah's Arkive, College of Veterinary Medicine, The University of Georgia.)*

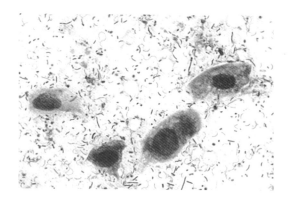

Fig. 7-161 **Swine dysentery, colon, pig.** This impression smear contains a few enterocytes and numerous bacteria. Note the spiral bacteria consistent with *Brachyspira* spp. Diff-Quik stain. *(Courtesy Dr. H. Gelberg, College of Veterinary Medicine, Oregon State University.)*

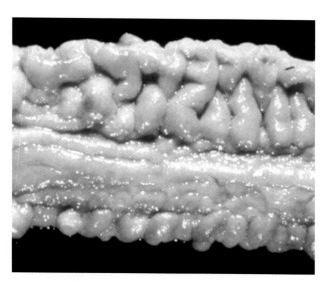

Fig. 7-162 **Proliferative enteritis, ileum, pig.** Note the marked mucosal expansion, the result of *Lawsonia*-induced epithelial hyperplasia. *(Courtesy Dr. H. Gelberg, College of Veterinary Medicine, Oregon State University.)*

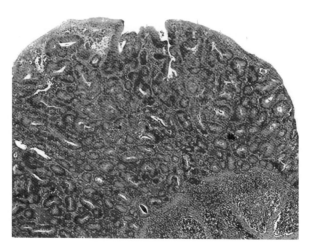

Fig. 7-163 *Lawsonia* **enteritis, ileum, pig.** There is notable hyperplasia of enterocytes, resulting in distortion of normal architecture and "collision necrosis" of tightly packed proliferating enterocytes. H&E stain. *(Courtesy Dr. W. Crowell, College of Veterinary Medicine, The University of Georgia; and Noah's Arkive, College of Veterinary Medicine, The University of Georgia.)*

lesions progress to necrosis of the proliferating crypt cells with hemorrhage (Fig. 7-164). Thus the morphologic appearance of the lesions varies from case to case. The mechanism of lesion production is not well understood. Infection results in immunosuppression with a reduction in CD8+ T lymphocytes and B lymphocytes. In the proliferative form of the disease, the causative bacteria may be seen in apical cytoplasm of enterocytes. The enterocyte hyperplasia that results may cause release of cytokines that attract macrophages. With severe disease, bacteria are present in macrophages in the lamina propria. This may cause release of tumor necrosis factor-α, resulting in vascular permeability and hemorrhage.

Morbidity within a herd is 10% to 15%; mortality is around 50%. In fatal cases, affected pigs usually die within a day of the appearance of clinical signs. Pigs that recover are generally "poor-doers." At clinical and necropsy examination, variable amounts of blood and intestinal casts are present in the feces. Microscopically the comma-shaped bacteria are made visible with special stains, such as Steiner's, within the mitotically active cells of the small intestinal villous crypts (Fig. 7-165). The massive mitoses of crypt cells and resultant cryptal crowding and necrosis prevent maturation to absorbent villous enterocytes. There is resultant villous shortening. Mitosis can be so intense that the histologic features suggest neoplasia and a diagnosis of "intestinal adenomatosis." A similar organism and associated intestinal proliferation are found in young miniature horses, hamsters, ostriches, cervids, and macaques.

Glasser's disease. Glasser's disease is characterized by fibrinous polyserositis (pleuritis, pericarditis, peritonitis, arthritis, and leptomeningitis). Although not generally a diarrheal disease, it causes inflammation of the intestinal serosa (serositis). Lesions range from arthritis to peritonitis to leptomeningitis depending on the serous surface infected. Glasser's disease generally occurs in 5- to 12-week-old pigs. Mortality of affected animals within a herd is high, but morbidity is low. Although classic Glasser's disease is caused either by *Haemophilus suis* or *Haemophilus parasuis*, porcine polyserositis can be caused by *Mycoplasma hyorhinis*,

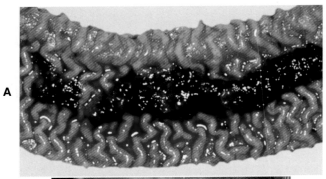

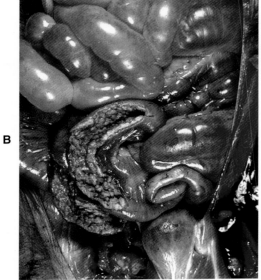

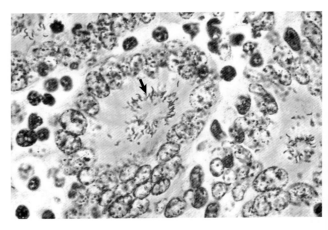

Fig. 7-165   Proliferative enteritis, ileum, pig. Curved *Lawsonia* spp. bacteria *(arrow)* are present in the apical cytoplasm of enterocytes. There is proliferation of crypt enterocytes. **Warthin-Starry stain.** *(Courtesy Dr. H. Gelberg, College of Veterinary Medicine, Oregon State University.)*

Fig. 7-164   *Lawsonia* enteritis, ileum, pig. A, Hemorrhagic bowel form. Note the prominent folds of hyperplastic mucosa and the concurrent hemorrhage forming a lumenal cast. **B,** Necroproliferative form. Note the prominent necrosis of the ileal mucosa and its overlying diphtheritic membrane formed by cellular debris and inflammatory exudate. *(**A,** Courtesy Dr. D.D. Harrington, School of Veterinary Medicine, Purdue University; and Noah's Arkive, College of Veterinary Medicine, The University of Georgia. **B,** Courtesy Dr. A.R. Doster, University of Nebraska; and Noah's Arkive, College of Veterinary Medicine, The University of Georgia.)*

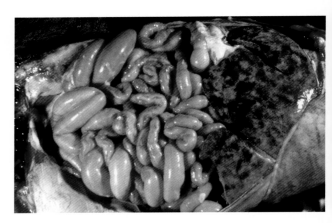

Fig. 7-166   Fibrinous polyserositis, abdomen, pig. Strands and clumps of fibrin are scattered throughout serosal surfaces. A milk-spotted liver is also present. *(Courtesy Dr. H. Gelberg, College of Veterinary Medicine, Oregon State University.)*

Streptococcus suis type II (zoonotic), septicemic salmonellosis, and septicemic *Escherichia coli* (Fig. 7-166).

Miscellaneous

Chlamydia infection.   Chlamydia has been found in enterocytes of normal pigs and pigs with diarrhea. In gnotobiotic pigs, *Chlamydia trachomatis* and *Chlamydia suis* infection results in villous atrophy and villous-tip necrosis. These lesions are most severe in the distal jejunum and ileum. Colonic infection has also been reported.

Intestinal emphysema.   Intestinal emphysema (pneumatosis cystoides intestinalis) of pigs and rabbits translates to gas-dilated lymphatics of the intestinal serosa and mesentery. The cause of this condition is unknown, and it is not associated with clinical disease (Fig. 7-167).

INTESTINAL DISEASES OF CARNIVORES
Viral

Parvovirus enteritis.   Parvovirus enteritis of dogs and cats is a severe, usually fatal disease. Because the target cells are those that are rapidly dividing in the intestine, the crypt cells are principally affected. This tropism is called radiomimetic. Identical crypt lesions are sometimes associated with FeLV infection. Initial virus replication occurs in lymphoid tissue. Although there is much overlap in the disease syndrome

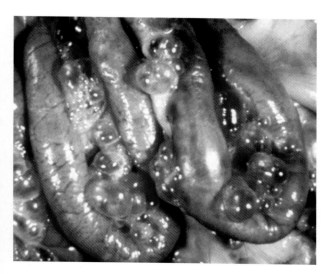

Fig. 7-167   **Intestinal emphysema, intestines, pig.** Gas bubbles dilate serosal and mesenteric lymphatics. *(Courtesy Dr. H. Gelberg, College of Veterinary Medicine, Oregon State University.)*

in dogs and cats, the dissimilarities warrant independent discussion of each species.

In the cat, mink, and raccoon, panleukopenia, cat distemper, feline enteritis, and mink enteritis are synonyms for this important disease. The clinical disease is characterized by dehydration, depression, and vomiting. Because the bone marrow is a rapidly dividing tissue, panleukopenia dominates the clinical pathologic findings.

Early lesions in the course of the disease are lymphoid depletion and thymic involution. Later, lesions include flaccid, segmentally reddened intestine with serositis. Lesions are generally limited to the small intestine, but colitis occurs in some cats. Villous atrophy occurs secondary to crypt cell destruction (Fig. 7-168). Basophilic intranuclear inclusion bodies are present in enterocytes and lymphocytes early in infection. In germ-free cats with a low enterocyte turnover, the disease caused by feline parvovirus is much less severe. Intrauterine infection causes congenital cerebellar hypoplasia of kittens. The virus, as described previously, is cytolytic and infects dividing cells and thus alters the differentiation of layers in the cerebellum during organogenesis.

Canine parvovirus enteritis first appeared in Europe and the United States in 1978. The disease was initially recognized because of the gross and microscopic lesions that were identical to those of feline parvovirus enteritis. Panleukopenia vaccines were effective in preventing this disease in dogs and were used extensively until canine-specific parvovirus vaccines were developed. Rottweilers and Doberman pinschers, which are genetically related, are at increased risk for parvovirus disease even if properly vaccinated.

Canine parvovirus disease initially was described as occurring in three distinct syndromes. Puppies younger than 2 weeks of age had generalized disease with focal areas of virus-induced necrosis in those tissues with rapidly dividing cells. Thus multiple organs and tissues, such as the liver, kidney, heart, vessel, bone marrow, intestine, and lung are affected. Puppies 3 to 8 weeks of age would sometimes have myocarditis develop for the same reason. Often initial infection would go undetected, and these animals would die unexpectedly up to 5 months later because of myocardial scarring and conduction failure. In puppies 8 weeks or older, the disease is identical to that in the cat. Cerebellar hypoplasia has not been induced in puppies.

At necropsy, the dilated, fluid-filled, flaccid, hemorrhagic, small intestine with serositis similar to that of panleukopenia is quite characteristic (Fig. 7-169, *A*). The contents of the small intestine are brown to red-brown and fluid with a fibrinous exudate, with or without hemorrhage (Fig. 7-169, *B*). Mesenteric lymphadenomegaly with variable hemorrhage is present. The bone marrow is depleted. Dogs, but not cats, may have coagulative lymphadenitis associated with severe lymphoid infection.

The intestinal lesion is necrosis of crypt epithelial cells. Surviving epithelial cells are not targets of the virus, but their morphology changes to squamoid to cover the surface of the denuded crypts and later to temporarily cover the denuded villous basement membrane, as replacement cells are not being produced, even though

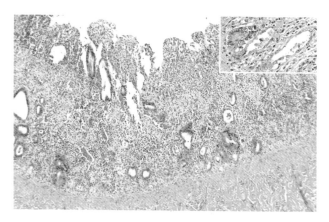

Fig. 7-168   **Panleukopenia virus enteritis, small intestine, cat.** Villi are denuded of epithelium and are atrophic. Some crypts are dilated. Note the squamoid epithelial cells in some crypts and hyperplasia in others, all indicative of attempts at epithelial repair and regeneration. Chronic inflammatory cells are present in the lamina propria. H&E stain. *Inset:* Higher magnification of crypts showing viral-induced degeneration, necrosis, and sloughing of epithelial cells. H&E stain. (***Figure*** and ***Inset,*** *Courtesy Dr. H. Gelberg, College of Veterinary Medicine, Oregon State University.)*

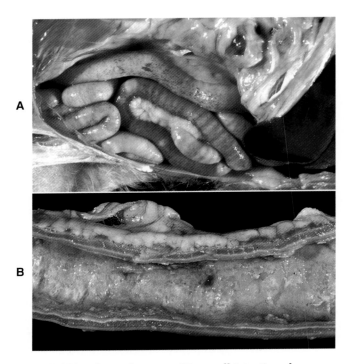

Fig. 7-169   Parvovirus enteritis, small intestine, dog.
A, Segments of the small intestine are diffusely reddened (active hyperemia of the mucosa), and the serosal surface is roughened, faintly granular, and petechiated. **B,** The mucosa of the small intestine is necrotic. Note the roughened, granular, focally petechiated, and focally sloughing mucosa. (**A,** *Courtesy College of Veterinary Medicine, University of Illinois.* **B,** *Courtesy Department of Veterinary Biosciences, College of Veterinary Medicine, The Ohio State University; and Noah's Arkive, College of Veterinary Medicine, The University of Georgia.*)

population, but disease is only diagnosed sporadically. The virus is spread via the oronasal route. Fetal death and embryo absorption occur between 25 and 35 days of gestation. Microscopically, intestinal lesions consist of enterocyte hyperplasia with eosinophilic or amphophilic intranuclear inclusion bodies in the enterocytes of the villous tips of the duodenum and jejunum. Crypt necrosis characteristic of canine parvovirus type 2 infection is not present.

Feline infectious peritonitis.   Feline infectious peritonitis (FIP) is a uniformly fatal disease of cats. Although it affects cats of all ages, the disease is principally found in the young and old. Twelve percent of feline deaths are associated with FIP. The cause of the disease is a coronavirus related to the coronavirus of transmissible gastroenteritis of pigs. After entry into the body, the first round of viral replication takes place in the lymphoid system. Macrophages are infected and carry the virus systemically. Endothelial cells are activated secondary to up-regulation of major histocompatibility complex II. Recent observations suggest that activated monocytes are critical for development of vasculitis. Lesions are multifocal and most organs, including the central nervous system, may be affected. The lesions in the vasculature of the eye are sometimes useful in making a tentative diagnosis of FIP in the live cat, but other diseases, such as toxoplasmosis and systemic fungi, may cause similar lesions. The "wet form" of the disease is characterized by fibrinous polyserositis (Fig. 7-170); the "dry form" is without the effusive process. Why one form develops rather than the other

senile epithelial extrusion continues to occur from the villous tips. Severe lesions consist of partially denuded villi over debris-filled crypts, some of which lack an epithelial lining. Because the villous basement membrane is exposed during the continuing extrusion process, villous fusion occurs, resulting in lack of a scaffold for enterocyte replacement once the crypts recover and in permanent villous distortion and atrophy. Hyperplastic crypt epithelium may therefore be present. Inclusion bodies are not present in lymphoid tissue. In bone marrow, erythropoiesis is normal, but granulopoiesis is reduced. Necrotizing colitis may occur but is much less important than the small intestinal lesions.

Dogs with hemorrhagic parvovirus enteritis have bloody diarrhea and die from shock within 24 hours. Secondary bacterial infections with endotoxemia are believed to be associated with this syndrome.

Minute virus of canids.   Canine parvovirus type 1 produces myocarditis and respiratory disease in young pups. The virus is widely distributed in the canine

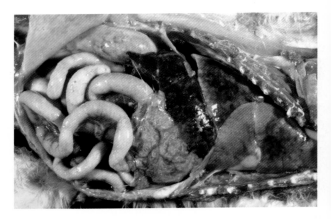

Fig. 7-170   Fibrinous polyserositis, abdomen, cat. Fibrin strands between viscera and mats of fibrin on organ surfaces are characteristic of the "wet form" of feline infectious peritonitis. The mesentery (below and left of the liver) has numerous white linear serpentine tracts, which are inflamed (type III hypersensitivity, immune complex) capillaries and venules. Note the small nodules (pyogranulomas) on the intestinal serosa and on the surface of the kidney. (*Courtesy Dr. H. Gelberg, College of Veterinary Medicine, Oregon State University.*)

is not completely understood, but may relate to the major type of immune effector cell. The disease often clusters in households, and virus spreads among cats by saliva on shared bowls and utensils or by mutation of an endogenous coronavirus.

Because of the presence of a nonneutralizing antibody, immune complexes develop and Arthus reactions localize in the vasculature. Complement is fixed, and inflammatory cell chemoattractants are produced. Vasculitis results in protein effusion. Thus lesions are vasocentric. The prodromal course of FIP is shortened, and the development and extent of lesions are accelerated in seropositive cats. FIP is usually characterized by progressive wasting because of protein loss. It is unusual for a virus to result in pyogranulomatous lesions, but in FIP the vasocentric deposition of immune complexes results in pyogranulomas. These lesions are single to multiple, white, and raised. On the surface of the kidney, they often are linear, clearly following the renal surface vasculature. In its "wet form," FIP is characterized by variable of amounts of thick, stringy, high-protein effusion in body cavities. When placed between gloved fingers, this transudate may be drawn out in strings as the fingers are separated. The transudate is sterile, eliminating most other causes of fibrinous peritonitis. The granulomas are translucent and less than 2 mm in diameter. The "dry form" of the disease is identical to the wet, but contains only pyogranulomas and not the exudates.

Bacterial

Histiocytic ulcerative colitis.   Because of its occurrence in boxer dogs and the genetically related French bulldog, this disease has been called boxer colitis. Granulomatous colitis is another term for this disease, although true granulomas are not present. It generally occurs in dogs younger than 2 years. Dogs can have soft feces, but often no diarrhea or weight loss is observed. In some cases, mucus and blood appear in the stool. The lesions, which are visible by proctoscopy, are raised ulcerative nodules (Fig. 7-171). Microscopically the colon is ulcerated and has marked infiltration by macrophages containing PAS-positive material.

Large macrophages with abundant foamy eosinophilic cytoplasm are present in the colonic lamina propria and submucosa early in the disease process. There may be lesser numbers of smaller, mononuclear inflammatory cells, principally lymphocytes and plasmacytes. The PAS-positive material in macrophages has been visualized by tissue Gram stains, electron microscopy, and immunohistochemistry. They likely contain bacteria and the phagolysosomal remnants of digested cells. Evidence suggests that the bacteria are probably *Escherichia coli*. The massive numbers of engorged macrophages within the lamina propria results in a

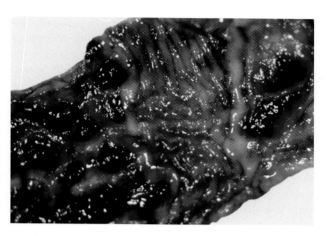

Fig. 7-171   Histiocytic ulcerative colitis, colon, boxer dog. There are numerous round and coalescing ulcers in the colon in this case of "boxer colitis." Recent research suggests *Escherichia coli* as the causative agent of boxer colitis. *(Courtesy Dr. H. Gelberg, College of Veterinary Medicine, Oregon State University.)*

space-occupying lesion that affects the overlying enterocytes. Enterocyte necrosis results in colonic erosion and ulceration. There is lymphadenopathy, both regional and generalized, characterized by an influx of foamy macrophages in the lymphatic sinuses.

***Citrobacter freundii* enteritis.**   Bacteremia and septicemia associated with *Citrobacter freundii* have been reported to cause mucohemorrhagic diarrhea in dogs with hemorrhagic lesions in the small intestine and colon. It is believed to be a condition of puppies and immunocompromised dogs. Being bacteremic and/or septicemic, many organs and tissues are affected besides the gut. The condition is more common in humans as a nosocomial infection with a high mortality rate. In humans, the route of infection is through the urinary tract, gallbladder, gastrointestinal tract, or cutaneous wounds. *Citrobacter* infections should be considered potentially zoonotic.

Fungal

Canine histoplasmosis.   Canine histoplasmosis occurs most often in the Ohio and Mississippi River valleys. This zoonotic systemic fungus can infect the intestine, but pneumonia is more common. Thus the route of infection is inhalation or ingestion. The reservoir is believed to be soil and bird feces. The yeast invades tissue, causes necrosis, and replicates in macrophages. Granulomatous lesions may be present in pulmonary, intestinal, lymphoid, hepatic, and other tissue. Signs of intestinal histoplasmosis in the dog include intractable chronic diarrhea with anorexia and its attendant weight loss, lethargy, poor pelage, and anemia. Respiratory signs and peripheral lymphadenitis may be present. At necropsy or biopsy, the intestine has a thickened and corrugated mucosa with ulceration. There is hepatomegaly and mesenteric lymphadenopathy and lymphadenomegaly. Scattered pulmonary granulomas may be present.

In the affected ileum and colon, the lamina propria is widened by macrophages that contain *Histoplasma capsulatum* (Fig. 7-172). With time, infection may extend transmurally through the intestine and to the lymphoid system. There is hyperplasia of regional lymph nodes, and lymphoid sinuses contain numerous macrophages. Multifocal granulomas with intracellular fungi are in the liver, presumably arriving via the portal vein.

Rickettsial

Salmon poisoning.   This acute and fatal hemorrhagic granulomatous enterocolitis of the dog and fox results from consuming salmon carrying the fluke *Nanophyetus salmincola*. When this trematode harbors *Neorickettsia helminthoeca*, a 0.3-μm coccoid rickettsia, disease may result. Six to eight days after eating parasitized fish, affected canids become febrile and depressed. There is an oculonasal discharge, severe diarrhea, emesis, anorexia, and splenolymphadenopathy characterized by enlarged tonsils, spleen, and lymph nodes. The mesenteric lymph nodes are often more severely affected than peripheral nodes. Unless treated, affected animals die within 10 days. Lesions may extend from the pylorus to the anus. The enteric lesions consist of hemorrhage at sites of GALT necrosis, especially near the ileocecal valves. In the small intestine, trematodes may be embedded in the mucosa. Diagnosis is confirmed by visualizing macrophages in many tissues, including the brain, containing Giemsa-stained elementary bodies.

Parasitic

Canine multifocal eosinophilic gastroenteritis. Canine multifocal eosinophilic gastroenteritis is an uncommon disease of dogs generally younger than 4 years. It is caused by migrating larvae of *Toxocara canis*. Therefore this disease occurs in association with poor parasite management. Chronic diarrhea, moderate weight loss, intermittent or persistent eosinophilia, and elevated serum β-globulin concentrations characterize this disorder. Serum albumin concentration, absorption tests, and small bowel contrast radiographs usually are normal.

Larvae of *Toxocara canis* are ingested, invade the mucosa of the stomach and small intestine, and then become trapped and localized in their self-induced inflammation. Dormant larvae migrate into the uterus and fetuses during late pregnancy. Postpartum, larvae are secreted in the milk of the bitch or ingested from environmental feces. Ingested larvae penetrate the gastric and small intestinal mucosa, enter lymph vessels or the portal vein, and travel to the liver and lungs. They then develop into third-stage larvae and are coughed up and swallowed. In the gastrointestinal tract, they mature to adult ascarids. In the majority of puppies, ascarid larvae complete their life cycle in several weeks. Alternatively the larvae are enveloped in granulomas that kill the parasite secondary to immune reactivity. These granulomas may occur anywhere along the parasite's migration tracts, including most abdominal organs, eyes, brain, and the lungs. Eosinophils are a prominent component of the inflammatory reaction and are attracted to the site of parasite entrapment by the waste products of the larvae. There may be subsequent mineralization of larvae, or they may remain viable for up to 4 years. This condition is especially common in aberrant host species and is called visceral

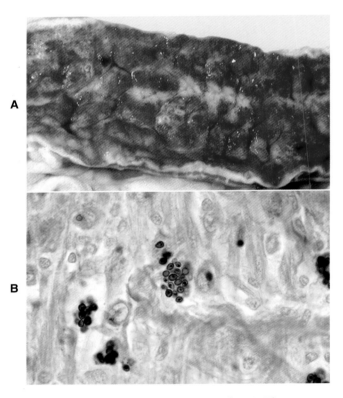

Fig. 7-172   Histoplasmosis, intestine, dog. A, The mucosa is greatly thickened and congested due to granulomatous inflammation that expands the lamina propria. **B,** Clusters of 3- to 5-μm *Histoplasma capsulatum* organisms with a central nucleoid are located in macrophages within the granulomatous inflammatory cells shown in Fig. 7-172, A. Grocott-Gomori's methenamine silver stain. (**A,** *Courtesy Dr. R. Panciera, School of Veterinary Medicine, Oklahoma State University; and Noah's Arkive, College of Veterinary Medicine, The University of Georgia.* **B,** *Courtesy Dr. H. Gelberg, College of Veterinary Medicine, Oregon State University.*)

larval migrans. It is an environmental danger where children play in sand or dirt contaminated by feces of infected animals. The ova are relatively resistant to environmental extremes.

Lesions are microscopic to macroscopic, may be quite numerous, and may be grossly visible. As in other inflammatory diseases, there may be regional lymphadenopathy with or without nodules that vary from principally granulomatous to eosinophilic or a mix of the two. Larvae, when present, are surrounded by an eosinophilic, amorphous, fringed material that stains PAS-positive (the Splendore-Hoeppli phenomenon). In general, canine multifocal eosinophilic gastroenteritis is asymptomatic.

Immunologic

Inflammatory bowel disease. In dogs and cats, this disease is microscopically a lymphoplasmacytic enteritis. Diagnosis is made by biopsy. Breeds with a predilection for this disease include the basenji and the German shepherd. The cause is unknown, but the presence of numerous lymphocytes and plasma cells suggests an immunologic problem. Malabsorption and chronic protein-losing enteropathy can result from the marked infiltrate of lymphocytes and plasmacytes in the lamina propria. In dogs, there are increased numbers of both B and T lymphocytes in the lamina propria of the small intestine (Fig. 7-173). In cats, but not dogs, dietary antigens cause some cases of inflammatory bowel disease; therefore control of the disease can be achieved by regulation of the diet. Anecdotal evidence suggests that lymphocytic plasmacytic enteritis in the cat can be a prelude to intestinal lymphosarcoma.

Diffuse eosinophilic gastroenteritis. Although this type of eosinophilic gastroenteritis has a predilection for the German shepherd breed, it occurs in other breeds of dogs and in cats. It is characterized by recurrent episodes of diarrhea associated with tissue and circulating eosinophilia. The increased concentration of eosinophils in the circulation and within lesions suggests a hypersensitivity reaction to some ingested substance or to parasites. The cause has not been identified. There are no gross lesions. Eosinophils, along with lymphocytes and plasma cells, heavily infiltrate all layers of the mucosa of the stomach and intestine.

Wheat-sensitive enteropathy of Irish setters. This hereditary condition, similar to gluten-sensitive enteropathy of human beings, is the first described dietary-induced enteropathy of dogs. It is characterized initially by increased numbers of intraepithelial lymphocytes and goblet cells and later by partial villous atrophy, particularly of the jejunum. Dietary therapy is palliative.

Idiopathic

Feline ulcerative colitis. Feline ulcerative colitis is grossly and histologically analogous to its canine counterpart, histiocytic ulcerative colitis (Fig. 7-174). The causative agent is unknown.

Canine senile gastrointestinal amyloidosis. Amyloid located in and around vessels of the submucosal and muscular layers of the alimentary tract and within the mesentery has been reported in dogs. The mechanism and chemical nature of the amyloid deposition has not been determined. Dysfunction of the alimentary tract has not been reported to occur with this condition.

PARASITIC ENTERITIDES

Parasites of the intestinal tract are legion in the various domestic animal species. Refer to a parasitology

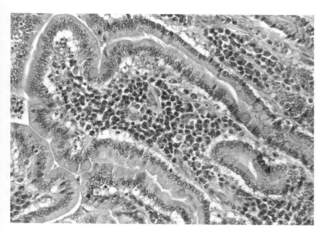

Fig. 7-173 **Lymphoplasmacytic enteropathy, intestine, dog.** The lamina propria is widened with lymphocytes and plasma cells. H&E stain. *(Courtesy Dr. H. Gelberg, College of Veterinary Medicine, Oregon State University.)*

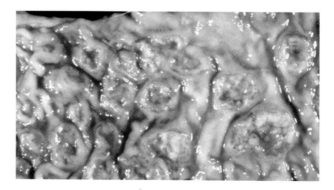

Fig. 7-174 **Feline ulcerative colitis, colon, cat.** There are numerous round ulcers in the mucosa. *(Courtesy Dr. H. Gelberg, College of Veterinary Medicine, Oregon State University.)*

textbook for specific information regarding the life cycles and identification of the various species. Diagnosis of enteric parasitism is generally performed via fecal flotation or intestinal scrapings.

AMEBIASIS

Entamoeba spp. are obligate intracellular parasites with a direct life cycle. The portal of entry is oral. Trophozoites are produced that dwell in the intestinal lumen. They may also invade through the intestinal wall and go to many other organs, such as the liver, brain, and lung, especially in humans, in whom microabscesses may form. Cysts are excreted with formed feces and continue their life cycle when ingested by another host. Trophozoites are more likely seen in diarrheic feces. Because cysts are the infective form, diarrheic feces of dogs are not usually considered to be especially dangerous to humans or other animals. The trophozoites vary from 12 to 30 μm in diameter, and the cysts vary from 10 to 20 μm with four nuclei. Contact of ameba and host cells is likely mediated by adhesins. Soluble factors produced by the parasite mediate pathogenicity.

Entamoeba histolytica is zoonotic in human beings, other primates, dogs, cats, and other animals. Disease is serious in humans. Lesions include colonic congestion, petechia, and ulceration (ulcerative colitis). This colitis may be acute or chronic, bloody or mucoid. In tissue, the amebas may be as large as 50 μm and often form typical flask-shaped ulcers spanning the mucosa and submucosa of the colon.

TRICHOMONIASIS

Tritrichomonas foetus is a sexually transmitted pathogen of cattle. Cats, especially those less than a year of age housed in groups, have a tendency toward large bowel diarrhea when infected with this flagellate. Diagnosis is often made by visualization of motile flagellates on fecal wet mounts. Histologic diagnosis is most accurate when at least six biopsy sections of colon containing surface mucus are examined. PCR on paraffin-embedded tissue has also been successful, even in the absence of histologic evidence of the parasite. Infection occurs in the ileum, cecum, and colon. Lesions include mild to moderate colitis, with microabscesses and occasional extension of infection into the lamina propria. There may be colonic enterocyte attenuation and/or increased mitotic activity in the crypts. The 5 μm by 7 μm teardrop-shaped parasites can often been seen in surface mucus, within colonic glands, and occasionally within macrophages and lymphatics. Thus the parasite is at least enteroinvasive under certain circumstances. Flagella are not visible on H&E staining. There is no effective treatment. The diarrheal disease in cats generally resolves within 2 years of onset.

COCCIDIOSIS

Coccidia are exquisitely host- and tissue-specific protozoa. They are obligate intracellular pathogens. Lesions vary from proliferative in sheep and goats (Fig. 7-175), to hemorrhagic in dogs, cats, and cattle (Fig. 7-176). In pigs, a fibrinonecrotic pseudomembrane, without blood, in 5- to 7-day-old animals is characteristic of enteric coccidiosis (Fig. 7-177). Most species of *Eimeria* and *Isospora* infect villous or crypt epithelial cells, more rarely lacteals, the lamina propria, and regional lymph nodes. The coccidia undergo one or more asexual reproductive cycles within enterocytes. The resulting sporozoites produce schizonts containing merozoites, which infect additional enterocytes.

Merozoites, produce gamonts that differentiate into microgametes and macrogametes. Microgametes fertilize macrogametes, producing zygotes that develop into oocysts. When a small number of coccidia parasitize the intestine of otherwise healthy young growing animals, little disease results. However, when animals are in crowded conditions associated with poor sanitation, fecal-oral transmission of large numbers of organisms can occur. It is in these circumstances, compounded by malnutrition and intercurrent infections or parasitism, that clinical disease results. Enterocyte rupture occurs in all stages of the parasite's life cycle. Clinical disease is dependent on parasitic load and varies by animal species. Because of diminished epithelial turnover in young animals, they are most susceptible to disease.

"Poor doing" associated with diarrhea is characteristic of clinical coccidiosis. Depending on the host species and the region of intestine that is affected, infected fresh blood may be present in the feces. The presence of tenesmus is variable. Oocysts are demonstrable in the feces.

Gross lesions of coccidiosis are variable by host species, parasite species, and intestinal location. Bleeding is variably present both within species and

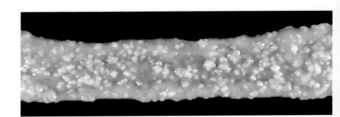

Fig. 7-175   Multifocal proliferative enteritis, small intestine, goat. Proliferative nodules in the small intestinal mucosa are characteristic of ovine and caprine coccidiosis. Sporozoites and merozoites infect enterocytes and replicate, resulting in physical expansion of the cell (hypertrophy). *(Courtesy Dr. H. Gelberg, College of Veterinary Medicine, Oregon State University.)*

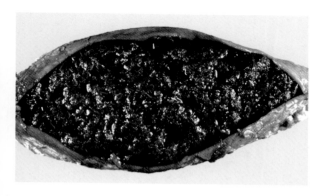

Fig. 7-176   Necrohemorrhagic enteritis, small intestine, calf. Coccidiosis in dogs, cats, and cattle is characterized by intestinal hemorrhage, or hemorrhagic diarrhetic feces may be visible on the perineum and hind legs. In severe cases there may be anemia, which will be evident as pale external mucous membranes. *(Courtesy College of Veterinary Medicine, Cornell University.)*

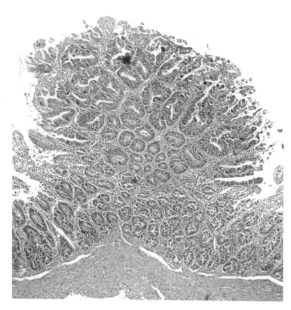

Fig. 7-178   Proliferative enteritis, small intestine, goat. Coccidia-induced enterocyte hyperplasia results in nodule formation. Note the hyperplastic enterocytes lining crypts. **H&E stain.** *(Courtesy Dr. H. Gelberg, College of Veterinary Medicine, Oregon State University.)*

among species. Coccidiosis in sheep and goats is characterized by enterocyte proliferation that is visible grossly as mucosal nodules (Fig. 7-178). The large schizonts of some species are sometimes grossly visible as well.

CRYPTOSPORIDIOSIS

Cryptosporidium parvum is a ubiquitous protozoan pathogen of mammals. Often waterborne, it is a significant cause of municipal water contamination. Although it causes a self-limiting infection in immunocompetent animals, the very young or immunocompromised individuals, such as AIDS patients, suffer from intractable diarrhea. When treating calves, veterinarians and veterinary students are at particular risk for infection. Cryptosporidia attach to surface epithelial cells of the stomach, small intestine, or colon. The protozoa displace the microvilli and are enclosed by surface

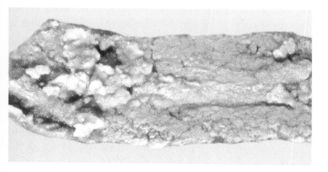

Fig. 7-177   Fibrinonecrotic enteritis, small intestine, pig. Pseudomembranes are characteristic of porcine coccidiosis. *(Courtesy Dr. H. Gelberg, College of Veterinary Medicine, Oregon State University.)*

cell membranes, but do not reside within a vacuole. Thus the parasite lives in a unique environment described as intracellular, but extracytoplasmic (Fig. 7-179). Microgametes, macrogametes, schizonts, trophozoites, meronts, merozoites, and oocysts can be demonstrated in the intestine adjacent to, or attached to, epithelial cells. Oocysts are 4 to 5 μm in diameter and are shed in the feces. Recent studies have indicated that there are species-specific tropisms or biotypes of cryptosporidia. Previously, fecal contamination of water supplies by ruminants was believed to be the cause of most human outbreaks. Molecular typing of the organism has shown in many disease outbreaks that contamination with human feces causes human epidemics.

Oocysts can be identified in feces by Sheather's sucrose flotation and a modified acid-fast stain. Cryptosporidiosis causes subacute or chronic, sometimes bloody, watery diarrhea. There is associated dehydration and electrolyte loss. Although the disease can be fatal, particularly in the presence of other pathogens, it is often self-limiting in immunocompetent individuals. In these cases, the illness resolves spontaneously in about a week. Affected portions of the gastrointestinal tract are diffusely reddened and have fluid contents. The organisms appear as tiny blue (hematoxylinophilic) dots attached to the epithelial cells of affected segments. In addition to the dot forms, ring- and banana-shaped organisms are

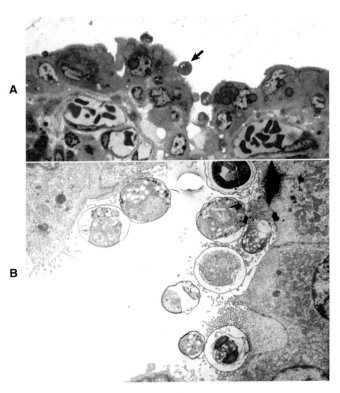

Fig. 7-179   Cryptosporidiosis, small intestine. A, Cow. Cryptosporidia *(arrow)* are attached to the microvillus border of the enterocyte membrane. Plastic-embedded, toluidine blue–stained section. **B,** Rabbit. The cryptosporidia form a trilaminated enveloping membrane upon fusion with the enterocyte membrane. Their location is thus intracellular, but extracytoplasmic. Microvilli are effaced. TEM. Uranyl acetate and lead citrate stain. *(A, Courtesy Dr. A.R. Doster, University of Nebraska; and Noah's Arkive, College of Veterinary Medicine, The University of Georgia. B, Courtesy Dr. H. Gelberg, College of Veterinary Medicine, Oregon State University.)*

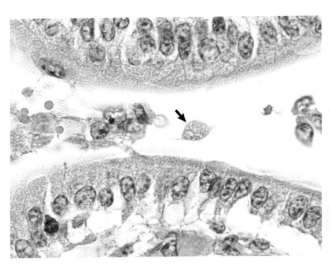

Fig. 7-180   Giardiasis, small intestine, dog. A single pear-shaped flagellated protozoa is readily visible in the intestinal lumen *(arrow)*. H&E stain. *(Courtesy Dr. J.F. Zachary, College of Veterinary Medicine, University of Illinois.)*

readily seen in Giemsa-stained sections. The lesions of enteritis or colitis consist of decreased mucosal (villous) height, irregular mucosal thickness, crypt necrosis, hyperemia, and an increase in lymphocytes and plasma cells in the lamina propria. Villous atrophy and fusion of the villi of the small intestine are the end result. Due to the intracellular, extracytoplasmic location of the parasite, chemotherapeutic intervention is ineffective. There are a few chemicals that can decontaminate the environment. Clorox, for example, is used experimentally to purify the parasites.

GIARDIASIS

Giardiasis has been reported in many species, including human beings, dogs, cats, horses, cattle, rabbits, guinea pigs, hamsters, rats, mice, chinchillas, and parakeets. In clinical veterinary practice, giardiasis is frequently recognized in puppies and kittens and causes concern among owners because of its zoonotic potential. Giardiasis is caused by a pear-shaped protozoan with posterior flagella, a ventral sucker, and four nuclei, two of which resemble eyes (Fig. 7-180). *Giardia lamblia* parasitizes the small intestine, particularly the duodenum. *Giardia* attach to the microvillous border of epithelial cells, producing membrane damage. Although generally asymptomatic, diarrhea may result in very young animals or in animals otherwise immunologically deficient.

In large numbers, the parasites decrease the absorption of simple sugars and disaccharides secondary to microvillous destruction. Ingesta are then fermented by bacterial flora, creating gas and osmotically drawing water into the intestinal lumen. Clinical cases of giardiasis have brown, fluid diarrhea, abdominal discomfort without fever, weight loss, melena, and/or steatorrhea. The diagnosis is made by demonstrating *Giardia* in preparations of fresh feces or in histologic sections by identifying the organisms either with H&E or Giemsa stains.

ASCARIASIS

Ascarids are easily recognized as proximal-intestinal, luminal nematodes that are smooth and white. They are round on cross section, thus giving them the appellation of roundworms together with the other nematodes. They vary greatly in length; the larger the host species, the larger the ascarids. They are 3 to 4 cm long in small animals and attain lengths of 40 to 50 cm in pigs and horses. Ascarids of domestic animals belong to the genera *Ascaris* (pigs), *Parascaris* (horses), and *Toxocara* (dogs, cats, and humans). The young of these species acquire larval ascarids by intrauterine transmission during the last 7 to 10 days of gestation, through the milk of the dam, and later in life through parasite ova contamination of the environment. After ingestion, infective larvae penetrate the intestine and migrate to the liver via the portal circulation. From there the larvae migrate via the caudal vena cava to the lungs. After leaving the circulation and entering the alveoli, the larvae undergo development, and are coughed into the pharynx and swallowed. Development to adults occurs in the intestine. Ova passed in the feces complete the life cycle.

Alternatively, *Toxascaris leonia* of canids and felids is ingested via an intermediate host. Hepatopulmonary migration does not occur. Lesions produced by ascarid larval migration include canine multifocal eosinophilic gastroenteritis and visceral larval migrans. Animals affected with heavy ascarid burdens lose weight, grow poorly as a result of competition for nutrients between luminal parasites and the host, and often have a pear-shaped abdomen when held vertically. Adult worms may be vomited or passed in the diarrheic feces. A hacking cough termed "thumping" is a sign of pulmonary larva migrans, especially in pigs. Anthelmintic administration can cause a rapid die off of adult ascarids, resulting in intestinal occlusion. Ascarids continue to migrate after the death of the host and may be found in aberrant locations such as the bile duct, stomach, oral cavity, pancreatic duct, and abdomen (Fig. 7-181).

HOOKWORM DISEASE

Parasitism by hookworms varies from asymptomatic to fatal based on the challenge dose of parasites, the host's

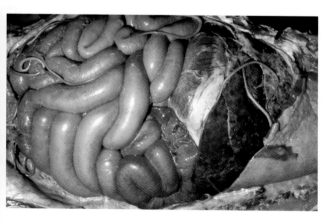

Fig. 7-181 **Fibrinous peritonitis, abdomen, pig.** The presence of fibrin along with ascarids in this pig's abdomen indicates that the intestinal rupture occurred antemortem. *(Courtesy Dr. M.D. McGavin, College of Veterinary Medicine, University of Tennessee.)*

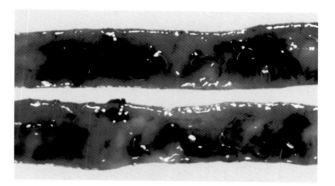

Fig. 7-182 **Hookworms, hemorrhagic enteritis, small intestine, dog.** Where hookworms have detached, hemorrhage is present. *(Courtesy Dr. H. Gelberg, College of Veterinary Medicine, Oregon State University.)*

age, nutritional status, and likely its immunologic state. Death, when it occurs, is by exsanguination because hookworms are blood eaters (Fig. 7-182). Challenge dosage is often exacerbated by poor nutritional and sanitary conditions, mild climatic conditions, and moisture. Hookworms are generally small nematodes, 1 to 1.5 cm long. Their habitat is usually the proximal small intestine. Genera include *Ancylostoma* and *Uncinaria* in dogs, *Bunostomum* in ruminants, *Globocephalus* in pigs, and *Ancylostoma* and *Necator* in humans. *Ancylostoma caninum* in dogs has zoonotic potential. Environmental contamination occurs from the large number of eggs produced in the intestine. The first- through third-stage larvae feed on environmental bacteria. Third-stage larvae are infective and enter the host either by ingestion or direct dermal penetration. From either point of entry, they migrate through the pulmonary system, through somatic tissue to the uterus, or through mucosal tissue. Larvae may also be present in colostrum. The final destination is the intestine, where eggs are produced, completing the life cycle.

Because prenatal infections with hookworms do not become patent for 11 days, fecal examinations may be negative. Otherwise, fecal examination, especially in young animals with anemia is diagnostic of this disease. Adult hookworms bury into the villous, ingesting tissue, mucus, and blood (Fig. 7-183). When the worm moves to another attachment site, blood may continue to flow from the wound for 30 minutes.

TRICHURIASIS

Trichurids, or whipworms, are long and slender at their anterior ends and may be numerous within the cecum and colon. Trichurids have a direct life cycle. The name *Trichuris* translates to "whip-tail," which is a misnomer because the parasite actually has a "whip-head" that invades and attaches to the mucosa of the cecum,

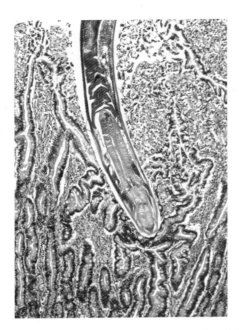

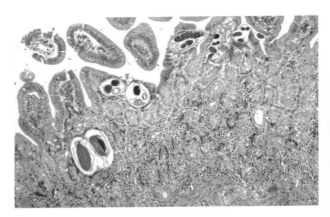

Fig. 7-184   **Strongyloidosis, small intestine, horse.** Cross sections of the parasite (*Strongyloides westeri*) are present in the superficial mucosa. Note the mild chronic inflammatory response with some eosinophils in the lamina propria. H&E stain. (*Courtesy Dr. C.S. Patton, College of Veterinary Medicine, University of Tennessee.*)

Fig. 7-183   **Hookworm enteritis, intestine, dog.** A hookworm has burrowed deep into and attached to the mucosa. H&E stain. (*Courtesy College of Veterinary Medicine, Cornell University.*)

colon, and rectum. Although the parasite ingests blood, anemia is rarely a clinical symptom. Bloody diarrhea may be present. Different species are parasites of carnivores, ruminants, pigs, and humans. The disease in each species is similar. The horse does not have a whipworm.

Trichuris eggs are elongate, or football-shaped, with an operculum at either end, and are very resistant to environmental conditions. Most infections are asymptomatic and the complete life cycle may take up to 3 months. Therefore repeated dewormings are necessary to eliminate infection, even in the absence of fecal ova. Symptoms may be vague, with only paroxysmal diarrhea. Gross enteric lesions vary from mild to erosive and ulcerative.

STRONGYLOIDOSIS

Strongyloides spp. are unique in having free-living and parasitic forms. Rhabditiform larvae may develop parthenogenetically. Free-living parasites are both male and female and undergo sexual reproduction. Enteritis can be severe; larvae or larvated eggs are in the feces of infected animals.

Strongyloides stercoralis of dogs is zoonotic. *Strongyloides* spp. also infect horses, pigs, and cats. Geographic differences in parasite populations account for differences in virulence within host species. Hyperinfection and autoinfection may occur, adding to the parasite burden. Larvae may enter the host by skin penetration, or less

often by ingestion. *Strongyloides* spp. infection may be acquired in utero and through colostrum and milk. Larvae migrate to the blood stream and lungs. When they gain access to alveoli, they subsequently migrate to airways, where they are carried, via the mucociliary elevator, to the pharyngeal cavity and are swallowed. Small intestinal parasitism is characterized by larvae residing within superficial mucosa (Fig. 7-184). Epithelial destruction by the parasites may result in villous atrophy and crypt hyperplasia. The nonspecific clinical signs include diarrhea, hypoproteinemia, weight loss, and dehydration. Rhabditiform dermatitis may also occur.

TRICHOSTRONGYLOSIS

Trichostrongyles are small nematodes that parasitize the small intestine of ruminants. Mild climates promote clinical disease. These parasites have a direct life cycle. Third-stage larvae are rendered infective in the acid environment of the abomasum. The larvae burrow in between crypt enterocytes, but do not generally penetrate the basement membrane. Paradoxically, crypt hyperplasia is followed by villous atrophy. As with most other parasitisms, crowding, poor sanitation, and inadequate nutrition potentiate disease. Protein leakage into the intestinal lumen together with absorptive enterocyte loss leads to diarrhea, cachexia, and its metabolic consequences, which can be severe and widespread through many organ systems.

NEMATODIROSIS

Nematodirus nematodes are parasites of the cranial small intestine of ruminants. The life cycle is direct. Unlike the case with other strongyles, *Nematodirus* larvae within ova are resistant to cold temperatures.

In fact, the ova must overwinter to be infective. This is evolutionarily interesting because it allows for a new crop of susceptible hosts, particularly lambs and calves each year. Fourth- and fifth-stage larvae reside in deeper layers of the mucosa than do the trichostrongyles. Villous atrophy of the cranial small intestine is the predominant histologic lesion. *Nematodirus* spp. do not generally cause disease except in association with other parasites. Signs include green diarrhea, weight loss, and hypoproteinemia secondary to weight loss and inappetence.

COOPERIOSIS

Also a small intestinal parasite of ruminants, *Cooperia* nematodes—unlike other trichostrongyles—do not burrow into the intestine. Rather, they reside between villi, causing pressure necrosis. Their life cycle and clinical signs are similar to that of the other strongyles already described.

OESOPHAGOSTOMUM

The nodular worms of ruminants (*Oesophagostomum columbianum, Oesophagostomum radiatum*) and pigs (*Oesophagostomum dentatum*) cause subserosal mineralized nodules that are characteristic of the disease. These nodules generally are of no clinical significance, but they make the intestines unsuitable for use as sausage casings. Occasionally, they are associated with, and can be the cause of, intussusceptions.

Third-stage larvae of *Oesophagostomum columbianum* of sheep are ingested, penetrate deeply into the small intestinal wall, excyst, and molt to fourth-stage larvae, which mature in the colon. They may encyst in the colonic wall and become mineralized subserosal nodules or may mature to adults. Disease is more severe in nutritionally debilitated animals. Most infestations are asymptomatic. *Oesophagostomum radiatum* of cattle may produce inappetence, hypoproteinemia from damaged enterocyte tight junctions, and anemia and hemorrhage from consumptive coagulopathy induced by the parasites. Nodules may also form, as in sheep. Oesophagostomiasis in pigs is usually asymptomatic, although ill thrift and malaise secondary to typhlocolitis may occur.

PINWORMS

Oxyuris equi is the most common pinworm of domestic animals. The parasites occupy the lumen of the distal intestine of horses and occasionally cause rectal pruritus by laying their eggs on the perineal region. *Enterobius vermicularis* is the pinworm of primates and great apes. It is not zoonotic and is generally of little clinical consequence.

CESTODES

Tapeworms, although frequently found in the alimentary system, are generally of little clinical significance.

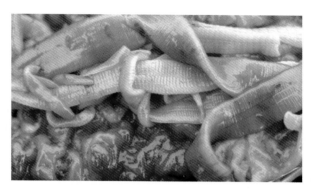

Fig. 7-185   Cestodiasis, small intestine, fur seal. Segmented tapeworms are present in this otherwise normal intestine. *(Courtesy Dr. H. Gelberg, College of Veterinary Medicine, Oregon State University.)*

They require two and sometimes three hosts to complete their life cycles. Tapeworms attach to the gut wall by means of their anterior scolex, which may have hooks in addition to four suckers (Fig. 7-185). Although they can cause some damage at the site of attachment, generally they compete with the host for nutrients. Lacking an alimentary system, they absorb nutrients through their surface. Tapeworms are flat, segmented, and hermaphroditic, reproducing by addition of segments or proglottids. Examples of tapeworms are *Anoplocephala* spp. in horses, *Moniezia* spp. in ruminants, and *Diphyllobothrium* and *Dipylidium* spp. in dogs and cats. *Mesocestoides* spp. can infect dogs. In some cases, this parasite can perforate through the intestine and proliferate in the peritoneal cavity.

Taenia and *Echinococcus* spp. are the most destructive of the cestodes. Although carnivores are the definitive hosts, the larval forms reside in the viscera and body cavities of the intermediate hosts, usually ruminants, pigs, horses, or rodents. Human beings can also become infected, sometimes taking 20 or 30 years for clinical disease to appear. The damage in the intermediate hosts may be quite severe.

TREMATODES

Trematodes are uncommon parasites of the alimentary tract. *Nanophyetus salmincola* uses a snail and a fish as intermediate hosts. It carries the rickettsia responsible for salmon poisoning in the Northwestern United States. Lesions of the intestine are hemorrhagic enteritis.

Alaria spp. can attach to the small intestine of dogs and cats, but are generally innocuous. The mesocercariae can cause tissue damage during their migrations through body organs of the host. Paratenic hosts are frogs, snakes, and mice.

Schistosomiasis of ruminants, pigs, horses, and dogs can cause granulomatous intestinal lesions with protein loss secondary to the parasite's presence in mesenteric veins after migration through the liver. Parasites are acquired by direct penetration of the skin by cercariae.

ACANTHOCEPHALANS

The thorny-headed worm of pigs, *Macracanthorhynchus hirudinaceus*, is a small-intestinal parasite with an arthropod intermediate host. They are occasionally misidentified as tapeworms, which they superficially resemble. However, they are not truly segmented parasites. They occasionally penetrate the bowel wall at the site of parasite attachment, causing peritonitis.

Prosthenorchis spp. are acanthocephalids of primates. Cockroaches are the intermediate hosts.

INTESTINAL NEOPLASIA

Neoplasms of various types occur in the gastrointestinal system of domestic animals. Those of the oral cavity and stomach have already been discussed. Intestinal neoplasms are diagnosed most frequently in dogs and cats, in large part because of their longer life span. Additionally, pets live in close harmony with their human companions, and thus it is possible that some of the same environmental factors that cause human cancer may also cause similar problems in animals.

In dogs, benign neoplasms of the intestinal tract are most commonly adenomas or polyps, and their malignant counterparts adenocarcinomas. Smooth muscle neoplasms termed leiomyomas and leiomyosarcomas arise from existing intestinal muscular layers. Lymphosarcoma can be solitary, metastatic, or multicentric. In cats, the most common neoplasms include alimentary lymphosarcoma (Fig. 7-186); mastocytomas (Fig. 7-187), which are associated with ulceration; adenomas; adenocarcinomas; and carcinoids. In canids, 5% to 7% of lymphomas are gastrointestinal. Those of the

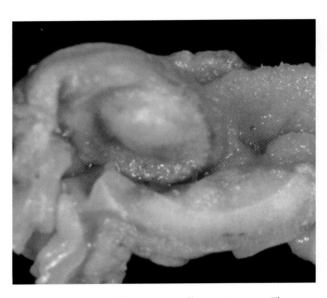

Fig. 7-187   Mast cell tumor, small intestine, cat. The submucosal nodule contains neoplastic mast cells. *(Courtesy Dr. H. Gelberg, College of Veterinary Medicine, Oregon State University.)*

gastrointestinal tract are epitheliotropic and primarily T lymphocyte in origin. In humans, most gastrointestinal lymphomas are of B-cell origin. In sheep, adenocarcinomas of the intestine are fairly common and are virus-induced. In cows, alimentary lymphosarcoma is most common. Horses rarely have intestinal neoplasms develop.

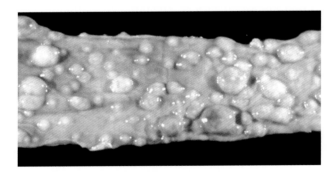

Fig. 7-186   Lymphoma (lymphosarcoma), colon, cat. Numerous submucosal nodules contain neoplastic lymphocytes. Note that the mucosal epithelium is intact (smooth and shiny) and not ulcerated. *(Courtesy Dr. H. Gelberg, College of Veterinary Medicine, Oregon State University.)*

▲ SUGGESTED READINGS

Altekruse SF, Tollefson LK: Human campylobacteriosis: a challenge to the veterinary profession, *J Am Vet Med Assoc* 223: 445-452, 2003.

Bacciarilni LN, Boerliln P, Straub R et al: Immunohistochemical localization of *Clostridium perfringens* β-2 toxin in the gastrointestinal tract of horses, *Vet Pathol* 40:376-381, 2003.

Bland AP, Frost AJ, Lysons RJ: Susceptibility of porcine ileal enterocytes to the cytotoxin of *Serpulina hyodysenteriae* and the resolution of epithelial lesions: an electron microscopic study, *Vet Pathol* 32:24-35, 1995.

Bowman DD: *Georgi's parasitology for veterinarians*, ed 7, Philadelphia, 1999, Saunders.

Cooper DM, Gebhart CJ: Comparative aspects of proliferative enteritis, *J Vet Med Assoc* 212:1446-1451, 1998.

Dennison AC, VanMetre DC, Callen RJ et al: Hemorrhagic bowel syndrome in dairy cattle: 22 cases (1997-2000), *J Am Vet Med Assoc* 221:686-689, 2002.

Dubielzig RR, Goldschmidt MH, Brodey RS: The nomenclature of periodontal epulides in dogs, *Vet Pathol* 16:209-214, 1979.

Dutra F, Schuch LFD, Delucchi E et al: Equine monocytic ehrlichiosis (Potomac horse fever) in horses in Uruguay and southern Brazil, *J Vet Diag Invest* 13:433-437, 2001.

Hoet AE, Nielsen PR, Hasoksuz M et al: Detection of bovine torovirus and other enteric pathogens in feces from diarrhea cases in cattle, *J Vet Diag Invest* 15:205-2123, 2003.

Kanter M, Mott J, Ohashi N et al: Analysis of 16S rRNA and 51-kilodalton antigen gene and transmission in mice of *Ehrlichia risticii* in virulgate nematodes from *Elimia livescens* snails in Ohio, *J Clin Microbiol* 38:3349-3358, 2000.

MacIntyre N, Smith DGE, Shaw DJ et al: Immunopathogenesis of experimentally produced proliferative enteropathy in pigs, *Vet Pathol* 40:421-432, 2003.

McCue ME, Davis EG, Rush BR et al: Dexamethasone for treatment of multisystemic eosinophilic epitheliotropic disease in a horse, *J Am Vet Med Assoc* 223:1320-1323, 2003.

Meyerholz DK, Stabel TJ: Comparison of early ileal invasion by *Salmonella enterica* serovars *cholerasuis* and *typhimurium*, *Vet Pathol* 40:371-375, 2003.

Moon HW: Intestine. In Cheville NF, editor: *Cell pathology*, ed 2, Ames, 1983, Iowa State University Press.

O'Toole D, Li H, Sourk C et al: Malignant catarrhal fever in a bison (*Bison bison*) feedlot, 1993-2000, *J Vet Diag Invest* 14:183-193, 2002.

Sanchez A, Lee MD, Harmon BG et al: Animal issues associated with *Escherichia coli* O157:H7, *J Am Vet Med Assoc* 221:1122-1126, 2002.

Santos RL, Zhang S, Tsolis RM et al: Morphologic and molecular characterization of *Salmonella typhimurium* infection in neonatal calves, *Vet Pathol* 39:200-215, 2002.

Songer JG: Clostridial enteric diseases of domestic animals, *Clin Microbiol Rev* 216-234, 1996.

Yaeger M, Funk N, Hoffman L: A survey of agents associated with neonatal diarrhea in Iowa swine including *Clostridium difficile* and porcine reproductive and respiratory virus syndrome, *J Vet Diag Invest* 14:281-287, 2002.

8

Liver, Biliary System, and Exocrine Pancreas*

JOHN M. CULLEN

INTRODUCTION

LIVER AND BILIARY SYSTEM

NORMAL ANATOMY

DEVELOPMENT

Early in embryogenesis, the origins of the liver are evident. The hepatic diverticulum, also termed the liver bud, arises from embryonic endoderm as a hollow outpouching of the primitive duodenum. Primitive hepatic epithelial cells of the hepatic diverticulum extend into the adjacent mesenchymal stroma and surround the vessels that form the vitelline venous plexus, a complex of vessels that drain the yolk sac. This relationship between the epithelial cells of the liver and the small-caliber vitelline vessels is the earliest developmental form of the hepatic sinusoids. The caudal part of the hepatic diverticulum will develop into the gallbladder and the cystic duct. Hepatic connective tissue is derived from the septum transversum, a sheet of cells that incompletely separates the pericardial and peritoneal cavity, and an ingrowth of mesenchymal cells from the coelomic cavity.

The biliary epithelium also arises from the hepatic diverticulum. Intrahepatic ducts develop from a structure, termed the limiting plate, which is composed of hepatoblasts that surround the portal vein branches and ensheathe the mesenchyme of the primitive portal tract. A second discontinuous outer layer of primitive hepatoblasts forms subsequently, and the two-cell thick regions remodel into tubules and become the intrahepatic biliary ductular system. Development of the ducts

begins at the porta hepatis and extends to the margins of the liver until the later stages of gestation. The residual portion of the hollow outpouching of the hepatic diverticulum persists to become the extrahepatic bile ducts.

It is known that the hepatocytes and the biliary epithelial cells share a common embryonic origin, but the factors that lead to the final characteristic morphology of the primitive hepatoblasts are not well understood. Epithelial-mesenchymal interactions are believed to play a role. Primitive hepatic epithelial cells in contact with vascular endothelium are destined to become hepatocytes, and those in contact with the developing mesenchyme of the portal tracts develop into bile ducts.

STRUCTURE

The liver is the largest internal organ in the body. In adult carnivores, the liver constitutes 3% to 4% of the body weight. In adult omnivores, it is about 2% of body weight and about 1% of the body weight in herbivores. In the neonate of all species, the liver is a larger percentage of body weight than in the adult. In monogastric animals, the liver abuts the diaphragm and occupies the central area of the cranial abdomen. In ruminants the liver is displaced to the right side of the cranial abdominal cavity. A series of ligaments maintain the liver in its position. The coronary ligament attaches the liver to the diaphragm near the esophagus. The falciform ligament attaches the midline of the liver to the ventral midline of the abdomen. The round ligament, a remnant of the umbilical vein, is embedded within the falciform ligament. The liver is supplied with blood from two sources. The portal vein drains the digestive tract and provides 60% to 70% of the total afferent hepatic blood flow. The hepatic artery provides the remainder of hepatic blood flow. Blood leaves the liver via the hepatic vein, which is very short, and enters the caudal

*Previous chapters on this subject in earlier editions were written or partially written by Dr. N. J. MacLachlan, School of Veterinary Medicine, University of California-Davis.

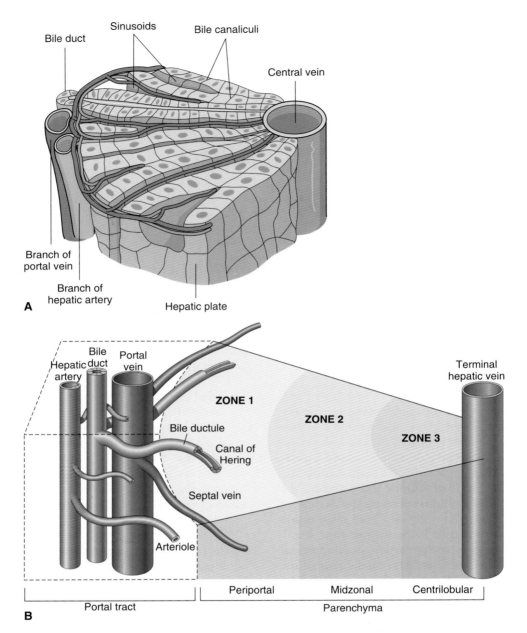

Fig. 8-1   **Schematic views of the microscopic and functional organization of the liver.**
A, Microscopic organization of the liver. A central vein is located in the center of the lobule
with plates of hepatocytes arranged radially. Branches of the portal vein and hepatic artery are
located on the periphery of the lobule, and blood from both perfuses the sinusoids. Peripherally
located bile ducts drain the bile canaliculi that run between hepatocytes. **B,** Functional organization of the liver. Both the lobule and the acinus are represented. The lobule is a hexagonal
unit with portal areas at the margin and a terminal hepatic vein (central vein) at the center.
The lobule is divided into the periportal, midzonal, and centrilobular areas. The acinus is a
diamond-shaped structure with the distributing branches of the vessels from the portal areas as
the center of the structure. Zone 1 of the acinus is closest to the afferent blood supply, and
zone 3 is at the tip of the diamond-shaped structure, close to the terminal hepatic vein. Zone 2
is between zones 1 and 3. (*A, From McCance KL, Huether SE: Pathophysiology: the biologic basis for diseases
in adults and children, ed 4, Mosby, 2002, St Louis. B, From Kumar V, Abbas AK, Fausto N: Robbins & Cotran
pathologic basis of disease, ed 7, Philadelphia, 2005, Saunders.*)

vena cava. The liver has a smooth capsular surface and the parenchyma consists of friable red-brown tissue that is divided into lobes. Gross subdivision of the liver into lobes differs among the domestic species. At the periphery, the lobes taper to a sharp edge.

The classical functional subunit of the liver is the hepatic lobule, a hexagonal structure, 1 to 2 mm wide. At the center, the lobule has a central vein (also termed the terminal hepatic venule), which is a tributary of the hepatic vein, and at the angles of the hexagon, it has portal tracts (Fig. 8-1). The portal tracts contain bile ducts, branches of the portal vein, the hepatic artery, nerves, and lymph vessels, all supported by a collagenous stroma (Fig. 8-2). The limiting plate, a discontinuous border of hepatocytes, forms the outer boundary of

the portal tract. Blood flows into the sinusoids from the terminal distributing branches of the hepatic artery and portal veins that leave the portal tracts and form an outer perimeter of the lobule (Fig. 8-2). Portal blood and hepatic arterial blood mix in the sinusoids. Blood drains from the sinusoids into the central veins and to progressively larger sublobular veins and then into the hepatic veins.

Alternatively, when the liver is viewed as a bile-secreting gland, the acinus is the anatomic subunit of the hepatic parenchyma. Terminal afferent branches (penetrating vessels) of the portal vein and hepatic artery project into the parenchyma, like branches from the trunk of a tree, forming the long axis of the diamond-shaped acinus. Thus terminal afferent branches

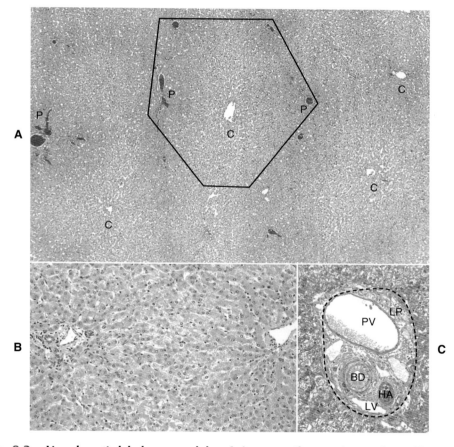

Fig. 8-2 **Liver, hepatic lobules, normal dog. A,** Low magnification. A central vein (C) is located in the center of the lobule. Branches of the portal vein, hepatic artery, bile duct, and lymphatic vessels are located on the periphery of the lobule in portal tracts (P) (also Fig. 8-2, C). H&E stain. **B,** Higher magnification. Plates of hepatocytes arranged radially between a central vein (C) to portal tracts (P). H&E stain. **C,** Higher magnification, portal tract. The normal portal tract contains the hepatic artery (HA), bile duct (BD), portal vein (PV), and several lymphatic vessels (LV). These structures are surrounded by a collagenous extracellular matrix that forms an abrupt border with a circumferential row of hepatocytes, termed the limiting plate (LP—*dotted line*). Note that the profile of the portal vein is typically larger than those of the hepatic artery and bile duct. H&E stain. (**A** *and* **C,** *Courtesy Dr. J.M. Cullen, College of Veterinary Medicine, North Carolina State University.* **B,** *Courtesy Dr. J.F. Zachary, College of Veterinary Medicine, University of Illinois.*)

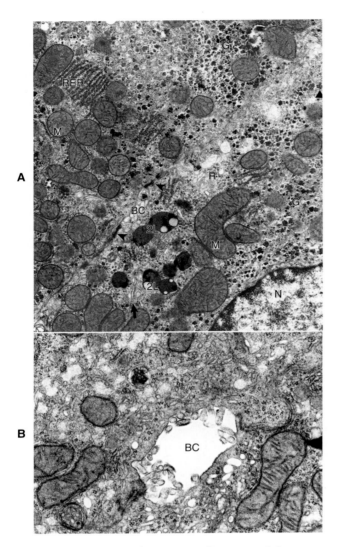

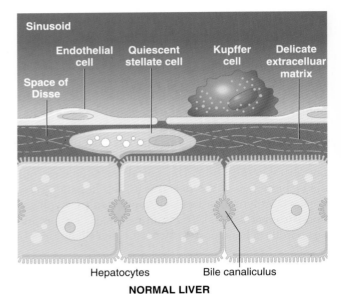

Fig. 8-4   Schematic diagram of the hepatic sinusoid. The vascular lumen is lined by discontinuous capillaries. Kupffer cells rest on the endothelial cells and project into the sinusoid. Between the endothelial cells and the hepatocytes is a gap called the space of Disse. Microvilli extending from the luminal aspect of the hepatocytes are found in this space. Hepatic stellate cells are situated within the space of Disse and extend between hepatocytes. *(Schematic based on concepts presented in Friedman SL: J Biol Chem 275:2247-2250, 2000; and Crawford JM: Curr Op Gastroenterol 13:175-185, 1997.)*

Fig. 8-3   Hepatocyte, ultrastructure, liver, normal dog. **A,** Features to note are the nucleus *(N)*, mitochondria *(M)*, secondary lysosomes *(2L)*, glycogen *(G)*, rough endoplasmic reticulum *(RER)*, Golgi *(arrow)*, bile canaliculus *(BC)*, and free ribosomes *(R)*. Note desmosomes on both sides of the bile canaliculus *(arrowheads)*. TEM. Uranyl citrate and lead acetate stain. **B,** Higher magnification of bile canaliculus *(BC)*. Note the microvilli projecting into the lumen of the canaliculus. TCM Uranyl citrate and lead acetate stain. *(A and B, Courtesy Dr. V. Meador, Eli Lilly Co.)*

of the portal vein and hepatic artery are at the center of the acinus and the terminal hepatic venule is located at the periphery. Each terminal hepatic venule (central vein) receives blood from several acini. There are three zones within the acinus. Zone 1 is closest to the afferent blood coming from the hepatic artery and the portal vein. Zone 2 is peripheral to zone 1, and zone 3 borders the terminal hepatic venule (Fig. 8-1). In this anatomic unit, bile flows from the hepatocytes through the bile canaliculi in zone 3 into the bile ductules at the termination of zone 1 at the portal area and then into bile ducts in the portal areas.

The ultrastructural appearance of hepatocytes reflects the cell's active metabolism, bile secretion, and close contact with the plasma (Fig. 8-3). The surface of the hepatocyte that faces the lumen of the sinusoids contains an abundance of microvilli, which increase the hepatocytic surface area and facilitate uptake of plasma-borne substances, such as bilirubin and amino acids, and the secretion of products of hepatic metabolism, such as lipoproteins and clotting factors. Basolateral aspects of hepatocytes are characterized by the presence of canaliculi, modified portions of the cell membrane in two adjacent hepatocytes, which form a lumen for bile secretion. The cytoplasm contains glycogen and a variety of organelles, including numerous mitochondria, lysosomes, and abundant smooth and rough endoplasmic reticulum.

Within the liver, hepatocytes are arranged in one-cell thick branching plates, which extend radially from the terminal hepatic venule. Hepatic plates are separated by vascular sinusoids. Blood from the terminal afferent branches of the hepatic artery and portal vein mixes in the hepatic sinusoids and flows to the terminal

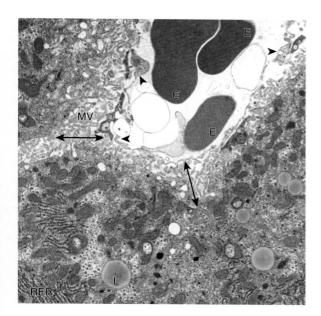

Fig. 8-5 **Hepatic sinusoids, liver, normal dog.** A sinusoid containing erythrocytes (E) can be seen in the upper right-hand portion of the figure. The margins of the sinusoid are lined with discontinuous capillaries *(arrowheads)*. The space of Disse *(double-headed arrows)* lies between the endothelial cells and the hepatocytes. Microvilli *(MV)* project from the hepatocytes into the space of Disse. Rough endoplasmic reticulum *(RER)* and lipid droplets *(L)* can be seen in the hepatocyte cytoplasm. TEM. Uranyl citrate and lead acetate stain. *(Courtesy Dr. V. Meador, Eli Lilly Co.)*

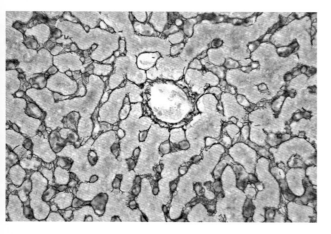

Fig. 8-6 **Reticulin fibers (reticulin stain), hepatic extracellular matrix, liver, normal dog.** This stain reveals "reticulin" *(black)*, composed of extracellular matrix and the type 3 collagen found within the space of Disse that forms the scaffolding of the hepatic parenchyma. Note the radial arrangements of the hepatic plates and the single hepatocyte thickness of the plates. A central vein is evident in the center of the image. Gordon and Sweet's reticulum stain with a nuclear fast red counterstain. *(Courtesy Dr. M.D. McGavin, College of Veterinary Medicine, University of Tennessee.)*

hepatic venule. Hepatic sinusoids differ from capillaries in that they are lined by discontinuous capillaries that lack a typical basement membrane (Fig. 8-4), whereas capillaries have a continuous endothelial lining and are ensheathed in the basement membrane. The sinusoids are critical for appropriate hepatic function. The architecture of the sinusoids enables efficient uptake of plasma constituents by hepatocytes and facilitates hepatocellular secretion. A fine scaffold of electron lucent basement membrane that contains collagen types III, IV, and XVIII, and other extracellular matrix components supports the sinusoidal endothelial cells (Figs. 8-4 and 8-5). These elements collectively make up the "reticulin" of the liver (Fig. 8-6).

Although blood cells are normally excluded from the space of Disse because they are too large to pass through endothelial gaps, the modified endothelial cells and basement membrane permit plasma to pass freely into a gap between the endothelial cells and the hepatocytes (Fig. 8-4). This critical anatomic feature of the liver is termed the space of Disse. Within this space, plasma constituents come into contact with the luminal surface of the hepatocytes. This surface of the hepatocytes is characterized by the presence of numerous microvilli, which increase the surface area of the hepatocytes and facilitate uptake of a variety of plasma-borne substances, as well secretion of synthesized products. Any damage to this area has significant impact on hepatic function.

The lumen of the sinusoids contains hepatic macrophages, termed Kupffer cells (Fig. 8-7). These cells are members of the monocyte-macrophage system, and they clear infectious agents and senescent cells, such as erythrocytes, particulate material, endotoxin, and other

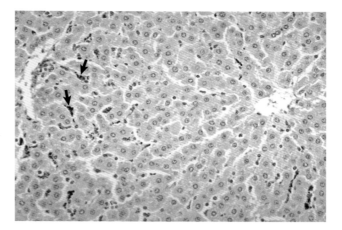

Fig. 8-7 **Kupffer cells, carbon particle uptake, liver, normal calf.** Carbon particles injected into the portal vein have been phagocytosed by Kupffer cells *(arrows)*, making them more easily detectable along the sinusoids of the liver. Nuclear fast red stain. *(Courtesy Dr. M.D. McGavin, College of Veterinary Medicine, University of Tennessee.)*

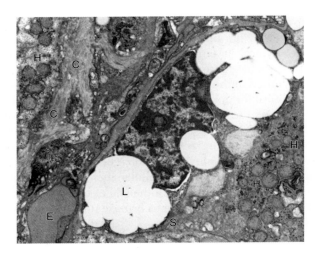

Fig. 8-8   Liver, normal dog. A hepatic stellate cell *(S)* with its characteristic cytoplasmic lipid vacuoles *(L)* is found adjacent to hepatocytes *(H)* and within the space of Disse. Bundles of collagen *(C)* are found at the margins of the cells. Erythrocytes *(E)* are within the sinusoidal lumen. TEM. Uranyl citrate and lead acetate stain. *(Courtesy Dr. V. Meador, Eli Lilly Co.)*

substances from the sinusoidal blood. They are mobile and able to migrate along the sinusoids and into areas of tissue injury and regional lymph nodes. Kupffer cells are involved in cytokine-driven interactions with hepatocytes, endothelial cells, and the stellate cells discussed later. They can express class II histocompatibility antigens and function as antigen-presenting cells, although they are not as efficient as the macrophages in other tissue. Phagocytosis and clearance of immune complexes are the primary roles of Kupffer cells. Kupffer cells are derived from in situ replication and recruitment of blood-borne monocytes.

Hepatic stellate cells (also termed lipocytes or Ito cells) are found within the space of Disse and between hepatocytes at the edge of the space of Disse (Fig. 8-8). Normally, hepatic stellate cells are primarily responsible for storing vitamin A in their characteristic cytoplasmic vacuoles. During hepatic injury, hepatic stellate cells alter their morphology and their function. These activated hepatic stellate cells lose their vitamin A content and synthesize collagen and other extracellular matrix components that lead to hepatic fibrosis.

Bile flows within the lobule in the opposite direction to blood flow, which facilitates the concentration of bile. The biliary system commences as canaliculi within the centrilobular (periacinar) areas of the hepatic lobule. The walls of canaliculi are formed entirely by the cell membranes of adjacent hepatocytes. Just outside the limiting plate, canaliculi drain into cholangioles (also known as the canals of Hering) that are lined by low cuboidal epithelium. The cholangioles converge into interlobular bile ducts that are lined with cuboidal epithelium and located in the portal areas. Bile then flows into the right and left hepatic ducts that unite to form the hepatic duct. The confluence of the common hepatic duct and the cystic duct from the gallbladder form the common bile duct by which bile is carried to the duodenum. The gallbladder is responsible for storage and concentration of bile in most species. It is absent in the horse and rat.

Both sympathetic and parasympathetic nerves running along the portal vein and the hepatic artery innervate the liver. The nerve fibers enter the liver at the hilus and ramify to the level of the portal tracts and then extend along the sinusoids. Nerve supply is believed to affect sinusoidal blood flow, the balance of hepatic blood flow from the portal vein and the hepatic artery, and metabolic functions of the liver.

NORMAL FUNCTION

The liver performs many critical functions, including the following:
- Bilirubin metabolism
- Bile acid metabolism
- Carbohydrate metabolism
- Lipid metabolism
- Xenobiotic metabolism
- Protein synthesis
- Immune function

Bilirubin metabolism

Excretion of bile is the main exocrine function of the liver. Bile is composed of water, cholesterol, bile acids, bilirubin, inorganic ions, and other constituents. Bile formation is continuous, but the rate of secretion can vary significantly. There are three major purposes for bile synthesis. The first purpose is excretory; many of the body's waste products, such as surplus cholesterol, bilirubin, and metabolized xenobiotics are eliminated in bile. The second purpose is the facilitation of digestion; bile acids secreted into the intestine aid in the digestion of lipids within the intestine. The third is to provide buffers to neutralize the acid pH of the ingesta.

Bilirubin, a major component of bile, is produced from the metabolic degradation of hemoglobin, and to a lesser extent, other heme proteins including myoglobin and the hepatic hemoproteins, such as cytochromes (Fig. 8-9). The majority of bilirubin is derived from normal extrahepatic breakdown of senescent erythrocytes in cells of the monocyte-macrophage phagocytic cell series. Senescent erythrocytes normally are phagocytosed by macrophages of the spleen, bone marrow, and liver. Within the phagocyte, the globin portion is degraded and the constituents are returned to the amino acid pool. The heme iron is transferred to iron-binding proteins such as transferrin for recycling. The remaining

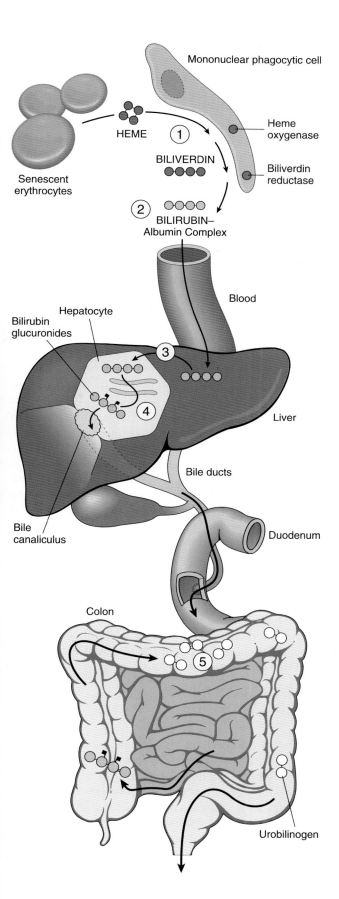

portion of heme is first oxidized by heme oxygenase to biliverdin. In the next metabolic step, biliverdin reductase converts biliverdin to bilirubin. Subsequently the bilirubin, which is poorly soluble in an aqueous medium, is then released into the blood in its unconjugated form and bound to albumin to increase its solubility in plasma.

The process of bilirubin elimination can be divided into three phases: uptake, conjugation, and secretion. Uptake refers to the process by which hepatocytes remove the bilirubin bound to albumin from the circulation. Unconjugated bilirubin is separated from albumin at the sinusoidal surface and bilirubin is taken up by hepatocytes by a carrier-mediated process. In the second phase of bilirubin metabolism, bilirubin is conjugated, principally with glucuronic acid, by bilirubin UDP-glucuronyltransferase in the endoplasmic reticulum. Following conjugation, bilirubin becomes water soluble and less toxic. It is then excreted, in the third phase of bilirubin metabolism, into the bile by active transport through specialized portions of hepatocyte membranes that form the margins of the bile canaliculi. The excretion phase is the rate-limiting step in most species.

Within the gastrointestinal tract, conjugated bilirubin is converted to urobilinogen by bacteria and a fraction of this is reabsorbed into the portal blood, a process called enterohepatic circulation, and returned to the liver. The majority of urobilinogen that is absorbed from the gastrointestinal tract is resecreted into bile. Urobilinogen has a small molecular weight and is freely filtered through the glomerulus, and small amounts are normally found in the urine. Urobilinogen that is not absorbed from the intestine becomes oxidized to stercobilin, which is responsible for the color of the feces.

Bile acid metabolism

The three principal functions of bile acids, important constituents of bile, are maintenance of cholesterol homeostasis, stimulation of bile flow and digestion, and absorption of fats and fat-soluble vitamins. Bile acids

---

Fig. 8-9   Schematic diagram of bilirubin metabolism and elimination (as depicted in human beings). *1,* Normal bilirubin production from heme (0.2 to 0.3 g per day) is derived primarily from the breakdown of senescent circulating erythrocytes, with a minor contribution from degradation of tissue heme-containing proteins. *2,* Extrahepatic bilirubin is bound to serum albumin and delivered to the liver. *3,* Hepatocellular uptake and *4,* glucuronidation in the endoplasmic reticulum generate bilirubin monoglucuronides and diglucuronides, which are water soluble and readily excreted into bile. *5,* Gut bacteria deconjugate the bilirubin and degrade it to colorless urobilinogens. The urobilinogens and the residue of intact pigments are excreted in the feces, with some reabsorption and excretion into urine. *(From Kumar V, Abbas AK, Fausto N: Robbins & Cotran pathologic basis of disease, ed 7, Philadelphia, 2005, Saunders.)*

are synthesized in the liver from cholesterol and are conjugated to glycine or taurine to facilitate their interaction with other components of bile and to prevent precipitation into calculi when they are secreted into the bile. The major bile acids are cholic acid and chenodeoxycholic acid, but there are various types and proportions of bile acids found in different species. Bile acids are actively secreted into the bile canaliculi from the hepatocyte cytoplasm by specific intramembranous molecular pumps against a concentration gradient, which creates an osmotic gradient, stimulating the inflow of water and solutes into the bile canaliculi. Conjugated bile acids are, therefore, the principal physiologic stimulus for bile production through a process termed bile acid–dependent flow. Bile acids are effective detergents that assist in the digestion of lipids within the intestine, and increasing the solubility of lipids secreted into the bile. The quantities of bile acids required far exceed the liver's capacity to produce them. For this reason, bile acids are avidly reabsorbed from the ileum, extracted from the portal blood, and resecreted into bile via a process known as enterohepatic circulation. This is a very efficient system. As much as 95% of secreted bile acids are recycled, and the proportion of reabsorbed bile acids in the liver greatly exceeds that of recently synthesized bile acids; bile acids may be recycled 15 times a day. Interruption of this process results in fat malabsorption and a deficiency of fat-soluble vitamins.

Carbohydrate metabolism

The liver has an important role in the regulation of plasma glucose concentrations. After eating, the liver removes carbohydrates (i.e., glucose, fructose) from the plasma and stores them as glycogen or fatty acids. In periods of need, energy balance is maintained by glycolysis of stored glycogen or by gluconeogenesis. Production of energy by oxidative phosphorylation and β-oxidation of fatty acids in hepatic mitochondria is used to sustain the activities of the hepatocyte.

Lipid metabolism

The liver plays a central role in lipid metabolism. It is involved in the production and degradation of plasma lipids, such as cholesterol, triglycerides, phospholipids, and lipoproteins. Cholesterol is synthesized, secreted, and degraded by hepatocytes. Hepatocytes can synthesize fatty acids when energy levels are high, and they can oxidize fatty acids as an energy source when necessary.

Xenobiotic metabolism

Foreign substances (xenobiotics), such as many therapeutic drugs, insecticides, and endogenous substances—such as steroids that are lipophilic—require conversion to water-soluble forms for elimination from the body. The cytochrome p450 enzymes of the smooth endoplasmic reticulum of the hepatocytes serve as the major site of metabolism of these substances in preparation for excretion in bile or urine. This process is discussed in detail in the section on toxic liver injury.

Protein synthesis

Synthesis of the majority of plasma proteins, mainly within the rough endoplasmic reticulum, is a principal function of the liver. Proteins produced in the liver include plasma proteins, such as albumin; a variety of transport proteins; lipoproteins; clotting factors II, V, and VII-XIII; fibrinolysis proteins; some acute phase proteins; and components of the complement system. The liver is responsible for synthesis of approximately 15% of body proteins.

The liver is also the principal site of ammonia metabolism. Highly toxic ammonia is generated through catabolism of amino acids. Metabolic conversion of ammonia into urea, a far less toxic compound, occurs through the urea cycle, which occurs almost exclusively in the liver.

Immune function

The liver has a significant immune function. It is involved in systemic, local, and mucosal immunity. It participates in the response to systemic inflammation through the synthesis and release of acute phase proteins. It contains, perhaps, the largest pool of mononuclear phagocytes and natural killer cells in the body in most species. The Kupffer cells lining the sinusoids provide the first line of defense against infectious agents, endotoxin, and foreign material absorbed from the intestines before they gain access to the systemic circulation. Most blood-borne foreign material is cleared by Kupffer cells in all domestic species, except members of the family Artiodactyla (pigs, goats, and cattle), in which this function is performed by intravascular macrophages in the pulmonary alveolar capillaries. The liver is also involved in transport from plasma cells and recirculation of secretory immunoglobulin A (IgA), the primary immunoglobulin of the mucosal surfaces, into the biliary tree and intestine.

HEPATOBILIARY INJURY AND DEGENERATION
PORTALS OF ENTRY

The liver and biliary systems are exposed to infectious or otherwise injurious substances via three main routes: hematogenous, biliary, and direct penetration (Box 8-1). The liver receives the entire flow of the portal vein and as a consequence is bathed in potentially injurious microbes, which inhabit and penetrate the digestive system, and toxic substances that have been ingested or produced by the intestinal flora. The distribution of blood from the portal vein to the different lobes

Box **8-1**

Portals of Entry

	Liver	Biliary System	Exocrine Pancreas
DIRECT EXTENSION			
Penetrating trauma through the abdominal wall or rib cage	Yes	Yes	Yes
Penetrating trauma through the lumen of the gastrointestinal tract	Yes	Yes	Yes
HEMATOGENOUS			
Localization within the sinusoids via the portal vein, hepatic artery, or umbilical vein in neonates	Yes	No	No
Localization within Kupffer cells	Yes	No	No
Localization within capillary beds of the wall of the gallbladder or arteriolar rete of the biliary tree	No	Yes	No
Localization within capillary beds of the pancreatic parenchyma	No	No	Yes
RETROGRADE BILIARY TRANSPORT			
Ascending bacterial or parasitic infections gain access to the organ	Yes	Yes	No
RETROGRADE PANCREATIC DUCTULAR TRANSPORT			
Ascending bacterial or parasitic infections gain access to the organ	No	No	Yes

of the liver is most likely nonuniform. So-called portal streaming refers to the differential flow of portal blood from one segment of the digestive tract to particular lobes of the liver. This explains why some lobes of the liver are more severely affected by toxins that are absorbed by the small intestine rather than the large intestine. Examples of this include the preponderance of injury to the left liver lobe of sheep that ingest the mycotoxin sporidesmin. Systemic infections or intoxications can also affect the liver through the blood from the hepatic artery. Neonates and fetal animals are also as risk from infections ascending the umbilical vein. Infectious agents, such as enteric bacteria and parasites, can also gain access to the liver through the biliary tree that is in direct connection with the duodenum and enteric bacteria. Finally, direct penetration of the body cavity or from the digestive tract (i.e., traumatic reticuloperitonitis or foreign bodies in the reticulum) can deliver infectious or traumatic insults.

DEFENSES

The liver is well defended from blood-borne injury by the Kupffer cells, the fixed macrophages that are distributed intermittently throughout the lumen of the sinusoids on the surface of endothelial cells (Box 8-2). They actively ingest and degrade bacteria and other organisms, senescent cells such as erythrocytes and particulate matter in the sinusoidal blood. They are very efficient and are able to clear virtually all particulate

matter in a single pass through the liver. Kupffer cells are particularly important in the removal of endotoxin from the portal blood.

The biliary tree, like the upper gastrointestinal tract, is defended from infection by secreted IgA as part of mucosal immunity (Box 8-2). The majority of biliary IgA is synthesized by gastrointestinal plasma cells. The majority of released IgA is taken into lymph and from there it enters the blood stream. Hepatocytes in many species can transport IgA from blood across their cell membranes via a secretory component–mediated endocytosis. Subsequently, IgA molecules reach the bile by secretion into canaliculi. Concentrations of bile IgA are maintained by enterohepatic circulation. Within the biliary tree, IgA provides defense from infectious agents and clearance of harmful antigens as antibody-antigen complexes. In addition, the biliary tree is protected by the sphincter at the terminal end of the common bile duct, which provides a physical barrier to the ascent of enteric bacteria and the continuous flow of bile that assists in flushing bacteria out of the ducts.

The liver is protected from direct penetration by its anatomic location within the protection of the rib cage. The wall of the digestive tract also provides a certain degree of protection from penetration by ingested foreign bodies.

The high metabolic rate of hepatocytes renders them highly susceptible to metabolic disturbances that lead to cellular degeneration and necrosis (Box 8-3).

Box **8-2**

Defense Mechanisms against Injury and Infectious Agents

	Liver	Biliary System	Exocrine Pancreas
STRUCTURAL AND FUNCTIONAL BARRIER			
Skin	Yes	Yes	Yes
Rib cage	Yes	Yes	Yes
Omentum (barrier that limits access of injurious material to the organ)	Yes	Yes	Yes
IMMUNOLOGIC RESPONSES			
Kupffer cells	Yes	No	No
Resident and migrating cells (recruited monocytes), which are part of the monocyte-macrophage system	Yes	No	No
Innate and adaptive immunologic responses (including secretory immunoglobulin A), which form the body's overall immune system	Yes	Yes	Yes
BIOCHEMICAL DEFENSES			
Enzyme inhibitors that reduce the risk of **premature enzyme activation** and tissue injury	No	No	Yes

This section will consider the patterns of hepatic degeneration, responses of the liver to injury, and inflammation of the liver.

HEPATOBILIARY INJURY
Necrosis and apoptosis

The epithelial cells of the liver, hepatocytes, and biliary epithelium are the principal targets of most liver diseases. Sublethal injury to hepatocytes is characterized by cell swelling (hydropic degeneration), steatosis, or atrophy. Cells that have sustained a sublethal injury often remove damaged organelles by forming autophagosomes. Material than cannot be digested further is retained as lipofuscin, which is why after sublethal injury this pigment can often be found in affected cells and associated phagocytes.

Box **8-3**

Mechanisms of Liver Injury

- Metabolic bioactivation of chemicals via cytochrome P450 to reactive species
- Stimulation of autoimmunity
- Stimulation of apoptosis
- Disruption of calcium homeostasis leading to cell surface blebbing and lysis
- Canalicular injury
- Mitochondrial injury

Data from Lee W: *N Engl J Med* 349:474-485, 2003.

By convention, cell death has been divided into two distinct processes. These are necrosis, characterized by cytoplasmic swelling, destruction of organelles, and disruption of the plasma membrane, and apoptosis or programmed cell death, characterized by one of several active processes involving caspases that lead to cell shrinkage and an intact cell membrane. Necrosis is triggered by lethal injury. Necrotic cells typically exhibit karyorrhexis and fragmentation of the cell body. Coagulative necrosis results from sudden denaturation of hepatocytes and produces swollen hepatocytes with a preserved eosinophilic cytoplasmic outline and karyorrhexis or karyolysis. Lytic necrosis is characterized by a loss of hepatocytes and an influx of erythrocytes into the vacant space or condensation of the reticular connective tissue (collagen and other extracellular matrix) scaffolding of the liver that once supported the hepatocytes.

Classical apoptosis is triggered by an interaction between tumor necrosis factor-α or Fas ligand and specific receptors on the cell membrane leading to caspase activation, although other pathways, including those involving mitochondrial cytochrome-c, have been identified. Apoptosis is recognized by the formation of acidophilic bodies, which are brightly eosinophilic, homogeneous, round structures that can be found between hepatocytes, within the lumen of sinusoids, or within macrophages or hepatocytes. A detailed review of cell death is beyond the scope of this section but is covered in Chapter 1. However, recent evidence reveals that there may some overlap between necrosis and apoptosis, depending on the cell type and the type and dose of injurious agent. Thus both hepatic necrosis and apoptosis can be produced by the same agent and can occur in the same liver.

Patterns of hepatocellular degeneration and necrosis

Although the liver is subjected to a wide variety of different insults, the cellular degeneration and/or necrosis that results invariably occurs in one of three morphologic patterns:

- Random hepatocellular degeneration and/or necrosis
- Zonal hepatocellular degeneration and/or necrosis
- Massive hepatocellular degeneration and/or necrosis

Random hepatocellular degeneration. Random hepatocellular degeneration and/or necrosis is characterized by the presence either of single cell necrosis throughout the liver or multifocal areas of necrotic hepatocytes. These areas are scattered randomly throughout the liver; there is no predictable location within a lobule. This pattern is typical of many infectious agents, including viruses, bacteria, and certain protozoa. Lesions may be obvious grossly as discrete, pale or less often dark red foci that are sharply delineated from the adjacent parenchyma (Fig. 8-10, *A*). The size of such foci is variable, ranging from tiny (<1 mm) to several millimeters. Hepatocytes in affected areas are either degenerated or necrotic because of the injurious effects of the infectious agents and the stage of the process (Fig. 8-10, *B*).

Zonal hepatocellular degeneration and/or necrosis. Zonal hepatocellular degeneration and/or necrosis or, as it is more simply termed, zonal change, affects hepatocytes within defined areas of the hepatic lobule. The zones are centrilobular (periacinar), midzonal (between centrilobular and periportal areas), or periportal (centroacinar) areas. Extensive zonal change within the liver, regardless of location within the lobule, typically produces a liver that is pale and modestly enlarged with rounded margins, has increased friability, and characteristically has an enhanced lobular pattern on the capsular and cut surface of the organ (Fig. 8-11). Degenerated hepatocytes swell and, when the majority of hepatocytes in a zone are affected, that portion of the lobule appears pale. In contrast, once the hepatocytes in a particular zone of the lobule have become necrotic, this results in dilation and congestion of sinusoids so that the affected zone appears red. Although zonal change typically produces an enhanced lobular pattern, microscopic examination is usually required to determine the type of zonal change. Specific forms of zonal change are described next.

Centrilobular degeneration and necrosis. Centrilobular degeneration and necrosis of hepatocytes is particularly common (Fig. 8-12), as this portion

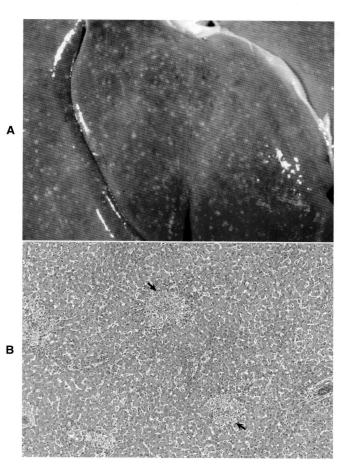

Fig. 8-10   Random hepatocellular injury, liver. A, Equine herpes virus infection, foal. Random foci of viral-induced lytic necrosis. **B,** Salmonellosis, focal necrosis and inflammation, pig. The random pattern (*arrows*) of hepatocellular necrosis and inflammation caused by septicemic *Salmonella* spp. can also be seen within the hepatic lobules. H&E stain. (*A, Courtesy Drs. J. King and L. Roth, College of Veterinary Medicine, Cornell University. B, Courtesy Dr. J.M. Cullen, College of Veterinary Medicine, North Carolina State University.*)

of the lobule receives the least oxygenated blood and is therefore susceptible to hypoxia, and it has the greatest enzymatic activity (mixed-function oxidases) capable of activating compounds into toxic forms. Centrilobular necrosis can result from a precipitous and severe anemia or right side heart failure. Similarly, passive congestion of the liver results in hypoxia as a result of stasis of blood and produces atrophy of centrilobular hepatocytes.

Paracentral (periacinar) cellular degeneration. Paracentral (periacinar) cellular degeneration involves only a wedge around the central vein because only the periphery of one acinus is affected, typically reflecting the action of a direct-acting toxin that requires bioactivation (Fig. 8-13) or severe, acute anemia. As several

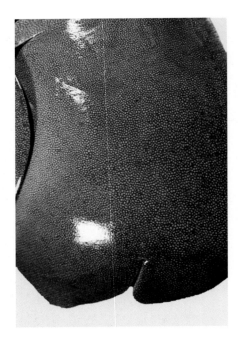

Fig. 8-11 Zonal hepatocellular injury, liver, horse. Accentuation of the normal lobular pattern is evident on the capsular surface of the liver. This is not a specific change, as it may be associated with zonal hepatocellular degeneration and/or necrosis (regardless of lobular location), passive congestion, or diffuse cellular infiltration of the portal and periportal areas (often reflecting hepatic involvement of hematopoietic neoplasms, such as lymphoma and myeloproliferative disorders). *(Courtesy Dr. J. King, College of Veterinary Medicine, Cornell University.)*

acini border on a single central vein (terminal hepatic venule), changes induced by hypoxia may not be present equally in all acini, and thus hepatocytes at the periphery of one acinus can have more severe change than those in adjacent acini.

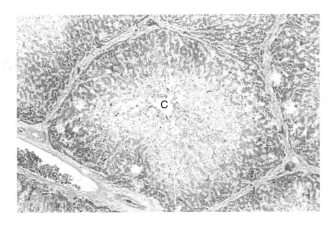

Fig. 8-12 Centrilobular necrosis, zonal hepatocellular injury, liver, pig. Centrilobular necrosis (periacinar or zone 3) is characterized by a circumferential zone of hepatocellular necrosis surrounding the terminal hepatic venule (central vein [C]). H&E stain. *(Courtesy Dr. M.D. McGavin, College of Veterinary Medicine, University of Tennessee.)*

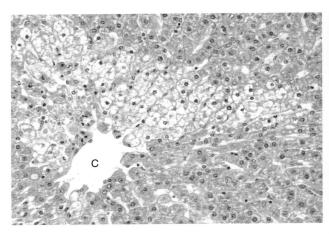

Fig. 8-13 Paracentral degeneration and necrosis, zonal hepatocellular injury, liver, cow. Rather than a pattern of complete circumferential necrosis, a wedge-shaped area of hepatocytes is damaged. In this case, the paracentral lesion consists of necrotic hepatocytes to the left and other hepatocytes with hydropic degeneration. This wedge is the apex of the diamond-shaped liver acinus (zone 3) and reflects the partitioning of the lobule based on the inflow of blood from each of the individual portal tracts that surround the lobule. This change can be seen as an early manifestation of hepatic hypoxia in animals with anemia or right-sided heart failure and precedes centrilobular necrosis. C, Central vein. H&E stain. *(Courtesy Dr. M.D. McGavin, College of Veterinary Medicine, University of Tennessee.)*

Midzonal degeneration and necrosis. Midzonal degeneration and necrosis are unusual lesions in domestic animals but have been reported in pigs and horses with aflatoxicosis and cats exposed to hexachlorophene (Fig. 8-14).

Periportal degeneration and necrosis. Periportal degeneration and necrosis are also uncommon but may

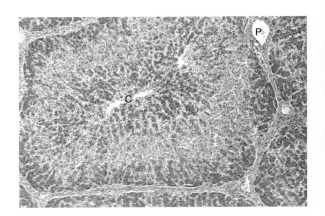

Fig. 8-14 Midzonal necrosis, zonal hepatocellular injury, liver, pig. Midzonal necrosis is the least common pattern of hepatic injury. Hepatocytes in the middle portion of the lobule (zone 2) are affected and hepatocytes in the other regions are spared. C, Central vein; P, portal vein. H&E stain. *(Courtesy Dr. M.D. McGavin, College of Veterinary Medicine, University of Tennessee.)*

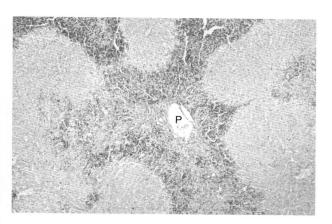

Fig. 8-15   Periporta l necrosis, zonal hepatocellular injury, liver, horse. Periportal (periacinar or zone 1) necrosis is an uncommon pattern of hepatocellular injury. Hepatocytes surrounding the portal tracts (*P*) are affected. H&E stain. *(Courtesy Dr. M.D. McGavin, College of Veterinary Medicine, University of Tennessee.)*

occur following exposure to toxins, such as phosphorus, that do not require metabolism by mixed function oxidases (most active in the centrilobular hepatocytes) to cause injury (Fig. 8-15). Some of these compounds may be metabolized to injurious intermediates by cytoplasmic enzymes found in periportal hepatocytes. Alternatively, some of these toxins may not require metabolism and produce hepatocyte injury in the first hepatocytes that they encounter as they flow from the portal areas.

Bridging necrosis.   Bridging necrosis is the result of confluence of areas of necrosis. Bridging may link centrilobular areas (central bridging) or centrilobular areas to periportal areas (Fig. 8-16).

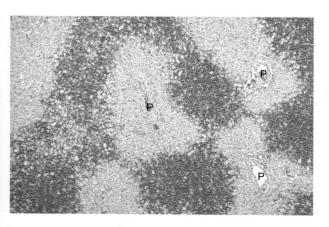

Fig. 8-16   Bridging necrosis, zonal hepatocellular injury, liver. *Bridging necrosis* refers to a pattern characterized by connection of areas of necrosis between different lobules. Three patterns of bridging necrosis are recognized: central to central, as seen here; portal to portal; and central to portal. *P*, Portal area. H&E stain. *(Courtesy Dr. M.D. McGavin, College of Veterinary Medicine, University of Tennessee.)*

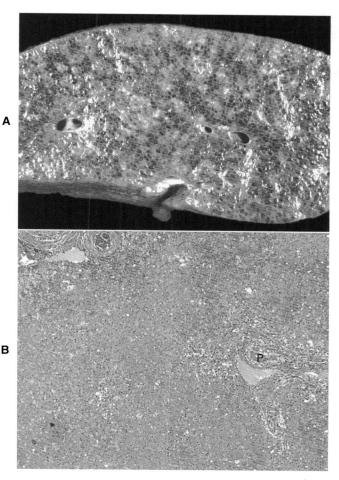

Fig. 8-17   Massive necrosis, liver. A, Pig, cut surface. *Massive necrosis* refers to a pattern of necrosis that involves an entire hepatic lobule, as seen here. **B,** Dog. The entire population of hepatocytes within the lobule has undergone necrosis. *P*, Portal area. H&E stain. *(**A,** Courtesy Dr. D. Cho, College of Veterinary Medicine, Louisiana State University; and Noah's Arkive, College of Veterinary Medicine, The University of Georgia. **B,** Courtesy Dr. J.M. Cullen, College of Veterinary Medicine, North Carolina State University.)*

Massive necrosis.   Massive necrosis is not necessarily, as the name might be taken to imply, necrosis of the entire liver, but rather the term describes necrosis of an entire hepatic lobule or contiguous lobules (Fig. 8-17, *A*). All hepatocytes within affected lobules are necrotic. The gross appearance of the liver varies with the maturity of the lesion. If, in acute cases, the majority of the parenchyma is affected, the liver may initially be modestly increased in size with a smooth external surface and dark parenchyma because of extensive congestion. At first, necrotic hepatocytes lyse and the residual stroma becomes condensed. Regeneration does not occur because virtually all hepatocytes in the lobule are affected. Microscopically, affected areas consist of blood-filled spaces within a connective tissue stroma devoid of hepatocytes (Fig. 8-17, *B*). Later in the course of the process, stellate cells or other extracellular matrix-producing cells from the portal and centrilobular areas that may survive or migrate to the site of injury contribute new collagen (collagen I, in particular). The final result is collapse of the lobule and replacement of the lost hepatic parenchyma with a scar consisting of condensed stroma, including variable amounts and types of collagen. Grossly the liver may be smaller than normal with a wrinkled capsule. Partial involvement of the liver is characterized by depressed areas of parenchymal necrosis and vascular congestion scattered throughout the organ.

MORPHOLOGIC CLASSIFICATION OF HEPATOBILIARY DISEASE

The nature and distribution of inflammatory lesions in the liver are usually dictated by the route of entry, the host inflammatory response, the nature of the infectious agent (e.g., virus, bacterium, fungus), and any predilection they have for involvement with a particular cell type in the liver. The hematogenous route of infection tends to cause a random multifocal distribution of lesions. Infections, usually bacterial, that ascend the biliary tract are typically centered in the bile ducts. Severe infections may affect the entire portal tract and extend into the adjacent parenchyma. Penetrating wounds cause discrete areas of inflammation with or without necrosis that are evident on the capsule and extend into the hepatic parenchyma. Liver injury should be characterized by: the pattern of involvement (multifocal random, zonal, or massive), type of inflammatory cells involved (neutrophils, lymphocytes, plasma cells, eosinophils, or macrophages), evidence of necrosis or fibrosis, severity of these processes, evidence of regeneration, and the presence of an etiologic agent or agents. The type of inflammatory response and the duration of the injury can help identify the infectious agents.

ACUTE HEPATITIS

Inflammation of the liver parenchyma is termed hepatitis. Acute hepatitis is characterized by inflammation, hepatocellular necrosis, and apoptosis. The proportion and type of inflammatory cells involved varies considerably depending on the cause of inflammation, the host response, and the stage or age of the lesion. Characterization of the type of inflammation usually requires microscopic evaluation. In many forms of acute hepatitis, particularly bacterial and protozoal infections, neutrophils accumulate in response to the usual chemotactic stimuli. Random foci of neutrophilic hepatitis, as a consequence of embolic localization of bacteria, are relatively common in all species. In neonates—especially calves, lambs, and foals—bacteria, such as *Escherichia coli*, usually seed the liver via the umbilical veins or less often the portal venous or hepatic arterial systems.

Acute hepatitis produced by viral infections, such as herpesvirus infection in many species, is more frequently characterized by a random distribution of necrosis and apoptosis with minimal inflammation or infiltrations of lymphocytes.

CHRONIC HEPATITIS

Chronic hepatitis results when there is continued inflammation as a result of persistence of an antigenic stimulus. In the absence of such a stimulus, inflammation rapidly resolves. Chronic hepatitis is characterized by fibrosis; accumulation of mononuclear inflammatory cells, including lymphocytes, macrophages, and plasma cells; and, frequently, regeneration. Neutrophils often are present in chronic unresolved hepatic inflammation such as that which characterizes some forms of canine chronic hepatitis. The proportion and distribution of each of these elements varies with the inciting cause and host response. Local variation within the liver can also occur.

Different terms are used to distinguish separate types of chronic hepatitis. Granulomatous hepatitis may be obvious grossly if it produces discrete granulomas of sufficient size. These may be focal or diffuse. Chronic suppurative hepatitis is usually manifested as discrete or multiple abscesses. Focal lesions, such as abscesses or granulomas, often are sufficiently localized so that they do not alter hepatic function. In contrast, diffuse and severe chronic hepatitis, as seen in dogs, usually leads to loss of hepatic parenchyma and architectural distortion of the liver as a consequence of fibrosis and nodular parenchymal regeneration. This process can proceed to end-stage hepatic disease with hepatic failure and its associated constellation of clinical signs. The form of chronic hepatitis that has been referred to as chronic active hepatitis is discussed in a separate section next.

NONSPECIFIC REACTIVE HEPATITIS

Nonspecific reactive hepatitis is a diffuse process distributed throughout the liver in response to some systemic illness, most often the gastrointestinal tract, or is the residuum of prior liver inflammation. Typically, there is a mild inflammatory infiltrate in the portal tract and possibly the parenchyma without evidence of necrosis. In acute cases, there is a minimal to mild infiltrate of neutrophils within the connective tissue of the portal tracts that may vary in intensity. Mononuclear cells, primarily lymphocytes and plasma cells, predominate in more chronic manifestations. Pigmented macrophages containing hemosiderin, lipofuscin, or both may be scattered throughout the parenchyma. Mononuclear inflammatory cells may also be evident within the hepatic parenchyma and at the periphery of central veins. Kupffer cells are usually reactive (i.e., they appear somewhat swollen because of abundant cytoplasm and display prominent nuclei as well).

CHOLANGITIS

Cholangitis is characterized by inflammation that is centered on the biliary tract. The inflammatory cell population and the degree of fibrosis will vary with the type and duration of injury. Cholecystitis refers to inflammation of the gallbladder.

CHOLANGIOHEPATITIS

Inflammation that affects the biliary ducts and hepatic parenchyma is termed cholangiohepatitis. In most cases of intrahepatic disease, the primary focus of inflammation can be identified as affecting either the hepatocytes or the biliary tree, but on occasion both components of the liver are affected, usually as an extension of biliary disease to involve the periportal hepatocytes, and in that circumstance the term *cholangiohepatitis* should be used.

DISTURBANCES OF BILE FLOW AND ICTERUS

Hepatic injury is frequently manifested as an increased concentration of conjugated or unconjugated bilirubin in blood called hyperbilirubinemia. High concentrations of bilirubin (> approximately 2 mg/dl) can produce jaundice (icterus), a yellow discoloration of tissue that is especially evident in tissue rich in elastin, such as the aorta and sclera (Fig. 8-18). This concentration is within the reference range for horses, so horses may not be hyperemic at this level because their reference range reaches that concentration. However, in other species, hyperbilirubinemia can occur once the concentration exceeds 0.5 mg/dl (dog) and therefore the patient is hyperbilirubinemic, but icterus will not be detected until it exceeds 2 mg/dl. Maximal accumulation of bilirubin in tissues takes about 2 days and explains why some animals with acute hepatic failure may have only slight icterus.

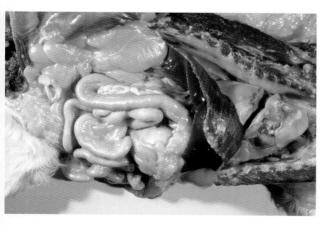

Fig. 8-18   **Icterus, dog.** Icterus and jaundice are terms that refer to the yellow discoloration of tissue, by bilirubin, in this case evident in the fat and serosa. *(Courtesy Dr. M.D. McGavin, College of Veterinary Medicine, University of Tennessee.)*

The causes of hyperbilirubinemia include the following:

1. Overproduction of bilirubin as a consequence of hemolysis, particularly severe intravascular hemolysis, which overwhelms the liver's capacity to remove bilirubin from the plasma and to secrete conjugated bilirubin into bile. The destruction of damaged red blood cells by extravascular hemolysis can also increase the burden of bilirubin presented to the liver. Hypoxia secondary to anemia may also play a role. Secretion of conjugated bilirubin into bile canaliculi is an energy-dependent process and is the rate-limiting step in bilirubin excretion in most species.

2. Decreased uptake, conjugation, or secretion of bilirubin by hepatocytes arising as a consequence of severe, diffuse hepatic disease, whether acute or chronic.

3. Reduced outflow of bile (cholestasis). Cholestasis is defined as a defect in bile secretory mechanisms that leads to an accumulation in the blood of substances normally excreted into the bile. Cholestasis occurs as a consequence of either obstruction of the biliary ducts (extrahepatic cholestasis) or impairment of bile flow within canaliculi (intrahepatic cholestasis).

Obviously, hepatic dysfunction is not the only cause of hyperbilirubinemia and icterus. In fact, icterus in ruminants is usually a consequence of severe intravascular hemolysis and less often a sequel to hepatic damage. Horses often manifest icterus with acute hepatic dysfunction, but icterus may or may not occur in horses with chronic hepatic disease. Interestingly, "physiologic icterus" is also common in the horse, and horses deprived of feed for several days can become icteric because uptake of bilirubin from the plasma by hepatocytes is decreased. Icterus in carnivores occurs as a consequence of either hemolysis or hepatic dysfunction. Inherited metabolic abnormalities can also lead to abnormal concentrations of serum bilirubin. In Southdown sheep with certain mutations, bile is ineffectively taken up from the circulation and a persistent unconjugated bilirubinemia develops, although icterus is rarely apparent because there is sufficient excretion despite the mutation. Corriedale sheep may have a mutation that leads to deficient conjugated bilirubin excretion. Affected sheep have persistently elevated plasma bilirubin concentration, but jaundice is not apparent. Other compounds that are normally excreted through conjugation also accumulate in the liver of affected sheep. The livers are dark and discolored due to accumulated polymerized catecholamine metabolites that accumulate in lysosomes. These residues resemble lipofuscin histologically.

Cholestasis can be divided into two types: intrahepatic and extrahepatic. Intrahepatic cholestasis can result from (1) wide spectrum of liver injury affecting the ability of hepatocytes to metabolize and excrete bile,

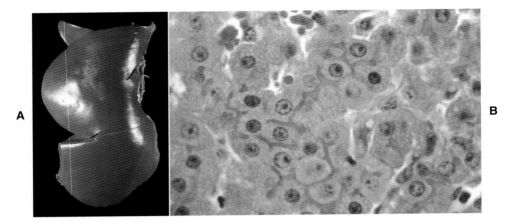

Fig. 8-19   Hepatic bilirubin retention, icterus, liver. A, Cat. The liver is markedly yellowed by retained bilirubin. **B,** Canalicular bilirubin, acute hemolytic anemia, calf. Acute hemolysis caused by babesiosis has led to a dramatic increase in bilirubin production and distention of canaliculi, clearly demonstrating the location of canaliculi between hepatocytes. H&E stain. (**A,** *Courtesy College of Veterinary Medicine, University of Illinois.* **B,** *Courtesy Dr. M.D. McGavin, College of Veterinary Medicine, University of Tennessee.*)

(2) hemolysis, which produces an abundance of bilirubin for excretion and diminishes the supply of oxygen for hepatocyte metabolism, or (3) inherited abnormalities of bile synthesis that inhibit the excretion of bile. Extrahepatic obstruction is produced by obstruction of the extrahepatic bile ducts. This can occur by intraluminal obstruction (calculi or possibly parasites) or extraluminal means, including neoplasia or adjacent inflammation, often involving the pancreas. Cholestasis, if sufficiently severe, can produce a greenish brown discoloration to the liver (Fig. 8-19, *A*).

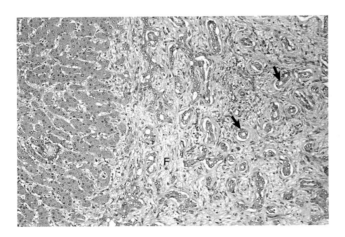

Fig. 8-20   Chronic extrahepatic cholestasis, cholelithiasis, liver, horse. There is reduplication of bile ducts (*arrows*) and extensive fibrosis (*F*) throughout the portal tract (biliary fibrosis) as a consequence of prolonged stasis and subsequent leakage of bile. H&E stain. *(Courtesy Dr. J.M. Cullen, College of Veterinary Medicine, North Carolina State University.)*

Histologically, acute intrahepatic cholestasis is characterized by formation of bile plugs within canaliculi (Fig. 8-19, *B*). As intrahepatic cholestasis becomes more chronic, bile that has been released from hepatocytes is taken up by Kupffer cells and can be detected within their cytoplasm.

Acute extrahepatic obstruction is characterized by edema of the portal areas, a mild neutrophilic inflammatory cell infiltrate, and a proliferative reaction by the biliary epithelium of the bile ducts. In chronic extrahepatic biliary obstruction, portal areas are enlarged by deposition of fibrosis, and there is a prominent laminar, circumferential fibrosis of bile ducts (Fig. 8-20). Biliary hyperplasia characterized by proliferation of small-caliber bile ducts is often prominent. Pigmented macrophages, containing bile, and mixed inflammatory infiltrates are also present. In severe cases, bridging fibrosis connecting portal tracts may develop.

Complete biliary obstruction leads to maldigestion of fats and a characteristic clay-colored stool termed acholic feces because of the lack of normal dark pigment, stercobilin, the bilirubin-derived pigment produced by bacterial metabolism (Fig. 8-21).

RESPONSE OF THE LIVER TO INJURY

Following destruction of hepatic parenchyma, regeneration of parenchyma, replacement by fibrosis, and biliary hyperplasia may occur. The outcome of a given hepatic insult depends on the nature and duration of the insult, and survival of the host.

REGENERATION

A characteristic feature of the liver is the ability to rapidly and efficiently regenerate lost hepatic mass.

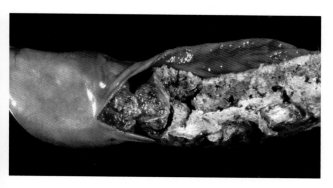

Fig. 8-21   Intrahepatic biliary obstruction, intestine, dog. In cases of complete biliary obstruction, bile is unable to reach the intestine and as a result stool(s) lacks the characteristic dark color produced by bile pigments. *(Courtesy College of Veterinary Medicine, North Carolina State University.)*

Experimentally, as much as two thirds of the liver can be excised from a healthy animal without signs of hepatic dysfunction, and the liver is rapidly regenerated. In addition to replication of hepatocytes, there is a wave of replication in bile duct epithelium, endothelium, and sinusoidal lining cells that is coordinated with hepatocyte replication.

Regeneration usually takes place by replication of mature hepatocytes. In most circumstances, this leads to an increase in the size of existing lobules; however, recent data suggest that some new lobule formation can also occur through subdivision of existing lobules. Following removal of liver lobes only, the remaining liver lobes persist, and no new lobe formation occurs.

Individual cell necrosis leads to local proliferation by regeneration of adjacent hepatocytes. Scattered foci of necrotic hepatocytes are quickly replaced through cell division of adjacent hepatocytes. Necrosis in the centrilobular area of the lobule leads to a wave of hepatocyte proliferation in the hepatocytes in the remaining areas of the lobule, particularly the periportal hepatocytes. In some circumstances, such as necrosis of nearly all hepatocytes or exposure to certain chemical toxins that inhibit replication of mature hepatocytes, replacement of hepatocytes lost by necrosis occurs through proliferation of hepatocyte stem cells or oval cells. This process is most often observed in experimental manipulations of laboratory rodents, but probably occurs in naturally occurring cases of hepatotoxicity also. These cells reside in the connective tissue of the portal tracts and have the ability to differentiate into hepatocyte or bile duct epithelium. Histologically, they are identified as small basophilic cells with an oval shape. They are not apparent in most circumstances of hepatic regeneration, but can be abundant in experimental studies of hepatic regeneration.

The body carefully orchestrates hepatic regeneration to replace lost hepatocyte mass along with bile ducts and vessels without producing excess liver. A variety of growth factors, including transforming growth factor-α and hepatocyte growth factor, stimulate hepatocyte replication. Once normal hepatic mass has been established, macrophages release transforming growth factor-β, which in concert with other less well characterized factors stops hepatic parenchymal cell proliferation.

Extensive hepatic necrosis is usually followed by parenchymal regeneration without scarring as long as the normal extracellular matrix (reticulin) scaffolding of the affected portion remains intact and has not collapsed, as in massive hepatic necrosis. However, repetitive injury or massive necrosis can disrupt the normal lobular architecture, and there may be parenchymal collapse after removal of the dead hepatocytes and/or stromal collapse with repair by collagen synthesis (postnecrotic scarring) (Fig 8-22). Even when necrosis of hepatocytes is continuous, the liver will attempt to regenerate its functional mass. However, prolonged regenerative effort with damage to the normal extracellular matrix scaffolding of the liver often results in nodular proliferations of parenchyma, which architecturally distort the liver. Although regenerative nodules may reconstitute a proportionately large amount of hepatic mass, adequate function is rarely attained. Blood flow into the regenerative nodules and bile flow out of the nodules is abnormal and as a result, hepatic function cannot be reestablished. As the nodules develop, the portal tract vessels and the central veins develop communications within the fibrous septa between nodules, which leads to vascular shunts between the portal vein and the central vein that bypass hepatocytes within the nodules.

FIBROSIS

Fibrosis is one of the more common manifestations of chronic liver injury. The pattern of fibrosis is frequently a useful indicator of the type of insult that produces the lesion. The significance of fibrosis depends on its effect on hepatic function and its reversibility. Despite the considerable regenerative capacity of the liver, hepatic fibrosis, when sufficiently severe, can be lethal.

In the normal liver, fibrillar collagens I and III are confined primarily to the connective tissue of the portal tracts and immediately around the terminal hepatic venule (central vein). Collagen IV is the most abundant collagen type in the reticulin framework of the sinusoids, but it is present in only small amounts. A delicate scaffolding of collagen and other extracellular matrix components, which are produced by stellate cells, endothelial cells and hepatocytes, make up the normal framework of the sinusoid. This stroma in the space of Disse supports the endothelial cells and maintains their relationship to the hepatocytes.

Hepatic fibrosis is an overall increase in the extracellular matrix within the liver. In a fibrotic liver, there is an increase in the amount of extracellular matrix and a

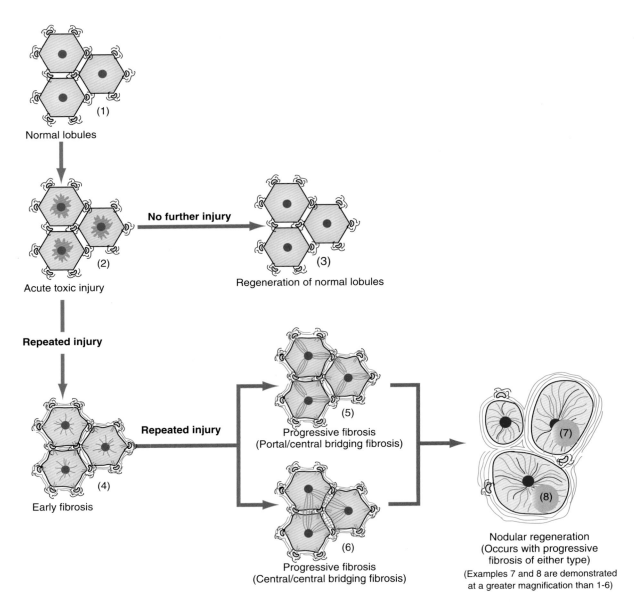

Fig. 8-22   Schematic diagram of the effects of hepatic injury on the development of fibrosis. Acute hepatic centrilobular injury *(2)* that occurs only once usually resolves, and normal liver architecture returns *(1, 3)*. Repeated bouts of injury or severe injury can initiate hepatic fibrosis *(4)*. In the earliest stages, fibrosis may be reversible, but as fibrosis progresses it reaches a point at which repair is not likely. Fibrosis starts as fine branches of collagen deposition between portal areas or central areas or dissecting into the hepatic parenchyma *(5, 6)*. Over time, greater amounts of collagen and other extracellular matrix are deposited and the lobular architecture becomes progressively distorted. In the end-stage liver, nodular regeneration *(7, 8)* and extensive, circumferential fibrosis are typical. The regenerative nodules shown here *(7, 8)* are at an early stage of regeneration. As shown Fig. 8-24, they will regenerate to form nodules that will commonly exceed the size of normal hepatic lobules. These nodules will often compress *(7)* the central vein(s) of hepatic lobules within and adjacent to those from which they arose.

change in the types of collagen and their site of deposition. A severely fibrotic liver can contain up to six times as much collagen and proteoglycan as a normal liver. Hepatic fibrosis is characterized by an increase of fibrillar collagens, type I and type III, and nonfibrillar collagen XVIII within the space of Disse, the portal areas, and the area surrounding the central veins. In addition to an increase in collagens, there is also a commensurate increase in the extracellular matrix components, proteoglycans, fibronectin, and hyaluronic acid.

The stellate cells (Ito cells and lipocytes) have a central role in hepatic fibrosis, although it should be noted that there are myofibroblastic cells with similar capabilities found within the connective tissue of the portal areas and connective tissue surrounding the central vein. In the normal liver, stellate cells occupy the space of Disse (a subendothelial position in the sinusoid) nestled between hepatocytes. They are characterized by the presence of large lipid-containing vacuoles in their cytoplasm (Fig. 8-8). The vacuoles are a primary storage site for retinyl esters, including vitamin A. Stellate cells are positioned in the space of Disse around the circumference of the endothelium of the sinusoids and have been likened to pericytes in other organs, such as the mesangial cells of the renal glomerulus. Hepatic stellate cells have been shown to have a role in the control of the diameter of the sinusoids and consequently the flow of blood through the sinusoids.

When the liver is injured, these cells go through a progressive phenotypic change from the typical lipid-storing cell to a cell with a myofibroblastic appearance (Fig. 8-23). When they are activated, they express smooth muscle actin and desmin, a marker usually found in muscle cells. Once these cells have switched phenotype to the myofibroblast phenotype, they begin synthesis of collagen types I, III, and IV. They also produce other extracellular matrix components, including laminin and chondroitin sulfate proteoglycans. Hepatocytes synthesize few or no matrix proteins, and the large sum of matrix proteins is derived from the hepatic stellate cells. The type of hepatic injury does not seem to be important in the genesis of hepatic fibrosis. Chemical injury, biliary obstruction, and iron overload produce similar patterns of activation of hepatic stellate cells.

The site in which collagen is deposited in the liver has a significant impact on liver function. Perisinusoidal fibrosis can have a severe effect on hepatic function. In addition to collagen and extracellular matrix deposits, there is a loss of gaps in the endothelial cells and a loss of microvilli on the luminal surface of the hepatocytes. These changes have been termed capillarization of the sinusoids because the alterations in the sinusoids result in a vascular structure that more closely resembles a capillary than a sinusoid. The functional effect of this microanatomic change is profound. The ability of the liver to carry out its synthetic, catabolic, and excretory roles is severely compromised by the reduced exposure of hepatocytes to plasma.

Within the hepatic lobule, the site of fibrosis can be indicative of the type of insult. Most often, chronic toxic injury produces centrilobular (periacinar) fibrosis. This region is affected because the centrilobular hepatocytes are the site of metabolism for most drugs. Long-standing right side heart failure can cause fibrosis in this site as well. Periportal (centroacinar) fibrosis can result from

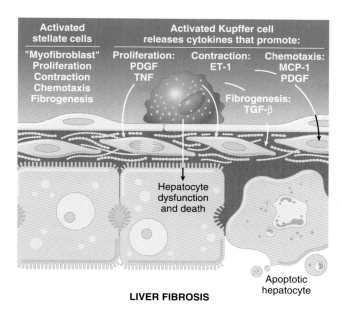

LIVER FIBROSIS

Fig. 8-23   Schematic diagram of a fibrotic hepatic sinusoid. Contact between the plasma and the hepatocytes is dramatically reduced. The sinusoidal endothelial cells have lost their gaps. The space of Disse contains abundant collagen type I fibers that have been synthesized by activated hepatic stellate cells. The hepatic stellate cells have eliminated the lipid vacuoles and assumed a myofibroblastic morphology with cell extensions that often surround the endothelial cells (not shown here). Hepatocyte microvilli have been lost on the apoptotic hepatocyte, and this loss begins with the onset of hepatocyte disfunction and degeneration. *ET-1,* Endothelin-1; *MCP-1,* macrophage chemotactic protein-1; *PDGF,* platelet-derived growth factor; *TGF-β,* transforming growth factor-β; *TNF,* tumor necrosis factor. *(Schematic based on concepts presented in Friedman SL: J Biol Chem 275:2247-2250, 2000; and Crawford JM: Curr Op Gastroenterol 13:175-185, 1997.)*

chronic inflammatory conditions or a small group of toxins that affect the periportal hepatocytes because they do not require metabolism by the cytochrome p450 enzymes to produce an injurious metabolite. Fibrosis may be limited to individual lobules, but in more severe injuries the areas of fibrosis can be more extensive. Bridging fibrosis, which is analogous to bridging necrosis, implies fibrosis that extends from one portal tract to another or from portal tracts to central veins. Bridging fibrosis is more likely to impair hepatic function than focal forms of hepatic fibrosis; however, all forms of hepatic fibrosis, if sufficiently severe, lead to impaired hepatic function. However, because of the enormous reserve capacity of the liver, fibrosis is usually quite extensive before there are clinical signs of hepatic dysfunction.

A single event of widespread hepatocellular necrosis is sometimes followed, not by the usual regenerative response, but by fibrosis and condensation of the preexisting connective tissue stroma that results in formation of bands of dense connective tissue. This process is referred to as postnecrotic scarring.

Other patterns of hepatic fibrosis can occur, including biliary fibrosis (centered on bile ducts in the portal triads), focal or multifocal hepatic fibrosis (randomly scattered throughout the hepatic parenchyma)—which is produced, for example, by migrating nematode larvae—and diffuse hepatic fibrosis (affects all regions of the lobule and is present throughout the liver). Diffuse fibrosis with hyperplastic nodule formation is by definition cirrhosis. Different hepatic insults may produce different patterns of fibrosis, but when fibrosis is severe (end-stage liver disease), it frequently is impossible to determine either the cause or the initial pattern of fibrosis.

BILIARY HYPERPLASIA

Biliary hyperplasia, which is proliferation of new biliary ducts within the portal areas and periportal regions, can be a relatively nonspecific response to a variety of insults to the liver. The mechanism responsible for this proliferation is unknown. Biliary hyperplasia can occur swiftly, particularly in young animals, but is usually regarded as a lesion seen in long-standing hepatic injury. Biliary hyperplasia occurs particularly after diseases that obstruct normal bile drainage.

END-STAGE LIVER OR CIRRHOSIS

The best accepted definition for cirrhosis was pronounced by the World Health Organization in 1977 and is as follows: "a diffuse process characterized by fibrosis and the conversion of the normal liver architecture into structurally abnormal lobules (Fig. 8-24)." As it is the final, irreversible result of any one of several different hepatic diseases, the term *end-stage liver* is appropriate, particularly because the term *cirrhosis* is neither descriptive nor precise in meaning and originally meant "tawny yellow." Another authority states that the hallmark is the total absence of any normal lobular architecture. The architecture of the liver is altered by loss of hepatic parenchyma, condensation of reticulin framework, and formation of tracts of fibrous connective tissue. Regeneration of hepatic tissue between fibrous bands leads to the formation of variably sized regenerative nodules (Fig. 8-25). The entire liver is thus distorted and consists of nodules of regenerating parenchyma separated by fibrous bands, which appear as depressions on the surface (Fig. 8-24).

Lobular dissecting hepatitis is a form of cirrhosis usually seen in young dogs. The condition is frequently fatal and has no known cause. Affected livers tend to be smooth and small, rather than the multinodular livers seen in typical cirrhosis. Histologically the livers are characterized by fine septa with increased fibrosis that

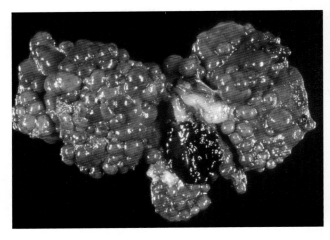

Fig. 8-24   End-stage liver (cirrhosis), dog. End-stage liver from a dog that had received phenobarbital for many years. The liver is small, firm, and irregular with nodules of regenerative parenchyma separated by tracts of fibrous connective tissue. *(Courtesy Dr. J.M. Cullen, College of Veterinary Medicine, North Carolina State University.)*

dissect the hepatic plates, distort the lobular architecture, and isolate small aggregates or individual hepatocytes (Fig. 8-26). Inflammation in the tissue is usually mild to moderate, and the inflamed area contains mononuclear cell infiltrates.

Profound vascular abnormalities with serious consequences for the health of affected patients occur in this condition, including multiple abnormal vascular anastomoses between the portal vein and the systemic vasculature, as a consequence of the increased portal pressure. Also, venous shunts between the central veins and the portal veins, and arteriovenous shunts between the hepatic arteries and the central veins, can occur within the regenerative nodules.

The potential causes of an end-stage (cirrhotic) liver are numerous (Box 8-4). Chronic toxic insult results from the continued ingestion of any hepatotoxin (e.g., herbivores ingesting toxic plants, such as those that contain pyrrolizidine alkaloids, and the long-term administration of anticonvulsant drugs, such as primidone for dogs). Chronic extrahepatic biliary obstruction and cholestasis leads to extensive fibrosis, which primarily affects the portal triads, but the fibrosis can eventually extend into the adjacent hepatic parenchyma. Chronic inflammation of the liver (hepatitis) or biliary tract (cholangitis) may lead to an end-stage liver. Although infection of the liver typically is focal or multifocal, diffuse hepatitis and subsequent fibrosis occurs in disease entities such as so-called canine chronic (chronic-active) hepatitis. Chronic passive hepatic congestion eventually leads to fibrosis near central veins, which is sometimes termed cardiac sclerosis and which can progress to

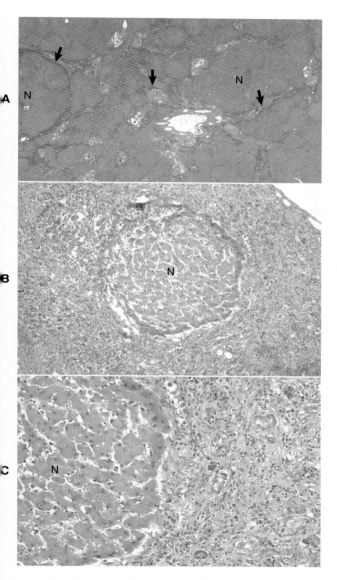

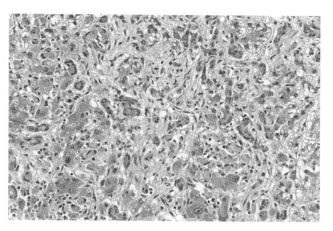

Fig. 8-26   Lobular dissecting hepatitis, liver, dog. Lobular dissecting hepatitis is a form of end-stage liver characterized microscopically by fine septa of extracellular matrix (chiefly collagen) that divide hepatocyte plates into small clusters of individual hepatocytes. Because of the disruption of blood flow through the liver and the failure of hepatocytes to come in contact with blood, there is profound hepatic dysfunction. **H&E stain.** *(Courtesy Dr. J.M. Cullen, College of Veterinary Medicine, North Carolina State University.)*

Fig. 8-25   End-stage, liver, dog. A, Histologic appearance of end-stage liver disease. Nodules of regenerative parenchyma *(N)* are separated by tracts of collapsed reticulin and fibrous connective tissue *(arrows)*, which also contains numerous blood vessels and bile ducts. H&E stain. **B,** A single regenerative hepatic nodule *(N)* is surrounded by haphazardly arranged bands of fibrous connective tissue that contains numerous blood vessels and hypertrophied and hyperplastic bile ducts. H&E stain. **C,** Higher magnification of Fig. 8-25, *B*. Note the regenerative nodule *(N)*, bands of fibrous connective tissue, hyperplastic bile ducts, and chronic inflammatory cells. H&E stain. *(A, Courtesy Dr. J.M. Cullen, College of Veterinary Medicine, North Carolina State University. B and C, Courtesy College of Veterinary Medicine, University of Illinois.)*

cardiac cirrhosis. The actual amount of fibrosis is usually small. Abnormal storage or metabolism of metals, such as copper, as occurs in Dalmatians and Bedlington and West Highland white terriers with hereditary copper accumulations, may produce an end-stage liver. A variety of more poorly defined disease entities can lead to progressive hepatocellular injury and hepatic fibrosis resulting in end-stage hepatic disease.

The end-stage liver obviously cannot perform its normal functions, so the clinical manifestations of hepatic failure invariably occur in affected animals. However, the cause of the hepatic damage that leads to the end-stage liver frequently cannot be determined at the time signs of hepatic failure are observed.

HEPATIC FAILURE

The liver has considerable functional reserve and regenerative capacity. In healthy animals, more than two thirds of the hepatic parenchyma can be removed without significant impairment of hepatic function and normal hepatic mass can be regenerated in a matter of days. This process of tissue removal can be repeated several times, particularly in younger animals, and function is retained. In all species, clinical signs from hepatic

Box **8-4**		

Causes of End-Stage Liver

Chronic toxicity (therapeutic agents or naturally occurring toxins)
Chronic cholangitis and/or obstruction
Chronic congestion (right side heart failure)
Inherited disorders of metal metabolism (copper or iron)
Chronic hepatitis
Idiopathic

derangement are similar, regardless of their cause. These are manifest, however, only when the liver's considerable reserve and regenerative capacity are depleted or when biliary outflow is obstructed. Only lesions that affect the majority of the hepatic parenchyma are likely to produce the signs of hepatic failure because focal lesions rarely destroy sufficient parenchyma to deplete the liver's reserve. The term *hepatic failure* implies loss of adequate hepatic function as a consequence of either acute or chronic hepatic damage; however, all hepatic functions are not usually lost at the same time. The potential consequences of hepatic dysfunction and failure include: (1) hepatic encephalopathy; (2) disturbances of bile flow with a resultant hyperbilirubinemia; (3) a variety of metabolic disturbances; (4) vascular and hemodynamic alterations, such as shunting of portal blood into the systemic circulation bypassing the hepatocytes; and (5) cutaneous manifestations, such as epidermal necrosis in dogs and photosensitization in herbivores.

Hepatic encephalopathy

Hepatic failure can result in a metabolic disorder of the central nervous system termed hepatic encephalopathy (synonyms: hepatic coma or portosystemic encephalopathy). Neurologic manifestations range from depression and other behavioral changes to mania and convulsions. Affected horses may walk aimlessly. The central feature of this disorder is abnormal neurotransmission in the central nervous system and the neuromuscular system. Undetermined as yet are the specific metabolites that cause the neurologic dysfunction, but increased concentrations of plasma ammonia derived from amines absorbed from the gastrointestinal tract may be responsible. Normally, amines are absorbed from the intestines into the portal blood and metabolized by the liver. If they bypass the liver and gain access to the systemic circulation, they can exert toxic effects on the brain. These toxic products can enter the systemic circulation by two mechanisms. Blood can be shunted to the systemic circulation before it reaches the liver as a result of congenital portosystemic shunts or secondary to portal vein hypertension. Shunting of more than 10% to 15% of portal flow away from the liver is considered abnormal. Alternatively the toxic products may not be fully eliminated by the liver if there is sufficient liver disease. However, abnormal ammonia concentrations are not the only possible cause of hepatic encephalopathy. An altered balance of inhibitory and excitatory amino acid neurotransmitters, γ-aminobutyric acid, and L-glutamate, respectively, and increased brain concentrations of endogenous benzodiazepines are other possible explanations. Hepatic encephalopathy is common in ruminants and horses with hepatic failure, dogs and cats with congenital portosystemic shunts, and animals with end-stage liver

(hepatic fibrosis and nodular regeneration) that leads to shunting of blood within regenerative nodules.

Metabolic disturbances of hepatic failure

Hepatic failure can be manifested by a variety of metabolic disturbances. The type and duration of the hepatic disorder may influence the nature of the metabolic perturbation.

Bleeding tendencies. Bleeding tendencies (hemorrhagic diathesis) sometimes accompany hepatic failure. Impaired synthesis of clotting factors, reduced clearance of the products of the clotting process, and metabolic abnormalities affecting platelet function can affect normal clotting, individually or in combination. All clotting factors, with the possible exception of factor VIII, are synthesized in the liver. In acute liver failure, diminished synthesis of clotting factors with a short half-life, such as factors V, VII, IX, and X, impairs the ability of blood to coagulate. In chronic liver disease, factor II (prothrombin) deficiency also contributes to diminished coagulation of blood. Diminished clearance of fibrin degradation products (FDPs), activated coagulation factors, and plasminogen factors by the damaged liver also perturbs clotting. Metabolic disturbances resulting from liver failure can affect platelet function and lead to synthesis of abnormal fibrinogen, a condition termed dysfibrinogenemia. Obstruction of the biliary system prevents the release of bile into the intestinal tract. The resulting impaired fat absorption limits vitamin K uptake from the intestine, which leads to an inactivity of factors II, VII, IX, and X. Acute hepatic failure may also precipitate disseminated intravascular coagulation, which can itself cause hemorrhagic diathesis. Impaired removal of activated clotting factors by the damaged liver is one potential mechanism for this. Acute hepatic failure in the horse and perhaps other species is sometimes accompanied by severe intravascular hemolysis, the cause of which is unknown.

Hypoalbuminemia. Hypoalbuminemia, as a consequence of hepatic dysfunction, usually reflects severe and chronic liver disease rather than acute disease. This is because of the relatively long half-life of plasma albumin (which ranges from 8 days in the dog to 21 days in cattle), which masks, for a period of time, the diminished albumin synthesis of the diseased liver. Severe diffuse liver disease can obstruct portal vein inflow, leading to portal hypertension, which accelerates the formation of ascites in affected animals. Loss of albumin in ascetic fluid or into the intestinal tract accentuates the loss of intravascular albumin, and widespread edema can result.

Vascular and hemodynamic alterations of hepatic failure

Chronic hepatic injury typically is accompanied by extensive diffuse fibrosis of the liver, which increases resistance to blood flow through the liver. This in turn elevates pressure within the portal vein (portal hypertension). With time, collateral vascular channels open to allow blood in the portal vein to bypass the abnormal liver (acquired portosystemic vascular anastomoses, which connect the portal vein and its tributaries to the systemic venous circulation). Shunting of portal vein blood directly to the central vein can also occur within the fibrous septa formed in the liver. In addition, the increased pressure within the hepatic vasculature causes transudation of fluid (modified transudate) into the peritoneal cavity to produce ascites in several species, except in most cases horses. Transudation of fluid into the peritoneal cavity can be enhanced by hypoalbuminemia because there is a decreased colloid osmotic pressure in plasma. Hypoalbuminemia and reduced plasma colloid osmotic pressure can arise as a consequence of accelerated albumin loss into the lumen of the intestines as a result of portal hypertension or because of reduced hepatic synthesis of albumin and other plasma proteins by the diseased liver. Ascites associated with hepatic fibrosis in chronic liver disease (end-stage liver) or other causes of portal hypertension, such as right side heart failure, occurs most commonly in the dog and cat, occasionally in sheep, and rarely in horses and cattle.

Cutaneous manifestations of hepatic failure

Hepatocutaneous syndrome (necrolytic migratory erythema, superficial necrolytic dermatitis). Hepatocutaneous syndrome is a syndrome of chronic

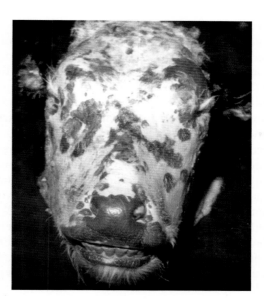

Fig. 8-28   **Cutaneous necrosis, photosensitization, skin, cow.** When the liver of herbivores fails and can no longer remove the photodynamic pigment phylloerythrin from the portal blood, skin with little pigment or hair covering, exposed to ultraviolet light, initially becomes acutely inflamed and may be followed by necrosis, as seen on the face of this cow. *(Courtesy Dr. H. Gelberg, College of Veterinary Medicine, Oregon State University.)*

hepatic injury and skin disease. The central diagnostic elements include crusting, erosions, and ulceration of the epidermis of the muzzle, mucocutaneous areas of the face, footpads, and pressure points of the skin in some dogs with severe hepatic disease (Fig. 8-27). The mechanism of cutaneous injury is not understood, but affected animals have characteristic multinodular livers, often with little fibrosis between the nodules. It seems likely that this histologically distinctive skin disorder results from abnormal hepatic metabolism. Typically the cutaneous lesion are parakeratosis, edema of the superficial epithelium, and basal cell hyperplasia.

Photosensitization.   Injury to the skin resulting from activation of photodynamic pigments by ultraviolet light in the sun's rays is called photosensitization. Cutaneous lesions display hair loss, erythema, and necrosis (Fig. 8-28). Lesions are typically limited to hairless skin and to lightly or nonpigmented areas of skin. The sources of photodynamic pigments that can induce photosensitization include plants, certain drugs, and products of inherited disorders of porphyrin metabolism. The mechanism of tissue injury is not well characterized but is presumed to involve oxidative injury when photodynamic pigments that have been activated by the radiant energy of ultraviolet light subsequently release their energy to adjacent tissue. Hepatic dysfunction is only responsible for one form of photosensitization termed secondary (hepatogenous) photosensitization.

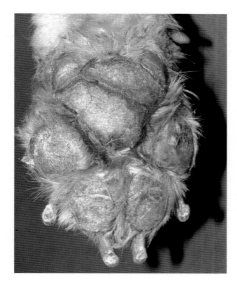

Fig. 8-27   **Cutaneous necrosis, hepatocutaneous syndrome, foot pads, dog.** In some cases of hepatic failure, there is a syndrome of associated cutaneous necrosis termed hepatocutaneous syndrome. Footpads as well as areas of haired skin can be affected. *(Courtesy Dr. T. Olivry, College of Veterinary Medicine, North Carolina State University.)*

Primary photosensitization. Primary photosensitization occurs after a primary (preformed) photodynamic agent is ingested, absorbed into the blood, and deposited in tissue. Certain plants, such as St. John's wort (*Hypericum perforatum*) and buckwheat (*Fagopyrum esculentum*), and pharmaceutical agents, such as tetracycline or phenothiazine, contain compounds that are photodynamic.

Secondary photosensitization. Secondary or hepatogenous photosensitization occurs in herbivores when hepatic dysfunction or biliary obstruction impairs normal excretion of phylloerythrin in bile. Phylloerythrin, a photodynamic agent, is produced by chlorophyll contained in ingested plants by gastrointestinal bacteria of herbivores. Phylloerythrin is normally absorbed from the intestines, taken up by hepatocytes, and excreted in bile, using the same pathway as bilirubin. Thus hepatocellular dysfunction or biliary obstruction prevents normal excretion and allows high concentrations of phylloerythrin to accumulate in blood and cutaneous tissue. Most often, secondary photosensitization occurs in animals with chronic liver disease and loss of 80% or more of normal hepatic function, but it can also occur in animals with acute liver disease or inflammatory or obstructive disorders of the biliary tree. Mutant Corriedale sheep have an inherited inability to excrete conjugated bilirubin and are also susceptible to secondary photosensitization because phylloerythrin concentrations are increased in these sheep.

Congenital porphyria. Congenital porphyria is a metabolic disorder involving the liver that occurs in several species, including cattle and cats. This disorder is caused by abnormal metabolism of heme, leading to abnormal excretion and an accumulation of porphyrins, which are themselves photodynamic.

Immunologic manifestations of hepatic failure

Chronic liver failure leads to an impairment of normal hepatic immune function. As a consequence, the affected patient frequently develops endotoxemia and an increased risk of systemic infection. For the most part, this impairment is manifest as a reduction of blood filtration by Kupffer cells, which is primarily a result of shunting of portal blood rather than reduced phagocytic activity of the Kupffer cells.

GALLBLADDER STRUCTURE AND FUNCTION

The structure of the gallbladder and major ducts of the biliary system is similar in all species (the gallbladder is absent in the horse, the rat, and the elephant). It consists of a muscular wall (tunica muscularis) and a mucosa lined by simple columnar epithelium. The epithelium and muscularis are separated only by the lamina propria because the gallbladder lacks a muscularis mucosae. Right and left hepatic ducts carry bile from

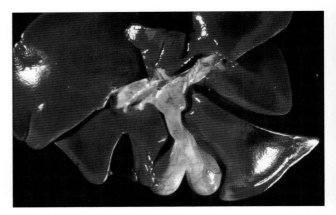

Fig. 8-29   Bilobed gallbladder, liver, cat. Bilobed gallbladders are developmental anomalies that have little or no clinical significance and are found most often in cats. (*Courtesy College of Veterinary Medicine, University of Illinois.*)

different lobes of the liver; these ducts and the cystic duct from the gallbladder unite to form the common bile duct. Location of the opening of the common bile duct into the intestine differs somewhat among the domestic species; it is as little as 2 cm from the pylorus in the pig to as much as 70 cm from the pylorus in the cow.

The gallbladder stores and concentrates bile. Considerable concentration (twentyfold to thirtyfold) of bile by active transport of sodium and anions across the

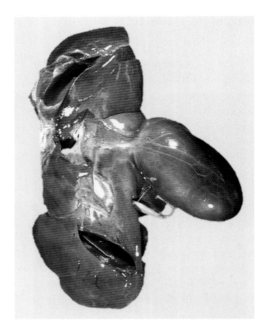

Fig. 8-30   Distended gallbladder, calf. Note the distended gall bladder, which is common in all species following a prolonged period of fasting, because there is no stimulus for emptying the gallbladder. Thus they are frequently seen at necropsy of sick animals. (*Courtesy Dr. J. King, College of Veterinary Medicine, Cornell University.*)

gallbladder epithelial cells occurs in dogs and cats, whereas little concentration occurs in pigs and ruminants. The horse lacks a gallbladder and continuously releases bile into the duodenum.

Developmental anomalies of the gallbladder may be most common in the cat, of bilobed and occasionally trilobed gallbladders can occur (Fig. 8-29). There is no reported clinical significance of these anomalies.

Animals that have not eaten in 24 to 48 hours or that are starving or cachectic can have notably enlarged gallbladders. The reason is that these animals lack the paracrine stimulus (i.e., cholecystokinin), and a number of other neural and hormonal stimuli, to contract the gallbladder and relax the sphincter at the termination of the common bile duct, which regulates flow of bile into the duodenum (Fig. 8-30).

EXOCRINE PANCREAS

NORMAL ANATOMY

DEVELOPMENT

The embryonic origin of the pancreas begins as a dorsal and a ventral bud of the duodenum. These buds fuse during embryogenesis to give rise to the entire pancreas. The major pancreatic duct arises from fusion of the ventral duct and the distal portion of the dorsal duct.

STRUCTURE

The pancreas is a lobulated, pink to gray, tubuloalveolar gland, a large portion of which is located in the mesentery immediately adjacent to the duodenum. The blood vessels, nerves, and lymph vessels that serve the pancreas are located within the delicate connective tissue septa that separate the lobules of pancreatic tissue. The pancreas contains both endocrine and exocrine elements, the endocrine portion being the islets of Langerhans. The exocrine portion constitutes the majority of the pancreas, up to 80% to 85% of the organ, and consists of acini composed of columnar to triangular secretory cells. The acinar cells have basally located oriented nuclei and cytoplasm with a deeply basophilic basal margin and eosinophilic, granular zymogen granules occupying the apical portion of the cytoplasm. When the cells are appropriately signaled, the zymogen granules, containing the digestive enzymes of the pancreas, are released into the lumen of the acinus. The ductal system, in which secretions of the exocrine pancreas are conveyed to the intestinal tract, commences as fine radicals within acini and progresses to intralobular and interlobular ducts. These small ducts eventually drain into the main pancreatic duct or ducts. The arrangement of the major pancreatic ducts and how they empty into the duodenum varies among the domestic species. It is particularly variable in the dog, in which at least five different anatomic arrangements are recognized.

In the cat, the major pancreatic duct enters the duodenum in close proximity to the common bile duct, and this may predispose the cat to pancreatic injury.

NORMAL FUNCTION

The exocrine pancreas produces secretions that contribute to digestion. The secretions contain a variety of enzymes that break down dietary lipids (lipase and phospholipase), proteins (trypsin and chymotrypsin), and carbohydrates (amylase). The secretions also contain electrolytes, which maintain the pH of the intestinal contents within a range that is optimal for enzymatic activity. Pancreatic enzymes act on the products of gastric digestion after they enter the duodenum. These enzymes often are released into secretions as inactive precursors (proenzymes), which helps prevent degradation of the pancreas by its own digestive enzymes. These are activated within the intestine. In addition, inhibitors of pancreatic enzymes are present in the pancreatic tissue. Secretion is controlled by neural stimulation regulated by the vagus nerve and by humoral factors. Secretin is one of the more important hormones involved in pancreatic secretion, and it stimulates water and bicarbonate secretion by duct cells. It is produced by neuroendocrine cells within the duodenal epithelium. The efflux of acid from the stomach and the presence of fatty acids in the duodenum stimulate its release. Cholecystokinin, another important hormone, stimulates the release of digestive enzymes from the acinar cells. It is produced by neuroendocrine cells of the duodenum in response to the presence of fatty acids, peptides, and amino acids.

CONSEQUENCES OF DYSFUNCTION OF THE EXOCRINE PANCREAS

The exocrine pancreas has considerable functional reserve; thus only disorders that affect significant portions of this organ can cause the maldigestion that characterizes exocrine pancreatic insufficiency. Maldigestion as a consequence of exocrine pancreatic insufficiency is most common in the dog. In dogs pancreatic exocrine deficiency is usually the result of either exocrine pancreatic atrophy or chronic pancreatitis. However, pancreatic exocrine deficiency does occur sporadically in other species, including cats and in cattle, specifically calves with pancreatic hypoplasia. Exocrine pancreatic insufficiency in small animals and calves is clinically characterized by steatorrhea, diarrhea, and weight loss despite polyphagia. In contrast, horses with very little functional pancreatic tissue may develop hypoinsulinism, but rarely develop the clinical signs that characterize exocrine pancreatic insufficiency in other species.

PORTALS OF ENTRY

Portals of entry into the exocrine pancreas are listed in Box 8-1.

DEFENSE MECHANISMS

Defense mechanisms for the exocrine pancreas are listed in Box 8-2.

DISEASES OF THE LIVER AND BILIARY SYSTEM

DEVELOPMENTAL ANOMALIES AND INCIDENTAL FINDINGS

Developmental anomalies of the liver occur in domestic animals, although most are of little consequence.

CONGENITAL BILIARY CYSTS

These cysts are found within the livers of dogs, cats, and pigs, but presumably all domestic species can be affected. The cysts are usually an incidental finding. They are usually single, have a thin wall lined by a single layer of biliary epithelium, and are filled with clear fluid. The predominant origin of congenital biliary cysts is thought to be through abnormal development of intrahepatic bile ducts. They can be found in animals of any age. Congenital cysts must be distinguished from parasitic cysts, particularly cysticerci, because they also have a thin wall and are fluid-filled. The presence of the larval cestode within parasitic cysts assists in distinguishing the two structures.

Cysts that occur within the liver of cats, pigs, and to a lesser extent dogs, which typically are multiple and affect extensive areas of the liver, are thought to be developmental anomalies of the intrahepatic bile ducts, although they are considered to be benign cystic biliary neoplasms by some (Fig. 8-31). Congenital polycystic liver disease, characterized by numerous epithelial-lined cysts in the liver and kidneys, occurs in dogs. Cairn terriers and West Highland white terriers are predisposed to the disease as are cats, with Persian cats believed to have a higher risk for the disorder, and goats. Affected animals can die of either liver or renal failure.

HEPATIC DISPLACEMENT

Displacement of the liver into the thoracic cavity, called a diaphragmatic hernia, can occur when there is a defect in the diaphragm. A congenital malformation that leaves an opening in the diaphragm or a traumatic event that ruptures the diaphragm can cause this condition.

TENSION LIPIDOSIS

Discrete, pale areas of parenchyma at the liver margins are common in cattle and horses (Fig. 8-32). These foci typically occur adjacent to the insertion of a ligament (serosal) attachment, and it is proposed that these

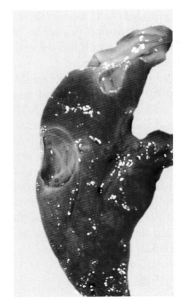

Fig. 8-31   Biliary cysts, liver, pig. Multiple biliary cysts within the liver of a pig. Unilocular cysts replace a portion of the parenchyma in the affected portion of the liver. *(Courtesy Dr. J. King, College of Veterinary Medicine, Cornell University.)*

attachments impede blood supply to the subjacent hepatic parenchyma by exerting tension on the capsule. Affected hepatocytes most probably accumulate fat within their cytoplasm (lipidosis) as a consequence of hypoxia. The lesions are of no functional significance.

CAPSULAR FIBROSIS

Discrete fibrous tags or plaques are frequently present on the diaphragmatic surface of the liver and on

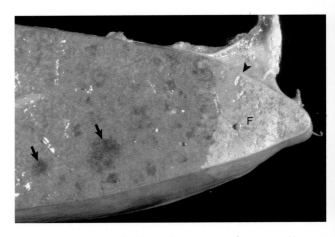

Fig. 8-32   Tension lipidosis, liver, cut surface, cow. Note the area of fatty infiltration (*F*), the ligamentous attachment adjacent to the affected portion (*arrowhead*), and the areas of telangiectasis (*arrows*). *(Courtesy College of Veterinary Medicine, North Carolina State University.)*

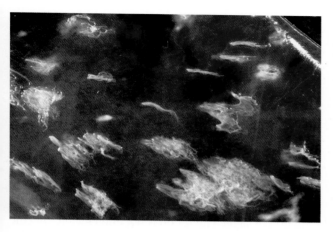

Fig. 8-33   Capsular fibrosis, liver, horse. Numerous fibrous tags are present on the diaphragmatic surface of the liver. These tags are thought to be attributed to reparative fibrosis of the migration tracts of *Strongylus* spp. larvae. *(Courtesy College of Veterinary Medicine, North Carolina State University.)*

the adjacent diaphragm of the horse (Fig. 8-33). Resolution of nonseptic peritonitis, possibly as a result of contact between the diaphragm and the adjacent liver capsule, rather than of parasitic nematode migration tracts, has been proposed as the cause of these regions of capsular fibrosis.

POSTMORTEM CHANGE

Autolysis of the liver occurs rapidly and can be advanced before it is obvious in most other tissue. At or just before death, bacteria are released from the gastrointestinal tract into the portal circulation and reach the liver where they proliferate rapidly after death. This process is especially rapid in large animals during hot weather—particularly cattle, in which fermentation in the adjacent rumen produces heat—and in pigs, which are often well insulated by fat. Pale areas appear on the capsular surface as bacterial degradation begins. In time, the organ becomes green-blue as bacteria degrade blood pigments to iron sulfide. The liver in contact with the gallbladder is quickly discolored by bile pigment, which passes through the wall of the gallbladder. The consistency of the organ becomes puttylike and gas bubbles may form beneath the capsule and in the parenchyma from bacterial fermentation. Postmortem changes are covered in detail in Chapter 1.

CIRCULATORY DISORDERS

DISTURBANCES OF OUTFLOW

PASSIVE CONGESTION (ACUTE AND CHRONIC)

Passive congestion of the liver can occur in any species and is almost always the consequence of cardiac dysfunction. Right side heart failure produces elevated pressure within the caudal vena cava that later involves the hepatic vein and its tributaries. Chronic passive congestion is particularly common in aged dogs and occurs secondary to endocardiosis (mucoid degeneration) of the right atrioventricular valve. Acute passive congestion, on the other hand, can occur as a consequence of acute right side heart failure, which has a wide variety of causes.

The appearance of the liver differs with the duration and severity of the congestion. Passive congestion initially causes distention of central veins and centrilobular sinusoids. Persistent centrilobular hypoxia leads to atrophy or loss of hepatocytes and eventually to centrilobular fibrosis. Fibrosis of the central vein (phlebosclerosis) may also occur.

Acute congestion of the liver produces slight enlargement of the organ, and blood flows freely from any cut surface. The intrinsic lobular pattern of the liver may be slightly more pronounced, particularly on the cut surface, because centrilobular areas are congested (dark red) in contrast to the more normal color of the remainder of the lobule.

Diffuse enlargement and rounded edges of liver lobes are the main features of chronic passive congestion (Fig. 8-34). Chronic passive congestion leads to persistent hypoxia in centrilobular areas and, because of oxygen and nutrient deprivation, the centrilobular hepatocytes atrophy, degenerate, or eventually may undergo necrosis. As a result, sinusoids in these areas are dilated and congested and grossly appear red, whereas periportal hepatocytes frequently undergo lipidosis (fatty degeneration) because of hypoxia, thereby causing this area of the lobule to appear yellow. The result is accentuation of the lobular pattern of the liver, referred to as an enhanced lobular or reticular pattern. It is especially evident on

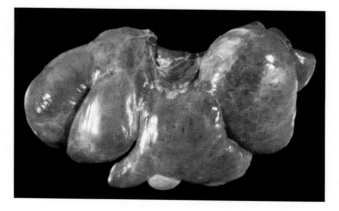

Fig. 8-34   Chronic passive congestion, liver, dog. Chronic passive hepatic congestion in the liver of a dog with a heart base tumor that impeded venous return to the heart. The liver is enlarged with rounded margins. *(Courtesy College of Veterinary Medicine, North Carolina State University.)*

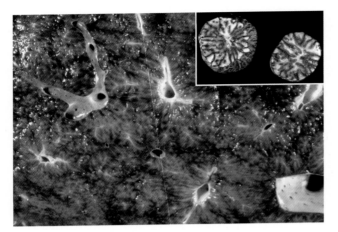

Fig. 8-35   *Chronic passive congestion (nutmeg liver), liver, cut surface, cow.* The congestion in the centrilobular areas and the peripheral lipid accumulation give the liver a characteristic appearance that has been likened to that of the cut surface of a nutmeg, hence the term *nutmeg liver*. *Inset:* Cut surface of a nutmeg for comparison. (*Figure,* Courtesy Dr. D.A. Mosier, College of Veterinary Medicine, Kansas State University. *Inset,* Courtesy Dr. M.O. Howard, College of Veterinary Medicine, Iowa State University; and Noah's Arkive, College of Veterinary Medicine, The University of Georgia.)

the cut surface of the liver, and the enhanced lobular pattern that occurs with severe chronic passive congestion has been likened to the appearance of the cut surface of a nutmeg, and so is termed nutmeg liver (Fig. 8-35). This pattern is not unique to passive congestion, however, and is encountered with other processes, such as zonal hepatic necrosis. In addition to an enhanced lobular pattern, chronic passive congestion is characterized by focal fibrous thickening of the capsule, and, in severe cases, widespread hepatic fibrosis that bridges between central veins (Fig. 8-36).

HEPATIC VENO-OCCLUSIVE DISEASE

Intimal thickening and occlusion of the central vein by fibrous connective tissue characterize the distinctive lesions of this syndrome. The consequence is passive hepatic congestion and resultant hepatic injury, which may progress to hepatic failure and its associated constellation of signs. The lesion is not etiologically specific but can follow pyrrolizidine alkaloid or aflatoxin-induced hepatic injury. An extremely high incidence is recognized in captive exotic cats, such as cheetahs, possibly because of the ingestion of large amounts of vitamin A, although the mechanism for this lesion is not known.

DISTURBANCES OF BLOOD FLOW INTO THE LIVER
ANEMIA

The centrilobular (periacinar) regions of the lobule receive blood last; thus it is the least oxygenated, and the effects of hypoxia are usually manifested first in this area. Acute severe anemia, regardless of cause, can cause centrilobular or paracentral degeneration and even necrosis of hepatocytes (Fig. 8-37). This typically occurs in severe anemias of precipitous onset. Chronic anemia can cause atrophy of centrilobular hepatocytes, which results in dilation, and congestion of sinusoids.

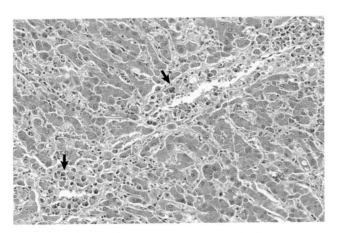

Fig. 8-36   *Chronic passive congestion, liver, dog.* The liver is firm because of hepatic fibrosis that is most severe in centrilobular areas (*arrows*). The central vein is surrounded by a mild amount of connective tissue from which fine fibrous septa extend out into the lobule. Note the macrophages containing hemosiderin, the result of erythrocyte breakdown in this area as a result of chronic congestion. H&E stain. (*Courtesy Dr. J.M. Cullen, College of Veterinary Medicine, North Carolina State University.*)

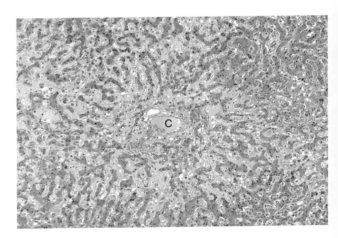

Fig. 8-37   *Centrolobular hepatocyte atrophy, liver, dog.* In chronic anemia, centrilobular hepatocytes, which are the last hepatocytes in the lobule to receive oxygenated blood, become atrophic, and as a consequence, their sinusoids are more dilated. C, Central vein. H&E stain. (*Courtesy Dr. J.M. Cullen, College of Veterinary Medicine, North Carolina State University.*)

Livers from animals with severe anemia, whether acute or chronic, typically have an enhanced lobular pattern that is evident on both the capsular and cut surfaces of the organ (see description of enhanced lobular pattern later).

CONGENITAL PORTOSYSTEMIC SHUNTS

A congenital portosystemic shunt is an abnormal vascular channel that allows blood within the portal venous system to bypass the liver and to drain into the systemic circulation. A congenital shunt can be either intrahepatic or extrahepatic in location but is usually limited to a single relatively large-caliber vessel (Fig. 8-38, A). A variety of different shunts have been described. Typically, intrahepatic portosystemic shunts involve failure of

closure of the ductus venosus at birth. The ductus venosus is a normal fetal vessel that conducts blood from the portal vein to the caudal vena cava. These shunts, such as the ductus venosus, are most often located in the left side of the liver. This anomaly occurs most often in large breed dogs. Extrahepatic congenital shunts, such as portal vein to caudal vena cava anastomoses and portal vein to azygous vein anastomoses, occur more often in small breeds of dogs. Shunts have been described in several species but occur most commonly in the dog and cat. Affected animals are typically stunted and frequently develop signs of hepatic encephalopathy. The liver is small and may have a characteristic histologic appearance of lobular atrophy and reduplication of arterioles and small or absent portal veins within the portal tracts (Fig. 8-38, B). The portal vein pressure is normal in congenital shunts and ascites does not occur. Abnormal vascular anastomoses are often difficult to identify without benefit of antemortem imaging studies. Affected dogs frequently have abnormal plasma ammonia concentrations and, as a consequence, pass ammonium biurate crystals in their urine (Fig. 8-39). It should be noted that the liver has a stereotypic response to inadequate portal vein perfusion. Thus the histologic appearance of congenital portosystemic shunts and other vascular anomalies of the liver (discussed later) have considerable overlap. Clinical data, such as the presence or absence of shunt vessels and the determination of portal vein pressure, may be necessary to achieve a final diagnosis.

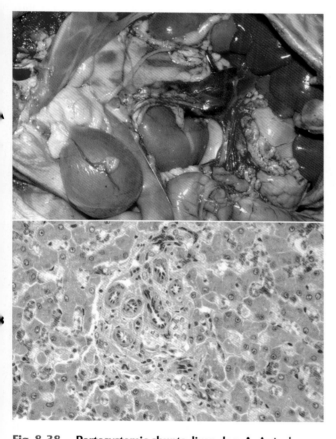

Fig. 8-38   **Portosystemic shunts, liver, dog. A,** A single anomalous vessel that connects the portal circulation with the systemic circulation is the characteristic lesion of congenital portosystemic shunt. Note the small size but normal color of the liver (up under the rib cage). **B,** Congenital portosystemic shunt. Portal areas are abnormal because they lack a portal vein and contain numerous small-caliber arterioles. H&E stain. (**A,** *Courtesy Dr. J. Sagartz, College of Veterinary Medicine, The Ohio State University; and Noah's Arkive, College of Veterinary Medicine, The University of Georgia.* **B,** *Courtesy Dr. J.M. Cullen, College of Veterinary Medicine, North Carolina State University.*)

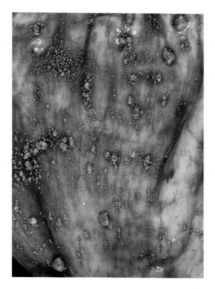

Fig. 8-39   **Ammonium biurate crystals, urinary bladder, dog.** The bladder contains ammonium biurate crystals. These crystals can result from abnormal ammonia metabolism in dogs with portosystemic vascular anastomoses. (*Courtesy College of Veterinary Medicine, North Carolina State University.*)

PORTAL HYPERTENSION

Increased pressure within the portal vein can arise from disturbances of venous blood flow in any of following three sites:

- Prehepatic
- Intrahepatic
- Posthepatic

Prehepatic portal hypertension is relatively uncommon and occurs when blood flow through the portal vein is impaired before it enters the liver. Portal vein thrombosis can be induced by damage to the portal vein, by local inflammatory disorders including pancreatitis, or by hypercoagulable states. Tumor emboli can also obstruct the portal vein. External compression by tumors or abscesses can restrict or obstruct portal vein flow as well. Portal vein hypoplasia affecting the extrahepatic segment of the portal vein is another cause.

Intrahepatic portal hypertension arises from increased resistance to blood flow to, or within, the sinusoids. Chronic liver disease that typically results in bridging collagenous septa, loss of normal lobular architecture, and regenerative nodule formation is the most common intrahepatic cause of portal hypertension. Sinusoidal fibrosis from diseases such as lobular dissecting hepatitis is another cause. Disorders such as veno-occlusive disease, amyloidosis, and schistosomiasis and other granulomatous disease processes can also produce intrahepatic portal hypertension. Arteriovenous fistulae (discussed later) within the hepatic parenchyma can also lead to intrahepatic portal hypertension.

Posthepatic causes of portal hypertension are uncommon and include any abnormalities that lead to increased resistance to venous outflow in the hepatic vein or adjacent vena cava. Partial or complete thrombosis of the hepatic veins (Budd-Chiari syndrome) or of the adjacent caudal vena cava are the most likely, although uncommon, causes of posthepatic portal hypertension. Congestive heart failure can lead to portal hypertension.

Regardless of cause, persistent portal hypertension can lead to acquired portosystemic shunts with the exception of passive congestion, which rarely, if ever, results in the development of shunt vessels. These shunts are usually numerous and composed of distended thin-walled veins, which may connect the mesenteric veins and the caudal vena cava (Fig. 8-40). Ascites is common in conditions that develop acquired shunts because of the associated portal hypertension.

Vascular anomalies that may produce portal hypertension

Intrahepatic arteriovenous shunts (anastomoses).   Arteriovenous shunts, either acquired or congenital, occur in the dog and cat and are direct

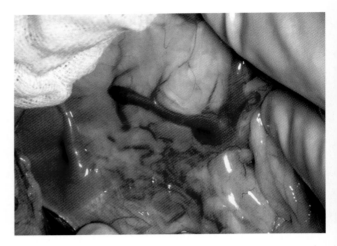

Fig. 8-40   Acquired portosystemic anastomoses, abdomen, dog. Acquired portosystemic anastomoses secondary to portal hypertension (in this case as a consequence of chronic hepatitis in a dog). The numerous prominent veins that are present over the surface of the kidney allow blood within the portal venous system to bypass the liver and directly enter the systemic circulation. *(Courtesy Dr. L. Hardy, College of Veterinary Medicine, North Carolina State University.)*

communications between the hepatic artery and branches of the portal vein. They may occur anywhere within the liver. Affected portions of the liver contain convoluted thick-walled arteries and distended portal vein branches. Shunting of blood may lead to portal hypertension or reversal of the direction of portal blood flow, subsequent development of acquired portocaval shunts and ascites. Clinical signs vary in intensity, most likely in relationship to the caliber of vessels that are affected, and are probably the result of the degree of portosystemic shunting of blood that results.

Portal vein hypoplasia (microvascular dysplasia, noncirrhotic portal hypertension).   Portal vein hypoplasia is a congenital vascular anomaly that occurs in dogs and occasionally in cats. It is characterized by abnormally small extrahepatic or intrahepatic portal veins, which result in diminished hepatic perfusion by the portal vein blood flow and the potential for portal hypertension. Typically, affected animals have small livers and the typical histologic pattern of portal vein hypoperfusion, small or absent portal veins, proliferated hepatic arterioles (so-called reduplication), and hepatocyte atrophy. This disorder resembles portosystemic shunts histologically, but affected animals often have portal hypertension and resultant ascites. Portal fibrosis and biliary hyperplasia occur in about half of the cases. Because of the histologic similarities between portal vein hypoplasia and congenital portosystemic shunts, clinical data, such as imaging studies to

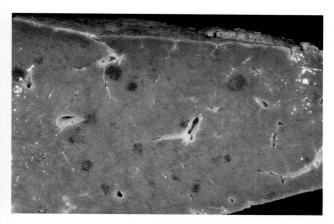

Fig. 8-41   Telangiectasia, liver, cut surface, cow.
Telangiectasia is a condition in which hepatic sinusoids become dilated and filled with blood. These lesions can be seen as dark red areas on the cut and capsular surface of the liver. *(Courtesy Dr. M.D. McGavin, College of Veterinary Medicine, University of Tennessee.)*

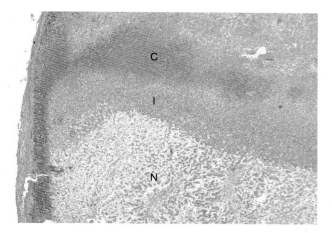

Fig. 8-42   Hepatic infarction, liver, dog. Hepatic infarction is uncommon and usually occurs at the margins of the liver where the terminal divisions of the blood supply are found. Infarction of the liver is characterized by a zone of coagulative necrosis (**N**) rimmed with inflammatory cells (**I**) and an outer zone of congestion (**C**) in the viable liver. H&E stain. *(Courtesy Dr. J.M. Cullen, College of Veterinary Medicine, North Carolina State University.)*

determine the presence of a shunt vessel, are often required to make final diagnosis from biopsy material.

INCIDENTAL VASCULAR DISORDERS
TELANGIECTASIS

Telangiectasis is the notable dilation of sinusoids in areas where hepatocytes have been lost. Grossly, these areas appear as variably sized dark blue foci within the liver that vary from pinpoint to several centimeters in size (Fig. 8-41). Telangiectasis is particularly common in cattle and apparently is of no clinical significance. It also occurs in old cats, in which it can be mistaken for vascular tumors such as hemangioma or hemangiosarcoma. Histologically, there is ectasia of the sinusoidal space and a loss of hepatocytes. There is no evidence of inflammation or fibrosis associated with this lesion.

INFARCTION

Infarction of the liver occurs infrequently because of the organ's dual blood supply from the hepatic artery and portal vein. Infarcts are usually sharply delineated and may be either dark red when acute or pale as they age. They tend to occur at the margins of the liver, the terminal end of parenchymal perfusion, and can affect small wedges of only a few centimeters in length or larger portions of a lobe. Histologically, infarcted liver is characterized by a zone of coagulative necrosis bordered by a basophilic band of inflammatory cells and an outer band of hyperemia (Fig. 8-42). Torsion of individual lobes of the liver, which occurs infrequently, can result in vascular occlusion and infarction of the affected lobe.

METABOLIC DISTURBANCES AND HEPATIC ACCUMULATIONS
HEPATOCELLULAR LIPIDOSIS OR FATTY LIVER (STEATOSIS)

Lipids are normally transported to the liver from adipose tissue and the gastrointestinal tract in the form of either free fatty acids or chylomicrons, respectively. Within hepatocytes, free fatty acids are esterified to triglycerides that are complexed with apoproteins to form low-density lipoproteins, and these are released into the plasma as a readily available energy source for use by a variety of tissues. Some oxidation of fatty acids for energy production occurs within hepatocytes, and some fatty acids are converted to phospholipid and cholesterol esters. With the exception of ruminants, the liver also actively produces lipids from amino acids and glucose.

The presence of excessive lipid within the liver is termed hepatocellular lipidosis (steatosis) or fatty liver and occurs when the rate of triglyceride accumulation within hepatocytes exceeds either their rate of metabolic degradation or their release as lipoproteins. Hepatocellular lipidosis is obviously not a specific disease entity but can occur as a sequel to a variety of perturbations of normal lipid metabolism. The potential mechanisms responsible for excessive accumulation of fat within the liver include the following:

1. Excessive entry of fatty acids into the liver, which occurs as a consequence of excessive dietary intake of fat or increased mobilization of triglycerides from

adipose tissue because of increased demand (e.g., lactation, starvation, and endocrine abnormalities).

2. Abnormal hepatocyte function leads to accumulation of triglycerides within hepatocytes as a result of decreased energy for oxidation of fatty acids within hepatocytes.

3. Excessive dietary intake of carbohydrates results in the synthesis of increased amounts of fatty acids with formation of excessive triglycerides within hepatocytes.

4. Increased esterification of fatty acids to triglycerides in response to increased concentrations of glucose and insulin, which stimulate the rate of triglyceride synthesis from glucose or from prolonged increases in dietary chylomicrons.

5. Decreased apoprotein synthesis and subsequent decreased production and export of lipoprotein from hepatocytes.

6. Impaired secretion of lipoprotein from the liver because of secretory defects produced by hepatotoxins or drugs.

It must be stressed that these are potential mechanisms (some being more significant than others, depending on the condition of the animal) and that more than one defect might occur in any given hepatic disorder. Regardless of cause, the gross appearance of the hepatocellular lipidosis is highly characteristic. With progressive accumulation of lipid, the liver enlarges and becomes yellow (Fig. 8-43, A). In mild cases, lipids may only accumulate in specific portions of each lobule, such as centrilobular regions, thereby imparting an enhanced lobular pattern to the liver. In extreme cases, the entire liver is affected, and the organ may become considerably enlarged and have an extremely greasy texture. Lipid vacuoles are readily detected within the cytoplasm of hepatocytes (Fig. 8-43, B).

Specific causes and syndromes of hepatocellular lipidosis in domestic animals include the following:

1. Dietary causes of hepatocellular lipidosis include simple dietary excess in monogastric animals, such as a high-fat and/or high-cholesterol diet. Hepatocellular lipidosis is especially common in ruminants with high-energy demands, such as those in peak lactation or late gestation, and reflects increased mobilization of lipids from adipose tissue. Obese animals are particularly predisposed to develop hepatocellular lipidosis, such as occurs when dietary intake is restricted. Deficiencies of cobalt and vitamin B_{12} have been implicated as causes of fatty liver in sheep and goats.

2. Toxic and anoxic causes of hepatocellular lipidosis are common. Sublethal (reversible) injury to hepatocytes frequently results in accumulation of lipid within the affected cell. Injury to hepatocytes can

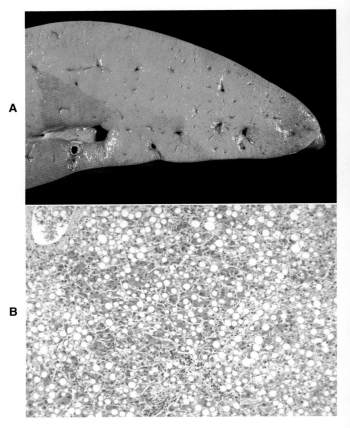

Fig. 8-43   Fatty liver syndrome (hepatic lipidosis). A, Cut surface, cow. The liver is swollen and yellow because of notable infiltration of lipid into hepatocytes. **B,** Steatosis or fatty degeneration, cat. Diffuse cytoplasmic accumulation of lipid is evident within the hepatocytes throughout the liver. H&E stain. (*A, Courtesy Dr. M.D. McGavin, College of Veterinary Medicine, University of Tennessee. B, Courtesy Dr. J.M. Cullen, College of Veterinary Medicine, North Carolina State University.*)

lead to accumulation of lipids because of decreased formation and/or export of lipoproteins by hepatocytes and decreased oxidation of fatty acids within hepatocytes.

3. Ketosis is a metabolic disease that results from impaired metabolism of carbohydrate and volatile fatty acids. In times of energy demand, free fatty acids are released from body fat stores, and the free fatty acids are esterified into fatty acyl CoA in the liver. Ketone bodies (acetoacetic acid and β-hydroxybutyric acid) are derived from fatty acyl CoA by oxidation in the mitochondria. In pregnant and lactating animals, there is a continuous demand for glucose and amino acids, and ketosis results when fat metabolism, which occurs in response to the increased energy demands, becomes excessive. Ketosis is characterized by increased concentrations

of ketone bodies in blood (hyperketonemia), hypoglycemia, and low concentrations of hepatic glycogen. Ketosis is common in ruminants and usually occurs during peak lactation, whereas ketosis of sheep usually occurs in late gestation, particularly in ewes carrying twins; this latter disease is known as pregnancy toxemia.

4. Bovine fatty liver syndrome, also known as fatty liver disease, is mechanistically similar to ketosis. In dairy cattle, the disease is usually encountered in obese animals within a few days after parturition and is often precipitated by an event that causes anorexia, such as retained placenta, metritis, mastitis, abomasal displacement, or parturient paresis. Typically, affected beef cattle are obese and the disease occurs within a few days before parturition. Accumulation of lipid within the liver is the result of both increased mobilization of lipids from adipose tissue, which results in increased influx of fatty acids to the liver, and defective hepatocytic function, which results in decreased export of lipoprotein from the liver.

5. Feline fatty liver syndrome is a distinct syndrome of idiopathic hepatocellular lipidosis recognized in cats. Typically affected cats are obese and anorectic and have no other diseases that could cause hepatocellular lipidosis. Cats with this type of hepatocellular lipidosis frequently develop hepatic failure, icterus, and subsequently hepatic encephalopathy.

6. Hepatocellular lipidosis occurs in ponies, miniatures horses, and donkeys. Shetland ponies are predisposed. The condition usually occurs in overweight pregnant or lactating mares, characteristically after an event that causes stress or anorexia. In addition to notable hepatocellular lipidosis, affected ponies are usually hyperlipemic and may also manifest signs of renal failure and hepatic rupture. In severe cases, hepatic encephalopathy and/or terminal disseminated intravascular coagulation can occur.

7. Endocrine disorders, such as diabetes mellitus and hypothyroidism, can produce hepatocellular lipidosis in a variety of species. In these cases, hepatocellular lipidosis is obviously but one manifestation of abnormal metabolism. The accumulation of lipids in the liver in the diabetic animal is the result of increased fat mobilization and decreased use of lipids by injured hepatocytes.

GLYCOGEN ACCUMULATION

Glucose is normally stored within hepatocytes as glycogen and is often present in large amounts after feeding. Excessive hepatic accumulation of glycogen occurs with the metabolic perturbations involving glucose regulation, including diabetes mellitus and the glycogen storage diseases. In these instances, hepatic involvement is just one manifestation of a systemic disease process.

Glucocorticoid-induced hepatocellular degeneration is a specific disorder characterized by excessive hepatic accumulation of glycogen (Fig. 8-44, A). Excessive amounts of endogenous or exogenous glucocorticoids cause extensive swelling of hepatocytes from the accumulation of glycogen. Glucocorticoids induce glycogen synthetase and so enhance hepatic storage of glycogen. Glycogen accumulation leads to pronounced swelling of hepatocytes (up to 10 times normal volume), particularly those in the midzonal areas (Fig. 8-44, B). In severe cases of glucocorticoid-induced hepatocellular degeneration (often referred to as steroid-induced hepatopathy), the liver is enlarged and pale but otherwise unremarkable. The disorder occurs in dogs, and frequently is iatrogenic, but can also be a consequence of hyperadrenocorticism. The diagnosis can be confirmed on the basis of the characteristic microscopic

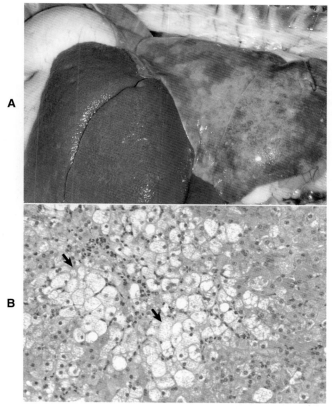

Fig. 8-44   Glucocorticoid-induced hepatopathy, liver, dog. A, In dogs with glucocorticoid excess (Cushing's disease) from endogenous or exogenous sources, an extensive accumulation of glycogen in hepatocytes results in an enlarged, pale-brown to beige liver. Note also the pulmonary edema. **B,** Note the swollen hepatocytes *(arrows)* with extensive cytoplasmic vacuolation from glycogen accumulation. H&E stain.
(**A,** *Courtesy Dr. K. Bailey, College of Veterinary Medicine, University of Illinois.* **B,** *Courtesy Dr. J.M. Cullen, College of Veterinary Medicine, North Carolina State University.)*

appearance of the liver and identification of the source of the excess glucocorticoids.

AMYLOIDOSIS

Hepatic amyloidosis occurs in most species of domestic animals. Amyloidosis is not a single disease entity but a term used for various diseases that lead to the deposition of proteins that are composed of β-pleated sheets of nonbranching fibrils. Affected livers are enlarged, friable, and pale (Fig. 8-45, A). Histologically, hepatic amyloid appears as bright eosinophilic amorphous deposits that are usually found in the space of Disse along the sinusoids but can be found in the portal tracts and within blood vessel walls (Fig. 8-45, B). Amyloid's physical properties are responsible for its birefringence and characteristic apple green appearance in Congo red stained sections viewed under polarized light. As many as 15 distinct amyloid proteins have been identified, but the hepatic amyloid is usually derived from one of three types. In primary amyloidosis, the amyloid fibril is designated AL (amyloid light chain) and is composed of immunoglobulin light chains derived from the amino terminal variable region of κ- and λ-light chains synthesized by plasma cell neoplasms. Secondary or reactive amyloidosis occurs as a consequence of prolonged inflammation, such as chronic infection or tissue destruction. In secondary amyloidosis, by far the most common type to occur in veterinary medicine, the fibrils are composed of amyloid A (AA). The precursor protein is serum amyloid–associated (SAA) protein, an apolipoprotein which is an acute phase protein synthesized by the liver. Inherited or familiar amyloidosis is uncommon in animals but occurs in Shar-Pei dogs and Abyssinian, Siamese, and other Oriental breeds of cats.

Regardless of its cause, amyloid can accumulate in more than one pattern. It may accumulate in vessel walls in the portal area, within the connective tissue of the portal area, and in the space of Disse, where it impairs the normal access of plasma to hepatocytes. Amyloid deposits can produce varying degrees of hepatomegaly, and extensive accumulations cause the liver to appear pale. In severe cases, affected animals may have clinical signs of either hepatic dysfunction or failure because the liver is more fragile; liver rupture and exsanguinations may occur, especially in the horse. Frequently, amyloid is also deposited within the kidneys, particularly the glomeruli. Renal failure often occurs before signs of hepatic dysfunction are manifested.

COPPER ACCUMULATION

Copper poisoning is included as a metabolic disorder because hepatic injury in copper poisoning of domestic animals frequently is the result of progressive accumulation of copper within the liver. This occurs in domestic animals, especially sheep, in which storage of copper is poorly regulated. Also, hereditary disorders of copper metabolism have been described in dogs.

Copper is an essential trace element of all cells, but even a modest excess of copper can be life threatening because copper must be properly sequestered to prevent toxicosis. Normally, serum copper is bound to ceruloplasmin and hepatic copper is bound to metallothionein. In cases of excess, the copper distribution is initially diffuse throughout the hepatic cytoplasm, but in later stages it is concentrated within lysosomes. Excess copper, like excess iron, can lead to the production of reactive oxygen species that initiate destructive lipid peroxidation reactions that affect the mitochondria and other cellular membranes. In domestic animals, copper toxicosis usually occurs as a consequence of one of the following:

1. Simple dietary excess in ruminants, particularly sheep, and pigs occurring, for example, because of excessive dietary supplementation as an overcorrection for copper deficiency or from contamination of the pasture with copper from sprays or fertilizer.

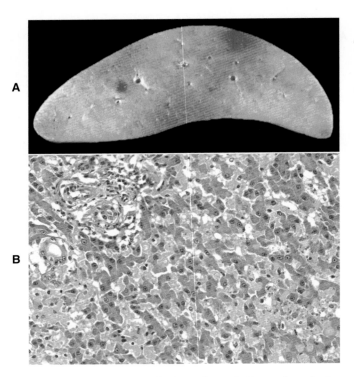

Fig. 8-45   **Hepatic amyloidosis, liver. A,** Cut surface, duck. Hepatic amyloidosis has imparted a firm, waxy appearance and a pale brownish hue to the affected liver. **B,** Dog. The perisinusoidal spaces of Disse adjacent to the sinusoids are lined with a glassy eosinophilic (hyaline) material–amyloid. H&E stain. (*A, Courtesy Drs. J. King and L. Roth, College of Veterinary Medicine, Cornell University. B, Courtesy Dr. J.M. Cullen, College of Veterinary Medicine, North Carolina State University.*)

It also occurs in sheep that have access to copper-containing mineral blocks formulated for cattle.

2. Grazing animals on pastures with normal concentrations of copper but with inadequate concentrations of molybdenum, which antagonizes copper uptake.

3. Pasturing herbivores on fields with plants that contain hepatotoxic phytotoxins, usually pyrrolizidine alkaloids. *Heliotropium*, *Crotalaria*, and *Senecio* species are common examples of such plants. Pyrrolizidines prevent hepatocellular proliferation by their toxic action on the spindle during mitosis. This failure to replace necrotic hepatocytes leads to an ever-increasing copper load in surviving hepatocytes because these hepatocytes take up the copper released by the dying cells. Copper is excreted in the bile, and hepatic diseases that result in cholestasis are particularly likely to produce excessive accumulation of copper within the liver, even when dietary intake of copper is not excessive.

4. Hereditary disorders of copper metabolism, as occur in Dalmatians and Bedlington and West Highland white terriers. The disorder is best characterized in Bedlington terriers that have an autosomal recessive inheritance that leads to impaired biliary excretion of copper, which results in progressive accumulation within the liver.

The consequences of excessive accumulation of copper within the liver of domestic animals are species-dependent. In ruminants, particularly sheep, copper accumulates within the liver over a period of time (for one of the first three reasons listed previously), but some event triggers a sudden release of copper, which is followed by acute, severe intravascular hemolysis and hepatocellular necrosis, mostly because of acute anemia. Necrosis of the liver is extensive and affects centrilobular and midzonal regions most consistently because of hypoxia, but massive necrosis can occur in severe cases. Despite the acute and fulminant nature of the terminal event, this process is referred to as chronic copper poisoning to distinguish it from disease caused by simple copper intoxication that causes gastroenteritis. In contrast, copper continues to accumulate in the livers of Bedlington terriers shown to have a mutation (deletion of exon 2) or mutations in the *MURR1* gene, which encodes a chaperone protein involved in copper excretion by hepatocytes. Copper accumulates in the centrilobular regions of the liver and leads to ongoing necrosis of hepatocytes, chronic inflammation, replacement fibrosis, and eventually to an end-stage liver and signs of hepatic failure (Fig. 8-46). Excessive concentrations of hepatic copper may be present in other breeds of dog including the Dalmatian, West Highland white terrier, Skye terrier, Doberman pinscher, American and English cocker spaniel, and Labrador retriever, although the significance or role of copper in the hepatic disease

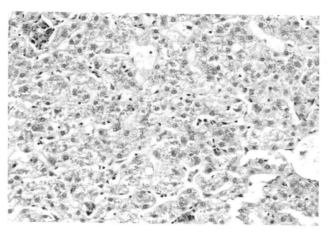

Fig. 8-46   Hepatic copper, liver, dog. The red-brown copper-containing granules are indicative of excess copper in the lysosomes of hepatocytes. Copper is not readily visible with H&E staining but can be confirmed by special stains. Rhodanine stain. *(Courtesy Dr. J.M. Cullen, College of Veterinary Medicine, North Carolina State University.)*

of these breeds of dog is uncertain. These diseases are discussed in the section on canine chronic hepatitis.

PIGMENT ACCUMULATION

Pigments are colored substances, some of which are normal cellular constituents, whereas others accumulate only in abnormal circumstances. They are covered in detail in Chapter 1.

BILE PIGMENTS

Bile pigments may accumulate in excessive amounts as a consequence of either extrahepatic or intrahepatic cholestasis and typically produce icterus and green discoloration of the liver.

HEMOSIDERIN

Hemosiderin is an iron-containing, golden-brown, granular pigment derived from ferritin, the initial iron-storage protein. As iron accumulates within the cell, aggregates of ferritin molecules form hemosiderin (Fig. 8-47). Most hemosiderin in Kupffer cells and other macrophages located in tissues throughout the body is derived from the breakdown of erythrocytes, whereas most hepatocellular hemosiderin is derived from iron present in transferrin and to a lesser extent hemoglobin. Hemosiderin forms in the liver when there is local or systemic excess of iron, such as when erythrocytic breakdown is excessive (e.g., hemolytic anemia), and within areas of hepatic necrosis. An excessive systemic load of iron that is characterized by abundant hemosiderin in a variety of tissues without impairment of

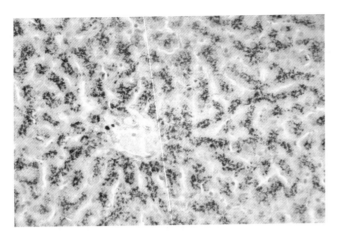

Fig. 8-47   Hemosiderosis, liver, dog. Dark blue granules, indicative of iron, stored as hemosiderin in hepatocytes are confirmed by the Prussian blue reaction. *(Courtesy Dr. J.M. Cullen, College of Veterinary Medicine, North Carolina State University.)*

organ function is called hemosiderosis. In contrast, hemochromatosis is an abnormally increased storage of iron within the body that can cause hepatic dysfunction. Notable accumulation of iron can produce a dark brown or even a black liver.

LIPOFUSCIN

Lipofuscin is an insoluble pigment that is yellow-brown to dark brown and is derived from incomplete oxidation of lipids, such as those in cell membranes (Fig. 8-48). Lipofuscin is progressively oxidized with time; thus it actually is a group of lipid pigments, all of which consist of polymers of lipid, phospholipids,

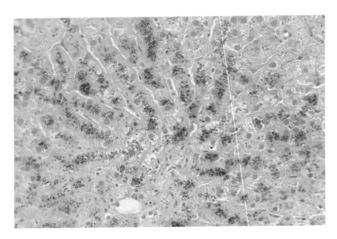

Fig. 8-48   Lipofuscinosis, liver, dog. Lipofuscin can be detected by a variety of special stains. In these hepatocytes, lipofuscin granules in lysosomes are dark gray-blue to green. **Schmorl's stain.** *(Courtesy Dr. J.M. Cullen, College of Veterinary Medicine, North Carolina State University.)*

protein (and minimal carbohydrate in early forms). Amounts of lipofuscin present in the liver tend to increase with age.

MELANIN

Melanin is an endogenous pigment that is dark brown or black. Benign disorders of melanin pigmentation are usually designated as melanosis. Congenital melanosis of the liver occurs in pigs and ruminants and produces variably sized areas of discoloration of the liver. Acquired "melanosis" of sheep has been described in Australia and is associated with the ingestion of certain plants, but the pigment has not been proven to be melanin and may be derived from a component of the ingested plants.

PARASITE HEMATIN

Liver flukes specifically produce very dark excreta that contain a mixture of iron and porphyrin. These excreta produce the characteristic discoloration that occurs in fascioliasis (*Fasciola hepatica*), and is especially pronounced in the migratory tracts produced by *Fascioloides magna* in bovine livers.

INFECTIOUS DISEASES OF THE LIVER
VIRAL DISEASES
INFECTIOUS CANINE HEPATITIS

Infectious canine hepatitis is, as the name implies, a viral infection of the liver of dogs and other canids, including foxes and coyotes, that produces acute necrosis and inflammation. The disease is caused by canine adenovirus 1. The majority of infections are asymptomatic, and infections that result in disease may not be fatal. The virus has a predilection for hepatocytes, vascular endothelium, and renal epithelium; fulminant disease is characterized by hepatic necrosis and widespread hemorrhage that can affect a variety of organs.

Exposure of susceptible dogs is most often via the oral route by contact with urine from infected dogs. Viremia last for 4 to 8 days, but virus is shed in the urine of infected dogs for prolonged periods. Virus multiplication initially occurs in the tonsils and produces tonsillitis with spread to local lymph nodes and then to the systemic circulation via the thoracic duct. Viremia is associated with leukopenia and fever. Spread of virus to the liver, endothelial cells, and mesothelial cells follows. Infection of Kupffer cells may precede hepatocytic injury. Adenoviruses are cytolytic and cause necrosis of infected cells.

Lesions of infectious canine hepatitis include widespread petechiae and ecchymoses, accumulation of clear fluid in the peritoneal and other serous cavities, the presence of fibrin strands on the surface of the liver, and enlargement and reddening of the tonsils and lymph nodes (Fig. 8-49, A). The liver is moderately enlarged and friable and may contain small foci of hepatocellular necrosis centered on centrilobular areas. An enhanced lobular pattern is sometimes evident because of the centrilobular hepatic necrosis. Characteristically the wall of the gallbladder is thickened by edema.

The severity of microscopic lesions present in individual dogs may reflect the duration of the disease.

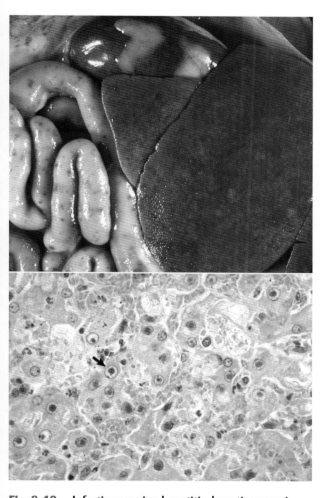

Fig. 8-49   Infectious canine hepatitis, hepatic necrosis, liver, dog. A, The liver from a dog infected with infectious canine hepatitis (ICH) can be slightly enlarged and friable with a blotchy yellow discoloration. Sometimes fibrin is evident on the capsular surface. Note the petechiae on the serosal surface of the intestines caused by vascular damage from canine adenovirus type I infection. **B,** Infection of hepatocytes and endothelial cells with canine adenovirus type I produces characteristic basophilic intranuclear inclusions surrounded by a clear zone that separates them from the marginated chromatin (*arrow*). H&E stain. (**A,** *Courtesy Dr. W. Crowell, College of Veterinary Medicine, The University of Georgia; and Noah's Arkive, College of Veterinary Medicine, The University of Georgia.* **B,** *Courtesy Dr. M.D. McGavin, College of Veterinary Medicine, University of Tennessee.*)

Susceptible puppies rapidly succumb to infection and have only scattered foci of hepatocellular necrosis, whereas fulminant disease in older dogs often produces both randomly scattered foci of hepatocellular necrosis and widespread centrilobular necrosis. The predilection for centrilobular necrosis is more likely to be related to the virus's penchant for infection and necrosis of endothelial cells that may lead to vascular stasis and local hypoxia than to any increased propensity for the virus to damage centrilobular hepatocytes. Large amphophilic intranuclear inclusions are found in vascular endothelium and hepatocytes (Fig. 8-49, B). Zonal necrosis may reflect ischemic injury and not direct virus-mediated destruction of hepatocytes. Virus-induced endothelial damage may lead to disseminated intravascular coagulation and hemorrhagic diathesis, which contribute to the hemorrhage observed in affected dogs. Some dogs recovering from infectious canine hepatitis develop an immune-complex uveitis (type III hypersensitivity), which produces degeneration and necrosis of the corneal endothelium and resultant corneal edema clinically known as "blue eye."

HERPESVIRUS INFECTIONS

Herpesvirus infections of the liver typically occur in neonates or fetuses. A variety of abortigenic herpesviruses are described, each animal species being affected by a specific virus. Examples of these viruses include the abortigenic equine herpesvirus (equine herpesvirus 1), infectious bovine rhinotracheitis virus (bovine herpesvirus 1), caprine herpesvirus, canine herpesvirus (canine herpesvirus 1), feline viral rhinotracheitis virus, and pseudorabies virus.

Infection can occur via several routes, including transplacental exposure, passage through the birth canal, contact with infected littermates, and contact with oronasal secretions from the dam. In neonates, initial infection often occurs in the oronasal epithelium where virus replication first takes place. After local replication, the virus enters the blood stream via infected mononuclear phagocytic cells. Viremia leads to dissemination of the virus to a variety of organs, and viral infection is cytolytic.

The abortigenic herpesviruses characteristically induce multifocal, randomly distributed, small (<1 mm) areas of necrosis in several fetal organs, including the liver (Fig. 8-50, A). Similar lesions occasionally are present in neonates infected with herpesviruses.

Histologically, herpesvirus can produce multifocal hepatic necrosis with scant inflammation in fetuses and neonates (Fig. 8-50, B). The liver is often affected, but foci of necrosis are more consistently present in the kidneys, lungs, and spleen. The virus most often affects neonates in the first 2 weeks of life and is most severe before they develop competent thermoregulation.

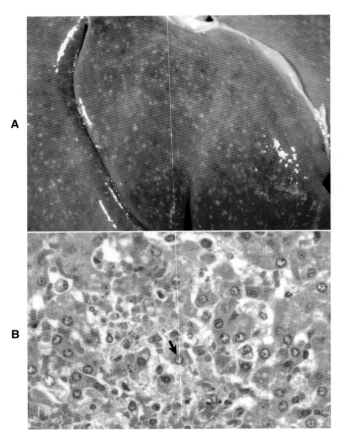

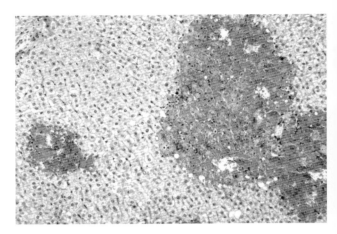

Fig. 8-51   Focal hepatic necrosis, Rift Valley fever, liver, sheep. This disease produces randomly distributed focal areas of necrosis in the liver of lambs and fetuses, often with a central area of older necrosis surrounded by a rim of hepatocytes, which have been killed at a later stage in the infection. H&E stain. *(Courtesy Armed Forces Institute of Pathology.)*

Fig. 8-50   Equine herpesvirus hepatitis, hepatic necrosis, liver, foal. A, Note the randomly distributed gray-to-white foci of random hepatocellular necrosis caused by equine herpesvirus. **B,** Infection of hepatocytes with equine herpesvirus produces characteristic acidophilic intranuclear inclusions surrounded by a clear zone that separates them from the marginated chromatin *(arrow)*. Note the individual cell necrosis. H&E stain. *(A, Courtesy Drs. J. King and L. Roth, College of Veterinary Medicine, Cornell University. B, Courtesy Dr. J.M. Cullen, College of Veterinary Medicine, North Carolina State University.)*

Animals that are able to maintain a normal body temperature are less likely to be affected.

RIFT VALLEY FEVER

This is an acute, arthropod (mosquito)-transmitted zoonotic viral disease that principally affects ruminants, causing extensive mortality among calves and lambs, and abortion of pregnant ewes and cows. The causative virus is a member of the family Bunyaviridae, genus *Phlebovirus.* The disease occurs throughout much of Africa, and it is especially prevalent after periods of unusually high rainfall.

Hepatic involvement is consistently present in fulminant cases, typically in neonates, and is characterized by hepatic enlargement and yellow-orange discoloration.

Areas of congestion may be present. In older animals, pale foci of hepatocellular necrosis that are randomly scattered throughout the parenchyma impart a mottled appearance and sometimes an enhanced lobular pattern because of the centrilobular hepatic necrosis. Diffuse petechiae and ecchymoses are also characteristic of the disease, as are edema and hemorrhages of the wall of the gallbladder. Disseminated intravascular coagulation probably contributes to the hemorrhagic diathesis and perhaps to the development of zonal hepatic necrosis.

Microscopic lesions are characterized by the presence of both randomly distributed foci of hepatocellular necrosis and more widespread zonal necrosis, which ranges from centrilobular to massive (Fig. 8-51). These lesions, particularly random hepatic necrosis, are more severe and widespread in young animals and aborted fetuses. Eosinophilic intranuclear inclusion bodies may be present in degenerate hepatocytes in areas of necrosis.

WESSELSBRON DISEASE

This disease, like Rift Valley fever, is a zoonotic arthropod (mosquito)-transmitted viral disease that occurs in Africa; the virus occasionally causes disease in newborn lambs and abortion in ewes. The causative agent is a member of the Flaviviridae. Affected lambs have multifocal areas of hepatocellular necrosis, and icterus develops occasionally. Canalicular cholestasis may be apparent. Infected adult sheep usually survive infection, although they may develop focal areas of hepatocellular necrosis.

OTHER VIRAL INFECTIONS

Certain viral diseases may involve the liver, but the hepatic involvement either does not occur invariably or it may be but one manifestation of a systemic process. Such diseases include feline infectious peritonitis that is characterized by foci of pyogranulomatous vasculitis or perivascular accumulations of lymphocytes and plasma cells within multiple organs, sometimes including the liver. Subacute and chronic forms of equine infectious anemia are characterized by cellular accumulations, particularly lymphocytes, in sinusoids and the space of Disse. Systemic adenoviral infection of lambs, calves, and goat kids may produce multifocal areas of hepatocellular necrosis, cholangitis, and necrosis of biliary epithelium. Porcine circovirus type 2 injures hepatocytes and Kupffer cells and can cause mild to severe necrosis.

BACTERIAL DISEASES
LIVER ABSCESSES AND GRANULOMAS

Bacteria can reach the liver via a number of different routes and form abscesses (Figs. 8-52 through 8-54). Routes include the following:

- The portal vein
- The umbilical veins from umbilical infections in newborn animals
- The hepatic artery, as part of a generalized bacteremia
- Ascending infection of the biliary system
- Parasitic migration
- Direct extension of an inflammatory process from tissues immediately adjacent to the liver, such as the reticulum

Both gram-positive and gram-negative organisms can cause hepatic abscesses. In adult small animals, hepatic

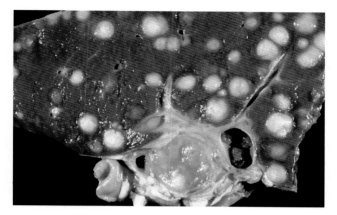

Fig. 8-53   Hepatic abscesses, *Rhodococcus equi*, liver, goat. Disseminated hepatic abscesses in a goat caused by *Rhodococcus equi*. This lesion is more commonly found in foals. (*Courtesy Dr. P. Stromberg, College of Veterinary Medicine, The Ohio State University.*)

abscesses are often caused by *Yersinia* spp., *Nocardia asteroides*, and *Actinomyces* spp. Bacterial infections of the liver and subsequent formation of hepatic abscesses are especially common in feedlot cattle. This usually occurs as a sequel to toxic rumenitis because damage to the ruminal mucosa allows ruminal microflora, particularly *Fusobacterium necrophorum*, to enter the portal circulation. After initially localizing within the liver, bacteria proliferate and produce focal areas of hepatocellular necrosis and hepatitis that can, in time, develop into hepatic abscesses (Fig. 8-55). Liver abscesses of cattle frequently are incidental lesions, but they can cause weight loss and decreased milk production.

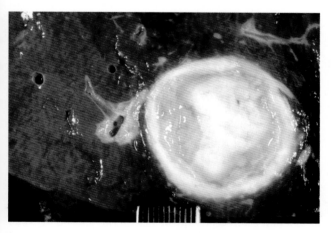

Fig. 8-52   Chronic hepatic abscesses, *Corynebacterium pseudotuberculosis*, liver, sheep. Note the thick fibrous capsule and the pale caseous exudate characteristic of pus produced by *Corynebacterium pseudotuberculosis* in sheep. (*Courtesy College of Veterinary Medicine, North Carolina State University.*)

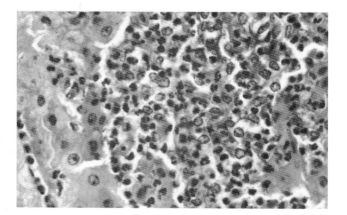

Fig. 8-54   Hepatic abscess, liver, cow. An abscess in the liver is similar to those in other tissues and consists of an infiltrate of neutrophils, degenerating neutrophils, and necrotic tissue debris. H&E stain. (*Courtesy Dr. M.D. McGavin, College of Veterinary Medicine, University of Tennessee.*)

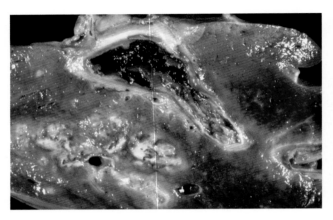

Fig. 8-55   Hepatic abscess, *Fusobacterium necrophorum*, liver, cow. Foci of necrosis and abscess formation. Abscesses such as this one can erode the wall of a hepatic vein or the caudal vena cava, rupture, and release their contents into the blood stream. *(Courtesy Dr. P. Stromberg, College of Veterinary Medicine, The Ohio State University.)*

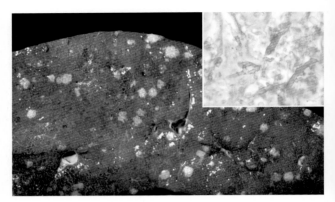

Fig. 8-57   Multiple necrotic foci, disseminated fungal infection (*Mucor* spp.), liver, cow. *Mucor* spp. enter the portal blood following ulcerative rumenitis and cause focal necrosis and inflammation in the liver. *Inset:* The hyphae of the causative organism *(pink)* are usually evident within the granuloma. Periodic acid-Schiff reaction. *(**Figure,** Courtesy College of Veterinary Medicine, University of Illinois. **Inset,** Courtesy Dr. M.D. McGavin, College of Veterinary Medicine, University of Tennessee.)*

Less commonly, a hepatic abscess encroaches on the lumen of either a hepatic vein or the caudal vena cava. This can cause phlebitis that results in mural thrombosis, and because of the obstruction of the outflow to the venous drainage of the liver, passive congestion of the liver and portal hypertension can occur (Fig. 8-56). Detachment of portions of these mural thrombi can produce septic thromboemboli that lodge in the lungs. Rupture of hepatic abscesses directly into the hepatic vein or into the caudal vena cava occurs sporadically in cattle and may result in fatal septic embolization of

the lungs. Sometimes death can be sudden from the blockage of large areas of pulmonary capillaries by the exudate. Hepatic abscesses derived from bacteria arriving via the portal vein may not be evenly distributed throughout the liver, possibly because of selective distribution of portal blood into different liver lobes, termed portal streaming. Occasionally, fungi such as *Mucor* sp. that proliferate in areas of ruminal ulceration invade the portal circulation and are carried to the liver and there cause extensive areas of necrosis and inflammation (Fig. 8-57).

Tuberculosis (*Mycobacterium bovis*) has been eradicated from almost all of the United States, but its occurrence in other countries varies with the effectiveness of control efforts. The primary site of the disease is pulmonary with subsequent dissemination to other organs including the liver. Other domestic animal species can be infected with *Mycobacterium bovis*, and it is also a zoonotic microbe. *Mycobacterium avium-intracellulare* complex can occur in domestic animals, especially dogs in the southern areas of the United States. Granulomas are randomly distributed (i.e., hematogenous spread) in the liver. They have a central core of cell debris, caseation, and granulomatous inflammation surrounded by a fibrous capsule (Fig. 8-58).

BACILLARY HEMOGLOBINURIA

Bacillary hemoglobinuria is an acute and highly fatal disease of cattle and sheep that occurs in various areas of the world, typically in those regions in which liver fluke (*Fasciola hepatica*) infection also occurs. Spores of *Clostridium haemolyticum*, the causative agent of bacillary hemoglobinuria, are ingested and come to reside within

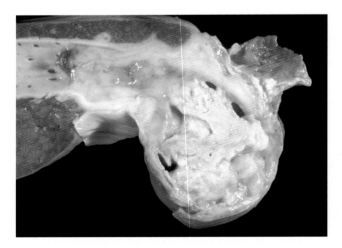

Fig. 8-56   Hepatic abscess, caudal vena cava, cow. A hepatic abscess has eroded the wall of the vena cava, ruptured, and released its contents into the caudal vena cava. *(Courtesy College of Veterinary Medicine, North Carolina State University.)*

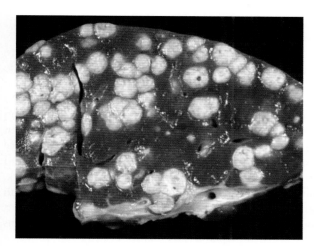

Fig. 8-58 **Multiple caseous granulomas, tuberculosis,** ***Mycobacterium bovis,*** **liver, cow.** Hepatic tuberculosis is characterized by random multifocal pale white to yellow caseous granulomas on the capsular and cut surfaces. *(Courtesy Dr. M. Domingo, Autonomous University of Barcelona; and Noah's Arkive, College of Veterinary Medicine, The University of Georgia.)*

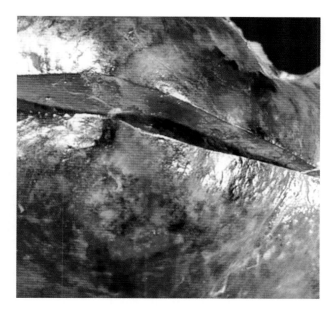

Fig. 8-59 **Focal hepatic necrosis,** ***Clostridium haemolyticum*** **(bacillary hemoglobinuria), liver, cut surface, cow.** These large areas of necrosis are sharply delineated from the adjacent parenchyma, are usually pale, and are surrounded by an intensely hyperemic zone of acute inflammation. *(Courtesy Dr. J. King, College of Veterinary Medicine, Cornell University.)*

Kupffer cells, but they proliferate only in areas of low oxygen tension. Migration of immature liver flukes, or less commonly other parasites, or an event such as liver biopsy produces a nidus of necrotic hepatic parenchyma in which bacterial spores can germinate. Bacteria proliferate and release toxins, the most important of which is phospholipase C, that induce the hepatocellular necrosis and intravascular hemolysis that characterize the disease. Grossly, these foci, which have been misnamed infarcts, are sharply delineated from the adjacent parenchyma, and usually are pale and surrounded by an intensely hyperemic zone (Fig. 8-59). Migration tracts of the immature flukes that typically precipitate the disease may be present. Serous cavities (pleura, peritoneum, and pericardium) often contain excessive accumulation of red or straw-colored fluid that is sometimes flecked with fibrin. The liver contains one or more discrete foci of hepatic necrosis in which causative organisms may be visible in histologic sections. Affected animals have icterus, hemoglobinemia, and hemoglobinuria.

INFECTIOUS NECROTIC HEPATITIS

Also known as black disease, infectious necrotic hepatitis is most common in sheep and cattle but also occurs in pigs and horses. This disease is somewhat analogous to bacillary hemoglobinuria in that dormant spores of *Clostridium novyi* (usually type B) germinate in areas of lowered oxygen tension and release toxins that produce discrete foci of coagulation necrosis within the liver and eventually death of the host. Germination of spores is usually initiated by hepatic necrosis caused by

the migration of immature liver flukes; however, a variety of other initiating factors that produce low oxygen tension within the liver parenchyma have been described. Parasitic migration tracts are usually present within the affected liver. Other lesions that may be present include diffuse venous congestion and accumulation of fluid within the pericardial sac and pleural and peritoneal cavities. Affected animals typically have one or more areas of hepatocellular necrosis, which usually manifests as discrete, pale areas of variable size. A zone of intense hyperemia often surrounds these foci. The carcass of affected animals typically putrefies rapidly because of high fever before death.

TYZZER'S DISEASE

This disease is caused by *Clostridium piliforme* (formerly *Bacillus piliformis*), a gram-negative staining obligate intracellular parasite. It is well recognized in laboratory animals but occurs only sporadically in domestic animals. Infection is most common in foals, but has been described in calves, cats, and dogs and other species. Typically, only very young or immunocompromised animals are affected. The bacteria are found in the intestinal tract of rodents. Infection is most likely through the oral route. The mechanisms of attachment and entry into host cells are unknown. After colonization of the gastrointestinal tract, organisms penetrate into the portal venous drainage and enter the liver. The disease is characterized by enlarged, edematous, and hemorrhagic abdominal lymph nodes, hepatic enlargement, and the presence of randomly distributed, pale foci of hepatocellular necrosis surrounded by a variably intense inflammatory infiltrate of neutrophils and mononuclear cells (Fig. 8-60, A). Diagnosis requires the demonstration of the characteristic, elongated large bacilli within viable hepatocytes at the margins of necrotic foci (Fig. 8-60, B). Silver stains, such as Warthin-Starry or Gomori's silver stain, are frequently used for this purpose (Fig. 8-60, C).

LEPTOSPIROSIS

This disease is caused by infection with the thin, spiral, motile bacterium of the genus *Leptospira*. There are several species, and each species consists of several serovars. Each serovar can differ with respect to the species affected, organs affected, and severity of disease. Leptospires enter the body through the mucous membranes or through the skin if its barrier functions have been disrupted. Contaminated water, bedding, and soil are common sources of infection, as the organism is shed in urine. Fetuses can develop transplacental infection. Infection can involve red blood cells, kidney, liver, and a number of other tissues depending on the infecting serovar. The liver is often involved in acute, severe leptospirosis of all domestic species. This is because a number of serovars cause intravascular hemolytic anemia leading to ischemic injury to centrilobular areas. Furthermore, organisms are present in large numbers in the liver, although the direct effects of leptospira toxins on hepatocytes are less well established.

Gross lesions include icterus when animals are infected with serovars that produce hemolysis. Hepatic hemorrhage and ascites can occur depending on the course of infection and the serovar involved. In some cases, acute infection can cause focal necrosis in addition to or instead of centrilobular necrosis. A common but nonspecific change in the liver of infected dogs is dissociation of hepatocytes. Affected cells become rounded and have eosinophilic granular cytoplasm and dark, shrunken hyperbasophilic nuclei. Bile casts in canaliculi are often apparent. Kupffer cells may contain abundant hemosiderin. Infection of dogs with *Leptospira interrogans serovar Grippotyphosa* has been reported to produce chronic (chronic-active) hepatitis, but it is unlikely that leptospira are involved in the pathogenesis of the majority of spontaneous cases of chronic hepatitis.

OTHER BACTERIAL INFECTIONS

These diseases are grouped together because they all arise from a bacteremia that occurs during a systemic infection. A comprehensive list of systemic infections that may produce hepatocellular necrosis and hepatitis is beyond the scope of this chapter, but examples include *Yersinia pseudotuberculosis*, *Salmonella* spp. (lesions present within the liver are discrete accumulations of mixed mononuclear inflammatory cells, which often are referred to as "paratyphoid nodules") and *Brucella* spp. infection in many species (Fig. 8-61, A and B). *Haemophilus agni*

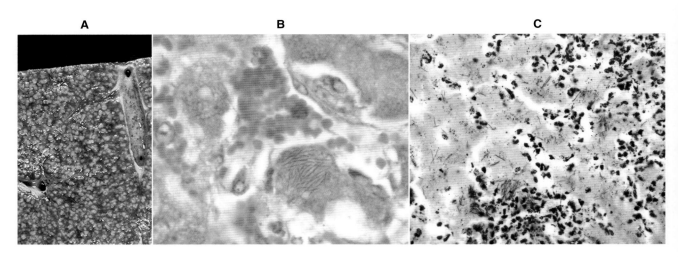

A **B** **C**

Fig. 8-60 **Tyzzer's disease (*Clostridium piliforme*). A,** Liver, horse. Disseminated gray-white 1- to 2-mm foci of necrosis surrounded by suppurative inflammation. **B,** Foal. *Clostridium piliforme* can be identified by the haphazard distribution of filamentous bacteria in the cytoplasm of hepatocytes. Giemsa stain. **C,** Foal. *Clostridium piliforme* can be readily seen with special stains such as Giemsa and Warthin-Starry stains. Warthin-Starry stain. (*A, Courtesy Dr. R.C. Giles, University of Kentucky; and Noah's Arkive, College of Veterinary Medicine, The University of Georgia. B and C, Courtesy Dr. M.D. McGavin, College of Veterinary Medicine, University of Tennessee.*)

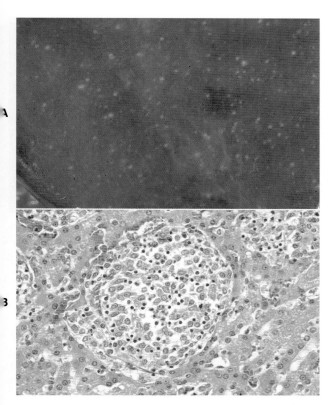

Fig. 8-61 **Hepatic salmonellosis, liver. A,** Diaphragmatic surface, cow. Random 1- to 2-mm foci of focal necrosis in a cow with *Salmonella* septicemia. Multiple pale subcapsular foci of necrosis are evident. **B,** Pig. Later in the disease process, the necrotic foci are infiltrated by macrophages and form discrete granulomas termed paratyphoid nodules. H&E stain. (**A,** *Courtesy Dr. M.D. McGavin, College of Veterinary Medicine, University of Tennessee.* **B,** *Courtesy Dr. J. Simon, College of Veterinary Medicine, University of Illinois.*)

and *Pasteurella haemolytica* can present as infections in sheep. Other infections include *Arcanobacter pyogenes* (*Actinomyces pyogenes*) of the bovine fetus and neonate, *Campylobacter fetus* ssp. *fetus* in fetal and neonatal lambs, *Actinobacillus equuli* infection of neonatal foals, and *Nocardia asteroides* infection of dogs. *Yersinia tularensis* (*Francisella tularensis*), the cause of tularemia, can occur in cats and dogs. Bacterial infections such as these may produce lesions within the liver that range from small foci of hepatic necrosis to multiple, large abscesses. Determination of the specific causative agent is often dependent upon bacterial isolation and characterization.

PROTOZOAL DISEASES

The liver can be involved in systemic infections with *Toxoplasma gondii* or *Neospora* sp. Liver lesions are usually characterized by multifocal necrosis and inflammation.

Inflammatory cells include neutrophils, macrophages, and smaller numbers of other inflammatory cells. Free tachyzoites or cysts containing bradyzoites can be found within necrotic areas or adjacent to them. Although there are subtle physical differences between the organisms, immunologic testing, such as immunohistochemical staining, is a more reliable means to separate the two organisms.

DIMORPHIC FUNGAL DISEASES

Histoplasmosis is a fungal disease that is endemic in the United States and Canada and can occur occasionally in other areas. It is caused by *Histoplasma capsulatum*, a soil-dwelling organism. Dogs are affected most often. The route of infection is primarily through inhalation, although ingestion is also a possible route. In some circumstances pulmonary infections become disseminated and affect a variety of visceral organs, including the liver. Lesions in the liver consist of a multifocal distribution of granulomas with intralesional yeast forms of the organism. Numerous yeast forms can be found in the cytoplasm of macrophages and can be readily stained with the periodic acid–Schiff reaction. (Fig. 8-62, A and B).

PARASITIC DISEASES
NEMATODES

Migration of larvae through the liver is a common component of a nematode's life cycle in domestic animals. As larvae travel through the liver, they produce local tracts of hepatocellular necrosis that are accompanied by inflammation. These tracts are eventually replaced with connective tissue that matures into fibrous scars and which are especially prominent on the capsular surface (Fig. 8-63). These capsular scars appear as pale areas, and the term "milk spotted liver" has been used to describe livers in pigs scarred by migrating larvae of *Ascaris suum*. Larvae occasionally become entrapped within the liver or its capsule and are walled off within abscesses or granulomas. Examples of chronic hepatitis or hepatic scarring as a consequence of larval migration include migration of ascarids in several species of domestic animals, such as *Stephanurus dentatus* in pigs, and *Strongylus* sp. in the horse. Infection of the liver with adult nematodes is considerably less common than larval migration. *Capillaria hepatica* occasionally may be found in the hepatic parenchyma of dogs and cats.

Dogs with heartworm infection (*Dirofilaria immitis*) occasionally develop vena caval syndrome, also known as the postcaval syndrome, which is characterized by disseminated intravascular coagulation, intravascular hemolysis, and acute hepatic failure. The syndrome typically occurs in dogs with large numbers of adult worms in the vena cava and their more usual location

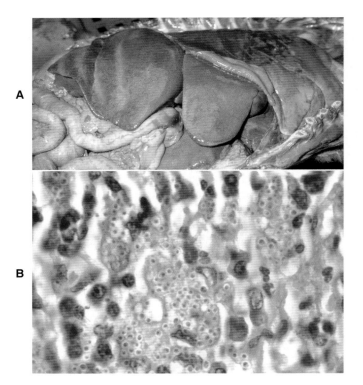

Fig. 8-62 **Hepatic histoplasmosis, liver, dog. A,** In disseminated cases, *Histoplasma capsulatum* can involve the liver. Affected livers tend to be enlarged and pale mahogany from the diffuse hypertrophy and proliferation of Kupffer cells and macrophages. **B,** Note the yeast form of *Histoplasma* in the cytoplasm of Kupffer cells and macrophages. H&E stain. (**A,** *Courtesy College of Veterinary Medicine, University of Illinois.* **B,** *Courtesy Dr. J. Simon, College of Veterinary Medicine, University of Illinois.*)

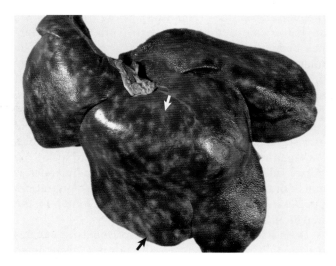

Fig. 8-63 **Capsular and portal fibrosis (milk-spotted liver), Ascaris suum larval migration, liver, diaphragmatic surface, pig.** Fibrous tissue *(scars)* has been deposited in the migration tracks of the ascarid larvae and in adjacent portal areas *(arrows)*. *(Courtesy Dr. M.D. McGavin, College of Veterinary Medicine, University of Tennessee.)*

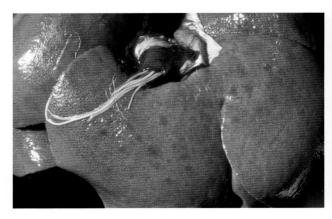

Fig. 8-64 **Dirofilariasis, vena caval syndrome, caudal vena cava at the level of the liver, dog.** Large collections of adult *Dirofilaria immitis* are present in the caudal vena cava. The condition is rapidly fatal unless the nematodes are removed. *(Courtesy Dr. C.S. Patton, College of Veterinary Medicine, University of Tennessee.)*

within the right side of the heart and pulmonary artery (Fig. 8-64). The liver is engorged with blood as a consequence of severe passive congestion from the partial blockage of the caudal vena cava. It is proposed that mechanical factors produced by the presence of large numbers of worms in the right atrium or caudal vena cava are the cause of intravascular hemolysis, which characterizes vena caval syndrome, although other theories suggest that there may be a hypersensitivity reaction to antigens released by the worms.

CESTODES

A number of cestodes occur within the hepatobiliary system of domestic animals. Those cestode parasites of greatest clinical significance develop encysted forms within the liver of the intermediate hosts. The most important are larval cestodes of the genus *Taenia*, adults of which inhabit the gastrointestinal tract of carnivores and which usually are innocuous to their definitive host. The ova ingested by an intermediate host develop into embryos, which penetrate the wall of the gut and then are distributed via the blood to virtually any site in the body. Parasitic cysts develop within the tissue of the intermediate host, and the life cycle of the parasite is completed when the cysts are ingested by the definitive host. Although the liver is but one organ in the intermediate host that may be affected, hepatic involvement is common because portal blood, in which embryos migrate, drains into the liver before flowing to the systemic circulation.

The adult cestode *Taenia hydatigena* shows up in dogs, whereas its intermediate stage, *Cysticercus tenuicollis*, appears in the peritoneal cavity of a variety of species, including horses, ruminants, and pigs (Fig. 8-65).

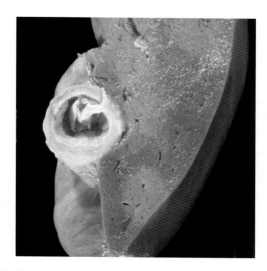

Fig. 8-65   Cysticercosis, liver, cut surface, sheep. The thick fibrous capsule usually indicates the death of the larva. *(Courtesy Dr. K. Read, College of Veterinary Medicine, Texas A&M University; and Noah's Arkive, College of Veterinary Medicine, The University of Georgia.)*

Immature cysticerci migrate in the liver and can induce extensive damage if infection is heavy; lesions present are comparable to those induced by migration of immature *Fasciola hepatica.*

Hydatid liver disease is common in some countries. *Echinococcus granulosus* is a cestode that parasitizes canids as the definitive host, and hydatid cysts can develop in many different intermediate host animal species, including humans. The dog-sheep cycle is most important in many geographic areas. Pastured cattle are also commonly affected in other geographic locations. Adult worms in the intestines of dogs pass proglottids into the dog's stool and thereby contaminate pastures. Ova are then ingested by sheep, cattle, or other species. Embryos may develop into hydatid cysts in virtually any organ in the intermediate host, but the liver and lungs are commonly affected. These cysts are usually less than 10 cm in diameter but can attain quite a spectacular size, particularly in humans. Hydatid cysts, even when present in large numbers, rarely cause overt clinical signs of disease in domestic animals.

Cestode adults occurring within the hepatobiliary system include *Stilesia hepatica*, *Stilesia globipunctata*, and *Thysanosoma actinoides*, all of which can inhabit the bile duct of ruminants. Infections with these parasites may result in chronic inflammation of the biliary tract, but they usually do not produce clinical signs of hepatic dysfunction.

TREMATODES

Liver fluke disease of sheep and cattle, and occasionally other species, most commonly is caused by *Fasciola hepatica.* Hepatic fascioliasis occurs throughout the world in areas where climatic conditions, typically in low swampy areas, are suitable for the survival of aquatic snails, which serve as intermediate hosts for the parasites. Adult *Fasciola hepatica* are leaf-shaped parasites that inhabit the biliary system; their eggs pass via the bile to the intestinal tract and eventually are passed in the feces. Larvae then must develop in the snail intermediate host (genus *Lymnaea*). Cercariae that leave the snail, encyst on herbage where they develop into infectious metacercariae. Metacercariae are ingested by the ruminant host and penetrate the wall of the duodenum to enter the peritoneal cavity and subsequently enter the liver. They migrate within the liver before taking up residence within the bile ducts. Migration of immature flukes through the liver produces hemorrhagic tracts of necrotic liver parenchyma. These tracts are grossly visible and in acute infection are dark red, but with time become paler than the surrounding parenchyma. Repair is often by fibrosis. A variety of untoward sequelae can follow these migrations, including acute peritonitis; hepatic abscesses; death of the host as a consequence of acute, widespread hepatic necrosis produced by a massive infiltration of immature flukes; and the proliferation of spores of *Clostridium haemolyticum* or *Clostridium novyi* in necrotic tissue, which causes the subsequent development of bacillary hemoglobinuria or infectious necrotic hepatitis, respectively.

Mature flukes reside in the larger extrahepatic and intrahepatic bile ducts and cause cholangitis. Chronic cholangitis and bile duct obstruction lead to ectasia and stenosis of the ducts, and periductular fibrosis that thickens the walls so that the ducts become increasingly prominent. Obstruction of the ducts leads to cholestasis. Animals with chronic liver fluke disease are often in poor body condition.

Fasciola gigantica and *Fascioloides magna* are important causes of liver fluke disease of ruminants in some parts of the world. The adults of *Fasciola gigantica* and *Fasciola hepatica* reside in the bile ducts (Fig. 8-66). In contrast, adult *Fascioloides magna*, whose normal hosts are elk and white-tailed deer, reside in the hepatic parenchyma in aberrant hosts, such as cattle and sheep. In cattle, the immature *Fascioloides magna* flukes cause extensive tissue damage as they migrate through the liver (Fig. 8-67), but the adults are enclosed by fibrous connective tissue in cysts containing a black fluid. In sheep and goats, the flukes continuously migrate through the liver, causing extensive damage and eventual death.

Other trematodes that may inhabit the bile ducts include *Dicrocoelium dendriticum* in horses, ruminants, pigs, dogs, and cats; *Eurytrema pancreaticum* and *Eurytrema coelomaticum* in ruminants; *Opisthorchis tenuicollis* in pigs, dogs, and cats, and *Opisthorchis viverrini* in dogs and cats; *Pseudamphistomum truncatum, Metorchis conjunctus, Metorchis albidus, Parametorchis complexus, Concinnum procyonis,* and *Platynosomum fastosum* in dogs and cats.

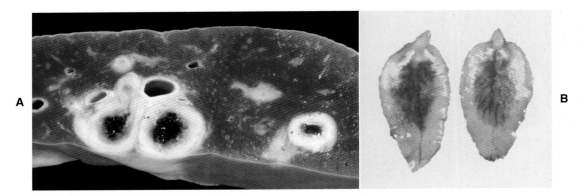

Fig. 8-66 *Fasciola hepatica* **infection. A,** Chronic intrahepatic cholangitis (*Fasciola hepatica*), liver, cow. When *Fasciola hepatica* metacercariae are ingested, they migrate to the liver and then take up residence within the bile ducts. Mature flukes reside in the larger extrahepatic and intrahepatic bile ducts and cause chronic cholangitis and bile duct obstruction that lead to ectasia and stenosis of the ducts and periductular fibrosis that thickens the walls so that the ducts become increasingly prominent, as shown here. **B,** Adult *Fasciola hepatica*. Adult *Fasciola hepatica* are leaf-shaped flukes that inhabit the biliary system; their eggs pass via the bile into the intestinal tract and eventually are passed in the feces. (*A, Courtesy Dr. K. Read, College of Veterinary Medicine, Texas A&M University; and Noah's Arkive, College of Veterinary Medicine, The University of Georgia. B, Courtesy Dr. T. Boosinger, College of Veterinary Medicine, Auburn University; and Noah's Arkive, College of Veterinary Medicine, The University of Georgia.*)

All are capable of inducing changes similar to but usually considerably milder than those caused by *Fasciola hepatica*. In addition, they occasionally cause obstruction of the biliary ducts.

Cats, and less often dogs, can develop pronounced chronic cholangitis from infections with flukes, most often Opisthorchiidae. Microscopically, larger intrahepatic bile ducts are dramatically thickened by concentric fibrosis and the duct lumen is usually dilated, often with papillary projections of biliary epithelium into the lumen (Fig. 8-68). A mild to moderate inflammatory infiltrate of neutrophils and macrophages is often found in and around the ducts, and the portal tracts are infiltrated by neutrophils, lymphocytes, and plasma cells. Eosinophils are generally uncommon. It is often difficult to detect adult flukes or ova in affected animals.

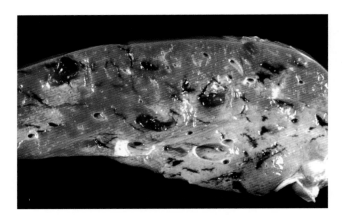

Fig. 8-67 **Fluke migration tracts, fascioloidiasis, liver, cow.** Migration of *Fascioloides magna* through the bovine liver produces extensive parenchymal damage. A black excretory pigment deposited by the fluke discolors the migration tracks black. (*Courtesy Dr. J. Wright, College of Veterinary Medicine, North Carolina State University; and Noah's Arkive, College of Veterinary Medicine, The University of Georgia.*)

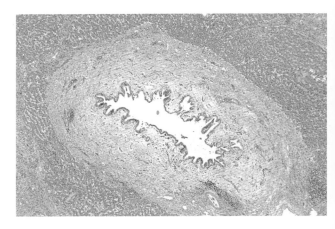

Fig. 8-68 **Chronic intrahepatic cholangitis, liver, cat.** Fluke infections of the biliary tree of cats produce a characteristically pronounced periductular fibrosis, dilated bile duct, and papillary projections of biliary epithelium, although flukes may be difficult to find. H&E stain. (*Courtesy Dr. J.M. Cullen, College of Veterinary Medicine, North Carolina State University.*)

Dogs can be infected with the schistosome *Heterobilharzia americana*, which is normally a parasite in raccoons. Ova shed into water by infected raccoons release miracidia, which penetrate host snails. Dogs become infected when their skin is penetrated by cercariae, which are released from the intermediate snail hosts. Granulomatous lesions of the liver, and pancreas, intestines and mesentery result when ova released by adult schistosomes lodge in affected tissue and incite an inflammatory reaction.

INFLAMMATORY DISORDERS OF THE BILIARY TRACT

NEUTROPHILIC CHOLANGITIS

Inflammation of the biliary ducts (either intrahepatic or extrahepatic) is termed cholangitis. There are several patterns of inflammation of the biliary tree that can be recognized. Neutrophilic (suppurative) cholangitis is the most common type of cholangitis. It is characterized by the presence of neutrophils within the lumen or the epithelium (Fig. 8-69). Acute and chronic forms of this process can occur. Rupture of affected bile ducts can lead to hepatic abscess formation. Most neutrophilic cholangitis is believed to be caused by ascending bacterial infections from the intestine.

LYMPHOCYTIC CHOLANGITIS

This disorder occurs most often in cats. Affected cats are usually older than 4 years of age and often have icterus as a consequence of intrahepatic cholestasis. The inflammatory cells can involve bile ducts directly,

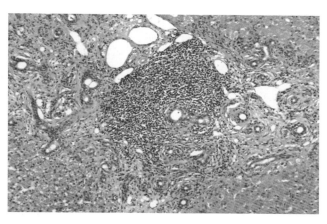

Fig. 8-70   Feline lymphocytic cholangitis, liver, cat. Large numbers of lymphocytes surrounding bile ducts and biliary hyperplasia in portal areas are the hallmarks of this disease. The inflammation most often affects the periphery of the bile ducts and could be termed a pericholangitis, but the syndrome is referred to as cholangitis. H&E stain. *(Courtesy Dr. J.M. Cullen, College of Veterinary Medicine, North Carolina State University.)*

making it difficult to identify the original bile duct within an affected portal tract, but usually the inflammatory cells are arrayed at the periphery of the ducts. Often by the time a biopsy is obtained, the liver is characterized by extensive aggregations of inflammatory cells, typically lymphocytes and plasma cells in portal tracts, particularly around numerous small bile ducts (Fig. 8-70). Inflammation usually is accompanied by bile duct proliferation, hepatic or biliary fibrosis, and intrahepatic cholestasis. The cause or causes of this syndrome are unknown. The disease might have an immunologic basis. Chronic lymphocytic cholangitis should be distinguished from suppurative cholangitis, which is caused most often by ascending bacterial infection of the biliary tree.

DESTRUCTIVE CHOLANGITIS

Destructive cholangitis is an uncommon syndrome characterized by necrosis of the epithelium of bile ducts (Fig. 8-71). Inflammation is often present around the areas of biliary destruction, but within the portal area. Certain chemicals, such as trimethoprim sulfa, have been implicated in this syndrome in dogs.

NUTRITIONAL DISEASES OF THE LIVER

HEPATOSIS DIETETICA

Hepatosis dietetica (nutritional hepatic necrosis) is a syndrome of acute hepatic necrosis that occurs in young, rapidly growing pigs. This is but one manifestation of a variety of disorders that are likely to be, at least in part, caused by deficiency of vitamin E

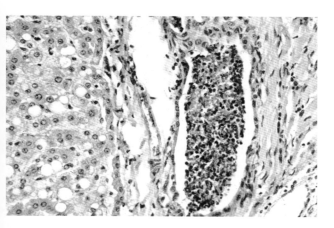

Fig. 8-69   Suppurative cholangitis (intrahepatic), liver, cat. This condition is characterized by the presence of degenerate neutrophils within the lumen or the walls of bile ducts in the portal areas. Ascending bacterial infection from the intestine via the common bile duct is the most common cause. H&E stain. *(Courtesy Dr. M.D. McGavin, College of Veterinary Medicine, University of Tennessee.)*

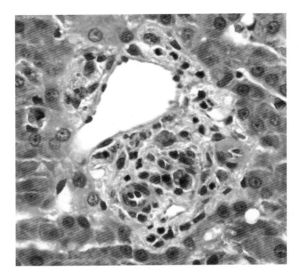

Fig. 8-71   Destructive cholangitis, liver, dog. This condition is an uncommon disorder characterized by the destruction of bile duct epithelium, followed by regeneration in some instances. Necrotic or absent biliary epithelium, pigmented macrophages, and small numbers of mononuclear inflammatory cells in portal tracts are the typical histologic findings. **H&E stain.** *(Courtesy Dr. J.M. Cullen, College of Veterinary Medicine, North Carolina State University.)*

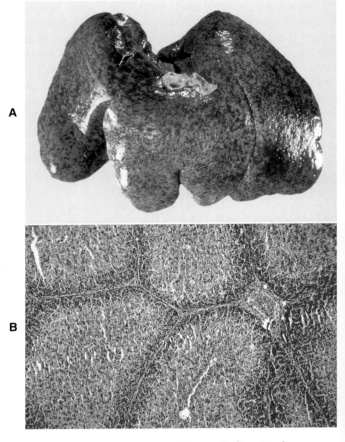

Fig. 8-72   Massive necrosis, *Hepatosis dietetica*, liver, pig. A, Areas of hemorrhagic centrilobular necrosis and massive necrosis appear as dark regions of different size scattered throughout the liver. **B,** Acute centrilobular necrosis is the principal lesion of this disorder. *(**A,** Courtesy Dr. R. Michel, College of Veterinary Medicine, University of Tennessee. **B,** Courtesy College of Veterinary Medicine, North Carolina State University; Dr. A.R. Doster, University of Nebraska; and Noah's Arkive, College of Veterinary Medicine, The University of Georgia.)*

and/or selenium. The pathogenesis of hepatosis dietetica is incompletely defined. Although it is apparent that affected animals respond to the provision of vitamin E or selenium, it has been difficult, on an experimental basis, to produce the syndrome consistently by feeding diets deficient in vitamin E and selenium. Because vitamin E and selenium-containing enzymes are antagonists of free radical formation and are therefore important for the maintenance of stability and integrity of cellular membranes, it is believed that oxidative injury leads to hepatocyte necrosis.

Regions of massive necrosis in the affected liver will initially be distended, deep red, and friable. Hepatosis dietetica is characterized by hemorrhagic centrilobular to massive hepatic necrosis (Fig. 8-72, A and B). The appearance of the liver reflects the extent of hepatic necrosis, the severity of the hemorrhage, and the duration of the deficiency. Later, in animals that survive the acute disease, parenchymal collapse and dense tracts of connective tissue (postnecrotic scarring) are usually evident.

WHITE LIVER DISEASE

White liver disease derives its name from the pale, fatty livers in sheep that develop from a nutritional deficiency caused by insufficient cobalt intake. Animals grazing on soil that is depleted in cobalt either by natural deficiency or previous use of the area for

plants, such as potatoes, that deplete soil of cobalt are affected. Cobalt is a necessary cofactor in the synthesis of vitamin B_{12} and other enzymes. Deficiency of vitamin B_{12} can lead to anemia, and the liver lesions may be attributed to the effects of anemia.

TOXIN-INDUCED LIVER DISEASE

The liver is subjected to toxic injury more often than any other organ. This is not surprising because the portal vein blood that drains from the absorptive surface of the intestinal tract flows directly to the liver. Thus the liver is exposed to virtually all ingested substances, including plant, fungal, and bacterial products, and metals, minerals, and other chemicals that are absorbed into the portal blood. Hepatotoxic injury can range along a spectrum from pure hepatocellular injury to pure biliary injury and a mixed pattern of injury that involves both components of the liver.

Hepatotoxic drugs can be divided into two basic categories. Predictable hepatotoxins are those that affect the large majority of animals that are exposed, and the effect is evident within a similar dose range. A partial list of predictable hepatotoxins is presented in Table 8-1. The majority of recognized hepatotoxins in veterinary medicine fall into this category; carbon tetrachloride and pyrrolizidine alkaloids are examples

Table **8-1** **Common Hepatotoxic Plants of Veterinary Importance**

Plant Family	Species Affected	Toxic Principle	Characteristic Injury	Miscellaneous
Compositae *Xanthium* spp.	Cattle, pigs	Carboxyatractyloside	Centrilobular necrosis	Hypoglycemia and ascites occur in acute intoxication in pigs.
Myoporaceae *Myoporum* spp.	Sheep, cattle, horses, pigs	Furanosesquiterpenoid oils (ngaione)	Usually centrilobular to variable zonal necrosis	Sheep also develop pulmonary injury.
Verbenaceae *Lantana camara,* *Lippia* spp.	Cattle, sheep, occasionally goats	Triterpenes (lantadene A & B)	Megalocytosis, canalicular cholestasis, focal hepatocellular necrosis	Icterus and photosensitization is common. Renal and myocardial injury also occur.
Compositae *Senecio* spp.	Pigs, horses, cattle, sheep, goats	Pyrrolizidine alkaloids	Megalocytosis, fibrosis, biliary hyperplasia	Pulmonary and renal injury also occur.
Leguminosae *Crotalaria* spp.		Pyrrolizidine alkaloids	Megalocytosis, fibrosis, biliary hyperplasia	
Boraginaceae *Heliotropium* spp. *Echium* spp.		Pyrrolizidine alkaloids	Megalocytosis, fibrosis, biliary hyperplasia	
Leguminosae *Cassia* spp.	Cattle	Unknown	Centrilobular necrosis	Myocardial and skeletal muscle injury predominate in *Cassia occidentalis* intoxication.
Zygophyllaceae *Tribulus terrestris*	Sheep	Unknown	Crystalline material in bile ducts	Interaction with mycotoxin sporidesmin necessary to produce characteristic photosensitization (geeldikkop).
Ulmaceae *Trema aspera*	Cattle, sheep, goats	Trematoxin	Centrilobular necrosis	Neuromuscular toxins also. Usually acute disease.
Solanaceae *Cestrum parqui*	Cattle, sheep	Saponins	Centrilobular necrosis	Gallbladder edema and hemorrhage. Usually acute disease.
Asteraceae *Tetradymia glabrata*	Sheep	Tetradymol	Centrilobular necrosis	Photosensitization is common.
Cycadales Zamiaceae Cycadaceae Stangeriaceae	Cattle, sheep, goats, dogs	Methylazoxymethanol	Centrilobular necrosis, megalocytosis, cholestasis	Toxin split from nontoxic glycoside. Neurotoxins also present. Chronic ingestion causes paralysis in cattle.
Fabaceae *Indigofera linnaei*	Cattle, dogs	Indospicine	Centrilobular necrosis	Dogs can be intoxicated by eating meat from horses ingesting *Indigofera.*
Cyanophyceae (Blue-green algae) *Microcystis* *Aphanizomenon*	Cattle, sheep, horses, goats, dogs	Microcystins and others	Centrilobular to massive necrosis	Blue-green algae are not considered to be plants, but cyanobacteria. Multiple toxins are present. Can cause death by neuromuscular injury.

Table **8-2**   **Selected Therapeutic Agents with Potential to Cause Hepatic Injury in Domestic Animals**

Acetaminophen
Amiodarone
Aspirin
Carprofen
Diazepam
Diethylcarbamazine-oxibendazole
Glucocorticoids
Griseofulvin
Halothane
Ketoconazole
Lomustine (CCNU)
Manganese chloride
Mebendazole
Megestrol acetate
Methoxyflurane
Naproxen/ibuprofen
Nitrofurantoin
Phenazopyridine
Phenobarbital
Phenylbutazone
Phenytoin
Primidone
Stanozolol
Tetracycline
Thiacetarsemide
Trimethoprim-sulfa

of predictable hepatotoxins. Toxic injury, even with predictable toxins, is not always uniform, however. A variety of factors influence the severity of injury induced by a toxin; these factors include age, sex, diet, endocrine function, genetic constitution, and diurnal factors. It is therefore not surprising that responses of individual animals exposed to the same toxin can vary considerably.

Idiosyncratic drug reactions are characterized as responses seen in only a small minority of exposed individuals. There are a number of possible mechanisms for idiosyncratic drug reactions, including atypical metabolism as a result of inheritance of rare genes encoding enzymes involved in drug metabolism or deletions of genes encoding certain enzymes or immunologic responses to drugs or modified hepatocyte proteins. A list of selected idiosyncratic hepatotoxic drugs is listed in Table 8-2. Interactions with other drugs or effects of diet and health status can also play a role. Diazepam toxicity in cats is an example of an idiosyncratic toxicity.

The response of the liver to acute hepatotoxic injury depends on the mechanism and site of toxic insult. By far, the most common pattern of acute liver toxicity is centrilobular necrosis. The mechanisms for this pattern of injury involve metabolism by the cytochrome p450 system and are discussed later. Certain chemicals that are uncommonly encountered these days produce periportal necrosis. These chemicals are able to produce a toxic effect without metabolism by the cytochrome p450 system and include phosphorus (once used as a rodenticide) and allyl alcohol.

It should be kept in mind that a single episode of nonlethal hepatotoxic injury in an otherwise healthy animal will be difficult to detect histologically within a few days after the episode. Within 48 to 72 hours, macrophages will clear cell debris, and hepatocytes will begin to undergo mitosis to replace the lost cells. Within a week or less, the liver regains a normal histologic appearance, unless there is massive necrosis, which can lead to collapse of the hepatic connective tissue scaffolding and subsequent fibrosis surrounding the central vein. Chronic toxic liver injury, manifest either as repeated bouts of toxin exposure or more consistent daily exposure (e.g., through dietary contamination) can lead to activation of hepatic stellate cells within the space of Disse or related myofibroblasts in the portal areas and the connective tissue of the central vein area, which may then initiate synthesis of extracellular matrix leading to hepatic fibrosis. In addition, chronic liver injury can lead to disruption of the normal framework that supports the hepatic architecture and leads to hepatic fibrosis. Sufficient injury also can produce nodules of regenerative hepatocytes that are surrounded by bands of fibrosis that connect central vein areas to each other, connect portal tracts to each other, or bridge portal tracts to centrilobular areas. This pattern is recognized as cirrhosis.

Hepatocytes are not the only cell type in the liver that can be affected by toxic drugs. The biliary epithelium (trimethoprim-sulfa, sporidesmin), Kupffer cells (endotoxin), endothelial cells (arsenicals), and the hepatic stellate cells (vitamin A excess) can all suffer chemically induced damage or, in the case of stellate cells, activation. Bile duct necrosis or proliferation can disrupt bile flow. Activated Kupffer cells can release cytokines that affect the type and degree of inflammation within the liver. Hepatic stellate cells play a central role in hepatic fibrosis as will be discussed later. Damage to endothelial cells can affect blood flow through the liver.

Hepatotoxic liver injury can be classified into six categories based on the cellular target involved:

1. The most frequent mechanism of hepatocellular injury involves production of injurious metabolites by the cytochrome p450 system. This family of enzymes is located in the smooth endoplasmic reticulum of hepatocytes primarily, although they are also found in many other cells of the body. A major

role of cytochrome p450 enzymes is to metabolize lipid-soluble chemicals into water-soluble compounds for excretion from the body in bile or urine. In the first step of this three-step process, termed biotransformation, chemicals are bioactivated to a high-energy reactive intermediate molecule, termed phase I, in preparation for the second step, phase II, which involves formation of covalent bonds with polar molecules, such as glucuronic acid. This conjugation forms a water-soluble metabolite that can be excreted. Phase III involves the transport of these molecules across the cell membrane into the lumen of the canaliculus by molecular pumps.

In some circumstances, such as an overdose, the high-energy reactive metabolites can form covalent bonds with other cellular constituents, such as proteins, and nucleic acids termed adducts. In acute toxicity, adducts with essential cellular enzymes may lead to cell injury or death. Toxic hepatocellular injury of this category occurs most often in the centrilobular area of the liver because this is the region of the liver with the highest concentration of cytochrome p450 enzymes. For instance, carbon tetrachloride is metabolized by cytochrome p450 enzymes to $CCl_3\cdot$, a free radical that is responsible for the toxicity of the parent compound. Lesions induced by carbon tetrachloride are most severe in the centrilobular (periacinar) areas, where the active form of the chemical is present in greatest concentration. Acetaminophen toxicity in dogs and cats and the many plant toxicities in herbivores are examples of injury produced by this mechanism.

2. Adduct formation between drugs and cellular enzymes, other proteins, or nucleic acids can alter the cellular constituents sufficiently that they become neoantigens, as may be the case with halothane toxicity. These neoantigens, like other foreign antigens, can be processed in the cytoplasm, transported to the cell surface, presented as antigens, and recognized by the immune system. Consequently the immune system may develop an inflammatory response toward hepatocytes or biliary epithelium that contain the adducts. Both cellular and humoral immunity can be involved. Injury can occur through direct cellular cytotoxicity and antibody-dependent cellular cytotoxicity. Although this mechanism is not well characterized in clinical veterinary medicine, it is likely to occur on occasion.

3. Certain toxins, including retained or excess hydrophobic bile acids, can trigger apoptosis (individual cell necrosis), by direct stimulation of proapoptotic pathways in the hepatocytes. Alternatively, apoptosis can be stimulated by immune-mediated events, such as those discussed previously, which lead to the release of tumor necrosis factor-α or activate Fas pathways.

4. Injury that damages cell membranes and disables enzymes responsible for calcium homeostasis, as seen in carbon tetrachloride toxicity, can lead to an influx of calcium. One consequence of the increased intracellular calcium is activation of proteases that damage actin filaments. Blebbing and lysis of the cell membranes can result.

5. Chemicals that bind to and disrupt the molecular pumps that secrete bile constituents into the canaliculi, such as estrogen and erythromycin, can produce cholestasis. More extensive hepatocellular injury that affects canalicular pumps and hepatocytes may produce cholestasis by disrupting the actin filaments situated around the bile canaliculi and preventing the normal pulsatile contractions that move bile through the canalicular system to the bile ducts.

6. Hepatocyte injury or death can follow mitochondrial damage, as seen with some toxic antiviral nucleosides or intravenous tetracycline administration because the mitochondria are the powerhouse of the cell. Chemical or reactive oxygen species–induced injury to mitochondrial membranes, enzymes, or DNA can inhibit or disrupt mitochondrial function. Interference with mitochondrial β-oxidation of lipid leads to accumulation of free fatty acids and triglycerides producing a characteristic microvesicular steatosis. Disruption of the electron transport chain can release reactive oxygen species, which can produce widespread cellular damage. Also, damaged mitochondria do not produce sufficient adenosine triphosphate (ATP) to power the essential functions of the hepatocytes. In addition, release of cytochrome-c through damaged mitochondrial membranes can trigger apoptosis. Hepatocytic oxidative phosphorylation (ATP generation) and β-oxidation of lipids are reduced once the mitochondria are damaged, which leads to intrahepatic lipid accumulation (microvesicular steatosis), diminished energy production, and generation of reactive oxygen species, such as superoxide. Damaged mitochondria may release cytochrome-c, triggering apoptosis, or if disruption of mitochondrial function is sufficient, hepatocyte necrosis ensues.

HEPATOTOXIC AGENTS
BLUE-GREEN ALGAE

Blue-green algae are now classified in the phylum Monera, division Cyanophyta; are considered to be more closely related to bacteria; and are no longer considered members of the plant family. Several genera of blue-green algae, including *Anabaena*, *Aphanizomenon*, and *Microcystis*, can cause lethal poisoning of livestock and less commonly small animals, such as dogs and cats. Algal blooms usually occur in late summer or early fall because of the warm temperatures, long hours of sunlight, and abundance of essential nutrients. Dead and dying algae, which contain preformed toxins, such as microcystin LR, a cyclic heptapeptide, accumulate on the surface of bodies of water and are ingested by livestock. Secondary bacterial growth in dying algae may contribute to toxin formation. Signs develop rapidly and include diarrhea, prostration, and death. Gross lesions include hemorrhagic gastroenteritis and a red, swollen, hemorrhagic liver. Histologically, zonal, or even massive, hepatic necrosis and hemorrhage is evident. Animals that survive the acute manifestations may develop clinical signs of chronic liver disease. Other preformed toxins that affect different organ systems, including the nervous system, have also been identified in blue-green algae.

TOXIC PLANTS

Toxic plants of great variety cause hepatic injury in domestic animals. A comprehensive discussion of each is beyond the scope of this chapter. The phytotoxins (Table 8-1) to be discussed represent two distinct types. The first of these, represented by pyrrolizidine alkaloids, must be metabolized to an active form in the liver. The second type of toxin is deconjugated by bacteria within the digestive tract to release a factor that is subsequently bioactivated in the liver.

Pyrrolizidine alkaloids are found in many plant families, including Compositae, Leguminosae, and Boraginaceae, that occur throughout much of the world. The most important genera are *Senecio, Cynoglossum, Amsinckia, Crotalaria, Echium, Trichodesma,* and *Heliotropium.* Approximately 100 different alkaloids are recognized; toxic effects depend upon which alkaloids are present within ingested plants. Ingested alkaloids are converted to pyrrolic esters by hepatic cytochrome p450 enzymes. These esters are alkylating agents, which react with cytosolic and nuclear proteins and nucleic acids. Pigs are particularly susceptible to pyrrolizidine alkaloid intoxication, sheep considerably less so, and cattle and horses are intermediate in susceptibility. Most cases of intoxication arise from chronic intoxication and the gross lesion is typically hepatic fibrosis (Fig. 8-73, A). The characteristic histologic lesions of pyrrolizidine alkaloid intoxication are the megalocytes, which are hepatocytes with enlarged nuclei and increased cytoplasmic volume. Megalocytes may be many times the size of normal hepatocytes (Fig. 8-73, B). Megalocytes are the result of the antimitotic effects of pyrrolizidine alkaloids, which prevent cell division but not DNA synthesis because the hepatocytes attempt to divide to replace those that have undergone necrosis. This change, although indicative of pyrrolizidine alkaloid intoxication, is not pathognomonic, because it occurs with other toxins, such as aflatoxins and

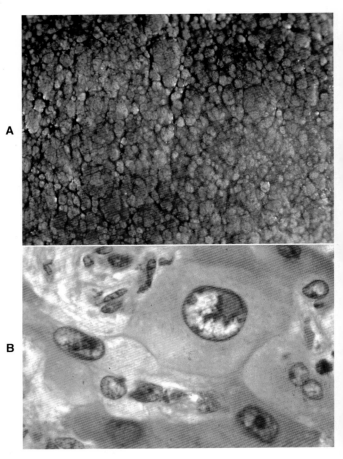

Fig. 8-73 **Chronic pyrrolizidine hepatotoxicity, cow.** **A,** Chronic pyrrolizidine intoxication produces a fibrotic and sometimes distorted liver with an irregular capsular surface. **B,** Greatly enlarged hepatocytes (megalocytes) in the persisting parenchyma are typical of pyrrolizidine toxicity. H&E stain. (*A* and *B, Courtesy Dr. P. Carbonell, School of Veterinary Science, Melbourne.*)

nitrosamines. Typically, chronic pyrrolizidine intoxication is accompanied by hepatic fibrosis, biliary proliferation, and in some circumstances nodular regeneration of parenchyma. Nodular regeneration does not always occur because hepatocyte proliferation can be inhibited by pyrrolizidines; however, exposure is not likely to be constant, and there may be periods during which hepatocyte replication can occur, such as the end of the dry season when more desirable plant species reappear. Species differences may also have an effect on the hepatic response to pyrrolizidines because cattle have regenerative nodules more often than horses. Chronic hepatic damage can lead to hepatic failure and its associated constellation of signs (described in detail earlier).

Cycads are primitive palmlike plants that inhabit tropical and subtropical regions. They contain cycasin, a nontoxic glycoside, which following ingestion is deconjugated by intestinal bacteria to release a toxic metabolite, methylazoxymethanol. Following absorption into the portal vein, hepatic metabolism of this compound yields alkylating agents, leading to acute or chronic liver injury. Chronic hepatic lesions in cattle include hepatocellular megalocytosis caused by the mitoinhibitory effects of alkylating agents and nuclear hyperchromasia, and varying degrees of hepatic fibrosis. Chronic cycad poisoning in cattle causes a nervous disease with progressive proprioceptive deficits in the hind legs because of "dying back" of axons in the dorsal funiculus and the spinocerebellar and corticospinal tracts. Acute intoxication is more common in sheep than in other species and produces acute gastrointestinal dysfunction and centrilobular hepatic necrosis. Dogs can also be intoxicated by cycads.

MYCOTOXINS

Mycotoxins are secondary metabolites of fungi; that is, their production is not necessary for the survival of the fungus. The amount of toxin synthesized by a given strain of fungus reflects the genetic constitution of the particular strain, presence of appropriate substrate, temperature, humidity, and available nutrients. There are several hepatotoxic mycotoxins of veterinary significance.

AFLATOXIN

Aflatoxins are produced by the fungus *Aspergillus flavus*. Aflatoxin B_1 is the most common form and is also the most potent toxin and carcinogen. Aflatoxins are usually elaborated during storage of fungus-contaminated feed, particularly in humid conditions, and may be present in many crops, including corn, peanuts, and cottonseed. Aflatoxins are converted to toxic intermediates by hepatic cytochrome p450 enzymes. Carcinogenic, toxic, and teratogenic effects of aflatoxins reflect binding of the toxic intermediates to cellular DNA, RNA, or proteins. Pigs, dogs, horses, cattle and ducks, especially younger animals, are sensitive to the toxic effects of aflatoxins, whereas sheep are more resistant. Acute aflatoxin intoxication is rare in horses and cattle because an inordinately large amount of contaminated feed would have to be ingested to achieve a sufficient dose. Acute aflatoxicosis in dogs is characterized by hemorrhagic central to massive necrosis. Lipidosis and biliary proliferation also may occur. Chronic intoxication is more common than acute intoxication and results in ill-thrift, increased susceptibility to infection, and occasionally signs of hepatic failure. Affected livers are firm and pale and microscopically are characterized by lipidosis and necrosis of hepatocytes, biliary hyperplasia, centrilobular to bridging fibrosis, and cellular atypia of hepatocytes, characterized by variable cells size and variable nuclear size (Fig. 8-74, *A* and *B*).

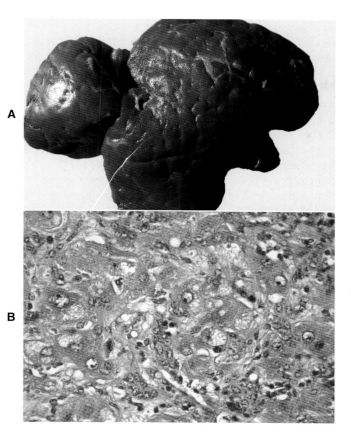

Fig. 8-74   **Chronic hepatic aflatoxicosis. A,** Postnecrotic scarring, pig. Chronic aflatoxicosis produces a shrunken and fibrotic liver from collapse of areas of massive necrosis and condensation of the fibrous stroma. **B,** Histologic appearance. Chronic aflatoxicosis is characterized by variable amounts of fatty change, biliary hyperplasia, and cellular atypia in hepatocytes. H&E stain. (**A,** *Courtesy Dr. M.D. McGavin, College of Veterinary Medicine, University of Tennessee.* **B,** *Courtesy Dr. J. Simon, College of Veterinary Medicine, University of Illinois.*)

SPORIDESMIN

The mycotoxin sporidesmin is produced by *Pithomyces chartarum*, a fungus that grows particularly well in dead rye grass (*Lolium perenne*), a common pasture plant in New Zealand and Australia. Ingestion of sufficient amounts of the toxin produces necrosis of the epithelium of large intrahepatic and extrahepatic biliary ducts in sheep and less so in cattle. Cholestasis with a concurrent failure to excrete phylloerythrin frequently leads to photosensitization with skin lesions predominantly on the head, thus the common name facial eczema. Acute cases are characterized by a bile-stained liver with prominent small-caliber bile ducts. These are dilated by bile in the lumens and surrounded by periductal edema. In chronic cases of facial eczema, the bile ducts become thickened by fibrosis secondary to biliary epithelial necrosis and subsequent inflammation (chronic cholangitis). Perhaps because of streaming of blood in the portal vein, the left lobe of the liver (although this lobe occupies the ventral portion of the ruminant liver), which may have an increased proportion of blood draining from the small intestine, is usually most severely affected and in severe cases undergoes atrophy and fibrosis.

A similar disease, Geeldikkop, which is characterized by hepatogenous photosensitization, occurs in sheep in South Africa that ingest puncture vine (Tribulus terrestris). It was previously thought to be caused by a mycotoxin, but recent studies have revealed that it is caused by ingestion of steroidal sapogenins that can damage or obstruct the bile ducts.

PHOMOPSINS

Phomopsins are toxic metabolites of the fungus Phomopsis leptostromiformis. The fungus grows on lupine (Lupinus sp.), and cattle, sheep, and occasionally horses that graze contaminated lupine stubble develop hepatic injury. Hepatic dysfunction is usually chronic, and the liver is atrophic and fibrotic. The microscopic appearance of affected livers is characterized by diffuse scattered hepatocyte necrosis with a background of mitotic figures, often appearing to be arrested in metaphase. Later in the course of the disease, diffuse fibrosis and biliary hyperplasia predominate. Signs of hepatic failure, including photosensitization, may occur in affected animals. This mycotoxicosis should not be confused with the condition known as lupinosis, which is caused by naturally occurring alkaloids in lupines that are capable of inducing skeletal deformities, but not obvious hepatic injury.

MUSHROOMS

Poisonous mushrooms, such as Amanita species and others, can cause acute fatal liver necrosis. Intoxication by Amanita phalloides, known as the death cap, is caused by a group of toxins termed toxic cyclopeptides. This species is particularly toxic; a single gram of this mushroom is sufficient to kill a human, and even smaller amounts are likely to prove fatal to dogs. Amatoxin, an octapeptide, is in particular responsible for hepatocellular injury. The mechanism of injury is attributed to inhibition of RNA polymerase II function disrupting DNA and RNA transcription. Gross lesions usually consist of hepatic hemorrhage and a shrunken liver because of the loss of hepatocytes. Hepatocellular lipidosis, hemorrhage, and centrilobular to massive necrosis are the typical lesions. Death from liver failure may occur 3 to 4 days after the onset of clinical signs. Phalloidin, a toxic heptapeptide found in Amanita species, causes disruption of intracellular actin filaments, leading to cell injury or death. It is a less significant toxin in natural exposure because of the limited absorption from the digestive tract. Other mushroom species contain different toxic agents.

HEPATOTOXIC CHEMICALS
PHOSPHORUS

Phosphorus occurs in two forms: red phosphorus and white phosphorus. Red phosphorus is unimportant as a toxin, but white phosphorus was previously used as a rodenticide. The mechanism of phosphorus toxicity is unclear, although it apparently is directly toxic. Poisoning is first indicated by signs of gastroenteritis and subsequently by microscopic lesions of lipidosis of hepatocytes and periportal necrosis. The pattern of periportal necrosis is unusual because most toxic liver injury occurs in the centrilobular region of the liver. This is explained by the fact that white phosphorus does not require metabolic transformation to a reactive intermediate by cytochrome p450 enzymes, which are most concentrated in the centrilobular region of the liver lobule.

CARBON TETRACHLORIDE

Carbon tetrachloride is the classic example of a hepatotoxin that must be bioactivated by the mixed-function oxidase system to produce a toxic intermediate form. Although once used widely, it is only occasionally used as an anthelmintic. Carbon tetrachloride produces centrilobular hepatic necrosis and lipidosis of surviving hepatocytes (see Chapter 1).

CRESOLS

Cresols once were incorporated in clay pigeons and asphalt shingles. If pigs ingest cresols, centrilobular to massive hepatic hemorrhage and necrosis result, a pattern that can also be seen in pigs with hepatosis dietetica or in those that ingest cotton seed meal.

METALS

Several metals can cause toxic hepatic injury. Copper toxicity may present as an acute intravascular hemolytic anemia in ruminants or as chronic hepatic injury and end-stage hepatic disease in dogs. Excessive iron supplementation in dogs and cats may result in excessive storage of iron and subsequently hepatic disease caused by iron overload, termed hemochromatosis. Two specific syndromes of iron poisoning are iron-dextran intoxication of piglets and ferrous fumarate (a component of a specific dietary supplement) intoxication of newborn foals. Severe cases of these two toxicities are characterized by massive hepatic necrosis. Intoxication of foals with ferrous fumarate occurred following its use as a component of a specific dietary supplement, and was characterized by massive necrosis and also a remarkable amount of hyperplasia of bile ducts and cholangioles, possibly with oval cell proliferation, despite the short clinical course of the disease. Iron-dextran is frequently administered intramuscularly to suckling pigs to prevent anemia, but administration of iron-dextran has occasionally resulted in significant mortality, and affected pigs die soon after injection.

HEPATOTOXIC THERAPEUTIC DRUGS

There are a variety of drugs that have a proven therapeutic application, but can cause significant acute or chronic hepatic injury in some animals. Clearly, these drugs would not be used if the proportion of injured animals was high, but it is important to keep in mind that many drugs have the potential to cause hepatic injury in some patients. The mechanisms by which these drugs cause injury vary by species and by individual. Some therapeutic drugs are predictable toxins, and all members of a particular species are susceptible to liver injury if a sufficient dose is given. But because the therapeutic effect occurs at a lower dose than the toxic dose, liver injury occurs only when overdoses are ingested. Hepatic metabolism (bioactivation) of these compounds is likely to be involved because the site of liver injury is typically centrilobular. Cats are more susceptible than dogs to intoxication by many chemicals because they are relatively deficient in hepatic glucuronyltransferase activity. This phase II enzyme forms conjugates between bioactivated (phase I) xenobiotics and glutathione. When phase II metabolism is overwhelmed, injurious bioactivated products cause liver injury. Cats are more sensitive to acetaminophen intoxication than dogs because of this relative enzyme deficiency. Other therapeutic drugs are idiosyncratic toxins, and they affect only a small minority of patients. The mechanism of injury is not known but may be a consequence of inherited differences in hepatic enzyme content and activity, or atypical immune reactions to drug metabolites, or novel antigens created when drug metabolites bind to cellular proteins may play a role. For example, the anti-inflammatory drug carprofen can occasionally cause acute hepatic necrosis in a variety of dogs, but certain breeds of dogs, such as Labrador retrievers, are affected more often than others. The tranquilizer diazepam can cause acute fatal hepatic injury in some cats, but the majority of treated cats are unaffected, and dogs do not seem to be adversely affected.

Chronic liver toxicity has been described in dogs receiving any of the anticonvulsants, primidone, phenytoin, and phenobarbital for prolonged periods. The mechanism of hepatotoxicity is unknown. Only a small proportion of dogs receiving these drugs are affected, and these dogs frequently have signs of hepatic failure. The liver is small and has widespread hepatic fibrosis and nodular regeneration (end-stage liver).

DISEASES OF UNCERTAIN CAUSE
EQUINE SERUM HEPATITIS

This disease was first described by Theiler in South Africa at the beginning of the twentieth century, but now is recognized in many countries. It occurs frequently, but not invariably, in horses that have received an injection of a biologic that contains equine serum; for instance, equine antisera, such as tetanus antitoxin or pregnant mare serum gonadotropin. It appears that an infectious agent is responsible, although none has been identified. The incubation period is prolonged, but the clinical course of the disease is very rapid and is invariably fatal. Affected horses typically have hepatic failure, which manifests as hepatic encephalopathy and icterus. Intravascular hemolysis occurs in the terminal stages of the disease. The livers of affected animals are typically small, flabby, and discolored greenish brown to dark brown (Fig. 8-75, A). The liver of affected animals is small and friable, with an enhanced lobular pattern because of diffuse centrilobular degeneration and necrosis of hepatocytes and subsequent congestion of these necrotic areas (Fig. 8-75, B). Frequently, only narrow rims of hepatocytes around portal areas (periportal hepatocytes) survive, and these sometimes are accompanied by proliferating tubules or columns of cells, which are speculated to have arisen from the cholangioles and probably are a regenerative response.

CANINE CHRONIC HEPATITIS (CHRONIC-ACTIVE HEPATITIS)

Chronic hepatitis in dogs is a poorly understood, in most cases, persistent inflammation of the liver. The terminology of this entity, in keeping with the inflammatory process, has been a persistent topic of dispute. Chronic-active hepatitis is a descriptive term that has been used to identify a particular pattern of inflammation in the human liver. Originally the purpose of this classification was to identify hepatic lesions, regardless of cause, that were predictive of a progressive course of inflammation and fibrosis. This term was adopted by veterinary pathologists and used to indicate hepatic disorders of the dog that have microscopic changes similar to those seen in human livers. Based on usage, the term *chronic active hepatitis* has incorrectly evolved from a morphologic description into a disease entity. The appropriateness and usefulness of this designation is conjectural in human beings and in dogs. Recent publications in the medical literature have argued that this terminology should be abandoned because it is no longer regarded as useful in predicting the course of liver disease, and it ignored the cause of the liver inflammation. Accordingly the term chronic hepatitis is preferred to describe this entity in dogs.

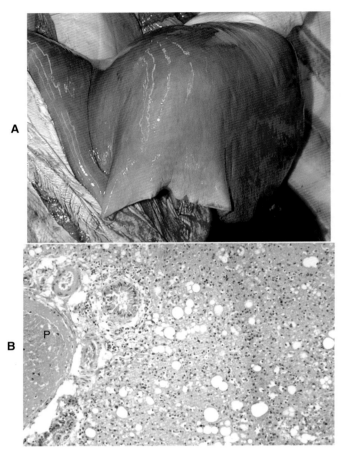

Fig. 8-75   Equine serum hepatitis, liver, horse. A, Livers from horses affected with equine serum hepatitis can be small, flabby and pale or discolored by bile pigment. **B,** In horses with equine serum hepatitis, most hepatocytes are necrotic, although there may be a few remaining hepatocytes with lipid-containing vacuoles in the periportal regions *(P)*. Inflammation consists of mononuclear cells predominantly. H&E stain. (**A,** *Courtesy Dr. K. Bailey, College of Veterinary Medicine, University of Illinois.* **B,** *Courtesy Dr. J.M. Cullen, College of Veterinary Medicine, North Carolina State University.*)

The term *chronic hepatitis*, with modifiers indicating the type and degree of inflammation and fibrosis, is used to fully characterize the activity and stage of the lesion. If the cause of the inflammation is known, it should be included in the diagnosis. The cause of most of the spontaneous cases of canine chronic (chronic-active) hepatitis is undetermined, although some cases have been hypothesized to be caused by leptospira infection or experimental canine adenovirus I infection. Progressive chronic hepatitis has been described in cases of hereditary copper toxicosis of Dalmatians and Bedlington and West Highland white terriers and was described earlier under Metabolic Disturbances and

Hepatic Accumulations. Familial chronic hepatitis also is usually characterized by excessive hepatic accumulation of copper in the Doberman pinscher (females are predisposed), Skye terrier, cocker spaniel, and Labrador retriever. Although abnormal concentrations of hepatic copper in at least some of these breeds have been attributed to cholestasis and decreased excretion of copper in bile, the actual mechanism of copper retention remains unclear. Many dogs with chronic hepatitis do not have elevated liver concentrations of hepatic copper, and a wide range of hepatic copper concentrations is present in clinically normal dogs. Thus the precise role of copper in mediating chronic hepatic disease in breeds of dogs other than the Bedlington terrier and Dalmatian remains uncertain.

The liver in cases of chronic hepatitis is usually small, often with an accentuated lobular pattern; severely affected livers are characterized by architectural distortion, which ranges from a coarsely nodular texture to an end-stage liver (Fig. 8-76, *A*). Chronic hepatitis, depending on the duration of inflammation and injury, is characterized by portal and periportal mononuclear cell inflammation, intrahepatic cholestasis, and fibrosis of portal areas that may extend into adjacent periportal areas of the lobule, leading to the prominent lobular pattern (Fig. 8-76, *B*).

HEPATIC INJURY AS A CONSEQUENCE OF SYSTEMIC DISEASE

A variety of extrahepatic disorders, usually affecting the gastrointestinal tract, can result in hepatocellular injury and hepatic dysfunction. Acute hemorrhagic pancreatitis of dogs, for example, sometimes is accompanied by icterus and increased activities of hepatic enzymes in serum. Release of various toxins and inflammatory mediators from the injured pancreas into the portal vein showers the liver with a variety of injurious substances. Similarly, movement of hepatotoxic substances, such as endotoxins, into the portal vein can occur as a consequence of diseases that disrupt the mucosal barrier of the intestine. Some cases of chronic inflammation of the colon can result in chronic hepatic inflammation as well. Accumulation of inflammatory cells within the portal triads may accompany blood-borne infection or abdominal sepsis (nonspecific reactive hepatitis).

The liver is particularly susceptible to the effects of hypoxia; thus any disease that causes anemia can produce centrilobular or paracentral degeneration and necrosis. Also, the hepatocytes in hemolytic anemias must remove and conjugate the increased amounts of circulating bilirubin and hemoglobin, and Kupffer cells must remove either erythrocytes during extravascular hemolysis or erythrocytic fragments during intravascular hemolysis.

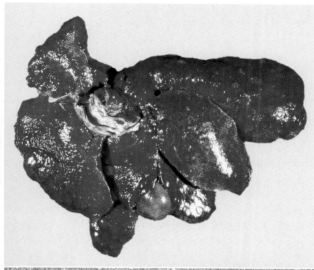

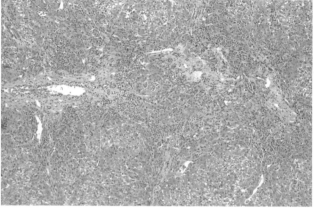

Fig. 8-76   Chronic active hepatitis. A, Liver, diaphragmatic surface, dog. The liver is characterized by scattered regenerative nodules of different sizes and extensive fibrosis that gives the liver an irregular surface. **B,** End-stage liver with chronic hepatitis. The liver lobular architecture is replaced by irregular nodules of regenerative parenchyma separated by tracts of connective tissue with an inflammatory infiltrate and pigment accumulation. H&E stain. (**A,** *Courtesy College of Veterinary Medicine, University of Illinois.* **B,** *Courtesy Dr. J.M. Cullen, College of Veterinary Medicine, North Carolina State University.*)

PROLIFERATIVE LESIONS OF THE LIVER
HEPATOCELLULAR NODULAR HYPERPLASIA

Hepatocellular nodular hyperplasia is common only in the dog. The incidence increases with age, starting around 6 years of age, without predilection for either sex or breed. Nodular hyperplasia is not the result or the cause of significant hepatic dysfunction, but nodular hyperplasia should be distinguished from regenerative nodules and hepatic neoplasms, with which they are often confused. Multiple hyperplastic nodules are frequently present. Nodules that can be seen on the capsular surface are typically raised and hemispherical, yellow to tan (although they can be dark red when congested), 0.5 to 3 cm in diameter, and are more friable than normal liver. On incision, the hyperplastic nodules are well demarcated from normal parenchyma and usually compress adjacent parenchyma (Fig. 8-77, A and B). Hyperplastic nodules contain all the elements of normal liver, but the lobular pattern is distorted. The lobules in areas of nodular hyperplasia contain an increased proportion of hepatocytes and decreased numbers of portal tracts and central veins compared with a normal liver. Hepatocytes are variably sized and frequently contain cytoplasmic lipid or glycogen-containing vacuoles (Fig. 8-77, C).

REGENERATIVE NODULES

Regenerative nodules are another type of nodular hepatocellular lesion. Regenerative nodules are unlikely to be related to nodular hyperplasia, because regenerative nodules arise from the proliferation of hepatocytes in response to loss of hepatocytes, and the incidence is not related to age. Often the insult is unknown, but the response of some dogs to anticonvulsant drugs, such as phenobarbital or phenytoin, is a well-recognized cause. Regenerative nodules are readily distinguished from nodular hyperplasia because the process occurs in the presence of significant fibrosis and disruption of normal hepatic parenchymal architecture. Because these lesions result from the outgrowth of surviving hepatocytes, there is usually only a single portal tract apparent in sections of the regenerative nodules.

CHOLANGIOCELLULAR (BILE DUCT) HYPERPLASIA

Hyperplasia of biliary ductules commonly occurs as a nonspecific response to a variety of hepatic injuries and has been described under Response of the Liver to Injury. Reactive proliferation of the bile ductules of the liver must be distinguished from neoplastic proliferations.

HEPATIC NEOPLASIA

Primary neoplasms of the hepatobiliary system can arise from epithelial elements, including hepatocytes, biliary epithelium of bile ducts or the gallbladder, and mesenchymal elements, such as connective tissue and blood vessels. The liver is a common site of metastasis for many malignant tumors; in fact, the majority of neoplasms within the liver are metastases from other organs.

HEPATOCELLULAR ADENOMA

Hepatocellular adenomas are benign neoplasms of hepatocytes. Hepatocellular adenomas have been described most commonly in young ruminants.

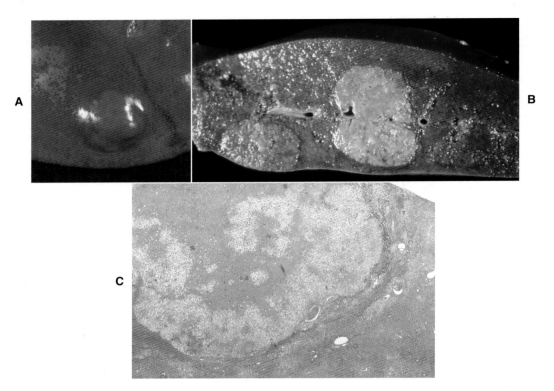

Fig. 8-77 **Hepatic nodular hyperplasia, Liver, dog. A,** A nodule protrudes above the surface of the adjacent, normal parenchyma. **B,** Nodular hyperplasia, cut surface of liver. Two hyperplastic nodules are shown. **C,** A hyperplastic nodule compresses adjacent hepatocytes, and the hepatocytes of the nodule can be prominently vacuolated as in this case. H&E stain. (**A,** *Courtesy Dr. M.D. McGavin, College of Veterinary Medicine, University of Tennessee.* **B,** *Courtesy Dr. R. Fairley, Lincoln University.* **C,** *Courtesy Dr. J.M. Cullen, College of Veterinary Medicine, North Carolina State University.*)

The neoplasms usually are single, unencapsulated, variably sized, red or brown masses that compress adjacent parenchyma. They are typically spherical, but may be pedunculated (Fig. 8-78). They are composed of well-differentiated hepatocytes, which form uniform plates

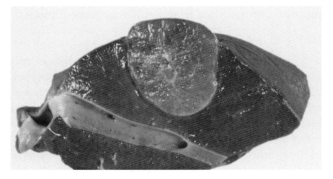

Fig. 8-78 **Hepatocellular adenomas, liver, dog.**
Hepatocellular adenomas form discrete masses of hepatocytes that compress adjacent normal parenchyma. (*Courtesy Dr. J.M. Cullen, College of Veterinary Medicine, North Carolina State University.*)

that may be two to three cells thick. Hepatic plates in adenomas tend to abut normal adjacent hepatocytes at right angles. Portal tracts and central veins are scarce within the neoplasm, if they can be found at all. Diagnostic criteria to distinguish hepatocellular adenomas from hepatocellular nodular hyperplasia can be somewhat subjective because both arise in livers with no background abnormality, unlike regenerative nodules that arise in damaged livers. Histologically, adenomas are characterized by only one or very few portal tracts, whereas hyperplastic nodules retain normal lobular architecture elements, although the portal tracts are more separated than normal. In other cases, it may be difficult to distinguish hepatocellular adenomas from well-differentiated hepatocellular carcinomas.

HEPATOCELLULAR CARCINOMA

Hepatocellular carcinomas are malignant neoplasms of hepatocytes. They are uncommon in all domestic species but may occur more frequently in ruminants, particularly sheep. These neoplasms are often solitary, frequently involve an entire lobe, and are well demarcated. They typically consist of friable, gray-white or yellow-brown tissue, which is subdivided into lobules by multiple fibrous bands (Fig. 8-79, A). Malignant hepatocytes characteristically form irregular plates (trabeculae) three or more cells thick, and vascular spaces are present between the trabeculae (Fig. 8-79, B). Crude acini forming a pseudoglandular pattern of neoplastic cells are sometimes present. Within an individual tumor, trabecular, pseudoglandular, and solid patterns may be found. Cells present in the neoplasm range from well-differentiated hepatocytes to atypical or bizarre forms. In the absence of metastasis, which is obviously indicative of malignancy, distinction of well-differentiated carcinoma from adenoma can be difficult, although invasion by malignant hepatocytes at the margin of the adjacent compressed normal hepatocytes and hepatocellular atypia are useful indicators of malignancy.

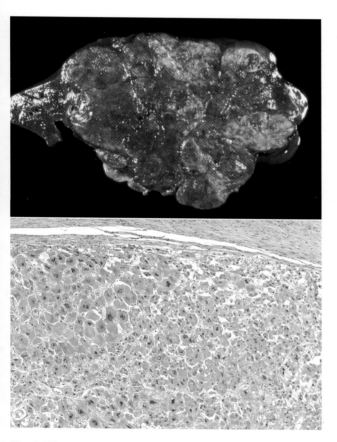

Fig. 8-79 Hepatocellular carcinoma, liver, dog.
A, A multilobular carcinoma has replaced much of the normal liver. **B,** Hepatocellular carcinomas contain pleomorphic hepatocytes that can form trabeculae, a glandular-like pattern or solid sheets of cells, as in this case. H&E stain. (**A,** *Courtesy College of Veterinary Medicine, North Carolina State University.* **B,** *Courtesy Dr. J.M. Cullen, College of Veterinary Medicine, North Carolina State University.*)

Metastasis to a variety of sites may occur, particularly to lymph nodes within the cranial abdomen, lungs, and seeding into the tissue of the peritoneal cavity. Some hepatocellular carcinomas extensively spread within the liver (intrahepatic metastasis).

CHOLANGIOCELLULAR (BILE DUCT) ADENOMA

Adenomas of the biliary ducts are uncommon in most species but may be the most common primary hepatic neoplasm in cats. They are usually discrete, firm, gray or white masses consisting of well-differentiated biliary epithelium. Cholangiomas are glandlike structures formed by tubules lined with cuboidal epithelium and moderate amounts of stroma. The tubules may have narrow lumens or may be distended by fluid-forming cystic structures of variable sizes. Cystic variants, biliary cystadenomas, typically have a nonencapsulated, multilocular cystic structure. Hepatocytes are usually compressed at the margins or may on occasion be entrapped by expanding cysts. The stroma of the cyst wall consists of fibrovascular tissue with moderate amounts of collagen. Cysts are lined with benign biliary epithelium (simple cuboidal to flattened). The lining epithelium tends to be more flattened in the biliary cystadenomas, presumably because of compression. Biliary epithelial cells may form papillary projections extending into the cystic spaces.

In cats, large cystic cavities that are lined with flattened biliary epithelium are regarded as adenomas or cystadenomas by some investigators, but it may be more appropriate to consider them to be congenital malformations. Congenital biliary cysts are multiloculated and can involve extensive areas of the liver. Typically, they have flattened epithelium and varying amounts of fibrous tissue, and islands of hepatocytes are often scattered between the cysts.

CHOLANGIOCELLULAR (BILE DUCT) CARCINOMA

Cholangiocellular carcinomas are malignant neoplasms of biliary epithelium, which usually arise from the intrahepatic ducts, but extrahepatic bile ducts can be affected. These neoplasms occur in all species. A large single mass or multiple nodules may be present within the liver; these typically are firm, raised, often with a central depression (umbilicated), pale gray to tan, and unencapsulated (Fig. 8-80, A). The tumors are composed of cells that retain a resemblance to biliary epithelium. Characteristically, well-differentiated carcinomas are organized into a tubular or acinar arrangement. In less differentiated neoplasms, some acinar arrangements can be detected among solid masses of neoplastic cells. Poorly differentiated carcinomas are composed of packets, islands, or cords, and areas of squamous differentiation can occur. The epithelial components of the neoplasms are usually separated by fibrous connective

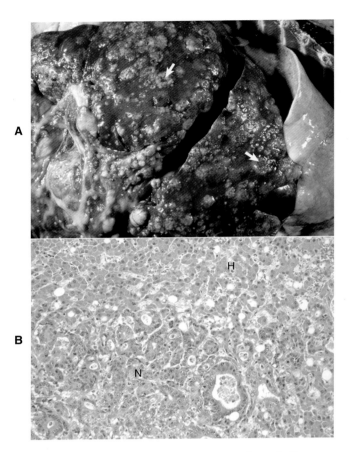

Fig. 8-80 **Cholangiocellular carcinoma, liver. A,** Dog. Multiple nodules of tumor, some of which are umbilicated *(arrows).* **B,** Cat. Cords and acini of neoplastic bile duct epithelial cells *(N)* are invading the adjacent normal hepatic parenchyma *(H).* H&E stain. *(A, Courtesy Dr. M.D. McGavin, College of Veterinary Medicine, University of Tennessee. B, Courtesy Dr. J. Simon, College of Veterinary Medicine, University of Illinois.)*

tissue (Fig. 8-80, *B*). The amount of connective tissue varies among tumors, but an abundant deposition of collagen, termed a scirrhous response, is relatively common and is responsible for the firm texture of these neoplasms. The margins of cholangiocarcinomas are characterized by multiple sites of local invasion by tumor cells of surrounding hepatic parenchyma. Multiple sites of hepatic necrosis are also common in the adjacent parenchyma.

Metastasis to extrahepatic sites is common, particularly to the adjacent lymph nodes of the cranial abdomen, lungs, or by seeding into the abdominal cavity. Metastasis into the peritoneal cavity can produce variably sized nodules within the mesentery and on the serosal surface of the abdominal viscera.

CARCINOIDS

Carcinoids are uncommon tumors that are believed to arise from neuroendocrine cells that lie within the biliary epithelium. They can form within the intrahepatic

or extrahepatic biliary system. Often they form a single mass, but multiple nodules can occur, probably secondary to intrahepatic metastasis. Cells tend to be small, elongated, or spindle-shaped and form ribbons or rosettes (Fig. 8-81). Immunohistochemical detection of neuroendocrine markers, such as chromogranin A, can be used to confirm the diagnosis.

MISCELLANEOUS PRIMARY MESENCHYMAL NEOPLASMS OF THE LIVER

Primary neoplasms can arise from any of the cellular constituents of the liver, including mesenchymal neoplasms derived from the liver's connective tissue (fibrosarcoma, leiomyosarcoma, and osteosarcoma) and endothelium (hemangioma and hemangiosarcoma). Primary hepatic hemangiosarcoma is well recognized in dogs, although it is a relatively uncommon site of origin for this neoplasm as compared with the skin and spleen. Primary mesenchymal neoplasms of the liver must be distinguished from metastases; the presence of disseminated masses throughout the liver is more typical of metastatic sarcomas than of primary hepatic sarcomas.

METASTATIC NEOPLASMS

The liver and the lung are the two most common sites for metastatic spread of malignant neoplasms. Metastatic neoplasms must be distinguished from primary hyperplasia or neoplasia of the hepatobiliary tissue. It is important, therefore, when evaluating a neoplasm within the liver to determine if a neoplasm is present at some extrahepatic site that might be the primary neoplasm. The animal's medical history should also be reviewed to determine if masses have been removed previously.

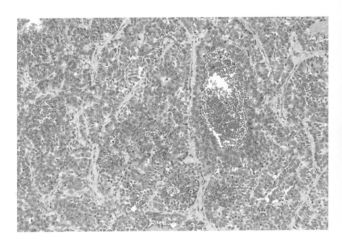

Fig. 8-81 **Neuroendocrine tumors, carcinoid, liver, dog.** Carcinoids are malignant neoplasms of neuroendocrine cells of the liver or bile ducts. Histologically the tumor is composed of small elongated or spindle-shaped basophilic cells that form ribbons or rosettes and contain numerous vascular spaces. H&E stain. *(Courtesy Dr. J.M. Cullen, College of Veterinary Medicine, North Carolina State University.)*

Malignant lymphoma is the most common metastatic neoplasm found in the liver of most, if not all, species.

Some metastatic neoplasms have a typical appearance within the liver; for example, melanomas frequently are black because of the presence of melanin, and hemangiosarcomas are usually dark red to brown because of blood. Hematopoietic neoplasms, such as lymphoma and the myeloproliferative disorders, can diffusely expand the liver and can have diffuse infiltrative (Fig. 8-82, *A*) and nodular (Fig. 8-82, *B*) variants, thus producing hepatomegaly and an enhanced lobular pattern on the cut surface, or they may have a nodular appearance. This characteristic appearance of diffuse involvement is attributable to centrilobular hepatocellular degeneration because of anemia in both lymphoma and myeloproliferative disorders and because of the specific location of accumulations of neoplastic cells; locations include portal and periportal for lymphomas (Fig. 8-82, *C*) and sinusoidal for myeloproliferative disorders. Metastatic carcinomas often have an umbilicated appearance, similar to that seen with cholangiocellular carcinomas, but umbilication is rarely a feature of sarcomas.

DISEASES OF THE GALLBLADDER
CHOLELITHIASIS

Choleliths, or gallstones as they are commonly called, occur infrequently in all the domestic species, but they are especially well described in ruminants. Choleliths are concretions of normally soluble components of bile (Fig. 8-83). They form when these components become supersaturated and precipitate. Choleliths in the gallbladder usually do not become clinically significant unless they migrate and obstruct the extrahepatic bile ducts.

CHOLECYSTITIS

Cholecystitis is inflammation of the gallbladder and can be acute or chronic. Acute inflammation of the gallbladder may be produced by viral infections, such as Rift Valley fever in ruminants and infectious canine hepatitis and produces characteristic edema and hemorrhage in the gallbladder. Fibrinous cholecystitis may occur in calves with acute salmonellosis, particularly that caused by *Salmonella enteritidis* serotype *dublin* (Fig. 8-84). Other bacteria, either derived from the blood or ascended from the intestine, can cause acute or chronic cholecystitis. Chronic cholecystitis typically accompanies prolonged bacterial infection of the biliary tree, or ongoing irritation from choleliths or parasites of the gallbladder. Rupture of the gallbladder is rare but can occur as a result of acute or chronic infection. The resultant release of bile, with or without accompanying bacteria, can cause life-threatening peritonitis because of the irritating effect of bile on the serosal surfaces of the abdomen.

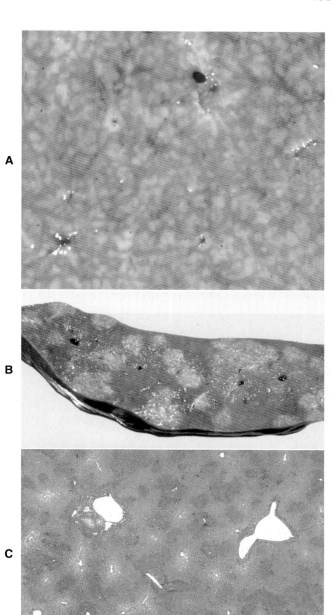

Fig. 8-82   Hepatic lymphoma (lymphosarcoma), liver.
A, Cut surface, high magnification, dog. The entire liver is enlarged (not shown here), and there are multiple pale foci caused by infiltrating neoplastic lymphocytes. The regular distribution of neoplastic foci apparent on the cut surface is due to the preferential infiltration of the portal tracts by neoplastic cells. **B,** Cow. As shown here, hepatic lymphoma can have a nodular rather than a diffuse pattern, as seen in Fig. 8-82, A. **C,** Dog. Neoplastic lymphocytes are typically distributed within and around the portal tracts and central veins (Fig. 8-82, A). H&E stain. (*A and C, Courtesy Dr. J.M. Cullen, College of Veterinary Medicine, North Carolina State University. B, Courtesy College of Veterinary Medicine, University of Illinois.*)

the dog and cat. This type of anomaly, normal tissue in an abnormal location, is termed a choristoma.

PACINIAN CORPUSCLES

Pacinian corpuscles are normally present within the interlobular connective tissue of the pancreas and mesentery of the cat, and appear as discrete 1- to 3-mm nodules (Fig. 8-88). The corpuscles should not be mistaken for abnormal structures.

AUTOLYSIS

Autolysis of the pancreas is very rapid after death, particularly if the pancreas is traumatized. Postmortem release and activation of pancreatic proteolytic enzymes within the pancreas can hasten tissue breakdown. Thus autolysis may be advanced in the pancreas before it is evident in other organs. As autolysis progresses, the color of the gland may change from its normal pink to dark red or green. The metabolic activity of intestinal bacteria, which can easily gain access to the pancreas, can contribute to the discoloration of the pancreas through hemolysis and tissue decomposition.

PANCREATIC CALCULI

The formation of concretions or "stones" within the pancreatic duct system is termed pancreolithiasis, and occurs uncommonly in cattle. It is usually an incidental finding at slaughter, and apparently is slightly more common in cattle older than 4 years of age than in younger animals.

STROMAL FAT CELL INFILTRATION

Fat cell infiltration of the interstitial connective tissue of the pancreas occurs occasionally, especially in obese cats. The pancreas itself is usually unaffected, so

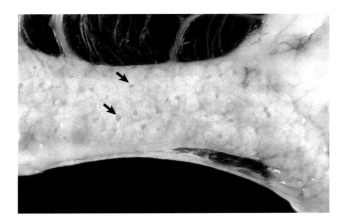

Fig. 8-88 Pacinian corpuscles (arrows), pancreas, cat. The feline pancreas contains numerous Pacinian corpuscles, which may be visible grossly as about 1-mm clear foci. (*Courtesy College of Veterinary Medicine, North Carolina State University.*)

exocrine pancreatic function is normal, but the dispersion of the parenchyma creates the impression that the pancreas has been replaced by adipose tissue.

PANCREATIC DEGENERATION AND ATROPHY

Degeneration of the acinar cells of the exocrine pancreas is a nonspecific process that can occur as a consequence of a variety of local and systemic diseases. For instance, starvation results in loss of zymogen granules within the cytoplasm of acinar cells of the exocrine pancreas because the rate of synthesis of the granules is diminished, and available protein is used to maintain serum protein concentrations when dietary protein is limited. Obstruction of the pancreatic ducts, whatever the cause, can also cause degeneration and atrophy of the exocrine pancreas. Obstruction of the pancreatic duct(s) can be caused by neoplasms or chronic inflammation and associated fibrosis that compress the duct, or by foreign bodies, such as parasites or pancreoliths, that occlude the ductal lumen. Exocrine pancreatic atrophy also may occur secondary to widespread interstitial fibrosis of the pancreas, as occurs for example, in dogs with chronic pancreatitis.

PANCREATIC PSEUDOCYSTS

Pancreatic pseudocysts are fluid-filled nonepithelialized fibrous sacs containing cellular debris and pancreatic enzymes that form within the pancreas or adjacent to the organ following pancreatic inflammation. They are described in dogs and cats. They should be distinguished from abscesses and cystic neoplasms.

ACUTE PANCREATITIS/ACUTE PANCREATIC NECROSIS

Acute pancreatitis is a condition characterized primarily by necrosis and varying degrees of inflammation of the pancreas. In fact, the predominance of necrosis over inflammation supports using the term *acute pancreatic necrosis* over acute pancreatitis for dogs and cats in most instances. Obese, sedentary bitches are especially predisposed. Acute pancreatitis occurs less often in cats than dogs, but more often in cats than most other species. Acute pancreatitis has been described in a variety of species, although the cause usually is different in each species.

PATHOGENESIS

The routes of injury for the pancreas include the duct system, which normally drains the organ. Obstruction of the duct(s) by migration of ascarids or flukes into the duct system, which can occur in a variety of animal species, or by pancreatic calculi, which occurs in ruminants most often, can trigger pancreatitis. Pancreatitis or acute pancreatic necrosis can also be produced by blood-borne delivery of some toxins and presumably some therapeutic drugs, notably corticosteroids. Direct trauma to the organ can also trigger pancreatitis.

There are three major proposed mechanisms of pancreatitis:

- Obstruction of the duct(s)
- Direct injury to acinar cells
- Disturbances of enzyme trafficking within the cytoplasm of acinar cells.

Obstruction of ductal flow by calculi or parasites can lead to interstitial edema that compresses small-caliber vessels and compromises local blood flow leading to ischemic damage to acinar cells. Direct damage to acinar cells can be caused by a few specific agents in animals, including compounds found in *Cassia occidentalis* and T-2 toxin, a trichothecene mycotoxin that affects pigs, and zinc toxicosis of dogs, veal calves, and sheep. Certain therapeutic drugs, such as sulfonamides and potassium bromide–phenobarbital combinations, can damage the pancreas in dogs, and other species are probably similarly affected. Ischemia to the pancreas from a variety of causes may also produce direct injury to the acinar cells. A third mechanism involves aberrant transport of proenzymes within the acinar cells, leading to inappropriate activation of the enzymes within the cells. The association between corticosteroid administration in dogs and an increased risk of acute pancreatitis could possibly be explained by this mechanism. However, many cases of acute pancreatitis commonly occur after dogs have consumed a meal high in fat or some other dietary indiscretion, and the specific mechanism triggering the disease remain unclear. Pancreatitis is occasionally initiated by trauma, usually in dogs and cats as a consequence of some accidental crushing or impact trauma to the abdomen or surgical trauma. Leakage of enzymes from the pancreas initiates necrosis, followed by trauma and inflammation of the pancreas and adjacent tissue in the same manner as previously described for pancreatitis in the dog.

Acute pancreatitis in dogs occurs as a consequence of release of activated pancreatic enzymes into the pancreatic parenchyma and adjacent tissue producing autodigestion. Trypsin is believed to be a key player in pancreatitis. Once activated, trypsin in turn can activate proelastase and prophospholipase into elastase and phospholipase A. These enzymes digest pancreatic tissue and adjacent fat, and damage blood vessels. Trypsin also activates prekallikrein, leading to involvement of the kinin system, complement, and clotting cascades in affected tissue. These in turn amplify the process, promote thrombosis and hemorrhage, and attract inflammatory cells.

The pancreas is protected by the continuous flow of secretions into the duodenum, which prevents reflux of duodenal contents. The normal secretion of the pancreas contains trypsin, chymotrypsin, elastase, aminopeptidases, lipase, phospholipases, amylase, and nucleases. Trypsin is a critical enzyme because it has a role in the activation of several of the other pancreatic enzymes. Several mechanisms exist to protect the healthy pancreas from the effects of digestive enzymes it produces. Before secretion, enzymes are isolated from the acinar cell cytoplasm in membrane-bound zymogen granules. Most enzymes, except amylase and lipase, are secreted as proenzymes to prevent pancreatic injury. In particular, trypsin activation is tightly controlled because of its central role in activation of other enzymes. Consequently, the proenzyme trypsinogen is not normally activated until it enters the lumen of the duodenum through duodenal enteropeptidase. In addition, the chance of inappropriate trypsin activation in acinar cells or ducts of the pancreas is reduced by secretion of protective trypsin inhibitors. In circumstances in which trypsin or other enzymes are inappropriately activated, there are several other defenses in place. Acinar cells have an innate resistance to several of the digestive enzymes. Intrapancreatic release of active enzymes triggers the release of other enzymes that will degrade the offending digestive enzymes, and lysosomal enzymes can degrade the zymogen granules when the pancreatic secretion is disturbed, reducing the burden of potentially injurious enzymes.

Direct trauma to the pancreas is uncommon, except during surgical manipulations, because the organ has a central location within the abdomen and is protected from all but serious physical trauma.

The gross lesions of acute pancreatitis are referable to proteolytic degradation of pancreatic parenchyma, vascular damage and hemorrhage, and necrosis of peripancreatic fat by lipolytic enzymes of the pancreas. Mild cases of pancreatitis are characterized by edema of the interstitial tissue of the pancreas. Acute hemorrhagic pancreatitis is more severe, and characteristically the pancreas is edematous and contains areas that are gray-white, the result of coagulation necrosis, and other areas that are dark red or blue-black, which are hemorrhagic (Fig. 8-89, A). Areas of fat necrosis are manifest as chalky-white foci as a result of saponification of necrotic adipose tissue in the mesentery adjacent to the pancreas. Portions of normal pancreatic parenchyma may be interspersed between affected portions. The peritoneal cavity frequently contains blood-stained fluid, which may contain droplets of fat in the early stage. Peritonitis is manifest by fibrinous adhesions between the affected portions of the pancreas and adjacent tissues.

The microscopic appearance of acute hemorrhagic pancreatitis reflects the gross lesions just described. Characteristic lesions include focally extensive areas of hemorrhage, influx of leukocytes, and coagulation necrosis of the pancreatic parenchyma, accumulation of fibrinous exudate in the interlobular septa, and

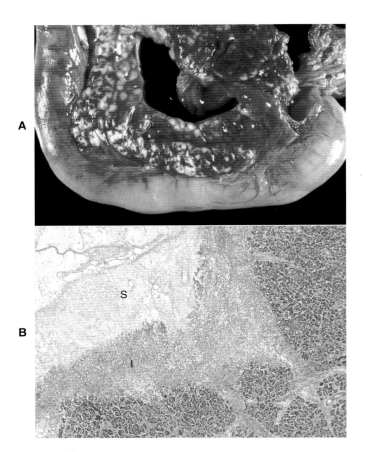

Fig. 8-89 **Acute pancreatic necrosis, acute pancreatitis, pancreas, dog. A,** Note the expansion of the pancreas by areas of hemorrhage and edema. **B,** Acute pancreatitis (histologic appearance of the pancreas depicted in Fig. 8-89, A). Note the accumulation of fibrinous exudate and edema within the interlobular septa (*S*) and inflammatory cell infiltrate (*I*). H&E stain. (**A,** *Courtesy Dr. R. Fairley.* **B,** *Courtesy Dr. J.M. Cullen, College of Veterinary Medicine, North Carolina State University.*)

necrosis and inflammation of fat in the mesentery adjacent to the affected portions of pancreas (Fig. 8-89, B).

Species differences in acute pancreatitis are recognized. For example, in cats there appears to be two distinct syndromes of acute pancreatitis, one characterized by an acute pancreatic necrosis and a distinct suppurative pancreatitis that is most likely the consequence of ascending bacterial infection.

Acute pancreatitis is usually characterized by vomiting, diarrhea, anorexia, and abdominal tenderness. Acute, severe pancreatitis also produces systemic effects in affected dogs. The release of inflammatory mediators and activated enzymes from the damaged pancreas may produce widespread vascular injury and subsequent widespread hemorrhage, shock, and disseminated intravascular coagulation. The liver also is affected in many cases of pancreatitis, as indicated by increased concentrations of serum hepatic enzymes (such as alanine aminotransferase), and sometimes, focal hepatic necrosis.

The pancreas possesses modest regenerative capacity following acute pancreatitis with necrosis of pancreatic exocrine epithelial cells, although more robust regeneration following partial pancreatectomy has been shown. Acinar cells can undergo replication in cases of limited injury, and precursor cells arise from cells within or adjacent to ductal epithelium in more severe injury. Following acute pancreatic injury, there is usually little evidence of regeneration of the exocrine pancreas if there has been sufficient tissue destruction. Fibrosis is the principal response to exocrine pancreatic injury. Proliferated ductules and atrophic exocrine pancreatic lobules are also found following significant pancreatic injury.

Acute pancreatitis sufficient to cause clinical disease apparently is considerably less common in species other than the dog and cat. Acute pancreatic necrosis and pancreatitis have been described in the horse, but the pathogenesis of pancreatitis in this species differs from that in the dog and cat. Necrosis and inflammation are the result of migration of strongyle larvae through the pancreas, which results in the release of pancreatic enzymes and enzymatic digestion of the pancreas and surrounding tissue.

CHRONIC PANCREATITIS

Chronic pancreatitis is typically accompanied by fibrosis and parenchymal atrophy. It can occur in all species as a consequence of obstruction of the pancreatic ducts and presumably all of the other mechanisms associated with acute pancreatitis. Chronic inflammation of the pancreas, characterized by lymphoplasmacytic infiltrates, is most common and important in the dog, but does occur in the cat, horse, and cattle, in which it is rarely of clinical significance. In the dog, pancreatic fibrosis and chronic pancreatitis are the result of progressive destruction of the pancreas by repeated mild episodes of acute pancreatic necrosis and pancreatitis. The pancreas has modest regenerative capacity and responds to injury with replacement fibrosis and atrophy of persisting parenchyma. Thus ongoing destruction of pancreatic tissue will cause progressive loss of glandular tissue without replacement (Fig. 8-90). If a significant portion of the pancreas is affected, dogs may develop signs of exocrine pancreatic insufficiency, with or without signs of endocrine pancreatic insufficiency (diabetes mellitus). Grossly the pancreas in affected animals is a distorted, shrunken, nodular mass with fibrous adhesions to adjacent tissue. Destruction of pancreatic tissue frequently is not of sufficient magnitude

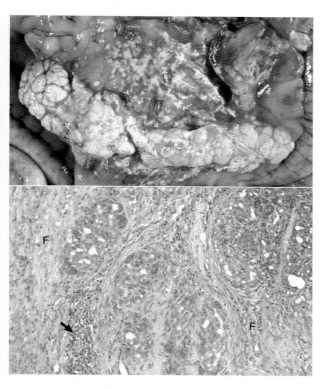

Fig. 8-90   Chronic pancreatitis, pancreas, dog. A, Lobules are more prominent due to fibrosis, and the pancreas is paler than normal. The white, raised, granular areas in the pancreas and mesentery are foci of fat necrosis that result from enzymatic digestion of lipids that then become mineralized. **B,** Remaining exocrine pancreatic cells are separated into small lobules by abundant fibrous connective tissue *(F)*, which contains chronic inflammatory cells *(arrow)*. H&E stain. *(**A,** Courtesy College of Veterinary Medicine, North Carolina State University. **B,** Courtesy Dr. J.M. Cullen, College of Veterinary Medicine, North Carolina State University.)*

to cause exocrine pancreatic insufficiency, and pancreatic fibrosis is sometimes found as incidental lesions at necropsy of dogs with apparently normal digestive function. Fibrosis of the exocrine pancreas also occurs with some frequency in cats and following the necrosis of exocrine pancreatic cells from zinc toxicosis in sheep. Ectasia of the pancreatic ducts with cyst formation also is relatively common in cats with interstitial pancreatic fibrosis.

Chronic pancreatitis and replacement fibrosis occurs sporadically in the horse, usually as a consequence of either parasitic migration or from ascending bacterial infection of the pancreatic ducts. In addition, pancreatitis may occur in horses with chronic eosinophilic gastroenteritis. However, chronic pancreatitis usually is not clinically apparent in the horse, as signs of exocrine pancreatic insufficiency rarely, if ever, occur in this species.

PARASITIC INFECTIONS

A variety of parasites may inhabit the pancreatic ducts of domestic animals. Parasitic infections of the pancreatic ducts are important if they occlude the ducts, either by direct physical obstruction or by inducing inflammation within and around ducts. Examples include flukes of the families Opisthorchiidae *(Opisthorchis tenuicollis, Opisthorchis viverrini, Clonorchis sinensis, Metorchis albidus, Metorchis conjunctus)* and Dicrocoeliidae *(Eurytrema pancreaticum, Concinnum procyonis, Dicrocoelium dendriticum)*, which may inhabit the pancreatic ducts of a variety of animal species. Nematodes, particularly ascarids, and cestodes are common gastrointestinal parasites of the domestic species; occasionally, they may lodge within the pancreatic ducts.

HYPERPLASIA AND NEOPLASIA
PANCREATIC NODULAR HYPERPLASIA

Nodular hyperplasia of the exocrine pancreas occurs in dogs, cats, and cattle. It is especially common in older dogs and cats. The lesion is of no clinical significance, but it must be distinguished from neoplasms of the endocrine and exocrine pancreas.

These hyperplastic nodules typically are multiple, raised, smooth, and a uniform gray or white on a cut surface (Fig. 8-91, *A*). The nodules may be firmer than the adjacent normal pancreas. Microscopically, these nodules consist of unencapsulated aggregates of acinar cells that may lack zymogen granules or contain an abundance of them (Fig. 8-91, *B*). Some nodules contain a mixture of the two types of acinar cells. The distinction between hyperplasia and adenoma of the exocrine pancreas is poorly defined in domestic animals.

PANCREATIC ADENOMA

Adenomas of the exocrine pancreas are extremely rare but have been described in the cat. Those of acinar cell origin share all the features of hyperplastic nodules, but are single and larger than normal pancreatic lobules, whereas hyperplastic nodules are not larger than normal lobules; this distinction clearly is somewhat arbitrary.

PANCREATIC CARCINOMA

Carcinoma of the ductular epithelium or acinar cells of the exocrine pancreas is uncommon in all species. It is most often reported in the dog and cat. The neoplasms may consist of single or multiple nodules of variable size within the pancreas, each of which consists of gray or yellow tissue. Lesions may consist of a single nodule or affect the organ diffusely. Tumors are typically grayish-white to pale yellow with a firm to hard consistency (Fig. 8-92, *A*). Tumors are often gritty when cut. Areas of hemorrhage, mineralization, or necrosis may be present within the neoplasm. The neoplasm is usually firmer than the adjacent pancreas because of proliferation of fibrous connective tissue. Adhesion of the affected pancreas to adjacent tissue may occur. This neoplasm often invades adjacent tissue and seeds the peritoneal cavity. Peritoneal implants form nodules over the mesentery, omentum, and serosa of the abdominal viscera. Metastasis to the regional lymph nodes (pancreatoduodenal, which is inconstantly present and the right hepatic lymph node) is also common, and some carcinomas metastasize widely.

Microscopic features of carcinomas of the exocrine pancreas range from well-differentiated adenocarcinomas with tubular patterns to undifferentiated carcinomas with solid patterns. The amount of fibrous stroma varies considerably, and usually is greatest in poorly differentiated neoplasms (Fig. 8-92, *B*). Zymogen granules similar to those present in normal acinar cells of the pancreas are often absent within the cytoplasm of the neoplastic cells. Mitotic figures are common.

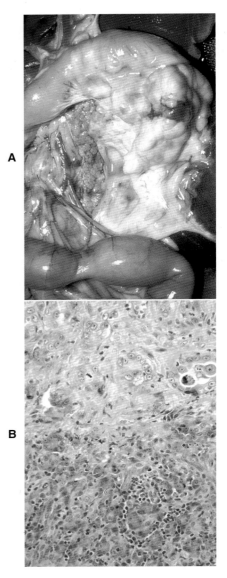

Fig. 8-92   Pancreatic carcinoma. A, Stomach and pancreas *(center),* ventral-dorsal view, dog. Pancreatic carcinoma has invaded the mesentery, wall of the stomach, and gastrosplenic ligament. Note the lobulated appearance of the mass, which is formed by neoplastic exocrine pancreatic epithelial cells and scirrhous connective tissue. Proximal duodenum *(bottom),* liver *(top),* and spleen *(right [left anatomically]).* **B,** Pancreas, cat. Pancreatic carcinoma tends to form crude acini or tubules that aggressively invade adjacent normal tissue. Prominent fibrosis, termed scirrhous response, is commonly caused by this type of tumor. H&E stain. *(**A,** Courtesy College of Veterinary Medicine, University of Illinois. **B,** Courtesy Dr. M.D. McGavin, College of Veterinary Medicine, University of Tennessee.)*

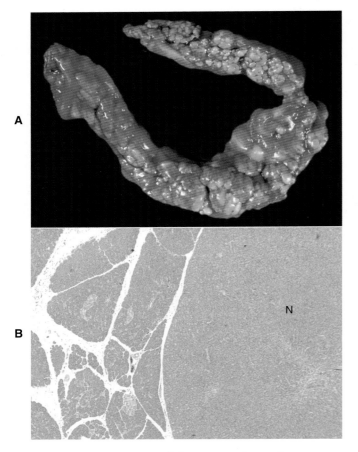

Fig. 8-91   Pancreatic nodular exocrine hyperplasia, pancreas, dog. A, Hyperplastic nodules are pale beige to white and project above the surface. **B,** Microscopically hyperplastic nodules *(N)* are composed of numerous small acini, most of which, in this case, lack typical zymogen granules. H&E stain. *(**A,** Courtesy Dr. M.D. McGavin, College of Veterinary Medicine, University of Tennessee. **B,** Courtesy Dr. J.M. Cullen, College of Veterinary Medicine, North Carolina State University.)*

SUGGESTED READINGS

Anthony PP, Ishak KG, Nayak NC et al: The morphology of cirrhosis: definition, nomenclature, and classification, *Bull WHO* 55:521-540, 1977.

Bedossa P, Paradis V: Liver extracellular matrix in health and disease, *J Pathol* 200:504-515, 2003.

Bunch SE: Hepatotoxicity associated with pharmacologic agents in dogs and cats, *Vet Clin North Am Small Anim Pract* 23:659-670, 1993.

Cullen JM, Popp JA: Tumors of the liver and gall bladder, In DJ Meuten, editor: *Tumors in domestic animals*, ed 4, Ames, 2002, Iowa State Press.

Head KW, Cullen JM, Dubielzig RR et al: Histological classification of tumors of the alimentary system of domestic animals, Second series, vol X. In World Health Organization international histologic classification of tumors of domestic animals, 2003.

Hill RC, Van Winkle TJ: Acute necrotizing pancreatitis and acute suppurative pancreatitis in the cat: a retrospective study of 40 cases (1976-1989), *J Vet Int Med* 7: 25-33, 1993.

Jubb KVF: The pancreas. In Jubb KVF, Kennedy PC, Palmer N, editors: *Pathology of domestic animals*, ed 4, New York, 1985, Academic Press.

Kelly WR: The liver and biliary system. In Jubb KVF, Kennedy PC, Palmer N, editors: *Pathology of domestic animals*, ed 4, New York, 1985, Academic Press.

Kingsbury JM: *Poisonous plants of the United States and Canada*, Englewood Cliffs, NJ, 1964, Prentice-Hall.

Lee W: Drug-induced hepatotoxicity, *N Engl J Med* 349:474-485, 2003.

MacSween RNM, Burt AD, Portmann BC et al, editors: *Pathology of the liver*, ed 4, New York, 2002, Churchill Livingstone.

Pearson E: Liver disease in the mature horse, *Equine Vet Educ* 11:87-96, 1999.

Seawright AA: Directly toxic effects of plant chemicals which may occur in human and animal foods, *Nat Toxins* 3:227-232, 1995.

Thornburg LP: A perspective on copper and liver disease in the dog, *J Vet Diagn Invest* 12:101-110, 2000.

van den Ingh TS, Rothuizen J, Meyer HP: Circulatory disorders of the liver in dogs and cats, *Vet Q* 17:70-76, 1995.

9

Respiratory System

ALFONSO LÓPEZ

INTRODUCTION

Diseases of the respiratory system are some of the leading causes of morbidity and mortality in animals and a major source of economic losses. Thus veterinarians are routinely called to diagnose, treat, and implement health management practices to reduce the impact of these diseases. In companion animals, diseases of the respiratory tract are also common and, although of little economic significance, are important to the health of the animals and thus to clinicians and owners.

STRUCTURE AND FUNCTION

To facilitate the understanding of the structure and function, it is convenient to arbitrarily divide the respiratory system into conducting, transitional, and gas exchange systems (Fig. 9-1). The conducting system includes nasal cavity, paranasal sinuses, pharynx, larynx, trachea, and extrapulmonary and intrapulmonary bronchi, all of which are largely lined by pseudostratified, ciliated columnar cells plus a variable proportion of secretory goblet (mucous) and serous cells (Figs. 9-2, 9-3, and 9-4). The transitional system of the respiratory tract is composed of bronchioles, which serve as a transition zone between the conducting system (ciliated) and the gas exchange (alveolar) system (Fig. 9-1). The disappearance of cilia in the transitional system is not abrupt; the ciliated cells in the proximal bronchiolar region become scarce and progressively attenuated, until the point where distal bronchioles no longer have ciliated cells. Normal bronchioles also lack goblet cells, but instead have other types of secretory cells, notably Clara and neuroendocrine cells. Clara cells contain numerous biosynthetic organelles that play an active role in detoxification of xenobiotics (foreign substances), similar to the role of hepatocytes. In carnivores and monkeys, and to a much lesser extent in horses and human beings, the terminal portions of bronchioles are not only lined by cuboidal epithelium but also by

segments of alveolar capillaries. These unique bronchioloalveolar structures are known as respiratory bronchioles (Fig. 9-1). The gas exchange system of the respiratory tract in all mammals is formed by alveolar ducts and millions of alveoli (Fig. 9-5). Alveoli are superficially lined by two distinct types of epithelial cells known as type I pneumonocytes (membranous) and type II pneumonocytes (granular) (Fig. 9-6).

All three—the conducting, transitional and exchange systems of the respiratory system—are vulnerable to injury because of constant exposure to a myriad of microbes, particles and fibers, and toxic gases and vapors present in the air. Vulnerability of the respiratory system to aerogenous (airborne) injury is primarily because of (1) the extensive area of the alveoli, which are the interface between the respiratory system and inspired air;

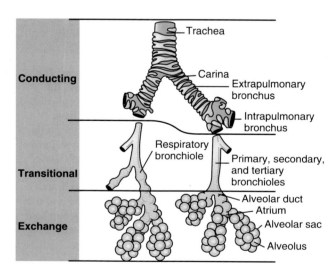

Fig. 9-1 **Schematic diagram of airways from the trachea to the alveoli.** Conducting, transitional, and exchange components of the respiratory system. The transitional zone (bronchioles) is not present or as equally well developed in all species.
(From Banks WJ: Applied veterinary histology, ed 3, St Louis, 1993, Mosby.)

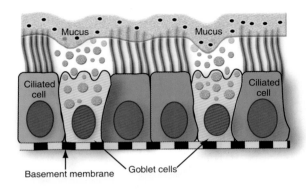

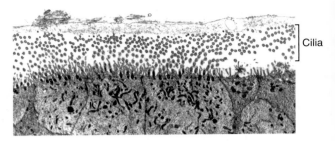

Fig. 9-2 Schematic representation of the mucociliary carpet that covers the conducting system. Both ciliated and goblet cells rest on the basement membrane. Mucus produced and released by goblet cells forms a carpet on which inhaled particles (*dots*) are trapped and subsequently expelled into the pharynx by the mucociliary apparatus. (*Courtesy Dr. A. López, Atlantic Veterinary College.*)

Fig. 9-4 Normal ciliated epithelium, trachea, cow. This trachea was specially fixed to preserve the mucous layer, which consists of an internal, clear, hypophase-fluid layer (not visible here) surrounding microvilli and kinocilia and an external mucous epiphase at the level of the tips of the kinocilia (cut in both transverse and longitudinal section here). TEM. Uranyl acetate and lead citrate stain. (*From Sims DE, Westfall JA, Kiorpes AL, Horne MM:* Biotech Histochem 66:173-180, 1991.)

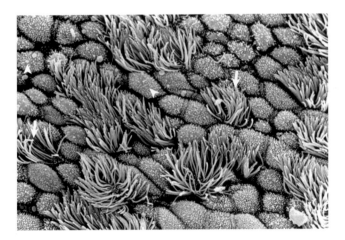

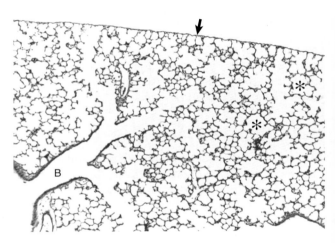

Fig. 9-3 Normal bronchial mucosa, bronchus, rat. The mucous layer was removed before fixation to expose the external surface of the epithelium. Mucosa consists of ciliated cells and nonciliated secretory cells. Ciliated cells have numerous slender cilia (*arrows*). Nonciliated secretory cells have a dome-shaped surface with abundant microvilli (*arrowheads*). The proportion of ciliated to nonciliated cells varies depending on the level of airways. Ciliated cells are more abundant in proximal airways, whereas secretory cells are more numerous in distal portions of the conducting and transitional systems. Scanning electron micrograph. Carbon sputter coating method. (*Courtesy Dr. A. López, Atlantic Veterinary College.*)

Fig. 9-5 Lung, rat. Lungs were fixed by intratracheal perfusion of fixative to retain normal distention of airways. Note the dichotomous branching of the bronchioles and the slender visceral pleura covering the surface of the lungs. *B*, Branching bronchioles; ***, alveoli; *arrow*, visceral pleura. H&E stain. (*Courtesy Dr. J. Martínez-Burnes, Atlantic Veterinary College.*)

(2) the large volume of air passing continuously into the lungs; and (3) the high concentration of noxious elements that can be present in the air (Table 9-1). For human beings, it has been estimated that the surface of the pulmonary alveoli is approximately 200 m², roughly the area of a tennis court. It has also been estimated that the volume of air reaching the human lung every day is around 9000 L. The surface of the equine lung is estimated to be around 2000 m².

Lungs are also susceptible to blood-borne (hematogenous) microbes, toxins, and emboli. This fact is not surprising because the entire cardiac output of the right ventricle goes into the lungs, and approximately 9% of the total blood volume is within the pulmonary vasculature. Also the pulmonary capillary bed is the largest in the body, with a surface area of 70 m² in the

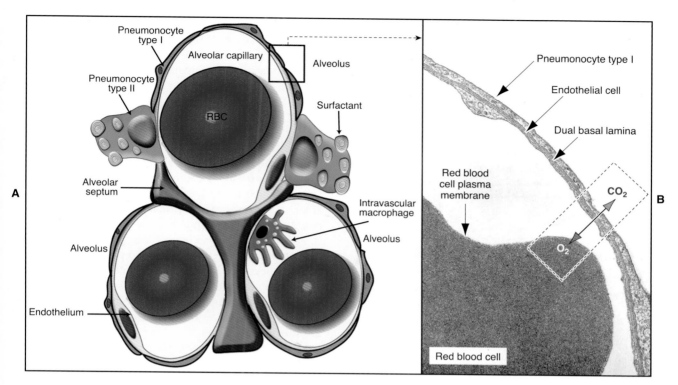

Fig. 9-6   The blood-air barrier. A, In this schematic diagram, note the thin membrane separating the blood compartment from the alveoli. Type I alveolar cells (membranous pneumonocytes) are remarkably thin and cover most of the alveolar wall. Note the endothelial cells lining the alveolar capillary. Alveolar interstitium supports the alveolar epithelium on one side and the endothelium on the other side of the blood-air barrier. Type II (granular) pneumonocytes appear as large cuboidal cells with lamellar bodies (surfactant) in the cytoplasm. A pulmonary intravascular macrophage, a component of the monocyte-macrophage system, is depicted on the wall of an alveolar capillary. A red blood cell *(RBC)* is present inside the lumen of the alveolar capillary. **B,** Alveolar wall. The blood-air barrier consists of cytoplasmic extensions of (1) type I alveolar cells (membranous pneumonocytes); (2) a dual basal lamina synthesized by type I alveolar cells; (3) cytoplasmic extensions of endothelial cells.   TEM. Uranyl acetate and lead citrate stain. (**A,** *Courtesy Dr. A. López, Atlantic Veterinary College.* **B,** *From Kierszenbaum AL: Histology and cell biology, St Louis, 2002, Mosby.)*

adult human being; this area is equivalent to a length of 2400 km of capillaries, with 1 ml of blood occupying up to 16 km of capillary bed.

NORMAL FLORA OF THE RESPIRATORY SYSTEM

The respiratory system has its own normal bacterial flora, as does any other body system in contact with the external environment. If a sterile swab is passed deep into the nasal cavity of any healthy animal and cultured for microbes, many species of bacteria are recovered, such as *Mannheimia (Pasteurella) haemolytica* in cattle; *Pasteurella multocida* in cats, cattle, and pigs; and *Bordetella bronchiseptica* in dogs and pigs. The organisms that

constitute the normal flora of the respiratory tract are restricted to the most proximal (rostral) region of the conducting system (nasal cavity, pharynx, and larynx). The thoracic portions of the trachea, bronchi, and lungs are considered to be essentially sterile. The types of bacteria present in the nasal flora vary considerably among animal species and in different geographic regions of the world. Some bacteria present in the nasal flora are pathogens that can cause important respiratory infections. For instance, *Mannheimia (Pasteurella) haemolytica* is part of the bovine nasal flora, yet this bacterium causes a devastating disease in cattle–pneumonic mannheimiosis (shipping fever). Experimental studies have established that microorganisms from the nasal flora are continuously carried into the lungs via

Table **9-1**   **Common Pathogens, Allergens, and Toxic Substances Present in Inhaled Air**

Microbes	Viruses, *Chlamydophila*, bacteria, fungi, protozoa
Plant dust	Grain, flour, cotton, wood
Animal products	Dander, feathers, mites, insect chitin
Toxic gases	Ammonia (NH_3), hydrogen sulfide (H_2S), nitrogen dioxide (NO_2), sulfur dioxide (SO_2), chlorine
Chemicals	Organic and inorganic solvents, herbicides, asbestos, nickel, lead

Box **9-1**

Portals of Entry into the Respiratory System

Aerogenous (air)	Virus, bacteria, *Chlamydophila*, fungi, toxic gases, and pneumotoxicants
Hematogenous (blood)	Virus, bacteria, fungi, parasites, toxins, and pneumotoxicants
Direct extension	Penetrating wounds, migrating awns, bites, and ruptured esophagus or perforated diaphragm (hardware)

tracheal air. In spite of this constant bacterial bombardment from the nasal flora and from contaminated air, normal lungs remain sterile because of their remarkably effective defense mechanisms.

PORTALS OF ENTRY INTO THE RESPIRATORY SYSTEM

Microbes, toxins, and pneumotoxicants can gain access into the respiratory system by the following routes (Box 9-1):

1. Aerogenous—Pathogens, such as bacteria, mycoplasmas, and viruses, along with toxic gases and foreign particles, including food, can gain access to the respiratory system via inspired air. This is the most common route in the transmission of most respiratory infections in domestic animals.
2. Hematogenous—Some viruses, bacteria, parasites, and toxins can enter the respiratory system via the circulating blood. This portal of entry is commonly seen in septicemias, sepsis, protozoal infections, and viruses that target endothelial cells. Also, circulating leukocytes may release infectious organisms such as retroviruses and *Listeria monocytogenes* while traveling through the lungs.

3. Direct extension—In some instances pathogenic organisms can also reach the pleura and lungs through penetrating injuries, such as gunshot wounds, migrating awns, bites, or by direct extension from a ruptured esophagus or perforated diaphragm.

DEFENSE MECHANISMS OF THE RESPIRATORY SYSTEM

It is axiomatic that a particle, microbe, or toxic gas must first gain entry to a vulnerable region of the respiratory system before it can have a pathologic effect. The characteristics of size, shape, dispersal, and deposition of particles present in inspired air are studied in aerobiology. It is important to recognize the difference between deposition and retention of inhaled particles. Deposition is the process by which particles of various sizes and shapes are trapped within specific regions of the respiratory tract. Clearance is the process by which deposited particles are destroyed, neutralized, or removed from the mucosal surfaces. The main mechanisms involved in clearance are sneezing, coughing, mucociliary transport, and phagocytosis (Box 9-2). The difference between what is deposited and what is cleared from the respiratory tract is referred to as retention. Abnormal retention of particles resulting from increased deposition, decreased clearance, or a combination of both, is the underlying pathogenetic mechanism in many pulmonary diseases (Fig. 9-7).

The anatomic configuration of the nasal cavity and bronchi in the conducting system plays a unique role in preventing or reducing the penetration of noxious material into the lungs, especially into the alveolar region, which is the most vulnerable portion of the respiratory system. The narrow nasal meatuses and the coiled arrangement of the nasal conchae generate enormous turbulences of airflow and, as a result, physical forces are created that forcefully impact particles larger than

Box **9-2**

Main Defense Mechanisms of the Respiratory System

Conducting system (nose, trachea and bronchi)	Mucociliary clearance, antibodies, lysozyme, mucus
Transitional system (bronchioles)	Clara cells, antioxidants, lysozyme, antibodies
Exchange system (alveoli)	Alveolar macrophages (inhaled pathogens), intravascular macrophages (circulating pathogens), opsonizing antibodies, surfactant, antioxidants

Bacterial Retention in Lung

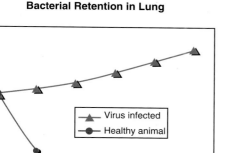

Fig. 9-7   **Pulmonary clearance and retention of bacteria following inhalation of an experimental aerosol of bacteria.** When large numbers of bacteria are inhaled, the normal defense mechanisms promptly eliminate these microorganisms from the lungs *(blue line)*. However, when the defense mechanisms are impaired by a viral infection, lung edema, stress, etc., the inhaled bacteria are not eliminated but colonize and multiply in the lung *(red line)*. *(Courtesy Dr. A. López, Atlantic Veterinary College.)*

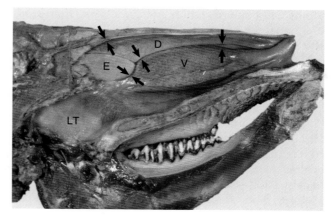

Fig. 9-8   **Dorsal (D), ventral (V), and ethmoidal (E) conchae, midsagittal section of head, cow.** These narrow meatuses *(spaces between arrows)* and the air turbulence produced in the meatuses by the coiled arrangement of the conchae cause suspended particles to impact on the mucus covering the surface of the nasal mucosa. These particles are then moved caudally by the mucociliary escalator and finally swallowed. Note the abundant lymphoid tissue *(LT)* in the nasopharynx. *(Courtesy Dr. R.G. Thomson, Ontario Veterinary College.)*

10 μm onto the surface of the nasal mucosa (Fig. 9-8). Although particles smaller than 10 μm could escape trapping in the nasal cavity, these medium-sized particles meet a second barrier at the tracheal and bronchial bifurcations. Here, abrupt changes in the direction of air (inertia), which occurs at the branching of major airways, cause particles in the 2- to 10-μm size range to collide with the surface of bronchial mucosa (Fig. 9-1). Because the velocity of inspired air at the level of the small bronchi and bronchioles has become rather slow, inertial and centrifugal forces no longer play a significant role in the trapping of inhaled particles. Here, in the transitional (bronchiolar) and exchange (alveolar) regions, particles 2 μm or smaller may come into contact with the mucosa by means of sedimentation because of gravitation or by diffusion as a result of Brownian movement. Infective aerosols containing bacteria and viruses are within the size ranges (0.01 to 2 μm) that gain access to the bronchioloalveolar region.

In addition to size, other factors, such as shape, length, electrical charge, and humidity, play an important role in mucosal deposition, retention, and pathogenicity of inhaled particles. For instance, particles longer than 200 μm may also reach the lower respiratory tract, provided their mean aerodynamic diameter is less than 1 μm. Asbestos is a good example of a large but slender fiber that can bypass the filtrating mechanisms by traveling

parallel to the airstream. Once in the lungs, asbestos fibers cause asbestosis, a serious pulmonary disease in human beings. In summary, the anatomic features of the nasal cavity and airways provide an effective barrier, preventing the penetration of most large particles into the lungs.

Once larger particles are trapped in the mucosa of conducting airways and small particles are deposited on the surface of the bronchioalveolar mucosa, it is crucial that these exogenous materials be removed to prevent or minimize injury to the respiratory system. For these purposes, the respiratory system is equipped with several defense mechanisms, all of which are provided by specialized cells operating in a remarkably well-coordinated manner.

DEFENSE MECHANISMS OF THE CONDUCTING SYSTEM (NOSE, TRACHEA, AND BRONCHI)

Mucociliary clearance is the physical unidirectional movement and removal of deposited particles and gases dissolved in the mucus from the respiratory tract. Mucociliary clearance is provided by the mucociliary blanket (mucociliary escalator) and is the main defense mechanism of the conducting system (nasal cavity, trachea, and bronchi) (Figs. 9-2 and 9-4). Mucus is a complex mixture of water, glycoproteins, immunoglobulins, lipids, and electrolytes produced by goblet (mucous) cells, serous cells, submucosal glands, and fluid from transepithelial ion and water transport. Once serous fluid and mucus are secreted onto the surface of the respiratory mucosa, a thin, double-layer film of mucus is formed on top of the cells. The outer layer of this film is in a viscous gel phase, whereas the inner layer, which is in a fluid or sol phase, is directly in contact with cilia (Fig. 9-4). A healthy human being produces around 100 ml of mucus per day. Each ciliated cell in the conducting system has around 250 cilia (6 μm long), beating metachronously (forming a wave) at approximately 1000 strokes per minute, and in a horse, for instance, mucus moves longitudinally up to 20 mm per minute. Rapid and powerful movement of cilia creates a series of waves that, in a continuous and synchronized manner, propel the mucus, exfoliated cells, and trapped particles out of the respiratory tract. The mucus is finally swallowed, or when present in large amounts, it is coughed up out of the conducting system. If mucus flow were to move at the same rate in all levels of a conducting system, a "bottleneck" effect would be created in major airways as the minor but more numerous airways enter the bronchi. For this reason, the mucociliary transport in proximal (rostral) airways is physiologically faster than that of the distal (caudal) ones.

The mucociliary blanket of the nasal cavity, trachea, and bronchi also plays an important role in preventing injury from toxic gases. If a soluble gas contacts the mucociliary blanket, it mixes with the mucus, thus reducing the concentration of gas reaching deep into the alveoli. In other words, mucus acts as a "scavenger system," whereby gases are solubilized and subsequently cleared from the respiratory tract via mucociliary transport. If ciliary transport is reduced (loss of cilia) or mucus production is excessive, coughing becomes an important mechanism for clearing the airways.

In addition to the physical transport provided by the mucociliary escalator, other cells closely associated with ciliated epithelium contribute to the defense mechanism of the conducting system. Among the most notable ones are the M cells ("microfold cells"), which are modified epithelial cells covering the bronchial associated lymphoid tissue (BALT), both of which are strategically located at the corner of the bifurcation of bronchi and bronchioles, where inhaled particles often collide with the mucosa because of inertial forces. From here, inhaled particles and soluble antigens are phagocytosed and transported by macrophages, dendritic cells, and other professional "antigen-presenting cells" (APCs) into the BALT, thus providing a unique opportunity for B and T lymphocytes to enter into close contact with inhaled pathogenic substances. Pulmonary lymphocytes are not quiescent in the BALT but are in continual traffic to other organs and contribute to both cellular (cytotoxic, helper, suppressor T lymphocytes) and humoral

immune responses. Immunoglobulin (Ig)A, produced by mucosal plasma cells, and to a lesser extent, IgG and IgM play important roles in the local immunity of the conducting system, especially with regard to preventing attachment of pathogens to the mucociliary blanket. Chronic airway diseases, especially those due to infection—such as those caused by mycoplasmas or retroviruses—are often accompanied by severe hyperplasia of the BALT.

The mucociliary clearance terminates at the pharynx, where mucus, propelled caudally from the nasal cavity and cranially from the tracheobronchial tree, is eventually swallowed and thus eliminated from the conducting system of the respiratory tract. Some respiratory pathogens such as *Rhodococcus equi* can infect the intestines after having been removed and swallowed from the respiratory tract into the alimentary system.

DEFENSE MECHANISMS OF THE EXCHANGE SYSTEM (ALVEOLI)

Alveoli lack ciliated and mucus-producing cells; thus the defense mechanism against inhaled particles in the alveolar region cannot be provided by mucociliary clearance. Instead the main defense mechanism of alveoli (exchange system) is phagocytosis provided by the pulmonary alveolar macrophages (Fig. 9-9). These highly phagocytic cells are derived largely from blood monocytes and, to a much lesser extent, from a slowly dividing population of interstitial macrophages. After a temporary adaptive stage within pulmonary interstitium, blood monocytes reduce their glycolytic and

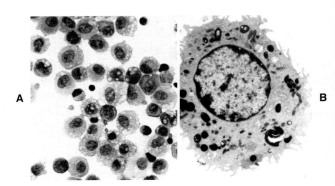

Fig. 9-9 Pulmonary alveolar macrophages. A, Bronchoalveolar lavage, healthy pig. Alveolar macrophages characterized by abundant and vacuolated cytoplasm are the predominant cell in lavages from healthy lungs. **B,** Alveolar macrophage, rat. Note abundant cytoplasm with numerous phagolysosomes and elongated pseudopods extending from the cell surface. TEM. Uranyl acetate and lead citrate stain. (**A,** *Courtesy Dr. L.A. Rijana-Ludbit, Tübingen.* **B,** *Courtesy Dr. A. López, Atlantic Veterinary College.*)

increase their oxidative metabolism to function in an aerobic rather than in an anaerobic environment. Pulmonary alveolar macrophages rapidly attach and phagocytose bacteria and any other particle reaching the alveolar region. The number of macrophages in the alveolar space is closely related to the number of inhaled particles reaching the lungs. This ability to increase, within hours, the number of available phagocytic cells is vital in protecting the distal lungs against foreign material, particularly when the inhaled particle load is high. Unlike that of tissue macrophages, the life span of alveolar macrophages in the alveoli is notably short, only a few days, and thus they are continuously being replaced.

Alveolar phagocytosis plays a prominent role in the innate defense mechanism against inhaled bacteria without the need of an inflammatory reaction. Bacteria reaching the alveoli are rapidly phagocytosed, and bactericidal enzymes present in lysosomes are discharged into the phagosome containing the bacteria (Fig. 9-9). Except for some facultative pathogens that are resistant to intracellular killing (e.g., *Mycobacterium tuberculosis*, *Listeria monocytogenes*, *Brucella abortus*, some *Salmonella* spp.), most bacteria reaching the lungs are rapidly destroyed by activated alveolar macrophages. Similarly, inhaled particles, such as dust, pollen, spores, carbon, or erythrocytes from intraalveolar hemorrhage, are all phagocytosed and eventually removed from alveoli by pulmonary alveolar macrophages. Most alveolar macrophages leave the alveoli by migrating toward the bronchiolar (transitional) region until the mucociliary blanket is reached. Once there, pulmonary macrophages are removed in the same way as any other particle, which is, along the mucociliary flow to the pharynx and swallowed.

Destruction and removal of inhaled microbes and particles by alveolar macrophages is a well-orchestrated mechanism that engages many cells and pulmonary secretions in the lung. The cell-to-cell interactions are complex and involve pulmonary alveolar macrophages, pneumonocytes, endothelial cells, lymphocytes, plasma cells, and dendritic cells. Antibodies are also important in the protection (acquired immune response) of the respiratory tract against inhaled pathogens. IgA is the most abundant antibody in the nasal and tracheal secretions and prevents the attachment and absorption of antigens (immune exclusion). IgG, and to a lesser extent IgE and IgM, promote the uptake and destruction of inhaled pathogens by phagocytic cells (immune elimination). IgG is the most abundant antibody in the alveolar surface and acts primarily as an opsonizing antibody for alveolar macrophages and neutrophils. In addition to antibodies, there are several secretory products locally released into the alveoli that constitute the alveolar lining material and contribute to the pulmonary

defense mechanisms. The most important of these antimicrobial products are transferrin, anionic peptides, and pulmonary surfactant (Table 9-2).

To facilitate phagocytosis and discriminate between "self" and "foreign" antigens, pulmonary alveolar macrophages are furnished with a wide variety of specific receptors on their cell surfaces. Among the most important ones are Fc receptors for antibodies; complement receptors (C3b, C3a, C5a); tumor necrosis factor (TNF) receptor; and CD40 receptors, which facilitate phagocytosis; and destruction of opsonized particles. Toll-like receptors recognize microbial components, and

Table 9-2 Defense Mechanisms Provided by Some Cells and Secretory Products Present in the Respiratory System

Cell/Secretory Product	Action
Alveolar macrophage	Phagocytosis, main line of defense against inhaled particles and microbial pathogens in the alveoli
Intravascular macrophage	Phagocytosis, removal of particles, endotoxin, and microbial pathogens in the circulation
Ciliated cells	Expel mucus and inhaled particles and microbial pathogens by ciliary action
Clara cells	Detoxification of xenobiotics (mixed function oxidases) and protective secretions against oxidative stress and inflammation
Mucus	Traps inhaled particles and microbial pathogens and neutralizes soluble gases
Surfactant	Protects alveolar walls and enhances phagocytosis
Lysozyme	Antimicrobial enzyme
Transferrin and lactoferrin	Inhibition and suppression of bacterial growth
α_1-Antitrypsin	Protects against the noxious effects of proteolytic enzymes release by phagocytic cells; also inhibits inflammation
Interferon	Antiviral agent and modulator of the immune and inflammatory responses
Interleukins	Chemotaxis, up-regulation of adhesion molecules
Antibodies	Prevent microbe attachment to cell membranes, opsonization
Complement	Chemotaxis; enhances phagocytosis
Antioxidants*	Prevent injury caused by superoxide anion, hydrogen peroxide, and free radicals generated during phagocytosis, inflammation, or by inhalation of oxidant gases (ozone, NO_2, SO_2)

*Superoxide dismutase, catalase, glutathione peroxidase, oxidant free radical scavengers (tocopherol, ascorbic acid).

FAS receptors are involved in apoptosis and in the phagocytosis of apoptotic cells in the lung. "Scavenger receptors," which are responsible for the recognition and uptake of foreign particulates, such as dust and fibers, are also present on pulmonary alveolar macrophages.

DEFENSE MECHANISMS AGAINST BLOOD-BORNE PATHOGENS (INTRAVASCULAR SPACE)

Lungs are also susceptible to hematogenously borne microbes, toxins, or emboli. In dogs, laboratory rodents, and human beings, the hepatic (Kupffer cells), and splenic macrophages are the primary cells responsible for removing circulating bacteria and other particles from the blood. In contrast, the cell responsible for the removal of circulating particles, pathogenic bacteria, and endotoxin from the blood of ruminants, cats, pigs, and horses, is mainly the pulmonary intravascular macrophage, a distinct population of phagocytes normally residing within the pulmonary capillaries (Fig. 9-6). In pigs, 16% of the pulmonary capillary surface is lined by pulmonary intravascular macrophages. In ruminants, 95% of intravenously injected tracer particles or bacteria are rapidly phagocytosed by these intravascular macrophages. Recent studies showed that an abnormally reduced number of Kupffer cells in diseased liver results in proliferation of pulmonary intravascular macrophages, even in animal species in which these phagocytic cells are normally absent from the lung.

DEFENSE MECHANISMS AGAINST OXIDANT-INDUCED LUNG INJURY

Existing in an oxygen-rich environment and being the site of numerous metabolic reactions, the lungs also require an efficient defense mechanism against oxidant-induced cellular damage (oxidative stress). This form of damage is caused by inhaled oxidant gases (e.g., nitrogen dioxide, ozone, sulfur dioxide, tobacco smoke), and by xenobiotic toxic metabolites produced locally or by reaching the lungs via the blood stream (e.g., 3-methylindole and paraquat), or by free radicals (reactive oxygen species) released by phagocytic cells during inflammation. Oxygen and free radical scavengers, such as catalase, superoxide dismutase, and vitamin E, are largely responsible for protecting pulmonary cells against peroxidation. These scavengers are present in alveolar and bronchiolar epithelial cells and in the extracellular spaces of the lung.

In summary, the defense mechanisms are so effective in trapping, destroying, and removing bacteria that, under normal conditions, animals can be exposed to aerosols containing massive numbers of bacteria without any ill effects. If defense mechanisms are impaired, inhaled bacteria colonize and multiply in bronchi, bronchioles, and alveoli, and produce infection, which can result in fatal pneumonia. Similarly, when airborne and blood-borne pathogens, inhaled toxicants, or free radicals overwhelm the protective defense mechanisms, cells of the respiratory system are likely to be injured, often causing serious respiratory diseases.

IMPAIRMENT OF DEFENSE MECHANISMS IN THE RESPIRATORY SYSTEM

For many years, factors such as stress, viral infections, and pulmonary edema have been implicated in predisposing human beings and animals to secondary bacterial pneumonia. There are many pathways by which the defense mechanisms can be impaired; only those relevant to veterinary species are discussed.

VIRAL INFECTIONS

Viral agents are notorious in predisposing human beings and animals to secondary bacterial pneumonias by what is known as viral-bacterial synergism. A good example of this synergistic effect of combined virus-bacterial infections is documented from epidemics of human beings with influenza virus in which the mortality rate was significantly increased from secondary bacterial pneumonia. The most common viruses incriminated in predisposing animals to secondary bacterial pneumonia include influenza virus in pigs and horses; bovine herpesvirus 1 (BHV-1), parainfluenza-3 (PI-3), and bovine respiratory syncytial virus (BRSV) in cattle; and canine distemper virus in dogs. The mechanism of the synergistic effect of viral-bacterial infections was previously believed to be the destruction of the mucociliary blanket and a concurrent reduction of mucociliary clearance, but in experimental studies, viral infections did not significantly reduce the physical removal of particles or bacteria out of the lungs. Now it is known that 5 to 7 days after a viral infection, the phagocytic function of pulmonary alveolar macrophages is notably impaired. Other mechanisms by which viruses impair defense mechanisms are multiple and remain poorly understood (Box 9-3). Immunization against viral infections in many cases prevents or reduces the synergistic effect of viruses and thus the incidence of secondary bacterial pneumonia.

TOXIC GASES

Certain gases also impair respiratory defense mechanisms, rendering animals more susceptible to secondary bacterial infections. For instance, hydrogen sulfide and ammonia, frequently encountered on farms—especially in buildings with poor ventilation—can impair pulmonary defense mechanisms and increase susceptibility to bacterial pneumonia. The effects of environmental

Box **9-3**

Postulated Mechanisms by Which Viruses May Impair the Defense Mechanisms of the Respiratory Tract

Changes in mucociliary clearance
Injured epithelium enhances attachment for bacteria
Enhanced bacterial attachment predisposes to colonization
Decreased mucociliary clearance prolongs resident time of bacteria favoring colonization
Injured epithelium prevent mucociliary clearance and physical removal of bacteria
Lack of secretory products facilitate further cell injury
Break down the antimicrobial barrier in mucus and cells (β-defensins and anionic peptides)
Ciliostasis caused by inflammation or by some pathogenic organism (mycoplasmas)
Dysfunction of pulmonary alveolar macrophages and lymphocytes
Consolidation of lung cause hypoxia resulting in decreased phagocytosis
Infected macrophages fail to release chemotactic factors for other cells
Infected macrophages fail to attach and ingest bacteria
Lysosomes become disoriented and fail to fuse with phagosome-containing bacteria
Intracellular killing or degradation is decreased because of biochemical dysfunction
Reduced cytokines and secretory products impair bacterial phagocytosis
Viral induced apoptosis of alveolar macrophages
Altered CD4 and CD8 lymphocytes

pollutants on the defense mechanisms of human beings and animals living in crowded and polluted cities remain to be determined.

IMMUNODEFICIENCY

Immunodeficiency disorders, whether acquired or congenital, are often associated with increased susceptibility to viral, bacterial, and protozoal pneumonias. For instance, human beings with acquired immunodeficiency syndrome (AIDS) are notably susceptible to pneumonia caused by proliferation of *Pneumocystis carinii*. This ubiquitous organism, which under normal circumstances is not considered pathogenic, is also found in the pneumonic lungs of immunosuppressed pigs, foals, dogs, and rodents. Pigs infected with the porcine reproductive and respiratory syndrome (PRRS) virus frequently develop *Pneumocystis carinii* infection. Arabian foals born with combined immunodeficiency disease easily succumb to infectious diseases, particularly adenoviral pneumonia. Also, large doses of chemotherapeutic agents, such as steroids and alkylating agents, cause immunosuppression

in dogs, cats, and other animals, increasing susceptibility to secondary bacterial infections.

OTHER CONDITIONS THAT PREDISPOSE TO SECONDARY BACTERIAL PNEUMONIA

Uremia, endotoxemia, dehydration, starvation, hypoxia, acidosis, pulmonary edema, anesthesia, ciliary dyskinesia, and stress are only some of the many conditions that have been implicated in impairing respiratory defense mechanisms and consequently predisposing animals to develop secondary bacterial pneumonia. The mechanisms by which each of these factors suppresses pulmonary defenses are diverse and sometimes not well understood. For instance, hypoxia and pulmonary edema decrease phagocytic function of pulmonary alveolar macrophages and alter the production of surfactant by type II pneumonocytes. Dehydration is thought to increase the viscosity of mucus, reducing or stopping mucociliary movement. Anesthesia induces ciliostasis with concurrent loss of mucociliary function. Ciliary dyskinesia, an inherited defect in cilia, causes abnormal mucus transport; starvation, hypothermia, and stress can reduce humoral and cellular immune responses.

EXAMINATION OF THE RESPIRATORY TRACT

POSTMORTEM

The respiratory tract should always be examined in a systematic fashion. To determine whether negative pressure is present in the thoracic cavity, the diaphragm is punctured through the abdominal cavity before the thoracic cavity has been opened. When the diaphragm is punctured in a fresh carcass, the loss of negative pressure in the thorax causes the diaphragmatic cupola to drop back caudally toward the abdominal cavity, and at the same time, it makes an audible sound caused by the inrush of air into the thorax. Lack of this movement may be an indication of advanced pneumothorax, pleural effusion, or the presence of noncollapsible lungs because of pulmonary edema, pneumonia, fibrosis, or emphysema. In carcasses that have been dead for a long time, pulmonary air and gas produced by saprophytic bacteria leak into the pleural cavity, reducing pressure and collapsing the lung.

The rib cage must be removed by cutting along the costosternal joints and along the neck of the ribs (close to the costovertebral joints) in such a way that pleural adhesions and abnormal thoracic contents can be observed and grossly quantified (e.g., 200 ml of clear, yellow fluid). The tongue, pharynx, esophagus, larynx, trachea, and thoracic viscera (lungs, heart, and thymus) should be removed as a unit (often called the pluck) and placed on the postmortem table.

The pharynx and esophagus are opened starting at the pharynx by a single cut with scissors along the dorsal midline and inspected for ulcers, foreign bodies, and neoplasms. The larynx and trachea must be examined by opening both along the dorsal midline from cranial to caudal ends and then extending the incision into the large bronchi of the caudal lung lobes. Normal tracheo-bronchial mucosa has a smooth and glistening pearl-colored surface with empty lumina in airways. The presence of foamy fluid in airways indicates pulmonary edema. Feed particles may suggest aspiration; however, careful examination of the mucosa is required because aspiration of ingesta from stomach or rumen into the lungs commonly takes place at death or can be displaced into these areas when the carcass is moved.

The lungs should be examined before incision. Normal lungs have a pink color (Fig. 9-10). External changes include the presence of rib imprints on the pleural surface when lungs fail to collapse. In addition, the lungs should be inspected for changes in color and texture and distribution of lesions. Color changes can be various shades of red, indicating hypostatic congestion, hyperemia (acute pneumonia), and hemorrhage; dark blue collapsed lobules or areas are indicative of atelectasis; pale pink to white lungs indicate notable anemia, fibrosis, or emphysema; and uniformly or patchy yellow-brown lungs indicate chronic passive congestion and pulmonary fibrosis likely secondary to chronic heart failure. Lungs from exsanguinated animals are generally paler than the normal pink color because of reduced blood in the pulmonary tissue. A covering of yellowish material on the pleural surface indicates accumulation of fibrin. Because it is impossible to describe the texture of normal lungs,

repeated palpation is required to understand the actual texture of a normal lung. Texture is determined by gently palpating the surface and parenchyma of the lungs. Normal texture can change to firm, hard, elastic (rubbery), or crepitus (with a crackling sound or feeling). For a detailed description of lung texture, see Classification of Pneumonias. Palpation of the lungs, which should be gentle, also permits detection of nonvisible nodules or abscesses in the parenchyma. Knowing the distribution of a lesion in the lungs also facilitates diagnosis because particular etiologic agents cause lesions with specific distribution. Distribution of lesions is generally described as focal, multifocal, locally extensive, or diffuse. According to their topography, pulmonary lesions can also be classified as cranioventral, dorsocaudal, and so on.

Postmortem reports must also contain an estimate of the extent of the pulmonary lesions, preferably expressed as a percentage of the volume of the lungs affected. For instance, a report may read "cranioventral consolidation involving 40% of the lungs." If the lungs have focal lesions, a rough estimate of the number should also be included in the report. For instance, "numerous (approximately 25), small (1 to 2 cm in diameter), hard nodules were randomly distributed in all lung lobes."

Two methods are used to examine the nasal structures. The first is making a midsagittal cut through the head and removing the nasal septum; the second is making several transverse sections of the nose at the level of the second premolar teeth. This latter method is preferred when examining pigs suspected of having atrophic rhinitis or animals suspected of having nasal neoplasms.

HISTOPATHOLOGY AND BIOPSIES

Microscopic examination of pulmonary tissue is routinely done in diagnostic laboratories. Samples of normal and abnormal lungs, along with other appropriate tissue, should always be submitted in 10% buffered-neutral formalin for histopathologic evaluation. Lung biopsy specimens are taken only sporadically because complications often outweigh the diagnostic value. However, the use of new techniques, such as endoscopic-directed biopsies, has notably reduced some of these complications. Biopsies of the lungs are recommended in cases of chronic persistent pulmonary disease unresponsive to treatment or intrathoracic masses of undetermined origin. Endoscopic-directed biopsies of the nasal and bronchial mucosa are routinely used in clinical practice and generally have a much better diagnostic value.

BRONCHOALVEOLAR LAVAGE AND TRACHEAL ASPIRATES

Two valuable diagnostic tools in human medicine, bronchoalveolar lavage (BAL) and tracheal aspirates, have in recent years become more widely used in veterinary clinical diagnosis of respiratory ailments in

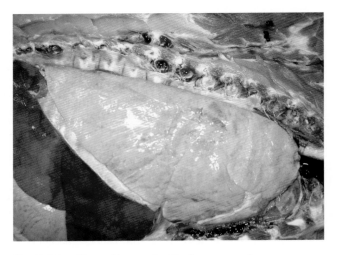

Fig. 9-10 **Normal lung, pig.** The lung parenchyma appears homogenously pink. The pale pink appearance of these normal lungs is due to exsanguination. The appearance of normal unexsanguinated lungs is bright pink to red. (*Courtesy Dr. A. López, Atlantic Veterinary College.*)

animals, particularly in horses, dogs, and cats. The basis of BAL is sampling to determine the cellular and biochemical composition of the lung in a live animal by infusing and retrieving sterile fluid via the trachea. BAL is done by inserting a tube directly through the larynx into a bronchus, or transtracheally by inserting a tube through a needle percutaneously into the cervical trachea. Microscopic examination of properly collected, stored, and processed samples may reveal many erythrocytes and siderophages in pulmonary hemorrhage or left side heart failure; inclusion bodies or syncytial cells in viral pneumonias; increased number of leukocytes in pulmonary inflammation; abundant mucus in asthma or equine heaves (chronic obstructive pulmonary disease [COPD]); presence of pulmonary pathogens, such as parasites, fungi and bacteria; or tumor cells in cases of pulmonary neoplasia.

DISEASES OF THE RESPIRATORY SYSTEM

NASAL CAVITY AND SINUS MUCOSA

PATTERN OF INJURY AND HOST RESPONSE

The conducting portion of the respiratory system is lined by pseudostratified columnar ciliated epithelium (most of the nasal cavity, paranasal sinuses, part of the larynx, and all of the trachea and bronchi), olfactory epithelium (part of the nasal cavity, particularly ethmoidal conchae), and squamous epithelium (nasal vestibulum and parts of the larynx). The pattern of injury, inflammation, and host response is characteristic for each of these three types of epithelium and independent of its anatomic location.

Pseudostratified ciliated epithelium, which lines most of the nasal cavity and nasopharynx, part of the larynx, and all of the trachea and bronchi, is exquisitely sensitive to injury. When these cells are irreversibly injured, whether caused by a viral infection, trauma, or inhalation of toxic gases, ciliated cells swell, typically lose their attachment to underlying basement membrane, and rapidly exfoliate (Fig. 9-11). A transient and mild exudate of plasma proteins and neutrophils covers the ulcer. In the absence of complications or secondary bacterial infections, a specific type of progenitor cell known as "nonciliated secretory cells" that is normally present in the mucosa migrates and undergoes mitosis to cover the denuded basement membrane, eventually differentiating into new ciliated epithelial cells (Fig. 9-11). Cellular migration, proliferation, and attachment are regulated by locally released growth factors and extracellular matrix proteins, such as collagen, integrins,

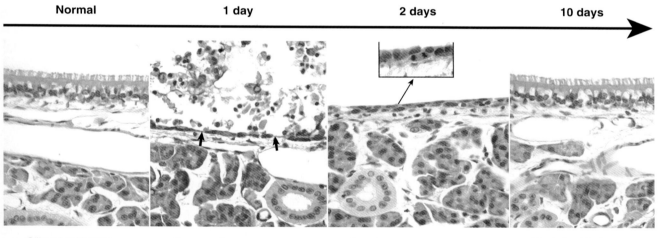

Normal	1 day	2 days	10 days
• Ciliated epithelium	• Degeneration	• Repair	• Healed epithelium
• ~250 cilia/cell	• Loss of attachment	• Preciliated cells	• Normal function
• Highly vascularized	• Necrosis	• Mitosis	
• Abundant glands	• Exfoliation	• Cell differentiation	

Fig. 9-11 **Normal and injured mucosa, nasal conchae, rats.** Normal ciliated epithelium composed of tall columnar cells with numerous cilia. Day 1. Nasal epithelium following exposure to air containing an irritant gas (hydrogen sulfide). Note detachment and exfoliation of ciliated cells, leaving a denuded basement membrane *(arrows)*. This same type of lesion is seen in viral or mechanical injury to the mucosa of the conducting system. Two days after exposure, the basement membrane is lined by rapidly dividing preciliated cells, some of which exhibit mitotic activity *(arrow)*. Ten days after injury, the nasal epithelium is completely repaired. H&E stain. *(From López A, Prior M, Yong S et al: Am J Vet Res 49:1107-1111, 1988.)*

and fibronectin. The capacity of ciliated epithelium to repair itself is remarkably effective. For instance, complete restoration of an uncomplicated ulcer of the tracheal mucosa can be completed in only 10 days. This sequence of cell degeneration, exfoliation, ulceration, mitosis, and repair is typically present in many viral infections in which viruses replicate in nasal, tracheal, and bronchial epithelium. Examples of transient infections of this type include human colds (rhinoviruses), infectious bovine rhinotracheitis (bovine herpesvirus 1), feline rhinotracheitis (feline herpesvirus 1), and canine infectious tracheobronchitis (canine adenovirus 2 and canine parainfluenza-2).

If damage to the mucociliary blanket becomes chronic, goblet cell hyperplasia results in excessive mucus production (hypersecretion) and reduced mucociliary clearance, and when there is loss of basement membrane, repair is by fibrosis and granulation tissue (scarring). In the most severe cases, prolonged injury causes squamous metaplasia, which together with scarring is an impediment to mucociliary clearance. In laboratory rodents, hyperplastic and metaplastic changes, such as those seen in nasal polyps and squamous metaplasia, are considered a prelude to neoplasia.

The second type of epithelium lining the conducting system is the sensory olfactory epithelium, present in parts of the nasal mucosa, notably in the ethmoidal conchae. The patterns of degeneration, exfoliation, and inflammation in the olfactory epithelium are similar to those of the ciliated epithelium, except that olfactory epithelium has only limited capacity for regeneration. When olfactory epithelium has been irreversibly injured, olfactory cells swell, separate from adjacent sustentacular cells, and finally exfoliate into the nasal cavity. Once the underlying basement membrane of the olfactory epithelium is exposed, cytokines are released by leukocytes and endothelial cells, and inflammatory cells move into the affected area. When damage is extensive, ulcerated areas of olfactory mucosa are replaced by ciliated and goblet cells or squamous epithelium, or by fibrous tissue, all of which eventually cause reduction or loss of olfactory function (anosmia).

Squamous epithelium, located in the vestibular region of the nose (mucocutaneous junctions), is the third type of epithelium present in the nasal passages. Compared with ciliated and olfactory epithelia, nasal squamous epithelium is quite resistant to all forms of injury.

ANOMALIES OF THE NASAL CAVITY

Localized congenital anomalies of the nasal cavity are rare in domestic animals and are often merely part of a more extensive craniofacial deformity (e.g., cyclops) or a component of generalized malformation (e.g., chondrodysplasia). Congenital anomalies involving the nasal cavity and sinuses, such as choanal atresia, some types of chondrodysplasia, and osteopetrosis, are incompatible with life. Examples of nonfatal congenital anomalies include cystic nasal conchae, deviation of nasal septum, cleft upper lip (harelip, cheiloschisis), hypoplastic turbinates, and cleft palate (palatoschisis) (see Fig. 7-1). Bronchoaspiration and aspiration pneumonia are common sequelae to cleft palate. Nasal and paranasal sinus cysts are slowly growing and expansive lesions that mimic neoplasia and cause severe cranial deformations in horses. These large cysts presumably originate congenitally from dentigerous tissue. As in other organs or systems, it is extremely difficult to determine the actual cause (genetic versus congenital) of anomalies based on pathologic evaluation.

METABOLIC DISTURBANCES OF THE NASAL CAVITY

Metabolic disturbances affecting the nasal cavity and sinuses are also rare in domestic animals. Amyloidosis, the deposition of amyloid protein (fibrils with a β-pleated configuration) in various tissues, has been sporadically reported in the nasal cavity of horses and human beings. Microscopic lesions are similar to those seen in other organs and consist of a deposition of hyaline amyloid material in nasal mucosa that is confirmed by a histochemical stain, such as Congo red. Unlike amyloidoses in other organs of domestic animals where amyloid is generally of the reactive type (amyloid AA), equine nasal amyloidosis appears to be of the immunocytic type (amyloid AL). Affected horses with large amyloid masses have difficulty breathing, epistaxis, and reduced athletic performance; on clinical examination, large, firm nodules resembling neoplasms (amyloidoma) can be observed in the alar folds, rostral nasal septum, and floor of nasal cavity.

CIRCULATORY DISTURBANCES OF THE NASAL CAVITY
CONGESTION AND HYPEREMIA

The nasal mucosa is well vascularized and is capable of rather dramatic variation in blood flow, whether passively a result of interference with venous return (congestion) or actively because of vasodilation (hyperemia). Congestion of the mucosal vessels is a nonspecific lesion commonly found at necropsy and presumably associated with the circulatory failure preceding death (e.g., heart failure, bloat in ruminants where the increased intraabdominal pressure causes increased intrathoracic pressure impeding the venous return from the head and neck). Hyperemia of the nasal mucosa is seen in early stages of inflammation, whether caused by irritations (e.g., ammonia, regurgitated feed), viral infections, secondary bacterial infections, allergy, or trauma.

HEMORRHAGE

Epistaxis is the clinical term used to denote blood flow from the nose (nosebleed) regardless of whether blood originates from the nasal mucosa or from deep in the lungs. Unlike blood in the digestive tract, where the approximate anatomic location of the bleeding can be estimated by the color the blood imparts to fecal material, blood in the respiratory tract is always red. This fact is due to the rapid transport of blood out of the respiratory tract by the mucociliary blanket and during breathing. Hemorrhages into the nasal cavity can originate from local trauma, erosions of submucosal vessels by inflammation (e.g., guttural pouch mycosis), or neoplasms. Hemoptysis refers to the presence of blood in sputum or saliva (coughing or spitting blood), and it is most commonly the result of pneumonia, lung abscesses, ulcerative bronchitis, pulmonary thromboembolisms, and pulmonary neoplasia.

Ethmoidal (progressive) hematomas are important in older horses and are characterized clinically by chronic, progressive, often unilateral nasal bleeding. Grossly or endoscopically, an ethmoidal hematoma appears as a single, soft, tumorlike, pedunculated, expansive, dark red mass arising from the mucosa of the ethmoidal conchae (Fig. 9-12). Microscopic examination reveals a capsule lined by epithelium and hemorrhagic stromal tissue infiltrated with abundant macrophages, some of which are siderophages.

INFLAMMATION OF THE NASAL CAVITY

Inflammation of the nasal mucosa is called rhinitis and that of the sinuses, sinusitis. These conditions usually occur together, although mild sinusitis can be undetected. Clinically, rhinosinusitis is characterized by nasal discharge.

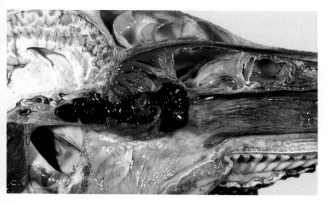

Fig. 9-12   Ethmoidal hematoma, midsagittal section of head, horse. A large amount of dark-red hemorrhage overlying the ethmoid conchae conceals an underlying hematoma in these conchae. *(Courtesy Dr. J.M. King, College of Veterinary Medicine, Cornell University.)*

The occurrence of infectious rhinitis presupposes an upset in the balance of the normal microbial flora of the nasal cavity. Innocuous bacteria present normally protect the host through a process called competitive exclusion, whereby potential pathogens are kept at harmless numbers. Disruption of this protective mechanism can be caused by respiratory viruses, pathogenic bacteria, fungi, irritant gases, environmental changes, immunosuppression, local trauma, stress, or prolonged antibacterial therapy.

Based on the nature of exudate, rhinitis can be classified as serous, catarrhal, purulent, fibrinous, or granulomatous. These types of inflammatory reactions can progress from one to another (i.e., serous to catarrhal to purulent), or in some instances exudates can be mixed, such as those seen in mucopurulent, fibrinohemorrhagic, or pyogranulomatous rhinitis. Microscopic examination of impression smears and bacterial or fungal cultures are generally required in establishing the cause of the exudate. Other results are hemorrhage, ulcers, and mucosal hyperplasia in inflamed nasal mucosa. Rhinitis also can be classified according to the age of the lesions as acute, subacute, or chronic; to the severity of the insult as mild, moderate, or severe; and to the etiologic agent as viral, allergic, bacterial, mycotic, traumatic, or toxic.

SEROUS RHINITIS

Serous rhinitis is the mildest form of inflammation and is characterized by hyperemia and increased production of a clear fluid locally manufactured by serous glands present in the nasal submucosa. Serous rhinitis is of clinical interest only. It is caused by mild irritants or cold air, and it occurs during the early stages of viral infections, such as the common cold in human beings and upper respiratory tract infections in animals, or in mild allergic reactions.

CATARRHAL RHINITIS

Catarrhal rhinitis is a slightly more severe process and has, in addition to serous secretions, a substantial increase in mucus production by increased activity of goblet cells and mucous glands. A mucous exudate is a thick, translucent, or slightly turbid viscous fluid, sometimes containing a few exfoliated cells, leukocytes, and cellular debris. In chronic cases, catarrhal rhinitis is characterized microscopically by notable hyperplasia of goblet cells. As the inflammation becomes more severe, the mucus is infiltrated with neutrophils giving the exudate a cloudy mucopurulent appearance. This exudate is referred to as mucopurulent.

PURULENT (SUPPURATIVE) RHINITIS

This inflammation, characterized by a neutrophilic exudate, occurs when the nasal mucosa suffers a more severe injury that generally is accompanied by mucosal necrosis and secondary bacterial infection. Cytokines, leukotrienes, complement activation, and bacterial products cause exudation of leukocytes, especially neutrophils, which mix with nasal secretions including mucus. Grossly the exudate in suppurative rhinitis is thick and opaque, but it can vary from white to green to brown, depending on the types of bacteria and type of leukocytes (neutrophils or eosinophils) present in the exudate (Fig. 9-13). In severe cases, the nasal passages are completely blocked by the exudate. Microscopically, neutrophils can be seen in the submucosa and mucosa and form plaques of exudate on the mucosal surface. Neutrophils are commonly found attached to the vessels and between epithelial cells in their migration to the surface of the mucosa.

FIBRINOUS RHINITIS

This reaction occurs when nasal injury causes a severe increase in vascular permeability, resulting in abundant exudation of plasma fibrinogen, which coagulates into fibrin. Grossly, fibrin appears like a yellow, tan, or gray rubbery mat on nasal mucosa. Fibrin accumulates on the surface and forms a distinct film of exudate sometimes referred to as pseudomembrane (Fig. 9-14). If this fibrinous exudate can be removed, leaving an intact underlying mucosa, it is termed a croupous or pseudodiphtheritic rhinitis. Conversely, if the pseudomembrane is difficult to remove and leaves an ulcerated mucosa, it is referred to as diphtheritic or fibrinonecrotic rhinitis. The term *diphtheritic* was derived from human diphtheria, which causes a severe and destructive inflammatory process of the

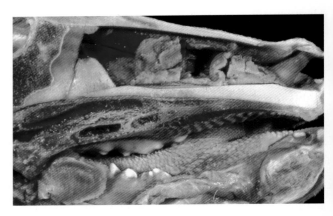

Fig. 9-14   Fibrinous rhinitis, midsagittal section of head, calf. Infectious bovine rhinotracheitis (IBR; bovine herpesvirus 1). The nasal septum has been removed to expose nasal conchae. The nasal mucosa is covered by diphtheritic yellow membranes consisting of fibrinonecrotic exudate. Removal of these fibrinous membranes reveals focal ulcers in the underlying mucosa. *(Courtesy Dr. Scott McBurney, Atlantic Veterinary College.)*

nasal, tonsillar, pharyngeal and laryngeal mucosa. Microscopically the lesions include a perivascular edema with fibrin, a few neutrophils infiltrating the mucosa, and superficial plaques of exudate consisting of fibrin strands mixed with leukocytes and cellular debris covering a necrotic and ulcerated epithelium. Fungal infections, such as aspergillosis, can cause a severe fibrinonecrotizing rhinitis.

GRANULOMATOUS RHINITIS

This reaction in the nasal mucosa and submucosa is characterized by infiltration of numerous activated macrophages mixed with few lymphocytes and plasma cells. In some cases, inflammation leads to the formation of polypoid nodules that, in severe cases, are large enough to cause obstruction of the nasal passages (Fig. 9-15). Granulomatous rhinitis is generally associated with chronic allergic inflammation or infection with specific organisms, such as those of systemic mycoses (see Lungs), tuberculosis, rhinosporidiosis, and with foreign bodies. In some cases, the cause of granulomatous rhinitis cannot be determined.

Inflammatory processes in the nasal cavity are not life threatening and usually resolve completely. However, some adverse sequelae in cases of infectious rhinitis include bronchoaspiration of exudate leading to bronchopneumonia. Chronic rhinitis often leads to destruction of the nasal conchae (turbinates), deviation of the septum, and eventually craniofacial deformation. Also, nasal inflammation may extend into the sinuses causing sinusitis, into facial bones causing osteomyelitis, through the cribriform plate causing meningitis, along the eustachian tubes causing otitis media and interna, and

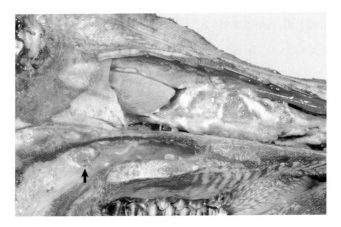

Fig. 9-13   Suppurative rhinitis, midsagittal section of head, calf. The nasal septum has been removed to expose nasal conchae. The nasal mucosa is covered by yellow-white purulent exudate. There is also a large, round ulcer in mucosa of the nasopharynx (*arrow*). *(Courtesy Western College of Veterinary Medicine.)*

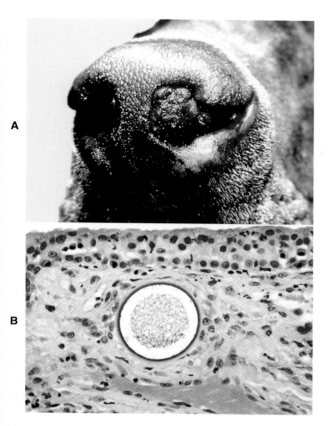

Fig. 9-15 **Granulomatous rhinitis (*Rhinosporidium seeberi*), nasal cavity and nostril, dog. A,** A polypoid granulomatous mass fills the rostral part of the left nasal cavity. **B,** Nasal granuloma containing a single large sporangium of *Rhinosporidium seeberi*. H&E stain. (***A,*** *Courtesy Dr. C. Bridges, College of Veterinary Medicine, Texas A&M University; and Dr. J.M. King, College of Veterinary Medicine, Cornell University.* ***B,*** *Courtesy Dr. A. López, Atlantic Veterinary College.*)

vestibular syndrome (abnormal head tilt and abnormal gait), which in severe cases may lead to emaciation.

SINUSITIS

Sinusitis occurs sporadically in domestic animals and is frequently combined with rhinitis (rhinosinusitis) or occurs as a sequela to penetrating or septic wounds of the cranium; improper dehorning in cattle, which exposes the frontal sinus; or tooth infection in horses and dogs (maxillary sinus). Based on the type of exudate, sinusitis are classified as serous, catarrhal, fibrinous (rare), purulent, and granulomatous (Fig. 9-16). Paranasal sinuses have poor drainage; therefore exudate tends to accumulate, causing mucocele (accumulation of mucus), or empyema (accumulation of pus). Chronic sinusitis may extend into the adjacent bone (osteomyelitis) or through the ethmoidal conchae into the meninges and brain (meningitis and encephalitis).

SPECIFIC DISEASES OF THE NASAL CAVITY AND SINUSES
EQUINE NASAL DISEASES
Equine viral infections

Viruses such as equine viral rhinopneumonitis virus, influenza virus, adenovirus, and rhinovirus cause mild and generally transient respiratory infections in horses. The portal of entry for these respiratory viruses is typically aerogenous. All these infections are indistinguishable clinically; signs consist mainly of malaise, fever, coughing, and nasal discharge varying from serous to purulent. Viral respiratory infections are common medical problems in adult horses.

Equine viral rhinopneumonitis (EVR). This disease, caused by two ubiquitous equine herpesvirus (EHV-1 and EHV-4), may be manifested as a mild respiratory disease in weanling foals and young racehorses or as abortion in mares. The portal of entry for the respiratory form is typically aerogenous and the disease is generally transient; thus, the primary viral-induced lesions in the nasal mucosa and lungs are rarely seen at necropsy unless complicated by secondary bacterial rhinitis, pharyngitis, or bronchopneumonia. Studies with polymerase chain reaction (PCR) techniques have demonstrated that, like other herpesvirus, EHV-1 and EHV-4 persist latently in the trigeminal ganglia for long periods of time. Reactivation because of stress or immunosuppression and subsequent shedding of the virus are the typical source of infection for susceptible animals on the farm.

Equine influenza. This disease is a common, highly contagious, self-limiting upper respiratory infection of horses caused by aerogenous exposure to type A strains of influenza virus (A/equi-1 and A/equi-2). Equine influenza has high morbidity (outbreaks) but low mortality, and it is clinically characterized by fever, conjunctivitis, and serous nasal discharge. It occurs mainly in 2- to 3-year-old horses at the racetrack. As with human influenza, equine influenza is usually a mild disease, but occasionally it can cause severe bronchointerstitial pneumonia with pulmonary edema. In some horses, impaired defense mechanisms caused by the viral infection is complicated by a secondary bacterial bronchopneumonia caused by opportunistic organisms (*Streptococcus zooepidemicus; Staphylococcus aureus; Bacteroides* sp.) found in the normal flora of the upper respiratory tract. Uncomplicated cases of equine influenza are rarely seen in the postmortem room.

Other equine respiratory viruses. Equine rhinovirus, adenovirus, and parainfluenza virus produce mild and transient upper respiratory infections (nasopharynx and trachea) in horses, unless complicated by secondary pathogens. In addition to reduced athletic performance, infected horses may have a temporary

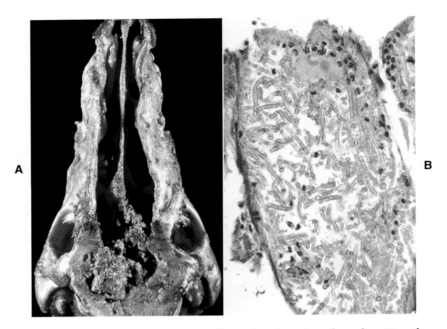

Fig. 9-16   **Fibrinonecrotic sinusitis, aspergillosis, dorsal section of nasal cavities, dog.**
A, The nasal conchae have been destroyed by chronic granulomatous inflammation.
Mycotic exudate remaining in the caudal aspect of the nasal cavity is yellow-green and granular.
B, Hyphae of *Aspergillus* spp. were isolated from the granulomatous inflammatory exudate.
Note the neutrophils at the periphery of the fungal matt. H&E stain. (**A,** *Courtesy College of Veterinary
Medicine, University of Illinois.* **B,** *Courtesy Dr. M.A. Wallig, College of Veterinary Medicine, University of Illinois.*)

suppression of cell-mediated immunity leading to opportunistic infections, such as *Pneumocystis carinii* pneumonia. Fatal adenoviral infections with severe pneumonia or enteritis occur commonly in immuno-compromised horses, particularly in Arabian foals with inherited combined immunodeficiency disease.

Equine bacterial infections: strangles, glanders, and melioidosis

Strangles, glanders, and melioidosis of horses are all systemic bacterial diseases that cause purulent rhinitis and suppuration in various organs. These diseases are grouped as upper respiratory diseases because nasal discharge is often the most notable clinical sign.

Strangles.   This infectious and highly contagious disease of Equidae is caused by *Streptococcus equi* ssp. *equi* (*Streptococcus equi*). It is characterized by suppurative rhinitis and lymphadenitis (mandibular and retropharyngeal) with occasional hematogenous dissemination to internal organs. Unlike *Streptococcus equi* ssp. *zooepidemicus* (*Streptococcus zooepidemicus*) and *Streptococcus dysgalactiae* ssp. *equisimilis* (*Streptococcus equisimilis*), *Streptococcus equi* is not part of the normal nasal flora. Infection occurs when susceptible horses come into contact with feed, exudate, or air droplets containing the bacterium. After penetrating through the nasopharyngeal mucosa, *Streptococcus equi*

drains to the regional lymph nodes—mandibular and retropharyngeal lymph nodes—via lymphatic vessels. The gross lesions in horses with strangles (mucopuru-lent rhinitis) correlate with clinical findings and consist of copious amounts of mucopurulent exudate in the nasal passages with notable hyperemia of nasal mucosa. Affected lymph nodes are enlarged and contain thick purulent exudate (purulent lymphadenitis). The term "bastard strangles" is used in cases where hematoge-nous dissemination of *Streptococcus equi* results in metastatic abscesses in such organs as the lungs, liver, spleen, kidneys, brain, or in the joints. This form of strangles is often fatal.

Common sequelae to strangles include broncho-pneumonia due to aspiration of nasopharyngeal exudate; laryngeal hemiplegia ("roaring"), resulting from compres-sion of the recurrent laryngeal nerves by enlarged retropharyngeal lymph nodes; facial paralysis and Horner syndrome caused by compression of sympathetic nerves; and purpura hemorrhagica as a result of vasculitis caused by deposition of *Streptococcus equi* antigen-anti-body complexes in arterioles, venules, and capillaries of the skin and mucosal membranes. In severe cases, nasal infection extends directly into the paranasal sinuses or to the guttural pouches via the eustachian tubes, causing inflammation and accumulation of pus (guttural pouch empyema). Rupture of abscesses in the mandibular and retropharyngeal lymph nodes leads to suppurative inflammation of adjacent subcutaneous tissue (cellulitis).

Strangles can affect horses of all ages, but it is most commonly seen in foals and young horses. It is clinically characterized by cough, nasal discharge, conjunctivitis, and painful swelling of regional lymph nodes. Some horses become carriers and a source of infection to other horses.

Glanders.   This infectious disease of Equidae is caused by *Burkholderia mallei (Pseudomonas mallei)* and can be transmitted to carnivores by consumption of infected horse meat. Human beings are also susceptible, and the untreated infection is often fatal. This bacterium has been listed as potential agent for biological warfare and bioterrorism. In the past, *Burkholderia mallei* was found throughout the world, but today glanders has been eradicated from most countries, except for some areas in North Africa, Asia, and Eastern Europe. There also have been some sporadic outbreaks reported in Brazil. The pathogenesis of glanders is not fully understood. Results from experimental infections suggest that infection occurs via the ingestion of contaminated feed and water and, very rarely, via inhalation of infectious droplets. The portals of entry are presumed to be the oropharynx or intestine, where bacteria penetrate the mucosa and spread via lymph vessels to regional lymph nodes, then to the blood stream, and thus hematogenously to the internal organs, particularly the lungs.

Lesions in the nasal cavity start as pyogranulomatous nodules in the submucosa; these lesions subsequently ulcerate, releasing copious amounts of *Burkholderia mallei*-containing exudate into the nasal cavity. Finally, ulcerative lesions in conchal mucosa heal and are replaced by typical stellate (star-shaped), fibrous scars. In some cases the lungs also contain numerous gray, hard, small (2 to 10 mm), miliary nodules (resembling millet seeds), randomly distributed in one or more pulmonary lobes because of the hematogenous route. Microscopically, these nodules are typical chronic granulomas composed of a necrotic center, with or without calcification, surrounded by a thick band of connective tissue infiltrated with numerous macrophages, some giant cells, lymphocytes, and plasma cells. Cutaneous lesions, often referred to as equine farcy, are the result of severe suppurative lymphangitis characterized by nodular thickening of extended segments of lymph vessels in the subcutaneous tissue of the legs and ventral abdomen. Eventually affected lymph vessels rupture and release large amounts of purulent exudate through sinuses to the surface of the skin.

Melioidosis (pseudoglanders).   This important, life-threatening disease of human beings, horses, cattle, sheep, goats, pigs, dogs, cats, and rodents is caused by *Burkholderia pseudomallei (Pseudomonas pseudomallei)*. This disease in horses is clinically and pathologically similar to glanders, hence the name *pseudoglanders*. In human beings, this infection can cause severe sepsis and septic shock, and has also been considered to have potential for biologic welfare. Melioidosis is currently present in Southeast Asia and, to a much lesser extent, in some European countries and Northern Australia, where the causative organism is frequently found in rodents, feces, soil, and water. Ingestion of contaminated feed and water appears to be the main route of infection; direct transmission between infected animals and insect bites has also been postulated as a possible mechanism of infection. After gaining entrance to the animal, *Burkholderia pseudomallei* is disseminated by the blood stream and causes suppuration and abscesses in most internal organs, such as nasal mucosa, joints, brain and spinal cord, liver, spleen, and lymph nodes. The exudate is creamy or caseous and yellow to green. The pulmonary lesions in melioidosis are those of an embolic bacterial pneumonia with formation of pulmonary abscesses. Focal adhesive pleuritis develops where abscesses rupture through the pleura and heal.

Other causes of equine rhinitis

Rhinosporidium seeberi causes nasal infection in human beings, horses, mules, cattle, dogs, and cats. Gross lesions vary from barely visible granulomas to large expansive polypoid nodules that may be mistaken as tumors. These granulomatous nodules are detected by direct observation when present in the nasal mucosa close to the nares or by rhinoscopy when located in the deep nasal cavity. The offending organism, *Rhinosporidium seeberi*, is readily visible in histologic preparations and in impression smears, appearing as a large (400 μm), oval sporangium containing thousands of endospores (Fig. 9-15). *Rhinosporidium seeberi* used to be considered a mycotic agent, but recent phylogenetic investigations suggest that it is an aquatic protistan parasite of the class Mesosmycetozoea.

BOVINE NASAL DISEASES
Infectious bovine rhinotracheitis (IBR; "rednose")

This disease is of great importance in the cattle industry because of the synergism of the IBR virus with *Mannheimia haemolytica* producing pneumonia. The causative agent, bovine herpesvirus 1 (BHV-1), has probably existed as a mild venereal disease in cattle in Europe since at least the mid-1800s, but the respiratory form was not reported until intensive management feedlot systems were first introduced in North America around the 1950s. Typically the disease is manifested as a transient, acute, febrile illness, which only in very severe cases results in inspiratory dyspnea caused by obstruction of airflow by exudate. Other forms of BHV-1 infection include ulcerative rumenitis, enteritis, and multifocal hepatitis in neonatal calves, nonsuppurative meningoencephalitis, infertility, and, in experimental infections, mastitis, mammillitis, and ovarian necrosis. Except for the encephalitic form, the type of disease caused by BHV-1 depends more on the site of entry than the viral strain. Like other herpesviruses, BHV-1 also can remain latent in nerve ganglia, with recrudescence following stress or immunosuppression. This virus also causes bovine abortion, systemic infections of calves, and genital infections, such as infectious pustular vulvovaginitis (IPV) and infectious balanoposthitis (IBP).

The respiratory form of IBR is characterized by severe hyperemia and focal necrosis of nasal, pharyngeal, laryngeal, tracheal (Figs. 9-14 and 9-17), and sometimes bronchial mucosa. As in other respiratory viral infections, IBR lesions are microscopically characterized by necrosis and exfoliation of ciliated cells followed by repair. Secondary bacterial infections of these areas of necrosis result in the formation of a thick layer of fibrinonecrotic material (diphtheritic) in the airway. Intranuclear inclusion bodies, commonly seen in herpesvirus infections, are rarely seen in field cases because inclusion bodies occur only during the early stages of the disease.

The most important sequela to IBR is pneumonia, which is caused either by direct aspiration of exudate from airways or as a result of an impairment in pulmonary defense mechanisms, thus predisposing the animal to secondary bacterial infection, most frequently *Mannheimia haemolytica* (see pneumonic mannheimiosis discussion). Postmortem diagnosis of IBR is confirmed by isolation of the virus or its identification by immunohistochemistry or PCR.

Other bovine rhinitis

Nasal granulomas occur in cattle presumably as a result of repeated exposure to as yet unidentified inhaled antigens. Nasal granulomas (atopic rhinitis) are reported mainly in cattle in Australia, South Africa, and the United Kingdom, where affected cattle develop multiple, small, pink or red, polypoid nodules, starting in the nasal vestibule which in time, extend into the caudal aspect of the nasal septum. These nodules are composed of fibrovascular tissue mixed with lymphocytes (granulation tissue) superficially lined by hyperplastic epithelium with abundant mast cells and eosinophils in the lamina propria (nasal eosinophilia). The microscopic features suggest that hypersensitivity type I (immediate),

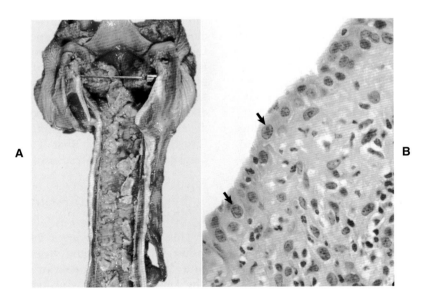

Fig. 9-17   Subacute fibrinous laryngitis and tracheitis, longitudinal (dorsal) section of larynx and trachea, calf. Infectious bovine rhinotracheitis (IBR; bovine herpesvirus 1). **A,** Thick plaques of fibrinonecrotic exudate cover the laryngeal and tracheal mucosae. **B,** Note the intranuclear inclusion (*arrows*), characteristic of herpes virus infection, in a tracheal mucosal epithelial cell. Chronic inflammation is also present in the subjacent connective tissue. (**A,** *Courtesy Dr. J.M. King, College of Veterinary Medicine, Cornell University.* **B,** *Courtesy College of Veterinary Medicine, University of Illinois.*)

type III (immune complex), and IV (delayed) may be involved in nasal granulomas of cattle. Bovine (idiopathic) nasal granuloma must be differentiated from nasal mycetomas, nasal rhinosporidiosis, and nasal schistosomiasis, which also cause the formation of nodules in the nasal mucosa of cattle. An eosinophilic material consistent with the Splendore-Hoeppli phenomenon is occasionally observed in bovine mycotic granulomas. This phenomenon seen in some mycotic or bacterial infections is microscopically characterized by a deeply eosinophilic homogenous material surrounded by bacteria or mycelia. It is thought to result from a localized antigen-antibody response in tissue.

OVINE AND CAPRINE NASAL DISEASE

Oestrus ovis (Diptera: Oestridae; nasal bot) is the brownish fly, about the size of a honeybee that deposits its first-stage larvae in the nostrils of sheep in most parts of the world. Microscopic larvae mature into large bots (maggots), which spend most of their larval stages in nasal passages and sinuses, causing irritation, inflammation, and obstruction of airways. Matured larvae drop to the ground and pupate into flies. This type of parasitism in which living tissues are invaded by larvae of flies is known as myiasis (Fig. 9-18). Although *Oestrus ovis* is a primarily nasal myiasis of sheep, it sporadically affects goats, dogs, and sometimes human beings (shepherds). The presence of the larvae in nasal passages causes chronic irritation and erosive mucopurulent rhinitis and sinusitis; bots of *Oestrus ovis* can be found easily if the head is cut to expose the nasal passages. Rarely, larvae of *Oestrus ovis* penetrate the cranial vault through the ethmoidal plate, causing direct or secondary bacterial meningitis.

Infectious rhinitis is only sporadically reported in goats and most of these cases are caused by *Pasteurella multocida* or *Mannheimia haemolytica*. The lesions range from a mild serous to catarrhal or mucopurulent inflammation.

PORCINE NASAL DISEASES
Inclusion body rhinitis

This disease of young pigs, with high morbidity and low mortality, is caused by a porcine cytomegalovirus (herpesvirus) and is characterized by a mild rhinitis. This virus commonly infects the nasal epithelium of piglets younger than 5 weeks. Because this disease is seldom fatal, lesions are seen only incidentally or in euthanized animals. In uncomplicated cases, the gross lesion is hyperemia of the nasal mucosa, but with secondary bacterial infections, mucopurulent exudate can be abundant. Microscopic lesions are typical and consist of a necrotizing, nonsuppurative rhinitis with giant, basophilic, intranuclear inclusion bodies in the nasal epithelium and glands (Fig. 9-19). Immunosuppressed piglets can develop a systemic cytomegalovirus infection

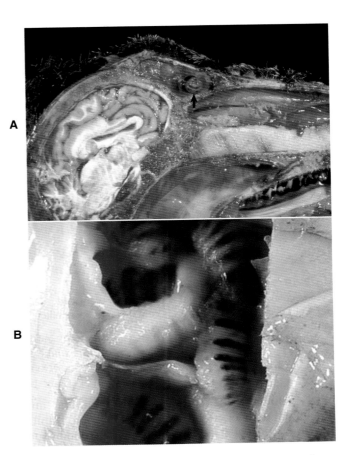

Fig. 9-18 **Oestrus ovis, sheep. A,** Frontal sinus. Note the parasitic (fly) larvae in the frontal sinus (*arrow*). **B,** Nasal cavity. Close-up view of larvae of *Oestrus ovis* in a nasal cavity. (**A,** *Courtesy Dr. M.D. McGavin, College of Veterinary Medicine, University of Tennessee.* **B,** *Courtesy Drs. M. Sierra and J. King, College of Veterinary Medicine, Cornell University.*)

characterized by necrosis of the liver, lungs, adrenal glands, and brain with intralesional inclusion bodies. Inclusion body rhinitis is clinically characterized by a mild and transient rhinitis, causing sneezing, nasal discharge, and excessive lacrimation.

Atrophic rhinitis

A common worldwide disease of pigs, atrophic rhinitis (progressive atrophic rhinitis) is characterized by inflammation and atrophy of nasal conchae (turbinates). In severe cases, atrophy of the conchae may cause a striking facial deformity in growing pigs because of deviation of the nasal septum and nasal bones. The etiopathogenesis of atrophic rhinitis is complex and has been a matter of controversy for many years. Pathogens historically associated with atrophic rhinitis include *Bordetella bronchiseptica*, *Pasteurella multocida*, *Haemophilus parasuis*, and viral infections such as porcine cytomegalovirus (inclusion body rhinitis). In addition, predisposing factors

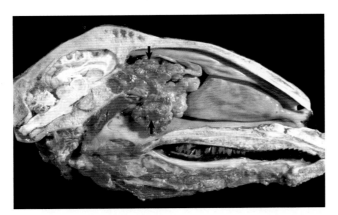

Fig. 9-23   Nasal adenocarcinoma (arrows), midsagittal section of the head, sheep. The tumor has occluded the right nasal passage and choanae. The location (ethmoturbinates) and type of tumor (carcinoma) are typical of retrovirus-induced "enzootic nasal carcinoma." *(Courtesy Dr. D.L. Craig, College of Veterinary Medicine, University of Tennessee.)*

eustachian tubes. The pathogenesis of these benign growths is uncertain, although many cases follow chronic rhinitis or sinusitis. Grossly, polyps appear as firm, pedunculated nodules of various sizes protruding from the nasal mucosa into the nasal passages; the surface may be smooth, ulcerated, secondarily infected, and hemorrhagic. Microscopically, polyps are characterized by a core of well-vascularized stromal tissue that contains inflammatory cells and are covered by pseudostratified or squamous epithelium.

Nasal and paranasal sinus cysts are common in horses and are of great medical importance because they clinically mimic neoplasms or infections. Although not considered a neoplastic growth, cysts are expansive and cause deformation or destruction of the surrounding bone. These cysts are typically composed of an epithelial cell capsule filled with yellow or hemorrhagic fluid, and do not recur after surgical removal. Ethmoidal hematomas also resemble nasal tumors in horses.

PHARYNX, GUTTURAL POUCHES, LARYNX, AND TRACHEA
PATTERNS OF INJURY AND HOST RESPONSE

The laryngeal mucosa is formed by columnar ciliated epithelium with goblet cells (mucociliary blanket) and squamous epithelium, whereas the trachea is exclusively lined by columnar ciliated epithelium. The pattern of injury and host response in the larynx and trachea is similar to those in the nasal mucosa (see Defense Mechanisms of the Conducting System). The pharyngeal mucosa, composed of squamous epithelium, has similar patterns of necrosis and inflammation as the oral mucosa (see Chapter 7).

ANOMALIES

Congenital anomalies of this region are rare in all species. Depending on their location and severity, they may be inconsistent with postnatal life, pose little or no problem, interfere with quality of life, or manifest themselves in later life. If clinical signs of respiratory distress, such as stridor, coughing, dyspnea, or gagging, do occur, they are usually exacerbated by excitement, heat, stress, or exercise.

BRACHYCEPHALIC AIRWAY SYNDROME

This clinical term refers to respiratory impairment caused by stenotic external nostrils and an excessive length of soft palate. These abnormalities are present in brachycephalic canine breeds, such as bulldogs, boxers, Boston terriers, pugs, Pekingese, and others. The defects are a result of a mismatch of the ratio of soft tissue to cranial bone and the obstruction of airflow by excessive length of the palatine soft tissue. Secondary changes, such as nasal and laryngeal edema caused by forceful inspiration, eventually lead to severe upper airway obstruction, respiratory distress, and exercise intolerance.

HYPOPLASTIC EPIGLOTTIS, EPIGLOTTIC ENTRAPMENT, AND DORSAL DISPLACEMENT OF THE SOFT PALATE

These anomalies are important causes of respiratory problems and reduced athletic performance in horses. An undersized epiglottis is prone to entrapment below the arytenoepiglottic fold, causing an equine syndrome known as epiglottic entrapment. This syndrome also occurs in horses with lateral deviation and deformity of epiglottis, epiglottic cysts, or necrosis of the tip of the epiglottis. Hypoplastic epiglottis also occurs in pigs. Dorsal displacement of the soft palate, particularly during exercise, creates narrowing of the nasopharynx and abnormal air turbulence in the conducting system of horses. Epiglottic entrapment is clinically characterized by airway obstruction, exercise intolerance, respiratory noise, and cough.

SUBEPIGLOTTIC AND PHARYNGEAL CYSTS

These types of anomalous lesions are occasionally seen in horses. These cysts vary in size (1 to 9 cm) and occur most commonly in the subepiglottic area and to a lesser extent in the dorsal pharynx, larynx, and soft palate. Cysts are lined by squamous or pseudostratified epithelium and contain thick mucus. Large cysts cause airway obstruction, reduced exercise tolerance, or dysphagia and predispose to bronchoaspiration of food.

TRACHEAL AGENESIS AND TRACHEAL HYPOPLASIA

Tracheal hypoplasia occurs most often in English bulldogs and Boston terriers; the tracheal lumen is decreased throughout its length.

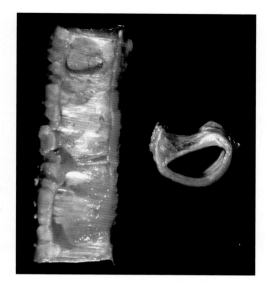

Fig. 9-24   Tracheal collapse, trachea, pony. *Left specimen:* The dorsal surface of the trachea is flattened dorsoventrally, the dorsal ends of the C-shaped tracheal rings are widely separated, and the dorsal ligament between the two ends is lengthened and thinned. *Right specimen* (transverse section): The ends of the tracheal rings are widely separated, and the dorsal wall of the trachea is formed by the lengthened and thinned dorsal ligament. *(Courtesy Dr. C.S. Patton, College of Veterinary Medicine, University of Tennessee.)*

TRACHEAL COLLAPSE AND TRACHEAL STENOSIS

Tracheal collapse with reduction in tracheal patency occurs in toy and miniature breeds of dogs, in which the condition is also called tracheobronchial collapse or central airway collapse. The defect also occurs in horses (Fig. 9-24), cattle, and goats. By radiographic, endoscopic, or gross examination, there is dorsoventral flattening of the trachea with concomitant widening of the dorsal tracheal membrane, which may then prolapse ventrally into the lumen. Most commonly, the defect extends the entire length of the trachea and only rarely affects the cervical portion alone. Affected segments with a reduced lumen contain froth and even are covered by a diphtheritic membrane. In horses, the so-called scabbard trachea is characterized by lateral flattening, so the tracheal lumen is a narrow vertical slit.

Segmental tracheal collapse causing stenosis has been associated with congenital and acquired abnormalities. In severe cases, abnormal cartilaginous glycoproteins and loss of elasticity of tracheal rings causes the trachea to collapse. In some other cases, it is an acquired tracheal lesion that follows trauma, compression caused by extraluminal masses, peritracheal inflammation, and flawed tracheotomy or transtracheal aspirate techniques.

Other tracheal anomalies include tracheoesophageal fistula, which is most commonly found in human beings and sporadically in dogs and cattle. It can occur at any site of the cervical or thoracic segments of the trachea. Acquired tracheoesophageal fistula can be a complication of improper intubation, tracheotomy, or esophageal foreign body.

DEGENERATIVE DISEASES
LARYNGEAL HEMIPLEGIA (PARALYSIS)

This disease, sometimes called *roaring* in horses, is a common, but obscure, disease characterized by atrophy of the dorsal and lateral cricoarytenoid muscles (abductor and adductor of the arytenoid cartilage), particularly on the left side. Muscular atrophy is most commonly caused by a primary denervation (recurrent laryngeal neuropathy) of unknown cause (idiopathic axonopathy) and to a much lesser extent, secondary nerve damage. Idiopathic laryngeal hemiplegia is an incurable axonal disease (axonopathy) of the cranial laryngeal nerve that affects mostly larger horses. Secondary laryngeal hemiplegia is rare and occurs after nerve damage caused by other pathologic processes, such as compression or inflammation of the left recurrent laryngeal nerve. The medial retropharyngeal lymph nodes are located immediately ventral to the floor of the guttural pouches. As a result of this close anatomic relationship, swelling or inflammation of the guttural pouches and retropharyngeal lymph nodes often results in secondary damage to the laryngeal nerve. Common causes of secondary nerve damage (Wallerian degeneration) include guttural pouch mycosis, retropharyngeal abscesses, inflammation because of iatrogenic injection into the nerves, neck injury, and metastatic neoplasms involving the retropharyngeal lymph nodes (e.g., lymphosarcoma).

Grossly the affected laryngeal muscle in a horse with laryngeal hemiplegia is pale and smaller than normal (muscle atrophy) (Fig. 9-25). Microscopically, muscle fibers have lesions of denervation atrophy (see Chapter 15). Atrophy of laryngeal muscles also occurs in dogs as an inherited condition (Siberian husky and Bouvier des Flandres), as a degenerative neuropathy in older dogs, secondary to laryngeal trauma in all species (e.g., choke chain damage), or to hepatic encephalopathy in horses.

The abnormal inspiratory sounds (roaring) during exercise in horses with laryngeal hemiplegia are caused by paralysis of the left dorsal and lateral cricoarytenoid muscles, which cause incomplete dilation of the larynx, obstructing of airflow, and vibration of vocal cords.

CIRCULATORY DISTURBANCES
LARYNGEAL AND TRACHEAL HEMORRHAGES

Hemorrhages in these sites occur as mucosal petechiae and are most commonly seen in coagulopathies,

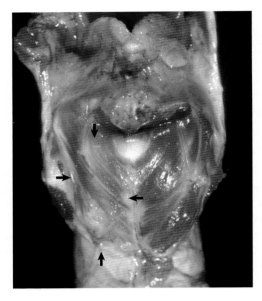

Fig. 9-25   Laryngeal hemiplegia, larynx, dorsal surface, 2-year-old horse. The left cricoarytenoideus dorsalis muscle is pale and atrophic *(arrows)*, whereas the right cricoarytenoideus dorsalis muscle is normal. *(Courtesy Dr. A. López, Atlantic Veterinary College.)*

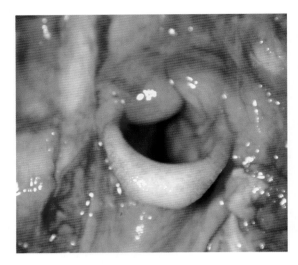

Fig. 9-26   Laryngeal edema, larynx, mature cow. Note the edematous thickening of the laryngeal mucosa of the vocal cords, which can cause respiratory distress due to the narrowing of the laryngeal lumen (rima glottidis). *(Courtesy Dr. J. Andrews, College of Veterinary Medicine, University of Illinois.)*

inflammation, and sepsis, particularly in pigs with classical swine fever (hog cholera) or salmonellosis. Severe dyspnea and asphyxia before death can cause congestion, ecchymosis, and petechiae in the laryngeal and tracheal mucosa; this lesion must be differentiated from postmortem imbibition of hemoglobin in autolyzed carcasses (see Chapter 1).

LARYNGEAL EDEMA

This lesion is a common feature of acute inflammation, but it is of particular importance because of its potential to obstruct the laryngeal orifice, resulting in asphyxiation. Laryngeal edema occurs in pigs with edema disease, in horses with purpura hemorrhagica, in cattle with acute interstitial pneumonia, in cats with systemic anaphylaxis, and in all species as a result of trauma, improper endotracheal tubing, inhalation of irritant gases (e.g., smoke), local inflammation, and allergic reactions. Grossly the laryngeal mucosa is thickened and swollen, often protrudes dorsally onto the epiglottis, and has a gelatinous appearance (Fig. 9-26).

TRACHEAL EDEMA

Also known as the "honker syndrome" or "tracheal edema syndrome of feeder cattle," this entity is a poorly documented, acute disease of unknown cause, most often seen during the summer months. Severe edema and a few hemorrhages are present in the mucosa and

submucosa of the dorsal surface of the trachea, extending caudally from the midcervical area to as far as the tracheal bifurcation. On a cut section, the tracheal mucosa is diffusely thickened and gelatinous. Clinical signs include inspiratory dyspnea that can progress to oral breathing, recumbency, and death by asphyxiation in less than 24 hours.

INFLAMMATION
PHARYNGITIS, LARYNGITIS, AND TRACHEITIS

Inflammation of the pharynx, larynx, and trachea are important because of their potential to obstruct airflow and to lead to aspiration pneumonia. The pharynx is commonly affected by diseases of the upper respiratory and upper digestive tracts, and the trachea can be involved by extension from both the lungs and larynx.

Intraluminal foreign bodies in the pharynx, such as medicament boluses, apples, or potatoes, can obstruct the larynx and trachea. Also, pharyngeal obstruction can be caused by masses in surrounding tissue, such as neoplasms of the thyroid gland, thymus, and parathyroid glands.

PHARYNGEAL PERFORATION

A number of nonspecific insults can cause lesions and clinical signs. Trauma may take the form of penetrating wounds in any species: perforation of the caudodorsal wall of the pharynx from the improper use of drenching or balling guns in sheep, cattle, or pigs: choking injury because of use of collars in dogs and cats; and the shearing forces of bite wounds. The results of the trauma may be minimal (local edema and inflammation) or as serious as fatal exudate. Foreign bodies may be trapped anywhere in the pharyngeal region; the location and size determine the occurrence of dysphagia, regurgitation, dyspnea, or asphyxiation. Pigs have a unique structure known as the pharyngeal diverticulum (4 cm long in adult pigs), which is located in the pharyngeal wall rostral and dorsal to the esophageal entrance. It is important because barley awns may lodge in the diverticulum, causing an inflammatory swelling that affects swallowing. The diverticular wall may be perforated by awns or drenching syringes, which results in an exudate that can extend down the tissue planes between muscles of the neck and even into the mediastinum. The pharynx of the dog may also be damaged by trauma from chicken bones, sticks, and needles, resulting in the formation of a pharyngeal abscess.

EQUINE PHARYNGEAL LYMPHOID HYPERPLASIA (PHARYNGITIS WITH LYMPHOID FOLLICULAR HYPERPLASIA)

This lesion is a common cause of partial upper airway obstruction in horses, particularly in 2- and 3-year-old racehorses. Lymphoid hyperplasia is also seen in healthy horses as part of a response to chronic pharyngitis, which in many instances tends to regress with age in older animals. The cause is undetermined, but chronic bacterial infection combined with environmental factors may cause excessive antigenic stimulation and lymphoid hyperplasia. The gross lesions, visible endoscopically or at necropsy, consist of variably sized white foci located on the dorsolateral walls of the pharynx and extend into the openings of the guttural pouches and onto the soft palate. In severe cases, lesions may appear as pharyngeal polyps. Microscopically, the lesion is hyperplastic lymphoid nodules. Clinical signs consist of stertorous inspiration, expiration, or both.

INFLAMMATION OF GUTTURAL POUCHES

The guttural pouches of horses are large diverticula (300 to 500 ml) of the ventral portion of the auditory (eustachian) tubes. These diverticula are therefore exposed to the same pathogens as is the pharynx and have drainage problems similar to those of sinuses. Although it is probable that various pathogens including viruses can infect them, the most common pathogens are fungi, which cause guttural pouch mycosis and guttural pouch empyema. Because of the close anatomic proximity of guttural pouches to the internal carotid arteries, cranial nerves (VI, IX, X, XI, and XII), and atlantooccipital joint, disease of these diverticula may involve these structures and cause a variety of clinical signs in horses.

Guttural pouch mycosis occurs primarily in stabled horses and is caused by *Aspergillus fumigatus* and other *Aspergillus* species. Infection is usually unilateral and

presumably starts with the inhalation of spores from moldy hay. Grossly the mucosal surfaces of the dorsal and lateral walls of the guttural pouch mucosa are covered by a diphtheritic, fibrinonecrotic exudate. Microscopically the lesions are severe necrotic inflammation of the mucosa and submucosa with widespread vasculitis and intralesional fungal hyphae. The characteristic necrosis of this mycotic disease and its proximity to the internal carotid artery explain why guttural pouch mycosis can lead to vascular erosion with leakage of blood into the guttural pouch and epistaxis. Invasion of the internal carotid artery causes arteritis, which can also lead to formation of an aneurysm and fatal bleeding into the guttural pouches. In other cases, the fungi may be angioinvasive, leading to the release of mycotic emboli into the internal carotid artery, generally resulting in multiple cerebral infarcts. Dysphagia, another clinical sign seen in guttural pouch mycosis, is associated with damage to the pharyngeal branches of the vagus and glossopharyngeal nerves, which lie on the ventral aspect of the pouches. Horner's syndrome results from damage to the cranial cervical ganglion and sympathetic fibers located in the caudodorsal aspect of the pouches. Finally, equine laryngeal paralysis (hemiplegia) can result from damage to the laryngeal nerves as previously described in Degenerative Disease, Laryngeal Hemiplegia (Paralysis).

Empyema of guttural pouches is a sequela to suppurative inflammation of the nasal cavities, most commonly from *Streptococcus equi* infection (strangles). In severe cases, the entire guttural pouch can be filled with purulent exudate (Fig. 9-27). The sequelae are similar to those of guttural pouch mycosis except that there is no erosion of the internal carotid artery. It is clinically characterized by nasal discharge, enlarged retropharyngeal lymph nodes, parotid swelling, dysphagia, and respiratory distress.

NECROTIC LARYNGITIS (CALF DIPHTHERIA, OROLARYNGEAL NECROBACILLOSIS)

Necrotic laryngitis is a common disease of feedlot cattle and cattle affected with other diseases, with nutritional deficiencies, or housed under unsanitary conditions. It also occurs in sheep. Necrotic laryngitis, caused by *Fusobacterium necrophorum*, is part of the syndrome termed orolaryngeal necrobacillosis, which can include lesions of the tongue, cheeks, palate, and pharynx. An opportunistic pathogen, *Fusobacterium necrophorum* produces several exotoxins and endotoxins after gaining entry either through lesions of viral infections, such as IBR and exudative stomatitis in cattle, or after traumatic injury produced by feed or careless use of specula or balling guns.

The gross lesions, regardless of location in the mouth or larynx (most common in the mucosa overlying the laryngeal cartilages), consist of well-demarcated, dry,

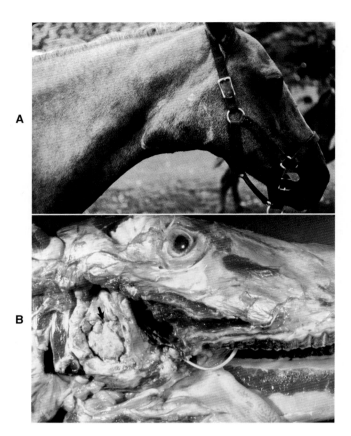

Fig. 9-27   Guttural pouch empyema, guttural pouch, horse.
A, Note the swollen right neck (*outlined in yellow*) in this horse
with guttural pouch empyema. **B,** The guttural pouch is
filled with masses of inspissated purulent exudate (*arrow*).
(**A,** *Courtesy College of Veterinary Medicine, University of Illinois.* **B,** *Courtesy
Dr. M.D. McGavin, College of Veterinary Medicine, University of Tennessee.*)

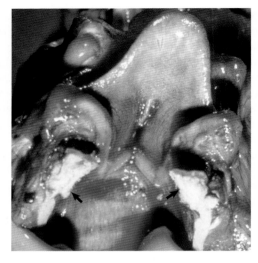

**Fig. 9-28   Necrotic laryngitis, calf diphtheria (*Fusobacterium
necrophorum*), larynx, calf.** Plaques of fibrinopurulent exudate
are present on the mucosa of the arytenoid cartilages (*arrows*).
Pieces of the exudate can be aspirated into the lungs and cause
bronchopneumonia. (*Courtesy Ontario Veterinary College.*)

yellow-gray, thick-crusted, fibrinonecrotic exudate
(Fig. 9-28) that, in the early stages, is bounded by a zone
of active hyperemia. Deep ulceration develops, and if
the lesion does not result in death, healing is by granulation tissue formation. Microscopically the necrotic
foci are first surrounded by hyperemic borders, then by
a band of leukocytes, and finally the ulcers heal by
granulation tissue and collagen (fibrosis). The lesions
can extend deep into the submucosal tissue. Numerous
bacteria are evident at the advancing edge.

There are numerous and important sequelae to calf
diphtheria, the most serious being death because of toxemia or fusobacteremia. Sometimes the exudate may be
copious enough to cause asphyxiation or be aspirated
and cause bronchopneumonia. The clinical signs of
necrotic laryngitis are fever, anorexia, depression, halitosis, moist painful cough, dysphagia, and inspiratory dyspnea and ventilatory failure because of fatigue of the
respiratory muscles (diaphragm and intercostal).

LARYNGEAL CONTACT ULCERS

Ulcerative lesions in the larynx are commonly
found in feedlot cattle. Grossly the laryngeal mucosa
reveals circular ulcers (up to 1 cm in diameter), which
may be unilateral or bilateral and sometimes deep
enough to expose the underlying arytenoid cartilages.
The cause has not been established, but causal agents
such as viral, bacterial, and traumatic have been proposed along with increased frequency and rate of closure of the larynx (excessive swallowing and
vocalization) when cattle are exposed to market and
feedlot stresses, such as dust, pathogens, and interruption of feeding. Contact ulcers predispose a calf to
diphtheria (*Fusobacterium necrophorum*) and laryngeal
papillomas. Ulceration of the mucosa and necrosis of
the laryngeal cartilages have also been described in
calves, sheep, and horses under the term *laryngeal
chondritis*. Laryngeal abscesses involving the mucosa
and underlying cartilage occur as a herd or flock problem in calves and sheep, presumably caused by a secondary infection with *Arcanobacterium pyogenes*
(*Actinomyces pyogenes*; *Corynebacterium pyogenes*).

TRACHEITIS

The types of injury and host inflammatory responses
in the trachea are essentially the same as those described
for the nasal mucosa. Although tracheal mucosa is prone
to aerogenous injury and necrosis, it has a remarkable
capacity for repair. The most common causes of tracheitis
are viral infections, such as those causing infectious

bovine rhinotracheitis (IBR) (Fig. 9-17), equine virus rhinopneumonitis (EVR), canine distemper, and feline rhinotracheitis. Viral lesions are generally mild and transient, but often become complicated with secondary bacterial infections.

Chemical tracheitis is also commonly seen following aspiration. Also, inhalation of fumes during barn fires can cause extensive injury and necrosis of the tracheal mucosa. In forensic cases, the presence of carbon pigment in the mucosal surface of trachea, bronchi, and bronchioles indicates that the burned animal was alive during the fire.

According to the exudate, tracheitis in all animal species is classified as catarrhal, purulent, fibrinous, or granulomatous. Chronic polypoid tracheitis occurs in dogs and cats, probably secondary to chronic infection.

Canine infectious tracheobronchitis (kennel cough)

This highly contagious infection is clinically characterized by an acute onset of coughing notably exacerbated by exercise. The term is nonspecific, much like "common cold" in human beings or "pneumonic mannheimiosis" in cattle. The infection occurs commonly as a result of mixing dogs from different origins, such as occurs at commercial kennels, animal shelters, and veterinary clinics. Between bouts of coughing, most animals appear normal, although some have rhinitis, pharyngitis, tonsillitis, or conjunctivitis; and some with secondary pneumonia become quite ill.

The cause of canine infectious tracheobronchitis is complex, and many pathogens and environmental factors have been incriminated. *Bordetella bronchiseptica*, canine adenovirus 2 (CAV-2), and canine parainfluenza virus (CPV) are most commonly implicated. The severity of the disease is increased when more than one agent is involved or extreme environmental conditions (e.g., poor ventilation) add additional stresses. For example, dogs asymptomatically infected with *Bordetella bronchiseptica* are more severely affected by superinfection with CAV-2 than those not carrying the bacterium. Other agents sometimes isolated but of lesser significance include CAV-1 (infectious canine hepatitis virus), reovirus type 1, canine herpesvirus, and *Mycoplasma* species.

Depending on the agents involved, gross and microscopic lesions are completely absent or they vary from catarrhal to mucopurulent tracheobronchitis, with enlargement of the tonsils and retropharyngeal and tracheobronchial lymph nodes. In dogs with *Bordetella bronchiseptica* infection, the lesions are suppurative or mucopurulent rhinitis and tracheobronchitis, and suppurative bronchiolitis. In contrast, when lesions are purely viral, microscopic changes are focal necrosis of the tracheobronchial epithelium. Sequelae can include spread either proximally or distally into the respiratory tract, the latter sometimes inducing chronic bronchitis and bronchopneumonia.

PARASITIC DISEASES OF THE LARYNX AND TRACHEA

Parasitic infections of the larynx and trachea can have dramatic obstructive consequences, but burdens sufficient to cause such effects are not commonly seen in veterinary practice.

BESNOITIOSIS (*BESNOITIA BENNETTI*; *BESNOITIA BESNOITI*)

This apicomplexan coccidian parasite, whose life cycle is still unknown, can cause pedunculated lesions in the skin, sclera, nasal cavity, and larynx of horses and donkeys, cattle, and wild animals. Besnoitiosis has been reported from Africa, Central and South America, and Britain. Grossly, pale, round, exophytic nodules up to 2 cm in diameter can be observed protruding from mucosal surfaces. These nodules microscopically consist of fingerlike projections covered by hyperplastic and sometimes, ulcerated epithelium containing numerous thick-walled parasitic cysts with little inflammatory response.

MAMMOMONOGAMUS LARYNGEUS (*SYNGAMUS LARYNGEUS*)

This nematode is seen attached to the laryngeal mucosa of cattle in tropical Asia and South America, and cats (gapeworm) in the Caribbean and Southern United States. Occasionally, human beings with a persistent cough or asthmalike symptoms have the parasite in the larynx or bronchi.

OSLERUS (*FILAROIDES*) OSLERI

This parasite of dogs and other Canidae causes characteristic protruding nodules into the lumen at the tracheal bifurcation. They are readily seen on endoscopic examination or at necropsy. In severe cases, these nodules can extend 5 cm cranially or caudally from the tracheal bifurcation and even into primary and secondary bronchi. The disease occurs worldwide, and *Oslerus osleri* is considered the most common respiratory nematode of dogs.

The gross lesions are variably sized, up to 1 cm, submucosal nodules that extend up to 1 cm into the tracheal lumen (Fig. 9-29). Microscopically a mild mononuclear cell reaction is present when parasites are alive, but with the death of the parasite, an intense foreign body reaction develops with neutrophils and giant cells. Clinically, it can be asymptomatic, although it most often causes a chronic cough that can be exacerbated by exercise or excitement. Severe infestations can result in dyspnea, exercise intolerance, cyanosis, emaciation, and even death in young dogs.

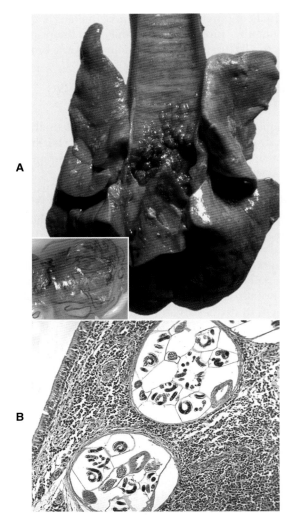

Fig. 9-29   **Parasitic tracheobronchitis (*Oslerus osleri*), trachea and main bronchi, dog. A,** Note the numerous large parasitic nodules on the mucosal surface of the distal trachea and main bronchi. These nodules cause clinical signs only in severe infections. *Inset:* Filarial forms of *Oselrus osleri* can be seen in the nodule. **B,** Filarial forms of *Oselrus osleri* can be seen in the lamina propria of the tracheal mucosa. Numerous chronic inflammatory cells are also present. H&E stain. (*A, Courtesy Dr. M.D. McGavin, College of Veterinary Medicine, University of Tennessee. Inset and B, Courtesy College of Veterinary Medicine, University of Illinois.*)

NEOPLASMS OF GUTTURAL POUCHES, LARYNX, AND TRACHEA
NEOPLASMS OF THE GUTTURAL POUCHES

These occur rarely in horses and are usually squamous cell carcinomas.

NEOPLASMS OF THE LARYNX AND TRACHEA

Laryngeal neoplasms are rare in dogs and extremely so in other species, although they have been reported in cats and horses.

The most common laryngeal neoplasm in dogs is squamous cell carcinoma. Other less common tumors are laryngeal rhabdomyoma previously referred to as laryngeal oncocytoma, and chondromas and osteochondromas. Lymphoma involving the laryngeal tissue is sporadically seen in cats.

When large enough to be obstructive, neoplasms may cause a change or loss of voice, cough, or respiratory distress with cyanosis, collapse, and syncope. Other signs include dysphagia, anorexia, and exercise intolerance. The neoplasm is sometimes visible from the oral cavity and causes swelling of the neck. The prognosis is poor, as most lesions recur after excision.

Tracheal neoplasms are even more uncommon than those of the larynx. The tracheal cartilage or mucosa can be the site of an osteochondroma, leiomyoma, osteosarcoma, mast cell tumor, and carcinoma. Lymphosarcomas in cats can extend from the mediastinum to involve the trachea.

LUNGS
SPECIES DIFFERENCES

Each lung is subdivided into various numbers of pulmonary lobes. In the past, these were defined by anatomic fissures. However, in current anatomy, lobes are defined by the ramification of the bronchial tree. Following this criterion, the left lung of all domestic species is composed of cranial and caudal lobes, whereas the right lung, depending on species, is composed of cranial, middle (absent in horse), caudal, and accessory lobes. Each pulmonary lobe is further subdivided by connective tissue into pulmonary lobules, which in some species are rather prominent and in others are much less conspicuous. From a practical point of view, identification of the lungs among different species could be achieved by carefully observing the degree of lobation (external fissures) and the degree of lobulation (connective tissue between lobules). Cattle and pigs have well-lobated and well-lobulated lungs; sheep and goats have well-lobated but poorly lobulated lungs; horses have both poorly lobated and poorly lobulated lungs and resemble human lungs; finally, dogs and cats have well-lobated but not well-lobulated lungs. The degree of lobulation determines the degree of air movement between the lobules. In pigs and cattle, movement of air between lobules is practically absent because of the thick connective tissue wall separating individual lobules. This movement of air between lobules and between adjacent alveoli (pores of Kohn) constitutes what is referred to as collateral ventilation. This collateral ventilation is poor in cattle and pigs and good in dogs. The functional implications of collateral ventilation are discussed under Pulmonary Emphysema.

The lungs have an interconnecting network of stromal tissue supporting the blood and lymphatic vessels, nerves, bronchioles, and alveoli. For purposes of simplicity, the pulmonary interstitium can be anatomically divided into contiguous compartments: (1) bronchovascular interstitium, where main bronchi and pulmonary vessels are situated; (2) interlobular interstitium separating pulmonary lobules and supporting small blood and lymph vessels; and (3) alveolar interstitium supporting the alveolar walls that contain pulmonary capillaries and alveolar epithelial cells (no lymphatic vessels here) (see blood-air barrier discussion under Alveoli). Pulmonary changes, such as edema and emphysema, may affect one or more of these interstitial compartments.

CONGENITAL ANOMALIES

Congenital anomalies of the lungs are rare in all species but are most commonly reported in cattle and sheep. Compatibility with life largely depends on the type of structures involved and the proportion of functional tissue present at birth. Accessory lungs are one of the most common anomalies and consist of distinctively lobulated masses of incompletely differentiated pulmonary tissue present in the thorax, abdominal cavity, or subcutaneous tissue virtually anywhere in the trunk. Large accessory lungs can cause dystocia. Ciliary dyskinesia (immotile cilia syndrome; Kartagener's syndrome) is characterized by defective ciliary movement, which results in reduced mucociliary clearance because of a defect in the microtubules of all ciliated cells and, most importantly, in the ciliated respiratory epithelium and spermatozoa. Primary ciliary dyskinesia often associated with *situs inversus* has been reported in dogs, which as a result usually have chronic recurrent rhinosinusitis, pneumonia, and infertility. Pulmonary agenesis, pulmonary hypoplasia, abnormal lobulation, congenital emphysema, lung hamartoma, and congenital bronchiectasis are occasionally seen in domestic animals. Congenital melanosis is a common incidental finding in pigs and ruminants and is usually seen at slaughter (Fig. 9-30). It is characterized by black spots, often a few centimeters in diameter, in various organs, mainly the lungs, meninges, intima of the aorta, and caruncles of the uterus. Melanosis has no clinical significance, and the texture of pigmented lungs remains unchanged.

METABOLIC DISTURBANCES
PULMONARY CALCIFICATION ("CALCINOSIS")

Calcification of the lungs occurs in some hypercalcemic states, generally secondary to hypervitaminosis D or from ingestion of toxic (hypercalcemic) plants, such as *Solanum malacoxylon* (Manchester wasting disease) that contain vitamin D analogs. It is also a common sequela to uremia and hyperadrenocorticism in dogs and to pulmonary necrosis (dystrophic calcification) in

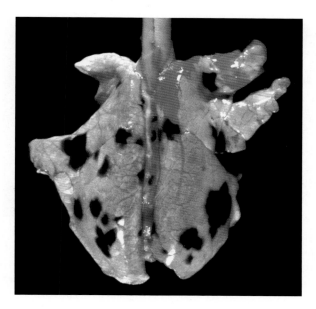

Fig. 9-30   Pulmonary melanosis, lungs, pig. Note the areas of black (melanin pigment) discoloration of the pleural surface. This pigmentation extends into the lungs and is an incidental finding that has no clinical or pathological significance. It is most common in "black-face" breeds. *(Courtesy College of Veterinary Medicine, University of Illinois.)*

most species. Calcified lungs may fail to collapse when the thoracic cavity is opened and have a characteristic "gritty" texture (Fig. 9-31). Microscopically, lesions vary from calcification of the alveolar basement membranes (Fig. 9-31) to heterotopic ossification of the lungs. In most cases, pulmonary calcification in itself has little clinical significance, although its cause (e.g., uremia or vitamin D toxicosis) may be very important.

ABNORMALITIES OF INFLATION

To achieve gaseous exchange, a balanced ratio of the volumes of air to capillary blood must be present in the lungs (ventilation/perfusion ratio), and the air and capillary blood must be in close proximity across the alveolar wall. A ventilation-perfusion mismatch occurs if pulmonary tissue is either collapsed (atelectasis) or overinflated (hyperinflation and emphysema).

ATELECTASIS (CONGENITAL AND ACQUIRED)

The term *atelectasis* means incomplete distention of alveoli and is used to describe lungs that have failed to expand with air at the time of birth (congenital atelectasis) or lungs that have collapsed after inflation has taken place (acquired atelectasis) (Figs. 9-32 and 9-33).

During fetal life, lungs are not fully distended, contain no air, and are partially filled with a locally produced fluid known as fetal lung fluid. Not surprisingly,

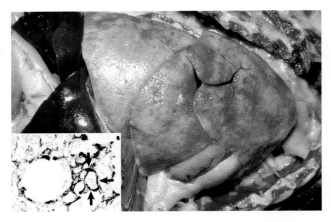

Fig. 9-31   Uremic pneumopathy from chronic renal failure, lung, 4-year-old dog. The lungs have failed to collapse when the thorax was opened because of extensive mineralization of alveolar walls. *Inset:* Calcification of alveolar septa. Note the linear deposits of mineral in the alveolar septa *(arrows).* von Kossa stain with nuclear fast red counterstain. (**Figure** and **Inset,** *Courtesy Dr. A. López, Atlantic Veterinary College.*)

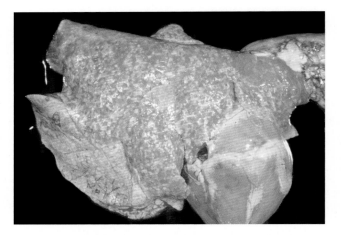

Fig. 9-32   Multifocal neonatal atelectasis, lung, 1-day-old calf. Prominent mosaic pattern of normally inflated *(light)* and atelectatic, uninflated *(dark)* lobules. Atelectasis is due to aspiration of amniotic fluid, meconium, and squamous epithelial cells, causing obstruction of small bronchi and bronchioles at the time of birth. All pulmonary lobes are involved. Although focal lobular atelectasis is commonly seen in neonates, this lesion suggests that the fetus was acidotic and aspirated amniotic fluid. *(From López A, Bildfell R: Vet Pathol 29:104-111, 1992.)*

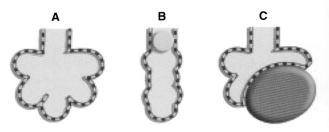

Fig. 9-33   Schematic representation of the types of atelectasis. A, Normal alveolar distention. **B,** Obstructive atelectasis; obstruction of airways (i.e., exudate or parasite) affecting airflow and causing alveolar collapse. **C,** Compressive atelectasis; mass (i.e., abscess or tumor) compressing the lung parenchyma and causing alveolar collapse. (**A, B,** and **C,** *Redrawn with permission from Dr. A. López, Atlantic Veterinary College.*)

occurs in newborns who fail to inflate their lungs after taking their first few breaths of air; it is caused by obstruction of airways, often as a result of aspiration of amniotic fluid and meconium (described under meconium aspiration syndrome) (Fig. 9-32). Congenital atelectasis also develops when alveoli cannot remain distended following initial aeration because of an alteration in quality and quantity of pulmonary surfactant produced by type II pneumonocytes and Clara cells. This form of congenital atelectasis is referred to in human neonatology as "acute respiratory distress syndrome" or as "hyaline membrane disease" because of the clinical and microscopic features of the disease. It commonly occurs in babies who are premature or born to diabetic or alcoholic mothers and is occasionally found in animals, particularly in foals and piglets. The pathetic, gasping attempts of affected foals and pigs to breathe have prompted the use of the name "barkers;" foals that survive may have brain damage from cerebral hypoxia (see Chapter 14) and are referred to as "wanderers," owing to their aimless behavior and lack of a normal sense of fear.

Acquired atelectasis is much more common and occurs in two main forms: compressive and obstructive (Fig. 9-33). Compressive atelectasis has two main causes: space-occupying masses in the pleural cavity, such as abscesses and tumors, or from the transferred pressures, such as that caused by bloat, hydrothorax, hemothorax, chylothorax, and empyema (Fig. 9-34). Another form of compressive atelectasis occurs when the negative pressure in the thoracic cavity is lost because of pneumothorax. This form generally has massive atelectasis and thus is also referred to as lung collapse.

Obstructive (absorption) atelectasis occurs when there is a reduction in the diameter of the airways caused by mucosal edema and inflammation, or when the lumen of the airway is blocked by mucus plugs, exudate,

lungs of aborted and stillborn fetuses sink when placed in water, whereas those from animals that have breathed float. At the time of birth, fetal lung fluid is rapidly reabsorbed and replaced by inspired air, leading to the normal distention of alveoli. Congenital atelectasis

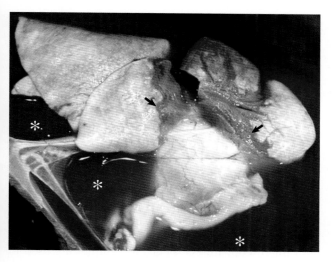

Fig. 9-34 **Atelectasis and hydrothorax, lungs, dog.** Atelectatic lung appears as dark depressed pulmonary tissues (*arrows*). Also note a large volume of transudate in the ventral pleural cavity (***). (*Courtesy Atlantic Veterinary College.*)

aspirated foreign material, or lungworms (Fig. 9-33). When the obstruction is complete, trapped air in the lung eventually becomes reabsorbed. Unlike the compression type, obstructive atelectasis often has a lobular pattern as a result of blockage of the airway supplying that lobule. This lobular appearance of atelectasis is more common in species with poor collateral ventilation, such as cattle and sheep. The extent and location of obstructive atelectasis depends largely on the size of the affected airway (large versus small) and on the degree of obstruction (partial versus complete).

Atelectasis also occurs when large animals are kept recumbent for prolonged periods, such as during anesthesia (hypostatic atelectasis). The factors contributing to hypostatic atelectasis are a combination of blood-air imbalance, shallow breathing, airway obstruction because of mucus and fluid that has not been drained from bronchioles and alveoli, and from inadequate local production of surfactant. Atelectasis can also be a sequel to paralysis of respiratory muscles and prolonged use of mechanical ventilation or general anesthesia in intensive care.

In general, the lungs with atelectasis appear depressed below the surface of the normally inflated lung. The color is generally dark blue and the texture is flabby or firm; they are firm if there is concurrent edema or other processes, such as can occur in "shock" lungs (see Pulmonary Edema). Distribution and extent vary with the process, being patchy (multifocal) in congenital atelectasis, lobular in the obstructive type, and of various degrees in between in the compressive type.

Microscopically the alveoli are collapsed or slitlike and the alveolar walls appear parallel and close together, giving prominence to the interstitial tissue even without any superimposed inflammation.

PULMONARY EMPHYSEMA

Pulmonary emphysema, often simply referred to as emphysema, is an extremely important primary disease in human beings, whereas in animals it is always a secondary condition resulting from a variety of pulmonary lesions. In human medicine, emphysema is strictly defined as an abnormal permanent enlargement of airspaces distal to the terminal bronchiole, accompanied by destruction of alveolar walls (alveolar emphysema). This definition separates it from simple air space enlargement or hyperinflation, in which there is no destruction of alveolar walls and which can occur congenitally (Down syndrome) or be acquired with age (aging lung, sometimes misnamed "senile emphysema"). The pathogenesis of emphysema in human beings is still controversial, but current thinking overwhelmingly suggests that destruction of alveolar walls is largely the result of an imbalance between proteases released by phagocytes and antiproteases produced in the lung as a defense mechanism (the protease-antiprotease theory). The destructive process is markedly accelerated by any factor, such as cigarette smoking, pollution, or defects in the synthesis of antiproteases in human beings that increases the recruitment of macrophages and leukocytes in the lungs. This theory originated when it was found that human beings with homozygous α_1-antitrypsin deficiency were remarkably susceptible to emphysema, and that proteases (elastase) inoculated intratracheally into the lungs of laboratory animals produced lesions similar to those found in the disease. More than 90% of the problem relates to cigarette smoking, and airway obstruction is no longer considered to play a major role in the pathogenesis of emphysema in human beings.

Primary emphysema does not occur in animals, and thus no animal disease should be called simply emphysema. In animals, this lesion is always secondary to obstruction of outflow of air or is agonal at slaughter. Secondary pulmonary emphysema occurs frequently in animals with bronchopneumonia, in which exudate plugging bronchi and bronchioles causes an airflow imbalance where the volume of air entering exceeds the volume leaving the lung. This airflow imbalance is often promoted by the so-called one-way valve effect caused by the exudate, which allows air into the lung during inspiration but prevents movement of air out of the lung during expiration.

Depending on the area of the lung affected, emphysema can be classified as alveolar or interstitial. Alveolar emphysema characterized by distention and rupture of the alveolar walls, forming variably sized air bubbles in pulmonary parenchyma, occurs in all species (Fig. 9-35). Interstitial emphysema occurs mainly in cattle, presumably because of their wide interlobular septa, and lack of collateral ventilation in these species does not permit air to move freely into adjacent pulmonary lobules. As a result, accumulated air penetrates the alveolar and bronchiolar walls and forces its way into the interlobular connective tissue, causing notable distention of the interlobular septa. It is also suspected that forced respiratory movements predispose to interstitial emphysema when air at high pressure breaks into the loose connective tissue of the interlobular septa (Fig. 9-35). Sometimes these bubbles of trapped air in alveolar or interstitial emphysema

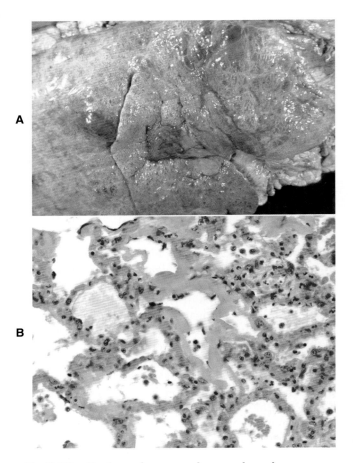

Fig. 9-35   Bovine pulmonary edema and emphysema (fog fever), lung, cow. A, Emphysema, edema, and interstitial pneumonia involving all pulmonary lobes. Note the variably sized air bubbles in the interlobular septa and pulmonary parenchyma. The texture of these lungs would be notably crepitus due to the accumulation of air in pulmonary parenchyma. **B,** Note the thick eosinophilic hyaline membranes lining the alveoli. The alveoli are dilated and also contain some edema fluid, occasional pulmonary macrophages, and necrotic alveolar cells. H&E stain. (**A,** *Courtesy Western College of Veterinary Medicine.* **B,** *Courtesy Dr. A. López, Atlantic Veterinary College.*)

become confluent, forming large (several centimeters in diameter) pockets of air that are referred to as bullae (singular: bulla); the lesion is then called bullous emphysema. This lesion is not a specific type of emphysema and does not indicate a different disease process, but rather is a larger accumulation of air at one focus. In the most severe cases, air moves from the interlobular septa into the connective tissue surrounding the main stem bronchi and major vessels (bronchovascular bundles), and from here air leaks into the mediastinum causing pneumomediastinum first, and eventually into the cervical and thoracic subcutaneous tissue causing subcutaneous emphysema.

It should be noted that mild and even moderate alveolar emphysema is difficult to judge at necropsy and by light microscopy unless special techniques are used to prevent collapse of the lung when the thorax is opened. These techniques include plugging of the trachea or intratracheal perfusion of fixative (10% neutral-buffered formalin) before the thorax is opened to prevent collapse of the lungs. Important diseases that cause secondary pulmonary emphysema in animals include small airway obstruction (such as heaves) in horses and pulmonary edema and emphysema (fog fever) in cattle (Fig. 9-35) and exudates in bronchopneumonia.

CIRCULATORY DISTURBANCES OF THE LUNGS

Lungs are extremely well-vascularized organs with a dual circulation provided by pulmonary and bronchial arteries. Disturbances in pulmonary circulation have a notable effect on gaseous exchange, which may result in life-threatening hypoxemia and acidosis. In addition, circulatory disturbances in the lungs can have an impact on other organs, such as the heart and liver. For example, impeded blood flow in the lungs because of chronic pulmonary disease results in cor pulmonale, which is caused by pulmonary hypertension followed by cardiac dilation, right heart failure, chronic passive congestion of the liver (nutmeg liver), and generalized edema (anasarca).

HYPEREMIA AND CONGESTION

Hyperemia is an active process that is part of acute inflammation, whereas congestion is the passive process resulting from decreased outflow of venous blood, as occurs in congestive heart failure (Fig. 9-36). In the early acute stages of pneumonia, the lungs appear notably red, and microscopically, blood vessels and capillaries are engorged with blood from hyperemia. Pulmonary congestion is most frequently caused by heart failure, which results in stagnation of blood in pulmonary vessels, leading to edema and egression of erythrocytes into the alveolar spaces. As with any other foreign particle, erythrocytes in alveolar spaces are rapidly phagocytosed (erythrophagocytosis) by pulmonary

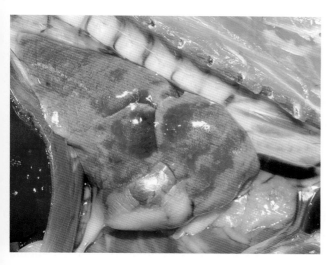

Fig. 9-36   Acute pulmonary congestion, lungs, dog. The lung parenchyma is red because of congestion of pulmonary vasculature and alveolar capillaries. *(Courtesy Dr. A. López, Atlantic Veterinary College.)*

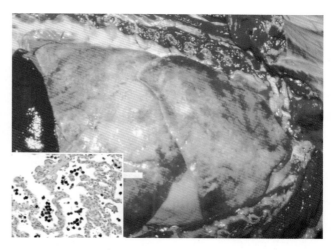

Fig. 9-37   Chronic congestion and edema, because of chronic heart failure (dilative cardiomyopathy), lungs, 5-year-old dog. The lungs have failed to collapse (fibrosis) and have a mottled and brownish appearance (hemosiderosis). *Inset:* Microscopic view of alveoli. Large numbers of macrophages containing hemosiderin (heart failure cells) are present in alveoli. During heart failure, red blood cells gain access to alveoli where they are rapidly phagocytozed by pulmonary macrophages and the iron of the hemoglobin molecule is converted to hemosiderin. Hemosiderin gives a positive reaction for iron with the Prussian blue reaction. Prussian blue (iron) reaction with nuclear fast red counterstain. *(**Figure** and **Inset,** Courtesy Dr. A. López, Atlantic Veterinary College.)*

alveolar macrophages. When extravasation of erythrocytes is severe, large numbers of macrophages with brown cytoplasm may accumulate in the bronchoalveolar spaces. The brown cytoplasm is the result of accumulation of considerable amounts of hemosiderin; these macrophages filled with iron pigment (siderophages) are generally referred to as heart failure cells (Fig. 9-37). The lungs of animals with chronic heart failure usually have a patchy red appearance with foci of brown discoloration because of accumulated hemosiderin. In severe and persistent cases of heart failure, the lungs fail to collapse because of edema and pulmonary fibrosis. Terminal pulmonary congestion (acute) is frequently seen in animals euthanized with barbiturates and should not be mistaken for an antemortem lesion.

Hypostatic congestion is another form of pulmonary congestion that results from the effects of gravity and poor circulation on a highly vascularized tissue, such as the lung. This type of gravitational congestion is characterized by buildup of blood in the lower side of the lung of animals in lateral recumbency, particularly horses and cattle. The affected portions of the lung appear dark red and can have a firmer texture. In animals and particularly human beings that have been prostrated for extended periods of time, hypostatic congestion may be followed by hypostatic edema, and hypostatic pneumonia as edema interferes locally with the bacterial defense mechanisms.

PULMONARY HEMORRHAGE

Pulmonary hemorrhages can occur as a result of trauma, coagulopathies, pulmonary thromboembolism

from jugular thrombosis or from embolisms of exudate from a hepatic abscess that has ruptured into the vena cava (cattle), disseminated intravascular coagulation, vasculitis, or sepsis. A gross finding that resembles pulmonary hemorrhage and often leads to an erroneous diagnosis is the aspiration of blood after the carotid arteries and trachea have been cut at the time of slaughter. Affected lungs have numerous, focal (1 to 10 mm) areas of red discoloration scattered randomly throughout the lungs.

Rupture of a major pulmonary vessel with resulting massive hemorrhage occurs occasionally in cattle when a growing abscess in a lung invades and disrupts the wall of a major pulmonary artery or vein (Fig. 9-38). In most cases, animals die rapidly, often with spectacular hemoptysis, and on postmortem examination, bronchi are filled with blood (Fig. 9-38).

"Exercise-induced pulmonary hemorrhage" (EIPH) is a specific form of pulmonary hemorrhage in racehorses following exercise and clinically is characterized by epistaxis. Because only a small percentage of horses with bronchoscopic evidence of hemorrhage have clinical epistaxis, it is likely that EIPH goes undetected in many cases. The pathogenesis is still controversial, but current literature suggests laryngeal paralysis, bronchiolitis,

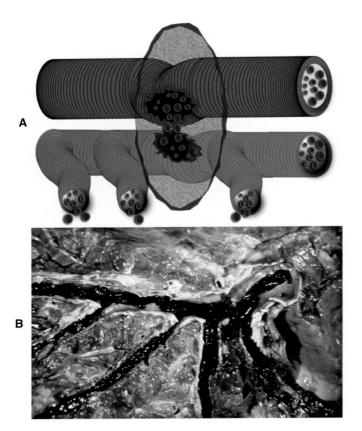

Fig. 9-38   **Fatal pulmonary hemorrhage. A,** Schematic of an abscess *(green)* eroding the wall of a major pulmonary artery *(red)* and causing bleeding into the airways *(blue).* **B,** Cut surface of lung, cow. Major bronchi and the trachea are filled with clotted blood. This cow died unexpectedly, with severe respiratory distress and blood coming from the nose and mouth. A large abscess in the lung had eroded through the wall of a major pulmonary vessel. (*A, Courtesy Dr. A. López, Atlantic Veterinary College. B, Courtesy Dr. R. Curtis, Atlantic Veterinary College.*)

extremely high pulmonary vascular pressures during exercise, alveolar hypoxia, and preexisting pulmonary injury as possible causes. EIPH is seldom fatal; postmortem lesions in the lungs of horses that have been affected with several episodes of hemorrhage are characterized by large areas of dark brown discoloration, largely in the caudal lung lobes. Microscopically, lesions are alveolar hemorrhages, abundant alveolar macrophages containing hemosiderin (siderophages), and mild interstitial fibrosis.

PULMONARY EDEMA

In normal lungs, fluid from the vascular space slowly but continuously passes into the interstitial tissue where it is rapidly drained by the pulmonary and pleural lymphatic vessels. Recent investigations demonstrated that alveolar fluid clearance across the alveolar epithelium

is also a major mechanism of fluid removal from the lung. Edema develops when the rate of fluid transudation from pulmonary vessels into interstitium or alveoli exceeds that of lymphatic and alveolar removal. Pulmonary edema can be physiologically classified as cardiogenic (hydrostatic; hemodynamic) and noncardiogenic (permeability) types.

Hydrostatic (cardiogenic) pulmonary edema develops when there is an elevated rate of fluid transudation because of increased hydrostatic pressure in the vascular compartment or decreased osmotic pressure in the blood. Once the lymph drainage has been overwhelmed, fluid accumulates in the perivascular spaces, causing distention of the bronchovascular bundles and alveolar interstitium, and eventually leaks into the alveolar spaces. Causes of hemodynamic pulmonary edema include congestive heart failure (increased hydrostatic pressure), iatrogenic fluid overload, disorders in which blood osmotic pressure is reduced, such as in the hypoalbuminemia seen in some hepatic diseases, nephritic syndrome, and protein-losing enteropathy. Hemodynamic pulmonary edema also occurs when lymph drainage is impaired and is generally secondary to neoplastic invasion of lymph vessels.

Permeability edema (inflammatory) occurs when there is excessive opening of endothelial gaps or damage to the blood-air barrier (endothelial cells or type I pneumonocytes). This type of edema is an integral and early part of the inflammatory response, primarily because of the effect of inflammatory mediators, such as leukotrienes, platelet-activating factor, cytokines, and vasoactive amines released by neutrophils, macrophages, mast cells, lymphocytes, and endothelial cells. These inflammatory mediators increase the permeability of the blood-air barrier. In other cases, permeability edema results from direct damage to the endothelium and pneumocytes, allowing plasma fluids to move freely from the vascular space into the alveolar lumen (Fig. 9-39). Because type I pneumonocytes are highly vulnerable to some pneumotropic viruses (influenza, BRSV), toxicants (NO_2, SO_2, H_2S, 3-methylindole), and particularly to free radicals, it is not surprising that alveolar edema commonly accompanies many viral or toxic pulmonary diseases. A permeability edema also occurs when endothelial cells in the lung are injured by bacterial toxins (sepsis), disseminated intravascular coagulation (DIC), anaphylactic shock, milk allergy, paraquat toxicity, and adverse drug reactions.

The concentration of protein in edematous fluid is greater in permeability edema (exudate) than in hemodynamic edema (transudate); this difference has been used clinically in human medicine to differentiate one type of pulmonary edema from another. Microscopically, edema fluid tends to stain more intensely eosinophilic in lungs with inflammation or damage to the blood-air

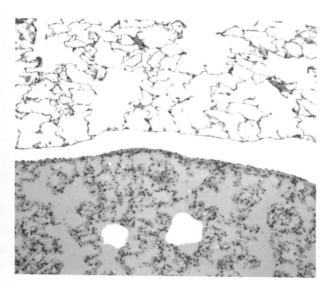

Fig. 9-39   Pulmonary edema, lung, rat. Normal lung with alveoli filled with air *(top)* and lung with severe pulmonary edema characterized by transudation of protein-rich fluid (deeply eosinophilic) filling the alveoli and congested alveolar septa *(bottom)*. H&E stain. *(Courtesy Dr. A. López, Atlantic Veterinary College.)*

barrier, because of its higher protein concentration than the fluid of hydrostatic edema from heart failure.

Grossly the edematous lungs—independent of the cause—are wet and heavy (Fig. 9-40); the color varies depending on the degree of congestion or hemorrhage; and fluid may be present in the pleural cavity. If edema is severe, bronchi and trachea contain considerable amounts of foamy fluid, which originates from the mixing of edema fluid and air. On cut surfaces, the lung parenchyma oozes fluid like a wet sponge. In cattle and pigs, the lobular pattern becomes rather accentuated because of edematous distentions of lymphatic vessels in the interlobular septa (Fig. 9-40). Severe pulmonary edema may be impossible to differentiate from peracute pneumonia; this fact is not surprising because pulmonary edema occurs in the very early stages of inflammation. Careful observation of the lungs at the time of necropsy is critical because diagnosis of pulmonary edema cannot be reliably performed microscopically. This is due in part to the loss of the edema fluid from the lungs during fixation with 10% neutral-buffered formalin and in part to the fact that the fluid itself stains very poorly or not at all with eosin because of its low protein content (hemodynamic edema). A protein-rich (permeability) edema is easier to visualize microscopically because it is deeply eosinophilic in

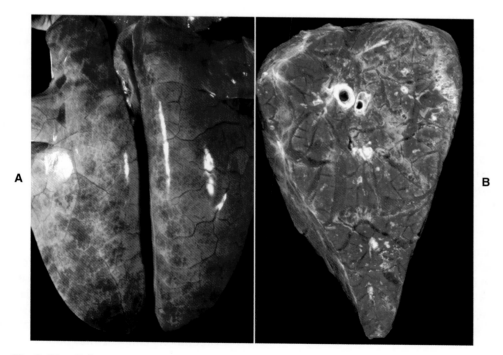

Fig. 9-40   Pulmonary edema, lungs, pig. A, The lungs are distended by edema fluid, which has resulted in rounded edges and edematous distention of the interlobular septa. **B,** The cut surface is wet and the interlobular septa are markedly distended with edema fluid. Lung lobules are also congested. (**A** and **B,** *Courtesy College of Veterinary Medicine, University of Illinois.*)

hematoxylin and eosin (H&E) stained sections (Fig. 9-39), particularly if a fixative—such as Zenker's solution, which precipitates protein—is used.

Acute (adult) respiratory distress syndrome (ARDS; shock lung) is an important condition in human beings characterized by pulmonary hypertension, intravascular aggregation of neutrophils in the lungs, diffuse alveolar damage, permeability edema, and formation of hyaline membranes, which are a mixture of plasma proteins, fibrin, surfactant, and cellular debris. The pathogenesis is complex and multifactorial but in general terms can be defined as diffuse alveolar damage that results from lesions in distant organs, from generalized systemic diseases, or from direct injury to the lung. Sepsis, major trauma, aspiration of gastric contents, extensive burns, and pancreatitis are some of the disease entities known to trigger ARDS. All these conditions provoke "hyperreactive macrophages" to directly or indirectly generate overwhelming amounts of cytokines (mainly TNF-α, interleukin [IL]-1, IL-6, and IL-8). Some of these cytokines prime neutrophils stationed in the lung capillaries to release enzymes and free radicals, thus causing diffuse endothelial and alveolar damage that culminates in a fulminating pulmonary edema. A syndrome analogous to ARDS occurs in domestic animals and explains why pulmonary edema is one of the most common lesions found in many animals dying of sepsis, toxemia, aspiration of gastric contents, and pancreatitis, for example.

Neurogenic pulmonary edema is another distinctive, but poorly understood form of lung edema in human beings that follows increased intracranial pressure (i.e., head injury, brain edema, brain tumors, or cerebral hemorrhage). This type of pulmonary edema can be experimentally reproduced in laboratory animals by injecting fibrin into the fourth ventricle. It involves both hemodynamic and permeability pathways presumably from massive sympathetic stimulation and overwhelming release of catecholamines. Neurogenic pulmonary edema has sporadically been reported in animals with brain injury or severe seizures or following severe stress and excitement.

PULMONARY EMBOLISMS

With its vast capillary bed and position in the circulation, the lungs act as a safety net to catch emboli before they reach the brain and other tissues. However, this positioning is often to its own detriment. The most common pulmonary emboli in domestic animals are thromboemboli, septic (bacterial) emboli, fat emboli, and tumor cell emboli.

Pulmonary thromboembolism generally originates from a thrombus present elsewhere in the venous circulation (Fig. 9-41). Fragments released inevitably reach the lungs and become trapped in the pulmonary

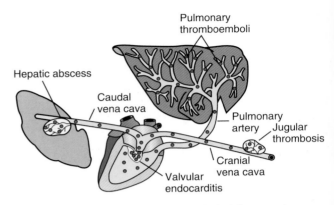

Fig. 9-41   **Sources of pulmonary emboli.** Schematic diagram of pulmonary emboli *(red dots)* arising from: (1) rupture of a hepatic abscess into the caudal vena cava; (2) vegetative valvular endocarditis (tricuspid valve); and (3) jugular thrombosis. Pulmonary infarcts are rare and often of little clinical significance because of the lung's dual arterial circulation (i.e., pulmonary and bronchial arteries). *(Redrawn with permission from Dr. A. López, Atlantic Veterinary College.)*

vasculature (Fig. 9-41). Small sterile thromboemboli are generally of little clinical or pathologic significance because they can be rapidly degraded and disposed of by the fibrinolytic system. Parasites such as *Dirofilaria immitis* and *Angiostrongylus vasorum*, endocrinopathies such as hyperadrenocorticism and hypothyroidism, glomerulopathies, and hypercoagulable states can be responsible for pulmonary arterial thrombosis and pulmonary thromboembolism in dogs. Pieces of thrombi breaking free from a jugular vein thrombus can cause pulmonary thromboembolism. This outcome is particularly evident in animals undergoing long-term intravenous catheterization (Fig. 9-42).

Septic emboli, pieces of thrombi contaminated with bacteria or fungi and broken free from infected mural or valvular thrombi in the heart and vessels, eventually become entrapped in the pulmonary circulation. These emboli originate most commonly from bacterial endocarditis (right side) and jugular thrombophlebitis in all species, hepatic abscesses that have eroded and discharge their contents into the caudal vena cava in cattle, and septic arthritis and omphalitis in farm animals (Fig. 9-41). When present in large numbers, septic emboli may cause unexpected death because of massive pulmonary edema; survivors generally develop pulmonary arteritis and thrombosis and embolic (suppurative) pneumonia, which may lead to pulmonary abscesses.

Fat emboli can form after bone fractures or surgical interventions of bone. These are not as significant a problem in domestic animals as they are in human beings. Brain emboli (i.e., pieces of brain tissue) in the pulmonary vasculature reported in severe cases of head

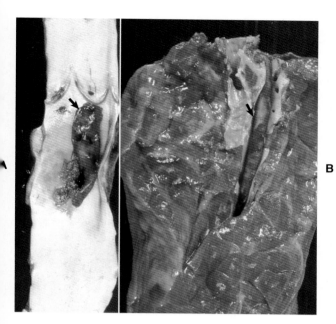

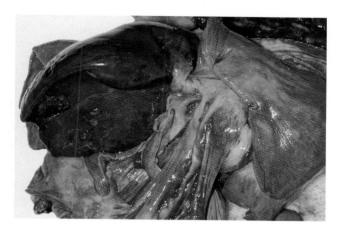

B

Fig. 9-43   Lobe torsion, lung and heart, dog. The right middle lung lobe is markedly congested and hemorrhagic from complete torsion. Although the right middle lobe is most frequently affected, other lobes can also rotate and undergo torsion. *(Courtesy Dr. R. Fredrickson, College of Veterinary Medicine, University of Illinois.)*

Fig. 9-42   Jugular thrombophlebitis and pulmonary thromboembolism, jugular vein and lung cut surface, cow. A, The jugular vein has a large thrombus *(arrow)* attached to the wall at the site of prolonged catheterization. **B,** The pulmonary artery contains a large thrombus *(arrow)*, presumably a thromboembolus that has broken off the jugular mural thrombus. Note that the pulmonary thromboembolus is not attached to the wall of the pulmonary artery. *(A and B, Courtesy Dr. A. López, Atlantic Veterinary College.)*

injury in human beings has recently been recognized in the bovine lung following pneumatic stunning at slaughter. Although obviously not important as an antemortem pulmonary lesion, brain emboli are intriguing as a potential risk for public health in bovine spongiform encephalopathy (BSE). Hepatic emboli formed by circulating pieces of fragmented liver occasionally become trapped in the pulmonary vasculature following severe trauma and hepatic rupture. Tumor emboli (e.g., osteosarcoma and hemangiosarcoma in dogs and uterine carcinoma in cattle) can be numerous and striking and the ultimate cause of death in malignant neoplasia. In experimental studies, cytokines released during pulmonary inflammation are chemotactic for tumor cells and promote pulmonary metastasis.

PULMONARY (LUNG) INFARCTS

Because of a dual arterial supply to the lung, pulmonary infarction is rare and generally asymptomatic. However, pulmonary infarcts can be readily caused when pulmonary thrombosis and embolism are superimposed on an already compromised pulmonary circulation, such as occurs in congestive heart failure. It also occurs in dogs with torsion of a lung lobe (Fig. 9-43).

The gross features of infarcts vary considerably depending on the stage, and they can be red to black, swollen, firm, and cone or wedge shaped. In the early acute stage, microscopic lesions are severely hemorrhagic, and this is followed by necrosis. In 1 to 2 days, a border of inflammatory cells develops, and a few days later, a large number of siderophages are present in the necrotic lung. If sterile, pulmonary infarcts heal as fibrotic scars; if septic, an abscess may form surrounded by a thick fibrous capsule.

PATTERNS OF INJURY AND HOST RESPONSE IN THE LUNGS
BRONCHI

The patterns of necrosis, inflammation, and repair in intrapulmonary bronchi are similar to those previously described for the nasal and tracheal epithelium. In brief, injury to ciliated bronchial epithelium may result in degeneration, detachment, and exfoliation of necrotic cells. Under normal circumstances, cellular exfoliation is promptly followed by inflammation, mitosis, cell proliferation, cell differentiation, and finally by repair (Fig. 9-44). Depending on the type of exudate, bronchitis can be fibrinous, catarrhal, purulent, fibrinonecrotic (diphtheritic), and sometimes granulomatous. When epithelial injury becomes chronic, production of mucus is increased via goblet cell hyperplasia (chronic catarrhal inflammation). This form of chronic bronchitis is well illustrated in habitual smokers who continuously need to cough out excessive mucus secretions (sputum). Unfortunately, in some cases excessive mucus cannot be effectively cleared from airways, and this leads to chronic obstructive bronchitis (Fig. 9-45).

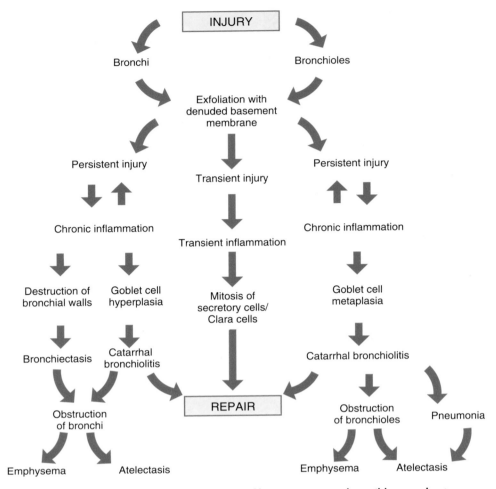

Fig. 9-44   Schematic diagram of the patterns of host response and possible sequelae to bronchial and bronchiolar injury. *(Redrawn with permission from Dr. A. López, Atlantic Veterinary College.)*

Chronic bronchial irritation can also cause squamous metaplasia, in which highly functional but vulnerable ciliated epithelium is replaced by nonfunctional, but more resistant, squamous epithelium. Squamous metaplasia has a calamitous effect on pulmonary clearance because it causes a structural loss and functional breakdown in the mucociliary escalator.

Bronchiectasis is one of the most devastating sequela that follows chronic bronchitis. It consists of a pathologic and permanent dilation of a bronchus as a result of the accumulation of exudates in the lumen and partial rupture of bronchial walls. Destruction of walls occurs, in part, when proteolytic enzymes released from phagocytic cells during chronic inflammation degrade and weaken the smooth muscle and cartilage that help to maintain normal bronchial diameter. Bronchiectasis may be saccular when destruction affects only a small

localized portion of the bronchial wall or cylindrical when destruction involves a large segment of a bronchus. Grossly, bronchiectasis is manifested by prominent lumps in the lungs (bosselated appearance or having rounded eminences) resulting from distention of bronchi with exudate, which results in a concurrent obstructive atelectasis of surrounding parenchyma (Fig. 9-46). The cut surfaces of dilated bronchi are filled with purulent exudates; for this reason, bronchiectasis is often mistaken for pulmonary abscesses. Careful inspection, usually requiring microscopic examination, will confirm that exudate is contained and surrounded by remnants of a bronchial wall lined by squamous epithelium and not by a pyogenic membrane (connective tissue) as it is in the case of a pulmonary abscess. The squamous metaplasia further interferes with the normal function of the mucociliary escalator.

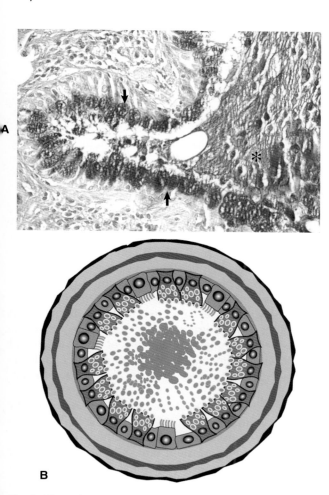

Fig. 9-45   Chronic obstructive pulmonary disease (heaves), recurrent airway obstruction, goblet cell metaplasia, bronchiole, lung, horse. A, This horse had a 3-year history of recurrent dyspnea and terminal pulmonary emphysema. Numerous goblet cells *(arrows)* in the bronchiolar epithelium are discharging mucus *(*)* into the lumen, causing complete obstruction of the bronchiole. The majority of the mucus has stained blue with alcian blue. Healthy bronchioles do not have goblet cells or mucus. PAS reaction-Alcian blue stain. **B,** Schematic diagram of goblet cell metaplasia in chronic obstructive pulmonary disease. Note how the mucus has obstructed the bronchiole. *(A and B, Courtesy Dr. A. López, Atlantic Veterinary College.)*

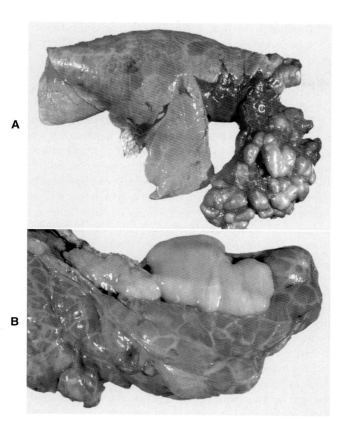

Fig. 9-46   Severe bronchiectasis with chronic bronchopneumonia, right lung, calf. A, Note the segmentally distended (bosselated) bronchi supplying the ventral portion of the cranial lung lobe. The lumens of affected bronchi are filled with purulent exudate. The surrounding lung parenchyma supplied by these bronchi is atelectatic *(C)*. Bronchiectatic bronchi resemble pulmonary abscesses, but unlike abscesses, which are lined by a pyogenic membrane, the exudate in bronchiectasis is lined by the remnants of the bronchial wall. **B,** These distended bronchi are filled with purulent exudate. *(A, Courtesy Ontario Veterinary College. B, Courtesy Dr. M.D. McGavin, College of Veterinary Medicine, University of Tennessee.)*

BRONCHIOLES

The epithelial lining of the bronchiolar region (transitional zone) is exquisitely susceptible to injury, particularly to that caused by some respiratory viruses (PI-3, adenovirus, BRSV, canine distemper), oxidant gases (NO_2, SO_2, O_3), and toxic substances (3-methylindole). The precise explanation as to why bronchiolar epithelium is so prone to injury is still not clear, but it is presumably due in part to (1) its high vulnerability to oxidants and free radicals; (2) the presence of Clara cells rich in mixed-function oxidases, which locally generate toxic metabolites; and (3) the tendency for pulmonary alveolar macrophages and leukocytes to accumulate in this region of the lungs.

Once injury to the cells becomes irreversible, bronchiolar ciliated cells degenerate and exfoliate into the bronchiolar lumen, leaving a denuded basement membrane. Repair in the bronchiolar region is similar to, but less effective than that in the tracheal or nasal mucosa. Under normal circumstances, recruited phagocytic cells remove exudate and cell debris from the lumina of affected bronchioles, thus preparing the basement membrane to be repopulated with new, undifferentiated cells originating from a rapidly dividing pool of Clara cells. After several days, these proliferating cells fully differentiate into normal bronchiolar ciliated cells (Fig. 9-44).

Depending on the types of injury and inflammatory response, bronchiolitis is classified as necrotizing, suppurative, catarrhal (mucous metaplasia), or granulomatous. In severe injury, exudate cannot be removed from the basement membrane of bronchioles. The exudate becomes infiltrated by fibroblasts, which form small masses of fibrovascular tissue and develop into well-organized, microscopic polyps inside the bronchiolar lumen. Their external surface eventually becomes covered by ciliated cells. This lesion is referred to as bronchiolitis obliterans and the polyps may become so large as to cause severe interference in airflow. Peribronchiolar proliferation of lymphocytes (BALT hyperplasia) is also a common microscopic lesion seen in chronic bronchiolitis.

On the other hand, if bronchiolar injury is mild but persistent, goblet cells normally absent from bronchioles proliferate from basal cells, resulting in goblet cell metaplasia and causing a profound alteration in the physicochemical properties of bronchiolar secretions (Fig. 9-45). The normally serous bronchiolar fluid released by Clara cells becomes a tenacious material when mucus produced by goblet cells is added. As a result of increased viscoelasticity of the mucus, bronchiolar secretions cannot be removed effectively by ciliary action, leading to plugging and obstruction of distal airways. Under such conditions, often grouped as chronic obstructive pulmonary disease, coughing is required to clear mucus from obstructed bronchioles. Pulmonary emphysema and atelectasis are further sequelae to bronchiolar metaplasia and mucous hypersecretion blocking or partially blocking the lumens of these bronchioles. These two inflation abnormalities are characteristically present in chronic obstructive pulmonary disease (COPD), such as "heaves" in horses.

COPD of horses (heaves, recurrent airway obstruction, chronic bronchiolitis-emphysema complex, chronic small airway disease, alveolar emphysema, and "broken wind") is a common clinically asthmalike syndrome of horses and ponies, characterized by recurrent respiratory distress, chronic cough, poor athletic performance, airway neutrophilia, and mucus hypersecretion. The pathogenesis is still obscure, but genetic predisposition, T_H2 (allergic) immune response, and the exceptional sensitivity of airways to environmental allergens (hyperreactive airway disease) have been postulated as the basic underlying mechanisms. What makes small airways hyperreactive to allergens is still a matter of controversy. Epidemiologic and experimental studies suggest

that it could be the result of preceding bronchiolar damage caused by viral infections, ingestion of pneumotoxicants (3-methylindole), or prolonged exposure to organic dust, endotoxin, and environmental allergens (molds). Most recently, it has been postulated that sustained inhalation of dust particles, whether antigenic or not, up-regulates the production of cytokines (TNF-α, IL-8, and monokine-inducible protein [MIP-2]) by alveolar macrophages, attracting neutrophils into the bronchioloalveolar region and promoting leukocyte-induced bronchiolar injury.

The lungs of horses with heaves are grossly unremarkable, except for extreme cases in which alveolar emphysema may be present. Microscopically the lesions include goblet cell metaplasia in bronchioles; plugging of bronchioles with mucus mixed with a few eosinophils (Fig. 9-45); peribronchiolar infiltration with lymphocytes, plasma cells, and variable numbers of eosinophils; and hypertrophy of smooth muscle in bronchi and bronchioles. In severe cases, accumulation of mucus leads to the complete obstruction of bronchioles and alveoli, and resultant alveolar emphysema characterized by enlarged "alveoli" from the destruction of alveolar walls.

"Airway hyperresponsiveness" (hyperreactive airway disease) is another sequela of bronchiolar injury. It develops in human beings and animals (experimentally) following a transient and often innocuous viral infection of the lower respiratory tract or from exposure to certain allergens. Experimental work has shown that airway hyperreactivity in postviral bronchiolitis is associated with increased expression of Toll-like receptors and unusual susceptibility to inhaled endotoxin. Hyperreactive animals typically have an increased number of mast cells, eosinophils, and T lymphocytes in the airway mucosa. Clinically, airway hyperresponsiveness is characterized by an exaggerated bronchoconstriction following exposure to mild stimuli, such as cold air, or after animals are exposed to aerosols of histamine or methacholine.

Feline asthma (feline asthma syndrome; feline allergic bronchitis)

Feline asthma, also known as feline allergic bronchitis, is a clinical syndrome in cats of any age characterized by recurrent episodes of bronchoconstriction, cough, or dyspnea. The pathogenesis is not well understood, but is presumed to originate, as in human asthma, as a type I hypersensitivity (IgE–mast cell reaction) to inhaled allergens. Dust, cigarette smoke, plant and household materials, and parasitic proteins have been incriminated as possible allergens. This self-limited allergic disease responds well to steroid therapy; thus it is rarely implicated as a primary cause of death except when suppressed defense mechanisms result in secondary bacterial pneumonia. Bronchial biopsies from affected cats at the early stages reveal mild to moderate inflammation characterized by mucosal edema and infiltration of leukocytes, particularly eosinophils. Increased numbers of circulating eosinophil leukocytes (blood eosinophilia) are present in some, but not all, cats with feline asthma. In the most advanced cases, chronic bronchoconstriction and excess mucus production may result in smooth muscle hyperplasia and obstruction of the bronchi and bronchioles, and infiltration of the airway mucosa by eosinophils. A syndrome known as canine asthma has been reported in dogs but is not as well characterized as the feline counterpart.

ALVEOLI

Because of their extremely delicate structure, alveoli are quite vulnerable to injury once defense mechanisms have been overwhelmed. The alveolar wall is thin and has three layers composed of vascular endothelium, basal lamina (alveolar interstitium), and alveolar epithelium. These three layers of the alveolar septum constitute what is customarily referred to as the blood-air barrier (Fig 9-6). The epithelial side of the alveolus is primarily lined by rather thin type I pneumonocytes, which are arranged as a very delicate continuous membrane extending along the alveolar surface (Fig. 9-6). Type I pneumonocytes are particularly susceptible to noxious agents that reach the alveolar region either aerogenously or hematogenously. Injury from type I pneumonocytes causes swelling and vacuolation of these cells. When cellular damage has become irreversible, type I cells detach, resulting in denudation of the basement membrane, increased alveolar permeability, and alveolar edema. Alveolar repair is possible as long as the basement membrane remains intact and lesions are not complicated by further injury or infection. Within 3 days, cuboidal type II (granular) pneumonocytes, which are the precursor cells and more resistant to injury, undergo mitosis and provide a large pool of new undifferentiated cells. These new cells repave the denuded alveolar basement membrane and finally differentiate in type I pneumonocytes. When alveolar injury is diffuse, proliferation of type II pneumonocytes becomes so spectacular that the microscopic appearance of the alveolus resembles that of a gland or fetal lung; the lesion has been termed epithelialization or fetalization. Although it is part of the normal alveolar repair, hyperplasia of type II pneumonocytes can interfere in gas exchange and cause hypoxemia. In uncomplicated cases, type II pneumonocytes eventually differentiate into type I pneumonocytes, thus completing the last stage of alveolar repair.

Type I pneumonocytes are one of the three structural components of the blood-air barrier, so when these epithelial cells are damaged there is an increase in alveolar capillary permeability and transient leakage of plasma fluid, proteins, and fibrin into the alveolar lumen. Under normal circumstances, these fluids are rapidly cleared from the alveolus by alveolar and lymphatic absorption, and necrotic pneumonocytes (type 1) and fibrin strands are phagocytosed and removed by pulmonary alveolar macrophages. When there is persistent and severe injury, fibroblasts may proliferate in the alveolar walls (alveolar interstitium) causing alveolar fibrosis, whereas in other forms of severe injury, fibroblasts actively migrate from the interstitium into the alveolar spaces, causing intraalveolar fibrosis. These two types of alveolar fibrosis are most commonly seen in toxic and allergic pulmonary diseases, which have a devastating effect of lung function.

On a minute-to-minute basis, the pulmonary defense mechanisms deal effectively with noxious stimuli and mild tissue injury without the need for an inflammatory response. However, if normal defense mechanisms are ineffective or insufficient (overwhelmed), the inflammatory process is rapidly turned on as a second line of defense.

GENERAL ASPECTS OF LUNG INFLAMMATION

In the past two decades, an information explosion has increased the overall understanding of pulmonary inflammation, with so many proinflammatory and antiinflammatory mediators described to date that it would be impossible to review them all here (see Chapter 3).

Pulmonary inflammation is a highly regulated process that involves a complex interaction between cells imported from the blood (neutrophils, eosinophils, mast cells, and lymphocytes) and pulmonary cells (type I and II pneumonocytes and endothelial, Clara, and stromal interstitial cells). Blood-borne leukocytes, platelets, and plasma proteins are brought into the areas of inflammation by an elaborate network of chemical signals emitted by pulmonary cells and resident leukocytes. Long-distance communication between pulmonary cells and blood cells is largely done by soluble cytokines; once in the lung, imported leukocytes communicate with pulmonary and vascular cells through adhesion and other inflammatory molecules. The best known inflammatory mediators are the complement system (C3a, C3b, C5a), coagulation factors (factors V, VII), arachidonic acid metabolites (leukotrienes and prostaglandins), cytokines (interleukins, monokines, chemokines), adhesion molecules (ICAM, VCAM), enzymes and enzyme inhibitors (elastase, antitrypsin), oxygen metabolites ($O_2^{\cdot}$, $OH^{\cdot}$, H_2O_2), antioxidants (glutathione), and nitric oxide (Table 9-3). Acting in concert, these and many other molecules send positive or negative signals to initiate, maintain, and hopefully resolve

Table **9-3**   **Main Chemical Mediators Involved in Pulmonary Inflammation**

Name	Source	Function in the Lung
Histamine	Mast cells, basophils, monocytes	Increase vascular permeability, pain
Prostaglandins and leukotrienes	Cell membranes	Increase permeability, platelet aggregation, vasoconstriction or vasodilation, lung edema, pain
L-selectin	Neutrophils, monocytes	Leukocyte attachment and migration, homing to areas of pulmonary inflammation
P-, E-selectins; ICAM-1, ELAM-1	Venules and capillary endothelium	Leukocyte attachment and migration to areas of pulmonary inflammation
IL-1	Alveolar macrophages	Endothelial-leukocyte adherence (ELAMs), leukocyte chemotaxis
IL-6	Macrophages	Lymphocyte and fibroblast activation in the lung; down-regulates TNF and reduces inflammation
IL-8	Macrophages, fibroblasts	Leukocyte and lymphocyte chemotaxis
IL-9	Macrophages, alveolar cells	Decreases cytokine production in pulmonary alveolar macrophages
Tumor necrosis factor (TNF-α)	Alveolar macrophages	Endothelial-leukocyte attachment (ELAMs), vascular permeability, lung edema; fever and acute-phase proteins, apoptosis
Eotaxin and IL-5	Lymphocytes	Eosinophil chemotaxis, airway eosinophilia, asthma, pulmonary allergies
Epithelial secretory proteins	Type I and II pneumonocytes, Clara cells	Modulation of lung inflammation; regulation of fibroblasts, fibrosis, and NO
Surfactant A, B (collectins)	Type II pneumonocyte and Clara cells	Chemotaxis, phagocytosis, immunomodulation, regulation of NO
Nitric oxide (NO)	Pneumonocytes, macrophages, endothelium	Decreases cytokine production in pulmonary alveolar macrophages; modulation of apoptosis
Transforming growth factors (TGF-α and TGF-β)	Pneumonocytes, macrophages	Lung remodeling, deposition of connective tissue, fibrosis

ELAM, Endothelial adhesion molecule; *ICAM*, intercellular adhesion molecule; *IL*, interleukin.

the inflammatory process without causing injury to the lung.

Pulmonary macrophages (alveolar, intravascular, and interstitial), which have an immense biologic armamentarium, are the single most important effector cell and source of cytokines for all stages of pulmonary inflammation. These all-purpose phagocytic cells modulate the recruitment and trafficking of blood-borne leukocytes in the lung through the secretion of chemokines (Table 9-3).

Before reviewing how inflammatory cells are recruited in the lungs, three significant features in pulmonary injury must be remembered: (1) Leukocytes can exit the vascular system through the alveolar capillaries, unlike in other tissues, where postcapillary venules are the sites of leukocytic diapedesis (extravasation); (2) the intact lung contains within alveolar capillaries a large pool of resident leukocytes (marginal pool); and (3) additional neutrophils are sequestered within alveolar capillaries within minutes of local or systemic inflammatory response. These three pulmonary idiosyncrasies, along with the enormous length of the capillary network in the lung, explain why recruitment and migration of leukocytes into alveolar spaces develops so rapidly. Experimental studies with aerosols of endotoxin or gram-negative bacteria have shown that within minutes of exposure, there is a significant increase in capillary leukocytes, and by 4 hours the entire alveolar lumen is filled with neutrophils. Not surprisingly, the BAL fluid collected from patients with acute pneumonia contains large amounts of inflammatory mediators such as TNF-α, IL-1, and IL-8. Also, the capillary endothelium of patients with acute pneumonia has increased "expression" of adhesion molecules, which facilitate the migration of leukocytes from capillaries into the alveolar interstitium and from there into the alveolar lumen. In allergic pulmonary diseases, eotaxin and IL-5 are primarily responsible for recruitment and trafficking of eosinophils in the lung (Table 9-3).

Movement of plasma proteins into the pulmonary interstitium and alveolar lumen is a common but poorly understood phenomenon in pulmonary inflammation.

Leakage of fibrinogen and plasma proteins can be caused by direct physical damage to the blood-air barrier. This leakage is also promoted by some types of cytokines that enhance procoagulant activity, whereas others reduce fibrinolytic activity. Excessive exudation of fibrin into the alveoli is particularly common in ruminants and pigs. The fibrinolytic system plays a major role in the resolution of pulmonary inflammatory diseases. In some cases, excessive plasma proteins leaked into alveoli mix with necrotic type I pneumonocytes and pulmonary surfactant, forming microscopic eosinophilic bands (membranes) along the lining of alveolar septa. These membranes, known as "hyaline membranes," are found in specific types of pulmonary diseases, particularly in ARDS, and in cattle with acute interstitial pneumonias such as bovine pulmonary edema and emphysema and extrinsic allergic alveolitis (Fig. 9-35).

In the last few years, nitric oxide has been identified as a major regulatory molecule of inflammation in a variety of tissues, including the lung. Produced locally by macrophages, pulmonary endothelium, and pneumonocytes, nitric oxide regulates the vascular and bronchial tone, modulates the production of cytokines, controls the recruitment and trafficking of neutrophils in the lung, and switches on/off genes involved in inflammation and immunity. Experimental work has also shown that pulmonary surfactant up-regulates the production of nitric oxide in the lung, supporting the current view that pneumonocytes are also pivotal in amplifying and down-regulating the inflammatory and immune responses in the lung (Table 9-3).

As the inflammatory process becomes chronic, the types of cells making up cellular infiltrates in the lung change from mainly neutrophils to largely mononuclear cells. This shift in cellular composition is accompanied by an increase in specific cytokines, such as IL-4, interferon-γ (IFN-γ), and interferon-inducible protein (IP-10), which are chemotactic for lymphocytes and macrophages. Under appropriate conditions, these cytokines activate T lymphocytes, regulate granulomatous inflammation, and induce the formation of multinucleated giant cells, such as in mycobacterial infections.

Inflammatory mediators locally released from inflamed lungs also have a biologic effect in other tissue. For instance, pulmonary hypertension and right side heart failure (cor pulmonale) often follows chronic alveolar inflammation, not only as a result of increased pulmonary blood pressure but also from the effect of inflammatory mediators on the contractibility of smooth muscle of the pulmonary and systemic vasculature. Cytokines, particularly TNF-α, which are released during inflammation are associated, both as cause and effect, with the systemic inflammatory response syndrome (SIRS), sepsis, severe sepsis with multiple organ dysfunction, and septic shock (cardiopulmonary collapse).

As it occurs in any other sentinel system where many biologic promoters and inhibitors are involved (coagulation, the complement and immune systems), the inflammatory cascade could go into an "out-of-control" state, causing severe damage to the lungs. ARDS, extrinsic allergic alveolitis, pulmonary fibrosis, and asthma are archetypical diseases that ensue from an uncontrolled production and release of cytokines.

As long as alveolar injury is transient and there is no interference with the normal host response, the entire process of injury, degeneration, necrosis, inflammation, and repair can occur in less than 1 week. On the other hand, when alveolar injury becomes persistent or when the capacity of the host for repair is impaired, lesions can progress to an irreversible stage in which restoration of alveolar structure is no longer possible. In diseases such as extrinsic allergic alveolitis, the constant release of proteolytic enzymes and free radicals by phagocytic cells perpetuates alveolar damage in a vicious circle. In other cases, such as in paraquat toxicity, the magnitude of alveolar injury can be so severe that type II pneumonocytes, basement membranes, and alveolar interstitium are so disrupted that the capacity for alveolar repair is lost. Fibronectins and transforming growth factors released from macrophages and other mononuclear cells at the site of chronic inflammation regulate the recruitment, attachment, and proliferation of fibroblasts. In turn, these cells synthesize and release considerable amounts of extracellular matrix (collagen, elastic fibers, proteoglycans), eventually leading to fibrosis and total obliteration of normal alveolar architecture. In summary, in diseases in which there is chronic and irreversible alveolar damage, lesions invariably progress to a stage of terminal alveolar fibrosis.

CLASSIFICATION OF PNEUMONIAS

Few subjects in veterinary pathology have caused so much debate as the classification of pneumonias. Historically, pneumonias in animals have been classified or named based on (1) presumed cause, with names such as viral pneumonia, *Pasteurella* pneumonia, distemper pneumonia, verminous pneumonia, chemical pneumonia, and hypersensitivity pneumonitis; (2) type of exudation, with names such as suppurative pneumonia, fibrinous pneumonia, and pyogranulomatous pneumonia; (3) morphologic features, with names such as gangrenous pneumonia, proliferative pneumonia, and embolic pneumonia; (4) distribution of lesions, with names such as focal pneumonia, cranioventral pneumonia, diffuse pneumonia, and lobar pneumonia; (5) epidemiologic attributes, with names such as enzootic pneumonia, contagious bovine pleuropneumonia, and pneumonic mannheimiosis pneumonia; (6) geographic regions, with names such as Montana progressive pneumonia; and finally, (7) miscellaneous attributes, with names such as atypical pneumonia, cuffing pneumonia, progressive pneumonia, aspiration pneumonia, pneumonitis, farmer's lung, and extrinsic allergic alveolitis. Until a universal and systematic nomenclature for animal pneumonias are established, veterinarians should be acquainted with this heterogeneous list of names and should be well aware that one disease may be known by different names. In pigs, for instance, enzootic pneumonia, virus pneumonia, and *Mycoplasma* pneumonia all refer to the same disease caused by *Mycoplasma hyopneumoniae.*

The word *pneumonitis* has been used by some as a synonym for pneumonia; however, others have restricted this term to chronic proliferative inflammation generally involving the alveolar interstitium and with little or no evidence of exudate. In this chapter, the word *pneumonia* is used for any inflammatory lesion in the lungs, regardless of whether it is exudative or proliferative, alveolar, or interstitial.

Pneumonias in domestic animals can be classified based on texture, distribution, appearance and exudation into four morphologically distinct types: bronchopneumonia, interstitial pneumonia, embolic pneumonia,

and granulomatous pneumonia. By using this classification, it is possible to predict with some degree of certainty the likely cause (virus, bacteria, fungi, parasites), routes of entry (aerogenous versus hematogenous), and possible sequelae to which each of these types of pneumonia may progress if the animal were to survive. However, overlapping of these four types of pneumonias is possible, and sometimes two morphologic types may be present in the same lung.

The criteria used to classify pneumonias into bronchopneumonia, interstitial pneumonia, embolic pneumonia, and granulomatous pneumonia are based on morphologic changes, including distribution, texture, color, and appearance of the affected lungs (Table 9-4). According to distribution of the inflammatory lesions in the lungs, pneumonias can be cranioventral, as in most bronchopneumonias; multifocal, as in embolic pneumonias; diffuse, as in interstitial pneumonias; or locally extensive, as in granulomatous pneumonias (Fig. 9-47). Texture of pneumonic lungs can be firmer or harder (bronchopneumonias), more elastic (rubbery) than normal lungs (interstitial pneumonias), or have a nodular feeling (granulomatous pneumonias). Describing in words the palpable difference between the texture of a normal lung compared with the firm or hard texture of a consolidated lung can be a difficult undertaking.

Table **9-4** **Morphologic Types of Pneumonias in Domestic Animals**

Type of Pneumonia	Port of Entry (e.g., Pathogens)	Distribution of Lesions	Texture of Lung	Grossly Visible Exudate	Disease Example	Common Pulmonary Sequelae
Bronchopneumonia:						
Suppurative (lobular)	Aerogenous (bacteria and mycoplasmas)	Cranioventral consolidation	Firm	Purulent exudate in bronchi	Enzootic pneumonia	Cranioventral abscesses, adhesions bronchiectasis,
Fibrinous (lobar)	Aerogenous (bacteria and mycoplasmas)	Cranioventral consolidation*	Hard	Fibrin in lung and pleura	Pneumonic mannheimiosis	BALT hyperplasia, "sequestra," pleural adhesions, abscesses
Interstitial pneumonia	Aerogenous or hematogenous (virus, toxin, allergen, sepsis)	Diffuse	Elastic with rib imprints	Not visible, trapped in alveolar septa	Influenza, extrinsic allergic alveolitis, PRRS, ARDS	Edema, emphysema, type II alveolar hyperplasia, alveolar fibrosis
Granulomatous pneumonia	Aerogenous or hematogenous (*Mycobacteria,* systemic mycoses)	Multifocal	Nodular	Pyogranulomatous, caseous necrosis, calcified nodules	Tuberculosis, blastomycosis, cryptococcosis	Dissemination of infection to lymph nodes and distant organs
Embolic pneumonia	Hematogenous (septic emboli)	Multifocal	Nodular	Purulent foci surrounded by hyperemia	Vegetative endocarditis, ruptured liver abscess	Abscesses randomly distributed in all pulmonary lobes

ARDS, Adult respiratory distress syndrome; *BALT,* bronchial associated lymphoid tissue; *PRRS,* Porcine reproductive and respiratory syndrome.
*Porcine pleuropneumonia is an exception because it often involves the caudal lobes.

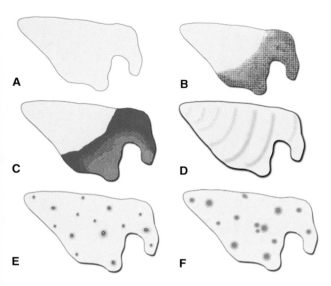

Fig. 9-47   Schematic diagram of the patterns of pneumonia. A, Normal lung. **B,** Suppurative bronchopneumonia showing cranioventral consolidation and accentuated lobular pattern. **C,** Fibrinous bronchopneumonia showing cranioventral consolidation and fibrin on pleura (*yellow*). **D,** Interstitial pneumonia showing diffuse distribution and rib imprints in all pulmonary lobes. **E,** Embolic pneumonia showing multifocal distribution involving all pulmonary lobes. **F,** Granulomatous pneumonia showing multifocal nodules in all pulmonary lobes. (*A through F,* *Redrawn with permission from Dr. A. López, Atlantic Veterinary College.*)

An analogy illustrating this difference based on touching the parts of the face with the tip of your finger has been advocated by some pathologists. The texture of a normal lung is comparable to the texture of the center of the cheek. Firm consolidation is comparable to the texture of the tip of the nose, and hard consolidation is comparable to the texture of the forehead. The term *consolidation* is frequently used to describe a firm or hard lung filled with exudate.

Changes in the appearance of pneumonic lungs include abnormal color, presence of nodules or exudate, fibrinous or fibrous adhesions, and presence of rib imprints on serosal surfaces (Fig. 9-47). On cut surfaces, pneumonic lungs may have exudate, hemorrhage, edema, necrosis, abscesses, bronchiectasis, granulomas or pyogranulomas, and fibrosis, depending on the stage.

Palpation and careful observation of the lungs are essential in the diagnosis of pneumonia. (For details, see Examination of the Respiratory Tract, Postmortem.)

BRONCHOPNEUMONIA

Bronchopneumonia refers to a particular type of pneumonia in which injury and the inflammatory process take place primarily in the bronchial, bronchiolar, and alveolar lumens. Bronchopneumonia is undoubtedly the most common type of pneumonia seen in domestic animals and is, with few exceptions, characterized by cranioventral consolidation of the lungs (Fig. 9-48). The reason why bronchopneumonias in animals are almost always restricted to the cranioventral portions of the lungs is not well understood. Possible factors contributing to this topographic selectivity within the lungs include (1) gravitational sedimentation of the exudate; (2) greater deposition of infectious organisms; (3) inadequate defense mechanisms; (4) reduced vascular perfusion; (5) shortness and abrupt branching of airways; and (6) regional differences in ventilation.

The term *cranioventral* of veterinary anatomy is the equivalent of "anterosuperior" of human anatomy. The latter is defined as "in front (ventral) and above (cranial)." Thus applied to the lung of animals, "cranioventral"

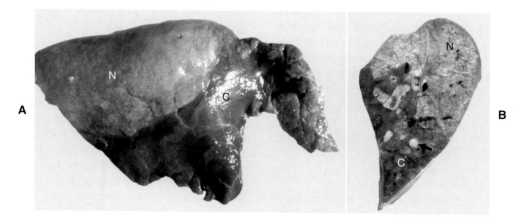

Fig. 9-48   Suppurative bronchopneumonia, enzootic pneumonia, lung, calf. A, Cranioventral consolidation (C) of the lung involves approximately 40% of pulmonary parenchyma. Most of the caudal lung is normal (N). **B,** Cut surface. Consolidated lung is dark red to mahogany (C), and a major bronchus contains purulent exudate (*arrow*). N, Normal. (*A and B,* *Courtesy Ontario Veterinary College.*)

means the ventral portion of the cranial lobe. However, by common usage in veterinary pathology, the term *cranioventral* used to describe the location of lesions in pneumonias has come to mean "cranial and ventral." Thus it includes pneumonias affecting not only the ventral portion of the cranial lobe (true cranioventral) but also those cases in which the pneumonia has involved the ventral portions of adjacent lung lobes—initially the middle, and then caudal on the right and the caudal lobe on the left side.

Bronchopneumonias are generally caused by bacteria and mycoplasmas, by bronchoaspiration of feed or gastric contents, or by improper tubing. As a rule, the pathogens causing bronchopneumonias arrive in the lungs via inspired air (aerogenous), either from infected aerosols or from the nasal flora. Before establishing infection, pathogens must overwhelm or evade the pulmonary defense mechanism. The initial injury in bronchopneumonias is centered on the mucosa of bronchioles; from there, the inflammatory process can spread downward to distal portions of the alveoli and upward to the bronchi. Typically for bronchopneumonias, the inflammatory exudates collects in the bronchial, bronchiolar, and alveolar lumina leaving the alveolar interstitium reasonably unchanged. Through the pores of Kohn, the lesions and exudate can spread centripetally to adjacent alveoli until part or all of the alveoli in an individual lobule are involved. If the inflammatory process cannot control the inciting cause of injury, the lesions spread rapidly from lobule to lobule through alveolar pores and destroyed alveolar walls, until an entire lobe or large portion of a lung is involved. The lesion tends to spread centrifugally, with the older lesions being in the center, and exudate can be coughed up and then aspirated into other lobules, where the inflammatory process starts again.

At the early stages of bronchopneumonia, the pulmonary vessels are engorged with blood (active hyperemia) and the bronchi, bronchioles, and alveoli contain some fluid (permeability edema). In cases in which pulmonary injury is mild to moderate, cytokines locally released in the lung cause rapid recruitment of neutrophils and alveolar macrophages into bronchioles and alveoli (Fig. 9-49). When pulmonary injury is much more severe, proinflammatory cytokines induce more pronounced vascular changes by further opening endothelial gaps, thus increasing vascular permeability resulting in fibrinous exudates and sometimes hemorrhage in the alveoli. Alterations in permeability can be further exacerbated by structural damage to pulmonary capillaries and vessels directly caused by microbial toxins. The final result of these functional and structural changes is that blood vessels become notably permeable and allow substantial leakage of plasma fluid and proteins (fibrinogen) into the alveoli. Filling of alveoli, bronchioles,

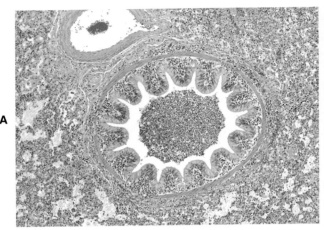

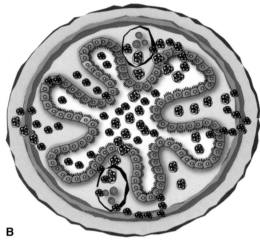

Fig. 9-49   Suppurative bronchopneumonia, lung, pig. **A,** Note the bronchiole plugged with purulent exudate. The alveoli are filled with leukocytes and some edematous fluid. H&E stain. **B,** Schematic diagram of acute bronchiolitis. Note the neutrophils exiting the submucosal capillaries (leukocyte adhesion cascade; see Chapter 3) and moving into the walls of the bronchioles and then into the bronchiolar lumen. (**A** *and* **B,** *Courtesy Dr. A. López, Atlantic Veterinary College.*)

and small bronchi with inflammatory exudate progressively obliterates airspaces, and as a consequence of this process, portions of severely affected (consolidated) lungs sink to the bottom of the container when placed in fixative. The replacement of air by exudate also changes the texture of the lungs, and depending on the severity of bronchopneumonia, the texture varies from firmer to harder than normal.

The term *consolidation* is used when the texture of pneumonic lung becomes firmer or harder than normal as a result of loss of airspaces because of exudation and atelectasis. (For details, see the discussion of lung texture in Classification of Pneumonias.)

Inflammatory consolidation of lungs has been referred to in the past as "hepatization," because the affected lung had the appearance and texture of liver. The process was referred to as "red hepatization" in acute cases in which there was notable active hyperemia with little exudation of neutrophils; conversely, the process was referred to as "gray hepatization" in those chronic cases in which hyperemia was no longer present, but there was abundant exudation of neutrophils and macrophages. This terminology, although used and applicable to human pneumonias, is rarely used in veterinary medicine primarily because the evolution of pneumonic processes in animals does not necessarily follow the red-to-gray hepatization pattern.

Bronchopneumonias can be arbitrarily subdivided into suppurative bronchopneumonia if the exudate is predominantly composed of neutrophils, and fibrinous bronchopneumonia if fibrin is the predominant component of the exudate (Table 9-4). It is important to note that some pathologists use the term *fibrinous pneumonia* or *lobar pneumonia* as a synonym for fibrinous bronchopneumonia, and *bronchopneumonia* or *lobular pneumonia* as a synonym for suppurative bronchopneumonia. Currently, the term *bronchopneumonia* is widely used for both suppurative and fibrinous consolidation of the lungs, because both forms of inflammation have essentially the same pathogenesis in which the pathogens reach the lung by the aerogenous route, injury occurs initially in the bronchial and bronchiolar regions, and the inflammatory process extends centrifugally deep into the alveoli. It must be emphasized that it is the severity of pulmonary injury that largely determines whether bronchopneumonia becomes suppurative or fibrinous. In some instances, however, it is difficult to discriminate between suppurative and fibrinous bronchopneumonia because both types can coexist (fibrinosuppurative bronchopneumonia), and one type can progress to the other.

Suppurative bronchopneumonia is characterized by cranioventral consolidation of lungs (Figs. 9-47 and 9-48), with typical presence of purulent or mucopurulent exudate in the airways. This exudate can be best demonstrated by expressing intrapulmonary bronchi, thus forcing exudate out of the bronchi (Fig. 9-48). The inflammatory process in suppurative bronchopneumonia is generally confined to individual lobules, and, as a result of this distribution, the lobular pattern of the lung becomes notably emphasized. This pattern is particularly obvious in cattle and pigs because these species have prominent lobulation of the lungs. The gross appearance often resembles an irregular checkerboard because of an admixture of normal and abnormal (consolidated) lobules (Fig. 9-48). Because of this typical lobular distribution, suppurative bronchopneumonias are also referred to as lobular pneumonias.

Different inflammatory phases occur in suppurative bronchopneumonia where the color and appearance of consolidated lungs varies considerably depending on the virulence of offending organisms and chronicity of the lesion. The typical phases of suppurative bronchopneumonia could be summarized as follows: During the first 12 hours when bacteria are rapidly multiplying, the lungs become hyperemic and edematous. Soon after neutrophils start filling the airways and by 48 hours the parenchyma starts to consolidate and becomes firm in texture. Three to 5 days later, hyperemic changes are less obvious, but the bronchial, bronchiolar, and alveolar spaces continue to fill with neutrophils and macrophages, and the affected lung sinks when placed in formalin. At this stage, the affected lung has a gray-pink color, and on cut surface purulent exudate can be expressed from bronchi. In favorable conditions where the infection is under control of the host defense mechanisms, the inflammatory processes begin to regress, a phase known as resolution. Complete resolution in favorable conditions could take 1 to 2 weeks. In animals in which the lung infection cannot be rapidly contained, inflammatory lesions can progress into a chronic phase. Around 7 to 10 days after infection, the lungs become pale gray and take a "fish flesh" appearance. This appearance is the result of purulent and catarrhal inflammation, obstructive atelectasis, mononuclear cell infiltration, lymphoid hyperplasia, and early fibrosis. Complete resolution is unusual in chronic bronchopneumonia, and lung scars, such as fibrosis, bronchiectasis, atelectasis, adhesions, and abscesses, may remain unresolved for a long time. "Enzootic pneumonias" of ruminants and pigs are typical examples of chronic suppurative bronchopneumonias.

Microscopically, suppurative bronchopneumonias are characterized by abundant neutrophils, macrophages, and cellular debris within the lumen of bronchi, bronchioles, and alveoli (Fig. 9-49). Recruitment of leukocytes is promoted by cytokines, complement, and other chemotactic factors that are released in response to alveolar injury or by the chemotactic effect of bacterial toxins, particularly endotoxin. In most severe cases, purulent or mucopurulent exudates completely obliterate the entire lumen of bronchi, bronchioles, and alveoli.

If suppurative bronchopneumonia is merely the response to a transient pulmonary injury or a mild infection, lesions resolve uneventfully. Within 7 to 10 days, cellular exudate can be removed from the lungs via the mucociliary escalator, and complete resolution may take place within 4 weeks. In other cases, if injury or infection is persistent, suppurative bronchopneumonia can become chronic with goblet cell hyperplasia, an important component of the inflammatory process. Depending on the proportion of pus and mucus, the exudate in chronic suppurative bronchopneumonia varies from mucopurulent to mucoid. A mucoid exudate is found in the more chronic stages when the consolidated lung has a "fish flesh" appearance.

Hyperplasia of BALT is another change commonly seen in chronic suppurative bronchopneumonias; it appears grossly as conspicuous white nodules (cuffs) around bronchial walls (cuffing pneumonia). This hyperplastic change merely indicates a normal reaction of lymphoid tissue to infection. Further sequelae of chronic suppurative bronchopneumonia include bronchiectasis (Fig. 9-46), pulmonary abscesses, and pleural adhesions (from pleuritis), and atelectasis and emphysema from completely or partially obstructed bronchi or bronchioles (e.g., bronchiectasis).

Clinically, suppurative bronchopneumonias can be acute and fulminating, but are often chronic, depending on the etiologic agent, stressors affecting the host, and immune status. The most common pathogens causing suppurative bronchopneumonia in domestic animals include *Pasteurella multocida*, *Bordetella bronchiseptica*, *Arcanobacterium* (*Actinomyces*) *pyogenes*, *Streptococcus* spp., *Escherichia coli*, and several species of mycoplasmas. Most of these organisms are secondary pathogens requiring a preceding impairment of the pulmonary defense mechanisms to colonize the lungs and establish an infection. Suppurative bronchopneumonia can also result from aspiration of bland material (e.g., milk). Pulmonary gangrene may ensue when the bronchopneumonic lung is invaded by saprophytic bacteria.

Fibrinous bronchopneumonia is similar to suppurative bronchopneumonia except that the predominant exudate is fibrinous rather than neutrophilic. With only a few exceptions, fibrinous bronchopneumonias also have a cranioventral distribution (Figs. 9-47, C and 9-50). However, exudation is not restricted to the boundaries of individual pulmonary lobules, as is the case in suppurative bronchopneumonias. Instead the inflammatory process in fibrinous pneumonias involves numerous contiguous lobules and the exudate moves quickly through pulmonary tissue until the entire pulmonary lobe is rapidly affected. Because of the involvement of the entire lobe and pleural surface, fibrinous bronchopneumonias are also referred to as lobar pneumonias or pleuropneumonias. In general terms, fibrinous bronchopneumonias are the result of more severe pulmonary injury and thus are more life threatening than suppurative bronchopneumonias. Even in cases in which fibrinous bronchopneumonia involves 30% or less of the total area, clinical signs and death can occur as a result of severe toxemia.

The gross appearance of fibrinous bronchopneumonia depends on the age and severity of the lesion and on whether the lung is observed externally or on a cut surface. Externally, early stages of fibrinous bronchopneumonias are characterized by severe congestion and hemorrhage, giving the affected lungs a characteristically intense red discoloration. A few hours later, fibrin starts to accumulate on the pleural surface, giving the pleura a ground glass appearance and eventually forming plaques of fibrinous exudate over a red, dark lung (Fig. 9-50). At this stage, a yellow fluid starts to accumulate in the thoracic cavity. The color of fibrin deposited over the pleural surface is also variable

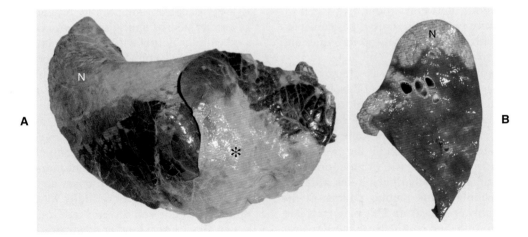

Fig. 9-50   **Fibrinous bronchopneumonia (pleuropneumonia), right lung, steer. A,** The pneumonia has a cranioventral distribution that extends into the middle and caudal lobes and affects approximately 80% of the lung parenchyma. The lung is firm, swollen, and covered with yellow fibrin (*). The dorsal portion of the caudal lung is normal (N). **B,** Cut surface. Affected parenchyma appears dark and hyperemic as compared with a normal (N) lung. This type of lesion is typical of *Mannheimia haemolytica* infection in cattle (shipping fever). (*A* and *B*, Courtesy Ontario Veterinary College.)

depending on the proportion of red blood cells, hemoglobin, and leukocytes. It can be yellow when the exudate is formed primarily by fibrin, tan when fibrin is mixed with blood, and gray when a large number of leukocytes are part of the fibrinous plaque. Because of the tendency of fibrin to deposit on the pleural surface, some pathologists use the term *pleuropneumonia* as a synonym for fibrinous bronchopneumonia.

On the cut surface, early stages of fibrinous bronchopneumonia appear as simple red consolidation (Fig. 9-50). In more advanced cases (24 hours), fibrinous bronchopneumonia is generally accompanied by notable dilation and thrombosis of lymph vessels and edema of interlobular septa. This distention of the interlobular septa gives affected lungs a typical marbled appearance. Distinct focal areas of coagulative necrosis in the pulmonary parenchyma are also common in fibrinous bronchopneumonia, such as in shipping fever pneumonia and contagious bovine pleuropneumonia. In animals that survive the early stage of fibrinous bronchopneumonia, pulmonary necrosis often develops into pulmonary "sequestra," which are isolated pieces of necrotic lung encapsulated by connective tissue. Pulmonary sequestra result from extensive necrosis of lung tissue caused either by severe ischemia or by the effect of necrotizing toxins released by pathogenic bacteria. Sequestra in veterinary pathology should not be confused with "bronchopulmonary sequestration," a term used in human pathology to describe a congenital malformation in which whole lobes or parts of the lung develop without normal connections to the airway or vascular systems.

Microscopically, in the initial stage of fibrinous bronchopneumonia, there is massive exudation of plasma proteins into the bronchioles and alveoli, and as a result most of the airspaces become obliterated by fluid and fibrin. Leakage of fibrin and fluid into alveolar lumina is because of extensive disruption of the integrity and increased permeability of the blood-air barrier. Fibrinous exudates can move from alveolus to alveolus through the pores of Kohn. Because fibrin is chemotactic for neutrophils, these types of leukocytes are always present a few hours after the onset of fibrinous inflammation. As inflammation progresses (3 to 5 days), fluid exudate is gradually replaced by a fibrinocellular exudates composed of fibrin, neutrophils, macrophages, and necrotic debris (Fig. 9-51). In chronic cases (after 7 days), there is notable fibrosis of the interlobular septa and pleura.

In contrast to suppurative bronchopneumonia, fibrinous bronchopneumonia rarely resolves completely, thus leaving noticeable scars in the form of pulmonary fibrosis and pleural adhesions. The most common sequelae found in animals surviving an acute episode of fibrinous bronchopneumonia include bronchiolitis obliterans,

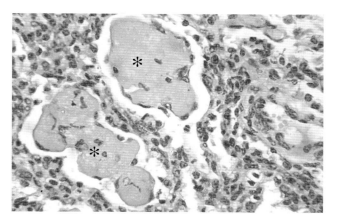

Fig. 9-51   **Fibrinous bronchopneumonia, chronic, lung, calf.** Note large aggregates of condensed fibrin (*) surrounded and infiltrated by phagocytic cells. H&E stain. *(Courtesy Dr. A. López, Atlantic Veterinary College.)*

in which organized exudate becomes attached to the bronchiolar lumen; gangrene, when saprophytic bacteria colonize necrotic lung; pulmonary sequestra; pulmonary fibrosis; abscesses; and chronic pleuritis with pleural adhesions. In some cases, pleuritis can be so extensive that fibrous adhesions extend onto the pericardial sac. Pathogens causing fibrinous bronchopneumonias in domestic animals include *Mannheimia (Pasteurella) haemolytica* (pneumonic mannheimiosis), *Histophilus somni* (formerly *Haemophilus somnus*), *Actinobacillus pleuropneumoniae* (porcine pleuropneumonia), *Mycoplasma bovis*, and *Mycoplasma mycoides* ssp. *mycoides* small colony type (contagious bovine pleuropneumonia). Fibrinous bronchopneumonia and pulmonary gangrene can also be the result of bronchoaspiration of irritant materials, such as gastric contents.

Fulminating hemorrhagic bronchopneumonia can be caused by highly pathogenic bacteria, such as *Bacillus anthracis*. Although the lesions in anthrax are primarily related to a severe septicemia and sepsis, anthrax should always be suspected in animals with sudden death and exhibiting severe acute fibrinohemorrhagic pneumonia, splenomegaly, and multisystemic hemorrhages. Animals are considered good sentinels for anthrax in cases of bioterrorism.

INTERSTITIAL PNEUMONIA

Interstitial pneumonia refers to a particular type of pneumonia in which injury and the inflammatory process take place primarily in any of the three layers of the alveolar walls (endothelium, basement membrane, and alveolar epithelium) and the contiguous bronchiolar interstitium. This type of pneumonia is perhaps the most difficult to diagnose at necropsy and generally requires microscopic confirmation. The pathogenesis of interstitial pneumonia is complex and can result from aerogenous injury to the alveolar epithelium (type I and II pneumonocytes) or from hematogenous injury to the alveolar capillary endothelium or alveolar basement membrane.

Aerogenous inhalation of toxic gases (i.e., ozone, NO_2), toxic fumes (smoke inhalation), and infection with pneumotropic viruses (influenza, IBR, EVR, canine distemper) are just a few of the different agents that can damage the alveolar epithelium. Hematogenous injury to the vascular endothelium occurs in septicemias (i.e., sepsis), in disseminated intravascular coagulation (DIC), from microembolism, from circulating larva migrans (*Ascaris suum*), from toxins absorbed in the alimentary tract (endotoxin) or toxic metabolites locally generated in the lungs (3 methylindole, paraquat), from release of free radicals in alveolar capillaries (ARDS), and from infections with endotheliotropic viruses (canine adenovirus and classical swine fever [hog cholera]). Damage to the alveolar wall can also occur when inhaled antigens, such as fungal spores, combine with circulating antibodies and form deposits of antigen-antibody complexes (type III hypersensitivity) in the alveolar wall, which initiate a cascade of inflammatory responses and injury (allergic alveolitis). As are interstitial pneumonias in human beings, those of the domestic animals are subdivided, based on some morphologic features, into acute and chronic. It should be kept in mind, however, that not all acute interstitial pneumonias are fatal and that they do not necessarily progress to the chronic form.

Acute interstitial pneumonias begin with injury to either type I pneumonocytes or alveolar capillary endothelium, which provokes a disruption of the blood-air barrier and a subsequent exudation of plasma proteins into the alveolar space. This leakage of proteinaceous fluid into the alveolar lumen constitutes the exudative phase of acute interstitial pneumonia. In some cases of diffuse alveolar damage, exuded plasma proteins mix with lipids and other components of pulmonary surfactant and form elongated membranes that become partially attached to the alveolar and bronchiolar walls. These membranes are referred to as hyaline membranes because they have a hyaline appearance (eosinophilic, homogenous, and amorphous) on microscopic examination (Fig. 9-35). In addition to intraalveolar exudation of fluid, inflammatory edema and neutrophils accumulate in the alveolar interstitium and cause thickening of the alveolar walls. This acute exudative phase is generally followed a few days later by the proliferative phase of acute interstitial pneumonias characterized by hyperplasia of type II pneumonocytes to replace the lost type I alveolar cells. Type II pneumonocytes are, in fact, progenitor cells that differentiate and replace necrotic type I pneumonocytes

(see General Aspects of Lung Inflammation). As a consequence, the alveolar walls become increasingly thickened. This process is in part the reason why lungs become rubbery on palpation, what prevents their normal collapse after the thorax is opened, and why the cut surface of the lung has a "meaty appearance."

Acute interstitial pneumonias are often mild and transient, especially those caused by some respiratory viruses, such as those responsible for equine and porcine influenza. These mild forms of pneumonia are rarely seen in the postmortem room because they are not fatal and do not leave significant sequelae (see Defense Mechanisms of the Exchange System [Alveoli]). In severe cases of acute interstitial pneumonias, animals may die of respiratory failure, usually as a result of diffuse alveolar damage, a profuse exudative phase (leakage of proteinaceous fluid) leading to a fatal pulmonary edema. Examples of this type of fatal acute interstitial pneumonia are bovine pulmonary edema and emphysema, and ARDS in all species.

In contrast to bronchopneumonias, in which distribution of lesions is generally cranioventral, in acute or chronic interstitial pneumonias lesions are more diffusely distributed and generally involve all pulmonary lobes, or in some cases they appear to be more pronounced in the dorsocaudal aspects of the lungs. Three important gross features of interstitial pneumonia are the failure of lungs to collapse when the thoracic cavity is opened, the occasional presence of rib impressions on the lung's pleural surface indicating poor deflation, and the lack of visible exudates in airways unless complicated with secondary bacterial pneumonia (Figs. 9-47, D and 9-52). The color of affected lungs varies from diffusely red to diffusely pale gray to a mottled red, pale appearance. Pale lungs are caused by severe obliteration of alveolar capillaries (reduced blood-tissue ratio), especially when there is fibrosis. The texture of lungs with uncomplicated interstitial pneumonia is typically elastic or rubbery, but definitive diagnosis based on texture alone is difficult because of the intrinsic subjectivity of palpation. On a cut surface, the lungs may appear more "meaty" (having the texture and appearance of raw meat) and have no evidence of exudate (Fig. 9-52). It should be remembered, however, that acute interstitial pneumonias, particularly in cattle, are frequently accompanied by pulmonary edema (exudative phase) and interstitial emphysema secondary to partial obstruction of bronchioles by edema fluid and strenuous air gasping before death. Because edema tends to gravitate into the cranioventral portions of the lungs, and emphysema is often more obvious in the dorsocaudal aspects, acute interstitial pneumonias in cattle occasionally have a gross cranioventral-like pattern that may resemble that of bronchopneumonia generally. Lungs are notably heavy because of the edema and the infiltrative and proliferative changes.

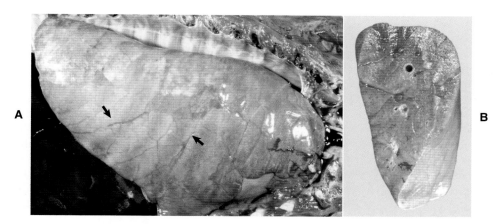

Fig. 9-52   Interstitial pneumonia, lung, feeder pig. A, The lung is heavy, pale, and rubbery in texture. It also has prominent costal (rib) imprints *(arrows)*, a result of hypercellularity of the interstitium and the failure of the lungs to collapse when the thorax was opened. **B,** Transverse section. The pulmonary parenchyma has a "meaty" appearance and some edema, but no exudate is present in airways or on the pleural surface. This type of lung change in pigs is highly suggestive of a viral pneumonia. *(A and B, Courtesy Dr. A. López, Atlantic Veterinary College.)*

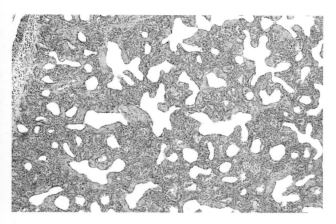

Fig. 9-53   Interstitial pneumonia, lung, aged ewe. The alveolar septa are notably thickened by severe interstitial infiltration of lymphocytes and mononuclear cells. H&E stain. *(Courtesy Western College of Veterinary Medicine.)*

When the source of alveolar injury persists, the proliferative and infiltrative lesions of acute interstitial pneumonia can progress into a different morphologic stage referred to as chronic interstitial pneumonia. The hallmark of chronic interstitial pneumonias is fibrosis of the alveolar walls (with or without intraalveolar fibrosis), and in some cases accumulation of mononuclear inflammatory cells in the interstitium (Fig. 9-53) and persistence of hyperplastic type II pneumonocytes. It should be emphasized again that, although the lesions in interstitial pneumonia are centered in the alveolar walls and its interstitium, a mixture of desquamated epithelial cells, macrophages, and mononuclear cells are usually present in the lumen of bronchioles and alveoli. Other, concurrent changes that can accompany some forms of chronic interstitial pneumonia are formations of microscopic granulomas and hyperplasia of smooth muscle in airways or pulmonary vasculature. Ovine progressive pneumonia, hypersensitivity pneumonitis in cattle and dogs, and silicosis in horses are good veterinary examples of chronic interstitial pneumonia. Pneumoconioses (silicosis, asbestosis), paraquat toxicity, pneumotoxic antineoplastic drugs (bleomycin), and extrinsic allergic alveolitis (farmer's lung) are well-known examples of diseases that lead to chronic interstitial pneumonias in human beings. Massive pulmonary migration of ascaris larvae in pigs also causes interstitial pneumonia (Fig. 9-54).

The term *bronchointerstitial pneumonia* has been introduced into veterinary pathology to describe cases in which pulmonary lesions share some histologic features of both bronchopneumonia and interstitial pneumonia. This combined-type pneumonia is, in fact, frequently seen in many viral infections in which viruses replicate and cause injury in bronchial, bronchiolar, and alveolar cells. Damage to the bronchial and bronchiolar epithelium causes influx of neutrophils similar to that of bronchopneumonias, and damage to alveolar walls causes proliferation of type II pneumonocytes, similar to that which takes place in the proliferative phase of acute interstitial pneumonias. Examples of bronchointerstitial pneumonia include uncomplicated cases of respiratory syncytial virus infections in cattle and lambs, canine distemper, and influenza in pigs and horses.

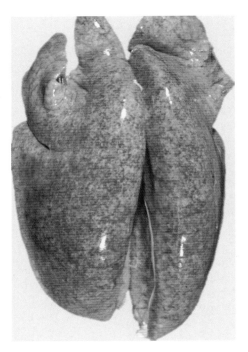

Fig. 9-54   Interstitial pneumonia, edema, and hemorrhages, lungs, pig. This pig had migrating *Ascaris suum* larvae. The lungs are heavy and wet and failed to collapse when the thorax was opened, due to pulmonary edema. The mottled appearance of lungs is due to the presence of numerous petechiae scattered in the pulmonary parenchyma. Petechiae are likely alveolar hemorrhages caused by migrating larvae. Larvae leave the blood stream to enter the alveoli by penetrating and rupturing alveolar capillaries and thus damage the blood-air barrier in alveolar septa. *(Courtesy Dr. J.M. King, College of Veterinary Medicine, Cornell University.)*

EMBOLIC PNEUMONIA

Embolic pneumonia refers to a particular type of pneumonia in which injury is hematogenous, and the inflammatory response is typically centered in pulmonary arterioles and alveolar capillaries. Lungs act as a biologic filter for circulating particulate matter. Sterile thrombi, unless extremely large, are rapidly dissolved and removed from the pulmonary vasculature by fibrinolysis, causing little if any ill effects. Experimental studies have confirmed that most types of bacteria when injected intravenously (bacteremia) generally are phagocytosed by pulmonary intravascular macrophages, or bypass the lungs and are finally trapped in the liver, spleen, joints, or other organs. To cause pulmonary infection, circulating bacteria must first attach to the pulmonary endothelium with specific binding proteins or simply attach to intravascular fibrin and then evade phagocytosis by intravascular macrophages or leukocytes. Infected thrombi because of their size facilitate entrapment of bacteria in the pulmonary vessels and provide a

favorable environment to escape phagocytosis. Once trapped in the pulmonary vasculature, usually in small arterioles or alveolar capillaries, offending bacteria disrupt endothelium and basement membranes, spread from the vessels to the interstitium and then to the surrounding lung, forming finally a new nidus of infection.

Embolic pneumonia is characterized by multifocal lesions randomly distributed in all pulmonary lobes because of entrapment of septic emboli (Fig. 9-47, E). Early lesions in embolic pneumonia are characterized grossly by the presence of very small (1 to 10 mm), white foci in the lungs surrounded by a discrete, red, hemorrhagic halo (Fig. 9-55). Unless emboli arrive in massive numbers, causing fatal pulmonary edema, embolic pneumonia is seldom fatal; therefore these acute lesions are rarely seen at postmortem examination. In most instances, acute lesions if unresolved rapidly progress to the formation of pulmonary abscesses that are randomly distributed in all pulmonary lobes and are not restricted to the cranioventral aspects of the lungs, as is the case of abscesses developing from suppurative bronchopneumonia. The early inflammatory lesions in embolic pneumonias are always focal (Fig. 9-56); thus they differ from those of endotoxemia or septicemia, in which endothelial damage and interstitial reactions (interstitial pneumonia) are diffusely distributed in the lungs.

When embolic pneumonia or its sequelae (abscesses) are encountered, careful postmortem evaluation is

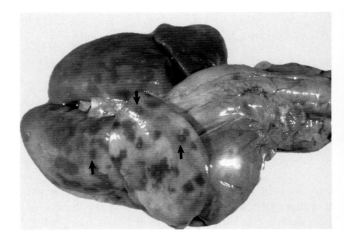

Fig. 9-55   Embolic pneumonia, lungs, 6-week-old puppy. Large hemorrhagic foci are scattered relatively uniformly throughout all pulmonary lobes *(arrows)*. These hemorrhagic foci are the sites of lodgment of *Pseudomonas aeruginosa* emboli (septic) which originated from necrotizing enteritis. Note the multifocal distribution of the inflammatory foci, which is typical of embolic pneumonia. Septic emboli were also present in the liver. *(Courtesy Atlantic Veterinary College.)*

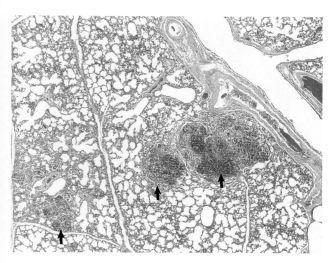

Fig. 9-56   Embolic pneumonia, lung, cow. Foci of necrosis and infiltration of neutrophils (*arrows*) resulting from septic emboli. Note the multifocal distribution of the lesion, which is typical of embolic pneumonia. Vegetative endocarditis involving the tricuspid valve was the source of septic emboli in this cow. H&E stain. *(Courtesy Dr. A. López, Atlantic Veterinary College.)*

required to locate the source of septic emboli. Most common causes include rupture of hepatic abscesses into the caudal vena cava in cattle, omphalophlebitis in farm animals, chronic bacterial skin or hoof infections, and infected jugular catheter in all species (Fig. 9-41). Valvular or mural endocarditis in the right side of the heart is also a usual source of septic emboli and embolic pneumonia in all species. Most frequently, bacterial isolates from septic pulmonary emboli in domestic animals are *Arcanobacterium (Actinomyces) pyogenes, Fusobacterium necrophorum, Erysipelothrix rhusiopathiae, Streptococcus suis* type II, *Staphylococcus aureus,* and *Streptococcus equi.*

GRANULOMATOUS PNEUMONIA

Granulomatous pneumonia refers to a particular type of pneumonia in which aerogenous or hematogenous injury is caused by organisms or particles that cannot be normally eliminated by phagocytosis and that evoke a local inflammatory reaction with numerous alveolar and interstitial macrophages, lymphocytes, a few neutrophils, and sometimes giant cells. The term *granulomatous* is used here to describe an anatomic pattern of pneumonia typically characterized by the presence of pulmonary granulomas.

The pathogenesis of granulomatous pneumonia shares some similarities with that of interstitial and embolic pneumonias. Not surprisingly, some pathologists group granulomatous pneumonias within one of these types of pneumonias (e.g., granulomatous interstitial pneumonia). What makes granulomatous pneumonia

a distinctive type is not so much the portal of entry or site of initial injury in the lungs, but the unique type of inflammatory response that results in the formation of granulomas, which can be easily recognized at gross and microscopic examination. The portal of agent entry into lungs can be aerogenous or hematogenous. As a rule, agents causing granulomatous pneumonia are resistant to intracellular killing by phagocytic cells and to the acute inflammatory response and persist in affected tissue for a long time.

The most common causes of granulomatous pneumonia in animals include systemic fungal diseases, such as cryptococcosis (*Cryptococcus neoformans*), coccidioidomycosis (*Coccidioides immitis*), histoplasmosis (*Histoplasma capsulatum*), and blastomycosis (*Blastomyces dermatitidis*). In most of these fungal diseases, the port of entry is aerogenous and from the lungs the fungi disseminate systemically to other organs, particularly the lymph nodes, liver, and spleen. Granulomatous pneumonia is also caused by some bacterial diseases, such as tuberculosis (*Mycobacterium bovis*) in all species, and inhaled foreign material (starch). Sporadically, aberrant parasites such as *Fasciola hepatica* in cattle and aspiration of foreign bodies can also cause granulomatous pneumonia. Feline infectious peritonitis is one of a few viral infections of domestic animals that result in granulomatous pneumonia. Lesions are caused by the deposition of antigen-antibody complexes in the vasculature of many organs, including the lungs, and subsequent vasculitis.

Granulomatous pneumonia is characterized by the presence of variable numbers of caseous or noncaseous granulomas randomly distributed in the lungs (Figs. 9-47, F and 9-57). On palpation, lungs have a typical nodular character given by well-circumscribed, variably sized nodules that, generally, have a firm texture, especially if calcification has occurred. During postmortem examination, granulomas in the lungs occasionally can be mistaken for neoplasms. Microscopically, pulmonary granulomas are composed of a center of necrotic tissue, surrounded by a rim of macrophages (epithelioid cells) and giant cells and an outer delineated layer of connective tissue commonly infiltrated by lymphocytes and plasma cells (Fig. 9-58). Unlike other types of pneumonias, the causative agent in granulomatous pneumonia can, in many cases, be identified microscopically in sections stained by PAS reaction or by Grocott-Gomori's methenamine silver (G-GMS) stains for fungi or the acid-fast stain for mycobacteria.

SPECIES-SPECIFIC PNEUMONIAS
PNEUMONIAS OF HORSES

Viral infections of the respiratory tract, particularly equine viral rhinopneumonitis and equine influenza, are important diseases of horses around the world. The effects of these and other respiratory viruses on the

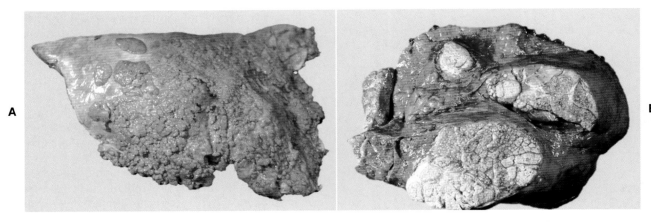

Fig. 9-57   Pulmonary tuberculosis, lung, aged cow. A, Multifocal, coalescing granulomatous pneumonia involves most of the lung, except for the dorsal portion of the caudal lung lobe. **B,** Transverse section. Large multifocal to confluent caseating granulomas are present in the pulmonary parenchyma. Note the caseous ("*cheesy*," *pale yellow-white*) appearance of the granulomas, which is typical of bovine tuberculosis. (**A,** *Courtesy Facultad de Medicina Veterinaria, UNAM, México.* **B,** *Courtesy Dr. J.M. King, College of Veterinary Medicine, Cornell University.*)

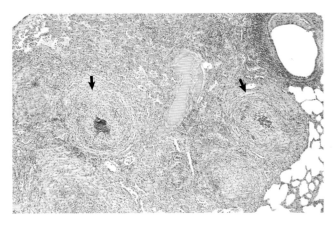

Fig. 9-58   Granulomatous pneumonia, lung, cow.
There are several noncaseous granulomas (*arrows*), each with a small necrotic center filled with neutrophils, surrounded by histiocytes and mononuclear cells, and with an outer rim of connective tissue. H&E stain. (*Courtesy Western College of Veterinary Medicine.*)

horse can be manifested in three distinct ways. First, as pure viral infections, their severity may range from mild to severe, making them a frequent interfering factor in training and athletic performance. Second, superimposed infections by opportunistic bacteria such as *Streptococcus* spp., *Escherichia coli*, *Klebsiella pneumoniae*, *Rhodococcus equi*, and various anaerobes can cause fibrinous or suppurative bronchopneumonias. Third, it is possible, but yet unproven, that viral infections may also predispose horses to "airway hyperresponsiveness" and "chronic obstructive pulmonary disease."

Equine influenza

Equine influenza is an important and highly contagious flulike respiratory disease of horses characterized by high morbidity and low mortality, and explosive outbreaks occur in susceptible populations of horses. Two antigenically unrelated subtypes of equine influenza viruses have been identified (A/equi-1 and A/equi-2). The course of the disease is generally mild and transient, and its importance is primarily because of its economic impact on horse racing. The types of injury and host response in the conducting system are described under Specific Diseases of Nasal Cavity and Sinuses (see Equine Nasal Diseases). Uncomplicated lesions in the lungs are those of mild and self-limiting bronchointerstitial pneumonia. The influenza virus antigen can be readily demonstrated in ciliated cells and alveolar macrophages. Clinical signs are characterized by fever, cough, abnormal lung sounds (crackles and wheezes), anorexia, and depression. Secondary bacterial infections (*Streptococcus equi, Streptococcus zooepidemicus, Streptococcus aureus*) commonly complicate equine influenza.

Equine viral rhinopneumonitis (EVR, equine herpesvirus infection)

This respiratory disease of young horses is particularly important in weanlings between 4 and 8 months of age and to a much lesser extent in young foals and adult horses. The causative agent is a ubiquitous equine herpesvirus (EHV-1 and EHV-4) that, in addition to respiratory disease, can cause abortion in pregnant mares and neurologic diseases in horses of all ages (see also EVR under Equine Nasal Diseases).

The respiratory form of EVR is a mild and a transient bronchointerstitial pneumonia seen only by pathologists when complications with secondary bacterial infections cause a fatal bronchopneumonia (*Streptococcus equi, Streptococcus zooepidemicus, Staphylococcus aureus*). Uncomplicated lesions in EVR are seen only in aborted fetuses or in foals that die within the first few days of life. They consist of focal areas of necrosis (0.5 to 2 mm) in various organs, including liver, adrenal glands, and lungs. In some cases intranuclear inclusion bodies are microscopically observed in these organs. Recent outbreaks of interstitial pneumonia in donkeys have been attributed to novel strains of equine (asinine) herpesvirus. Clinically, horses affected with the respiratory form of EVR exhibit fever, anorexia, conjunctivitis, cough, and nasal discharge.

Equine viral arteritis (EVA)

This pansystemic disease of foals and horses, caused by an arterivirus, occurs sporadically throughout the world, sometimes as an outbreak. This virus infects and causes severe cellular injury in macrophages and endothelial cells. Gross lesions consist of hemorrhage and edema in many tissues, including pulmonary edema, voluminous hydrothorax and hydroperitoneum, and edematous distention of the intestinal walls, scrotum, and periorbital tissues. Fibrinoid necrosis and inflammation of the vessel walls (vasculitis), particularly the small muscular arteries (lymphocytic arteritis), are the underlying microscopic lesions that explain most of the clinical and pathologic features. Pulmonary lesions are those of interstitial pneumonia with hyperplasia of type II pneumonocytes and vasculitis with distended pulmonary lymphatic vessels and abundant fluid in the bronchoalveolar spaces. Viral antigen can be detected by immunoperoxidase techniques in the walls and endothelial cells of affected pulmonary vessels and in alveolar macrophages.

Clinical signs are respiratory distress, fever, abortion, diarrhea, colic, and edema of the limbs and ventral abdomen. Respiratory signs are frequently seen and consist of serous or mucopurulent rhinitis and conjunctivitis with palpebral edema. Like most viral respiratory infections, EVA can predispose horses to opportunistic secondary bacterial pneumonias.

African horse sickness

This vector-borne disease of horses, mules, and donkeys is caused by an orbivirus (family Reoviridae) and is characterized by respiratory distress or cardiovascular failure. It has a high mortality rate—up to 95% in the native population of horses in Africa, the Middle East, India, Pakistan, and most recently Spain. Although the virus is transmitted primarily by insects (*Culicoides*) to horses, other animals such as dogs can be infected by eating infected equine flesh. The pathogenesis of African horse sickness remains unclear, but this equine orbivirus has an obvious tropism for pulmonary and cardiac endothelial cells, and to a lesser extent mononuclear cells. Based on clinical signs (not pathogenesis), African horse sickness is arbitrarily divided into four different forms—namely pulmonary, cardiac, mixed, and mild.

The pulmonary form is characterized by severe respiratory distress and rapid death because of massive pulmonary edema, presumably from viral injury to the pulmonary endothelial cells. Grossly, large amounts of froth are present in the airways, lungs fail to collapse, subpleural lymph vessels are distended, and the ventral parts of the lungs are notably edematous. In the cardiac form, recurrent fever is detected, and heart failure results in subcutaneous and interfascial edema, most notably in the neck and supraorbital region. The mixed form is a combination of the respiratory and cardiac forms. Finally, the mild form, rarely seen in postmortem rooms, is characterized by fever and clinical signs resembling those of equine influenza; it is, in most cases, transient and followed by a complete recovery. This mild form is most frequently seen in donkeys, mules, and zebras and in horses with some degree of immunity. Detection of viral antigen for diagnostic purposes could be done by immunohistochemistry in paraffin-embedded tissues.

Equine *Morbillivirus* (Hendra virus)

Fatal cases of a novel respiratory disease in horses and human beings suddenly appeared around 1994 in Hendra, a suburb of Brisbane, Australia. This outbreak was attributed to a newly recognized virus that was tentatively classified as equine *Morbillivirus* and is currently referred to as Hendra virus, a new member of the subfamily Paramyxoviridae. The involvement of fruit bats (flying foxes) in the transmission of this viral disease has been suggested. The lungs of affected horses are severely edematous with gelatinous distention of pleura and subpleural lymph vessels. Microscopically the lungs have diffuse alveolar edema associated with vasculitis, capillary thrombosis, distention of lymphatic vessels, and presence of multinucleated syncytial cells typical of *Morbillivirus* infections in the endothelium of small pulmonary blood vessels and alveolar capillaries. The characteristic inclusion bodies seen in other *Morbillivirus* infections are not seen in horses; however, the virus can be easily detected by immunohistochemistry in pulmonary endothelial cells and alveolar epithelial cells. Clinical signs are nonspecific and include fever, anorexia, respiratory distress, and nasal discharge.

Rhodococcus equi

Rhodococcus equi, formerly known as *Corynebacterium equi*, is an important cause of morbidity and mortality in foals around the world. It is a facultative intracellular gram-positive bacterium that causes two major forms of disease—one involves the intestine, causing ulcerative enterocolitis, and the other affects the respiratory tract, resulting in a severe and often fatal bronchopneumonia. Although half of foals with pneumonia have ulcerative enterocolitis, it is rare to find animals with intestinal lesions alone. Occasionally, infection is disseminated to lymph nodes, joints, bones, genital tract, and other organs. Because *Rhodococcus equi* is present in soil and feces of herbivores (particularly foals), it is not unusual for the disease to become enzootic on farms where the organism has been shed earlier by infected foals. Serologic evidence of infection in horses is widespread, yet clinical disease is sporadic and largely restricted to young foals or to adult horses with severe immunosuppression. Virulence factors encoded by plasmids (virulence-associated proteins) appear to be responsible for the survival of *Rhodococcus equi* in macrophages, thus determining the evolution of the disease. This bacterium also has been sporadically incriminated with infections in cattle, goats, pigs, dogs, and cats, and quite often in immunocompromised human beings—for example, those infected with the AIDS virus, after organ transplantation, or undergoing chemotherapy.

It is still debatable whether natural infection starts as a bronchopneumonia (aerogenous route) from which *Rhodococcus equi* reaches the intestine via swallowed sputum, or whether infection starts as an enteritis (oral route) with subsequent bacteremia into the lungs. The results of experimental studies suggest that natural infection with this organism likely starts from inhalation of infected dust or aerosols. Once in the lung, *Rhodococcus equi* undergoes rapid phagocytosis by alveolar macrophages, but because of defective phagosome-lysosome fusion and premature lysosomal degranulation, bacteria survive and multiply, eventually leading to the destruction of the macrophage. Interestingly, *Rhodococcus equi* appears to be easily killed by neutrophils but not macrophages. Released cytokines and lysosomal enzymes and bacterial toxins are responsible for extensive caseous necrosis of the lungs and the recruitment of large numbers of neutrophils, macrophages, and giant cells containing intracellular gram-positive organisms in their cytoplasm.

Depending on the stage of infection and the immune status and age of affected horses, pulmonary lesions induced by *Rhodococcus equi* can vary from suppurative bronchopneumonia to granulomatous pneumonia with caseated necrosis. In young foals, the infection starts as a suppurative cranioventral bronchopneumonia, which progresses within a few days into small variable-size pulmonary abscesses. These abscesses

rapidly transform into pyogranulomatous nodules some of which become confluent and form large masses of caseous exudate (Fig. 9-59). Microscopically the early lesion starts with neutrophilic infiltration, followed by an intense influx of alveolar macrophages into the bronchoalveolar spaces. This type of histiocytic inflammation tends to persist for a long period of time because *Rhodococcus equi* is a facultative intracellular organism that survives the bactericidal effects of equine alveolar macrophages. In the most chronic cases, the pulmonary lesions culminate with the formation of large necrotic masses with extensive fibrosis of the surrounding pulmonary parenchyma. PCR analysis of tracheal aspirates has successfully been used as an alternative to bacteriologic culture in the diagnosis of *Rhodococcus equi* infection in live foals.

Clinically, *Rhodococcus equi* infection can be acute, with rapid death caused by severe bronchopneumonia, or chronic, with depression, cough, weight loss, and respiratory distress. In either form, there may be diarrhea, arthritis, or subcutaneous abscess formation.

Other pneumonias of horses

Chlamydophila (Chlamydia) psittaci, an obligatory intracellular pathogen, can cause systemic infection in many mammalian and avian species; in horses, it also causes keratoconjunctivitis, rhinitis, pneumonia, abortion, polyarthritis, enteritis, hepatitis, and encephalitis. Serologic studies suggest that infection without apparent disease is common in horses. Horses experimentally infected with *Chlamydophila psittaci* develop mild and transient bronchointerstitial pneumonia. Detection of chlamydial organisms in affected tissue is not easy and requires special laboratory techniques, such as PCR and fluorescent antibody tests.

Horses are susceptible to mycobacteriosis (*Mycobacterium avium* complex, *Mycobacterium tuberculosis*, and *Mycobacterium bovis*). The intestinal tract and associated lymph nodes are usually affected, suggesting ingestion, but with hematogenous dissemination, the lungs are involved (Fig. 9-60). The tubercles (granulomas) definitely differ from those in ruminants and pigs, being smooth, gray, solid nodules without grossly visible caseous necrosis or calcification; they typically appear more like sarcomas. Microscopically, the tubercles are composed of macrophages, epithelioid cells, and multinucleated giant cells. Fibrosis increases with time, accounting in part for the sarcomatous appearance.

Adenovirus infections occur commonly in Arabian foals with combined immunodeficiency (CID), a hereditary lack of B and T lymphocytes. In cases of adenoviral infection, large basophilic or amphophilic inclusions are present in the nuclei of tracheal, bronchial, bronchiolar, alveolar, renal, and intestinal

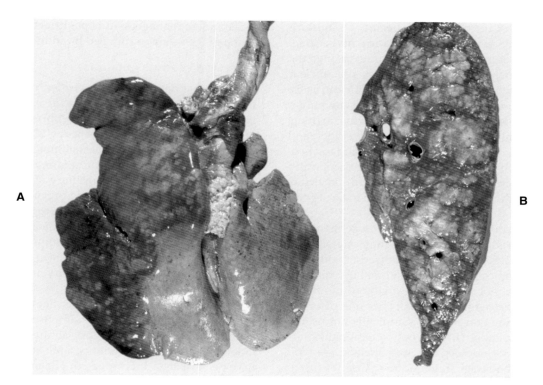

Fig. 9-59   Granulomatous pneumonia (*Rhodococcus equi*), lungs, foal. A, Cranioventral consolidation of the lungs with subpleural granulomas. Note that the pneumonic lesions in this foal are unilateral. This was an experimental case in which a foal was intratracheally inoculated with a suspension of *Rhodococcus equi*. **B,** Cut surface. Note the large, confluent, caseated granulomas. (**A** *and* **B,** *Courtesy Drs. J. Yager and J.Prescott, Ontario Veterinary College.*)

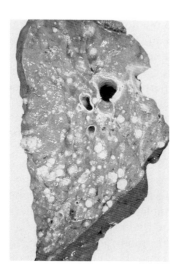

Fig. 9-60   Multifocal granulomatous pneumonia, tuberculosis (*Mycobacterium avium-intracellulare*), lung, cut surface, aged horse. Note the large numbers of non-caseating granulomas scattered throughout the pulmonary parenchyma. In horses, tuberculous granulomas often resemble sarcomatous nodules. (*Courtesy Western College of Veterinary Medicine.*)

epithelial cells. As it occurs in other species, infection with a unique fungal pathogen known as *Pneumocystis carinii* typically occurs in immunosuppressed or immunoincompetent individuals, such as Arabian foals with CID. Diagnosis of *Pneumocystis carinii* requires microscopic examination of lungs and special stains (see under Pneumonias of Pigs).

Diffuse proliferative interstitial pneumonias of undetermined cause that can progress to pulmonary fibrosis have been reported in North American horses. The gross and microscopic lesions are reminiscent of those of bovine pulmonary edema and emphysema with hyperplasia of type II pneumonocytes. The cause of this form of equine interstitial pneumonia is not known, but toxic and viral causes have been proposed.

Aspiration pneumonia is often a devastating sequela to improper gastric tubing of horses, particularly exogenous lipid pneumonia from mineral oil delivered into the trachea in treatment of colic. Gross and microscopic lesions are described in detail in the section Aspiration Pneumonias of Cattle.

Parasitic pneumonias of horses. *Parascaris equorum* is a large nematode (roundworm) of the small intestine of horses; the larval stages migrate through the lungs as ascarid larvae do in pigs. It is still unclear whether migration of *Parascaris equorum* larvae can cause significant pulmonary lesions under natural conditions. Experimentally, migration of larvae results in coughing, anorexia, weight loss, and small necrotic foci and petechial hemorrhages in the liver, hepatic and tracheobronchial lymph nodes, and lungs. Microscopically, eosinophils are prominent in the interstitium and airway mucosa during the parasitic migration and in focal granulomas caused by dead larvae in the lung.

Dictyocaulus arnfieldi is not a very pathogenic nematode, but it should be considered if there are signs of coughing in horses that are pastured together with donkeys. Donkeys are considered the natural hosts and can tolerate large numbers of parasites without ill effects. *Dictyocaulus arnfieldi* does not usually become patent in horses, so examination of fecal samples is not useful; bronchoalveolar lavage (BAL) is only occasionally diagnostic because eosinophils, but not parasites, are typically found in the lavage fluid. Mature parasites (up to 8 cm in length) cause obstructive bronchitis, edema, and atelectasis particularly along the dorsocaudal lung. The microscopic lesion is an eosinophilic bronchitis similar to the less acute infestations seen in cattle and sheep with their *Dictyocaulus* species.

PNEUMONIAS OF CATTLE
Bovine respiratory disease (BRD) complex; acute undifferentiated respiratory disease

These two general terms are often used by clinicians to describe acute and severe bovine respiratory illness of clinically undetermined cause. The BRD complex and acute undifferentiated respiratory disease are clinical terms that do not imply any particular type of pneumonia and therefore should not be used in pathology reports. Clinically, the BRD complex includes enzootic pneumonia of calves (multifactorial etiology); pneumonic mannheimiosis (*Mannheimia haemolytica*); respiratory histophilosis (*Histophilus somni*), previously known as respiratory hemophilosis (*Haemophilus somnus*); respiratory viral infections such as infectious bovine rhinotracheitis (IBR/BHV-1), parainfluenza-3 (PI-3 virus), and bovine respiratory syncytial virus (BRSV); and noninfectious interstitial pneumonias such as bovine pulmonary edema and emphysema, reinfection syndrome, and many others.

Enzootic pneumonia, sometimes simply referred to as "calf pneumonia," is a disease caused by a variety of etiologic agents that produces an assortment of lung lesions in young, intensively housed calves. Morbidity is often high (up to 90%), but fatalities are uncommon (>5%) unless management is poor or unless new, virulent pathogens are introduced by additions to the herd.

Bovine enzootic pneumonia

Enzootic pneumonia is also called viral pneumonia because it often begins with an acute respiratory infection with PI-3 virus, BRSV, or possibly with one or more of several other viruses (adenoviruses, BHV-1, reoviruses, and rhinoviruses). Mycoplasmas, notably *Mycoplasma dispar*, *Mycoplasma bovis*, *Ureaplasma*, and possibly *Chlamydophila* may also be primary agents. Following infection with any of these agents, opportunistic bacteria such as *Pasteurella multocida*, *Arcanobacterium (Actinomyces) pyogenes*, *Histophilus somni*, *Mannheimia haemolytica*, and *Escherichia coli* cause a secondary suppurative bronchopneumonia, the most serious stage of enzootic pneumonia. The pathogenesis of the primary invasion and how it predisposes the host to invasion by the opportunists are poorly understood, but it is likely that there is impairment of pulmonary defense mechanisms. Environmental factors, including air quality (poor ventilation), high relative humidity, and animal crowding have been strongly incriminated. The immune status of the calf also plays an important role in the development and severity of enzootic pneumonia. Calves with bovine leukocyte adhesion deficiency (BLAD), which prevents the migration of neutrophils from the capillaries, are highly susceptible to bronchopneumonia.

Lesions are variable and depend largely on the agents involved and on the duration of the inflammatory process. In the acute phases, lesions caused by viruses are those of bronchointerstitial pneumonia, which are generally mild and transient, and therefore are seen only sporadically at necropsy. Microscopically the lesions are necrotizing bronchiolitis, necrosis of type I pneumonocytes with hyperplasia of type II pneumonocytes, and mild interstitial and alveolar edema.

In the case of PI-3 and BRSV infection, intracytoplasmic inclusion bodies and the formation of large multinucleated syncytia, resulting from the fusion of infected bronchiolar epithelial cells, can also be observed in the lungs (Fig. 9-61).

The mycoplasmas also can cause bronchiolitis, bronchiolar and alveolar necrosis, and an interstitial reaction, but in contrast to viral-induced pneumonias, mycoplasmal lesions tend to progress to a chronic stage characterized by striking peribronchiolar lymphoid hyperplasia (cuffing pneumonia). When complicated by secondary bacterial infections (e.g., *Pasteurella multocida*, *Arcanobacterium pyogenes*), viral or mycoplasmal lesions change from a pure bronchointerstitial to a suppurative bronchopneumonia (Fig. 9-62). In late stages of bronchopneumonia, the lungs contain a creamy-mucoid exudate in the airways and often have pulmonary abscesses or bronchiectasis (Fig. 9-46). Airway hyperreactivity has been recently described in neonatal calves following BRSV infection; however, the significance of this syndrome in relation to enzootic pneumonia of calves is still under investigation.

It should be noted that the same viruses and mycoplasmas involved in the enzootic pneumonia complex can also predispose cattle to other diseases,

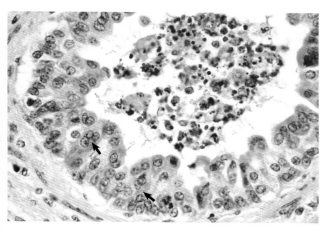

Fig. 9-61   Necrotizing bronchiolitis, bovine respiratory syncytial virus, lung, 5-week-old calf. This is the reparative stage of necrotizing bronchiolitis and is characterized by epithelial hyperplasia and exfoliation of necrotic cells into the bronchiolar lumen. Epithelial cells are swollen, and the cytoplasm of some cells contains eosinophilic inclusion bodies surrounded by a clear halo *(arrows)*. Many of these hyperplastic bronchiolar cells eventually undergo apoptosis during the last stage of bronchiolar repair. H&E stain. *(Courtesy Dr. A. López, Atlantic Veterinary College.)*

such as pneumonic mannheimiosis (*Mannheimia haemolytica*). Clinically, enzootic pneumonia is usually mild, but fatal cases are occasionally seen even in farms with optimal health management.

Pneumonic mannheimiosis (shipping fever)

Shipping fever (transit fever) is a vague clinical term used to denote acute respiratory diseases that occurred in cattle several days or weeks after shipment. The disease is characterized by a severe fibrinous bronchopneumonia, reflecting the fact that death generally occurs early or at an acute stage. Because *Mannheimia haemolytica* (formerly *Pasteurella haemolytica*) is typically isolated from affected lungs, the names pneumonic mannheimiosis and pneumonic pasteurellosis have been used synonymously. It is known that pneumonic mannheimiosis can occur in animals that have not been shipped and that organisms other than *Mannheimia haemolytica* can cause similar lesions. Therefore, the term *shipping fever* should be relinquished in favor of more specific names such as pneumonic mannheimiosis or respiratory histophilosis (hemophilosis).

Pneumonic mannheimiosis (shipping fever) is the most important respiratory disease of cattle in North America, particularly in feedlot animals that have been through the stressful marketing and assembly processes. *Mannheimia haemolytica* biotype A, serotype 1 is the etiologic agent responsible for the severe pulmonary lesions. A few investigators still consider that *Pasteurella multocida* and other serotypes of *Mannheimia haemolytica* are also causes of this disease.

Even after many years of intense investigation, from the gross lesions to the molecular aspects of the disease, the pathogenesis of pneumonic mannheimiosis

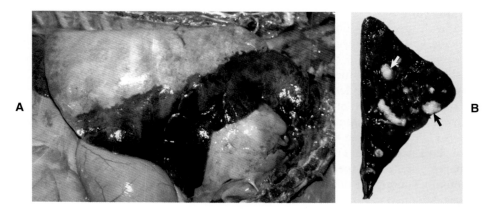

Fig. 9-62   Suppurative bronchopneumonia, right lung, calf. A, Approximately 40% of the lung parenchyma is consolidated and includes most of the cranial lung lobe and the ventral portions of the middle and caudal lung lobes, a distribution often designated as cranioventral. Note the dark color of the consolidated lung and the normal appearance of the dorsal portion of the caudal lung lobe. **B,** Transverse section of the cranial lung lobe showing bronchi filled with purulent exudate. *(arrows).* *(A and B, Courtesy Ontario Veterinary College.)*

remains incompletely understood. Experiments have established that *Mannheimia haemolytica* A1 alone is usually incapable of causing disease because it is rapidly cleared by pulmonary defense mechanisms. These findings may explain why *Mannheimia haemolytica*, in spite of being present in the nasal cavity of healthy animals, only sporadically causes disease. For *Mannheimia haemolytica* to be established as a pulmonary infection, it is first required that stressors impair the defense mechanisms and allow the bacteria to colonize the lung (see Impairment of Defense Mechanisms). These stressors include weaning, transport, fatigue, crowding, mixing of cattle from various sources, inclement weather, temporary starvation, and viral infections. Horizontal transmission of viruses and *Mannheimia haemolytica* occurs during crowding and transportation of cattle.

Viruses that most commonly predispose cattle to pneumonic mannheimiosis include BHV-1, PI-3, BRSV, and several others. Once established in the lungs, *Mannheimia haemolytica* causes lesions by means of different virulence factors, which include endotoxin, lipopolysaccharide, and outer membrane proteins, but the most important is probably the production of a leukotoxin (exotoxin), which binds and kills bovine macrophages and neutrophils. The fact that this toxin exclusively affects ruminant leukocytes probably explains why *Mannheimia haemolytica* is a respiratory pathogen in cattle and sheep but not in other species. During *Mannheimia haemolytica* infection, alveolar macrophages, neutrophils, and mast cells release maximum amounts of proinflammatory cytokines, particularly TNF-α, IL-1, IL-8, adhesion molecules, histamine, and leukotrienes. By locally releasing enzymes and free radicals, leukocytes further contribute to the injury and necrosis of bronchiolar and alveolar cells.

The gross lesions of acute and subacute pneumonic mannheimiosis are the prototype of fibrinous (lobar) bronchopneumonia, with prominent fibrinous pleuritis (Fig. 9-63) and pleural effusion. Lesions are always cranioventral and usually ventral to a horizontal line through the tracheal bifurcation. The interlobular septa are distended by yellow, gelatinous edema and fibrin. The "marbling" of lobules is the result of areas of coagulation necrosis, interlobular interstitial edema, and congestion (Fig. 9-64). The necrotic areas are typically bordered by a rim of elongated cells often referred to as "swirling macrophages" or "oat-shaped cells," now known to be degenerating neutrophils mixed with a few alveolar macrophages. Edema and fibrin are the major components of the exudate in alveoli and interlobular septa (Fig. 9-64). The extensive deposition of fibrin is the result of increased permeability of alveolar capillaries exacerbated by altered platelet function, increased procoagulant activity, and diminished profibrinolytic

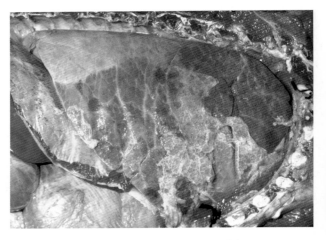

Fig. 9-63 **Fibrinous bronchopneumonia (pleuropneumonia), pneumonic mannheimiosis (*Mannheimia haemolytica*), right lung, steer.** Note the cranioventral pneumonia involving approximately 85% of the lung parenchyma. The lung is firm and swollen, and the pleura is covered with a thick layer of fibrin. *(Courtesy College of Veterinary Medicine, University of Illinois.)*

activity in the lungs. The trachea and bronchi can have considerable amounts of blood and exudate transported by the mucociliary escalator or coughed up from deep within the lungs, but their walls are not particularly involved. Because of the necrotizing process, sequelae to pneumonic mannheimiosis can be serious and can include abscesses, sequestra (isolated piece of necrotic lung), chronic pleuritis, fibrous pleural adhesions, and bronchiectasis.

Clinically, pneumonic mannheimiosis is characterized by a severe toxemia that can kill animals even when considerable parts of the lungs remain functional and structurally normal. Cattle usually become depressed, febrile (104° to 106° F/40° to 41° C), and anorexic and have a productive cough, encrusted nose, mucopurulent nasal exudate, shallow respiration, or an expiratory grunt.

Hemorrhagic septicemia

Pneumonic mannheimiosis should not be confused with hemorrhagic septicemia (septicemic pasteurellosis) of ruminants caused by inhalation or ingestion of serotypes B and E of *Pasteurella multocida*. This disease does not occur in North America and currently is reported only from some countries in Asia and Africa. In contrast to pneumonic mannheimiosis, in which lesions are always confined to the lower respiratory tract, the bacteria in hemorrhagic septicemia always disseminates hematogenously to other organs. Hemorrhagic septicemia is clinically characterized by

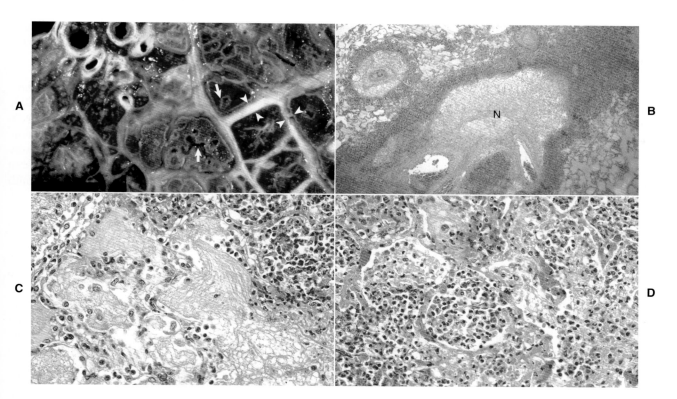

Fig. 9-64   Pneumonic mannheimiosis (*Mannheimia haemolytica*), lung, steer. A, Cut surface. Interlobular septa (*arrowheads*) are notably distended by edema and fibrin. In the lung parenchyma are irregular areas of coagulative necrosis (*arrows*) surrounded by a rim of inflammatory cells. **B,** Note a large area of necrosis (*N*) of the pulmonary parenchyma. Typically these necrotic areas are surrounded by an outer dense layer of inflammatory cells. Alveoli in the bottom right corner are edematous; those in the top left corner are relatively normal. H&E stain. **C,** Note alveoli filled with fibrin (*center*) and with neutrophils and macrophages (*top right*). H&E stain. **D,** *Mannheimia haemolytica* produces leukotoxin (cytotoxic for ruminant leukocytes) and lipopolysaccharide. Note the accumulation of cells, chiefly neutrophils, in the alveoli. Also note the active hyperemia of acute inflammation of the alveolar capillaries. H&E stain. (**A,** *Courtesy Dr. A. López, Atlantic Veterinary College.* **B, C,** *and* **D,** *Courtesy Dr. J.F. Zachary, College of Veterinary Medicine, University of Illinois.*)

a severe, acute septicemia, high fever, and rapid death. At necropsy, typically, generalized petechiae are present on the serosal surfaces of the intestine, heart, lungs, and in skeletal muscles. Superficial and visceral lymph nodes are swollen and hemorrhagic. Variable lesions include edematous and hemorrhagic lungs with or without consolidation, hemorrhagic enteritis, blood-tinged fluid in the thorax and abdomen, and subcutaneous edema of the head, neck, and ventral abdomen. Bacteria can be cultured from blood and tissue.

Respiratory histophilosis (hemophilosis)

Respiratory hemophilosis is part of the *Histophilus somni* (*Haemophilus somnus*) disease complex, which has different clinicopathologic forms, each one involving different organs. This complex includes septicemia, encephalitis (known as thrombotic meningoencephalitis [TME]), pneumonia (respiratory histophilosis [hemophilosis]), pleuritis, myocarditis, arthritis, ophthalmitis, conjunctivitis, otitis, and abortion. The portals of entry for the different forms of histophilosis have not been properly established.

The respiratory form of bovine histophilosis is the result of the bacterium's capacity to produce both suppurative and fibrinous bronchopneumonia. The latter is in some cases indistinguishable from that of pneumonic mannheimiosis. The pathogenesis of respiratory histophilosis is still poorly understood, and the disease cannot be reproduced consistently by administration of *Histophilus somni* alone. Like *Mannheimia haemolytica*, it requires predisposing factors, such as stress or a preceding viral infection. *Histophilus somni* is often isolated from the lungs of calves with enzootic pneumonia. The capacity of *Histophilus somni* to cause septicemia and localized infections in the lungs, brain, eyes, ear, heart, mammary gland, male and female genital organs, or placenta is perhaps attributable to specific virulence factors, such as immunoglobulin binding proteins (IgBPs). Also, *Histophilus somni* has the ability to undergo structural and antigenic variation, evade phagocytosis by promoting leukocytic apoptosis, inhibit intracellular killing, reduce transferrin concentrations, and induce endothelial apoptosis in affected calves. Mixed pulmonary infections of *Histophilus somni*, *Mannheimia haemolytica*, *Pasteurella multocida*, and mycoplasmas are fairly common in calves.

Contagious bovine pleuropneumonia

Contagious bovine pleuropneumonia is of historical interest in veterinary medicine, as the object of early national control programs for infectious disease. It was eradicated from North America in 1892 and from Australia in the 1970s, but it is still enzootic in large areas of Africa, Asia, and Eastern Europe. The etiologic agent, *Mycoplasma mycoides* ssp. *mycoides* small colony type, was the first *Mycoplasma* isolated and is one of the most pathogenic of those that infect domestic animals. Portal of entry is aerogenous, and infections occur when a susceptible animal inhales infected droplets. The pathogenic mechanisms are still inadequately understood but are suspected to involve toxin production, unregulated production of TNF-α, ciliary dysfunction, immunosuppression, and immune-mediated vasculitis. Vasculitis and thrombosis of blood vessels lead to lobular infarction.

The name of the disease is a good indication of the gross lesions. It is a severe, fibrinous bronchopneumonia (pleuropneumonia) similar to that of pneumonic mannheimiosis but having a more pronounced "marbling" of the lobules because of extensive lymphatic thrombosis and interlobular edema (different stages of inflammation), 60% to 79% of lesions in the caudal lobes (not cranioventrally), and more frequent and larger pulmonary sequestra (necrotic lung encapsulated by connective tissue). Microscopically the appearance again is like that of pneumonic mannheimiosis, except that vasculitis and thrombosis of pulmonary arterioles and capillaries are much more obvious and are clearly the major cause of the infarction and thrombosis of lymphatic vessels in interlobular septa. *Mycoplasma mycoides* ssp. *mycoides* small colony type remains viable in the sequestra for many years, and under stress (e.g., starvation), the fibrous capsule may break down, and the mycoplasma are released into the airways and become a source of infection for other animals. Vaccination is highly effective in preventing the disease.

Bovine tuberculosis

Tuberculosis is an ancient, communicable, worldwide, chronic disease of human beings and domestic animals. It continues to be a major problem in human beings in underdeveloped countries, and it is on the rise in some industrialized nations, largely because of the immunosuppressive effects of AIDS, immigration, and movement of infected animals across borders. The World Health Organization (WHO) estimated that 30 million people, mostly in developing countries, died of tuberculosis between 1990 and 1999. *Mycobacterium tuberculosis* is transmitted between human beings, but where unpasteurized cow's milk is consumed, *Mycobacterium bovis* from the milk of cattle with mammary tuberculosis is also important.

Cattle can be infected with *Mycobacterium bovis*, *Mycobacterium tuberculosis*, and *Mycobacterium avium-intracellulare* complex (*Mycobacterium avium* ssp. *avium*, *Mycobacterium avium* ssp. *silvaticum*, *Mycobacterium avium* ssp. *paratuberculosis*, and *Mycobacterium avium* ssp. *intracellulare*) by several routes, but infection of the lungs by inhalation of *Mycobacterium bovis* is the most common in adult animals, whereas ingestion of infected milk is more predominant in young animals.

Respiratory infection usually starts when inhaled bacilli reach the alveoli and are phagocytosed by pulmonary alveolar macrophages. If these cells are successful in destroying the bacteria, infection is averted. However, *Mycobacterium bovis*, being a facultative pathogen of the monocytic-macrophagic system, may multiply intracellularly, kill the macrophage, and initiate infection. From this first nidus of infection, bacilli spread aerogenously via airways within the lungs and eventually via the lymph vessels to tracheobronchial and mediastinal lymph nodes.

The initial focus of infection at the portal of entry (lungs) plus the involvement of regional lymph nodes is termed the primary (Ghon) complex of tuberculosis. If the infection is not contained within this primary complex, bacilli disseminate via the lymph vessels to distant organs and other lymph nodes by the migration of infected macrophages. Hematogenous dissemination occurs sporadically when the inflammatory process containing the mycobacteria erodes the walls of blood vessels and causes vasculitis. If bacterial dissemination is sudden and massive, numerous small foci of infection develop in many tissues and organs and is referred to as miliary tuberculosis (like millet seeds). The host becomes hypersensitive to the mycobacterium, which enhances the cell-mediated immune defenses in early or mild infections but can result in host-tissue destruction in the form of caseous necrosis. The evolution and dissemination of the pulmonary infection are closely regulated by cytokines and TNF-α production by alveolar macrophages.

Unlike abscesses that tend to grow rather fast, granulomas evolve slowly at the site of infection. The lesion starts with few macrophages and neutrophils ingesting the offending organism, but because mycobacterium organisms are resistant to phagocytosis, infected macrophages eventually die, releasing viable bacteria, lipids, and cell debris. Cell debris accumulates in the center of the lesion, whereas viable bacteria and bacterial lipids attract additional macrophages and a few lymphocytes at the periphery of the lesion. Some of these newly recruited macrophages are activated by local lymphocytes and become large phagocytic cells with abundant cytoplasm resembling epithelial cells, thus the term *epithelioid cells*. Multinucleated macrophages also appear at the edges of the lesion, and finally the entire focal inflammatory process becomes surrounded by fibroblasts and connective tissue. It may take weeks or months for a granuloma to be grossly visible.

Bovine tuberculosis, the prototype for granulomatous pneumonia, is characterized by the presence of a few or many caseated granulomas (Fig. 9-57). The early gross changes are small foci (tubercles) most frequently seen in the dorsocaudal, subpleural areas. With progression, the lesions enlarge and become confluent with the formation of large areas of caseous necrosis. Calcification of the granulomas is a typical finding in bovine tuberculosis. Single nodules or clusters occur on the pleura and peritoneum, and this presentation has been termed pearl disease. Microscopically the tubercle is composed of mononuclear cells of various types. In young tubercles, which are noncaseous, epithelioid and Langhans' giant cells are at the center, surrounded by lymphocytes, plasma cells, and macrophages. Later, caseous necrosis is at the center, secondary to the effects of cell-mediated hypersensitivity, enclosed by other cell types and fibrosis at the periphery. Acid-fast organisms may be numerous but, more often are difficult to find in histologic section or smears.

Clinically the signs relate to the dysfunction of a particular organ system or to general debilitation, reduced milk production, and emaciation. In the pulmonary form, which is more than 90% of bovine cases, a chronic, moist cough can progress to dyspnea. Enlarged tracheobronchial lymph nodes can contribute to the dyspnea by impinging on airways, and the enlargement of caudal mediastinal nodes can compress the caudal thoracic esophagus and cause bloating.

Mycoplasma bovis pneumonia

Mycoplasma bovis is the most common *Mycoplasma* sp. isolated from pneumonic lungs of cattle in Europe and North America. Pulmonary infection is exacerbated by stress or any other adverse factor (e.g., viral infection) that depresses the pulmonary defense mechanisms.

Lung lesions are those of a chronic necrotizing bronchopneumonia. The microscopic lesions consist of distinct areas of pulmonary necrosis surrounded by a rim of neutrophils, macrophages, and fibroblasts. The diagnosis is confirmed by isolation or immunohistochemical labeling of tissue sections for *Mycoplasma* antigens. *Mycoplasma bovis* has also been incriminated in arthritis, otitis, mastitis, abortion, and keratoconjunctivitis.

Interstitial pneumonias of cattle

Atypical interstitial pneumonia (AIP) is a vague clinical term well entrenched in veterinary literature, but one that has led to enormous confusion among veterinarians. It was first used to describe acute or chronic forms of bovine pneumonia that did not fit in any of the "classical" forms because of the lack of exudate and lack of productive cough. Microscopically the criteria for diagnosis of AIP in cattle were based on the absence of obvious exudate and the presence of edema, interstitial emphysema (see Pulmonary Emphysema), hyaline membranes, hyperplasia of type II pneumonocytes, and interstitial fibrosis with cellular infiltrates. At that time, any pulmonary disease or pulmonary syndrome that had a few of the above lesions was traditionally diagnosed as AIP, and grouping all these different syndromes together was inconsequential because their etiopathogenesis were then unknown.

Field and laboratory investigations have demonstrated that most of the bovine syndromes previously grouped under AIP have rather different causes and pathogeneses (Fig. 9-65). Further, what was "atypical" in the past has become so routine that it is fairly common nowadays to find "typical cases" of AIP. For all these reasons, investigators, largely from Britain, proposed that all these syndromes previously clustered into AIP should be named according to their specific cause or pathogenesis. The most common bovine syndromes characterized by edema, emphysema, hyaline membranes, and hyperplasia of type II pneumonocytes include bovine pulmonary edema and emphysema (fog fever), "extrinsic allergic alveolitis" (hypersensitivity pneumonitis), "reinfection syndrome" (hypersensitivity to *Dictyocaulus* sp. or BRSV), milk allergy, ingestion of moldy potatoes, and others.

Acute bovine pulmonary edema and emphysema (fog fever).   Acute bovine pulmonary edema and emphysema (ABPE), known in Britain as fog fever (no association with atmospheric conditions), occurs in cattle usually grazing "fog" pastures (that is, aftermath or foggage, regrowth after a hay or silage has been cut). Epidemiologically, ABPE usually occurs in adult beef cattle in the fall when there is a change in pasture, from a short, dry grass to a lush, green grass. It is generally accepted that L-tryptophan present in the pasture is metabolized in the rumen to 3-methylindole, which in turn is absorbed into the blood stream and carried to

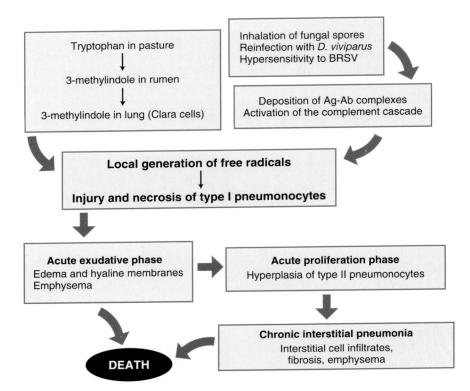

Fig. 9-65   Schematic diagram of the pathogenesis of toxic and allergic pneumonias ("atypical interstitial pneumonia") in cattle. *BRSV,* Bovine respiratory syncytial virus. *(Redrawn with permission from Dr. A. López, Atlantic Veterinary College.)*

the lungs. Mixed function oxidases present in the non-ciliated bronchiolar epithelial (Clara) cells metabolize 3-methylindole into a highly pneumotoxic compound that causes extensive necrosis of bronchiolar cells and type I pneumonocytes (Fig. 9-65), and increases alveolar permeability leading to edema, interstitial pneumonia, and alveolar and interstitial emphysema.

The gross lesions are those of a diffuse interstitial pneumonia with severe alveolar and interstitial edema and interlobular emphysema (Fig. 9-35). The lungs are enlarged, pale, and rubbery in texture, and the lesions are most notable in the caudal lobes. Microscopically the lesions are alveolar and interstitial edema and emphysema, formation of hyaline membranes within alveoli, and in those animals that survive for several days, hyperplasia of type II alveolar epithelial cells.

Clinically, severe respiratory distress develops within 2 weeks of the pasture change, and cattle develop expiratory dyspnea, oral breathing, and evidence of emphysema within the lungs and even subcutaneously along the back. Experimentally, reducing ruminal conversion of L-tryptophan to 3-methylindole prevents the development of ABPE.

A number of other agents cause virtually the same clinical and pathologic syndrome as is seen in ABPE. The pathogenesis is assumed to be similar, although presumably other toxic factors will be specific for each syndrome. One of these pneumotoxic factors is 4-ipomeanol, which is found in moldy sweet potatoes contaminated with the fungus *Fusarium solani*. Mixed-function oxidases in the lungs activate 4-ipomeanol into a potent pneumotoxicant capable of producing irreversible injury to type I pneumonocytes and bronchiolar epithelial cells. Similarly, purple mint (*Perilla frutescens*), stinkwood (*Zieria arborescens*), and rapeseed and kale (*Brassica* species) also cause pulmonary edema, emphysema, and interstitial pneumonia.

Extrinsic allergic alveolitis. Extrinsic allergic alveolitis (hypersensitivity pneumonitis), one of the most common allergic diseases in cattle, is seen mainly in housed, adult dairy cows in the winter. This disease shares many similarities with its human counterpart known as farmer's lung, which results from a type III hypersensitivity reaction to inhaled organic antigens most commonly fungal spores, mainly of the thermophilic actinomycete, *Saccharopolyspora rectivirgula* (*Micropolyspora faeni*), commonly found in moldy hay. This is followed by an antibody response to inhaled fungal spores and local deposition of antigen-antibody complexes (Arthus reaction) in the lungs (Fig. 9-65). Because it occurs only in a few animals of the herd or a sporadic farmer, it is presumed that intrinsic host factors such as dysregulation of IgG, interleukins, IFN-γ, and T lymphocytes are involved in the pathogenesis of the disease. Clinically, it can be acute or chronic; the latter has a cyclical pattern of exacerbation during winter months. Weight loss, coughing, and poor exercise tolerance are clinical features.

Grossly the postmortem lesions vary from subtle, gray, subpleural foci (granulomatous inflammation) to severe, in which the lungs are firm and heavy and have a "meaty appearance" because of alveolar epithelial hyperplasia, lymphocytic infiltration, and interstitial fibrosis. Characteristically, discrete noncaseous granulomas formed in response to the deposition of antigen-antibody complexes are scattered throughout the lungs. Chronic cases of extrinsic allergic alveolitis can eventually progress to diffuse fibrosing alveolitis. Full recovery can occur if it is recognized and treated at the early stages of the disease.

Hypersensitivity to reinfection with larvae of *Dictyocaulus viviparus* is another allergic syndrome manifested in the lungs that cause signs and lesions indistinguishable from ABPE, with the exception of a component of eosinophils and possibly larvae seen microscopically in the alveolar exudate. It has been suggested that emphysema with diffuse proliferative alveolitis and formation of hyaline membranes can also occur in the late stages of BRSV infection in cattle. Presumably, this disease shares many similarities with "atypical" infections occasionally seen in children with respiratory syncytial virus (RSV human strain), in which a hypersensitivity to the virus or virus-induced augmentation of the immune response results in allergic interstitial pneumonia (Fig. 9-65).

Other forms of bovine interstitial pneumonia. Milk allergy, a type of systemic anaphylaxis (type I hypersensitivity) in cows sensitized to their own milk casein and lactalbumin, can cause acute pulmonary congestion, edema, and even hemorrhage and emphysema. Occasionally, adverse drug reactions can induce a similar allergic response in the lung.

Inhalation of manure ("pit") gases, such as hydrogen sulfide (H_2S), ammonia (NH_3), and nitrogen dioxide (NO_2) from silos, can be a serious hazard to animals and human beings. At toxic concentrations, these gases cause necrosis of bronchiolar cells and type I pneumonocytes, a fulminating pulmonary edema that causes asphyxiation, and rapid death (Fig. 9-39). Like other oxidant gases, inhalation of NO_2 also causes bronchiolitis, edema, and interstitial pneumonia and in survivors, bronchiolitis obliterans ("silo filler's disease").

Smoke inhalation resulting from barn or house fires is sporadically seen by veterinarians and pathologists. In addition to skin burns and asphyxiation, animals involved in fire accidents suffer extensive thermal injury produced by the heat on the nasal and laryngeal mucosa, and severe chemical irritation caused by inhalation of combustion gases and particles in the lung. Animals that survive or are rescued from fires frequently develop nasal, laryngeal, and tracheal edema, and pulmonary hemorrhage and alveolar edema, which are caused by chemical injury to the blood-air barrier. Microscopic examination of the lungs often reveals carbon particles (soot) on mucosal surfaces of the conducting system.

Parasitic pneumonias of cattle

Verminous pneumonia (*Dictyocaulus viviparus*). Pulmonary lesions in parasitic pneumonias (the word is used here in its restricted sense to mean helminth infestations of the lungs) vary from interstitial in larval migration to chronic bronchitis, which is caused by some intrabronchial adult parasites, to granulomatous pneumonia, which is caused by dead larvae, aberrant parasites, or eggs of parasites. In many cases, an "eosinophilic syndrome" in the lungs is characterized by infiltrates of eosinophils in the pulmonary interstitium and bronchoalveolar spaces and by blood eosinophilia. Atelectasis and emphysema secondary to the obstruction of airways are also common findings in parasitic pneumonias. The severity of these lesions relates to the numbers and size of the parasites and the nature of the host reaction, which sometimes includes hypersensitivity reactions. A common general term for all of these diseases is verminous pneumonia, and the adult nematodes are often visible grossly in the airways (Fig. 9-66).

Dictyocaulus viviparus is an important pulmonary nematode (lungworm) responsible for a disease in

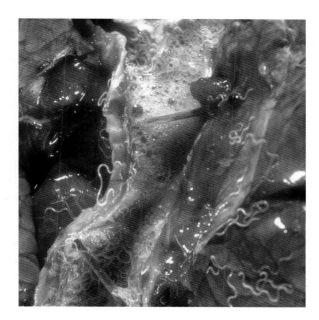

Fig. 9-66   Verminous pneumonia (*Dictyocaulus viviparus*), bronchus, calf. The bronchus contains numerous slender lungworms and large amounts of clear foamy fluid, indicative of pulmonary edema. (*Courtesy Ontario Veterinary College.*)

cattle referred to as verminous pneumonia or verminous bronchitis. Adult parasites live in the bronchi of cattle, mainly in those of the caudal lobes of the lungs. Adult parasites cause severe bronchial irritation, bronchitis, and pulmonary edema, which in turn is responsible for lobular atelectasis and interstitial emphysema. Atelectasis is clearly confined to the lobules of the lungs ventilated by the obstructed bronchi (dorsocaudal). Interstitial emphysema (interlobular) is caused by forced expiratory movements against a partially obstructed single bronchus. In addition to the inflammation of bronchial mucosa, bronchoaspiration of larvae and eggs also causes an influx of leukocytes into the bronchoalveolar space (alveolitis). Verminous pneumonia is most commonly seen in calves during their first summer grazing pastures that are used repeatedly from year to year, particularly in regions of Europe that have a moist, cool climate. The parasite can overwinter in pastures, even in climates as cold as Canada's, and older animals may be carriers for a considerable length of time.

At necropsy, lesions appear as large, dark or gray, depressed, wedge-shaped areas of atelectasis present usually along the dorsocaudal aspect of the lungs. On a cut surface, edematous foam and mucus mixed with white, slender (up to 80-mm long) nematodes are visible in the bronchi (Fig. 9-66). In most severe cases, massive numbers of nematodes fill the bronchial tree. Microscopically the bronchial lumens are filled with parasites admixed with mucus because of goblet cell hyperplasia, and there is also squamous metaplasia of the bronchial and bronchiolar epithelium because of chronic irritation. There is also alveolar edema; hyperplasia of BALT caused by a persistent immunologic stimulus; hypertrophy and hyperplasia of bronchiolar smooth muscle because of increased contraction and decreased muscle relaxation; and a few eosinophilic granulomas around the eggs and dead larvae. These granulomas, grossly, are gray, noncaseated nodules (2 to 4 mm in diameter) and may be confused with those caused by tuberculosis.

The clinical signs (coughing) vary with the severity of infection, and severe cases can be confused clinically with interstitial pneumonias. Expiratory dyspnea and death can occur with heavy parasitic infestations when there is massive obstruction of airways.

A different form of bovine pneumonia, an acute allergic reaction known as reinfection syndrome, occurs when previously sensitized adult cattle are exposed to large numbers of larvae (*Dictyocaulus viviparus*). Lesions in this syndrome are those of a hypersensitivity pneumonia as previously described.

Other lung parasites.   *Ascaris suum* is the common intestinal roundworm of pigs; larvae cannot complete their life cycle in calves, but the larvae can cause severe pneumonia and death within 2 weeks if calves are housed in places where infested pigs were previously kept. Pigs, the natural host, also can be killed if exposed to an overwhelming larval migration. Clinical signs because of migration of larvae through the lungs include cough and expiratory dyspnea to the point of oral breathing. The gross lesions are of a diffuse interstitial pneumonia with hemorrhagic foci, atelectasis, and interlobular edema and emphysema (Fig. 9-54). Microscopically, there are focal intraalveolar hemorrhages caused by migratory larvae, which in some cases can be seen in bronchioles and alveoli admixed with edematous fluid and cellular exudate (including eosinophils). The alveolar walls are thickened because of edema and few inflammatory cells.

Hydatid cysts, the intermediate stage of *Echinococcus granulosus*, can be found in the lungs and liver and other viscera of sheep and to a lesser extent in cattle, pigs, goats, horses, and human beings. The adult stage is a tapeworm that parasitizes the intestine of Canidae. Hydatidosis is still an important zoonosis in some countries, and perpetuation of the parasite life cycle results from animals being fed uncooked offal from infected sheep and consumption of uninspected meat. Hydatid cysts are generally 5 to 15 cm in diameter and numerous cysts can be found in the viscera of affected animals (Fig. 9-67); they have little clinical significance in animals but are of economic importance because of carcass condemnation.

Aspiration pneumonias of cattle

The inhalation of regurgitated ruminal contents or iatrogenic deposition of medicines or milk into the trachea can cause severe and often fatal aspiration pneumonia.

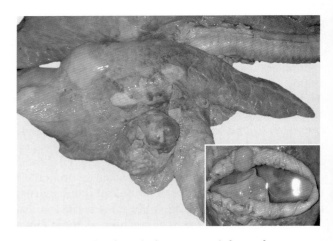

Fig. 9-67   Hydatidosis (echinococcosis), lung, sheep.
A large hydatid cyst is present in the pulmonary parenchyma. *Inset:* Hydatid cyst, cut-open section. The cyst contains fluid and larvae and is often enclosed by a fibrous capsule. (***Figure*** and ***Inset***, *Courtesy Dr. Manuel Quezada, Universidad de Concepción, Chile.*)

Bland substances such as mineral oil may incite only a mild suppurative or histiocytic bronchopneumonia, whereas some "home remedies" or ruminal contents are highly irritating and cause a fibrinous, necrotizing bronchopneumonia. The right lung tends to be more severely affected because the right cranial bronchus is closest to the trachea. However, the distribution may vary when animals aspirate while in lateral recumbency. In some severe cases, pulmonary necrosis can be complicated by infection with saprophytic organisms present in ruminal contents, causing fatal gangrenous pneumonia. Aspiration pneumonia should always be considered in animals with cleft palate or in those whose swallowing has been compromised because of disorders such as hypocalcemia (milk fever). On the other hand, neurological diseases such as encephalitis (e.g., rabies) or encephalopathy (e.g., lead poisoning) should be investigated in animals in which the cause of aspiration pneumonia could not be explained otherwise. Depending on the nature of the aspirated material, histopathologic evaluation generally reveals foreign particles such as vegetable cells, milk droplets, and large numbers of bacteria in bronchi, bronchioles and alveoli. Vegetable cells and milk typically induce an early neutrophilic response followed by a histocytic reaction with "foreign body" multinucleated giant cells. Special stains are used for the microscopic confirmation of aspirated particles in the lung (e.g., PAS for vegetable cells and O-red oil for oil or milk droplets).

PNEUMONIAS OF SHEEP AND GOATS

In the past, *Pasteurella haemolytica* was incriminated in four major ovine diseases known as acute ovine pneumonic pasteurellosis (shipping fever), enzootic pneumonia (nonprogressive chronic pneumonia), fulminating septicemia, and mastitis. Under the new nomenclature, *Mannheimia haemolytica* (biotype A) is now responsible for ovine pneumonia resembling shipping fever in cattle (ovine pneumonic mannheimiosis), septicemia in young lambs (under 3 months of age), and ovine enzootic pneumonia and sporadic severe gangrenous mastitis in ewes. *Pasteurella trehalosi* (formerly *Pasteurella haemolytica* biotype T) is the agent incriminated with septicemia in lambs 5 to 12 months old.

Ovine pneumonic mannheimiosis

Ovine pneumonic mannheimiosis is one of the most common and economically significant diseases in most areas where sheep are raised. It is caused by *Mannheimia haemolytica* (biotype A) and has pathogenesis and lesions similar to those of pneumonic mannheimiosis of cattle. Colonization and infection of lungs are facilitated by stressors such as changes in weather, handling, deworming, dipping, and by viral infections such as PI-3

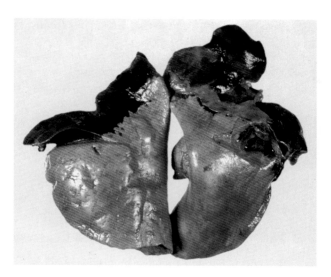

Fig. 9-68 **Acute fibrinous bronchopneumonia (pleuropneumonia), pneumonic mannheimiosis (*Mannheimia haemolytica*), lungs, lamb.** The cranioventral aspects of the lung are red, swollen, and very firm (consolidated) with some fibrin on the pleural surface. Note that the consolidated lung resembles liver, hence the previous name of "lung hepatization." *(Courtesy Ontario Veterinary College.)*

virus, RSV, adenovirus, and probably chlamydia and *Bordetella parapertussis*. Lesions are characterized by a severe fibrinous bronchopneumonia (lobar, cranioventral) with pleuritis (Fig. 9-68). Subacute to chronic cases appear as a fibrinopurulent bronchopneumonia, and sequelae include abscesses and fibrous pleural adhesions.

Chronic enzootic pneumonia

In sheep, this entity is a multifactorial disease complex that, in contrast to ovine pneumonic mannheimiosis, causes only a mild to moderate pneumonia, and it is rarely fatal. It generally affects animals younger than 1 year of age. Significant costs associated with chronic enzootic pneumonia include reduction of weight gain, labor costs, veterinary fees, and slaughterhouse waste. The modifier "chronic" is used here to avoid any confusion with pneumonic mannheimiosis ("acute enzootic pneumonia"). It is also sometimes called atypical pneumonia, chronic nonprogressive pneumonia, proliferative pneumonia, or other names.

Chronic enzootic pneumonia is a clinicoepidemiologic term and does not imply a single causal agent, but a combination of infectious, environmental, and managerial factors. The list of infectious agents involved in ovine enzootic pneumonia includes *Mannheimia haemolytica*, *Pasteurella multocida*, PI-3, adenovirus, reovirus, RSV, chlamydia, and mycoplasmas (*Mycoplasma ovipneumoniae*).

In the early stages of the disease, a cranioventral bronchointerstitial pneumonia is characterized by

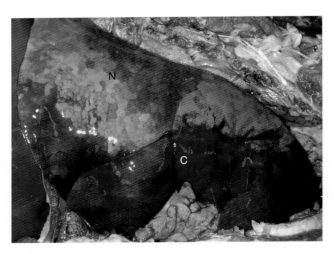

Fig. 9-69   **Acute fibrinosuppurative bronchopneumonia (*Pasteurella multocida*), lung, sheep.** The ventral portions of the cranial, middle, and caudal lobes are consolidated (C), involving approximately 50% of the lung. The dorsal portion of the caudal lung is relatively normal (N) but is multifocally congested and edematous. (*Courtesy Dr. J. Andrews, College of Veterinary Medicine, University of Illinois.*)

moderate thickening of alveolar walls because of hyperplasia of type II pneumonocytes. In some cases, when further colonization of the lungs with secondary pathogens such as *Pasteurella multocida* takes place it may progress to fibrinous or suppurative bronchopneumonia (Fig. 9-69). One might expect some specific evidence pointing to the infectious agents (for example, large intranuclear inclusion bodies in epithelial cells with adenoviral infection), but such is often not the case, either because examination is seldom done at the acute stage when the lesions are still present or because secondary bacterial infections mask the primary lesions. In the late stages, chronic enzootic pneumonia is characterized by hyperplastic bronchitis, atelectasis, alveolar and bronchiolar fibrosis, and severe peribronchial lymphoid hyperplasia (cuffing pneumonia).

Septicemic pasteurellosis

This condition is a common ovine disease caused by *Pasteurella trehalosi* (biotype T) in animals 5 months or older, or by *Mannheimia haemolytica* (biotype A) in lambs younger than 2 months of age. Both organisms are carried in the tonsils and oropharynx of normal sheep; but, under abnormal circumstances, bacteria can invade adjacent tissues, enter the blood stream, and cause septicemia, particularly in association with stresses such as dietary or environmental changes. Affected animals die after a short illness and only rarely have clinical signs such as dullness, recumbency, and dyspnea. Gross lesions

include a distinctive necrotizing pharyngitis and tonsillitis, severe congestion and edema of the lungs, focal hepatic necrosis, infarcts and petechiae in the tongue, esophagus, and intestine, but particularly in the lungs and pleura. Microscopically, the hallmark lesion is a disseminated intravascular thrombosis often associated with the presence of bacterial colonies in the capillaries of affected tissues. *Mannheimia haemolytica* and *Pasteurella trehalosi* are readily isolated from many organs.

Contagious caprine pleuropneumonia

This disease in goats is the counterpart of contagious bovine pleuropneumonia in cattle; sheep do not have a corresponding disease. The etiopathogenesis and geographic distribution of contagious caprine pleuropneumonia are yet to be determined. Three mycoplasmas, namely *Mycoplasma mycoides* ssp. *mycoides* large colony type, *Mycoplasma mycoides* ssp. *capri*, and *Mycoplasma capricolum* ssp. *capripneumoniae*, have been associated with respiratory infections in goats; however, only the last is considered as the etiologic agent of typical contagious caprine pleuropneumonia.

Caprine pleuropneumonia is important in Africa, the Middle East, and parts of Asia but is also seen elsewhere. *Mycoplasma mycoides* ssp. *mycoides* large colony type and *Mycoplasma mycoides* ssp. *capri* are present in North America and have been isolated from respiratory diseases of goats. Although it is unwise to speak in absolute terms when dealing with many aspects of biology, transmission from goats to sheep or cattle does not occur to any significant degree.

Clinically the disease is similar to contagious bovine pleuropneumonia, with high morbidity and mortality, fever, cough, dyspnea, and increasing distress and debility. The gross lesions caused by *Mycoplasma capricolum* ssp. *capripneumoniae* are similar to those in the bovine disease and consist of a severe fibrinous bronchopneumonia and pleuritis; however, distention of the interlobular septa and formation of pulmonary sequestra are less obvious than in the bovine disease. Fibrinous polyarthritis, septicemia, meningitis, mastitis, peritonitis, and abortion are other possible manifestations of disease caused by *Mycoplasma mycoides* ssp. *mycoides* large colony type and *Mycoplasma mycoides* ssp. *capri*. The pathogenicity of other mycoplasmas such as *Mycoplasma ovipneumoniae*, *Mycoplasma arginini*, and *Mycoplasma capricolum* ssp. *capricolum* in sheep and goats is still being defined, and specific description of the lesions would be premature. These organisms probably cause disease only in circumstances similar to those for enzootic pneumonia, where host, infectious, and environmental factors play a complex interaction in the pathogenesis of the disease. Most recently, it has been suggested that IgG antibodies directed against ovine mycoplasmal antigens cross-react with ciliary proteins causing inflammation and ciliary dysfunction, a condition in lambs referred to as "coughing syndrome."

Maedi (maedi-visna)

This entity is an important, lifelong, persistent viral disease of sheep and occurs in most countries, except Australia and New Zealand. Maedi means "shortness of breath" in the Icelandic language, and it is known as Graaff-Reinet disease in South Africa, Zwoegerziekte in The Netherlands, la bouhite in France, and ovine (Montana or Marsh's) progressive pneumonia (OPP) in the United States. More recently, the disease has also been referred to as ovine lentivirus-induced lymphoid interstitial pneumonia or simply, lymphoid interstitial pneumonia (LIP).

Maedi is caused by a nononcogenic retrovirus of the lentivirus subfamily (ovine lentivirus) antigenically related to the retrovirus causing caprine arthritis-encephalitis. Seroepidemiologic studies indicate that infection is widespread in the sheep population, yet the clinical disease seems to be rare. The pathogenesis is incompletely understood, but it is known that transmission occurs largely through ingestion of infected colostrum and to a lesser extent by close contact between infected and susceptible sheep. Once in the body, the ovine lentivirus remains for long periods of time within monocytes and macrophages, including alveolar and pulmonary intravascular macrophages; clinical signs do not develop until after a long incubation period of 2 years or more.

Pulmonary lesions at the time of death are a severe interstitial pneumonia, and the lungs fail to collapse when the thorax is opened. Notable rib imprints, indicators of expanded lungs, are often present on the pleural surface. The lungs are pale and mottled (Fig. 9-70) and typically heavy (2 to 3 times normal weight), and the tracheobronchial lymph nodes are enlarged. Microscopically, the interstitial pneumonia is characterized by BALT hyperplasia and thickening of alveolar walls and peribronchial interstitial tissue by heavy infiltration of lymphocytes, largely T lymphocytes (Fig. 9-53). Recruitment of mononuclear cells into the pulmonary interstitium is presumably the result of sustainable production of cytokines by retrovirus-infected pulmonary macrophages and lymphocytes. Hyperplasia of type II pneumonocytes is not a prominent feature of maedi, but there is some fibrosis and smooth muscle hypertrophy in bronchioles. Secondary bacterial infections often confound the microscopic lesions of the disease. Enlargement of regional lymph nodes (tracheobronchial) is because of severe lymphoid hyperplasia, primarily of B lymphocytes. The virus also can infect many other tissues, causing nonsuppurative encephalitis (visna), lymphocytic arthritis, lymphofollicular mastitis, and vasculitis.

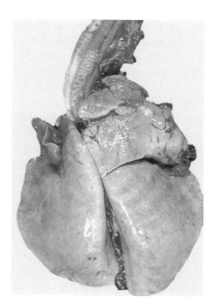

Fig. 9-70   **Interstitial pneumonia (unknown etiology), lung, sheep.** The lung is heavy, rubbery, and shows costal (rib) imprints on the pleural surface. The diffuse distribution is typical of interstitial pneumonia. The trachea contains some edema fluid. *(Courtesy Western College of Veterinary Medicine.)*

Maedi is clinically characterized by dyspnea and an insidious, slowly progressive emaciation despite good appetite. Death is inevitable once clinical signs are present, but may take many months.

Caprine arthritis-encephalitis (CAE)

This retroviral disease of goats (lentivirus) has a pathogenesis remarkably similar to that of maedi-visna in sheep. It was first described in the United States in the 1970s, but also occurs in Canada, Europe, Australia, and probably elsewhere. This disease has two major clinicopathologic forms: One involves the central nervous system of goat kids and young goats and is characterized by a nonsuppurative leukoencephalomyelitis; the other form involves the joints of adult goats and is characterized by a chronic, nonsuppurative arthritis-synovitis. In addition, infection with CAE virus can cause chronic lymphocytic interstitial pneumonia.

The lentivirus of CAE is closely related to the maedi-visna virus, and, in fact, cross infection with CAE virus in sheep has been achieved experimentally. Similar to maedi, CAE infection presumably occurs during the first weeks of life when the doe transmits the virus to her offspring through infected colostrum or milk. Horizontal transmission between infected and susceptible goats has also been described. After coming into contact with mucosal cells at the portal of entry, the virus initially replicates in monocytes-macrophages. Infected macrophages are disseminated hematogenously to the central nervous system, joints, lungs, and mammary glands. Like maedi, there is some evidence that the recruitment of lymphocytic cells results from dysregulation of cytokine production by infected macrophages and lymphocytes in affected tissues. It can take several months before serum antibodies can be detected in infected goats. Recent reports indicate that CAE antibodies cross-react with HIV retroviruses.

Grossly a diffuse interstitial pneumonia tends to be most severe in the caudal lobes. The lungs are gray-pink and firm in texture with numerous, 1- to 2-mm, gray-white foci on the cut surface (Fig. 9-71). The tracheobronchial lymph nodes are consistently enlarged. Microscopically, thickening of the alveolar wall is present because of infiltration of lymphocytes and conspicuous hyperplasia of type II pneumonocytes. One important difference between CAE pneumonia and maedi is that pulmonary lesions in goats may be accompanied by accumulation of proteinaceous eosinophilic material in the alveoli, which in electron micrographs has structural features of pulmonary surfactant. The pulmonary form of CAE can be mistaken for parasitic pneumonia (*Muellerius capillaris*), as these two diseases share some macroscopic similarities and the two diseases can coexist in the same goat.

Clinically, goats are active and afebrile but progressively lose weight in spite of normal appetite. The encephalitic or arthritic signs tend to obscure the respiratory signs, which are only evident on exertion. Secondary bacterial infections are common in affected animals.

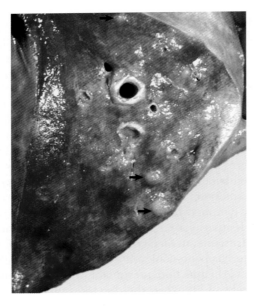

Fig. 9-71 Interstitial pneumonia with alveolar proteinosis, lung, cut surface sheep. Note the gray nodules (*arrows*) and meaty appearance of the lung. These lesions are seen in sheep with the caprine arthritis-encephalitis-pneumonia disease complex. (*Courtesy Dr. J.M. King College of Veterinary Medicine, Cornell University.*)

Tuberculosis

This disease is uncommon in sheep and goats, but infection with *Mycobacterium bovis* or with the *Mycobacterium avium* complex does occur when the disease is prevalent in other species in the locality. The pulmonary form, similar to that seen in cattle, is characterized by a granulomatous pneumonia with multiple, large, caseous, calcified, and well-encapsulated granulomas scattered throughout the lungs. Intralesional acid-fast organisms within macrophages are not as abundant as in bovine tuberculosis.

Parasitic pneumonias of sheep and goats

Dictyocaulus filaria is a serious, worldwide, parasitic disease of the lungs, most commonly of lambs and goat kids, but occurring in adults as well. The life cycle and lesions are similar to those of *Dictyocaulus viviparus* of cattle. The clinical signs (cough, moderate dyspnea, and loss of condition) and lesions relate mainly to obstruction of the small bronchi by adult worms and filaria. As seen in cattle with *Dictyocaulus viviparus*, areas of atelectasis secondary to bronchiolar obstruction are present particularly along the dorsal caudal lungs. Microscopically, affected lungs are characterized by a catarrhal, eosinophilic bronchitis, with peribronchial lymphoid hyperplasia, thickening of alveolar interstitium as a result of hyperplasia of type II pneumonocytes, and focal infiltration of lymphocytes. Bronchioles and alveoli contain edematous fluid, eosinophils, and parasitic larvae and eggs. Anemia of undetermined pathogenesis and secondary bacterial pneumonia are common in small ruminants with this parasitic disease.

Muellerius capillaris, also called the nodular lungworm, occurs in sheep and goats in most areas of the world and is the most common lung parasite of sheep in Europe and Northern Africa. It requires slugs or snails as intermediate hosts. Clinical signs are usually not apparent. The lesions in sheep are typically multifocal, subpleural nodules that tend to be most numerous in the dorsal areas of the caudal lung lobes (Fig. 9-72). These nodules are soft and hemorrhagic in the early stages, but later become gray-green and hard or even calcified. Microscopically, a focal, eosinophilic, and granulomatous reaction occurs in the subpleural alveoli where the adults, eggs, and larvae reside.

Goats differ from sheep by having diffuse interstitial rather than focal lesions, and the reaction to the parasites seen microscopically varies from almost no lesions to a severe interstitial pneumonia with heavy infiltrates of mononuclear cells in alveolar walls resembling CAE or mycoplasmal infections. Secondary effects of *Muellerius capillaris* infection in sheep and goats include decreased weight gain and, possibly, secondary bacterial infections.

Protostrongylus rufescens is a worldwide parasite of sheep and goats. It requires a snail as an intermediate host.

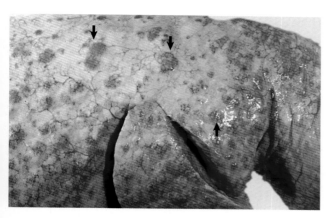

Fig. 9-72   Multifocal granulomatous pneumonia, lungworms (*Muellerius* spp.), lungs, sheep. Multiple gray nodules (granulomas) (*arrows*) are scattered throughout the pulmonary parenchyma. On palpation, the lungs have a nodular texture. (*Courtesy Dr. J. Edwards, Texas A&M University, Olafson Short Course, Cornell Veterinary Medicine.*)

Infection is usually subclinical, but *Protostrongylus rufescens* can be pathogenic for lambs and goat kids, and can cause anorexia, diarrhea, weight loss, and mucopurulent nasal discharge. The adult parasite lives in bronchioles as *Dictyocaulus* spp., but it causes pulmonary nodules similar to those of *Muellerius capillaris*.

PNEUMONIAS OF PIGS

Porcine pneumonias are unequivocally a major component of the problems facing the contemporary swine industry. The incidence, prevalence, and mortality rates of pneumonias in pigs are dependent on a series of complex, multifactorial interactions. Among the most commonly recognized elements linked to porcine pneumonias are the following:
- Host (age, genetic makeup, immune status)
- Infectious agents (viruses, bacteria, mycoplasmas)
- Environmental determinants (humidity, temperature, ammonia concentrations)
- Management practices (crowding, mixing of animals, air quality, nutrition, stress)

Because of the nature of these multifactorial interactions, it will become obvious in the following paragraphs that more often than not a specific type of pneumonia frequently progresses to, or coexists with, another one.

Swine influenza

It is generally accepted that this pig disease resulted from adaptation of the type A influenza virus, the cause of the human influenza pandemic during World War I. Swine influenza is enzootic worldwide and is known to infect human beings who are in close contact with sick pigs. Infection between pigs occurs mainly by aerosols

or oral route; however, the virus can also be transmitted by lungworms and the common earthworm (when ingested). The infection of epithelial cells spreads rapidly throughout the nasal, tracheal, and bronchial mucosa, with the more severe outbreaks reflecting more involvement of intrapulmonary airways and secondary infection with *Pasteurella multocida*, *Arcanobacterium pyogenes*, or *Haemophilus* spp.

Pulmonary lesions caused by influenza virus alone are rarely seen in the postmortem room because this disease has very low mortality unless complicated with secondary bacterial infections. Grossly a copious catarrhal to mucopurulent inflammation extends from the nasal passages to the bronchioles, the volume of mucus being sufficient to plug small airways and cause a lobular or multilobular atelectasis in the cranioventral regions of the lungs. The appearance can be quite similar grossly, though not microscopically, to that of *Mycoplasma pneumoniae*. Fatal cases have severe alveolar and interstitial pulmonary edema. Microscopically the lesions in uncomplicated cases are typical of a virus-induced, necrotizing bronchitis-bronchiolitis, which in severe cases extends into the alveoli as bronchointerstitial pneumonia. It is characterized by thickening and infiltration of the alveolar wall with mononuclear cells, and aggregates of macrophages, neutrophils, mucus, and some necrotic cells within the alveolar lumen. If these changes are extensive enough, the lumen of bronchioles can be occluded by exudate, causing lobular atelectasis. Viral antigen can be demonstrated in infected epithelial cells by immunoperoxidase techniques. In the later stages of alveolar inflammation, neutrophils are progressively replaced by intraalveolar macrophages, unless the pneumonia is complicated by secondary bacterial infections. Recent serologic surveys indicate that infection is also prevalent in wild pigs.

Clinically a sudden onset of painful and often paroxysmal coughing is followed by respiratory distress, nasal discharge, high fever, stiffness, and weakness or even prostration in most or the entire herd, including animals of all age groups. The outbreak subsides virtually without mortality within a week; the clinical appearance is much more alarming than the pathologic changes, unless the pigs have secondary infection with bacteria. Infection can be confirmed using PCR in secretions collected with nasal swabs. The most important effect of most outbreaks of influenza is severe weight loss, but pregnant sows also abort or give birth to weak piglets.

Porcine reproductive and respiratory syndrome (PRRS)

A novel disease named "mystery disease of swine" was first recognized in the United States in 1987. In 1990 it was also seen in Europe, and since then the disease has been reported in many Latin American and

Asian countries. In 1991 Dutch investigators isolated a virus as the etiologic agent, which is currently classified under the *Arterivirus* group.

As its name implies, porcine reproductive and respiratory syndrome is characterized by late-term abortions and stillbirths and respiratory problems in young pigs. The respiratory form generally seen in nursing or young pigs is clinically characterized by anorexia, dyspnea, cough, and occasional death. Some piglets develop severe cyanosis of the abdomen and ears, which explains why this syndrome when first described in Europe was named "blue ear disease." The pathogenesis has not been completely elucidated, but it is presumed that there is a mucosal portal of entry with virus replication in local macrophages, followed by transient viremia and finally dissemination of phagocytic cells to the lungs and other organs, such as the thymus, liver (Kupffer cells), spleen, all lymph nodes, and intestine. The PRRS virus is known to induce apoptosis as a mechanism of cell destruction and persistent infection as a mechanism of dissemination. Although clinical evidence suggests that the PRRS virus also inhibits pulmonary defense mechanisms, experimental studies have been inconsistent in producing dual infections with other, secondary pathogens. Detection of porcine parvovirus and circovirus in pigs with PRRS has created controversy regarding the pathogenesis of this disease (see Postweaning Multisystemic Wasting Syndrome).

On postmortem examination, pulmonary lesions vary from very mild changes characterized by failure of the lung to collapse when the thorax is opened and the presence of rib imprints (Fig. 9-52) to severe changes manifested by consolidation of the lung in cases that have been complicated with bacterial pneumonia. Tracheobronchial and mediastinal lymph nodes are enlarged. Microscopically, pulmonary changes are those of interstitial pneumonia characterized by thickening of alveolar walls by infiltrating macrophages and lymphocytes and mild hyperplasia of type II pneumonocytes. Necrotic cells are scattered in the alveolar lumens. Unlike some other viral infections, bronchiolar epithelium appears not to be affected. Diagnosis of PRRS in tissue collected at the postmortem room can be confirmed by immunohistochemistry and PCR techniques. Infected pigs may become carriers and transmit the infection through body fluids and semen.

Postweaning multisystemic wasting syndrome (PMWS)

Another newly recognized porcine syndrome, characterized clinically by progressive emaciation in weaned pigs, has been recently described in Canada, the United States, and Europe. Because of the clinical signs and lesions in many organs, this syndrome was named postweaning multisystemic wasting syndrome

(PMWS); a porcine circovirus-2 (PCV-2) has been incriminated as the etiologic agent.

At necropsy, affected pigs are in poor body condition, and the most remarkable changes, not considering other possible secondary infections, are enlargement of the superficial and visceral lymph nodes and a mild interstitial pneumonia characterized by failure of the lungs to collapse when the thorax is opened. Jaundice is occasionally observed. Microscopically the lymph nodes show necrosis of lymphoid follicles, depletion of lymphocytes, and notable proliferation of follicular macrophages, some of which fuse and form syncytial cells (granulomatous lymphadenitis). In many cases, large basophilic inclusion bodies resembling grapes are often present in the cytoplasm of macrophages, particularly in Peyer's patches, spleen, and lymph nodes. The lungs show thickening of the alveolar walls because of hyperplasia of type II pneumonocytes and interstitial infiltrates of mononuclear cells, some of which may contain intracytoplasmic inclusion bodies. Circovirus antigen can be confirmed in affected tissue by immunohistochemical or PCR techniques.

Secondary infections with *Pneumocystis carinii* are commonly seen in pigs with PRRS and PMWS. Characteristically, alveoli are filled with a distinctive foamy exudate, which contains the organism not visible in H&E stain but easily demonstrated with Gomori's methenamine silver stain (Fig. 9-73). In human beings, *Pneumocystis carinii* pneumonia (pneumocystosis) is one of the most common and often fatal complications in AIDS patients. As in AIDS patients, in foals and pigs, abnormal populations of CD4$^+$ and CD8$^+$ T lymphocytes

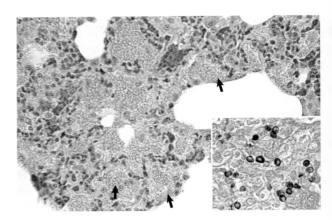

Fig. 9-73   **Pneumocystosis (*Pneumocystis carinii*), lung, pig.** Alveoli are filled with a foamy eosinophilic proteinaceous material in which numerous punctiform organisms (*arrows*) are present. *Inset*: Silver stained oval bodies typical of *Pneumocystis carinii*. Pneumocystosis is generally a microscopic diagnosis because this condition does not cause remarkable gross lesions. Gomori's methenamine silver stain. (***Figure*** and *Inset*, Courtesy Dr. A. López, Atlantic Veterinary College.)

have been incriminated as the underlying mechanism leading to pneumocystosis.

Porcine enzootic pneumonia (mycoplasmal pneumonia of pigs)

This highly contagious disease of pigs caused by *Mycoplasma hyopneumoniae* is grossly characterized by suppurative or catarrhal bronchopneumonia (Fig. 9-74). When its worldwide prevalence and deleterious effect on feed conversion are taken into account, this disease is probably the most economically significant respiratory disease of pigs. Although an infectious disease, it is very

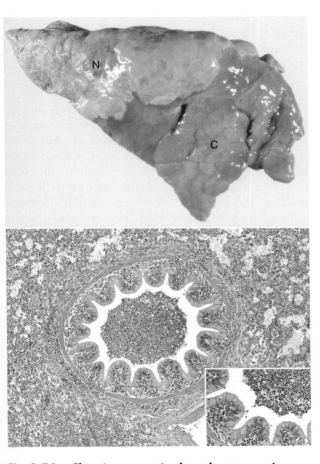

Fig. 9-74   Chronic suppurative bronchopneumonia (enzootic pneumonia), lung, pig. A, Cranioventral consolidation of 40% to 50% of pulmonary parenchyma. Consolidated lung (C) is firm, and the outlines of the lobules are accentuated by edema of the interlobular septa. N, Normal lung. **B,** The bronchiole and alveoli contain numerous neutrophils and macrophages. Some of the neutrophils are migrating from the capillaries of the lamina propria of the bronchiole into its lumen. Alveoli are edematous and contain similar inflammatory cells. Alveolar septa are also widened by inflammation. *Inset:* Higher magnification of wall of bronchiole Fig. 9-74, **B.** H&E stain. (**A,** *Courtesy Ontario Veterinary College.* **B** and **Inset,** *Courtesy Dr. A. López, Atlantic Veterinary College.*)

much influenced by immune status and management factors, such as crowding (airspace and floor space), ventilation (air exchange rate), concentrations of noxious gases in the air (ammonia, hydrogen sulfide), relative humidity, temperature fluctuations, and mixing of stock from various sources. It has been recently demonstrated with PCR technique that *Mycoplasma hyopneumoniae* is present in the air of infected farms.

The cause of porcine enzootic pneumonia remained unclear for many years, and so the disease was mistakenly known as "virus pneumonia of pigs" based on the assumption that if the agent was hard to find it must be a virus. The causative agent, *Mycoplasma hyopneumoniae*, is a fastidious organism and very difficult to grow; thus the final diagnosis is frequently based on interpretation of lesions alone, or supported by ancillary tests to detect this mycoplasma in affected lungs by immunohistochemical, immunofluorescence, enzyme-linked immunosorbent assay (ELISA), or PCR techniques. The bronchopneumonic lesions of porcine enzootic pneumonia are in most cases mild to moderate, and thus mortality is low unless complicated with secondary pathogens, such as *Pasteurella multocida, Arcanobacterium pyogenes, Bordetella bronchiseptica, Haemophilus* spp., *Mycoplasma hyorhinis,* and other mycoplasmas and ureaplasmas. Although the pathogenesis of porcine enzootic pneumonia is not completely elucidated, it is known that *Mycoplasma hyopneumoniae* first adheres to the cilia of the bronchi by means of a unique adhesive protein, produces ciliostasis, and finally colonizes the respiratory system by firmly attaching to the ciliated epithelial cells of the trachea and the bronchi of the cranioventral regions of the lungs. Once attached to the respiratory epithelium, it provokes an influx of neutrophils into the tracheobronchial mucosa, causes extensive loss of cilia (deciliation), stimulates an intense hyperplasia of lymphocytes in the BALT, and attracts mononuclear cells into the peribronchial, bronchiolar, and alveolar interstitium. Additional virulence factors include the ability of *Mycoplasma hyopneumoniae* to reduce the phagocytic activity of neutrophils in the lung and change the chemical composition of mucus, predisposing the lung to secondary bacterial infections.

The lesions caused by *Mycoplasma hyopneumoniae* start as a bronchointerstitial pneumonia microscopically characterized by mononuclear infiltrates in the alveolar walls and a few macrophages and neutrophils in bronchiolar and alveolar lumens. This inflammatory reaction progresses to a suppurative or mucopurulent bronchopneumonia once secondary pathogens, such as *Pasteurella multocida, Bordetella bronchiseptica,* or *Arcanobacterium pyogenes,* are involved (commonly seen at necropsy). In most pigs, gross lesions affect only portions of the cranial and accessory lobe, but in more severely affected pigs, lesions involve 50% or more of the cranioventral portions of the lungs (Fig. 9-74). The affected lungs are dark red in the early stages and have a homogeneous pale-gray ("fish flesh") appearance in the more chronic stages of the disease. On the cut surface, exudate can easily be expressed from airways, and depending on the stage of the lesions and secondary infections, the exudate varies from purulent to mucopurulent to mucoid. Microscopic lesions are characterized by an influx of macrophages and neutrophils into the bronchi, bronchioles, and alveoli with notable BALT hyperplasia. In some cases, accumulation of exudate can be severe enough to cause occlusion of bronchioles and atelectasis of their lobules (Fig. 9-74). The suppurative bronchopneumonia may be accompanied by a mild fibrinous pleuritis, which is often more severe if other organisms, such as *Mycoplasma hyorhinis*, *Pasteurella multocida*, or *Actinobacillus pleuropneumoniae*, are also involved. Abscesses and pleural fibrous adhesions can be long-term sequelae of chronic complicated infections.

Clinically, enzootic pneumonia occurs as a herd problem in two disease forms. A newly acquired infection of a previously clean herd causes disease in all age groups, resulting in acute respiratory distress and low mortality. In a chronically infected herd, the mature animals are immune, and clinical signs are usually apparent only in growing pigs at times of particular stress, such as at weaning. In such herds, coughing and reduced rate of weight gain are the most notable signs.

Porcine pasteurellosis

This infectious disease complex with unclear pathogenesis includes primary infections caused by *Pasteurella multocida* alone, or more frequently, as a secondary infection when the opportunistic bacterium colonizes the lung only after the defense mechanisms are impaired (porcine pneumonic pasteurellosis). In some rare cases, *Pasteurella multocida* causes acutely fatal septicemias in pigs. It is important to remember that *Pasteurella multocida* serotypes A and D are both part of the normal nasal flora and are also causative agents of bronchopneumonia in pigs.

Pasteurella multocida is a secondary pathogen frequently isolated from the lungs of pigs with porcine influenza, PRRS, porcine circovirus-2 infection, pseudorabies, classical swine fever (hog cholera), enzootic pneumonia, and porcine pleuropneumonia. Secondary infections with *Pasteurella multocida* notably change the early and mild bronchointerstitial reaction of enzootic and viral pneumonias into a severe suppurative bronchopneumonia with multiple abscesses and sometimes pleuritis. The other important role for *Pasteurella multocida* in porcine pneumonias is as a cause of a fulminating, cranioventral, fibrinous bronchopneumonia (pleuropneumonia) following influenza virus infection or stress associated with poor management

practices, such as faulty ventilation with high levels of ammonia in the air. The nature of the lesion and the predisposing factors of poor management or coexisting viral infections suggest that fulminating porcine pasteurellosis has a pathogenesis similar to that of pneumonic mannheimiosis of cattle. Pharyngitis with subcutaneous cervical edema, fibrinohemorrhagic polyarthritis, and focal lymphocytic interstitial nephritis are also associated with porcine pneumonic pasteurellosis. Whether this disease is a separate form of pasteurellosis (septicemic) or a change to bronchopneumonia needs to be elucidated. Sequelae of porcine pneumonic pasteurellosis include fibrous pleuritis and pericarditis, pulmonary abscesses, socalled sequestra, and usually death. In contrast to responses in ruminants, *Mannheimia haemolytica* is not a respiratory pathogen for pigs, but in some instances it can cause abortion in sows.

Porcine pleuropneumonia

This entity is a highly contagious, worldwide disease of pigs, caused by *Actinobacillus pleuropneumoniae* (*Haemophilus pleuropneumoniae*), which is characterized by a severe, often fatal, fibrinous bronchopneumonia with extensive pleuritis (pleuropneumonia). Survivors generally develop notable residual lesions and become carriers of the organisms. Porcine pleuropneumonia is an increasingly important cause of acute and chronic pneumonias, particularly in intensively raised pigs (2 to 5 months old). Transmission of *Actinobacillus pleuropneumoniae* occurs by the respiratory route, and the disease can be reproduced experimentally by intranasal inoculation of the bacterium. Considered as a primary pathogen, *Actinobacillus pleuropneumoniae* can sporadically produce septicemia in young pigs and otitis media and otitis interna with vestibular syndrome in weaned pigs. Twelve serotypes of the organism, most of which can cause the disease, have been identified. The pathogenesis is not yet well understood, but specific virulence factors, such as capsular factors, fimbriae and adhesins, lipopolysaccharide, hemolysins, cytotoxins, and permeability factors have been identified. These factors allow *Actinobacillus pleuropneumonia* to attach to cells; produce pores in cell membranes; damage capillaries and alveolar walls, resulting in vascular leakage and thrombosis; impair phagocytic function; and elicit failure of clearance mechanisms.

The gross lesions in the acute form consist of a fibrinous bronchopneumonia characterized by severe consolidation and a fibrinous exudate on the pleural surface. Although all lobes can be affected, a common site is the dorsal area of the caudal lobes. In fact, a large area of fibrinous pleuropneumonia involving the caudal lobe of a pig's lung is considered almost diagnostic for this disease (Fig. 9-75). On the cut surface, consolidated lungs

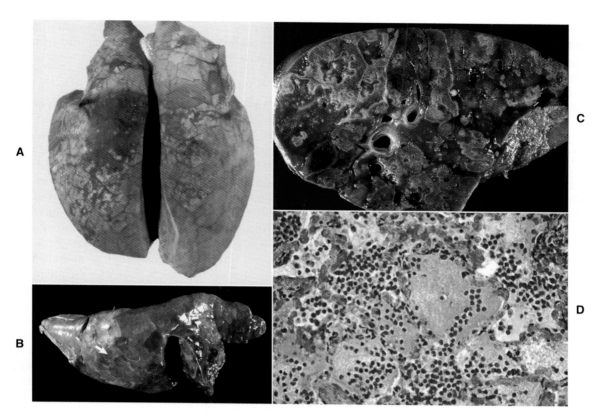

Fig. 9-75   **Porcine pleuropneumonia** *(Actinobacillus pleuropneumoniae)*, **lung, pig. A,** In peracute porcine pleuropneumonia the pneumonic lesions are locally extensive in the dorsal aspects of the caudal lung lobes. There is lobular congestion, consolidation, and interlobular edema. **B,** As the disease progresses and becomes acute to subacute, the lesions expand in size and severity. Note the large area of hemorrhagic necrotizing fibrinous bronchopneumonia. Fibrin is abundant *(arrow)* on the pleural surface and in interlobular septa. **C,** The cut surface has numerous discrete and coalescing zones of lobular inflammation and necrosis *(upper left),* which are pale pink to white and often surrounded by a white margin (inflammation). There is extensive congestion (active hyperemia) and hemorrhage throughout the section. **D,** Alveoli are filled with fibrin, edema fluid, and neutrophils. Capillaries in alveolar septa are congested (active hyperemia), and in many cases there is necrosis of alveolar septa (not visible at this magnification). **(A,** *Courtesy Dr. A. López, Atlantic Veterinary College.* **B,** *Courtesy Dr. J. Render, College of Veterinary Medicine and Animal Health Diagnostic Laboratory, Michigan State University; and Noah's Arkive, College of Veterinary Medicine, The University of Georgia.* **C** *and* **D,** *Courtesy Dr. A.R. Doster, University of Nebraska; and Noah's Arkive, College of Veterinary Medicine, The University of Georgia.*

have notably dilated interlobular septa and irregular, but well-circumscribed areas of coagulative necrosis caused by potent cytotoxins produced by *Actinobacillus pleuropneumoniae.* Except for the distribution, pulmonary lesions of porcine pleuropneumonia are identical to those of pneumonic mannheimiosis of cattle. The microscopic lesions are also very similar to those of bovine pneumonic mannheimiosis and include areas of necrosis surrounded by a thick cluster of "streaming (oat-shaped) leukocytes," and a notable distention of the interlobular septa because of severe edema and lymph vessel thrombosis. Pigs with the chronic form have

multiple pulmonary abscesses and large pieces of necrotic lung encapsulated by connective tissue (sequestra), changes frequently seen in slaughter houses.

Clinically, porcine pleuropneumonia can vary from an acute form with unexpected death and blood-stained froth at the nostrils and mouth to a subacute form characterized by coughing and dyspnea accompanied by clinical signs of sepsis such as high fever, hypoxemia, anorexia, and lethargy. A chronic form is characterized by decreased growth rate and persistent cough. Animals that survive often carry the organism in the tonsils, shed the organism, and infect susceptible pigs.

Haemophilus pneumonia

In addition to Glasser's disease characterized by polyserositis (pericarditis, pleuritis, peritonitis, polyarthritis and meningitis), some serotypes of *Haemophilus parasuis* (originally *Haemophilus parasuis suis*) can also cause suppurative bronchopneumonia that, in some severe cases, can be fatal. The causal organism, *Haemophilus parasuis*, is usually carried in the nasopharynx of normal pigs and requires abnormal circumstances such as those following stress (weaning, cold weather) or viral infections (swine influenza or porcine circovirus-2). Specific pathogen-free (SPF) pigs seem to be particularly susceptible to Glasser's disease (arthritis and serosis) but not to pulmonary infection (bronchopneumonia).

Streptococcal pneumonia

Streptococcus suis type II is a common cause of porcine disease worldwide and a serious zoonosis capable of causing death by septic shock or meningitis and residual deafness in butchers, veterinarians, and pig farmers. Typically, *Streptococcus suis* type II gains entrance to the susceptible young pig through the oropharyngeal mucosa and it can be carried in the tonsils, nasal mucosa, and mandibular lymph nodes of healthy animals, particularly in survivors of an outbreak. Infected sows can abort or vertically transmit the infections to their offspring. Some serotypes of *Streptococcus suis* cause neonatal septicemia, and this can result in suppurative meningitis, arthritis, polyserositis, myocarditis, valvular endocarditis, and embolic pneumonia. Other serotypes may reach the lung by the aerogenous route and cause suppurative bronchopneumonia, generally in combination with *Pasteurella multocida*, *Escherichia coli*, or *Mycoplasma hyopneumoniae*, and fibrinous bronchopneumonia when *Streptococcus suis* infection occurs in combination with *Actinobacillus pleuropneumoniae*.

Tuberculosis

Tuberculosis is an important disease in pigs, which, in many countries, including those in North America, has a much greater prevalence in pigs than in cattle or other domestic mammals. Porcine tuberculosis is attributed to infection with *Mycobacterium bovis* and *Mycobacterium avium-intracellulare* complex. A common scenario in small mixed-farming operations is the diagnosis of avian tuberculosis at the time that pigs are slaughtered, the source being ingestion of tuberculous chickens or contaminated litter. As would be expected, granulomas are found in the mesenteric, mandibular, and retropharyngeal lymph nodes, and to a lesser extent in the intestine, liver, and spleen, and only in rare cases in the lung. The route of infection in pulmonary tuberculosis of pigs is most often hematogenous after oral exposure and intestinal infection. The microscopic lesions are basically those of tubercles, but the degree of encapsulation, caseation, and calcification varies with the type of mycobacterium, age of the lesion, and host immune response.

Other infectious pneumonias of pigs

Porcine respiratory coronavirus (PRCV) is sporadically incriminated in pneumonia in pigs. This viral pneumonia is generally mild, and most pigs fully recover if the pneumonia is not complicated with other infections. Lesions in the lung are those of bronchointerstitial pneumonia with necrotizing bronchiolitis. Interestingly, infections with porcine and other respiratory coronaviruses have been used to investigate the pathogenesis of severe acute respiratory syndrome (SARS), an emerging and highly contagious condition recently reported in human beings and attributed to a novel human coronavirus (SARS-CoV). The relationship between SARS and animal coronavirus is still under investigation.

Septicemias in pigs often cause petechial hemorrhages in the lung and pulmonary edema, and these features may be a part of African swine fever, classical swine fever (hog cholera), pseudorabies, and other diseases. *Salmonellae*, *Escherichia coli*, and *Listeria monocytogenes* can cause severe interstitial pneumonia as part of a septicemic process in very young animals. *Salmonella choleraesuis* causes a necrotizing fibrinous pneumonia, and *Salmonella typhisuis*, a chronic suppurative bronchopneumonia.

Foreign body granulomatous pneumonia occurs frequently in pigs following inhalation of vegetable material (starch pneumonia), presumably from dusty (nonpelleted) feed. Lesions are clinically silent but are often mistaken for other pneumonic processes during inspection at slaughter houses. Microscopically, pulmonary changes are typical of foreign body granulomatous inflammation in which variably sized feed particles are surrounded by macrophages and neutrophils, and often are found in multinucleated giant cells. Feed (vegetable) particles appear as thick-walled polygonal cells that stain positive with PAS because of their rich carbohydrate (starch) content.

Parasitic pneumonias of pigs

Metastrongylus apri (elongatus), *Metastrongylus salmi*, and *Metastrongylus pudendotectus* (lungworms) of domestic and feral pigs occur throughout most of the world and require earthworms as intermediate hosts for transmission. Lungworms may transmit the virus of swine influenza. The importance of pig lungworms is mainly because of growth retardation of the host. Clinical signs include coughing because of parasitic bronchitis.

The gross lesions, when noticeable, consist of small gray nodules, particularly along the ventral borders of the caudal lobes. The adult worms are grossly visible in

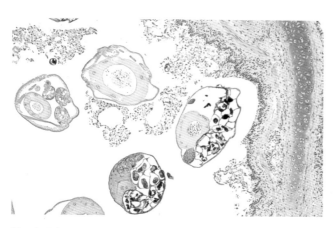

Fig. 9-76 **Acute verminous bronchitis (*Metastrongylus apri*), bronchus, cross section, pig.** Several sections of nematodes (*Metastrongylus apri*) admixed with mucus, neutrophils, and eosinophils (not visible at this magnification) are present in the lumen of the bronchus. H&E stain. *(Courtesy Armed Forces Institute of Pathology and Dr. G. Conboy, Atlantic Veterinary College.)*

bronchi, and microscopically, the parasites cause a catarrhal inflammation with infiltration of eosinophils and lobular atelectasis (Fig. 9-76).

During migration through the lungs of pigs, larvae of *Ascaris suum* can cause edema, focal subpleural hemorrhages, and interstitial inflammation (Fig. 9-54). Hemorrhages also occur in the liver, and after fibrosis they become the large, white "milk spots" seen so frequently as incidental findings at necropsy. It has recently been reported that *Ascaris suum* may cause immunosuppression in severely affected pigs.

PNEUMONIAS OF DOGS

In general, inflammatory diseases of the lungs are less of a problem in dogs than in food-producing species and can be subdivided in two major groups, infectious and noninfectious pneumonias. Of the infectious causes, two account for most cases: infectious tracheobronchitis (kennel cough), which was discussed previously, and canine distemper. Uremia and paraquat toxicity are perhaps the two most notable noninfectious causes of pulmonary disease in dogs.

Canine distemper

Canine distemper is an important and ubiquitous infectious disease of dogs, other Canidae, wild Felidae, Mustelidae, and marine mammals around the world. It is caused by a morbillivirus that is antigenically related to the human measles, rinderpest, and "peste de petit ruminants" viruses. Distemper virus invades through the upper respiratory tract and conjunctiva, proliferates in regional lymph nodes, becomes viremic, and, in dogs with an inadequate antibody response, infects nearly

all body tissues (pantropic), particularly the epithelial cells. During viremia, distemper virus hampers the immune response and appears to down-regulate cytokine production. This virus can target the lungs either directly as a viral pneumonia or by its immunosuppressive effects rendering the lungs susceptible to secondary bacterial infections.

Gross lesions in the acute stages include serous to catarrhal to mucopurulent nasopharyngitis and conjunctivitis. The lungs are edematous and have a diffuse interstitial pneumonia (Fig. 9-77) microscopically characterized by necrotizing bronchiolitis, necrosis and exfoliation of pneumonocytes, mild alveolar edema, and several hours later, thickening of the alveolar walls because of interstitial mononuclear cell infiltrates and hyperplasia of type II pneumonocytes. Secondary infections with *Bordetella bronchiseptica* and mycoplasmas are common and induce life-threatening suppurative bronchopneumonia. The thymus may be small relative to the age of the animal because of viral-induced lympholysis.

Microscopically, eosinophilic inclusions are present in the epithelial cells of many tissues, in the nuclei or cytoplasm, or in both (Fig. 9-77). They appear early in the bronchiolar epithelium, but are most prominent in the epithelium of the lung, stomach, renal pelvis, and urinary bladder, making these tissues good choices for diagnostic examination. The suppurative secondary bronchopneumonias often hinder the detection of viral lesions in the lung, particularly because bronchiolar cells containing inclusion bodies exfoliate and mix with the neutrophils recruited by the bacterial infection.

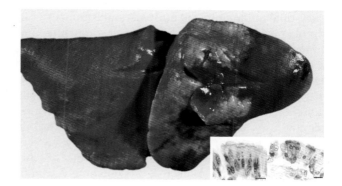

Fig. 9-77 **Interstitial pneumonia, canine distemper, lungs, dog.** The lungs are heavy, edematous, and rubbery, with costal (rib) imprints on the pleural surface. *Inset, left:* Bronchial epithelium contains intracytoplasmic eosinophilic inclusion bodies. H&E stain. *Inset, right:* Immunoperoxidase stain revealing canine morbillivirus antigen in the cytoplasm and apical borders of bronchial epithelial cells. Immunoperoxidase stain. Bars = 20 μm. *(**Figure** and **Inset,** From Berrocal A, López A: J Vet Diagn Invest 15:292-294, 2003.)*

Distemper virus antigens can be readily demonstrated in infected cells by the immunoperoxidase technique (Fig. 9-77). This technique can also be used in skin biopsies for the antemortem diagnosis of canine distemper.

Distemper virus also has a tendency to affect developing tooth buds and ameloblasts, causing enamel hypoplasia in dogs that recover from infection. Of all distemper lesions, demyelinating encephalomyelitis, which develops late, is the most devastating (see Chapter 14). Sequelae to distemper include the nervous and pneumonic complications mentioned previously and such various systemic infections as toxoplasmosis and sarcocystosis because of depressed immunity. Persistent viral infection occurs in some animals that survive the disease.

Clinical signs consist of biphasic fever, diarrhea, vomiting, weight loss, mucopurulent oculonasal discharge, coughing, respiratory distress, and possible loss of vision. Weeks later, hyperkeratosis of foot pads ("hard pad") and the nose are observed, along with nervous signs including ataxia, paralysis, convulsions, or residual myoclonus (muscle twitches, tremors, and "tics"). Distemper virus is transmitted to susceptible puppies through infected body fluids.

Canine adenovirus type 2 (CAV-2) infection

This entity is a common, but transient contagious disease of the respiratory tract of dogs, causing mild fever, oculonasal discharge, coughing, and poor weight gain. The portal of entry is generally by inhalation of infected aerosols followed by viral replication in pneumonocytes. Pulmonary lesions are initially those of a bronchointerstitial pneumonia, with necrosis and exfoliation of bronchiolar and alveolar epithelium and edema, and a few days later, proliferation of type II pneumonocytes, mild infiltration of neutrophils and lymphocytes in alveolar interstitium, and hyperplastic bronchitis and bronchiolitis. Large basophilic intranuclear viral inclusions are typically seen in bronchiolar and alveolar epithelial cells. The disease is sometimes associated or may be confused with the infectious tracheobronchitis complex (kennel cough). The infection with canine adenovirus is clinically mild unless complicated with a secondary bacterial infection. Experimental work suggests CAV-2 reinfection may lead to hyperreactive airways. However, it is not clear if this outcome is true in natural infections.

Canine herpesvirus 1 (CHV-1)

This viral infection can cause fatal generalized disease in newborn puppies, and it is probably part of the variety of factors that result in the "fading puppy syndrome." Hypothermia has been suggested as a pivotal component in the pathogenesis of fatal infections in puppies. CHV-1 also causes necrotizing rhinotracheitis and secondary bronchopneumonia in older animals. Many dogs are seropositive, suggesting that transient or subclinical infections are more common than realized; the virus remains latent in ganglia and can be reactivated following stress, resulting in asymptomatic transmission of CHV-1 virus to offspring via the placenta, resulting in abortion or stillbirths.

Canine influenza (canine flu)

Canine influenza is an emerging contagious respiratory infection of dogs that has been recently described in the United States. It has a high morbidity (close to 100%), but the mortality, as with most other influenza infections, is relatively low (less than 8%). The disease is caused by a novel influenza-A virus that appears to be a mutation from a previously recognized strain of equine influenza virus, presumably the H3N8 strain, and is clinically manifested by severe cough. It must be distinguished from kennel cough. Pulmonary lesions are generally mild and transient, but infected dogs are susceptible to secondary bacterial bronchopneumonia. The most relevant lesions in dogs dying unexpectedly from canine influenza are pleural and pulmonary hemorrhages. Microscopically, there is necrotizing bronchitis and bronchiolitis with exudation of neutrophils and macrophages. Influenza antigen can be demonstrated by immunohistochemistry in airway epithelium and alveolar macrophages.

Bacterial pneumonias of dogs

Dogs generally have bacterial pneumonias when the pulmonary defense mechanisms have been impaired. *Pasteurella multocida*, *Streptococcus* spp., *Escherichia coli*, *Klebsiella pneumoniae*, and *Bordetella bronchiseptica* can be involved in pneumonia secondary to distemper or after aspiration of gastric contents (Fig. 9-78). *Streptococcus zooepidemicus* also causes acute and fatal hemorrhagic pleuropneumonia with hemorrhagic pleural effusion in dogs. Death is generally a consequence of severe sepsis or generalized bacterial embolisms affecting the lungs, liver, brain, and lymph nodes. The primary source of the infection cannot be determined in most cases. Dental disease in dogs may be a source of systemic and pulmonary infection, which is not a new concept, as it has recognized in human medicine for many years. The role of mycoplasmas in canine pneumonia is still uncertain, as these organisms are frequently isolated from normal nasopharyngeal flora.

Tuberculosis is uncommon in dogs, as these animals appear to be quite resistant to infection; most cases occur in immunocompromised dogs or in dogs living with infected human beings. Dogs are susceptible to the *Mycobacterium tuberculosis*, *Mycobacterium bovis*, and *Mycobacterium avium* complex strains, and therefore canine infection presupposes contact with human or

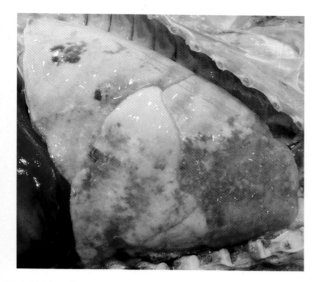

Fig. 9-78   Aspiration pneumonia, bronchopneumonia, right lung, dog. The cranioventral portions of the lung are firm and contain purulent exudate *(yellow areas)*. Aspiration pneumonia starts as an acute necrotizing bronchitis and bronchiolitis caused by aspiration of irritant materials such as gastric acid or a caustic material administered by mouth. The aspirate also contains potentially pathogenic bacteria, and because the mucociliary apparatus is damaged and these bacteria are not removed, they settle into the ventral portions of the lung (from gravity) and provoke a fibrinosuppurative bronchopneumonia. *(Courtesy Dr. A. López, Atlantic Veterinary College.)*

animal tuberculosis. The clinicopathologic manifestation is pulmonary after inhalation or alimentary after oral exposure, but in most cases infection is disseminated to lymph nodes and visceral organs. The gross pulmonary lesions are multifocal, firm, usually calcified nodules with necrotic centers, most often seen in the lungs, lymph nodes, kidneys, and liver. Diffuse granulomatous pleuritis and pericarditis with copious serofibrinous or sanguineous effusion are common. Microscopically, granulomas are formed by closely packed macrophages, but with very little connective tissue.

Mycotic pneumonias of dogs

These are serious diseases seen commonly in animals in some areas. There are two main types: those caused by opportunistic fungi and those caused by a group of fungi associated with systemic "deep" mycoses. All these fungi affect human beings and most domestic animals but are probably not transmitted between species.

Opportunistic fungi, such as *Aspergillus fumigatus*, are important in birds, but in domestic animals they mainly affect immunosuppressed animals or those animals on prolonged antibiotic therapy. The pulmonary lesion is a multifocal, nodular, pyogranulomatous, or granulomatous pneumonia. Microscopically, the fungal hyphae are present, and there is usually necrosis, vasculitis, neutrophilic infiltrates, macrophages and lymphocytes, and fibroblasts, eventually leading to encapsulation of the granulomas.

Systemic (deep) mycoses are caused by *Blastomyces dermatitidis*, *Histoplasma capsulatum*, *Coccidioides immitis*, and *Cryptococcus neoformans* (Fig. 9-79). Blastomycosis mainly affects dogs and is discussed here, whereas cryptococcosis is discussed in the section Pneumonias of Cats. In contrast to other fungi such as *Aspergillus* spp., organisms of the systemic mycosis group are all primary pathogens of human beings and animals and thus do not necessarily require a preceding immunosuppression to cause disease. These fungi have virulence factors that favor hematogenous dissemination and evasion of immune and phagocytic responses. In general, cytological evaluation of affected tissues is very rewarding in the antemortem diagnosis of all systemic mycoses. Systemic dissemination is often exacerbated by the administration of immunosuppressant drugs such as corticosteroids.

Blastomycosis occurs in many countries of the American continent, Africa, and the Middle East and occasionally in Europe. In the United States, it is most prevalent in the Atlantic, St. Lawrence, and Ohio-Mississippi River Valley states, as compared with the Mountain-Pacific region. *Blastomyces dermatitidis* is a dimorphic fungus (mycelia-yeast) seen mainly in young dogs and occasionally in cats. This fungus is present in the soil, and inhalation of spores is considered the principal route of infection; thus it most frequently affects outdoor and hunting dogs. From the lung, infection is disseminated hematogenously to other organs, mainly bone, skin, brain, and probably the eyes.

Pulmonary lesions are characterized by multifocal to coalescing granulomatous pneumonia, generally with firm nodules (pyogranulomas) scattered throughout the lungs (Fig. 9-80). Microscopically, nodules are granulomas with numerous macrophages (epithelioid cells), some neutrophils, multinucleated giant cells, and thick-walled yeasts (Figs. 9-79, A and 9-80). Yeasts are 5 to 25 μm in diameter and are much better visualized when they are stained with PAS reaction or Gomori's methenamine silver stain. Nodules can also be present in other tissues, chiefly lymph nodes, skin, spleen, liver, kidneys, bones, testes, prostate, and eyes. This fungus can be easily identified in properly prepared and stained transtracheal washes or lymph node aspirates.

Clinical signs can reflect involvement of virtually any body tissue; pulmonary effects include cough, decreased exercise tolerance, and terminal respiratory distress.

Coccidioidomycosis (San Joaquin Valley fever), caused by the dimorphic fungus *Coccidioides immitis*,

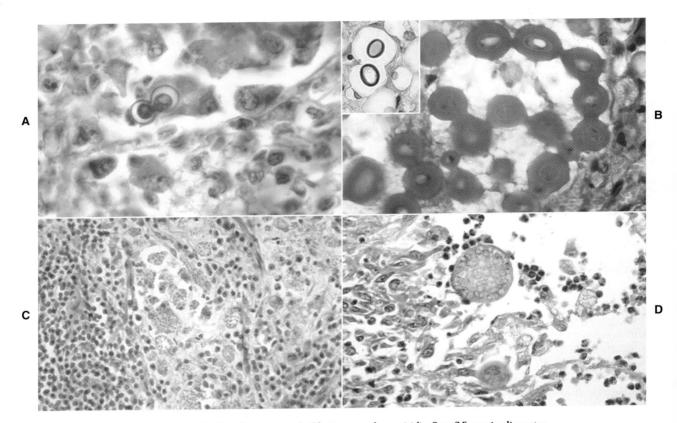

Fig. 9-79   Systemic (deep) mycoses. A, *Blastomyces dermatitidis,* 8 to 25 μm in diameter, broad-based budding spherical yeastlike organisms, intracellular or extracellular location. H&E stain. **B,** *Cryptococcus neoformans,* spherical, 2 to 10 μm in diameter, usually surrounded by a thick mucus capsule, which can increase the overall diameter up to 30 μm, intracellular or extracellular location. The mucus capsule does not stain with H&E (*inset*) but is stained by mucicarmine. With routine mountants, the capsule shrinks and distorts, but this effect has been prevented here by using an aqueous mounting medium. Mayer's mucicarmine stain, aqueous mounting medium. *Inset:* In H&E stained sections, the capsule is not visible but appears as a halo around the cell body. H&E stain. **C,** *Histoplasma capsulatum,* located intracellularly, is spherical to slightly elongated, 5 to 6 μm in diameter. H&E stain. **D,** *Coccidioides immitis,* spherules, 20 to 30 μm in diameter, containing endospores (<5 μm in diameter), intracellular or extracellular location. H&E stain. (*A, B, C,* and *Inset, Courtesy Dr. M.D. McGavin, College of Veterinary Medicine, University of Tennessee.* *D, Courtesy College of Veterinary Medicine, University of Illinois.*)

occurs mainly in animals living in arid regions of the southwestern United States, Mexico, and Central and South America. It is a primary respiratory tract (aerogenous) infection commonly seen at slaughterhouses in clinically normal feedlot cattle. In dogs, coccidioidomycosis also has an aerogenous portal of entry and then disseminates systemically to other organs. Clinical signs relate to the location of lesions, so there can be respiratory distress, lameness, generalized lymphadenopathy, or cutaneous lesions, among others.

The lesions caused by *Coccidioides immitis* consist of focal granulomas or pyogranulomas that can have suppurative or caseated centers. The fungal organisms are readily seen in histologic or cytologic preparation as large (10 to 80 μm in diameter), double-walled and highly refractile spherules (Fig. 9-79, *D*).

Histoplasmosis is a systemic infection that results from inhalation of another dimorphic fungus, *Histoplasma capsulatum.* Histoplasmosis occurs sporadically in dogs and human beings, and to a lesser extent, in cats and horses. Bats often eliminate *Histoplasma capsulatum* in the feces, and droppings from bats and birds heavily promote the growth and survival of this fungus in the soil of enzootic areas.

Pulmonary lesions are grossly characterized by variably sized, firm, well-encapsulated granulomas,

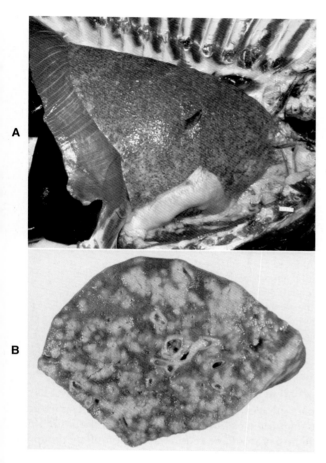

Fig. 9-80   Granulomatous pneumonia, blastomycosis (*Blastomyces dermatitidis*), right lung, dog. A, The lung contains large numbers of small granulomas distributed throughout all pulmonary lobes. **B,** The cut surface of the lung shows multiple discrete and coalescing gray-white granulomas distributed randomly throughout the lung. (**A,** *Courtesy Dr. R.G. Thomson, Ontario Veterinary College.* **B,** *Courtesy College of Veterinary Medicine, University of Illinois.*)

and, sometimes, more diffuse involvement of the lungs. Microscopically, granulomatous tissue typically has many macrophages filled with small (1 to 3 μm), punctiform, intracytoplasmic, dark oval bodies (yeasts), and best demonstrated with PAS reaction (Fig. 9-79, C) or Gomori's methenamine silver stain. Similar nodules can be present in other tissues, chiefly lymph nodes, spleen, intestines, and liver.

Aspiration pneumonia in dogs

This disease is an important form of pneumonia in dogs when vomited or regurgitated materials are aspirated into the lungs or when drugs or radiographic contrast media is accidentally introduced into the airways. As in other animal species, aspiration pneumonia may be unilateral or may more severely affect the right cranial lobe (Fig. 9-81). The severity of lesions depends very much on the chemical and microbiologic composition of the aspirated material. In general, aspiration in monogastric animals, particularly in dogs and cats, is more severe because of the low pH of the gastric contents (chemical pneumonitis). In severe cases, dogs and cats die rapidly from septic shock and ARDS, which is microscopically characterized by diffuse alveolar damage, protein-rich pulmonary edema, neutrophilic alveolitis, and formation of typical hyaline membranes along the alveolar walls (Fig. 9-81). In animals that survive the acute stages of aspiration, pulmonary lesions progress to bronchopneumonia. Aspiration pneumonia is a common sequela to cleft palate, and megaesophagus in dogs secondary to either myasthenia gravis or persistent right aortic arch. It is also an important complication of anesthesia.

Toxic pneumonias in dogs

Paraquat, a broad-spectrum herbicide widely used in gardening and agriculture, can cause severe and often fatal toxic interstitial pneumonia (pneumonitis) in dogs, cats, human beings, and other species. Following ingestion or inhalation, this herbicide selectively accumulates in the lung and paraquat metabolites are produced by Clara cells. These metabolites promote local release of free radicals in the lung, which cause extensive injury to Clara cells and to the blood-air barrier, presumably through lipid peroxidation of type I and II pneumonocytes and alveolar endothelial cells. Paraquat toxicity has been used experimentally as a model of oxidant-induced alveolar injury and pulmonary fibrosis. Soon after poisoning, the lungs are heavy, edematous, and hemorrhagic because of extensive necrosis of epithelial and endothelial cells in the alveolar walls. The lungs of animals that survive acute paraquat toxicosis are pale, fail to collapse when the thorax is opened, and have interstitial emphysema, bullous emphysema, and pneumomediastinum. Microscopic findings in the acute and subacute phases include necrosis of type I pneumonocytes, interstitial and alveolar edema, intraalveolar hemorrhages, and proliferation of type II pneumonocytes. In the chronic stages (4 to 8 weeks later), the lesions are typically characterized by severe interstitial and intraalveolar fibrosis.

Uremic pneumonopathy (pneumonitis) is one of the many extrarenal lesions seen in dogs with chronic uremia. Lesions are characterized by a combination of pulmonary edema and calcification of vascular smooth muscle and alveolar basement membrane. In severe cases, alveolar calcification prevents lung collapse when the thorax is opened.

Grossly, the lungs appear diffusely distended, pink or red in color, and show a rough pleural surface with rib imprints (Fig. 9-31). On palpation, the pulmonary

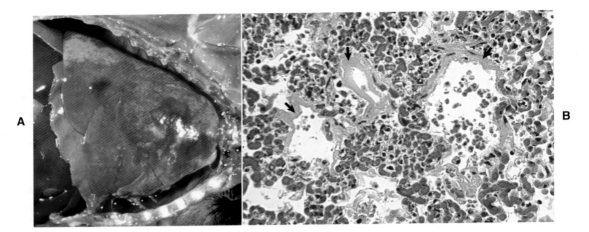

Fig. 9-81   Acute hemorrhagic bronchopneumonia, acute respiratory distress syndrome (ARDS), lungs, 4-week-old puppy. A, Note that the lungs did not collapse when the thorax was opened (loss of negative pressure) and as a result fill almost the entire thoracic cavity. The cranioventral aspects of the lung are consolidated with diffuse hemorrhage. **B,** Alveolar capillary congestion, thick hyaline membranes along the alveolar septa *(arrows),* and intraalveolar hemorrhage. These microscopic changes are typical of the diffuse alveolar damage seen in lungs with ARDS. H&E stain. *(**A** and **B,** Courtesy Dr. A. López, Atlantic Veterinary College.)*

parenchyma has a typical "gritty" texture because of mineralization of the alveolar and vascular walls which is best visualized microscopically by using special stains such as von Kossa (Fig. 9-31). Because this is not primarily an inflammatory lesion, the term *pneumonitis* should be avoided.

Parasitic pneumonias of dogs

Toxoplasmosis is a worldwide disease caused by the obligate intracellular, protozoal parasite *Toxoplasma gondii.* Cats and other Felidae are the definitive host where the mature parasite divides sexually in the intestinal mucosa. Human beings, dogs, cats, and many wild mammals can become intermediate hosts following accidental ingestion of fertile oocysts shed in cat feces, or fetuses can be infected transplacentally from an infected dam. In most instances, the parasite infects many cells of different tissues, induces an antibody response (seropositive animals), but does not cause clinical disease. Toxoplasmosis is often triggered by immunosuppression, such as that caused by canine distemper virus. Toxoplasmosis is characterized by focal necrosis of epithelial cells around the protozoan.

Pulmonary lesions are severe, multifocal necrotizing interstitial pneumonia with notable proliferation of type II pneumonocytes and infiltrates of macrophages and neutrophils. Other lesions in disseminated toxoplasmosis include focal necrotizing hepatitis, myocarditis, splenitis, myositis, encephalitis, and ophthalmitis. The parasites appear microscopically as small (3 to 6 μm) basophilic cysts that can be found free in affected tissues

or within the cytoplasm of many epithelial cells and macrophages. Similar findings can be seen sporadically in dogs infected with *Sarcocystis canis* and immunohistochemistry would be required to differentiate that protozoal organisms from *Toxoplasma gondii.*

Pneumocystis carinii has also been reported as a sporadic cause of chronic interstitial pneumonia in dogs with a compromised immune system (see Equine Pneumonias).

Filaroides hirthi, a lungworm of the alveoli and bronchioles of dogs, has long been known as a cause of mild subclinical infection in large colonies of beagle dogs in the United States. However, it can on occasion cause severe and even fatal disease in individual pets, presumably as a result of immunosuppression. Clinical signs may include coughing and terminal respiratory distress. Grossly, the lesions are multifocal subpleural nodules, often with a green hue because of eosinophils, scattered throughout the lungs. Microscopically, these nodules are eosinophilic granulomas associated with larvae or dead worms, as little reaction develops to the live adults.

Crenosoma vulpis is a lungworm seen commonly in foxes and sporadically in dogs with access to the intermediate hosts—slugs and snails. The adult lungworms live in small bronchi and bronchioles, causing eosinophilic and catarrhal bronchitis manifested grossly as gray areas of inflammation and atelectasis in the caudal lobes. In some animals, *Crenosoma vulpis* causes bronchiolar goblet cell metaplasia and mucous obstruction.

Paragonimus kellicotti in North America and *Paragonimus westermani* in Asia are generally asymptomatic fluke infections in fish-eating species; cats and dogs acquire it in

North America by eating crayfish. Gross lesions include pleural hemorrhages when the metacercariae migrate into the lungs. Later, multifocal eosinophilic pleuritis, and cysts up to 7 mm long containing pairs of adult flukes, are found along with eosinophilic granulomas around clusters of eggs. Like many other parasitic pneumonias, lesions and scars are more frequent in the caudal lubes. Pneumothorax can occur if a cyst that communicates with an airway ruptures to the pleural surface.

Angiostrongylus vasorum and *Dirofilaria immitis* are parasites of the pulmonary arteries and right ventricle and, depending on the stage, can produce different forms of pulmonary lesions. Adult parasites can cause chronic arteritis that leads to pulmonary hypertension, interstitial (eosinophilic) pneumonia, pulmonary interstitial fibrosis, congestive right side cardiac failure, and eventually caudal vena caval syndrome. Other lesions include pleural petechial hemorrhages, and in later stages, diffuse pulmonary hemosiderosis, parasitic granulomas and multifocal pulmonary infarcts. Larvae cause also alveolar injury, thickening of the alveolar walls with eosinophils and lymphocytes (interstitial pneumonia) and multifocal granulomas with giant cells.

PNEUMONIAS OF CATS

Although upper respiratory tract infections are common and important in cats, pneumonias are uncommon except when there is immunosuppression or aspiration of gastric contents. Viral infections such as feline rhinotracheitis and calicivirus may cause lesions in the lungs, but unless there is secondary invasion by bacteria, they do not usually pose a problem (see Specific Diseases of the Nasal Cavity, Feline Diseases).

Feline pneumonitis

This mild, subclinical bronchointerstitial pneumonia is caused by *Chlamydophila (psittaci) felis.* The term *feline pneumonitis* is a misnomer because the major lesions from chlamydial infections are a severe conjunctivitis and rhinitis (see Nasal Cavity and Sinuses), but pneumonia is mild and transient. Pulmonary lesions are characterized by neutrophilic bronchiolitis, thickening of the alveolar septa because of edema, infiltration of neutrophils and mononuclear cells, type II pneumonocyte hyperplasia, and alveolar histiocytosis. The elucidation of the importance of feline viral rhinotracheitis and feline calicivirus has removed *Chlamydophila felis* from its previously overstated importance.

Bacterial pneumonias of cats

Bacteria from the nasal flora such as *Pasteurella multocida* and *Pasteurella*-like organisms are occasionally associated with secondary bronchopneumonia in cats (Fig. 9-82). *Pasteurella multocida* also causes otitis media

and meningitis, but its role as a respiratory pathogen is mainly associated with pyothorax. Interestingly, there are reports of *Pasteurella multocida* pneumonia in older or immunosuppressed human beings acquired through contact with domestic cats. Mycoplasmas are often isolated from the lungs of cats with pulmonary diseases, but are not definitively established as primary pathogens in feline pneumonias.

Cats are susceptible to three types of mycobacterial infections: classical tuberculosis, feline leprosy, and atypical mycobacteriosis. Classical tuberculosis in cats is rare and generally caused by *Mycobacterium bovis,* but also to a lesser extent by *Mycobacterium tuberculosis* and *Mycobacterium avium.* The usual route of infection for feline tuberculosis is oral, through infected milk or meat, so the lesions are mainly in the alimentary tract from where they may disseminate to other organs. The solid and noncaseated appearance of tuberculous nodules is grossly similar to that of neoplasms, so they must be differentiated from pulmonary neoplasms (e.g., lymphosarcoma). Classic tuberculosis with dermal lesions in cats should be differentiated from feline leprosy (localized skin granulomas) caused by *Mycobacterium lepraemurium* and other nonculturable species of acid-fast bacilli. Atypical mycobacteriosis is caused by contamination of a skin wound with saprophytic mycobacteria such as those of the *Mycobacterium avium-intracellulare* complex.

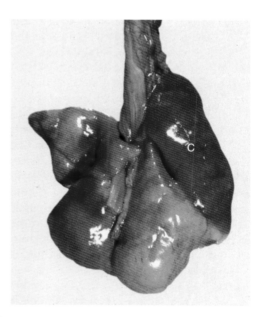

Fig. 9-82   Fibrinopurulent bronchopneumonia, lungs, kitten, 5-month-old kitten with history of conjunctivitis, rhinitis, and bacterial pneumonia. Cranioventral consolidation (C) of the right lung involves approximately 40% of lung parenchyma. The consolidated lung is firm, and on the cut surface some exudate is present in major bronchi. *(Courtesy Dr. S. McBurney, Atlantic Veterinary College.)*

Advances in PCR techniques have notably reduced the time required for etiological diagnosis of mycobacteriosis in veterinary diagnostic laboratories.

Mycotic pneumonias of cats

Cryptococcosis (pulmonary *Cryptococcus neoformans*) is the most frequent systemic mycosis in cats, and lesions are akin to those discussed under Pneumonias of Dogs, Mycotic Pneumonias (see Chapter 14). It occurs worldwide in all species but is diagnosed most frequently in cats, horses, dogs, and human beings. Some healthy dogs and cats harbor *Cryptococcus neoformans* in the nasal cavity and become asymptomatic carriers. Cats that are immunologically compromised such as by feline leukemia virus infection (FeLV), feline immunodeficiency virus (FIV), malnutrition, or corticosteroid treatment, are most susceptible to clinical infection. Lesions can occur in nearly any tissue, resulting in a wide variety of clinical signs. However, granulomatous rhinitis, sinusitis, otitis, pneumonia, ulcerative dermatitis, and meningoencephalitis are most common.

The pulmonary lesion in cryptococcosis is a multifocal granulomatous pneumonia and, like those occurring in other internal organs, they are small, gelatinous, white foci. The gelatinous appearance is because of the broad mucous capsule around the yeast (Fig. 9-79, *B*). Microscopically, lesions contain great numbers of fungal organisms (4 to 10 μm in diameter without capsule) and only a few macrophages, lymphocytes, and multinucleated giant cells. This thick polysaccharide capsule does not stain well with H&E, and thus there is a large empty space or halo around the yeast.

Other pneumonias of cats

Endogenous lipid (lipoid) pneumonia. This condition is an obscure, subclinical pulmonary disease of cats and occasionally of dogs, which is unrelated to aspiration of foreign material. Although the pathogenesis is not understood, it is presumed that lipids from pulmonary surfactant and from degenerated cells accumulate within alveolar macrophages. The gross lesions are multifocal, white, firm nodules scattered throughout the lungs. Microscopically, the alveoli are filled with foamy, lipid-laden macrophages accompanied by interstitial infiltration of lymphocytes and plasma cells, fibrosis, and alveolar epithelialization.

Lipid (lipoid) pneumonia occurs frequently in the vicinity of cancerous lung lesions in human beings, cats, and dogs. The reason for this association remains unknown and frequently unrecognized by pathologists. Recent investigations suggest that lipids are the breakdown products of neoplastic cells.

Exogenous lipid pneumonia. Another form of lipid pneumonia occurs accidentally in cats given mineral oil by their owners in attempts to remove hairballs.

Aspiration pneumonias. This condition is common in cats as a result of vomiting, regurgitation, dysphagia, anesthetic complication, or following accidental administration of food, oral medicaments, or contrast media into the trachea (iatrogenic); pulmonary lesions are similar to those described for dogs (see Aspiration Pneumonia in Dogs).

Parasitic pneumonias of cats

Aelurostrongylus abstrusus, known as "feline lungworm," is a parasite that occurs in cats wherever the necessary slug and snail intermediate hosts are found. It can cause chronic respiratory disease with coughing and weight loss and, sometimes, severe dyspnea and death, particularly if there are secondary bacterial infections. The gross lesions are multifocal, amber, subpleural nodules up to 1 cm in diameter throughout the lungs. On incision, these granulomatous nodules typically contain eggs, larvae, and turbid, viscous exudate. Microscopically, the parasites and their eggs and larvae are in the bronchioles and alveoli where they cause catarrhal bronchiolitis, hyperplasia of submucosal glands and later, granulomatous alveolitis, alveolar fibrosis, and fibromuscular hyperplasia. During routine examination of feline lungs, it is quite common to find fibromuscular hyperplasia in bronchioles and arterioles in otherwise healthy cats. It was alleged in the past that this fibromuscular hyperplasia was a long-term sequela of subclinical infection with *Aelurostrongylus abstrusus*. However, this view has been challenged and thus the pathogenesis and significance of pulmonary fibromuscular hyperplasia in healthy cats remains uncertain.

Toxoplasma gondii, *Paragonimus kellicotti*, and *Dirofilaria immitis* can also affect cats (see Parasitic Pneumonias of Dogs).

FETAL AND PERINATAL PNEUMONIAS
FETAL PNEUMONIAS

Pneumonia is one of the most frequent lesions found in fetuses submitted for postmortem examination, particularly in foals and food-producing animals. Because of autolysis, lack of inflation, and the lungs being at various stages of development, lesions are often missed or misdiagnosed. In the nonaerated fetal lung, the bronchoalveolar spaces are filled with a viscous, locally produced fluid known as "lung fluid" or "lung liquid." It has been estimated that each hour an ovine fetus produces about 2.5 ml of "lung fluid" per kilogram of body weight. In the fetus, this fluid normally moves along the tracheobronchial tree, reaching the oropharynx, and is swallowed or discharged into the amniotic fluid. At the time of birth, the lung fluid is rapidly reabsorbed from the lungs by alveolar absorption and lymphatic drainage.

Aspiration of amniotic fluid contaminated with meconium and bacteria from placentitis is the most common route by which microbial pathogens reach the fetal lungs. This form of pneumonia is secondary to fetal hypoxia and acidosis ("fetal distress"), which cause the fetus to relax the anal sphincter, release meconium into the amniotic fluid, and in the terminal stages inspire deeply with open glottis, resulting in the aspiration of contaminated fluid (Fig. 9-83). Gross lesions are only occasionally recognized, but microscopic changes are similar to those of a bronchopneumonia. Microscopically, bronchoalveolar spaces contain variable numbers of neutrophils, macrophages, and pieces of meconium that appear as bright yellow material because of its bile content. In contrast to postnatal bronchopneumonia, lesions in fetuses are not restricted to the cranioventral aspects of the lungs, but involve all pulmonary lobes.

In cattle, *Brucella abortus* and *Arcanobacterium (Actinomyces) pyogenes* are two of the most common bacteria isolated from the lungs of aborted fetuses. These bacteria are usually present in large numbers in the amniotic fluid of cows with bacterial placentitis. Inflammation of the placenta interferes with oxygen exchange between fetal and maternal tissue, inducing fetal hypoxia and predisposing the fetus to "breathe" with an open glottis and aspirate inside the amniotic sac. *Aspergillus* spp. (mycotic abortion) and *Ureaplasma diversum* cause sporadic cases of placentitis, which results in fetal pneumonia and abortion.

In addition to aspiration of bacteria, pathogens can also reach the lungs via fetal blood and cause interstitial pneumonia. Listeriosis (*Listeria monocytogenes*), salmonellosis (*Salmonella* spp.), and chlamydiosis (*Chlamydophila psittaci*) are the best known examples of blood-borne diseases that cause fetal pneumonia in farm animals. Gross lesions in the lungs are generally undetected, but microscopic lesions include focal necrotizing interstitial pneumonia, and focal necrosis in the liver, spleen, or brain. Fetal bronchointerstitial pneumonia occurs also in some viral abortions, such as those caused by infectious bovine rhinotracheitis virus and PI-3 virus in cattle and equine viral rhinopneumonitis in horses. Fetal pneumonias in dogs and cats are infrequently described, perhaps because aborted puppies and kittens are rarely submitted for postmortem examination. With advancements in molecular biology techniques, the etiological diagnosis of abortions and their association with pulmonary fetal lesions is rapidly improving.

NEONATAL PNEUMONIAS AND SEPTICEMIAS

These entities are rather common in newborn animals lacking passive immunity from hypogammaglobulinemia because of the lack of either ingestion or absorption of maternal colostrum (failure of passive transfer). In addition to septicemias causing interstitial pneumonia, farm animals with hypogammaglobulinemia can develop bronchopneumonia by inhalation of bacterial pathogens. These include *Histophilus somni* and *Pasteurella multocida* in calves, *Streptococcus* spp. in foals, and *Escherichia coli*, *Listeria monocytogenes*, and *Streptococus suis* in pigs.

MECONIUM ASPIRATION SYNDROME (MAS)

This is an important but preventable condition in human babies that originates when amniotic fluid contaminated with meconium is aspirated during labor or immediately after birth. The pathogenesis of MAS is basically the same as in fetal bronchopneumonia and abortion (Fig. 9-83). Fetal hypoxia, a common event during dystocia or prolonged parturition, causes the fetus to release meconium into the amniotic fluid. Aspiration can occur directly from aspirating contaminated amniotic fluid before delivery (respiratory movements with an open glottis), or immediately after delivery when the meconium lodged in the nasopharynx is carried into the lung with the first breath of air. This latter form of aspiration is prevented in delivery rooms by routine suction of the nasopharynx in meconium-stained babies. MAS is well known in human babies, but the occurrence and significance in animals remains largely unknown. Although pulmonary lesions are generally mild and transient, aspiration of meconium can be life threatening for newborn babies because it is accompanied by neonatal hypoxia and acidosis, and may be followed by pulmonary hypertension and possibly airway hyperreactivity.

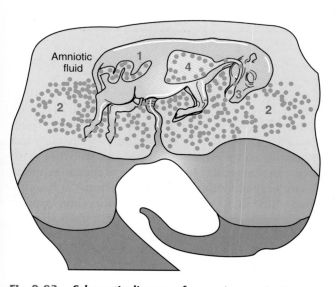

Fig. 9-83   Schematic diagram of meconium aspiration resulting from intrauterine hypoxia. *1,* Increased peristalsis and relaxation of anal sphincter. *2,* Meconium contamination of amniotic fluid. *3,* Meconium in the oropharynx. *4,* Intrauterine gasping with open glottis causing aspiration of meconium and amniotic fluid into fetal lung. *(Redrawn with permission from Dr. J. Martínez-Burnes, Facultad de Medicina Veterinaria y Zootecnia, Universidad Autónoma de Tamaulipas, México.)*

In the most severe cases of MAS, focal (patchy) atelectasis can be observed grossly in the lung, indicating failure of the lungs to be fully aerated because of the mechanical obstruction and the chemical effect of meconium on pulmonary surfactant (Fig. 9-32). Microscopically, meconium and keratin exfoliated from skin into the amniotic fluid are present in bronchi, bronchioles, and alveoli, accompanied by mild alveolitis characterized by infiltration of leukocytes followed by alveolar macrophages and occasional giant cells.

NEOPLASMS OF THE LUNGS
GENERAL CONSIDERATIONS

Lung cancer in animals is rare, unlike in human beings where the incidence is alarming and continues to be the number one cause of cancer deaths in Canada, the United States, and Europe. Interestingly, prostatic and breast cancers, so much feared by men and women, are a distant second. To say that cigarette smoking is responsible for this epidemic of lung cancer is superfluous. Although dogs have been proposed as valuable "sentinels" for environmental hazards, such as exposure to passive smoking, asbestos, dyes, and insecticides, it is not known if the prevalence of canine lung tumors has increased in the last few years. Alterations in genes (oncogenes) and chromosomes, and changes in biologically active molecules have been linked to lung cancer in recent years.

As with many other forms of cancer, epidemiologic studies indicate that the incidence of pulmonary neoplasms increase with age, but there are still insufficient data to confirm that particular canine or feline breeds have a higher predisposition to spontaneous lung neoplasms.

A standard nomenclature of pulmonary neoplasms in domestic animals is lacking, and as a consequence, multiplicity of names and synonyms occur in the veterinary literature. Some classifications are based on the primary site, whereas others emphasize more the histomorphologic type. The most common types of benign and malignant pulmonary neoplasms in domestic mammals are listed in Table 9-5.

Clinically the signs of pulmonary neoplasia vary with the degree of invasiveness, the amount of parenchyma involved, and locations of metastases. Signs may be vague, such as cough, lethargy, anorexia, weight loss, and perhaps dyspnea. In addition, paraneoplastic syndromes, such as hypercalcemia, endocrinopathies, and pulmonary hypertrophic osteoarthropathy (see Chapter 16) have been associated with pulmonary neoplasms.

PRIMARY NEOPLASMS OF THE LUNGS

Primary neoplasms of the lungs arise from cells normally present in the pulmonary tissue and can be epithelial or mesenchymal, although the latter are rare.

Table 9-5 Classification of Pulmonary Neoplasms

PRIMARY EPITHELIAL ORIGIN

Benign

Papillary adenoma
Bronchiolar-alveolar adenoma

Malignant

Adenocarcinoma (acinar or papillar)
Squamous cell carcinoma
Adenosquamous carcinoma
Bronchiolar-alveolar carcinoma
Small cell and large cell carcinomas
Anaplastic (undifferentiated) carcinoma
Carcinoid tumor (neuroendocrine)
Ovine (retroviral) pulmonary carcinoma

PRIMARY MESENCHYMAL ORIGIN

Benign

Hemangioma

Malignant

Osteosarcoma, chondrosarcoma
Hemangiosarcoma
Malignant histiocytosis
Lymphomatoid granulomatosis
Granular cell tumor
Mesothelioma

SECONDARY (METASTATIC) LUNG TUMORS

Any malignant tumor metastatic from another body location (e.g., osteosarcoma in dogs, uterine carcinoma in cows, malignant melanoma in horses)

Primary benign neoplasms of the lungs, such as pulmonary adenomas, are highly unusual in domestic animals. Most primary neoplasms are malignant and appear as solitary masses of variable size that, with time, can metastasize to other areas of the lungs and to distant organs. Without a diligent necropsy, it is sometimes difficult to differentiate primary lung cancer from pulmonary metastasis resulting from malignant neoplasms elsewhere in the body.

It is often difficult to determine the precise topographic origin of a neoplasm within the lungs—for instance, whether it originates in the conducting system (bronchogenic carcinoma), transitional system (bronchiolar carcinoma), exchange system (alveolar carcinoma), or bronchial glands (bronchial gland carcinoma). According to the literature, pulmonary carcinomas in animals arise generally from Clara cells or type II pneumonocytes of the bronchioloalveolar region, in contrast to those in human beings, which are mostly bronchogenic.

Tumors located at the hilus generally arise from major bronchi and tend to be a solitary large mass with occasional small metastasis to the periphery. In contrast, tumors arising from the bronchioloalveolar region are often multicentric with numerous peripheral metastases in the lung parenchyma. Because of histologic architecture and irrespective of their site of origin, many malignant epithelial neoplasms are frequently classified by the all encompassing term of pulmonary adenocarcinomas.

Dogs and cats are the species most frequently affected with primary pulmonary neoplasms, largely carcinomas, generally in older animals. The mean age for primary lung tumors is 11 years for dogs and 12 years for cats. Pulmonary carcinomas in other domestic animals are less common, possibly because fewer are allowed to live a natural life span. These neoplasms can be invasive or expansive, have varying color (white, tan, or gray) and texture (soft or firm), and often have areas of necrosis and hemorrhage, which result in a "craterous" or "umbilicate" appearance. This umbilicate appearance is frequently seen in rapidly growing carcinomas in which the center of the tumoral mass undergoes necrosis as a result of ischemia. Some lung neoplasms mimic pulmonary consolidation or large granulomas. Cats with moderately differentiated neoplasms had significantly longer survival time (median, 698 days) than cats with poorly differentiated neoplasms (median, 75 days). Dogs with primary lung neoplasms, grades I, II, and III, had survival times of 790, 251, and 5 days, respectively.

Ovine pulmonary carcinoma (pulmonary adenomatosis)

This disease, also known as pulmonary adenomatosis and jaagsiekte (from the South African Afrikaans word for "driving sickness"), is a transmissible, retrovirus-induced neoplasia of ovine lungs. It occurs in sheep around the world, with the notable exception of Australia and New Zealand; its incidence is great in Scotland, South Africa, and Peru and unknown, but probably low, in North America. This pulmonary carcinoma behaves very much like a chronic pneumonia, and the "Jaagsiekte sheep retrovirus" shares many epidemiologic similarities with the ovine lentivirus responsible for Maedi and the retrovirus responsible for enzootic nasal carcinoma in ruminants. Pulmonary adenomatosis has been transmitted to goats experimentally, but is not known to be a spontaneous disease in that species.

This disease affects mainly mature sheep but can occasionally affect young stock. Intensive husbandry probably facilitates horizontal transmission by the copious nasal discharge and explains why the disease occurs in Iceland as devastating epizootics with 5% to 80% mortality. Differential diagnosis between maedi and pulmonary adenomatosis often proves difficult because both diseases often coexist in the same flock or in the same animal. Death is inevitable after several months of the initial onset of respiratory signs, and a specific humoral immune response to the Jaagsiekte sheep retrovirus is undetectable in affected sheep.

During the early stages of ovine pulmonary carcinoma, the lungs are enlarged, heavy, and wet and have several firm, gray, variably sized nodules that tend to be located in the cranioventral lobes (Fig. 9-84, A). In the later stages, the nodules become confluent, and large segments of both lungs are diffusely, but not symmetrically, infiltrated by neoplastic cells. On cross section, edematous fluid and a copious mucoid secretion are present in the airways (Fig. 9-84, B). Microscopically the

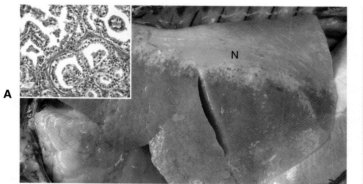
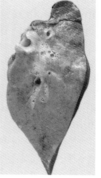

Fig. 9-84   **Ovine pulmonary carcinoma (pulmonary adenomatosis, jaagsiekte), lung, 3-year-old sheep. A,** Neoplastic cell infiltration involving the cranial and ventral portions of the lung and mainly sparing the dorsal portions of the caudal lung lobe (*N*). The affected lung is enlarged and firm. *Inset:* Papillary proliferation of cuboidal epithelial cells (presumed type II pneumonocytes). H&E stain. **B,** Transverse section of the cranial lobe. Note the solid appearance of the ventral portion (*bottom*) of the lung and the frothy fluid (edema) that originates in the alveolar walls. (**A, Inset,** *and* **B,** *Courtesy Dr. M. Heras, Facultad de Veterinaria, Universidad de Zaragoza, Spain.*)

nodules consist of cuboidal or columnar epithelial cells lining airways and alveoli and forming papillary or acinar (glandlike) structures (Fig. 9-84, C). Because the cells have been identified ultrastructurally as originating from both type II alveolar epithelial cells and Clara cells, the neoplasm is considered a "bronchiolo-alveolar" carcinoma. Sequelae often include secondary bronchopneumonia, abscesses, and fibrous pleural adhesions. Metastases occur to tracheobronchial and mediastinal lymph nodes and to a lesser extent to other tissues, such as pleura, muscle, liver, and kidneys.

Clinically, pulmonary adenomatosis is characterized by a gradual loss of condition, sometimes coughing, and respiratory distress, especially after exercise (such as herding or "driving"). Appetite and temperature are normal, unless there are secondary bacterial infections. An important differentiating feature from maedi (interstitial pneumonia) can be observed if the animals are raised by their hind limbs; copious, thin, mucoid fluid, produced by neoplastic cells in the lungs, pours from the nostrils of some animals with pulmonary adenomatosis.

Carcinoid (neuroendocrine tumor) of the lungs

This neoplasm, presumably arising from neuroendocrine cells, is sporadically seen in dogs as multiple, large, firm pulmonary masses close to the main stem bronchi. It has also been reported in the nasal cavity of horses. Tumor cells are generally polygonal with finely granular, pale, or slightly eosinophilic cytoplasm. Nuclei are small, and mitotic figures are absent or rare.

Lymphomatoid granulomatosis

This is a rare but interesting disease of human beings, dogs, and cats characterized by nodules or large solid masses in one or more lung lobes. These frequently metastasize to lymph nodes, kidneys, and liver. Microscopically, tumors are formed by large pleomorphic mononuclear (lymphomatoid) cells with a high mitotic rate and frequent formation of binucleated or multinucleated cells. Tumor cells have a distinct tendency to grow around blood vessels and destroy the vascular walls. Lymphomatoid granulomatosis has some resemblance to lymphomas, and phenotypic marking confirms that neoplastic cells are a mixed population of plasma cells, B and T lymphocytes, and histiocytes.

SECONDARY NEOPLASMS OF THE LUNGS

These are all malignant by definition because they are the result of metastasis to the lungs from malignant neoplasms elsewhere. Because the pulmonary capillaries are the first filter met by tumor emboli released into the vena cava, secondary neoplasms in the lung are relatively common in comparison to primary ones.

Secondary tumors can be of epithelial or mesenchymal origin, also. Common metastatic tumors of epithelial origin are mammary, thyroid (Fig. 9-85), and uterine carcinomas; tumors of mesenchymal origin are osteosarcoma (Fig. 9-86, A), and hemangiosarcoma (Fig. 9-86, B), malignant melanoma in dogs, malignant lymphoma in cows, pigs, dogs, and cats (Fig. 9-87); and the recently reported vaccination-site fibrosarcoma in cats. Usually, secondary pulmonary neoplasms are multiple, scattered throughout all pulmonary lobes (hematogenous dissemination), of variable size, and according to the growth pattern, can be nodular, diffuse, or radiating.

The appearance of metastatic neoplasms differs according to the type of neoplasm. For instance, dark red cystic nodules containing blood are indicative of hemangiosarcoma; dark black solid nodules, melanoma; and hard solid nodules (white, yellow, or tan color) with bone spicules, osteosarcoma. The gross appearances of metastatic carcinomas are generally similar to the primary neoplasm and sometimes have umbilicated centers. Proper diagnoses of pulmonary neoplasms in live animals require history, clinical signs, radiographs, cytologic analysis of BAL fluid, and when necessary a lung biopsy. Identification of a specific lineage of neoplastic

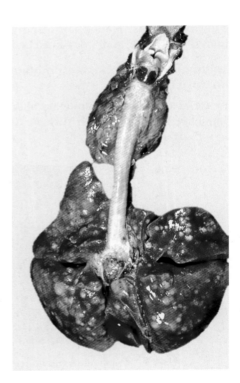

Fig. 9-85   Metastatic thyroid carcinoma, lungs, adult dog. The lungs contain multiple randomly distributed metastatic nodules, which originated from the enlarged and neoplastic left thyroid gland. *(Courtesy Dr. J.M. King, College of Veterinary Medicine, Cornell University.)*

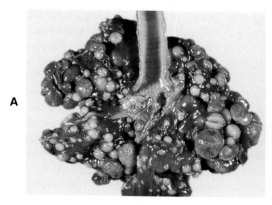
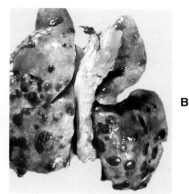

Fig. 9-86   Lung, dog. A, Metastatic sarcoma (primary site unknown). Large numbers of metastatic nodules are randomly distributed throughout all lung lobes. **B,** Metastatic hemangiosarcoma. Note the red to dark red masses throughout the lung parenchyma. If these masses were black, metastatic melanoma would be the likely diagnosis. (**A,** *Courtesy Dr. J.M. King College of Veterinary Medicine, Cornell University.* **B,** *Courtesy College of Veterinary Medicine, University of Illinois.*)

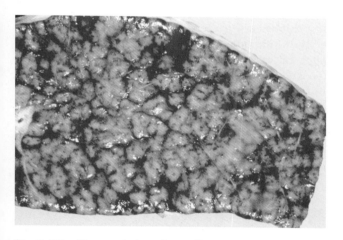

Fig. 9-87   Metastatic lymphoma (lymphosarcoma), lungs, cut surface, cow. Note the numerous discrete and confluent metastatic nodules with the smooth texture and gray color characteristic of lymphoma. (*Courtesy College of Veterinary Medicine, University of Illinois.*)

cells in biopsy or postmortem specimens is often difficult and requires electron microscopy or immunohistochemical techniques. Electron microscopy allows identification of distinctive cellular components, such as osmophilic lamellar phospholipid nephritic bodies in alveolar type II epithelial cells or melanosomes in melanomas. Immunohistochemical staining of intermediate filaments is also helpful in identifying tumor cells, for instance, a metastatic neurofibrosarcoma can be distinguished from an anaplastic hemangiosarcoma by the presence of S-100 protein and factor VIII–related markers.

PLEURA AND THORACIC CAVITY

The thoracic wall, diaphragm, and mediastinum are lined by the parietal pleura, which reflects onto the lungs at the hilum and continues as the visceral pleura, covering the entire surface of the lungs except at the hilus where the bronchi and blood vessels enter. The space between these two pleurae (pleural space) is only minimal and under normal conditions, contains only traces of clear fluid with a few exfoliated cells. Samples of this fluid are obtained by thoracocentesis, a simple procedure in which a needle is passed into the pleural cavity. Volumetric, biochemical, and cytologic changes in this lubricant fluid are routinely used in veterinary diagnostics.

ANOMALIES

Congenital defects are rare and generally of little clinical significance. Cysts within the mediastinum of dogs can be large enough to compromise pulmonary function or mimic neoplasia in thoracic radiographs. These cysts may arise from the thymus (thymic branchial cysts), perinephric tissue (perinephric pseudocyst), bronchi, or from remnants of the branchial pouches and are generally lined by epithelium and surrounded by a capsule of stromal tissue. Anomalies of the thoracic duct cause some cases of chylothorax.

DEGENERATIVE DISTURBANCES
PLEURAL CALCIFICATION

This disorder is commonly found in dogs with chronic uremia. Lesions appear as linear white streaks in parietal pleura, mainly over the intercostal nephritic muscles of the cranial part of the thoracic cavity. The lesions are not functionally significant but indicate a severe underlying renal problem. Vitamin D toxicity (hypervitaminosis D) and ingestion of hypercalcemic substances, such as vitamin D analogs, can also cause calcification of the pleura and other organs.

PNEUMOTHORAX

This disorder is the presence of air in the thoracic cavity where there should normally be negative pressure to facilitate inspiration. Human beings have a complete and strong mediastinum so that pneumothorax is generally unilateral and thus not a serious problem. In dogs the barrier is variable, but in general less complete, so often some communication exists between left and right sides.

There are two main forms of pneumothorax. In spontaneous pneumothorax, air leaking into the pleural cavity occurs without any known underlying disease or trauma. In secondary pneumothorax, movement of air into the pleural cavity results from an underlying pulmonary or thoracic wall disease. Most common causes of secondary pneumothorax in veterinary medicine are penetrating wounds to the thoracic wall, ruptured esophagus, iatrogenic trauma to thorax and lung during a transthoracic lung biopsy or thoracoscopy, tracheal rupture from improper intubation, and rupture of emphysematous bullae or parasitic pulmonary cysts (*Paragonimus* spp.) that communicate with the thoracic cavity. Pneumothorax and pneumomediastinum due to high air pressure (barotrauma) are also well documented in cats after equipment failure during anesthesia. Clinical signs of pneumothorax include respiratory distress, and the lesion is simply a collapsed, atelectic lung. The air is readily reabsorbed from the cavity if the site of entry is sealed.

CIRCULATORY AND LYMPHATIC DISTURBANCES
PLEURAL EFFUSION

This general term is used to describe accumulation of any fluid (transudate, modified transudate, exudate, blood, lymph, or chyle) in the thoracic cavity. Cytologic and biochemical evaluations of pleural effusions are sometimes helpful in suggesting a possible pathogenesis. Based on protein concentration and total numbers of nucleated cells, pleural effusions are cytologically divided into transudates, modified transudates, and exudates.

HYDROTHORAX

When the fluid is serous, clear, and odorless, and fails to coagulate when exposed to air, the condition is referred to as hydrothorax (transudate). Causes of hydrothorax are the same as those involved in edema formation in other organs: increased hydrostatic pressure (heart failure), decreased oncotic pressure (hypoproteinemia, as in liver disease), alterations in vascular permeability (ANTU toxicity), or obstruction of lymph drainage (neoplasia). In cases where the leakage is

corrected, if the fluid is a transudate, it is rapidly reabsorbed. If the fluid persists, it irritates the pleura and causes mesothelial hyperplasia and fibrosis, which thickens the pleura.

In severe cases, the amount of fluid present in the thoracic cavity can be considerable. For instance, a medium size dog can have 2 L of fluid, and a cow may accumulate 25 L or more. Excessive fluid in the thorax causes compressive atelectasis, resulting in respiratory distress (Fig. 9-34). Hydrothorax is most commonly seen in cattle with right side heart failure or cor pulmonale; dogs with congestive heart failure, chronic hepatic disease (hepatic hydrothorax) (Fig. 9-88) or nephrotic syndrome; pigs with mulberry heart disease; and horses with African horse sickness.

HEMOTHORAX

Blood in the thoracic cavity is called hemothorax, but the term has been used for exudate with a sanguineous component. Causes include rupture of a major blood vessel as a result of severe thoracic trauma (e.g., hit by car), erosion of a vascular wall by malignant cells or inflammation (e.g., aortitis caused by *Spirocerca lupi*), or ruptured aortic aneurysms, clotting defects (coagulopathies as in warfarin toxicity), disseminated intravascular coagulation (consumption coagulopathy), and thrombocytopenia due to bone marrow suppression. Hemothorax is generally acute and fatal. On gross examination, the thoracic cavity can be filled with blood, and the lungs are partially or completely atelectatic (Fig. 9-89).

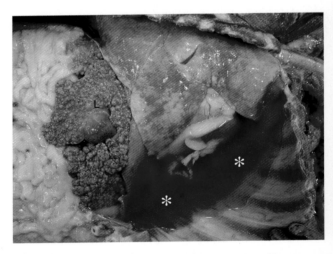

Fig. 9-88   Hydrothorax (hepatic hydrothorax) and hepatic cirrhosis, pleural cavity, 8-year-old dog. The pleural cavity contains a large amount of dark yellow transudate (*) (ventrally). The lungs show focal lobular atelectasis. Fluid in the thoracic cavity can compress the ventral portions of the lung. Also note the nodular surface of the cirrhotic liver (L). (*Courtesy Dr. S. McBurney, Atlantic Veterinary College.*)

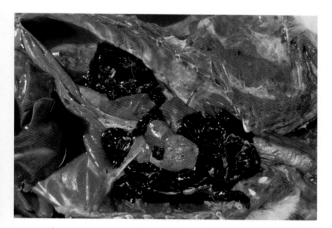

Fig. 9-89   Hemothorax, right pleural cavity, dog. The right pleural cavity is filled with a large clot of blood from a ruptured thoracic aortic aneurysm, which caused unexpected death. Canine aortic aneurysms are associated with migration of *Spirocerca lupi* larvae along the aortic wall before their final migration into the wall of the adjacent esophagus. (*Courtesy Dr. A. López, Atlantic Veterinary College.*)

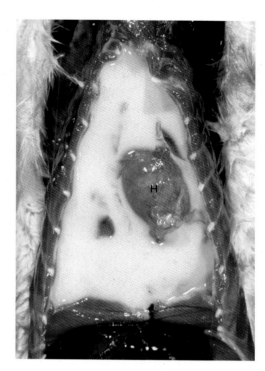

Fig. 9-90   Chylothorax (cause unknown), thoracic (pleural) cavity, mink. Lymph (chyle) fills both the left and right pleural cavities. The heart (*H*) and pericardium are essentially normal because the chyle does not adhere to the outer surface of the pericardial sac, as typically happens with suppurative and fibrinous exudates in the thoracic cavity. (*Courtesy Western College of Veterinary Medicine.*)

CHYLOTHORAX

The accumulation of chyle (lymph rich in triglycerides) in the thoracic cavity (Fig. 9-90) is a result of the rupture of major lymph vessels, usually the thoracic duct or the right lymphatic duct. The clinical and pathologic effects of chylothorax are similar to those of the other pleural effusions. Causes include thoracic neoplasia (the most common cause in human beings, but a distant second to idiopathic cases in dogs), trauma, congenital lymph vessel anomalies, fungal infections, dirofilariasis, and iatrogenic rupture of the thoracic duct during surgery. The source of the leakage of chyle is rarely found at necropsy. When the leakage of chyle occurs in the abdominal cavity, the condition is referred to as chyloabdomen.

INFLAMMATION OF THE PLEURA

Pleural tissue is readily susceptible to injury caused by direct implantation of an organism through a penetrating thoracic or abdominal wound, by hematogenous dissemination of infectious organisms in septicemias, or by direct extension from an adjacent inflammatory process, such as in fibrinous bronchopneumonia or from a perforated esophagus. Chronic injury typically results in serosal fibrosis and tight adhesions between visceral and parietal pleurae. In severe cases, these adhesions can obliterate the pleural space.

PLEURITIS OR PLEURISY

Inflammation of the visceral or parietal pleurae is called pleuritis and, according to the type of exudate, can be fibrinous, suppurative, granulomatous, hemorrhagic,

or a combination of exudates. When suppurative pleuritis results in accumulation of purulent exudate in the cavity, the lesion is called pyothorax or thoracic empyema (Fig. 9-91). Clinically, pleuritis causes considerable pain, and in addition, empyema can result in severe toxemia. Pleural adhesions and fibrosis are the most common sequelae of chronic pleuritis and can notably interfere with inflation of the lungs.

Pleuritis can occur as an extension of pneumonia, particularly in fibrinous bronchopneumonias (pleuropneumonia), or it can occur alone, without obvious pulmonary involvement (Fig. 9-92). Bovine and ovine pneumonic mannheimiosis and porcine and bovine pleuropneumonia are good examples of pleuritis associated with fibrinous bronchopneumonias. Polyserositis in pigs and pleural empyema, particularly in cats and horses, are examples of pleural inflammation in which involvement of the lungs may not accompany the pleurisy. Pleuritis is most frequently caused by bacteria, which cause polyserositis reaching the pleura hematogenously. These bacteria include *Haemophilus parasuis* (Glasser's disease), *Streptococcus suis* type II, and some

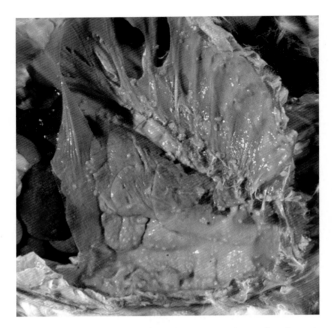

Fig. 9-91   Pyothorax (Pasteurella multocida), right pleural cavity, cat. Large amounts of purulent exudate cover the visceral and parietal pleurae. This lesion is also referred to as pleural empyema. *(Courtesy Dr. A. López, Atlantic Veterinary College.)*

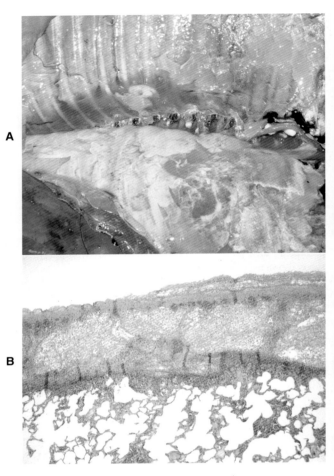

Fig. 9-92   Fibrinous pleuritis, right pleural cavity, horse. **A,** Large masses of yellow fibrin cover the visceral and parietal pleurae. The lungs are normal. **B,** The visceral pleura is covered by a thick layer of fibrin. Subjacent alveoli are essentially normal. H&E stain. *(**A,** Courtesy Dr. A. López, Atlantic Veterinary College. **B,** Courtesy College of Veterinary Medicine, University of Illinois.)*

strains of *Pasteurella multocida* in pigs; *Streptococcus equi* ssp. *equi.* and *Streptococcus zooepidemicus* ssp. *zooepidemicus* in horses; *Escherichia coli* in calves; and *Mycoplasma* spp. and *Haemophilus* spp. in sheep and goats. Contamination of pleural surfaces can be the result of extension of a septic process (e.g., puncture wounds of the thoracic wall and in cattle traumatic reticulopericarditis) and ruptured pulmonary abscesses (e.g., *Arcanobacterium [Actinomyces] pyogenes*).

In dogs and cats, bacteria (such as *Nocardia, Actinomyces,* and *Bacteroides*) can cause pyogranulomatous pleuritis, characterized by accumulation of blood-stained pus ("tomato soup") in the thoracic cavity. This exudate usually contains yellowish flecks called "sulfur granules" (Fig. 9-93), although these are less common in nocardial empyema in cats. Many species of bacteria, such as *Escherichia coli, Arcanobacterium pyogenes, Pasteurella multocida,* and *Fusobacterium necrophorum,* can be present in pyothorax of dogs and cats. These bacteria occur alone or in mixed infections. The pathogenesis of pleural empyema in cats is still debatable, but bite wounds or penetration of foreign material (migrating grass awns) are likely. Pyogranulomatous pleuritis with empyema occurs occasionally in dogs, presumably associated with inhaled small plant material, penetrating (migrating) grass awns, and nasal flora microorganisms. Because of their physical shape (barbed) and assisted by the respiratory movement, aspirated grass awns can penetrate airways, move through the pulmonary parenchyma, and eventually perforate the visceral pleura causing pyogranulomatous pleuritis.

Cats with the noneffusive ("dry") form of feline infectious peritonitis frequently have focal pyogranulomatous pleuritis, in contrast to those with the "wet" or "effusive" form, in which thoracic involvement is primarily that of a pleural effusion. Cytologic evaluation of the effusion typically shows a high cellularity with many degenerated leukocytes, lymphocytes, macrophages, and mesothelial cells, and a pink granular background as a result of the high protein content.

Pleuritis is also an important problem in horses. *Nocardia asteroides* and *Nocardia brasiliensis* can cause fibrinopurulent pneumonia and pyothorax with characteristic sulfur granules. Although *Mycoplasma felis* can be isolated from the respiratory tract of normal horses, it is also isolated from horses with pleuritis and pleural effusion, particularly during the early stages of infection.

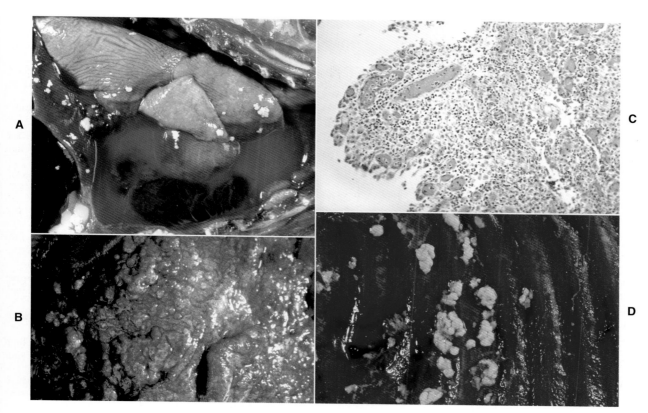

Fig. 9-93   Nocardiosis. A, Chronic pleuritis *(Nocardia asteroides)*, pleural cavity, cat. The pleural cavity holds abundant red-brown exudate ("tomato soup"). Once considered to be pathognomonic of *Nocardia* infection, it is no longer regarded as being diagnostic of nocardiosis. The fluid contains granulomatous inflammatory cells and sulfur granules. **B,** Chronic pleuritis *(Nocardia asteroides)*, visceral pleura, dog. The thickened pleura has a granular appearance because of granulomatous inflammation and the proliferation of fibrovascular tissue of the pleura. **C,** Chronic pleuritis *(Nocardia asteroides)*, thoracic cage, dog. The pleura has been thrown up into villouslike projections composed of abundant fibrovascular tissue and granulomatous inflammation. Leakage from the neocapillaries of the fibrovascular tissue is responsible for the hemorrhagic appearance of the pleural exudate. H&E stain. **D,** Chronic pleuritis *(Nocardia asteroides)*, parietal pleura, cat. Large pieces of exudate, which contain sulfur granules, are present on the thickened pleura. *(A, B, and C, Courtesy Dr. M.D. McGavin, College of Veterinary Medicine, University of Tennessee. D, Courtesy College of Veterinary Medicine, University of Illinois.)*

NEOPLASMS

The pleural surface of the lung is often involved in neoplasms that have metastasized from other organs to the pulmonary parenchyma and rupture of the visceral pleura to seed the pleural cavity. Mesothelioma is the only primary neoplasm of the pleura.

MESOTHELIOMA

This rare neoplasm of the thoracic, pericardial, and peritoneal mesothelium of human beings and most domestic animals is seen most commonly in calves, in which it can be congenital. In human beings, it has long been associated with inhalation of certain types of asbestos fibers (asbestos mining, ship building) alone or with cigarette smoking as a probable cocarcinogen; no association between the incidence of mesothelioma and exposure to asbestos has been made convincingly in domestic animals. In animals, there may be pleural effusion with resulting respiratory distress, cough, and weight loss.

Mesothelioma frequently starts causing a thoracic effusion, but cytological diagnosis can be difficult because of the morphologic resemblance of malignant and reactive mesothelial cells. During inflammation, mesothelial cells become reactive and not only increase in number, but also become pleomorphic and form multinucleated cells that may be cytologically mistaken for a carcinoma.

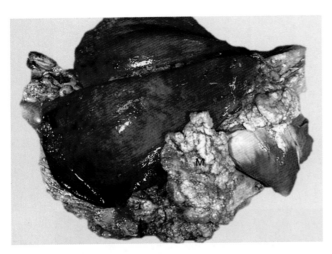

Fig. 9-94   Mesothelioma (M), lungs and heart, horse. The tumor has proliferated and extended over the ventral parietal pleura and pericardium. The pericardial sac has been opened, and the epicardium appears essentially normal, indicating that the tumor did not invade the pericardial sac. *(Courtesy Dr. J.M. King College of Veterinary Medicine, Cornell University.)*

Grossly, mesothelioma appears as multiple, discrete nodules or arborescent, spreading growths on the pleural surface (Fig. 9-94). Microscopically, either the mesothelial covering cells or the supporting tissue can be the predominant malignant component, so the neoplasm can appear microscopically as a carcinoma or as a fibrosarcoma. Although considered malignant, mesotheliomas rarely metastasize.

Secondary tumors may also spread into the visceral and parietal pleura. Thymomas are rare neoplasms that grow in the cranial mediastinum of adult or aged dogs, cats, pigs, cattle, and sheep. Thymomas are composed of thymic epithelium and lymphocytes (see Chapter 13).

ACKNOWLEDGMENT

I thank Dr. William Yates (Canadian Food Inspection Agency) for having provided the basis of this chapter; all pathologists at the Atlantic Veterinary College for providing case material; Dr. Julio Martínez-Burnes, University of Tamaulipas, Mexico, for his suggestions; and Dr. Shannon Martinson, Atlantic Veterinary College, for reviewing the text. Finally, I acknowledge Dr. Reginald G. Thomson (deceased), former Dean of the Atlantic Veterinary College, for years of advice, and Rosalie and Adriana for their support.

SUGGESTED READINGS

Allan GM, McNeilly F, Kennedy S et al: Isolation of porcine circovirus–like viruses from pigs with a wasting disease in the USA and Europe, *J Vet Diagn Invest* 9:3-9, 1998.

Arceneaux KA, Taboada J, Hosgood G: Blastomycosis in dogs: 115 cases (1980-1995), *J Am Vet Med Assoc* 213:658-664, 1998.

Beech J: *Equine respiratory disorders*, Philadelphia, 1991, Lea & Febiger.

Birks EK, Durando MM, McBride S: Exercise-induced pulmonary hemorrhage, *Vet Clin North Am Equine Pract* 9: 87-90, 2003.

Boy MG, Sweeney CR: Pneumothorax in horses: 40 cases (1980-1997), *J Am Vet Med Assoc* 216:1955-1959, 2000.

Brogden KA, Lehmkuhl HD, Cutlip RC: *Pasteurella haemolytica* complicated respiratory infections in sheep and goats, *Vet Res* 29:233-254, 1998.

Crawford PC, Dubovi EJ, Castleman WL et al: Transmission of equine influenza virus to dogs, *Science* 310(5747):482-485, 2005.

Davenport-Goodall CL, Parente EJ: Disorders of the larynx, *Vet Clin North Am Equine Pract* 19:169-187, 2003.

De la Concha-Bermejillo A: Maedi-visna and ovine progressive pneumonia, *Vet Clin North Am Food Anim Pract* 13:13-33, 1997.

De las Heras M, Gonzalez L, Sharp JM: Pathology of ovine pulmonary adenocarcinoma, *Curr Top Microbiol Immunol* 275:25-54, 2003.

Delclaux C, Azoulay E: Inflammatory response to infectious pulmonary injury, *Eur Respir J Suppl* 42:10s-14s, 2003.

Demetriou JL, Foale RD, Ladlow J et al: Canine and feline pyothorax: a retrospective study of 50 cases in the UK and Ireland, *J Small Anim Pract* 43:388-394, 2002.

Dixon PM, McGorum BC, Railton DI et al: Laryngeal paralysis: a study of 375 cases in a mixed-breed population of horses, *Equine Vet J* 33:452-458, 2001.

Dungworth DL: The respiratory system. In Jubb KVF, Kennedy PC, Palmer N, editors: *Pathology of domestic animals*, ed 3, vol 2, Toronto, 1993, Academic Press.

Hahn KA, McEntee MF: Prognosis factors for survival in cats after removal of a primary lung tumor: 21 cases (1979-1994), *Vet Surg* 27:307-311, 1998.

Johnson LR, Herrgesell EJ, Davidson AP et al: Clinical, clinicopathologic, and radiographic findings in dogs with coccidioidomycosis: 24 cases (1995-2000), *J Am Vet Med Assoc* 222: 461-466, 2003.

Johnson LR, Lappin MR, Baker DC: Pulmonary thromboembolism in 29 dogs: 1985-1995, *J Vet Intern Med* 13:338-345, 1999.

Jones DJ, Norris CR, Samii VF et al: Endogenous lipid pneumonia in cats: 24 cases (1985-1998), *J Am Vet Med Assoc* 216: 1437-1440, 2000.

King LG: *Respiratory diseases of dogs and cats*, Philadelphia, 2004, Saunders.

Krohne SG: Canine systemic fungal infections, *Vet Clin North Am Small Anim Pract* 30:963-990, 2000.

Mellanby RJ, Villiers E, Herrtage ME: Canine pleural and mediastinal effusions: a retrospective study of 81 cases, *J Small Anim Pract* 43:447-451, 2002.

Ruffin DC: Mycoplasma infections in small ruminants, *Vet Clin North Am Food Anim Pract* 17:315-332, 2001.

Thacker EL: Diagnosis of *Mycoplasma hyopneumoniae*, *Anim Health Res Rev* 5:317-320, 2004.

Tremaine WH, Clarke CJ, Dixon PM: Histopathological findings in equine sinonasal disorders, *Equine Vet J* 31:296-303, 1999.

Wilson DW, Dungworth DL: Tumors of the respiratory system. In Meuten DJ, editor: *Tumors in domestic animals*, ed 4, Ames, 2002, Iowa State Press.

10

Cardiovascular System

JOHN F. VAN VLEET • VICTOR J. FERRANS

PROPERTY OF
DIAGNOSTIC CENTER FOR
POPULATION & ANIMAL HEALTH
4125 BEAUMONT ROAD
LANSING, MI 48910-8104

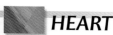

HEART

INTRODUCTION

NORMAL MORPHOLOGY

The heart is a conical, muscular organ that in mammals and birds has evolved into a four-chambered pump with four valves. During early fetal development, the heart is converted from an elongated muscular tube into a C-shaped structure by a process termed looping. Subsequently, septation occurs to produce the right and left atrial and ventricular chambers and separation of the common truncus arteriosus into the aorta and pulmonary artery. The heart lies within a fibroelastic sac, the pericardium, which normally contains a small amount of clear, serous fluid. The heart is interposed as a pump into the vascular system, with the right side supplying the pulmonary circulation and the left side the systemic circulation.

The wall of the heart is composed of three layers: the epicardium, the myocardium, and the endocardium. The epicardium, the outermost layer of the heart, is the visceral pericardium, which is continuous at the cardiac base, with the parietal pericardium. The entire inner surface of the pericardial cavity is covered by mesothelium. The subepicardial layer is attached to the myocardium and consists of a thin layer of fibrous connective tissue, variable but generally abundant amounts (in well-nourished animals) of adipose tissue, and numerous blood vessels, lymph vessels, and nerves (Fig. 10-1).

The myocardium is the muscular layer of the heart. It consists of cardiac muscle cells (myocytes) arranged in overlapping spiral patterns. These sheets of cells are anchored to the fibrous skeleton of the heart, which surrounds the atrioventricular valves and the origins of the aorta and pulmonary artery. The myocardial thickness is related to the pressure present in each chamber; thus the atria are thin walled and the ventricles are thicker.

The thickness of the left ventricular free wall is approximately threefold that of the right ventricle, measured in a transverse section across the middle of the ventricles, because the pressure is greater in the systemic circulation than in the pulmonary circuit.

The endocardium is the innermost layer of the heart and lines the chambers and extends over projecting structures, such as the valves, chordae tendineae, and papillary muscles. The endocardium of the atria is thicker than that of the ventricles and thus normally appears more pale at gross examination. The surface of the endocardium is endothelium that lies on a thin layer of connective tissue; the subendocardial layer contains blood vessels, nerves, and connective tissue. Purkinje fibers are distributed in the subendocardium throughout both ventricles.

The arterial supply to the heart is the left and right coronary arteries, which arise from the aorta at the sinuses of Valsalva behind the left and right cusps of the aortic valves. The arteries course over the heart in the subepicardium and give off perforating intramyocardial arteries that supply a rich capillary bed throughout the myocardium. Extensive anastomoses occur between the capillaries that tend to run parallel to the elongated cardiac muscle cells. The ratio of the area of capillaries to that of muscle cells is approximately 1:1, a fact evident when the myocardium is viewed in cross section.

The cardiac conduction system is infrequently examined in animals because it is a labor-intensive process. Exceptions are cases with documented electrocardiographic alterations of undetermined origin. Components include (1) the sinoatrial (SA) node at the junction of the cranial vena cava and the right atrium; (2) the atrioventricular (AV) node located beneath the septal leaflet of the tricuspid valve, and the AV bundle traversing the lower atrial septum onto the dorsal portion of the muscular interventricular septum; and (3) the right and left bundle branches that descend on each side of the muscular interventricular septum and eventually ramify in the ventricular myocardium as the Purkinje fiber network.

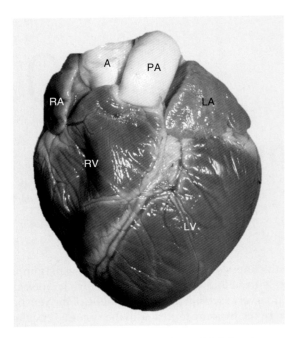

Fig. 10-1   Normal heart, pig. A, Aorta; *LA,* left atrium; *LV,* left ventricle; *PA,* pulmonary artery; *RA,* right atrium; *RV,* right ventricle. *(Courtesy School of Veterinary Medicine, Purdue University.)*

The cardiac valves (tricuspid valve [right atrioventricular valve], mitral valve [left atrioventricular valve], aortic valve, and pulmonary valve) are attached to fibrous rings and have thin avascular cusps. The valves open and close to regulate blood flow through the heart. During embryogenesis, endocardial cushions (mesenchymal tissue covered by endothelium) are precursors of the valve cusps. By remodeling, growth, and elongation, the cushions become thin mature cusps composed of connective tissue with an endothelial covering.

Occasionally, normal features in animal hearts can be misinterpreted as lesions. The epicardial lymph vessels, especially in cattle, can appear as prominent white streaks that could be interpreted as areas of necrosis. The septal cusp of the tricuspid valve in dogs is normally rather tightly attached to the ventricular septum. In young ruminants up to 2 to 3 weeks of age, the ductus arteriosus and foramen ovale can be probe patent, but unless the openings are large, no significant shunting of blood is likely to occur during life. The overall shape of normal hearts can vary from the elongated conical profile in the horse to the somewhat rounded shape in the dog. Cardiac weights vary greatly among species and breeds; pigs have relatively small hearts (approximately 0.3% of body weight) and dogs have relatively large hearts (from 0.75% of body weight in nonathletic breeds to 1.25% in athletic breeds).

Postmortem alterations in hearts must be recognized and correctly interpreted. Rigor mortis occurs in myocardium much as in skeletal muscles and produces contracted, rigid ventricular walls, which empties the more muscular left ventricle. After rigor passes, the ventricular walls relax.

Postmortem blood clotting produces red ("currant jelly") clots in the atria, right ventricle, and large vessels at the base of the heart. Postmortem blood clots are found in these anatomic structures because they lack contractile elements (large vessels) or have less muscle mass (atria, right ventricle) to undergo contraction during rigor mortis. In postmortem evaluations of the heart, it is important to note the presence (or absence) of blood clots in the ventricles and their appearance ("currant jelly" versus "chicken fat") (Fig. 10-2). Under normal conditions, because of its larger chamber volume and thinner walls, a blood clot will be found in the right ventricle, whereas little or no blood clot will be found in the left ventricle because of its smaller chamber volume and thicker walls. Animals with prolonged heart disease may lack adequate glycogen reserves in

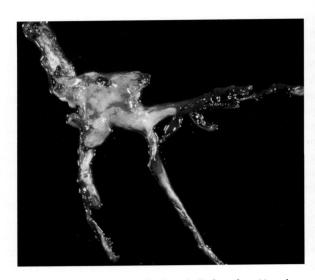

Fig. 10-2   Postmortem "chicken fat" clot, dog. Note how the clot conforms to the shape of the lumens of the vessels from which it was removed. Chicken fat clots consist primarily of clotted plasma and fibrin and other proteins of the coagulation cascade. They are often indicative of anemia; however, in all animals their formation by the separation of the red blood cells from the rest of the components of blood depends on the erythrocyte sedimentation rate (ESR). Separation can occur in all animals in response to systemic inflammation, which increases the ESR, but the horse normally has a high ESR because equine erythrocytes clump together in rouleau formation, which increases the ESR. Thus depending on the ESR, postmortem clots may be pale white to yellow ("chicken fat" clot) or shiny red ("currant jelly" clot) or sometimes a mixture. *(Courtesy Dr. R.K. Myers, College of Veterinary Medicine, Iowa State University.)*

cardiac myocytes. As a result, the ventricular chambers may fail to contract during rigor mortis, allowing a blood clot to form in the left ventricle.

Occasionally, pale "chicken fat" clots that contain reduced numbers of erythrocytes form in animals with severe anemia, systemic inflammatory disease, leukemia, or after prolonged agonal periods. Horses more often have pale clots because of a rapid erythrocyte sedimentation rate termed rouleaux formation. Postmortem lysis of erythrocytes followed by imbibition of hemoglobin produces diffuse red staining of the endocardium and epicardium and simulates the appearance of hemorrhage.

Other potentially misleading findings at necropsy of young dogs and horses include diffuse or patchy myocardial pallor that subsequently fails to correlate with any detectable microscopic alterations. Also, the intracardiac injection of euthanasia solution and other substances can cause hemopericardium and myocardial pallor from tissue dissolution and from crystalline deposits at the site of solution deposition (Fig. 10-3).

Cardiac muscle cells are surrounded by interstitial components, which include blood and lymph vessels, nerves, and connective tissue cells such as fibroblasts, histiocytes, mast cells, pericytes, primitive mesenchymal stem cells and extracellular matrix elements of connective tissue, including collagen fibrils, elastic fibers, and acid mucopolysaccharides. Cardiac muscle cells can be divided into two populations: the working myocytes and the specialized fibers of the conduction system. The working myocyte is a cross-striated branching fiber of an irregular cylindrical shape that measures 60 to 100 μm in length and 10 to 20 μm in diameter, with centrally located, elongated nuclei. Myocytes in young animals are smaller and have small amounts of sarcoplasm. Atrial myocytes are smaller than ventricular myocytes. Adjacent myocytes are joined end-to-end by specialized junctions known as intercalated disks and less frequently by side-to-side connections termed lateral junctions. Multinucleated fibers with nuclei arranged in central rows are frequently seen in hearts of growing pigs (Fig. 10-4, A).

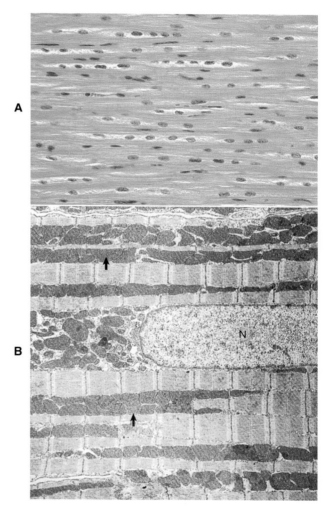

Fig. 10-4   Normal cardiac muscle. A, Left ventricular myocardium, longitudinal section, normal young pig. The multiple nuclei in a myocyte are readily seen and evaluated in a longitudinal section. H&E stain. **B,** Heart, left ventricular myocytes, longitudinal section, normal rat. Numerous dense mitochondria (*arrows*) lie between myofibrils, which have prominent bands. N, Nucleus. TEM. Uranyl acetate and lead citrate stain. (*A and B, Courtesy School of Veterinary Medicine, Purdue University.*)

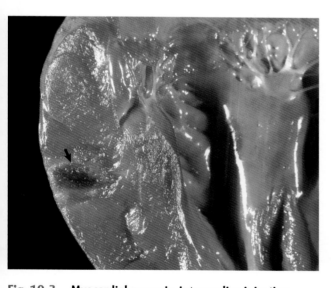

Fig. 10-3   Myocardial necrosis, intracardiac injection, euthanasia solution, left ventricle, dog. Injections of barbiturates and other euthanasia solutions into the myocardium itself will cause localized hemorrhage and myocardial destruction at the injection site (*arrow*). Injections into the ventricle will cause endocardial hemorrhage and necrosis (not shown). (*Courtesy College of Veterinary Medicine, University of Illinois.*)

The myocytes of old animals commonly have large polyploid nuclei. The cytoplasm (sarcoplasm) of myocytes is largely occupied by the contractile proteins that are highly organized into sarcomeres, the repeating contractile units of the myofibril. Myofibrils are formed by end-to-end attachment of many sarcomeres. The cross-striated or banded appearance of myocytes is the result of sarcomeric organization into A bands composed of myosin in the form of "thick" filaments (12 to 16 nm in diameter), I bands composed of actin in the form of "thin" filaments (5 to 8 nm in diameter), and dense Z bands at the end of each sarcomere. Thick and thin filaments interdigitate and provide the basis for the sliding mechanism of muscle contraction. Myocytes are enclosed by the sarcolemma, which consists of the plasma membrane and the covering basal lamina (external lamina). Other important components of cardiac muscle cells are generally only apparent in electron micrographs and include abundant mitochondria, a highly organized network of intracellular tubules termed the sarcoplasmic reticulum, cylindrical invaginations of the plasma membrane called T tubules, ribosomes, cytoskeletal filaments, glycogen particles, lipid droplets, Golgi complexes, atrial granules (contain atrial natriuretic factor), lysosomes, and residual bodies (Fig. 10-4, B).

The morphologic features of the cardiac muscle cells of the specialized conduction tissues, including the sinoatrial node, atrioventricular node, atrioventricular bundle (bundle of His), and bundle branches, vary greatly at different sites and among animal species but generally are thin fibers surrounded by abundant fibrous connective tissue and have only small amounts of contractile material. The Purkinje fibers are distinguished by their large diameters (in horse, ox) and abundant pale eosinophilic sarcoplasm rich in glycogen and poor in myofibrils.

REACTION TO INJURY

Cardiac muscle cells respond to injury by a limited spectrum of reactions. Reversible morphologic alterations include cellular growth disturbances that lead to atrophy or hypertrophy (Fig. 10-5). Various sublethal injuries or degenerations, such as fatty degeneration, lipofuscinosis, vacuolar degeneration, and myocytolysis, result in distinctive myocyte alterations (Fig. 10-6). Lethal injury to myocytes results in necrosis or apoptosis (Fig. 10-7).

Necrosis of cardiac muscle cells is generally followed by leukocytic invasion and phagocytosis of sarcoplasmic debris. The end result is persistence of collapsed sarcolemmal "tubes" of basal lamina surrounded by condensed interstitial stroma and vessels. Lesions with severe disruption of the myocardium have residual changes of fibroblastic proliferation and collagen deposition to form scar tissue. Regeneration of cardiac muscle cells generally does not occur, except in less evolved animals, such as amphibians and fish, and in certain inbred mouse strains. The continual contraction of intact cardiac muscle cells impairs the mechanisms for regeneration. Also, in hearts of neonatal animals and more often in avian hearts, a limited amount of myocyte regeneration has been reported. Recent studies indicate

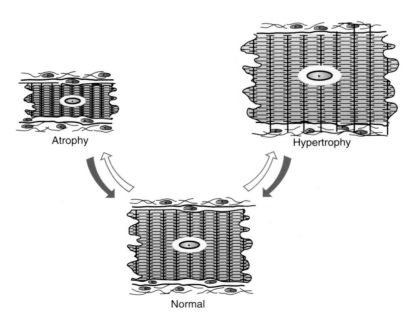

Fig. 10-5   Schematic diagram of cardiac muscle cells. Growth disturbances of atrophy and hypertrophy. *(Redrawn with permission from School of Veterinary Medicine, Purdue University.)*

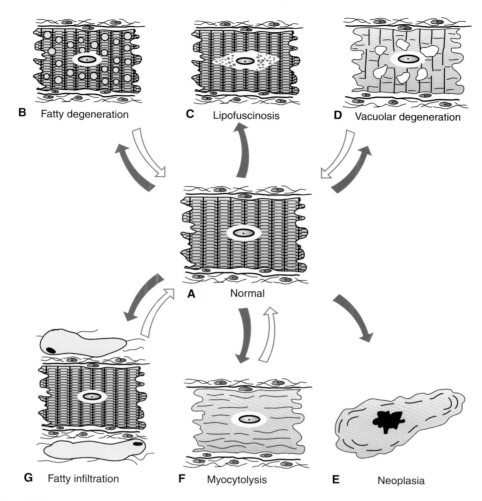

Fig. 10-6   Schematic diagram of various sublethal cardiac muscle cell injuries. A, Normal muscle cell. **B,** Fatty degeneration. **C,** Lipofuscinosis. **D,** Vacuolar degeneration. **F,** Myocytolysis. Also illustrated is fatty infiltration of interstitium (**G**) and neoplastic transformation of myocytes (**E**). (**A** *through* **G,** *Redrawn with permission from School of Veterinary Medicine, Purdue University.*)

that stem cells exist in adult animal and human hearts and, with myocardial injury, these cells may differentiate into cardiac muscle cells. However, the extent of myocyte regeneration is probably minimal. Hyperplasia of myocytes is a normal component of cardiac growth in the first several months of life. Then proliferation ceases. Normal growth then is the result of hypertrophy of myocytes until cell sizes normal for the species are reached.

Apoptosis (programmed cell death of myocytes) is increasingly recognized for its role in the development of various myocardial lesions and cardiac diseases. These conditions include cardiac development, ischemic injury, several types of experimentally induced heart failure (ischemia-reperfusion, hypoxia, pressure-overload hypertrophy), and cardiotoxicity. In some cell systems,

apoptosis can be triggered by the presence of excessive amounts of oxygen free radicals. Cells dying by apoptosis shrink and form apoptotic bodies. In contrast to cell death by necrosis, apoptosis is not accompanied by an inflammatory reaction and fibrosis.

Histopathologic study of sections of the myocardium is substantially limited in respect to specific diagnoses and only rarely can an etiologic diagnosis be made from the morphologic alterations. This inadequacy exists because the spectrum of pathologic reactions is a limited one, and many agents that damage the heart produce similar lesions. Myocardial necrosis can be confused with myocardial inflammation with secondary necrosis because both lesions have substantial leukocytic infiltration. Some animals that die peracutely from cardiac failure lack detectable microscopic alterations and are

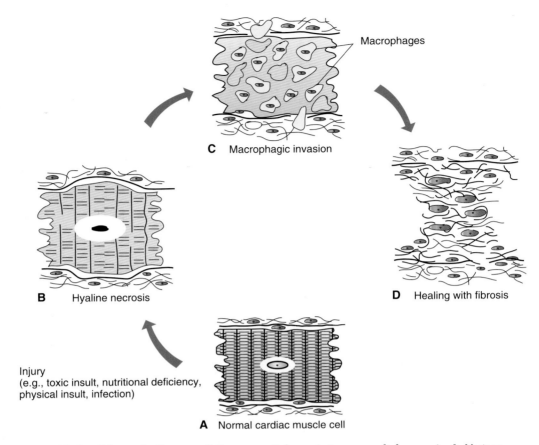

Fig. 10-7 **Schematic diagram of the sequential events in myocardial necrosis. A,** Various injuries lead to **(B)** hyaline necrosis or apoptosis of myocyte. **C,** Healing with phagocytosis of cellular debris by macrophages, and **(D)** subsequent healing with fibrosis, rather than by regeneration. (**A** through **D,** *Redrawn with permission from School of Veterinary Medicine, Purdue University.*)

presumed to have suffered from an arrhythmic episode resulting in syncope. Hearts with long-standing myocardial damage have foci of fibrosis, regardless of the cause of the loss of myocytes. Correlation between the severity of clinical cardiac disease and the severity of myocardial injury can be poor: a small lesion at a critical site, such as a portion of the conduction system can be fatal, whereas a widespread myocardial lesion, such as myocarditis, can be asymptomatic.

CARDIAC PATHOPHYSIOLOGY

The results of normal cardiac function include the maintenance of adequate blood flow, called cardiac output, to peripheral tissues that provide delivery of oxygen and nutrients, the removal of carbon dioxide and other metabolic waste products, the distribution of hormones and other cellular regulators, and the maintenance of adequate thermoregulation and glomerular filtration pressure (urine output). The normal heart has

a threefold to fivefold functional reserve capacity, but this capacity can eventually be lost in cardiac disease and the result is impaired function. Compensatory mechanisms operate in both normal and diseased hearts in an attempt to meet both the short-term and long-term demands for adequate cardiac output. These mechanisms include cardiac dilation, myocardial hypertrophy, increase in heart rate, increase in peripheral resistance, increase in blood volume, and redistribution of blood flow. These compensatory mechanisms can maintain cardiac output that is adequate for some time, even in animals with rather severe cardiac disease sufficient to compromise cardiac function from loss of myocardial contractility, sustained pressure overload, or sustained volume overload.

Cardiac dilation can occur as a terminal lesion in many cardiac diseases (Fig. 10-8, A). As a compensatory response to achieve increased cardiac output, dilation allows stretching of cardiac muscle cells to increase contractile force according to the Frank-Starling

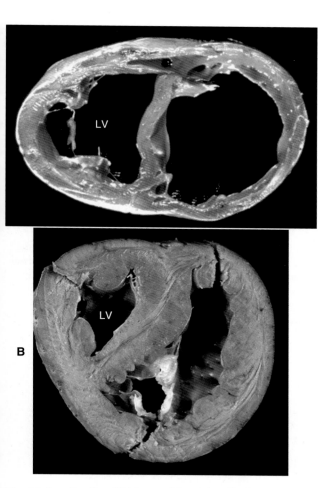

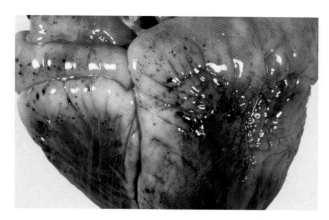

Fig. 10-9   Epicardial hemorrhage, petechiae and ecchymoses, endotoxemia, heart, cow. Note the epicardial and subepicardial hemorrhages in the fat of the coronary groove (a common site). Petechiae and ecchymoses are often attributable to severe septicemia, endotoxemia, anoxia, or electrocution. In this case, the hemorrhage resulted from injury to the endothelium from endotoxin (component of the cell wall of gram-negative bacteria). The smaller, pinpoint hemorrhages (1 to 2 mm) are petechiae. The larger hemorrhages (3 to 5 mm) are ecchymoses. *(Courtesy Dr. M.D. McGavin, College of Veterinary Medicine, University of Tennessee.)*

Fig. 10-8   Cardiac dilation and hypertrophy, heart, transected ventricles, dog. A, Cardiac dilation. Note the thin walls of both dilated ventricles. *LV,* Left ventricle. **B,** Cardiac hypertrophy (fixed tissue). Note that the right ventricular and left ventricular *(LV)* walls are approximately the same thickness, indicating that there is right ventricular hypertrophy. *(**A,** Courtesy Dr. Y. Niyo, College of Veterinary Medicine, Iowa State University; and Noah's Arkive, College of Veterinary Medicine, The University of Georgia. **B,** Courtesy College of Veterinary Medicine, University of Florida; and Noah's Arkive, College of Veterinary Medicine, The University of Georgia.)*

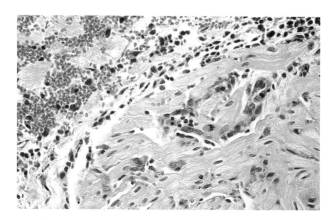

Fig. 10-10   Epicardial hemorrhage, minoxidil cardiotoxicity, heart, left atrium, pig. Note epicardial hemorrhage *(upper left)* and prominent small blood vessels with swollen endothelial cells. H&E stain. *(Courtesy School of Veterinary Medicine, Purdue University.)*

phenomenon, and increased stroke volume is the result. However, stretching beyond certain limits decreases contractile strength.

Myocardial hypertrophy is an important long-term compensatory response of the heart to maintain adequate cardiac output in the face of increased pressure or volume overload (see Myocardial Diseases) (Fig. 10-8, *B*).

CIRCULATORY DISTURBANCES

Hemorrhage is a frequent lesion of the epicardium, endocardium, and myocardium. Hemorrhages vary in size from petechiae (1- to 2-mm diameter), to ecchymoses

(2- to 10-mm diameter), to suffusive (diffuse). Animals dying from septicemia, endotoxemia, anoxia, or electrocution often have prominent epicardial (Figs. 10-9 and 10-10) and endocardial (Fig. 10-11) hemorrhages. Horses dying of any cause usually have agonal hemorrhages on the epicardial and endocardial surfaces.

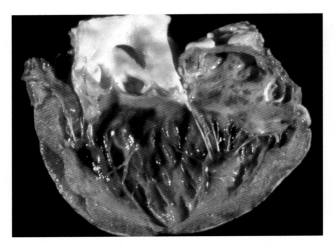

Fig. 10-11   Endocardial suffusive hemorrhage, heart, left ventricle, calf. A red to dark-red sheet of suffusive hemorrhage is present in the endocardium of the left ventricle. Suffusive hemorrhage is often attributed to severe septicemia, endotoxemia, anoxia, or electrocution. *(Courtesy College of Veterinary Medicine, University of Illinois.)*

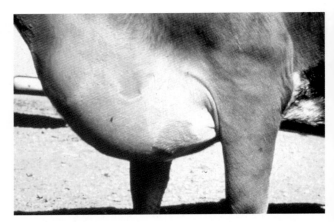

Fig. 10-12   Subcutaneous edema, high altitude disease with congestive heart failure ("brisket disease"), presternal, sternal, and caudal sternocephalic regions (brisket), cow. The extensive subcutaneous edema is the result of chronic congestive heart failure. *(Courtesy School of Veterinary Medicine, Purdue University.)*

A distinctive example of a specific disease with cardiac hemorrhage is mulberry heart disease, associated with selenium–vitamin E deficiency in growing pigs. In these pigs, hydropericardium accompanies severe myocardial hemorrhage that results in a red, mottled (mulberry-like) appearance of the heart.

SYNDROMES OF CARDIAC FAILURE OR DECOMPENSATION (TABLE 10-1)

Cardiac syncope, an acute expression of cardiac disease, is characterized clinically by collapse, loss of consciousness, and extreme changes in heart rate and blood pressure, and with or without demonstrable lesions. Syncope can be caused by massive myocardial necrosis, ventricular fibrillation, heart block, arrhythmias, and reflex cardiac inhibition (e.g., that associated with high intestinal blockage).

Congestive heart failure usually develops slowly from gradual loss of cardiac pumping efficiency associated with either pressure or volume overload or myocardial damage (Figs. 10-12 and 10-13; also see Figs. 8-34 and 8-35). Pathogenetically, congestive heart failure is initiated by development of cardiac disease (myocardial, valvular, congenital, etc.) or increased workload associated with pulmonary, renal, or vascular disease leading to loss of cardiac reserve and development of decreased blood flow to peripheral tissue (forward failure) and accumulation of blood behind the failing chamber (backward failure). Reduced renal blood flow creates hypoxia in the kidneys and increases renin release

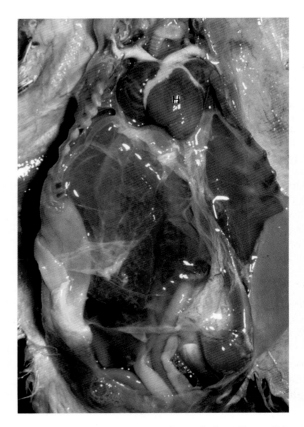

Fig. 10-13   Ascites, congestive heart failure, furazolidone cardiotoxicity, heart and liver, duckling. Note prominent accumulations of serous fluid in the abdomen and fibrin deposits over the liver. The heart (*H*) is dilated.
(Courtesy School of Veterinary Medicine, Purdue University.)

Table 10-1   Experimental Models of Heart Failure

Experimental Model	Experimental Method	Species
Pressure loading	Pulmonary artery banding	Rat, dog, pig, sheep, pony
	Aortic constriction	Rat, rabbit, dog, sheep
	Supravalvular aortic constriction	Dog
	Aortic valve stenosis	Rabbit, dog
	Pulmonary valve stenosis	Dog
	Experimental hypertension	Rat, dog
Volume loading	Fluid overload	Baboon
	Aorta-to-vena cava fistula	Rat, dog
	Aortic valve incompetence	Rat, rabbit
	Atrial septal defect	Cat
Myocardial infarction	Sustained atrial pacing	Dog
	Coronary ligation	Dog, pig
	Controlled occlusion—subclavian-to-carotid shunt	Dog
	Coronary embolism	Dog, calf, pig
	Thrombus generation	Dog
	Chronic hypoxia	Rat
Cardiomyopathy and other conditions	Left ventricular Dacron patch	Dog
	Spontaneous cardiomyopathy	Hamster, mouse, cattle, rat, turkey, cat, dog
	Barbiturate overdose	Dog
	Furazolidone cardiomyopathy	Turkey, duckling
	Adriamycin cardiomyopathy	Rat, dog, mouse, pig
	Isoprenaline	Rat
	Noradrenaline	Dog
	Amphetamine	Rat
	Cobalt chloride	Rat, pig
	Vitamin E deficiency	Rat, mouse, calf, lamb
	Alcohol intoxication	Rat
	Coxsackie viral myocarditis	Mouse
	Viral encephalomyocarditis	Mouse
	Altered cardiac development and/or function	Transgenic mice

Modified from Smith HJ, Nuttall A: *Cardiovasc Res* 19:181-186, 1985.

from the juxtaglomerular apparatus, resulting in stimulation of aldosterone release from the zona glomerulosa of the adrenal cortex. Sodium and water retention are the results of the action of aldosterone on the renal tubules; increased plasma volume follows, as does accumulation of edema fluid (mainly in body cavities). Hypoxia also stimulates increased erythropoiesis in bone marrow and extramedullary organs, such as the spleen, causing polycythemia and thus increased viscosity of the blood. The hypervolemia from aldosterone-induced water retention increases the workload on the already failing heart. Thus a vicious cycle of cardiac decompensation is initiated that will lead to death from cardiac failure unless therapeutic intervention occurs. Cardiac dilation, hypertrophy, and increased heart rate can provide some compensation for the increased workload.

Acute left side heart failure is manifested by pulmonary congestion and edema, whereas chronic left side heart failure is manifested by chronic passive pulmonary congestion, chronic edema, hemosiderosis ("heart failure cells"), and fibrosis. The most common causes are (1) myocardial contractility loss associated with myocarditis, myocardial necrosis, or cardiomyopathy; (2) dysfunction of the mitral or aortic valves; and (3) several congenital heart diseases.

Acute right side heart failure results in acute passive congestion leading to hepatomegaly and splenomegaly, whereas chronic right side heart failure results in hepatic congestion (nutmeg liver) and more severe sodium and water retention than in left side heart failure. Edema is evident predominantly as ventral subcutaneous edema in horses and ruminants (Fig. 10-12), ascites in dogs, and hydrothorax in cats. Causes of right-sided failure include (1) pulmonary hypertension, (2) cardiomyopathy, and (3) disease of the tricuspid and pulmonary valves. (See Chapters 8 and 9 for further details on hepatic and pulmonary lesions, respectively, associated with congestive heart failure.)

A wide variety of experimental animal models of heart failure exist (Table 10-1). The models have been used to develop an understanding of human cardiac diseases.

CLINICAL DIAGNOSTIC PROCEDURES

The array of diagnostic tools available to the veterinarian to evaluate changes in cases of cardiac disease has grown dramatically in the past decade as many procedures have been adapted from use in human medicine. Procedures include physical examination, radiography, electrocardiology, echocardiography, angiocardiography, and cardiac catheterization. Cardiac damage can be detected by increased activity of serum enzymes and isoenzymes, such as creatine phosphokinase, lactate dehydrogenase, troponin T, and aspartate aminotransferase, which are specifically released from injured cardiac muscle cells. Also, increased plasma concentrations of plasma natriuretic peptides (A type [atrial], B type [brain], and C type) may indicate cardiac disease because these hormones are synthesized by cardiac muscle cells. In research studies of cardiac diseases in animals, endomyocardial biopsies have been used to assess the light microscopic and ultrastructural alterations during the course of the disease.

EXAMINATION OF THE HEART AT NECROPSY AND TISSUE SAMPLING FOR HISTOPATHOLOGIC EVALUATION

Following the removal of the rib cage and exposure of the thoracic organs, the pericardial sac should be incised and observations made on the presence of pericardial thickening and adhesions and the nature and amount of pericardial fluid present. The heart and lungs should be removed together and examined. The great vessels are transected, and the entire heart is examined to determine its overall shape, size, and color.

The hearts of most animals are dissected to expose the endocardium and the four valves. A systematic approach should be followed; usually the heart is opened in the direction of blood flow with incisions through the right atrium and right ventricle to the right ventricular apex and then along the right ventricular wall adjacent to the interventricular septum into the pulmonary outflow tract. The left side is incised from the atrium to the left ventricular apex to expose the endocardial surfaces and mitral valve; subsequently, the mitral valve leaflet is incised to expose the outflow tract into the aorta.

After all observed lesions and the weight of the heart are entered in the written record, the heart is placed in fixative solution.

The hearts of small animals, such as rodents, birds, puppies, and kittens, are often collected and placed intact in the fixative solution.

Other procedures that can be performed on hearts before fixation to quantitate hypertrophy and dilation include measurements of ventricular wall thicknesses, determination of weights of individual cardiac chambers and septum, and measurements of atrioventricular valve ring circumferences.

After fixation for at least 24 hours, tissue samples should be removed from standard sites for histopathologic evaluation (Fig. 10-14). If gross lesions are apparent, representative samples should be taken of those lesions. In small-sized hearts, the fixed specimen is bisected perpendicular to the long axis of the septum to provide a sample for histopathologic study that includes sections of all four chambers and interventricular and interatrial septa.

Special sampling procedures are available for comprehensive evaluation of the cardiac conduction tissue.

DISEASES OF THE HEART

CONGENITAL ANOMALIES

The complex events involved in the embryologic development of the heart and great vessels allow substantial opportunities for congenital anomalies to develop. The functional significance of these anomalies varies widely. Animals with the most extreme defects will be unable to survive in utero, and those with the mildest lesions could have no clinical signs of disease during life. However, animals with defects of intermediate severity are most likely to be presented to a veterinarian because of gradually developing signs of cardiac failure, including poor exercise tolerance, cyanosis, and stunted body growth. The most frequently observed cardiovascular anomalies in domestic animals are listed in Table 10-2.

The causes of congenital cardiovascular anomalies are varied. Most animal species have a low background frequency of spontaneous cardiac malformations. In many species, especially in dogs, these defects are heritable and can be attributed to either single or multiple gene effects. Under experimental conditions, cardiovascular congenital defects can be elicited by exposure of pregnant dams to various chemicals and drugs, physical agents, toxins, or nutritional deficiencies. Chemical compounds implicated include thalidomide, ethanol, salicylates, griseofulvin, and cortisone. Prenatal exposure to x-irradiation or fetal hypoxia can induce defects. Maternal nutritional deficiencies of

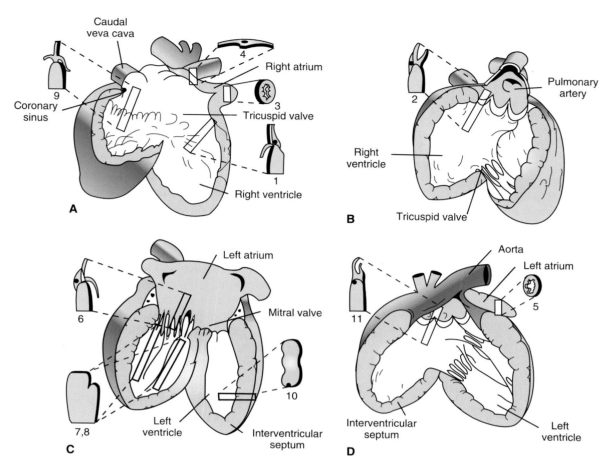

Fig. 10-14 **Schematic diagram of the gross and microscopic examination of the heart.** Diagrams **A** to **D** illustrate the heart opened. The numbers indicate the area and the shape of the blocks of tissue removed for histopathology. **A,** Right ventricle and right atrium. **B,** Right ventricular cavity and pulmonary outflow tract. **C,** Left ventricle and left atrium. **D,** Left ventricle and aortic outflow tract. *1,* Right ventricular free wall, atrioventricular valve, and atrium. *2,* Pulmonic valve, right ventricular outflow tract, and pulmonary artery. *3,* Right auricular appendage. *4,* Sinoatrial node. *5,* Left auricular appendage. *6,* Left atrioventricular valve, ventricle, and atrium. *7 and 8,* Left ventricular free wall and papillary muscles. *9,* Atrioventricular node, right atrioventricular valve, and atrium. *10,* Interventricular septum. *11,* Aortic valve, left aortic outflow tract and aorta. (**A** through **D,** *From Bishop SP: Necropsy techniques for the heart and great vessels. In Fox P, Sisson D, Moise N, editors: Textbook of canine and feline cardiology, ed 2, Philadelphia, 1999, Saunders.*)

vitamin A, pantothenic acid, riboflavin, or zinc and excess intake of vitamin A, retinoic acid, or copper can result in cardiovascular anomalies in newborn animals.

Sites of the major cardiovascular anomalies in the dog are shown in Fig. 10-15.

ANOMALIES FROM FAILURE OF CLOSURE OF FETAL CARDIOVASCULAR SHUNTS

Patent ductus arteriosus is a frequent anomaly in poodle, collie, Pomeranian, Chihuahua, Maltese, English springer spaniel, keeshond, bichon frise, and Shetland sheepdog breeds (Fig. 10-16). In poodles, it is an inherited lesion. Female dogs have a greater incidence. This vascular channel between the pulmonary artery and aorta allows blood to bypass the lungs during fetal life and normally is converted to the solid ligamentum arteriosum postnatally. It remains patent in dogs with this anomaly. Generally, blood is shunted from the left to the right ventricle, resulting in pulmonary hypertension.

An atrial septal defect could represent the failure of closure of the foramen ovale, which is an interatrial septal shunt that allows blood to bypass the lungs of the fetus, or it can be the result of true septal defects at

Table **10-2**   **Most Common Cardiovascular Anomalies in Several Domestic Animal Species**

DOG
Patent ductus arteriosus
Pulmonic stenosis
Subaortic stenosis
Persistent right aortic arch

CAT
Endocardial cushion defects
Mitral malformation
Ventricular septal defect
Endocardial fibroelastosis
Patent ductus arteriosus

COW
Atrial septal defect
Ventricular septal defect
Transposition of aorta and pulmonary artery
Valvular hematomas

PIG
Subaortic stenosis
Endocardial cushion defect

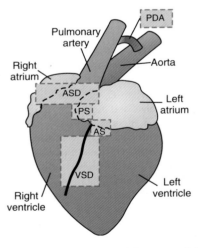

Fig. 10-15 **Schematic diagram of the sites of the major cardiovascular anomalies of the dog.** *AS,* aortic stenosis; *ASD,* atrial septal defect; *PDA,* patent ductus arteriosus; *PS,* pulmonic stenosis; *VSD,* ventricular septal defect. *(Redrawn with permission from School of Veterinary Medicine, Purdue University.)*

another site because of faulty development of the interatrial septum (Fig. 10-17). Dog breeds with greatest frequency of this defect are the boxer, Doberman pinscher, and Samoyed.

A ventricular septal defect indicates failure of complete development of the interventricular septum and allows the shunting of blood between the ventricles (Fig. 10-18). The defect occurs in many species and more commonly in the upper, membranous portion of the interventricular septum rather than in the lower, muscular septum. Among breeds of dogs, the greatest frequency has been observed in the English bulldog, English springer spaniel, and West Highland white terrier.

The tetralogy of Fallot is a complicated cardiac anomaly with four lesions (Fig. 10-19). The three primary defects are a ventricular septal defect located high in the septum, pulmonic stenosis (see later discussion), and dextroposition of the aorta (see later discussion). The fourth defect, which develops secondarily, is hypertrophy of the right ventricular myocardium. This complex anomaly is inherited in keeshond dogs and is frequent in English bulldogs. Cyanosis is often an associated clinical sign. The anomaly is one of the most common cardiac abnormalities seen in hearts of human beings (so-called blue babies). By genetic and pathologic studies of keeshond dogs, the basic defect has been determined to be hypoplasia and malpositioning of the conotruncal septum. Wide variability in the severity of the lesions has been observed.

ANOMALIES FROM FAILURE OF NORMAL VALVULAR DEVELOPMENT

Pulmonic stenosis has been recognized as a frequently occurring anomaly in dogs and is inherited in such breeds as the beagle, English bulldog, and Chihuahua (Fig. 10-20). Other breeds in which this lesion is frequent are basset hound, boxer, Chow chow, cocker spaniel, Labrador retriever, mastiff, Newfoundland, Samoyed, schnauzer, and terriers. Several types of valvular lesions have been described and include formation of a circumferential band of fibrous or muscular tissue beneath the valve (subvalvular stenosis) or malformation of the valve (valvular stenosis), with a small central orifice in a dome of thickened valvular tissue. Notable concentric hypertrophy (see Myocardial Diseases, Growth Disturbances) of the right ventricle will develop from the resulting pressure overload.

Subaortic stenosis is a cardiac anomaly frequently observed in pigs and dogs. It apparently is inherited in Newfoundland, boxer, and German shepherd dogs (Fig. 10-21). The lesion is also observed in the German shorthair pointer, golden retriever, Great Dane, rottweiler, Samoyed, and bull terrier breeds. In clinical cases, the stenosis is produced by the presence of a thick zone of endocardial fibrous tissue that encircles the left ventricular outflow tract below the valve. In mild cases, often subclinical, the lesion is limited to white nodules on the ventricular septum immediately below the valve. Microscopically the altered endocardial tissue can contain proliferated mesenchymal cells,

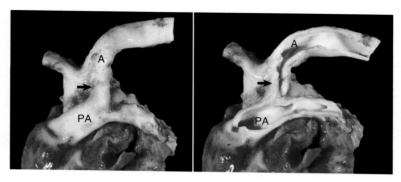

Fig. 10-16   Patent ductus arteriosus, heart, neonatal animal. Note the prominent ductus arteriosus *(arrow)* between the pulmonary artery *(PA)* and the aorta *(A)* in the undissected *(left)* and dissected vessels *(right)*. *(Courtesy Dr. D.D. Harrington, School of Veterinary Medicine, Purdue University; and Noah's Arkive, College of Veterinary Medicine, The University of Georgia.)*

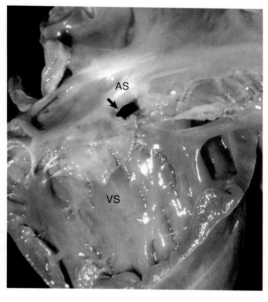

Fig. 10-17   Atrial septal defect, heart, opened right side, pig. The prominent opening *(arrow)* low in the atrial septum *(AS)* and just above the arterioventricular valve is the atrial septal defect. *VS,* Ventricular septum. *(Courtesy School of Veterinary Medicine, Purdue University.)*

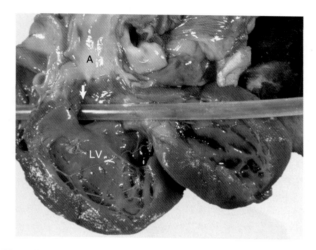

Fig. 10-18   Ventricular septal defect (high defect), heart, opened left side, calf. Note the large opening in the basal portion of the ventricular septum *(arrow)* immediately below the aortic valve through which the tube has been passed. *A,* Aorta; *LV,* left ventricle. *(Courtesy Dr. M. D. McGavin, College of Veterinary Medicine, University of Tennessee.)*

mucinous ground substance, and foci of metaplastic cartilage. Other cardiac lesions develop as a result of the altered left ventricular outflow; these include left ventricular concentric hypertrophy, disseminated foci of myocardial necrosis, fibrosis in the inner left ventricular wall, and thickening of the walls of intramyocardial arteries.

Valvular hematomas (hematocysts) frequently are observed on the atrioventricular valves of postnatal ruminants (Fig. 10-22, A). These lesions, which generally regress spontaneously by the time the animals are several months of age, do not produce any functional abnormalities. Lesions are bulging, blood-filled cysts, several millimeters in diameter, on the edges of the atrioventricular valves.

Valvular lymphocysts may also occur and appear as yellow serum-filled cysts on the atrioventricular valve cusps (Fig. 10-22, B).

Other valvular developmental anomalies include endocardial cushion defects (persistent atrioventricular canal) in pigs and cats, mitral dysplasia in cats and dogs, and tricuspid dysplasia in cats and dogs.

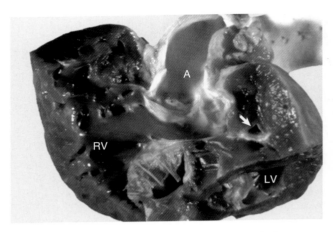

Fig. 10-19   Tetralogy of Fallot, heart, dissected, dog. Above the large basal ventricular septal defect is an overlying, straddling aorta (*A*). There is also severe pulmonic stenosis (*arrow*) with massive right ventricular hypertrophy. *LV,* Left ventricle; *RV,* right ventricle. (*Courtesy School of Veterinary Medicine, Purdue University.*)

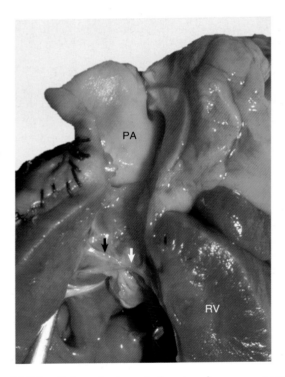

Fig. 10-20   Pulmonic stenosis, heart, pulmonary artery, dog. Note the prominent right ventricular (*RV*) hypertrophy and the white, thick mass of fibrous connective tissue (*arrows*) lining and constricting the outflow tract beneath the pulmonary valve. The pulmonary artery (*PA*) above the stenotic valve is dilated because the narrowing of the valve lumen forces the blood through the narrow lumen, resulting in a "jetlike" stream of blood that strikes the surface of the pulmonary artery, leading to roughening, deformation, and eventual dilation. (*Courtesy School of Veterinary Medicine, Purdue University.*)

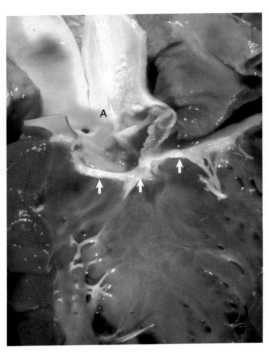

Fig. 10-21   Subaortic stenosis, heart, opened left side, dog. A thick, white, broad band of fibrous connective tissue (*arrows*) encircles the left ventricular outflow tract below the aortic valve. The force of the blood ejected through the stenotic lesion is responsible for the "jet lesions" in the overlying aorta (*A*) (*right half*—roughened surface; *left half*—dilation [note the gray area]). (*Courtesy College of Veterinary Medicine, University of Illinois.*)

ANOMALIES FROM MALPOSITIONING OF GREAT VESSELS

Persistent right aortic arch occurs in dogs; German shepherd, Irish setter, and Great Dane dogs are predisposed (Fig. 10-23). This defect arises because the right fourth aortic arch, rather than the left, develops and ascends on the right side of the midline so that the ligamentum arteriosum forms a vascular ring over the esophagus and trachea. This arrangement eventually results in esophageal obstruction and proximal dilation (megaesophagus) as the animal matures and consumes solid feed.

Transposition of the aorta and pulmonary artery are severe anomalies, of which there are several types.

OTHER CARDIAC ANOMALIES

Ectopia cordis is the congenital development of the heart at an abnormal site outside of the thoracic cavity. In cattle, cases in healthy adult animals have been described in which the heart was located subcutaneously in the caudoventral neck area.

Endocardial fibroelastosis in animals has been most recognized as a primary cardiac defect in Burmese and Siamese cats. In this heritable disease, the heart has

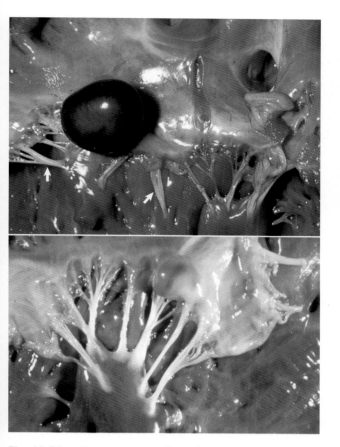

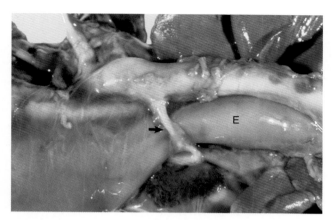

Fig. 10-23   Persistent right aortic arch, ligamentum arteriosum, megaesophagus, calf. Because during embryogenesis the aorta was formed from the right aortic arch instead of the left one, the aorta is now on the right. Thus in order for the ligamentum arteriosum (*arrow*) to connect the aorta with the pulmonary artery, it has to pass dorsally over the esophagus and trachea. The ligamentum, together with the aorta and pulmonary artery, form a vascular ring that constricts the esophagus (*E*), which is dilated cranial to the constriction. *(Courtesy Dr. S. Snyder, College of Veterinary Medicine, Colorado State University; and Noah's Arkive, College of Veterinary Medicine, The University of Georgia.)*

Fig. 10-22   Hematocysts and lymphocysts, calf. A, Valvular hematocyst, heart, opened left side, mitral valve, postnatal calf. A dark, blood-filled cyst protrudes from a cusp of the mitral valve. Arrows indicate chordae tendinae. Hematocysts usually occur in ruminants, do not cause any functional abnormality, and usually regress within a few months of birth. **B,** Valvular lymphocyst, heart. A lymph-filled cyst is on a cusp of the atrioventricular valve. Like hematocysts, lymphocysts usually occur in ruminants, do not cause any functional abnormality, and usually regress within a few months of birth. (**A,** *Courtesy Dr. M.D. McGavin, College of Veterinary Medicine, University of Tennessee.* **B,** *Courtesy College of Veterinary Medicine, University of Illinois.*)

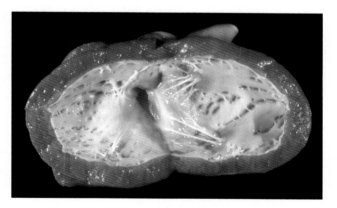

Fig. 10-24   Subendocardial fibroelastosis, heart, left ventricle, dog. The endocardium is opaque because increased amounts of collagen and elastic fibers were deposited in the subendocardium secondary to turbulence of blood flow within the ventricles. This dog had a persistent ductus arteriosus. This lesion may have a hereditary basis in Burmese cats and is often a sequela to turbulence within ventricles in cardiac disease. *(Courtesy College of Veterinary Medicine, University of Illinois.)*

prominent, white, thickened endocardium, especially of the left ventricle, because of the proliferation of fibroelastic tissue (Fig. 10-24).

Peritoneopericardial diaphragmatic hernias occur in dogs with incomplete development of the diaphragm. Abdominal viscera can be located in the pericardial sac.

PERICARDIAL DISEASES

FLUID ACCUMULATIONS IN THE PERICARDIAL SAC

Hydropericardium is the accumulation of clear to light yellow, watery, serous fluid (i.e., transudate) in the pericardial sac, which becomes distended (Fig. 10-25).

In cases associated with vascular injury, such as "mulberry heart disease" (dietary microangiopathy of pigs), a few fibrin strands are present, and the fluid could clot following exposure to air. The pericardial surfaces are smooth and glistening in acute cases, but in chronic

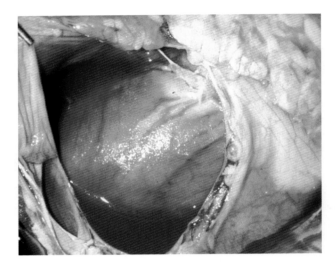

Fig. 10-25   Hydropericardium, pericardial sac, pig. The thin-walled pericardial sac contains serous fluid that has accumulated secondary to alterations in hydrostatic pressure between the pericardial cavity, circulatory system, and lymphatic system. *(Courtesy College of Veterinary Medicine, University of Illinois.)*

cases the epicardium becomes opaque because of mild fibrous thickening and can appear roughened and granular when there is villous proliferation of fibrous tissue, especially over the atria.

Hydropericardium occurs in those diseases that have generalized edema. Thus ascites and hydrothorax often occur concurrently with hydropericardium. Congestive heart failure is an important mechanism of hydropericardium and is usually due to primary myocardial, valvular, congenital, or neoplastic diseases. Common specific diseases include dilated cardiomyopathy of dogs and cats and "ascites syndrome" of poultry. Hydropericardium can also accompany pulmonary hypertension (e.g., "brisket disease" or "high-altitude disease" of cattle), renal failure, and hypoproteinemia from various chronic debilitating diseases. Hydropericardium can also occur in various systemic diseases with vascular injury, such as septicemia in pigs, "heartwater" (*Cowdria ruminantium* infection) in small ruminants, African horse sickness, and bovine ephemeral fever.

Hydropericardium of rapid onset and of sufficient volume leads to development of cardiac tamponade or compression, which interferes with cardiac filling (especially of the atria) and venous return to the heart. In cases with slow development, stretching of the pericardium allows accumulation of a large volume of fluid without tamponade. Hydropericardium can be reversed if the underlying cause is removed. However, many cases are associated with progressive cardiac diseases, and death is the outcome.

Hemorrhagic pericardial effusion of unknown cause is frequently seen in dogs. Large or giant breeds, such as the Great Dane, Saint Bernard, Great Pyrenees, German shepherd, and golden retriever are most often affected. The preferred treatment for the condition is pericardectomy. Similar effusions have occurred in

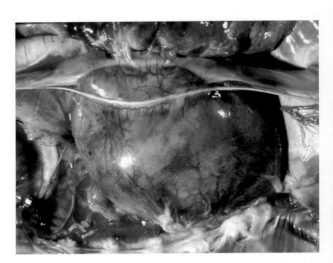

Fig. 10-26   Hemopericardium (cardiac tamponade), right atrial hemangiosarcoma. heart, dog. The pericardium is distended and dark blue because it contains whole blood secondary to rupture of an atrial hemangiosarcoma. Hemopericardium can cause death if it is sudden and is of sufficient volume to compress the heart and thus reduce cardiac output, a condition known as cardiac tamponade. On clinical examination, heart sounds are muffled. *(Courtesy College of Veterinary Medicine, University of Illinois.)*

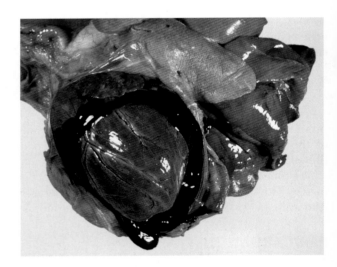

Fig. 10-27   Hemopericardium, heart, dog. The pericardial sac is filled with clotted blood. Hemorrhage into a body cavity results in pooling of coagulated or noncoagulated blood within that cavity. *(Courtesy Dr. D.A. Mosier, College of Veterinary Medicine, Kansas State University.)*

dogs with cardiac hemangiosarcomas and heart base tumors, common cardiac neoplasms in this species. These diseases will be discussed later in this chapter.

Hemopericardium is an accumulation of whole blood in the pericardial sac (Figs. 10-26 and 10-27). Death often occurs suddenly from cardiac tamponade, a condition with compression of the heart caused by blood or fluid accumulation in the pericardial sac leading to reduced cardiac output. Bleeding into the pericardial sac can result from spontaneous atrial rupture in dogs, atrial rupture in dogs with hemangiosarcoma, rupture of the intrapericardial aorta in horses, or as a complication of intracardiac injections.

METABOLIC ALTERATIONS

Serous atrophy of fat is readily identified by the gray gelatinous appearance of epicardial fat deposits (Fig. 10-28). Healthy animals normally have abundant white or yellow epicardial fat deposits, especially along the atrioventricular junction. Microscopically, lipocytes are atrophic and edema fluid is present in interstitial tissue. Serous atrophy of epicardial fat occurs rapidly during anorexia, starvation, or cachexia as fat is catabolized to maintain energy balance.

Epicardial mineralization (cardiac calcinosis) is a striking lesion of certain inbred strains of mice (Fig. 10-29, *A* and *B*). In this inherited disorder, white, firm, mineralized

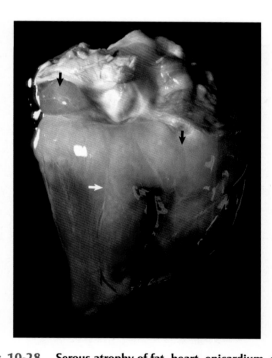

Fig. 10-28   Serous atrophy of fat, heart, epicardium, cow. The epicardial fat deposits are gray and gelatinous (*arrows*), indicating that fat has been catabolized, for example as in the early stages of starvation. (*Courtesy Dr. M.D. McGavin, College of Veterinary Medicine, University of Tennessee.*)

plaques are present, especially over the right ventricular epicardium. The lesion, arising by dystrophic calcification, does not tend to cause cardiac dysfunction.

Urate deposits on the pericardium occur in birds and snakes with visceral gout. The affected serosal surface appears thickened and white from the accumulations of uric acid crystals (Fig. 10-30).

INFLAMMATION

The various portals of entry and defense mechanisms involved in pericardial inflammation are summarized in Box 10-1 and Box 10-2. Fibrinous pericarditis, the most common type of pericardial inflammation in

---

Box 10-1

Portals of Entry for the Cardiovascular System

PERICARDIUM

Hematogenous dissemination
Foreign body penetration from reticulum (cattle)

ENDOCARDIUM

Hematogenous dissemination
Parasitic migration
Intravenous and intracardiac catheters (long-term placement)
Uremia-induced vascular damage and secondary endocardial ulceration (dog, left atrium)

MYOCARDIUM

Hematogenous dissemination
Embolic dissemination of infective material fragments from vegetative endocarditis lesions into coronary arterial tree

ARTERIES

Hematogenous dissemination
Local extension of suppurative and necrotizing inflammatory processes
Immune-mediated arterial injury
Parasitic migration

VEINS

Hematogenous dissemination
Local extension of severe inflammatory processes
Intravenous injections and indwelling catheters
Parasitic migration
Immune-mediated venous injury

LYMPH VESSELS

Hematogenous dissemination
Local extension of severe inflammatory processes
Parasitic migration

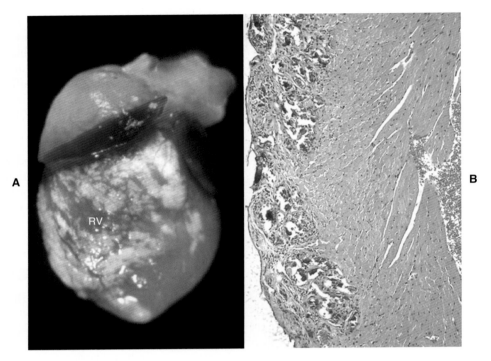

Fig. 10-29   Epicardial calcification, heart, right ventricle, mouse. A, Note the prominent white mineral deposits over the right ventricle *(RV)*. **B,** The basophilic mineral deposits are present epicardially and in the outer myocardium *(left)*. H&E stain. *(**A** and **B,** Courtesy School of Veterinary Medicine, Purdue University.)*

Box **10-2**

Defense Mechanisms in the Cardiovascular System

PERICARDIUM

Immunologic responses—humoral and innate

ENDOCARDIUM

Constant blood flow through cardiac chambers
Immunologic responses—humoral and innate

MYOCARDIUM

Immunologic responses—humoral and innate

ARTERIES

Constant blood flow through arteries
Immunologic responses—humoral and innate

VEINS

Constant blood flow through veins
Immunologic responses—humoral and innate

LYMPH VESSELS

Constant lymph flow through lymph vessels
Immunologic responses—humoral and innate

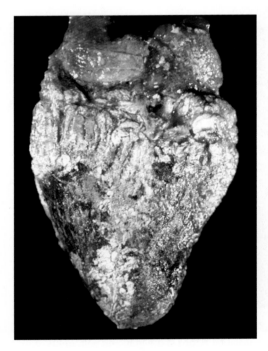

Fig. 10-30   Visceral gout, heart, pericardium, chicken.
White urate deposits are present on the epicardial surface.
(Courtesy College of Veterinary Medicine, The Ohio State University; and Noah's Arkive, College of Veterinary Medicine, The University of Georgia.)

animals, is usually the result of hematogenously spread infection. Specific diseases with this lesion include those in cattle (pasteurellosis, blackleg, coliform septicemias, and sporadic bovine encephalomyelitis), pigs (Glasser's disease, streptococcal infections, pasteurellosis, enzootic mycoplasmal pneumonia, and salmonellosis), horses (streptococcal infections), and birds (psittacosis). Grossly, both the visceral and parietal pericardial surfaces are covered by variable amounts of yellow fibrin deposits, which can result in adherence between the parietal and visceral layers. When the pericardial sac is opened upon necropsy, these attachments are torn away (so-called bread-and-butter heart) (Fig. 10-31). Microscopically an eosinophilic layer of fibrin with admixed neutrophils lies over a congested pericardium (Fig. 10-32).

The outcome of fibrinous pericarditis varies. Early death is frequent because many of these lesions result from infection by highly virulent bacteria and concurrent septicemia. When survival is prolonged, fibrous adhesions form between the pericardial surfaces after fibrous organization of the exudate.

Suppurative pericarditis is seen mainly in cattle as a complication of traumatic reticuloperitonitis ("hardware disease"). Foreign bodies, such as nails or pieces of wire that accumulate in the reticulum, occasionally penetrate the reticular wall and diaphragm, enter the adjacent pericardial sac, and introduce infection. Some affected cattle survive for weeks to months until death ensues from congestive heart failure and septicemia. Grossly the pericardial surfaces are notably thickened by white, often rough, shaggy-appearing masses of fibrous connective tissue that enclose an accumulation of white to gray, thick, foul-smelling, purulent exudate (Fig. 10-33).

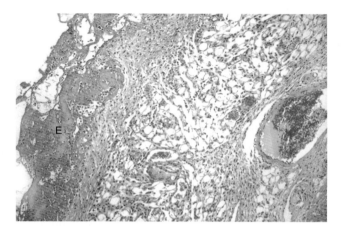

Fig. 10-32 **Fibrinous pericarditis, heart, epicardium, pig.** Note eosinophilic fibrin deposits (*left*) on the epicardial surface (*E*). This lesion commonly occurs with septicemias of bacteria that cause vasculitis. H&E stain. (*Courtesy School of Veterinary Medicine, Purdue University.*)

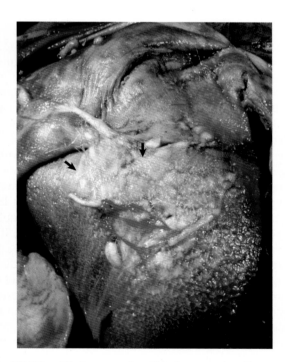

Fig. 10-31 **Fibrinous pericarditis, heart, epicardium, horse.** The epicardium is covered dorsally by a thick, yellow layer of fibrin (*arrows*) and ventrally by granulation tissue (finely granular surface), thus indicating the chronicity of the inflammatory process. The apposing parietal pericardium (not shown) was also covered with fibrin. This lesion commonly occurs in horses with *Streptococcus zooepidemicus* septicemia causing vasculitis. (*Courtesy Dr. M.D. McGavin, College of Veterinary Medicine, University of Tennessee.*)

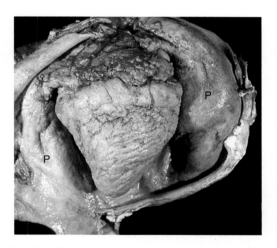

Fig. 10-33 **Chronic suppurative pericarditis, traumatic reticuloperitonitis ("hardware disease"), heart, pericardial sac (opened), cow.** The exposed epicardial and parietal surfaces are notably thickened by fibrous connective tissue and covered by a fibrinopurulent exudate. On clinical examination, heart sounds are muffled. *P,* Reflected parietal pericardium. (*Courtesy Dr. J. King, College of Veterinary Medicine, Cornell University.*)

Constrictive pericarditis is a chronic inflammatory lesion of the pericardium accompanied by extensive fibrous proliferation and eventual formation of fibrous adhesions between the surfaces of the visceral and parietal pericardium. The condition is seen in some cases of suppurative pericarditis in cattle. Severe lesions obliterate the pericardial sac and constrict the heart with fibrous tissue and can interfere with cardiac filling and thus cardiac output. Compensatory myocardial hypertrophy can result in diminished ventricular chamber volumes and contribute to the eventual development of congestive cardiac failure.

ENDOCARDIAL DISEASES

DEGENERATION

Endocardial mineralization and endocardial fibrosis can occur singly or together. Mineralization occurs from intake of excessive amounts of vitamin D and from intoxication by calcinogenic plants (*Cestrum diurnum, Trisetum flavescens, Solanum malacoxylon, Solanum torvum*) that contain vitamin D analogs. These plant-induced syndromes of cattle have been called by different names in various areas of the world, such as "Manchester wasting disease" in Jamaica, "enzootic calcinosis" in Europe, "naahelu disease" in Hawaii, "enteque seco" in Argentina, and "espichamento" in Brazil. Multiple, large, white, rough, firm plaques of mineralized fibroelastic tissue are present in the endocardium and intima of large elastic arteries. Fibrosis, with or without mineralization, occurs in chronically dilated hearts, in hearts of debilitated cattle with Johne's disease (Fig. 10-34), in dogs with healed lesions of left atrial ulcerative endocarditis

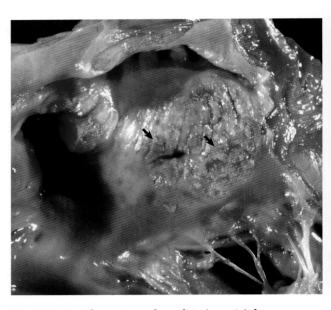

Fig. 10-35   Ulcerative endocarditis (uremia), heart, endocardium of left atrium, dog. Note the white-red, thick, wrinkled area (*arrows*) of endocarditis, mineralization, and fibrous tissue (scar) formation caused by uremia in this dog with chronic renal failure. (*Courtesy Dr. K. Read, College of Veterinary Medicine, Texas A&M University; and Noah's Arkive, College of Veterinary Medicine, The University of Georgia.*)

associated with a prior uremic episode (Fig. 10-35), and in the so-called jet lesions produced by the trauma of refluxed blood in valvular insufficiencies.

Valvular endocardiosis is an important age-related cardiac disease of middle-aged to old dogs, especially small and toy breeds, associated with degeneration of valvular collagen. Other names for this disease include valvular fibrosis and myxomatous or mucoid valvular degeneration. This disease, the most common cause of congestive heart failure in old dogs, appears to have a polygenic basis. Males of certain breeds are most frequently affected. The cavalier King Charles spaniel breed has a unique susceptibility, with more than 50% prevalence by 4 years of age and 100% prevalence by 10 years of age. Other breeds with high incidence include the cocker spaniel, beagle, dachshund, poodle, Pomeranian, schnauzer, Chihuahua, Doberman pinscher, fox terrier, Boston terrier, Pekingese, deerhound, and wolfhound. Lesions occur most frequently on the mitral valve, less commonly on the tricuspid, and infrequently on the aortic and pulmonary valves. Affected valves are shortened and thickened (nodular), either focal or diffusely, and appear smooth and shiny (Fig. 10-36, A and B) rather than rough and granular as is usual in cases of valvular endocarditis. These lesions result in valvular insufficiency with subsequent atrial dilation and development of atrial "jet lesions." The jet lesion is a raised, rough, firm streak of endocardial fibrosis resulting from

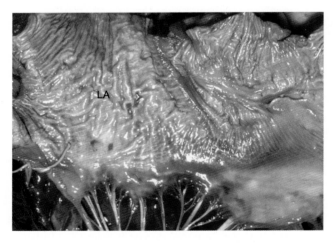

Fig. 10-34   Endocardial mineralization, Johne's disease, heart, left atrial endocardium, cow. The left atrial (*LA*) endocardium is white, thick, and wrinkled from mineralization. (*Courtesy School of Veterinary Medicine, Purdue University.*)

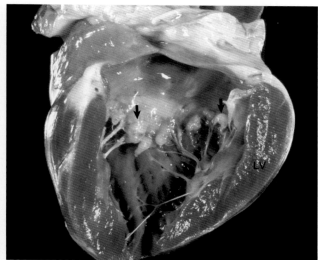

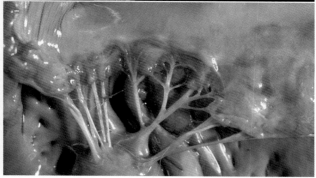

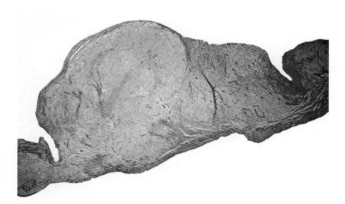

Fig. 10-37   Valvular endocardiosis, cusp of right atrioventricular valve, heart, dog. The valve is thickened and nodular from an increase in myxomatous tissue supported by a fibrous stroma. H&E stain. (*Courtesy School of Veterinary Medicine, Purdue University.*)

Fig. 10-36   Valvular endocardiosis, left atrioventricular valve, heart, dog. A, The cusps of the mitral valve are thickened by white, smooth nodules (*arrows*). *LV,* Left ventricular free wall. **B,** Note the characteristic smooth and shiny (endocardial) surface of the valve and nodules. This differentiates endocardiosis from the rough and granular surface of chronic bacterial endocarditis. The pink staining of the valve is caused by postmortem inbibition of hemoglobin. (**A,** *Courtesy Dr. J. Wright, College of Veterinary Medicine, North Carolina State University; and Noah's Arkive, College of Veterinary Medicine, The University of Georgia.* **B,** *Courtesy Dr. M.D. McGavin, College of Veterinary Medicine, University of Tennessee.*)

long-term trauma by a jet of blood leaking through the damaged valve in the closed position. Other complications of valvular endocardiosis include occasional rupture of the chordae tendineae and occasional splitting or rupture of the left atrial wall. Microscopically the thickened valves have notably increased fibroblastic proliferation and deposition of acid mucopolysaccharides (Fig. 10-37). Frequent accompanying myocardial alterations include arteriosclerosis of intramyocardial arteries and multifocal myocardial necrosis and fibrosis.

CIRCULATORY DISTURBANCES

Atrial thrombosis is a frequent lesion in aged Syrian hamsters and in certain strains of mice and has been

found in the failing hearts of dogs and cats with idiopathic cardiomyopathies. In affected hamsters and mice, the atria are swollen, firm, mottled and have gray-to-tan, laminated masses of fibrin. Fibroblastic organization occurs rapidly in the thrombi. Etiologic factors include aging, and genetic and dietary influences. Susceptible strains fed a thrombogenic diet (high fat, low protein, and hypolipotropic) have a high incidence of atrial thrombosis.

INFLAMMATION

The various portals of entry and defense mechanisms involved in endocardial inflammation are summarized in Box 10-1 and Box 10-2. Endocarditis is usually the result of bacterial infections, except for lesions produced by migrating *Strongylus vulgaris* larvae in horses and an occasional case of mycotic infection. The lesions are often very large by the time of death and are present on the valves (valvular endocarditis), although some lesions extend to the adjacent wall (mural endocarditis). Grossly the affected valves have large, adhering, friable, yellow-to-gray masses of fibrin termed "vegetations," which can largely occlude the valvular orifice (Fig. 10-38,). In chronic lesions, the fibrin deposits are organized by fibrous connective tissue to produce irregular nodular masses termed "verrucae" (wartlike lesions). Microscopically the lesion consists of accumulated layers of fibrin and numerous embedded bacterial colonies underlain by a zone of infiltrated leukocytes and granulation tissue (Fig. 10-39). Relative frequency of valvular involvement with endocarditis in animals is mitral > aortic > tricuspid > pulmonary.

The pathogenesis of endocarditis is complicated and frequently incompletely understood, but the components

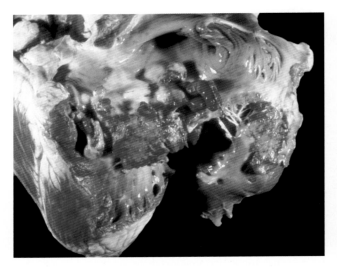

Fig. 10-38   Vegetative valvular endocarditis, tricuspid valve, heart, calf. Multiple, large, raised, friable, yellow-red thrombotic masses are attached to cusps of the tricuspid valve. The roughened and granular surface of the valve leaflets is attributable to fibrin, platelets, and trapped bacteria (Fig. 10-39) and erythrocytes. This calf had an indwelling jugular catheter, presumed to be the source of the infection. *(Courtesy College of Veterinary Medicine, University of Illinois.)*

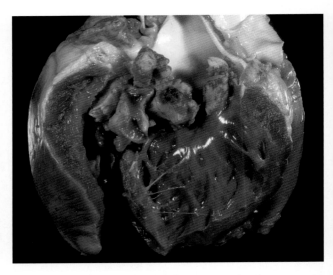

Fig. 10-40   Valvular endocarditis, erysipelas, heart, aortic valve, pig. Note the reddish-brown friable exudate thickening the valve cusps. *(Courtesy Dr. M.D. McGavin, College of Veterinary Medicine, University of Tennessee.)*

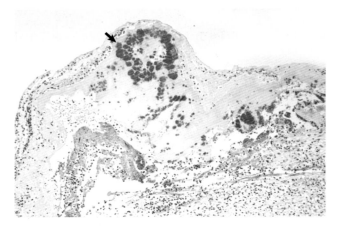

Fig. 10-39   Vegetative valvular endocarditis, bacterial infection, heart, tricuspid valve, cow. Note abundant masses of fibrin and bacterial colonies *(arrow)*. H&E stain. *(Courtesy Dr. M.D. McGavin, College of Veterinary Medicine, University of Tennessee.)*

of Virchow's triad in thrombogenesis—endothelial injury, turbulence, and hypercoagulability—are involved. Affected animals often have preexisting extracardiac infections, such as gingivitis or dermatitis, that have resulted in one or more bouts of bacteremia. Turbulent intracardiac blood flow associated with congenital anomalies, or the presence of intracardiac devices, such

as catheters, is contributory to initiation of the lesion. Focal trauma-induced endothelial disruption on the surface of the normally avascular valves allows bacteria to adhere, proliferate, and initiate an inflammatory reaction that results in subsequent deposition of masses of fibrin. Bacteria frequently recovered from the vegetative lesions are *Arcanobacter pyogenes* in cattle, *Streptococcus* spp. and *Erysipelothrix rhusiopathiae* in pigs (Fig. 10-40), and *Streptococcus* spp. and *Escherichia coli* in dogs and cats. Death is the result of cardiac failure from valvular dysfunction or the effects of bacteremia. In some animals, septic emboli lodge in organs such as the heart and kidneys, leading to infarction and localized inflammation or abscess formation.

Ulcerative endocarditis of the left atrium is a distinctive red hemorrhagic lesion acutely associated with acute renal insufficiency in dogs. Grossly, after the initial ulcer heals, the area is replaced by raised, white plaques of fibrous and mineralized tissue.

Major cardiac valvular lesions are summarized in Fig. 10-41.

MYOCARDIAL DISEASES

GROWTH DISTURBANCES

Hypertrophy of the myocardium represents an increase in muscle mass, the result of an increase in size of cardiac muscle cells. Hypertrophy is generally secondary and is the result of a compensatory response to increased workload; it is usually reversible on removal of the cause. However, primary hypertrophy also occurs,

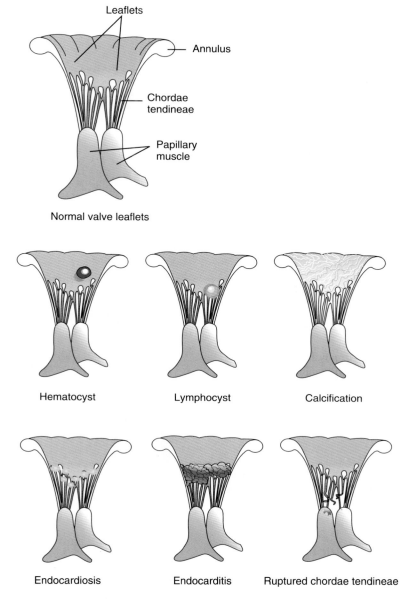

Fig. 10-41 Schematic diagram of the major types of cardiac atrioventricular valvular disease. *(Redrawn with permission from School of Veterinary Medicine, Purdue University.)*

as in cats and dogs with idiopathic hypertrophic cardiomyopathy (see later discussion) and is not reversible. Two anatomic forms of hypertrophy are recognized. Eccentric hypertrophy results in a heart with enlarged ventricular chambers and walls of normal to somewhat decreased thickness; it is produced by lesions that increase blood volume load, such as valvular insufficiencies and septal defects. In concentric hypertrophy the heart is characterized by small ventricular chambers that have thick walls; it results from lesions that increase pressure load, such as valvular stenosis, systemic hypertension,

and pulmonary disease. Some cats with hyperthyroidism have a cardiac hypertrophy that is mediated by enhanced production of myocardial contractile proteins under the influence of increased concentration of circulating thyroid hormones (Fig. 10-42). The hypertrophy is reversible on return to euthyroidism.

STAGES OF MYOCARDIAL HYPERTROPHY

Three stages of myocardial hypertrophy are recognizable: (1) initiation, (2) stable hyperfunction, and (3) deterioration of function associated with degeneration of

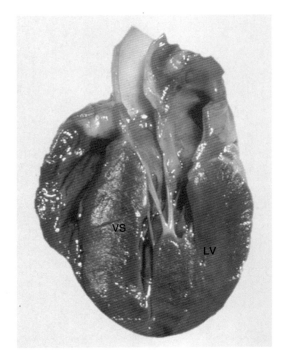

Fig. 10-42   **Left ventricular hypertrophy, hyperthyroidism, heart, bisected, cat.** Note prominent thickening of the left ventricular *(LV)* free wall. The ventricular septum *(VS)* is also thickened. *(Courtesy School of Veterinary Medicine, Purdue University.)*

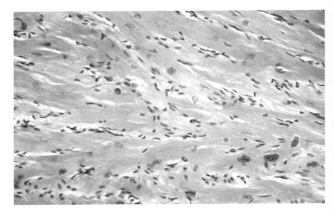

Fig. 10-43   **Hypertrophic cardiomyopathy, myocyte hypertrophy, heart, myocardium, cat.** Cardiac myocytes are hypertrophied, and there is an increase in interstitial fibroblasts. H&E stain. *(Courtesy School of Veterinary Medicine, Purdue University.)*

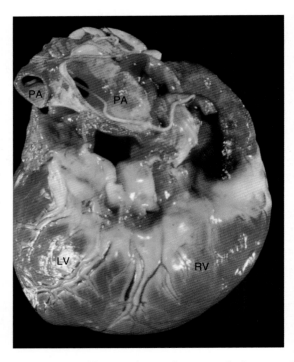

Fig. 10-44   **Dirofilariasis, heart, dog.** Note the hypertrophy of the right ventricle *(RV)* and adult *Dirofilaria immitis* in the pulmonary artery and its branches *(PA)*. *LV*, Left ventricle. *(Courtesy Dr. K. Read, College of Veterinary Medicine, Texas A&M University; and Noah's Arkive, College of Veterinary Medicine, The University of Georgia.)*

hypertrophied myocytes. Microscopically, in myocardial hypertrophy, the myocytes are enlarged and have large nuclei (Fig. 10-43).

Right ventricular hypertrophy

Diseases that produce right ventricular hypertrophy include dirofilariasis (Fig. 10-44) and congenital pulmonic stenosis in dogs, "brisket disease" ("high-altitude disease") in cattle, and chronic alveolar emphysema ("heaves") in horses. Cattle maintained under the hypoxic conditions that exist at altitudes above 7000 feet above sea level develop pulmonary hypertension and subsequent right side heart failure with subcutaneous edema, chronic passive congestion of the liver (nutmeg liver), and right ventricular hypertrophy. Exposure to certain poisonous plants (*Oxytropis* spp. and *Astragalus* spp.) increases the severity of the disease.

In the United States, dirofilariasis (heartworm disease) may occur in 35% to 45% of dogs and 2% of cats in areas of high infection rates, such as within 150 miles of the Atlantic and Gulf coasts from Texas to New Jersey and along the Mississippi River and its major tributaries. The extent of cardiac alterations is related to the numbers of adult parasites present. Initially the parasites accumulate in the pulmonary arteries

(Figs. 10-45 and 10-46), and as the numbers increase, they are present in the right ventricle, then in the right atrium, and finally may occupy the vena cavae. Pulmonary hypertension results from vascular blockage and pulmonary vascular lesions produced by the parasites and right ventricular hypertrophy follows.

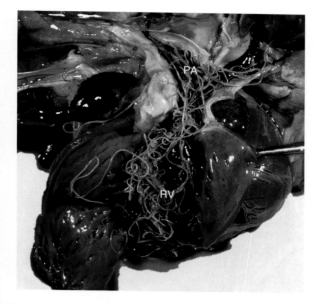

Fig. 10-45   Dirofilariasis, heart, opened right ventricle, right atrium, and pulmonary artery, dog. Numerous adult *Dirofilaria immitis* are present in the right ventricle *(RV)*, right atrium, and pulmonary artery *(PA)*. *(Courtesy Dr. M.D. McGavin, College of Veterinary Medicine, University of Tennessee.)*

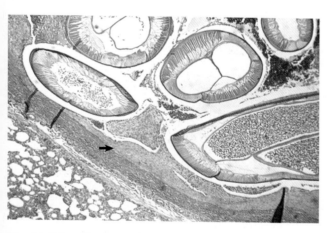

Fig. 10-46   Chronic endarteritis, dirofilariasis, lung, pulmonary artery, dog. Several intact adult *Dirofilaria immitis* are in the lumen. Note the thickened fibrotic intima *(arrow)*. H&E stain. *(Courtesy School of Veterinary Medicine, Purdue University.)*

Right side heart failure may eventually develop. Dogs with massive adult parasite loads may suffer acute collapse from caval syndrome, characterized by shock, intravascular hemolysis, and hepatic and renal failure.

Left ventricular hypertrophy

Left ventricular hypertrophy occurs in dogs with congenital subaortic stenosis, in cats with hyperthyroidism, and in dogs and cats with systemic hypertension. Systemic hypertension tends to be associated with hyperthyroidism and chronic renal failure in cats, and with chronic renal failure and hyperadrenocorticism in dogs. Affected animals may have ocular lesions secondary to damage to retinal vessels.

Biventricular hypertrophy

Biventricular hypertrophy can occur with hypertrophic cardiomyopathy and various congenital cardiac anomalies. Eccentric hypertrophy develops in the late stages of diseases that initially cause concentric hypertrophy as cardiac dilation is superimposed.

The appearance of cardiac hypertrophy and dilation is summarized in Fig. 10-47.

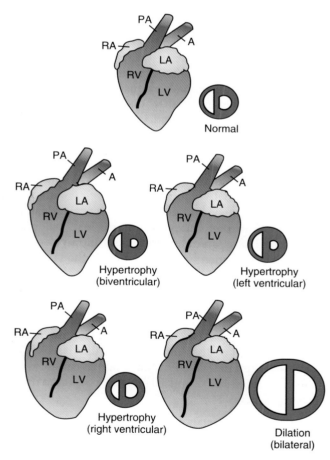

Fig. 10-47   Schematic diagram of the types of myocardial hypertrophy and dilation. Left lateral view and midventricular cross section (not drawn to same scale). *A,* Aorta; *LA,* left atrium; *LV,* left ventricle; *PA,* pulmonary artery; *RA,* right atrium; *RV,* right ventricle. *(Redrawn with permission from School of Veterinary Medicine, Purdue University.)*

INFILTRATION

Fatty infiltration is the presence of increased numbers of lipocytes interposed between myocardial fibers. The lesion is associated with obesity and appears as abundant epicardial and myocardial deposits of adipose tissue.

DEGENERATION

Fatty degeneration (fatty change) is the accumulation of abundant lipid droplets in the sarcoplasm of myocytes. Grossly the myocardium is pale and flabby. Microscopically, affected myocytes have numerous variably sized spherical droplets that appear as empty vacuoles in paraffin sections but stain positively for lipids with lipid-soluble stains in frozen sections. This lesion occurs with systemic disorders, such as severe anemia, toxemia, and copper deficiency, but is seen much less often in the heart than in the liver and kidneys.

Hydropic degeneration, a distinctive microscopic alteration in cardiac muscle cells, is associated with chronic administration of anthracyclines, a group of antineoplastic drugs. Chronic passive congestion with ascites and cardiac dilation may result (Figs. 10-48 and 10-49). Affected fibers have extensive vacuolization of sarcoplasm that is initiated by distention of elements of sarcoplasmic reticulum and, eventually, ends in lysis of contractile material (Figs. 10-50 and 10-51).

Lipofuscinosis (brown atrophy) of the myocardium occurs in aged animals and in animals with severe cachexia, but it also has been described as a hereditary lesion in healthy Ayrshire cattle. Severely affected hearts appear brown and microscopically have clusters of yellow-brown granules at the nuclear poles of myocytes. These granules represent intralysosomal accumulation of membranous and amorphous debris (residual bodies).

Myofibrillar degeneration (myocytolysis) represents a distinctive sublethal injury of cardiac muscle cells. Affected fibers have pale eosinophilic sarcoplasm and lack cross striations. Ultrastructurally, myofibrils have a variable extent of dissolution (myofibrillar lysis). This lesion has been described in furazolidone cardiotoxicity in birds (Figs. 10-52 and 10-53) and potassium deficiency in rats.

NECROSIS AND MINERALIZATION

Myocardial necrosis can result from a number of causes, including nutritional deficiencies, chemical and plant toxins, ischemia, metabolic disorders, heritable diseases, and physical injuries (Box 10-3). From this large list of causes of myocardial injury, some of the most frequently observed current examples are ionophore toxicity in horses and ruminants, vitamin E–selenium

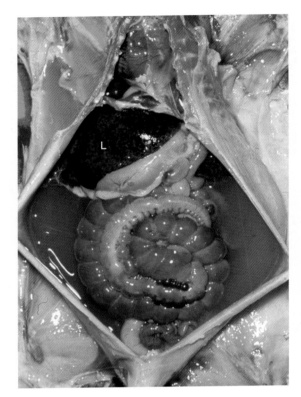

Fig. 10-48 **Chronic passive congestion, doxorubicin cardiotoxicity, congestive heart failure, liver, ascites, peritoneal cavity, rabbit.** Note the light-red stained transparent fluid in the peritoneal cavity (ascites) and the mottled liver (*L*) characteristic of chronic passive congestion. *(Courtesy School of Veterinary Medicine, Purdue University.)*

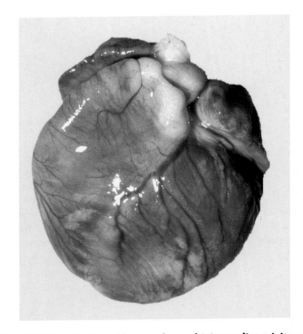

Fig. 10-49 **Cardiac dilation, doxorubicin cardiotoxicity, heart, rabbit.** All cardiac chambers are dilated. *(Courtesy School of Veterinary Medicine, Purdue University.)*

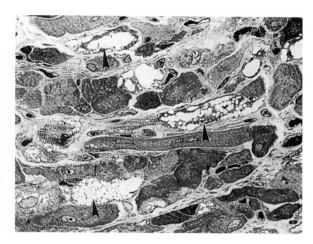

Fig. 10-50   **Myocardial vacuolar degeneration, chronic doxorubicin cardiotoxicity, heart, section of myocardium, dog.** The affected myocytes have prominent sarcoplasmic vacuolation (*arrowheads*). Plastic-embedded, toluidine blue–stained section. (*Courtesy School of Veterinary Medicine, Purdue University.*)

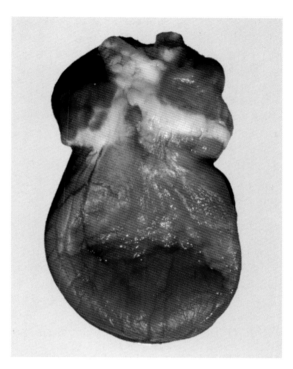

Fig. 10-52   **Ventricular dilation, furazolidone cardiotoxicity, heart, duckling.** Note that the dilated ventricles have collapsed once the blood was removed. (*Courtesy School of Veterinary Medicine, Purdue University.*)

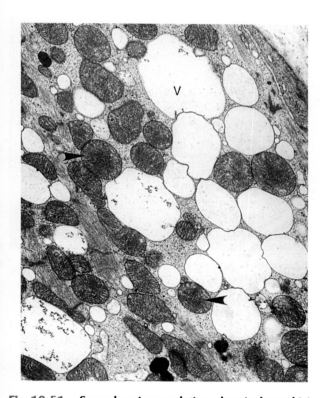

Fig. 10-51   **Sarcoplasmic vacuolation, chronic doxorubicin cardiotoxicity, heart, section of myocardium, dog.** The prominent sarcoplasmic vacuolation (*V*) is produced by distention of elements of sarcoplasmic reticulum. Even though the myofibrils have extensive lysis, mitochondria (*arrowheads*) are intact. TEM. Uranyl acetate and lead citrate stain. (*Courtesy School of Veterinary Medicine, Purdue University.*)

Box **10-3**

Causes of Myocardial Necrosis in Animals

NUTRITIONAL DEFICIENCIES

Selenium–vitamin E, potassium, copper, thiamine, magnesium

TOXICITIES

Cobalt, catecholamines, vasodilator antihypertensives, methylxanthines (theobromine, theophylline, caffeine), ionophores (monensin, lasalocid, salinomycin, narasin), vitamin D and calcinogenic plants (*Cestrum diurnum, Trisetum flavescens, Solanum malacoxylon, Solanum torvum*), other poisonous plants (*Acacia georginae, Gastrolobium* spp., *Oxylobium* spp., *Dichapetalum cymosum, Persea americana, Cassia occidentalis, Cassia obtusifolia, Karwinskia humboldtiana, Ateleia glazioviana*), blister beetles (*Epicauta*), high-erucic-acid rapeseed oil, brominated vegetable oils, gossypol, T-2 mycotoxin, uremia

PHYSICAL INJURIES AND SHOCK

Central nervous system lesions and trauma ("heart-brain syndrome"), gastric dilation and volvulus, stress, overexertion, electrical defibrillation, hemorrhagic shock

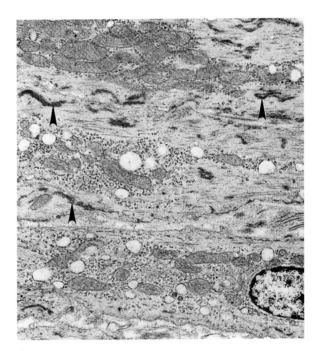

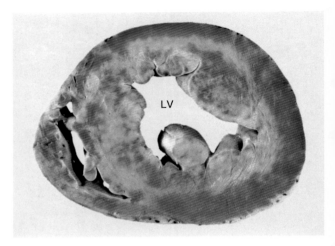

**Fig. 10-54   Myocardial necrosis, "heart-brain syndrome,"
heart, transverse section of ventricles, dog.** Necrotic areas
are pale beige to white and are concentrated in the inner
half of the wall of the left ventricle (*LV*) and in the ventricular
septum. (*Courtesy School of Veterinary Medicine, Purdue University.*)

**Fig. 10-53   Myofibrillar lysis, furazolidone cardiotoxicity,
heart, ventricular myocardium, duckling.** Affected myocytes
have extensive dissolution of myofibrils with scattered free
myofilaments and dense clumps of Z-band material (*arrowheads*). Other organelles appear normal. TEM. Uranyl acetate
and lead citrate stain. (*Courtesy School of Veterinary Medicine, Purdue
University.*)

deficiency in the young of all species, "heart-brain
syndrome" of dogs (Fig. 10-54), anthracycline toxicity
in dogs, and gossypol toxicosis in pigs. In various localized areas throughout the world, numerous deaths in
ruminants have resulted from consumption of poisonous plants, such as *Acacia georginae* and *Dichapetalum
cymosum.*

Cardiotoxicity has emerged as a significant clinical
entity in veterinary medicine in recent years with the
growing use of antineoplastic drugs in small animal
practice and the widespread use of growth promotants
in ruminants (Fig. 10-55). The mechanisms of cardio-
toxicities include (1) exaggerated pharmacologic action
of drugs acting on cardiovascular tissues, (2) exposure to
substances that depress myocardial function, (3) direct
injury of cardiac muscle cells by chemicals, and
(4) hypersensitivity reactions.

Grossly, affected areas appear pale initially, and some
progress to prominent yellow to white (Fig. 10-55), dry
areas made gritty by dystrophic mineralization. The
lesions are focal, multifocal, or diffuse. The most frequent
sites of focal lesions are the left ventricular papillary
muscles and the subendocardial myocardium, especially

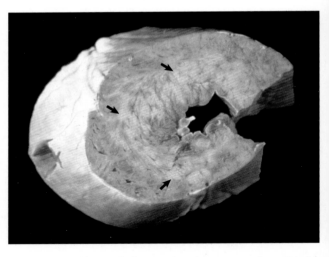

**Fig. 10-55   Myocardial necrosis, acute monensin toxicosis,
heart, cross section, left ventricular myocardium, calf.** Note
the pale, mottled, necrotic areas (*arrows*) distributed throughout
the ventricular myocardium. (*Courtesy School of Veterinary Medicine,
Purdue University.*)

when such lesions are related to transient reduction of
vascular perfusion. These lesions can be overlooked at
necropsy unless multiple incisions are made in the ventricular myocardium. In diseases with diffuse cardiac
necrosis, such as white muscle disease of calves and lambs
due to selenium–vitamin E deficiency, the discrete

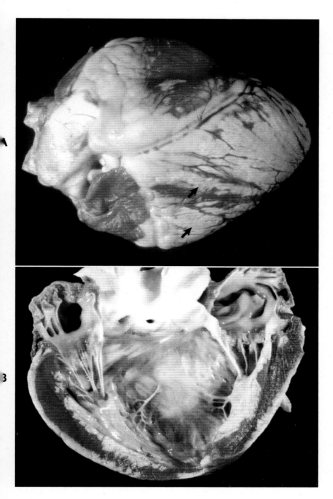

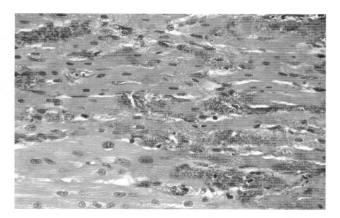

Fig. 10-57   Acute myocardial necrosis with mineralization, minoxidil cardiotoxicity, heart, ventricular myocardium, pig. The darker red myocytes are necrotic, and some are mineralized *(purplish areas)*. **H&E stain.** *(Courtesy School of Veterinary Medicine, Purdue University.)*

Fig. 10-56   Myocardial necrosis, selenium–vitamin E deficiency, heart, left ventricular myocardium, calf. A, Note the prominent white chalky areas of necrosis with mineralization *(arrows)* of the myocardium. **B,** Similar necrosis is subepicardially and subendocardially in the sectioned free walls of the left ventricle and subendocardially in the myocardium of the ventricular septum *(center)*. **(A,** *Courtesy School of Veterinary Medicine, Purdue University.* **B,** *Courtesy Dr. P.N. Nation, Animal Pathology Services; and Noah's Arkive, College of Veterinary Medicine, The University of Georgia.)*

can be confirmed by electron microscopy (Fig., 10-58). In a second pattern of necrosis, affected myocytes have a "shredded" appearance because of hypercontraction and the formation of multiple transversely oriented bars of disrupted contractile material (often termed contraction band necrosis) (Fig. 10-59). A third pattern is seen in necrotic myocytes in large areas of ischemic necrosis (infarcts). These myocytes have features of coagulation necrosis and have relaxed rather than hypercontracted contractile elements.

Within 24 to 48 hours after injury, necrotic areas are infiltrated by inflammatory cells, mainly macrophages and a few neutrophils; these phagocytose and lyse the

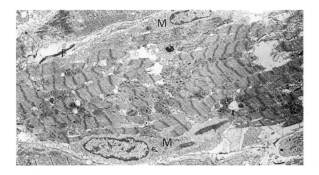

Fig. 10-58   Myocardial necrosis, monensin toxicosis, necrotic myocyte, heart, longitudinal section, calf. The necrotic myocyte *(center)* has disrupted myofibrils, damaged mitochondria with matrical densities, and several invading macrophages *(M)*. **F,** Fibrin. **TEM. Uranyl acetate and lead citrate stain.** *(Courtesy School of Veterinary Medicine, Purdue University.)*

white lesions can be readily observed on the epicardial and endocardial surfaces (Fig. 10-56, *A* and *B*).

Microscopically the appearance depends on the age of the lesions. Fibers in areas of recent necrosis often appear swollen and hypereosinophilic (hyaline necrosis). Striations are indistinct, and nuclei are pyknotic. Necrotic fibers often have scattered basophilic granules (Fig. 10-57) that represent calcified mitochondria and

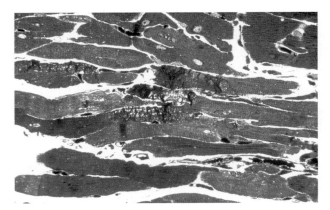

Fig. 10-59 **Myocardial necrosis, electric shock overdose by defibrillator, heart, dog.** The dark shredded segments of myocytes are due to acute contraction band necrosis. The time interval between defibrillation and the fixation of the heart was 24 hours. Plastic-embedded, toluidine blue–stained section. *(Courtesy School of Veterinary Medicine, Purdue University.)*

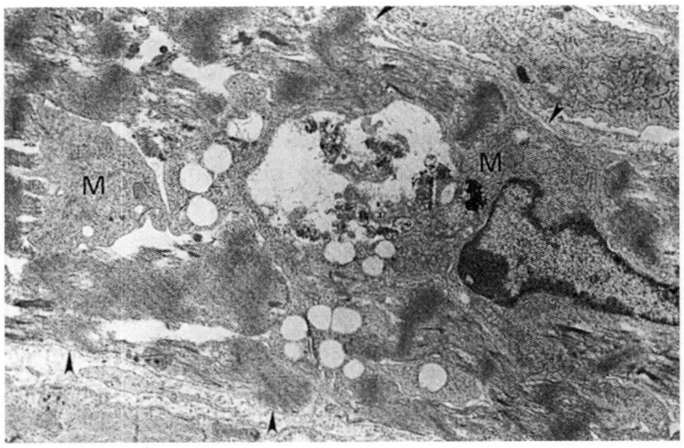

Fig. 10-60 **Myocardial necrosis, monensin toxicosis, heart, section of myocardium, calf.** Necrotic myocyte has disrupted contractile material invaded by a macrophage *(M)*. The basal lamina of the necrotic myocyte is noted by arrowheads. TEM. Uranyl acetate and lead citrate stain. *(Courtesy School of Veterinary Medicine, Purdue University.)*

necrotic cellular debris (Fig. 10-60). In early stages of healing of necrosis, it is often difficult to distinguish the lesions from those found in some types of myocarditis (see later discussion). Later, when necrosis has progressed somewhat, lesions consist of persistent stromal tissue (interstitial fibroblasts, collagen, and capillaries) and empty "tubes" of basal laminae formally occupied by necrotic myocytes (see Chapter 15). The healing phase is characterized by proliferation of connective tissue cells (fibroblasts) (Fig. 10-61) and by deposition of connective tissue products (collagen and elastic tissue and acid mucopolysaccharides). Grossly, these areas with healing of myocardial necrosis appear as white, firm, contracted scars.

The outcome of myocardial necrosis varies depending on the extent of the damage:
1. Many animals die unexpectedly of acute cardiac failure if the myocardial damage is extensive.
2. Early deaths from necrosis-related arrhythmias also occur when cardiac conduction is disrupted.
3. Some cases eventually develop cardiac decompensation and die with cardiac dilation, scarring, and lesions of chronic congestive failure.

Hearts with minimal damage have only microscopically detectable myocardial fibrosis when death eventually occurs from other diseases.

Myocardial mineralization is a prominent feature in several diseases, such as hereditary calcinosis in mice, cardiomyopathy in hamsters, vitamin E–selenium deficiency in sheep and cattle (Fig. 10-62), vitamin D toxicity in several species, calcinogenic plant toxicosis in cattle ("Manchester wasting disease"), and spontaneous myocardial calcification in aged rats and guinea pigs.

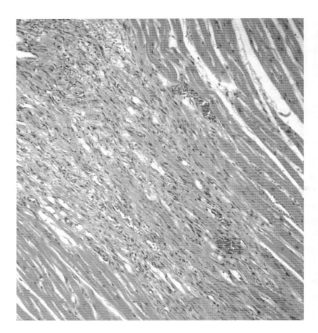

Fig. 10-61 **Healing, postmyocardial necrosis, heart, ventricle, dog.** The necrotic myocytes have been removed by phagocytosis by macrophages (not seen here), and the area is now undergoing fibrosis. H&E stain. *(Courtesy College of Veterinary Medicine, University of Illinois.)*

CARDIOMYOPATHIES

Primary and secondary cardiomyopathies (Table 10-3) represent important generalized myocardial diseases of either idiopathic or known causation.

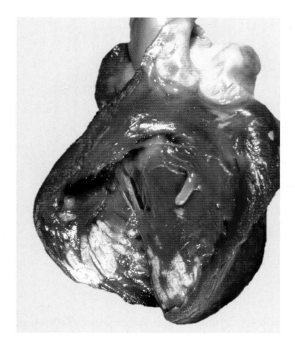

Fig. 10-62   Calcification, selenium-vitamin E deficiency, myocardial necrosis, heart, right ventricle, lamb. The multiple white subendocardial lesions are areas of calcified necrotic cardiac myocytes. *(Courtesy Dr. M.D. McGavin, College of Veterinary Medicine, University of Tennessee.)*

Table 10-3   Cardiomyopathies in Animals

PRIMARY CARDIOMYOPATHIES (IDIOPATHIC)

Hypertrophic: cat, dog, rat, pig
Dilated (congestive): cat, dog, hamster, turkey, pig, cow
Restrictive: cat

SECONDARY CARDIOMYOPATHIES (SPECIFIC HEART MUSCLE DISEASES)

Heritable (known or suspected): hereditary cardiomyopathy of hamsters, mice, rats, turkeys, and cattle; Duchenne's type, x-linked muscular dystrophy of golden retriever dogs with dystrophin deficiency; glycogenoses
Nutritional deficiencies: see list in Box 10-3; other examples include taurine deficiency in cats and foxes
Toxic: see list in Box 10-3; other examples include anthracycline toxicity, furazolidone toxicity, NaCl toxicity
Physical injuries and shock: see list in Box 10-3
Endocrine disorders: hyperthyroidism, acromegaly (hypersomatotropism), hypothyroidism, glucocorticoid excess, functional pheochromocytoma, diabetes mellitus
Infections: see list in Box 10-6
Neoplastic infiltration: malignant lymphoma
Systemic hypertension in cats: spontaneous or associated with chronic renal disease, hyperthyroidism, diabetes mellitus, acromegaly, primary aldosteronism

Primary or idiopathic cardiomyopathies are progressive cardiac diseases. These diseases affect cats, dogs, cattle, rats, mice, hamsters, turkeys, and several wild animal species and resemble some diseases of human beings. These diseases are divided into three morphologic types: hypertrophic, dilated, and restrictive cardiomyopathies.

Hypertrophic cardiomyopathy occurs frequently in cats, especially in middle-aged males (1 to 3 years old), and is seen infrequently in dogs, usually affecting males of large breeds. Cats usually have congestive heart failure, and approximately 10% to 20% have posterior paresis from concurrent thromboembolism of the caudal abdominal aorta ("saddle thrombosis") secondary to left atrial thrombosis. The occurrence of clusters of cases in Persians, American shorthairs, and Maine coon cat breeds suggests heritability of the disease in some cases. Some dogs die unexpectedly as the only clinical expression of the disease. This clinical presentation also is often seen in humans with the disease. In both cats and dogs, the hearts are enlarged and have prominent hypertrophy of the left ventricle and interventricular septum (Fig. 10-63, A and B). The left ventricular cavity is small and the left atrium is dilated. In a few cases, the interventricular septum is disproportionately hypertrophied in relation to the remainder

of the myocardium. Microscopically the lesions of the myocardium are prominent disarrays or disorganizations of myocytes, with interweaving rather than

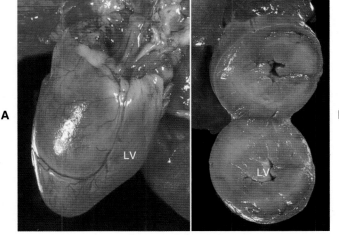

Fig. 10-63   Hypertrophic cardiomyopathy, heart, cat. A, Note the thickened left ventricular wall (*LV*). **B,** The thickened left ventricular free wall and septum have markedly reduced the lumen of the left ventricle (*LV*). *(A and B, Courtesy Dr. W. Crowell, College of Veterinary Medicine, The University of Georgia; and Noah's Arkive, College of Veterinary Medicine, The University of Georgia.)*

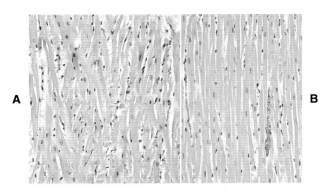

Fig. 10-64   Hypertrophic cardiomyopathy, heart, ventricular myocardium, cat. A, Note the pattern of interwoven cardiac myocytes, indicating myofiber disarray, and the hypertrophic myocytes (compare with Fig. 10-64, B). There is also an increase increase in interstitial fibroblasts. H&E stain. B, Normal cardiac myocytes arranged in parallel bundles. H&E stain. *(Courtesy Dr. L. Borst, College of Veterinary Medicine, University of Illinois.)*

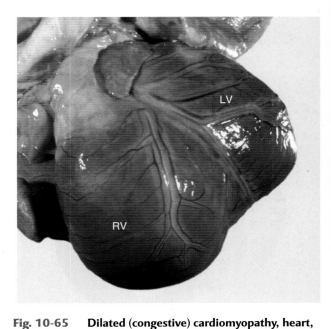

Fig. 10-65   Dilated (congestive) cardiomyopathy, heart, left ventricle (*LV*) and right ventricle (*RV*), dog. Biventricular dilation has resulted in the heart having a double apex. *(Courtesy Dr. T. Boosinger, College of Veterinary Medicine, Auburn University; and Noah's Arkive, College of Veterinary Medicine, The University of Georgia.)*

parallel arrangement of fibers (Fig. 10-64). Myocyte hypertrophy, various degenerative alterations in myocytes, and interstitial fibrosis also are present.

Dilated or congestive cardiomyopathy is an important cause of congestive heart failure in cats and dogs. Many affected cats and some dogs have low tissue concentrations of taurine, and supplementation of cats with taurine has reversed the clinical signs of cardiac failure. Routine taurine supplementation of feline commercial diets has resulted in a dramatic reduction in cases of dilated cardiomyopathy. Taurine-deficient foxes also develop cardiac failure. Cattle with dilated cardiomyopathy in Switzerland and Japan have an autosomal recessive mode of inheritance.

Affected cats often are middle-aged males, and affected dogs often are males of large breeds such as Doberman pinschers, Portuguese water dogs, Dalmatians, Scottish deerhounds, Irish wolfhounds, Saint Bernards, Afghan hounds, Newfoundlands, Old English sheepdogs, Great Danes, and boxers, although smaller breeds, such as English cocker spaniels, may be affected. The disease often has a familial pattern in the affected breeds and appears to be inherited as an autosomal recessive or x-linked recessive trait. Some cats also develop aortic thromboembolism. At necropsy, lesions of congestive heart failure are present and the hearts are rounded because of biventricular dilation (Figs. 10-65 and 10-66). The dilated cardiac chambers often have a diffusely white, thickened endocardium. Microscopic and ultrastructural alterations are nonspecific, can be either mild or absent, and may include interstitial fibrosis and fatty infiltration and changes of myocyte degeneration, including the occurrence of so-called attenuated wavy fibers.

Restrictive cardiomyopathy occurs infrequently. It occurs in cats as one of two types of endocardial lesions that result in impaired ventricular filling. In one type, the left ventricular endocardium has diffuse notable fibrosis. Available evidence suggests that the fibrotic lesion is preceded by endomyocarditis. The second type results from excessive moderator bands that traverse the left ventricular cavity. Other examples of restrictive cardiomyopathy in animals include endocardial fibrosis in certain strains of aged rats and congenital endocardial fibroelastosis in Burmese cats (Fig. 10-24).

Secondary cardiomyopathies (Table 10-3) (also termed specific heart muscle diseases) are generalized myocardial diseases of known cause.

Our understanding of the molecular mechanisms of the hereditary cardiomyopathies is developing rapidly. In human patients with familial hypertrophic cardiomyopathy inherited in an autosomal dominant manner, a variety of single-gene mutations have been documented. The mutations affect genes that encode sarcomeric proteins of cardiac myocytes. Altered cardiac proteins include cardiac β-myosin heavy chain, cardiac troponin T, cardiac troponin I, α-tropomyosin, actin, ventricular myosin essential light chain, ventricular myosin regulatory light chain, and cardiac myosin-binding protein C. It remains unclear how these mutant

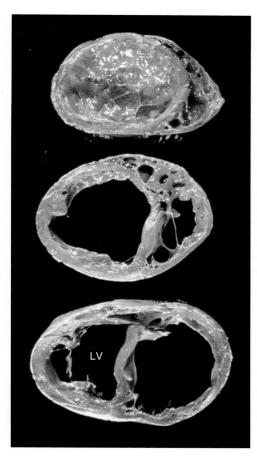

Fig. 10-66   Dilated cardiomyopathy (congestive cardiomyopathy), heart, ventricles, cross section, dog. The left ventricle *(LV)* and right ventricle have thin walls, dilated chambers, and white fibrotic endocardium. *(Courtesy Dr. Y. Niyo, College of Veterinary Medicine, Iowa State University; and Noah's Arkive, College of Veterinary Medicine, The University of Georgia.)*

INFLAMMATION

The various portals of entry and defense mechanisms involved in myocardial inflammation are summarized in Box 10-1 and Box 10-2. Myocarditis generally is the result of infections spread hematogenously to the myocardium and occurs in various systemic diseases. Infrequently, the heart is the primary location in affected animals and responsible for their death. Types of inflammation provoked by infectious agents that produce myocarditis include suppurative, necrotizing, hemorrhagic, lymphocytic, and eosinophilic. Suppurative myocarditis results from localization of pyogenic bacteria in the myocardium. These often originate from the vegetations of vegetative valvular endocarditis on the mitral and aortic valves. Septic infarcts with pale, disseminated lesions are present grossly in the myocardium. These foci consist of neutrophils and necrotic myocytes that form abscesses. Necrotizing myocarditis is a frequent lesion of toxoplasmosis, a common disease of cats and dogs. Hemorrhagic myocarditis occurs together with the hemorrhagic inflammation typically found in skeletal muscle of cattle with blackleg (*Clostridium chauvoei*) (Fig. 10-67). Lymphocytic myocarditis is usually a lesion of viral infections and is well illustrated by the lesions of parvoviral myocarditis of puppies (Fig. 10-68, *A* and *B*). Dogs with parvoviral myocarditis die unexpectedly and have generalized lesions of acute congestive heart failure but lack lesions in the intestine, the primary site of viral damage in approximately 95% of clinical cases. The heart is pale and flabby and has disseminated

proteins result in functional and structural alterations of cardiac muscle cells. However, recent studies suggest that shortening of telomeres (structures that cap the ends of chromosomes) triggers apoptosis of cardiac muscle cells and may explain the end-stage finding of myocardial fibrosis in heart failure of various causes including cardiomyopathy. It is expected that similar gene mutations and altered proteins will be discovered in the various heritable cardiomyopathies of animals.

Also, a portion of cases of dilated cardiomyopathy in human patients appears to be inherited. In these patients, alterations in several myocytic proteins, including dystrophin, actin, desmin, troponin T, β-myosin heavy chain, lamin, and taffazin, and alterations in the cardiac calcium regulating protein phospholamban have been documented.

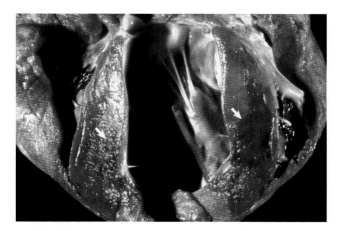

Fig. 10-67   Necrohemorrhagic myocarditis, heart, steer. Note the area of hemorrhagic myocarditis *(arrows)* in the wall of the ventricular myocardium. This disease is caused by *Clostridium chauvoei*, and lesions are most common in skeletal muscle. *(Courtesy Dr. J. Simon, College of Veterinary Medicine, University of Illinois.)*

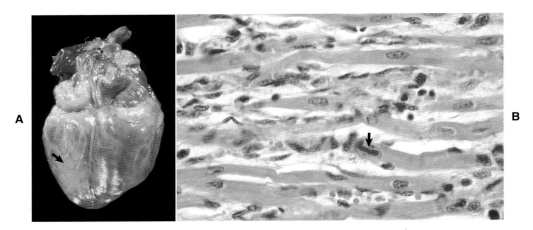

Fig. 10-68 **Parvovirus myocarditis, heart, dog. A,** Note the multifocal pale areas *(arrow)* in the ventricular myocardium. **B,** Parvovirus infection, section of myocardium. An intranuclear basophilic inclusion body is in a myocyte *(arrow)*. H&E stain. *(**A,** Courtesy Dr. B. Weeks, College of Veterinary Medicine, Texas A&M University; and Noah's Arkive, College of Veterinary Medicine, The University of Georgia. **B,** Courtesy School of Veterinary Medicine, Purdue University.)*

interstitial lymphocytic infiltrations and scattered myocytes with large, basophilic, intranuclear viral inclusion bodies in dogs that survive fibrosis (Fig. 10-68, A and B). East Coast fever is a tick-transmitted protozoal disease of cattle in Africa caused by *Theileria parva,* which causes myocardial necrosis and inflammation (Fig. 10-69). Eosinophilic myocarditis and the accumulation of eosinophils in the inflammatory response is the result of some parasitic infections, such as sarcocystosis. The various infectious diseases that cause myocarditis in animals are summarized in Table 10-4.

The pathogenesis and expected outcome of cases of myocarditis remain an important area of research because of the severity of this lesion in cardiac failure in human beings. The sequelae to myocarditis include (1) complete resolution of lesions, (2) scattered residual myocardial scars, or (3) progressive myocardial damage with acute or, in some cases, chronic cardiac failure as secondary dilated (congestive) cardiomyopathy. In experimental studies of myocarditis induced in mice by coxsackie B virus, the severity of myocarditis was influenced by the virulence of the virus and mouse strain and was enhanced by host factors such as young age, male sex, pregnancy, poor nutrition, whole-body ionizing radiation, cold environmental temperatures, alcohol ingestion, exercise, and cortisone administration. Much of the myocardial damage in coxsackie B virus infection is induced by immunologic reactions (with T lymphocyte involvement) rather than by direct viral injury.

The appearance of the heart with major myocardial diseases is illustrated in Fig. 10-70.

CONDUCTION SYSTEM DISEASES

Conduction system disorders have been described mainly in dogs and horses, probably because clinical cardiologic evaluations are done most frequently in these species. Few pathologic evaluations of the tissue of the conduction system have been reported.

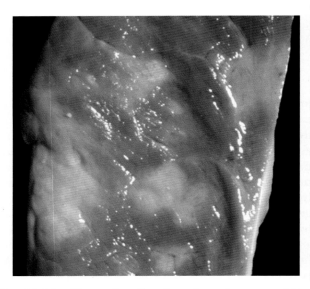

Fig. 10-69 **Myocarditis, East Coast fever, heart, cow.** The multiple pale areas in the left ventricular wall are infiltrates of mononuclear inflammatory cells. *(Courtesy School of Veterinary Medicine, Purdue University.)*

Table 10-4   Diseases That Cause Myocarditis in Animals

VIRAL

Canine parvovirus, encephalomyocarditis, foot-and-mouth disease, pseudorabies, canine distemper, cytomegalovirus, Newcastle disease, avian encephalomyelitis, Eastern and Western equine encephalomyelitis

BACTERIAL

Blackleg (*Clostridium chauvoei*), listeriosis (*Listeria monocytogenes*), Tyzzer's disease (*Bacillus piliformis*), necrobacillosis (*Fusobacterium necrophorum*), tuberculosis (*Mycobacterium* spp.), caseous lymphadenitis (*Corynebacterium pseudotuberculosis*), disseminated infections by *Actinobacillus equuli*, *Staphylococcus* sp., *Corynebacterium kutscheri*, *Pseudomonas aeruginosa*, and *Streptococcus pneumoniae*

PROTOZOAN

Toxoplasmosis (*Toxoplasma gondii*), sarcocystosis (*Sarcocystis* sp.), neosporosis (*Neospora caninum*), encephalitozoonosis (*Encephalitozoon cuniculi*), trypanosomiasis (Chagas' disease [*Trypanosoma cruzi*])

PARASITIC

Cysticercosis (*Cysticercus cellulosae*), trichinosis (*Trichinella* spp.)

IDIOPATHIC

Eosinophilic myocarditis

Specific presumably inherited diseases in dogs include: (1) unexpected death in Doberman pinscher dogs associated with focal degeneration of the bundle of His; (2) syncope in pug dogs with lesions of the bundle of His; (3) intermittent sinus arrest in deaf Dalmatian dogs, presumably associated with lesions in the sinus node; (4) sinoatrial syncope (sick sinus syndrome) in female miniature schnauzers; and (5) inherited ventricular arrhythmia and sudden unexpected death in German shepherds. Other arrhythmias in dogs and horses are atrial fibrillation and heart block. Dogs with atrial fibrillation usually have short survival times and have atrial dilation with mitral insufficiency, but some horses survive longer and at necropsy have atrial myocardial fibrosis. Heart block of the first degree (incomplete), second degree (incomplete with dropped beats), and third degree (complete) has been associated with myocardial lesions such as areas of scarring in horses and dogs. However, some investigators consider second-degree heart block in horses a normal phenomenon.

Persistent atrial standstill (silent atria, atrioventricular myopathy) is a progressive cardiac disease of English springer spaniels and Siamese cats characterized by notable atrial dilation and fibrosis.

Atrial fibrillation occurs in cattle in association with right atrial dilation and fibrosis and alterations in the sinoatrial mode. Also, sudden cardiac death is described in racehorses with right atrial myocardial fibrosis, fibrosis of the upper ventricular septum, and arteriosclerosis of intramyocardial arteries.

NEOPLASTIC DISEASES

Various primary and secondary neoplasms develop either in or near the heart. The primary neoplasms include rhabdomyoma, rhabdomyosarcoma, schwannoma, and hemangiosarcoma. Rhabdomyomas and rhabdomyosarcomas are rare in animals and form gray nodules in the myocardium that often project into the cardiac chambers. Congenital rhabdomyomatosis in pigs and guinea pigs is really a nonneoplastic hamartoma (i.e., malformation often resembling a neoplasm that is composed of an overgrowth of mature cells and tissues that normally occur in the affected organ). Multiple, pale, poorly circumscribed areas are scattered in the myocardium and are composed of large glycogen-laden myocytes. Schwannomas involve cardiac nerves in cattle and appear as single or multiple white nodules detected as incidental findings at slaughter.

Cardiac hemangiosarcoma is an important neoplasm of dogs and can arise either in the heart (primary) or by metastasis (secondary) from sites such as the spleen. This neoplasm is usually seen in the wall of the right atrium and only occasionally involves the right ventricle. Grossly, protruding red to red-black blood-containing masses are located on the epicardial surface (Fig. 10-71) and may also protrude into the atrial lumen. Rupture produces fatal hemopericardium and cardiac tamponade. Microscopically the neoplasms are composed of scattered, elongated, plump neoplastic endothelial cells, which may or may not form vascular spaces containing blood (Fig. 10-72). Pulmonary metastases are frequent.

Malignant lymphoma (lymphosarcoma) often causes lesions in the hearts of cattle, and these can be severe enough to cause death from cardiac failure. Cardiac lesions may also be present in dogs and cats with malignant lymphoma. The neoplastic cell infiltration can be diffuse or nodular and involve the myocardium and pericardium. Lymphomatous tissue appears as white masses that resemble deposits of fat (Fig. 10-73, *A*, and *B*). Microscopically, extensive infiltrations of neoplastic lymphocytes are present between myocytes (Fig. 10-74).

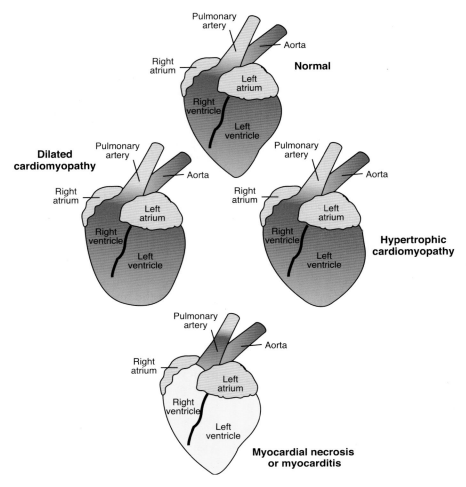

Fig. 10-70   Schematic diagram of the major myocardial diseases. *(Redrawn with permission from School of Veterinary Medicine, Purdue University.)*

Other generalized neoplasms, such as malignant melanomas, occasionally have metastatic lesions in the heart.

Heart base tumors are primary neoplasms of extracardiac tissues in dogs, but they arise at the base of the heart and can produce vascular obstruction and cardiac failure. The most common neoplasm arising at this location is the aortic body tumor or chemodectoma (paraganglioma), but occasionally ectopic thyroid or parathyroid tissue gives origin to neoplasms in this area. The aortic body is a chemoreceptor organ. In some cases, aortic body tumors become large, white, firm masses that surround and compress the great vessels and atria (Fig. 10-75). Brachycephalic dog breeds are most frequently affected. Microscopically the neoplastic cells are polyhedral with vacuolated cytoplasm and are supported by an abundant, fine connective tissue stroma.

The most common cardiac diseases in the dog and cat are summarized in Table 10-5. The appearance of the heart with major neoplastic diseases is illustrated in Fig. 10-76.

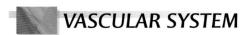

VASCULAR SYSTEM

INTRODUCTION

NORMAL MORPHOLOGY

The vascular system is subdivided into arterial, capillary, venous, and lymph segments. The arteries are classified into three types: elastic arteries, muscular arteries, and arterioles. The venous vessels are termed venules and veins. The lymph vasculature includes lymph capillaries and lymph vessels. Interposed

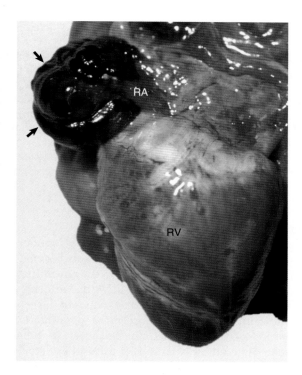

Fig. 10-71   Hemangiosarcoma, heart, right atrium, dog. A dark-red hemangiosarcoma protrudes from the wall of the right atrium *(RA)*, a predilection site in the dog for this tumor *(arrows)*. *RV*, Right ventricle. *(Courtesy College of Veterinary Medicine, University of Illinois.)*

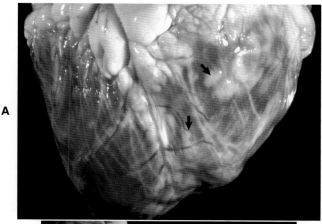

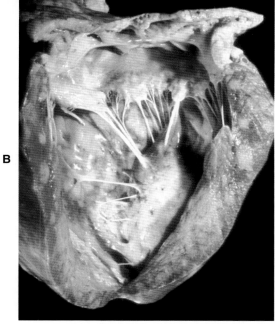

Fig. 10-73   Lymphosarcoma, heart, myocardium, cow. **A,** Sites of infiltrating neoplastic lymphocytes in the ventricular myocardium are evident as numerous white areas and nodules *(arrows)*. **B,** Similar white areas of tumor are visible in the section of the left ventricular wall and subendocardially in the ventricular septum. *(**A** and **B,** Courtesy College of Veterinary Medicine, University of Illinois.)*

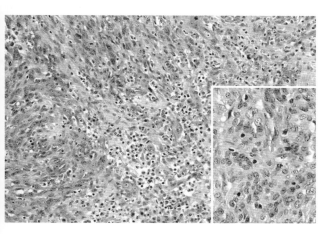

Fig. 10-72   Hemangiosarcoma, heart, right atrium, dog. The tumor consists of spindle cells with large, round-to-oval nuclei and numerous mitotic figures *(inset)*. In this case, these cells have formed poorly delineated and haphazardly arranged vascular channels. The golden-brown pigment is hemosiderin that forms secondary to erythrophagocytosis of damaged or effete erythrocytes. H&E stain. *(**Figure** and **Inset,** courtesy Dr. J.F. Zachary, College of Veterinary Medicine, University of Illinois.)*

between the arterial and venous segments are the capillary beds. A vascular segment termed the microcirculation includes arterioles, capillaries, and venules and is the major area of exchange between the circulating blood and the peripheral tissue.

The overall design of the blood and lymph vessels is similar, except that luminal diameter, wall thickness, and the presence of other anatomic features, such as valves, vary between the different segments. The luminal surface of all vessels is lined by longitudinally

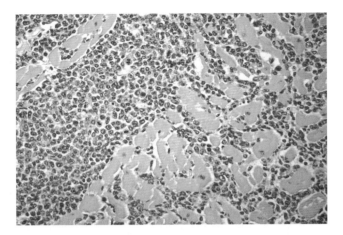

Fig. 10-74   Lymphosarcoma, heart, section of myocardium, cow. Neoplastic lymphocytes have extensively infiltrated between the cardiomyocytes. Extensive infiltration can result in myocyte atrophy and loss. H&E stain. (*Courtesy School of Veterinary Medicine, Purdue University.*)

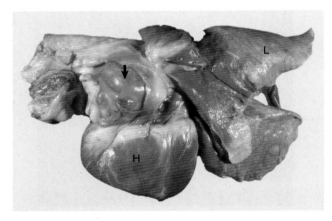

Fig. 10-75   Chemodectoma (heart base tumor), aortic body, dog. Note the large mass (*arrow*) at the base of the heart (**H**). **L**, Lungs. (*Courtesy College of Veterinary Medicine, University of Illinois.*)

Table 10-5   Most Common Cardiac Diseases in the Dog and Cat

Dog	Cat
1. Valvular endocardiosis	1. Hypertrophic cardiomyopathy
2. Congenital heart disease	2. Dilated cardiomyopathy
3. Dilated cardiomyopathy	3. Hyperthyroidism-associated hypertrophy
4. Hemorrhagic pericardial effusion	4. Congenital heart disease

lamina, and (3) an outer tunica adventitia layer composed of collagen and elastic fibers and connective tissue cells with penetrating blood vessels, termed the vasa vasorum, supplying nutrients to the adventitia and the outer half of the media. In muscular arteries and arterioles, the tunica media is composed largely of smooth muscle cells arranged in a circumferential pattern. Arterioles are the smallest arterial channels and are generally less than 100 μm in diameter and with one to three layers of smooth muscle cells in the tunica media.

Capillaries are 5 to 10 μm in diameter, and their endothelium is one of three types: (1) continuous, (2) fenestrated (as in the endocrine glands), and (3) porous (as in renal glomeruli). The endothelium rests on an external lamina surrounded by pericytes. Pericytes are located abluminally to capillaries and postcapillary venules and because of their location, contractility, and cytoskeletal proteins may play a role in regulating capillary and venular blood flow. Lesions of the endothelium might not be evident by light microscopy, and electron microscopy is required for characterization.

Veins have thin walls in relation to their luminal size when compared with those of arteries, in which blood pressure is greater. The adventitia is the thickest layer. Valves are present to prevent retrograde blood flow (i.e., away from the heart).

Lymph capillaries lack a basal lamina. Large lymph vessels are similar in structure to veins and generally have large lumina, thin walls, and intimal valves, but contain lymph.

REACTIONS TO INJURY

The response of vessels to injury involves a complex interaction among the cellular and noncellular elements of the vessel wall and the cellular and noncellular elements of the blood. The key cells of vessels in these reactions are endothelial cells and smooth muscle cells. Endothelial cells are metabolically active and provide a thromboresistant monolayer at the interface of

aligned endothelial cells lying over a basal lamina. Vessel walls are divided into three layers or tunics: intima, media, and adventitia. However, some of the layers can be deleted or all of the layers can be thinned in some segments of the vascular system, depending on the intravascular pressures. The large elastic arteries, such as the aorta, have (1) an intima composed of endothelium and subendothelial connective tissue, (2) a very thick tunica media composed of fenestrated elastic laminae with interposed smooth muscle cells and ground substance and bordered internally by the internal elastic lamina and externally by the external elastic

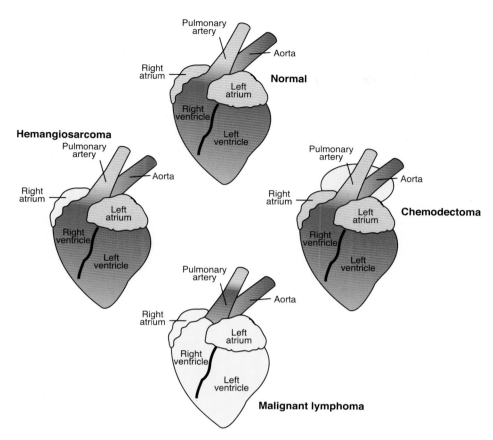

Fig. 10-76   Schematic diagram of the locations of the major cardiac neoplasms. *(Redrawn with permission from School of Veterinary Medicine, Purdue University.)*

blood and the vessel wall. Key functions of endothelial cells include prostacyclin production, macromolecular transport, and recruitment of inflammatory cells. Injury of endothelial cells is followed by separation from the underlying basement membrane and increased permeability to movement of plasma proteins into the subendothelium. Necrosis of endothelium will expose subendothelial collagen and elicit thrombus formation. Endothelial cells at the margin of denuded areas proliferate and reendothelialize the damaged area. The arterial intima has regional differences in the uptake of macromolecules, as well as other unique structural and functional features that result in lesion-prone areas of the vasculature. Bilirubin staining of the intima results in yellow discoloration in jaundiced animals (Fig. 10-77).

The other major cellular component of vessels involved in reaction to injury is the smooth muscle cell. These cells have important functions, including production of extracellular components such as collagen, elastin, and proteoglycans; maintenance of vascular tone; blood monocyte recruitment; lipoprotein metabolism;

production of bioactive lipids, such as prostaglandins; and formation of oxygen-free radicals. These functions are regulated by a wide variety of biochemical mediators, such as various growth factors, cytokines, and inflammatory mediators.

POSTMORTEM ALTERATIONS

Usually 12 to 24 hours after death, erythrocytes lyse, and the resultant imbibition of hemoglobin produces red discoloration of the normally white intima of blood vessels. Postmortem clotting must be differentiated from thrombosis. Postmortem clots, found in veins and large elastic arteries as red "currant jelly" type or occasionally as pale "chicken fat" type, are readily removed by traction or gentle flushing at necropsy, in contrast to thrombi, which are adherent. Postmortem contraction of muscular arteries because of rigor mortis extrudes blood. Microscopically, these muscular arteries are devoid of blood, and their internal elastic lamina is wavy in cross sections of the contacted vessel.

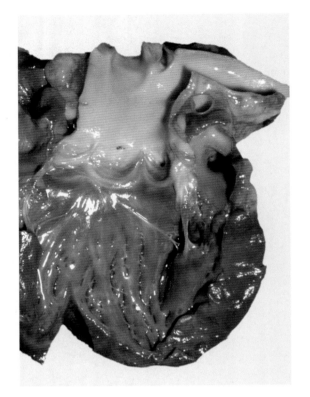

Fig. 10-77   Jaundice, heart, aorta, dog. Note yellow discoloration of the aortic intima. (*Courtesy School of Veterinary Medicine, Purdue University.*)

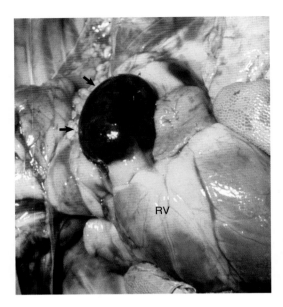

Fig. 10-78   Dissecting aneurysm, copper deficiency, heart, pulmonary artery, right ventricle (*RV*), pig. The dark, blood-filled, bulging segment of the wall of the pulmonary artery (*arrows*) has resulted from disruption of elastic fibers. (*Courtesy School of Veterinary Medicine, Purdue University.*)

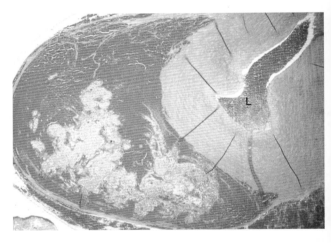

Fig. 10-79   Dissecting aneurysm, aorta, turkey. Blood has dissected through the tunica media (in a nearby section of the aorta) and in this section has come to lie in the outer layers of the tunica media and adventia. *L,* Vessel lumen. H&E stain. (*Courtesy School of Veterinary Medicine, Purdue University.*)

ARTERIAL DISEASES

ANEURYSMS AND RUPTURES

An aneurysm is a localized dilation or outpouching of a thinned and weakened portion of a vessel. Usually arteries are affected, especially large elastic arteries, but the lesion can also occur in veins. Known causes include copper deficiency in pigs (Fig. 10-78), as copper is necessary for normal development of elastic tissue, and damage from infection with *Spirocerca lupi* in dogs or *Strongylus vulgaris* in horses. Most cases are idiopathic. Dissecting aneurysms are infrequent but have been seen in birds (Fig. 10-79). They result from disruption of the intima, which allows entry of blood into the media, and this dissects along the wall. Aneurysms can rupture. Usually the consequences are rapidly fatal, as rather large arteries typically are involved.

Aortic rupture and rupture of large arteries can be the sequela of severe trauma or occur spontaneously. Sudden rupture of the ascending aorta in horses is associated with notable exertion and severe trauma to the ventral thorax from falling. Death ensues rapidly from cardiac tamponade, as the tear is in that portion of the aorta within the pericardial sac. In horses, the internal carotid artery can rupture into the adjacent guttural pouch, with subsequent epistaxis. This is a consequence of deep mycotic infection of the guttural pouch. Rupture of the middle uterine artery may occur during parturition in mares and with uterine torsion or prolapse in cows. Aortic rupture, with or without dissection, is an important cause of death in male turkeys.

GROWTH DISTURBANCES

Arterial hypertrophy is a response to sustained increases in pressure or volume loads. Affected vessels are generally muscular arteries, and the increase in wall thickness is predominantly because of hypertrophy (and, to some degree, hyperplasia) of smooth muscle cells of the tunica media. Muscular pulmonary arteries of cats are frequently affected, and the lesion has been associated with infection by several parasites, including *Aelurostrongylus abstrusus* (the lungworm of cats), *Toxocara* sp., and *Dirofilaria immitis* (Fig. 10-80). However, the lesions often occur in the absence of parasitic infections (Fig. 10-81). Often, no clinical disease is associated with the lesion in cats, but asthmatic signs have been seen in cats with these parasitic infections. Similar hypertrophy of muscular pulmonary arteries occurs in cattle with hypoxia-induced pulmonary arterial vasoconstriction and subsequent pulmonary hypertension associated with right side heart failure from exposure to high altitudes (so-called high-altitude disease or "brisket disease") (see Stages of Myocardial Hypertrophy and Myocardial Diseases). Also, animals with cardiovascular anomalies that shunt blood left to right result in pulmonary hypertension and have hypertrophy of the muscular pulmonary arteries. Uterine arteries in pregnant animals also are hypertrophic.

DEGENERATION AND NECROSIS

Generalized vascular degenerative diseases in animals are classified into three principal groups: arteriosclerosis, atherosclerosis, and arterial medial calcification.

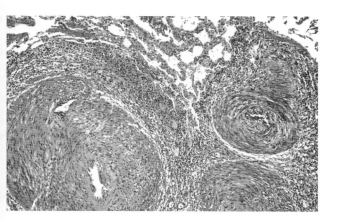

Fig. 10-80 Medial hypertrophy, periarteritis, dirofilariasis, lung, small pulmonary arteries, cat. Note the massively thickened tunica media of the small branches of the pulmonary arteries and their periarterial cuff of chronic inflammatory cells and some eosinophils. H&E stain. *(Courtesy School of Veterinary Medicine, Purdue University.)*

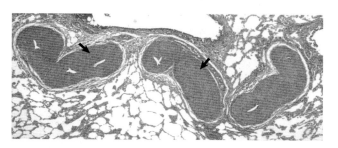

Fig. 10-81 Medial hypertrophy, lung, small pulmonary arteries, cat. Proliferation of smooth muscle cells *(arrows)* has resulted in marked thickening of the tunica media. Note luminal narrowing. H&E stain. *(Courtesy School of Veterinary Medicine, Purdue University.)*

Arteriosclerosis is characterized by intimal fibrosis of large elastic arteries, atherosclerosis is characterized by intimal and medial lipid deposits in elastic and muscular arteries, and arterial medial calcification has characteristic mineralization of the walls of elastic and muscular arteries.

Arteriosclerosis is an age-related disease that occurs frequently in many animal species but rarely causes clinical signs. The disease develops as chronic degenerative and proliferative responses in the arterial wall and results in loss of elasticity ("hardening of the arteries") and luminal narrowing. The abdominal aorta is most frequently affected, but other elastic arteries and peripheral large muscular vessels may be involved. Lesions are often localized around the orifices of arterial branches. Etiologic factors in the development of arteriosclerosis are not well defined, but the significant role of hemodynamic influences is suggested by the frequent involvement at arterial branching sites, where blood flow is turbulent. Grossly the lesions are seen as slightly raised, firm, white plaques. Microscopically, initially the intima is thickened by accumulation of mucopolysaccharides and later by the proliferation of smooth muscle cells in the tunica media and fibrous tissue infiltration into the intima. Splitting and fragmentation of the internal elastic lamina are common.

Atherosclerosis, the vascular disease of greatest importance in human beings, occurs only infrequently in animals and rarely leads to clinical disease, such as infarction of the heart or brain. The principal alteration is accumulation of deposits (atheroma) of lipid, fibrous tissue, and calcium in vessel walls, which eventually results in luminal narrowing. Many studies have established that the pig, rabbit, and chicken are susceptible to the experimental disease produced by the feeding of a high-cholesterol diet; the dog, cat, cow, goat, and rat are resistant. Lesions of the naturally occurring disease have been detected in aged pigs and birds and in dogs

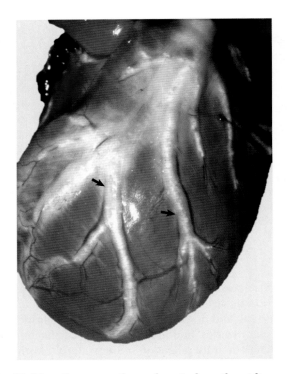

Fig. 10-82   Coronary atherosclerosis, hypothyroidism, heart, left ventricle, dog. The affected coronary arteries are prominent and cordlike (*arrows*) with thickened walls. The diffuse and focal yellow areas in the walls of the arteries are the sites of atheromatous deposits. *(Courtesy School of Veterinary Medicine, Purdue University.*

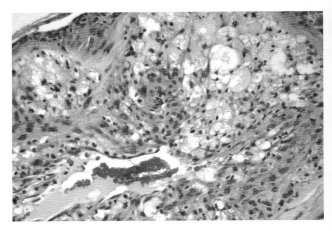

Fig. 10-83   Atherosclerosis, meningeal artery, horse. Note extensive accumulation of lipid-laden (clear vacuoles) "foam cells" throughout the thickened media. H&E stain. *(Courtesy School of Veterinary Medicine, Purdue University.)*

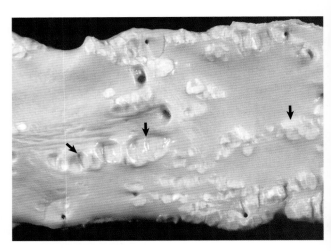

Fig. 10-84   Johne's disease, arteriosclerosis, aorta, cow. Multiple prominent, white, mineralized foci are in the tunica intima and media (*arrows*). *(Courtesy College of Veterinary Medicine, University of Illinois.)*

with hypothyroidism that develop an accompanying hypercholesterolemia. Arteries of the heart, mesentery, and kidneys are prominently thickened, firm, and yellow-white (Fig. 10-82). Microscopically, lipid globules accumulate in the cytoplasm of smooth muscle cells and macrophages, often termed "foam cells," in the media and intima (Fig. 10-83). Necrosis and fibrosis develop in some arterial lesions.

Arterial medial calcification is a frequent lesion in animals that often have concurrent endocardial mineralization and involves both elastic and muscular arteries. The causes of arterial medial calcification include calcinogenic plant toxicosis, vitamin D toxicosis, renal insufficiency, and severe debilitation, as seen in cattle with Johne's disease (Fig. 10-84). Medial calcification occurs spontaneously in rabbits and in aged guinea pigs and rats with chronic renal disease. Affected arteries, such as the aorta, have a unique gross appearance; they appear as solid, dense, pipelike structures with raised, white, solid intimal plaques (Fig. 10-85). Microscopically, in elastic arteries prominent basophilic granular mineral deposits are present on elastic fibers of the media, but in muscular arteries they form a complete ring of mineralization in the tunica media (Fig. 10-86). Siderocalcinosis (so-called iron rings), the result of deposition of both iron and calcium salts, occurs in the cerebral arteries of aged horses. Lesions in the surrounding brain tissue are generally absent. Siderocalcinosis lesions are considered incidental.

Arterial intimal calcification (intimal bodies) are distinctively small, mineralized masses within the subendothelium in small muscular arteries and arterioles of horses (Fig. 10-87). They have no deleterious effect.

Hyaline degeneration, fibrinoid necrosis, and amyloidosis are vascular lesions of small muscular arteries and arterioles and occur in all animal species.

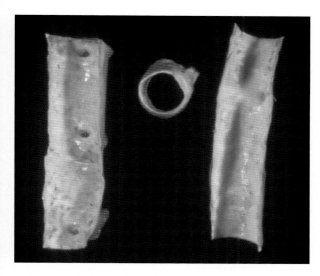

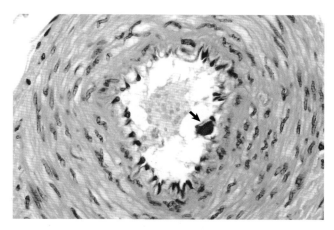

Fig. 10-87   Intimal body (*arrow*), intestine, muscular artery, horse. Intimal bodies are distinctive small, mineralized masses within the subendothelium of small muscular arteries and arterioles of horses. They are an incidental finding and have no pathologic significance. H&E stain. *(Courtesy Dr. M.D. McGavin, College of Veterinary Medicine, University of Tennessee.)*

Fig. 10-85   Calcification, vitamin D toxicosis, aorta, rabbit. The aorta is firm and inelastic because of the calcium deposits in the tunica intima and media. *(Courtesy School of Veterinary Medicine, Purdue University.)*

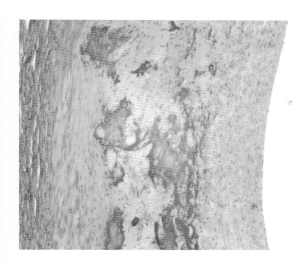

Fig. 10-86   Medial calcification, aorta, cow. Note the layer of mineralization in the middle of the tunica media. H&E stain. *(Courtesy Dr. M.D. McGavin, College of Veterinary Medicine, University of Tennessee.)*

These lesions are generally not detected grossly, but in some diseases with fibrinoid necrosis of vessels, hemorrhages and edema are seen in affected organs at necropsy. The microscopic feature shared by these lesions is the formation of a homogeneous eosinophilic zone in the vessel wall. Special stains allow differentiation into three types: (1) amyloid confirmed by Congo red and methyl violet; (2) fibrinoid deposits, positive by the periodic acid–Schiff technique; and (3) negative staining of hyaline deposits by these stains.

Amyloidosis and hyaline degeneration are often observed in small muscular arteries of the myocardium, lungs, and spleen of old dogs. Lesions in the intramyocardial arteries can cause small foci of myocardial infarction.

Fibrinoid necrosis of arteries is associated with endothelial damage and is characterized by entry and accumulation of serum proteins followed by fibrin polymerization in the vessel wall. These materials form an intensely eosinophilic collar that obliterates cellular detail. This lesion is frequent in many acute degenerative and inflammatory diseases of small arteries and arterioles. It is particularly frequent in pigs and is an important diagnostic feature in cases of selenium–vitamin E deficiency (heart), edema disease (gastric submucosa), cerebrospinal angiopathy, and organic mercury toxicosis (meninges). Fibrinoid necrosis is seen frequently in dogs with uremia and in dogs with hypertension, although hypertension is an uncommon finding in animals compared with human beings.

In pigs with selenium–vitamin E deficiency, the vascular fibrinoid necrosis produces gross lesions of cardiac hemorrhage ("mulberry heart disease") (Figs. 10-88 and 10-89) and massive hemorrhagic hepatic necrosis (hepatosis dietetica) (see Fig. 8-72). With either form of the disease, fibrinoid necrosis of small muscular arteries and arterioles is widespread and is accompanied by endothelial damage and fibrin thrombi in capillaries, especially capillaries of the myocardium. (Figs. 10-90 and 10-91). This complex of vascular lesions has been termed dietary microangiopathy. Similar capillary lesions of endothelial damage and occlusion by fibrin thrombi are seen in the cerebellum

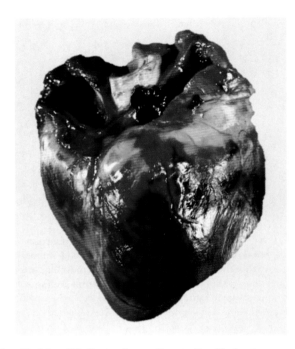

Fig. 10-88   "Mulberry heart disease," suffusive hemor-rhage, epicardium, right ventricle, heart, pig. Red areas of suffusive hemorrhage ("mulberry-like") are present on the epicardial surface of the right ventricle. *(Courtesy Dr. M.A. Miller, College of Veterinary Medicine, University of Missouri; and Noah's Arkive, College of Veterinary Medicine, The University of Georgia.)*

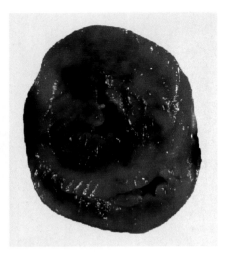

Fig. 10-89   "Mulberry heart disease," hemorrhage, left (top) and right ventricular myocardium, transverse section, pig. Dark red areas are caused by myocardial hemorrhage secondary to vascular fibrinoid necrosis originating from a diet deficient in selenium-vitamin E. *(Courtesy Department of Comparative Pathobiology, School of Veterinary Medicine, Purdue University.)*

THROMBOSIS AND EMBOLISM

Thrombosis represents the process of intravascular coagulation during life. Predisposing factors to thrombosis include (1) endothelial damage, (2) turbulence or stasis of blood flow, and (3) hypercoagulative states. Endothelial damage can be a feature of many arterial diseases. It is frequently present in arteritis but is uncommon in most of the degenerative arterial diseases, such as fibrinoid necrosis and atherosclerosis. Alterations in blood flow occur with vascular or cardiac

of ischemia-induced encephalomalacia of vitamin E–deficient chicks and in the skin and skeletal muscles of selenium–vitamin E–deficient chicks with exudative diathesis.

Cerebrospinal angiopathy in pigs is characteristically sporadic in pigs with signs of nervous system disease. Vascular lesions, such as fibrinoid necrosis, are present consistently in arteries of the central nervous system. Similar lesions occur in the arteries of the gastric submucosa of pigs with edema disease, a form of colibacillosis, and many researchers believe that cerebrospinal angiopathy represents a subacute form of edema disease (Figs. 10-92 and 10-93).

Medial necrosis and hemorrhage is a distinctive lesion produced in muscular arteries and arterioles of dogs and rats by a wide variety of vasoactive drugs. These vascular lesions, detected during evaluations of new compounds, produce grossly apparent hemorrhage, especially in the epicardium. Microscopically, acute damage is evident as necrosis of smooth muscle cells in the tunica media with surrounding erythrocytes. Healing lesions will have fibrosis of the vessel wall and perivascularly.

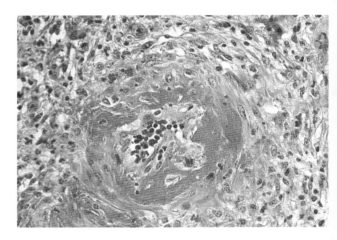

Fig. 10-90   Selenium–vitamin E deficiency ("mulberry heart disease"), fibrinoid necrosis, myocardial arteriole, heart, pig. Note the circumferential eosinophilic deposits in the wall of the arteriole. H&E stain. *(Courtesy Dr. J. Simon, College of Veterinary Medicine, University of Illinois.)*

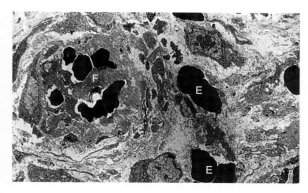

Fig. 10-91 **Fibrinoid necrosis, "mulberry heart disease," selenium–vitamin E deficiency, heart, section of myocardium, pig.** The affected arteriole *(left)* has intraluminal masses of fibrin *(F)* and entrapped erythrocytes. Fibrin masses are also present in the vessel wall, and the adjacent interstitium has edema and hemorrhage. Note scattered erythrocytes *(E)*. TEM. Uranyl acetate and lead citrate stain. *(Courtesy School of Veterinary Medicine, Purdue University.)*

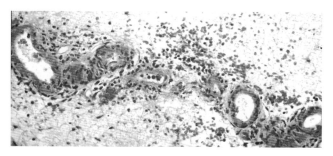

Fig. 10-93 **Fibrinoid necrosis of small arteries, edema disease, stomach, submucosa, pig.** Note the circumferential eosinophilic material in the walls of the arterioles and the extensive edema and mild hemorrhage in surrounding submucosa. H&E stain. *(Courtesy School of Veterinary Medicine, Purdue University.)*

valvular lesions that cause turbulence; stasis of blood flow can accompany congestive cardiac failure and cardiovascular collapse, as occurs in systemic shock. Hypercoagulative states have occurred in dogs with amyloidosis and some types of renal disease.

Examples of arterial thrombosis frequently observed in animals include caudal aortic thromboembolism in cats and dogs with primary cardiomyopathy (Fig. 10-94), thrombosis of mesenteric and intestinal arteries in horses with verminous arteritis from migrating larvae of strongylosis (Fig. 10-95), thrombosis of the pulmonary arteries in dogs with dirofilariasis, and aortoiliac thrombosis in horses. In these diseases, because large arteries can be affected, ischemia results in the peripheral tissue unless adequate collateral circulation exists. Recently formed

mural thrombi appear as yellow, firm masses of fibrin adhered focally to the arterial intima (Fig. 10-96). Fibroblastic proliferation and organization develop within days in thrombi.

Thrombosis or embolism of the coronary arteries can result in myocardial infarction (Fig. 10-97) and cardiac failure. These lesions are much less common in animals than in human beings. Affected animals generally have

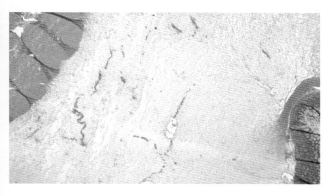

Fig. 10-92 **Submucosal edema, edema disease, stomach, submucosa, pig.** The submucosa is distended with edema fluid. H&E stain. *(Courtesy School of Veterinary Medicine, Purdue University.)*

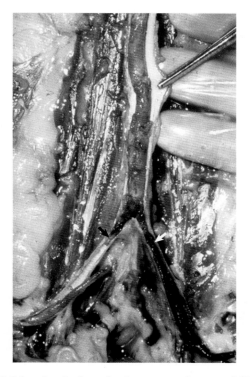

Fig. 10-94 **Aortic thrombosis, aorta and external iliac arteries, dog.** The tan thrombus occluding the caudal abdominal aorta is a cranial extension of the red saddle thrombus at the aortic bifurcation and in the external iliac arteries *(arrows)*. *(Courtesy School of Veterinary Medicine, Purdue University.)*

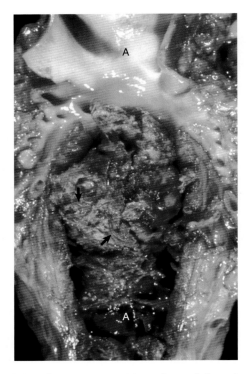

Fig. 10-95 **Verminous arteritis and mural thrombosis, strongylosis, abdominal aorta (A) and cranial mesenteric artery, horse.** A pale friable thrombotic mass, in which several *Strongylus vulgaris* larvae *(arrows)* are embedded, is attached to the wall of the cranial mesenteric artery. *(Courtesy College of Veterinary Medicine, University of Illinois.)*

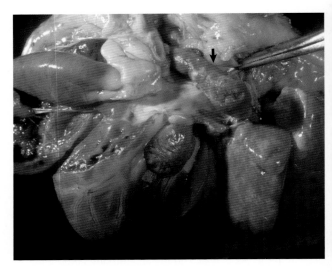

Fig. 10-96 **Arterial thrombus, pulmonary artery, dog.** Arterial thrombi are composed primarily of platelets and fibrin because the rapid flow of blood tends to exclude erythrocytes from the thrombus, and thus arterial thrombi are usually pale beige to gray *(arrow)*. *(Courtesy Dr. D.A. Mosier, College of Veterinary Medicine, Kansas State University.)*

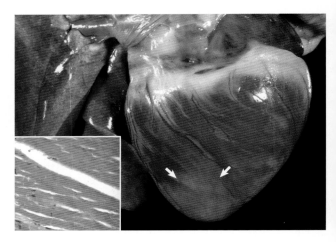

Fig. 10-97 **Myocardial infarction, heart, left and right ventricles, dog.** Pale, necrotic, circumscribed areas *(arrows)* are present in the ventricular walls and are most prominent at the apex. *Inset:* The cardiac myocytes are eosinophilic (ischemic necrosis) and have lost their nuclei (karyolysis). *(**Figure** and **Inset,** courtesy Dr. M.D. McGavin, College of Veterinary Medicine, University of Tennessee.)*

one of several types of coronary arterial disease, including atherosclerosis, arteriosclerosis, or periarteritis. In atherosclerosis associated with hypothyroidism (discussed previously), severe lesions are present in the extramural (epicardial) coronary arteries of dogs, but this only rarely leads to thrombosis and myocardial infarction. In contrast, severe arteriosclerosis of intramural cardiac arteries in aged dogs can cause small multifocal myocardial infarcts. Affected dogs often also have valvular endocardiosis, also an age-related disease.

Disseminated intravascular coagulation, initiated by a variety of causes, results in formation of widespread clotting within arterioles and blood capillaries. This clotting phenomenon is due largely to (1) endothelial damage with exposure of subendothelial collagen and subsequent platelet aggregation and (2) intravascular activation of the coagulation process. Diseases that can be accompanied by disseminated intravascular coagulation include bacterial endotoxemias; certain viral infections, such as feline infectious peritonitis and infectious canine hepatitis; dirofilariasis; certain neoplastic diseases, such as hemangiosarcoma and leukemia; shock; hemolysis; and extensive tissue necrosis, such as occurs in animals with burns. Extensive clotting depletes

coagulation factors (termed consumption coagulopathy), which results in widespread hemorrhages. Hemorrhagic lesions produced by this mechanism include hemorrhagic renal cortical necrosis (Shwartzman-like reaction) or hemorrhagic adrenal gland necrosis in cases of septicemia. Microscopically, organs with disseminated

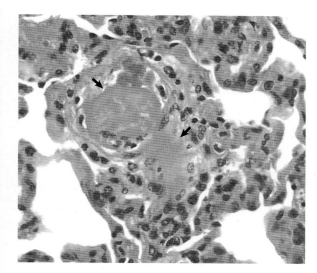

Fig. 10-98   Fibrin thrombi, disseminated intravascular coagulation, lung, alveolar septal capillaries, horse. Fibrin thrombi *(arrows)* occlude two alveolar capillaries. H&E stain. *(Courtesy School of Veterinary Medicine, Purdue University.)*

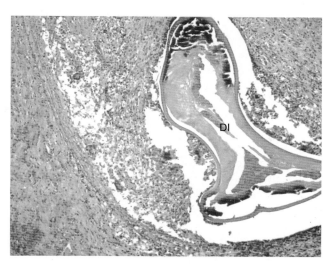

Fig. 10-99   Verminous arteritis, dirofilariasis, pulmonary artery, dog. A dead adult *Dirofilaria immitis* (*DI*) parasite in the lumen of the pulmonary artery is surrounded by pyogranulomatous inflammatory cells adhered to the wall (left) of the artery. Note the loss of the endothelial cells on the left side of the artery. H&E stain. *(Courtesy School of Veterinary Medicine, Purdue University.)*

intravascular coagulation have numerous fibrin thrombi in arterioles and capillaries (Fig. 10-98). Fibrinolysis, an intravascular enzymatic process to lyse clots, can continue to be active following the death of the animal and can lead to failure to observe fibrin thrombi in autolyzed tissue.

Embolism is the occlusion of arteries by lodgment of foreign materials, such as disrupted fragments of thrombi (thromboemboli), neoplastic cells, and bacteria. Thromboemboli originating from thrombotic lesions are either bland (sterile) or septic. Septic emboli most often originate from lesions of vegetative endocarditis. Right-sided lesions are disseminated to the lungs and left-sided lesions to the myocardium, kidneys, spleen, joints, and leptomeninges. Nonseptic emboli include air bubbles or hair fragments forced into the circulation during intravenous injections, release of fat from the bone marrow into the vasculature from fractures, release of fragments of dead intravascular parasites such as *Dirofilaria immitis* into the pulmonary circulation of carnivores following administration of adulticidal drugs (Fig. 10-99), and introduction of fragments of fibrocartilage into spinal arteries of dogs and less frequently other species (pig, human beings, horse, cat, and turkey) from disruption of degenerated intervertebral disk material (Fig. 10-100).

Animals with fibrocartilaginous embolism of the spinal vasculature develop infarction of the spinal cord, with resulting posterior paresis or paralysis. Affected dogs are typically middle-aged large or giant breeds, but occurrence in young Irish wolfhounds has been reported. The mechanism of formation of the arterial emboli is still unclear, but retrograde movement within the spinal

vasculature of fibrocartilaginous fragments from degenerated intervertebral disks is generally considered to underlie the presence of these unusual emboli.

Thromboembolism of the pulmonary arterial tree, often life threatening, occurs in dogs and cats. A wide variety of predisposing conditions that may result in altered blood flow, hypercoagulability, or endothelial

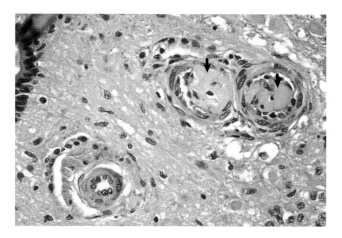

Fig. 10-100   Fibrocartilaginous emboli, spinal cord, pig. The basophilic masses *(arrows)* occluding small arteries (cross sections) in the spinal cord gray matter adjacent to the central canal *(top left margin)* are fibrocartilaginous emboli. H&E stain. *(Courtesy School of Veterinary Medicine, Purdue University.)*

damage includes sepsis, immune-mediated hemolytic anemia, protein-losing nephropathy or enteropathy, disseminated intravascular coagulation, cardiac disease, neoplastic disease, hyperadrenocorticism, dirofilariasis, amyloidosis, and use of intravenous catheters.

Thrombosis of the femoral artery, with resulting partial to complete occlusion, has been reported in cavalier King Charles spaniels. The condition may share a common etiopathogenesis with valvular endocardiosis, which is frequent in this breed, through a genetically mediated connective tissue disorder. Affected dogs generally do not develop hindlimb ischemia, in contrast to human patients with this condition, because of extensive collateral circulation.

In cattle, thrombosis of the caudal vena cava occurs in association with rupture of hepatic abscesses into either the hepatic vein or the caudal vena cava.

INFLAMMATION

The various portals of entry and defense mechanisms involved in arterial inflammation are summarized in Box 10-1 and Box 10-2. Arteritis occurs as a feature of many infections and immune-mediated diseases (Table 10-6). Often, all types of vessels are affected rather than only arteries, and then vasculitis or angiitis is the term applied to the lesions. In inflamed vessels,

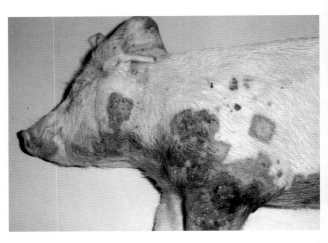

Fig. 10-101   Cutaneous infarcts, diamond skin disease, *Erysipelothrix rhusiopathiae* septicemia, skin, pig. Emboli of *Erysipelothrix rhusiopathiae* have lodged in cutaneous vessels and caused a localized vasculitis, which has resulted in thrombosis followed by ischemia and cutaneous infarction. *(Courtesy Dr. M.D. McGavin, College of Veterinary Medicine, University of Tennessee.)*

leukocytes are present within and surrounding the walls, and damage to the vessel wall is evident as fibrin deposits or necrotic endothelial and smooth muscle cells. As a result of endothelial damage, thrombosis which can result in ischemic injury or infarction in the circulatory field may be present. The "diamond skin" lesions of porcine erysipelas caused by *Erysipelothrix rhusiopathiae* is an example of cutaneous infarction (Fig. 10-101).

Arteritis and vasculitis can develop from endothelial injury caused by either infectious agents or immune-mediated mechanisms or may be caused by local extension of suppurative and necrotizing inflammatory processes. Equine viral arteritis is a systemic viral infection with a tropism for vascular endothelial cells. In this disease, affected small muscular arteries have lesions of fibrinoid necrosis, extensive edema, and leukocytic infiltration (Fig. 10-102). Grossly the vascular injury is reflected by severe edema of the intestinal wall and mesentery accompanied by notable accumulation of serous fluids in body cavities.

Arteritis is a prominent feature of several parasitic diseases. In canine dirofilariasis (heartworm infection), maturation of adult parasites occurs in the pulmonary arteries and right atrium and ventricle. The pulmonary arteries containing parasites initially have an infiltration of the intima (termed endarteritis) by eosinophils, with subsequent development of an irregular fibromuscular proliferation of the intima visible grossly as a rough granular or shaggy appearance of the luminal surface (Fig. 10-99). Live or dead parasites can be present within these vascular lesions and be accompanied

Table 10-6   Diseases That Cause Vasculitis in Animals

VIRAL

Equine viral arteritis, malignant catarrhal fever, hog cholera, feline infectious peritonitis, bluetongue, African swine fever, equine infectious anemia, bovine virus diarrhea

BACTERIAL

Salmonellosis, erysipelas (*Erysipelothrix rhusiopathiae*), Hemophilus spp. infections (*Hemophilus suis, Hemophilus somnus, Hemophilus parasuis*)

MYCOTIC

Phycomycosis, aspergillosis

PARASITIC

Equine strongylosis (*Strongylus vulgaris*), dirofilariasis (*Dirofilaria immitis*), spirocercosis (*Spirocerca lupi*), onchocerciasis, elaeophoriasis (*Elaeophora schneideri*), filariasis in primates, aelurostrongylosis, angiostrongylosis

IMMUNE-MEDIATED

Canine systemic lupus erythematosus, rheumatoid arthritis, Aleutian mink disease, polyarteritis nodosa, lymphocytic choriomeningitis, drug-induced hypersensitivity

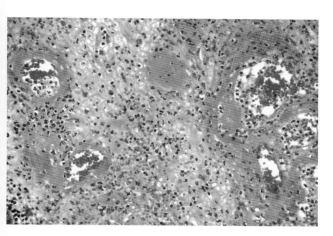

Fig. 10-102   Acute arteritis, equine viral arteritis, small intestine, submucosa, horse. Small arteries have fibrinoid degeneration (circumferential eosinophilic material) of the tunica media with leukocytic infiltration. The surrounding loose connective tissue is edematous and also infiltrated by numerous leukocytes. H&E stain. *(Courtesy School of Veterinary Medicine, Purdue University.)*

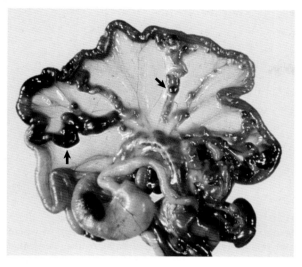

Fig. 10-103   Polyarteritis nodosa, mesenteric arteries, rat. The affected segments of the arteries are thick, red, hemorrhagic and tortuous *(arrows)*. *(Courtesy School of Veterinary Medicine, Purdue University.)*

by thromboembolism and pulmonary infarction. Infection of horses by *Strongylus vulgaris* is now less common because of widespread use of highly efficacious antiparasitic drugs. During its larval development, the parasite migrates through the intestinal arteries, and the most severe lesions are generally found in the cranial mesenteric artery. The affected vessel is enlarged, and its wall is firm and fibrotic. The intimal surface often has an adhering thrombus admixed with larvae. Microscopically the affected vessel has extensive infiltration of inflammatory cells and proliferation of fibroblasts throughout the wall. As a consequence, thromboembolism of the intestinal arteries frequently occurs and can produce colic, but the abundant collateral circulation to the equine intestinal tract makes intestinal infarction an unusual event.

Polyarteritis is a disease that occurs sporadically in many animal species and is an important disease of aged rats (Fig. 10-103). Many recent reports have described the occurrence of polyarteritis in a disease termed idiopathic necrotizing polyarteritis involving the coronary and meningeal arteries in pet and laboratory beagle dogs ("beagle pain syndrome"). Clinically, affected dogs typically show recurrent episodes of fever, body weight loss, and occasionally cervical pain manifested by a still gait and stiff neck with a hunched body posture. However, some affected dogs will not display clinical signs of disease. The lesions are usually attributed to an immune-mediated vascular injury. Medium-sized muscular arteries in a wide variety of organs, including the heart and meninges, are selectively involved and grossly appear thick and tortuous, have associated focal hemorrhage, and develop aneurysms and thrombosis.

Microscopically the early lesions include fibrinoid necrosis and leukocytic invasion of the intima and media (Fig. 10-104). In chronic lesions, inflammatory cells and fibrosis involve all layers of the vascular wall.

NEOPLASTIC DISEASES

Neoplasms arising from vascular endothelial cells develop in many different organs. Hemangiomas are benign neoplasms often found in the skin of dogs (Fig. 10-105). These red, blood-filled masses are well circumscribed. The malignant neoplasm hemangiosarcoma occurs frequently in the spleen and the right atrium

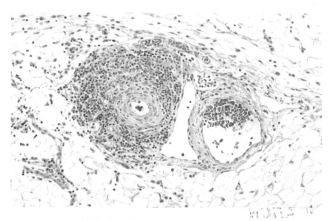

Fig. 10-104   Periarteritis and arteritis (polyarteritis—"beagle pain syndrome"), beagle dog. Note the accumulation of lymphocytes and macrophages around the arteriole. H&E stain. *(Courtesy Dr. P.W. Snyder, School of Veterinary Medicine, Purdue University.)*

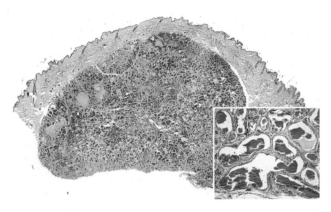

Fig. 10-105   Cutaneous hemangioma, skin, dog. The subcutis contains a well-demarcated mass formed by vascular channels lined by a single layer of well-differentiated endothelial cells. *Inset:* Higher magnification of the well-differentiated endothelial cells lining the vascular channels. H&E stain. (***Figure*** *and* ***Inset,*** *courtesy Dr. M.D. McGavin, College of Veterinary Medicine, University of Tennessee.*)

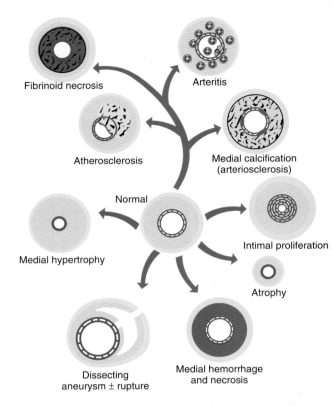

Fig. 10-106   Schematic diagram of the major arterial diseases. (*Redrawn with permission from School of Veterinary Medicine, Purdue University.*)

of dogs. This neoplasm is also generally a red mass, but microscopically the neoplastic cells are pleomorphic and may not form distinct vascular spaces. Another neoplasm of vascular origin is the hemangiopericytoma of the canine skin. The distinctive microscopic feature is a laminated arrangement of elongated, plump neoplastic pericytes around small blood vessels.

Metastasis of primary sarcomas to distant sites often occurs after invasion of blood vessels. The major arterial diseases are illustrated in Fig. 10-106.

VENOUS DISEASES

CONGENITAL ANOMALIES

Portocaval shunts occur in dogs and, because blood bypasses the liver, can result in signs of nervous system disease associated with failure of hepatic degradation of nitrogenous products such as ammonia (resulting in hyperammonemia). The resulting nervous system syndrome is termed hepatic encephalopathy. Specifically the shunts represent retained fetal vascular structures, as in persistent ductus venosus, or arise from prominent dilation of various portosystemic shunts that normally are quite small vessels. See Chapter 8 on diseases of the liver for further details.

DILATION

A venous dilation from weakened vascular walls is termed a varicosity (localized involvement) or phlebectasia (generalized alteration). Although a frequent lesion in the superficial veins of the legs in women, it is rather

uncommon in animals. The pampiniform plexus in the spermatic cord in aged rams and bulls can be affected.

INFLAMMATION

The various portals of entry and defense mechanisms involved in venous inflammation are summarized in Box 10-1 and Box 10-2. Phlebitis is a common vascular lesion and is often complicated by thrombosis. The vascular lesion arises from (1) systemic infections, (2) local extension of infection, and (3) a faulty intravenous injection procedure. Systemic infections with phlebitis as a lesion include salmonellosis in several species and feline infectious peritonitis. In pigs with various septicemias, such as salmonellosis and colibacillosis, the gastric fundic mucosa is often severely congested and hemorrhagic because of venous endothelial damage and thrombosis. In severe local infections, such as in metritis or hepatic abscesses, inflammation extends into the walls of adjacent veins and produce phlebitis, with or without thrombosis. Intravenous injections of irritant solutions, injecting solutions into the vascular wall, or intimal trauma produced by indwelling venous

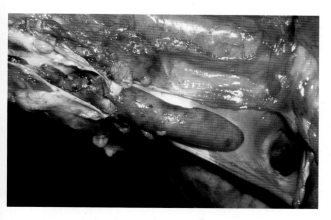

Fig. 10-107 **Thrombus (mural), jugular vein (opened), dog.** Note the nodular mural thrombus *(left)* in the jugular vein. This thrombus likely occurred at a site of venipuncture and a subsequent phlebitis. The smooth-surfaced reddish-tan thrombus *(right)* extending toward the heart is a trailing thrombus, connected to the mural thrombus. *(Courtesy School of Veterinary Medicine, Purdue University.)*

catheters result in vascular damage and create an opportunity for localization and proliferation of infectious agents and development of phlebitis and thrombosis (Fig. 10-107). Animals with phlebitis complicated by thrombosis have the additional risk of septic embolism, which can cause endocarditis and pulmonary abscesses.

Omphalophlebitis ("navel ill") is inflammation of the umbilical vein and often occurs in neonatal farm animals because of bacterial contamination of the umbilicus immediately following parturition. Bacteria from this site can cause septicemia, suppurative polyarthritis, hepatic abscesses (the umbilical vein drains into the liver), and umbilical abscesses.

Cats with feline infectious peritonitis often develop phlebitis in various abdominal organs. This lesion appears to result from deposition of immune complexes, which subsequently induce an inflammatory reaction in affected vessels. Occasionally, in some cattle with hepatic abscesses, infection extends into the adjacent large hepatic veins and results in formation of a septic thrombus in the caudal vena cava. Rupture and release of the contents of the abscess into the lumen can cause multiple septic emboli in the pulmonary capillaries and unexpected death of the affected animal.

Several parasitic diseases important in tropical regions of the world are characterized by presence of parasites in the lumens of veins. These diseases include schistosomiasis (blood fluke infection–*Schistosoma* spp.) and infection of cats in South America by *Gurltia paralysans*. Affected cats have spinal cord damage from thrombophlebitis in the lumbar veins, associated with

the presence of adult parasites in affected vessels. In schistosomiasis, adult parasites are present in the mesenteric and portal veins, and the resulting phlebitis is characterized by intimal proliferation and thrombosis.

LYMPH VESSEL DISEASES

CONGENITAL ANOMALIES

Hereditary lymphedema has been described in dogs, Ayrshire calves, and pigs. Affected animals have prominent subcutaneous edema that, in calves, often causes severe swelling of the tips of the ears. Interference with lymph drainage results from defective development of the lymph vessels that are aplastic or hypoplastic.

DILATION AND RUPTURE

Lymphangiectasis is dilation of lymph vessels. The cause may be a congenital anomaly (Fig. 10-108) or due to obstruction of lymph drainage by invading masses of malignant neoplasms (Fig. 10-109). Another example is intestinal lymphangiectasis, an important disease of dogs in which there is a protein-losing enteropathy. Lacteals in the intestinal villi are prominently dilated, and lymph vessels throughout the wall of the bowel and the mesentery are distended. The role of obstruction of lymph vessels in the pathogenesis of this disease is still unclear. Many diseases with severe acute inflammatory alterations accompanied by vascular damage, as with the pneumonia of bovine pasteurellosis, have prominently dilated lymph vessels.

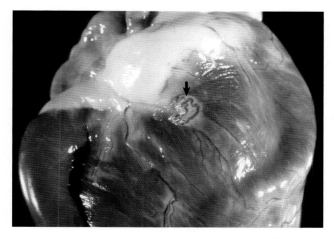

Fig. 10-108 **Congenital lymphangiectasia, epicardium, young horse.** Note the tortuous appearance of the epicardial lymphatic vessel *(arrow)*. In congenital lymphangiectasia, lymph vessels fail to make connections with other vessels or are obstructed because of anomalous development. *(Courtesy College of Veterinary Medicine, University of Illinois.)*

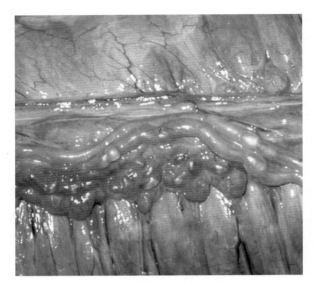

Fig. 10-109 **Acquired lymphangiectasia, lymphoma (lymphosarcoma), mesentery, horse.** Note the distended lymphatics on the serosal surface of the large colon, the result of impeded lymph flow through the mesenteric lymph nodes at the root of the mesentery, due to obstruction of flow in the lymph node secondary to compression of the lymphatic cortical and medullary lymph sinuses by neoplastic lymphocytes. *(Courtesy College of Veterinary Medicine, University of Illinois.)*

Table 10-7 **Diseases That Cause Lymphangitis in Animals**

BACTERIAL

Porcine anthrax (*Bacillus anthracis*), Johne's disease (*Mycobacterium paratuberculosis*), tuberculosis (*Mycobacterium* spp.), actinobacillosis (*Actinobacillus lignieresii*), glanders (farcy) (*Pseudomonas mallei*), cutaneous streptothricosis (*Dermatophilus congolensis*), bovine farcy, ulcerative lymphangitis of horses, sporadic lymphangitis of horses

MYCOTIC

Epizootic lymphangitis of horses (*Histoplasma farciminosum*), sporotrichosis (*Sporothrix schenckii*)

PARASITIC

Brugia spp. infection of dogs and cats

Rupture of the thoracic duct, either as a result of trauma or from spontaneous disruption, causes chylothorax in dogs and cats (see Fig. 9-90). However, many cases of chylothorax occur without injury to the thoracic duct and have been attributed to lesions that interfere with central venous return or produce obstruction of the thoracic duct (right side heart failure, neoplasms, granulomas, cranial vena cava thrombosis, dirofilariasis) or that are idiopathic.

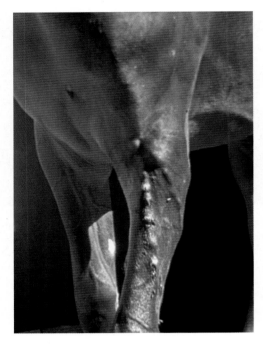

Fig. 10-110 **Lymphangitis, forelimb, lymphatic vessels, horse.** Note the multiple swellings (cordlike) of the afferent lymphatics in the skin. These lymphatics lie in the subcutis and empty into the caudal superficial cervical (prescapular) lymph node. *(Courtesy School of Veterinary Medicine, Purdue University.)*

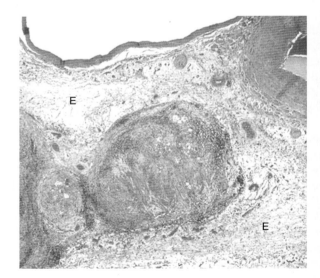

Fig. 10-111 **Granulomatous lymphangitis, Johne's disease, mesenteric lymph vessel, sheep.** The lymphatic is occluded by a fibrinous thrombus secondary to the destruction of the endothelium by inflammatory cells including macrophages. Early proliferating fibrous tissue and extensive edema (E) surround the lymph vessel. The adjacent artery and vein are unaffected. H&E stain. *(Courtesy School of Veterinary Medicine, Purdue University.)*

INFLAMMATION

The various portals of entry and defense mechanisms involved in lymph vessel inflammation are summarized in Box 10-1 and Box 10-2. Lymphangitis is a feature of many diseases (Table 10-7). The affected vessels are often located in the distal limbs and are thick, cord-like structures (Fig. 10-110). Lymphedema also can be present. Nodular suppurative lesions of lymphangitis often ulcerate and discharge pus onto the surface of the skin. In Johne's disease, the mesenteric lymph vessels are often prominent because of granulomatous lymphangitis, an extension of the enteric infection producing a granulomatous enteritis and lymphangitis (Fig. 10-111).

NEOPLASTIC DISEASES

Lymphangioma represents a rare benign neoplasm composed of lymph channels. Lymphangiosarcoma occurs more often than the benign neoplasm. Vascular spaces contain lymph rather than the blood. Lymph vessels are frequently invaded by primary carcinomas and are a common route of metastasis.

■ SUGGESTED READINGS

Anversa P, Leri A, Beltrami C et al: Myocyte death and growth in the failing heart, *Lab Invest* 78:767-786, 1998.

Ayers KM, Jones SR: The cardiovascular system. In Benirschke K, Garner FM, Jones TC, editors: *Pathology of laboratory animals*, vol I, New York, 1978, Springer-Verlag.

Beardow AW, Buchanan JW: Chronic mitral valve disease in cavalier King Charles spaniels: 95 cases (1987-1991), *J Am Vet Med Assoc* 203:1023-1029, 1993.

Bishop SP: Necropsy techniques for the heart and great vessels. In Fox P, Sisson D, Moise N, editors: *Textbook of canine and feline cardiology*, ed 2, Philadelphia, 1999, Saunders.

Bonagura JD, Lehmkuhl LB: Congenital heart disease. In Fox P, Sisson D, Moise N, editors: *Textbook of canine and feline cardiology*, ed 2, Philadelphia, 1999, Saunders.

Buchanan JW: Prevalence of cardiovascular disorders. In Fox P, Sisson D, Moise N, editors: *Textbook of canine and feline cardiology*, ed 2, Philadelphia, 1999, Saunders.

Calvert CA, Hall G, Jacobs G et al: Clinical and pathologic findings in Doberman pinschers with occult cardiomyopathy that died suddenly or developed congestive heart failure: 54 cases (1984-1991), *J Am Vet Med Assoc* 210:505-511, 1997.

Calvert CA, Rawlings C, McCall J: Canine heartworm disease. In Fox P, Sisson D, Moise N editors: *Textbook of canine and feline cardiology*, ed 2, Philadelphia, 1999, Saunders.

Everett R, McGann J, Wimberly H: Dilated cardiomyopathy of Doberman pinschers: retrospective histomorphologic evaluation of heart from 32 cases, *Vet Pathol* 36:221-227, 1999.

Fox PR: Feline cardiomyopathies. In Fox P, Sisson D, Moise N, editors: *Textbook of canine and feline cardiology*, ed 2, Philadelphia, 1999, Saunders.

Gandini G, Cizinauskas S, Lang J et al: Fibrocartilaginous embolism in 75 dogs: clinical findings and factors influencing the recovery rate, *J Small Anim Pract* 44:76-80, 2003.

Johnson LR, Lappin MR, Baker DC: Pulmonary thromboembolism in 29 dogs: 1985-1995, *J Vet Int Med* 13:338-345, 1999.

Kerns W, Roth L, Hosokawa S: Idiopathic canine polyarteritis. In Mohr U, Carlton W, Dungworth D et al, editors: *Pathobiology of the aging dog*, vol 2, Ames, 2001, Iowa State University Press.

King JM, Roth L, Haschek WM: Myocardial necrosis secondary to neural lesions in domestic animals, *J Am Vet Med Assoc* 180:144-148, 1982.

Leferovich J, Bedelbaeva K, Samulewicz S et al: Heart regeneration in adult MRL mice, *Proc Nat Acad Sci* 98:9830-9835, 2001.

Lewis W, Silver MD: Adverse effects of drugs on the cardiovascular system. In Silver MD, Gotlieb AI, Schoen FJ, editors: *Cardiovascular pathology*, New York, 2001, Churchill Livingstone.

Liu S, Fox PR: Cardiovascular pathology. In Fox P, Sisson D, Moise N, editors: *Textbook of canine and feline cardiology*, ed 2, Philadelphia, 1999, Saunders.

Louden C, Morgan DG: Pathology and pathophysiology of drug-induced arterial injury in laboratory animals and its implications on the evaluation of novel chemical entities for human clinical trials, *Pharm Toxicol* 89:158-170, 2001.

Palate BM, Denol SR, Roba JL: A simple method for performing routine histopathological examination of the cardiac conduction tissue in the dog, *Toxicol Pathol* 23:56-62, 1995.

Pion PD, Kittleson MD, Rogers QR et al: Myocardial failure in cats associated with low plasma taurine: a reversible cardiomyopathy, *Science* 237:764-768, 1987.

Schmitt J, Kamisago M, Asahi M et al: Dilated cardiomyopathy and heart failure caused by a mutation in phospholamban, *Science* 299:1410-1413, 2003.

Schwartz CJ, Sprague EA, Valente AJ et al: Cellular mechanisms in the response of the arterial wall to injury and repair, *Toxicol Pathol* 17:66-71, 1989.

Sisson D, Kvart C, Darke PGG: Acquired valvular heart disease in dogs and cats. In Fox P, Sisson D, Moise N, editors: *Textbook of canine and feline cardiology*, ed 2, Philadelphia, 1999, Saunders.

Sisson D, O'Grady M, Calvert C: Myocardial diseases of dogs. In Fox P, Sisson D, Moise N, editors: *Textbook of canine and feline cardiology*, ed 2, Philadelphia, 1999, Saunders.

Sisson D, Thomas W: Pericardial disease and cardiac tumors. In Fox P, Sisson D, Moise N, editors: *Textbook of canine and feline cardiology*, ed 2, Philadelphia, 1999, Saunders.

Van Vleet JF, Ferrans VJ: Characterization of myocardial toxicity caused by agents that affect the myocytes. In Bishop SP, Kerns WD, editors: *Comprehensive toxicology: cardiovascular toxicology*, vol 6, New York, 1997, Elsevier.

Van Vleet JF, Ferrans VJ: Myocardial disease of animals, *Am J Pathol* 124:98-178, 1986.

Van Vleet JF, Ferrans VJ, Herman E: Cardiovascular and skeletal muscular systems. In Haschek WM, Rousseaux CG, Wallig MA editors: *Handbook of toxicologic pathology*, ed 2, Academic Press, 2002, New York.

Van Vleet JF, Ferrans VJ, Weirich WE: Pathologic alterations in congestive cardiomyopathy of dogs, *Am J Vet Res* 42:416-424, 1981.

Van Vleet JF, Ferrans VJ, Weirich WE: Pathologic alterations in hypertrophic and congestive cardiomyopathy of cats, *Am J Vet Res* 41:2037-2048, 1980.

11

Urinary System

SHELLEY J. NEWMAN • ANTHONY W. CONFER • ROGER J. PANCIERA

INTRODUCTION

KIDNEY

Mammalian kidneys are paired organs present in the retroperitoneum, ventrolateral and adjacent to the lumbar vertebral bodies and their corresponding transverse processes. These complex organs, which function in excretion, metabolism, secretion, and regulation, are susceptible to disease insults that affect the four major anatomic structures of the kidney: the glomeruli, tubules, interstitium, and vasculature. Because of the limited ways that renal tissue can respond to injury, the patterns of injury and outcomes that initially may be distinctive in severe and prolonged diseases will result in a similar end point—chronic renal disease and failure. Interdependence between components of the nephron also are responsible for producing a narrow range of repeatable injury patterns, which students can come to recognize on gross or histologic assessment.

STRUCTURE AND FUNCTION
MACROSCOPIC STRUCTURE

Kidneys are organized functionally and anatomically into lobules. Each lobule represents collections of nephrons separated by the medullary rays (Fig.11-1). Renal lobules should not be confused with renal lobes. Each lobe is represented by a renal pyramid (Fig.11-1). Among domestic animals, carnivores and horses have unilobar (or unipyramidal) kidneys. Porcine and bovine kidneys are multilobar (or multipyramidal), but only bovine kidneys have external lobation (Fig.11-2). Kidneys are covered by a diffuse fibrous capsule that in normal kidneys can be easily removed from the renal surface. The renal parenchyma is divided into a cortex and medulla (Fig.11-3). The corticomedullary ratio is usually approximately 1:2 or 1:3 in domestic animals. The ratio varies among species; for example, those adapted to the desert have a far larger medulla and thus a corticomedullary ratio that can approach 1:5.

Normally the cortex is radially striated and dark red-brown except in mature cats, in which the cortex is often yellow because of the large lipid content of tubular epithelial cells. The renal medulla is pale gray and has either a single renal papilla, as in cats; a fused, crestlike papilla (renal medullary crest), as in dogs, sheep, and horses; or multiple renal papillae, as in pigs and cattle. The medulla generally can be subdivided into an outer zone, that portion of the medulla close to the cortex, and an inner zone, that portion closer to the pelvis. Papillae are surrounded by minor calyces that coalesce to form major calyces, which empty into the renal pelvis, where urine collects before entry into the ureters.

Knowledge of the normal renal blood supply is important in understanding the pathogenesis and distribution of various renal lesions. The kidneys receive blood

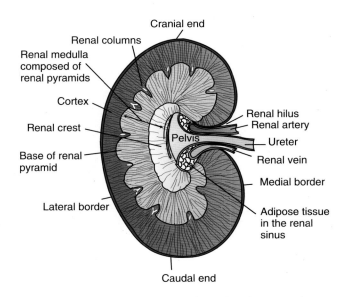

Fig. 11-1   Schematic diagram, kidney, dorsal section, dog.
(Based on Schaller O, Enke F, Stuttgart V, editors: Illustrated veterinary anatomical nomenclature, Kinderhook, NY, 1992, IBD Ltd.)

primarily through the renal artery. An interlobar artery extends along the boundary of each renal lobe (renal column) and then branches at right angles to form an arcuate artery that runs along the corticomedullary junction (Fig.11-4). Interlobular arteries branch from

the arcuate artery and extend into the cortex. They have no anastomoses, making them susceptible to focal ischemic necrosis (infarct) as in any organ with end arteries.

MICROSCOPIC STRUCTURE

The functional unit of the kidney is the nephron, which includes the renal corpuscle (glomerulus within Bowman's capsule), and a tubular system that includes the proximal convoluted tubules, the loop of Henle, and the distal convoluted tubule, which empties into the collecting tubule (Fig. 11-5).

The glomerulus is a complex, convoluted tuft of fenestrated endothelial-lined capillaries held together by a supporting structure of cells in a glycoprotein matrix, the mesangium (Fig. 11-6). The capillary tuft is covered by the visceral epithelial cells (podocytes) and is contained within a membranous "cap," called Bowman's capsule, which is lined by parietal epithelial cells (resembling squamous epithelium) (Fig. 11-6). The fluid that filters through the glomerulus into the capsular space (also referred to as Bowman's space) is called glomerular filtrate and it arises after passage through the glomerular filtration membrane (composed of fenestrated endothelial cells, basement membrane, and filtration slits located between visceral epithelial cells or podocytes). This ultrafiltrate of plasma (primary urine), which contains water, salts, ions, glucose, and albumin, passes into the capsular space (Bowman's space) and then empties into the proximal convoluted tubule at the urinary pole.

The glomerular filtration barrier is composed of podocytes, fenestrated endothelium, and basal lamina, the last produced by both endothelial and epithelial

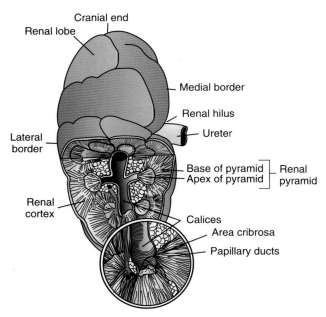

Fig. 11-2 Schematic diagram, kidney, dorsal surface and partial dorsal section, cow. In the Nomina Anatomica Veterinaria (NAV), the dorsal plane or dorsal section is parallel to the dorsum (back). *(Based on Schaller O, Enke F, Stuttgart V, editors: Illustrated veterinary anatomical nomenclature, Kinderhook, NY, 1992, IBD Ltd.)*

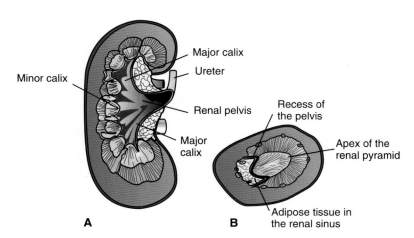

Fig. 11-3 Schematic diagram, kidney. A, Dorsal section through hilus, pig. **B,** Transverse section through hilus, dog. *(A and B, Based on Schaller O, Enke F, Stuttgart V, editors: Illustrated veterinary anatomical nomenclature, Kinderhook, NY, 1992, IBD Ltd.)*

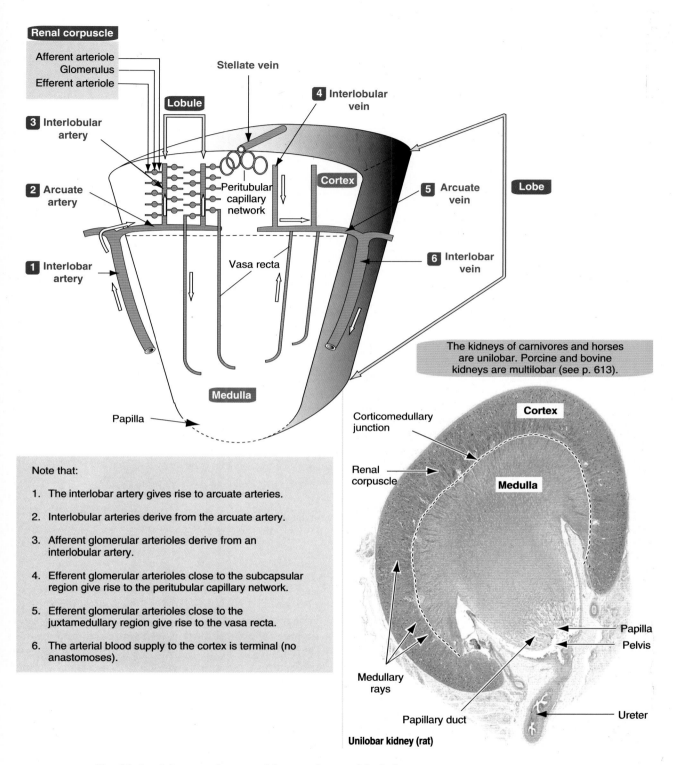

Renal corpuscle
Afferent arteriole
Glomerulus
Efferent arteriole

Stellate vein

4 Interlobular vein

Lobule

3 Interlobular artery

2 Arcuate artery

Peritubular capillary network

Cortex

5 Arcuate vein

Lobe

1 Interlobar artery

Vasa recta

6 Interlobar vein

Medulla

Papilla

The kidneys of carnivores and horses are unilobar. Porcine and bovine kidneys are multilobar (see p. 613).

Note that:

1. The interlobar artery gives rise to arcuate arteries.

2. Interlobular arteries derive from the arcuate artery.

3. Afferent glomerular arterioles derive from an interlobular artery.

4. Efferent glomerular arterioles close to the subcapsular region give rise to the peritubular capillary network.

5. Efferent glomerular arterioles close to the juxtamedullary region give rise to the vasa recta.

6. The arterial blood supply to the cortex is terminal (no anastomoses).

Corticomedullary junction

Cortex

Renal corpuscle

Medulla

Papilla

Pelvis

Medullary rays

Papillary duct

Ureter

Unilobar kidney (rat)

Fig. 11-4   **Schematic diagram of the vasculature of the kidney.** *(From Kierszenbaum AL:* Histology and cell biology: an introduction to pathology, *St Louis, 2002, Mosby.)*

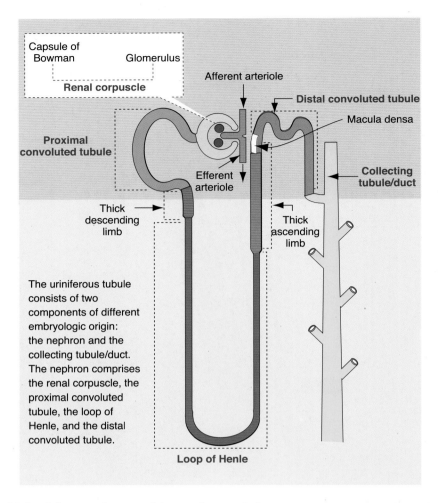

Capsule of
Bowman
Glomerulus
Renal corpuscle

Afferent arteriole

Distal convoluted tubule

Macula densa

**Proximal
convoluted tubule**

Efferent
arteriole

**Collecting
tubule/duct**

Thick
descending
limb

Thick
ascending
limb

The uriniferous tubule
consists of two
components of different
embryologic origin:
the nephron and the
collecting tubule/duct.
The nephron comprises
the renal corpuscle, the
proximal convoluted
tubule, the loop of
Henle, and the distal
convoluted tubule.

Loop of Henle

Fig. 11-5   Schematic diagram of the uriniferous tubule. *(From Kierszenbaum AL:* Histology and cell
biology: an introduction to pathology, *St Louis, 2002, Mosby.)*

cells (Fig. 11-7). The glomerular basement membrane has a thick, dense central layer, the lamina densa, which is covered by thinner, more electron-lucent inner and outer layers, the lamina rara interna and lamina rara externa, respectively. The basement membrane has a network of type IV collagen, which forms a tetrameric porous infrastructure. Numerous glycoproteins, such as acidic proteoglycans and laminin, together with the collagen fibers form the complete structure of the membrane. Visceral epithelial cells (podocytes), aligned on the external surface of the basement membrane, are responsible for synthesis of basement membrane components and have special cytoplasmic processes (foot processes) that are embedded in the lamina rara externa. Negatively charged glycoproteins overlying the endothelial cells and the podocytes contribute to the charge differential of the glomerular basement membrane.

Foot processes from adjacent visceral epithelium interdigitate to form filtration slits between them. Filtration slit diaphragms are composed of nephrin, a cell adhesion molecule of the immunoglobulin superfamily, which controls slit size by its connection to podocyte actin (Fig. 11-7). The glomerular filtration barrier selectively filters molecules based on size (<70,000 Da), electrical charge (the more cationic, the more permeable), and capillary pressure. In summary, both size-dependent and charge-dependent filtration is possible because of the porous structure of capillary walls, which is a function of endothelial fenestrations, a basement membrane formed of type IV collagen, basement membrane anionic glycoproteins, and filtration slits of the visceral epithelium. The entire glomerular tuft is supported by mesangial matrix that is secreted by the mesangial cells, a type of modified pericyte (Fig. 11-8). Mesangial cells are

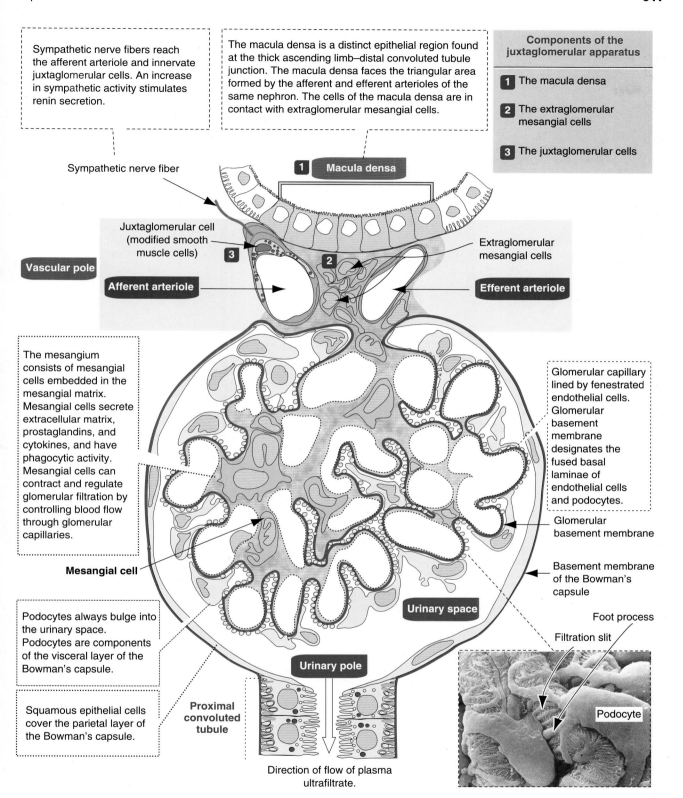

Sympathetic nerve fibers reach the afferent arteriole and innervate juxtaglomerular cells. An increase in sympathetic activity stimulates renin secretion.

The macula densa is a distinct epithelial region found at the thick ascending limb–distal convoluted tubule junction. The macula densa faces the triangular area formed by the afferent and efferent arterioles of the same nephron. The cells of the macula densa are in contact with extraglomerular mesangial cells.

Components of the juxtaglomerular apparatus

1 The macula densa

2 The extraglomerular mesangial cells

3 The juxtaglomerular cells

Sympathetic nerve fiber

1 Macula densa

Juxtaglomerular cell (modified smooth muscle cells) 3

Extraglomerular mesangial cells

Vascular pole

Afferent arteriole

2

Efferent arteriole

The mesangium consists of mesangial cells embedded in the mesangial matrix. Mesangial cells secrete extracellular matrix, prostaglandins, and cytokines, and have phagocytic activity. Mesangial cells can contract and regulate glomerular filtration by controlling blood flow through glomerular capillaries.

Glomerular capillary lined by fenestrated endothelial cells. Glomerular basement membrane designates the fused basal laminae of endothelial cells and podocytes.

Glomerular basement membrane

Basement membrane of the Bowman's capsule

Mesangial cell

Urinary space

Podocytes always bulge into the urinary space. Podocytes are components of the visceral layer of the Bowman's capsule.

Urinary pole

Foot process

Filtration slit

Podocyte

Squamous epithelial cells cover the parietal layer of the Bowman's capsule.

Proximal convoluted tubule

Direction of flow of plasma ultrafiltrate.

Fig. 11-6 **Schematic diagram of the renal corpuscle.** *(From Kierszenbaum AL: Histology and cell biology: an introduction to pathology, St Louis, 2002, Mosby. Scanning electron micrograph from Kessel RG, Kardon RH: Tissues and organs, New York, 1979, WH Freeman.)*

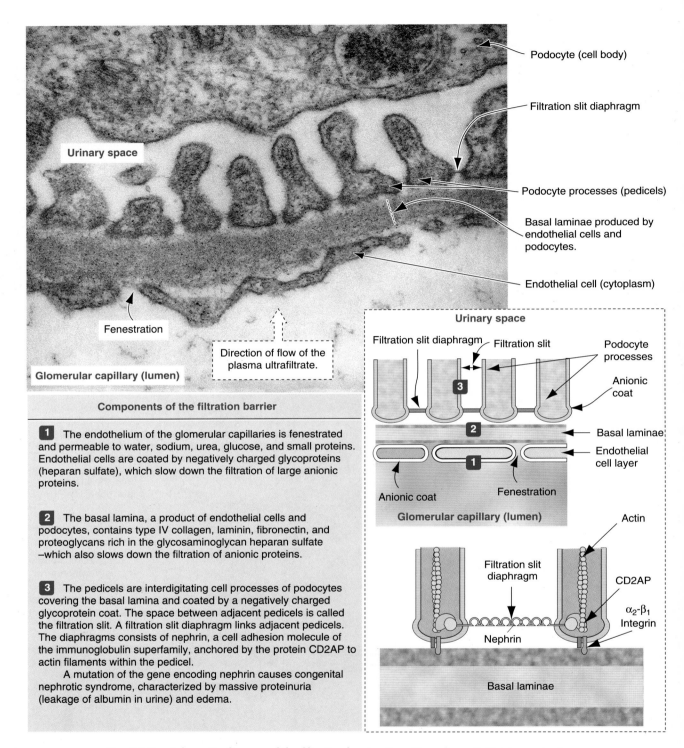

Components of the filtration barrier

1 The endothelium of the glomerular capillaries is fenestrated and permeable to water, sodium, urea, glucose, and small proteins. Endothelial cells are coated by negatively charged glycoproteins (heparan sulfate), which slow down the filtration of large anionic proteins.

2 The basal lamina, a product of endothelial cells and podocytes, contains type IV collagen, laminin, fibronectin, and proteoglycans rich in the glycosaminoglycan heparan sulfate –which also slows down the filtration of anionic proteins.

3 The pedicels are interdigitating cell processes of podocytes covering the basal lamina and coated by a negatively charged glycoprotein coat. The space between adjacent pedicels is called the filtration slit. A filtration slit diaphragm links adjacent pedicels. The diaphragms consists of nephrin, a cell adhesion molecule of the immunoglobulin superfamily, anchored by the protein CD2AP to actin filaments within the pedicel.

A mutation of the gene encoding nephrin causes congenital nephrotic syndrome, characterized by massive proteinuria (leakage of albumin in urine) and edema.

Fig. 11-7   **Schematic diagram of the filtration barrier.** *(From Kierszenbaum AL: Histology and cell biology: an introduction to pathology, St Louis, 2002, Mosby.)*

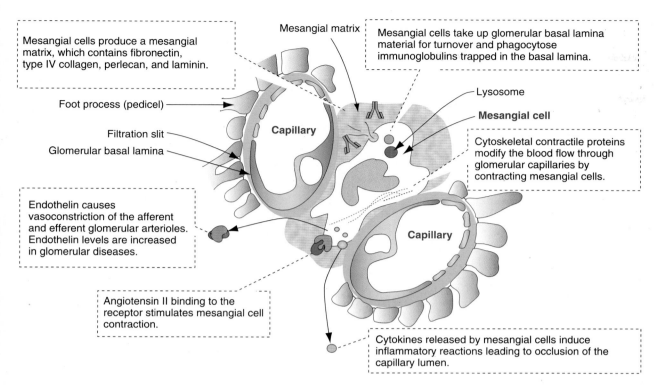

Mesangial cells produce a mesangial matrix, which contains fibronectin, type IV collagen, perlecan, and laminin.

Mesangial matrix

Mesangial cells take up glomerular basal lamina material for turnover and phagocytose immunoglobulins trapped in the basal lamina.

Foot process (pedicel)

Filtration slit

Glomerular basal lamina

Capillary

Lysosome

Mesangial cell

Cytoskeletal contractile proteins modify the blood flow through glomerular capillaries by contracting mesangial cells.

Endothelin causes vasoconstriction of the afferent and efferent glomerular arterioles. Endothelin levels are increased in glomerular diseases.

Capillary

Angiotensin II binding to the receptor stimulates mesangial cell contraction.

Cytokines released by mesangial cells induce inflammatory reactions leading to occlusion of the capillary lumen.

Fig. 11-8 Schematic diagram of the functions and organization of the mesangium. *(From Kierszenbaum AL: Histology and cell biology: an introduction to pathology, St Louis, 2002, Mosby.)*

pluripotential mesenchymal cells that are contractile and phagocytic, which besides being capable of synthesizing collagen and mesangial matrix, also secrete inflammatory mediators.

In addition to the principal glomerular function of plasma filtration, glomerular functions also include regulation of blood pressure by means of secreting vasopressor agents and/or hormones, regulation of peritubular blood flow, regulation of tubular metabolism, and removal of macromolecules from circulation by the glomerular mesangium. Integral to these functions is the juxtaglomerular apparatus, which functions in tubuloglomerular feedback by autoregulating renal blood flow and glomerular filtration rate. The juxtaglomerular apparatus is composed of four components: (1) an afferent arteriole whose smooth muscle is modified to form myoepithelial cells, which are the juxtaglomerular cells that secrete renin; (2) an efferent arteriole; (3) the macula densa; and (4) the extraglomerular mesangium (Fig. 11-9). Renin, produced by cells of the juxtaglomerular apparatus, stimulates the production of angiotensin I from circulating angiotensinogen. The angiotensin-converting enzyme in the macula densa converts angiotensin I to angiotensin II, which then functions to constrict afferent renal arterioles; maintain renal blood

pressure; stimulate aldosterone secretion from the adrenal gland, thus increasing sodium reabsorption; and stimulate antidiuretic hormone (ADH) release. ADH principally increases the permeability of collecting tubules to water and increases the permeability of the medullary region to urea.

The proximal and distal convoluted tubules are linked by the loop of Henle, which is divided into a descending and an ascending limb. The wall of the descending limb and initial portion of the ascending limb is thin (permeable), whereas the cortical portion of the ascending limb is thick (impermeable) (Fig. 11-5). The uriniferous tubule is the name given to the nephron and the collecting duct.

The proximal tubule is lined by columnar epithelial cells that have a microvillous (brush) border, which greatly increases their absorptive surface. A major function of the proximal tubules is to reabsorb sodium, chloride, potassium, albumin, glucose, water, and bicarbonate. This is facilitated by luminal brush border, basolateral infoldings, magnesium-dependent sodium and potassium pumps, and transport proteins. The proximal tubule is continuous with the loop of Henle that is in close physiologic and anatomic association with the peritubular capillary network (within the cortex) and

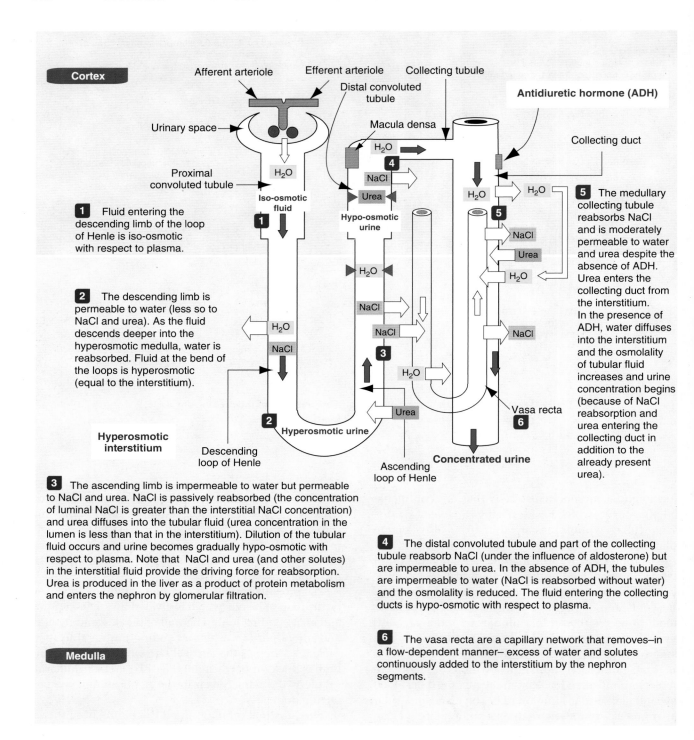

Cortex

Afferent arteriole   Efferent arteriole   Collecting tubule

Distal convoluted tubule

Antidiuretic hormone (ADH)

Urinary space

Macula densa

Collecting duct

Proximal convoluted tubule

H_2O

Iso-osmotic fluid

1 Fluid entering the descending limb of the loop of Henle is iso-osmotic with respect to plasma.

H_2O

H_2O

H_2O

4

NaCl

Urea

Hypo-osmotic urine

H_2O

NaCl

Urea

H_2O

5

NaCl

5 The medullary collecting tubule reabsorbs NaCl and is moderately permeable to water and urea despite the absence of ADH. Urea enters the collecting duct from the interstitium. In the presence of ADH, water diffuses into the interstitium and the osmolality of tubular fluid increases and urine concentration begins (because of NaCl reabsorption and urea entering the collecting duct in addition to the already present urea).

2 The descending limb is permeable to water (less so to NaCl and urea). As the fluid descends deeper into the hyperosmotic medulla, water is reabsorbed. Fluid at the bend of the loops is hyperosmotic (equal to the interstitium).

H_2O

NaCl

H_2O

NaCl

NaCl

3

H_2O

H_2O

NaCl

Hyperosmotic interstitium

2

Urea

Hyperosmotic urine

Descending loop of Henle

Ascending loop of Henle

Urea

Vasa recta

6

Concentrated urine

3 The ascending limb is impermeable to water but permeable to NaCl and urea. NaCl is passively reabsorbed (the concentration of luminal NaCl is greater than the interstitial NaCl concentration) and urea diffuses into the tubular fluid (urea concentration in the lumen is less than that in the interstitium). Dilution of the tubular fluid occurs and urine becomes gradually hypo-osmotic with respect to plasma. Note that NaCl and urea (and other solutes) in the interstitial fluid provide the driving force for reabsorption. Urea is produced in the liver as a product of protein metabolism and enters the nephron by glomerular filtration.

4 The distal convoluted tubule and part of the collecting tubule reabsorb NaCl (under the influence of aldosterone) but are impermeable to urea. In the absence of ADH, the tubules are impermeable to water (NaCl is reabsorbed without water) and the osmolality is reduced. The fluid entering the collecting ducts is hypo-osmotic with respect to plasma.

6 The vasa recta are a capillary network that removes–in a flow-dependent manner– excess of water and solutes continuously added to the interstitium by the nephron segments.

Medulla

Fig. 11-9   Schematic diagram of the counter-current multiplier and exchanger. *(From Kierszenbaum AL: Histology and cell biology: an introduction to pathology, St Louis, 2002, Mosby.)*

the vasa recta (within the medulla). The loop of Henle, via a countercurrent mechanism and sodium and potassium ATPase pumps, absorbs Na+ and Cl– ions, producing a hypotonic filtrate that flows into the next portion of the nephron–the distal convoluted tubule.

Here, water is reabsorbed from the tubule into the interstitium because of a solute concentration gradient and by the effects of antidiuretic hormone. The filtrate is further concentrated in the collecting ducts by water and sodium reabsorption by a sodium-potassium

ATPase pump and additional water reabsorption into the medullary interstitium by a urea gradient. Intercalated cells of the collecting tubule regulate acid-base balance and reabsorb potassium. Thus the final excretory product, urine, is formed (Fig. 11-10).

The interstitium consists of a relatively scant connective tissue stroma, primarily present as a reticular meshwork found around and between uriniferous tubules. Blood vessels, nerves, and lymphatics are also present in the renal interstitium.

Interlobular arteries have small branches that become afferent glomerular arterioles, which enter the renal corpuscle and subsequently exit at the vascular pole as efferent glomerular arterioles (Fig.11-4).

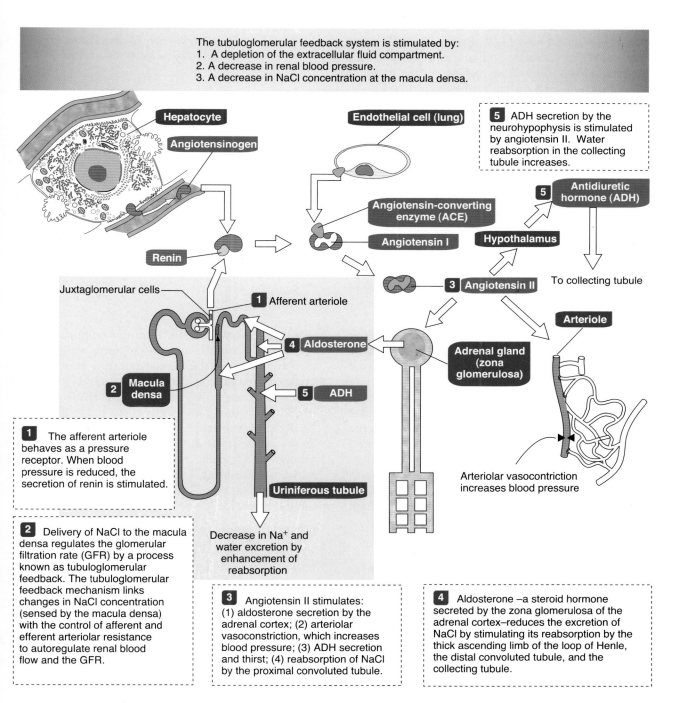

The tubuloglomerular feedback system is stimulated by:
1. A depletion of the extracellular fluid compartment.
2. A decrease in renal blood pressure.
3. A decrease in NaCl concentration at the macula densa.

Hepatocyte

Angiotensinogen

Endothelial cell (lung)

5 ADH secretion by the neurohypophysis is stimulated by angiotensin II. Water reabsorption in the collecting tubule increases.

Angiotensin-converting enzyme (ACE)

Renin

Angiotensin I

5 Antidiuretic hormone (ADH)

Hypothalamus

Juxtaglomerular cells

3 Angiotensin II

To collecting tubule

1 Afferent arteriole

Arteriole

4 Aldosterone

Adrenal gland (zona glomerulosa)

2 Macula densa

5 ADH

1 The afferent arteriole behaves as a pressure receptor. When blood pressure is reduced, the secretion of renin is stimulated.

Uriniferous tubule

Arteriolar vasocontriction increases blood pressure

2 Delivery of NaCl to the macula densa regulates the glomerular filtration rate (GFR) by a process known as tubuloglomerular feedback. The tubuloglomerular feedback mechanism links changes in NaCl concentration (sensed by the macula densa) with the control of afferent and efferent arteriolar resistance to autoregulate renal blood flow and the GFR.

Decrease in Na$^+$ and water excretion by enhancement of reabsorption

3 Angiotensin II stimulates: (1) aldosterone secretion by the adrenal cortex; (2) arteriolar vasoconstriction, which increases blood pressure; (3) ADH secretion and thirst; (4) reabsorption of NaCl by the proximal convoluted tubule.

4 Aldosterone –a steroid hormone secreted by the zona glomerulosa of the adrenal cortex–reduces the excretion of NaCl by stimulating its reabsorption by the thick ascending limb of the loop of Henle, the distal convoluted tubule, and the collecting tubule.

Fig. 11-10 Schematic diagram of the renin-angiotensin-aldosterone system. (*From Kierszenbaum AL: Histology and cell biology: an introduction to pathology, St Louis, 2002, Mosby.*)

Efferent arterioles supply the blood for the extensive network of capillaries that surround the cortical and medullary tubular system of the kidneys, known as the peritubular capillary network. The latter surrounds cortical segments of the tubules and then drains into the interlobular vein, arcuate vein, interlobar vein, and ultimately the renal vein. Additionally, the vasa recta are formed from the deeper portions of the peritubular network and descend into the medulla and around the lower portions of the loops of Henle before ascending to the cortex and emptying into venous vessels that connect to the interlobular and arcuate veins. The vasa recta parallel the descending and ascending limbs of the loop of Henle and the collecting ducts (Fig. 11-5).

RENAL FUNCTION

Renal function can be summarized into five basic components:

1. Formation of urine for the purpose of elimination of metabolic wastes.
2. Acid-base regulation, predominantly through reclamation of bicarbonate from the glomerular filtrate.
3. The conservation of water through reabsorption by the proximal convoluted tubules, the countercurrent mechanism of the loop of Henle, antidiuretic hormone activity in the distal tubules, and the urea gradient in the medulla. The tubular system is capable of absorbing up to 99% of the water in the glomerular filtrate.
4. The maintenance of normal extracellular potassium ion concentration through passive reabsorption in the proximal tubules and tubular secretion in the distal tubules under the influence of aldosterone.
5. Endocrine function through three hormonal axes: renin-angiotensin (Fig. 11-9), most importantly, but also erythropoietin and vitamin D. Erythropoietin, produced in the kidneys in response to reduced oxygen tension, is released into the blood and stimulates bone marrow to produce erythrocytes. Vitamin D is converted in the kidneys to its most active form (1,25-dihydroxycholecalciferol [calcitriol]), which facilitates calcium absorption by the intestine.

PORTALS OF ENTRY

The renal system can be exposed to injurious stimuli and agents (e.g., bacteria by various routes, including ascension from the exterior via the urethra, urinary bladder, and ureters hematogenously and by exposure to preformed or locally metabolized substances that are excreted through the renal tubular system (Box 11-1). The first of these is relatively unique in that few body systems have an opening to the exterior, and these are rarely blind-ended as in the urinary system. Hence, ascending infection from the exterior can localize and be perpetuated in the kidneys. Common etiologic agents

---

Box **11-1**

Portals of Entry to the Kidney

ASCENSION

- Extension from lower urinary tract secondary to gastrointestinal content contamination (diarrhea) (females primarily)
- Extension from lower urinary tract secondary to genital tract contamination (pyometra) (females exclusively)
- Extension from lower urinary tract secondary to dermal contamination (perivulvar dermatitis)

HEMATOGENOUS

- Localization within corticomedullary vessels
  - Septic–embolic nephritis
  - Nonseptic necrosis with infarction
- Localization within large renal vasculature
  - Massive infarction
- Localization within glomerular tufts
- Localization within interstitial vessels

METABOLIC PROCESSING IN RENAL TUBULES

- Activation of products in proximal tubules–necrosis
- Presence of heavy metal–mercury, cadmium
- Crystalline oversaturation
- Direct toxic action–cisplatin

---

in this process, such as bacteria, may originate from the exterior skin surface and the adjacent orifices of the intestinal tract or the genital tract. As in all visceral organs, the sustaining blood supply can provide a portal of hematogenous entry for infectious organisms, which in the case of the kidney leads to arterial or glomerular localization. Substances secreted into the filtrate, such as crystalline salts, can produce localized trauma to tubular lining cells. Additionally, filtered toxins or metabolized substances processed by the tubular lining epithelium exert their effect principally on the proximal tubular epithelium.

DEFENSE MECHANISMS

Defense mechanisms unique to the renal system have evolved to counteract the typical forms of injury (Box 11-2). The most notable of these includes barrier systems, such as those of the tubular basement membranes and more importantly the glomerular filtration membranes (Fig. 11-8). The latter is structurally adept at separating substances based on size and charge. Additionally, the glomerulus is equipped with its own clearance mechanism, a function of mesangial cells (Fig. 11-9). Finally, innate humoral and cellular responses by the immune system contribute to protection, but can also be responsible for renal damage.

Box **11-2**

Defense Mechanisms against Injury and Infectious Agents

- Barrier system–glomerular basement membrane
- Monocyte-macrophage system–glomerular mesangium
- Immune system
  - Innate responses
  - Humoral responses
  - Cellular responses

RESPONSES TO INJURY

The response of the urinary system to injury is the response of each of its components–kidneys, ureters, urinary bladder, and urethra–to injury. This will be described sequentially in this chapter and is summarized in Box 11-3. It is important to remember that the functional unit of the kidney is the nephron and that damage to any component of the nephron (renal corpuscle and tubules) results in diminished function and progressive damage to the kidney. Renal disease can be best summarized by dividing it into general tissue responses that affect the primary anatomic components: glomeruli, tubules, interstitium, and vasculature. In the early stages of diseases, specific anatomic components may be targeted by specific insults: glomeruli in immune-mediated disease and tubules in toxin-induced necrosis. But in the more chronic stages of disease, the kidney undergoes changes related to nephron loss that are not specific to the original cause but are considered common end-stage responses to many injurious stimuli.

Primary glomerular damage often occurs as a result of deposition of immune complexes, entrapment of thromboemboli and bacterial emboli, or direct viral or bacterial infection of glomerular components. Such insults are reflected morphologically by necrosis, proliferation of glomerular cells or membranes, or infiltration of leukocytes, and functionally by reduced vascular perfusion or increased vascular permeability, the latter of which is characterized by leakage of large quantities of plasma proteins and other molecules (bicarbonate ions and chloride) into the glomerular filtrate. Continued or severe injury can result in chronic changes characterized at first by atrophy and fibrosis of the glomerular tuft and secondarily by atrophy of renal tubules. Similar chronic glomerular changes can result from reduced blood flow or chronic loss of tubular function.

Box **11-3**

Renal Responses to Injury

GLOMERULI

Necrosis
Glomerular cell proliferation
Glomerular basement membrane proliferation
Mesangial cell proliferation
Infiltration of leukocytes
Reduced vascular perfusion
Increased vascular permeability
Atrophy of the glomerular tuft
Fibrosis of the glomerular tuft

TUBULES

Cell degeneration
Cell necrosis
Cell apoptosis
Cell atrophy
Basement membrane rupture
Basement membrane thickening
Cell regeneration
Compensatory hypertrophy

INTERSTITIUM

Edema
Hemorrhage
Inflammation
Fibrosis

VASCULATURE

Thrombosis
Sclerosis
Basement membrane thickening
Endothelial cell hypertrophy

Renal tubular epithelial cells can respond to injury by undergoing degeneration, necrosis, apoptosis, and/or atrophy. The basement membrane can respond by rupture or thickening. Tubular disease occurs as a result of tubular epithelial damage from the following:
1. Blood-borne infections (innocent bystander effect)
2. Ascending infections (intratubular pathogens)
3. Direct damage from toxins (intratubular effects)
4. Ischemia

When nephrons are lost because of injury, remaining tubules can undergo compensatory hypertrophy in an attempt to maintain overall renal function, but there is no regeneration of nephrons. In many instances of tubular epithelial cell necrosis, particularly as a response to toxins, tubular epithelium can regenerate and contribute to restoration of function. Severe damage to or loss of tubular basement membranes, as occurs following ischemic damage, results in necrosis and loss of tubular segments, failure of functional repair, and permanent loss of function of the entire nephron. Tubular atrophy can occur secondary to the following:

1. External compression
2. Interstitial fibrosis
3. Intratubular obstruction
4. Diminished glomerular perfusion and filtration
5. Reduced oxygen tension

The renal interstitium is the fibrovascular stroma that surrounds the nephron and is significantly involved in renal diseases, whether or not this is of primary interstitial origin or subsequent to tubular damage, it is often referred to as tubulointerstitial disease. Interstitial inflammation occurs as the result of ascending urinary tract infections (pyelonephritis), systemically derived infections of tubules and interstitium, and secondary to injury of tubules or glomeruli. Common acute lesions of the interstitium include edema, hemorrhage, and inflammation characterized by infiltration of neutrophils. As lesions become subacute to chronic, neutrophils become less prominent, and in several diseases, infiltrates of macrophages, lymphocytes, and plasma cells predominate. With chronic injury to or following atrophy of nephrons, fibrosis of the interstitium can be severe, resulting in notable reduction in nephron function and perpetuation of the renal disease.

Injury to or obstruction of any component that significantly decreases or blocks renal function can result in major systemic effects, including azotemia; uremia; plasma protein loss; water, electrolyte, and acid-base imbalances; retention of drugs; and hyperparathyroidism and osteodystrophy of renal origin.

LOWER URINARY TRACT

STRUCTURE AND FUNCTION

The lower urinary tract is the conduit for the transport of urinary waste from the kidney to the exterior through paired ureters, the urinary bladder, and the urethra. The ureters enter the bladder wall obliquely and are covered by a mucosal flap, the vesicoureteral valve, which is an important structure because it normally prevents reflux of urine from the bladder into the ureter and renal pelvis. At death, the urinary bladder can contract to such a degree that the normal bladder wall appears thick on necropsy. The normal mucosa of the lower urinary tract should be smooth and glistening. Urine should be clear except in horses, where it is cloudy because of the normal presence of mucus and crystalline material produced by the branched tubuloalveolar mucous glands in the submucosa of the renal pelvis and proximal ureter.

The renal pelvis, ureters, and urinary bladder are lined by transitional epithelium, whereas the urethra is lined by transitional epithelium cranially and stratified squamous epithelium immediately cranial to or at the urethral orifice. Histologically the ureteral mucosa is folded longitudinally; there are poorly defined internal and external longitudinal muscle layers, a prominent middle circular muscle layer, and externally either adventitia or peritoneal serosa. As in other mucous membranes, the lamina propria has small lymphoid follicles which, following inflammation or antigenic stimulation, can be large enough to be seen grossly as discrete, circular, white foci (1 to 2 mm) in the mucosa. The function of the ureter is to propel urine from the kidney to the bladder by peristalsis. Histologically the bladder is an expanded ureter, lined by pseudostratified transitional epithelium ranging from 3 to 14 cells thick, depending on the species and degree of distention. The urinary bladder stores urine, and in concert with the urethra, expels it. During continence, the bladder is relatively flaccid and the urethra acts as a valve. During micturition, contraction of the detrusor muscle (the urinary bladder musculature) pumps urine through the relaxed urethra.

PORTALS OF ENTRY

The lower urinary system can be exposed to injurious stimuli by various routes including the following:

1. Ascension from the external urinary and genital orifices
2. Exposure to preformed, variably concentrated toxins excreted in the urine
3. Following hematogenous spread of infectious organisms, principally bacteria and viruses (Box 11-4)

Damage secondary to ascension of injurious stimuli is a distinct mechanism because the lower urinary tract

---

Box **11-4**

Portals of Entry into Lower Urinary System

ASCENSION FROM EXTERIOR

Extension from exterior secondary to contamination from the gastrointestinal tract

Extension from exterior secondary to contamination from the genital tract

Extension from exterior secondary to contamination from the dermis

HEMATOGENOUS

Localization within transmural vasculature

METABOLIC PROCESSING

Accumulation of toxic levels due to stasis and collection

Urinary tract calculi formation

represents a tubular system that is blind-ended and has only one exit to the exterior, unlike the intestinal system, which is a continuous tubular system. This predisposes to bacterial ascension and entrapment, especially in females. In males, end-stage obstruction is due to the narrow diameter and length of the urethra. Etiologic agents, such as bacteria, may originate from the exterior skin surface or the closely located openings of the intestinal tract and the female genital tract. Bacteria with adhesion capabilities may overcome peristalsis and periodic urine flushing. Regular complete emptying will minimize risks of pathologic changes, in contrast to stasis, retention of urine, and infrequent urinations, which predispose to ascending disease. Concentration of excreted urinary substances can damage the surface of the lower urinary system and predispose it to infection, secondary hyperplasia, or neoplastic responses. The importance of blood supply cannot be overlooked as a portal of entry to the lower urinary tract. The vasculature provides sustenance to the lower urinary system, but compression of thin-walled veins predisposes the urinary bladder to hypoxia and spread of organisms, such as bacteria and viruses.

DEFENSE MECHANISMS

Defense mechanisms unique to the lower urinary system have evolved to counteract the typical forms of injury (Box 11-5). The most notable of these are as follows:
1. The flushing action of urine
2. Peristalsis
3. Inhospitable environment for bacterial growth controlled by urine pH
4. Protective urothelial mucus coating
5. Innate humoral immune response
6. Cellular immune responses

Box **11-5**

Defense Mechanisms against Injury and Infectious Agents

- Urine flow–flushing
- Peristalsis
- pH control
- Urothelial cell protective mucus coat
- Immune system
  - Innate responses
  - Humoral responses
  - Cellular responses

DISEASES OF THE KIDNEY

DEVELOPMENTAL ABNORMALITIES

RENAL APLASIA, HYPOPLASIA, AND DYSPLASIA

Renal aplasia (agenesis) is the failure of development of one or both kidneys, such that there is no recognizable renal tissue present. In these cases, the ureter may be present or absent. If present, the cranial extremity of the ureter begins as a blind pouch. A familial tendency for renal aplasia has been observed in Doberman pinscher and beagle dogs. Because life can be sustained when more than one fourth of renal function is maintained, unilateral aplasia is compatible with life, provided that the other kidney is normal. Unilateral aplasia can go unnoticed during life and be recognized at necropsy. Bilateral aplasia is obviously incompatible with life and occurs sporadically.

Renal hypoplasia designates incomplete development of the kidneys, such that fewer than normal nephrons are present at birth. Renal hypoplasia has been documented as an inherited disease of purebred or cross-bred Large White pigs in New Zealand and described in foals of various breeds, as well as in dogs (Fig. 11-11, *A*) and cats (Fig. 11-11, *B*). Hypoplasia can be unilateral (Fig. 11-11, *B*) or bilateral; it is rare, and it is difficult to diagnose subtle cases at necropsy or microscopically. In cattle and pigs, the number of renal papillae in the hypoplastic kidney can be compared with those in a normal kidney. Hypoplastic kidneys from pigs and foals have a notable reduction in the number of glomeruli. In foals, for example, 5 to 12 glomeruli are present per low-power field in affected kidneys compared with 30 to 35 glomeruli per low-power field in normal adult kidneys. Unless significant renal mass is compromised by this condition, hypoplasia is clinically silent.

Occasionally, some bovine kidneys are found to have reduced numbers of external lobes, but these kidneys are not hypoplastic and are microscopically and functionally normal; the reduction in external lobes merely represents fusion of the lobes. The shrunken, pitted kidneys in young animals, particularly dogs, are often diagnosed as hypoplastic. However, in most of these cases, these small kidneys are due to the following:
1. Renal fibrosis, resulting from renal disease developing at an early age
2. Dysplasia
3. Progressive juvenile nephropathy

Renal dysplasia is an abnormality of altered structural organization resulting from abnormal differentiation and the presence of structures not normally present in nephrogenesis. Cystic renal dysplasia has been described in sheep and is inherited as an autosomal dominant trait. Renal dysplasia occurs infrequently and, like renal

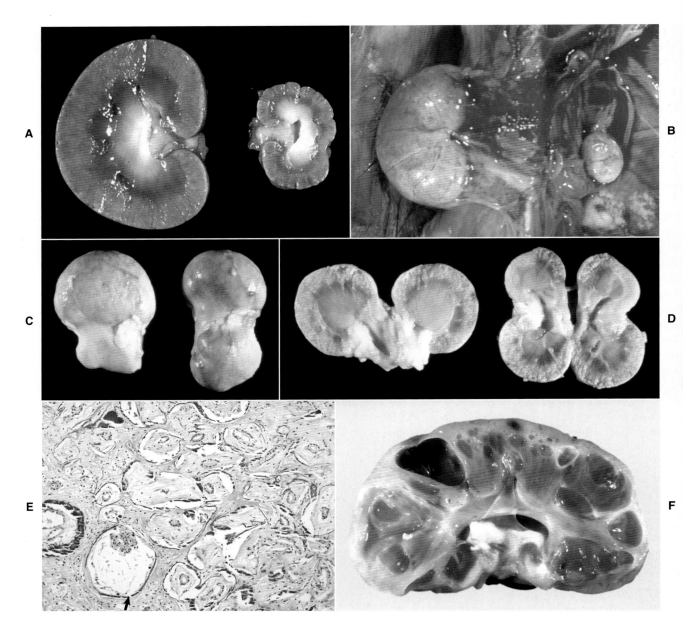

Fig. 11-11 **Types of congenital developmental anomalies, kidney. A,** Unilateral hypoplastic kidney, dorsal sections, young dog. Grossly, the affected right kidney is nearly identical structurally to the left kidney but smaller in size (hypoplasia). **B,** Unilateral hypoplastic kidney, young cat. The left kidney (ventral-dorsal view) is normal in shape and structure but reduced in overall size. **C,** Juvenile progressive nephropathy, young dog. Bilateral abnormally shaped firm kidneys. **D,** Juvenile progressive nephropathy, dorsal sections, dog. Section of the kidneys from Fig 11-11, C. **E,** Juvenile progressive nephropathy, chronic, dog. Note the interstitial fibrosis, tubular atrophy, dilated urinary space, and mineralization. H&E stain. **F,** Polycystic disease, dorsal section, cat. Numerous variably sized tubular cysts are present in the cortex and medulla and affect approximately 60% of the kidney. The cysts contain clear colorless fluid. This condition is hereditary, and Persian cats are predisposed. (*A, Courtesy Dr. B. Weeks, College of Veterinary Medicine, Texas A&M University; and Noah's Arkive, College of Veterinary Medicine, The University of Georgia. B, Courtesy Dr. M. Miller, College of Veterinary Medicine, University of Missouri; and Noah's Arkive, College of Veterinary Medicine, The University of Georgia. C and D, Courtesy College of Veterinary Medicine, University of Illinois. E, Courtesy Dr. S. J. Newman, College of Veterinary Medicine, University of Tennessee. F, Courtesy Dr. A. Confer, College of Veterinary Medicine, Oklahoma State University.*)

hypoplasia, must be differentiated from renal fibrosis and progressive juvenile nephropathy. Dysplastic changes can be unilateral or bilateral and can involve much of an affected kidney or occur only as focal lesions. Dysplastic kidneys can be small, misshapen, or both. Microscopically, five primary features of dysplasia are described as follows:

1. Asynchronous differentiation of nephrons inappropriate for the age of the animal—aggregates of small hypercellular glomeruli in the cortex
2. Persistence of primitive mesenchyme such that the interstitial connective tissue has a myxomatous appearance
3. Persistence of metanephric ducts
4. Atypical (adenomatoid) tubular epithelium
5. The presence of cartilaginous and/or osseous tissue

Interstitial fibrosis, renal cysts, and a few enlarged hypercellular glomeruli (compensatory hypertrophy) are changes seen secondarily to the primary dysplastic changes. The number of nephrons, lobules, and calyces are normal. Bilateral renal dysplasia characterized by persistent mesenchyme and atypical tubular development has been described in foals.

Progressive juvenile nephropathy (familial renal disease) of Lhaso apso, Shih Tzu, golden retriever dogs, and perhaps other canine breeds could be examples of renal dysplasia (Fig. 11-11, *C, D,* and *E*). Asynchronous differentiation is often seen and to a lesser extent several other features of dysplasia. However, until these hereditary lesions of dogs are better characterized, it is probably best to retain the diagnostic term of progressive juvenile nephropathy.

ECTOPIC AND FUSED KIDNEYS

Ectopic kidneys are misplaced from their normal sublumbar location because of abnormal migration during fetal development. Ectopic kidneys occur most frequently in pigs and dogs and usually involve only one kidney. Ectopic locations often include the pelvic cavity or inguinal position. Although ectopic kidneys are usually structurally and functionally normal, malposition of the ureters predisposes them to obstruction, which results in secondary hydronephrosis.

Fused (horseshoe) kidneys result from the fusion of the left and right cranial or left and right caudal poles of the kidneys during nephrogenesis. This fusion results in the appearance of one large kidney with two ureters. The histologic structure and function of the fused kidneys are usually normal.

RENAL CYSTS

Renal cysts are spherical, thin-walled, variably sized distentions principally of the cortical or medullary renal tubules and are filled with clear, watery fluid. Congenital renal cysts can occur as a primary entity or in cases of renal dysplasia. The pathogenesis of primary renal cysts is not entirely understood. Cysts are likely derived from normal or noncystic segments of the nephron, most commonly the renal tubules, the collecting ducts, and Bowman's (uriniferous) space. Although genetic mechanisms can be involved in the pathogenesis of renal cysts, experiments with toxic chemicals indicate that genetic predisposition is not a requirement. Four mechanisms of renal cyst formation are considered plausible:

1. Obstruction of nephrons can cause increased luminal pressure and secondary dilation.
2. Modifications in extracellular matrix and cell-matrix interactions result in weakened tubular basement membranes allowing saccular dilation of tubules.
3. Focal tubular epithelial hyperplasia with production of new basement membranes, increased tubular secretion, and increased intratubular pressure causes development of enlarged, dilated tubules.
4. Dedifferentiation of tubular epithelial cells results in loss of polarity of cells with abnormal cell arrangements in tubules, reduced tubular fluid absorption, increased intratubular pressure, and dilation of tubules.

These mechanisms are not mutually exclusive, and several mechanisms often work in concert to create renal cysts.

Cysts range in size from barely visible to several centimeters in diameter. Cysts are usually spherical, delineated by a thin fibrous connective tissue wall lined by flattened epithelium, and are filled with clear watery fluid. The sources of fluid are glomerular filtrate, transepithelial secretions, or both. When viewed from the renal surface, the cyst wall is pale gray, smooth, and translucent. Cysts can arise anywhere along the nephron and be located in either cortex or medulla. Kidneys can have single or multiple cysts. Some cysts cause no alteration in renal function and therefore are considered incidental findings. Such incidental renal cysts are common in pigs and calves and must be differentiated from hydronephrosis. Acquired renal cysts can occur as a result of renal interstitial fibrosis or other renal diseases that cause intratubular obstruction. These cysts are usually small (1 to 2 mm in diameter) and occur primarily in the cortex.

Polycystic kidneys have many cysts that involve numerous nephrons. Congenital polycystic kidneys occur sporadically in many species, but can be inherited as an autosomal dominant lesion in pigs and lambs and can be inherited along with cystic biliary disease in Cairn and West Highland white terriers. The lesion, termed polycystic kidney disease (PKD), is inherited as an autosomal dominant trait in families of Persian cats and bull terriers. Although less well characterized in animals than in human beings, this autosomal dominant, high penetrance, heritable condition is thought to be related to mutations in one or more genes (PKD-1 and/or PKD-2) and altered function of the related proteins, principally polycystin-1 and polycystin-2. Manifestation of tubular cysts occurs following mutation of both alleles of these genes, the first of which is a germ-line mutation, and the second of which, is somatic. Polycystin-1 is a cell membrane–associated protein with a large extracellular domain. Polycystin-1, the product of PKD-1, is involved in normal cell proliferation and apoptosis pathways. Although the exact mechanisms for cyst formation are not known, polycystin-1 mutations allow cells either to enter a differentiation pathway that results in tubule formation or to become susceptible to apoptosis. Additionally, polycystin 1 is known to be important in both cell adhesion and cell signaling because it is an essential component of desmosomes. Loss of polycystin-1 from its basolateral location may alter critical pathways controlling normal tubulogenesis, thus contributing to cyst formation. Similarly, polycystin-2 functions principally as a localized plasma membrane calcium channel. Further study of these mutated proteins will allow us to narrow the mechanistic pathway of the inherited form, and potentially extrapolate to the acquired and sporadic congenital cystic lesions documented. A polycystic renal disease with cysts arising from glomeruli has been described in collie puppies. The gross appearance of the cut surface of a polycystic kidney has been described as a "Swiss cheese" (Fig. 11-11, F). As cysts enlarge, they compress the adjacent parenchyma. When extensive regions of renal parenchyma are polycystic, renal function can be impaired.

INHERITED ABNORMALITIES IN RENAL TUBULAR FUNCTION

Inherited abnormalities in tubular metabolism, in transport, or in reabsorption of glucose, amino acids, ions, and proteins have been described in dogs. Primary renal glucosuria, an inherited disorder in Norwegian elkhounds and of sporadic occurrence in other dog breeds, occurs when the capacity of tubular epithelial cells to reabsorb glucose is significantly reduced. Gross and histologic lesions are not expected, as this is a functional disorder. Glucosuria most commonly results from diabetes mellitus, acromegaly, or catecholamine release and predisposes dogs to the following:
1. Bacterial infections of the lower urinary tract
2. Urinary bladder emphysema, secondary to splitting of glucose molecules by bacteria (principally *Escherichia coli, Clostridium perfringens,* and rarely with *Candida* yeasts), with release of CO_2 into the bladder lumen and absorption of gas into bladder lymphatics (Fig. 11-12)

A hereditary generalized defect in tubular reabsorption similar to the Fanconi syndrome in human beings has been described in basenji dogs. The underlying tubular defect appears to be abnormal membrane structure of the proximal tubular epithelial cell brush borders because of altered lipid content in the

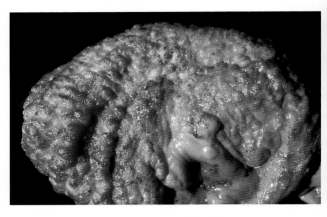

Fig. 11-12 **Emphysema, urinary bladder mucosa, cow.** The multiple "nodules" are mucosal gas bubbles that expand the mucosa and are secondary to bacterial infections of the lower urinary tract (principally by *Escherichia coli, Clostridium perfringens,* and rarely *Candida* yeasts), which result in splitting of glucose molecules to release CO_2 into the bladder lumen, from where the gas can be absorbed into bladder lymphatics. This animal was injected with calcium borogluconate as a calcium source to treat milk fever. Following intravenous injection, calcium ions readily dissociate from the parent molecule, and the resulting gluconate provides a sugar source for resident urinary bacteria. *(Courtesy Dr. M.D. McGavin, College of Veterinary Medicine, University of Tennessee.)*

cell membrane. Gross lesions are not identifiable in the early stages. Histopathologic changes in the kidneys are initially minimal, consisting of irregularly sized tubular epithelial cells in the convoluted tubules and loops of Henle. With time, dogs with Fanconi syndrome develop progressive renal insufficiency and associated renal fibrosis. Aminoaciduria, glucosuria, proteinuria, increased phosphaturia, metabolic acidosis, and multiple endocrine abnormalities characterize this disease clinically.

The excretion of large quantities of cystine in the urine (cystinuria) is a sex-linked inherited disease seen occasionally in purebred and mongrel male dogs. It is of importance because it predisposes affected dogs to calculus formation and obstruction of the lower urinary tract (see Urolithiasis).

GLOMERULAR DISEASES

All functions of the glomerulus include the following:
1. Plasma ultrafiltration
2. Blood pressure regulation
3. Peritubular blood flow regulation
4. Tubular metabolism regulation
5. Circulating macromolecule removal

These are affected by processes that target this structure in disease. Damage to the glomerular filtration barrier can result from several causes and produce a variety of clinical signs. The major clinical finding of glomerular disease is the leakage of various low molecular weight (small molecule size) proteins, such as albumin, into the glomerular filtrate. As a result, large quantities of albumin overload the protein reabsorption capabilities of the proximal convoluted tubular epithelium to such an extent that protein-rich glomerular filtrate accumulates in the variably dilated tubular lumina and protein subsequently appears in the urine. In such diseases, the proximal tubular cells often have microscopic eosinophilic intracytoplasmic bodies referred to as hyaline droplets, which represent accumulations of intracytoplasmic protein absorbed from the filtrate.

Renal diseases that result in proteinuria are called protein-losing nephropathies. Protein-losing nephropathy is one of several causes of severe hypoproteinemia in animals. Prolonged, severe renal protein loss results in hypoproteinemia, reduced plasma colloid osmotic (oncotic) pressure, and loss of antithrombin III. The nephrotic syndrome is further characterized by generalized edema, ascites, pleural effusion, and hypercholesterolemia.

The pathophysiologic mechanisms of glomerular injury from infectious or chemical insults have been summarized by three theories:
1. Intact nephron hypothesis
2. Hyperfiltration hypothesis
3. The theory of complex deposition

The intact nephron hypothesis proposes that damage to any portion of the nephron affects the entire nephron function. This is seen when glomerular damage interferes with peritubular blood flow and results in decreased tubular resorption or secretion. Not all nephron damage is irreversible, but nephrons are not capable of regeneration and thus outcomes vary from hypertrophy to repair.

Unlike the intact nephron hypothesis, the hyperfiltration hypothesis helps explain the progressive nature of glomerular disease. Glomerular hyperfiltration is a result of increased hydrostatic pressure that damages delicate glomerular capillaries and in cases of prolonged hypertension produces a sustained repeating deleterious effect on the glomerulus, ultimately resulting in glomerulosclerosis. Increased dietary protein can produce a transient increase in glomerular hyperfiltration and if persistent can result in glomerulosclerosis. There may be a species effect, as dogs that undergo experimental hyperfiltration are much less prone to development of progressive glomerular disease than are rats.

The theory of complex deposition is derived from the fact that glomeruli are the primary site for removal of macromolecules (principally immune complex) from the circulation. Complexes may be deposited in subepithelial, subendothelial, or mesangial locations. These immune complexes are capable of triggering a sequence of inflammatory events including the following:

1. Recruitment and localization of inflammatory cells at the site
2. Release of inflammatory mediators and enzymes
3. Destruction of glomerular structures
4. Further compromise of nephron function
5. Continuing damage by altered transglomerular hyperfiltration and perfusion shifts between nephron populations

Different forms of glomerulonephritis including bacterial, viral, chemical, and immune-mediated will be discussed in the next section.

SUPPURATIVE GLOMERULITIS (EMBOLIC NEPHRITIS)

Suppurative glomerulitis, which can also be referred to as acute embolic nephritis, is the result of a bacteremia, in which bacteria lodge in random glomeruli and to a lesser extent in interstitial capillaries, and cause the formation of multiple foci of inflammation (microabscesses) throughout the renal cortex (Fig. 11-13). A specific example of embolic nephritis is actinobacillosis of foals caused by *Actinobacillus equuli*. These foals usually die within a few days of birth and have small abscesses in many visceral organs, especially the renal cortex. Embolic nephritis also occurs commonly in the bacteremias of pigs infected with *Erysipelothrix rhusiopathiae* or sheep and goats infected with *Corynebacterium pseudotuberculosis*.

Grossly, multifocal random, raised, tan pinpoint foci are seen subcapsularly and on the cut surface throughout the renal cortex. Microscopically, glomerular capillaries contain numerous bacterial colonies intermixed with necrotic debris and extensive infiltrates of neutrophils that often obliterate the glomerulus. Glomerular or interstitial hemorrhage can occur as well. As with many other inflammatory diseases, if the affected animal survives, the neutrophilic infiltrates will either persist as focal residual abscesses or be progressively replaced by increasing numbers of lymphocytes, plasma cells, and macrophages; reactive fibroblasts; and ultimately coalescing scars.

VIRAL GLOMERULITIS

Glomerulitis, caused by a direct viral insult to the glomerulus, occurs in acute systemic viral diseases, such as acute infectious canine hepatitis, equine arteritis virus infection, hog cholera, avian Newcastle disease, and neonatal porcine cytomegalovirus infection. The lesions are mild, usually transient, and result from viral replication in capillary endothelium. Acute viral glomerulonephritis produces the following gross lesions:
1. Kidneys are often slightly swollen.
2. Renal capsular surface is smooth.
3. Kidneys are normal color or pale.
4. Glomeruli are visible as pinpoint red dots on the cut surface of the cortex.

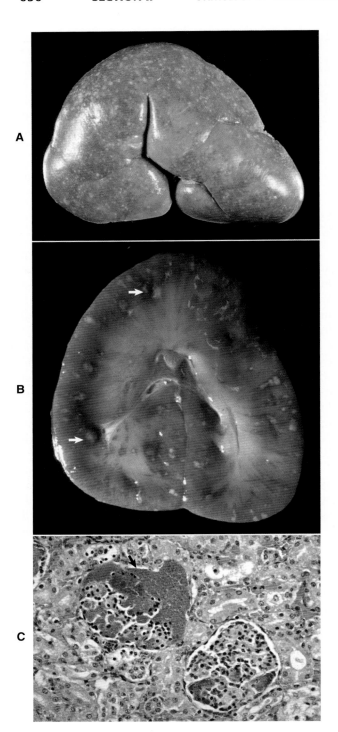

Viral-induced intranuclear inclusions are present in glomerular capillary endothelium from viremias of infectious canine hepatitis and cytomegalovirus infections. The inclusions of each disease are similar and are usually large, basophilic to magenta, and either fill the nucleus or are separated from the nuclear membrane by a clear halo. In the other diseases (equine arteritis, hog cholera, and avian Newcastle), viral antigens can be demonstrated in endothelium, epithelium, or mesangial cells by immunofluorescence or immunohistochemistry. In cases of viral glomerulitis, lesions include endothelial hypertrophy, a thickened and edematous mesangium, hemorrhages, and necrosis of endothelium. Clinically, animals are systemically ill from the viral infection, but the glomerular signs are specifically those of a transient proteinuria.

CHEMICAL GLOMERULONEPHRITIS

Although much less common than the immune-mediated forms of glomerulonephritis, chemically induced glomerular disease occurs in a variety of different ways. Chemicals typically induce glomerular injury by any of the following:
1. Direct injury to glomerular epithelial cells
2. Direct injury to endothelial cells of the glomerulus
3. Altered renal blood flow
4. Induction of immunologic reactions and inflammatory responses, which may occur following:
   a. Incorporation of drugs into immune complexes
   b. The formation and targeted deposition of antigen-antibody complexes
   c. The formation of antinuclear antibodies
   d. The formation of antibasement membrane antibodies within the glomerular tuft

Puromycin aminonucleoside, adriamycin, and histamine-receptor antagonists all induce proteinuria through targeted damage to glomerular epithelial cells. The immunosuppressive drug, cyclosporine A,

Fig. 11-13   Embolic nephritis (suppurative glomerulitis), kidney, horse. A, Multiple, small pale white necrotic foci and abscesses are present subcapsularly. **B,** Dorsal section. Variably sized abscesses are scattered throughout the cortex (*arrows*). **C,** Causative bacteria (*arrow*) enter the kidney via the vasculature (bacteremia) and lodge in the capillaries of glomeruli, where they replicate and induce necrosis and inflammation. H&E stain. (*A, Courtesy Dr. A. Confer, College of Veterinary Medicine, Oklahoma State University. B, Courtesy Dr. M.D. McGavin, College of Veterinary Medicine, University of Tennessee. C, Courtesy Dr. W. Crowell, College of Veterinary Medicine, The University of Georgia; and Noah's Arkive, College of Veterinary Medicine, The University of Georgia.*)

alters renal perfusion and ultimately the glomerular filtration rate by damaging glomerular endothelial cells. Examples of foreign substances capable of producing immune complexes include injectable hyperimmune serum, gold, and d-penicillamine. Procainamide and hydralazine result in production of antinuclear antibodies, and occupational exposure to hydrocarbon solvents can create antibasement membrane antibodies. Often drug-induced lesions lead to irreversible nephron loss and compensatory cellular and functional hypertrophy of other nephrons. The continuing physical loss of nephrons sets up a cycle for an increase in glomerular hypertension and hyperfiltration, which results in glomerulosclerosis, progressive nephron loss, and interstitial fibrosis.

IMMUNE-MEDIATED GLOMERULONEPHRITIS

Glomerulonephritis most often results from immune-mediated mechanisms, most notably following the deposition of soluble immune complexes within the glomeruli and less commonly following the formation of antibodies directed against antigens within the glomerular basement membrane. Antibodies to the basement membrane (antibasement membrane disease) bind and damage the glomerulus through fixation of complement and resulting leukocyte infiltration. This mechanism of glomerulonephritis has been well documented in human beings and nonhuman primates but only rarely in other domestic animals. To confirm the diagnosis of antibasement membrane disease, immunoglobulin (Ig) and complement (C3) must be demonstrated within glomeruli. Antibodies must be eluted from the kidneys and found to bind to normal glomerular basement membranes of the appropriate species.

Immune-complex glomerulonephritis occurs in association with persistent infections, or other diseases that characteristically have a prolonged antigenemia that enhances the formation of soluble immune complexes. In domestic animals, immune-complex glomerulonephritis occurs most commonly in dogs and cats. Immune-complex glomerulonephritis is associated with specific viral infections, such as feline leukemia virus or feline infectious peritonitis virus; chronic bacterial infections, such as pyometra or pyoderma; chronic parasitism, such as dirofilariasis; autoimmune diseases, such as canine systemic lupus erythematosus; and neoplasia (Box 11-6). In addition to the role of persistent infections, a familial tendency for development of immune-complex glomerulonephritis has been described in a group of related Bernese mountain dogs.

Immune-complex glomerulonephritis is initiated by the formation of soluble immune complexes

---

Box **11-6**

Diseases with Immune-Complex Glomerulonephritis

HORSES
Equine infectious anemia
Streptococcus sp.

CATTLE
Bovine viral diarrhea
Trypanosomiasis

SHEEP
Hereditary hypocomplementemia in Finnish Landrace lambs

PIGS
Hog cholera
African swine fever

DOGS
Infectious canine hepatitis
Chronic hepatitis
Chronic bacterial diseases
Endometritis (pyometra)
Pyoderma
Prostatitis
Dirofilariasis
Borreliosis (Lyme disease)
Systemic lupus erythematosus
Polyarteritis
Autoimmune hemolytic anemia
Immune-mediated polyarthritis
Neoplasia—mastocytoma
Hereditary C3 deficiency

CATS
Feline leukemia virus infection
Feline infectious peritonitis
Feline immunodeficiency virus
Progressive polyarteritis
Neoplasia
Progressive membranous glomerulonephritis

(antigen-antibody complexes) in the presence of antigen-antibody equivalency or slight antigen excess, which then do the following:
1. Selectively deposit in the glomerular capillaries
2. Stimulate complement fixation with formation of C3a, C5a, and C567, which are chemotactic for neutrophils
3. Damage the basement membrane through neutrophil release of proteinases, arachidonic acid metabolites (such as thromboxane), and oxidants, particularly oxygen-derived free radicals and hydrogen peroxide

4. Continue to damage the glomeruli by the release of biologically active molecules from monocyte infiltrations in the later stages of inflammation (Fig. 11-14, *A*)

Although circulating immune complexes may contribute to this process, antibody binding to endogenous glomerular antigens or entrapped nonspecific antigens is more common. Direct action of C5b-C9 on the glomerular components results in activation of both glomerular epithelial cells and mesangial cells to produce damaging mediators, such as oxidants and proteases.

Many specific factors determine the extent of deposition of soluble immune complexes in the glomerular capillary walls. These include persistence of appropriate quantities of immune complexes in the circulation, glomerular permeability, the size and molecular charge of the soluble complexes, and the strength of the bond between the antigen and antibody (avidity). Small or intermediate complexes are the most damaging, because large complexes are removed from circulation through phagocytosis by cells of the monocyte-macrophage system in the liver and spleen. An increase in local glomerular vascular permeability is necessary for immune complexes to leave the microcirculation and deposit in the glomerulus. This process is usually facilitated via vasoactive amine release from mast cells, basophils, or platelets (Fig. 11-14, *A*). Mast cells or basophils release vasoactive amines as a result of the interaction of the immune complexes with antigen-specific IgE on the surface of these cells, by stimulation of the mast cells or basophils by cationic proteins released from neutrophils, or by the anaphylatoxin activity of C3a and C5a. Platelet-activating factor (PAF) is released from immune complex–stimulated mast cells, basophils, or macrophages and causes platelets to release vasoactive amines.

Localization of the complexes within the various levels of the basement membrane or in subepithelial

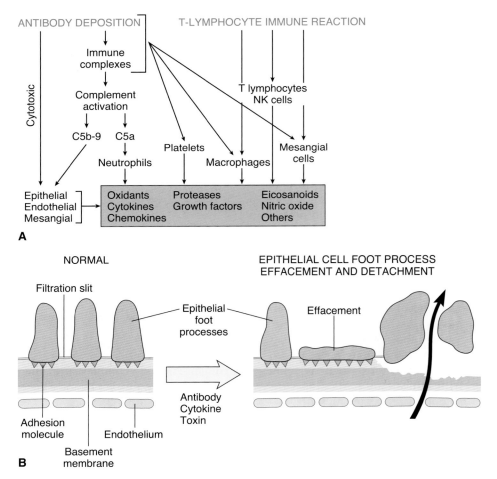

Fig. 11-14   **Schematic diagram of the mediators of immune glomerular injury and epithelial cell injury. A,** Mediators of immune glomerular injury. **B,** Epithelial cell injury. The postulated sequence is a consequence of antibodies to epithelial cell antigens, with subsequent toxins, cytokines, or other factors causing injury and detachment of epithelial cells, resulting in protein leakage through the defective glomerular basement membrane and filtration slits. (*A* and *B, From Kumar V, Abbas AK, Fausto N: Robbins & Cotran pathologic basis of disease, ed 7, Philadelphia, 2005, Saunders.*)

locations depends on their molecular charge and avidity. Once small, soluble immune complexes are deposited within the capillary wall, they can become greatly enlarged as a result of interactions of immune complexes with free antibodies, free antigens, complement components, or other immune complexes.

After immune-complex deposition, glomerular injury can also occur from the aggregation of platelets and activation of Hageman factor, which results in the formation of fibrin thrombi that produce glomerular ischemia. Furthermore, glomerular epithelial cell and extracellular matrix damage can result directly from the terminal membrane attack complex of the activated complement cascade (C5 to C9). This can result in epithelial detachment (causing proteinuria) and, glomerular basement membrane thickening subsequent to up-regulation of epithelial cell receptors for transforming growth factor (Fig. 11-14, *B*). Cell-mediated cytotoxic responses (from sensitized T lymphocytes) to glomerular antigens or complexes may exacerbate

renal lesions. Complexes themselves may modulate the immune response through interaction with receptors on various cells (Box 11-7).

Finally, if exposure of the glomerulus to immune complexes is short lived, as in a transient infection, such as infectious canine hepatitis, glomerular immune complexes will be phagocytosed by macrophages or mesangial cells and removed, and the glomerular lesions and clinical signs may resolve. Conversely, continual exposure of glomeruli to soluble immune complexes such as in persistent viral infections (e.g., feline leukemia virus infection) and chronic heartworm disease (Fig. 11-15) can produce progressive glomerular injury, with severe lesions and clinical manifestation of glomerular disease.

Ultrastructurally, immune complexes either in the glomerular basement membrane or in a subepithelial location appear as electron-dense bodies (Figs. 11-15 and 11-16). Complexes that are poorly soluble, fairly large, or of high avidity often enter the mesangium, where they can be phagocytosed by macrophages and

Box **11-7**

Progression of Glomerular Immune-Complex Deposition

Deposition affected by:
1. Appropriate quantities of immune complexes in the circulation
2. Glomerular permeability
3. The size and molecular charge of the soluble complexes
4. Strength of the bond between antigen and antibody

Glomerular permeability affected by:
1. Release of vasoactive amines from mast cells, basophils or platelets
   a. Immune complexes interact with antigen-specific immunoglobulin E on surface of mast cells or basophils
   b. Cationic proteins from neutrophils stimulate release of vasoactive amines from mast cells and basophils
   c. C3a and C5a cause release of vasoactive amines
   d. Platelets release vasoactive amines following release of platelet-activating factor from immune-complex stimulated mast cells, basophils, and macrophages

Glomerular progression affected by:
1. Aggregation of platelets, activation of Hageman factor, fibrin thrombi formation, and glomerular ischemia
2. Terminal membrane active complex of activated complement cascade damages glomerular epithelial cells and extracellular matrix resulting in epithelial cell detachment and basement membrane thickening
3. Cell mediated cytotoxic responses from T lymphocytes sensitized to glomerular antigens or complexes may exacerbate renal lesions

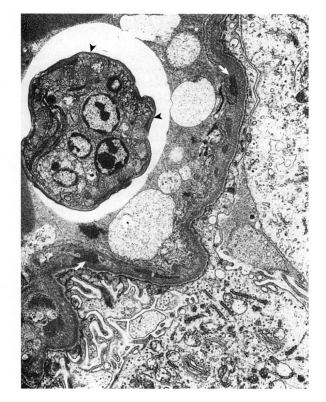

Fig. 11-15 **Immune-complex glomerulonephritis, kidney, glomerulus, dog.** Transmission electron photomicrograph of a glomerulus with immune-complex deposits due to dirofilariasis. A heartworm microfilaria is present in the capillary lumen (*arrowheads*). The basement membrane is irregularly thickened and contains granular, electron-dense deposits (*arrows*). The podocytic foot processes are fused. TEM. Uranyl acetate and lead citrate stain. (*Courtesy Dr. N. Cheville, College of Veterinary Medicine, Iowa State University.*)

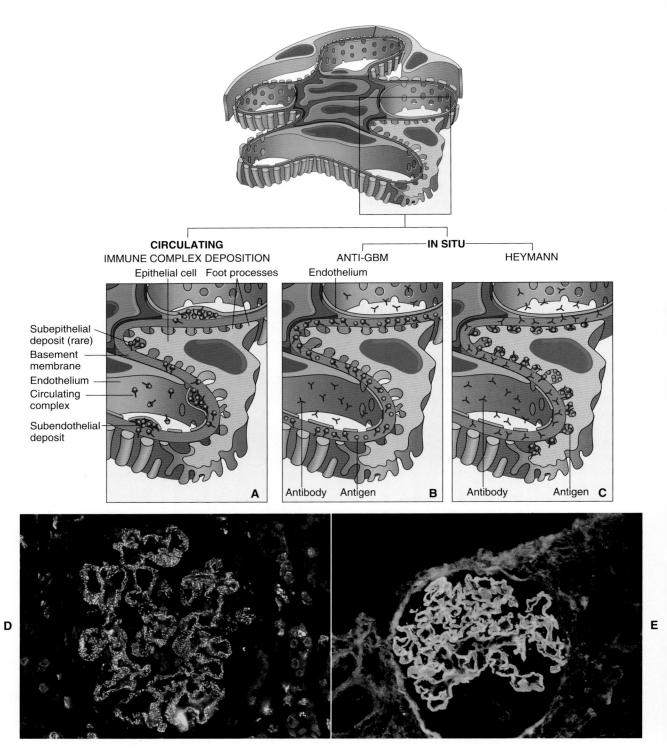

Fig. 11-16 **Schematic diagrams of the antibody-mediated glomerular injury.** Antibody-mediated glomerular injury can result either from the deposition of circulating immune complexes (**A**) or from formation of complexes in situ (**B** and **C**). Antiglomerular basement membrane (*anti-GBM*) disease (**B**) or antitubular deposits (**C**) are characterized by linear immunofluorescence patterns, whereas lesions caused by immune complexes reveal granular patterns. **D** and **E**, Two patterns of deposition of immune complexes as seen by immunofluorescence microscopy: granular, characteristic of circulating and in situ immune complex nephritis (**D**); and linear, characteristic of classic anti-GBM disease (**E**). (*A* through *E, From Kumar V, Abbas AK, Fausto N:* Robbins & Cotran pathologic basis of disease, *ed 7, Philadelphia, 2005, Saunders.*)

appear ultrastructurally as dense granular deposits within the mesangial stroma or within macrophages. Other ultrastructural changes commonly seen are loss or effacement of visceral epithelial cell foot processes, cytoplasmic vacuolation, retraction and detachment of visceral epithelium, and infiltrates of neutrophils and monocytes within the mesangium.

A diagnosis of immune-mediated glomerulonephritis can be made by immunofluorescent or immunohistochemical demonstration of immunoglobulin and complement components, usually C3, in glomerular tufts. In dogs, IgG or IgM are the most common isotypes demonstrated in glomerulonephritis; however, combinations of IgG, IgM, and IgA also occur in the glomeruli of some dogs. In one study, IgA was the only immunoglobulin found in three dogs with immune-complex glomerulonephritis. Both Ig and C3 are usually demonstrated in a granular ("lumpy-bumpy") pattern using immunofluorescent or immunohistochemical techniques (Fig. 11-17); however, in antibasement membrane disease, as reported in human beings and horses, the antibody deposits have a linear distribution conforming to the basement membranes (Fig. 11-16). It is important to remember that fluorescing deposits indicate the presence of immunoglobulin or complement but do not specifically indicate the presence of disease. Additionally, immunofluorescence may be negative when all reactive binding sites are occupied, thus complicating diagnosis of this condition.

The diagnosis of preformed immune-complex glomerulonephritis can be confirmed only by demonstrating that the antibodies from the immune complexes, eluted from glomeruli, are not capable of binding to normal glomerular elements and hence represent deposition of preformed circulating complexes. Once this has been done, the ideal situation would be to identify the causative antigen present in the immune complexes. This process is accomplished by eluting antibodies from diseased glomeruli and attempting to identify their specificity for suspected antigens. For example, antibodies eluted from the glomeruli of dogs with glomerulonephritis associated with severe heartworm disease bind to several *Dirofilaria immitis* antigens, including the body wall of adult worms, parasitic uterine fluid, and microfilaria. In most cases of immune-complex glomerulonephritis, the specific causative antigen usually escapes determination. Demonstration of electron-dense deposits in mesangial, subepithelial, or subendothelial locations by electron microscopy is also supportive of the diagnosis of immune-mediated glomerulonephritis.

Gross lesions of acute immune-complex glomerulonephritis are usually subtle. The kidneys are often slightly swollen, have a smooth capsular surface, are of normal color or pale, and have glomeruli that are visible as pinpoint red dots on the cut surface of the cortex (Fig. 11-18). The normal glomeruli of horses are usually visible, so this feature of pinpoint red dots for glomeruli cannot be used for diagnosis in that species. If lesions do not resolve but become subacute to chronic, the renal cortex becomes somewhat shrunken and the capsular surface has a generalized fine granularity. On cut surface, the cortex can be thinned and granular, and glomeruli can appear as pinpoint pale gray dots. With time, more severe scarring can develop throughout the cortex (see Renal Fibrosis).

Microscopically, immune-complex glomerulonephritis has several histopathologic forms. Although various classifications of glomerulonephritis have been published,

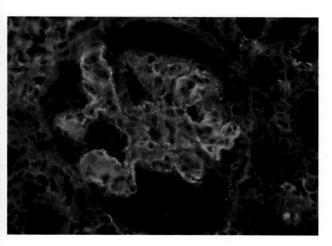

Fig. 11-17   Immune-complex glomerulonephritis, kidney, glomerulus, mink. Intraglomerular immunoglobulin deposits demonstrated by immunofluorescence. Note the granular ("lumpy-bumpy") pattern of fluorescence in this case of Aleutian mink disease. Immunofluorescence microscopy. *(Courtesy Dr. S.J. Newman, College of Veterinary Medicine, University of Tennessee.)*

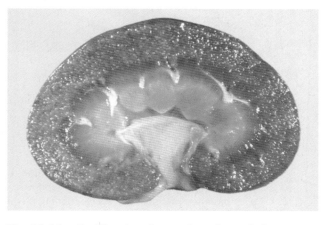

Fig. 11-18   Proliferative glomerulonephritis, kidney, dorsal section, dog. The small, white, round foci in the cortex are enlarged glomeruli. *(Courtesy Dr. S.J. Newman, College of Veterinary Medicine, University of Tennessee.)*

the following simple classification is well understood among veterinary pathologists. Lesions in glomeruli may be described as proliferative, membranous, or membranoproliferative (Figs. 11-19 and 11-20). Glomerular lesions can be distributed diffusely, when most of the glomeruli are involved; focally, when only a certain proportion of glomeruli are involved; globally, when an entire glomerular tuft is involved; and segmentally, when only a portion of the glomerular tuft is affected. Most of the lesions in immune-complex glomerulonephritis are diffuse, but within an individual affected glomerulus, the lesions can be either global or segmental.

Microscopic details of each type of glomerular disease are outlined in the next section.

PROLIFERATIVE GLOMERULONEPHRITIS

Proliferative glomerulonephritis is a form of immune-complex glomerular disease characterized by increased cellularity of the glomerular tufts caused by proliferation of glomerular endothelial, epithelial, and mesangial cells and an influx of neutrophils and other leukocytes and

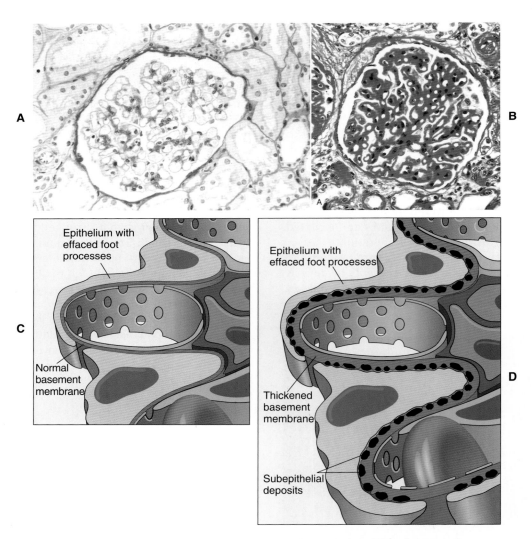

Fig. 11-19   **Schematic diagram of lupoid nephrosis (A and C) and membranous glomerulonephritis (B and D). A,** Lupoid nephrosis. The glomerulus appears normal, with a thin basement membrane. PAS reaction. **B,** Membranous glomerulonephritis. The glomerular basement membrane is diffusely thickened. PAS reaction. **C,** Lupoid nephrosis. Diffuse loss of foot processes of visceral epithelial cells. **D,** Membranous glomerulonephritis is characterized by subepithelial deposits, which by transmission electron microscopy are electron dense, and by loss of foot processes. *(A through D, From Cotran RS, Rennke H, Kumar V: The kidney and its collecting system, ed 7, Philadelphia, 2002, Saunders.)*

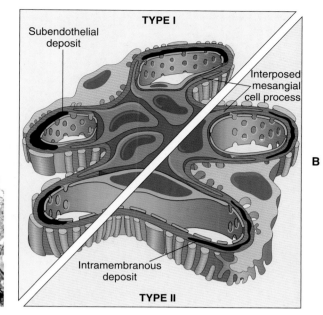

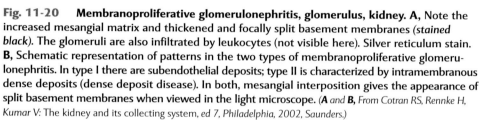

Fig. 11-20   **Membranoproliferative glomerulonephritis, glomerulus, kidney. A,** Note the increased mesangial matrix and thickened and focally split basement membranes *(stained black).* The glomeruli are also infiltrated by leukocytes (not visible here). Silver reticulum stain. **B,** Schematic representation of patterns in the two types of membranoproliferative glomerulonephritis. In type I there are subendothelial deposits; type II is characterized by intramembranous dense deposits (dense deposit disease). In both, mesangial interposition gives the appearance of split basement membranes when viewed in the light microscope. *(**A** and **B**, From Cotran RS, Rennke H, Kumar V: The kidney and its collecting system, ed 7, Philadelphia, 2002, Saunders.)*

involves both the capillary loops and the mesangium (Fig. 11-21, *A*).

MEMBRANOUS GLOMERULONEPHRITIS

Membranous glomerulonephritis is characterized by diffuse glomerular capillary basement membrane thickening because of the presence of subepithelial immunoglobulin deposits, as the predominant change (Figs. 11-21, *B*; 11-19; and 11-20). These deposits are separated by protrusions of glomerular basement membrane matrix that eventually encompass these deposits. Following removal of the deposited material, cavities are left in the glomerular basement membrane and later these fill with glomerular basement membrane-like material, which results in sclerotic change within the glomerular tuft. This is characterized by increased deposition of (periodic acid–Schiff) positive material and a lesser amount of fibrosis. This variation is the most common form of immune-complex glomerulonephritis in cats.

MEMBRANOPROLIFERATIVE GLOMERULONEPHRITIS

Membranoproliferative glomerulonephritis (mesangioproliferative, mesangiocapillary) is characterized by hypercellularity following proliferation of glomerular

cells and thickening of the capillary basement membrane and mesangium (Figs. 11-19 and 11-20). This variant appears to be the most common morphologic form of immune-complex glomerulonephritis in the dog. Light microscopy fails to detect differences evident by immunofluorescent and electron microscopy. The latter allows subcategorization of membranoproliferative glomerulonephritis into type I and type II (Fig. 11-19). Type I is characterized by the presence of subendothelial deposits and a granular pattern following deposition of C3 and lesser quantities of IgG, C1q, and C4. Type I disease appears to be secondary to deposition of circulating immune complexes. Type II is also referred to as dense deposit disease because electron-dense material of unknown composition, and smaller quantities of C3, form an irregular deposit within the subendothelial space and the lamina densa. Type II disease appears to be a form of autoimmune disease, but its pathogenesis is not clear.

Several other changes in the glomerulus and Bowman's capsule usually accompany the lesions discussed previously. These changes include adhesions between the epithelial cells of the glomerular tuft and Bowman's capsule (synechiae; singular = synechia), hypertrophy and hyperplasia of the parietal epithelium

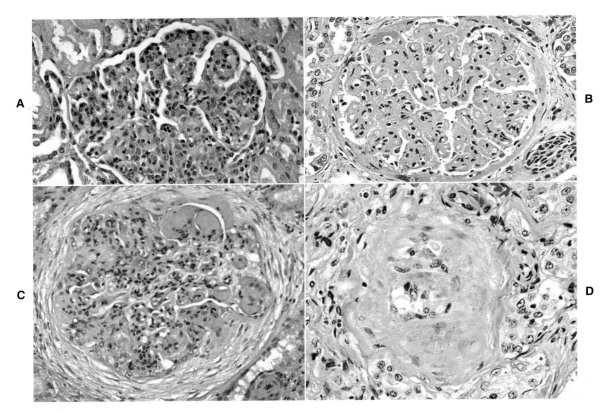

Fig. 11-21   Types of glomerulonephritis. A, Proliferative glomerulonephritis, pig. The lesion is characterized principally by hypercellularity of the glomerulus due to increased numbers of mesangial cells. H&E stain. **B,** Membranous glomerulonephritis, dog. The lesion is characterized by generalized hyaline thickening of glomerular capillary basement membranes. It can occur in dogs with dirofilariasis. H&E stain. **C,** Membranoproliferative glomerulonephritis, horse. Membranoproliferative glomerulonephritis has histologic features of both proliferative glomerulonephritis and membranous glomerulonephritis. Abundant periglomerular fibrosis surrounds this hypercellular glomerulus (mesangial cells). Mesangial matrix is prominent in the top-right area of the glomerulus. H&E stain. **D,** Glomerulosclerosis, dog. Note the hypocellularity, shrinkage, and hyalinization due to an increase in fibrous connective tissue and mesangial matrix and almost complete loss of glomerular capillaries. In glomerulosclerosis (the end stage of chronic glomerulonephritis), glomeruli are essentially nonfunctional. H&E stain. (**A** and **C,** *Courtesy Dr. W. Crowell, College of Veterinary Medicine, The University of Georgia; and Noah's Arkive, College of Veterinary Medicine, The University of Georgia.* **B** and **D,** *Courtesy Dr. S.J. Newman, College of Veterinary Medicine, University of Tennessee.*)

lining Bowman's capsule, deposition of fibrinogen and fibrinous thrombi in glomerular capillaries, secondary to or as a result of the glomerular damage, and dilated renal tubules filled with homogeneous proteinaceous fluid. An increase in mesangial matrix is often also present. If the damage is mild and the cause is removed, glomeruli can heal without obvious or with minimal residual lesions. However, if the lesion is severe and prolonged, subacute to chronic glomerular changes develop. Bowman's capsule can become thickened, hyalinized, and reduplicated. In severe cases, proliferation of parietal epithelium, an influx of monocytes, and deposition of fibrin can occur within Bowman's capsule, resulting in the formation of a

semicircular, hypercellular, intraglomerular lesion known as a glomerular crescent (Fig. 11-21, *C*). The glomerular crescent can also undergo fibrosis, and if Bowman's capsule ruptures, glomerular fibrosis can become continuous with interstitial fibrosis. Interstitial and periglomerular fibrosis, foci of interstitial lymphocytes, and plasma cells and glomerulosclerosis may be present in chronic glomerulonephritis.

GLOMERULOSCLEROSIS

In chronic glomerulonephritis, severely affected glomeruli shrink and become hyalinized because of an increase in both fibrous connective tissue and mesangial matrix and a loss of glomerular capillaries (Fig. 11-21, *D*).

These glomeruli are hypocellular and essentially nonfunctional. This process is referred to as glomerulosclerosis. Glomerulosclerosis can be diffuse, involving all glomeruli, or multifocal. In addition, glomerulosclerosis can involve a whole glomerular tuft (global) or only portions of the tuft (segmental) thus appearing as a nodular or segmental hyalinized thickening in affected glomeruli. Because tubules receive their blood supply from the vasa recta, derived from the glomerular efferent arteriole, glomerulosclerosis reduces the blood flow through the vasa recta, thus decreasing oxygen tension in the tubules. The resulting hypoxia is responsible for tubular epithelial cell death via apoptosis and results in tubular atrophy and flattening of the remaining tubular epithelium. In addition, chronic proteinuria often accompanies glomerulosclerosis and has been reported to stimulate tubular epithelial cell loss through apoptosis.

Numerous factors are associated with and accelerate glomerulosclerosis. These factors include the following:
1. Unrestricted protein in the diet
2. Increased glomerular capillary pressure in functional glomeruli
3. Cytokines
4. Platelet-derived growth factors
   These factors have the following effects:
1. Alter cellular components of the functional glomerular tufts
2. Cause hypertension and transglomerular hyperfiltration with resultant damage to endothelium
3. Activate mesangial cells to proliferate
4. Increase mesangial matrix production
5. Accelerate visceral epithelial cell loss, which allows synechiae (i.e., adhesions between visceral and parietal epithelial cell layers in the glomerulus) to form
   Glomerulosclerosis is not only the end-stage of glomerulonephritis but also can develop in any chronic disease in which severe damage to nephrons or loss of nephron function occurs. Mild multifocal glomerulosclerosis of unknown cause is often an incidental finding in aged animals. Glomerulosclerosis has been reported occasionally in animals with hypertension and diabetes mellitus. In these cases, global or nodular eosinophilic glycoprotein material (hyaline material) is deposited in the glomerular mesangium.

GLOMERULAR AMYLOIDOSIS

Amyloid, an insoluble fibrillar protein with a β-pleated sheet conformation, is produced after incomplete proteolysis of several soluble amyloidogenic proteins. Amyloid deposits in patients with plasma cell myelomas or other B-lymphocyte dyscrasias (called AL amyloidosis) are composed of fragments of the light (L) chains of immunoglobulins. In domestic animals, spontaneously occurring amyloidosis is usually an example of what is called reactive amyloidosis (AA amyloidosis). This form of the disease is often associated with chronic inflammatory diseases; the amyloid deposits are composed of fragments of a serum acute-phase reactant protein called serum amyloid–associated (SAA) protein. Amyloid fibrils from either source are deposited in tissue along with a glycoprotein called amyloid P-component.

Glomeruli are the most common renal sites for deposition of amyloid in most domestic animal species, although the medullary interstitium is a common site in cats, particularly in Abyssinian breeds. Renal amyloidosis commonly occurs in association with other diseases, particularly chronic inflammatory or neoplastic diseases. However, idiopathic renal amyloidosis (i.e., amyloidosis in which an associated disease process is not recognized) is also described in dogs and cats. The underlying pathogenic mechanisms of idiopathic renal amyloidosis are not known. In a recent study, 23% of dogs that presented with proteinuria had renal amyloidosis. A hereditary predisposition for the development of reactive amyloidosis (AA) has been found in Abyssinian cats and Chinese Shar-Pei dogs. A familial tendency is suspected in Siamese cats, English foxhounds, and beagle dogs. In cattle, renal amyloidosis is nearly always due to chronic systemic infectious disease. Glomerular amyloidosis is responsible for many cases of protein-losing nephropathy in animals that have notable proteinuria and uremia. It can, like immune-complex glomerulonephritis, result in the nephrotic syndrome. Long-standing glomerular amyloidosis results in diminished renal blood flow through the glomeruli and the vasa recta. Such reduced renal vascular perfusion can lead to renal tubular atrophy, degeneration, diffuse fibrosis and in severe cases, renal papillary necrosis. Medullary amyloidosis is usually asymptomatic unless it results in papillary necrosis.

Kidneys affected with glomerular amyloidosis are often enlarged, pale, and increased in consistency, and have a smooth to finely granular capsular surface (Fig. 11-22). Amyloid-laden glomeruli may be visible grossly as fine translucent dots on the capsular surface. Similarly, the cut surface of the cortex can have a finely granular appearance (Fig. 11-22). Treatment of kidneys with an iodine solution, such as Lugol's iodine, in many cases results in red-brown staining of glomeruli, which become purple when exposed to dilute sulfuric acid (Fig. 11-23). This technique provides a rapid presumptive diagnosis of renal amyloidosis. Medullary amyloidosis is usually not grossly recognizable.

Microscopically, glomerular amyloid is deposited in both the mesangium and subendothelial locations. Amyloid is relatively acellular and can accumulate segmentally within glomerular tufts; thus a portion of the normal glomerular architecture is replaced by eosinophilic, homogeneous to slightly fibrillar

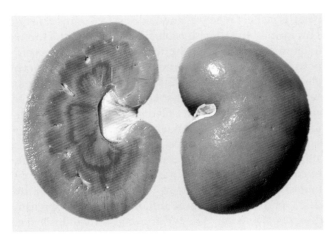

Fig. 11-22   Amyloidosis, kidney, dog. Grossly, kidneys affected by amyloid deposition are diffusely tan, waxy (firm), and of normal size or slightly enlarged. Affected glomeruli are not grossly visible in this specimen, unlike in advanced cases of glomerular amyloidosis or chronic glomerulonephritis. In advanced cases of amyloidosis, glomeruli may be visible as pinpoint, glistening, round, cortical foci. In cats and Shar-Pei dogs, amyloid is deposited in the medullary interstitium, not in the glomeruli. There are also multiple foci of medullary crest necrosis (*yellowish-green*). *(Courtesy Dr. G.K. Saunders, The Virginia-Maryland Regional College of Veterinary Medicine; and Noah's Arkive, College of Veterinary Medicine, The University of Georgia.)*

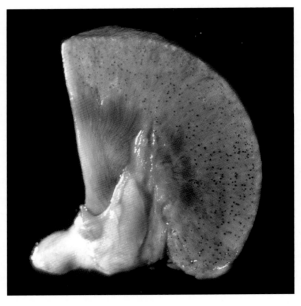

Fig. 11-23   Amyloidosis, kidney, transverse section, dog. On the cut surface of fresh kidney treated with Lugol's iodine followed by dilute sulfuric acid, glomeruli containing amyloid are visible as multiple dark blue dots in the cortex. Lugol's iodine treatment. *(Courtesy Dr. M.D. McGavin, College of Veterinary Medicine, University of Tennessee.)*

material (Fig. 11-24, *A*). When amyloidosis involves the entire glomerular tuft, the glomerulus is enlarged, capillary lumina become obliterated, and the tuft can appear as a large hypocellular, eosinophilic hyaline sphere (Fig. 11-24, *B*). Amyloid can be present in renal tubular basement membranes, and these membranes are hyalinized and thickened. Additionally, in cases of glomerular amyloid deposition, secondary changes may be present in renal tubules, which are usually markedly dilated, have variably atrophic epithelium, and contain proteinaceous and cellular casts. Amyloid is confirmed microscopically by staining with Congo red stain (Fig. 11-24, *C*). When viewed with polarized light, amyloid has a green birefringence (Fig. 11-24, *D*). Loss of Congo red staining after treatment of a section of affected kidney with potassium permanganate suggests the amyloid is AA-amyloid (i.e., of acute-phase reactant protein origin).

MISCELLANEOUS GLOMERULAR LESIONS

Glomerular lipidosis, characterized by small aggregates of lipid-laden foamy macrophages in glomerular tufts, is an occasional incidental finding in dogs. A similar but more extensive glomerular lipidosis has been described in cats with inherited hyperlipoproteinemia, which is a generalized disease characterized by hyperchylomicronemia, atherosclerosis, and xanthogranulomas in numerous parenchymatous organs, including the kidneys (see Granulomatous Nephritis). Microscopically, glomeruli contain foamy macrophages, characteristic of glomerular lipidosis, as well as increased mesangium and thickened Bowman's capsule.

An idiopathic renal glomerular vasculopathy and cutaneous vasculopathy occurs in greyhounds. The cause of this disease is unknown, but renal lesions are similar to those seen in disseminated intravascular coagulation, thrombotic thrombocytopenic purpura, and hemolytic-uremic syndrome in human beings. At necropsy, kidneys from affected dogs are swollen and congested and show cortical petechiae (Fig. 11-25, *A*). Microscopically, numerous glomeruli have segmental or global fibrinous thrombi, hemorrhage, and necrosis (Fig. 11-25, *B*). At the glomerular vascular pole, the walls of afferent arterioles have fibrin deposits and foci of necrosis. Affected greyhounds have multifocal erythematous and ulcerated skin lesions and distal limb edema. Variable systemic signs of uremia often accompany the cutaneous lesions. Thrombocytopenia is frequently seen.

In canine hyperadrenocorticism or as a result of excessive exogenous glucocorticoid therapy, proteinuria often develops. The cause of this lesion is unknown; however, hypertension has been postulated because of its occurrence with increased plasma glucocorticoid concentrations. Glomerular lesions consist of mild

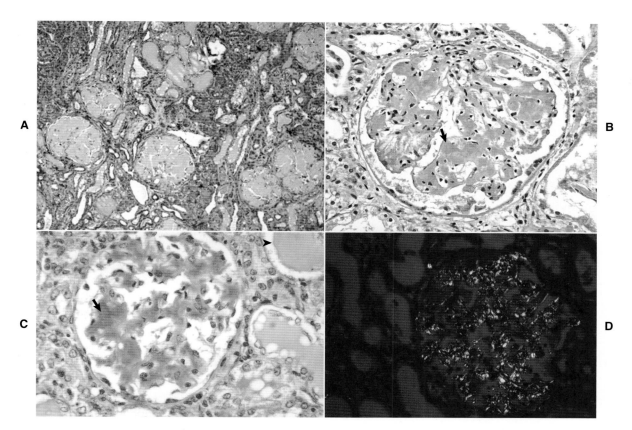

Fig. 11-24   Amyloidosis, glomerulus, kidney, dog. A, All glomerular tufts are diffusely and notably expanded by amyloid (pale eosinophilic homogeneous deposits), with the result that they are relatively acellular. H&E stain. **B,** Amyloid, the pale eosinophilic homogeneous hyalinized deposits, expands the mesangium of the glomerulus (*arrow*). H&E stain. **C,** Amyloid stains orange with Congo red staining (*arrow*), a technique used to confirm it. Note the proteinaceous casts in tubular lumina (*arrowhead*), a consequence of glomerular damage allowing leakage of proteins into the filtrate (protein-losing nephropathy). Congo red stain. **D,** Congo red–stained amyloid deposits. These deposits have a light-green (often called apple green) birefringence when viewed under polarized light. Polarized light microscopy. (**A,** *Courtesy Dr. B.C. Ward, College of Veterinary Medicine, Mississippi State University; and Noah's Arkive, College of Veterinary Medicine, The University of Georgia.* **B,** *Courtesy Dr. S.J. Newman, College of Veterinary Medicine, University of Tennessee.* **C,** *Courtesy Dr. M.D. McGavin, College of Veterinary Medicine, University of Tennessee.* **D,** *Courtesy Dr. W. Crowell, College of Veterinary Medicine, The University of Georgia; and Noah's Arkive, College of Veterinary Medicine, The University of Georgia.*)

mesangial hypercellularity, synechiae, thickened basement membranes, and effacement of epithelial foot processes. Lesions are devoid of immunoglobulin.

DISEASES OF THE TUBULES AND INTERSTITIUM

AZOTEMIA AND UREMIA

Assays for plasma or serum concentrations of urea, creatinine, and the nitrogenous waste products of protein catabolism, are routinely used as indices of diminished renal function. The intravascular increase of these nitrogenous waste products is referred to as azotemia. Renal failure can result in the following:

1. Intravascular accumulation of other metabolic wastes, such as guanidines, phenolic acids, and large molecular weight alcohols (example: myoinositol)
2. Reduced blood pH (metabolic acidosis)
3. Alterations in plasma ion concentrations, particularly potassium, calcium, and phosphate
4. Hypertension

The result of renal failure is a toxicosis called uremia. Uremia can therefore be defined as a

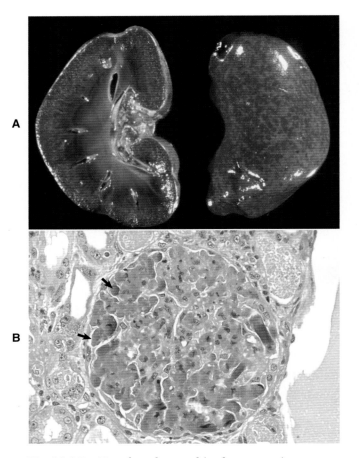

Fig. 11-25 **Vasculopathy, renal (and cutaneous) vasculopathy syndrome, glomerulus, kidney, dog, greyhound.** **A,** The fine white dots in the cortex (both on the capsular and cut surfaces) are glomeruli with extensive glomerular capillary thrombosis. **B,** Necrotic glomerular endothelial cells and extensive glomerular capillary thrombosis (*arrows*) are typical of idiopathic glomerular (and cutaneous) vasculopathy syndrome in greyhound dogs. H&E stain. (*A, Courtesy Dr. B. Weeks, College of Veterinary Medicine, Texas A&M University; and Noah's Arkive, College of Veterinary Medicine, The University of Georgia. B, Courtesy Dr. B.W. Fenwick, Virginia Tech.*)

Table 11-1   Nonrenal Lesions of Uremia

Lesion	Mechanism
Pulmonary edema	Increased vascular permeability
Fibrinous pericarditis	Increased vascular permeability
Ulcerative and hemorrhagic gastritis	Ammonia secretion and vascular necrosis
Ulcerative and necrotic stomatitis	Ammonia secretion in saliva and vascular necrosis
Atrial and aortic thrombosis	Endothelial and subendothelial damage
Hypoplastic anemia	Increased erythrocyte fragility and lack of erythropoietin production in the kidney
Soft-tissue mineralization	Altered calcium-phosphorus metabolism (stomach, lungs, pleura, kidneys)
Fibrous osteodystrophy	Altered calcium-phosphorus metabolism
Parathyroid hyperplasia	Altered calcium-phosphorus metabolism

syndrome associated with multisystemic lesions and clinical signs because of renal failure.

Nonrenal lesions of uremia identified clinically or at necropsy are useful indicators of renal disease (Table 11-1). The severity of nonrenal lesions of uremia is dependent on the length of time that the animal has survived in the uremic state. Therefore in acute renal failure, nonrenal lesions are few, whereas in chronic renal failure many lesions can be present. Typically, lesions can be attributed to either of the following:

1. Endothelial degeneration and necrosis, resulting in vasculitis with secondary thrombosis and infarction in a variety of tissues

2. Caustic injury to epithelium of the oral cavity and stomach secondary to the production of large concentrations of ammonia following splitting of salivary or gastric urea by bacteria

Systemic lesions of uremia include the following:

1. Ulcerative and necrotic stomatitis characterized by a brown, foul-smelling, mucoid material adherent to the eroded and ulcerated lingual and oral mucosa; ulcers are most commonly present on the underside of the tongue (Fig. 11-26)

2. Ulcerative and hemorrhagic gastritis in dogs and cats (Fig. 11-27), often with secondary midzonal mineralization (Fig. 11-28)

3. Ulcerative and hemorrhagic colitis in horses and cattle. Large areas of the gastric or colonic mucosa are often edematous and dark red because of hemorrhage. The gastrointestinal contents can be bloody and smell of ammonia. Microscopically, coagulative necrosis, hemorrhage, and a neutrophilic infiltrate occur in the mucosa. Degeneration, necrosis, and mineralization of the arteriolar intima and media are often present in the gastric mucosa and submucosa (Fig. 11-28).

4. Fibrinous pericarditis characterized by fine granular fibrin deposits on the epicardium (visceral pericardium)

5. Diffuse pulmonary edema. In the latter, alveoli contain fibrin-rich fluid and often a mild infiltrate of macrophages and neutrophils. This lesion is called uremic pneumonitis. These lesions result secondary to increased vascular permeability from the associated vasculitis.

6. Mucoarteritis characterized grossly by finely granular roughened plaques

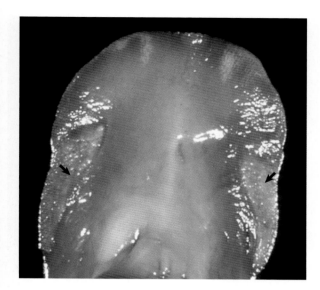

Fig. 11-26 Ulcerative glossitis, uremia, tongue, ventral surface, cat. Bilaterally symmetrical ulcers *(arrows)* are present on the rostrolateral borders of the ventral surface of the tongue. *(Courtesy Dr. M.D. McGavin, College of Veterinary Medicine, University of Tennessee.)*

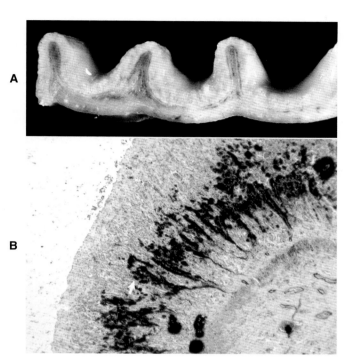

Fig. 11-28 Uremic gastritis, stomach, dog. A, There is accentuation of the gastric rugae and calcification in the deep mucosa. **B,** The mucosa has laminar mineralization of gastric glands *(arrow).* von Kossa stain. *(**A,** Courtesy Dr. J. King, College of Veterinary Medicine, Cornell University. **B,** Courtesy Dr. M.D. McGavin, College of Veterinary Medicine, University of Tennessee.)*

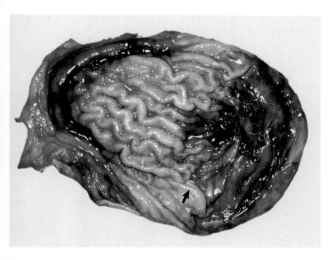

Fig. 11-27 Uremic gastritis, stomach *(right),* dog. Because of uremia, the stomach wall is hemorrhagic and the contents contain blood and mucus (not shown here). Note the edematous mucosal thickening *(arrow).* *(Courtesy Dr. A. Confer, College of Veterinary Medicine, Oklahoma State University.)*

In the uremic animal, focal subendothelial degeneration can occur in the left atrial endocardium and less frequently in the endothelial surface of the proximal aorta and pulmonary trunk. Mucoarteritis in conjunction with loss of the anticoagulant antithrombin III by glomerular leakage is conducive to the formation of large mural thrombi at these sites.

Chronic renal failure often results in hematologic and biochemical alterations. In the diseased kidney, production of erythropoietin, a stimulant of erythropoietic maturation, is reduced and contributes to nonregenerative anemia, as does uremia-associated increased erythrocytic fragility. Most animals in renal failure have hyperphosphatemia and low to normal calcium levels, although variations exist depending on species and stage of the disease. Alterations in calcium-phosphorus metabolism in the uremic animal are a hallmark of chronic renal failure and result from a complex set of events as outlined below:

1. When the glomerular filtration rate is chronically reduced to less than 25% of normal, phosphorus is no longer adequately secreted by the kidneys and hyperphosphatemia results.
2. Because of the mass law interactions between serum calcium and phosphorus, ionized calcium concentration in serum is reduced as a result of precipitation of calcium and phosphorus.
3. Reduced ionized serum calcium stimulates parathyroid hormone secretion, causing calcium release from the readily mobilizable calcium stores in the bone and from osteoclastic bone resorption.
4. These changes in calcium-phosphorus metabolism are made more severe by the reduced ability of the

diseased kidneys to hydroxylate 25-hydroxychole-calciferol to the more active 1,25-dihydroxychole-calciferol (calcitriol), resulting in decreased intestinal absorption of calcium.

5. Calcitriol production is further inhibited by hyperphosphatemia.

6. In addition, calcitriol normally suppresses parathyroid hormone secretion; therefore reduced calcitriol production further increases parathyroid hormone secretion. With time, these events lead to parathyroid chief cell hyperplasia (renal secondary hyperparathyroidism), fibrous osteodystrophy (renal osteodystrophy), and soft tissue calcification.

7. Renal secondary hyperparathyroidism is further thought to perpetuate and enhance renal disease by stimulating nephrocalcinosis (Fig. 11-29), the process by which renal tubular epithelium is damaged by an increase in intracellular calcium. Calcium is precipitated in mitochondria and in tubular basement membranes.

8. Soft tissue calcification associated with uremia occurs in numerous sites and represents both dystrophic and metastatic calcification.

A characteristic lesion of uremic mineralization, particularly in dogs, is calcification of the subpleural connective tissue of the cranial intercostal spaces (Fig. 11-30). These lesions are white-gray granular pleural thickenings with a horizontal "ladderlike" arrangement. The intercostal muscles are only superficially calcified. Patchy or diffuse pulmonary calcification of the lungs results in their failure to collapse, areas of paleness, and mild to moderate firmness and crunchiness and can occur occasionally in conjunction with the lesions of uremic pneumonitis. Microscopically the alveolar septa are calcified and can focally rupture, causing small emphysematous bullae. Although usually not visible at necropsy, calcification occurs in the kidneys. The kidneys can be gritty when cut because of calcification of tubular basement membranes, Bowman's capsules, and necrotic tubular epithelium, especially in the medulla and inner cortex. The gastric wall can be gritty when cut because of calcification of the inner and middle layers of the mucosa, and the submucosal arterioles. Necrotic arterioles (uremic vasculitis) throughout the body are particularly susceptible to dystrophic calcification following uremic injury.

Animals that die of acute renal failure often do so because of the cardiotoxicity of elevated serum potassium, metabolic acidosis, and/or pulmonary edema. Hyperkalemia results from decreased filtration, decreased tubular secretion, and decreased tubular sodium transport. Cell lysis and the extracellular shift of fluid in acidic environments also contribute to the increased serum potassium concentrations.

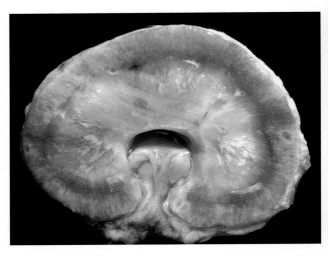

Fig. 11-29   Nephrocalcinosis, kidney, dorsal section, dog. Note the white streaks in the cortex and medulla attributable to mineralization of the interstitium, basement membranes, and tubules. This lesion results from diseases that increase plasma calcium concentrations (e.g., hyperparathyroidism). Renal tubular epithelium is damaged by an increase in intracellular calcium, which is initially precipitated in mitochondria and tubular basement membranes. *(Courtesy Dr. M.D. McGavin, College of Veterinary Medicine, University of Tennessee.)*

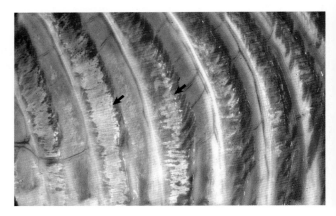

Fig. 11-30   Thoracic cavity, parietal pleura, cat. Horizontally oriented streaks *(arrows)* of mineral (intercostal mineralization) are present in the subpleural intercostal connective tissue as a result of chronic uremia. *(Courtesy Dr. J. King, College of Veterinary Medicine, Cornell University.)*

ACUTE RENAL FAILURE

When renal functional capacity is abruptly impaired (loss of 75%), such that the kidneys fail to carry out their normal metabolic and endocrine functions, acute renal failure can ensue. It is important to remember that the glomerulus, tubules, collecting ducts, and capillary blood supply in each nephron are closely interrelated, both anatomically and functionally. Alterations in tubular structure or function influence glomerular structure and function and vice versa. For example, necrosis or atrophy of renal tubules results in loss of function of the affected nephrons and secondary atrophy of the glomerulus. In addition, because most of the capillary blood supply to tubules is through postglomerular capillaries, a reduction in glomerular blood flow consequently reduces the blood supply to the tubules.

Acute renal failure can be caused by prerenal (compromised renal perfusion), intrarenal (compromised kidney function), or postrenal (obstruction of the urinary tract) factors. Prerenal factors include reduced renal blood flow, whether secondary to circulatory collapse (shock, severe hypovolemia) or local obstruction of vascular supply (thrombus or lodgment of embolus).

Prerenal and intrarenal factors are most responsible for episodes of acute renal failure, with prerenal azotemia and ischemic tubular damage actually being a continuum. Intrarenal disease can target tubules by three main mechanisms:
1. Ascending disease, such as pyelonephritis
2. Intraluminal toxic metabolites
3. Ischemia

Postrenal obstructive diseases will be discussed in the lower urinary tract section.

Acute renal failure occurs when the kidney fails to excrete waste products and to maintain fluid and electrolyte homeostasis. The four main pathologic alterations in acute renal failure are as follows:
1. Decreased ultrafiltration
2. Intratubular obstruction
3. Fluid back leak
4. Intrarenal vasoconstriction

These can occur following many insults, including the following:
1. Decreased renal perfusion
2. Decreased glomerular filtration
3. Ischemic tubular damage
4. Toxic tubular damage
5. Obstructive renal tubular damage
6. Tubulointerstitial inflammation, edema, or fibrosis

ACUTE TUBULAR NECROSIS

Acute tubular necrosis is the single most important cause of acute renal failure. Acute tubular degeneration and necrosis, often referred to as nephrosis, lower nephron nephrosis, tubular nephrosis, tubular dysfunction, or acute cortical necrosis, is principally the result of nephrotoxic damage to the renal tubular epithelial cells or ischemia.

Nephrotoxins preferentially damage kidneys because 20% to 25% of cardiac output goes to the kidney and because of the concentration of the toxin or its metabolites within the renal tubular lumens. Nephrotoxins can directly damage renal epithelial cells, particularly those of the proximal convoluted tubules, following their intracellular conversion to reactive metabolites. Additionally, reactive metabolites in the tubular filtrate or less commonly in the intertubular capillaries can cause renal tubular epithelial necrosis following reabsorption or diffusion, respectively. Additionally, many of these metabolites can indirectly stimulate vasoconstriction and ischemia, which further compromises renal function. In nephrotoxin-associated ischemia, one of the first events in renal tubular cell damage is altered ion transport at the luminal surface. This process results in decreased sodium absorption and increased sodium ions in the lumens of the distal tubules, which stimulate the renin-angiotensin mechanism, causing vasoconstriction and reduced blood flow that result in ischemia and tubular cell damage. Nephrotoxins usually do not damage the tubular basement membranes, and thus regeneration (repair) of tubules can occur in an orderly and expeditious manner. The intact basement membrane acts as a scaffold over which regenerating epithelial cells may slide. Exposure to a variety of nephrotoxins, either from the vasculature (including certain chemicals [glycoaldehyde, glycolic acid and glyoxylic acid] or excessive metabolites, such as glycogen or fat) or from the tubular lumen (including certain antibiotics [aminoglycosides], pigments [hemoglobin], metals [lead], or chemicals [ethylene glycol–induced calcium oxalate crystals]), cause cells to undergo degeneration followed by necrosis and sloughing into the tubular lumen. Cell death results from decreased adenosine triphosphate (ATP) production, which is central to many of the secondary metabolic derangements, including calcium ion influx, purine depletion, metabolic acidosis, and generation of oxygen radicals. Increased intracellular calcium is associated with degenerative changes in renal tubular cells, smooth muscle cells, and mesangial cells (Table 11-2). Oxygen radicals activate phospholipase, which subsequently increases membrane permeability. Because mitochondrial respiration is disrupted, further cell membrane damage occurs.

Notably reduced renal perfusion from any cause can result in tubular necrosis. Severe hypotension associated with shock results in preglomerular vasoconstriction and reduced glomerular filtration. The resulting renal ischemia can produce sublethal tubular cell injury and dysfunction or cause cell death by necrosis or apoptosis. Following less severe insults and within different portions of the renal tubule, apoptosis may occur in lieu of necrosis.

Table **11-2**   **Causes of Ischemic Acute Renal Failure in Small Animals**

INTRAVASCULAR VOLUME DEPLETION

Dehydration
Vomiting
Diarrhea
Sequestration or shock
Thermal burns
Blood loss
Trauma
Surgery
Hypoalbuminemia
Hypoadrenocorticism
Hyponatremia (nondilutional)

DECREASED CARDIAC OUTPUT

Congestive heart failure
Low output
Restrictive pericardial disease
Tamponade
Arrhythmia
Positive-pressure ventilation
Prolonged resuscitation after cardiac arrest

ALTERED RENAL AND SYSTEMIC VASCULAR RESISTANCES

Renal vasoconstriction
Circulating catecholamines
Renal sympathetic nervous stimulation
Vasopressin
Angiotensin II
Hypercalcemia
Amphotericin B
Hypothermia
Myoglobinuria
Hemoglobinuria
Systemic vasodilation
Arteriolar or mixed vasodilator therapy
Anaphylaxis
Gaseous anesthesia
Sepsis
Heatstroke

INCREASED BLOOD VISCOSITY

Multiple myeloma
Polycythemia (absolute or relative)

INTERFERENCE WITH RENAL AUTOREGULATION DURING HYPOTENSION

Nonsteroidal antiinflammatory drugs

WARM OR COLD ISCHEMIA

Modified from Chew D, DiBartola S: Diagnosis and pathophysiology of renal disease. In Ettinger SJ, editor: *Textbook of veterinary internal medicine*, ed 3, vol 2, Philadelphia, 1989, Saunders.

The apoptotic pathway can be triggered by the following:

1. Binding of ligands to the tumor necrosis factor (TNF) superfamily
2. Deficiency of cellular growth factors
3. Imbalance between proapoptotic and antiapoptotic oncogenes
4. Alteration of other mediators of apoptotic signaling pathways, such as reactive oxygen metabolites, caspases, and ceramide

Proximal tubular epithelium has a microvillous border, which amplifies absorptive surface area and cellular junctional complexes that structurally polarize the cell such that membrane phospholipids and specialized proteins remain in the appropriate domains. The integrity of these cellular structures is critical to absorption and secretion. Early structural changes following ischemic insult include formation of apical blebs, loss of brush border, loss of cellular polarity, disruption of tight junctions, and sloughing of cells, which result in intratubular cast formation (Figs. 11-31 and 11-32).

Damage to the cellular cytoskeleton modifies cell polarity, cell-to-cell interactions and cell-matrix interactions. Initially, ischemic damage modifies cell polarity by disruption of the terminal web and disassembly of the microvillar actin cores. This is followed by conversion of G actin to F actin and its redistribution from the apical cell component to form diffuse aggregates throughout the cytoplasm (Figs. 11-33 and 11-34). Cells are attached to each other by junctional complexes, tight junctions and adherens junctions, and to the extracellular matrix by integrins. Several mechanisms contribute to tight junction disruption, which is manifested as alteration in cellular permeability and cell polarity. The contributing mechanisms include redistribution of membrane lipids and proteins, such as Na^+K^+-ATPase, to the apical membrane following alteration of the actin cytoskeleton and redistribution of integrins to the apical cell surface, such that cell desquamation occurs. The former results in deranged sodium handling by the proximal tubular cell.

Animals with severe tubular necrosis have accompanying functional derangements of vascular, tubular, and/or glomerular origin. Vascular derangements include the following:

1. Afferent arteriolar constriction
2. Efferent arteriolar dilation
3. Loss of autoregulation of renal blood flow

Prolonged ischemia can produce a paradoxical response of the autoregulatory system, where increased glomerular capillary resistance from tubular fluid stasis results in activation of afferent arteriolar vasoconstriction. Decreased production of or response to vasodilative factors, such as prostaglandin and atrial natriuretic peptide, also contribute. Afferent arteriole vasoconstriction,

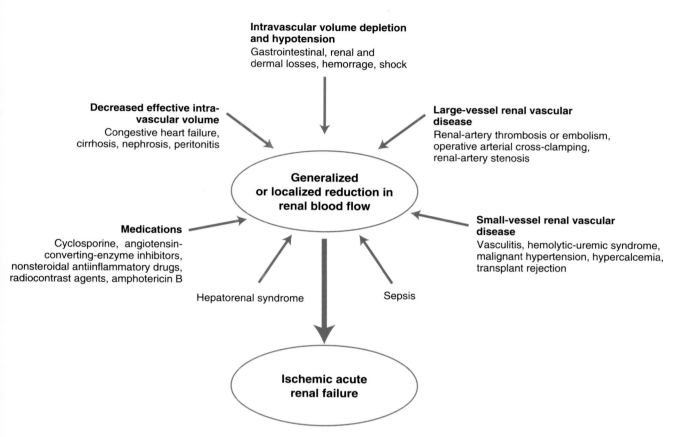

Fig. 11-31   **Schematic diagram of ischemic renal failure.** A wide spectrum of clinical conditions can result in a generalized or localized reduction in renal blood flow, thus increasing the likelihood of ischemic acute renal failure. The most common condition leading to ischemic acute renal failure is severe and sustained prerenal azotemia. Kidney ischemia and acute renal failure are often the result of a combination of factors. *(Redrawn from Thadhani R, Pascual M, Bonventre JV: N Engl J Med 334(22):1448-1460, 1996.)*

back leak of fluid, and tubular obstruction account for decreased glomerular filtration rate (GFR) (Fig. 11-35).

Tubuloglomerular feedback is the mechanism by which GFR is matched to the solute load and the solute handling characteristics of the tubules. Because of altered sodium handling, increased levels reach the macula densa, and activation of the renin-angiotensin system occurs. This is followed by intrarenal vasoconstriction, particularly affecting outer cortical nephrons, and results in decreased glomerular blood flow, decreased filtration, and reduced formation of urine. Tubular metabolic demand is concurrently reduced. Tubular fluid flow can be negligible due to renal tubular epithelial cell swelling and tubular cast formation, and there may be accompanying back leak of glomerular filtrate, as a result of either loss of integrity of the tight junctions or an altered distribution of β-1 integrins, such that cell sloughing and tubular

obstruction result. Fluid present in the interstitium further increases intratubular pressure and compromise of the intertubular capillaries. A vicious cycle ensues.

If the insult to the renal tubules is not lethal and is removed, some forms of acute tubular necrosis are reversible. The success of reparative regeneration is affected by several variables including severity of necrosis:

1. Single cell loss (apoptosis) from the tubular epithelial lining is handled efficiently by adjacent viable tubular epithelial cells, which by mitotic division, fill the epithelial gap. The cells that are lost slough into the lumen to form cellular casts within the lumens of renal tubules (Fig. 11-36).
2. More severe generalized loss of tubular epithelial lining cells is repaired by proliferation of the remaining viable epithelial cells over an intact tubular basement membrane to form a low cuboidal rather than

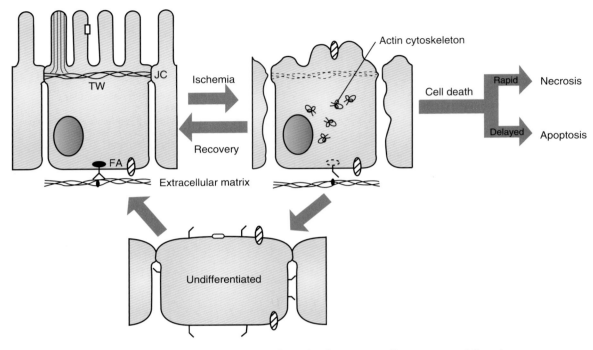

Fig. 11-32   Schematic diagram of the effect of ischemia on cell structure and function.
A polarized renal proximal tubule cell with a well-developed actin cortical cytoskeleton is
shown on the left. Also shown is attachment to the extracellular matrix via integrins. Following
ischemic injury there is extensive disruption, redistribution, and aggregation of the actin
cytoskeleton resulting in loss of microvilli structure, blebbing of microvilli into the lumen,
detachment of cells from the extracellular matrix, and opening of junctional complexes (*JC*).
Injured proximal tubule cells can undergo primary repair and recover directly into a polarized
epithelial cell. Cells can also go through an undifferentiated phase followed by redifferentiation,
or cells can die either rapidly via necrosis or in a much slower programmed fashion known as
apoptosis. The primary route of cellular repair involves direct recovery. The percentage of cells
reverting to an undifferentiated state or dying depends on the severity of the injury and the
location within the kidney. *FA,* Focal adhesions; *TW,* terminal web. *(Redrawn from Molitoris BA,
Marrs J: Am J Med 106:583-592, 1999.)*

a mature columnar epithelial lining. This appears
as an ectatic proximal tubule. Restitution of renal
function eventually results, despite the presence of
replacement low cuboidal epithelium, which is not
identical to the tubular lining cell (with microvilli)
present before the injury. The exact mechanism
of this return to function is not entirely known. The
main determinant of this regenerative ability is
the viability of tubular basement membranes, which
are retained more consistently following toxic rather
than ischemic insults.

Because the regenerative process is reliant on many
factors for its success, things often go awry. Examples
include the following:

1. Focal loss of basement membrane scaffolding
   allows for a bulge defect to occur where the regenerative population of proliferating tubular epithelial
   cells coalesce to form well-differentiated syncytial
   cells (giant cells) at certain levels of the tubule.

2. Regenerative epithelial cells fail to regain all cytoplasmic structural aspects of the original columnar
   epithelial cells (e.g., microvilli and luminal enzymes)
   because of a failure to fully differentiate, and thus
   function may be affected.

3. If there is excessive tubular epithelial loss, the potential for regeneration is lost and repair proceeds by
   replacement fibrosis and scarring.

4. Reperfusion is necessary for cell viability following
   ischemia, but reperfusion injury occurs when activated endothelial cells produce proinflammatory
   mediators such as reactive oxygen species, proteolytic
   enzymes, and cytokines, which result in further renal
   injury.

Recent evidence indicates that epidermal growth
factor secreted by distal convoluted tubules mediates
the tubular repair process. The sequence of events in
tubular regeneration following necrosis have been well
documented in experimental model systems using

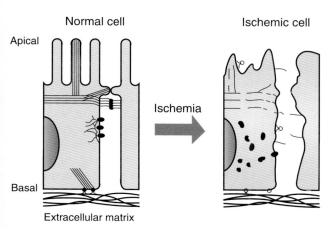

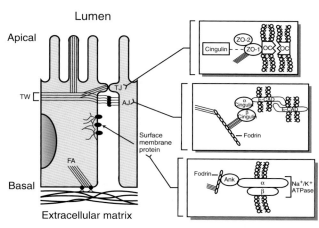

Fig. 11-33   **Schematic diagram of the effect of ischemia on the actin cytoskeleton and the cytoskeletal-surface membrane interactions in proximal tubule cells.** During ischemia, alterations in the actin cytoskeleton involve disruption of the actin cytoskeleton with redistribution and aggregation of actin throughout the cytoplasm. Consequently, notable alterations occur in cytoskeletal-surface membrane interactions. Loss of cell-cell adhesion, cell-matrix adhesion, and polarity of surface membrane proteins during ischemia play a role in the diminished glomerular filtration rate that is the hallmark of ischemic acute renal failure. *(Redrawn from Sutton TA, Molitoris BA: Sem Nephr 18(5):490-497, 1998.)*

Fig. 11-34   **Schematic diagram of the actin cytoskeleton and the cytoskeletal-surface membrane interactions in proximal tubule cells.** Microvillar F-actin filaments extend into the apical actin network termed the terminal web *(TW)* and are bound together by villin and attached to the surface membrane by myosin and ezrin to form the structural core of the apical microvilli. The actin cytoskeleton associates with junctional complexes involved in cell-cell interactions, including the tight junction and the adherens junction. More detailed schematics of the tight junction *(TJ)* and the adherens junction *(AJ)* appear to the right and demonstrate the interaction of F-actin filaments with TJ and AJ protein complexes. *OC* represents occludin in the schematic of the TJ, and *E-CAD* represents E-cadherin in the schematic of the AJ. The cortical actin network associates with surface membrane proteins, such as the sodium-potassium adenosinetriphosphatase, which is demonstrated by the detailed schematic to the lower right. *Ank* represents ankyrin in this schematic. Finally the actin cytoskeleton associates with structures involved in cell-matrix interactions, including focal adhesions *(FA)*. F-actin filaments (stress fibers) possibly bundled together by myosin II associate with a protein complex at sites where integrins bind to the extracellular matrix. *(Redrawn from Sutton TA, Molitoris BA: Sem Nephr 18(5):490-497, 1998.)*

mercuric chloride in mice, rats, and rabbits. In that system, morphologic evidence of regeneration of proximal convoluted tubules is seen within 3 days after a toxic dose. At this time, basement membranes are partially covered with low cuboidal to flattened and elongated epithelial cells that are more basophilic than normal because of the increased concentrations of cytoplasmic ribosomes and rough endoplasmic reticulum producing protein for repair. Nuclei are hyperchromatic and mitotic figures are present. Regenerating tubules do not function normally because they lack both a brush border and normal tubular membrane function, and this is evident clinically as polyuria. Normal-appearing tubular epithelium subsequently reappears between 7 and 14 days after toxin exposure. Normal renal structure without residual evidence of tubular damage is restored between 21 and 56 days after exposure to the nephrotoxin. Similar time frames for tubular regeneration have been described through sequential renal biopsies from human patients naturally exposed to inorganic mercury and in experimental systems using other nephrotoxins.

The alternative to regeneration is tubular loss, and this can occur following either an ischemic insult or exposure to a limited number of nephrotoxins. The ultimate result is replacement fibrosis/scarring. This is seen most commonly if:

1. The toxin is not removed.
2. The basement membrane does not remain intact.
3. Adequate tubular epithelium does not survive the toxic dose to allow for complete repair.

A characteristic histologic lesion of ischemic tubular necrosis is disruption of the tubular basement membranes, referred to as tubulorrhexis (Fig. 11-37). Tubular repair in these kidneys is imperfect because regenerating epithelial cells do not have their normal scaffolding. Tubules that remain in an affected site are nonfunctional, can be dilated and lined by flattened epithelium, or are notably atrophic, appearing shrunken

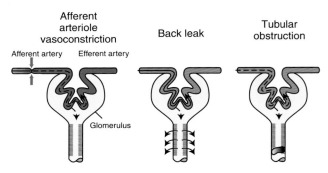

Fig. 11-35 Schematic diagram of the mechanisms of decreased glomerular filtration rate (GFR) during ischemic acute renal failure. Proposed mechanisms for the decrease in GFR that occurs during ischemic acute renal failure include afferent arteriole vasoconstriction, back leak of glomerular filtrate, and tubular obstruction. All three of these mechanisms relate to ischemia-induced alterations in proximal tubule cells. Deranged proximal tubule handling of sodium leads to a high delivery of sodium to the macula densa, which in turn causes afferent arteriole vasoconstriction via tubuloglomerular feedback. Afferent arteriole vasoconstriction reduces glomerular capillary pressure and therefore GFR. Altered cell-cell adhesion results in an open tight junction that leads to increased paracellular permeability and subsequent back leak of glomerular filtrate from the tubular lumen into the extracellular space and ultimately into the blood stream. Disrupted cell-matrix adhesion and abnormal cell-cell adhesion leads to cellular cast formation, which obstructs the tubular lumen and causes increased tubular pressure resulting in diminished or no GFR. *(Redrawn from Sutton TA, Molitoris BA: Sem Nephr 18(5):490-497, 1998.)*

with a collapsed lumen lined by flattened epithelium. Hence the failure to heal by regeneration results in tubular atrophy and interstitial fibrosis.

On gross necropsy, the recognition of acute tubular necrosis is often difficult. Nevertheless, initially the cortex is swollen, pale mahogany to beige and with a slightly translucent smooth, thinned, capsular surface. The cut surface of the renal cortex bulges and is excessively moist; striations are muted or accentuated by radially oriented opaque, white streaks. The medulla is either pale or diffusely congested.

The microscopic appearance of kidneys with acute tubular necrosis can be variable, depending on the following:
1. The severity of the injury
2. The duration of exposure to the damaging agent
3. The length of time between the injury and death

Initially, tubular necrosis is randomly distributed in nephrons, but the proximal convoluted tubules are most severely affected (Fig. 11-38). Prolonged ischemia can produce necrosis of epithelium of the proximal and distal convoluted tubules, the loops of Henle, and

the collecting ducts throughout the cortex, and to a lesser extent, the medulla. Glomeruli are resistant to ischemia and often remain morphologically normal, even when ischemia is prolonged. Initially, proximal tubular epithelium is swollen, and the cytoplasm is vacuolated or granular and intensely eosinophilic, all features indicative of coagulation necrosis. In such cells, the nuclear changes are pyknosis, karyorrhexis, or karyolysis. Necrotic tubular epithelium is subsequently sloughed into tubular lumens resulting in dilated, notably hypocellular tubules that contain necrotic cellular debris and hyalinized or granular casts.

Acute tubular necrosis induces clinical oliguria (decrease in urine production) or anuria (absence of urine production) by one or several mechanisms. These mechanisms include the following:
1. Leakage of tubular ultrafiltrate from damaged tubules across disrupted basement membranes into the renal interstitium
2. Intratubular obstruction resulting from sloughed necrotic epithelium

The latter mechanism is less well accepted, but both mechanisms result in decreased glomerular filtration rate.

The balance of this section will deal with specific disease processes that produce acute tubular necrosis and include the following:
- Pigments
  - Hemoglobin/myoglobin
  - Bile/bilirubin
- Heavy metals
- Antibiotics
  - Aminoglycosides
  - Oxytetracycline
  - Amphotericin B
  - Sulfonamides
  - Monensin
- Nonsteroidal antiinflammatory drugs
- Fungal toxins
- Plant toxins
- Antifreeze (ethylene glycol)
- Vitamins
- Hydrocarbons
- Bacterial toxins

A set of events leading to ischemic tubular necrosis frequently occurs in hypoperfused kidneys complicated by hemoglobinuria or myoglobinuria. Hemoglobinuria accompanies episodes of hemoglobinemia seen secondary to severe intravascular hemolysis as observed in the following:
1. Chronic copper toxicity in sheep
2. Leptospirosis or babesiosis in cattle
3. Red maple toxicity in horses
4. Babesiosis or autoimmune hemolytic anemia in dogs

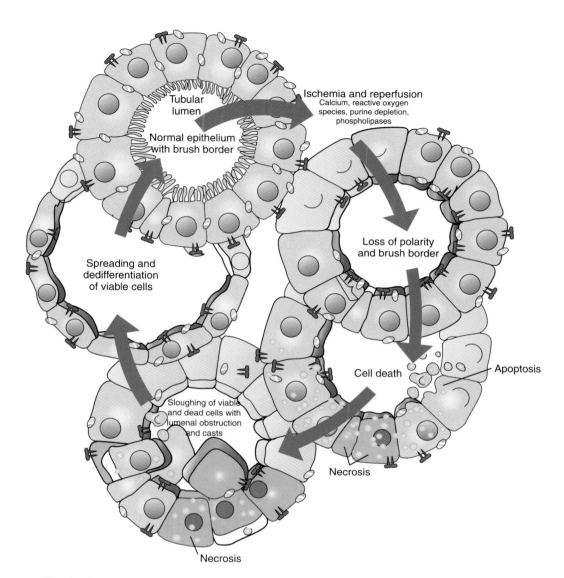

Fig. 11-36 **Schematic diagram of the effects of ischemia and reperfusion.** After ischemia and reperfusion, morphologic changes occur in the proximal tubules, including loss of the brush border, loss of polarity, and redistribution of integrins and sodium-potassium adenosinetriphosphatase to the apical surface. Calcium, reactive oxygen species, purine depletion, and phospholipases probably have a role in these changes in morphology and polarity and in the subsequent cell death that occurs as a result of necrosis and apoptosis. There is a sloughing of viable and nonviable cells into the tubular lumen, resulting in the formation of casts and luminal obstruction and contributing to the reduction in the glomerular filtration rate. The severely damaged kidney can completely restore its structure and function. Spreading and dedifferentiation of viable cells occur during recovery from ischemic acute renal failure, which duplicates aspects of normal renal development. A variety of growth factors probably contribute to the restoration of a normal tubular epithelium. *(Redrawn from Thadhani R, Pascual M, Bonventre JV:* N Engl J Med *334(22):1448-1460, 1996. Color from Molitoris BA, Finn WF, editors:* Acute renal failure: a companion to Brenner and Rector's the kidney, *Philadelphia, 2001, Saunders.)*

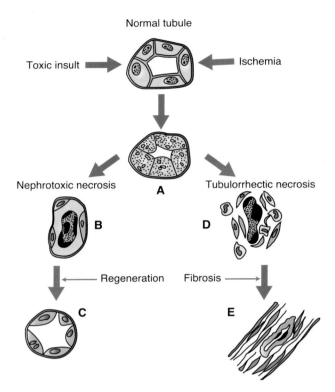

Fig. 11-37   **Schematic diagram of acute tubular necrosis, kidney, proximal tubules.** Acute tubular necrosis results from a nephrotoxin or ischemia. **A,** Both insults cause acute necrosis characterized by cellular swelling, pyknosis, karyorrhexis, and karyolysis. **B,** Subsequent to nephrotoxic necrosis, there is sloughing of necrotic epithelium into the tubular lumina. The basement membranes remain intact and act as a scaffold for (**C**) tubular epithelial regeneration to occur. **D,** Ischemia may result in tubulorrhexis. Necrotic epithelial cells slough into the tubular lumen, the basement membrane is disrupted, macrophages infiltrate, and fibroblasts proliferate. **E,** Fibrosis with tubular atrophy results.

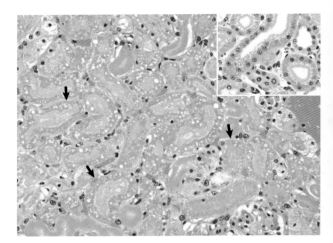

Fig. 11-38   **Acute tubular necrosis, kidney, proximal tubules, cat.** The lesion is characterized by coagulation necrosis of tubular epithelial cells (*arrows*), as demonstrated by nuclear karyolysis and intratubular nuclear and proteinaceous debris. Note that the nuclei, chiefly of endothelial cells of intertubular capillaries and fibroblasts are viable, which differentiates this lesion from an infarct in which all cells are dead. H&E stain. *Inset:* Normal proximal tubules, kidney. In this example, the proximal tubular epithelial cells lack both the nuclear and cytoplasmic changes characteristic of coagulation necrosis, as demonstrated in the main figure. H&E stain. (***Figure*** *and **Inset**, Courtesy Dr. S.J. Newman, College of Veterinary Medicine, University of Tennessee.)*

Myoglobinuria accompanies acute rhabdomyolysis as occurs in any extreme necrosis of muscle as seen with the following:

1. Azoturia ("Monday morning disease") of horses
2. Capture myopathy of exotic or wild animals
3. Severe direct trauma to muscle (i.e., traffic accident)

In these diseases, serum concentrations of hemoglobin or myoglobin are increased. These products pass into the glomerular filtrate, producing greatly increased intraluminal concentrations that cause hemoglobinuric nephrosis or myoglobinuric nephrosis. Hemoglobin attaches to a carrier haptoglobin for transportation, but the latter is too big to pass through the glomerulus. Hemoglobin is not excreted in the urine until supplies of the carrier molecule are depleted and hemoglobin becomes free in the plasma. Myoglobin does not use a carrier protein for transportation, and because it is a small molecule, excesses pass through the glomerular filter and are excreted in the urine. Hemoglobin and myoglobin are not nephrotoxic in themselves, and intravenous infusions of these compounds into healthy animals produce no recognizable lesions. However, large concentrations of hemoglobin or myoglobin in the glomerular filtrate can increase the tubular necrosis that occurs as a result of renal ischemia. In some of the diseases described previously (e.g., chronic copper toxicity in sheep, rhabdomyolysis in horses), affected animals often have renal ischemia secondary to hypovolemic shock or severe anemia. Hemoglobinuria and myoglobinuria can have an additive deleterious affect on tubular epithelium already undergoing ischemic necrosis.

At necropsy, the renal cortices of animals with severe hemoglobinuria or myoglobinuria are diffusely stained red-brown to blue-black and have intratubular hemoglobin or myoglobin casts (Figs. 11-39 and 11-40). These hemoglobin casts appear as a red-black stippling of the external surface and continue into the cortex as radially oriented, dark red streaks (Fig. 11-39, A). The medulla is diffusely dark red or has patchy red streaks. Classically, kidneys from sheep with chronic copper toxicity are diffusely, uniformly and strikingly

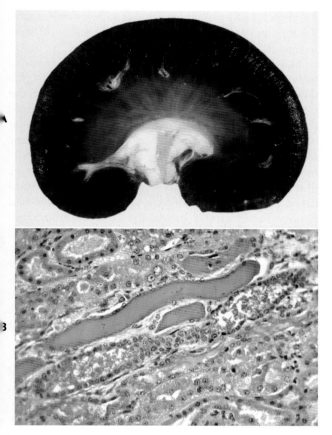

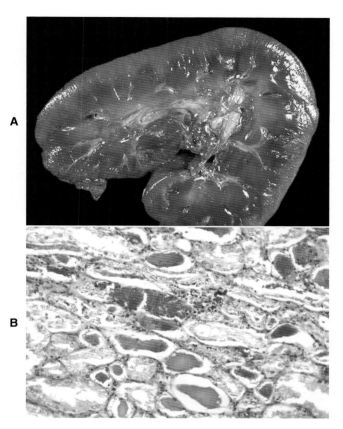

Fig. 11-39   Hemoglobinuric nephrosis, kidney. A, Dog. Severe diffuse hemoglobin staining of the cortex and medulla is secondary to hemoglobinemia from an acute intravascular hemolytic crisis. Note the yellow staining (jaundice) of the pelvic fat and the intima of cross sections of the arcuate artery at the corticomedullary junction. **B,** Sheep. Several distal tubules contain hyaline and coarsely granular hemoglobin casts that occurred following intravascular hemolysis (hemoglobinemia) from chronic copper toxicosis. H&E stain. (**A,** *Courtesy Dr. A. Confer, College of Veterinary Medicine, Oklahoma State University.* **B,** *Courtesy Dr. A.R. Doster, University of Nebraska; and Noah's Arkive, College of Veterinary Medicine, The University of Georgia.*)

Fig. 11-40   Myoglobinuric nephrosis, kidney, horse. A, Diffuse myoglobin staining of the cortex and medulla (*reddish-brown*) is secondary to myoglobinemia from severe rhabdomyolysis. **B,** Myoglobin casts are present in dilated distal tubules, which are lined by flattened epithelial cells. H&E stain. (**A,** *Courtesy Dr. W. Crowell, College of Veterinary Medicine, The University of Georgia; and Noah's Arkive, College of Veterinary Medicine, The University of Georgia.* **B,** *Courtesy Dr. M.D. McGavin, College of Veterinary Medicine, University of Tennessee.*)

blue-black and described as "gunmetal blue." Microscopically, proximal tubular epithelial degeneration and necrosis are severe and tubular lumens are filled by abundant orange-red granular refractile material, the characteristic appearance of a heme compound (Fig. 11-39, *B*).

Also, increased serum concentrations of bilirubin, as in young lambs, calves, and foals with immature hepatic conjugating mechanisms, can be associated with cellular swelling, degeneration, and brown-green pigmentation of the proximal tubular epithelial cells. The term *cholemic nephrosis* has been applied to this lesion;

however, its significance is doubtful. Acute tubular necrosis, when seen in association with severe bilirubinemia, the so-called hepatorenal syndrome, probably is not due to bile acid or bilirubin retention per se, but to ischemia from prerenal causes, such as constriction of renal vessels related to shock or catecholamine release.

Nephrotoxic tubular necrosis is caused by several classes of naturally occurring or synthetic compounds (Table 11-3). Inorganic arsenic and certain heavy metals, including inorganic mercury, lead, cadmium, and thallium, are nephrotoxins. Common sources of heavy metals for oral exposure include herbicides (arsenic), old paints (lead), batteries (lead), automobile components (lead), impure petroleum distillates, and other environmental contaminants. Acute tubular necrosis is due to the following:

1. Damage to membranes of proximal convoluted tubular epithelial cells

Table **11-3** **Common Nephrotoxins of Domestic Animals**

HEAVY METALS

Mercury
Lead
Arsenic
Cadmium
Thallium

ANTIBACTERIAL AND ANTIFUNGAL AGENTS

Aminoglycosides:
    Gentamicin
    Neomycin
    Kanamycin
    Streptomycin
    Tobramycin
Tetracyclines
Amphotericin B

GROWTH-PROMOTING AGENTS

Monensin

NONSTEROIDAL ANTIINFLAMMATORY DRUGS

Aspirin
Phenylbutazone
Carprofen
Flunixin meglumine
Ibuprofen
Naproxen

MYCOTOXINS

Ochratoxin A
Citrinin

PLANTS

Pigweed (*Amaranthus retroflexus*)
Oaks (*Quercus* sp.)
Isotropis sp.
Yellow wood tree (*Terminalia oblongata*)

OXALATES

Ethylene glycol (antifreeze)
Halogeton (*Halogeton glomeratus*)
Greasewood (*Sarcobatus vermiculatus*)
Rhubarb (*Rheum rhaponticum*)
Sorrel, dock (*Rumex* sp.)

VITAMIN D

Vitamin D supplements
Calciferol-containing rodenticides
Cestrum diurnum
Solanum sp.
Trisetum sp.

ANTINEOPLASTIC COMPOUNDS

Cisplatin

2. Mitochondrial damage produced by these toxins; damage is often related to the interaction of these metals with protein sulfhydryl groups

In mercury toxicosis, mercuric ions enter the proximal tubular cells both from the luminal side, because the ions are present in the glomerular filtrate, and from the peritubular side, where the mercuric ions diffuse from the capillary blood, traverse the interstitium and tubular basement membrane, and enter the tubular epithelium. Mercuric ions become concentrated in the rough endoplasmic reticulum and cause early tubular changes that include loss of brush borders and dispersion of ribosomes. These changes are followed by mitochondrial swelling and cellular death. Recently, cadmium has been reported to cause cell death in proximal convoluted tubules by apoptosis.

The specific metal involved in toxic tubular injury cannot be identified by the renal lesions alone. The exception is lead toxicity, in which the endothelial and epithelial cells of affected glomeruli and tubules, respectively, sometimes have acid-fast intranuclear inclusions composed of lead-protein complexes (Fig. 11-41).

Certain pharmaceutical agents are nephrotoxic and cause acute tubular necrosis when administered at excessive doses or too frequently. Cisplatin, a platinum-containing cancer chemotherapeutic agent, causes tubular necrosis by:

1. Direct tubular damage
2. Reducing renal blood flow via vasoconstriction mediated by the renin-angiotensin mechanism

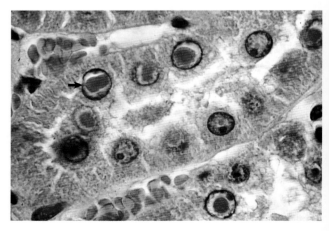

Fig. 11-41 **Nephrosis, lead toxicosis, kidney, cortex, rat.** Acid-fast intranuclear inclusion bodies (*arrow*) present in the proximal convoluted tubular epithelium are diagnostic of lead poisoning. Acid-fast stain with H&E counterstain. (*Courtesy Dr. J. King, College of Veterinary Medicine, Cornell University.*)

Aminoglycoside antimicrobials, such as gentamicin, neomycin, kanamycin, tobramycin, amikacin, and streptomycin are nephrotoxic by means of one of the mechanisms described later. Relative renal toxicity varies among the different aminoglycoside drugs and correlates with the concentration of the compound in the renal cortex. Neomycin, which is highly nephrotoxic, concentrates to the greatest extent in the renal cortex; streptomycin, the least nephrotoxic, does not concentrate appreciably in the renal cortex. Although gentamicin is intermediate in its nephrotoxicity between that of neomycin and streptomycin, tubular damage from gentamicin occurs with some frequency because it is a commonly used drug in veterinary medicine.

The susceptibility of animal species to the nephrotoxic effects of these drugs is variable and is related to differences in susceptibility of renal tubules and to differences in the rate of excretion or inactivation of the drug among animal species. Aminoglycosides become concentrated in lysosomes, and their toxic effects occur after release of large concentrations of the drugs from these organelles. Toxic levels of aminoglycosides:

1. Become concentrated in lysosomes
2. Subsequently escape from lysosomes to accumulate in the cytoplasm
3. Alter tubular cell membrane transport by the inhibition of sodium-potassium-ATPase, causing an intracellular influx of hydrogen, sodium ions, and water
4. Inhibit phospholipase activity so that phospholipids accumulate intracellularly
5. Alter mitochondrial function
6. Inhibit protein synthesis

These biochemical changes are responsible for acute swelling of proximal tubular epithelial cells, mitochondrial swelling, rupture of lysosomes, dilation of endoplasmic reticulum, shedding of the brush border, and cellular death.

Oxytetracycline is occasionally nephrotoxic in cattle and dogs. The mechanism of tubular damage has not been determined, but it is known that large concentrations of tetracycline antibiotics can inhibit protein synthesis in mammals. Renal failure occurs in oxytetracycline toxicosis and is likely the result of tubular obstruction caused by desquamated necrotic tubular epithelium.

Amphotericin B, an antifungal polyene antibiotic, is nephrotoxic by the direct disruption of cellular membranes; this membrane damage interferes with normal cholesterol-lipid interactions and causes potassium ion loss, intracellular hydrogen ion accumulation, acute cellular swelling, and necrosis. These renal changes are not confined to cases of an overdose of the drug but can occur in animals given the recommended therapeutic dosage.

Sulfonamide-induced tubular necrosis, a common entity in years past, occurs infrequently today because the presently used sulfonamides have greater solubility than those used in the past. Sulfonamides produce tubular epithelial cell necrosis most readily in dehydrated animals. Crystals form in tubules and necrosis is caused by direct toxicity to the renal tubular epithelium and to mechanical damage. Fine granular yellow crystalline deposits can be seen grossly in the medullary tubules of affected animals, but the crystalline deposits are dissolved during fixation in aqueous fixatives, such as 10% buffered neutral formalin, and during the processing of tissue for histologic sections.

Monensin is an ionophore antibiotic used as a feed additive to control coccidiosis and stimulate weight gains in poultry and cattle. Horses are particularly susceptible to toxicosis with monensin. Although necrosis of striated muscle is the major lesion of the toxicosis, renal tubular degeneration or necrosis can also be a result of altered ionic transport in renal tubular epithelial cells and possibly due to diminished transport of membrane proteins from the cytosol to the cell membrane.

Ingestion of nonsteroidal antiinflammatory drugs (NSAIDs), such as phenylbutazone, aspirin, carprofen, flunixin meglumine, ibuprofen, and naproxen, have been associated with acute renal failure in small animals, especially dogs. Concurrent dehydration often predisposes dogs to papillary necrosis. The mechanism of acute renal failure is related to the NSAIDs' decreasing synthesis of renal prostaglandins. Because prostaglandins are responsible for maintaining normal renal blood flow, NSAID administration results in afferent arteriolar constriction that decreases renal perfusion, resulting in acute tubular degeneration and necrosis and acute renal failure. The overall incidence of NSAID-induced renal failure in small animals is low and is seen most commonly in animals that ingest excessive amounts of the drug or have a concomitant disorder, such as dehydration, congestive heart failure, or chronic renal disease.

Naturally occurring nephrotoxins can originate from plants (ochratoxins and citrinins) or from fungal organisms (mycotoxins produced by *Aspergillus* sp. and *Penicillium* sp). Ochratoxin A is nephrotoxic for monogastric animals, particularly pigs, in which the lesions are tubular degeneration and necrosis. In addition, long-term ingestion results in diffuse renal fibrosis.

Nephrotoxic plant ingestion can result in acute tubular necrosis. Several species of pigweed, particularly *Amaranthus retroflexus*, can be responsible for acute tubular necrosis and perirenal edema in pigs and cattle. The toxic principle has not been identified. Ruminants develop tubular necrosis after ingestion of leaves, buds, or acorns from oak trees and shrubs (*Quercus* sp.). The toxic substances are metabolites of tannins; however, the mechanism of tubular damage is unknown. Acutely affected cattle often have swollen, pale kidneys that occasionally have cortical petechial hemorrhages (Fig. 11-42).

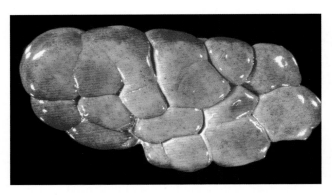

Fig. 11-42   Acute tubular necrosis, oak toxicity, kidney, cow. Ingestion of leaves, buds, or acorns from oak trees produces cortical petechiation, acute tubular necrosis, and perirenal edema. The toxic principal is a metabolite of oak tannins and creates acute tubular necrosis, which heals by scarring. *(Courtesy Dr. K. Read, College of Veterinary Medicine, Texas A&M University; and Noah's Arkive, College of Veterinary Medicine, The University of Georgia.)*

Perirenal edema is a common lesion, and the body cavities contain excessive amounts of a clear fluid. The kidneys show acute tubular necrosis and in chronic cases are fibrotic, pale tan, reduced in size with thinned pale cortices, and have a finely pitted or dimpled surface.

Ethylene glycol (antifreeze) ingestion is a common cause of acute tubular necrosis in dogs and cats. Ethylene glycol, the major constituent of antifreeze, is readily absorbed from the gastrointestinal tract, and a small percentage is oxidized by hepatic alcohol dehydrogenase to the toxic metabolites glycolaldehyde, glycolic acid, glyoxylate, and oxalate. Ethylene glycol and its toxic metabolic products are filtered by the glomeruli, and acute tubular necrosis is caused by the direct interaction of these toxic metabolites, especially glycolic acid, with tubular epithelium (Fig. 11-43, A and B). Of particular significance is that calcium oxalate precipitates as large numbers of pale yellow crystals in renal tubular lumens, tubular epithelial cells, and the interstitium (Fig. 11-43, C). These crystals cause intrarenal obstruction and degeneration and necrosis of tubular epithelium subsequent to a postulated direct effect and/or mechanical damage. Using polarized light, the microscopic identification of large numbers of these birefringent, round to pyramidal crystals arranged in rosettes or sheaves within renal tubules is virtually pathognomonic for ethylene glycol toxicity in dogs and cats (Fig. 11-43, D).

Oxalate-induced tubular necrosis also occurs in sheep and cattle after ingestion of toxic quantities of oxalates that accumulate in plants of various genera, such as *Halogeton, Sarcobatus, Rheum,* and *Rumex.* After absorption of these oxalates from the intestine, calcium oxalate

deposits form and precipitate in vessel walls and in renal tubules, where they cause obstruction and epithelial cell necrosis. Illness in oxalate poisoning occurs not only because of renal disease but also because of neuromuscular dysfunction, the result of the hypocalcemia produced by chelation of serum calcium by oxalates. Recently, an oxalate-induced nephrosis was described in Tibetan spaniels with an inherited hyperoxaluria.

Vitamin D given as multiple excessive doses (vitamin D intoxication [vitamin D nephropathy]) or by accidental ingestion of calciferol-containing rodenticides can cause nephrosis in dogs and cats. In livestock, chronic ingestion of plants, such as *Cestrum diurnum* in the southern United States or *Solanum* sp. or *Trisetum* sp. in other countries, each of which contains a chemical with vitamin D–like biologic activity, can also cause nephrosis. Ingestion of excessive amounts of vitamin D can induce hypercalcemia. The subsequent tubular necrosis is the consequence of renal ischemia resulting from vasoconstriction and of tubular epithelial cell absorption of calcium, causing mitochondrial calcification, mitochondrial dysfunction, and cellular death. Tubular and glomerular basement membranes are also calcified (Fig. 11-29). Development of lesions depends on the length of time between exposure to rodenticides and death or the duration of continued exposure to vitamin D. In acute cases, the kidneys have a smooth capsular surface. Microscopically, tubular epithelium is necrotic and atrophic with a few calcific deposits in tubules scattered randomly throughout the cortex. In more chronic cases, the surface of the kidney is finely granular as a result of fibrosis. White, chalky calcific deposits can be seen within the cortex. Interstitial fibrosis, tubular dilation and atrophy, glomerular atrophy, and extensive calcification of tubular basement membranes are seen microscopically.

Natural gas condensate, a complex mixture of hydrocarbon compounds, has been reported to cause an acute nephrosis in exposed sheep. The mechanism of nephrotoxicity has not been identified, but it is not caused by heavy metal contaminants.

Bacterial toxins, such as the epsilon exotoxin, produced following notable enteric proliferation by *Clostridium perfringens* type D in small ruminants, can result in grossly recognizable bilateral renal lesions termed "pulpy kidney" (Fig. 11-44, A). The pulpy texture of the kidney is due to acute tubular epithelial degeneration and/or necrosis and interstitial edema and hemorrhage (Fig. 11-44, B).

INCIDENTAL LESIONS OF RENAL TUBULES

Pigment can be present in the renal tubules. The origin of hemosiderin pigment is most likely from degradation of hemoglobin resorbed from the glomerular filtrate by proximal tubular epithelium. However, a history

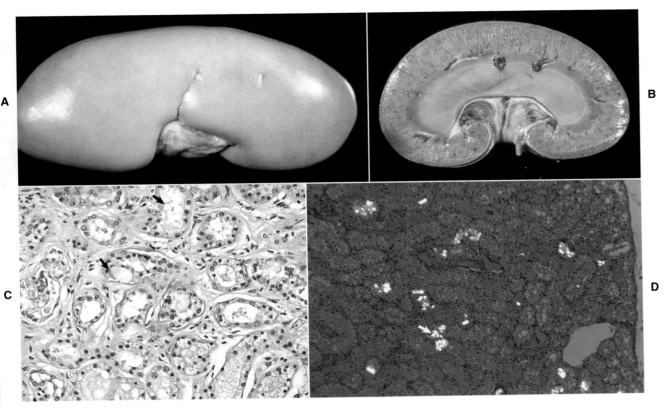

Fig. 11-43   Oxalate nephrosis, kidney. A, Pig. Oxalate nephrosis following ingestion of oxalate-containing plants. The kidney is diffusely pale beige and swollen. **B,** Dorsal section, dog. The cortex is pale beige and finely mottled due to the deposition of multiple small foci of oxalate crystals in the renal tubules. **C,** Dog. Tubular dilation, necrosis, and early regeneration (increased numbers of epithelial cells lining several tubules). Numerous tubules contain oxalate crystals (*arrows*) which have dilated the tubules and compressed their epithelium. H&E stain. **D,** Cat. Birefringent radiating sheaves of calcium oxalate crystals (*arrow*) in renal tubules. Polarized light. H&E stain. (*A, B,* and *D, Courtesy Dr. M.D. McGavin, College of Veterinary Medicine, University of Tennessee. C, Courtesy Dr. S.J. Newman, College of Veterinary Medicine, University of Tennessee.*)

or concurrent lesions of a prior hemolytic crisis are often lacking. In dogs, microscopic granules of hemosiderin are frequent incidental findings in the cytoplasm of proximal convoluted tubular epithelial cells in kidneys that are otherwise normal.

Fine golden granules of lipofuscin ("wear and tear pigment") can accumulate in renal proximal and distal convoluted tubules of old cattle and in striated muscle, resulting in lipofuscinosis. Grossly the renal cortex can have streaks of brown discoloration, but renal function is not affected.

Cloisonné kidneys, which occur in goats, are the result of tubular membrane thickening as a result of deposits of ferritin and hemosiderin. Grossly, these kidneys have diffuse, intense, black or brown discoloration of the cortex (Fig. 11-45). The medulla is spared. Although this lesion is striking, renal function is normal.

Other causes of incidental tubular changes include the following:
1. Vacuolation of renal tubular epithelium in the lysosomal storage diseases, such as feline sphingomyelinosis and ovine GM_1 gangliosidosis
2. Intranuclear eosinophilic crystalline pseudoinclusions (so called crystalloids), which occur in renal tubular epithelium of old dogs. These can be round or rectangular and often greatly distort the nuclei.

Klossiella equi is a sporozoan parasite of the horse, which has various stages of development in the kidney following oral infection. No gross lesions are noted. Various stages of schizogony can be found microscopically in proximal convoluted tubular epithelium and to a lesser extent in glomerular endothelium (Fig. 11-46). Stages of sporogony are present in the epithelial cells of

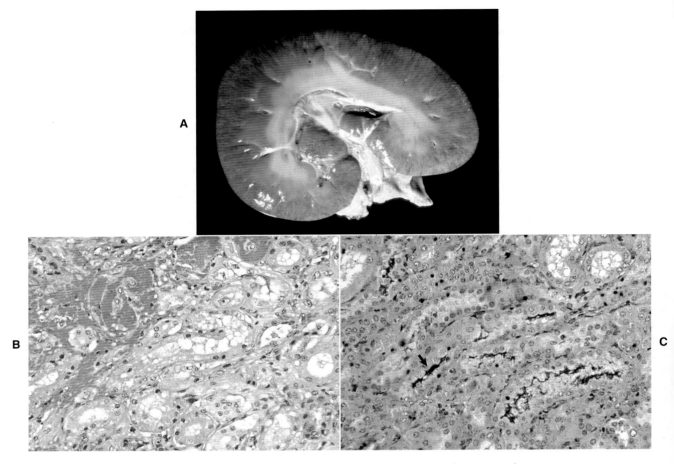

Fig. 11-47   Acute leptospirosis, kidney. A, Interstitial nephritis, acute leptospira infection, dorsal section, dog. Radiating pale streaks are caused by cortical tubular necrosis, and acute interstitial inflammatory infiltrates. The hilar fat and medulla are yellow from jaundice. **B,** Acute tubular necrosis, early regeneration, dog. Note the segments of tubular epithelium devoid of nuclei (coagulation necrosis) *(top left)* and the hemorrhage. At this early stage, there is an almost complete lack of inflammatory cells in the interstitium, but later in the subacute stage of leptospirosis there are interstitial infiltrates of lymphocytes and plasma cells, which tend to be near the corticomedullary junction. H&E stain. **C,** Leptospira, cow. Numerous leptospira *(arrow)* are present in the lumens of tubules. Leptospira colonization of tubule epithelial cells is typical of this bacterium. Warthin Starry silver stain. *(**A** and **C,** Courtesy Dr. M.D. McGavin, College of Veterinary Medicine, University of Tennessee. **B,** Courtesy Dr. S.J. Newman, College of Veterinary Medicine, University of Tennessee.)*

portions of the nephron as basophilic intranuclear viral inclusions

6. Persistence of virus in tubular epithelium for weeks to months
7. Production of tubular epithelial necrosis as a result of viral-induced cytolysis
8. Production of chronic lymphocytic, plasmacytic, and less commonly histiocytic interstitial nephritis

Infection with equine arteritis virus or porcine reproductive and respiratory syndrome virus often results in multifocal lymphohistiocytic chronic tubulointerstitial nephritis with interstitial edema. Lesions can involve any area of the cortex but are especially intense in the medulla and at the corticomedullary junction. A severe vasculitis, characterized by fibrinoid necrosis and lymphohistiocytic infiltrates that involve the adventitial and medial layers of cortical and medullary arteries and veins, is present. Virus can be found in endothelium and in macrophages.

Deposition of immune complexes in or interactions between antibasement membrane antibodies and tubular basement membranes can initiate immune-mediated tubulointerstitial disease in human beings and laboratory animals. Depositions of immunoglobulin (Ig) and complement have rarely been identified in renal

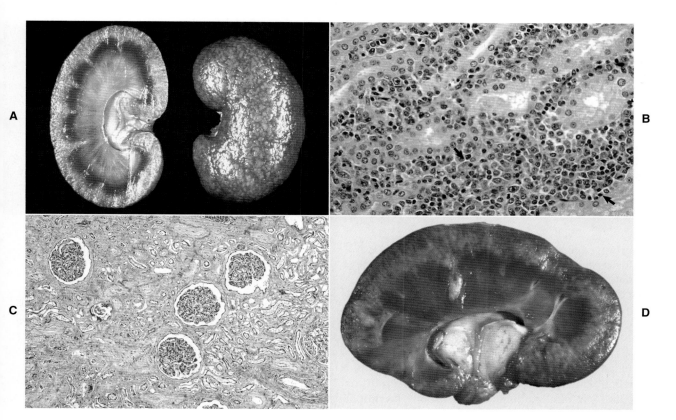

Fig. 11-48   Chronic tubulointerstitial nephritis. A, Kidney, dorsal surface and dorsal section, dog. Note the nodularity of the capsular surface (*right*) from cortical interstitial fibrosis and the reduced width of the cortex (atrophy). **B,** Kidney, dorsal section, dog. There is an intense lymphoplasmacytic interstitial infiltrate (*arrows*). H&E stain. **C,** Exotic zoo animal. This disease is characterized by cortical and medullary fibrosis, variable degrees of tubular atrophy, and mononuclear cell interstitial infiltrate. Masson trichrome stain. **D,** Leptospirosis, dog. The pale streaks and foci in the cortex are chiefly interstitial lymphoplasmacytic infiltrates.
(**A** *and* **C,** *Courtesy Dr. A. Confer, College of Veterinary Medicine, Oklahoma State University.* **B,** *Courtesy Dr. Abdy, College of Veterinary Medicine, The University of Georgia; and Noah's Arkive, College of Veterinary Medicine, The University of Georgia.* **D,** *Courtesy Dr. M.D. McGavin, College of Veterinary Medicine, University of Tennessee.*)

tubular basement membranes in domestic animals, but administration of preformed complexes (bovine serum albumin and antibody) to dogs demonstrated that these complexes interacted with renal tubules, not glomeruli. Damaged tubules respond with epithelial cell and basement membrane proliferation and peritubular fibrosis. At present, the role of immune-mediated mechanisms in tubulointerstitial nephritis in domestic animals is unclear.

Gross lesions of tubulointerstitial nephritis can be classified as acute, subacute, or chronic; chronic tubulointerstitial nephritis is discussed in more detail later (see Renal Fibrosis). The distribution of lesions can be diffuse as in canine leptospirosis (Figs. 11-47 and 11-48) or multifocal as in "white spotted kidneys" of calves because of *Escherichia coli septicemia* (Fig. 11-50),

infectious canine hepatitis, canine herpesvirus infection (Fig. 11-51), malignant catarrhal fever (Fig. 11-52), or porcine and bovine leptospirosis (Figs. 11-47 and 11-48). In diffuse tubulointerstitial nephritis, kidneys can be swollen and pale tan with a random gray mottling of the capsular surface. The cut surface bulges; gray infiltrates of varying sizes and intensities obscure the normal radially striated cortical architecture. These renal lesions usually are manifested as coalescing gray foci that are particularly intense in the inner cortex. Focal lesions of tubulointerstitial nephritis are less extensive and composed of more discrete gray areas in the cortex and outer medulla.

Microscopically, aggregates of lymphocytes, plasma cells, monocytes, and fewer neutrophils are randomly scattered or intensely localized throughout the

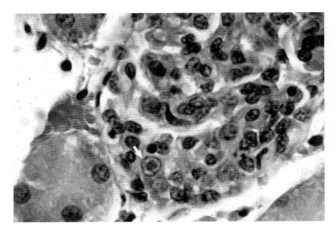

Fig. 11-49 **Infectious canine hepatitis, kidney, cortex, dog.** Renal glomerular endothelial cells contain intranuclear inclusion bodies *(arrow)*. H&E stain. *(Courtesy Dr. W. Crowell, College of Veterinary Medicine, The University of Georgia; and Noah's Arkive, College of Veterinary Medicine, The University of Georgia.)*

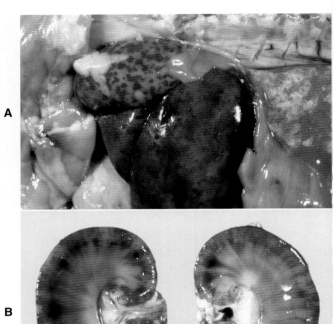

Fig. 11-51 **Canine herpesvirus nephritis (canine herpesvirus type I), kidney, neonatal puppy. A,** Abdominal viscera. Multifocal renal cortical hemorrhages are grossly characteristic of this disease. **B,** Dorsal sections. Multifocal cortical hemorrhages are due to viral-induced vasculitis with necrosis and secondary hemorrhage. (**A** and **B,** Courtesy Dr. M.D. McGavin, College of Veterinary Medicine, University of Tennessee.)

edematous interstitium. Tubular epithelial cells within severely inflamed areas can be degenerate, necrotic, or both, and profound tubular loss is usually accompanied by eventual replacement fibrosis.

GRANULOMATOUS NEPHRITIS

Granulomatous nephritis is a tubulointerstitial disease that often accompanies chronic systemic diseases that are characterized by multiple granulomas in various organs. In domestic animals, granulomatous nephritis has been associated with a variety of infectious agents, including viruses (feline coronavirus), bacteria (mycobacteria), fungi (*Aspergillus* sp.), and parasites

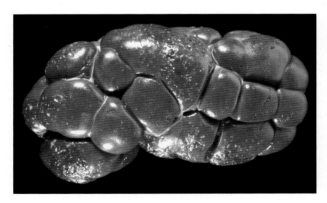

Fig. 11-50 **Multifocal interstitial nephritis (white-spotted kidney), kidney, calf.** Multiple pale-yellow to white 2- to 5-mm foci of inflammatory cells (usually neutrophils) are scattered randomly throughout and over the surface of the kidney (as shown here). *(Courtesy College of Veterinary Medicine, University of Illinois.)*

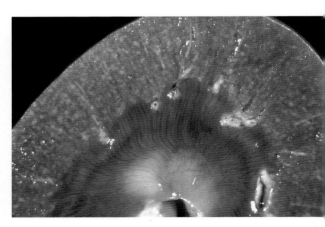

Fig. 11-52 **Interstitial nephritis, malignant catarrhal fever, kidney, dorsal section, gaur.** Multiple, pale-white to gray, discrete interstitial inflammatory cells (lymphoplasmacytic) have effaced some of the cortical striations in affected areas. *(Courtesy Dr. A. Confer, College of Veterinary Medicine, Oklahoma State University.)*

(*Toxocara* sp.). Common to each, however, is the formation of grossly visible granulomas randomly scattered throughout the kidneys, but especially in the cortex.

Cats with feline infectious peritonitis, particularly the noneffusive (dry) form, often have multifocal pyogranulomatous nephritis, secondary to the severe primary vasculitis. The pathogenesis of this lesion is thought to be related to a cell-mediated hypersensitivity (type IV) reaction to feline infectious peritonitis virus. The immune response causes a granulomatous necrotizing vasculitis and development of pyogranulomas. The renal lesions are characterized grossly by multiple, large, irregular, pale gray subcapsular cortical foci (Fig. 11-53, A) that are firm and granular on a cut surface (Fig. 11-53, B). These lesions are somewhat circumscribed and bulge from the capsular surface. They may be misinterpreted as neoplastic infiltrates, such as those associated with renal lymphosarcoma. Microscopically, extensive accumulations of macrophages interspersed with lymphocytes, plasma cells, and neutrophils (pyogranulomas) surround foci of necrotizing fibrinoid vasculitis (see Fig. 14-51).

Granulomatous nephritis is also caused by a variety of granuloma-inducing infectious agents including fungi such as *Aspergillus* sp., Phycomycetes, or *Histoplasma capsulatum*; algae such as *Prototheca* sp.; rickettsia such as *Ehrlichia canis*; protozoa such as *Encephalitozoon cuniculi*; and bacteria such as *Mycobacterium bovis*. Small, gray-white, granulomatous foci (2 to 5 mm) or larger nodules (up to 10 cm in diameter) can be scattered randomly throughout the kidneys of animals with granulomatous nephritis. These foci are white to tan, dry, and granular and can have calcified, caseous centers. Microscopically, lesions are characterized by central foci of necrosis surrounded by epithelioid macrophages, variable minerals, and giant cells that contain acid-fast bacteria.

In cattle, granulomatous nephritis is part of the multisystemic granulomatous disease caused by hairy vetch (*Vicia villosa*) toxicosis. Lesions are characterized by multifocal to coalescing cortical granulomas (Fig. 11-54, A). Microscopically, infiltrates of monocytes, lymphocytes, plasma cells, eosinophils, and multinucleated giant cells are seen primarily within the renal cortex (Fig. 11-54, B).

Migratory *Toxocara canis* larvae can induce small, gray to white granulomas (2 to 3 mm) randomly scattered throughout the subcapsular renal cortex of dogs (Fig. 11-55, A). Such lesions probably are due to cell-mediated immune responses to the migrating larvae and are composed of aggregates of macrophages, lymphocytes, and eosinophils surrounded by fibroblasts within concentrically arranged fibrous connective tissue (Fig. 11-55, B). In recently acquired lesions, nematode larvae can often be seen in the center of these lesions (Fig. 11-55, B). Following death, the larvae become

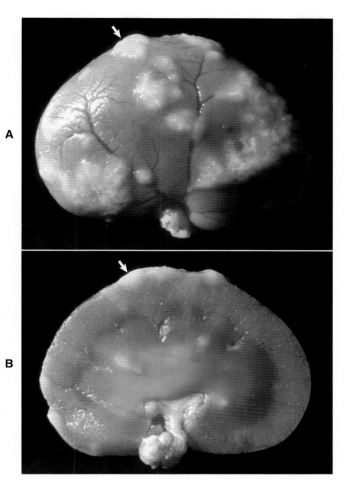

Fig. 11-53 **Granulomatous nephritis, feline infectious peritonitis, kidney, cat. A,** Lesions are typical of the noneffusive (dry) form of feline infectious peritonitis. There are multifocal, coalescing white to gray granulomas *(arrow)*, which can be confused with the nodular form of lymphosarcoma, thus warranting histologic examination. **B,** Dorsal section. Multifocal, coalescing white to gray granulomas extend into the cortical parenchyma *(arrow)*. The pathogenesis of this lesion is determined by the effectiveness and/or ineffectiveness of both humoral and cellular immune responses. Depending on the immune response, the pathogenesis can involve a primary immune complex vasculitis (type III hypersensitivity [effusive form]) and/or delayed hypersensitivity response (type IV hypersensitivity [noneffusive form]); thus the lesions are oriented around blood vessels (primarily capillaries and venules) and are granulomatous. *(A and B, Courtesy Dr. M.D. McGavin, College of Veterinary Medicine, University of Tennessee.)*

fragmented and the debris is either phagocytosed and eliminated or less commonly retained. Lesions heal by fibrosis, leaving a few finely pitted (contracted) foci on the capsular surface.

Cats with inherited hyperlipoproteinemia have xanthogranulomas in various organs, including the kidneys.

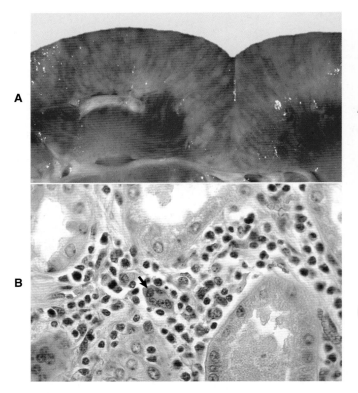

Fig. 11-54 Granulomatous nephritis, hairy vetch toxicosis, kidney, cow. A, Cortical striations are obliterated by coalescing granulomatous foci associated with hairy vetch toxicosis. **B,** Cortex. Lesions associated with hairy vetch toxicosis are characterized by a mixed cell interstitial inflammatory infiltrate (macrophages, lymphocytes, and occasional multinucleated giant cell *[arrow]*) with renal tubular atrophy. It is specifically known as an unusual poisoning because of its ability to induce granulomatous inflammation in addition to the necrosis. The kidney is not the primary organ affected. H&E stain. (*A, Courtesy Dr. J. King, College of Veterinary Medicine, Cornell University; and Dr. J. Edwards, College of Veterinary Medicine, Texas A&M University. B, Courtesy Dr. R. Panciera, College of Veterinary Medicine, Oklahoma State University.*)

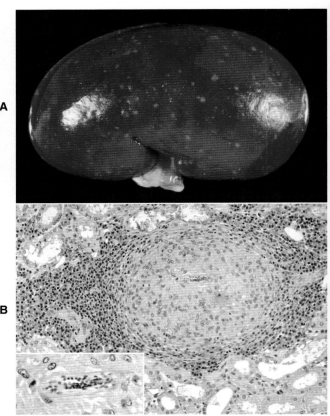

Fig. 11-55 Granulomatous nephritis, kidney, cortex, dog. A, Multiple subcapsular, cortical, tan, raised granulomas caused by migrating ascarid larvae. **B,** A mature granuloma composed of a central ascarid larva surrounded by epithelioid macrophages and concentrically arranged fibrous connective tissue and inflammatory cells. H&E stain. *Inset:* Ascarid larva. (*A, B, and Inset, Courtesy Dr. W. Crowell, College of Veterinary Medicine, The University of Georgia; and Noah's Arkive, College of Veterinary Medicine, The University of Georgia.*)

We have observed similar renal xanthogranulomas in dogs with hypothyroidism and severe atherosclerosis. These lesions are characterized by foamy, lipid-laden macrophages, lymphocytes, plasma cells, and fibrosis interspersed with cleftlike spaces typical of cholesterol deposits (cholesterol clefts).

DISEASES OF THE RENAL PELVIS

PYELONEPHRITIS

Although *pyelitis* refers to inflammation of the renal pelvis, pyelonephritis is inflammation of both the renal pelvis and renal parenchyma and is an excellent example of suppurative tubulointerstitial disease.

Each disease usually originates as an extension of a bacterial infection affecting the lower urinary tract that ascends the ureters to the kidneys and establishes an infection in the pelvis and inner medulla (Fig. 11-56). Rarely, pyelonephritis can result from descending bacterial infections, wherein bacterial infection of the kidneys occurs via the hematogenous route, that is, embolic nephritis. In human pathology, the term *pyelonephritis* is used to include both ascending and descending infections (Fig. 11-57). Ascending infection, however, is by far the most common cause of pyelonephritis in animals.

The pathogenesis of ascending pyelonephritis depends on the abnormal reflux of bacteria-contaminated urine from the lower tract to the renal pelvis and collecting ducts (vesicoureteral reflux). Normally, little vesicoureteral reflux occurs during micturition. Vesicoureteral reflux

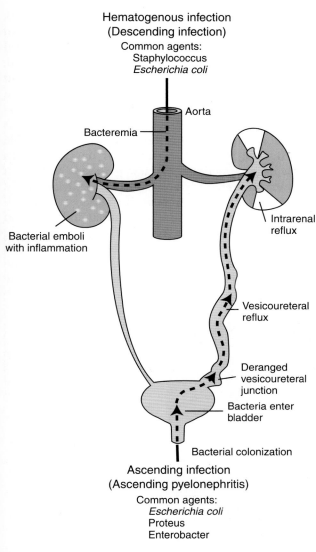

Hematogenous infection
(Descending infection)
Common agents:
Staphylococcus
Escherichia coli

Aorta

Bacteremia

Intrarenal
reflux

Bacterial emboli
with inflammation

Vesicoureteral
reflux

Deranged
vesicoureteral
junction

Bacteria enter
bladder

Bacterial colonization

Ascending infection
(Ascending pyelonephritis)
Common agents:
Escherichia coli
Proteus
Enterobacter

Fig. 11-56   Schematic diagram of the pathways of renal infection. Hematogenous infection results from bacteremia. More common is ascending infection, which results from a combination of urinary bladder infection, vesicoureteral reflux, and intrarenal reflux. *(From Kumar V, Abbas AK, Fausto N: Robbins & Cotran pathologic basis of disease, ed 7, Philadelphia, 2005, Saunders.)*

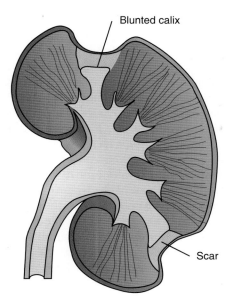

Blunted calix

Scar

Fig. 11-57   Schematic diagram of pyelonephritis, kidney, human being. Typical coarse scars of chronic pyelonephritis associated with vesicoureteral reflux. The scars are usually polar and with the loss of the renal papilla, the calyx underlying each scar is blunted. The cow and pig are the only domestic animals with calyces. *(From Kumar V, Abbas AK, Fausto N: Robbins & Cotran pathologic basis of disease, ed 7, Philadelphia, 2005, Saunders.)*

occurs more readily when pressure is increased within the urinary bladder, as with urethral obstruction. Bacterial infection of the lower urinary tract can enhance vesicoureteral reflux by several other mechanisms:

1. When the bladder wall is inflamed (cystitis), the normal competency of the vesicoureteral valve can be compromised, allowing greater opportunity for urine to reflux.
2. Endotoxin, liberated from gram-negative bacteria infecting the ureter and bladder, can inhibit normal ureteral peristalsis, increasing reflux.

The urinary tract has a number of protective features in place to help prevent bacterial colonization and these include the following:

1. Mucoproteins in the surface urothelial mucosal lining that prohibit bacterial adherence
2. Sloughing of superficial urothelial cells to minimize surface colonization
3. Goblet cell metaplasia
4. Phagocytosis by superficial mucosal urothelial cells
   Bacteria that colonize the pelvis can readily infect the inner medulla. The medulla is highly susceptible to bacterial infection because of the following:
1. Its poor blood supply
2. Its great interstitial osmolality or osmolarity that inhibits neutrophil function
3. Its large ammonia concentration that inhibits complement activation

Thus bacteria can infect and ascend collecting ducts, cause tubular epithelial necrosis and hemorrhage, and incite a notable inflammatory response. Bacterial infection can progressively ascend within tubules and the interstitium until the inflammatory lesions extend from pelvis to capsule. Chronic pyelonephritis may result from infection superimposed on conditions that result in recurrent obstructive disease or reflux (reflux nephropathy). Recurrent infections lead to recurrent bouts of inflammation that result in scarring.

Because most occurrences of pyelonephritis are ascending infections and because females are more susceptible to lower urinary tract infections, pyelonephritis occurs more frequently in females. *Escherichia coli*, especially uropathogenic strains that produce virulence factors such as α-hemolysin, adhesins, and P fimbria, is one of the most common causes of lower urinary tract disease and pyelonephritis. *Proteus* sp., *Klebsiella* sp., *Staphylococcus* sp., *Streptococcus* sp., and *Pseudomonas aeruginosa* are also common causes of lower urinary tract infection and pyelonephritis in all species. *Corynebacterium renale* and *Eubacterium (Corynebacterium) suis* are specifically pathogenic for the lower urinary tract of cattle and pigs, respectively, and are common causes of pyelonephritis. Recent or multiple catheterizations may be a predisposing factor.

A gross diagnosis of pyelonephritis is accomplished by recognizing the existence of pelvic inflammation with extension into the renal parenchyma (Fig. 11-58, A). Pyelonephritis can be unilateral, but it is often bilateral and most severe at the renal poles. The pelvic and ureteral mucous membranes can be acutely inflamed, thickened, reddened, roughened or granular, and coated with a thin exudate. The pelvis and ureters can be markedly dilated and have purulent exudate in the lumina (Fig. 11-58, B). The medullary crest (papilla) is often ulcerated and necrotic. Renal involvement is notable by irregular, radially oriented, red or gray streaks involving the medulla, extending toward and often reaching the renal surface (Fig. 11-58). Occasionally, inflammation extends through the surface of the kidneys to produce extensive subcapsular inflammation and localized peritonitis.

The renal lesions of chronic pyelonephritis, in which an active bacterial infection exists, include most of the elements of acute inflammation described previously

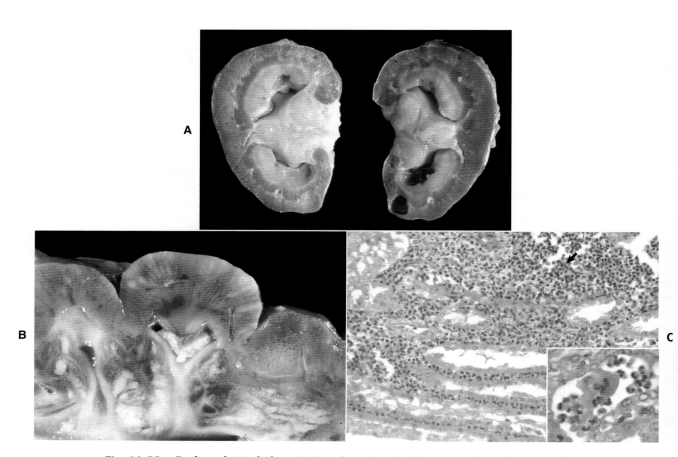

Fig. 11-58   **Pyelonephritis, kidney. A,** Dorsal section, dog. Extensive pelvic inflammation has destroyed areas of the inner medulla and extends focally into the outer medulla. **B,** Dorsal section, cow. Renal calyces in the cow contain suppurative exudate. **C,** Dog. There is both intratubular and interstitial inflammation, characterized by infiltrates of principally neutrophils **(arrow).** **Inset:** Higher magnification of intratubular neutrophils. H&E stain. (**A, C,** and **Inset,** *Courtesy Dr. M.D. McGavin, College of Veterinary Medicine, University of Tennessee.* **B,** *Courtesy Dr. K. Read, College of Veterinary Medicine, Texas A&M University; and Noah's Arkive, College of Veterinary Medicine, The University of Georgia.*)

and extensive necrosis of the medulla, patchy fibrosis in the outer medulla and cortex, and variable amounts of pelvic inflammatory exudates. Chronic pyelonephritis often produces a grossly visible deformity of the renal parenchyma because of extensive interstitial inflammation and scarring (Fig. 11-58).

Microscopically the most severe acute lesions of pyelonephritis are usually in the inner medulla. The transitional epithelium is usually focally or diffusely necrotic and desquamated. Necrotic debris, fibrin, neutrophils, and bacterial colonies can be adherent to the denuded surface. Medullary tubules are notably dilated, and their lumina contain neutrophils and bacterial colonies. Focally the tubular epithelium is necrotic. An intense neutrophilic infiltrate, present in the renal interstitium, can be accompanied by notable interstitial hemorrhages and edema (Fig. 11-58, C). If obstruction of vasa recta has occurred, coagulative necrosis of the inner medulla (papillary necrosis) can be severe. Similar tubular and interstitial lesions, although less severe, extend radially into the cortical tubules and interstitium. When the lesions become subacute, the severity of the neutrophilic infiltrates diminishes, and lymphocytes, plasma cells, and monocytes infiltrate the interstitium. Chronic lesions have severe fibrosis. If active bacterial infection persists or is untreated, an intense infiltrate of all inflammatory cell types interspersed with tubular necrosis and fibrosis can be seen. All stages of disease progression can occur in a single kidney.

HYDRONEPHROSIS

Hydronephrosis refers to dilation of the renal pelvis because of obstruction of urine outflow and is principally caused by a slow or intermittent increase in pelvic pressure. Abrupt increases in pressure, such as those associated with inadvertent surgical ligation of a ureter, more commonly result in a decline in filtration rate in the affected kidney and a lesser propensity to develop hydronephrosis.

Obstruction leading to hydronephrosis can occasionally be caused by congenital malformation of the ureter, vesicoureteral junction, or urethra or from congenitally malpositioned kidneys with secondary kinking of the ureter. The more common causes of hydronephrosis are as follows:
1. Ureteral or urethral blockage due to urinary tract calculi (see Lower Urinary Tract)
2. Chronic inflammation
3. Ureteral or urethral neoplasia
4. Neurogenic functional disorders

Hydronephrosis occurs in all domestic animals. Depending on the location of the obstruction, hydronephrosis can be unilateral (ureteral) or bilateral (both ureters, bladder trigone, or urethra). Unilateral hydronephrosis is caused by obstruction of the ureters anywhere throughout its length or at its entrance into the urinary bladder. Bilateral hydronephrosis can be caused by urethral obstruction, bilateral ureteral obstruction, or extensive urinary bladder lesions centered on the trigone. When hydronephrosis is unilateral, pelvic enlargement of the kidney can become extensive, even cystic, before the lesion is recognized clinically. If the obstructive process causes partial or intermittent blockage, bilateral hydronephrosis can become notable because of continual urine production and pooling of urine in the expanding pelvis. When obstruction is complete and bilateral, death as a result of uremia occurs before pelvic enlargement becomes extensive.

When the increase in intrapelvic pressure is substantial and sustained, the following occur:
1. Intratubular pressure is increased and results in microscopic renal tubular dilation.
2. Glomeruli remain functional, and even with complete obstruction, glomerular filtration does not stop completely and soon overwhelms tubular reabsorption pathways.
3. Much of the glomerular filtrate diffuses into the interstitium, where it is initially removed via lymphatic vessels and veins.
4. As intrapelvic pressure increases, the interstitial vessels collapse and renal blood flow is reduced, resulting in hypoxia, tubular atrophy, and, if the pressure increase is continued, interstitial fibrosis.
5. The glomeruli have a relatively normal morphologic appearance for a prolonged period, but they eventually become atrophic and sclerotic.

Early changes of hydronephrosis include dilation of the pelvis and calyces and blunting of the renal crest and papillae (Fig. 11-59). When pelvic dilation is progressive, the kidney silhouette is enlarged and rounder than normal, and the cortex and medulla are progressively thinned (Fig. 11-60). Interstitial vascular obstruction from compression produces an expanding front of medullary and later cortical ischemia and necrosis. The continued pelvic dilation causes loss of tubules by degeneration and atrophy, followed by condensation of interstitial connective tissue and fibrosis of the renal parenchyma. In its most advanced form, the hydronephrotic kidney is a thin-walled (2- to 3-mm-thick), fluid-filled sac. This sac is lined by flattened transitional epithelium, which is spared during lesion development. Occasionally, a severely hydronephrotic kidney becomes contaminated by bacteria and the thin-walled sac becomes filled with pus instead of urine. This lesion, referred to as pyonephrosis, is likely the result of blood-borne bacteria lodging in a hydronephrotic kidney.

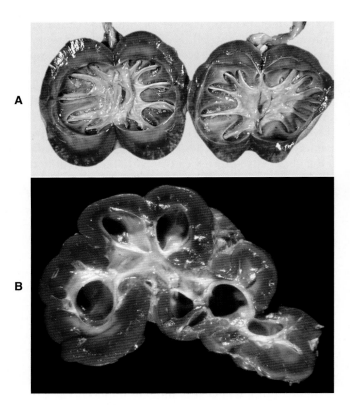

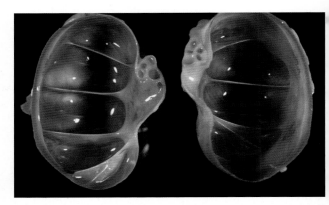

Fig. 11-60 Chronic hydronephrosis, kidney, dorsal section, cat. Advanced hydronephrosis is characterized by loss of medullary tissue and atrophy or even loss of the entire cortex in response to elevated pelvic fluid pressure. Note that this case was so severe that only the renal capsule, which contains clear yellow fluid, remains. *(Courtesy Dr. M.D. McGavin, College of Veterinary Medicine, University of Tennessee.)*

Fig. 11-59 Hydronephrosis, kidney, dorsal section. A, Sheep. The pelvis of each kidney is markedly dilated. **B,** Cow. Bovine kidneys are lobulated, and each lobule has its own renal papilla surrounded by a calyx, an extension of the pelvis. Thus in early hydronephrosis, each of these calyces is distended, and these distended calyces should not be confused with the cysts of a cystic or polycystic kidney. *(**A,** Courtesy Dr. J. King, College of Veterinary Medicine, Cornell University. **B,** Courtesy College of Veterinary Medicine, University of Illinois.)*

PARASITES

The giant kidney worm (*Dioctophyma renale*) is seen infrequently in dogs from temperate and cold countries worldwide. It is endemic in Canada and in northern regions of the United States. Because of a prolonged and complex life cycle, this nematode is seen only in dogs 2 years old or older. The adult nematode is red and cylindrical, with the females measuring 20 to 100 cm long and 4 to 12 mm in diameter, and the males measuring 14 to 45 cm long and 4 to 6 mm in diameter. This nematode resides in the renal pelvis where it causes severe hemorrhagic or purulent pyelitis, subsequent ureteral obstruction, and destruction of the renal parenchyma, resulting in a hydronephrotic kidney that appears as a cyst containing the nematode and purulent exudate.

In North America, the kidney worm (*Stephanurus dentatus*) is found most often in adult pigs in southern regions of the United States. The parasite is also a problem in other countries with warm climates. Adult worms normally encyst in perirenal fat; however, some parasites may reside in the kidney. Peripelvic cysts often communicate with the renal pelvis and ureter, and fibrosis and chronic granulation tissue can enclose the parasite. Occasionally, nematode eggs are present in the urine sediment.

Capillaria plica and *Capillaria feliscati* have been identified infrequently in dogs and cats worldwide. Typically, these nematodes are attached to the renal pelvis, ureter, or bladder of animals of various ages. Microscopically, inflammatory cells infiltrate and focal hemorrhages are associated with sites of attachment in the underlying submucosa. Clinical effects usually are not present, but hematuria and dysuria are produced occasionally.

RENAL FIBROSIS (SCARRING)

Renal fibrosis is the replacement of renal parenchyma, including tubules, glomeruli, and interstitium with mature fibrous connective tissue (Fig. 11-61). It can occur as a primary event, but more frequently is a manifestation of the healing phase of a preexisting tubular or glomerular lesion. It is the common end point of all reparative stages and results when conditions are not conducive for healing of the tubular epithelium by regeneration. Regeneration of nephrons as a whole is not possible. Renal fibrosis follows many renal lesions, including primary inflammation of glomeruli (glomerulonephritis), tubules, or interstitial tissue (tubulointerstitial nephritis) and necrosis of renal tubules. Its severity usually parallels the intensity of the primary renal disease. The mechanisms will be described next for glomerular disease, renal tubular necrosis, and tubulointerstitial disease.

The distribution of fibrosis secondary to glomerular disease is diffuse and primarily cortical. This is because most primary glomerular diseases involve all glomeruli throughout the renal cortex and ultimately result in glomerulosclerosis of some significance. Additionally, because the blood flow through glomerular capillaries is reduced in chronic glomerulonephritis and amyloidosis, the pattern of interstitial fibrosis is diffuse. Sustained proteinuria can also increase tubular epithelial cell apoptosis, leading to tubular atrophy and interstitial fibrosis. Because all components of the nephron are interdependent, glomerular fibrosis and loss of function ultimately results in secondary atrophy of cortical and medullary tubules and fibrosis of the cortical and to a lesser degree medullary interstitium.

Diffuse fibrosis with a finely granular pattern can occur subsequent to widespread necrosis of renal tubular epithelium (acute tubular necrosis). An example is oak poisoning of cattle (Fig. 11-42), in which severe tubular necrosis extends to the level of the renal tubular basement membrane, resulting in leakage of tubular contents. The loss of the continuity of the basement membrane prevents orderly tubular epithelial cell regeneration and this can be followed by interstitial fibrosis. Recent experimental studies have demonstrated that after severe nephrotoxin-induced tubular epithelial cell injury, the remaining cells undergo accelerated apoptosis resulting in tubular atrophy, interstitial fibroblast proliferation, and eventual fibrosis.

Different coarser patterns of renal fibrosis occur when the primary lesion is less evenly distributed in the kidneys. Fibrosis secondary to the tubulointerstitial inflammation of pyelonephritis follows the pattern of the acute disease (targeting the renal poles), and results in irregularly distributed, patchy scarring that is seen as deeply depressed regions on the renal capsular surface and linear areas extending through both the cortex and medulla to the pelvis (Fig. 11-62).

The scarring that follows embolic or thrombotic vascular obstruction and infarction is related to several variables, including the size of the ischemic area caused by vascular compromise. Ischemia resulting from obstruction of relatively large arterioles causes large areas of coagulative necrosis. Healing results in large, deeply depressed wedge-shaped scars that involve primarily the cortex, but can extend into the medulla. Obstruction of smaller arterioles results in smaller areas of more superficial coagulative necrosis that heal as small-diameter pits in the renal surface, which correspond to pale white, linear scars on the cut surface.

A coarser pattern of diffuse renal fibrosis occurs in chronic interstitial nephritis and certain progressive juvenile nephropathies of dogs. Both cortex and medulla

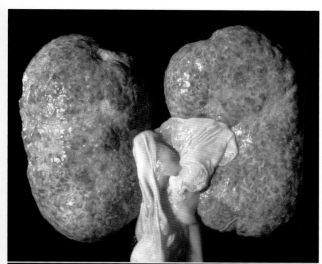

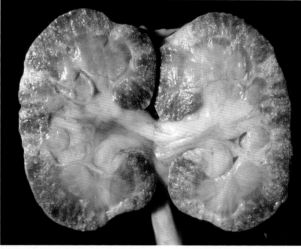

Fig. 11-61   Chronic interstitial nephritis, kidney, dog.
A, Diffuse interstitial fibrosis is responsible for the fine pitting of the capsular cortical surface, which is stippled red, the result of bands of fibrous tissue (*gray*) surrounding islands of renal cortex. **B,** Dorsal section. The cortex is pitted and granular because of multiple linear and focal scars, and it is also thinner than normal (atrophic). (*A* and *B*, *Courtesy Dr. M.D. McGavin, College of Veterinary Medicine, University of Tennessee.*)

by which fibrosis is induced are related to destruction and loss of nephron components by inflammatory or less commonly noninflammatory processes. Renal fibrosis is seen commonly following any number of renal insults and includes the following:

1. Infarction
2. Glomerulonephritis/amyloidosis
3. Tubulointerstitial disease/chronic pelvic diseases

Without careful attention to the pattern of resultant fibrosis, such kidneys can be indiscriminately termed as end-stage kidneys; however, fibrosis generally follows a pattern characteristic of the antecedent injury and

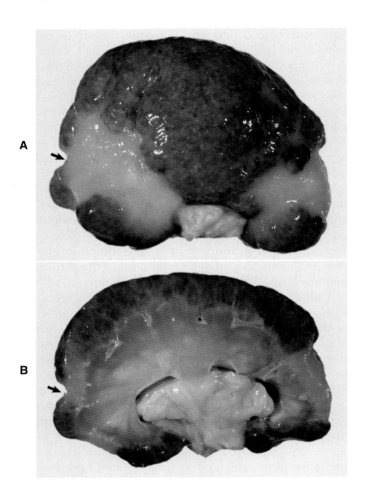

Fig. 11-62   Chronic pyelonephritis, kidney, dog. A, Note the two large polar scars visible as large indentations on the capsular surface *(arrow).* The fine gray spots are regions of chronic inflammatory infiltrates and fibrosis. **B,** Dorsal section. The cortical scars are localized to the renal poles *(arrow),* but there is a finely stippled pattern of nodularity and fibrosis in the remaining kidney. This polar pattern of scarring suggests previous pyelonephritis. *(A and B, Courtesy Dr. A. Confer, College of Veterinary Medicine, Oklahoma State University.)*

can be fibrotic; cortical striations are severely distorted or effaced; and the formation of multiple cortical cysts is common.

Specifically, renal fibrosis may manifest in a multitude of grossly recognizable forms as described previously. Generally, fibrotic kidneys are recognized grossly by the pale, tan-to-white, shrunken, pitted and firm consistency along with excessive adhesions of the capsule to the underlying cortex. Fibrosis can be diffuse and finely stippled with pinpoint dimpling and granularity on the capsular surface, or it can be coarser as seen by deep and irregularly shaped depressions of the capsular surface in either a diffuse, multifocal, or patchy

distribution. In addition to these changes of the capsular surface, the cut surface of the cortex is thinned beneath the capsular surface depressions, and these fibrotic areas are pale tan when compared with more normal parenchyma.

Microscopically, renal fibrosis is characterized by an increase in interstitial connective tissue and disappearance of renal tubules (Fig. 11-63, A). Remaining tubules are usually atrophic and have a reduced luminal diameter or can appear ectatic because they are lined by flattened epithelium, producing an enlarged luminal diameter. A thickened hyalinized basement membrane and a lining of flattened epithelium (squamous or low cuboidal) are also characteristic. Multiple acquired cysts can be present throughout the cortex and medulla and can be a result of either dilated Bowman's capsules and associated atrophic glomerular tufts or nephrons whose tubules have segments compressed by connective tissue (Fig. 11-63, B). Even in fibrotic lesions that are not the result of an infectious disease or inflammation, foci of lymphocytes and plasma cells can be seen randomly scattered throughout the interstitium (Fig. 11-63, C). In areas of severe interstitial fibrosis, glomerulosclerosis (as an end stage of isolated glomeruli) is common. Calcification of vessels, tubular basement membranes, Bowman's capsules, and degenerate tubular epithelium is common in fibrotic kidneys because of alterations in calcium-phosphorus metabolism associated with chronic renal failure (Fig. 11-29).

Renal fibrosis and chronic renal disease are the most frequently recognized renal pathologic processes in mature or aging domestic animals, particularly dogs and cats. When renal fibrosis and loss of nephrons are severe, these lesions can be manifested clinically as chronic renal failure and uremia. One of the most common expressions of this chronic disease is the inability of an animal to concentrate urine, resulting in frequent urination (polyuria) of dilute urine (isosthenuria). Polyuria is accompanied by dehydration and excessive water drinking (polydipsia). Hypoplastic anemia occurs as a result of the kidneys' failure to synthesize and secrete erythropoietin. Fibrous osteodystrophy can develop because of abnormal calcium-phosphorus metabolism and renal secondary hyperparathyroidism.

PROGRESSIVE JUVENILE NEPHROPATHY

The development of severe bilateral renal fibrosis has been described in young dogs of several breeds and referred to as progressive juvenile nephropathy or familial (hereditary) renal disease (Table 11-5). In many dogs, a familial tendency is demonstrated, but the mode of inheritance has been determined with certainty in only a few dog breeds. In Samoyeds, the lesion is sex-linked; in bull terriers, it is autosomal dominant;

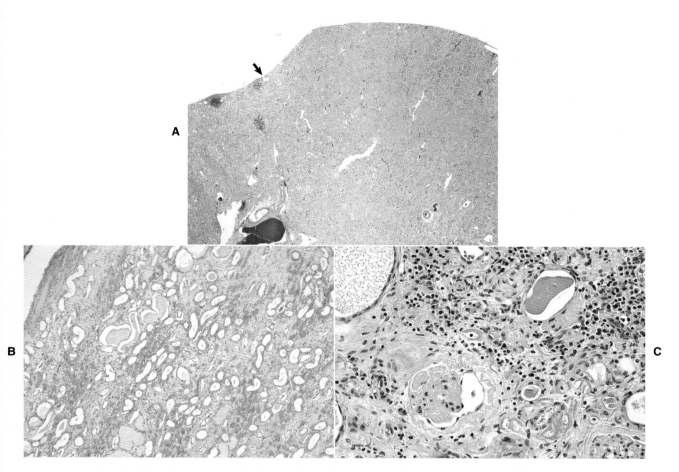

Fig. 11-63 **Chronic interstitial nephritis, kidney, dog. A,** Dorsal section, cortex. This lesion is characterized by interstitial fibrosis, tubular atrophy, and interstitial inflammatory cell (lymphocytes and plasma cell) infiltration. Note the depressed capsular surface as a result of scarring and the shrunken sclerotic glomeruli *(arrow).* H&E stain. **B,** Acquired cystic tubules are due to constriction of portions of the nephron by renal fibrosis. H&E stain. **C,** Cortex. Higher magnification of notable interstitial fibrosis, lymphocytic inflammatory infiltrates, sclerotic glomerular tufts, and ectatic tubules and Bowman's spaces. H&E stain. (***A*** *and* ***C,*** *Courtesy Dr. S.J. Newman, College of Veterinary Medicine, University of Tennessee.* ***B,*** *Courtesy Dr. M.D. McGavin, College of Veterinary Medicine, University of Tennessee.)*

and in the Shih Tzu, the disease appears to have a simple autosomal recessive inheritance. Recently, a progressive juvenile nephropathy, similar to that seen in dogs, was described in six young Japanese black cattle. The cattle had a common male ancestor, suggesting a familial basis.

Progressive juvenile nephropathy is a syndrome, the morphologic manifestations of which can be the result of any of several chronic pathologic processes. The main manifestations include the following:

1. Membranoproliferative glomerulonephritis
2. Tubular disease of unknown cause with tubular atrophy and interstitial fibrosis
3. Renal dysplasia

Gross renal lesions of progressive juvenile nephropathy are variable among affected breeds and among affected dogs within a breed. Generally, kidneys are notably shrunken, pale tan to white, and firm (Fig. 11-11, C and D). The renal surface can be diffusely pitted and have a fine granular pattern, particularly in those dogs in which glomerular disease is the primary event. In these cases of juvenile nephropathy that are of tubular origin or dysplastic, the renal surface can have patchy, deeply depressed areas of cortical scarring. On the cut surface, the cortex is thin and has linear radial scars. The medulla is usually diffusely fibrotic. Small (1 to 2 mm), variably sized cysts are seen often in the cortex and the medulla.

Table **11-5** Breeds of Dogs with Progressive Juvenile Nephropathy

American cocker spaniels
English cocker spaniels
Norwegian elkhounds
Samoyeds
Doberman pinschers
Lhasa apsos
Shih Tzus
Soft-coated Wheaten terriers
Bull terriers
Standard poodles
Alaskan malamutes
Miniature schnauzers
German shepherds
Keeshonds
Chow chows
Weimaraners
Golden retrievers

In the Doberman pinscher, the primary lesion is a glomerulopathy that appears microscopically as a membranoproliferative glomerulonephritis. Later in the clinical course of the disease, the lesions include extensive periglomerular fibrosis, tubular atrophy, and cystic dilation of Bowman's (urinary) space and tubules. In affected Samoyeds and English cocker spaniels, multilamellar splitting of the glomerular basement membrane is caused by inherited abnormalities in basement membrane collagen. These lesions progress to severe glomerulosclerosis.

In Norwegian elkhounds, a tubular disorder of unknown cause has been described and is characterized by progressive tubular atrophy, periglomerular and interstitial fibrosis, and glomerulosclerosis without any indication of a primary glomerular disease.

Progressive juvenile nephropathy has been described in Lhasa apsos, Shih Tzus, Wheaten terriers, standard poodles, and golden retrievers as a condition resembling renal dysplasia, defined as an abnormality of renal development as a result of anomalous differentiation. Small, shrunken, fetal-like glomeruli composed of small cells with dense nuclei, minimal mesangial tissue, and nonpatent capillaries can be seen interspersed with normal, sclerotic, or hypertrophied glomeruli. Other lesions include marked interstitial fibrosis and tubular dilation. Most of the kidneys have minimal lympho-plasmacellular interstitial cell infiltrates.

Although variations exist in gross and microscopic lesions (Fig. 11-11, *E*), as well as in the pathogenesis of progressive nephropathy among the different breeds, a typical case is a dog 4 months to 2 years of age that has polyuria, polydipsia, and uremia. The clinical presentation, gross lesions, and microscopic changes are identical to those of chronic renal disease and renal fibrosis in mature or aging dogs.

CIRCULATORY DISTURBANCES

HYPEREMIA AND CONGESTION

Hyperemia refers to an increase in arterial blood flow, and congestion is an increase in venous blood pooling within the vasculature of the kidney. Renal hyperemia is an active process usually secondary to acute renal inflammation. Renal congestion can be:
1. Physiologic
2. Passive
3. Secondary to hypovolemic shock
4. Secondary to cardiac insufficiency
5. Hypostatic

Hyperemic kidneys are darker red than normal, can be perceptibly swollen, and ooze blood from the cut surface. Congested kidneys are dark purple and ooze blood from the cut surface due to the accumulation unoxygenated blood in the renal venous system. At necropsy, unilateral renal hypostatic congestion is present in animals that die in lateral recumbency, following which the force of gravity pulls the unclotted blood downward. Microscopically the arterial and venous vessels are distended with blood, and if there has been sufficient time for the blood to clot, serum and blood cells may be present.

HEMORRHAGE AND THROMBOSIS

Hemorrhage occurs when red blood cells extend beyond the vessel walls. Large intrarenal hemorrhages can result from direct trauma, renal biopsy, and systemic bleeding disorders, such as factor VIII deficiency. Subcapsular and renal cortical hemorrhages occur in association with septicemic diseases, vasculitis, vascular necrosis, thromboembolism, and disseminated intravascular coagulation (DIC).

Petechial hemorrhages are commonly seen on the surface and throughout the cortex of kidneys from pigs that die of viremia or septicemia caused by diseases such as hog cholera (swine fever), African swine fever, erysipelas, streptococcal infections, salmonellosis, and other embolic bacterial diseases (Fig. 11-64). Renal cortical ecchymotic hemorrhages associated with multifocal tubular and vascular necrosis are salient and diagnostically important lesions of viremia in neonatal puppies infected with herpesvirus. Valvular endocarditis can predispose to renal thromboembolic damage in any species.

When DIC causes widespread thrombosis in the glomerular capillaries (Fig. 11-65), the interlobular arteries, and afferent arterioles, widespread cortical infarction results and is designated renal cortical necrosis. This lesion is not to be confused with ischemic acute

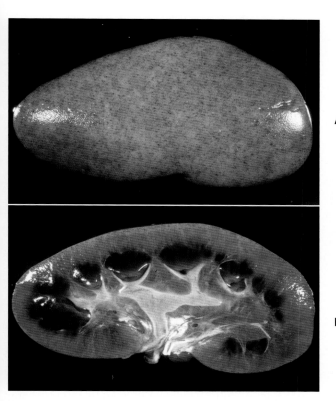

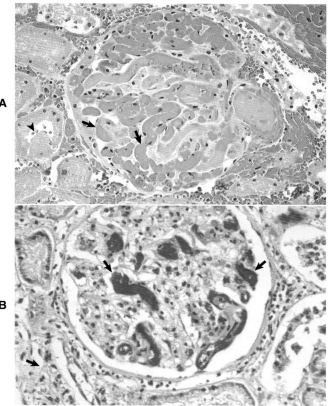

Fig. 11-64   Bacterial-induced septicemic renal cortical hemorrhages, erysipelas, kidney, pig. A, Petechial hemorrhages caused by septic emboli of *Erysipelothrix rhusiopathiae* are randomly scattered over the capsular surface of the kidney. **B,** Dorsal section. Similar petechiae are present on the cut surface of the renal cortex. (**A** and **B,** *Courtesy Dr. M.D. McGavin, College of Veterinary Medicine, University of Tennessee.*)

Fig. 11-65   Glomerular capillary thrombosis, kidney, glomerulus, dog. A, Microthrombi. Capillary lumens are occluded by microthrombi (*arrows*) caused by disseminated intravascular coagulation. Adjacent cortical tubular epithelial cells are undergoing coagulation necrosis with nuclei undergoing pyknosis and karyolysis (*arrowhead*), the result of ischemia from reduced blood flow to the peritubular capillaries, which are downstream from the glomerulus. H&E stain. **B,** Fibrinous microthrombi. A glomerulus similar to the one shown in Fig. 11-65, A stained to demonstrate fibrinous thrombi (*arrows*). Fibrin is red. Lendrum-Fraser stain for fibrin. (**A,** *Courtesy Dr. W. Crowell, College of Veterinary Medicine, The University of Georgia; and Noah's Arkive, College of Veterinary Medicine, The University of Georgia.* **B,** *Courtesy College of Veterinary Medicine, University of Illinois.*)

tubular necrosis discussed in this chapter (see Tubular Necrosis). Partial or complete renal cortical necrosis is usually a bilateral lesion that occurs in all animal species, especially in association with gram-negative septicemias or endotoxemias, and is related to the following:

1. Endotoxin-induced endothelial damage
2. Activation of the extrinsic clotting mechanism
3. Widespread capillary thrombosis

The lesion can be induced experimentally in animals by two endotoxin injections 24 hours apart and is a manifestation of the generalized Shwartzman reaction.

The resulting microthrombosis of vessels throughout the renal cortex results in widespread ischemia and small and large areas of coagulation necrosis and hemorrhage. The renal cortex can be diffusely pale with a zone of hyperemia separating the necrotic cortex from the viable medulla, or more often the cortex is a mosaic of large, irregular hemorrhagic areas, resembling hemorrhagic infarcts interspersed with large yellow-gray areas resembling pale infarcts. The necrotic tissue

can involve the full width of the cortex or only the outer portion. Thrombi are demonstrable in the renal vasculature.

INFARCTION

Renal infarcts are areas of coagulative necrosis that result from the local ischemia of vascular occlusion and usually are due to thromboembolism secondary to valvular endocarditis; endarteritis from parasitic diseases, such as heart worm or strongyles; mural thrombosis (atherosclerotic plaque); or aseptic emboli (neoplastic emboli).

Because of the high circulating blood volume (20% to 25% of cardiac output) through the kidney, renal infarcts from thromboemboli secondary to embolism from mitral or aortic valvular vegetative endocarditis or mural endocarditis are common in many species, especially in cats with left atrial thrombosis associated with cardiomyopathy. Rarely, emboli may occlude the renal artery, causing infarction of the entire kidney. Sometimes emboli occlude the interlobar arteries, causing infarction of variable segments of the cortex and medulla. Most commonly, emboli obstruct many smaller vessels (e.g., interlobular arteries), causing multiple smaller infarcts involving only the renal cortex. In general, renal infarction can occur because of thrombosis resulting from endothelial damage associated with a vascular disease (as in Alabama rot in greyhounds; Fig. 11-25) or with cardiovascular collapse and shock. Renal infarcts in horses can result from emboli lodging in the renal vasculature following mural thrombosis of the aorta, from aortic wall damage, and from migrating larvae of *Strongylus vulgaris*. Thrombosis of pulmonary, coronary, splenic, or renal arteries and resultant infarction are common in dogs with renal amyloidosis primarily because of loss of plasma anticoagulants, such as antithrombin III, through damaged glomeruli. Endotoxin-mediated arterial or capillary thrombosis is a common cause of infarction in association with gram-negative sepsis or endotoxic shock. Septic emboli, particularly those from bacterial valvular endocarditis, caused by *Arcanobacterium pyogenes* in cattle, *Erysipelothrix rhusiopathiae* in pigs, and *Staphylococcus aureus* in small animals can cause renal infarcts.

Grossly, renal infarcts appear red or pale white depending on several factors, including the interval after vascular occlusion (i.e., age of infarct) (Figs. 11-66 and 11-67). Occlusion of small interlobular arteries results in infarcts that are initially slightly swollen and red because of hemorrhage (Fig. 11-67, *A*) and which later become pale yellow-gray within 2 to 3 days because of lysis of erythrocytes and loss of hemoglobin (Fig. 11-67, *B*). Initially, large infarcts develop when an embolus lodges in the interlobular artery closer to its origin from the arcuate artery. These larger infarcts have a central area of pallor (coagulative necrosis) and are usually surrounded by a peripheral red zone of congestion and hemorrhage along with a pale margin because of a surrounding zone of leukocytes (Fig. 11-67, *C*). Because of the loss of parenchyma, healing infarcts are depressed below the cortical surface, and later become pale and shrunken as a result of fibrosis (Fig. 11-67, *D*).

Infarcts are often wedge-shaped in a cross section of kidney, with the base against the cortical surface and the apex pointing toward the medulla, conforming to a zone of cortical parenchyma supplied by the obstructed interlobular artery. Infarcts can involve the cortex only or the cortex and medulla depending on the size of the occluded vessel and the site of obstruction. For example, thrombosis of an arcuate artery, which supplies both cortex and medulla, would result in an infarct involving the cortex and extending partway into the medulla (Fig. 11-4). Thrombosis of a cortical interlobular artery, which supplies mainly the cortex, would result in an infarct of the cortex only (Fig. 11-4). Although less common, hypoxic renal necrosis due to venous occlusion and/or infarction are seen occasionally, and they retain their hemorrhagic appearance longer than infarcts resulting from arterial occlusion because of the continued arterial blood flow into the area.

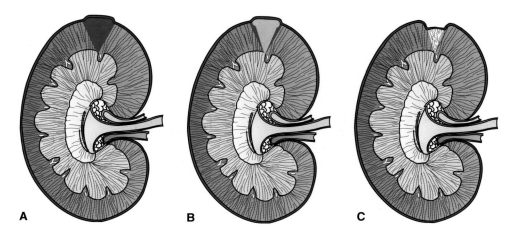

Fig. 11-66   Schematic diagram of renal infarction. The normal progression of renal infarcts is outlined. **A** and **B,** Acute renal infarcts. Initially, renal infarcts are swollen and hemorrhagic (**A**). In 2 to 3 days, infarcts become pale (**B**), surrounded by a zone of hyperemia and hemorrhage. **C,** Chronic infarcts are pale, shrunken, and fibrotic, resulting in distortion and depression of the renal contour. See Fig. 11-1 for identification of the anatomic components of the kidney.

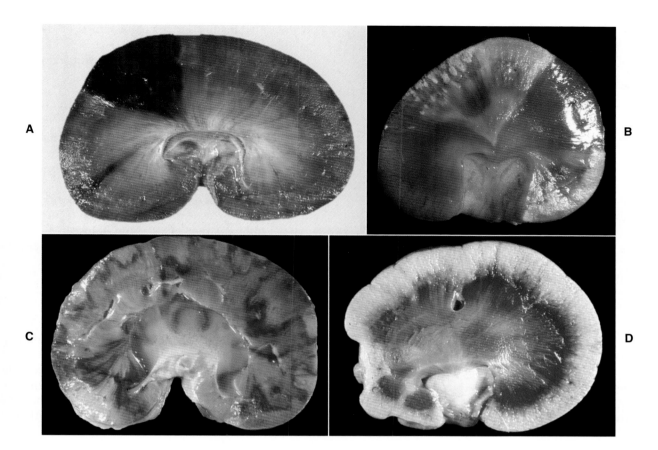

Fig. 11-67   Gross appearance of renal cortical infarcts with age, kidney, dorsal sections.
A, Acute (early) hemorrhagic infarct, dog. Focal wedge-shaped area of cortical necrosis. Note
how the infarct bulges above the capsular surface due to cell swelling and hemorrhage.
B, Acute pale infarcts, rabbit. There are two pale white to tan wedge-shaped infarcts *(top, lower*
right). Note how the infarct *(top)* bulges above the capsular surface, indicating cell swelling.
C, Subacute infarcts, dog. Multiple renal cortical infarcts are pale and surrounded by a red rim
of active hyperemia. The cortical surface of many, but not all, of the infarcts is even with that of
the adjacent unaffected cortex, indicating that cell swelling has subsided. **D,** Chronic infarct,
cat. A focal pale truncated wedge-shaped scar of fibrous connective tissue has replaced the
pole of the renal cortex. Note that the surface of the infarct is below that of the adjacent
normal kidney because of the loss of tissue, fibrosis, and contraction of the fibrous scar.
(**A,** *Courtesy Dr. W. Crowell, College of Veterinary Medicine, The University of Georgia; and Noah's Arkive, College of*
Veterinary Medicine, The University of Georgia. **B,** *Courtesy Dr. M.D. McGavin, College of Veterinary Medicine,*
University of Tennessee. **C,** *Courtesy Dr. K. Read, College of Veterinary Medicine, Texas A&M University; and Noah's*
Arkive, College of Veterinary Medicine, The University of Georgia. **D,** *Courtesy Dr. J. Sagartz, College of Veterinary*
Medicine, The Ohio State University; and Noah's Arkive, College of Veterinary Medicine, The University of Georgia.)

Microscopically, in an acute infarct, nephrons
(including tubules, glomeruli, and interstitium) in the
central zone of the infarct become necrotic (Fig. 11-68).
At the periphery of the infarct, only the proximal tubules,
because of their high metabolic rate, are necrotic; the
glomeruli tend to be spared. After a couple of days, the
margin of the necrotic zone contains an inflammatory
infiltrate consisting largely of neutrophils and fewer

macrophages and lymphocytes (Fig. 11-68). Capillaries
adjacent to the necrotic area are notably engorged with
blood. Healing of the infarcted area occurs by lysis and
phagocytosis of the necrotic tissue and replacement by
fibrous connective tissue, which matures to a discrete
scar. Scars range from linear to broad depending on the
size of the acute infarct. Septic infarcts are initially
hemorrhagic, but because of the presence of pyogenic

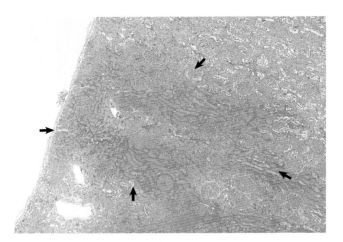

Fig. 11-68   Acute infarct, kidney, cortex, dog. Note the acute infarct with a central zone of coagulation necrosis surrounded by a zone of hyperemia and hemorrhage *(arrows)*. H&E stain. *(Courtesy Dr. S.J. Newman, College of Veterinary Medicine, University of Tennessee.)*

bacteria, the necrotic tissue undergoes liquefactive necrosis and the infarcts can eventually develop into abscesses and ultimately into substantial scars. Septic infarcts often fail to respect a solely cortical or medullary pattern of distribution due to the extensive local inflammation that they generate.

PAPILLARY (MEDULLARY CREST) NECROSIS

Necrosis of the renal papillae, or their counterpart, the medullary crest, is a response of the inner medulla to ischemia. Papillary necrosis can be a primary or secondary lesion. Papillary necrosis occurs as a primary disease in animals treated with nonsteroidal antiinflammatory analgesic drugs and is analogous to analgesic nephropathy in human beings. The primary disease occurs quite frequently in horses treated for prolonged periods with phenylbutazone or flunixin meglumine. It is of potential importance in dogs and cats because of accidental ingestion of or treatment with ibuprofen, aspirin, or acetaminophen at excessive dosages. Drugs associated with papillary necrosis are sometimes referred to as "papillotoxins." The medullary interstitial cells are the primary targets of papillotoxins. These cells have a key role in synthesis of prostaglandins, antihypertensive factors, and the glycosaminoglycan matrix of the medullary interstitium. Interstitial cell damage decreases prostaglandin synthesis, which reduces normal blood flow and causes ischemia, increases tubular transport, and modifies the interstitial matrix; the net effect is degenerative changes in tubular epithelial cells in the inner medulla. In addition to its inhibition of prostaglandin biosynthesis, acetaminophen also causes direct oxidative damage to medullary tubular epithelium after covalent binding

to the cells, further enhancing necrosis of the renal papillae.

Secondary papillary necrosis results from the following:
A. Reduced blood flow in vasa recta
   1. Glomerular lesions restricting blood flow—amyloid, hyalinization
   2. Compression of vasa recta—within the medulla
     a. Interstitial fibrosis—chiefly in the outer medulla, secondary to ischemia (see later discussion)
     b. Interstitial renal medullary amyloidosis (cats)
     c. Pyelitis—ascending tubular and interstitial inflammation, edema, and fibrosis
B. Compression of renal papilla by factors external to the kidney
   1. Intrapelvic pressure secondary to:
     a. Pelvic calculi
     b. Lower urinary tract obstruction
     c. Vesicoureteral reflux

The outer medulla and the cells of the thick ascending loop of Henle in particular are the least well perfused of any zones of the kidneys. This is because the medulla has little direct perfusion; instead, most of the medullary blood supply comes from the cortex, through the vasa recta. Because of this limited blood flow, in addition to the high metabolic medullary cellular demand, any lesion or disease process that further reduces medullary blood flow can cause ischemic necrosis (infarction) of the papillae. Additionally, the high metabolic demand for cell transport and the maintenance of an ion gradient to enhance urinary concentration makes this area particularly vulnerable. This is most evident following ischemic tubular damage where swollen endothelial and tubular epithelial cells, in conjunction with neutrophil adhesion in small vessels, upset the balance of oxygenation and energy demand by the outer medullary tubular cells. Medullary blood flow is ultimately balanced through levels of vasodilators, such as prostaglandin, nitric oxide, and adenosine, and vasoconstrictors, such as endothelin and angiotensin II.

Typically, acute lesions are irregular, discolored areas of necrotic inner medulla sharply delineated from the surviving medullary tissue (Fig. 11-69). The affected tissue, which is undergoing coagulation necrosis, is yellow-gray, green, or pink. With time, the necrotic tissue sloughs, resulting in a detached, friable, and discolored tissue fragment in the pelvis. The remaining inner medulla is usually narrowed and attenuated. Overlying cortex can be somewhat shrunken because of atrophy of some of the nephrons caused by blockage of the tubules secondary to the chronic medullary changes. Small pieces of sloughed necrotic medullary tissue pass inconsequentially into the ureter. However, large pieces of sloughed tissue can

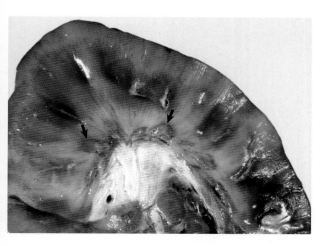

Fig. 11-69   Papillary (medullary crest) necrosis, chronic nonsteroidal antiinflammatory drug treatment, kidney, dorsal section, horse. Acute coagulation necrosis of the medullary crest and inner medulla (*greenish areas*). There is also hemorrhage of the outer medulla (*arrows*). The term *papillary necrosis* is retained for all animals, although only the pig and cow have distinct renal papillae. In other animals, these have fused to form the medullary crest. (*Courtesy Dr. A. Confer, College of Veterinary Medicine, Oklahoma State University.*)

obstruct the ureter, causing hydronephrosis, or form a nidus for precipitation of minerals, resulting in the formation of pelvic or ureteral calculi. Papillary necrosis is usually an incidental finding at necropsy and rarely leads to progressive renal damage and failure.

NEOPLASIA

The prevalence of primary renal neoplasms in domestic animals is less than 1% of the total neoplasms reported. They are usually unilateral and can be of epithelial, mesenchymal, or embryonal origin.

EPITHELIAL TUMORS

Renal adenomas are rare, benign, epithelial neoplasms consisting of proliferating renal cortical epithelial cells. They are incidental findings at necropsy and usually appear as a small (1 to 3 cm), white-to-yellow, solitary, well-circumscribed, nonencapsulated mass in the cortex. Microscopically, adenomas are composed of solid sheets, tubules, or papillary proliferations of cuboidal epithelial cells that are uniform in size and have granular eosinophilic cytoplasm and small, round to oval nuclei. Mitotic figures, necrosis, and fibrosis are rare. These incidental tumors are clinically asymptomatic.

Oncocytomas are rare benign epithelial tumors that can occur in a variety of tissues. Grossly, renal oncocytomas are tan, homogeneous, well-encapsulated masses composed of oncocytes. Histologically, they are composed of large eosinophilic granular round cells with condensed

round nuclei. Ultrastructurally, they are characterized by numerous prominent cytoplasmic mitochondria. Their origin in the kidney is speculated to be from the intercalated cells of the collecting ducts. These tumors are clinically asymptomatic.

Renal carcinomas are the most common primary renal neoplasms and occur most frequently in older dogs. The specific causes of renal adenocarcinomas in human beings are well determined compared with those in animal species, but several mechanisms have been proven in natural animal disease or experimental models. These include the following:
1. Viruses—herpesvirus oncogenes are known to play a major role in formation of virally induced adenocarcinoma (Lucke's tumor) in the kidney of frogs, and avian erythroblastosis virus [strain ES4] induces renal adenocarcinomas in chickens.
2. Chemical carcinogens—these have been postulated to be causative and typically exert their neoplastic influence by direct DNA damage or inhibition of DNA synthesis or repair.
3. Autosomal dominant gene mutations in Eker rats—these predispose these rats to bilateral renal cell carcinoma and a variety of other secondary cancers, resembling the human von Hippel-Lindau disease.

These neoplasms are usually large (up to 20 cm in diameter), spherical to oval, and firm. They often are pale yellow and contain dark areas of hemorrhage and necrosis and foci of cystic degeneration. The masses usually occupy and obliterate one pole of the kidney and grow by expansion, compressing the adjacent normal renal tissue (Fig. 11-70). Histologic types include papillary, tubular, and solid (Fig. 11-70, C), with solid variants being the most poorly differentiated. Metastasis to the lungs, lymph nodes, liver, and adrenal occur frequently. Renal carcinoma has been associated with paraneoplastic conditions, principally polycythemia. This is because of concurrent overexpression of erythropoietin, which increases bone marrow production of red blood cells.

A variant of the typical renal carcinoma has been seen in German shepherd dogs in conjunction with nodular dermatofibrosis. The lesions are hereditary and consist of multifocal, bilateral, renal cystadenomas or cystadenocarcinomas. Grossly, these resemble the adenocarcinomas described previously, but cysts are much more prominent. The neoplastic cells form solid sheets, tubules, or papillary growth patterns, and the cells in the carcinomas are more atypical and anaplastic. Cells vary in shape from cuboidal and columnar to polyhedral, vary in size, and have clear or granular eosinophilic cytoplasm. Nuclei range from small, round, granular, and uniform to large, oval, vesicular, and pleomorphic. Mitotic figures are numerous. These neoplasms have a moderate fibrovascular stroma.

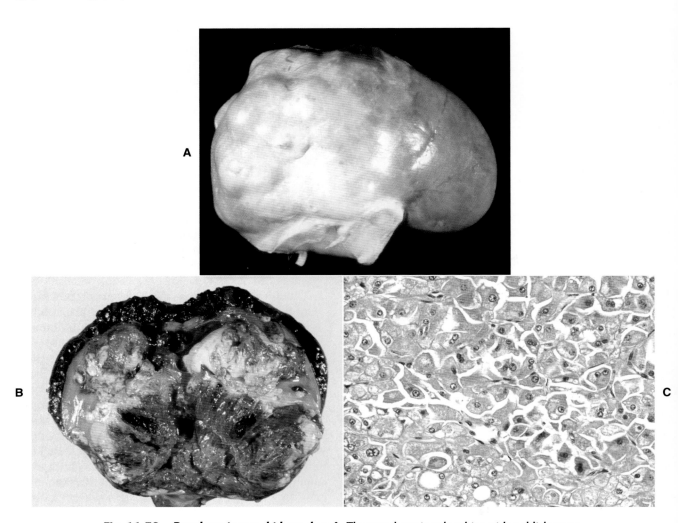

Fig. 11-70   Renal carcinoma, kidney, dog. A, The neoplasm is pale white with reddish areas, lobulated, and has infiltrated and replaced one pole of the kidney. **B,** Dorsal section. The normal architecture of the cranial half of the kidney has been obliterated by the tumor, which has hemorrhaged caudally into the adjacent kidney and subcapsularly. **C,** The tumor consists of anaplastic renal epithelial cells, typical of the solid, more poorly differentiated variant of renal carcinoma. H&E stain. *(A and B, Courtesy College of Veterinary Medicine, University of Illinois. C, Courtesy Dr. S.J. Newman, College of Veterinary Medicine, University of Tennessee.)*

Transitional cell papillomas and transitional cell carcinomas arise in the renal pelvis and lower urinary tract and, when large, can obstruct urinary outflow. Such carcinomas can invade into the kidney and typically carry a poor prognosis. The morphologic features of transitional cell neoplasms will be discussed later with the urinary bladder neoplasms (see Lower Urinary Tract).

MESENCHYMAL TUMORS

Occasionally, fibromas, fibrosarcomas, or hemangiosarcomas originate in the kidneys. Primary renal sarcomas are rare. Microscopically, in hemangiosarcomas, neoplastic spindle cells are arranged in solid interlacing bundles and whorls or as variable channels lined by neoplastic endothelium. Cellular pleomorphism and mitotic rate are relatively low.

METASTATIC TUMORS

Carcinomas and sarcomas (metastatic tumors) arising in other organs can metastasize to the kidneys and are characteristically composed of randomly scattered multiple nodules, usually involving both kidneys (Fig. 11-71). Renal lymphosarcoma occurs with some frequency in cattle and cats, particularly as part of generalized or multicentric lymphosarcoma, which is secondary to retrovirus infection. These neoplastic foci appear as single or multiple homogeneous gray-white nodules (Fig. 11-71, *B* and *E*) or as diffuse lymphomatous infiltrates that cause uniform enlargement and pale discoloration of the kidney (Fig. 11-71, *C*). In cats, renal lymphosarcoma must be differentiated histologically from the necrotizing, fibrinous, and granulomatous renal vasculitis of feline infectious peritonitis and less

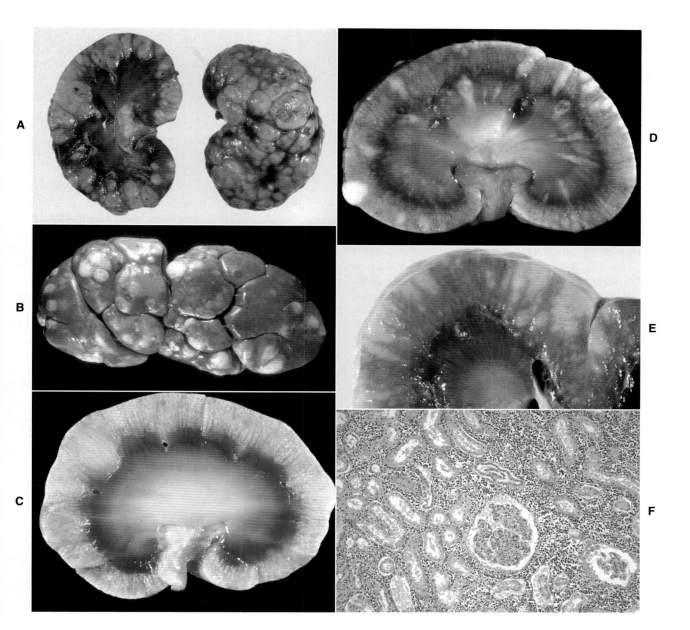

Fig. 11-71   Primary and metastatic renal tumors, kidney. A, Metastatic mast cell tumor, dorsal section, dog. Multiple pale tan, raised nodules are randomly scattered throughout the renal cortex. **B,** Lymphoma (lymphosarcoma), cow. Multifocal raised pale white nodules are typical of nodular renal lymphosarcoma. **C,** Lymphoma (lymphosarcoma), dorsal section, cat. Note the pale white areas in the cortex, which bulge from the surface. This lesion can be confused with the granulomatous vasculitis of renal feline infectious peritonitis, thus warranting histologic evaluation. **D,** Systemic cryptococcosis (*Cryptococcus neoformans*), cat. This is not a neoplasm, but the multiple pale, occasionally raised nodules can be confused with the nodular form of lymphoma (Fig. 11-71, *C*), thus requiring histologic examination. **E,** Lymphoma (lymphosarcoma), dorsal section, bovine. Multiple coalescing pale white nodules are present throughout the cortex. **F,** Lymphoma (lymphosarcoma), cow. Neoplastic lymphocytes infiltrate and distend the renal interstitium. H&E stain. (*A, Courtesy Dr. A. Confer, College of Veterinary Medicine, Oklahoma State University. B, Courtesy College of Veterinary Medicine, University of Illinois. C, Courtesy Dr. K. Read, College of Veterinary Medicine, Texas A&M University; and Noah's Arkive, College of Veterinary Medicine, The University of Georgia. D, Courtesy Dr. S.J. Newman, College of Veterinary Medicine, University of Tennessee. E, Courtesy Dr. J. King, College of Veterinary Medicine, Cornell University; and Dr. J. Edwards, College of Veterinary Medicine, Texas A&M University. F, Courtesy Dr. J. Simon, College of Veterinary Medicine, University of Illinois.*)

commonly systemic cryptococcosis (Fig. 11-71, *E*). Microscopically, neoplastic lymphocytes form obliterative sheets of cells within the renal parenchyma, unrelated to the vasculature (Fig. 11-71, *F*). Neoplastic lymphocytes have distinct cellular borders, moderate amounts of basophilic cytoplasm, and large round vesicular nuclei with variable prominence to the nucleoli. Lymphosarcoma of the kidney can be treated with some success with chemotherapeutics.

TUMORS OF EMBRYONAL ORIGIN

Nephroblastomas (embryonal nephroma or Wilms tumor) are common renal neoplasms of pigs and chickens, and are usually recognized as incidental findings at slaughter. They occur in cattle and dogs as well, but less frequently. These neoplasms arise from metanephric blastema and thus occur in young animals. It is speculated that neoplasms result from malignant transformation during normal nephrogenesis or from neoplastic transformation of nests of embryonic tissue that persist in the postnatal kidneys. At necropsy, nephroblastomas can be solitary or multiple masses that often reach a great size and in which recognizable renal tissue can be difficult to detect. They usually are soft to rubbery and gray with foci of hemorrhage. On a cut surface, they are often lobulated. Because nephroblastomas arise from primitive pluripotential tissue, histologic features vary but are morphologically similar to the developmental stages of embryonic kidneys. Characteristically, three components—including primitive, loose myxomatous mesenchymal tissue interspersed with primitive tubules lined by elongated, deeply staining cells and structures that resemble primitive glomeruli—are present. Nests of cells resembling the metanephric blastema can be present. Nephroblastomas also have mesenchymal components, such as cartilage, bone, skeletal muscle, and adipose tissue. Clinically, these are usually incidental findings, except in dogs, in which they rarely present as spinal dysfunction, the result of spread to the vertebral canal with secondary spinal cord compression.

DISEASES OF THE LOWER URINARY SYSTEM

DEVELOPMENTAL ANOMALIES

APLASIA AND HYPOPLASIA

Ureteral aplasia (agenesis) is the lack of formation of a recognizable ureter, and hypoplasia is the presence of a notably small-diameter ureter. Agenesis of the ureters is due to failure of the ureteral bud to form, and may be unilateral or bilateral. Both conditions are rare. If these defects occur alone, then there is disruption of urinary flow from the kidney to the urinary bladder, resulting in obstructive diseases such as hydronephrosis. If these defects occur with concurrent renal aplasia, then they are clinically silent when unilateral and life threatening when bilateral.

ECTOPIC URETERS

Ectopic ureters are ureters that may empty into the urethra, vagina, neck of the bladder, ductus deferens, prostate, or other secondary sex glands. There are two possible causes:
1. The ureteral bud arises too far craniad to be incorporated into the urogenital sinus.
2. The differential growth of the sinus is abnormal, and the ureter fails to migrate to its usual location.

Ectopic ureters are more subject to obstruction or infection, and thus they predispose animals to pyelitis and pyelonephritis. Otherwise, histologically these are normal. This condition is found most frequently in dogs and certain breeds, especially the Siberian husky, are at greater risk. Affected animals present clinically with urinary incontinence and consequent urine dribbling.

PATENT URACHUS

The most common malformation of the urinary bladder is patent urachus (pervious urachus). This lesion develops when the fetal urachus fails to close and therefore forms a direct channel between the bladder's apex and the umbilicus. Failure of the urachal remnant and the umbilical arteries and vein to involute is frequently observed in cases of "neonatal" omphalitis, in which abscess formation may result in a patent urachus. Patent urachus has also occurred because of congenital urethral obstruction. Increased bladder pressure because of the obstruction forces urine out into the urachus. Rupture of the urachus causes uroperitoneum. The condition must be differentiated from perinatal rupture of the bladder. Foals are affected most often and animals with this defect dribble urine from the umbilicus. Diverticula of the bladder may be primary or acquired and secondary to partial obstruction of the outflow of urine or the result of pressure changes exerted during normal contractions. Occasionally, during urachal closure, the mucosa closes but closure of the bladder musculature is incomplete. When this occurs, a bladder diverticulum (outpouching) of the apex of the bladder can develop. Urine stasis can occur in the diverticulum, predisposing the animal to cystitis or urinary calculi.

OBSTRUCTIVE DISEASES

UROLITHIASIS

Urinary calculi (uroliths) are concretions formed anywhere in the urinary collecting system, and although some clearly originate in the lower urinary tract or as microscopic calculi in the renal collecting tubules, the point of development of most is not known. Uroliths are commonly found in the ureter, followed by any portion of the lower urinary tract and least commonly in the renal pelvis (accounting for 1% to 4 % of canine uroliths). The diseases caused by uroliths are among the most important urinary tract problems of domesticated animals, especially cattle, sheep, dogs, and cats, and are of lesser importance in horses and pigs.

Calculi are grossly visible aggregations of precipitated urinary solutes, principally mineral admixed with urinary proteins and proteinaceous debris. Calculi typically are hard spheres or ovoids, with a central nidus, surrounded by concentric laminae ("stone"), an outer shell, and surface crystals. Many calculi contain significant quantities of "contaminants," such as calcium oxalates in "silica" calculi; few are relatively pure. Large renal pelvic calculi classically have a "staghorn" appearance because they take the shape of the renal calyces in animal species that have true calyces (Fig. 11-72). These calculi predispose affected animals to pyelitis and pyelonephritis. Urinary bladder calculi can be single or multiple, variable in size (2 mm to 10 cm), and sometimes are composed of a fine, sandlike material, which causes cloudy urine (Fig. 11-73). Calculi can have smooth or rough surfaces; and may be solid, soft, or friable. Calculi vary in color depending on their composition; however, color is variable among calculi even of the same composition. The calculi can be white to gray (e.g., struvite and oxalate), yellow (e.g., urate, cystine, benzocoumarin, and xanthine), or brown (e.g., silica, urate, and xanthine), depending on their composition.

Small calculi may be voided in the urine, but typically calculi cause urinary obstruction. This is more common in males because of their long and narrow-diameter urethra. The most common sites of lodgment of urethral calculi vary with the animal species. In male cattle, calculi lodge in the urethra at the ischial arch and at

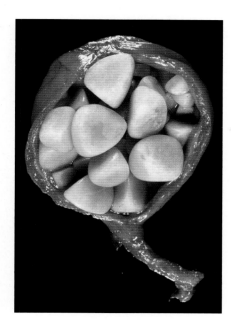

Fig. 11-73   Urolithiasis, urinary bladder, dog. Multiple smooth calculi are present in the urinary bladder. The bladder wall is diffusely thickened. *(Courtesy Dr. A. Confer, College of Veterinary Medicine, Oklahoma State University.)*

the proximal end of the sigmoid flexure; in rams and wethers, the urethral process (vermiform appendage) is the most common site (Fig. 11-74, A); and in dogs, calculi lodge proximal to the base of the os penis (Fig. 11-74, B). At the site where calculi lodge, there is local pressure necrosis, ulceration of the mucosa, and acute hemorrhagic urethritis. Because the urethral sites are prone to rupture, hydronephrosis following urethral obstruction is less common than with unilateral long-standing ureteral impaction. In cats, fine struvite crystals (sand) in a rubberlike protein matrix can fill the entire urethra, and such calculi are typical for the disease called feline urologic syndrome (Fig. 11-74, C). When obstruction or dysuria occurs in females, calculi are usually large and located in the renal pelvis or urinary bladder (Fig. 11-75).

Factors that are either important in predisposing to calculus formation or in precipitating disease include the following:

1. Calculus precursors material in urine in quantities sufficient to be precipitated.
2. Substance is metabolized in an unusual way, as is uric acid in Dalmatian dogs.
3. Substance may be processed abnormally by the kidney (hereditary defects), as with cystine or xanthine.
4. Abnormally high levels of a substance are encountered in the diet, such as the following:
   a. Silicic acid in native pastures

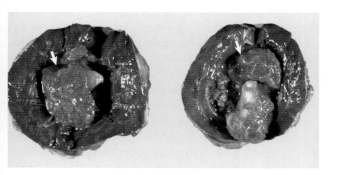

Fig. 11-72   Urolithiasis, kidney, dorsal section, dog. A calculus fills and distends the renal pelvis (*arrows*) and has caused pressure atrophy of the medulla. *(Courtesy Dr. M.D. McGavin, College of Veterinary Medicine, University of Tennessee.)*

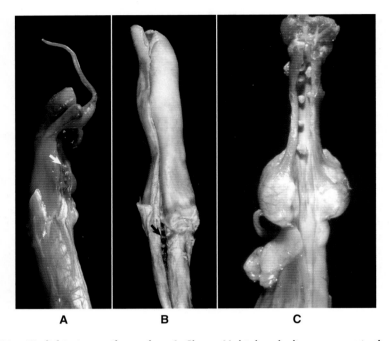

Fig. 11-74   Urolithiasis, penile urethra. A, Sheep. Multiple calculi are present in the penile urethra *(arrow)* and the urethral process (vermiform appendage). **B,** Ventral aspect, dog. Calculi have lodged in the urethra proximal to the caudal end of the os penis *(arrow)*. **C,** Cat. Calculi are present throughout the penile urethra, several just caudal to the external urethral orifice at tip of the penis. (**A** *and* **B,** *Courtesy Dr. M.D. McGavin, College of Veterinary Medicine, University of Tennessee.* **C,** *Courtesy College of Veterinary Medicine, University of Illinois.)*

b. Phosphate in milo or sorghum products (struvites)
c. Estrogens in subterranean clover (clover stones [benzocoumarin] or carbonates)
d. Magnesium in commercial dry cat food
e. Oxalate in oxalate-accumulating plants (oxalates)
5. Abnormally low levels of a substance are encountered in the diet, such as the following:
a. Vitamin A (equivocal evidence that vitamin A deficiency may produce metaplastic change in the urinary tract epithelium that creates a nidus of calculus formation following sloughing of epithelium)

Regardless of the type of calculus, certain factors are more or less important in calculus formation; these are as follows:
1. Urinary pH, in terms of its optimum for solute precipitation (oxalates at acid pH and struvites and carbonates at alkaline pH)
2. Reduced water intake, in relation to the degree of urine concentration and mineral supersaturation
3. Bacterial infection of the lower urinary tract (struvite calculi in dogs)
4. Obstruction
5. Structural abnormalities of the lower urinary system

6. Foreign bodies (suture, grass awn, catheter, needle), or a conglomerate of bacterial colonies, exfoliated epithelium, or leukocytes, which can serve as a nidus for precipitation of mineral constituents
7. Drugs excreted in the urine, which may act as a nidus for calculus formation (e.g., sulfonamides and tetracyclines)

Supersaturation of urine with respect to the components of stone-forming salts is the essential precursor to initiation of urolith formation (nucleation). Supersaturation may be in the unstable range where precipitation occurs spontaneously (homogeneous nucleation) or the metastable range where precipitation occurs by epitaxy (one type of crystal grows on the surface of another type; heterogeneous nucleation).

Although it was formerly thought that urinary proteins such as uromucoid, which make up 5% to 20% or more of some calculi, were preeminent initiators of crystal formation in the metastable range, it is now believed that in many cases either co-precipitation of proteins and minerals occurs or that proteins are adsorbed onto formed crystals. It is possible that crystals of one salt, for which urine is supersaturated in the unstable range, cause induction of crystals of another salt for which supersaturation is apparently stable.

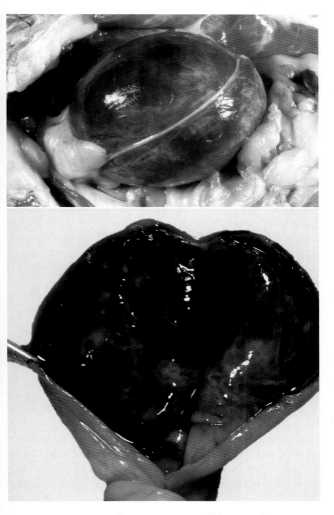

Fig. 11-75   Hemorrhagic urocystitis (feline urologic syndrome) urinary bladder, cat. A, Obstructive urolithiasis. The bladder is overdistended and turgid as the result of urethral obstruction. Note the serosal and intramuscular ecchymotic and suffusive hemorrhages at the neck and apex of the bladder. **B,** Urolithiasis, acute hemorrhagic cystitis. The severe diffuse transmural hemorrhage throughout the urinary bladder wall is secondary to blockage of the urethra by calculi and distension of the urinary bladder. (*A* and *B, Courtesy Dr. M.D. McGavin, College of Veterinary Medicine, University of Tennessee.*)

Crystals are much more common in urine than are calculi. Even though equine urine is normally supersaturated with calcium carbonate, and crystalluria is normal, horses experience a low prevalence of calculi. The factors, which promote or prevent crystal growth and crystal aggregation are poorly understood. Experimentally, high concentrations of urinary inorganic pyrophosphate and magnesium are important inhibitors of calcium phosphate and calcium oxalate crystallization. Pyrophosphate also inhibits aggregation of calcium phosphate crystals. Certain urinary macromolecules,

probably glycosaminoglycans, are also strong inhibitors of crystal aggregation in experimental systems. Deficiency of inhibitors of crystallization may be important in calcium oxalate and calcium phosphate calculogenesis (crystallization-inhibition theory of urolith initiation).

Discussion of calculogenesis for a few specific calculi of importance is warranted.

SILICA CALCULI

Silica calculi (75% silica dioxide) are very common in pastured ruminants. Certain grasses contain as much as 4% to 5% silica; most of the silica is insoluble except that which is in the cell sap (unpolymerized silicic acid). After absorption, silica is returned to the gut in digestive secretions; less than 1% of dietary silica is excreted in urine and up to 60% is resorbed from the filtrate. However, when urine production is very low, the concentration of silicic acid excretion in urine may reach five times the saturation level. Precipitation from solution requires other substances in the urine. Silica calculi are hard, white to dark-brown, radiopaque, often laminated, large-diameter stones and are a major cause of urinary tract obstruction. Calculus formation is reduced to subclinical levels by adding sodium chloride to the ration, acidifying the diet, or reducing the dietary calcium to phosphorus ratio.

STRUVITE CALCULI

Struvite is magnesium ammonium phosphate hexahydrate (Mg $NH_4PO_4.6H_2O$), formerly referred to by the misnomer "triple phosphate." Struvite calculi are important in dogs (the most common type of calculus), cats, and ruminants. Females are more commonly affected because of the common association of these stones (infection calculi) with lower urinary tract infections. Bacterial ureases can induce supersaturation of urine with struvite by increasing urine pH, which decreases struvite solubility and increases ionization of trivalent phosphate, both of which favor calculus formation. A high incidence of struvite calculi in miniature schnauzers may be related to a familial susceptibility to urinary tract infections. Struvite stones are white or gray, radiopaque, chalky, usually smooth, and easily broken. They may be single and large, or numerous and sandlike.

In cats, one manifestation of feline lower urinary tract disease (FLUTD) is struvite urolithiasis, occurring subsequent to feeding calculogenic diets containing 0.15% to 1.0% dry weight magnesium to normal cats. Coagulase-positive staphylococci and other bacteria may be cultured from the urine or calculi of some affected cats, and the formation of infection-induced struvite calculi is similar to that mentioned previously for dogs; these calculi are much less common than sterile struvite uroliths in cats.

Of considerably more importance than discrete calculi are the amorphous accumulations of protein, cellular debris, and struvite crystals that form sabulous (gritty or sandy) urethral plugs (a condition formerly referred to as feline urologic syndrome [FUS]) in middle-aged, castrated male cats. It is thought to result from concomitant occurrence of urinary tract inflammation and the presence of various types of urine crystals. The obstructive material may be either struvite "sand" and/or rubberlike protein matrix, the latter of which is composed of Tamm-Horsfall mucoprotein (secreted by the cells lining the ascending limb of the loop of Henle and the distal tubules), albumin, globulins, and cellular debris. The inflammatory component of plugs in cats may be the product of infection with the following:

1. Viruses, including feline cell-associated herpesvirus (a strain of bovine herpesvirus 4), feline syncytia-forming virus, and feline calicivirus
2. Bacteria
3. Fungi

The incidence of urethral plugs has decreased as more cats have been fed magnesium-restricted and/or low pH diets.

OXALATE CALCULI

Oxalate calculi occur as the calcium oxalates, whewellite (calcium oxalate monohydrate) and weddellite (calcium oxalate dihydrate). Their development is not well understood, but hypercalciuria and hyperoxaluria are involved. Oxalic acid is synthesized from glyoxylic and ascorbic acid, and oxalates may be ingested in certain foods and plants. Dietary magnesium and citrate inhibit the formation of calcium oxalate uroliths by forming soluble intestinal complexes with oxalate and calcium. Oxalate calculi are hard, heavy, white or yellow, and are typically covered with jagged spines, although some are smooth. They tend to be large and solitary stones in the bladder.

In ruminants, exposure to oxalate-containing plants predisposes these animals to oxalate nephrosis and unexpected death and thus only rarely results in oxalate uroliths in the lower urinary tract. The primary symptoms in ruminants result from the following:

1. Chelation of calcium to produce hypocalcemia
2. Calcification of vessel walls throughout the body, predisposing to widespread vascular infarction and hemorrhage
3. Calcification of renal tubules, resulting in tubular obstruction and renal failure

In dogs, oxalate calculi are second to struvite calculi in prevalence and are of increasing importance, but little is known of their origins. Calcium oxalate and calcium phosphate (hydroxyapatite or calcium apatite) calculi occur in dogs:

1. With primary hyperparathyroidism
2. With hypercalcemia
3. With hyperadrenocorticism
4. Following exogenous steroid administration

Males are more frequently affected than females, and calculi are seen more commonly in older animals. The miniature schnauzer, bichon frisé, Lhasa apso, Yorkshire terrier, Shih Tzu, and miniature poodle are breeds at increased risk.

The prevalence of oxalate uroliths in cats has increased notably from the early 1980s to the present. This increase has been accompanied by a notable decline in the prevalence of struvite uroliths. The underlying cause for oxalate uroliths in cats is unknown but is likely related to diet. Several dietary factors can contribute to calciuria (high levels of calcium in the urine) including the following:

1. High percentage of animal-source protein
2. Low magnesium
3. High sodium chloride
4. Diets formulated to acidify urine

Oxalate uroliths in cats have been associated with parathyroid neoplasia, as in dogs.

URIC ACID AND URATE CALCULI

Uric acid is a metabolite of purine metabolism. These calculi contain either ammonium urate with some uric acid and phosphate or sodium urate. Urate stones are most common in dogs, especially male Dalmatians, because they excrete high concentrations of uric acid in their urine. This is due to defective hepatocellular uptake of uric acid from the blood (hepatic uricase levels are normal), which results in incomplete conversion of uric acid to allantoin, a more soluble product of purine metabolism. This defect is an inherited autosomal recessive trait. Additionally, the defective transport system in the renal tubules, which prevents reabsorption of uric acid from glomerular filtrate, and the active tubular secretion both contribute to urine supersaturation.

Predisposing factors for urolith formation include the following:

1. Hyperuricemia
2. Hyperammonemia
3. Hyperuricosuria
4. Hyperammonuria
5. Aciduria
6. Genetic predisposition

Dogs with portosystemic shunts have ammonium biurate crystals in their urine, and they may have urate-containing calculi in the kidneys and bladder. These calculi are usually multiple, hard, concentrically laminated, brown-green, and moderately radiodense. In the bladder, they are frequently spherical and less than 5 mm in diameter.

XANTHINE CALCULI

Xanthine is another metabolite of purines. It seldom appears in urine because normally it is degraded by xanthine oxidase to uric acid. As in human beings, two pathogenic forms exist in dogs. The primary form is inherited as an autosomal recessive trait and is due to an inborn enzyme defect in xanthine oxidase. This hepatic enzyme catalyses two sequential steps in degradation of purines:

1. Conversion of hypoxanthine to xanthine
2. Conversion of xanthine to uric acid; this form has been noted most often in dachshunds and recently in a family of cavalier King Charles spaniels.

The secondary form (iatrogenic) is the more common in dogs, especially Dalmatians, and is usually the result of previous treatment with allopurinol, which binds to and inhibits the action of xanthine oxidase. Additionally, cases in sheep were circumstantially related to deficiency of molybdenum in unimproved pasture; molybdenum is a component of the xanthine oxidase enzyme.

CYSTINE CALCULI

Many cystine calculi consist of pure cystine; others may also contain calcium oxalate, struvite, brushite (calcium hydrogen phosphate dihydrate), and complex urates. Cystine stones occur in dogs and rarely in cats. Cystinuria occurs in both males and females, but cystine calculi and urinary obstruction occur almost exclusively in males. Predisposed breeds include Newfoundlands, dachshunds, bulldogs, mastiffs, basset hounds, and Tibetan spaniels. The mode of inheritance of cystinuria is unknown in most breeds of dogs, but it is transmitted as a simple autosomal recessive trait in Newfoundlands.

Although blood cystine concentrations are normal, an inborn error of metabolism in affected dogs results in high levels of urinary cystine because of defective proximal tubular reabsorption from glomerular filtrate. Many dogs with cystinuria also have high concentrations of other amino acids in their urine, but these are more soluble than cystine. Cystine precipitates in acid urine, but factors other than urinary pH probably are important in the genesis of cystine stones because dogs with crystalluria do not always form them. Cystine calculi are small and irregular, soft and friable, waxy, and light yellow to red-brown turning to green on exposure to daylight.

At necropsy, animals that have died of urinary obstruction have greatly distended (Fig. 11-76, *A*), turgid, or ruptured bladders and dilated ureters and renal pelves. The bladder wall is thin and often has mucosal

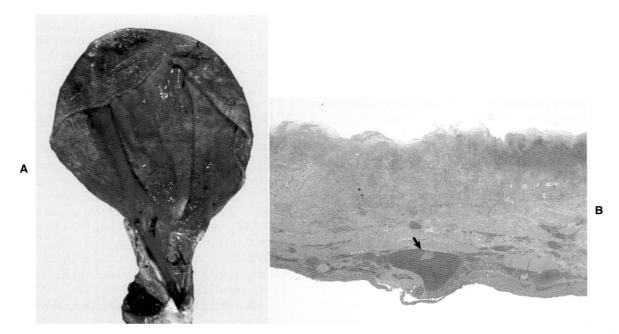

Fig. 11-76   **Acute cystitis, urinary bladder. A,** Mucosal and serosal surfaces, calf. Patchy areas of ulcerated mucosa are interspersed with areas of hemorrhagic mucosa. Note the subserosal hemorrhages *(top)*. **B,** The mucosa has been denuded of transitional epithelium. There are marked mucosal and submucosal infiltrates of neutrophils, which extend into the adjacent tunica muscularis. Congested vessels *(arrow)* and hemorrhages are in the outer tunica muscularis and subserosa. H&E stain. (**A,** *Courtesy Dr. A. Confer, College of Veterinary Medicine, Oklahoma State University.* **B,** *Courtesy Dr. S.J. Newman, College of Veterinary Medicine, University of Tennessee.*)

to transmural ecchymoses or diffuse hemorrhage (Fig. 11-76, *B*). When urine is released from the bladder, either because of rupture or incision at surgery or necropsy, the wall of the bladder is flaccid, the mucosa is often ulcerated, and the urine contains blood clots. Mucosal ulceration, localized lamina propria hemorrhage, and mucosal necrosis are usually present in the ureter, bladder, or urethra adjacent to an obstructive calculus. If the bladder ruptures antemortem, blood clots and fibrin are at the site of rupture, and in some cases there is an acute, localized chemical (urine-induced) peritonitis.

Microscopically, inflammation and hemorrhage are present in the lower urinary tract. Lesions are most severe in cases in which obstruction has been complete. The mucosa is usually ulcerated, and areas of hyperplastic transitional epithelium are interspersed with goblet cells. The lamina propria is usually infiltrated with inflammatory cells. Neutrophils are present at foci of ulceration, and lymphocytes and plasma cells infiltrate perivascularly or uniformly throughout the lamina propria. Hemorrhage is transmural, but is most evident in the mucosa and can cause separation of the smooth muscle bundles. Degeneration and necrosis of smooth muscle occurs in severe cases.

Urolithiasis can cause urinary obstruction or traumatic injury to the urinary bladder mucosa. Lesions of the urinary bladder are manifested clinically as difficult or painful urination (stranguria; dysuria), with or without hematuria. Small calculi may be voided in the urine, but typically calculi cause urinary obstruction. In males, dysuria can result from large calculi, but urinary tract obstruction with uremia most commonly occurs because of obstruction of the urethra with small calculi.

HYDROURETER AND HYDROURETHRA

Hydroureter and hydrourethra refer to dilation of the ureter and urethra, respectively, and are caused by obstruction of urine outflow by blockage of the ureter(s) or urethra by calculi, chronic inflammation, or luminal or intramural neoplasia. Hydroureter can be unilateral or bilateral. Depending on the location of the obstruction, hydronephrosis, hydroureter, and hydrourethra can occur concurrently (see Hydronephrosis). Histologic findings demonstrate little change except for a greater cross-sectional diameter of the ureter or urethra and compression of their lining epithelium. The clinical signs of these conditions are related to obstruction.

INFLAMMATORY DISEASES

ACUTE CYSTITIS

Inflammation of the urinary bladder (cystitis) is common in domestic animals. Because inflammation of the ureter (ureteritis) or urethra (urethritis) in the absence of cystitis is rare, this discussion concentrates on cystitis. The causes of acute cystitis are varied; however, for all animal species, bacterial infection is the most common cause. Cystitis may be acute or chronic. Normally the bladder is resistant to infection, and contaminating bacteria are quickly eliminated by the normal flow of normal urine. Predisposition to urinary tract infection (UTI) occurs when there is stagnation of urine because of obstruction, incomplete voiding at micturition, or urothelial trauma. Other risk factors for UTI include: catheterization, vaginoscopy, vaginitis, urinary incontinence, or prolonged administration of medications such as antibiotics that induce bacterial resistance. Bacterial cystitis is more common in females because their relatively short urethra provides a shorter barrier to ascending infections than the longer, narrow diameter of the male urethra. The bacterial species most commonly associated with cystitis are uropathogenic *Escherichia coli* (α-hemolysin–producing strains) in all animal species; *Corynebacterium renale* in cattle; *Eubacterium (Corynebacterium) suis* in pigs; and *Klebsiella* sp. in horses. In addition, *Proteus* sp., *Streptococcus* sp., and *Staphylococcus* sp. have been isolated from cases of cystitis in several animal species.

Except for the distal urethra, the lower urinary tract is normally free of bacteria. Sterility of the urinary bladder is maintained through normal repeated voiding of urine and because of the antibacterial properties of urine. These antibacterial properties are attributable to the following:
1. The acidic urine of carnivores
2. Secretory IgA
3. Secreted mucin that inhibits bacterial adhesion
4. The large concentration of urea and organic acids
5. High urine osmolality

Cystitis occurs when bacteria are able to overcome normal defense mechanisms and adhere to or invade (colonize) the urinary bladder mucosa. Several factors can enhance colonization and predispose animals to cystitis. Colonization is more likely for strains of bacteria that express molecules on their surfaces that enhance adhesion (e.g., the P and type 1 fimbriae of certain strains of *Escherichia coli*). Retention of urine as a result of obstruction or neurogenic causes such as spinal cord diseases often leads to cystitis.

Trauma to the urinary bladder mucosa due to calculi, faulty catheterization, or other causes can cause erosion and hemorrhage and predispose to bacterial invasion of the lamina propria. Hydrolysis of urea by urease-producing bacteria, such as *Corynebacterium renale* and *Eubacterium suis*, releases excessive ammonia that can damage the mucosa. Bacterial growth can be enhanced when glucosuria is present, such as in diabetes mellitus. Compromise of the host immune system as found with infection by the feline immunodeficiency virus can increase susceptibility to bacterial cystitis. Other bacterial virulence factors, such as the *Escherichia coli* hemolysin, enhance pathogenicity and help bacteria overcome antibacterial factors of the urinary bladder and urine.

Once bacteria gain access to the lamina propria, they cause vascular damage and inflammation. Acute cystitis is often grossly described as hemorrhagic, fibrinopurulent, necrotizing, or ulcerative, and these changes are often sequential over time. Vascular damage predisposes to hemorrhage, leakage of fibrin and if severe, ischemic necrosis of the bladder. This is often accompanied by mucosal ulceration. Neutrophils are present as a component of vascular damage and in any lesion with accompanying bacterial colonization. However, in each case, components of several of these processes are present. The urinary bladder wall often is thickened by edema and an inflammatory cell infiltrate and is diffusely or focally hemorrhagic. Hemorrhage is most common when obstruction is concurrently present or after direct trauma from catheterization. Urine in such cases is described as cloudy, flocculent, foul-smelling, and red-tinged. The mucosa can have foci of erosion or ulceration, patches or sheets of adherent exudate and necrotic debris, or adherent blood clots (Fig. 11-76, *A*).

Microscopically, acute cystitis is characterized by epithelial denudation with bacterial colonies present on the surface. The lamina propria is intensely edematous and has a diffuse neutrophilic infiltrate. Superficial hyperemia and hemorrhage are usually present (Fig. 11-76, *B*). A mild perivascular leukocytic infiltrate can occur in the tunica muscularis.

Clinically, dysuria, stranguria, and hematuria characterize acute onset of bacterial cystitis. An inflammatory sediment is detected on urinalysis, and bacteria can be grown in pure culture from urine samples.

Viral causes of acute cystitis are relatively rare in veterinary medicine. In cats a cell-associated herpesvirus has been found in some cases of mild cystitis. Hemorrhagic cystitis sometimes occurs in malignant catarrhal fever in cattle and deer and occasionally is the dominant gross feature in the disease.

Acute cystitis can result from several chemical causes. Active metabolites of cyclophosphamide, a drug used to treat neoplastic and immune-mediated diseases of dogs and cats, can cause a sterile hemorrhagic cystitis. Cantharidin toxicosis in horses results from ingestion of blister beetles (*Epicauta* sp.) in alfalfa hay, and hemorrhagic and necrotic cystitis develops from cantharidin excreted through the urinary tract. Chronic ingestion of bracken fern (*Pteridium aquilinum*) by cattle can result in the syndrome enzootic hematuria, which can be manifested as acute urinary bladder hemorrhage, chronic cystitis, or urinary bladder neoplasia.

CHRONIC CYSTITIS

Chronic cystitis presents as several forms based on the pattern and type of inflammatory response noted. These forms include diffuse, follicular, and polypoid variants. Diffuse variants reveal an irregularly reddened and usually thickened mucosa. There is some epithelial desquamation, and the submucosa is heavily infiltrated with mononuclear inflammatory cells; there are few neutrophils. In addition, there is often connective tissue thickening of the submucosa and hypertrophy of the muscularis layer.

Follicular variants reveal disseminated, nodular, submucosal lymphoid proliferations (2 to 4 mm in diameter) such that the mucosa has a cobblestone appearance (follicular cystitis) (Fig. 11-77). This response is particularly common when cystitis is associated with chronic urolithiasis. These white-gray lymphoid foci are often surrounded by a zone of hyperemia. Often, the lesions are a diffusely thickened, hyperplastic mucosa with goblet cell hyperplasia and a chronic lymphoplasmacytic infiltrate and fibrosis in the lamina propria. Hypertrophy of the tunica muscularis can be observed.

Polypoid masses (chronic polypoid cystitis), seen predominantly in female dogs, likely develops from inflammatory and hyperplastic responses secondary to

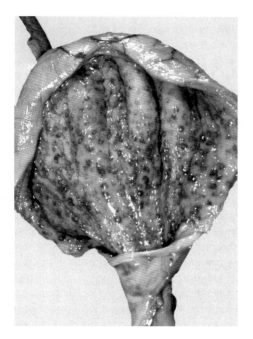

Fig. 11-77 **Chronic follicular cystitis, urinary bladder, mucosal surface, dog.** Multiple small raised red nodules are present on the mucosal surface. These nodules are hyperplastic lymphoid cells surrounded by hyperemia and hemorrhage. *(Courtesy Dr. A. Confer, College of Veterinary Medicine, Oklahoma State University.)*

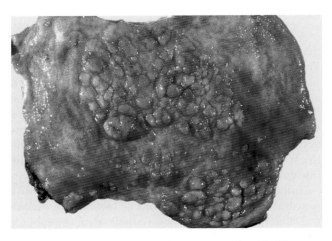

Fig. 11-78 Chronic polypoid cystitis, urinary bladder, mucosal surface, dog. This type of cystitis is characterized by multiple masses composed of proliferative nodules of connective tissue (polypoid) mixed with neutrophils and lymphocytes. *(Courtesy Dr. A. Confer, College of Veterinary Medicine, Oklahoma State University.)*

chronic irritation, which most often arises from persistent bacterial urinary tract infection or uroliths. These hyperplastic transitional epithelial responses are called cystitis cystica, cystitis glandularis, and Brunn's epithelial nests. Inflammation, epithelial proliferation, and development of a nonneoplastic mass occur most typically in the cranioventral bladder wall. The mucosa has single or multiple, nodular mucosal masses (Fig. 11-78) composed of fibrous connective tissue and infiltrated with neutrophils and mononuclear leukocytes. The masses are broad-based or pedunculated, ulcerated, or covered by hyperplastic epithelium with goblet cell metaplasia. Chronic polypoid cystitis is characterized by clinical hematuria.

MYCOTIC CYSTITIS

Mycotic cystitis is occasionally seen in domestic animals when opportunistic fungi, such as *Candida albicans* or *Aspergillus* sp., colonize the urinary bladder mucosa. Such fungal infections usually occur secondary to chronic bacterial cystitis, especially when animals are immunosuppressed or subjected to prolonged antibiotic therapy. Occasionally, blastomyces can produce lower urinary tract lesions in dogs. The urinary bladder is usually ulcerated with proliferation of underlying lamina propria; a generalized thickening of the urinary bladder wall is because of extensive inflammation consisting of neutrophils, lymphocytes, plasma cells, macrophages and edema, and fibrosis.

TOXIC CYSTITIS

There are rare proven veterinary examples of toxic cystitis (see Acute Cystitis). The most recognized is that of enzootic hematuria subsequent to ingestion of bracken fern.

ENZOOTIC HEMATURIA

Enzootic hematuria is a disease of cattle caused by chronic ingestion of bracken fern (*Pteridium aquilinum*). Bracken fern is a very common forage plant and one of the few to cause both cystitis and naturally occurring tumors in animals. There are two subspecies of bracken fern: *Pteridium aquilinum* ssp. *aquilinum*, containing eight varieties, and *Pteridium aquilinum* ssp. *caudatum*, containing four varieties, and it is not known whether all varieties are toxic. *Pteridium revolutum*, a species of bracken fern common in south Asia, and *Pteridium esculentum*, a bracken fern of Australia, also produce enzootic hematuria. In areas where bracken does not grow, other ferns, such as the Australian *Cheilanthes sieberi* (mulga or rock fern) are capable of producing enzootic hematuria.

Bracken fern contains several toxic substances, including a thiaminase, a variety of carcinogens (quercetin, shikimic acid, prunasin, ptaquiloside [braxin C], ptaquiloside Z, aquilide A, and others), a "bleeding factor" of unknown structure, and substances that act as immunosuppressants. Following administration of ptaquiloside to guinea pigs, hemorrhagic cystitis results, suggesting that this is one of the toxic principles in bracken fern hematuria.

The extent and persistence with which toxic ferns are grazed probably influences the incidence of bladder lesions. Cattle fed low levels of bracken fern develop microscopic, followed by macroscopic, hematuria. Microhematuria usually is associated with petechial, ecchymotic, or suffusive hemorrhages in the urothelium of the renal calyces, pelvis, ureter, and bladder, and, microscopically, ectasia and engorgement of capillaries are present. Altered vessels are prone to hemorrhage into the bladder wall or lumen, and nodular hemangiomatous lesions develop in affected areas. In a few animals, macroscopic hematuria is due solely to these nonneoplastic changes, but usually it is caused by development of tumors, which ulcerate and bleed into the lumen.

A large proportion of neoplasms are located on the ventral and lateral walls of the bladder, which are in constant contact with urine, although occasionally tumors also develop in the renal pelvis and ureter. Epithelial neoplasms appear to develop from the hyperplastic and metaplastic (squamous and mucous) changes in the urothelium, which often accompany the vascular lesions described previously. Additionally, Brunn's nests (solid or branched clusters of epithelial cells occurring in the submucosa of the ureter) in the mucosa may act as the site of origin for these neoplasms. Chronic cystitis usually accompanies the neoplastic changes.

Several types of epithelial and mesenchymal neoplasms may develop, including: transitional cell carcinoma, squamous cell carcinoma, papilloma, adenoma, hemangioma, hemangiosarcoma, leiomyosarcoma, fibroma, and fibrosarcoma. Multiple tumors of more than one type may be present, and in more than 50% of affected cattle, mixed epithelial-mesenchymal neoplasms develop. Malignant types may invade locally, and about 10% of epithelial malignancies metastasize to the medial iliac nodes or lungs.

Uroplakins are products of urothelial cell differentiation, which form a major portion of the asymmetric unit membrane and are more consistently expressed in the superficial transitional epithelium. There was a decrease in superficial positive immunohistochemical uroplakin staining in increasingly malignant urothelial tumors in cattle. Although not necessarily of use in prognosticating tumors, staining for this molecule may assist identification of metastatic urothelial cell clusters, and further characterize transitional cell differentiation in neoplasia.

NEOPLASIA

Neoplasms of the lower urinary tract occur predominantly in the urinary bladder. They are observed most frequently in dogs, occasionally in cats, and rarely in other species. Urinary bladder neoplasms comprise less than 1% of total canine neoplasms. Most occur in old dogs, without a sex predisposition.

Risk factors associated with bladder cancer in dogs include the following:
1. Topical insecticides
2. Exposure to marshes sprayed with chemicals for mosquitos
3. Environments with high industrial activity
4. Female gender
5. Obesity
6. Breed (e.g., Scottish terrier)

Retention of urine in the bladder and longer exposure of the epithelium to carcinogens results in a higher incidence of tumors in the urinary bladder. Many chemicals, including intermediate components of aniline dyes, aromatic hydrocarbons, and tryptophan metabolites, have been found experimentally or epidemiologically to induce urinary bladder neoplasms. Chemically induced and spontaneous tumors progress through a series of histologic stages from hyperplasia, squamous metaplasia, dysplasia, carcinoma in situ, papilloma, adenoma, and carcinoma. Lower urinary tract neoplasms occupy space and often cause mucosal ulceration, resulting in clinical signs of dysuria, hematuria, or obstruction. Urinary bladder neoplasms can invade or block the ureters, causing obstruction of ureteral urine flow, increased ureteral pressure, and hydronephrosis.

EPITHELIAL TUMORS

Epithelial neoplasms are by far the most common to involve the urinary system and are classified as transitional cell papillomas, transitional cell carcinomas, squamous cell carcinomas, adenocarcinomas, and undifferentiated carcinomas.
1. Papillomas have a papilliferous or pedunculated appearance. Microscopically, they have a papillary growth pattern consisting of multiple papilliferous fibrous cores covered by well-differentiated transitional epithelium.
2. Carcinomas are focal, raised nodules or diffuse thickening of the urinary bladder wall, most common in the trigone region of the bladder (Fig. 11-79, A). Transitional cell carcinomas are composed of pleomorphic to anaplastic transitional epithelium. Neoplastic transitional cells cover the mucosal surface as irregular layers, readily invade the lamina propria in the form of solid nests and acini, and are found within lymphatic vessels of the submucosal and muscle layers (Fig. 11-79, B).
3. Squamous cell carcinomas, adenocarcinomas, and unclassified carcinomas most likely arise from transitional epithelium. In the bitch, carcinomas are multicentric in origin, develop not only in the urinary bladder but also in the urothelium of the ureters, urethra, and renal pelvis and often extend to the vagina and vestibule.

Metastasis of urinary bladder carcinomas is most often first seen in regional lymph nodes adjacent to the aortic bifurcation, including the deep inguinal, medial iliac, and sacral lymph nodes. Other potential sites of metastasis include lungs and kidneys, with metastasis to other parenchymatous organs occurring later.

MESENCHYMAL TUMORS

Mesenchymal tumors including fibromas, fibrosarcomas, leiomyomas, leiomyosarcomas, rhabdomyosarcomas, lymphosarcomas, hemangiomas, and hemangiosarcomas occur in the lower tract. Primary fibrosarcomas, leiomyosarcomas, hemangiomas, and hemangiosarcomas are rare.
1. Leiomyomas are the most common neoplasms and are solitary or multiple, circumscribed, firm, pale white to tan masses in the urinary bladder wall. Leiomyomas have the macroscopic consistency and microscopic appearance of normal smooth muscle.
2. Fibromas arise from lamina propria connective tissue and project into the bladder lumen as solitary nodules.
3. Lymphosarcoma occasionally infiltrates the wall, not only of the bladder but also of the ureters and renal pelves in cattle with malignant lymphoma.

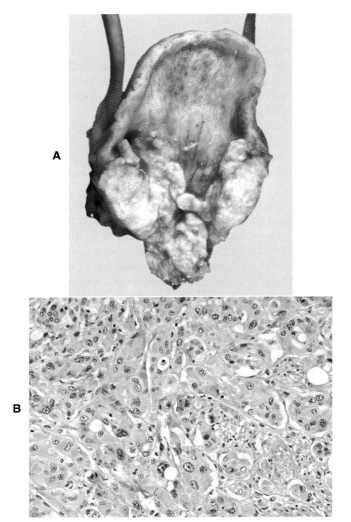

Fig. 11-79 **Transitional cell carcinoma, urinary bladder, dog.**
A, Transitional cell carcinomas are typically seen adjacent to the trigone (as here), where they can become large enough to obstruct the opening of a ureter or ureters and result in secondary hydroureter and/or hydronephrosis. **B,** Lamina propria. The tumor is anaplastic. Cells are grouped in small islands and clusters. Nuclei are vesicular with prominent nucleoli, and some nuclei show remarkable anisokaryosis. H&E stain.
(**A,** Courtesy Dr. A. Confer, College of Veterinary Medicine, Oklahoma State University. **B,** Courtesy Dr. S.J. Newman, College of Veterinary Medicine, University of Tennessee.)

4. Rhabdomyosarcomas are rare but occur in bladders and urethra of young large breed dogs (younger than 18 months old), suggesting an embryonal origin. The cell of origin is speculated to be embryonic myoblasts from the urogenital ridge. These masses are described as botryoid (grapelike) because they are large, fungating masses (4 to 18 cm in diameter) that protrude into the bladder lumen. Local invasion

and occasional metastasis to lymph nodes characterize the typical behavior. Microscopically the neoplasms are composed of sheets of fusiform cells interspersed with pleomorphic cells. Microscopic demonstration of cross striations typical of skeletal muscle or immunohistochemical demonstration of the intermediate filament desmin are useful to confirm the diagnosis of rhabdomyosarcoma. Clinical presentation includes hematuria, urinary obstruction, hydroureter, hydronephrosis, and hypertrophic osteopathy.

SELECTED READINGS

Bach PK, Thanh NTY: Renal papillary necrosis—40 years on, *Toxicol Pathol* 26:73-91, 1998.

Center SA, Smith CA, Wilkinson E et al: Clinicopathologic, renal immunofluorescent, and light microscopic features of glomerulonephritis in the dog: 41 cases (1975-1985), *J Am Vet Med Assoc* 190:81-90, 1987.

Cook AK, Cowgill LD: Clinical and pathological features of protein-losing glomerular disease in the dog: a review of 137 cases (1985-1992), *J Am Anim Hosp Assoc* 32:313-322, 1996.

DiBartola SP, Rutgers HC, Zack PK et al: Clinicopathologic findings associated with chronic renal disease in cats: 74 cases (1973-1984), *J Am Vet Med Assoc* 190:1196-1202, 1987.

DiBartola SP, Tarr MJ, Parker AT et al: Clinicopathologic findings in dogs with renal amyloidosis: 59 cases (1976-1986), *J Am Vet Med Assoc* 195:358-364, 1989.

Divers TJ: Diseases of the renal system. In BP Smith, editor. *Large animal internal medicine,* ed 2, St Louis, 1996, Mosby.

Divers TJ, Crowell, WA, Duncan JR et al: Acute renal disorders in cattle: a retrospective study of 22 cases, *J Am Vet Med Assoc* 181:694-699, 1982.

Elliott J, Barber PJ: Feline chronic renal failure: clinical findings in 80 cases diagnosed between 1992 and 1995, *J Small Anim Pract* 39:78-85, 1998.

Forrester SD, Troy GC: Renal effects of nonsteroidal antiinflammatory drugs, *Compendium* 21:910-919, 1999.

Grauer GF: Glomerulonephritis, *Semin Vet Med Surg* 7:187-197, 1992.

Howard JL, Smith RA: *Current veterinary therapy, food animal practice,* ed 4, Philadelphia, 1999, Saunders.

Kumar V, Abbas AK, Fausto N: *Robbins & Cotran pathologic basis of disease,* ed 7, Philadelphia, 2005, Saunders.

Ling GH: *Lower urinary tract disease of dogs and cats,* St Louis, 1995, Mosby.

Ling GV, Ruby AL, Johnson DL et al: Renal calculi in dogs and cats: prevalence, mineral type, breed, age, and gender interrelationships (1981-1993), *J Vet Intern Med* 12:11-21, 1998.

Maxie GM: The urinary system. In Jubb KVF, Kennedy PC, Palmer N, editors: *Pathology of domestic animals,* vol 2, ed 4, San Diego, 1993, Academic Press.

Mingeot-Leclercq MP, Tulkens PM: Aminoglycosides: nephrotoxicity, *Antimicrob Agents Chemother* 43:1003-1012, 1999.

Nagode LA, Chew DJ: Nephrocalcinosis caused by hyperparathyroidism in progression of renal failure: treatment with calcitriol, *Semin Vet Med Surg* 7:202-220, 1992.

Picut CA, Lewis RM: Comparative pathology of canine hereditary nephropathies: an interpretive review, *Vet Res Commun* 11:561-581, 1987.

Rebhun WC, Dill SG, Perdrizet JA et al: Pyelonephritis in cows: 15 cases (1982-1986), *J Am Vet Med Assoc* 194:953-955, 1989.

Robertson JL: Diseases of the tubules and interstitium. In Bovee KC, editor: *Canine nephrology,* Media, Pa, 1984, Harwal Pub Co.

Robertson JL: Immunologic injury to the kidney and the renal response. In Bovee KC, editor: *Canine nephrology,* Media, Penn, 1984, Harwal Pub Co.

Rosol TJ, Capen CC: Pathophysiology of calcium, phosphorus, and magnesium metabolism in animals, *Vet Clin North Am Small Anim Pract* 26:1155-1184, 1996.

Silva FG: Chemical-induced nephropathy: a review of the renal tubulointerstitial lesions in humans, *Toxicol Pathol* 32(2):71-84, 2004.

Woldemeskel M, Drommer W, Wendt M: Histology and ultrastructure of the urothelium lining the ureter and the renal pelvis in sows, *Anat Histol Embryol* 27:51-55,1998.

12

Endocrine System

KRISTA M.D. LA PERLE • CHARLES C. CAPEN

INTRODUCTION

Endocrine glands are collections of specialized cells that synthesize, store, and directly release their secretions, such as polypeptides, steroids, and amino acid derivatives—including catecholamines and thyroid hormones—into the blood stream, resulting in physiologic effects on target cells distant from the glands. They are sensing and signaling devices located in the extracellular fluid compartment that are capable of responding to changes in the internal and external environments to coordinate a multiplicity of activities that maintain homeostasis.

Signaling molecules are grouped into three general categories according to the source of the signal and the location of the target on which the signal has an effect (Fig. 12-1). In autocrine signaling, cells respond to signals that they themselves secrete. Molecules produced by one cell that act on a neighboring cell are characteristic of paracrine signaling. The final pattern of signaling, which is the focus of this chapter, is endocrine signaling whereby hormones produced by cells of endocrine organs are released into the circulation and act on distant target cells.

Endocrine cells that produce polypeptide hormones have a well-developed, rough endoplasmic reticulum that assembles the hormone, and a prominent perinuclear Golgi apparatus that packages the hormone into granules for intracellular storage and transport. Secretory granules are unique to polypeptide hormone- and catecholamine-secreting endocrine cells and provide a mechanism for intracellular storage of substantial amounts of preformed active hormone. When the cell receives a signal to secrete a hormone, secretory granules are moved to the periphery of the endocrine cell, most likely by the contraction of microfilaments. Following release of the peptides into the blood stream, they bind to receptors on the surface of target cells, activating a series of intracellular events often mediated by second messengers such as cyclic adenosine monophosphate (cAMP), protein kinases, or calcium.

Steroid hormone–secreting cells are characterized by large cytoplasmic lipid bodies that contain cholesterol and other precursor molecules. The lipid bodies are in close proximity to an extensive smooth endoplasmic reticulum and large mitochondria. The latter have hydroxylase and dehydrogenase enzyme systems that attach various side chains to the basic steroid nucleus. Steroid-producing cells lack secretory granules and do not store significant amounts of preformed hormone. They depend on continued biosynthesis to maintain the normal secretory rate of a particular hormone. Steroid hormones enter target cells by diffusion across the plasma membrane and then bind to nuclear or cytosolic receptors.

STRUCTURE AND FUNCTION

In general, endocrine organs are composed of islands of secretory epithelial cells delineated by a fine fibrovascular stroma, which is rich in capillaries. With the exception of thyroid follicular epithelial cells, endocrine cells are arranged in cords or packets. Endocrine cells that secrete polypeptide hormones and catecholamines typically contain abundant, lacy to finely granular, pale eosinophilic cytoplasm, which is immunoreactive for chromogranins and synaptophysin that are present in secretory granules and microvesicles, respectively. Steroid hormone–secreting endocrine cells also contain abundant cytoplasm that appears foamy because of the presence of abundant lipid vacuoles.

PITUITARY GLAND (HYPOPHYSIS)

The adenohypophysis consists of three portions: the pars distalis, pars tuberalis, and pars intermedia (Fig. 12-2). In many animal species, the adenohypophysis completely surrounds the pars nervosa of the neurohypophyseal system. The pars distalis is the largest and is composed of several different endocrine cell populations

693

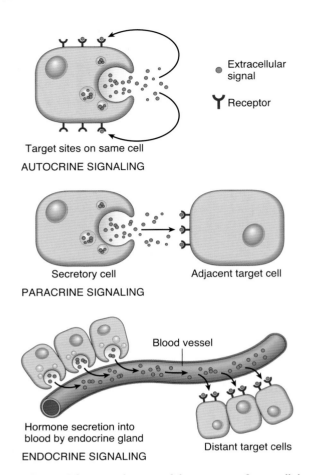

AUTOCRINE SIGNALING

Target sites on same cell

Extracellular signal

Receptor

PARACRINE SIGNALING

Secretory cell

Adjacent target cell

ENDOCRINE SIGNALING

Blood vessel

Hormone secretion into blood by endocrine gland

Distant target cells

Fig. 12-1   Schematic diagram of the patterns of intercellular signaling (see text). *(Modified from Lodish H, Baltimore D, Berk A et al, editors: Molecular cell biology, ed 3, New York, 1995, WH Freeman, with permission.)*

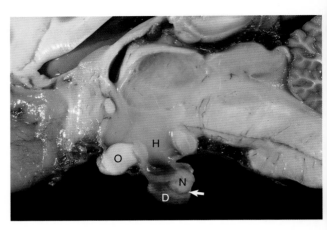

Fig. 12-2   **Pituitary gland and brain stem, normal dog.** Longitudinal section of the pituitary region illustrating the close relationship to the optic chiasm (*O*), hypothalamus (*H*), and overlying brain. The pars distalis (*D*) forms a major part of the adenohypophysis and completely surrounds the pars nervosa (*N*). The residual lumen of Rathke's pouch (*arrow*) separates the pars distalis and pars nervosa and is lined by the pars intermedia. *(Courtesy Dr. C. Capen, College of Veterinary Medicine, The Ohio State University.)*

that secrete pituitary trophic hormones (Fig. 12-3). The secretory cells are surrounded by abundant capillaries.

The pars tuberalis is an extension of the adenohypophysis and consists of dorsal projections of parenchymal cells along the infundibular stalk. It primarily functions as a scaffold for the capillary network of the hypophyseal portal system as it courses from the median eminence to the pars distalis. The pars intermedia is located between the pars distalis and pars nervosa; it lines the residual lumen of Rathke's pouch and has two populations of cells in certain species. In the dog, one of these cell types (B cell) synthesizes and secretes adrenocorticotropic hormone (ACTH).

A specific population of endocrine cells is present in the pars distalis (and also in the pars intermedia of dogs for ACTH secretion) that synthesizes, processes, and secretes each of the pituitary trophic hormones (Fig. 12-4). Secretory cells in the adenohypophysis are classified as acidophils, basophils, and chromophobes based on the reactions of their secretory granules with

pH-dependent histochemical stains. Based on contemporary specific immunohistochemical staining, acidophils can be further subclassified functionally into somatotrophs that secrete growth hormone (GH; somatotrophin), lactotrophs that secrete prolactin and ACTH-secreting corticotrophs. Their granules contain simple protein hormones. Basophils include both gonadotrophs that secrete luteinizing hormone (LH) and follicle-stimulating hormone (FSH) and thyrotrophs that secrete thyrotrophic hormone (thyroid-stimulating hormone [TSH]). Chromophobes are pituitary cells that by light microscopy lack stainable cytoplasmic secretory granules. They include the pituitary cells involved with the synthesis of ACTH and melanocyte-stimulating hormone (MSH) in some species, nonsecretory follicular (stellate) cells (Fig. 12-3), degranulated chromophils (acidophils and basophils) in the actively synthesizing phase of the secretory cycle, and undifferentiated stem cells of the adenohypophysis.

Each type of endocrine cell in the adenohypophysis is under the control of a specific releasing hormone or factor from the hypothalamus (Fig. 12-4). These releasing hormones are small peptides synthesized and secreted by neurons of the hypothalamus. They are transported by axonal processes to the median eminence, where they are released into capillaries and conveyed by the hypophyseal portal system to specific endocrine cells in the adenohypophysis. Each hormone stimulates the rapid release of secretory granules containing a specific preformed trophic hormone.

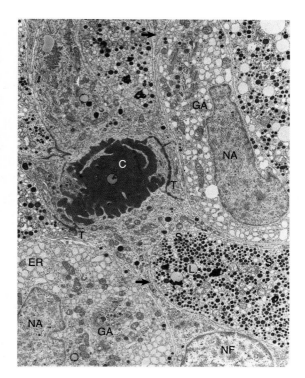

Fig. 12-3   Pituitary gland, pars distalis, normal dog.
Follicular cells *(NF)* in the pars distalis form a framework and extend cytoplasmic processes *(arrows)* around extracellular accumulations of colloid *(C)*. Adjacent follicular cells are joined by prominent terminal bars *(T)*. Acidophils in the storage phase of the secretory cycle contain numerous large, uniformly electron-dense secretory granules *(S)*, scattered lipofuscin *(L)* bodies, a small amount of endoplasmic reticulum *(ER)*, and a small Golgi apparatus. Hypertrophied acidophils *(NA)* have few mature secretory granules but many distended profiles of endoplasmic reticulum and large Golgi apparatuses *(GA)* associated with prosecretory granules in the process of formation. TEM. Uranyl acetate and lead citrate stain. *(Courtesy Dr. C. Capen, College of Veterinary Medicine, The Ohio State University.)*

The neurohypophysis is subdivided into three anatomic parts. The pars nervosa (posterior lobe) represents the distal component of the neurohypophyseal system. The infundibular stalk joins the pars nervosa to the overlying hypothalamus and is composed of axonal processes from neurosecretory neurons. It also has numerous capillaries, supported by modified glial cells or pituicytes, which are termination sites for the nonmyelinated axonal processes of neurosecretory neurons in the hypothalamus. The neurohypophyseal hormones, oxytocin and antidiuretic hormone (ADH) or vasopressin, are synthesized in the cell body of hypothalamic neurons, packaged into secretory granules, transported by long axonal processes of the hypothalamo-hypophyseal tract to axons in the pars nervosa, and released into the

capillary bed of the hypothalamohypophysial portal system (Fig. 12-4).

Neurosecretory neurons in the hypothalamus secrete hormone in response to neural input from higher centers, resulting in hormonal secretion. ADH and oxytocin are nonapeptides synthesized by neurons situated either in the supraoptic or paraventricular nuclei of the hypothalamus. ADH and its corresponding neurophysin appear to be synthesized as part of a common larger biosynthetic precursor molecule, termed propressophysin. The hormones are packaged with a corresponding binding protein (i.e., neurophysin) into membrane-limited neurosecretory granules and transported to the pars nervosa for release into the circulation.

ADRENAL GLAND
ADRENAL CORTEX

The adrenal glands of mammals consist of two distinct parts that differ not only in morphology and function but also in embryologic origin. Because of their close structural relationships, the outer cortex and inner medulla of the adrenal glands usually have been considered parts of one organ. The adrenal cortex develops from cells of the coelomic epithelium that are of mesodermal origin. The chromaffin tissue and sympathetic ganglion cells of the adrenal medulla are derived from ectoderm of the neural crest.

The adrenal cortex of normal dogs is firm, yellow, and of nearly uniform thickness. The soft, brown medulla is surrounded by the cortex. In normal dogs the cortical-to-medullary ratio is approximately 2:1. The adrenal glands are richly vascularized, and a sinusoidal network, which demarcates the cell columns of the adrenal cortex, empties into the venous tree at the periphery of the medulla.

The adrenal cortex microscopically and functionally is subdivided into three layers or zones, although the demarcation between zones often is not distinct. The zona glomerulosa or multiformis (outer zone) adjacent to the capsule is composed of columns of cells that have a sigmoid or arclike arrangement. It represents about 15% of the cortical volume and is responsible for the secretion of mineralocorticoid hormones. The secretory cells of the zona fasciculata (middle zone) are arranged in long anastomosing cords separated by numerous small capillaries. This zone constitutes about 80% of the cortical volume, is composed of cells that contain abundant cytoplasmic lipid, and is responsible for the secretion of the glucocorticoid hormones. The zona reticularis (inner zone) accounts for the remaining 5% of the cortical volume. The secretory cells, arranged in small groups surrounded by capillaries, are responsible for the secretion of sex steroids.

Mineralocorticoids are adrenal steroids that principally affect ion transport by epithelial cells and cause

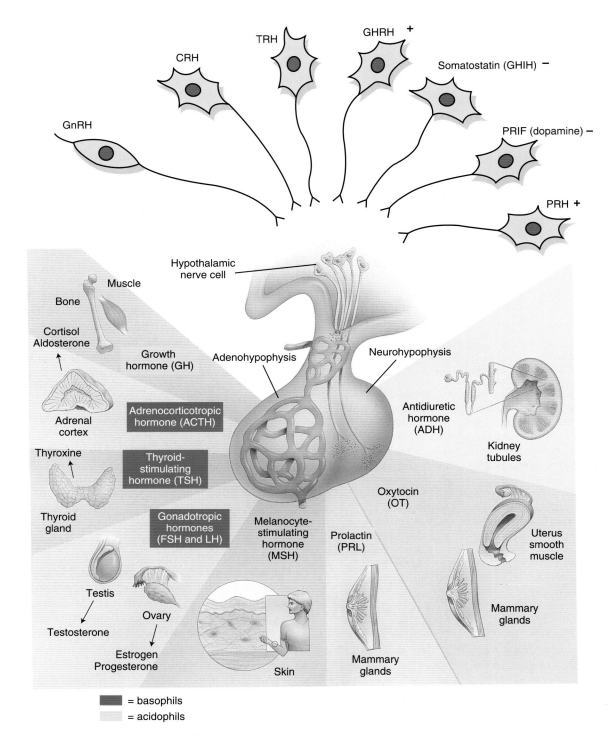

= basophils
= acidophils

Fig. 12-4 **Hypothalamic-pituitary-target gland axis.** Releasing hormones produced by the hypothalamus act on anterior or posterior portions of the pituitary gland to release trophic hormones. Trophic hormones act on specific endocrine glands, stimulating them to produce hormones that exert ultimate actions on downstream tissues. *CRH,* Corticotropin-releasing hormone; *FSH,* follicle-stimulating hormone; *GHIH,* growth hormone-inhibiting hormone; *GHRH,* growth hormone-releasing hormone; *GnRH,* gonadotropin-releasing hormone; *LH,* luteinizing hormone; *PRH,* prolactin-releasing hormone; *PRIF,* prolactin release-inhibiting factor; *TRH,* thyrotropin-releasing hormone. *(From Huether SE, McCance KL:* Understanding pathophysiology, *ed 2, St Louis, 2000, Mosby; and Squire L, Bloom F, McConnell S:* Fundamental neuroscience, *ed 2, San Diego 2003, Academic Press.)*

excretion of potassium and conservation of sodium. The most potent and important naturally occurring mineralocorticoid is aldosterone. Enzymatically controlled electrolyte pumps in epithelial cells of the renal tubule and sweat glands respond to mineralocorticoids by conserving sodium and chloride and by excreting potassium. In the distal convoluted tubule of the mammalian nephron, a cation-exchange mechanism is responsible for the resorption of sodium from the glomerular filtrate and secretion of potassium into the lumen (Fig. 12-5). These reactions are accelerated by mineralocorticoids but still proceed, although at a much slower rate in their absence. Lack of mineralocorticoid secretion, such as in the Addison's-like disease of dogs, can result in lethal retention of potassium and loss of sodium.

Cortisol and lesser amounts of corticosterone are the most important naturally occurring glucocorticoid hormones secreted by the adrenal glands in many animal species. In general, the actions of glucocorticoids on carbohydrate, protein, and lipid metabolism result in sparing of glucose, a tendency to hyperglycemia, and increased glucose production. In addition, glucocorticoids decrease lipogenesis and increase lipolysis in adipose tissue, which results in release of glycerol and free fatty acids.

Glucocorticoids also function to suppress both inflammatory and immunologic responses, thereby reducing the necrosis and fibroplasias that can occur with these responses. However, under the influence of increased concentrations of glucocorticoids, an animal has reduced resistance to bacteria, viruses, and fungi. Glucocorticoids can impair the immunologic response at any stage from the initial interaction and processing of antigens by cells of the monocyte-macrophage system through the induction and proliferation of immunocompetent lymphocytes and subsequent antibody production. Inhibition of a number of functions of lymphoid cells by glucocorticoids forms part of the basis for immunosuppression.

Glucocorticoids exert a profound negative effect on wound healing. Dogs with hypercortisolism can have wound dehiscence (Fig. 12-6). The basic mechanism is inhibition of fibroblast proliferation and collagen synthesis, leading to a decrease in scar tissue formation.

Sex hormones (e.g., progesterone, estrogens, and androgens) are synthesized in small amounts by secretory cells of the zona reticularis of the adrenal cortex. Excessive adrenal sex steroids secreted by a neoplasm arising in the zona reticularis can occur infrequently, resulting in clinical manifestations of virilism, precocious sexual development, or feminization (effects depend on which steroid is secreted in excess, the sex of the patient, and the age at onset).

ADRENAL MEDULLA

The adrenal medulla is derived from neuroectoderm of the neural crest and produces catecholamine hormones. The main biosynthetic pathway for catecholamines in mammals starts with tyrosine that is converted first to 1-dihydroxyphenylalanine (dopa) by tyrosine hydroxylase. Dopa is then decarboxylated by 3,4-amino acid decarboxylase to 3,4-dihydroxyphenylethylamine (dopamine), which subsequently undergoes

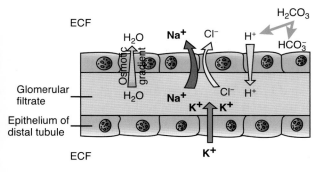

Action of aldosterone on the distal renal tubule

Fig. 12-5 **Aldosterone secreted by the zona glomerulosa of the adrenal cortex acts on the distal portions of the nephron to increase tubular excretion of potassium and increase resorption of sodium (and secondarily of chloride). The resulting osmotic gradient facilitates movement of water from the glomerular filtrate into the extracellular fluid (ECF).** *(Redrawn with permission from Dr. C. Capen, College of Veterinary Medicine, The Ohio State University.)*

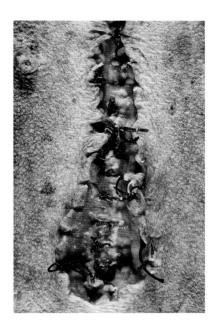

Fig. 12-6 **Dehiscence of surgical wound, skin, dog.** Wounds heal slowly in dogs with cortisol excess because of **an inhibition of fibroblastic proliferation.** *(Courtesy Dr. C. Capen, College of Veterinary Medicine, The Ohio State University.)*

β-hydroxylation by dopamine β-oxidase to form norepinephrine. In mammals the medulla is completely surrounded by the adrenal cortex, and venous blood from the cortex bathes the medullary cells. This blood has the greatest concentration of corticosteroids of any fluid in the body. This close anatomic association between the adrenal cortex and medulla in mammals is not fortuitous because the N-methylating enzyme, phenylethanolamine-N-methyl transferase, which converts norepinephrine to epinephrine, is corticosteroid hormone dependent.

THYROID GLAND
THYROID FOLLICULAR CELLS

The thyroid gland in most animal species has two lobes, one on each lateral surface of the trachea. In pigs, the main lobe of the thyroid gland is on the midline in the ventral cervical region with dorsolateral projections from each side. In dogs, the right lobe of the thyroid gland is situated slightly cranial to the left lobe and almost touches the caudal aspect of the larynx.

The thyroid gland is the largest of the endocrine organs that function exclusively as endocrine glands. The basic histologic structure of the thyroid gland is unique among endocrine glands and consists of follicles of varying size (20 to 250 μm), which contain colloid produced by the follicular cells. The follicular cells are cuboidal to columnar and are orientated so that their secretory pole is directed toward the lumen of the follicle. An extensive network of interfollicular and intrafollicular capillaries provides the follicular cells with an abundant blood supply. Follicular cells have extensive profiles of rough endoplasmic reticulum for synthesis and a large Golgi apparatus for packaging of substantial amounts of protein, which are then transported into the follicular lumen. The luminal side of follicular cells in contact with the colloid has numerous microvilli (Fig. 12-7).

The synthesis of thyroid hormones is unique among those of the endocrine glands because the final assembly of hormone occurs extracellularly within the follicular lumen. Follicular cells trap essential raw materials, such as iodide from the blood, by a sodium-iodide symporter in the basolateral plasma membrane and then transport them rapidly against a concentration gradient to the lumen, where the iodide is oxidized by thyroperoxidase in the microvilli to iodine (I_2) (Fig. 12-8). The assembly of thyroid hormones within the follicular lumen is made possible by a unique protein, thyroglobulin. Thyroglobulin is a high molecular weight (600,000 to 750,000 Da) glycoprotein synthesized in successive subunits on the ribosomes of the endoplasmic reticulum in follicular cells. The constituent amino acids (tyrosine and others) and carbohydrates (e.g., mannose, fructose, galactose) are derived from

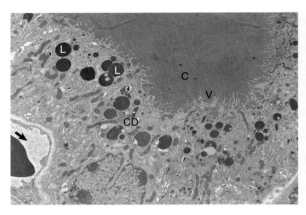

Fig. 12-7   Thyroid follicular cells, thyroid gland, normal dog. Thyroid follicular cells with long microvilli (*V*) that extend into the colloid (*C*) within the follicular lumen. Numerous lysosomes (*L*) and colloid droplets (*CD*) are present in the apical portion of the follicular cells. An interfollicular capillary (*arrow*) is present at the base of the follicle. TEM. Uranyl acetate and lead citrate stain. (*Courtesy Dr. C. Capen, College of Veterinary Medicine, The Ohio State University.*)

the circulation. Recently synthesized thyroglobulin (17S) leaves the Golgi apparatus and is packaged into apical vesicles that are extruded into the follicular lumen (Fig. 12-8). The amino acid tyrosine, an essential component of thyroid hormones, is incorporated within the molecular structure of thyroglobulin. Iodine is bound to tyrosyl residues in thyroglobulin at the apical surface of follicular cells to form monoiodotyrosine (MIT) and diiodotyrosine (DIT) (Fig. 12-8). The resulting MIT and DIT combine to form the two biologically active iodothyronines, T_4 and T_3, secreted by the thyroid gland.

The secretion of thyroid hormones into the blood stream from colloid is initiated by elongation of microvilli and formation of pseudopodia on the luminal surface of follicular cells. In response to TSH, these extend into the follicular lumen, and indiscriminately phagocytose the adjacent colloid. Colloid droplets within follicular cells fuse with numerous lysosomes. T_3 and T_4 are released from the thyroglobulin molecule, diffuse across the follicular cell basement membrane, and enter into adjacent capillaries. Negative feedback control of thyroid hormone secretion is accomplished by the coordinated response of the adenohypophysis and certain hypothalamic nuclei to concentrations of T_4 and T_3 in the blood.

TSH is delivered to thyroid follicular cells where it binds to the basilar aspect of the cell, activates adenyl cyclase, and increases the rate of all biochemical reactions concerned with the biosynthesis and secretion of thyroidal hormones. If the secretion of TSH is sustained (hours or days), thyroid follicular cells become

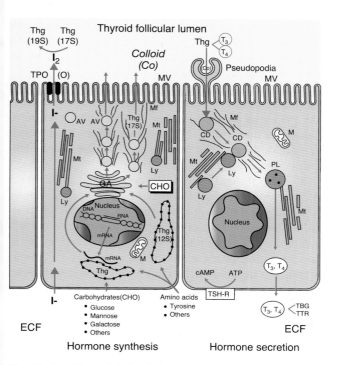

Fig. 12-8   **Thyroid follicular cells illustrating two-way traffic of materials from capillaries into the follicular lumen.** Raw materials, such as iodine, are concentrated by follicular cells and rapidly transported into the lumen *(left side of drawing).* Amino acids (tyrosine and others) and sugars are assembled by follicular cells into thyroglobulin *(Thg),* packaged into apical vesicles *(AV)* and released into the lumen. The iodination of tyrosyl residues with the thyroglobulin molecule to form thyroid hormones occurs within the follicular lumen. Elongation of microvilli *(MV)* and endocytosis of colloid *(Co)* by follicular cells occur in response to thyroid-stimulating hormone *(TSH)* stimulation *(right side of drawing).* The intracellular colloid droplets *(CD)* fuse with lysosomal bodies *(Ly),* active thyroid hormone is enzymatically cleaved from thyroglobulin, and free T_4 and T_3 are released into the circulation. *ATP,* Adenosine triphosphate; *cAMP,* cyclic adenosine monophosphate; *CHO,* carbohydrates; *ECF,* extracellular fluid; *GA,* golgi apparatus; *M,* mitochondrion; *Mf,* microfilaments; *Mt,* microtubules; *PL,* phagolysosome; *TBG,* thyroid binding globulin; *TPO,* thyroid peroxidase; *TSH-R,* thyroid-stimulating hormone receptor; *TTR,* transthyretin. *(From Capen CC: Pathophysiology of the thyroid gland. In Dunlop RH, Malbert C-H, editors:* Veterinary pathophysiology, *Ames, Iowa, 2004, Blackwell Publishing.)*

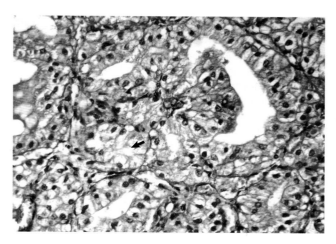

Fig. 12-9   **Hyperplasia, thyroid gland, sheep.** Follicular epithelial cells under prolonged thyroid-stimulating hormone stimulation are columnar, and many follicles are nearly depleted of colloid and are partially collapsed *(arrow).* **Periodic acid–Schiff reaction.** *(Courtesy Dr. C. Capen, College of Veterinary Medicine, The Ohio State University.)*

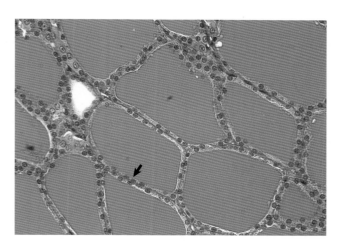

Fig. 12-10   **Atrophy, thyroid gland, dog.** Thyroid follicular epithelial cells *(arrow)* after long-term administration of exogenous thyroxine are cuboidal. Thyroid follicles are distended with dense colloid. Periodic acid–Schiff reaction. *(Courtesy Dr. C. Capen, College of Veterinary Medicine, The Ohio State University.)*

more columnar and follicular lumina become smaller as a result of increased uptake of colloid by endocytosis (Fig. 12-9). Numerous periodic acid–Schiff (PAS)-positive colloid droplets are present in the luminal aspect of the hypertrophied follicular cells. The converse occurs in the thyroid gland in response to increases in circulating T_4 and T_3, which cause a corresponding decrease in TSH. Thyroid follicles become enlarged and distended with colloid as a result of decreased TSH-mediated endocytosis of colloid. Follicular cells lining the involuted follicles become low cuboidal, with only a few endocytic vacuoles at the interface between the colloid and follicular cells (Fig. 12-10).

T_4 and T_3, once released into the circulation, act on many different target cells in the body. The overall functions of T_4 and T_3 are similar, although much of the biologic activity appears to be the result of monodeiodination of T_4 to 3,5,3′-triiodothyronine (T_3) before they interact with high-affinity nuclear receptors in target cells. In certain conditions such as protein starvation during the neonatal period, hepatic and renal disease, and fever, T_4 is preferentially monodeiodinated to 3,3′,5′-triiodothyronine (reverse T_3). Because reverse T_3 produced by target cells is biologically inactive, monodeiodination to form reverse T_3 provides a mechanism by which the overall metabolic effects of thyroid hormones are attenuated. The subcellular mechanism of action of thyroid hormones resembles that of steroids, in that free hormone enters target cells and binds initially to cytosol-binding proteins and subsequently to high-affinity nuclear receptors. Binding of thyroid hormone to receptors on the inner mitochondrial membrane is responsible for the early activation of energy metabolism and increased oxidative phosphorylation.

THYROID C (PARAFOLLICULAR) CELLS

Calcitonin is secreted by a second endocrine cell population, C or parafollicular cells, in the mammalian thyroid gland. These cells are situated either in the follicular wall, within the basement membrane between follicular cells (Fig. 12-11), or in small groups adjacent to interfollicular capillaries between follicles. C cells do not border the follicular colloid directly, and their secretory pole is oriented toward the interfollicular capillaries. The distinctive feature of C cells is the presence

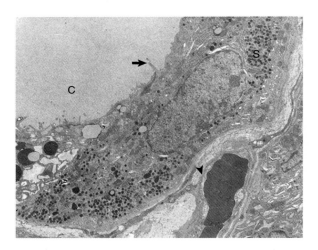

Fig. 12-11 Thyroid C cell, thyroid gland, normal dog.
Thyroid C (parafollicular) cell with numerous secretory granules *(S)* and moderate development of Golgi apparatus and rough endoplasmic reticulum. Microvilli from follicular cells *(arrow)* extend into the colloid of the follicular lumen *(C).* The secretory polarity of the C cell is directed toward an interfollicular capillary *(arrowhead)* with fenestrae. TEM. Uranyl acetate and lead citrate stain. *(Courtesy Dr. C. Capen, College of Veterinary Medicine, The Ohio State University.)*

of numerous small, membrane-limited secretory granules in their cytoplasm (Fig. 12-11). Immunohistochemical techniques have demonstrated calcitonin activity in these secretory granules.

Calcitonin is a polypeptide hormone, and the calcium ion concentration in plasma and extracellular fluids is the principal physiologic stimulus for the secretion of calcitonin by C cells. The rate of secretion of calcitonin is increased greatly in response to increased blood calcium concentrations.

C cells store substantial amounts of calcitonin in their cytoplasm, and the hormone is discharged rapidly into interfollicular capillaries in response to hypercalcemia (Fig. 12-12). C cells respond to long-term hypercalcemia by hyperplasia. When the blood calcium concentration is reduced, the stimulus for calcitonin secretion is diminished, and numerous secretory granules accumulate in the cytoplasm of C cells (Fig. 12-12). Calcitonin exerts its function by interacting with target cells located primarily in bone and kidneys. The actions of parathyroid hormone (PTH) and calcitonin are antagonistic on bone resorption, but synergistic in decreasing the renal tubular reabsorption of phosphorus.

PARATHYROID GLANDS

Parathyroid glands in most animal species consist of two pairs of glands situated in the cranial cervical region. The dog and cat have both external and internal parathyroid glands located near the thyroid gland. Other animal species, such as the pig and laboratory rat, have only a single pair of parathyroid glands cranial to the thyroid gland, embedded either in the thymus in young animals or in adipose connective tissue in adult animals. In cattle and sheep, the larger external parathyroid gland is located a considerable distance cranial to the thyroid gland in the loose connective tissue along the common carotid artery. The smaller internal parathyroid glands are situated on the dorsal and medial surface of the thyroid gland. In horses, the larger ("lower") parathyroid gland is located a considerable distance from the thyroid gland in the caudal cervical region, near the bifurcation of the bicarotid trunk at the level of the first rib, whereas the smaller ("upper") parathyroid gland is situated near the thyroid gland.

The parathyroid glands of animals and human beings are composed predominantly of chief cells in different stages of secretory activity or in transition to oxyphilic cells in certain species. Oxyphilic cells increase in number with advancing age and often form nodules in the parathyroid glands of aged animals. They are larger than chief cells, and their abundant cytoplasm is filled with numerous large, often bizarre-shaped mitochondria.

Biologically active PTH secreted by chief cells is a straight-chain polypeptide consisting of 84 amino acid

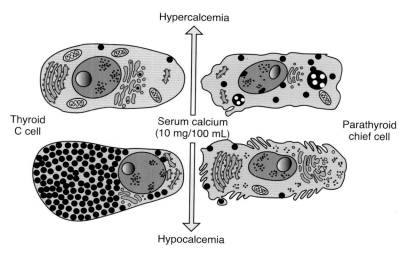

Fig. 12-12 **Response of thyroid C cells and parathyroid chief cells to hypercalcemia and hypocalcemia.** C cells accumulate secretory granules in response to hypocalcemia, whereas chief cells are nearly degranulated but have an increased development of synthetic and secretory organelles. In response to hypercalcemia, C cells are degranulated and parathyroid chief cells are predominantly in the inactive stage of the secretory cycle. *(Redrawn with permission from Dr. C. Capen, College of Veterinary Medicine, The Ohio State University.)*

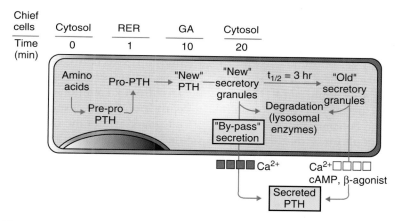

Fig. 12-13 **Bypass secretion of parathyroid hormone *(PTH)* in response to increased demand signaled by decreased blood calcium ion concentration.** Recently synthesized and processed active PTH can be released directly and not enter the storage pool of mature ("old") secretory granules in the cytoplasm of chief cells. PTH from the storage pool can be mobilized by cyclic adenosine monophosphate *(cAMP)* and β-agonists (such as epinephrine, norepinephrine, and isoproterenol) and by lowered blood calcium ion, whereas secretion from the pool of recently synthesized PTH can be stimulated only by a decreased calcium ion concentration. *RER,* Rough endoplasmic reticulum; *GA,* Golgi apparatus. *(Redrawn with permission from Dr. C. Capen, College of Veterinary Medicine, The Ohio State University.)*

residues, with a molecular weight of approximately 9500 Da. Secretory cells in the parathyroid glands of most animals store relatively small amounts of preformed hormone but are capable of responding to minor fluctuations in calcium ion concentration rapidly by altering the rate of hormonal secretion and, more slowly, by altering the rate of hormonal synthesis (Fig. 12-13). In contrast to most endocrine organs, which are under complex control, the parathyroid glands have a unique feedback control system based primarily on the concentration of calcium and, to a lesser extent, of magnesium ions in blood. Calcium ion concentration controls not only the rate of biosynthesis and secretion of PTH but also other metabolic and intracellular degradative processes within chief cells. Increased calcium ion concentration in extracellular fluids rapidly inhibits the uptake of amino acids by chief cells, and consequently synthesis of proPTH, its conversion to PTH, and secretion of stored PTH (Fig. 12-13).

PTH is the principal hormone involved in the minute-to-minute, fine regulation of blood calcium concentration (total and ionic calcium) in mammals. It does this by directly influencing the function of target cells located primarily in bone and the kidneys, and indirectly acting in the intestine to maintain plasma calcium concentration sufficient to ensure the optimal functioning of a wide variety of body cells. The overall action of PTH on bone is to mobilize calcium into extracellular fluids (Fig. 12-14). Bone responds to PTH by increasing the activity of osteoclasts and osteocytes existing in bone.

PTH has a rapid (within 5 to 10 minutes) and direct effect on renal tubular function, leading to decreased reabsorption of phosphorus and consequently the development of phosphaturia. The site of action where PTH blocks tubular reabsorption of phosphorus has been determined to be the proximal tubule. The ability of PTH to enhance the renal absorption of calcium also is of considerable importance in the maintenance of calcium homeostasis. This effect of PTH on tubular reabsorption of calcium appears to be a result of a direct action on the distal convoluted tubule. Calcitonin and PTH, acting in concert, provide a dual negative feedback control mechanism to maintain the concentration of calcium in extracellular fluids within narrow limits.

The third major hormone involved in the regulation of calcium metabolism and skeletal remodeling is cholecalciferol or vitamin D_3 (Fig. 12-14). Cholecalciferol is ingested in small amounts in the diet and can be synthesized in the epidermis from precursor molecules (e.g., 7-dehydrocholesterol) through a provitamin D_3 intermediate form in response to ultraviolet light. The active metabolites of vitamin D increase the absorption of calcium and phosphorus from the intestine and thereby maintain adequate concentrations of these electrolytes in the extracellular fluids as required for the appropriate mineralization of bone matrix. From a functional point of view, vitamin D brings about the retention of sufficient mineral ions to ensure mineralization of bone matrix, whereas PTH maintains the proper ratio of calcium to phosphorus in extracellular fluids. The major target tissue for $1,25\text{-}(OH)_2D_3$ is the mucosa of the small intestine, where it increases the active transcellular transport of calcium (cranial small intestine) and phosphorus (caudal small intestine).

PANCREATIC ISLETS

The endocrine function of the pancreas is performed by small groups of cells, the islets of Langerhans (Fig. 12-15), which are completely surrounded by acinar or exocrine cells that produce digestive enzymes. During embryonic development of the pancreas, a close relationship exists between the endocrine and exocrine portions. Evidence suggests that islet, acinar, and ductal cells arise from a common multipotential precursor cell. In early embryonic development, the endocrine cells are integrated within the exocrine matrix of the pancreatic bud. They subsequently accumulate in nonvascularized

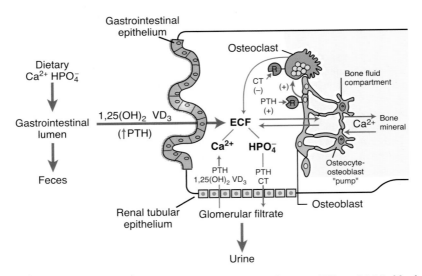

Fig. 12-14   Interrelation of parathyroid hormone *(PTH)*, calcitonin *(CT)*, and 1,25-dihydroxy-cholecalciferol *(1,25-[OH]₂VD₃)* in hormonal regulation of calcium and phosphorus in extracellular fluids *(ECF)*. *(Redrawn with permission from Dr. C. Capen, College of Veterinary Medicine, The Ohio State University.)*

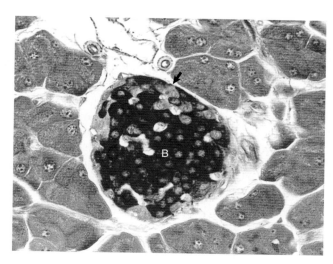

Fig. 12-15   **Pancreatic islet, normal dog.** Gomori's aldehyde fuchsin stains the centrally located β cells *(B)* surrounded by a thin rim of poorly staining α cells and δ cells *(arrow)* at the periphery. The islets are surrounded by the exocrine pancreas. Gomori's aldehyde fuchsin. *(Courtesy Dr. C. Capen, College of Veterinary Medicine, The Ohio State University.)*

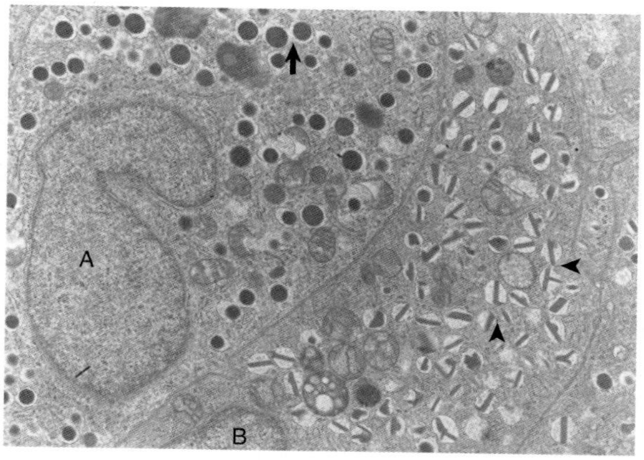

Fig. 12-16   **Pancreatic islet, normal dog.** Differences in secretion granules between β cells *(B)* and α cells *(A)*; the internal cores of secretion granules in β cells *(arrowheads)* are bar- or Y-shaped, with a prominent space between the limiting membrane and internal core. Secretion granules of the glucagon-secreting α cells have an electron-dense, circular, internal core with a narrow submembranous space *(arrow)*. TEM. Uranyl acetate and lead citrate stain. *(Courtesy Dr. C. Capen, College of Veterinary Medicine, The Ohio State University.)*

clusters and later become separated from the exocrine tissue and then independently vascularized.

The pancreatic islets of normal animals contain multiple types of cells. β Cells, the predominant secretory cell, function in the biosynthesis of insulin but co-secrete islet amyloid polypeptide. The glucagon-secreting α cells are less numerous than β cells. δ Cells and F or PP cells in the islets secrete somatostatin and pancreatic polypeptide, respectively. The different cell types of the endocrine pancreatic cells can be differentiated by cytochemical (Fig. 12-15) and immunohistochemical techniques, and by electron microscopy (Fig. 12-16). The α, β, and δ cells have well-developed rough endoplasmic reticulum and Golgi complexes that participate in the biosynthesis of polypeptide hormones, as well as numerous secretory granules in the cytoplasm. Each type of endocrine cell in the pancreatic islets has secretory granules with distinct morphologic characteristics, which can be used to identify the cell types (Fig. 12-16); however, immunohistochemical identification of the specific islet hormone is a more accurate method of identifying different cell types in the pancreatic islets.

The major physiologic stimulus for the release of insulin from β cells is glucose. An appropriate concentration of calcium ion in extracellular fluids is required for induction of insulin release from β cells. Insulin is a powerful hormone that has broad biologic influences and affects either directly or indirectly the structure and function of every organ in the body. Tissues especially responsive to insulin include skeletal and cardiac muscle, adipose tissue, fibroblasts, hepatocytes, leukocytes, mammary glands, cartilage, bone, skin, aorta, pituitary gland, and peripheral nerves. The principal function of insulin is to stimulate anabolic reactions involving carbohydrates, lipids, proteins, and nucleic acids. It catalyzes the formation of macromolecules used in cell structure, energy stores, and regulation of many cell functions. Hepatocytes, adipose cells, and muscle are three principal target sites for insulin. In general, insulin increases the transfer of glucose and certain other monosaccharides, some amino acids and fatty acids, and potassium and magnesium ions across the plasma membrane of target cells. In addition, it enhances glucose oxidation and glycogenesis, and stimulates lipogenesis and the formation of adenosine triphosphate, DNA, and RNA. Insulin also decreases the rate of lipolysis, proteolysis, ketogenesis, and gluconeogenesis.

Glucagon is a hormone that stimulates energy release from target cells and is secreted in response to a reduction in blood glucose concentration. It mobilizes stores of energy-yielding nutrients by increasing glycogenolysis, gluconeogenesis, and lipolysis, thereby increasing the blood concentration of glucose. At physiologic concentrations, glucagon increases both hepatic glycogenolysis and gluconeogenesis. Insulin and glucagon act in concert to maintain the concentration of glucose in extracellular fluids within relatively narrow limits. A glucose sensor in the pancreatic islets controls the relative proportion of these two biologic antagonists. Glucagon controls glucose influx into the extracellular space from the hepatocytes, and insulin controls glucose efflux from the extracellular space into such insulin-sensitive cells as adipocytes, myocytes, and hepatocytes.

PINEAL GLAND

The pineal gland is a neuroendocrine organ which influences circadian rhythm and is intimately associated with the brain. It is composed of loose neuroglial stroma containing nests of pinealocytes and scattered calcified bodies known as brain sand or corpora arenacea. Pinealocytes secrete the hormonelike compound melatonin during periods of darkness. In addition to its role in circadian rhythms, melatonin is thought to influence seasonal reproductive activity in mammals through inhibition of gonadotropin-releasing hormone (GnRH).

CHEMORECEPTOR ORGANS

Chemoreceptor tissue is present at several sites in the body, including the carotid body, aortic bodies, nodose ganglion of the vagus nerve, ciliary ganglion in the orbit, pancreas, bodies on the internal jugular vein below the middle ear, and glomus jugular along the recurrent branch of the glossopharyngeal nerve. The chemoreceptor organs are sensitive indicators of changes in the blood carbon dioxide content, pH, and oxygen tension, thereby aiding in the regulation of respiration and circulation. Carotid and aortic bodies can initiate an increase in the depth, minute volume, and rate of respiration via parasympathetic nerves, and an increase in heart rate and elevation of arterial blood pressure via the sympathetic nervous system. The bodies are composed of parenchymal (chemoreceptor) cells and stellate (sustentacular) cells. Nerve endings with synaptic vesicles as well as nerve fibers occur in close association with the chemoreceptor cells.

PORTALS OF ENTRY

The portals of entry for the inflammatory agents affecting endocrine glands include hematogenous spread and direct extension. Autoimmune and infectious inflammatory diseases affect various endocrine glands. The pathogenesis of autoimmune diseases typically involves autoreactive T lymphocytes and autoantibodies, both of which gain access to the endocrine gland via the blood. Bacterial, viral, and fungal diseases preferentially restricted to individual endocrine glands rarely occur; however, endocrine glands are equally vulnerable to involvement in systemic diseases. Endocrine glands, such as the pituitary and pineal glands and the thyroid and parathyroid glands, can also become secondarily

involved through direct extension from the meninges and larynx, respectively.

The endocrine system is unique in the fact that many of the disease processes affecting it involve disturbances of growth, such as hyperplasia and neoplasia. The histopathologic differentiation among nodular hyperplasia, adenoma, and carcinoma is often more difficult in endocrine glands than in most other organs of the body. However, criteria used to differentiate these proliferative lesions should be established and applied in a uniform manner in the evaluation of proliferative lesions in endocrine glands. For many endocrine glands (especially thyroid C cells, secretory cells of the adrenal medulla, thyroid follicular cells, parathyroid chief cells, endocrine cells of the pancreas, and specific trophic hormone–secreting cells of the adenohypophysis), there appears to be a continuous spectrum of proliferative lesions derived from a specific population of secretory cells between focal or nodular hyperplasia and adenomas.

Excessive focal growth of endocrine cells is the consequence of aberrant secretion of growth- and/or function-stimulating hormone(s) and has been referred to as nonneoplastic endocrine hyperplasia. Nodules arising in hyperplastic endocrine glands can be polyclonal and of clonal origin. Hyperfunction and cellular hypertrophy due to nonneoplastic endocrine hyperplasia are considered to be largely reversible upon cessation of the inciting stimulus; however, chronic and severe hyperplasia of endocrine tissues is not always fully reversible.

Endocrine glands, especially in laboratory rodents, appear predisposed to the development of an increased incidence of neoplasms following prolonged stimulation of a population of secretory cells. Long-continued stimulation can lead to the development of clones of cells within the hyperplastic endocrine glands that grow more rapidly than the remainder and are consequently more susceptible to genetic alterations, which can result in neoplastic transformation when exposed to the right combination of promoting agents.

DEFENSE MECHANISMS

The primary defense mechanism employed by the endocrine system is the hierarchy of hormonal regulation known as the hypothalamic-pituitary-target gland axis (Fig. 12-4). The hypothalamus produces a number of releasing and inhibitory hormones in response to sensory input from the central nervous system (CNS). These releasing and inhibitory hormones act on anterior or posterior portions of the pituitary gland to stimulate or prevent the release of trophic hormones. Trophic hormones act on specific endocrine glands, stimulating them to produce hormones that exert ultimate actions on downstream tissues. Under normal circumstances, the action of a hormone is self-limiting because of the existence of negative feedback loops for each hormone series in which secretion of a particular hormone ultimately leads to inhibition of its subsequent secretion. Negative feedback from target endocrine glands can be directed at the hypothalamus, the pituitary gland, or both.

PATHOGENIC MECHANISMS OF ENDOCRINE DISEASES

Many diseases of endocrine glands are characterized by dramatic functional disturbances and characteristic clinicopathologic alterations affecting one or more body systems. The affected animal can have changes primarily involving the skin (alopecia caused by hypothyroidism), nervous system (seizures caused by hyperinsulinism), urinary system (polyuria caused by diabetes mellitus, diabetes insipidus, and hyperadrenocorticism), or skeletal system (fractures induced by hyperparathyroidism). There are several mechanisms that can disrupt normal endocrine function, with the majority of processes resulting in insufficient or excessive hormone production.

PRIMARY HYPOFUNCTION OF AN ENDOCRINE GLAND

Hormone secretion is subnormal because of extensive destruction of secretory cells by a disease process, the failure of an endocrine gland to develop properly, or the result of a specific biochemical defect in the synthetic pathway of a hormone. In animals, immune-mediated injury causes hypofunction of several endocrine glands, including the adrenal cortex, thyroid gland, parathyroid glands, and pancreatic islets. Thyroiditis caused by this mechanism is characterized by notable infiltration of lymphocytes and plasma cells and deposition of electron-dense immune complexes along the follicular basement membranes with subsequent progressive destruction of secretory parenchyma.

Failure of development also results in primary hypofunction of an endocrine gland. The classic example of this mechanism in animals is the failure of oropharyngeal ectoderm to differentiate completely into trophic hormone–secreting cells of the adenohypophysis in dogs, resulting in pituitary dwarfism.

SECONDARY HYPOFUNCTION OF AN ENDOCRINE GLAND

In this mechanism a destructive lesion in one organ, such as the pituitary gland, interferes with the secretion of a trophic hormone. This results in hypofunction of the target endocrine gland. Large, endocrinologically

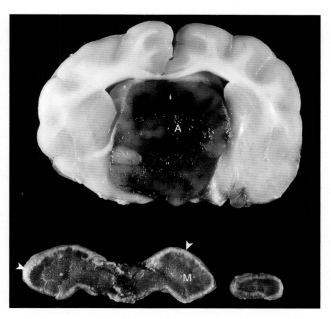

Fig. 12-17   Secondary hypofunction of an endocrine gland, brain, pituitary gland and adrenal glands, dog. A large nonfunctional chromophobe adenoma (*A*) has invaded and completely destroyed the adenohypophysis and hypothalamus, and infiltrated into the thalamus. Destruction of the adenohypophysis has resulted in a lack of secretion of thyrotropin, adrenocorticotropin, and other pituitary trophic hormones. This resulted in severe trophic atrophy of the adrenal cortex (*arrowheads*), especially the adrenocorticotropic hormone-dependent zona fasciculata and zona reticularis, and consequently, in a relatively more prominent medulla (*M*). *(Courtesy Dr. C. Capen, College of Veterinary Medicine, The Ohio State University.)*

inactive pituitary neoplasms in adult dogs, cats, and other animals can interfere with the secretion of multiple pituitary trophic hormones and result in clinically detectable hypofunction of the adrenal cortex (Fig. 12-17), follicular cells of the thyroid gland, and gonads.

PRIMARY HYPERFUNCTION OF AN ENDOCRINE GLAND

This is one of the most important pathologic mechanisms of endocrine disease in animals. The cells of a lesion, often a neoplasm derived from endocrine cells, autonomously synthesize and secrete a hormone at a rate in excess of the body's ability to use and degrade it, thereby resulting in a syndrome caused by hormone excess. Examples are summarized in Table 12-1. These include hyperfunction of secretory cells of the adrenal medulla, follicular cells and C (parafollicular) cells of the thyroid gland, parathyroid chief cells, and β cells of the pancreatic islets.

Table **12-1**   **Primary Hyperfunction of an Endocrine Gland**

Neoplasia	Hormone	Lesion/Sign
Acidophil adenoma (pituitary gland)	Growth hormone	Acromegaly
Adrenal cortical adenoma/carcinoma	Estrogen	Feminization
Pheochromocytoma (adrenal medulla)	Norepinephrine	Hypertension
Thyroid follicular cell adenoma	T_4, T_3	↑ Basal metabolic rate
C-cell adenoma/carcinoma (thyroid gland)	Calcitonin	Osteosclerosis
Parathyroid gland chief cell adenoma	Parathyroid hormone	Fibrous osteodystrophy
Pancreatic β-cell adenoma/carcinoma	Insulin	Hypoglycemia

SECONDARY HYPERFUNCTION OF AN ENDOCRINE GLAND

In this mechanism of endocrine disease, a lesion in one organ (e.g., adenohypophysis) secretes an excess of a trophic hormone that leads to long-term stimulation and hypersecretion of a hormone by a target organ. The classic example in animals is the ACTH-secreting neoplasm derived from pituitary corticotrophs in dogs (Fig. 12-18). The functional disturbances and lesions are the result primarily of increased blood cortisol concentrations resulting from the ACTH-stimulated hypertrophy and hyperplasia of the cells of the zona fasciculata and zona reticularis of the adrenal cortex. In some aging dogs, with notable adrenal cortical enlargement and functional disturbances of cortisol excess, no gross or histopathologic evidence of a neoplasm is present in the pituitary gland. These animals can have a change in negative feedback control due to an age-related increase in monoamine oxidase-β in the hypothalamus and increased metabolism of dopamine. This outcome results in reduced inhibition of ACTH production by the pars intermedia of the pituitary gland, leading to severe corticotroph hyperplasia, increased ACTH concentration in the blood, and long-term stimulation of the adrenal cortex, resulting in the syndrome of cortisol excess.

HYPERSECRETION OF HORMONES OR HORMONELIKE FACTORS BY NONENDOCRINE NEOPLASMS

Certain neoplasms of nonendocrine tissue in both animals and human beings either secrete new humoral substances or hormones that share chemical and/or biologic characteristics with the "native" hormones secreted by an endocrine gland. Most of the recently discovered humoral substances secreted by nonendocrine neoplasms are peptides rather than steroids, iodothyronines, or catecholamines. The nonpeptide hormones require more complex biosynthetic pathways and are infrequently produced by cancer cells. Pseudohyperparathyroidism or humoral hypercalcemia

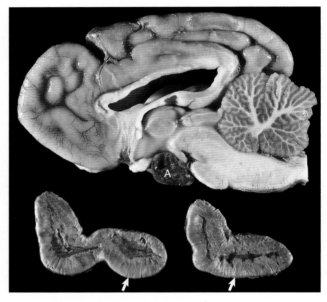

Fig. 12-18   Secondary hyperfunction of an endocrine organ, brain, pituitary gland and adrenal glands, dog. Corticotroph (adrenocorticotropic hormone [ACTH]-secreting) chromophobe adenoma **(A)** in the pituitary gland and bilateral enlargement of the adrenal glands. The chronic secretion of ACTH has resulted in hypertrophy and hyperplasia of secretory cells of the zona fasciculata and zona reticularis in the adrenal cortex *(arrows)* and excessive secretion of cortisol. *(Courtesy Dr. C. Capen, College of Veterinary Medicine, The Ohio State University.)*

of malignancy is a clinical syndrome primarily produced by the autonomous hypersecretion of parathyroid hormone–related peptide (PTH-rP) by cancer cells. PTH-rP interacts with the parathyroid hormone receptor in target cells (e.g., bone and kidneys) and results in persistent, often life-threatening hypercalcemia. A well-characterized example of this disease mechanism in animals is the adenocarcinoma of the apocrine glands of the anal sac in dogs. These neoplasms produce PTH-rP, which mimics the action of PTH and results in an accelerated mobilization of calcium from bone by osteoclasts leading to the development of persistent hypercalcemia. Serum PTH concentrations are lower in dogs with apocrine carcinomas than in controls, and PTH concentrations are undetectable in neoplastic tissue.

ENDOCRINE DYSFUNCTION DUE TO FAILURE OF TARGET CELL RESPONSE

This mechanism of endocrine disease is widely accepted now that there is a more complete understanding of how hormones interact with target cells to convey their biologic message. Failure of target cells to respond to a hormone can be due to a lack of adenyl cyclase in the cell membrane or to an alteration in hormone receptors on the cell surface. Hormone is secreted in normal or increased amounts by the cells of the endocrine gland. For example, insulin resistance in obese animals and human beings can result from a decrease or down-regulation of receptors on the surface of target cells. Receptor down-regulation develops in response to a chronic increase in insulin stimulated by the hyperglycemia resulting from excessive food intake. Secretory cells in the corresponding endocrine gland (i.e., pancreatic islets) undergo compensatory hypertrophy and hyperplasia in an attempt to secrete additional hormone.

An interesting form of hypoparathyroidism has been reported in human patients in whom the inability of target cells to respond is the result of a defect in the cAMP-mediated signal transduction that results from inactivating mutations of a specific nucleotide regulatory protein in the cell membrane. Human patients with pseudohypoparathyroidism develop hypocalcemia and hyperphosphatemia in spite of hyperplastic parathyroid glands and increased blood concentration of PTH.

ENDOCRINE HYPERACTIVITY DUE TO DISEASES OF OTHER ORGANS

The best characterized example of this is the hyperparathyroidism that develops as a result of chronic renal failure or nutritional imbalance. In the renal form, hyperphosphatemia occurs because of a decreased glomerular filtration rate, resulting in a reciprocal decline in serum calcium and parathyroid stimulation. Subsequently the progressive destruction of cells of the proximal convoluted tubules interferes with the metabolic activation of vitamin D by 1α-hydroxylase in the kidneys, leading to decreased intestinal calcium absorption and continued parathyroid stimulation. This rate-limiting step in the metabolism of vitamin D is controlled by multiple factors, including levels of PTH, serum phosphorus, and several other hormones. The intestinal absorption of calcium is impaired and results in the development of progressive hypocalcemia; the hypocalcemia leads to long-term parathyroid gland stimulation and subsequently to the development of

generalized demineralization of the skeleton. Nutritional hyperparathyroidism develops in animals fed abnormal diets that are either too low in calcium, too high in phosphorus, or deficient in cholecalciferol (e.g., in New World nonhuman primates).

Hyperfunction of an endocrine organ also can result from hormonal imbalances induced by xenobiotic chemicals. For example, in rodents undergoing chronic toxicity testing, hyperactivity of the pituitary gland can occur resulting in increased incidences of neoplasms in the gonads or mammary glands. Excess production of LH, usually because of disruption of negative feedback control by estrogen or testosterone, increases the incidence of tubulostromal adenomas and granulosa cell neoplasms in the ovaries of mice and of Leydig (interstitial) adenomas of the testes in rats.

ENDOCRINE DYSFUNCTION RESULTING FROM ABNORMAL HORMONE DEGRADATION
DECREASED DEGRADATION

The rate of secretion of a hormone by an endocrine gland can be normal with this mechanism, but because of the decreased rate of degradation, blood concentrations are persistently increased, thereby simulating a syndrome of hypersecretion. The classic example of this mechanism is the syndrome of feminization because of hyperestrogenism and from decreased hepatic degradation of estrogens in patients with cirrhosis. Hypercalcemia, due in part to a decrease in the ability of proximal convoluted tubular epithelial cells in the diseased kidneys to degrade PTH (along with a decrease in urinary excretion of calcium), is occasionally reported in dogs with chronic renal disease.

INCREASED DEGRADATION

The long-term administration of various xenobiotics, such as phenobarbital to laboratory rodents, results in the induction of hepatic enzymes (e.g., thyroxine [T_4] uridine diphosphate glucuronyl transferase) that increase the degradation rate of thyroxine. This chronic disruption of the thyroid-pituitary gland axis results in increased TSH secretion. In rodents, especially male rats, the development of thyroid follicular cell neoplasms often is increased in chronic toxicity and oncogenicity studies with certain new drugs and chemicals.

IATROGENIC SYNDROMES OF HORMONE EXCESS

The administration of an exogenous hormone can influence the activity of target cells either directly or indirectly and result in important functional disturbances. It is well recognized that the chronic administration of potent preparations of adrenal cortical steroids at inappropriately large daily doses (for the symptomatic treatment of various diseases) can produce most of the

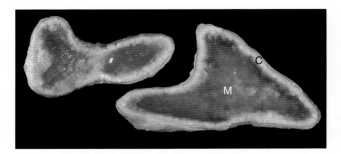

Fig. 12-19   Iatrogenic syndrome of hormone excess, adrenal glands, dog. Hyperadrenocorticism, caused by long-term administration of exogenous corticosteroids, has resulted in notable trophic atrophy of the adrenocorticotropic hormone–dependent zona fasciculata and zona reticularis of the adrenal cortex (C). The adrenal medulla (M) occupies a relatively greater percentage of the atrophic adrenal gland than of a normal adrenal gland. *(Courtesy Dr. C. Capen, College of Veterinary Medicine, The Ohio State University.)*

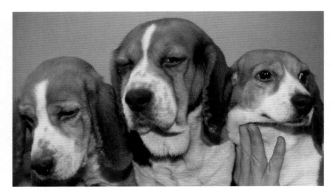

Fig. 12-20   Iatrogenic acromegaly, beagle, center (compared with unaffected littermates, left and right). Note the coarseness of the facial features and the marked thickening and folding of the skin of the face. These characteristic changes are the result of the protein anabolic effects of somatotropin (produced by hyperplastic ductular epithelial cells), which has been stimulated by the exogenous administration of medroxyprogesterone acetate. *(Courtesy Dr. P. Concannon, College of Veterinary Medicine, Cornell University.)*

functional disturbances that are secondary to an endogenous hypersecretion of cortisol. Increased concentrations of exogenous cortisol result in notable atrophy of the adrenal cortex, particularly the ACTH-dependent zona fasciculata and zona reticularis (Fig. 12-19). Similarly the administration of excessively large doses of insulin can result in hypoglycemia, and an excess of T_4 or triiodothyronine (T_3) can result in hyperthyroidism, especially in certain species, such as cats, which have limited capacities to conjugate T_4 with glucuronic acid and thus enhance its biliary excretion.

The administration of progestogens to dogs indirectly results in a syndrome of growth hormone excess. For example, the injection of medroxyprogesterone acetate for the prevention of estrus in dogs stimulates the expression of the growth hormone gene in the mammary glands and results in elevated circulating growth hormone concentrations, producing many of the clinical manifestations of acromegaly. The excessive skin folds (Fig. 12-20), expansion of interdigital spaces, and abdominal enlargement in dogs with iatrogenic acromegaly are related to the protein anabolic effects of growth hormone. Elongation of bones in response to exogenous progestogens requires functional growth plates and osteogenic surfaces.

DISEASES OF THE ENDOCRINE SYSTEM

DISORDERS OF THE ADENOHYPOPHYSIS

HYPOPITUITARISM

APLASIA AND PROLONGED GESTATION

Subnormal function of the fetal endocrine system, seen especially in ruminants, can disrupt normal fetal development and result in prolonged gestation. In Guernsey and Jersey cattle, a genetically determined failure of development (aplasia) of the adenohypophysis has been described, but the neurohypophysis develops normally. This aplasia results in a lack of fetal pituitary trophic hormone secretion during the last trimester and hypoplasia of target endocrine organs, namely the adrenal cortex, gonads, and follicular cells of the thyroid gland. Fetal development is normal up to approximately 7 months of gestation, but then fetal growth ceases irrespective of the length of time the viable fetus is retained in the uterus.

Prolongation of gestation occurs in ewes that ingest the plant *Veratrum californicum* between days 12 and 14 of gestation. *Veratrum californicum* contains potent alkaloids that inhibit neural tube development, resulting in cyclopia and extensive malformations of the CNS and hypothalamus in lambs. Arrhinencephalia and lack of development of nasal bones accompany the formation of a proboscis-like structure. Although the adenohypophysis may be present in some cases, it is unable to secrete normal amounts of trophic hormones (ACTH) because it lacks the necessary fine control derived from the hypothalamic-releasing hormones. Pregnancy is maintained until a cesarean section is performed or the lamb dies in utero. Although the lambs retained in the uterus continue to grow beyond the normal gestation period, target endocrine organs in the fetus are hypoplastic, and the adrenal cortex does not differentiate completely into the three distinctive zones that secrete corticosteroid hormones.

Two concepts have emerged from the study of prolonged gestation in cattle and sheep; (1) Fetal hormones are necessary for final growth and development of the fetus in certain animals, and (2) normal parturition at term in these species requires an intact fetal hypothalamic-pituitary-adrenocortical axis working in concert with trophoblasts of the placenta.

Although the presence or absence of functional adenohypophyseal tissue determines whether the fetus continues to grow in utero, the pathogenesis of prolongation of the gestational interval is similar in these two examples. The subnormal development of the fetal adrenal cortex in calves and lambs results in an inadequate secretion of cortisol and a failure to induce 17α-hydroxylase in the placenta, which converts precursor molecules, such as progesterone, to estrogen. Thus the dam's circulating progesterone is maintained near midgestational concentrations, and the notable increase in estrogens that normally occurs at term resulting in parturition is absent. The estrogen surge, when it occurs, stimulates prostaglandin synthesis in the uterus, which results in smooth muscle contractions and biochemical changes in collagen along the birth canal that normally permit delivery of the fetus.

PITUITARY CYSTS AND PITUITARY DWARFISM

Pituitary dwarfism in dogs is usually due to a failure of the oropharyngeal ectoderm of Rathke's pouch to differentiate into trophic hormone–secreting cells of the pars distalis. This results in a progressively enlarging, multiloculated cyst and an absence of the adenohypophysis (Fig. 12-21). Other cysts originating in the craniopharyngeal duct or the pharyngeal hypophysis can also become large enough to induce clinical signs.

Juvenile panhypopituitarism occurs most frequently in German shepherd dogs, but it has been reported in spitz, toy pinscher, and Carelian bear dogs. The dwarf pups appear normal from birth to about 2 months of age. Subsequently the slower growth, retention of puppy hair coat, and lack of primary guard hairs gradually become evident (Fig. 12-22). A bilaterally symmetric alopecia develops gradually and often progresses to complete alopecia except for the head and tufts of hair on the legs. There is progressive hyperpigmentation of the skin until the skin is uniformly brownish-black over most of the body. Adult German shepherd dogs with panhypopituitarism vary in size from as small as 2 kg to nearly half normal size, depending on whether the failure of formation of the adenohypophysis is partial or complete.

The mode of inheritance is simple autosomal recessive. The activity of somatomedin, also known as insulin-like growth factor (a non–species-specific, cartilage growth-promoting peptide whose production in the liver and plasma activity is controlled by somatotropin)

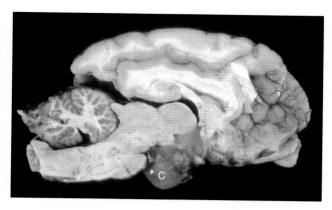

Fig. 12-21   **Cystic Rathke's pouch, brain, sagittal section, dog.** A large, multiloculated cyst (C) is noted on the ventral aspect of this brain where the adenohypophysis would normally be located. *(Courtesy College of Veterinary Medicine, University of Illinois.)*

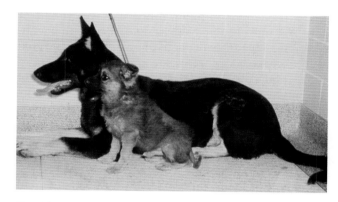

Fig. 12-22   **Panhypopituitarism ("pituitary dwarfism"), 5-month-old German shepherd and littermate.** The unaffected littermate weighed 27.3 kg, whereas the dwarf puppy weighed only 4 kg. The pituitary dwarf has retained its puppy hair coat. *(From Alexander JE: Can Vet J 3:83, 1962.)*

is low in dwarf dogs. Intermediate somatomedin activity is present in phenotypically normal ancestors suspected to be heterozygous carriers. Assays for somatomedin provide a useful indirect measurement of circulating growth hormone activity in dogs with suspected pituitary dwarfism if canine growth hormone assays are not available.

HYPERPITUITARISM AND NEOPLASMS OF THE ADENOHYPOPHYSIS
PARS INTERMEDIA ADENOMAS

Adenomas derived from cells of the pars intermedia are the most common type of pituitary gland neoplasm in horses and the second most common type in dogs, but they are rare in other species. Adenomas develop in older horses, more frequently in females. Nonbrachy-cephalic breeds of dogs have adenomas of the pars intermedia more often than brachycephalic breeds.

Adenomas of the pars intermedia in dogs are either functionally inactive and result in varying degrees of hypopituitarism and diabetes insipidus, or endocrinologically active and secrete excessive levels of ACTH, leading to bilateral adrenal cortical hyperplasia and a syndrome of cortisol excess. Endocrinologically active (ACTH-secreting) adenomas of the pars intermedia in dogs have prominent groups of corticotrophs that have abundant eosinophilic cytoplasm and more widely scattered follicles.

Two cell populations have been identified in the pars intermedia of normal dogs by immunohistochemistry. The predominant cell type (A cell) stains strongly for α-MSH, as in the pars intermedia of other species. A second cell type (B cell) in the canine pars intermedia stains intensely for ACTH but not for α-MSH. This second cell population accounts for the high bioactive ACTH concentration found in the pars intermedia of dogs and most likely gives rise to corticotroph adenomas of the pars intermedia in dogs with the syndrome of cortisol excess.

The clinical syndrome reported with neoplasms of the pars intermedia in horses is characterized by polyuria, polydipsia, polyphagia, muscle weakness, somnolence, intermittent hyperpyrexia, and generalized hyperhidrosis. The affected horses often develop hirsutism because of a failure to seasonally shed hair. The hair over most of the trunk and extremities is long (up to 10 to 12 cm), abnormally thick, wavy, and often matted (Fig. 12-23). Horses with larger neoplasms

sometimes have insulin-resistant hyperglycemia and glycosuria, probably due to the down-regulation of insulin receptors on target cells induced by chronic excessive intake of feed and hyperinsulinemia. The disturbances in carbohydrate metabolism, ravenous appetite, hypertrichosis, and hyperhidrosis are considered to be primarily a reflection of deranged hypothalamic function caused by compression of the overlying hypothalamus by the large pituitary neoplasms. The hypothalamus is the primary center for homeostatic regulation of body temperature, appetite, and cyclic shedding of hair.

In addition to their space-occupying effects, some adenomas of the pars intermedia are endocrinologically active. Plasma cortisol and immunoreactive adrenocorticotropin (iACTH, molecular weight 4500 Da) concentrations can be modestly elevated in horses with pars intermedia adenomas. The cortisol concentrations often lack normal diurnal rhythm and are not suppressed by either large or small doses of dexamethasone. The modest increases of plasma iACTH appear to be caused by the different processing of proopiomelanocortin (POMC) in neoplasms derived from cells of the pars intermedia. This could explain the normal or slightly increased blood cortisol concentrations and normal or mildly hyperplastic adrenal cortices observed in some horses with adenomas of the pars intermedia. The concentrations of ACTH in the neoplasm have been reported to be six times that of the normal pars intermedia and only approach the concentrations found in the pars distalis of normal horses. The plasma and neoplasm concentrations of pars intermedia-derived peptides (CLIP [corticotrophin-like intermediate lobe peptide], α-MSH, β-MSH, and β-endorphin [β-END]) are disproportionately increased (40 times or more) compared with those of ACTH, apparently as the result of selective posttranslational processing of POMC in a manner similar to that of the normal pars intermedia.

Adenomas of the pars intermedia have immunohistochemical staining similar to that of the nonneoplastic equine pars intermedia. The findings include a strong, diffuse cytoplasmic reaction for POMC, a moderately strong reaction for α-MSH and β-END, a weak reaction for ACTH, and negative immunostaining for prolactin, glial fibrillary acidic protein, and neuron-specific enolase. Two antisera directed against different parts of the N-terminal fragment of human (h) POMC differ in their immunoreactivity. Immunostaining of neoplastic cells was stronger with anti-h[1-48] N-POMC antisera than with anti-h[1-76] N-POMC antisera. These immunohistochemical findings support the biochemical studies that suggest horses with pituitary adenomas derived from the cells of the pars intermedia develop a unique clinical syndrome that is the result of hypothalamic and neurohypophyseal derangement and of an autonomous production of excess amounts of POMC-derived peptides.

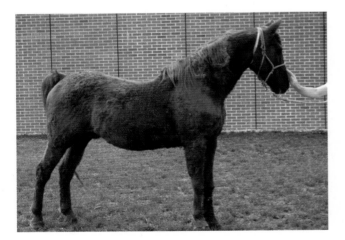

Fig. 12-23   Hirsutism, skin, horse. The hirsutism is the result of a failure to shed hair due to an adenoma of the pars intermedia. *(Courtesy Dr. C. Capen, College of Veterinary Medicine, The Ohio State University.)*

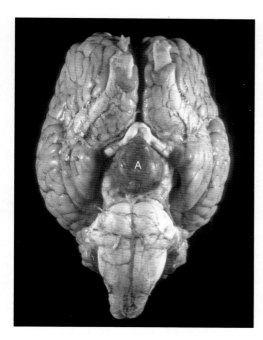

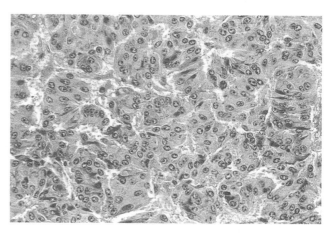

Fig. 12-25   **Adenoma, pituitary gland, pars intermedia, horse.** Adenoma composed of cords and ribbons of well-differentiated, tall cuboidal to columnar cells with ample amounts of granular basophilic cytoplasm. H&E stain. *(Courtesy Dr. C. Capen, College of Veterinary Medicine, The Ohio State University.)*

Fig. 12-24   **Adenoma, brain, pituitary gland, horse.** The pituitary gland is notably enlarged because of an adenoma **(A)** of the pars intermedia. *(Courtesy College of Veterinary Medicine, University of Illinois.)*

Although many of the functional disturbances in horses with pituitary adenomas (e.g., diabetes insipidus, polyphagia, hyperpyrexia, hyperhidrosis, and hirsutism) appear to be the result of hypothalamic or neurohypophyseal dysfunction, other behavioral signs (e.g., docility and diminished responsiveness to painful stimuli) could be related to increased plasma and cerebrospinal fluid concentrations of β-END. The clinical syndrome in horses with pituitary neoplasms is distinctly different from that of Cushing's disease in dogs, cats, and human patients.

In dogs, adenomas of the pars intermedia result in only a moderate enlargement of the pituitary gland. The pars distalis is readily identifiable and sharply demarcated from the anterior margin of the neoplasm, usually by an incomplete layer of condensed stroma. The neoplasm can extend across the residual hypophyseal lumen and result in compression atrophy, but it usually does not invade the pars distalis. The posterior lobe is incorporated within the neoplasm, but the infundibular stalk is intact. Histologically, canine pars intermedia adenomas are composed of numerous large colloid-filled follicles lined by partially ciliated simple columnar epithelium scattered among nests of variably sized chromophobic cells.

In horses, adenomas of the pars intermedia often are large neoplasms that extend out of the fossa hypophysialis

and severely compress the overlying hypothalamus (Fig. 12-24). The adenomas are yellow to white, are multinodular, and enclose the pars nervosa. When the neoplasm is incised, the pars distalis usually can be identified as a compressed subcapsular rim of tissue on the anterior margin. A sharp line of demarcation remains between the neoplasm and the compressed pars distalis. The neoplastic cells are arranged in cords and nests along the capillaries and connective tissue septa and are large, cylindrical, spindle-shaped, or polyhedral with oval hyperchromatic nuclei (Fig. 12-25). The pattern is often reminiscent of that of the prominent pars intermedia of normal horses. Ribbons of more cuboidal to columnar neoplastic cells occasionally form follicular structures that have dense eosinophilic colloid.

ACTH-SECRETING (CORTICOTROPH) ADENOMAS

Functional (endocrinologically active) neoplasms arising in the pituitary gland most likely are derived from corticotroph (ACTH-secreting) cells in the pars distalis but can also arise from the pars intermedia of dogs. These neoplasms cause a clinical syndrome of cortisol excess (Cushing's disease) resulting in gluconeogenic, lipolytic, protein catabolic, and antiinflammatory activities. These neoplasms are encountered most frequently in dogs, particularly in adult to aged boxers, Boston terriers, and dachshunds.

The pituitary gland is consistently enlarged (Fig. 12-18); however, neither the occurrence nor the severity of functional disturbances appear to be directly related to the size of the neoplasm. Because the diaphragma sellae are incomplete in the dog, the line of least resistance is dorsal and expansion of the gradually enlarging pituitary mass is in this direction. This results in invagination into the infundibular cavity, dilation of the infundibular recess and the third ventricle with eventual compression or replacement of the hypothalamus, and possible extension of the neoplasm into the thalamus (Fig. 12-17).

Bilateral enlargement of the adrenal glands occurs in dogs with functional corticotroph adenomas (Fig. 12-18). This enlargement is due to cortical hyperplasia, primarily of the zonae fasciculata and reticularis. Nodules of yellow-orange cortical tissue are often found outside the capsule and extending down into and compressing the adrenal medulla.

Pituitary corticotroph adenomas are composed of well-differentiated, large or small, chromophobic cells supported by fine connective tissue septa. The cytoplasm of the neoplastic cells usually is devoid of secretory granules, but stains immunohistochemically for ACTH and MSH. Hormone-containing secretory granules can be demonstrated by electron microscopy in functional corticotroph adenomas of dogs.

HYPOPITUITARISM AND NEOPLASMS OF THE ADENOHYPOPHYSIS
ENDOCRINOLOGICALLY INACTIVE CHROMOPHOBE ADENOMAS

Nonfunctional pituitary neoplasms occur in dogs, cats, laboratory rodents, and parakeets but are uncommon in other species. Although chromophobe adenomas seem endocrinologically inactive, they can cause significant functional disturbances and clinical signs by virtue of their compressing and causing atrophy of adjacent portions of the pituitary gland and also dorsal extension into the overlying brain (Fig. 12-26). The clinical disturbances result either from the lack of secretion of pituitary trophic hormones and diminished target organ function (e.g., adrenal cortex; Fig. 12-17) or from dysfunction of the CNS. Affected animals often have decreased spontaneous activity, incoordination and disturbances of balance, are weak, and sometimes collapse after exercise. Chronically affected animals are blind and have dilated and fixed pupils because of compression and disruption of the optic nerves by dorsal extension of the pituitary neoplasms (Fig. 12-26). Endocrinologically inactive pituitary adenomas often become large before they cause clinical signs or kill the animal (Figs. 12-17 and 12-26).

Clinical signs reported with nonfunctional pituitary adenomas and hypopituitarism are not specific and could be confused with other disorders of the CNS, such as brain neoplasms and encephalitis, or with chronic renal disease. There is no effect on body stature secondary to compression of the pars distalis and interference with growth hormone secretion because these

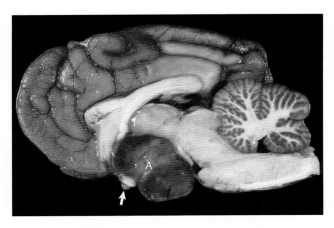

Fig. 12-26   Adenoma, pituitary gland, dog. A large pituitary adenoma (A) has extended dorsally and compresses the overlying brain. The optic chiasm (arrow) is also severely compressed. The adenohypophysis, neurohypophysis, and hypothalamus have been destroyed by the neoplasm.
(Courtesy Dr. C. Capen, College of Veterinary Medicine, The Ohio State University.)

neoplasms usually arise in adult animals that have already completed their growth. However, atrophy of the skin and loss of muscle mass could be related in part to a lack of the protein anabolic effects of growth hormone. Interference with the secretion of pituitary trophic hormones often leads to a reduced basal metabolic rate because of decreased TSH secretion and hypoglycemia secondary to trophic atrophy of the adrenal cortex (Fig. 12-17).

PITUITARY GLAND CARCINOMAS

Pituitary gland carcinomas are uncommon neoplasms compared with adenomas but have been seen in older dogs and cattle. They usually are endocrinologically inactive but can cause significant functional disturbances by destroying the pars distalis and neurohypophyseal system, leading to panhypopituitarism and diabetes insipidus. Carcinomas are large and invade extensively into the overlying brain, along the ventral aspect of the cranial cavity, and into the basisphenoid bone where they cause osteolysis. Metastases occur infrequently to cervical lymph nodes or distant sites, such as the spleen or liver. Carcinomas are highly cellular and often have large areas of hemorrhage and necrosis. Giant cells, nuclear pleomorphism, and mitotic figures are encountered more frequently than in adenomas.

CRANIOPHARYNGIOMAS (INTRACRANIAL GERM CELL TUMORS)

Craniopharyngiomas are benign neoplasms derived from epithelial remnants of the oropharyngeal ectoderm of the craniopharyngeal duct (Rathke's pouch). They often occur in animals younger than those with other types of pituitary neoplasms and are present in either suprasellar or infrasellar locations. Craniopharyngioma is one cause of panhypopituitarism and dwarfism in young dogs because it causes subnormal secretion of somatotrophin and other trophic hormones at an early age, before closure of the growth plates.

The reclassification of some pleomorphic neoplasms in the suprasellar region of younger dogs from craniopharyngiomas to germ cell tumors has recently been proposed. The diagnosis of germ cell tumors was based on three criteria: (1) midline suprasellar location, (2) presence within the tumor of several distinct cell types (one population resembles a seminoma or dysgerminoma and others suggest teratomatous differentiation into secretory glandular and squamous elements), and (3) positive staining for α-fetoprotein.

Craniopharyngiomas and suprasellar germ cell tumors often are large and grow along the ventral aspect of the brain, where they can surround several cranial nerves. In addition, they extend dorsally into the hypothalamus and thalamus (Fig. 12-27). The resulting clinical signs often occur because of a combination of the following:

- A lack of secretion of pituitary trophic hormones resulting in trophic atrophy and subnormal function

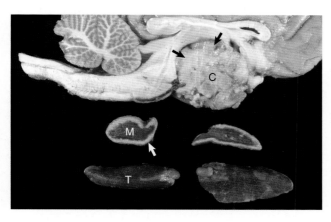

Fig. 12-27   Craniopharyngioma (C), pituitary area, adrenal glands, thyroid glands, dog. The neoplasm has extended dorsally through the hypothalamus and compressed the thalamus *(black arrows)*. The neoplasm has also destroyed the adenohypophysis and neurohypophysis, resulting in severe trophic atrophy of the adrenal cortex *(white arrow)*. The adrenal glands consist predominantly of medulla *(M)* surrounded by a thin rim of cortex (capsule plus zona glomerulosa). Although the thyroid follicular cells are atrophic, the overall gland *(T)* size is within normal limits because of colloid involution of the follicles. *(Courtesy Dr. C. Capen, College of Veterinary Medicine, The Ohio State University.)*

of the adrenal cortex and thyroid gland, atrophy of the gonads, and failure to attain somatic maturation because of a lack of secretion of growth hormone
- Disturbances in water metabolism (polyuria, polydipsia, low urine specific gravity, and osmolality) resulting from an interference in the synthesis and release of ADH by the large neoplasm
- Deficits in cranial nerve function
- CNS dysfunction due to extension into the overlying brain

Microscopically, craniopharyngiomas have alternating solid and cystic areas. The solid areas are composed of nests of cuboidal, columnar, or squamous epithelial cells with focal areas of mineralization. The cystic spaces are lined by either columnar or squamous cells and contain keratin debris and colloid.

DISORDERS OF THE NEUROHYPOPHYSIS
DIABETES INSIPIDUS

Diabetes insipidus results when inadequate ADH is produced (hypophyseal form) or when target cells in the kidneys lack the biochemical pathways necessary to respond to the secretion of normal or increased circulating concentrations of ADH (nephrogenic form). The hypophyseal form of diabetes insipidus results from compression and destruction of the pars nervosa, infundibular stalk, or supraoptic nucleus in the hypothalamus. The disruption of ADH synthesis or secretion in hypophyseal diabetes insipidus can be due to a large pituitary neoplasm, a dorsally expanding cyst, inflammatory granuloma, or traumatic injury to the skull with hemorrhage and glial proliferation in the neurohypophyseal tissue. Compression or disruption of the posterior lobe, infundibular stalk, and hypothalamus by neoplastic cells interrupts the transport of ADH in nonmyelinated axons from the site of production, primarily in the supraoptic nucleus of the hypothalamus, to the site of release in the capillary plexus of the pars nervosa.

Animals with diabetes insipidus excrete large volumes of hypotonic urine, which in turn necessitates the ingestion of large amounts of water to prevent dehydration and hyperosmolality of body fluids. Urine osmolality is decreased below normal plasma osmolality (approximately 300 mmol/L), in both hypophyseal and nephrogenic forms of diabetes insipidus. In response to water deprivation, urine osmolality still remains below that of the plasma in both forms of diabetes insipidus in contrast to increased osmolality observed in normal animals. Urine osmolality is increased above that of plasma in response to exogenous ADH in the hypophyseal form, but this increase does not occur in nephrogenic diabetes insipidus, a useful feature in differential diagnosis.

DISORDERS OF THE ADRENAL CORTEX

HYPOADRENOCORTICISM (ADDISON'S DISEASE)

Adrenal cortical insufficiency was the first recognized endocrine disease and is a common endocrinopathy in dogs. Clinical signs are a result of deficient production of any or all classes of corticosteroids (mineralocorticoids, glucocorticoids, and adrenal sex steroids). The synthesis and secretion of mineralocorticoids are reduced, resulting in marked alterations of serum potassium, sodium, and chloride concentrations (Fig. 12-5). Less potassium is excreted by the kidneys (hypokaliuria), resulting in severe hyperkalemia. Less sodium and chloride are reabsorbed from renal tubules, leading to varying degrees of hypernaturia and hyperchloriduria and a corresponding decline in blood concentrations of these ions. The severe hyperkalemia frequently produces notable cardiovascular disturbances. The pronounced bradycardia that develops in some dogs (heart rate of 50 or fewer beats per minute) does not change with exercise, but does predispose to weakness and circulatory collapse after minimal exertion.

A decreased production of glucocorticoids results in several characteristic functional disturbances of hypoadrenocorticism. A failure of gluconeogenesis and increased sensitivity to insulin contributes to the development of moderate hypoglycemia. Hyperpigmentation of the skin occurs in some dogs with long-standing adrenocortical insufficiency and is a common finding in human addisonian patients. This lesion results from a lack of negative feedback to the pituitary gland and the increased release of ACTH (and possibly MSH). The plasma cortisol concentrations in dogs with hypoadrenocorticism are low and range from 0.1 to 1.5 µg/dl. Because of the severe atrophy of the adrenal cortex, little or no increase in blood cortisol concentration results after the administration of ACTH.

ADRENALITIS

Bacterial and parasitic agents frequently localize in the adrenal glands and produce varying degrees of inflammation and necrosis. Focal inflammatory processes usually are suppurative, arising in the course of bacterial septicemias. The adrenal capsule provides an effective barrier against direct invasion by inflammatory reactions in adjacent tissue. Granulomatous adrenalitis due to *Histoplasma capsulatum*, *Coccidioides immitis*, or *Cryptococcus neoformans* occasionally occurs in dogs and cats. Multiple granulomas with central areas of necrosis and calcification can destroy nearly the entire adrenal cortex. *Toxoplasma gondii* produces necrosis with an infiltration of histiocytes in the adrenal cortex of many species of animals. Experimental evidence suggests that large local concentrations of antiinflammatory steroids in the adrenal cortex (e.g., cortisol and corticosterone) suppress local cell-mediated immunity and permit the progressive growth of certain fungi (e.g., *Histoplasma capsulatum*, *Coccidioides immitis*), protozoa (e.g., *Babesia darlingi*, *Babesia jellisoni*, or *Toxoplasma gondii*), and bacteria (e.g., *Mycobacterium tuberculosis*).

ADRENOCORTICAL HEMORRHAGE (WATERHOUSE-FRIDERICHSEN SYNDROME)

Massive, diffuse, often bilateral adrenal cortical hemorrhage, a condition known as Waterhouse-Friderichsen syndrome, is an uncommon but fatal consequence of overwhelming sepsis (Fig. 12-28). Although frequently seen in conjunction with endotoxic shock, Waterhouse-Friderichsen syndrome can also result from gram-positive organisms and noninfectious causes, such as anticoagulant therapy and trauma.

IDIOPATHIC ADRENOCORTICAL ATROPHY

Bilateral idiopathic adrenal cortical atrophy is an entity in young adult dogs that results in hypoadrenocorticism. The adrenal cortex is reduced to one tenth or less of its normal thickness because of a marked reduction of all layers of the cortex. It consists primarily of the

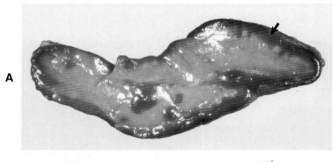

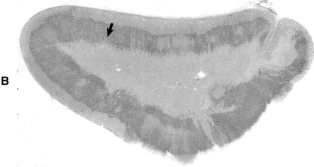

Fig. 12-28   **Adrenocortical hemorrhage (Waterhouse-Friderichsen syndrome), adrenal gland, horse. A,** Diffuse hemorrhage *(arrow)* affecting the adrenal cortex is frequently seen in endotoxic shock. **B,** Subgross of diffuse hemorrhage *(arrow)* affecting the adrenal cortex. H&E stain. (*A* and *B,* *Courtesy College of Veterinary Medicine, University of Illinois.*)

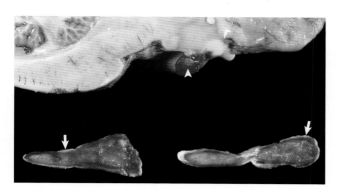

Fig. 12-29   Adrenal cortical atrophy, brain stem and pituitary gland, adrenal glands, dog. Bilateral atrophy of all three cortical layers *(arrows)* is characteristic of hypoadrenocorticism. The pituitary gland *(arrowhead)* was grossly normal with microscopic evidence of corticotroph hyperplasia. *(Courtesy Dr. C. Capen, College of Veterinary Medicine, The Ohio State University.)*

adrenal capsule (Fig. 12-29). Thus the adrenal medulla becomes relatively more prominent and, along with the capsule, makes up the bulk of the remaining adrenal gland. The precise pathogenesis of idiopathic adrenal cortical atrophy is unknown, but the lesion is most likely immune mediated. Early in the disease, multiple foci of lymphocytes and plasma cells are interspersed between the adrenal sinusoids and adrenal cortical cells. The capsule is thickened by condensation from the collapse of the adrenal cortex and fibroblastic proliferation. Pituitary gland lesions have not been observed in dogs with idiopathic adrenal cortical atrophy involving all three zones of the adrenal cortex, including the zona glomerulosa, which is not under ACTH control. By comparison, atrophy of the adrenal cortex due to a destructive pituitary gland lesion that decreases ACTH secretion is characterized by severe atrophy only of the two inner cortical zones (zona fasciculata and zona reticularis). The zona glomerulosa remains intact (Fig. 12-17), and thus these animals do not have electrolyte abnormalities because the secretion of aldosterone remains within normal limits.

HYPERADRENOCORTICISM (CUSHING'S SYNDROME OR DISEASE)

The clinical manifestations and lesions characteristic of the syndrome of hyperadrenocorticism result primarily from chronic overproduction of cortisol by hyperactive cells of the adrenal cortex. Affected dogs develop a spectrum of functional disturbances and lesions resulting from the combined glyconeogenetic, lipolytic, protein catabolic, and antiinflammatory effects of the glucocorticoid hormones on many organs. The disease is insidious

and slowly progressive. Cortisol excess or Cushing's syndrome is one of the most common endocrinopathies in adult and aged dogs but occurs infrequently in cats and rarely in other domestic animals.

The increase in circulating cortisol concentrations in dogs with hyperadrenocorticism can result from one of several different pathogenic mechanisms. The most common cause of Cushing's syndrome is Cushing's disease in which a functional corticotroph (ACTH-secreting) adenoma of the pituitary gland causes bilateral adrenal cortical hypertrophy and hyperplasia (Fig. 12-18). The cortex of each adrenal gland is widened considerably as a result of diffuse and nodular hyperplasia, primarily in the zona fasciculata. Functional adrenal gland neoplasms are an infrequent (10% to 15% of cases) cause of Cushing's syndrome in the dog. Many of the clinical signs and lesions of naturally occurring hyperadrenocorticism can be induced by the long-term, daily administration of large doses of corticosteroids. To accurately separate the different pathogenetic mechanisms responsible for cortisol excess, plasma cortisol concentrations must be evaluated with the animal in the basal state and then after dexamethasone (large or small dose) suppression and ACTH stimulation.

Appetite and food intake often are increased as a direct result of either the hypercortisolism or damage caused by compression of the hypothalamic appetite centers by a large, dorsally expanding pituitary gland neoplasm. The muscles of the extremities and abdomen are weakened and atrophied, resulting in gradual abdominal enlargement (Fig. 12-30), lordosis, muscle

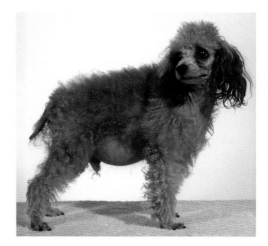

Fig. 12-30   Cushing's-like disease, hypercortisolism, dog, poodle. Hypercortisolism followed exogenous corticosteroid administration for the treatment of idiopathic adrenal cortical hyperplasia. Muscle asthenia is the cause of the pendulous abdomen. Note the alopecia of the skin of the abdomen, ventral cervical region, and tail. *(Courtesy Dr. C. Capen, College of Veterinary Medicine, The Ohio State University.)*

trembling, and a straight-legged, skeletal-braced posture assumed to support the body's weight. Hepatomegaly caused by increased deposits of lipid and glycogen (steroid hepatopathy; see Fig. 8-44) can contribute to the development of the distended, often pendulous, abdomen. The muscular asthenia and wasting are the result of increased catabolism of structural proteins combined with diminished protein synthesis in skeletal myocytes from the influence of long-term cortisol excess. Cutaneous lesions occur frequently in dogs with hyperadrenocorticism. The initial changes in the skin often are observed over points of wear (e.g., neck, flanks, behind the ears) and over bony prominences. These initial cutaneous changes spread in a bilaterally symmetric pattern to involve a significant percentage of the body surface (Fig. 12-30). Cutaneous lesions caused by excessive cortisol include atrophy of the epidermis and pilosebaceous units, combined with loss of collagen and elastin in the dermis and subcutis. Cutaneous calcification or calcinosis cutis is a characteristic lesion and occurs in up to 30% of dogs with hypercortisolism. Numerous calcium crystals are deposited along collagen and elastin fibers in the dermis and can penetrate through the atrophic and thinned epidermis. These calcium deposits occur in dogs with normal blood calcium and phosphorus concentrations. This manifestation of hypercortisolism is most likely related to the glyconeogenetic and protein catabolic action of cortisol, which results in the rearrangement of the molecular structure of such proteins as collagen and elastin, and the formation of an organic matrix that attracts and binds calcium. Severe calcification also occurs in other tissues, such as lungs, active skeletal muscle, and the stomach.

CONGENITAL ADRENAL HYPERPLASIA (ADRENOGENITAL SYNDROME)

Congenital adrenal hyperplasia is an entity of hypoadrenocorticism and hyperadrenocorticism. Affected individuals are deficient in an enzyme such as 21-hydroxylase, involved in both mineralocorticoid and glucocorticoid synthesis. As a consequence of reduced cortisol levels, there is a compensatory increase in ACTH secretion resulting in adrenal cortical hyperplasia. Subsequent steroid synthesis is diverted to the androgenic pathway, which is independent of 21-hydroxylase. Excessive androgen production leads to virilization and sexual ambiguity in newborns and premature closure of epiphyses. Hereditary adrenal hyperplasia occurs in rabbits of the IIIVO/ahj strain. The mode of inheritance, as in human beings, is autosomal recessive. Notable, bilateral adrenal enlargement is evident as early as day 19 of gestation. Although affected rabbit kits are viable, they die soon after birth. Pomeranians are predisposed to a congenital adrenal hyperplasia–like syndrome and associated dermatosis; however, no mutations in the

21-hydroxylase enzyme have been found in the small group of Pomeranians evaluated.

HYPERPLASIA AND NEOPLASIA OF ADRENAL CORTEX
Accessory adrenal tissue

Accessory or ectopic adrenal cortical tissue is common in the adrenal glands of adult to aged animals and can be found in the capsule, cortex, and medulla. Many of these nodules arise either as evaginations of the cortex into the capsule and surrounding periadrenal adipose tissue or invaginations of the cortex into the medulla.

Hyperplasia

Nodular hyperplasia is common in the adrenal glands as well-defined spherical nodules in the cortex or attached to the capsule (Fig. 12-31). Hyperplastic nodules are usually multiple, bilateral and yellow, and involve any of the three zones of the cortex. Histologically the nodules near the capsule resemble the zona glomerulosa and sometimes the zona fasciculata. The lipid content in these hyperplastic nodules is retained in circumstances that reduce the amount of lipid in the normal adrenal cortex. Hyperplastic cortical nodules are most common in older horses, dogs, and cats. Nodular hyperplasia of the zona reticularis has been seen in animals with functional disturbances suggestive of androgen excess (e.g., greater muscle mass, well-developed crest, clitoral hypertrophy, and mammary gland involution).

Diffuse cortical hyperplasia results in a uniform, usually bilateral, enlargement of the adrenal cortices. Notable hypertrophy and hyperplasia of cells of the zona fasciculata and zona reticularis occur in response to an autonomous hypersecretion of ACTH by a corticotroph adenoma of the pituitary gland (Fig. 12-18). The cytoplasm of the hyperplastic cells of the zona fasciculata is vacuolated because of the lipid content.

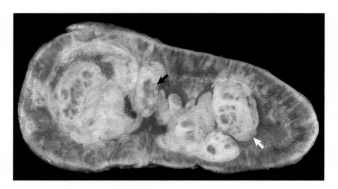

Fig. 12-31 **Nodular adrenal cortical hyperplasia, adrenal gland, dog.** Multiple discrete nodules (*arrows*) of cortical hyperplasia extend into the medulla. *(Courtesy Dr. C. Capen, College of Veterinary Medicine, The Ohio State University.)*

Cells of the outer zona glomerulosa can be compressed by the expansion of the inner two zones. Nodular hyperplasia can be present in a diffusely hyperplastic cortex.

Cortical adenomas

Adenomas of the adrenal cortex occur most frequently in older dogs and only sporadically in horses, cattle, and sheep. Castrated male goats have a greater incidence of cortical adenomas than intact males. Although these neoplasms are usually incidental findings at necropsy, they are occasionally endocrinologically active. Cortical adenomas are well demarcated and usually are a single, unilateral nodule. Larger cortical adenomas are yellow to red, distort the contour of the gland, compress the adjacent cortical parenchyma, and are partially or completely encapsulated (Fig. 12-32). Cortical adenomas often develop in an adrenal gland with multiple nodules of hyperplasia and can be difficult to differentiate grossly from hyperplastic nodules. However, these hyperplastic nodules consist of multiple small foci, usually in both adrenal glands, without encapsulation, and often with extracapsular nodules of hyperplastic cortical tissue. Cortical adenomas are composed of well-differentiated cells that resemble secretory cells of the normal zona fasciculata or zona reticularis. The cytoplasm of neoplastic cells is abundant and lightly eosinophilic and filled with lipid droplets. Adenomas are partially or completely surrounded by a fibrous connective tissue capsule of varying thickness and a rim of compressed cortical parenchyma.

Cortical carcinomas

Adrenal cortical carcinomas occur less frequently than adenomas and have been reported most often in

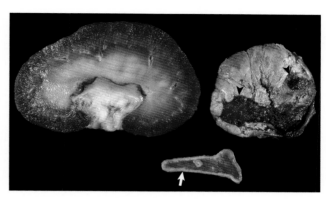

Fig. 12-33   Adrenocortical carcinoma and contralateral cortical atrophy, adrenal glands, dog. The adrenal gland (*right*) has a large adrenocortical carcinoma that is almost half the size of an adult kidney (*left*). Multifocal to coalescing areas of hemorrhage and necrosis are apparent (*arrowheads*) in this tumor. The cortex of the contralateral adrenal gland (*lower*) is notably thinned (*arrow*) because of severe trophic atrophy of the zona fasciculata and zona reticularis. (*Courtesy Dr. C. Capen, College of Veterinary Medicine, The Ohio State University.*)

cattle and older dogs, but they also occur infrequently in other species. Carcinomas develop in adult to older dogs. There is no apparent breed or sex prevalence. Adrenal carcinomas are larger than adenomas and are more likely to be bilateral. In dogs, they are composed of a variegated, yellow-red, friable tissue (Fig. 12-33) and can invade extensively into surrounding tissue, such as the wall of the caudal vena cava, resulting in thrombus formation. Carcinomas attain considerable size in cattle (up to 10 cm or more in diameter) and have multiple areas of calcification or ossification.

Carcinomas are composed of more highly pleomorphic secretory cells than adenomas and are subdivided by a fine fibrovascular stroma. The affected adrenal gland usually is completely obliterated by the carcinoma (Fig. 12-33). The growth pattern of neoplastic cells varies between neoplasms and within the same carcinoma, and can be trabecular, lobular, or focal. Neoplastic cells usually are large and polyhedral, and they have prominent nucleoli and densely eosinophilic or vacuolated cytoplasm.

Carcinomas and adenomas of the adrenal cortex in dogs occasionally are functional and secrete excessive amounts of cortisol. The clinical syndrome produced by excessive secretion by adrenal cortical carcinomas can be complicated by signs produced by compression of adjacent organs when the neoplasm is large; by invasion into the aorta or caudal vena cava, which can lead to intraabdominal hemorrhage; and by metastases to distant sites (e.g., liver, kidneys, mesenteric lymph nodes, and lungs). Functional cortical adenomas and carcinomas are responsible for severe atrophy of the contralateral adrenal

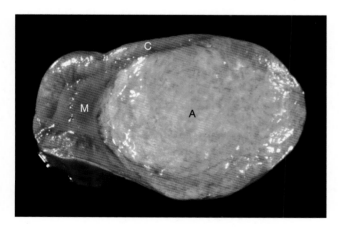

Fig. 12-32   Adrenocortical adenoma, adrenal gland, horse. Note the well-demarcated, large, yellowish-tan, adrenocortical adenoma (**A**) compressing the adjacent unaffected medulla (**M**). C, Adrenal cortex. (*Courtesy Dr. B. Weeks, College of Veterinary Medicine, Texas A&M University; and Noah's Arkive, College of Veterinary Medicine, The University of Georgia.*)

cortex because of negative feedback inhibition of pituitary ACTH secretion by the increased blood cortisol concentrations (Fig. 12-33). The atrophic cortex consists primarily of the adrenal capsule and zona glomerulosa. Atrophy is also present in the remnants of the adrenal cortex compressed by functional adenomas. Because of the lack of cortical tissue, the adrenal medulla appears more prominent (Fig. 12-33).

Functional proliferative lesions in ferrets

Adrenal gland neoplasms are the second most common neoplasm reported in ferrets, and they are being recognized with increasing frequency as more are being kept as pets and living longer. The adrenal gland enlargements are either bilateral (approximately 45%) as a result of diffuse (most frequent) or nodular hyperplasia, or unilateral (approximately 55%) as a result of adrenal cortical carcinoma or cortical adenoma. Adrenal gland neoplasms develop in adult ferrets (mean age 5 years) with females more frequently affected than males (sex ratio ≥2:1), and in animals gonadectomized at an early age (2 to 4 months). The latter finding is attributed to chronic trophic stimulation of the zona reticularis by LH.

A unique histologic feature of adrenocortical carcinomas in ferrets is the presence of a spindle cell component to the neoplastic cortical cells. These spindle cells express smooth muscle actin and arise from capsular or subcapsular smooth muscle cells, or they might represent a morphologically distinct adrenocortical cell. An emerging histologic variant of ferret adrenocortical carcinomas demonstrating increased invasiveness is characterized by myxoid differentiation (Fig. 12-34). In addition, immunoreactivity to the transcription factor GATA-4 has been identified as a marker of anaplasia in ferret adrenocortical tumors.

Clinical signs in ferrets with adrenal cortical neoplasms include vulvar enlargement, bilaterally symmetric alopecia (especially on the ventral abdomen and medial aspects of the rear legs), polyuria, polydipsia, and the presence of a palpable mass at the cranial pole of the kidneys (left side greater frequency than right). Other functional disturbances—including anemia and thrombocytopenia, pyometra, and endometrial hyperplasia in females, and squamous metaplasia of prostatic ductular epithelium and cystic prostatic disease in males—are changes consistent with an overproduction of estrogenic steroids by the adrenal gland neoplasms. Some of the functional disturbances resemble those seen in intact females with persistent or prolonged estrus; ferrets are seasonally polyestrous and are induced ovulators. About one third of ferrets with adrenal cortical neoplasms also have neoplasms derived from the insulin-producing B cells of the pancreatic islets. These neoplasms can produce increased concentrations of serum insulin resulting

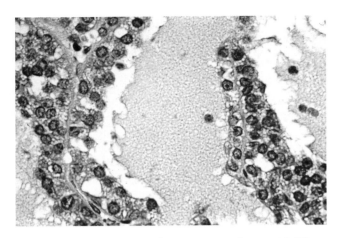

Fig. 12-34   Adrenocortical carcinoma with myxoid differentiation, adrenal gland, ferret. Note that the cystic spaces lined by neoplastic cells contain abundant mucinous material. Alcian blue stain. *(From Peterson RA, Kiupel M, Capen CC: Vet Pathol 40:136-142, 2003.)*

in hypoglycemia that can lead to seizures, episodic lethargy, ptyalism, ataxia, and hind leg weakness.

The most consistent endocrinologic change in ferrets with adrenal gland neoplasms is increased plasma concentrations of estradiol-17β. It is presumed that the estradiol-17β is produced directly by the neoplastic cells, but alternatively the adrenal gland neoplasms could secrete androgenic steroids that are aromatized in the skin and possibly elsewhere aromatized to estrogenic steroids. No increase in circulating estradiol-17β concentrations is found in response to exogenous ACTH, but plasma concentrations decrease after adrenalectomy. Plasma cortisol and corticosterone concentrations in ferrets with adrenal gland neoplasms are in the low to normal range and are not increased greatly in response to exogenous ACTH. Plasma cortisol is not decreased after unilateral adrenalectomy, and the contralateral adrenal cortex is not atrophic as would be expected if the adrenal gland neoplasm was secreting excess cortisol. The clinical signs in ferrets with adrenal cortical neoplasms can be effectively reversed by adrenalectomy (especially of the left side if there is no macroscopic enlargement) but not by chemotherapy with mitotane (o,p'-DDD). Complete regrowth of hair usually occurs by 2 to 3 months after adrenalectomy.

DISORDERS OF THE ADRENAL MEDULLA
PROLIFERATIVE LESIONS
ADRENAL MEDULLARY HYPERPLASIA

Diffuse or nodular adrenal medullary hyperplasia appears to precede the development of pheochromocytoma in bulls and human beings with C-cell neoplasms

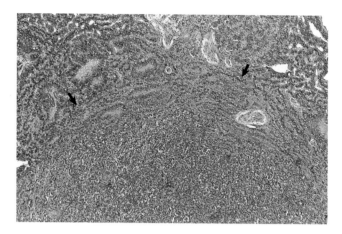

Fig. 12-35 **Hyperplasia, adrenal medulla, bull.** Bilateral diffuse hyperplasia of adrenal medulla in a bull with a concomitant C-cell carcinoma of the thyroid gland. The expanded adrenal medulla (*bottom*) has compressed the surrounding adrenal cortex (*arrows*). H&E stain. (*Courtesy Dr. C. Capen, College of Veterinary Medicine, The Ohio State University.*)

of the thyroid gland. The proliferated chromaffin cells are nonencapsulated but compress the surrounding adrenal cortex (Fig. 12-35). Hyperplastic cells are round to oval and have pale basophilic cytoplasm. Some bulls with prominent diffuse medullary hyperplasia often have a few small nodules of proliferated medullary cells. Medullary hyperplasia is diagnosed on the basis of the following criteria: an increased adrenal weight; a decrease in cortical to medullary ratio because of an increase in the size and number of medullary cells; and numerous mitotic figures in the adrenal medulla.

NEOPLASMS

Neuroblastomas and ganglioneuromas

Neuroblastomas usually occur in young animals, arise from primitive neuroectodermal cells, and form large intraabdominal masses. The tumors are composed of small neoplastic cells that have hyperchromatic nuclei and scant amounts of cytoplasm and resemble lymphocytes. Neoplastic cells tend to aggregate around blood vessels, forming pseudorosettes. Neurofibrils or unmyelinated nerve fibers can be demonstrated in neuroblastomas.

Ganglioneuromas are benign neoplasms composed of multipolar ganglion cells and neurofibrils, and have a prominent fibrous connective tissue stroma. The surrounding adrenal cortex is often severely compressed. Occasionally, neoplastic cells in adrenal medullary neoplasms differentiate into two cell lines, resulting in pheochromocytoma and ganglioneuroma in the same adrenal gland.

Pheochromocytomas

Pheochromocytomas are the most common neoplasms in the adrenal medullas of animals, occurring most often in cattle and dogs and infrequently in other species. Calcitonin-secreting C-cell neoplasms of the thyroid gland occasionally develop concurrently with pheochromocytomas in bulls and human beings. Extraadrenal pheochromocytomas, referred to as paragangliomas, also occur infrequently in the abdomen.

Pheochromocytomas often are large (10 cm or more in diameter) and replace most of the affected adrenal gland. Smaller neoplasms are completely surrounded by a thin, compressed rim of adrenal cortex (Fig. 12-36). Large pheochromocytomas are multilobular and variegated light brown to yellow-red as a result of areas of hemorrhage and necrosis. Malignant pheochromocytomas invade through the capsule of an adrenal gland into adjacent structures, such as the caudal vena cava (Fig. 12-37), and metastasize to distant sites including the liver, regional lumbar aortic, and renal lymph nodes or lungs. Histologically, neoplastic cells vary from small, round to polyhedral cells to large, pleomorphic cells with multiple hyperchromatic nuclei. The cytoplasm is lightly eosinophilic, finely granular, and often indistinct.

Functional pheochromocytomas composed of epinephrine- and/or norepinephrine-secreting cells have been reported infrequently in animals. Tachycardia, edema, and cardiac hypertrophy observed in several dogs and horses with pheochromocytomas were attributed to excessive catecholamine secretion. Arteriolar sclerosis and widespread medial hyperplasia of arterioles have been reported in dogs with pheochromocytomas and clinical signs suggestive of paroxysmal hypertension. Hypertension was detected in 43% of

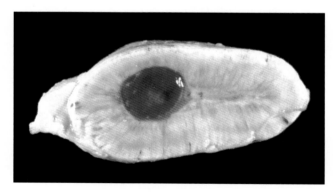

Fig. 12-36 **Pheochromocytoma, adrenal gland, horse.** A pheochromocytoma compressing the adjacent unaffected adrenal cortex. (*Courtesy College of Veterinary Medicine, University of Illinois.*)

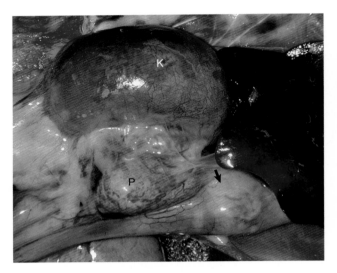

Fig. 12-37   Pheochromocytoma, kidney, adrenal gland, caudal vena cava, dog. A large pheochromocytoma (*P*) has obliterated the adrenal gland medial to the kidney (*K*) and has extensively invaded into the lumen of the caudal vena cava *(arrow)*. *(Courtesy Dr. April Paulman, College of Veterinary Medicine, University of Illinois.)*

dogs with pheochromocytomas; all hypertensive dogs had concurrent diseases that could have contributed to the increase in blood pressure. Infrequently, hyper-adrenocorticism occurs concurrently in dogs with pheochromocytoma and could contribute to the development of hypertension, particularly during digital manipulation of the affected adrenal gland during surgery.

Norepinephrine is the predominant catecholamine extracted from pheochromocytomas in dogs. This is similar to the finding in normal pups, in which norepinephrine is the predominant catecholamine; in adult dogs, epinephrine predominates in adrenal medullary tissues. The catecholamine content of pheochromocytomas in bulls with concurrent C-cell neoplasms of the thyroid gland is greater than in the normal adrenal medulla. Urinary excretion of free unconjugated catecholamines and metabolites of catecholamines, such as vanillylmandelic acid, are increased in bulls with pheochromocytomas.

DISORDERS OF THE THYROID GLAND
DEVELOPMENTAL DISTURBANCES
ACCESSORY THYROID TISSUE

The thyroid gland originates embryologically as a thickened plate of epithelium in the ventral aspect of the pharynx. The complex embryogenesis of the thyroid frequently leads to the formation of accessory thyroid tissue. This accessory thyroid tissue is most typically located in the mediastinum but can be located anywhere from the base of the tongue to the diaphragm. About 50% of adult dogs have nodules of accessory thyroid tissue embedded in the adipose around the base of the heart and the origin of the aorta. The follicular structure and function are the same as those of the main thyroid lobes. Attempts to induce hypothyroidism in the dog by surgical thyroidectomy are usually unsuccessful because the accessory thyroid tissue readily responds to the prompt increase in endogenous TSH secretion, and can undergo sufficient hyperplasia to sustain adequate hormone production. This accessory thyroid tissue can also undergo neoplastic transformation.

THYROGLOSSAL DUCT CYSTS

Thyroglossal duct cysts develop most frequently in dogs and pigs and are present occasionally in other animals. They form as a result of persistence of portions of the midline embryologic primordia of the thyroid gland, which migrates caudally from the ventral aspect of the primitive pharynx to form the thyroid lobes postnatally. These cysts are present in the ventral aspect of the cervical region in dogs and are fluctuant masses that can rupture and form a tract to the exterior. Their lining epithelium consists of multiple layers of follicular cells in which colloid-containing follicles are found occasionally. These cells sometimes undergo neoplastic transformation and give rise to papillary carcinomas.

HYPOTHYROIDISM

Hypothyroidism is a well-recognized and clinically important disease in dogs but is encountered only occasionally in other animals. Although the disease occurs in many adult purebred and mixed breed dogs, certain breeds such as the golden retriever, Doberman pinscher, dachshund, Shetland sheep dog, Irish setter, miniature schnauzer, cocker spaniel, and Airedale are more commonly affected. Hypothyroidism in dogs is usually the result of primary lesions in the thyroid gland, particularly idiopathic follicular collapse and lymphocytic thyroiditis. Less common causes of hypothyroidism include bilateral nonfunctional follicular cell neoplasms and severe iodine-deficient goiter. Hypothyroidism due to long-standing pituitary gland or hypothalamic lesions, which prevent the release of either TSH or thyrotropin-releasing hormone, is encountered infrequently in the dog. In these cases, the thyroid gland is moderately reduced in size and composed of colloid-distended follicles, lined by flattened follicular cells.

Many functional disturbances reported with hypothyroidism occur because of a reduction in basal metabolic rate. A gain in body weight without an associated change

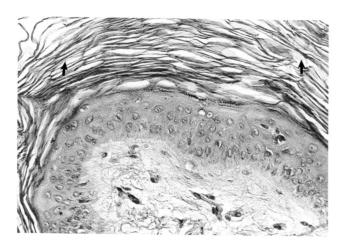

Fig. 12-38   Hypothyroidism, skin, dog. Hyperkeratosis (*arrows*) has resulted in thickening of the epidermis of the skin. H&E stain. (*Courtesy Dr. C. Capen, College of Veterinary Medicine, The Ohio State University.*)

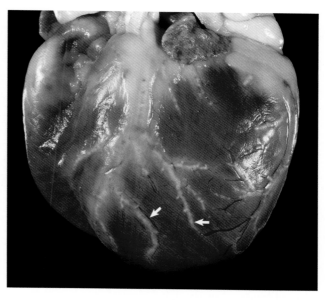

Fig. 12-39   Atherosclerosis, hypothyroidism with marked hyperlipidemia, heart, coronary arteries, dog. Note the atherosclerosis (*arrows*) of the coronary arteries which are thickened, firm, yellow-white, and often beaded. (*Courtesy Dr. C. Capen, College of Veterinary Medicine, The Ohio State University.*)

in appetite occurs in some hypothyroid dogs. Thinning of the hair coat is often accompanied by bilaterally symmetric alopecia. Areas affected initially by hair loss are those receiving frictional wear, such as the tail and cervical area.

Hyperkeratosis is a consistent finding in hypothyroidism and results clinically in an increased scaliness of the skin. When severe, it occurs as circular scaly patches resembling seborrhea. Microscopically, hyperkeratosis (Fig. 12-38) involves the external root sheath, resulting in follicular keratosis. Hyperpigmentation, especially in such localized areas of alopecia as the dorsal aspect of the nose and distal portion of the tail, occurs in many dogs with hypothyroidism. Myxedema may also develop because of the accumulation of glycosaminoglycans and hyaluronic acid in the dermis and subcutis. These substances bind considerable amounts of water, which results in notable thickening of the skin. Microscopically, mucins appear as granular or fibrillar material in hematoxylin and eosin (H&E) stained sections.

Reproductive abnormalities include lack of libido, reduced sperm count, abnormal or absent estrus cycles, and reduced conception rates. In chronic hypothyroidism, spermatogenic epithelium in the testes is often notably atrophic.

Hypothyroidism in dogs is accompanied by decreased circulating thyroidal hormone concentrations and decreased ^{131}I uptake by the thyroid gland. In dogs with hypothyroidism, the concentration of T_4 is usually below 0.8 µg/dl (normal 1.5 to 3.4 µg/dl) and that of T_3 is below 50 ng/dl (normal 48 to 150 ng/dl). In the euthyroid dog, T_4 concentrations will at least double 8 hours after intravenous or intramuscular injection

of TSH. In dogs with hypothyroidism, the T_4 concentrations do not change significantly after injection of TSH.

Serum cholesterol concentrations are often greatly increased (300 to 900 mg/dl) in many hypothyroid dogs (normal 40 to 80 mg/dl). The marked hypercholesterolemia in long-standing and severe hypothyroidism results in a variety of secondary lesions, including atherosclerosis, hepatomegaly, and glomerular and corneal lipidosis. Atherosclerosis of coronary (Fig. 12-39) and cerebral vessels develops in dogs that have severe hypothyroidism and long-standing hyperlipidemia.

IDIOPATHIC FOLLICULAR ATROPHY ("COLLAPSE")

In follicular atrophy, the loss of follicular epithelium and disruption of follicles is progressive and the gland is replaced by adipose connective tissue with only a minimal inflammatory response. The gland usually is smaller and lighter in color than normal. The early lesion in dogs with mild clinical signs of hypothyroidism appears to be confined to one part of the thyroid gland. The affected part is composed of small follicles that contain little colloid and are lined by tall columnar follicular cells. A more advanced form of follicular atrophy is present in dogs with clinical hypothyroidism and low blood concentrations of thyroidal hormones. These thyroid glands are notably reduced in size and are composed predominantly of adipose connective tissue with only a few clusters of small follicles containing vacuolated colloid.

LYMPHOCYTIC (IMMUNE-MEDIATED) THYROIDITIS

Lymphocytic thyroiditis in dogs, obese strains of chickens, nonhuman primates, and Buffalo rats closely resembles Hashimoto's disease of human beings. Although the exact pathogenetic mechanism in the dog is not completely established, evidence suggests a polygenic pattern of inheritance similar to that observed in human beings. The immunologic basis of the development of chronic lymphocytic thyroiditis in human beings and dogs appears to be through production of autoantibodies. These are usually directed against thyroglobulin or a microsomal antigen such as thyroperoxidase and infrequently against the TSH receptor, a nuclear antigen, or a second colloid antigen from thyroid follicular cells. Thyroglobulin autoantibodies have been found in 48% of pet dogs with hypothyroidism. Laboratory beagles with naturally occurring lymphocytic thyroiditis also have circulating thyroidal autoantibodies, but the focal thyroiditis usually is not severe enough to induce clinical signs of hypothyroidism.

Microscopic lesions consist of multifocal to diffuse infiltrates of lymphocytes, which occasionally form nodules, plasma cells, and macrophages. Thyroid follicles are small and lined by columnar epithelial cells; lymphocytes, macrophages, and degenerate follicular cells are often present in the colloid, which is vacuolated (Fig. 12-40). Thyroid C cells are present as small nests or nodules between follicles and often are more prominent than those in normal dogs. Some remaining follicular cells appear to be transformed into large oxyphilic cells with densely eosinophilic granular cytoplasm.

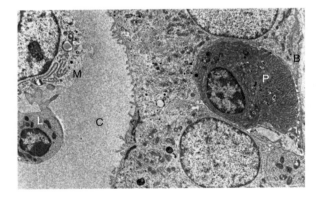

Fig. 12-40 **Lymphocytic thyroiditis in a dog with severe hypothyroidism.** A lymphocyte (*L*) and macrophage (*M*) are present in the colloid (*C*) of a thyroid follicle. A plasma cell (*P*) within the follicular basement membrane (*B*) is infiltrating between thyroid follicular cells. TEM. Uranyl acetate and lead citrate stain. (*From Gosselin SJ, Capen CC, Martin SL: Vet Immunol Immunopathol 3:185-201, 1982.*)

HYPERTHYROIDISM

Hyperthyroidism or thyrotoxicosis resulting from elevated circulating levels of T_4 and T_3 commonly occurs in middle-aged to older cats and rarely in dogs. The condition in cats is associated with a spectrum of functional proliferative lesions, whereas in dogs it is due to thyroid neoplasms.

Clinical signs result from an increased rate of basal metabolism. Consequently, animals are polyuric and polydipsic, and frequently lose weight despite a voracious appetite. Weakness and fatigue, nervousness or hyperexcitability, and hyperthermia and heat intolerance are also present. In addition, cardiac manifestations of hyperthyroidism, such as tachycardia and dysrhythmias, are well documented in animals; however, secondary hypertrophic cardiomyopathy characterized by concentric hypertrophy is primarily restricted to cats and rats.

In general, the likelihood of animals developing clinical hyperthyroidism secondary to thyroid neoplasms depends on (1) the capability of neoplastic cells to synthesize T_4 and T_3 (e.g., well-differentiated thyroid neoplasms that form follicles and produce colloid are more likely to synthesize thyroid hormones than poorly differentiated solid neoplasms), and (2) the extent of the increase in circulating concentrations of T_4 and T_3, which depends on a balance between the rate of secretion of thyroid hormones by the neoplasm, and the rate of degradation of thyroid hormones. Dogs have a much more efficient enterohepatic excretory mechanism for thyroid hormones, which is difficult to overload, than cats; therefore, clinical hyperthyroidism in dogs with functional thyroid follicular cell neoplasms is infrequent. Cats are very sensitive to phenol and phenol derivatives and have a poor ability to conjugate phenolic compounds such as T_4 with glucuronic acid and excrete the T_4 glucuronide into the bile. The capacity of conjugation of T_3 with sulfate is limited and easily overloaded in cats.

FUNCTIONAL PROLIFERATIVE LESIONS IN CATS

A spectrum of proliferative lesions that secrete excess thyroidal hormones (e.g., adenomas and multinodular hyperplasia) is common in the thyroid glands of adult and aged cats. Since the late 1970s, there has been a dramatic increase in the incidence of neoplasms and other focal proliferative lesions in the thyroid glands of cats and these have resulted in hyperthyroidism. Hyperthyroidism is one of the two most common endocrine diseases in adult to aged cats (diabetes mellitus being the other). Before 1980, clinical hyperthyroidism was infrequently diagnosed in cats. The reason for the apparently increased incidence is uncertain, but appears to be related in part to (1) a larger population of geriatric cats receiving veterinary medical care, (2) improved assays for thyroid hormones, (3) detailed characterization of the clinical syndrome, and (4) increased awareness by veterinary clinicians of its common occurrence in adult to aged cats. In addition, there does appear to be a real increase in the incidence of feline hyperthyroidism over the past 30 years. Potential risk factors that have been reported include a predominantly indoor environment, regular treatment with flea powders, exposures to herbicides and fertilizers, a diet primarily of canned food, and non-Siamese breeds (10 times greater occurrence). It has been suggested that wide variations (excessive to inadequate) in dietary iodine intake over prolonged periods could play a role in the pathogenesis of hyperthyroidism in cats.

The disease in cats is mechanistically different from that of Graves' disease in human patients in that hyperthyroid cats do not have increased concentrations of circulating thyroid-stimulating immunoglobulins, which are comparable to long-acting thyroid stimulator (LATS) in human beings (LATS is an autoantibody that binds to the TSH receptor and activates follicular cells). Purified immunoglobulin G, prepared from hyperthyroid cats, significantly increases ^{3}H-thymidine incorporation into DNA and stimulates thyroid follicular cell proliferation fifteenfold but does not stimulate intracellular cAMP production. The ^{3}H-thymidine incorporation can be completely inhibited by a specific TSH receptor blocking antibody. These data suggest that increased titers of thyroid growth-stimulating immunoglobulins are present in cats with hyperthyroidism and most likely act by the TSH receptor. In cats, the disease most closely resembles toxic nodular goiter in human patients with mutations in genes encoding for either the TSH receptor or the $G_{s\alpha}$ protein. Mutations in $G_{s\alpha}$ that correspond to the mutations in human beings have been reported in a small group of hyperthyroid cats. $G_{s\alpha}$ is a G protein that mediates cAMP-dependent TSH signaling. Follicular cell proliferation, differentiation, and secretion of thyroid hormone result from constitutive activation of TSH signaling. In a separate study, all cases of feline follicular hyperplasia and adenomas evaluated by immunohistochemistry demonstrated overexpression of the c-ras oncogene. As was the case for activating $G_{s\alpha}$ mutations, overexpression of c-ras results in constitutive mitogenesis of thyroid follicular epithelial cells. Hyperplastic and neoplastic thyroid tissue from cats is transplantable into athymic (nude) mice and continues to overproduce T_4 and T_3 in a subcutaneous location.

Follicular cell adenomas, which often develop in a thyroid gland with multinodular hyperplasia, are more common than thyroid carcinomas. Follicles in the rim of thyroid tissue around a functional adenoma are notably enlarged and distended with colloid (colloid involution). The follicular cells are low cuboidal and atrophic

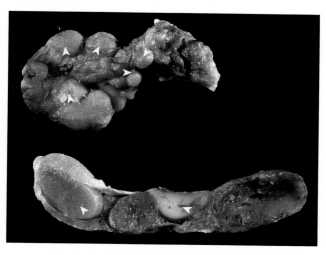

Fig. 12-41   **Hyperplasia, hyperthyroidism, thyroid glands, cat.** Multinodular follicular cell hyperplasia *(arrowheads)* involves both thyroid lobes. *(Courtesy Dr. C. Capen, College of Veterinary Medicine, The Ohio State University.)*

with little evidence of endocytic activity in response to the increased concentrations of circulating thyroid hormones. In cats with solitary adenomas, the opposite thyroid lobe should be examined carefully for evidence of nodular hyperplasia or microadenomas. These small foci of multinodular follicular cell hyperplasia can be the cause of hyperthyroidism recurring several months to a year or more after surgical removal of a functional adenoma.

Hyperthyroidism in cats also occurs in association with bilateral multinodular adenomatous hyperplasia (goiter), which usually causes only slight enlargement of the affected lobe(s) (Fig. 12-41). In contrast to adenomas, areas of nodular hyperplasia are not encapsulated and the adjacent thyroid tissue is not compressed. Microscopically, hyperplastic nodules are composed of irregularly shaped, colloid-filled follicles lined by cuboidal follicular cells and these nodules are considered a preneoplastic lesion as they can coalesce and form a thyroid follicular cell adenoma.

Cats with hyperthyroidism usually have notably increased serum T_4 and T_3 concentrations. The serum T_4 concentrations in cats with hyperthyroidism range from 3.4 to 30 μg/dL (normal 1.5 to 5 μg/dL), and serum T_3 concentrations range from 179 to 470 ng/dL (normal 60 to 200 ng/dL). Moderately increased serum enzyme activities, including serum alanine aminotransferase (ALT, SGPT), serum aspartate aminotransferase (AST, SGOT), and especially alkaline phosphatase, occur in hyperthyroid cats.

Hyperthyroid cats often have disturbances of calcium homeostasis and a concomitant diffuse chief cell hyperplasia in the parathyroid glands. Blood ionized calcium and plasma creatinine concentrations are significantly decreased, whereas plasma phosphorus and intact parathyroid hormone (PTH) concentrations are increased. Hyperparathyroidism occurs in 77% of hyperthyroid cats, with PTH concentrations elevated up to 19 times that of the upper limit of the reference range. Hyperphosphatemia is present in approximately 40% of hyperthyroid cats. The mechanisms for the development of hyperphosphatemia in feline hyperthyroidism are uncertain but could be related in part to polyphagia, resulting in increased intestinal phosphorus absorption, increased catabolism of muscle proteins, release of phosphorus because of the gluconeogenic effects of the increased thyroid hormone concentrations, and increased bone resorption with release of phosphorus into the blood. Hyperparathyroidism and chief cell hyperplasia appear to be related to the reciprocal decline in amounts of circulating ionized calcium in response to the hyperphosphatemia. Increased blood phosphorus concentrations also could decrease renal 1α-hydroxylase activity and decrease the production of the active form of vitamin D, thereby reducing intestinal calcium absorption. However, circulating concentrations of $1,25\text{-}(OH)_2$-dihydroxycholecalciferol were not decreased in a limited number of hyperthyroid cats evaluated.

HYPERPLASIA OF THYROID FOLLICULAR CELLS ("GOITER")

Goiter is a clinical term used to describe a nonneoplastic and noninflammatory enlargement of the thyroid gland. It develops in all domestic mammals, birds, and other submammalian vertebrates as a result of hyperplasia of follicular cells. Certain forms of thyroid hyperplasia, especially nodular, are difficult to differentiate from adenomas. The major pathogenetic mechanisms for the development of thyroid hyperplasia include iodine-deficient diets, goitrogenic compounds that interfere with thyroxinogenesis, excess dietary iodide, and genetically determined defects in the enzymes or thyroglobulin that are essential for the biosynthesis of thyroidal hormones. All these result in inadequate thyroxine synthesis and decreased blood concentrations of T_4 and $T_{3,}$ which are detected by the hypothalamus. This, in turn, stimulates the pituitary gland to increase the secretion of TSH, resulting in hypertrophy and hyperplasia of follicular cells.

DIFFUSE HYPERPLASTIC AND COLLOID GOITER

Dietary iodine deficiency that resulted in diffuse hyperplastic goiter was common in many areas of the world before the widespread addition of iodized salt to animal diets. Iodine-deficient goiter still occurs worldwide in domestic animals, but cases are sporadic and few animals are affected. Marginally iodine-deficient diets that contain goitrogenic compounds can cause severe thyroid follicular cell hyperplasia and goiter. Goitrogenic substances include thiouracil, sulfonamides, anions of the Hofmeister series, and a number of plants of the family Brassicaceae. Offspring of females fed iodine-deficient diets are likely to develop severe thyroidal follicular cell hyperplasia and have clinical signs of hypothyroidism. Both lateral lobes of the thyroid gland are uniformly enlarged in young animals as a result of diffuse hypertrophy and hyperplasia of follicular cells (Fig. 12-9). The enlargements, when extensive, result in palpable or visible swellings in the cranial ventral cervical area. The affected lobes are firm and dark red because an extensive interfollicular capillary network develops under the influence of long-term TSH stimulation.

Colloid goiter represents the involutionary phase of diffuse hyperplastic goiter in both young and adult animals. It develops either after sufficient amounts of iodide have been added to the diet or after the requirements for thyroid hormones have diminished as the animal ages. The notably hyperplastic follicular cells continue to produce colloid, but endocytosis of colloid from the lumen is decreased. This is a consequence of the diminished TSH concentrations produced in response to the return of blood T_4 and T_3 concentrations to normal. Both thyroid lobes are diffusely enlarged but are more translucent and lighter in color than in hyperplastic goiter. These differences in macroscopic appearances are the result of less vascularity in colloid goiter and development of macrofollicles distended with colloid. Follicles are progressively distended (Fig. 12-10) with densely eosinophilic colloid because of diminished TSH-induced endocytosis. As a result, follicular cells lining the macrofollicles are flattened and atrophic. The interface between the colloid and luminal surface of the follicular cells is smooth and the cells lack the endocytic vacuoles characteristic of actively secreting thyroid follicular cells. Some involuted follicles in colloid goiter have remnants of the papillary projections on follicular cells extending into their lumens.

The changes in diffuse hyperplastic and colloid goiters are uniform throughout the diffusely enlarged thyroid lobes. Follicles are irregular in size and shape in hyperplastic goiter because they contain varying amounts of colloid, which is lightly eosinophilic and vacuolated. Some follicles collapse because of the lack of colloid. Their lining epithelial cells are columnar and have deeply eosinophilic cytoplasm and small hyperchromatic nuclei, which are often situated in the basilar portions of the cells. The follicles are lined by single or multiple layers of hyperplastic follicular cells that, in some follicles, form papillary projections into the lumens (Fig. 12-42). Similar proliferative changes are present in ectopic thyroid tissue in the neck and mediastinum.

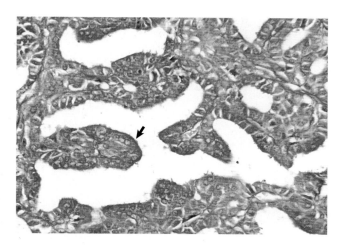

Fig. 12-42   Hyperplastic goiter, thyroid gland, dog.
Papillary projection *(arrow)* extends into the follicular lumen.
Note the partial collapse of the majority of the follicles.
Periodic acid–Schiff reaction. *(Courtesy Dr. C. Capen, College of Veterinary Medicine, The Ohio State University.)*

Although seemingly paradoxical, an excess of iodide in the diet also can result in thyroid hyperplasia in animals and human beings. Foals of mares fed dry seaweed containing excessive iodide develop thyroid hyperplasia and clinically evident goiter. The thyroid glands of suckling animals are exposed to greater blood iodide concentrations than those of the dam because iodide is concentrated first by the placenta and then by the mammary gland. Increased blood iodide interferes with one or more steps of thyroidal hormone synthesis and secretion, leading to lowered blood T_4 and T_3 concentrations and resulting in a compensatory increase in pituitary TSH secretion. Excess iodine blocks the release of T_3 and T_4 by interfering with proteolysis of colloid by lysosomal enzymes in thyroid follicular cells.

MULTIFOCAL NODULAR HYPERPLASIA

Multifocal nodular hyperplasia in thyroid glands occurs in old horses, cats, and dogs and appears as multiple, white to tan nodules of variable size (Fig. 12-41), giving affected lobes a moderately enlarged and irregular contour. Multifocal nodular goiter in most animals except cats is endocrinologically inactive and is an incidental lesion at necropsy. However, functional thyroid adenomas often develop in the thyroid glands of aged cats with hyperthyroidism and multinodular hyperplasia of follicular cells. In contrast to thyroid adenomas, the areas of nodular hyperplasia are not encapsulated and cause minimal to no compression of adjacent parenchyma. Thus nodular goiter consists of multiple foci of hyperplastic follicular cells that are sharply demarcated but not encapsulated from the adjacent thyroid tissue.

The microscopic appearance of nodular hyperplasia often varies. Some hyperplastic follicular cells form small follicles with little or no colloid. Other nodules are composed of larger, irregularly shaped follicles lined by one or more layers of columnar cells that form papillary projections into the lumen. Some of the follicles have undergone colloid involution and are filled with densely eosinophilic colloid. These changes appear to be the result of alternating periods of hyperplasia and colloid involution in the thyroid glands of aged animals.

CONGENITAL DYSHORMONOGENETIC GOITER

Congenital dyshormonogenetic goiter in sheep (Corriedale, Dorset Horn, Merino, and Romney breeds), Afrikander cattle, and Saanen dwarf goats is inherited as an autosomal recessive trait. The subnormal growth rate, absence of normal wool development or the presence of a rough, sparse hair coat, subcutaneous myxedematous swellings, weakness, and sluggish behavior suggest that the affected young are clinically hypothyroid. Most lambs with congenital goiter either die shortly after birth or are markedly sensitive to the effects of adverse environmental conditions, particularly cold.

Thyroid lobes are symmetrically enlarged at birth because of an intense diffuse hyperplasia of follicular cells (Fig. 12-43). Thyroid follicles are often collapsed because of lack of colloid resulting from the notable endocytic activity. Follicles are lined by tall columnar follicular cells, which have dilated profiles of rough endoplasmic reticulum, large mitochondria, and dense lysosomal granules associated with the Golgi apparatus, but have few thyroglobulin-containing apical vesicles near the luminal plasma membrane. Numerous long microvilli extend into the follicular lumen.

Although thyroidal uptake and turnover of ^{131}I are greatly increased compared with euthyroid controls, circulating T_4 and T_3 concentrations are consistently low. The lack of a defect in the iodide uptake or organification, plus an absence of normal 19S thyroglobulin in goitrous thyroids and only minute amounts of thyroglobulin-related antigens (0.01% of normal) suggest impaired thyroglobulin biosynthesis. A closely related or similar defect occurs in congenital goiter of sheep, cattle, and goats.

EPITHELIAL NEOPLASMS OF THE THYROID GLAND
FOLLICULAR CELL ADENOMAS

Adenomas usually are white to tan, small, solid nodules that are well demarcated from the adjacent thyroid parenchyma. The affected thyroid lobe is only moderately enlarged and distorted; usually only a single adenoma is present in a thyroid lobe. A distinct, white, fibrous connective tissue capsule of variable thickness

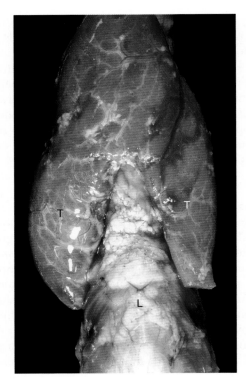

Fig. 12-43   Congenital dyshormonogenetic goiter, thyroid gland, lamb. The symmetrically enlarged thyroid *(T)* lobes are fused at the midline ventral to the larynx *(L)* and trachea. *(Courtesy Dr. C. Capen, College of Veterinary Medicine, The Ohio State University.)*

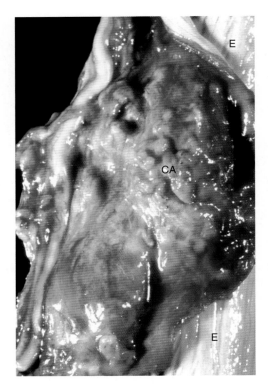

Fig. 12-44   Thyroid carcinoma, thyroid gland, dog. The poorly circumscribed and well-vascularized thyroid carcinoma *(CA)* is locally invasive and has extended into the wall of the esophagus. *E*, Esophageal mucosa. *(Courtesy College of Veterinary Medicine, University of Illinois.)*

separates the adenoma from the adjacent compressed parenchyma. Some thyroid adenomas are composed of thin-walled cysts filled with a yellow-red fluid. Their external surfaces are smooth and covered by an extensive network of blood vessels. Small masses of neoplastic tissue remain in the wall and form rugose projections into the cyst. Adenomas are classified as follicular and papillary types; the follicular type is more common in the thyroid gland of animals.

FOLLICULAR CELL CARCINOMAS

In dogs, thyroid carcinomas occur more often than adenomas, but in cats adenomas are more common. Boxers develop thyroid carcinomas more frequently than any other breed of dog, but beagles and golden retrievers have a higher risk of developing thyroid carcinomas. Approximately 60% of thyroid carcinomas in dogs are clinically detectable by palpation as a firm mass in the neck, and by evidence of respiratory distress caused by tracheal compression. Carcinomas become fixed in position as a result of extensive local invasion of adjacent structures, whereas localized adenomas are freely movable under the skin. Neoplasms of

thyroid origin also occur in accessory thyroidal tissue, located anywhere between the base of the tongue and the cranial mediastinum.

Thyroid carcinomas often grow rapidly and invade adjacent structures, such as the trachea, esophagus, and larynx (Fig. 12-44). The earliest and most frequent site of metastasis is to lungs because thyroid carcinomas, early in the course of development, invade branches of the thyroid vein. The retropharyngeal and caudal cervical lymph nodes are infrequent sites of metastases.

THYROID C (ULTIMOBRANCHIAL) CELL NEOPLASMS

Neoplasms derived from C cells of the thyroid gland occur most frequently in adult to aged bulls, certain strains of laboratory rats, occasionally in horses and dogs, and infrequently in other species. The incidence of C-cell neoplasms increases with advancing age in bulls that also typically have increased vertebral bone density. A high percentage of aged bulls fed calcium-rich diets develop C-cell neoplasms (30%) or hyperplasia of C cells and ultimobranchial derivatives (15% to 20%). The cause of C-cell neoplasms is unknown, but the chronic stimulation of C cells by large concentrations of calcium absorbed from the digestive tract can be responsible for their high incidence. A significant decline in the incidence of C-cell neoplasms occurs when the excessive calcium intake of bulls is reduced. Cows fed similar rations rarely develop proliferative lesions of C cells because of the greater physiologic requirements of pregnancy and lactation for calcium.

The syndrome of C-cell neoplasms in bulls is similar to the syndrome in human beings in that the tumors are commonly found in association with other endocrine neoplasms, especially bilateral pheochromocytomas and occasionally pituitary adenomas. There are two distinct forms of the familial cancer syndrome known as multiple endocrine neoplasia (MEN) in human beings. MEN1, also referred to as Werner syndrome, is due to a disease-causing mutation in the MEN1 gene and is characterized by primary hyperparathyroidism, pancreatic islet cell tumors that are predominantly gastrinomas, and pituitary tumors that are predominantly prolactinomas. Other lesions that can be associated with MEN1 include duodenal gastrinomas, carcinoids, thyroid adenomas, adrenocortical tumors, and lipomas. Mutations in the receptor tyrosine kinase RET result in MEN2. There are two subtypes, MEN2A (a.k.a. Sipple's syndrome) and MEN2B, both of which are associated with C-cell tumors, primary hyperparathyroidism, and pheochromocytomas. In addition, MEN2B patients frequently have mucosal neuromas and a marfanoid stature. There are increasing reports of multiple endocrine neoplasms in veterinary medicine in dogs, horses, a ferret, bulls, and Guernsey cattle. However, mutations in MEN1 or RET have never been documented in these cases. Furthermore, the tumors in animals are usually found in random endocrine organs, precluding definitive categorization as MEN1 or MEN2.

Both C-cell adenomas and carcinomas can contain deposits of amyloid. The source of the localized amyloid deposits in the neoplasms is uncertain, but the amyloid appears to be produced by the neoplastic cells, as amyloid deposits are not present in other organs. Amyloid deposition is consistently documented with medullary thyroid carcinoma in human beings, and amyloid has also been reported in certain other endocrine neoplasms. Amyloid in C-cell neoplasms is present between neoplastic cells, around vessels, and in the interstitium. Amyloid has been observed in bulls, horses, dogs, and laboratory rats, but in amounts varying (minimal to substantial) from case to case. Localized amyloid in C-cell tumors is derived from calcitonin.

Adenomas

C-cell adenomas occur as discrete, single, or multiple gray to tan nodules in one or both thyroid lobes. Adenomas are smaller (approximately 1 to 3 cm

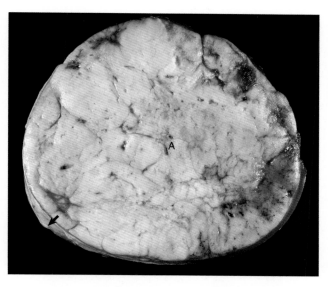

Fig. 12-45   C-cell adenoma, thyroid gland, horse. The adenoma (A) is confined by the thyroid capsule and a rim of compressed thyroid gland *(arrow)* at the periphery of the mass. *(Courtesy Dr. C. Capen, College of Veterinary Medicine, The Ohio State University.)*

in diameter) than carcinomas and are separated from the adjacent thyroid gland parenchyma, which is compressed by a thin, fibrous connective tissue capsule. Larger C-cell adenomas replace most of the thyroid lobe, but a rim of dark, brown-red thyroid gland often is present on one side (Fig. 12-45). Histologically, thyroid C-cell adenomas are discrete, expansive masses composed of cells larger than a colloid-distended follicle. The adenoma is well circumscribed or partially encapsulated, and adjacent follicles are compressed to varying degrees. The neoplastic C cells are well differentiated and have abundant to clear, pale eosinophilic cytoplasm.

Carcinomas

Thyroid C-cell carcinomas result in extensive multinodular enlargements of one or both thyroid lobes and can replace an entire thyroid gland. Thyroid C-cell neoplasms in bulls, other animal species, and human beings are firm, and in some areas the stroma consists of dense bands of fibrous connective tissue. Multiple metastases occur in the cranial cervical lymph nodes (Fig. 12-46). These nodes are usually large and have areas of necrosis and hemorrhage. Pulmonary metastases appear as discrete tan nodules and occur infrequently. C-cell carcinomas are composed of neoplastic cells that are more pleomorphic than cells of adenomas. The carcinomatous cells are poorly differentiated, polyhedral to spindle-shaped, and have pale eosinophilic, finely granular, indistinct cytoplasm.

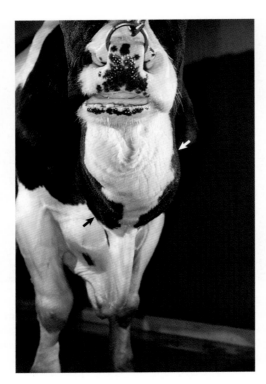

Fig. 12-46   C-cell carcinoma and metastases, thyroid and cervical lymph nodes, Holstein bull. Note the swellings in the neck *(arrows)* as a result of lymphadenopathy of the cranial cervical lymph nodes from metastases. *(Courtesy Dr. C. Capen, College of Veterinary Medicine, The Ohio State University.)*

Ultimobranchial neoplasms in the thyroid glands of bulls often have a more complex histologic structure than the typical C-cell (medullary) carcinoma in human beings, dogs, horses, and many strains of laboratory rats. The neoplasm is composed of differentiated C cells arranged as focal accumulations of neoplastic cells with abundant pale eosinophilic cytoplasm, either within the wall of the thyroid and ultimobranchial follicles or present as larger solid nodules. Ultimobranchial thyroid neoplasms often are accompanied by multifocal hyperplasia of C cells in other parts of the thyroid. The neoplastic C cells often are embedded in an increased amount of hyalinized stroma, and there are deposits of amyloid in some neoplasms. Portions of the thyroid neoplasm in bulls that are derived from less differentiated ultimobranchial remnants consist of follicle-like structures, cysts, and tubules composed of immature small basophilic cells. These neoplasms in bulls and other species closely resemble undifferentiated or stem cells of the normal ultimobranchial body that can differentiate into both C cells and follicular cells. Thyroid follicles and cribriform structures with colloidlike material formed by cells resembling differentiated follicular cells often are present in the neoplasms in close association with these more primitive ultimobranchial-derived structures. Histologically the structure of ultimobranchial neoplasms in bulls is heterogeneous and resembles a variant of thyroid carcinoma in human beings. This neoplasm, designated as an intermediate type of differentiated carcinoma, has structural and immunohistochemical characteristics of both C-cell (medullary) and follicular carcinomas.

DISORDERS OF THE PARATHYROID GLANDS

DEVELOPMENTAL DISTURBANCES

PARATHYROID (KÜRSTEINER'S) CYSTS

Small cysts within the parenchyma of the parathyroid glands or in the immediate vicinity of the glands occur frequently in dogs, but only occasionally in other animal species (Fig. 12-47). Parathyroid gland cysts are usually multiloculated, lined by a cuboidal to columnar, often ciliated epithelium, and are filled with a densely eosinophilic proteinaceous material. Parathyroid gland cysts appear to develop from persistent and dilated remnants of the duct that connects the parathyroid and thymic primordia during embryonic development. Parathyroid gland cysts are distinct from midline cysts derived from remnants of the thyroglossal duct. The latter are lined by multilayered thyroidogenic epithelium that often has colloid-containing follicles and are usually located near the midline, from the base of the tongue to the mediastinum.

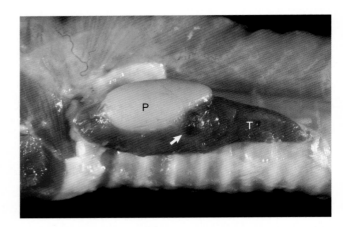

Fig. 12-47   Parathyroid cyst *(left)*, parathyroid gland, dog. The parathyroid cyst *(arrow)* was formed from the persistent and distended embryonic duct that connects parathyroid-thymic primordia in the III and IV pharyngeal pouches (Kürsteiner's cyst). Besides the parathyroid cyst, both parathyroid glands *(P)* are hyperplastic because of chronic renal failure. *T,* Thyroid gland. *(Courtesy Dr. C. Capen, College of Veterinary Medicine, The Ohio State University.)*

HYPOPARATHYROIDISM

In hypoparathyroidism, either the parathyroid glands secrete subnormal amounts of PTH or the hormone secreted is unable to interact with target cells. Hypoparathyroidism has been recognized in dogs, particularly in smaller breeds such as schnauzers and terriers, and infrequently in other animal species. Idiopathic hypoparathyroidism in adult dogs usually is caused by a diffuse lymphocytic parathyroiditis. Other infrequent causes of hypoparathyroidism include invasion and destruction of parathyroid glands by primary or metastatic neoplasms and trophic atrophy of parathyroid glands resulting from long-term hypercalcemia. In addition, the parathyroid glands are sometimes damaged or inadvertently removed during surgery involving the thyroid glands.

The functional disturbances and clinical manifestations of hypoparathyroidism primarily are the result of increased neuromuscular excitability and tetany. Because of the lack of PTH, bone resorption is decreased and blood calcium concentrations diminish progressively to 4 to 6 mg/dl (Fig. 12-48). Affected animals are restless, nervous, ataxic, weak, and have intermittent tremors of separate muscle groups. Tremors can progress to generalized tetany and convulsive seizures. Concurrently, blood phosphorus concentrations are increased because of increased renal tubular reabsorption.

LYMPHOCYTIC PARATHYROIDITIS

Lymphocytic parathyroiditis is characterized by extensive degeneration of chief cells and replacement fibrosis.

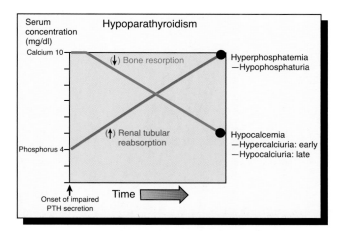

Fig. 12-48   Schematic diagram of the alterations in serum calcium and phosphorus concentrations in response to an inadequate secretion of parathyroid hormone *(PTH)*. A progressive increase in serum phosphorus concentration and a notable decline in the concentration of serum calcium resulted in increased neuromuscular excitability and tetany.
(Redrawn with permission form Dr. C. Capen, College of Veterinary Medicine, The Ohio State University.)

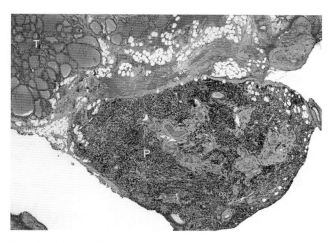

Fig. 12-49   Diffuse lymphocytic parathyroiditis, parathyroid gland, dog. The external parathyroid gland *(P)* has been completely replaced by lymphocytes, plasma cells, fibroblasts, and neocapillaries. *T,* Thyroid gland. H&E stain.
(Courtesy Dr. C. Capen, College of Veterinary Medicine, The Ohio State University.)

Mild lesions include infiltrates of lymphocytes and plasma cells and nodular hyperplasia of chief cells. Later the parathyroid gland is completely replaced by lymphocytes, fibroblasts, and neocapillaries with few remaining viable chief cells (Fig. 12-49). Lymphocytic parathyroiditis develops by an immune-mediated mechanism, as evidenced by the production of a similar destruction of parathyroid gland parenchyma and lymphocytic infiltration in dogs injected with emulsions of parathyroid gland in adjuvant.

HYPERPARATHYROIDISM
PRIMARY HYPERPARATHYROIDISM: FUNCTIONAL CHIEF CELL NEOPLASMS

Adenomas and carcinomas of parathyroid glands often secrete excessive amounts of PTH, resulting in a syndrome of primary hyperparathyroidism. Prolonged increased secretion of PTH accelerates osteolytic and osteoclastic bone resorption. Mineral is removed from the skeleton at an accelerated rate, and bone is replaced by immature fibrous connective tissue. The lesions of fibrous osteodystrophy are generalized throughout the skeleton but are accentuated in certain areas (e.g., maxilla, mandible, and subperiosteal areas of long bones).

Adenomas of parathyroid glands are encountered in older animals, particularly dogs and infrequently in certain strains of rats, but parathyroid carcinomas are uncommon. Chief cell adenomas usually cause considerable enlargement of a single parathyroid gland. This is light brown to red and located either in the cervical region by the thyroid gland or, infrequently, within the

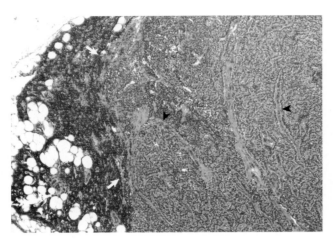

Fig. 12-50   Adenoma, parathyroid gland, dog. The adenoma consists of closely packed chief cells arranged in small groups separated by fine fibrous septa containing capillaries *(arrowheads)*. It is partially encapsulated and has compressed the adjacent, nonneoplastic parathyroid tissue *(arrows)*, which has undergone trophic atrophy. **H&E stain.** *(Courtesy Dr. C. Capen, College of Veterinary Medicine, The Ohio State University.)*

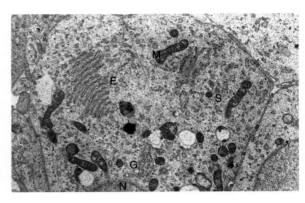

Fig. 12-51   Adenoma, parathyroid gland, dog. Active chief cells have large lamellar arrays of rough endoplasmic reticulum *(E)*, prominent Golgi apparatus *(G)*, and large mitochondria *(M)* but few secretory granules *(S)*. N, Nucleus of chief cell. **TEM. Uranyl acetate and lead citrate stain.** *(Courtesy Dr. C. Capen, College of Veterinary Medicine, The Ohio State University.)*

thoracic cavity near the base of the heart. Parathyroid adenomas are encapsulated and sharply demarcated from the adjacent thyroid gland.

Parathyroid gland adenomas are composed of small, closely packed groups of chief cells delineated by delicate vascular connective tissue septa that have many capillaries (Fig. 12-50). The neoplastic chief cells are round to polyhedral and have pale expanded eosinophilic cytoplasm in which are a few electron-dense secretory granules and prominent arrays of endoplasmic reticulum and Golgi complexes (Fig. 12-51).

The functional disturbances observed with endocrinologically active chief cell neoplasms are primarily the result of hypercalcemia and weakening of bones by excessive PTH-stimulated resorption of calcium. Cortical bone is thinned as a result of increased resorption by osteoclasts stimulated by the autonomous secretion of PTH (Fig. 12-52). Lameness can be due to fractures of long bones that occur after relatively minor physical trauma. Compression fractures occur in vertebral bodies, resulting in pressure on the spinal cord and nerves that leads to motor and/or sensory dysfunction. Facial hyperostosis due to extensive osteoblastic proliferation and deposition of poorly mineralized osteoid, and loosening or loss of teeth from alveolar sockets, has been observed in dogs with primary hyperparathyroidism. Hypercalcemia results in anorexia, vomiting, constipation, depression, polyuria, polydipsia, and generalized muscular weakness because of decreased neuromuscular excitability.

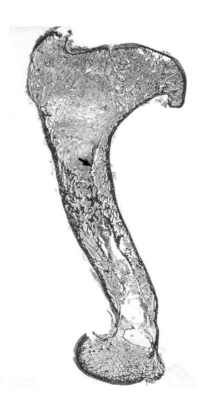

Fig. 12-52   Primary hyperparathyroidism, humerus, dog. Severe thinning of cortical bone and large resorptive cavities *(arrow)* have resulted from localized resorption of bone by osteoclasts. *(Courtesy Dr. C. Capen, College of Veterinary Medicine, The Ohio State University.)*

The most practical laboratory test to aid in the diagnosis of primary hyperparathyroidism is quantification of the concentrations of total blood calcium, phosphorus and circulating PTH (N-terminal or immunoradiometric [IRMA] assay). Dogs with primary hyperparathyroidism have greatly increased blood calcium concentrations (12 to 20 mg/dl or above). Blood phosphorus concentrations are low to normal (4 mg/dl or less) due to inhibition of renal tubular phosphorus reabsorption by the autonomous secretion of PTH. The urinary excretion of calcium and phosphorus is increased and this can predispose to the development of nephrocalcinosis and urolithiasis.

SECONDARY HYPERPARATHYROIDISM
Nutritional imbalances

Nutritional hyperparathyroidism occurs commonly in cats, dogs, certain nonhuman primates, horses, domestic and captive birds, and reptiles. The increased secretion of PTH is a compensatory mechanism induced by nutritional imbalances. Such imbalances occur in diets low in calcium, diets with an excess of phosphorus, and diets with normal or low content of calcium and in New World primates housed indoors and fed diets with inadequate amounts of vitamin D_3. The significant result is hypocalcemia, which stimulates the parathyroid glands. Blood phosphorus concentrations, when elevated, contribute indirectly to parathyroid stimulation by decreasing blood calcium.

In response to the diet-induced hypocalcemia, chief cells undergo hypertrophy and hyperplasia with increased amounts of lightly eosinophilic or vacuolated cytoplasm. The organelles involved with protein synthesis (endoplasmic reticulum) and packaging of secretory products (Golgi apparatus) are well developed. Many chronically stimulated chief cells with well-developed secretory organelles accumulate glycogen after 5 to 14 weeks.

The most frequent nutritional imbalance causing hyperparathyroidism is the ingestion of excessive amounts of phosphorus. Hyperphosphatemia stimulates the parathyroid gland indirectly by lowering blood calcium. Horses that develop the disease usually have been fed grain diets with below-average-quality roughage. Evidence of excessive phosphorus intake might be difficult to determine, as the excess phosphorus could have been supplied as a bran supplement to the grain ration. The disease in horses is commonly referred to as "big head" because of the fact that the fibrous osteodystrophy is typically hyperostotic and most severe in the mandible and maxilla (see Fig. 16-57). The diet is usually palatable and nutritious except for its excessive phosphorus and marginal or deficient calcium content. A diet deficient in calcium fails to supply the daily calcium requirement, and hypocalcemia develops even though a greater proportion of calcium ingested is absorbed. Changes in concentrations of calcium and phosphorus in urine are more consistent and useful in the clinical diagnosis of nutritional secondary hyperparathyroidism in horses than changes in blood concentrations of these minerals. The increased secretion of PTH acts on normal kidneys to notably increase urinary phosphorus excretion and to decrease calcium loss in the urine.

Renal disease

Hyperparathyroidism as a complication of chronic renal failure is characterized by excessive production of PTH in response to chronic hypocalcemia. When the renal disease is extensive enough to reduce the glomerular filtration rate, phosphorus is retained and hyperphosphatemia develops. The increased blood phosphorus concentration depresses ionized blood calcium concentration, resulting in parathyroid gland stimulation. Chronic renal disease also impairs the production of $1,25\text{-}(OH)_2D_3$ by the kidneys, thereby diminishing intestinal calcium transport and increasing mobilization of calcium from the skeleton. All parathyroid glands undergo notable chief cell hyperplasia, and the bones subsequently develop varying degrees of generalized fibrous osteodystrophy. The fibrous osteodystrophy that occurs with chronic renal failure is also most severe in the skull, but it is usually osteoporotic. Affected animals, especially dogs, have supple mandibles and/or maxillas known as "rubber jaws" (see Fig. 16-57).

PSEUDOHYPERPARATHYROIDISM: HUMORAL HYPERCALCEMIA OF MALIGNANCY

Hypercalcemia in animals is a common disorder with many causes. The most common form is cancer-associated hypercalcemia or humoral hypercalcemia of malignancy (HHM). Notable increases in serum calcium concentration resulting from an imbalance of calcium released from bones, excreted by the kidneys, or absorbed from the intestinal tract are reported with apocrine gland adenocarcinomas, metastases of solid neoplasms to bone, and hematologic malignancies, such as lymphosarcoma.

The clinical signs of hypercalcemia are similar regardless of the underlying cause and depend on the rapidity of onset of increased concentrations of serum ionized calcium. Animals with total serum calcium values in excess of 16 mg/dl (4 mmol/L) generally have the most severe clinical signs. Exceptions to this rule occur, and some animals with severe hypercalcemia have only mild clinical signs. Horses and rabbits have normal total serum calcium concentrations greater than those found in other domestic animals, which should be considered before hypercalcemia is diagnosed in these species. Metabolic acidosis enhances the severity of clinical signs because it results in an increase in the ionized fraction of serum calcium. Increased serum ionized calcium induces clinical signs relating to the gastrointestinal, neuromuscular, cardiovascular, and renal systems.

The parathyroid glands in animals with HHM are small and difficult to locate or undetectable grossly. The parathyroid glands respond to the persistent cancer-associated hypercalcemia by trophic atrophy. Atrophic parathyroid glands in dogs are characterized by narrow cords of inactive chief cells with an abundant fibrous connective tissue stroma and widened perivascular spaces. Thyroid C cells undergo either diffuse or nodular hyperplasia in response to the persistent elevation in blood calcium.

Renal calcification has been detected microscopically in approximately 90% of dogs with HHM caused by anal sac apocrine gland adenocarcinomas, particularly when the calcium × phosphorus product is ≥ 50. Tubular calcification is most pronounced near the corticomedullary junction but is also present in cortical and inner medullary tubules, Bowman's capsule, and glomerular tufts. Calcification also occurs in the fundic gastric mucosa and endocardium.

Excessive secretion of biologically active PTH-rP plays a central role in the pathogenesis of hypercalcemia in most forms of HHM; however, cytokines—such as interleukin-1 (IL-1), tumor necrosis factor-α, transforming growth factor-(TGF)-α and TGF-β or 1,25-dihydroxyvitamin D—can have synergistic or cooperative actions with PTH-rP. Before PTH-rP was identified, it was well understood that nonparathyroid neoplasms and humoral hypercalcemia of malignancy induced a syndrome that mimicked primary hyperparathyroidism because of secretion of a PTH-like factor that was antigenically unrelated to PTH. Purification of the substance with PTH-like activity from the adenocarcinoma derived from apocrine glands of the anal sac in dogs and multiple human neoplasms with documented HHM resulted in the discovery of PTH-rP. PTH-rP also can be demonstrated by immunohistochemical and biochemical analysis in a number of tissues, where it appears to function primarily as a paracrine factor.

APOCRINE GLAND ADENOCARCINOMA

A syndrome of HHM in aged, primarily female dogs with adenocarcinomas derived from apocrine glands of the anal sac has been characterized. These dogs have persistent hypercalcemia (mean 16.2 mg/dl) and often mild hypophosphatemia, both of which return to normal following surgical excision of the neoplasm. The hypercalcemia persists after removal of the parathyroid glands, suggesting that the humoral factor produced by neoplastic cells does not stimulate an increased secretion of PTH. Increased circulating concentrations of PTH-rP have been observed in hypercalcemic dogs

with anal sac apocrine gland adenocarcinomas. The neoplasms are malignant and most have metastasized to regional lumbar aortic lymph nodes at the time of initial presentation. Clinical signs include generalized muscular weakness, anorexia, vomiting, bradycardia, depression, polyuria, and polydipsia. These signs are primarily the result of severe hypercalcemia.

Apocrine gland adenocarcinomas develop as firm, usually unilateral masses, ventrolateral to the anus and close to the anal sac but not attached to the overlying skin (Fig. 12-53). The neoplasm arises in the wall of the anal sac and projects as a variably sized mass into the lumen (Fig. 12-54).

This adenocarcinoma forms glandular acini into whose lumens papillary projections of apical cytoplasm extend (Fig. 12-55). It is histologically distinct from the more common perianal (circumanal) gland tumor, which arises in hepatoid glands. The majority of neoplasms histologically contain glandular and solid areas. The solid pattern is characterized by sheets, microlobules, and packets separated by a thin fibrovascular stroma. Pseudorosettes are common in solid areas adjacent to small blood vessels.

NEOPLASMS METASTATIC TO BONE

Solid neoplasms that metastasize widely to bone and grow locally can produce hypercalcemia by inducing local

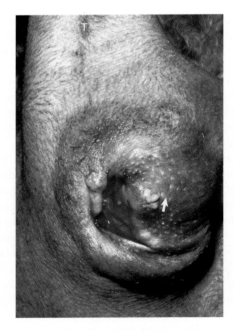

Fig. 12-53 **Adenocarcinoma, apocrine glands of right anal sac, anus, dog.** The right perianal region is distended by a small adenocarcinoma (*arrow*), which has compressed the right side of the anus. It also projects, as two nodules, on the dorsolateral margin of the anus. T, Tail. (*Courtesy Dr. C. Capen, College of Veterinary Medicine, The Ohio State University.*)

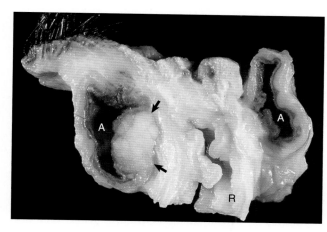

Fig. 12-54 **Adenocarcinoma, apocrine glands, anal sac, dorsal plane, formalin fixed specimen, dog.** A 1-cm-diameter nodule *(arrows)* derived from apocrine glands of the wall of the right anal sac (glands of the perianal sinus) protrudes into the lumen of the right anal sac. Anal sacs *(A)* are present on both sides of the rectum *(R)*. *(From Meuten DJ, Cooper BJ, Capen CC et al: Vet Pathol 18:454-471, 1981.)*

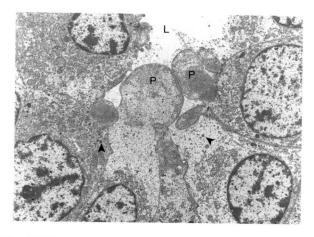

Fig. 12-55 **Adenocarcinoma, anal sac, dog.** Projections *(P)* of apical cytoplasm extend into the acinar lumen *(L)*. Small membrane-limited secretory granules *(arrowheads)* are present in the cytoplasm. TEM. Uranyl acetate and lead citrate stain. *(From Meuten DJ, Capen CC, Kociba GJ et al: Am J Pathol 107: 167-175, 1982.)*

bone resorption. This is not common in animals but is an important cause of HHM in human beings, particularly patients with metastatic breast and lung carcinomas.

The pathogenesis of enhanced bone resorption is not well understood, but the two primary mechanisms include (1) secretion of cytokines or factors that stimulate local bone resorption, and (2) indirect stimulation of bone resorption by tumor-induced cytokine secretion from local immune or bone cells. Cytokines or factors that are secreted by neoplastic cells and stimulate local bone resorption include PTH-rP, TGF-α and TGF-β, and prostaglandins, especially prostaglandin E_2.

LYMPHOSARCOMA

Lymphosarcoma is the most common neoplasm associated with hypercalcemia in dogs and cats. Estimates of the prevalence of hypercalcemia in dogs with lymphosarcoma vary from 20% to 40%. Peripheral lymph node enlargement is present in some cases; cranial mediastinal or visceral nodes usually are involved. The hypercalcemia results from the production of humoral substances by neoplastic cells and/or from physical disruption of trabecular bone by lymphosarcoma in bone marrow. Serum immunoreactive PTH concentrations are subnormal, and plasma prostaglandin E_2 concentrations are not different from those of controls.

Most dogs with lymphoma and HHM have significantly increased circulating PTH-rP concentrations, but these concentrations are lower (2 to 15 pmol) than in dogs with carcinomas and HHM; there is no correlation with serum calcium concentration. The latter indicates that PTH-rP is an important marker in dogs with HHM and lymphoma but is not the sole humoral factor responsible for the stimulation of osteoclasts and development of hypercalcemia. It is likely that cytokines such as IL-1 or tumor necrosis factor function synergistically with PTH-rP to induce HHM in dogs with lymphoma. Some dogs and human patients with lymphoma and hypercalcemia have increased serum 1,25-dihydroxyvitamin D concentrations that could be responsible for or contribute to the induction of hypercalcemia. PTH (N-terminal) concentrations in dogs with lymphoma and hypercalcemia usually are in the normal range; however, a few dogs have concentrations increased slightly above the normal range.

PARTURIENT HYPOCALCEMIA

Parturient paresis in dairy cattle is a complex metabolic disease characterized by the development of severe hypocalcemia and hypophosphatemia near the time of parturition and the initiation of lactation. The serum calcium concentration decreases to less than 50% of normal in spite of an increased secretion of PTH by the cow's parathyroid glands. Bone resorption remains minimal and few osteoclasts are present on bone surfaces. Biochemical and ultrastructural studies in cows indicate that the parathyroid glands are capable of responding to the acute hypocalcemia by increasing development of the cellular organelles responsible for hormonal synthesis and by increasing secretion of PTH.

The composition of the diet fed to dairy cows is a significant factor in the pathogenesis of parturient hypocalcemia. Diets with excessive calcium have been incriminated as significantly increasing the incidence of the disease. Conversely, diets low in calcium or diets supplemented with therapeutic doses of vitamin D reduce the incidence of parturient hypocalcemia. Calcium homeostasis in pregnant cows fed an excessive calcium diet appears to be maintained principally by intestinal calcium absorption (Fig. 12-56). This greater reliance on intestinal absorption rather than on PTH-stimulated bone resorption probably is a significant factor in the more frequent development of profound hypocalcemia near parturition in cows fed excessive calcium prepartal diets.

An increased prepartal secretion of calcitonin in cows that develop parturient hypocalcemia or milk fever, especially those fed excessive calcium diets, could be a factor contributing to the inability of increased PTH concentrations to mobilize calcium rapidly from skeletal reserves, and to maintain blood calcium concentrations during the critical periparturient period. The thyroidal content of calcitonin is reduced, many C cells are degranulated, and plasma concentrations of calcitonin often are increased in cows before the development of profound hypocalcemia.

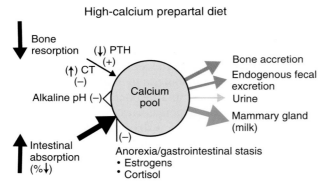

High-calcium prepartal diet

Total inflow < Total outflow

Fig. 12-56 **Schematic diagram of calcium homeostasis in cows fed a high-calcium prepartal diet.** In this case, calcium homeostasis is primarily dependent on intestinal calcium absorption. The rate of bone resorption is low, and parathyroid glands are inactive. Anorexia and gastrointestinal stasis that often occur near parturition interrupt the major inflow of calcium into the extracellular fluid calcium pool. Outflow of calcium with the onset of lactation exceeds the rate of inflow into the calcium pool, and cows develop a progressive hypocalcemia and paresis. *CT,* Calcitonin; *PTH,* parathyroid hormone. *(Redrawn with permission from Dr. C. Capen, College of Veterinary Medicine, The Ohio State University.)*

DISORDERS OF PANCREATIC ISLET CELLS

HYPOFUNCTION OF PANCREATIC ISLET CELLS: DIABETES MELLITUS

Diabetes mellitus is a metabolic disorder that results from a reduction of insulin available for normal function of many cells in the body. In some cases, increased concentrations of glucagon contribute to development of persistent hyperglycemia. Insulin unavailability could be due to degenerative changes in β cells of the pancreatic islets, reduced effectiveness of the hormone because of the formation of antiinsulin antibodies or inactive complexes, damage to β cells from immune-mediated islet cytotoxicity, or inappropriate secretion of hormones by neoplasms in other endocrine organs.

Diabetes mellitus is a common endocrinopathy in dogs, with a reported incidence of 1:200. Most cases of spontaneous diabetes occur in mature dogs and in females approximately twice as often as males. An increased incidence of diabetes mellitus has been observed in certain small breeds of dogs, such as miniature poodles, dachshunds, and terriers, but nearly all breeds of dogs can be affected.

Development of diabetes mellitus in young dogs is the result of idiopathic atrophy of the pancreas, acute pancreatitis with necrosis and hemorrhage, and aplasia of pancreatic islets. The pancreas with idiopathic atrophy is reduced to a third or less of its size. Hypoplasia of pancreatic islets in which the islets are absent but the pancreatic acini and ducts are present and functional has been a cause of diabetes mellitus in young dogs (2 to 3 months of age).

In the pathogenesis of diabetes mellitus, several factors are responsible for the decreased availability of insulin. Destruction of islets secondary to severe pancreatitis or the selective degeneration of islet cells are the most common causes in animals. In dogs, the pancreatic islets are often destroyed because of inflammation of the exocrine pancreas. Chronic relapsing pancreatitis with progressive loss of both exocrine and endocrine cells and replacement by fibrous connective tissue is a frequent cause of diabetes mellitus. In these dogs, the pancreas becomes firm, multinodular, and has scattered areas of hemorrhage and necrosis after a recent relapse (Fig. 12-57). Later in the course of the disease, all that remains of the pancreas is a thin fibrous band or nodule near the duodenum and stomach (Fig. 12-58).

Histologically, β cells are reduced in number and remaining cells have vacuolated cytoplasm (Fig. 12-59). The cytoplasm of β cells is distended by massive amounts of glycogen particles (Fig. 12-60). Hydropic degeneration with glycogen accumulation, especially in cats, appears to develop in β cells in response to

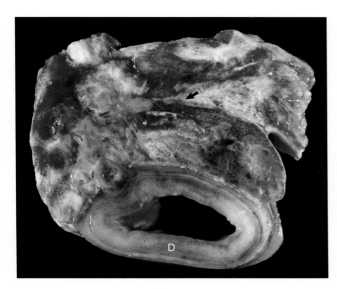

Fig. 12-57   Chronic relapsing pancreatitis, pancreas and duodenum, cross section, dog. The pancreas is multinodular and firm with areas of hemorrhage (*arrow*), fibrosis, and necrosis. *D,* Duodenum. *(Courtesy Dr. C. Capen, College of Veterinary Medicine, The Ohio State University.)*

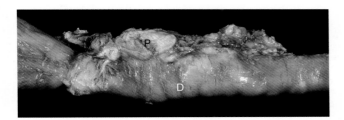

Fig. 12-58   Chronic pancreatitis, pancreas, dog. The pancreas (*P*) is markedly atrophied and its parenchyma almost completely replaced by fibrous connective tissue in "end-stage" pancreatitis. *D,* Duodenum. *(Courtesy Dr. C. Capen, College of Veterinary Medicine, The Ohio State University.)*

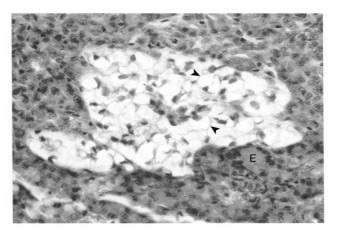

Fig. 12-59   Hydropic ("vacuolar") degeneration, pancreatic islet, cat. Discrete vacuoles (*arrowheads*) are present in the cytoplasm of β cells. *E,* Exocrine pancreas. H&E stain. *(Courtesy Dr. C. Capen, College of Veterinary Medicine, The Ohio State University.)*

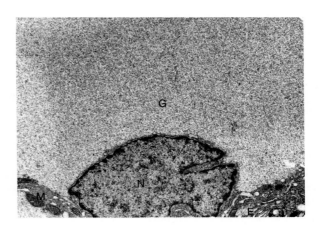

Fig. 12-60   Glycogen accumulation in the β cell, pancreatic islet, cat. The nucleus (*N*) and secretory organelles are displaced to the periphery of the β cell by the accumulation of glycogen (*G*) particles. *M,* Mitochondria; *E,* endoplasmic reticulum. TEM. Uranyl acetate and lead citrate stain. *(Courtesy Dr. C. Capen, College of Veterinary Medicine, The Ohio State University.)*

long-term overstimulation or exhaustion because of peripheral insulin resistance. When disease is chronic, the islets are difficult to find. Immune-mediated isletitis characterized by a progressive lymphoplasmacytic infiltration and selective destruction of β cells of the islets is another cause of diabetes mellitus (type 1) in human beings, rodent models, and occasionally in dogs.

Another common pancreatic change in cats with diabetes is the selective deposition of amyloid in islets, resulting in degenerative changes in α cells and β cells (Fig. 12-61). Scattered amyloid deposits in pancreatic islets that increase progressively with age occur in the pancreatic islets of many cats without clinically apparent diabetes mellitus. Islet amyloid polypeptide (IAPP)

(37 amino acids) and insulin are both secreted by β cells. The IAPP in cats, human beings, nonhuman primates, and raccoons has a unique amino acid sequence (amino acids 25 to 28: alanine, isoleucine, leucine, and serine), which is predisposed to polymerization and accumulation in pancreatic islets. As the insoluble amyloid fibers progressively accumulate in the islets, they disrupt β cells and surround islet capillaries, leading to the subsequent degeneration of islet cells.

Complete expression of the complex metabolic disturbances in diabetes mellitus appears to be the result

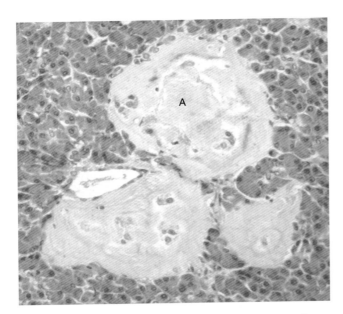

Fig. 12-61   Amyloidosis, pancreatic islets, cat. Note the deposits of amyloid (A) and degeneration and loss of islet cells. H&E stain. (*Courtesy College of Veterinary Medicine, University of Illinois.*)

of a bihormonal abnormality. Although a relative or absolute deficiency of insulin action in response to a rising extracellular glucose concentration has been long recognized as the sine qua non of diabetes mellitus, the importance of an absolute or relative increase of glucagon secretion in some forms of the disease in certain species has been appreciated only recently. Hyperglucagonemia in diabetic patients can be the result of increased secretion of pancreatic glucagon, enteroglucagon, or both. An increased blood glucagon concentration contributes to the severe endogenous hyperglycemia by mobilizing hepatic stores of glucose and to the development of ketoacidosis by increasing the oxidation of fatty acids by hepatocytes. The major glucoregulatory consequence of insulin deficiency is reduction in the movement of glucose into insulin-sensitive tissues (e.g., liver, adipose tissue, and muscle), with a corresponding increase in hepatic glucose production, resulting in notable endogenous hyperglycemia.

The onset of diabetes mellitus is insidious, and the clinical course is often chronic. Clinically, dogs with diabetes mellitus exhibit polydipsia, polyuria, weight loss in spite of polyphagia, bilateral cataracts, and weakness. The disturbances in water metabolism primarily have an osmotic basis. In dogs with persistent hyperglycemia and glycosuria, the renal tubular epithelium is unable to concentrate the urine effectively against the osmotic attraction of the glucose in the glomerular filtrate.

Diabetic animals have diminished resistance to bacterial and fungal infections, and diseases such as suppurative cystitis, prostatitis, bronchopneumonia, and dermatitis often become chronic or recurrent. This increased susceptibility to infection in patients with poorly controlled diabetes can be related in part to impaired chemotactic, phagocytic, and microbicidal functions and decreased adherence of polymorphonuclear leukocytes. The impaired microbicidal function of leukocytes can have a metabolic basis resulting from diminished production of cellular energy from glucose. Radiographic evidence of emphysematous cystitis is strongly suggestive of diabetes mellitus. Infections of the urinary bladder with glucose-fermenting organisms, such as *Proteus* sp., *Aerobacter aerogenes*, and *Escherichia coli* result in gas formation in the wall and lumen. Emphysema also develops in the wall of the gallbladder in some diabetic dogs.

Hepatomegaly occurs as a result of fatty degeneration. Lipids accumulate in the liver as the result of increased lipid mobilization, and hepatocytes injured by ketonemia have decreased usage of lipids. Individual hepatocytes are greatly enlarged by multiple droplets of lipid (Fig. 12-62). If the accumulation of lipids is extensive and long-standing, cirrhosis develops. The liver remains enlarged, and its surface becomes coarsely nodular because of extensive remodeling of hepatic parenchyma (Fig. 12-63). Individual hepatocytes degenerate and are replaced by regenerative and hyperplastic nodules and interlobular fibrosis. Icterus and bilirubinuria often accompany severe cirrhosis.

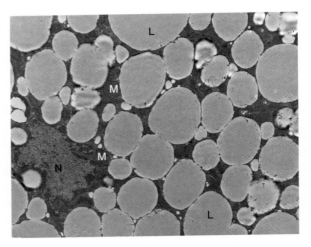

Fig. 12-62   Fatty degeneration, liver, dog. The cytoplasm contains multiple large lipid droplets (L) that have displaced the nucleus (N) peripherally and compressed cytoplasmic organelles, such as mitochondria (M). TEM. Uranyl acetate and lead citrate stain. (*Courtesy Dr. C. Capen, College of Veterinary Medicine, The Ohio State University.*)

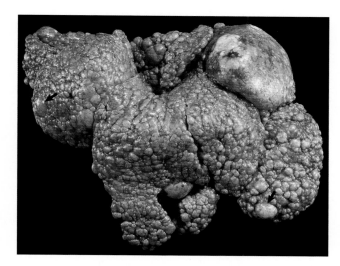

Fig. 12-63   Cirrhosis, liver, diaphragmatic surface, dog.
All lobes of the liver are considerably firm and have a coarsely
nodular surface. The nodules (*arrows*) represent areas of
regenerative hyperplasia of hepatocytes. (*Courtesy Dr. C. Capen,
College of Veterinary Medicine, The Ohio State University.*)

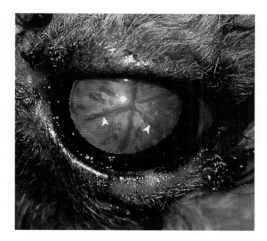

Fig. 12-64   Diabetes mellitus, eyeball, lens, dog. Early
stellate lesion (*arrowheads*) along the sutures of the lens.
In dogs (not in cats), cataracts (stellate lesions) can occur in
poorly regulated diabetes mellitus, because glucose is
metabolized in the lens by a sorbitol pathway, which leads
to edema of the lens. (*Courtesy Dr. C. Capen, College of Veterinary
Medicine, The Ohio State University.*)

Cataracts often develop in dogs with poorly controlled diabetes mellitus. They are stellate or asteroid in
shape (Fig. 12-64) and initially appear along the suture
lines of lenticular fibers. Cataract formation in the diabetic patient is related to the unique sorbitol pathway
by which glucose is metabolized in the lens. Glucose is

first converted to sorbitol by the enzyme aldose reductase and, subsequently, to fructose by sorbitol dehydrogenase. These sugar alcohols accumulate within the
lens and result in an intracellular accumulation of
solute and hypertonicity. The initial structural change
in the lens consists of swelling and hydropic degeneration of lenticular fibers. In long-standing cases of diabetes mellitus, swelling of lenticular fibers continues
until the majority of lenticular fibers are affected. Later,
macromolecular aggregation or precipitation of normally translucent lenticular proteins develops, accompanied by disruption of lenticular fibers and formation
of interfibrillar clefts. The result is diffuse, often bilateral lens opacity observed in animals with chronic diabetes mellitus.

Other extrapancreatic lesions of diabetes mellitus
such as chronic renal disease, blindness, and gangrene
are the result of microangiopathy characterized by
thickening of the capillary basement membrane. Dogs
with long-standing, poorly controlled, spontaneous diabetes mellitus develop nodular or diffuse glomerulosclerosis characterized by PAS-positive fibrillar
deposits of glycoprotein, which occasionally form
spherical nodules in the glomerular capillary tufts.
Other renal lesions include accumulation of glycogen
within cells of Henle's loop (intracytoplasmic) and
distal convoluted tubule (intranuclear) (Fig. 12-65).

HYPERFUNCTION OF PANCREATIC ISLET CELLS
β-CELL (INSULIN-SECRETING) NEOPLASMS (INSULINOMAS)

The neoplasms most frequently arising in pancreatic
islets are adenomas and carcinomas derived from β cells.

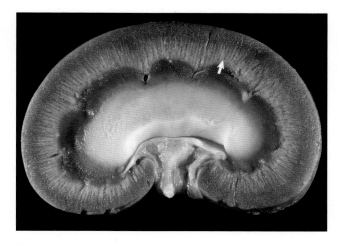

**Fig. 12-65   Glycogen "nephrosis," diabetes mellitus,
kidney, dog.** The radially arranged light areas in the inner
cortex of the kidney (*arrow*) represent tubules with abnormal
accumulations of glycogen. (*Courtesy Dr. C. Capen, College of
Veterinary Medicine, The Ohio State University.*)

These neoplasms are often endocrinologically active and produce dramatic functional disturbances. Other pancreatic neoplasms appear to be derived from multipotential ductal epithelial cells that differentiate into one of several other cell types in the pancreatic islets. β-Cell neoplasms are seen most frequently in dogs 5 to 12 years of age (mean 9 years). These neoplasms also occur in older cattle and can cause periodic convulsions. Carcinomas of the pancreatic islets are more common than adenomas in dogs and are commonly found in the duodenal (right) lobe of the pancreas. Carcinomas of the pancreatic islets can be differentiated grossly from adenomas by their larger size, multilobular appearance, extensive invasion of adjacent parenchyma and lymph vessels, and metastases to extrapancreatic sites, such as regional lymph nodes (e.g., duodenal, mesenteric, hepatic, and splenic), liver, mesentery, and omentum.

The clinical alterations observed with functional β-cell neoplasms are the result of excessive insulin secretion and the development of severe hypoglycemia. The clinical signs are not specific for the hyperinsulinism produced by β-cell neoplasms. Initial signs include weakness, fatigue after vigorous exercise, generalized muscular twitching and weakness, ataxia, mental confusion, and changes in temperament. Dogs are easily agitated and have intermittent periods of excitability and restlessness. Periodic convulsive seizures of the tonic-clonic type occur later in the disease and increase progressively in frequency and intensity.

The predominance of clinical signs relating to the CNS demonstrates the primary dependence of the brain on glucose metabolism for energy. The failure to recognize dogs with functional islet cell neoplasms when they have clinical signs suggestive of primary disease of the nervous system has frequently led to the misdiagnoses of idiopathic epilepsy, brain neoplasm, or other organic neurologic disease. Repeated episodes of prolonged and severe hypoglycemia result in neuronal necrosis and permanent neurologic disability with terminal coma and eventually death.

Adenomas of the β cells of the pancreatic islets typically exist as single, yellow to dark red, small (1 to 3 cm), spherical nodules. The neoplasms are of similar consistency to or slightly firmer than that of the surrounding pancreas. Adenomas occur as a single nodule or less often as multiple nodules in one or both lobes and/or body of the pancreas. Islet cell adenomas are sharply delineated and surrounded by a thin capsule of fibrous connective tissue (Fig. 12-66). Small nests of acinar epithelial cells are sometimes present throughout the neoplasm, but are more common at the periphery. Numerous connective tissue septa containing small capillaries radiate from the capsule into the neoplasm and subdivide the neoplasm into small lobules or packets.

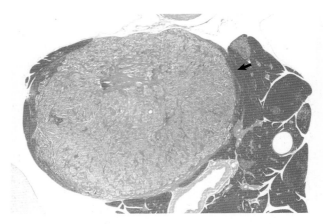

Fig. 12-66   β-**Cell adenoma, pancreatic islet, dog.** A solid islet adenoma, surrounded by a fibrous capsule of variable thickness has compressed the adjacent exocrine pancreas (*arrow*). **H&E stain.** (*Courtesy Dr. C. Capen, College of Veterinary Medicine, The Ohio State University.*)

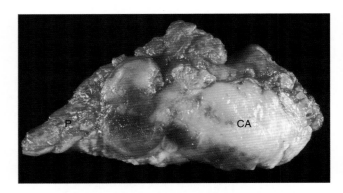

Fig. 12-67   β-**Cell carcinoma, pancreatic islet, dog.** The whitish-red carcinoma (*CA*) is well demarcated from the lobular exocrine pancreas (*P*). (*Courtesy Dr. C. Capen, College of Veterinary Medicine, The Ohio State University.*)

Well-differentiated neoplastic cells are round to polyhedral with distinct cell borders and pale eosinophilic, finely granular cytoplasm.

Islet cell carcinomas are consistently larger than adenomas, are multilobular, and invade into and through the fibrous capsule of the pancreas (Fig. 12-67). The dense bands of fibrous tissue that course through the neoplasm give rise to fine connective tissue septa containing capillaries that subdivide the neoplasm into small cords or lobules. Well-differentiated neoplastic cells in islet cell carcinomas are closely packed but are less uniform in size and shape than the cells in adenomas. They are round to polyhedral and have a granular eosinophilic cytoplasm. Mitotic figures are infrequent. Microscopic evidence of distinct local tissue invasion is the principal criterion for the diagnosis of islet cell carcinoma.

Cells composing functional islet cell neoplasms in dogs usually have histochemical and immunohistochemical characteristics of β cells. Ultrastructurally the neoplastic β cells are electron dense because of numerous cytoplasmic organelles.

NON-β (GASTRIN-SECRETING) ISLET CELL NEOPLASMS (GASTRINOMAS)

Gastrin-secreting, non-β islet cell neoplasms of the pancreas have been reported in human beings, dogs, and cats. The hypersecretion of gastrin in human beings results in the well-documented Zollinger-Ellison syndrome, consisting of hypersecretion of gastric acid and recurrent peptic ulceration in the gastrointestinal tract. The non-β islet cell neoplasms derived from ectopic APUD (*amine precursor uptake decarboxylase*) cells in the pancreas produce an excess of gastrin, which normally is secreted by cells of the antral and duodenal mucosa. The incidence of gastrin-secreting pancreatic neoplasms in dogs and cats is uncertain, but it appears to be uncommon compared with that of insulin-secreting β-cell neoplasms. In the comparatively few canine and feline cases studied, the clinical signs have included anorexia, vomiting of blood-tinged material, intermittent diarrhea, progressive weight loss, and dehydration, the result of the multiple ulcerations of the gastrointestinal mucosa because of gastrin-stimulated gastric acid hypersecretion (Zollinger-Ellison–like syndrome).

Animals with Zollinger-Ellison–like syndrome have single or multiple, variably sized neoplasms in the pancreas. These are firm, have increased amounts of fibrous connective tissue, and although partially encapsulated, the neoplasm usually extends into the surrounding pancreas.

Three histologic patterns of gastrin-secreting islet neoplasms in dogs are recognized: (1) the ribbon or trabecular pattern, (2) solid nests of cells with a delicate, highly vascularized stroma, and (3) an acinar pattern with cuboidal neoplastic cells arranged around a central lumen. The stroma is prominent and hyalinized in some gastrin-secreting neoplasms.

Canine gastrin-secreting islet cell neoplasms invade locally into the adjacent pancreas and often metastasize to regional lymph nodes and to the liver. These dogs have either single or multiple ulcerations of the gastric and/or duodenal mucosa, and blood in the gut lumen.

Other non-β islet cell neoplasms reported in animals are those of glucagon-secreting α cells. Glucagonomas have been reported rarely in dogs and are associated with superficial necrolytic dermatitis.

DISORDERS OF THE PINEAL GLAND
PINEALITIS

Pinealitis accompanying uveitis is well established in animal models of experimental autoimmune uveoretinitis following immunization with retinal antigens. Because the pineal gland is rarely, if ever, histologically examined during active uveitis in human beings with autoimmune uveitis, there is no direct evidence of concurrent pineal pathology, but it is suspected. However, there are reports documenting lymphocytic and eosinophilic pinealitis in horses with recurrent uveitis.

PINEAL TUMORS

Pineal tumors are exceedingly rare in both human beings and animals. The majority of cases in domestic animals involve laboratory rats, but there are isolated reports in a cow, goat, horse, cockatiel, and chicken. Tumors are classified as well-differentiated pinealocytomas, anaplastic pinealoblastomas, or mixed tumors. Immunoreactivity to synaptophysin has been shown to be the most consistent marker for pineal tumors.

DISORDERS OF THE CHEMORECEPTOR ORGANS
NEOPLASMS

Although chemoreceptor tissue appears to be widely distributed in the body, neoplasms develop principally in the aortic and carotid bodies. Aortic body chemodectomas are encountered more frequently in animals than those of the carotid body, but the reverse is true for human beings. These neoplasms develop primarily in dogs and infrequently in cats and cattle. Brachycephalic breeds of dogs, such as the boxer and Boston terrier, are highly predisposed to develop neoplasms of the aortic and carotid bodies.

NEOPLASMS OF THE AORTIC BODY

Aortic body neoplasms appear most frequently as a single mass or as multiple nodules near the base of the heart (Fig. 12-68). They vary considerably in size (from 0.5 to 12.5 cm) with carcinomas being larger than adenomas. Solitary small adenomas either are attached to the adventitia of the pulmonary artery and ascending aorta or are embedded in the adipose connective tissue between these major vessels. They have a smooth external surface and on cross section are white and mottled with red to brown areas. Larger adenomas are multilobular and can compress and indent the wall of the atria, displace the trachea, and partially surround the major vessels at the base of the heart. Aortic body carcinomas are less frequent than adenomas in dogs. Carcinomas infiltrate the wall of the pulmonary artery and form papillary projections into its lumen or invade

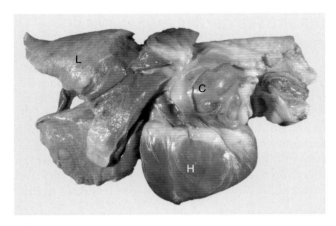

Fig. 12-68   Carcinoma, aortic body, dog. Note the large mass *(C)* at the base of the heart *(H)*. Contiguous portions of the right-middle and diaphramatic lung lobes are atelectatic. *L,* Lungs. *(Courtesy College of Veterinary Medicine, University of Illinois.)*

through the wall into the lumen of the atria. Although neoplastic cells often invade blood vessels, metastases to the lungs and liver occur infrequently in dogs.

Neoplasms of the aortic bodies in animals are not functional (i.e., they do not secrete excess hormone into the circulation), but as a space-occupying lesion they can produce a variety of functional disturbances. Larger aortic body adenomas and carcinomas put pressure on the atria, vena cava, or both and cause manifestations of cardiac decompensation. A higher percentage of aortic body neoplasms than carotid body neoplasms are benign. Aortic body carcinomas invade locally into the atria, pericardium, and adjacent vessels.

NEOPLASMS OF THE CAROTID BODY

Carotid body neoplasms arise near the bifurcation of the common carotid artery in the cranial cervical area. They are usually unilateral, only rarely bilateral, and are slow growing. Adenomas vary from approximately 1 to 4 cm in diameter, are well encapsulated, and have a smooth external surface. The bifurcation of the common carotid artery is incorporated in the mass, and neoplastic cells are firmly adhered to the tunica adventitia. Adenomas are firm, white with scattered areas of hemorrhage, and are extremely vascular.

Carotid body carcinomas are larger, more coarsely multinodular than adenomas, invade the capsule, and penetrate into the walls of adjacent blood and lymph vessels. The external jugular vein and some cranial nerves can be incorporated into the neoplasm. Metastases of carotid body carcinomas occur in approximately 30% of cases and have been found in the lungs, tracheobronchial and mediastinal lymph nodes, liver, pancreas, and kidneys. Multicentric neoplastic transformation of chemoreceptor tissue (aortic and carotid bodies) occurs frequently in brachycephalic breeds of dogs.

The microscopic features of chemoreceptor neoplasms ("chemodectomas") are essentially similar whether they are derived from the carotid or the aortic body. The neoplasm is subdivided into lobules by prominent branching trabeculae of connective tissue, which originate from the fibrous capsule. Neoplasms are further subdivided into smaller nests by fine septa of collagenous and reticulin fibers and small capillaries. Neoplastic cells are commonly aligned along and around small capillaries and are discrete, round to polyhedral, and closely packed and have pale eosinophilic, finely granular, and often vacuolated cytoplasm.

Although the cause of carotid and aortic body neoplasms is unknown, a genetic predisposition aggravated by chronic hypoxia could account for the greater risk of development in certain brachycephalic breeds, such as the boxer and Boston terrier. Carotid bodies of several mammalian species, including dogs, have developed hyperplastic foci when the animals were subjected to the chronic hypoxia of high altitude. Human beings living at high altitudes have 10 times the frequency of chemodectomas as those residing at sea level.

HEART-BASE NEOPLASMS DERIVED FROM ECTOPIC THYROID GLAND TISSUE

Adenomas and carcinomas derived from ectopic thyroid gland account for approximately 5% to 10% of "heart-base" neoplasms in dogs. They often compress or invade structures in the cranial mediastinum near the base of the heart (Fig. 12-69). Ectopic thyroid gland neoplasms have a compact cellular (solid) pattern that is difficult to distinguish histologically from that of

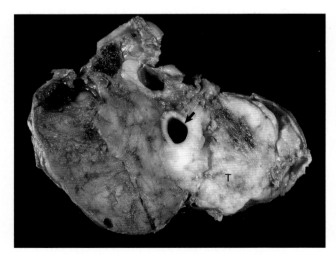

Fig. 12-69   Carcinoma, ectopic thyroid tissue, cranial mediastinum, cross section, dog. Neoplastic tissue *(T)* surrounds the trachea *(arrow)* and other structures in the cranial mediastinum. *(Courtesy Dr. C. Capen, College of Veterinary Medicine, The Ohio State University.)*

aortic body neoplasms. Cells of ectopic thyroid gland neoplasms generally are smaller than those of aortic body neoplasms and have more hyperchromatic nuclei and an eosinophilic cytoplasm. Thyroidal neoplasms of follicular cells are not consistently subdivided into small packets by fine strands of connective tissue. Giant cells are infrequent in ectopic thyroid gland neoplasms, and the stroma is not prominent. Usually, primitive follicular structures or colloid-containing follicles can be demonstrated in ectopic thyroid gland neoplasms, but not in aortic body neoplasms.

SUGGESTED READINGS

Barthez PY, Marks SL, Woo J et al: Pheochromocytomas in dogs: 61 cases (1984-1995), *J Vet Intern Med* 11:272-278, 1997.

Binns W, James LF, Shupe JL et al: A congenital cyclopean-type malformation in lambs induced by maternal ingestion of a range plant, *Veratrum californicum, Am J Vet Res* 24:1164-1175, 1963.

Black HE, Capen CC, Young DM: Ultimobranchial thyroid neoplasms in bulls. A syndrome resembling medullary thyroid carcinoma in man, *Cancer* 32:865-878, 1973.

Capen CC: Toxic responses of the endocrine system. In Klaassen CD, editor: *Casarett and Doull's toxicology: the basic science of poisons*, ed 6, New York, 2001, McGraw-Hill.

Capen CC: Tumors of the endocrine glands. In Meuten DJ, editor: *Tumors in domestic animals*, ed 4, Ames, Iowa, 2002, Blackwell Professional.

De Cock HE, MacLachlan NJ: Simultaneous occurrence of multiple neoplasms and hyperplasias in the adrenal and thyroid gland of the horse resembling multiple endocrine neoplasia syndrome: case report and retrospective identification of additional cases, *Vet Pathol* 36:633-636, 1999.

Doss JC, Gröne A, Capen CC et al: Immunohistochemical localization of chromogranin A in endocrine tissues and endocrine tumors of dogs, *Vet Pathol* 35:312-315, 1998.

Gosselin SJ, Capen CC, Martin SL: Histopathologic and ultrastructural evaluation of thyroid lesions associated with hypothyroidism in dogs, *Vet Pathol* 18:299-309, 1981.

Hammer KB, Holt DE, Ward CR: Altered expression of G proteins in thyroid gland adenomas obtained from hyperthyroid cats, *Am J Vet Res* 61:874-879, 2000.

Kalsow CM, Dubielzig RR, Dwyer AE: Immunopathology of pineal glands from horses with uveitis, *Invest Ophthalmol Vis Sci* 40:1611-1615, 1999.

O'Brien TD, Butler PC, Westernak P et al: Islet amyloid polypeptide: a review of its biology and potential roles in the pathogenesis of diabetes mellitus, *Vet Pathol* 30:317-332, 1993.

Peterson RA, Kiupel M, Capen CC: Adrenal cortical carcinomas with myxoid differentiation in the domestic ferret (*Mustel putorius furo*), *Vet Pathol* 39:136-142, 2003.

Rosol TJ, Capen CC: Biology of disease: mechanisms of cancer-induced hypercalcemia, *Lab Invest* 67:680-702, 1992.

Rosol TJ, Capen CC: Calcium-regulating hormones and diseases of abnormal mineral (calcium, phosphorus, magnesium) metabolism. In Kaneko JJ, Harvey JW, Bruss ML, editors: *Clinical biochemistry of domestic animals*, ed 5, New York, 1997, Academic Press.

Schaer M, Chen CL: A clinical survey of 48 dogs with adrenocortical hypofunction, *J Am Anim Hosp Assoc* 19:443-452, 1983.

Weiss CA, Williams BH, Scott JB et al: Surgical treatment and long-term outcome of ferrets with bilateral adrenal tumors or adrenal hyperplasia: 56 cases (1994-1997), *J Am Vet Med Assoc* 215:820-823, 1999.

13

Bone Marrow, Blood Cells, and Lymphatic System*

MICHAEL M. FRY • M. DONALD McGAVIN

INTRODUCTION

STRUCTURE AND FUNCTION

BONE MARROW AND BLOOD CELLS

Hematopoiesis, the term used to describe the process through which blood cells are made, is derived from *haima* (Gr., blood) and *poiein* (Gr., to make). Hematopoiesis is synonymous with hemopoiesis. The basic concepts below provide a framework for understanding the mechanisms of injury and diseases presented later in the chapter.

BASIC CONCEPTS

- Hematopoiesis occurs primarily in the bone marrow.
- Hematopoiesis may also occur elsewhere (extramedullary hematopoiesis), most commonly in the spleen.
- Hematopoietic tissue is highly proliferative; billions of cells per kilogram of body weight are produced each day.
- Pluripotent hematopoietic stem cells are a self-renewing population giving rise to cells with committed differentiation programs and are common ancestors of all blood cells. The process of hematopoietic differentiation is shown in Fig. 13-1.
- Hematopoietic cells undergo sequential divisions as they mature, so there are higher numbers of mature than immature cells. Cells also continue to mature after they have stopped dividing. Conceptually, it is helpful to consider cells in the bone marrow as belonging to mitotic and postmitotic compartments. Examples of developing hematopoietic cells are shown in Fig. 13-2.
- Mature cell types have different normal life spans, varying from hours (neutrophils), to days (platelets), to months (erythrocytes), to years (some lymphocytes).

- The hematopoietic system is under exquisite local and systemic control, and responds rapidly and predictably to various stimuli.
- Production and turnover of blood cells are balanced so that, in health, numbers are maintained within normal ranges (steady-state kinetics).
- Normally the bone marrow releases only mature cell types (and very low numbers of cells that are almost fully mature) into the circulation. In response to certain physiologic or pathologic stimuli, however, the bone marrow will release immature cells that are further back in the supply "pipeline."

DEVELOPMENT OF BONE MARROW AND BLOOD CELLS

Hematopoiesis is first evident as blood islands in the embryonic yolk sac. During gestation, the bulk of hematopoiesis shifts from the yolk sac to the liver and spleen, and eventually to the bone marrow. The distribution of hematopoietic cells changes with age. The general pattern is that hematopoietically active tissue (red marrow) regresses and is replaced with hematopoietically inactive tissue, mainly fat (yellow marrow). Thus, in newborns and very young animals, the bone marrow consists largely of hematopoietically active tissue, with relatively little fat. In adults, hematopoiesis occurs primarily in the pelvis, sternum, ribs, vertebrae, and the proximal ends of humeri and femora. Even within these areas of active hematopoiesis, fat may constitute a significant proportion of the marrow volume.

STRUCTURE AND FUNCTION OF BONE MARROW AND BLOOD CELLS

Hematopoietic microenvironment

Hematopoietic cells, supporting connective tissue cells, extracellular matrix components, and soluble factors form the bone marrow hematopoietic microenvironment.

---

*Previous chapters on this subject in earlier editions were written or partially written by Dr. G.P. Searcy, Western College of Veterinary Medicine, University of Saskatchewan.

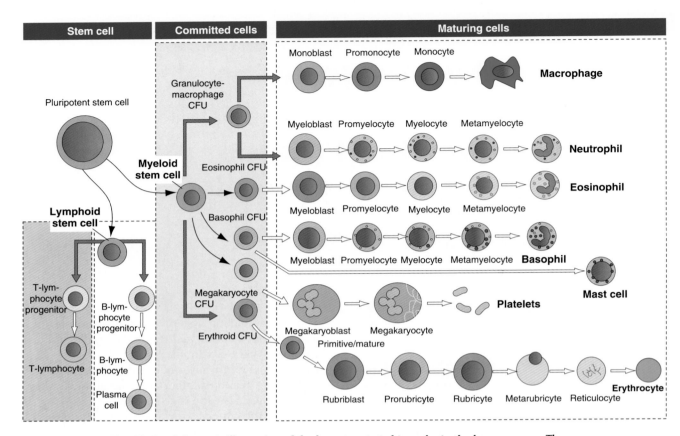

Fig. 13-1 **Schematic illustration of the hematopoietic hierarchy in the bone marrow.** The bone marrow consists of: (1) stem cells, pluripotent cells capable of self-renewal; (2) committed progenitor cells (myeloid and lymphoid progenitor cells); and (3) maturing cells. Maturing cells develop from cells called colony-forming units (CFUs). The myeloid stem cell gives rise to CFUs responsible for the regeneration of red blood cells (erythroid CFUs), platelets (megakaryocyte CFUs), basophils (basophil CFUs), and eosinophils (eosinophil CFUs). Monocytes and neutrophils are derived from a common committed progenitor cell (granulocyte-macrophage CFU). The lymphoid progenitor cell generates the B-lymphocyte progeny in the bone marrow and T-lymphocyte progeny in the thymus. *(From Kierszenbaum AL: Histology and cell biology: an introduction to pathology, St Louis, 2002, Mosby.)*

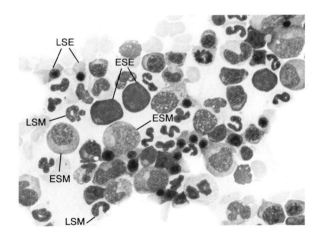

Fig. 13-2 **Normal hematopoiesis, canine bone marrow aspirate.** *ESE,* Early stage erythroid; *ESM,* early stage myeloid; *LSE,* late stage erythroid; *LSM,* late stage myeloid. Wright's stain. *(Courtesy Dr. M.M. Fry, College of Veterinary Medicine, University of Tennessee.)*

There is complex functional interplay among these components. Behavior of hematopoietic cells is influenced by direct cell-to-cell and cell-matrix interactions and by soluble mediators, such as cytokines and hormones, that interact both with cells and with matrix proteins. Cells localize to specific niches within the hematopoietic microenvironment via adhesion molecules, such as integrins, immunoglobulins (Igs), lectins, and other receptors, that recognize ligands on other cells or matrix components. Cells also express receptors for soluble molecules, such as chemokines (chemoattractant cytokines) and hormones, that influence cell trafficking and metabolism.

The marrow cavity is interlaced with venous sinuses composed of a luminal layer of specialized endothelial cells and an abluminal layer of specialized fibroblasts known as adventitial reticular cells (Figs. 13-3 and 13-4). Hematopoiesis takes place in the compartment

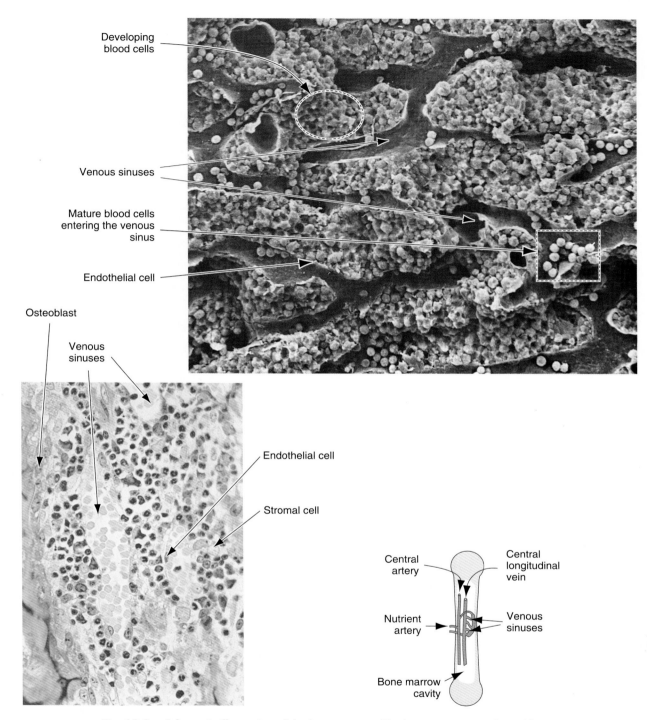

Fig. 13-3   Schematic illustration of the bone marrow. The bone marrow can be red because of the presence of hematopoietic elements, or yellow, owing to fat. Hematopoietic tissue may replace fat, or vice versa, depending on the demand for hematopoiesis. In the adult, red bone marrow is found in the skull, clavicles, vertebrae, ribs, sternum, pelvis, and ends of the long bones of the limbs. Blood vessels and nerves reach the bone marrow by piercing the bony shell. The nutrient artery enters the midshaft of a long bone and branches into central longitudinal arteries that connect with the venous sinuses. The venous sinuses empty into the central longitudinal vein, which runs parallel to the nutrient artery. The internal surface of the bone is lined by trabeculae projecting into the marrow cavity. The endosteum lines the bony surface. *(From Kierszenbaum AL: Histology and cell biology: an introduction to pathology, St Louis, 2002, Mosby. Scanning electron micrograph from Kessel RG, Kardon RH: Tissues and organs, New York, 1979, WH Freeman.)*

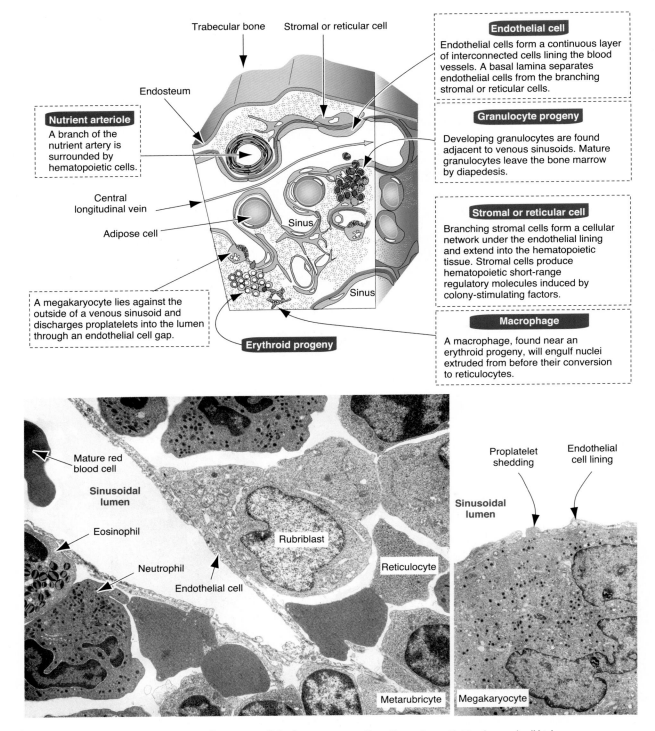

Endothelial cell
Endothelial cells form a continuous layer of interconnected cells lining the blood vessels. A basal lamina separates endothelial cells from the branching stromal or reticular cells.

Granulocyte progeny
Developing granulocytes are found adjacent to venous sinusoids. Mature granulocytes leave the bone marrow by diapedesis.

Stromal or reticular cell
Branching stromal cells form a cellular network under the endothelial lining and extend into the hematopoietic tissue. Stromal cells produce hematopoietic short-range regulatory molecules induced by colony-stimulating factors.

Macrophage
A macrophage, found near an erythroid progeny, will engulf nuclei extruded from before their conversion to reticulocytes.

Nutrient arteriole
A branch of the nutrient artery is surrounded by hematopoietic cells.

A megakaryocyte lies against the outside of a venous sinusoid and discharges proplatelets into the lumen through an endothelial cell gap.

Erythroid progeny

Trabecular bone
Stromal or reticular cell
Endosteum
Central longitudinal vein
Adipose cell
Sinus
Sinus

Mature red blood cell
Sinusoidal lumen
Eosinophil
Neutrophil
Endothelial cell
Rubriblast
Reticulocyte
Metarubricyte
Proplatelet shedding
Endothelial cell lining
Sinusoidal lumen
Megakaryocyte

Fig. 13-4   Schematic illustration of the bone marrow. *(From Kierszenbaum AL: Histology and cell biology: an introduction to pathology, St Louis, 2002, Mosby.)*

(hematopoietic spaces) between these venous sinuses. Sinusoidal endothelial cells perform a barrier function and regulate traffic of chemicals and particles between the intravascular and extravascular spaces. Reticular cells send cytoplasmic processes into the hematopoietic spaces, forming a scaffold that supports the hematopoietic cells. Adipocytes are a major component of marrow tissue. As discussed previously, the amount of fat increases with age, particularly in the long bones. Osteoblasts, osteoclasts, and elongated flat cells line the endosteum. Stromal cells, presumably of fibroblast origin, provide structural support and produce extracellular matrix components, such as proteoglycans, glycosaminoglycans, collagen, fibronectin, and others. Macrophages, lymphocytes, and plasma cells are also components of the hematopoietic microenvironment.

Regulation of hematopoiesis

Control of hematopoiesis is complex, with many redundancies, feedback mechanisms, and pathways that overlap with other physiologic and pathologic processes. Many cytokines influence cells of different lineages and stages of differentiation. The aim of this section is not to explain these regulatory pathways in detail, but rather to provide a broad overview, and thus a basic framework for understanding mechanisms of disease involving the hematopoietic system.

Erythropoiesis

Erythropoiesis—from *erythros* (Gr., red)—refers to the production of red blood cells (RBCs), or erythrocytes, whose main function is gas (O_2 and CO_2) exchange. The dominant regulator of erythropoiesis is a glycoprotein aptly named erythropoietin (Epo). Epo acts on early erythroid progenitor cells in concert with other cytokines, including interleukins (IL-3, IL-4, IL-9), granulocyte-macrophage colony-stimulating factor (GM-CSF), and insulin-like growth factor. Epo is synthesized primarily in the kidney, and exerts its effects by promoting proliferation and inhibiting apoptosis of developing erythroid cells that express Epo receptors. The stimulus for increased Epo production is hypoxia. Because erythrocytes are packed with hemoglobin, of which iron is a component, adequate iron availability is also essential to erythropoiesis. Physiologic systems exist to conserve and recycle iron, as discussed further later.

The earliest erythroid precursor identifiable by routine light microscopy is the rubriblast, which undergoes maturational division to produce 8 to 32 progeny cells. Late-stage erythroid precursors known as metarubricytes extrude their nuclei and become reticulocytes, the cells at the differentiation stage immediately preceding the mature erythrocyte. Reticulocytes start maturing in the bone marrow and finish maturing in the peripheral blood circulation and the spleen. (Horses are an exception in that they do not release reticulocytes into circulation, even in situations of increased demand.) The normal transit time from rubriblast to mature erythrocyte is on the order of approximately 1 week. Unlike mature erythrocytes, which lack organelles, reticulocytes still contain ribosomes and mitochondria, mainly to support completion of hemoglobin synthesis. These remaining organelles impart a bluish-purple cast (polychromasia) to reticulocytes on routine blood smear examination and, when stained with dye such as new methylene blue, precipitate to form irregular aggregates of dark-staining material (Fig. 13-5). Cats also release a more mature form of reticulocyte in circulation, the punctate reticulocyte, which has a much finer staining pattern when stained with new methylene blue and does not appear bluish-purple (polychromatophilic) on routine blood smear examination.

Mature erythrocytes circulate for a long time compared with other blood cells. Their mean life span varies between species: approximately 150 days in horses and cattle, 100 days in dogs, 70 days in cats. They therefore need to be highly resilient cells, built to withstand continual mechanical and biochemical stresses. In most mammalian species, erythrocytes have a biconcave disk shape, sometimes called the discocyte. This biconcavity is most pronounced in the dog. Species in which the

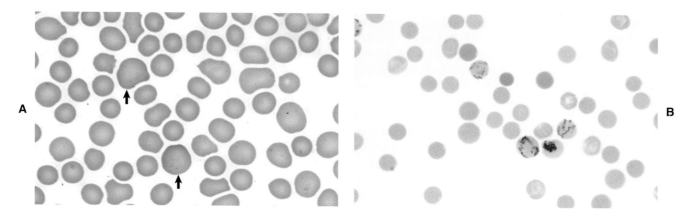

Fig. 13-5   Reticulocytosis, canine blood smears. A, Reticulocytes (*arrows*) appear polychromatophilic with routine staining. Wright's stain. **B,** Reticulocytes. Precipitated aggregates of RNA are stained blue with new methylene blue. (***A** and **B,** Courtesy Dr. M.M. Fry, College of Veterinary Medicine, University of Tennessee.)

discocyte is not the norm include goats (flat, irregularly shaped RBCs) camelids (oval RBCs), and some cervids (sickle-shaped RBCs). One of the key properties of erythrocytes is deformability; they change shape as they move through the microvasculature. This deformability is a function of interactions between the cell membrane, the cytoskeleton, and intracellular contents. Mature mammalian erythrocytes lack nuclei and organelles, and are thus incapable of transcription, translation, and oxidative metabolism. However, they do require energy for various functions—including maintenance of shape and deformability, active transport, and prevention of oxidative damage—and they generate this energy entirely through glycolysis (also known as the Embden-Meyerhof pathway). In addition to generating adenosine triphosphate (ATP), glycolysis generates nicotinamide adenine dinucleotide (NADH), a reducing agent in the pathway that converts the oxidized, nonfunctional form of hemoglobin, known as methemoglobin, back to its active reduced state. Another antioxidant erythrocyte metabolic pathway, the pentose shunt or hexose monophosphate shunt pathway, generates nicotinamide adenine dinucleotide plus hydrogen (NADPH) to maintain glutathione in the reduced state.

The concentration of circulating erythrocytes typically decreases postnatally and remains below normal adult levels during the period of rapid body growth. The age at which erythrocyte numbers begin to increase, and the age at which adult levels are reached, varies among species. In dogs, adult values are usually reached between 4 and 6 months of age; in horses, this occurs at approximately 1 year of age. In most species, erythrocytes are larger at birth, and their mean volume decreases as fetal erythrocytes are replaced.

Granulopoiesis and monocytopoiesis (myelopoiesis)

Granulocytes (neutrophils, eosinophils, basophils) and monocytes have key immunologic functions, including phagocytosis and microbicidal activity (neutrophils and monocyte-derived macrophages); parasiticidal activity and participation in allergic reactions (eosinophils and basophils); antigen processing and presentation; and cytokine production (macrophages). Many molecules influence production of these cell types, including cytokines such as granulocyte and granulocyte-monocyte colony-stimulating factors (G-CSF and GM-CSF, respectively) and interleukins (such as IL-3 and IL-6). Inflammatory mediators stimulate production of cytokines promoting granulopoiesis and monocytopoiesis.

Granulocytic and monocytic cells are sometimes referred to collectively as myeloid cells. (Note: This terminology can be confusing because "myeloid" also has other meanings. In the most general sense, it means

having to do with the bone marrow. In the context of hematology, "myeloid" is also sometimes used to mean any hematopoietic cell of a nonlymphoid origin, a distinction reiterated in the classification of leukemias as discussed later in the chapter. In neuroanatomy, the prefixes "myelo-" or "myel-" can refer to the spinal cord or myelin.) The earliest granulocytic or monocytic precursor identifiable by routine light microscopy is the myeloblast, which undergoes maturational division to produce 16 to 32 progeny cells. The normal transit time from myeloblast to mature neutrophil is approximately 5 days. In addition, a reserve of neutrophils is maintained in the bone marrow. The size of this so-called storage pool is species-dependent. (Species differences and clinical significance of the storage pool are discussed in more detail in the section on mechanisms of disease.) The concentration of granulocytes measured in the blood depends on the rate of production and release from the bone marrow, the proportions of cells circulating freely within the vasculature versus those transiently attached to the endothelial surface (marginated), and the rate of migration from the vasculature into tissues. Neutrophils normally are the predominant leukocyte type in blood of most domestic species. Ruminants usually have higher numbers of lymphocytes than neutrophils. Neutrophils are only in circulation for a short time (less than 12 hours).

Thrombopoiesis

Thrombopoiesis—from *thrombos* (Gr., clot)—refers to the production of platelets, which have a central role in primary hemostasis and also participate in coagulation and inflammatory pathways. Thrombopoietin (Tpo), synthesized primarily in the liver, is the dominant regulator of thrombopoiesis. Unlike Epo, which is up-regulated in response to hypoxia, Tpo is produced at a relatively constant rate (constitutively). The mechanism regulating production is therefore different. Platelets express the Tpo receptor, which binds Tpo in the plasma. When the platelet mass is decreased, less Tpo is bound to platelet receptors, and the increased concentration of Tpo free in the plasma stimulates thrombopoiesis.

Thrombopoiesis differs fundamentally from other forms of hematopoiesis. Platelets (sometimes called thrombocytes) are anucleate cells formed not by maturational division but by shedding of membrane-bound cytoplasmic fragments from precursor cells called megakaryocytes. (Side note: Birds and reptiles produce thrombocytes in the manner of other blood cells and their thrombocytes, and their erythrocytes, are nucleated.) As the name suggests, megakaryocytes are very large cells, much larger than any other hematopoietic cells (Fig. 13-6). Megakaryocytes arise from a progenitor cell and undergo endomitosis to become polyploid

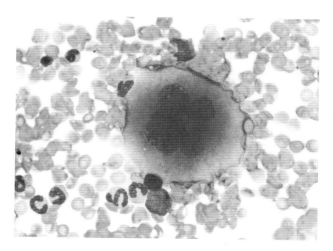

Fig. 13-6   **Megakaryocyte, canine bone marrow aspirate.** Note the cell's very large size, lobulated nucleus, and abundant granular cytoplasm. Wright's stain. *(Courtesy Dr. M.M. Fry, College of Veterinary Medicine, University of Tennessee.)*

(usually 8N-32N). As they mature, megakaryocytes increase in size and their cytoplasm becomes more abundant. They change in staining pattern (Wright's stain of aspirates) from intensely basophilic to eosinophilic, and their nuclei change from round to highly lobulated. Megakaryocytes extend cytoplasmic processes into the lumina of the bone marrow venous sinusoids, where they shed platelets into circulation. The life span of a platelet in circulation is approximately 6 days in the dog.

Lymphopoiesis

Lymphopoiesis refers to the production of new lymphocytes. T lymphocytes and B lymphocytes are the key effectors of cell-mediated and humoral immunity, respectively. Lymphopoiesis is discussed in more detail in Chapter 5, but a brief overview will be provided here. T lymphocytes originate in the bone marrow and migrate to the thymus, where they undergo differentiation, selection, and maturation processes before migrating to the peripheral lymphoid tissue as effector cells. B-lymphocyte development occurs in two phases, first in an antigen-independent phase in the bone marrow and ileal Peyer's patches (the site of B-lymphocyte development in ruminants), then in an antigen-dependent phase in peripheral lymphoid tissues (such as spleen, lymph nodes, and mucosal associated lymphoid tissue [MALT]). Trafficking of lymphocytes occurs under the direction of chemokine (chemoattractant cytokine) signals. Once they have migrated to the peripheral lymphoid tissue, lymphocytes may undergo clonal expansion in response to antigenic stimulation. Unlike other hematopoietic cells, which circulate only in the blood vessels, lymphocytes travel in both blood

and lymphatic vessels, continually recirculating between the two systems. In most species, the majority of lymphocytes in blood circulation are T lymphocytes. Lymphocytes normally are the predominant leukocyte type in blood of ruminants.

COAGULATION AND PLATELET FUNCTION

Hemostasis—from *haima* (Gr., blood) and *stasis* (Gr., "a standing still")—refers to the cessation of bleeding. The main components responsible for hemostasis are platelets, blood vessels, and the coagulation system. Bleeding disorders may result if any of these systems are perturbed. Although coagulation factors are mainly synthesized in the liver, they are included in this chapter because of their inextricable link with the hematopoietic system.

Physiologic hemostasis involves coordinated processes: formation of a platelet plug at the site of vascular damage (primary hemostasis), development of a cross-linked network of insoluble fibrin that provides further clot stability (secondary hemostasis) and retraction and enzymatic degradation of the clot (tertiary hemostasis). The main components of these processes are summarized in Figs. 2-14 through 2-19. Signalment, history, and clinical signs are important in evaluating any patient with a suspected bleeding tendency, but laboratory testing is required to definitively identify specific defects in hemostasis. Routine assays for assessing hemostasis are summarized in Appendix 13-1.

BLOOD VESSELS

Blood vessels have numerous functions in hemostasis. Endothelial cells produce and metabolize many molecules involved in promoting and regulating hemostasis (see Fig. 2-17). For example, they produce prothrombotic molecules, such as von Willebrand factor (vWF) and thromboxane A_2; antithrombotic molecules, such as prostacyclin (PGI_2), thrombomodulin, and nitric oxide; and fibrinolytic molecules, such as tissue plasminogen activator. When a blood vessel is damaged, a rapid, transient neuromechanical vasoconstriction occurs in response. Collagen underlying the damaged endothelium provides structural support for platelet adhesion and clot formation, and also acts as a key biochemical activator of platelets and the intrinsic pathway of the coagulation system (see next section).

COAGULATION SYSTEM

Stopping hemorrhage from a damaged blood vessel ultimately depends on the formation of a stable fibrin clot. This process depends on a number of plasma proteins, or clotting factors, that normally circulate in an inactive proenzyme state. These clotting factors, together with other molecules, including nonenzymatic proteins, calcium, and platelet phospholipids, are known collectively as the coagulation system. Activation of the coagulation system initiates a series of linked enzymatic reactions that result in the production of thrombin. Thrombin converts the soluble plasma protein fibrinogen to fibrin, which in turn is enzymatically cross-linked to form an insoluble clot. The coagulation system is conventionally considered to consist of three interrelated pathways for ease of understanding and interpretation of test results. These pathways—the intrinsic, extrinsic, and common pathways—are summarized in Fig. 2-15.

Anticoagulant and fibrinolytic pathways provide critical "checks and balances." These pathways are initiated simultaneously with activation of the coagulation system. Procoagulant and anticoagulant pathways are regulated at multiple levels, and normally maintained in a balance that avoids hypercoagulable or hypocoagulable states. Some key regulators of hemostasis are listed in Box 13-1. Counter-regulatory mechanisms are critical to the prevention of inappropriate or excessive clotting, and to the eventual dissolution of the clot (fibrinolysis) after it has formed. Fibrinolysis results from the action of plasmin on fibrin (see Figs. 2-15 and 2-16). The inactive proenzyme plasminogen is converted to plasmin by several molecules, including tissue plasminogen activator, factor XII, and thrombin. Note that some of these molecules (e.g., factor XII and thrombin) have both procoagulant and anticoagulant effects. There are also regulators of fibrinolysis, including inhibitors of plasminogen and plasmin. Fibrinolysis results in production of fibrin degradation products (FDPs). D-dimer is a specific type of FDP that results from the degradation of insoluble cross-linked fibrin. Fibrinolytic products (FDPs and D-dimer) in the blood are often measured to detect inappropriate coagulation and are also of clinical importance because they can impair hemostasis by inhibiting fibrin polymerization and platelet function.

Box 13-1

Key Regulators of Hemostasis

- Antithrombin (AT; formerly known as antithrombin III, ATIII)–inactivates thrombin; heparin potentiates activity of AT
- Protein C (with its cofactor, Protein S)–inactivates factors Va and VIIIa
- Thrombin–in addition to its procoagulant and platelet-activating activities, thrombin also: converts plasminogen to plasmin, which lyses fibrin; activates Protein C; and stimulates production of prostacyclin (PGI$_2$), a platelet inhibitor and vasodilator
- Thrombomodulin–binds thrombin, promotes thrombin-Protein C interactions

---

Platelets

Platelets normally circulate in a quiescent state, as flattened disks. Activation of platelets is triggered by soluble agonists, such as thrombin, or insoluble agonists, such as collagen. Platelets express surface receptors for fibrinogen, vWF, collagen, and other ligands. Other key features of platelets include a network of membrane invaginations known as the open canalicular system (not present in cattle), which facilitates the expansion of surface area and release of granule contents in response to activation; specialized endoplasmic reticulum known as the dense tubular system that acts as a reservoir for calcium; and cytoskeletal components involved in mediating shape change, release of granule contents, receptor interactions, and clot retraction. When activated, platelets change to more spherical forms with pseudopodia, and participate in a number of related processes at sites of vascular damage:

- Adhesion to exposed subendothelial collagen
- Secretion of bioactive granule contents (including calcium, adenosine diphosphate [ADP], fibrinogen, vWF, histamine, serotonin, and others)
- Aggregation with other platelets
- Eventual fusion with other platelets (a process known as viscous metamorphosis) to form a unified platelet plug

Phospholipids (e.g., phosphatidylserine) expressed on the surface of activated platelets also help to localize the clot to sites of vascular damage.

LYMPHATIC SYSTEM

Under the classification of the *Nomina Anatomica Veterinaria*, the thymus, spleen, lymph nodes, and lymph nodules are part of the lymphatic system. They are also part of the immune system. The thymus is one of the two primary lymphoid organs (the other is the bone marrow), and these are defined as the sites at which the cellular components of the immune system are formed. The spleen, lymph nodes, and lymph nodules are secondary lymphoid organs and thus are responsible for the immune responses (i.e., production of antibody and cell-mediated immunity). However, because the spleen and lymph nodes contain numerous cells of the monocyte-macrophage system, they also have functions outside those of the immune system, such as phagocytosis of nonantigenic materials like carbon, and in the case of the spleen, senescent and altered erythrocytes.

THYMUS

The thymus is classified as a component of the lymphatic system, but has also been called a lymphoepithelial organ because of its epithelial component. The thymus is essential for the development and function of the immune system, specifically for the development of T lymphocytes. Histologically it is divided into two portions, the stromal portion and the thymocytes portion (T lymphocytes at different stages of maturation). Unlike the spleen and lymph node, the stroma of the thymus consists of epithelial cells as well as macrophages and dendritic cells. The stromal portions of the thymus are derived embryologically from branchial pouches and the third pharyngeal cleft. The capsule, trabeculae, and blood vessels arise from the mesoderm of a branchial arch. The lymphoid component originates during gestation from hematopoietic progenitor cells, initially derived from the fetal liver and later from the bone marrow. The epithelial component consists of individual cells in the cortex and medulla and aggregates of epithelial cells in the medulla. The latter are called Hassall's corpuscles, a characteristic histological feature of the thymus. Cortical and medullary epithelial cells contribute to the microenvironment essential for T-lymphocyte development in neonate and adult thymuses. The thymus also contains reticular cells (a meshwork of specialized fibroblast-like cells with long interdigitating filamentous projections), macrophages interspersed among the reticular cells, and occasional myoid (smooth musclelike) cells.

The shape and location of the thymus vary among young domestic animals. In ruminants and pigs, the thymus has two lobes: cervical and thoracic. The cervical lobe is large and extends along the sides of the cervical trachea. The size of the cervical lobe varies in cats and horses but is usually small. Dogs do not have a cervical lobe. The thoracic lobe is present in all domestic animals and lies in the cranial mediastinum, ventrally in the horse, pig, and dog and dorsally in ruminants.

The thymus is divided into incomplete lobules each of which has a cortex and a medulla, with the medulla being confluent centrally (Fig. 13-7). On the basis of functional and epithelial components, three zones are recognized: a subcapsular zone, a cortex, and a medulla. Bone marrow–derived T-lymphocytes progenitor cells enter the circulation, travel to the thymus, and enter at the subcapsular zone (Fig. 13-8). Here they begin their maturation into T lymphocytes as they traverse the thymic cortex to the medulla. In the cortex, T lymphocytes that recognize self–major histocompatibility complex (MHC) molecules, but not self-antigens, are permitted to mature by a process called positive selection. Cells that do not recognize MHC molecules are removed by apoptosis. Those T lymphocytes that recognize both MHC molecules and self-antigens are removed by phagocytosis by macrophages at the corticomedullary junction, a process called negative selection. Approximately 95% of developing T lymphocytes are destroyed. The remaining mature T lymphocytes

leave the thymus through postcapillary venules in the corticomedullary region and are distributed to periarteriolar lymphoid sheaths in the spleen and cortical areas around germinal centers (paracortex) in lymph nodes. The critical balance between production and distribution of T lymphocytes is extremely important in immune homeostasis, so much so that immunodeficiency or autoimmunity may result from inadequate or overzealous activity of a particular subset.

The thymus attains its maximal mass relative to body weight at birth and involutes following sexual maturity; the lymphoid and epithelial components are gradually replaced by loose connective tissue and fat. T lymphocytes continually circulate through splenic and lymph node T-lymphocyte zones, arriving in the blood and departing in the lymph. Expansion of the antigen-specific T lymphocytes occurs subsequent to antigen presentation.

SPLEEN

The functions of the spleen are analogous to those of the lymph nodes. The spleen filters blood of foreign material and microorganisms and removes senescent and altered erythrocytes. It is the largest secondary lymphoid organ (a site at which immune responses occur). An additional function of the spleen in domestic species is to act as a reservoir for blood (reserve pool).

Thus the spleen has components of three anatomic systems—the monocyte-macrophage system, the lymphopoietic system, and the vasculature—and has the following functions:
- Red pulp
  - Removal of foreign material, particularly microorganisms and also senescent and altered erythrocytes (e.g., parasitized, immunocomplexed, or damaged by oxidative processes)
  - Storage of mature erythrocytes in the red pulp vascular spaces
  - Hematopoiesis under certain circumstances
- White pulp
  - Immunologic response with the production of B lymphocytes and plasma cells to produce antibody and memory lymphocytes

The spleen, suspended in the gastrosplenic ligament and covered by peritoneum, is located in the left cranial hypogastric region of the abdominal cavity between the diaphragm, stomach, and the body wall, except in domestic ruminants, where it is closely adhered to the left dorsolateral aspect of the rumen. The gross morphology (shape and size) of the spleen varies markedly among domestic animals, but in general it is a flattened, elongated organ.

The spleen is covered by a thick fibromuscular capsule from which numerous intertwining fibromuscular trabeculae extend into the parenchyma, forming the supporting stroma for the parenchymal components.

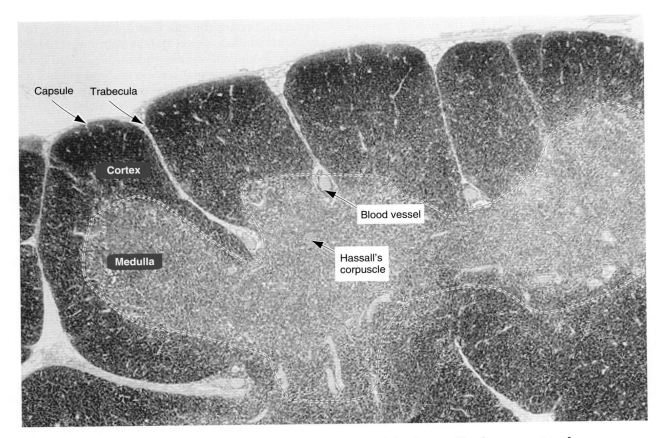

Fig. 13-7   **Schematic illustration of the organization of the thymus.** The thymus consists of several incomplete lobules. Each lobule contains an independent outer cortical region, but the central medullary region is shared by adjacent lobules. Trabeculae, extensions of the capsule down to the corticomedullary region, form the boundary of each lobule. The cortex consists of stromal cells and developing T lymphocytes (thymocytes), macrophages, and cortical epithelial cells. Major histocompatibility complex class I and II molecules are present on the surface of the cortical epithelial cells. The characteristic deep blue nucleus staining of the cortex in histological preparation reflects the predominant population of T lymphocytes as compared with the less basophilic medulla, which contains a lower number of thymocytes. Hassall's corpuscles are a characteristic component of the medulla. Hassall's corpuscles are not seen in the cortex.
(From Kierszenbaum AL: Histology and cell biology: an introduction to pathology, *St Louis, 2002, Mosby.)*

The splenic parenchyma, unlike that of many organs, does not have a cortex and medulla but is divided into two distinct structural and functional components: the red pulp and white pulp.

The artery supplying the spleen is the splenic artery, a branch of the celiac artery, which is a major branch of the abdominal aorta. The splenic artery penetrates the splenic capsule at the hilus, branches, and enters the fibromuscular trabeculae (Fig. 13-9). As these arteries leave the trabeculae, they become central arterioles of the white pulp, and each is surrounded by a cuff of lymphoid cells which forms the periarteriolar lymphoid sheath (PALS). After emerging from the PALS, the arteriole becomes the penicillar arteriole and in the horse, ox, pigs, and cat, its terminal branches empty into the reticular cell lined meshwork of the splenic cords. These spaces in the meshwork are referred to as red pulp vascular spaces or sometimes incorrectly, because they have no endothelium, as capillary beds. In dogs and human beings, branches of the central arteriole of the white pulp enter into venous sinusoids lined by discontinuous endothelium. These anatomic arrangements of opening into sinusoids or red pulp vascular spaces are known as closed and open systems, respectively.

The dog has both open and closed splenic circulations. In either case, the blood is exposed to macrophages and eventually empties into the splenic venules, then into the splenic veins, and ultimately into the portal vein, which drains the abdominal viscera

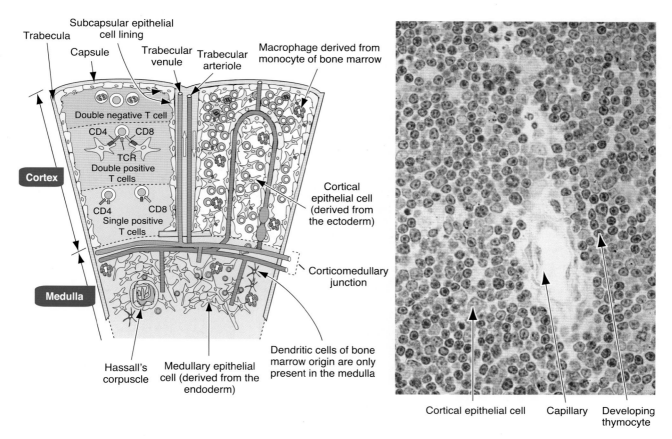

Fig. 13-8   **Schematic illustration of the histology of the thymus.** The functional thymus consists of two cell populations; the stromal cells and the thymocytes. The stromal cells include (1) the subcapsular epithelial cells also lining the trabeculae and perivascular spaces; (2) the cortical epithelial cells of ectodermal origin; (3) the medullary epithelial cells of endodermal origin that give rise to Hassall's corpuscles; (4) macrophages present in both cortex and medulla, involved in the removal of apoptotic thymocytes eliminated during clonal selection; and (5) dendritic cells of bone marrow origin, confined to the medulla. *TCR,* T-cell receptor. *(From Kierszenbaum AL: Histology and cell biology: an introduction to pathology, St Louis, 2002, Mosby.)*

and empties into the liver. Thus the vascular components of the red pulp vary among species depending on whether venous sinusoids are present or not. Understanding the blood flow through the spleen is helpful in understanding how blood comes in contact with the cells of the immune system (white pulp) to facilitate an immunologic response, and cells of the monocyte-macrophage system (red pulp) to enable phagocytosis of foreign materials.

The terminology used to characterize the type of splenic red pulp is confusing. The terms splenic sinuses and splenic sinusoids are both used, but because the endothelium is discontinuous, sinusoid is the correct term. Additionally, confusion arises when the spleen is incorrectly referred to as either sinusal or nonsinusal rather than correctly as sinusoidal or nonsinusoidal.

Splenic parenchyma

Red pulp.   This large sievelike vascular reservoir is formed by an interconnected network of splenic sinusoids and red pulp spaces in the dog and human being, which have a sinusoidal spleen. The spleens of the horse, ox, pigs, and cat lack sinusoids and are termed nonsinusoidal. Sinusoids are lined by elongated endothelial cells and are surrounded by macrophages whose cytoplasm may project through slits in the sinusoidal wall into the lumens of the sinusoids to facilitate phagocytosis. Splenic macrophages are responsible for the phagocytosis of blood-borne foreign material, senescent erythrocytes and damaged cells, such as in immune-mediated cytopenias. In nonsinusoidal spleens, the macrophages of the splenic cords of the red pulp perform these functions.

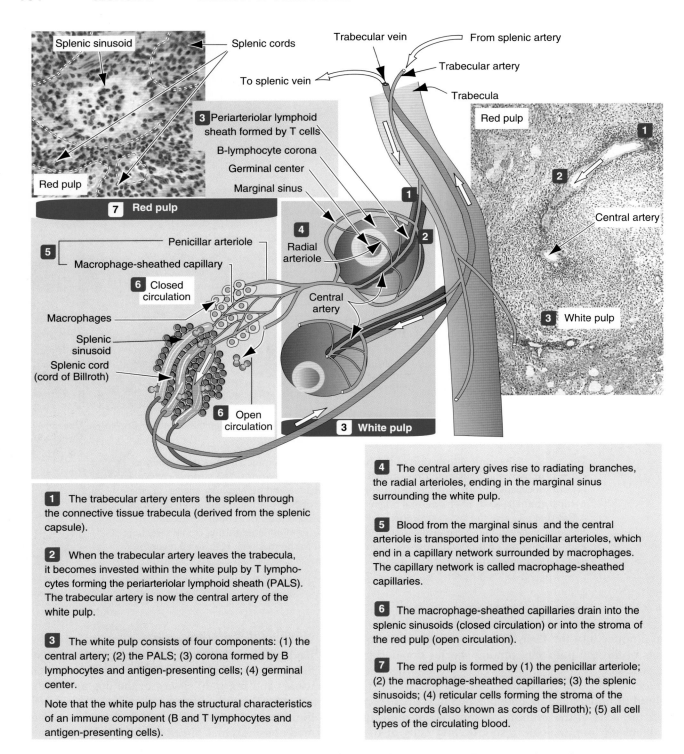

Fig. 13-9   Schematic representation of the human spleen. The blood flow depicted is applicable in domestic animals only to the canine spleen, which has splenic sinusoids. The other domestic animals do not have splenic sinusoids. *(From Kierszenbaum AL:* Histology and cell biology: an introduction to pathology, *St Louis, 2002, Mosby.)*

The sinusoidal and splenic cord macrophages are part of the monocyte-macrophage system (MMS). MMS cells are of bone marrow origin and include blood monocytes and monocytes that have migrated and differentiated into fixed macrophages in connective tissue throughout the body and within vascular beds of specific organs, such as the spleen (sinusoidal and splenic cord macrophages), lymph nodes (sinus histiocytes), liver (Kupffer cells), lung (pulmonary intravascular macrophages and alveolar macrophages), and brain (resident and perivascular microglial cells).

In the dog and human beings (species with sinusoidal spleens), macrophages can remove entire erythrocytes (erythrophagocytosis), portions of an erythrocyte's membrane and inclusions in erythrocytes, such as nuclear remnants, Heinz bodies, or rickettsial organisms. The process is called "pitting" in the case of nuclear debris and Heinz bodies. Indeed, the presence of large numbers of nuclear remnants in erythrocytes in blood smears may indicate splenic malfunction. The process of removal of senescent erythrocytes normally does not alter the size of the spleen, but when the spleen has to remove large numbers of defective erythrocytes, as in an acute hemolytic anemia, it is markedly enlarged.

Vasculature, storage, and defense spleens. Spleens have been classified as either storage or defense spleens. Human spleens have little storage capacity for blood and are classified as defense spleens. The spleens of domestic animals have both storage and defense functions and are classified as storage spleens. They have trabeculae and capsules with a high percentage of smooth muscle, which allows them to expand and contract. These are features of the equine, canine, and feline spleens, which have considerable capacity. It has been claimed that the canine spleen can store one third of the dog's erythrocytes while the animal sleeps. In contrast, spleens whose capsules and trabeculae have a low percentage of smooth muscle and elastic fibers, and thus cannot expand and contract (rabbit and human being), are designated as defense spleens. The spleens of ruminants and the pig are intermediate in the amount of smooth muscle. Storage spleens expand and contract quickly under the influence of the autonomic nervous system (sympathetic and vagal fibers; catecholamines, "flight or fight") and other circulatory perturbations, such as in hypovolemic and/or cardiogenic shock (see sections on small spleens and splenic contraction).

Hematopoiesis. Although hematopoiesis takes place in part in the spleen of the fetus, this ceases shortly after birth in most species. However, often but not necessarily under conditions of severe demand, for example in a severe and prolonged anemia, hematopoiesis can resume. This is called extramedullary hematopoiesis (EMH).

EMH is also present as an incidental finding in splenic nodular hyperplasia (see Splenic Nodules with Firm Consistency). Also, B lymphocytes in the germinal centers of splenic follicles are activated to proliferate and differentiate into antibody producing plasma cells, a form of lymphopoiesis. The marginal zone is the region between red and white pulp, the zone around the PALS and the splenic follicles. It is supplied by a branch of the central arteriole of the white pulp (Fig. 13-9) from which lymphocytes enter the spleen, and blood-borne antigens are taken up by dendritic cells and transported to the PALS for presentation to T lymphocytes. Other secondary lymphoid tissue, such as lymph nodes, do not have a marginal zone.

White pulp. The adaptive immune system component of the spleen consists of distinct organized foci of lymphoid tissue. These are the periarteriolar lymphoid sheaths (PALS, which are T-lymphocyte areas), which surround a so-called central artery of the white pulp, and splenic follicles (B-lymphocyte areas), which lie at the periphery of the PALS.

Normal foci of white pulp are so small that they are not usually visible on gross examination of a cut tissue section. However, if they are enlarged either by lymphoid hyperplasia as a result of a response to an antigenic stimulus or by a neoplastic process (e.g., lymphoma), these foci initially are evident on the cut surface as 0.5- to 1.0-mm white dots scattered through the red pulp. Also in animals with storage spleens (see previous discussion), the distention of the red pulp by blood may obscure white pulp that is enlarged.

The two primary functions of the splenic white pulp are trapping and phagocytosis of blood-borne foreign antigens and the presentation of antigens to T lymphocytes, which result in activation of T and B lymphocytes and the production of antibodies. Antibodies leave the spleen through the efferent lymphatics, which exit the spleen at the hilus, and then depending on the species, connect to the splenic, caudal mediastinal, or celiac lymph nodes. They then travel to the thoracic duct, which empties into the systemic circulation at the origin of the cranial vena cava or into one of its adjacent tributaries. Plasma cells after their formation in the germinal centers of the splenic follicles enter the red pulp and secrete antibody.

LYMPH NODES

Lymph nodes, along with the spleen and mucosal-associated lymphoid tissue (MALT), which includes tonsils, BALT (bronchus-associated lymphoid tissue), and GALT (gut-associated lymphoid tissue), are classified as secondary lymphoid organs—defined as the site of production of antibody and cells for cell-mediated immunity.

A lymph node includes components of two different anatomic systems, the monocyte-macrophage system and the hematopoietic (lymphopoietic) system. Its most important functions are filtration of lymph and immune responses.

The lymph node is enclosed almost completely by a fibrous capsule that is pierced by multiple afferent lymphatics, which empty into the subcapsular sinus. Efferent lymphatics exit and blood vessels enter and exit at the hilus.

In a cross section of lymph nodes, there are two main areas: cortex (outer) and a medulla (inner) (Fig. 13-10). The outer cortex contains the lymphoid follicles. The morphological and functional organization of the lymphoid follicle is identical to that of the splenic lymphoid follicle, except that the marginal zone is absent in the lymph node. Lymphoid follicles are almost absent from the lymph nodes of germ-free and unstimulated neonatal animals. Once lymph nodes are antigenically stimulated, lymphoid follicles form. These initially have no germinal centers and are termed primary lymphoid follicles. With continued antigenic stimulation, germinal centers—the site of proliferating B lymphocytes—develop, and these lymphoid follicles are designated secondary lymphoid follicles. The inner cortex (paracortex) consists of diffuse lymphoid tissue containing T lymphocytes and high endothelial venules (HEVs). T lymphocytes arrive in the blood and then migrate into the lymph node via the HEV.

Also in the cortex are trabeculae, which are collagenous bands extending radially inward from the capsule. They are often surrounded by trabecular (also called paratrabecular) sinuses, which are continuous with the subcapsular sinus and empty into the medullary sinuses (Fig. 13-10).

The medulla consists of two components: (1) medullary cords containing macrophages and lymphocytes—and in an immunologically stimulated lymph node, plasma cells actively secreting antibody; and (2) medullary sinuses surrounded by macrophages, which actively phagocytose foreign material and bacteria.

The porcine lymph node has a different structure. There is one afferent lymphatic that enters at the hilus and discharges lymph into the center of the node, from where it flows to the subcapsular sinus and then drains into several efferent lymphatics, which pierce the capsule.

All lymph nodes receive afferent lymphatic vessels from specific areas of the body. For example, peripheral lymph nodes, such as the popliteal and superficial inguinal, drain the hind leg. Central lymph nodes, such as the tracheobronchial and mesenteric lymph nodes (lymphocenters), drain the lungs and gastrointestinal tract, respectively. The term *lymphocenter* is used in veterinary anatomy for a lymph node or a group of lymph nodes that occur constantly in the same region and receive lymphatic vessels from the same region in all species.

LYMPHOID NODULES

This category includes so-called solitary and aggregated lymphoid nodules. Lymphoid nodules are present in the mucosal-associated lymphoid tissue (MALT), which includes the BALT (bronchus-associated lymphoid tissue), GALT (gut-associated lymphoid tissue), and lymphoid nodules at other sites, such as the tonsils and mucosa of the nasal cavity, conjunctiva, and urinary bladder. These lymphoid nodules consist of lymph follicles and some loose lymphoid tissue. The follicles, if antigenically stimulated can have active germinal centers. Peyer's patches in the small intestine and aggregated lymphoid nodules in the cecum and colon lie in the mucosa and are overlaid by a special epithelium known as the follicle-associated epithelium (FAE) in which there are numerous M cells. These M cells deliver macromolecules (including antigens), particles, pathogenic bacteria, and viruses across the epithelium to an area rich in dendritic cells, which are able to transport the material into the Peyer's patches. Live attenuated salmonella induce dendritic cells in the subepithelial tissue to migrate to the lymph follicle (B-lymphocyte) and parafollicular (T-lymphocyte) areas of Peyer's patches. Other pathogenic bacteria known or believed to enter via the M cells include *Listeria monocytogenes*, *Mycobacterium avium* ssp. *paratuberculosis*, and *Yersinia pseudotuberculosis*. The scrapie agent has been demonstrated to enter through M cells and accumulates in Peyer's patches. HIV and poliovirus are also believed to use this route.

HEMAL NODES

Although these are often considered to be unique to ruminants, they have also been found in horses and primates. Their architecture resembles that of a lymph node with lymph follicles and sinuses, except that the latter are filled with blood (Fig. 13-11). Some authors regard them as "miniature spleens." It was once thought that they had no afferent or efferent lymphatics, but these have been identified. As erythrophagocytosis can be present, it is presumed that hemal nodes can filter blood and remove senescent erythrocytes.

RESPONSES TO INJURY
BONE MARROW AND BLOOD CELLS

The main mechanisms of disease in the bone marrow and in blood cells are shown in Box 13-2, and are discussed in more detail next.

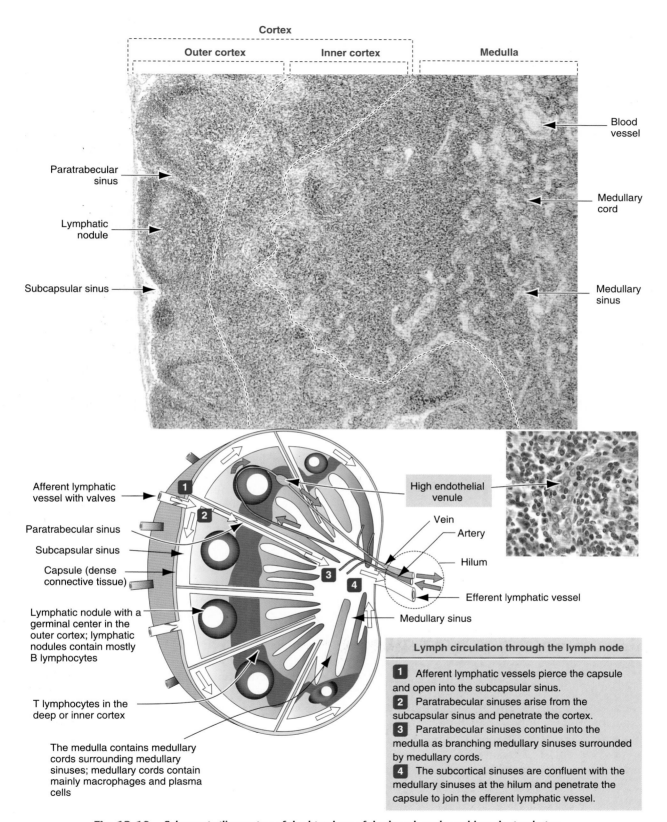

Fig. 13-10   Schematic illustration of the histology of the lymph node and lymph circulation.
(From Kierszenbaum AL: Histology and cell biology: an introduction to pathology, *St Louis, 2002, Mosby.)*

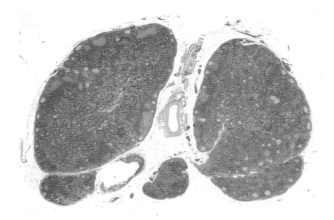

Fig. 13-11   Hemal node, ruminant. Hemal nodes resemble lymph nodes except that the sinuses are filled with blood. H&E stain. *(Courtesy Dr. M.D. McGavin, College of Veterinary Medicine, University of Tennessee.)*

Box **13-2**

Mechanisms of Disease in Bone Marrow and Blood Cells

BONE MARROW

Hypoplasia
Hyperplasia
Dysplasia
Aplasia
Neoplasia
Myelophthisis

BLOOD CELLS

Increased destruction
Hemorrhage (especially erythrocytes)
Consumption (platelets)
Neoplasia
Altered distribution
Abnormal function

ABNORMAL PROLIFERATION

The classic nomenclature for describing different types of abnormal cellular proliferations applies to the hematopoietic system, with some exceptions and modifications. Hyperplasia, an increase in cell number, may be an obviously appropriate response to a stimulus (e.g., erythroid hyperplasia in response to hypoxemia, or lymphoid hyperplasia in response to antigenic stimulation). In other situations, hyperplasia is a secondary phenomenon for which the specific stimulus is not clear—for example, a number of conditions (inflammation, neoplasia, iron deficiency, asplenia, and others)

are associated with reactive thrombocytosis, in which an increased concentration of circulating platelets reflects megakaryocytic hyperplasia. Sometimes hyperplasia is idiopathic. For example, splenic nodular hyperplasia, which often includes a hematopoietic component, is frequently an incidental finding.

Hypertrophy, an increase in cell size, is not a conventional description for hematopoietic cells or for bone marrow as an organ. Abnormally large hematopoietic cells are considered evidence of dysplasia, or altered cell formation (alterations to shape or organization of cells are also evidence of dysplasia). Dysplasia of hematopoietic cells, indicating dyshematopoiesis, may be primary (idiopathic) or secondary to a number of conditions, including infection, nutritional imbalance, and toxicosis. Unfortunately the terminology is sometimes confusing. For example, myelodysplastic syndromes are clonal hematopoietic stem cell disorders that are, in fact, neoplastic (see the later section titled Hematopoietic Neoplasia). Splenic hypertrophy is usually referred to as splenomegaly and may reflect processes other than hyperplasia or cellular hypertrophy. Similarly, lymph node enlargement is typically referred to as lymphadenopathy or lymphadenomegaly and may reflect lymphoid hyperplasia or other processes (e.g., neoplasia, inflammation, or edema).

Replacement of hematopoietic tissue in the bone marrow by abnormal tissue, usually fibrous tissue or malignant cells, is known as myelophthisis. The term *metaplasia*, describing the replacement of cells normally comprising a tissue with another well-differentiated cell type, is rarely used to describe hematopoietic tissues in veterinary medicine, although in human beings, the terms myeloid metaplasia and extramedullary hematopoiesis are sometimes used interchangeably. Similarly, the term *atrophy*—meaning a diminution in the size of a cell, tissue, organ, or part—is seldom used to describe bone marrow. Instead a decrease in bone marrow hematopoietic tissue is typically referred to as hypoplasia, as discussed later in the section on cytopenias. The absence of bone marrow hematopoietic tissue of a particular lineage is typically referred to as aplasia or, if affecting all lineages, by the misleading term *aplastic anemia*. An exception is a condition sometimes called "serous atrophy of fat," a condition associated with cachexia or starvation in which fat is catabolized and bone marrow reticular cells produce a mucoid ground substance. However, neither hematopoietic cells nor fat is necessarily absent from the bone marrow in this condition, and other names, such as "gelatinous transformation," have been suggested to describe it.

Neoplasia of bone marrow or lymphoid organs may be primary or due to metastasis (secondary). Hematopoietic neoplasia may arise from any hematopoietic lineage.

Leukemias are neoplasms arising from bone marrow hematopoietic cells, and are conventionally classified according to two criteria: as lymphocytic (lymphoid) or myelogenous (myeloid), based on the cell of origin; and as acute or chronic, based on the degree of differentiation of the neoplastic cells and on their biologic behavior. Myeloid leukemias encompass the range of leukemias of nonlymphoid origin. Chronic leukemias are characterized by well-differentiated cells and slowly progressive disease. Conversely, acute leukemias are characterized by poorly differentiated cells and an aggressive clinical course. This classification system is simplistic but facilitates communication and is useful for general understanding. Within each of the categories are subclassifications that may have different prognoses. Hematopoietic neoplasia may also originate from outside the bone marrow. For example, *lymphoma* (also known as malignant lymphoma or lymphosarcoma) refers to a group of malignant lymphoid neoplasms arising from lymphoid organs or tissues other than the bone marrow. Specific types of hematopoietic neoplasia (leukemias, lymphomas, and others) are covered later in this chapter.

ABNORMAL CONCENTRATIONS
Cytopenias

Cytopenia—from *kytos* (Gr., hollow vessel) and *penia* (Gr., poverty)—refers to a deficiency of blood cells, hence the terms neutropenia, thrombocytopenia, lymphopenia, and so on. Basic mechanisms causing cytopenias include decreased production (hypoplasia), increased destruction, blood loss, consumption, and altered anatomic distribution (e.g., shifts between marginated and circulating compartments in the blood, or between the spleen and the peripheral blood circulation). Most of these basic mechanisms may cause cytopenias of more than one lineage, and some processes affect multiple lineages simultaneously. Sustained decreased production of all three major bone marrow hematopoietic lineages results in pancytopenia (anemia, neutropenia, and thrombocytopenia). Pancytopenia may occur because of myelophthisis, in which normal bone marrow tissue is replaced by abnormal cells or tissue (as in the case of effacement by malignant cells or fibrous tissue) or because of an abnormality of hematopoietic cells themselves. Destruction of hematopoietic stem cells and progenitor cells causes a condition known as aplastic anemia, or aplastic cytopenia, which is discussed further in the section on specific diseases.

The pattern of development of cytopenias is partly a function of normal blood cell kinetics. Recall that the life span of different blood cells in circulation varies markedly (neutrophils, hours; platelets, days; erythrocytes, months). Thus severe neutropenia typically develops within 1 week after cessation of granulopoiesis, after the bone marrow storage pool of neutrophils is depleted, whereas severe thrombocytopenia typically develops in the second week after cessation of thrombopoiesis. Anemia develops much more slowly after the cessation of erythropoiesis, if at all, depending in part on how rapidly the marrow recovers from the insult and on species variation in the erythrocyte life span.

Anemia. *Anemia* refers to subnormal red blood cell mass (i.e., decreased erythrocyte concentration [usually expressed as RBC $\times 10^6/\mu$L], hematocrit [%], or packed cell volume [PCV, %]) or hemoglobin concentration (g/dL). (Note: Hematocrit [Hct] and PCV both express the proportion of blood volume that is occupied by erythrocytes, but the terms are not perfectly synonymous—Hct is a calculated value based on the number and size of RBCs, whereas PCV is a measured value based on centrifugation.) Anemia causes clinical signs referable to decreased oxygen-carrying capacity (pallor of mucous membranes, lethargy, weakness, exercise intolerance) and may also result in detectable abnormalities because of tissue hypoxia (e.g., increased liver enzyme activities as a result of hypoxia-induced damage to hepatocytes). Anemia also causes decreased viscosity of the blood, and in marked cases frequently causes heart murmurs as a result of a decrease in laminar blood flow.

Classifying anemia as regenerative or nonregenerative is clinically useful because it provides information about the mechanism of disease (Table 13-1). The hallmark of regenerative anemias, except in horses, is reticulocytosis (i.e., increased numbers of circulating reticulocytes [immature erythrocytes]), which is evident on examination of a blood smear as polychromasia. In ruminants, reticulocytosis is often accompanied by basophilic stippling (Fig. 13-12).

Reticulocytosis indicates increased bone marrow erythropoiesis and release of erythrocytes before they are fully mature (further back in the production "pipeline"). Reticulocytosis is an appropriate response to anemia. A strong regenerative response may produce an increased mean cell volume (MCV) and decreased mean cell hemoglobin concentration (MCHC) on the complete blood count (CBC), because reticulocytes are larger and have a lower hemoglobin concentration than mature erythrocytes. Horses are an exception to this classification scheme because they do not release reticulocytes into circulation even when their marrow is producing increased numbers of erythrocytes. Horses with a regenerative response may have an increased MCV and red cell distribution width (an index of variation in cell size). But definitive determination of regeneration in a horse requires either bone marrow examination, in which case the evidence of regeneration is erythroid hyperplasia, or sequential CBCs,

Table **13-1**   **Classification of Anemia**

	Regenerative		Nonregenerative
CBC hallmarks	Reticulocytosis (except horses) Polychromasia, anisocytosis ± ↑ MCV, ↓ MCHC		Absence of reticulocytosis ± ↓ MCV, ↓ MCHC (iron deficiency*)
	Hemorrhage	**Hemolysis**	
Causes	Trauma Hemostasis defect Neoplasia GI ulceration Parasitism	Extravascular: immune-mediated; hemoparasitism toxicosis; PK, PFK deficiencies Intravascular: immune-mediated; hemoparasitism; toxicity, enzymatic (e.g., bacterial phospholipases); hypophosphatemia; PFK deficiency (with alkalemia)	Anemia of chronic disease: ↓ iron availability; ↑ RBC turnover Altered humoral signaling: ↓ erythropoietin; endocrinopathies Ineffective erythropoiesis: immune-mediated; feline leukemia virus Primary production problem: toxicity; myelophthisis; pure red cell aplasia; pancytopenic disorders Iron deficiency*
Notes	Evaluate in concert with history, physical exam, other lab data. Fluid shift occurs within hours of hemorrhage. Regeneration takes approximately 3-4 days to become evident in blood, 7-10 days to reach maximum response.		Evaluate in concert with history, physical exam; other lab data may be indicated. Bone marrow evaluation may be indicated.

CBC, Complete blood count; *GI,* gastrointestinal; *MCHC,* mean cell hemoglobin concentration; *MCV,* mean cell volume; *PFK,* phosphofructokinase; *PK,* pyruvate kinase; *RBC,* red blood cell.
*Iron deficiency anemia is sometimes regenerative.

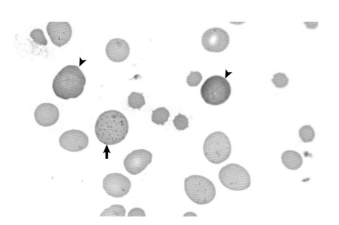

Fig. 13-12   Basophilic stippling and polychromasia, bovine blood smear. Erythrocytes from this cow with regenerative anemia include several cells with basophilic stippling *(arrow)* and two polychromatophilic cells (reticulocytes) *(arrowheads).* **Wright's stain.** *(Courtesy Dr. M.M. Fry, College of Veterinary Medicine, University of Tennessee.)*

in which case the evidence of regeneration is an increase in red cell mass over time. Punctate reticulocytes in cats are evident when blood is stained with new methylene blue, but they are not counted as reticulocytes on the CBC, and they have the same appearance as mature erythrocytes on routine blood smear examination.

Another finding that may accompany regeneration, in addition to reticulocytosis, is the presence of nucleated erythroid cells (nRBCs). However, the presence of circulating nRBCs is not in itself definitive evidence of regeneration, and in fact may signify dyserythropoiesis (e.g., because of lead poisoning or bone marrow disease) or splenic dysfunction. When nRBCs are present as part of a regenerative response to anemia, they should be in low numbers relative to the numbers of reticulocytes.

Recall that the stimulus for increased erythropoiesis is increased secretion of Epo in response to hypoxemia. Although the action of Epo on erythropoiesis is rapid, evidence of a regenerative response is not immediately apparent in a blood sample. One of the main effects of Epo is to expand the pool of early stage erythroid precursors, and it takes time for these cells to differentiate to the point where they are released into circulation. In a case of acute blood loss, for example, it typically takes 3 to 4 days until reticulocytosis is evident on the CBC, and several more days until the regenerative response peaks. A similar lag occurs in cases of acute hemolysis. The term "preregenerative" is sometimes used to describe anemia with a regenerative response that is impending but not yet apparent on the CBC. Confirming a regenerative response in such cases requires either evidence of erythroid hyperplasia in the bone marrow or emergence of a reticulocytosis on subsequent days.

Regenerative anemia occurs because of hemorrhage or hemolysis. Some find it useful to remember these as the "2 Hs" or, alternatively, the "2 Ls" (loss or lysis). In the case of hemorrhage, erythrocytes and the other components of blood escape from the vasculature. Hemorrhage may be acute or chronic, internal or external. Causes of hemorrhage include trauma, abnormal hemostasis, certain forms of parasitism, ulceration, and neoplasia. In general, regenerative anemias do not occur because of a problem with erythropoiesis but one that occurs after erythrocytes are made. However, it is important to note that chronic hemorrhage can deplete the body's iron stores, leading to iron-deficiency anemia, which may be either regenerative or nonregenerative. A regenerative response may occur when the deficiency is resolving or temporarily compensated (e.g., when hemorrhage ceases, or when a patient suddenly gains access to increased dietary or parenteral iron). Nonregenerative anemias, and iron-deficiency anemia specifically, are discussed in more detail later in this chapter.

Hemolysis may be intravascular—in which case erythrocytes release their contents, mostly hemoglobin, directly into the blood—or extravascular, in which case macrophages phagocytose erythrocytes, and little or no hemoglobin is released into the blood. Both forms (mostly extravascular hemolysis) occur as part of normal homeostasis and involve pathways to conserve iron and other reusable components in hematopoiesis. However, some diseases are associated with increased destruction of erythrocytes by one, or both, of these mechanisms. The next sections discuss basic mechanisms of intravascular and extravascular hemolysis in health and disease in more detail.

Mechanisms of hemolysis.   Normal turnover of erythrocytes occurs mainly by extravascular hemolysis, in which senescent erythrocytes are phagocytosed by macrophages in the spleen and to a lesser extent in other organs, such as liver (Kupffer cells) and bone marrow.

The exact controls are not clear, but factors that likely play a role include the following:
- Exposure of membrane components normally sequestered on the inner leaflet of the cell membrane, particularly phosphatidylserine (this mechanism is also important in apoptosis of other cell types)
- Decreased deformability
- Binding of IgG and/or complement
- Oxidative damage

Macrophages degrade erythrocytes into reusable constituents, such as iron and amino acids, and the waste product bilirubin. Intravascular hemolysis occurs normally at only very low levels. Hemoglobin is a tetramer that, when released from the erythrocyte into the blood, splits into dimers that bind to a plasma protein called haptoglobin. The hemoglobin-haptoglobin complex is taken up by hepatocytes and macrophages. This is the major pathway for handling free hemoglobin. However, free hemoglobin may also oxidize to form methemoglobin, which dissociates to form metheme and globin. Metheme binds to a plasma protein called hemopexin, which is taken up by hepatocytes and macrophages in a similar manner to hemoglobin-haptoglobin complexes. Free heme in the reduced form binds to albumin, from which it is taken up in the liver and converted into bilirubin.

In hemolytic anemia, erythrocytes are destroyed at an increased rate. Whether the mechanism is intravascular or extravascular, or a combination, depends on the specific disease process (specific diseases are discussed later in this chapter). A classic sequela of hemolytic anemias in general is hyperbilirubinemia, an increase in the plasma concentration of bilirubin. Bilirubin is a yellow pigment, which explains why hyperbilirubinemia, if severe enough, causes icterus—the grossly visible yellowing of serum or tissue (Fig. 13-13). Icterus of mucous membranes, skin, and other tissue is known as jaundice. Icterus is usually detectable when the plasma bilirubin concentration exceeds 2 mg/dL. In hemolytic diseases, hyperbilirubinemia is due to prehepatic disease (i.e., increased turnover of erythrocytes, as described earlier), but it is important to note that it can also be due to hepatic or posthepatic (cholestatic) disease.

Laboratory findings and clinical observations may point to a specific mechanism of hemolysis. In patients with extravascular hemolytic anemia, increased destruction of erythrocytes by splenic macrophages often results in splenomegaly (Fig. 13-14). Splenomegaly may also occur because of other conditions, as discussed elsewhere in this chapter. Intravascular hemolysis is grossly evident as hemoglobinemia, pink-tinged plasma or serum, if the concentration of extracellular hemoglobin is greater than approximately 50 mg/dL. Haptoglobin is saturated with dimeric hemoglobin at a concentration of approximately 150 mg/dL. When haptoglobin

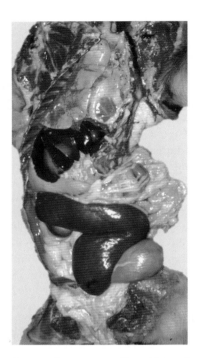

Fig. 13-13 **Icterus, immune-mediated hemolytic anemia, subcutaneous fat, splenomegaly, spleen, dog.** The marked yellow discoloration of tissues, most strikingly visible in the subcutaneous fat, is from high concentrations of serum bilirubin produced as a result of the hemolytic anemia. *(Courtesy Dr. J.A. Ramos-Vara, College of Veterinary Medicine, Michigan State University; and Noah's Arkive, College of Veterinary Medicine, The University of Georgia.)*

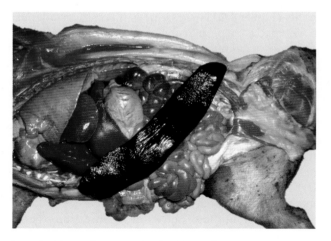

Fig. 13-14 **Splenomegaly, fatal hemolytic anemia,** ***Mycoplasma suis,* pig.** The spleen is extremely enlarged, meaty, and congested. *(Courtesy College of Veterinary Medicine, University of Illinois.)*

is saturated, any remaining free hemoglobin is of low enough molecular weight to pass through the renal glomerular filter into the urine (hemoglobinuria), imparting a pink or red discoloration to the urine. Thus extracellular hemoglobin can cause gross discoloration

of the plasma, where it is bound to haptoglobin, before becoming grossly visible in urine. The half-life of haptoglobin is markedly decreased when bound to hemoglobin, so when large amounts of haptoglobin-hemoglobin complex are formed, the concentration of haptoglobin in the blood decreases and hemoglobin can pass through the glomerulus at even lower concentrations. Although hemoglobin itself is not nephrotoxic, hemoglobinuria is a contributing factor in the renal tubular necrosis (hemoglobinuric nephrosis) that often occurs in cases of acute intravascular hemolysis (see Chapter 11). A similar lesion occurs in the kidneys of individuals with marked muscle damage and resulting myoglobinuria.

Hemoglobinuria cannot be distinguished grossly from hematuria (RBCs in the urine) or myoglobinuria, and both hemoglobin and myoglobin cause a positive reaction for "blood protein" on urine test strips. Comparing the colors of the plasma and the urine may be informative. In contrast to hemoglobin, myoglobin causes gross discoloration of the urine before the plasma is discolored. This is because myoglobin is a low molecular weight monomer, freely filtered by the glomerulus, and does not bind plasma proteins to a significant degree. Hematuria can be distinguished from hemoglobinuria on the basis of microscopic examination of urine sediment (RBCs will be detected in cases of hematuria).

CBC data is often useful in illuminating hemolytic mechanisms. Total hemoglobin concentration is conventionally measured by lysing all the erythrocytes and measuring the hemoglobin in solution spectrophotometrically. The value for mean cell hemoglobin (MCH) is calculated based on the total hemoglobin concentration and the concentration of erythrocytes. The value for MCHC is calculated based on the MCH and MCV. Thus although erythrocytes do not actually contain supranormal concentrations of hemoglobin, an excess of extracellular hemoglobin may cause an artifactual increase in the calculated MCH and MCHC. It is important to remember that similar increases may also occur artifactually because of interference with spectrophotometric measurement of hemoglobin, such as occurs with lipemia.

Extravascular hemolysis also often produces characteristic CBC abnormalities that may reflect the mechanism of disease. For example, spherocytosis and autoagglutination are hallmarks of immune-mediated hemolytic anemia. Spherocytes form when macrophages (mainly in the spleen) phagocytose part of an erythrocyte plasma membrane bound with autoantibody (Fig. 13-15). The remaining portion of the RBC assumes a spherical shape, thus preserving maximal volume. This change in shape results in decreased deformability of the cells. Erythrocytes must be extremely pliable to traverse the splenic red pulp

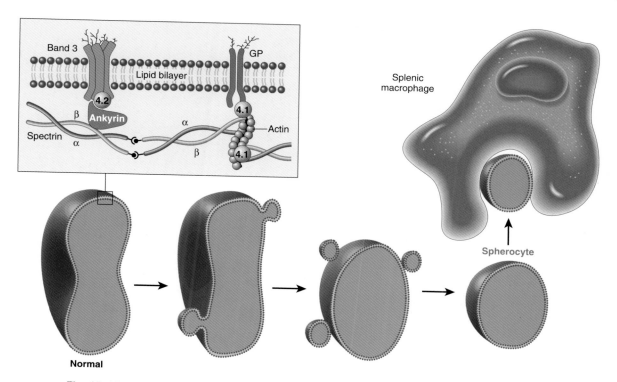

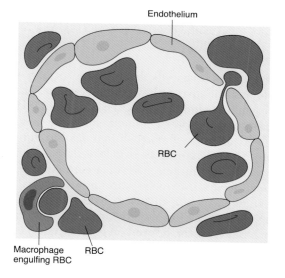

Fig. 13-15   Schematic representation of the mechanisms of spherocytosis and extravascular hemolysis (EVH). Hereditary spherocytosis occurs in human beings (as shown here) because of mutations that weaken the connections between cytoskeletal and membrane proteins. In cases of immune-mediated hemolytic anemia, the most frequent cause of spherocytes in animals, the underlying disease mechanism is different—spherocytes form when portions of the erythrocyte membrane bound with autoantibody are phagocytosed by macrophages—but the net result (spherocytosis and EVH) is similar to what is shown here. *GP*, Glycoprotein. *(From Kumar V, Abbas AK, Fausto N: Robbins & Cotran pathologic basis of disease, ed 7, Philadelphia, 2005, Saunders.)*

and sinusoidal walls (Fig. 13-16); spherocytes, therefore, tend to be retained in the spleen in close association with macrophages with risk of further injury and eventual destruction. In the dog, spherocytes appear smaller than normal and have uniform staining (Fig. 13-17, *A*), in contrast to normal RBCs, which have a region of central pallor imparted by their biconcave shape. This difference in staining between spherocytes and normal RBCs is not consistently discernible in many other domestic animals (including cats, horses, and cattle), whose erythrocytes differ from those of the dog in that they are smaller and have less pronounced biconcavity and therefore less pronounced central pallor. Autoagglutination occurs because of cross-linking of antibodies bound to erythrocytes. Autoagglutination is evident microscopically as clusters of erythrocytes, and macroscopically as blood with a grainy consistency (Fig. 13-17, *B*). Autoagglutination may also result in a falsely increased MCV and decreased RBC concentration when clustered cells are mistakenly counted as single cells by automated hematology analyzers.

Fig. 13-16   Schematic representation of a human splenic sinusoid. A red blood cell *(RBC)* is in the process of squeezing from the red pulp cords into the sinus lumen. Note the degree of deformability required for RBCs to pass through the wall of the sinus. *(From Kumar V, Abbas AK, Fausto N: Robbins and Cotran pathologic basis of disease, ed 7, Philadelphia, 2005, Saunders.)*

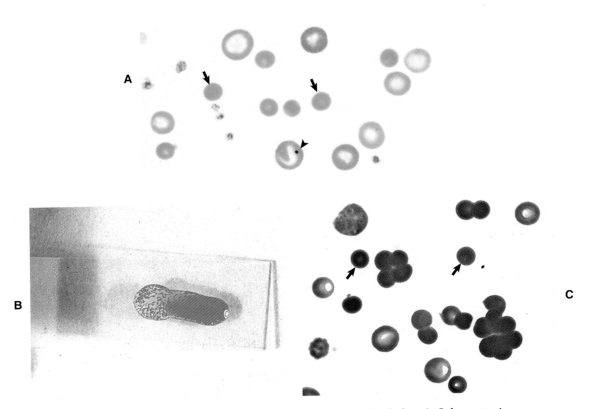

Fig. 13-17   **Immune-mediated hemolytic anemia, canine blood, dog. A,** Spherocytosis. Numerous spherocytes (*arrows*) and several polychromatophilic cells, one of which (*arrowhead*) contains a nuclear remnant known as a Howell-Jolly body, are visible. Wright's stain. **B,** Autoagglutination. Note the grossly visible agglutination. **C,** Spherocytosis and agglutination. Note the spherocytes (*arrows*) and microscopic agglutination of erythrocytes in a dog that received a blood transfusion. These abnormalities presumably indicate immune-mediated destruction of the donor erythrocytes. Wright's stain. (**A,** *Courtesy Dr. M.M. Fry, College of Veterinary Medicine, University of Tennessee.* **B** *and* **C,** *From Harvey JW:* Atlas of veterinary hematology: blood and bone marrow of domestic animals, *Philadelphia, 2001, Saunders.*)

Oxidative damage to erythrocytes occurs when normal antioxidative pathways that generate reducing agents (such as glutathione, NADH, and NADPH), are compromised or overwhelmed, and can result in hemolytic anemia, abnormal hemoglobin function, or both. Hemolysis due to oxidative damage may be extravascular or intravascular, or a combination (predominant forms of hemolysis are discussed further in the section on specific diseases). Evidence of oxidative damage to erythrocytes may be apparent on examination of a blood smear, or even on gross physical examination. Heinz bodies are foci of denatured globin that interact with the erythrocyte membrane. They are usually subtly evident on routine Wright's-stained blood smears as pale circular inclusions or blunt, rounded protrusions of the cell margin and are readily discernible on smears stained with new methylene blue (Fig. 13-18). Cats are particularly susceptible to Heinz body formation and may have low numbers of small

Heinz bodies normally. There is not unanimity of opinion, but some clinical pathologists believe that the presence of Heinz bodies in up to 10% of all RBCs in cats is within normal limits. This predisposition is believed to reflect unique features of the feline erythrocyte, whose hemoglobin has more sulfhydryl groups (preferential sites for oxidative damage) than do erythrocytes of other species and may also have lower intrinsic reducing capacity. It is also possible that the feline spleen, which is nonsinusoidal, does not have as efficient a "pitting" function as does a sinusoidal spleen, such as that of the dog (splenic structure and function are discussed in more detail earlier in this chapter). Eccentrocytes, evident as erythrocytes in which one side of the cell has increased pallor, are another manifestation of oxidative damage. They form because of cross-linking of membrane proteins, with adhesion of opposing areas of the cell's inner membrane leaflet, and displacement of most of the hemoglobin toward

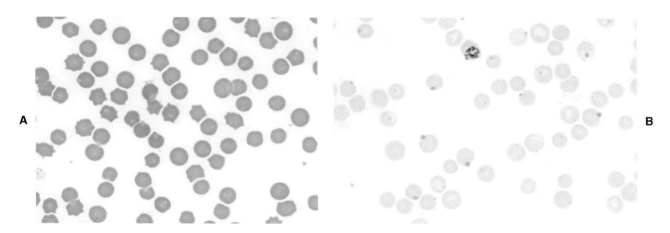

Fig. 13-18   Heinz bodies, blood smears. A, Feline blood smear. With routine staining, Heinz bodies appear as pale circular intraerythrocytic inclusions that may protrude from the margin of the cell. Wright's stain. **B,** Canine blood smear. Using a supravital stain, Heinz bodies are blue inclusions and easier to see. New methylene blue stain. (***A*** *and* ***B,*** *Courtesy Dr. M.M. Fry, College of Veterinary Medicine, University of Tennessee.*)

the other side (Fig. 13-19, *H*). Oxidative insult may also result in conversion of hemoglobin (iron in the Fe^{2+} state) to methemoglobin (iron in the Fe^{3+} state), which is incapable of binding oxygen. Methemoglobin is produced normally in small amounts, but reduced back to oxyhemoglobin by the enzyme cytochrome-b_5 reductase (also known as methemoglobin reductase). Methemoglobinemia results when methemoglobin is produced in excessive amounts (because of oxidative insult) or when the normal pathways for maintaining hemoglobin in the Fe^{2+} state are impaired (as in cytochrome-b_5 reductase deficiency). When present in sufficiently high concentration (approximately 10% of total hemoglobin), methemoglobin imparts a grossly discernible chocolate color to the blood.

Nonregenerative anemias are characterized by a lack of reticulocytosis on the CBC; however, reticulocytosis does not occur in horses even in the context of regeneration. Most often this is due to decreased production in the marrow (i.e., erythroid hypoplasia). Erythrocytes circulate for a long time (life span is approximately 100 days in dogs, 70 days in cats, 150 days in horses and cattle), so anemias caused by decreased production tend to develop slowly. The most common form of nonregenerative anemia is known as anemia of inflammation or anemia of chronic disease. In this form of anemia, RBCs are decreased in number, but are normal in mean size and hemoglobin concentration (so-called normocytic, normochromic anemia). It has long been known that patients with inflammatory or other chronic disease often become anemic, and that this condition is associated with increased iron stores in the bone marrow. Sequestration of iron may be a bacteriostatic

evolutionary adaptation because many bacteria require iron as a cofactor for growth. In recent years, investigators have begun to elucidate the molecular mechanisms underlying anemia of inflammation. Hepcidin, an acute phase protein synthesized in the liver that was first identified as an antimicrobial peptide, is a key mediator that acts by limiting iron availability. Hepcidin expression increases with inflammation, infection, or iron overload, and decreases with anemia or hypoxia. Anemia of inflammation almost certainly involves factors besides decreased iron availability. For example, experimentally induced sterile inflammation in cats resulted in a shortened erythrocyte life span, suggesting that anemia of inflammation is also a function of increased erythrocyte destruction.

True iron deficiency has long been recognized as a cause of anemia. Iron deficiency occurs most commonly because of chronic blood loss, and thus loss of iron in the form of hemoglobin, and less frequently is due to nutritional deficiency. Although iron deficiency often results in nonregenerative anemia, it is not always so, especially if caused by chronic hemorrhage and when nutritional iron is not a limiting factor. There are many underlying conditions that involve hemorrhage-induced iron deficiency anemia, including primary or secondary gastrointestinal disease (e.g., hookworms, neoplasia, ulceration) and marked ectoparasitism. The classic hematologic picture with iron deficiency is microcytic, hypochromic anemia. Microcytosis and hypochromasia are indicated on the CBC by abnormally low MCV and MCHC values, respectively. Microcytosis and hypochromasia may also be discernible on review of a blood smear as RBCs that are abnormally small, or

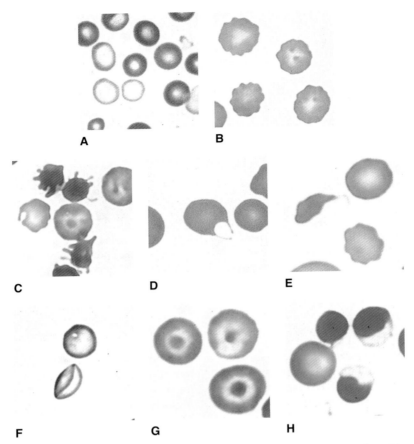

Fig. 13-19   Common erythrocyte morphologic abnormalities. A, Blood from a dog with a microcytic hypochromic iron-deficiency anemia was mixed with an equal volume of blood from a normal dog before blood smear was prepared. Because the hypochromic (pale-staining) cells are leptocytes (Fig. 13-19, *F*), they have diameters similar to normal cells even though they are microcytic cells. Wright-Giemsa stain. **B,** Echinocytes appear as erythrocytes with scalloped borders; consequently, the old term "crenation" from Latin meaning "notched" is used. Wright-Giemsa stain. **C,** Three acanthocytes with irregularly spaced, variably sized spicules in blood from a dog with hemangiosarcoma. Wright-Giemsa stain. **D,** A keratocyte, exhibiting what appears to be a ruptured "vesicle" in blood from a cat with hepatic lipidosis. Wright-Giemsa stain. **E,** A schistocyte *(left)*, discocyte *(top)*, and echinocyte *(bottom)* in blood from a dog with disseminated intravascular hemolysis. Wright-Giemsa stain. **F,** Two thin flat hypochromic-appearing erythrocytes (leptocytes), with increased membrane-to-volume ratios, are present in blood from a dog with severe iron-deficiency anemia. The bottom leptocyte is folded. Wright-Giemsa stain. **G,** Three codocytes in blood from a Cairn terrier with a regenerative anemia and hepatic hemochromatosis secondary to pyruvate kinase deficiency. These erythrocytes exhibit a central density or "bull's-eye" and are often referred to as target cells. Wright-Giemsa stain. **H,** Three eccentrocytes and a discocyte *(left)* in blood from a dog with oxidant injury induced by the administration of acetaminophen. The cell at top center appears spherical with a small tag of cytoplasm and may be referred to as a pyknocyte. Wright-Giemsa stain. *(A through H, From Harvey JW: Atlas of veterinary hematology: blood and bone marrow of domestic animals, Philadelphia, 2001, Saunders.)*

paler-staining because of their subnormal hemoglobin concentration, respectively. However, microscopic examination is not a reliable means of detection, especially in the case of mild abnormalities. Low hemoglobin concentration is believed to contribute to microcytosis because one of the feedback mechanisms signaling erythroid cells to stop dividing is reaching a threshold hemoglobin concentration. Abnormally low hemoglobin concentration during erythropoiesis thus results in extra cell divisions and smaller erythrocytes.

Other causes of decreased erythropoiesis include the following:

- Malnutrition
- Decreased hormonal stimulation

- Infection of erythropoietic cells
- Toxic insult to the bone marrow
- Other disease involving the bone marrow
- Immune-mediated destruction of erythroid precursors
- Inherited conditions

Specific examples of diseases causing nonregenerative anemia by these mechanisms are discussed later in this chapter. It is important to point out that nonregenerative anemia is not always caused by decreased erythropoiesis. For instance, immune-mediated hemolytic anemia (IMHA) is typically strongly regenerative, but there are also nonregenerative forms of IMHA. Bone marrow findings in dogs with severe nonregenerative immune-mediated hemolytic anemia range from a complete absence of erythropoiesis, known as pure red cell aplasia, to erythroid hyperplasia in a majority of patients in one study. The latter situation is an example of ineffective hematopoiesis (in this case, ineffective erythropoiesis), in which cells are being produced at normal or increased levels but are destroyed, presumably because of an immune-mediated mechanism, before they enter the circulation.

Neutropenia.   *Neutropenia* refers to a decrease in the concentration of neutrophils in circulating blood (usually expressed as cells $\times 10^3/\mu L$). Neutropenia may be due to decreased production, increased destruction, altered distribution, demand for neutrophils in inflamed tissue that exceeds the rate of granulopoiesis, or inherited disease. Decreased production is evident on bone marrow examination as granulocytic hypoplasia. This usually results from an insult that affects multiple hematopoietic lineages, such as chemical insult, radiation, neoplasia, infection, and fibrosis, but may also be due to a process that preferentially targets granulopoiesis. Immune-mediated neutropenia is a rare but recognized condition in veterinary literature. Bone marrow findings can range from granulocytic aplasia or hypoplasia to hyperplasia, depending on where the cells under immune attack are in their differentiation programs. Neutropenia with no evidence of decreased production, and in which other causes of neutropenia have been excluded, may be due to destruction of neutrophils before they leave the bone marrow, a condition known as ineffective granulopoiesis. Like other forms of ineffective hematopoiesis, this condition is often presumed to be immune mediated or, in cats, a result of infection of hematopoietic cells with the feline leukemia virus.

In marked contrast to erythrocytes, neutrophils have a very short life span in circulation. Once released from the bone marrow, a neutrophil is only in the blood stream for hours before migrating into the tissues. The fate of neutrophils after they leave the blood stream in normal conditions (i.e., not in the context of inflammation) is poorly understood. They migrate into the gastrointestinal and respiratory tracts, liver, and spleen and may be lost through mucosal surfaces or undergo apoptosis and be phagocytosed by macrophages. When neutrophil production ceases, a reserve of mature neutrophils in the bone marrow (discussed in more detail later) may be adequate to maintain normal numbers of circulating neutrophils for a few days; however, after the bone marrow storage pool is depleted, neutropenia rapidly ensues.

Neutrophils within the blood vasculature may be considered to consist of two compartments: a circulating pool, consisting of those cells flowing freely in the blood, and a marginated pool, consisting of those cells transiently associated with the endothelial surface. Circulating neutrophils are part of the blood sample collected during routine venipuncture and are thus counted in the CBC, whereas marginated neutrophils are not. (In reality, neutrophils are constantly shifting between these two pools, but the proportion of cells in either pool normally remains fairly constant in any given species.) *Pseudoneutropenia* refers to the situation in which there is an increased proportion of neutrophils in the marginated pool. This may occur because of decreased blood flow or in response to stimuli, such as endotoxemia, that increase expression of molecules promoting interaction between neutrophils and endothelial cells.

Neutropenia may also result from increased demand for neutrophils in the tissue. How rapidly such a situation develops depends not only on the magnitude of the inflammatory stimulus but also on the reserve of postmitotic neutrophils in the bone marrow. The size of this reserve, or storage pool, is species dependent. In dogs, this pool contains the equivalent of 5 days normal production of neutrophils. Cattle represent the other extreme in that they have a small storage pool, and thus are predisposed to becoming neutropenic more easily than are dogs. Horses and cats are somewhere between the two extremes, closer to cattle and dogs, respectively. It stands to reason that the clinical significance of neutropenia because of a supply and demand imbalance is also species dependent. In dogs, neutropenia due to inflammation is an alarming finding because it is evidence of a massive tissue demand for neutrophils that has exhausted the patient's storage pool and is exceeding the rate of granulopoiesis in the bone marrow, whereas in cows, neutropenia is commonly noted in a wide range of conditions involving acute inflammation and does not necessarily indicate an overwhelming demand.

Eosinopenia/basopenia.   In many laboratories, CBC reference values for eosinophils and basophils are as low as zero cells per microliter, precluding detection of eosinopenia or basopenia. When detectable, eosinopenia is often part of a stress (glucocorticoid-mediated) leukogram.

Thrombocytopenia. *Thrombocytopenia* refers to a decrease in the concentration of circulating platelets. Mechanisms of thrombocytopenia include decreased production, increased destruction, increased consumption, altered distribution, and hemorrhage. Decreased production may occur because of a condition affecting cells of multiple hematopoietic lineages, including platelets, or to one specifically depressing thrombopoiesis. In either case, decreased thrombopoiesis is evident on examination of a bone marrow sample as megakaryocytic hypoplasia. General causes of decreased hematopoiesis outlined earlier in the sections on anemia and neutropenia also apply to thrombocytopenia. Specific diseases causing thrombocytopenia will be covered later in this chapter. Immune-mediated thrombocytopenia is a fairly common disease in dogs and may also occur in other species. Increased consumption of platelets is a hallmark of disseminated intravascular coagulation (DIC), a syndrome in which hypercoagulability leads to increased consumption of both platelets and coagulation factors in the plasma, with subsequent hypocoagulability and susceptibility to bleeding. The spleen normally contains a significant proportion of total platelet mass (up to one third in some species), and abnormalities involving the spleen may result in changes in the number of circulating platelets. For example, splenic congestion may result in thrombocytopenia, and splenic contraction may result in thrombocytosis. Acute hemorrhage may result in mild to moderate thrombocytopenia. Potential mechanisms of thrombocytopenia due to hemorrhage include loss and consumption. Of course, thrombocytopenia can also be a cause of hemorrhage. In the absence of other complicating factors, marked to severe thrombocytopenia (less than 50,000 platelets/μL) is much more likely to be the cause of, rather than the result of, bleeding. Megakaryocytic hyperplasia on examination of a bone marrow sample is evidence of a regenerative thrombopoietic response, and an increase in the mean platelet volume (MPV) value on the CBC often accompanies such a response.

Lymphopenia. *Lymphopenia* refers to a decrease in the concentration of lymphocytes in blood circulation. It is a common CBC finding in sick animals. Usually the precise mechanism of lymphopenia is not clear. It is often presumed to be mediated at least in part by endogenous glucocorticoid excess. Lymphopenia may occur because of various mechanisms, including altered distribution of lymphocytes (increased trafficking of lymphocytes to, and decreased egress from, lymphoid tissues), lymphotoxicity (direct damage to lymphocytes or suppression of lymphopoiesis) of therapeutic or infectious agents, loss of lymphocyte-rich lymphatic fluid, or congenital disorders. Normal lymphocyte trafficking may be altered because of disruption of the normal architecture of lymphoid tissue (e.g., because of neoplasia or inflammation), or in response to cytokine signals. Glucocorticoid excess may cause lymphopenia via redistribution from the blood to lymphoid tissue, or via direct lymphotoxic effects. Anticancer treatments (chemotherapy or radiotherapy) and immunosuppressive drugs may also be lymphotoxic. Some hereditary immunodeficiencies (such as severe combined immunodeficiency or thymic aplasia) can cause lymphopenia.

Increased cell concentration

Increases in the concentration of many blood cells are indicated by the suffix, *-osis* (erythrocytosis, lymphocytosis, monocytosis, and thrombocytosis). Increases in granulocytes are indicated by the suffix, *-philia* (neutrophilia, eosinophilia, basophilia). Basic mechanisms causing increases in the concentration of blood cells vary considerably according to cell type, and are discussed in more detail later. Neoplasia can result in increased or decreased numbers of blood cells. In many kinds of hematopoietic neoplasia, especially leukemias, there are readily detectable numbers of neoplastic cells in the blood. Specific types of hematopoietic neoplasia are discussed later in this chapter. Increased concentrations of blood cells can also occur secondary to many forms of neoplasia (i.e., as a paraneoplastic syndrome), because of production of stimulatory cytokines by the tumor.

Veterinary laboratories typically provide species-specific hematology reference values based on a reference population of clinically normal adult animals. However, it is important to note that what is normal may vary not only between species but also as a function of other factors, such as age, breed, geographic location, and differences in laboratory methodology.

Erythrocytosis. An increase in the measured red cell mass above the normal range (i.e., the opposite of anemia) is known as erythrocytosis. The term *polycythemia* is often used interchangeably with erythrocytosis, but technically, and for the purposes of this chapter, *polycythemia* refers to a specific type of leukemia called primary erythrocytosis or polycythemia vera. Relative erythrocytosis occurs most frequently because of dehydration, when the decreased proportion of water in the blood results in hemoconcentration. A similar situation may occur as a result of epinephrine-mediated splenic contraction. Erythrocytosis due to splenic contraction occurs to the most pronounced degree in the horse, and may occur to a lesser extent in other species. In both of these cases, the total red blood cell mass is not in fact increased, but appears to be so because of other factors. *Secondary erythrocytosis* refers to a true, Epo-mediated increase in red cell mass, either as an appropriate response to hypoxemia (such as may be seen in patients with cardiopulmonary disease and severely impaired oxygenation, or cardiovascular defects causing

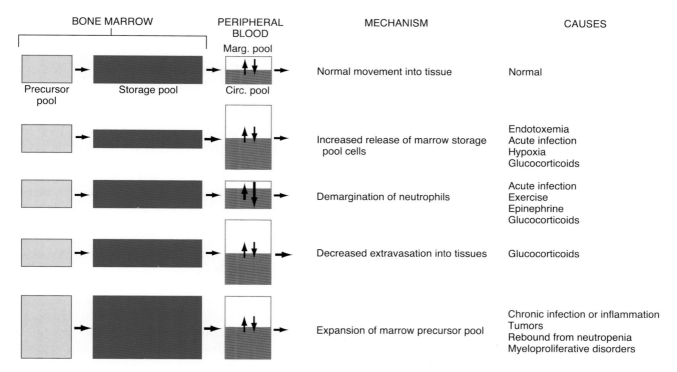

BONE MARROW   PERIPHERAL   MECHANISM   CAUSES
                     BLOOD

Fig. 13-20   Schematic illustration of the mechanism of neutrophilic leukocytosis.
Neutrophils and their precursors are distributed in five pools: a bone marrow precursor pool,
which includes progenitor cells and more committed, mitotically active precursors; a bone
marrow storage pool, consisting of mitotically inactive mature and slightly immature neutrophils
(band forms); a peripheral blood marginating pool (*Marg. pool*); a peripheral blood circulating
pool (*Circ. pool*); and a tissue pool. The relative size of each pool is represented by the size of
its corresponding box. The peripheral blood neutrophil count measures only the circulating
peripheral blood pool, which can be enlarged by increased release of cells from the marrow
storage pool, increased demargination, diminished extravasation into tissue, or expansion of
the marrow precursor cell pool. (*Modified from Finch SC:* Hematology, *ed 3, New York, 1983, McGraw-Hill.*)

right-to-left shunting) or in rare cases an Epo-secreting
tumor (inappropriate secondary erythrocytosis).
Polycythemia vera is diagnosed based on a marked
increase in red cell mass (hematocrit in normally
hydrated dogs from 65% to >80%), absence of hypoxemia,
absence of other tumors, and normal or decreased concentration of plasma erythropoietin concentration.
Absolute erythrocytosis, whether primary or secondary,
causes increased viscosity of the blood and resulting
impairment of blood flow and distention of the
microvasculature. Affected individuals are at increased
risk of tissue hypoxia and thrombosis or hemorrhage.
Related clinical signs (hyperviscosity syndrome) may
include erythematous mucous membranes and prolonged capillary refill time, prominent scleral vessels,
evidence of thrombosis or hemorrhage, and secondary
signs (e.g., neurologic and cardiovascular) related to
specific organ systems affected.

Neutrophilia.   Neutrophilia occurs in response
to a number of different stimuli, none of which are

mutually exclusive. Major mechanisms of neutrophilia
are shown in Fig. 13-20. Understanding the CBC findings characteristic of these responses is an important
part of clinical veterinary medicine. Inflammation can
result in neutropenia, as discussed earlier, or neutrophilia, as will be discussed next. However, before
moving on to a discussion of inflammatory neutrophilia
and the so-called left shift, it is important to mention
two other common causes of neutrophilia.

Glucocorticoid excess, either because of endogenous production or exogenous administration,
results in a CBC pattern known as the "stress leukogram," characterized by the following: mature neutrophilia (i.e., increased concentration of segmented
neutrophils), lymphopenia, and, especially in dogs,
monocytosis. Eosinopenia is another feature of the
stress leukogram, although in many situations this
is inapparent because the normal reference values for
eosinophils are so low (in some laboratories, the lower
reference value is zero). Mechanisms contributing to

glucocorticoid-mediated neutrophilia include the following:

- Increased release of mature neutrophils from the bone marrow storage pool
- Decreased margination of neutrophils within the vasculature, with a resulting increase in the circulating pool
- Decreased migration of neutrophils from the blood stream into tissues

The magnitude of neutrophilia tends to be species dependent, with dogs having the most pronounced response (up to 35,000 cells/μL) and, in decreasing order of responsiveness, cats (30,000 cells/μL), horses (20,000 cells/μL), and cows (15,000 cells/μL) having less marked responses. With long-term glucocorticoid excess, neutrophil numbers tend to normalize, whereas lymphopenia persists.

Epinephrine release results in a different pattern, known as "physiologic leukocytosis," characterized by mature neutrophilia (like the glucocorticoid response) and lymphocytosis (unlike the glucocorticoid response). This phenomenon is short lived (<1 hour). Neutrophilia occurs primarily because of a shift of cells from the marginated to the circulating pool. Physiologic leukocytosis is common in cats (especially when they are highly stressed during blood collection) and horses, less common in cattle, and uncommon in dogs.

Of course, neutrophilia may also indicate inflammation, and inflammatory stimuli of varying magnitude and duration produce different patterns of neutrophilia. A classic hematologic finding in patients with increased demand for neutrophils is the presence of immature forms in the blood, known as a "left shift." Not all inflammatory responses have a left shift, but the presence of a left shift almost always signifies active demand for neutrophils in the tissue. The magnitude of a left shift is assessed by the number of immature cells and their degree of immaturity. The mildest form is characterized by increased numbers of band neutrophils, the immediate predecessor to the segmented neutrophil normally found in circulation, with increasingly severe forms involving progressively immature predecessors. A left shift is considered orderly if the number of immature neutrophils in circulation decreases as they become progressively immature. The term "degenerative left shift" is sometimes used to describe cases where the number of immature forms exceeds the number of segmented neutrophils. As with glucocorticoid-mediated neutrophilia, the typical magnitude of neutrophilia due to inflammation varies by species, with dogs having the most pronounced response.

Marked neutrophilia may also occur because of an inherited condition known as leukocyte adhesion deficiency (LAD), in which leukocytes lack normal expression of an adhesion molecule required for migration from the blood stream into the tissue. This condition is described further in the section on specific diseases.

It might be useful to think of neutrophil kinetics in terms of a producer-consumer model in which the bone marrow is the factory, and the tissues (where the neutrophils eventually go) are the customers. The bone marrow storage pool is the factory inventory, the neutrophils in the blood stream are in delivery to the customer. Within the blood vessels, circulating neutrophils are on the highway, with marginated neutrophils temporarily pulled off to the side of the road. During health, there is an even flow of neutrophils from the factory to the customer. Thus the system is in steady state, and neutrophil numbers remain relatively constant and within the normal range. However, disease states may perturb this system at multiple levels. Decreased granulopoiesis is analogous to a factory working below normal production level. Ineffective granulopoiesis is analogous to goods being damaged during manufacturing and never leaving the factory. A left shift is analogous to the factory meeting increased customer demand by shipping out unfinished goods. Cases of persistent, established inflammation are characterized by bone marrow granulocytic hyperplasia and mature neutrophilia, analogous to a factory that has had time to adjust to increased demand and is meeting it more efficiently by increasing its output.

Eosinophilia/basophilia. Eosinophilia and, less commonly, basophilia (which, when present, often occurs in tandem with eosinophilia) may occur in response to parasitism, as part of an allergic response, as a paraneoplastic abnormality (because of production of cytokines by neoplastic cells or other inflammatory cells reacting to the neoplasm), or as an atypical response to nonparasitic infectious disease.

Thrombocytosis. Thrombocytosis, or concentration of platelets in the blood above normal reference values, is a relatively common nonspecific finding in veterinary patients. In the vast majority of cases, thrombocytosis is reactive—a response to another, often apparently unrelated, disease process. Examples of conditions associated with reactive thrombocytosis include inflammatory and infectious diseases, iron deficiency, hemorrhage, endocrinopathies, and neoplasia. Factors that may contribute to reactive thrombocytosis include increased plasma concentration of thrombopoietin, inflammatory cytokines (e.g., IL-6), or catecholamines. Thrombocytosis may also occur as part of a regenerative response in patients recovering from thrombocytopenia, or as a result of redistribution because of splenic contraction (especially in horses) or splenectomy. In these cases, thrombocytosis is transient. In the case of splenectomy, thrombocytosis may be marked, but normalizes after several weeks. Because the body's total platelet mass regulates thrombopoiesis, and a significant portion of the platelet mass is normally in the spleen, it makes sense that splenectomized animals develop thrombocytosis. However, the reason that the number of circulating platelets normalize in these individuals in the weeks after splenectomy is not clear. There is also a rare form of leukemia known as essential thrombocythemia, which is characterized by marked thrombocytosis.

Lymphocytosis.   *Lymphocytosis* refers to an increase in the concentration of lymphocytes in blood circulation. There are numerous causes of lymphocytosis. Young animals normally have higher numbers of lymphocytes than older animals, and normal healthy young animals may have counts that exceed adult reference values. As discussed earlier in the section on neutrophilia, lymphocytosis is also a feature of epinephrine-mediated physiologic leukocytosis, resulting from redistribution of lymphocytes into the blood circulating pool. Epinephrine-mediated lymphocytosis may be more marked than neutrophilia, particularly in cats (lymphocyte counts of >20,000/μL are not uncommon). Antigenic stimulation may result in lymphocytosis, even in rare cases in marked lymphocytosis (up to approximately 30,000 cells/μL in dogs, and 40,000/μL in cats): however, this is not usually the case, even when there is clear evidence of increased immunologic activity in lymphoid tissues. In cases of antigenic stimulation, it is common for a minority of lymphocytes to have a "reactive" morphology—larger in size than small, mature lymphocytes, and with more abundant, deeply basophilic cytoplasm and incompletely condensed chromatin (Fig. 13-21). Just as glucocorticoid excess can cause lymphopenia, glucocorticoid deficiency (hypoadrenocorticism) can cause lymphocytosis, or lack of lymphopenia under conditions of stress that typically result in glucocorticoid-mediated lymphopenia.

A condition known as persistent lymphocytosis (PL) occurs in approximately 30% of cattle infected with the bovine leukemia virus (BLV). The condition is defined as an increase in the blood concentration of lymphocytes above the reference interval for at least 3 months. This form of lymphocytosis is a nonneoplastic proliferation (hyperplasia) of B lymphocytes. In the absence of other disease, cattle with PL are asymptomatic. However, cattle infected with BLV, especially those animals with PL, are at increased risk to develop B-lymphocyte lymphoma. (BLV and lymphoma in cattle are discussed in more detail later in this chapter in the section on hematopoietic neoplasia.) As in most other forms of benign lymphocytosis, the morphology of most lymphocytes is within normal limits in cattle with PL.

ABNORMAL STRUCTURE OR FUNCTION IN RESPONSE TO INJURY

The preceding section focused on abnormalities in the number of blood cells. There are also various acquired and inherited conditions involving abnormal structure or function of hematopoietic cells or components of hemostasis. Primary disorders of blood cells and hemostasis are discussed later in the chapter in the section on specific diseases. However, abnormal structure or function may reflect disease and cause it. For example, morphologic abnormalities detected on routine microscopic examination of blood smears may provide important clues about underlying disease processes. Poikilocytosis is a broad term referring to the

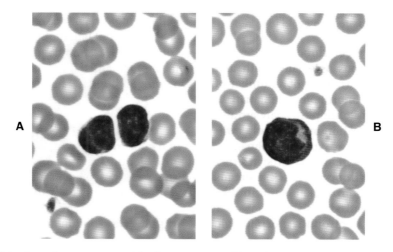

Fig. 13-21   Lymphocytes, canine blood smear. A, Small lymphocytes, the predominant type of lymphocyte in the blood under normal conditions. **B,** A reactive lymphocyte, characterized by mildly increased size and an increased amount of basophilic cytoplasm, from a recently vaccinated 16-week-old dog. Wright's stain. (**A** and **B,** *Courtesy Dr. M.M. Fry, College of Veterinary Medicine, University of Tennessee.*)

Monocyte-macrophage system

The spleen is a major site of cells of the monocyte-macrophage system, and these are responsible for "filtering" the blood through phagocytosis of bacteria, immune complexes, and altered cells, such as senescent erythrocytes and those containing hemotropic parasites (e.g., *Babesia*). Thus the spleen is able to mount a very strong response to blood-borne pathogens. In immunized rabbits injected intravenously with pneumococci, the blood was cleared of 98% of those bacteria within 15 minutes, and 100% of an inoculum of 1 billion bacteria was removed from the blood within an hour. Also the spleen removed 10 times the number of bacteria per gram as the liver. When 1 billion pneumococci per pound of body weight were injected into the splenic artery of a dog over a 5-minute period, all bacteria were removed from the blood in 65 minutes. After splenectomy, blood-borne organisms multiply rapidly and are disseminated widely in the body. Also it has been shown that the phagocytic function of the spleen is critical in the control of plasmodium and *Babesia* in human beings, and the same is true of hemotropic parasites in animals, for example in babesiosis in cattle. To facilitate filtering, all of the blood in the body passes through the spleen at least once in a day.

Sometimes the number of pathogenic bacteria arriving via the circulation at the spleen can be so large that it exceeds its capacity to overcome them immediately. The result will be abscesses or granulomas, depending on the microorganism, usually abscesses in response to bacteria, and granulomas in response to fungi and those bacteria that are intracellular facultative pathogens of macrophages (e.g., *Mycobacterium bovis*).

Lymphoid component of the spleen

The spleen is also a secondary lymphoid organ, the site of immune responses. The response of the white pulp (PALS and splenic follicles) is either hyperplasia or atrophy. Hyperplasia occurs in response to antigenic stimuli and results in the formation of antibodies, which are released into the efferent lymph and blood where they are available to combat hematogenously borne agents, including those arriving in the spleen. Atrophy occurs in response to lack of antigenic stimulation, toxins, antineoplastic chemotherapeutic agents, viruses, radiation, malnutrition, age, and wasting/cachectic diseases.

Vascular component of the spleen

Because of the contractility of the splenic capsule and trabeculae in the spleens of domestic animals, the spleen may either expand to store blood, or contract and expel the "reserve" of blood. Thus they may be either grossly enlarged and congested or small with a wrinkled surface and a dry parenchyma (see Uniform Splenomegaly and Small Spleens).

Lymph nodes

Like the spleen, lymph nodes contain elements of the monocyte-macrophage system and the lymphoid system, and their responses are similar (Box 13-6). Cells of the monocyte-macrophage system are the first line of defense against noxious agents. As most of these agents arrive in the afferent lymph, the sinus macrophages (histiocytes) are the first to respond. This is evidenced by an increase in their number (so-called sinus histiocytosis) in the subcapsular, trabecular, and medullary sinuses (Fig. 13-23). Additional inflammatory cells (e.g., neutrophils and monocytes) arrive in the blood and migrate to the parenchyma or into the sinuses.

Also, antigens from incoming material will be presented to cells of the germinal centers, which will produce immunoblasts that migrate to the medullary cords, mature into plasma cells, and secrete a specific antibody. The antibody will leave the lymph node through the efferent lymphatics, enter the blood circulation as a plasma protein, and be recirculated to the lymph node.

To understand the response of a lymph node, it is helpful to consider how molecules and cells arrive. This is accomplished in one of two ways: in the incoming lymph delivered by the afferent lymphatics to the subscapular sinus or via the arterial blood supply. T lymphocytes arrive by the latter route and migrate out of the high endothelial venules into the T-lymphocyte areas adjacent to the follicle (see Chapter 3). Particles and molecules in the lymph arriving at the lymph node enter the subcapsular sinus. Here hydrostatic pressure is low and particles tend to settle, facilitating phagocytosis by the sinus macrophages. Recent work has indicated that the pathway of particles and molecules whose diameters are greater than approximately 7 nm is different from that of molecules smaller than this. Larger molecules and particles flow from the

---

Box 13-6

Response of the Lymph Node to Injury

HYPERPLASTIC CHANGES

Cells of the monocyte macrophage system—sinus histiocytosis
Lymphoid tissue—hyperplasia with the production of antibody, immediate cell-mediated immunity

ATROPHIC CHANGES

Lymphoid atrophy

INFLAMMATION

Acute—microabscess and abscess formation
Chronic—abscesses and granulomas

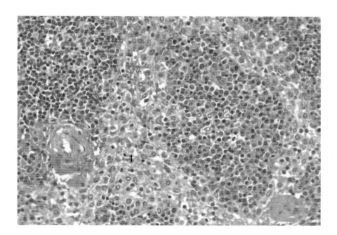

Fig. 13-23 Sinus histiocytosis, lymph node, medulla, dog. The sinuses (1) are filled with mostly macrophages and a few scattered neutrophils (small dark nuclei). Most of the macrophages are derived from the perisinusoidal macrophages, but some may arrive via the afferent lymphatics. The medullary cords (2) are filled with lymphocytes and plasma cells. Plasma cell precursors are formed in the germinal centers, mature into plasma cells, and migrate to the medullary cords. Thus the presence of large numbers of plasma cells in the medullary cords is indicative of ongoing production of antibody from an antigenic stimulus. *(Courtesy Dr. M.D. McGavin, College of Veterinary Medicine, University of Tennessee.)*

Box **13-7**

Response of Lymphoid Nodule to Injury

LYMPHOID ATROPHY

Viral Infections
Malnutrition
Cachexia
Aging
Antineoplastic chemotherapeutic drugs
Toxins
Irradiation

LYMPHOID HYPERPLASIA

Antigenic stimulus

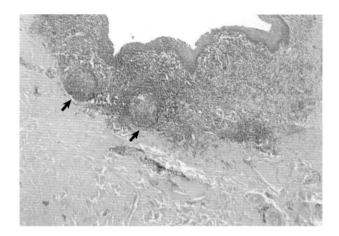

Fig. 13-24 Follicular lymphoid hyperplasia, conjunctiva, lymphoid nodules, cow. The diffuse lymphoid tissue has increased in size, and there are two follicles with germinal centers (*arrows*). This reaction is a frequent response to conjunctivitis from irritants and bacteria. H&E stain. *(Courtesy Dr. M.D. McGavin, College of Veterinary Medicine, University of Tennessee.)*

subcapsular into the trabecular sinuses and then into the medullary sinuses, where particles and bacteria are phagocytosed by the sinus histiocytes. This is well illustrated by the concentration of carbon in the medulla of the tracheobronchial lymph nodes of animals with anthracosis.

Lymph-borne soluble factors, such as chemokines, penetrate the floor of the subcapsular sinus and are carried along reticular fibers to the high endothelial venules, which is the site of migration of T lymphocytes into the cortex, thus bringing these molecules into close association with T lymphocytes and facilitating the production of specific antibodies from B lymphocytes.

LYMPHOID NODULES

The response of lymphoid nodules (Box 13-7) is similar to that of splenic and lymph node follicles. Thus with antigenic stimulation, there will be follicular hyperplasia, activation of germinal centers, and increased production of antibodies. The BALT can become markedly hyperplastic in chronic infections as in *Dictyocaulus* bronchitis or bronchiolitis in cattle, sheep, and goats; *Metastrongylus* bronchitis or bronchiolitis in pigs; and *Mycoplasma* bronchiolitis in calves. Hyperplastic lymphoid nodules can be so enlarged that they become grossly visible as white plaques or nodules (in the conjunctiva of the eyelids and the third

eyelid as in chronic conjunctivitis [Fig. 13-24] and in the pharyngeal mucosa in chronic pharyngitis). Presumably the enlargement of these lymph nodules from follicular hyperplasia is a reflection of the chronicity of the disease.

Atrophy of lymphoid tissues has the same causes as those affecting lymph nodes. These include lack of antigenic stimulus, cachexia, malnutrition, aging, and viral infections. The microscopic lesions of BVD infection of Peyer's patches are distinctive and consist of lysis of the cells of the lymphoid follicles.

PORTALS OF ENTRY

Portals of entry are summarized in Box 13-8.

Box 13-8

Portals of Entry into Bone Marrow and Lymphatic Organs

BONE MARROW
Hematogenously
Direct penetration (trauma)

THYMUS
Hematogenously

SPLEEN
Hematogenously
Direct penetration—rare

LYMPH NODE
Via afferent lymphatics
Hematogenously

LYMPHOID NODULE
Hematogenously
In the intestine, via M cells and dendritic cells to
    Peyer's patches

BONE MARROW AND BLOOD CELLS

Invading cells or microorganism gain access to the bone marrow or blood circulation either hematogenously or by trauma. Trauma may be as obvious as a gaping wound or as subtle as the bite of an insect.

LYMPHATIC SYSTEM
THYMUS

Toxic agents, such as aflatoxins and viruses, enter the thymus hematogenously.

SPLEEN

Noxious agents such as bacteria enter the spleen by two routes: hematogenously or by direct penetration. The spleen has no afferent lymphatics, and so this is not a possible route of entry of infection. Direct penetration is extremely rare. The capsule is thick, and thus inflammation from an adjacent peritonitis is unlikely to penetrate it. However, foreign bodies occasionally do. This is seen as a sequela to traumatic reticulitis in cattle, where a foreign body, usually a nail or wire is extruded through the left caudal reticulum wall by its contraction and enters the visceral surface of the ventral extremity of the spleen and often causes a splenic abscess. Most of these extruded foreign bodies usually travel cranially to penetrate the diaphragm and pericardium, causing traumatic reticulopericarditis. In horses, on rare occasions, splenic abscesses can develop secondary to perforation of the gastric wall. This can be caused by

gastric ulcers, *Gasterophilus intestinalis*, or by extension on the granulomatous inflammation around *Habronema* in the wall of the stomach.

LYMPH NODES

Noxious agents, including bacteria, viruses, and antigens, enter the lymph node by two routes: afferent lymphatics and the blood.

Afferent lymphatics

Noxious agents are transported in lymph to the regional lymph node or lymphocenter. Here some of these agents may escape removal by phagocytosis in that lymph node and then be transported in the efferent lymph to the next lymph node in the chain, where they can cause an inflammatory or immunologic response. If they are not removed by any of the lymph nodes in the chain, noxious agents may be eventually transported via the lymphatics to the circulating blood.

Blood

Agents can arrive hematogenously in septicemias and bacteremias. However, most pathogens arrive at lymph nodes via the afferent lymphatics.

Capsule

The lymph node is protected by a thick fibrous capsule, and thus direct penetration by inflammation, trauma, or neoplasms is extremely rare.

LYMPHOID NODULES

Lymphoid nodules also respond to antigens arriving hematogenously, but in many cases the agent or antigens will cross the mucous membrane, for example in chronic inflammation of nasal, oral, bronchial, gastrointestinal, or conjunctival mucous membranes. As described previously, M cells of Peyer's patches can transport infections agents.

METHODS FOR GROSS AND MICROSCOPIC EXAMINATION
BONE MARROW AND BLOOD CELLS

Routine diagnostic testing often provides great insight into disorders of the hematopoietic system. The complete blood count (CBC) is a cornerstone of diagnosis, part of routine evaluation of any sick patient. The CBC includes not only numerical data indicating the concentration of different cell types and hemoglobin in the blood, but also information gleaned from microscopic review of a blood smear, such as cell morphology and the presence of hemoparasites. (Note: Some parasites may be detected within blood cells, such as *Hepatozoon* organisms within circulating neutrophils or monocytes, but they mainly cause disease in other body systems and are therefore not discussed in this chapter.) Learning to evaluate blood smears is a valuable skill for any practicing veterinarian. The CBC also reports plasma protein concentration as measured with a refractometer. It is important to remember that changes in hydration status, and in the distribution of body fluids between the vascular and extravascular compartments, affect the concentration of both cells and proteins in the blood.

OTHER TESTS USED TO EVALUATE THE HEMATOPOIETIC SYSTEM

Other tests include the following:

- Bone marrow examination (aspiration or core biopsy). This is usually done to assess hematopoiesis when a patient has unexplained cytopenia(s) or atypical cells in circulation but also to look for neoplasia or, occasionally, infection. Preferred sites for collecting bone marrow samples are: in horses, the sternum; in cattle, the proximal ribs; and in dogs and cats, the proximal humerus, iliac crest, or proximal femur. Normal hematopoietic cellularity of the marrow is age-dependent (recall that the amount of fat increases with age). Cytologic evaluation of a Wright's-stained, air-dried smear of a bone marrow aspirate is the preferred method for evaluating cellular detail and in most cases provides a good estimate of overall marrow cellularity. Histopathologic evaluation of a hematoxylin and eosin (H&E) stained core biopsy is the most reliable way to assess marrow cellularity, because tissue architecture is preserved. In either case, bone marrow findings can only be interpreted fully along with a concurrent CBC. (Note: Hematopoietic tissue is highly susceptible to autolysis. This is more of a limitation with regard to cytology than histology. Postmortem samples are often not suitable for cytologic interpretation unless collected immediately [i.e., within minutes after death].) Bone marrow examination yields information about the production of cells of specific lineages (i.e., erythropoiesis, granulopoiesis, and thrombopoiesis) in addition to the overall cellularity of the marrow. Increased production is evident as hyperplasia; decreased production as hypoplasia. The proportion of different cell types varies somewhat by species, but as a rule there are similar numbers of erythroid and myeloid (granulocytic and monocytic) nucleated cells, and much higher numbers of late-stage than early-stage cells. The amount of iron in the marrow can also be estimated by microscopic examination. Hemosiderin, a water-insoluble form of storage iron (less readily accessible than ferritin, which is soluble), is found mainly in macrophages in the marrow, spleen, and liver, and appears as coarse yellow-brown granular material with routine stains. Staining the sample with an iron-specific stain, such as Prussian blue, can make it easier to assess marrow iron stores. Cats differ from other species in that their marrow normally does not contain stainable iron.

- Aspiration cytology and/or histopathology of other organs (e.g., to assess extramedullary hematopoiesis, increased destruction of erythrocytes, neoplasia, or infection). Evaluation of lymph nodes and spleen is discussed later.

- Tests to detect an autoantibody bound to the cell surface. The Coombs' test, or direct antiglobulin test, is the standard assay for immune-mediated hemolytic anemia. Flow cytometry and immunofluorescent antibody tests may also be used to detect autoantibody bound to erythrocytes or other cells.

- Immunophenotyping to identify cells based on expression of characteristic molecules (markers). Immunophenotyping may be done by immunohistochemistry, immunocytochemistry, or flow cytometry.

- Polymerase chain reaction (PCR) assays for infectious agents or clonal lymphocyte proliferations.

HEMOSTASIS

The CBC provides basic information about platelets, including numeric values for platelet concentration and mean platelet volume (MPV), subjective assessment of platelet morphology (size, shape, and granularity), and a rough estimation of platelet numbers based on examination of a blood smear. Some laboratories measure reticulated platelets (platelets recently released from the bone marrow), although this test is mostly used in the research setting at present. Increased MPV and increased numbers of reticulated platelets tend to indicate increased thrombopoiesis. Bone marrow examination is indicated with any unexplained cytopenia, including thrombocytopenia, to evaluate production.

Tests to evaluate the components of the hemostatic process are described and listed in Appendix 13-1 at the end of this chapter.

LYMPHATIC SYSTEM
THYMUS

Because the thymus involutes after sexual maturity, evaluating whether it is smaller than normal is difficult, unless the change is extreme or age-matched control animals are available. Before sexual maturity, the thymus is easily identified as a lobular organ, white to gray with a thin capsule. After sexual maturity, the gland is often indistinguishable from adipose connective tissue within the cranial mediastinum. An extremely small thymus in a neonatal animal should be considered abnormal and an indicator of a possible underlying primary or acquired immunodeficiency. Enlargement of the thymus is almost always due to tumors. The cut surface should be examined for tumors and hematomas.

Spleen

Spleens can be enlarged (splenomegaly), normal in size, or small. They can be uniform in shape or have a "lumpy-bumpy" to nodular surface. The appearance of the surface of the spleen varies among species of domestic animals, depending on the thickness of the capsule and consequently the visibility of the red pulp through it. In the pig, dog, and cat, the capsule is thin, and the red color of the red pulp is visible. The splenic capsules of horses and ruminants are thicker and appear gray because the color of the red pulp may not be visible through the capsule. However, if the capsule has thick and thin areas, it may be mottled gray and red.

The tenseness of the capsule of normal and diseased spleens depends on how much the splenic parenchyma is distended by stored blood or infiltrating inflammatory cells or neoplasms. Spleens devoid of stored blood can have a wrinkled surface. The spleens of ruminants have prominent trabeculae, which appear as gray bands in the red pulp. The ventral extremity of the canine spleen is expanded and is thus wider than the remainder of the spleen, which has approximately parallel sides. The parietal surface of the spleen is smooth, but the visceral surface has a longitudinal ridge, which is the hilus where arteries and veins enter and exit the spleen.

At necropsy, the pathologist has to evaluate the spleen based on whether there is splenomegaly, whether this is uniform or nodular, and whether the consistency is congested (bloody) or firm (meaty). The diseases associated with splenomegaly will be discussed using those criteria. The most common causes of splenomegaly are one or more of the following: storage of blood, increase in the cells of the monocyte-macrophage system, lymphoid hyperplasia, inflammation, or neoplasia. Occasionally, it can be due to stored material, such as occurs in lysosomal storage diseases or from extracellular deposits, such as amyloid.

Uniformly enlarged spleens (splenomegaly)

There are two basic types of splenomegaly: congestive and not congestive. The cut surface of severely congested spleens may be red to bluish-black and exude blood (congested or "bloody" spleens). Enlarged spleens that are not congested but firm are often called "meaty" because of their firmness and texture. Little blood oozes from their cut surfaces, and the color of this surface depends of how much of the normal red pulp has been replaced by neoplastic cells, inflammatory cells, or stored material. Table 13-3 lists the common causes of uniform splenomegaly.

Nodular spleens with or without splenomegaly

Nodular disorders are characterized by a spleen that has nodules that are randomly distributed, may be discrete or coalescent, are raised above the splenic surface, bulge from the cut surface, and have a variety of appearances and colors based on the cause of the lesion. Many of the disease processes causing a nodular splenomegaly are similar to those causing a uniform splenomegaly. Nodules can be abscesses, granulomas, hematomas, hyperplastic foci of lymphocytes, hematopoietic cells, or primary or metastatic neoplasms.

Lymph Nodes

Lymph nodes should be dissected free of fat and connective tissue. Gross examination includes determining the size and whether the capsule is intact (some very highly infiltrative neoplasms extend beyond the capsule) and an evaluation of the cut surface. For the latter, the visibility of the cortex and medulla, any lack of normal architecture, and the colors should be determined. Normal architecture can be completely or partially obliterated by tumor (e.g., lymphoma [lymphosarcoma]) or by diffuse granulomatous inflammation (e.g., in blastomycosis, histoplasmosis, or cryptococcosis). The cortex can be enlarged in lymphoid hyperplasia, and in extreme follicular lymphoid hyperplasia, follicles may be visible as nodules 1 to 2 mm in diameter. Because of the notable phagocytic activity of the medullary sinus macrophages, the medulla can be colored by phagocytosed material (e.g., black from carbon in anthracosis [tracheobronchial lymph nodes] and brown from hemosiderin as a result of draining a hemorrhagic area or a site of an intramuscular iron injection).

The cut surface can be red from acute hyperemia, as in acute lymphadenitis, or the sinuses can be red from blood drained from a hemorrhagic or inflamed area. Also, the cut surface can be excessively wet when the lymph node drains an edematous area.

It is essential that enlarged lymph nodes be examined microscopically. In the live animal, this is easily accomplished by cytologic evaluation of superficial lymph nodes. Cells are collected into a 22- to 25-gauge needle with gentle aspiration using a 6- or 12-mL syringe or by a nonsuction "pincushion" technique, and then they are gently expelled onto glass slides. The fragility of lymphocytes necessitates gentle spreading to prevent cellular distortion. Aspirates are stained with a Romanowsky's stain, such as Wright's, Wright-Giemsa, or Diff-Quik. The ease of lymph node sampling and staining provides veterinary clinicians with the opportunity to become proficient in the evaluation of lymph node cytology. Also, microorganisms, such as bacteria (e.g., streptococci, corynebacteria, and rhodococci), fungi (e.g., blastomyces and cryptococci), rickettsia (e.g., *Neorickettsia helmintheca*, the agent of salmon poisoning disease), and protozoa (e.g., leishmania) can be detected.

Table **13-3**   **Common Causes of Uniform Splenomegaly in Domestic Animals**

Animal	Congestive (Bloody) Spleen	Firm (Meaty) Spleen
Horse	Septicemia 　Anthrax 　Salmonellosis (peracute) Hemolytic disease 　EIA (acute)	Septicemia 　Salmonellosis Hemolytic diseases 　EIA 　Immune-mediated hemolytic anemia Neoplasms 　Lymphoma 　Metastatic neoplasms
Cattle and sheep	Septicemias 　Anthrax 　Salmonellosis (acute) Hemolytic disease 　Babesiosis (acute)	Septicemia 　Salmonellosis Hemolytic diseases 　Babesiosis (subacute) 　Anaplasmosis 　Trypanosomiasis 　Hemotropic mycoplasmosis Neoplasm 　Lymphoma
Pig	Septicemia 　Salmonellosis (peracute) Splenic torsion	Septicemias 　Salmonellosis 　Erysipelas Hemolytic disease 　Hemotropic mycoplasmosis Neoplasm 　Lymphoma
Dog and cats	Barbiturate euthanasia or anesthesia Gastric torsion Neoplasms 　Hemangioma (nodular) 　Hemangiosarcoma (nodular)	Hemolytic disease 　Immune-mediated hemolytic anemia Hematopoietic neoplasia 　Mast cell neoplasia (cat) 　Lymphoma 　Histiocytic sarcoma Granulomatous disease 　Histoplasmosis Lymphoid hyperplasia (nodular) Amyloidosis

EIA, Equine infectious anemia.

Aspirates provide excellent cellular detail, but for the study of architectural derangements, removal of the node for histologic evaluation is necessary. The surgeon must handle lymph nodes carefully to minimize artifacts. Any compression (e.g., squeezing with forceps) will cause artifacts and usually damage the nuclei. A portion of one end of the node should be removed and used to prepare impression smears. The remainder of the node should be placed in fixative fluid, with the capsule intact, for 1 hour. This period of fixation hardens the node and prevents artifactual bulging of the tissue from the cut surface when the lymph node is sliced. This is usually a problem when lymph nodes are cut without prior fixation. The lymph node, if large, should then be sliced transversely into parallel 2- to 3-mm thick sections to ensure penetration of the fixative fluid.

Cross sections of lymph node are preferred because they are usually sufficiently small to allow a full cross section, including both the cortex and medulla to fit onto a microscope slide. The exception is the porcine lymph node with its different anatomic arrangement. Because the location and amount of "cortical" and "medullary" matter varies with the direction of the cut, a longitudinal plane section is recommended as being the most representative. At a minimum, all lymph nodes should be incised at least once before being placed in a fixative; otherwise the time taken to penetrate the capsule will delay fixation.

Size of lymph nodes

Lymph nodes can be enlarged as a consequence of inflammatory (lymphadenitis) or noninflammatory (lymphadenopathy) processes. Clinically, lymph node enlargement can occur in several forms. First, all lymph nodes may be enlarged (systemic and/or generalized enlargement). This form of lymph node enlargement is generally attributed to systemic infectious, inflammatory, or neoplastic processes. If the regional lymph node (e.g., a lymph node draining one of the limbs or one side of the oral cavity) is enlarged, then infectious, inflammatory, or neoplastic processes must be considered in the area drained by that node. Finally, enlargement of the mesenteric lymph nodes or GALT suggests that the infectious, inflammatory, or neoplastic process originates within the gut.

The gross and histologic appearances of mesenteric lymph nodes are somewhat different from those of unstimulated peripheral lymph nodes. The mesenteric lymph nodes are continuously receiving a barrage of antigens and some bacteria via the afferent lymphatics, draining the gastrointestinal tract. This is reflected in their appearance. They are larger and have numerous well-developed lymphoid follicles (follicular lymphoid hyperplasia) with active germinal centers. Often the sinuses contain histiocytes (sinus histiocytosis), presumably in response to the need to phagocytose incoming material.

Enlargement of a lymph node is called lymphadenomegaly, although in common parlance it is often called lymphadenopathy. If a node(s) is congenitally small or absent, the condition is called lymph node hypoplasia or lymph node aplasia, respectively.

Enlargement may involve only an isolated lymph node, which is usually the result of a response to inflammatory products, infectious microbes, or neoplasms draining to a regional lymph node. Enlargement may also involve multiple nodes of a chain because infection or metastases spread up the lymphatics, from one lymph node to the next. Sometimes enlargement may be confined to superficial lymph nodes and on another occasion to visceral lymph nodes. Thus it is important that the clinician or prosector be familiar with the area drained by specific lymph nodes; for example, all lymph from the head drains to the medial retropharyngeal lymph nodes, and lymph from the foreleg drains to either the axillary or superficial cervical (prescapular) lymph node.

DISEASES OF THE BONE MARROW, BLOOD CELLS, AND LYMPHATIC SYSTEM

BONE MARROW AND BLOOD CELLS

This section focuses on diseases of bone marrow and blood cells. Some aspects of diseases covered in this section are discussed further in the Lymphatic System section later in the chapter.

STEM CELL DISORDERS AND PANCYTOPENIC DISORDERS
APLASTIC ANEMIA

Aplastic anemia is a rare condition characterized by aplasia or severe hypoplasia of all hematopoietic lineages in the bone marrow and resulting pancytopenia. The term is something of a misnomer because affected cells are not limited to the erythroid lineage (see the later discussion of pure red cell aplasia, with disorders of erythrocytes). Aplastic anemia is also known more accurately as aplastic pancytopenia. Destruction of hematopoietic stem cells or progenitor cells is recognized as a cause of the condition. Other proposed mechanisms include disruption of normal stem cell function because of mutation or perturbation of the hematopoietic microenvironment.

Many of the conditions reported to cause aplastic anemia in domestic animals do so only rarely, or idiosyncratically, and more frequently cause other hematologic or nonhematologic abnormalities. A partial list of reported causes of aplastic anemia in domestic animals includes the following:

- Chemical agents
  - Antimicrobial agents (dogs, cats)
  - Chemotherapeutic agents (dogs, cats)
  - Phenylbutazone (horses, dogs)
  - Bracken fern (cattle, sheep)
  - Estrogen (dogs)
  - Trichloroethylene (cattle, sheep)
  - Aflatoxin B_1 (horses, cattle, dogs, pigs)
- Infectious agents
  - Ehrlichiosis (dogs, cats)
  - Parvovirus (dogs, cats)
  - Feline leukemia virus (cats)
  - Feline immunodeficiency virus (cats)
  - Equine infectious anemia (horses)
- Idiopathic (horses, cattle, dogs, cats)

Aplastic anemia occurs in both acute and chronic forms. Most of the chemical causes result in acute disease. As discussed in the earlier section on mechanisms of disease, severe neutropenia typically develops within 1 week of an acute insult to the bone marrow, after the bone marrow storage pool is depleted, and severe thrombocytopenia in the second week. The development of anemia is more variable, depending in part on how rapidly the marrow recovers from the insult, and on the RBC life span of the particular species. Severe neutropenia and thrombocytopenia predispose affected individuals to infection and hemorrhage, respectively. In addition to aplasia, pathologic bone marrow findings in animals with aplastic anemia may include evidence of necrosis, degeneration of hematopoietic cells, and an increase in phagocytic macrophages. Fig. 13-25 shows bone marrow aspirates from a dog with acute 5-fluorouracil-induced pancytopenia, before and during recovery.

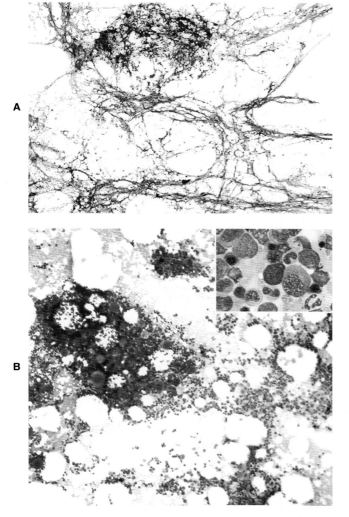

Fig. 13-25   Aplastic anemia, canine bone marrow. A, Bone marrow aspirate from a dog 8 days after ingestion of a toxic dose of 5-fluorouracil showing stromal cells but a lack of developing blood cells. **B,** Bone marrow aspirate from the same dog one week later, after resumption of hematopoiesis. *Inset,* Higher magnification of Fig. 13-25, *B* shows early- and late-stage erythroid and granulocytic precursors. Wright's stain. (**A, B,** and *Inset, Courtesy Dr. M.M. Fry, College of Veterinary Medicine, University of Tennessee.*)

Cyclic Hematopoiesis

Cyclic hematopoiesis (CH) is an inherited disorder of pluripotent hematopoietic stem cells, recognized in dogs and people. In dogs, the condition has an autosomal recessive inheritance pattern and is associated with dilute hair coat color. In dogs, CH (also known as lethal gray collie disease) is characterized by predictable fluctuations in concentrations of blood cells that occur in 14-day cycles. The pattern is cyclic marked neutropenia and in a different phase, cyclic reticulocytosis, monocytosis, and thrombocytosis. Production of key cytokines

involved in regulation of hematopoiesis is also cyclic. The specific lesion in CH is believed to involve defective intracellular signaling, but remains to be explained on the molecular level. Neutropenia predisposes affected animals to infection, and many die of infectious causes. Other related clinical manifestations include bleeding tendency, attributable at least in part to defective platelet function, and systemic amyloidosis, which occurs because of cyclic increases in concentration of acute phase proteins during phases of monocytosis.

DISORDERS OF ERYTHROCYTES

This section describes specific erythrocyte disorders and assumes an understanding of the basic mechanisms of anemia, erythrocytosis, and poikilocytosis, discussed previously. Hemorrhage is a common and important cause of anemia in veterinary species, but the list of potential causes of hemorrhage is almost limitless, including all the various forms of trauma and neoplasia. This chapter does not endeavor to cover them, except for commonly recognized disorders of hemostasis, which are discussed in a later section.

Immune-Mediated Disorders
Immune-mediated hemolytic anemia

Immune-mediated hemolytic anemia (IMHA) is a condition characterized by increased destruction of erythrocytes because of binding of immunoglobulin to cell surface antigens. It is a common, life-threatening condition in dogs and also has been described in horses, cattle, and cats. Although the clinical picture of IMHA is variable, it typically has an acute onset and causes severe anemia. Some studies have shown that certain dog breeds (cocker spaniels and others) are predisposed to develop IMHA, suggesting the possibility of a genetic component, and the disease is more common in young to middle-aged female dogs. In most cases the reactive antibody is IgG, and hemolysis is extravascular (i.e., RBCs with bound antibody are phagocytosed by macrophages, mainly in the spleen). IgM and/or complement proteins may also contribute to IMHA. Complement usually acts as an opsonin (C_3b) that promotes phagocytosis. However, formation of the complement membrane attack complex and resulting intravascular hemolysis is also a recognized mechanism and more likely to occur with IgM autoantibodies. Most immunoglobulins implicated in IMHA are reactive at body temperature (warm hemagglutinins). A smaller portion, usually IgM, are more reactive at lower temperatures and may lead to a condition known as cold hemagglutinin disease—ischemic necrosis at anatomic extremities (e.g., tips of the ears), where cooling of the circulation causes autoagglutination of erythrocytes and occlusion of the microvasculature. Typically, IMHA targets mature erythrocytes and is accompanied by a marked regenerative response. However, as discussed earlier in the chapter, immune-mediated destruction of immature erythroid cells in the bone marrow may also occur, resulting in nonregenerative anemia (ineffective erythropoiesis).

In veterinary medicine, IMHA is usually idiopathic (also called primary IMHA or autoimmune hemolytic anemia), and the specific trigger for the autoimmune reaction is not clear. Factors implicated in secondary IMHA include infection, drug administration, vaccination, neoplasia, and bee sting envenomation. Diagnosis of secondary IMHA is most often based on circumstantial evidence and exclusion of other known causes of hemolytic anemia, rather than on controlled experiments proving a direct causal relationship. Infectious agents affecting blood cells are discussed in more detail later. Drugs or chemicals associated with or suspected of causing IMHA in animals include antibiotics (cephalosporins, penicillin, sulfonamides), levamisole, propylthiouracil, and the insecticide pirimicarb. Most drug-induced IMHA is believed to occur because of drug or drug metabolite interacting with the erythrocyte plasma membrane. Other proposed mechanisms include binding of drug-antibody immune complexes to the erythrocyte membrane, or induction of a true autoantibody directed against an erythrocyte antigen. A case of suspected vaccine-associated IMHA has been reported in a cow. Certain vaccines used in cows have been incriminated in the development of a specific form of IMHA in newborn calves—neonatal isoerythrolysis, which is discussed later. Retrospective studies investigating the relationship between vaccination history and development of IMHA in dogs have yielded conflicting results.

Other common clinical findings in patients with IMHA include hyperbilirubinemia, splenomegaly, pyrexia, and inflammatory neutrophilia. These abnormalities vary in magnitude depending on the severity and duration of disease. Dogs with IMHA are also predisposed to develop hemostatic abnormalities (prolonged coagulation times, decreased plasma AT concentration, increased plasma concentration of FDPs/D-dimer, thrombocytopenia, and DIC). The severity of postmortem lesions in dogs with IMHA, including ischemic necrosis within vital organs (liver, kidney, heart, lung) and the spleen as a result of thromboembolic disease or hypoxia has been shown to correlate with the severity of leukocytosis. Intravascular hemolysis (IVH) plays a relatively insignificant role in most cases of IMHA, but evidence of IVH (hemoglobinemia, hemoglobinuria) is noted occasionally, presumably in those cases in which IgM and complement are major mediators of hemolysis.

Neonatal isoerythrolysis. A form of IMHA whose specific pathogenesis is well understood is neonatal isoerythrolysis (NI), a condition in which a newborn

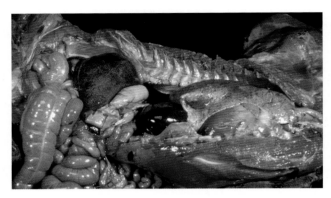

Fig. 13-26 **Neonatal isoerythrolysis, foal.** Note the enlarged spleen (also liver) and icterus. The newborn foal had colostrum-derived maternal antibodies, which reacted against its own erythrocytes. Macrophages in the splenic red pulp remove erythrocytes whose membranes have bound antibody. (*Courtesy College of Veterinary Medicine, University of Illinois.*)

has colostrum-derived maternal antibodies, which react against its own erythrocytes. NI is common in horses (Fig. 13-26) and has been reported in cattle, cats, and some other domestic and wildlife species. In horses, this situation occurs as a result of immunosensitization of the dam from exposure to an incompatible blood type inherited from the stallion (e.g., transplacental exposure to fetal blood during pregnancy or mixing of maternal and fetal blood during parturition). A previously mismatched blood transfusion will produce the same results. Some equine blood groups are more antigenic than others; in particular, types Aa and Qa are very immunogenic in mares. Severely affected foals become lethargic and weak as early as 8 to 10 hours after birth or at any time during the succeeding 4 to 5 days. They have pale, icteric mucous membranes and may have hemoglobinuria. Serum bilirubin concentrations are usually increased, and foals that die during a hemolytic crisis are notably icteric and have splenomegaly. In cattle, NI has been associated with vaccination with whole blood products or products containing erythrocyte membrane fragments. In cats, the recognized form of NI does not depend on prior maternal immunosensitization but on naturally occurring anti-A antibodies in queens with Type B blood. NI has been produced experimentally in dogs, but there are no reports of naturally occurring disease. NI can be prevented by typing the maternal and paternal blood and not allowing neonates from incompatible matings access to the mother's colostrum, or by not allowing animals with strongly incompatible blood types to breed.

Pure red cell aplasia

Pure red cell aplasia (PRCA) is a rare bone marrow disorder characterized by absence of erythropoiesis and severe nonregenerative anemia. Primary and secondary forms of PRCA have been described in dogs and cats. Primary PRCA is apparently caused by immune-mediated destruction of early erythroid progenitor cells, a presumption supported by the response of some patients to immunosuppressive therapy and by the detection of antibodies inhibiting erythroid colony formation in vitro in some dogs. Infection with feline leukemia virus subgroup C is associated with secondary erythroid aplasia in cats, probably because of infection of early stage erythroid precursors. Parvoviral infection has been suggested as a possible cause of secondary PRCA in dogs. Administration of recombinant human erythropoietin (rhEpo) has been identified as a cause of secondary PRCA in dogs, cats, and horses, presumably due to induction of antibodies against rhEpo that cross-react with endogenous erythropoietin. Experimentation with the use of species-specific recombinant erythropoietin has produced mixed results. Dogs treated with recombinant canine Epo have not developed PRCA. However, in experiments reported thus far involving cats treated with recombinant feline Epo, at least some animals have developed PRCA.

INFECTIOUS DISORDERS

Although various types of infections are associated with anemia of chronic disease, as discussed in the section on mechanisms of nonregenerative anemia, there are also a number of infectious agents that cause anemia directly by targeting erythrocytes. This section outlines important specific protozoal, bacterial, and viral causes of anemia in domestic animals.

Protozoal agents

***Babesia* species.** *Babesia* spp. are intraerythrocytic protozoal organisms (piroplasms) spread by arthropods (ticks, biting flies), transplacentally, and by blood transfusions. The apparent higher prevalence of babesiosis in some canine breeds has led to speculation that infection also may be transmitted by dog fighting. *Babesia* spp. cause hemolytic anemia in horses, cattle, dogs, cats, and various nondomesticated animals. *Babesia* organisms are typically classified as large or small form, based on routine light microscopic morphology. Examples of large and small form organisms are shown in Fig. 13-27. *Babesia equi* and *Babesia caballi* infect horses and other equids in tropical and subtropical areas worldwide (*Babesia equi*, which also infects lymphocytes, is not considered a true *Babesia*, but is phylogenetically more closely related to *Theileria* and *Cytauxzoon*). *Babesia bovis* and *Babesia bigemina* (small and large form organisms, respectively) are pathogenic *Babesia* spp. in cattle. These organisms have a worldwide distribution but have been eradicated in North America. Other, less pathogenic *Babesia* spp. may also

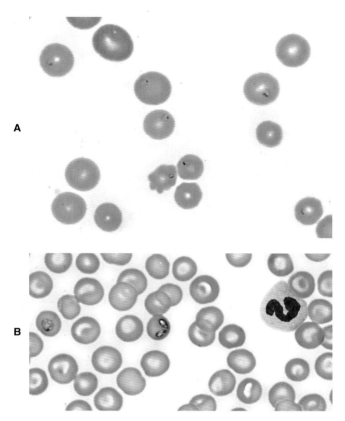

Fig. 13-27 **Babesiosis, canine blood smear. A,** Small form of *Babesia* (consistent with *Babesia gibsoni*). **B,** *Babesia canis* organisms infecting erythrocytes. Wright's stain. (**A** *and* **B,** *Courtesy Dr. M.M. Fry, College of Veterinary Medicine, University of Tennessee.*)

infect cattle. In dogs, the large form *Babesia canis* and at least three small forms, including *Babesia gibsoni* and other as yet unnamed species, cause hemolytic anemia. *Babesia canis* has three subtypes (*canis, rossi,* and *vogeli*). *Babesia canis vogeli*, considered the least pathogenic strain, is the most common one in the United States. In some areas, particularly the southeastern United States, the seroprevalence of *Babesia canis* is high, and many infected dogs are asymptomatic chronic carriers. A number of small form *Babesia* spp. (*Babesia cati, Babesia felis, Babesia herpailuri,* and *Babesia pantherae*) are reported to cause hemolytic anemia in domestic and wild cats in South America, Africa, and India.

Babesiosis may cause both intravascular and extravascular hemolysis, and is also associated with a wide range of other clinical signs. The wide variety of clinical signs is due to variations in pathogenicity of the organisms and susceptibility of the host. Infection with highly virulent strains may cause severe multisystemic disease. In these cases, massive immunostimulation and cytokine release cause circulatory disturbances, which may result in shock, induction of the systemic inflammatory response, and multiple organ dysfunction syndromes. Mechanisms of hemolysis may include direct damage to the erythrocyte by protozoal proteases, immune-mediated destruction, and oxidative damage. In animals with acute disease, signs often include fever, lethargy, pallor, hemoglobinuria, splenomegaly, and icterus. Animals are often thrombocytopenic, presumably due to immune-mediated destruction of platelets. They also may have lymphadenopathy. Less common signs include edema, ascites, signs of central nervous system dysfunction, renal failure, rhabdomyolysis, stomatitis, and gastroenteritis.

Babesia organisms can usually be detected on a routine blood smear in animals with acute disease. Infected erythrocytes may be more prevalent in capillary blood, so blood smears made from samples taken from the pinna of the ear or the nail bed may increase the likelihood of detecting organisms microscopically. Buffy coat smears also have an enriched population of infected RBCs. PCR testing is the most sensitive assay for detecting infection in animals with very low levels of parasitemia. At necropsy, animals dying of the acute disease have notable splenomegaly, jaundice, hemoglobinuria, swollen hemoglobin-stained kidneys, and subepicardial and subendocardial hemorrhages. The cut surface of the enlarged, congested spleen oozes blood. The gallbladder is usually distended with thick bile. A striking feature of *Babesia bovis* infections is congestion of gray matter throughout the brain, which is readily visible compared with the white matter. Parasitized erythrocytes are best visualized on impression smears of the kidney, brain, and skeletal muscle. Microscopic findings in the liver and kidney are typical of a hemolytic crisis and include anemia-induced degeneration and loss of periacinar hepatocytes and cholestasis, and hemoglobinuric nephrosis with degeneration of tubular epithelium. Erythroid hyperplasia is present in the bone marrow. In animals that survive the acute disease, there is hemosiderin accumulation in the liver, kidney, spleen, and bone marrow. In chronic cases, there is hyperplasia of macrophages in the red pulp of the spleen.

Cytauxzoon felis. *Cytauxzoon felis* is a protozoal organism causing severe, often fatal, disease in cats. Cytauxzoonosis in domestic cats is relatively common in the South Central United States, particularly during summer months. Bobcats (*Lynx rufus*), and perhaps other wild felids, are believed to be the reservoir host. They are usually asymptomatic, with persistent parasitemia and transient schizogony. *Cytauxzoon felis* is transmitted by a tick vector, *Dermacentor variabilis*, which is probably essential for infectivity of the organism. Cytauxzoonosis has a schizogenous phase involving macrophages throughout the body (especially liver, spleen, lung, lymph nodes, and bone marrow) that causes systemic illness, and an erythrocytic phase that

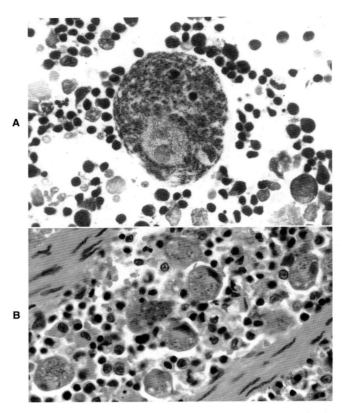

Fig. 13-28 **Cytauxzoonosis, cat. A,** Lymph node aspirate. A large macrophage is laden with schizonts of *Cytauxzoon felis.* Wright's stain. **B,** Splenic macrophages are filled with *Cytauxzoon* organisms. H&E stain. (**A,** *Courtesy Dr. D.F. Edwards, College of Veterinary Medicine, University of Tennessee.* **B,** *Courtesy Dr. A.R. Doster, University of Nebraska; and Noah's Arkive, College of Veterinary Medicine, The University of Georgia.*)

causes anemia of variable severity. Schizont-containing macrophages (Fig. 13-28) enlarge and accumulate within the walls of veins, eventually causing occlusion of the vessels. Merozoites are released and enter erythrocytes. Parasitemia develops relatively late in the course of infection. The signet ring–shaped erythrocytic inclusions (piroplasms) of *Cytauxzoon felis* closely resemble small form *Babesia* (Fig. 13-27, A) and some *Theileria* organisms. Affected cats typically become acutely ill with fever, pallor, and icterus and usually die within 2 to 3 days. For many years, cytauxzoonosis was considered to be almost always fatal. However, a recent report, in which numerous cats from a subregion of the endemic area in the United States survived infection with an organism with greater than 99% homology to *Cytauxzoon felis*, suggests the emergence of a less virulent strain. In affected cats, erythrophagocytosis is also often a prominent finding in tissue with the schizogenous phase.

***Theileria* species.** *Theileria* spp. are tick-borne protozoal organisms that infect many domestic and wild artiodactyls worldwide. Infection is characterized by intralymphocytic schizonts and pleomorphic intraerythrocytic piroplasms (merozoites and trophozoites). The latter stages closely resemble *Cytauxzoon* and small form *Babesia* spp. Recognized theilerial pathogens in cattle include *Theileria parva* (the cause of East Coast fever in Africa), *Theileria annulata* (the cause of tropical theileriosis in the Mediterranean regions, Middle East, and Asia), and *Theileria buffeli*, which has recently been documented as a cause of hemolytic anemia in the United States. Possible mechanisms of anemia in theileriosis include invasion of erythroid precursors by merozoite stages and associated erythroid hypoplasia (as occurs with *Theileria parva* infection), immune-mediated hemolysis, mechanical fragmentation because of vasculitis or microthrombi, enzymatic destruction by proteases, and oxidative damage. Clinical signs in a severely anemic cow infected with *Theileria buffeli* included recumbency, fever, pallor, tachycardia, and lymphadenopathy. Necropsy findings included splenic hemosiderosis, edema of lymph nodes and the subcutis, thoracic and peritoneal effusions, and pneumonia.

Trypanosoma **species.**   Trypanosomes are flagellated protozoa that normally survive and are nonpathogenic in wildlife reservoir hosts. They are transmitted by arthropod vectors. Some *Trypanosoma* spp. are recognized as causing hemolytic anemia in animals in tropical and subtropical regions outside of North America. *Trypanosoma brucei* and *Trypanosoma evansi* affect horses. *Trypanosoma congolense* and *Trypanosoma vivax* affect cattle. *Trypanosoma* spp. that causes anemia in other species includes *Trypanosoma simiae* in pigs and *Trypanosoma brucei* in camels and horses. Trypanosomes also cause nonhemolytic disease (e.g., *Trypanosoma cruzi*, the agent of Chagas' disease, or American trypanosomiasis) in many hosts, and nonpathogenic variants (e.g., *Trypanosoma theileri* in cattle worldwide) are also recognized. Trypanosomal organisms do not infect erythrocytes but rather exist as free trypomastigotes (flagellated forms with a characteristic undulating membrane) in the blood (Fig. 13-29, *A*) or as amastigotes in tissue. The mechanism of anemia is believed to be immune-mediated. Cattle with acute trypanosomiasis have significant anemia, which initially is regenerative, but less so with time. The extent of parasitemia is readily apparent with *Trypanosoma vivax* and *Trypanosoma theileri* infections because the organisms are present in large numbers in the blood. This is in contrast to *Trypanosoma congolense*, which localizes within the vasculature of the brain and skeletal muscle. Cattle with *Trypanosoma congolense* infections develop chronic debilitating disease; they have scruffy hair coats, appear "potbellied," and have fever, intermittent diarrhea, and exercise intolerance. Mortality is greater

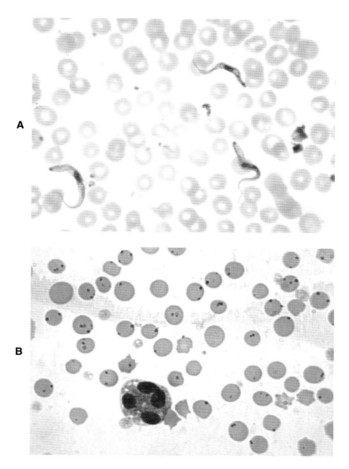

Fig. 13-29   Hemotropic parasites, bovine blood smear. A, Trypanosomiasis. Trypanosomes are flagellated protozoa characterized by an undulating membrane, kinetoplast, and nucleus. They may be identified in a wet mount made from the buffy coat portion of the packed cells. **B,** Anaplasmosis, *Anaplasma marginale.* Note the darkly stained organisms, most of which are located on the edges of the erythrocytes. Anaplasmosis causes anemia mainly by immune-mediated extravascular hemolysis. *(**A,** Courtesy Dr. M.D. McGavin, College of Veterinary Medicine, University of Tennessee. **B,** Courtesy Dr. J. Simon, College of Veterinary Medicine, University of Illinois.)*

with *Trypanosoma vivax* infections, usually because of intercurrent acute infectious diseases, such as salmonellosis. Necropsy findings in cattle with trypanosomiasis include cachexia, generalized edema with increased fluid in body cavities, and generalized lymph node enlargement. Bronchopneumonia, a flabby heart, and serous atrophy of pericardial fat may be present. Liver and kidneys are symmetrically enlarged. Lymph nodes are enlarged up to four times normal size because of lymphoid hyperplasia, and most of the fatty bone marrow is replaced by red hematopoietic tissue. The spleen is enlarged because of lymphoid hyperplasia and is firm when incised.

Bacterial and rickettsial agents

Anaplasma species.   *Anaplasma* spp. are rickettsial organisms that may be transmitted by arthropod vectors (ticks, biting flies) or by blood-contaminated needles. Anaplasmosis is a cause of hemolytic anemia in cattle in tropical and subtropical areas of many parts of the world. *Anaplasma marginale*, considered the more pathogenic species, has a worldwide distribution. *Anaplasma centrale* is found in South America, Africa, and the Middle East. The genus names reflect the typical locations of the organisms when detected on examination of a blood smear, either on the periphery or more centrally within infected erythrocytes. A related species, *Anaplasma ovis*, affects sheep and goats in tropical and subtropical areas worldwide. Wild animals such as deer, elk, and bison may be latently infected and serve as reservoir hosts for *Anaplasma marginale*. Anaplasma organisms infect erythrocytes intracellularly.

Anaplasmosis causes anemia mainly by immune-mediated extravascular hemolysis. The severity of disease in infected animals varies with age. Infected calves under 1 year of age rarely develop clinical disease, whereas cattle 3 years of age or older are more likely to develop severe, potentially fatal, illness. The reason for this discrepancy is not clear. In clinically affected animals, common signs include lethargy or recumbency, pallor, and icterus. Animals dying of acute anaplasmosis have blood of low viscosity, pale to icteric tissue, an enlarged turgid spleen, and an icteric liver with a distended gallbladder. In animals with acute disease, it is usually easy to detect *Anaplasma marginale* organisms on routine blood smear evaluation (Fig. 13-29, *B*). However, in recovering animals, the organisms may be difficult to find. Surviving cattle become chronic carriers (and thus reservoirs for infection of other animals) and develop cyclic parasitemia, which is typically not detectable on blood smears. Splenectomy of carrier animals results in marked parasitemia and acute hemolysis. PCR testing is the most sensitive means of identifying animals with low levels of parasitemia.

Clostridium species.   Certain *Clostridium* spp. may cause potentially fatal hemolytic anemias in animals. The mechanism of hemolysis involves a bacterial toxin (phospholipase C or lecithinase), which enzymatically degrades cell membranes, causing acute intravascular hemolysis. *Clostridium haemolyticum* and *Clostridium novyi* type D cause the disease in cattle known as bacillary hemoglobinuria. (The term *redwater* has also been used for this disease, and for hemolytic anemias in cattle caused by *Babesia* spp.) Similar naturally occurring disease has been reported in sheep and elk. In cattle, the disease is associated with liver fluke (*Fasciola hepatica*) migration in susceptible animals. Ingested clostridial spores may live in Kupffer cells of the liver for a long time without causing disease. However, when migrating flukes cause hepatic necrosis, the resulting anaerobic environment stimulates the clostridial organisms to proliferate and elaborate their hemolytic toxins. Bacillary hemoglobinuria has also been associated with liver biopsy in calves. *Clostridium perfringens* type A causes intravascular hemolytic anemia in lambs and calves—a condition known as yellow lamb disease, yellows, or enterotoxemic jaundice because of the characteristic jaundice. The organism is a normal inhabitant of the gastrointestinal tract in these animals, but may proliferate abnormally in response to some diets. *Clostridium perfringens* has also been associated with intravascular hemolytic anemia in horses with clostridial abscesses and in a ewe with clostridial mastitis.

Hemotropic mycoplasma species.   The term *hemotropic mycoplasmas,* or "hemoplasmas," encompasses a group of bacteria, formerly known as *Haemobartonella* or *Eperythrozoon* species, that commonly infect RBCs of many domestic, laboratory, and wild animals. Hemotropic mycoplasmas affecting common domestic species are listed in Table 13-4. The organisms are mainly transmitted by arthropods, but some cases of in utero transmission have been reported. Effects of infection vary from subclinical to fatal anemia, depending on the specific organism, dose, and host susceptibility. Anemia occurs mainly because of extravascular hemolysis. Although the pathogenetic mechanisms are not completely understood, an immune-mediated component is highly probable. Hemotropic mycoplasmas (and nonhemotropic mycoplasma ssp.) induce cold agglutinins in infected individuals, although it is not clear whether these particular antibodies are important in the development of hemolytic anemia. Like other mycoplasmas, hemotropic mycoplasmas are small (0.3 to 3 μm in diameter), are gram-negative, and

Table **13-4**   **Common Hemotropic Mycoplasmas in Domestic Animals**

Host	Organism
Cattle	*Mycoplasma wenyonii* (formerly *Eperythrozoon wenyonii*)
Dog	*Mycoplasma haemocanis* (formerly *Haemobartonella canis*)
Cat	*Mycoplasma haemofelis* (formerly *Haemobartonella felis* large form or Ohio variant)
Cat	Candidatus *Mycoplasma haemominutum* (formerly *Haemobartonella felis* small form or California variant)
Pig	*Mycoplasma suis* (formerly *Eperythrozoon suis*)
Alpaca	Candidatus *Mycoplasma haemolamae*

lack a cell wall. They are epicellular parasites, residing in indentations and invaginations of the RBC surface. When detected on routine blood smear evaluation, the organisms are variably shaped (cocci, small rods, or ring forms) and sometimes arranged in short, branching chains (especially *Mycoplasma haemocanis*). The organisms may also be noted extracellularly, in the background of the blood smear, especially if the smear is made after prolonged storage of the blood in an anticoagulant tube. Light and electron photomicrographs of hemotropic mycoplasma organisms are shown in Fig. 13-30.

Most hemotropic mycoplasma subspecies are more likely to cause acute illness in individuals that are immunocompromised or have concurrent disease. *Mycoplasma haemofelis* infection is an exception, causing

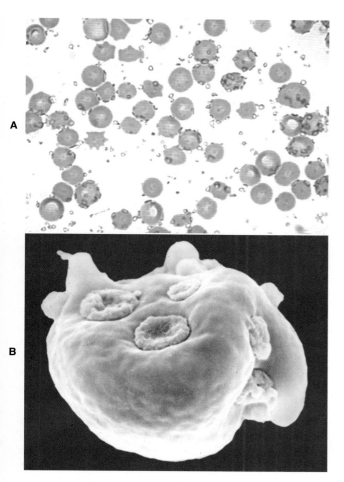

Fig. 13-30   Hemotropic mycoplasmosis. A, Blood smear from a splenectomized pig infected with *Mycoplasma suis* (formerly *Eperythrozoon suis*). Note the small oval- to ring-shaped organisms attached to the surface of the erythrocytes and free in the protein of the blood smear. Wright's stain. **B,** *Mycoplasma suis* attached to a porcine erythrocyte. Scanning electron micrograph. Carbon sputter coated method. (*A* and *B, Courtesy Dr. J.F. Zachary, College of Veterinary Medicine, University of Illinois.*)

acute hemolytic anemia in immunocompetent cats. The disease in sheep and pigs has a seasonal incidence corresponding to the peak occurrence of biting insects. However, it can also occur at other times of the year as a recrudescence in a carrier animal secondary to another disease. In both sheep and pigs, unexpected death of one or two animals is often followed by anemia in other animals within the herd. *Mycoplasma wenyonii* in cattle is less pathogenic than *Mycoplasma ovis* and *Mycoplasma suis* in sheep and pigs, respectively. Infection with *Mycoplasma wenyonii* appears to be widespread, but it rarely causes disease. Clinical signs in animals with acute disease include lethargy, fever, and pallor. Affected animals usually have mild to moderate hyperbilirubinemia and may be icteric. Animals probably remain chronically infected after recovery, even if treated with appropriate antibiotics. Chronically infected cattle, sheep, and pigs may have decreased production. Chronically infected dogs and cats are typically asymptomatic. In dogs, *Mycoplasma haemocanis* infection is usually subclinical in immunocompetent animals but causes acute hemolytic anemia when infected animals receive a splenectomy. Two forms of hemoplasmas are known to infect cats. As mentioned earlier, *Mycoplasma haemofelis*, the large form variant, causes acute hemolytic anemia in immunocompetent animals. Cats infected with the small form variant, which has the proposed name *Mycoplasma haemominutum*, are typically asymptomatic or have only mild disease. Organisms are often, but not always, detected on routine blood smear examination in acutely ill animals. PCR testing is the most sensitive means of detecting infection in animals with low levels of parasitemia. In animals dying of hemotropic mycoplasma infection, the findings are typical of extravascular hemolysis, with pallor, icterus, and splenomegaly, and distended gallbladder (Fig. 13-31). Microscopic lesions in the spleen include congestion, erythrophagia, macrophage hyperplasia, extramedullary hematopoiesis, and increased numbers of plasma cells. Bone marrow has varying degrees of erythroid hyperplasia, depending on the duration of hemolysis.

Leptospira **species.**   Leptospirosis is recognized as a cause of hemolytic anemia in calves, lambs, pigs, and black rhinoceros. Specific leptospiral organisms associated with hemolytic disease include *Leptospira interrogans* serovars *pomona* and *ictohaemorrhagica*. Proposed mechanisms of disease include immune-mediated (IgM cold agglutinin) extravascular hemolysis and enzymatic (phospholipase produced by the organism) intravascular hemolysis.

Leptospira organisms are ubiquitous in the environment. Infection occurs percutaneously and via mucosal surfaces and is followed by leptospiremia; organisms then localize preferentially in certain tissues (e.g., kidney, liver, and pregnant uterus). Leptospirosis can

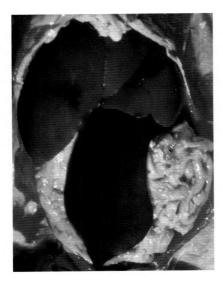

Fig. 13-31 *Mycoplasma haemofelis*, **cat.** Note the splenomegaly, hepatomegaly, and icterus caused by infection of erythrocytes with this hemotropic parasite. Splenomegaly and icterus are the result of increased destruction (extravascular hemolysis) of infected erythrocytes. *(Courtesy College of Veterinary Medicine, University of Illinois.)*

also cause many disease manifestations besides hemolysis (e.g., renal failure, liver failure, abortion, and other conditions) that are not discussed here.

In addition to anemia, common findings in animals with leptospirosis-induced hemolysis include hemoglobinuria and icterus. On necropsy, renal tubular necrosis, which occurs in part because of hemoglobinuria (hemoglobinuric nephrosis), may also be present.

Viral agents

Equine infectious anemia virus.   Equine infectious anemia virus (EIAV) is a lentivirus that infects cells of the mononuclear phagocyte system in horses (also ponies, donkeys, and mules) throughout the world. Natural transmission is by arthropods, and the virus can also be transmitted transplacentally. Disease occurs in both an acute, potentially fatal form after initial infection, as well as a chronic intermittent form associated with recurrent viremia. Recurrent episodes happen mostly in the first year after infection, and tend to decrease in frequency and severity with time. Infection is lifelong and animals may become asymptomatic carriers. Viral antigen is found mainly within liver, spleen, and serum of infected animals, and also in bone marrow, lymph nodes, thymus, circulating mononuclear cells, and other tissues. EIAV causes anemia by both immune-mediated hemolysis and decreased erythropoiesis. Hemolysis is typically extravascular but may have an intravascular component during the acute phase. Decreased erythropoiesis may result from direct

suppression of early-stage erythroid cells by the virus, as well as anemia of inflammation. Thrombocytopenia, likely due to secondary immune-mediated destruction, is also a classic feature of acute EIAV infection and recurring febrile episodes. Clinical findings associated with viremic episodes include fever, depression, icterus, petechial hemorrhages, lymph node enlargement, and dependent edema. EIA infection is diagnosed on the basis of the Coggins test, an agarose gel immunodiffusion test for the presence of the antibody against the virus.

Animals dying during hemolytic crises have icterus, anemia, and widespread hemorrhages. The spleen and liver are enlarged, dark and turgid, and they and other organs have superficial subcapsular hemorrhages. Petechiae are evident beneath the renal capsule and throughout the cortex and medulla. The bone marrow is dark red as a result of replacement of fat by hematopoietic tissue; the extent of replacement is an indication of the duration of the anemia. The severity of microscopic lesions is dependent on the chronicity of the disease, and they are most significant in the spleen, liver, and bone marrow. As would be anticipated, microscopic findings of the spleen are predominantly influenced by the number and activity of macrophages, which is a reflection of the duration of the disease and the frequency of hemolytic episodes. Hemosiderin-laden macrophages persist for months to years; therefore, large numbers are consistent with chronicity. Kupffer cell hyperplasia with hemosiderin stores and periportal infiltrates of lymphocytes are the most significant changes in the liver. Bone marrow histologic findings vary depending on the duration of the disease. In most animals, the marrow is cellular because of the replacement of fat by intense, orderly erythropoiesis. Granulocytes are relatively less numerous and plasma cells are increased. As in the spleen, hemosiderin-laden macrophages are present in large numbers in chronic cases. In more chronic cases, emaciated animals have serous atrophy of fat.

Feline leukemia virus.   Feline leukemia virus (FeLV) is an oncogenic, immunosuppressive lentivirus associated with hematologic abnormalities of widely varying type and severity, including anemia in most infected cats. Manifestations of disease due to FeLV infection vary depending on dose, viral genetics, and host factors, but normal hematopoiesis is probably suppressed to some degree in all cases. The virus infects hematopoietic precursor cells soon after the animal is exposed and continues to replicate in hematopoietic and lymphatic tissue of animals that remain persistently viremic. Persistently viremic cats are immunosuppressed and are prone to developing other diseases, including infectious diseases, bone marrow disorders, and lymphoma (lymphosarcoma).

FeLV-induced anemia is usually nonregenerative, presumably due to direct effects of the virus on infected erythroid cells. However, macrocytosis and metarubricytosis (the presence of nucleated RBC precursors in circulation) are often noted in the absence of significant reticulocytosis—findings consistent with dyserythropoiesis, although the exact mechanism is not clear. Bone marrow of cats with FeLV-induced anemia often has evidence of arrested or disordered maturation of hematopoietic precursors. The relatively uncommon subgroup C viruses are associated with erythroid aplasia, probably because of infection of early stage erythroid precursors. Regenerative anemia may also occur with FeLV infection, often because of coinfection with *Mycoplasma haemofelis*.

Feline immunodeficiency virus.   Feline immunodeficiency virus (FIV), another feline lentivirus, is associated with anemia in a minority of infected cats. Immunosuppressive effects of FIV from thymic depletion are discussed elsewhere. It is generally accepted that anemia does not result directly from FIV infection, but instead develops because of concurrent disease, such as co-infection with FeLV or hemotropic mycoplasma, other infection, or malignancy. The severity and type of anemia in FIV-infected cats depends on the other specific disease processes involved.

ACQUIRED AND INHERITED METABOLIC DISORDERS

This section discusses specific acquired and inherited metabolic disorders that cause anemia or impaired hemoglobin function.

Oxidative agents

Rather than presenting an exhaustive list, this section describes some of the more commonly recognized oxidants that cause hemolytic anemia or impaired hemoglobin function in common domestic species. Oxidative insult may result in extravascular hemolysis because of phagocytosis of damaged erythrocytes by splenic macrophages, or in intravascular hemolysis if the damage is severe enough. In horses, red maple (*Acer rubrum*) toxicity is a well-characterized, potentially fatal cause of acute intravascular hemolytic anemia and methemoglobinemia. Ingestion of sufficient amounts of wilted or dried leaves or bark causes Heinz body formation, eccentrocytosis, severe intravascular hemolysis, and methemoglobinemia. Common postmortem findings include notable icterus; splenic hemosiderosis; splenomegaly; brown discoloration and swollen liver; and swollen kidneys, which can be dark red to blue-black. Histologically the kidneys have characteristic red-brown tubular casts (hemoglobinuric nephrosis).

Phenothiazine can cause Heinz body formation in horses. In ruminants, *Brassica* spp. and rye grass are associated with Heinz body formation, and nitrite toxicity causes methemoglobinemia.

Copper toxicity is a well-known cause of acute intravascular hemolytic anemia in sheep, and may also occur in goats and calves. The condition occurs in animals that have accumulated large amounts of copper in the liver. The copper is released under conditions of stress (e.g., shipping, starvation) and is believed to cause hemolysis as a result of direct interaction with membrane proteins, lipid peroxidation, formation of reactive oxygen species, and enzyme inhibition. Affected animals are often markedly icteric, and hemoglobinuric nephrosis is a classic postmortem lesion.

Onions and garlic are most commonly recognized as a cause of Heinz body hemolytic anemia in dogs and cats but can cause oxidative damage to erythrocytes in other domestic animals, including horses and cattle. Other causes of Heinz bodies in dogs include acetaminophen, benzocaine, naphthalene, phenylhydrazine, vitamins K_1 and K_3, and zinc. Other causes of Heinz bodies in cats include acetaminophen, benzocaine, methionine, naphthalene, propofol, and propylene glycol.

Nutritional deficiencies

Severe malnutrition is probably a cause of nonregenerative anemia in all species due to combined deficiencies of molecular building blocks, energy, and essential cofactors. By far the most commonly recognized specific deficiency that results in anemia is iron deficiency. Iron deficiency is usually not a primary nutritional deficiency but rather occurs secondary to depletion of iron stores via chronic hemorrhage. The most common route of loss is through the gastrointestinal tract (e.g., due to neoplasia [especially gastrointestinal carcinoma or lymphoma] in older animals, or hookworm infection in puppies). Chronic hemorrhage may also be due to many other causes, including marked ectoparasitism (e.g., pediculosis in cattle, and massive flea burden in kittens and puppies), neoplasia in locations other than the GI tract, and bleeding diatheses. Rapidly growing nursing animals may be iron-deficient when compared with adults because milk is an iron-poor diet. In most cases, this is of little clinical significance (and in fact is normal). An important exception is piglets with no access to iron, which may cause anemia, failure to thrive, and increased mortality. Neonatal piglets are routinely given parenteral iron (intramuscular injection of iron dextran) for this reason.

Other specific nutritional deficiencies causing anemia in animals are uncommon or rare. Copper deficiency can cause iron deficiency in ruminants, and may occur because of copper-deficient forage or impaired usage of copper by high dietary molybdenum or sulfate. It is believed that copper deficiency impairs production of ceruloplasmin, a copper-containing enzyme involved in gastrointestinal iron absorption. Copper deficiency anemia, like iron deficiency anemia, is typically microcytic and hypochromic. Cobalamin (vitamin B_{12}) and folate deficiencies are recognized as causes of anemia in human beings but are rare in animals.

Hypophosphatemic hemolytic anemia

Marked hypophosphatemia is recognized as a cause of intravascular hemolytic anemia in postparturient dairy cows. Hypophosphatemia develops in these animals because of increased loss of phosphorus in their milk. Biochemical studies suggest that the mechanism of hemolysis involves decreased erythrocyte production of ATP, which may lead to compromised membrane and cytoskeletal integrity. An accompanying decrease in reducing capacity and increase in methemoglobin concentration have also been noted in experimental studies of hypophosphatemic hemolytic anemia in dairy cattle, suggesting that oxidative mechanisms may also contribute to anemia. Affected cows are anemic and hemoglobinuric. Gross postmortem findings include pallor, decreased viscosity of the blood, and discolored pale yellow and swollen liver and kidney. Renal tubular necrosis and hemoglobin pigment within the tubules is evident microscopically. Hemolysis has also been reported in association with hypophosphatemia in dogs and cats.

Water intoxication

Calves with sporadic access to water will sometimes drink excessively when water is available, to the point where their plasma becomes hypotonic and osmotic intravascular hemolysis occurs. Hemoglobinuria is commonly observed in affected animals. The condition is rarely fatal.

Enzyme deficiencies

Erythropoietic porphyrias. Porphyrias are inherited defects of enzymes involved in the synthesis of porphyrins, precursors of hemoglobin, and other heme proteins. Porphyrias result in accumulation of toxic porphyrin compounds. Congenital erythropoietic porphyria, transmitted as an autosomal recessive trait, occurs in Holstein and shorthorn cattle and is characterized by red-brown discoloration of teeth, bones, and urine caused by accumulation of porphyrins (see Fig. 1-74). Because of the circulation of the photodynamic porphyrins in blood, these animals have lesions of photosensitization of the nonpigmented skin and hemolytic anemia. All affected tissues, including erythrocytes, exhibit fluorescence with ultraviolet light. The premature destruction of developing and mature erythrocytes is caused by the accumulation within these cells of excess porphyrins. Bovine erythropoietic protoporphyria is an inherited disorder of heme synthetase, a terminal enzyme of the heme synthetic pathway, resulting in the accumulation of protoporphyrins in tissues and erythrocytes. It is inherited as an autosomal recessive trait and is confined to Limousin or Limousin-cross cattle. Photosensitivity is the only clinical manifestation of the disease; there is no anemia and no discoloration of teeth and bone. A congenital porphyria described in Siamese and domestic short-haired cats resembles congenital erythropoietic porphyria in cattle. These cats have brown teeth, photosensitization, and hemolytic anemia.

Pyruvate kinase deficiency. Pyruvate kinase (PK) deficiency is an inherited autosomal recessive condition in numerous dog breeds (most commonly in basenjis) and fewer cat breeds (Abyssinian, Somali, domestic shorthair). The glycolytic isoenzyme that is deficient in erythrocytes of affected animals normally catalyzes the last ATP-generating reaction in glycolysis. Thus in PK-deficient individuals there is decreased production of ATP, which results in loss of normal membrane function and decreased erythrocyte life span. The disease is characterized by moderate to severe extravascular hemolytic anemia that is strongly regenerative. In dogs, PK deficiency typically also involves progressive myelofibrosis, osteosclerosis, and hemosiderosis. Dogs with PK deficiency usually die from complications of the disease by 4 years of age. PCR tests to detect carrier and affected dogs are available for basenjis and West Highland white terriers (and probably Cairn terriers). In cats, PK deficiency is not associated with osteosclerosis, and the prognosis is more favorable.

Phosphofructokinase deficiency. Inherited autosomal recessive deficiency of another erythrocyte glycolytic enzyme, phosphofructokinase (PFK), is described in English springer spaniel and American cocker spaniel dogs. The enzyme is also deficient in muscle tissue of affected dogs. Erythrocytes in PFK-deficient dogs have decreased ATP and 2,3-diphosphoglycerate production, and increased fragility under alkaline conditions. The disease is characterized by chronic, extravascular hemolysis with marked reticulocytosis. The marked regenerative response may compensate for the ongoing hemolysis, and affected animals therefore are not necessarily anemic. However, acute intravascular hemolytic episodes may occur with hyperventilation and resulting alkalemia. There are three genes encoding PFK enzymes, designated M in muscle and erythrocytes, L in liver, and P in platelets. A point mutation in the gene coding for the M enzyme results in an unstable, truncated molecule. In English springer spaniels and related breeds, affected and carrier animals can be detected using PCR testing.

Other inherited erythrocyte disorders. Sporadic cases of other inherited deficiencies of enzymes, or other components of key erythrocyte metabolic pathways, have been reported. Deficiency of cytochrome-b₅ reductase (NADH-methemoglobin reductase), the enzyme that catalyzes the reduction of methemoglobin (Fe^{3+}) to hemoglobin (Fe^{2+}), has been recognized in a number of dogs and in a cat. Affected animals are not anemic, usually lack clinical signs of disease, and have normal life expectancies. Deficiency of the glycolytic enzyme glucose-6-phosphate dehydrogenase (G6PD), a common X-linked disease in people, has been reported in an American saddle bred colt with eccentrocytosis and persistent hemolytic anemia, and in a partially deficient male dog without anemia or clinical signs. Deficiency of erythrocyte flavin adenine dinucleotide (FAD) due to abnormal erythrocyte riboflavin metabolism was recently reported in a Spanish mustang mare with methemoglobinemia and eccentrocytosis.

Japanese black cattle lacking band 3, an integral membrane protein that connects to the cytoskeleton, have moderate hemolytic anemia and retarded growth. A heterogeneous group of conditions, known as hereditary stomatocytosis because of the characteristic slit-shaped area of central pallor in RBCs on stained blood smears, has been described in several dog breeds. The clinical manifestations vary in affected animals, and the specific underlying defects have not been identified. In all cases, however, erythrocytes have increased osmotic fragility and decreased survival. A condition characterized by increased erythrocyte osmotic fragility has been described in Abyssinian and Somali cats, although the specific defect has not been identified. Affected cats have chronic intermittent severe hemolytic anemia and often have other lesions secondary to hemolytic anemia (e.g., splenomegaly and hyperbilirubinemia). Other rare inherited or presumably inherited disorders of erythrocytes have also been described in animals.

DISORDERS OF GRANULOCYTES AND MONOCYTES/MACROPHAGES
DISORDERS OF GRANULOCYTES

Granulocytic ehrlichiosis

Ehrlichiae are small, pleomorphic, gram-negative, obligate intracellular bacteria that are transmitted by tick vectors. Some *Ehrlichia* spp. have a tropism for granulocytes, and morulae are sometimes found within the cytoplasm of neutrophils of affected animals (Fig. 13-32). Animals with granulocytic ehrlichiosis may be neutropenic, but the specific mechanism of neutropenia is not clear. Neutropenia is not a consistent finding in granulocytic ehrlichiosis, and clinical manifestations of infection are usually referable to other cell types (e.g., thrombocytopenia) or body systems (e.g., polyarthritis). Molecular analysis has shown that

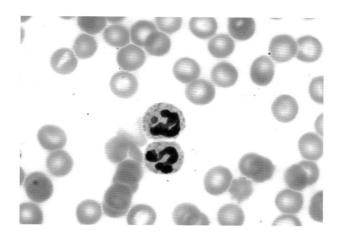

Fig. 13-32   Granulocytic ehrlichiosis, *Anaplasma phagocytophila*, canine blood smear. The top neutrophil contains an inclusion consistent with an *Anaplasma phagocytophila* morula. Wright's stain. (*Courtesy Dr. M.M. Fry, College of Veterinary Medicine, University of Tennessee.*)

Ehrlichia equi, the agent of human granulocytic ehrlichiosis, and *Ehrlichia phagocytophila* are genetically indistinguishable. All are now designated as *Anaplasma phagocytophila*. Granulocytic ehrlichiosis occurs naturally in horses (*Anaplasma phagocytophila*), dogs (*Anaplasma phagocytophila* and *Ehrlichia ewingii*), and cats (*Anaplasma phagocytophila*).

Leukocyte adhesion deficiency

Leukocyte adhesion deficiency (LAD) is an inherited fatal autosomal recessive condition characterized by deficiency of the common β₂ chain (a molecule also known as CD18) of leukocyte integrins. Without normal expression of this adhesion molecule, leukocytes have severely impaired ability to migrate from the blood stream into tissues. As a result, animals with LAD are highly susceptible to infections, and usually die at a young age. Infected foci are nonsuppurative because of the absence of infiltrating leukocytes. LAD is also characterized by very high concentrations of neutrophils in the blood. LAD has been recognized in Holstein cattle (known as bovine LAD, or BLAD) and Irish setter dogs.

Pelger-Huët anomaly

Pelger-Huët anomaly (PHA) is a condition characterized by lack of normal segmentation of the nuclei of mature granulocytes. This condition results in morphologic changes in granulocytes that are similar to those of granulocytes occurring in an inflammatory left shift; however, in the absence of any other disease process, animals with PHA should not have clinical signs or other laboratory findings indicative of inflammation. PHA cells can be distinguished from immature forms of otherwise normal granulocytes on the basis of their

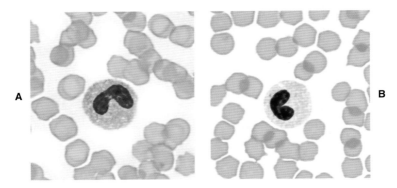

Fig. 13-33   Pelger-Huët anomaly, feline blood smear. Eosinophil (**A**) and neutrophil (**B**) have hyposegmented nuclei with mature, condensed chromatin. Wright's stain. (**A** *and* **B,** *Courtesy Dr. M.M. Fry, College of Veterinary Medicine, University of Tennessee.*)

mature chromatin pattern (Fig. 13-33). PHA has been described in dogs, cats, and rabbits, as well as in human beings. Prevalence is higher in certain dog breeds. In Australian shepherds, the mode of inheritance is autosomal dominant with incomplete penetrance. Most cases of PHA are the heterozygous form and probably of no clinical significance. In these cases, the shape of most granulocyte nuclei resembles those of band and metamyelocyte forms. A rare homozygous form of PHA has also been reported in rabbits and cats. It is associated with accompanying skeletal abnormalities and stillbirths or early mortality in these species (there are also rare reports of homozygous PHA in human beings, without associated skeletal abnormalities or shortened life span). In homozygous PHA cells, granulocyte nuclei are round or oval. An acquired, reversible condition mimicking PHA, known as pseudo–Pelger-Huët anomaly, is occasionally noted in animals with infectious disease, neoplasia, or in connection with drug administration.

Chédiak-Higashi syndrome

Chédiak-Higashi syndrome (CHS) is a rare autosomal recessive condition characterized by recurrent pyogenic infections, bleeding tendencies, ocular and cutaneous hypopigmentation, and prominent cytoplasmic inclusions in blood cells. CHS has been described in domestic (several breeds of cattle, Persian cats), wild (blue and silver foxes, Aleutian mink, an albino killer whale), and laboratory (beige mutant mice and rats) animals, as well as people. The mutated gene encodes a protein called beige or LYST (for lysosome trafficking regulator), the specific functions of which are still being investigated. Individuals with CHS have severely impaired cellular innate immunity because of neutropenia, impaired chemotaxis, and impaired killing by granulocytes and cytotoxic lymphocytes.

DISORDERS OF MONOCYTES/MACROPHAGES
Monocytic ehrlichiosis

Some ehrlichiae have a tropism for mononuclear cells, but clinical manifestations are usually referable to other cell types or body systems. Ehrlichial morulae may be found in mononuclear cells of infected animals on routine examination of blood smears, and examination of buffy coat smears increases the probability of detecting the organism. In horses, *Ehrlichia risticii*–the agent of Potomac horse fever (also known as equine monocytic ehrlichiosis)–infects monocytes and enterocytes and is primarily a diarrheal disease (see Chapter 7). In dogs, *Ehrlichia canis*, the agent of canine monocytic ehrlichiosis, infects mononuclear cells. Infection with *Ehrlichia chaffeensis*, the agent of human monocytic ehrlichiosis, has also been reported in dogs. Canine monocytic ehrlichiosis has acute and chronic forms. Acutely ill animals typically have a fever, lymph node enlargement, and splenomegaly. Thrombocytopenia and nonregenerative anemia are common findings. Untreated dogs recovering from acute disease develop a subclinical phase and may have persistent mild thrombocytopenia. A subset of these dogs develop chronic disease that may be debilitating and in some cases life threatening. Some studies indicate that German shepherd dogs with ehrlichiosis are predisposed to have particularly severe clinical disease. Severe cases are characterized by weight loss, lymph node enlargement, pyrexia, thrombocytopenia, and nonregenerative anemia. Thrombocytopenic animals may have severe bleeding tendencies. Some dogs with chronic disease develop pancytopenia. Necropsy findings vary with the stage of the disease. In the acute disease, there are widespread petechiae and ecchymoses, with splenomegaly and lymphadenomegaly. Chronically infected dogs are emaciated. The bone marrow is hyperplastic and red in the acute disease, but becomes hypoplastic and pale in animals with pancytopenia.

Histologic findings include generalized perivascular plasma cell infiltration, which is most pronounced in animals with chronic disease. Multifocal, nonsuppurative meningoencephalitis, interstitial pneumonia, and glomerulonephritis are present in most dogs with the disease. *Ehrlichia* organisms are difficult to detect histologically; examination of Wright-Giemsa–stained impression smears of lung, liver, lymph nodes, and spleen is a more effective method for detecting the morulae in macrophages. Ehrlichiosis is often diagnosed on the basis of serologic testing, but PCR testing is more sensitive.

Hemophagocytic syndrome

Hemophagocytic syndrome is a term used to describe proliferation of nonneoplastic (i.e., polyclonal), well-differentiated but highly erythrophagic macrophages. The condition is rare but has been recognized in dogs and cats. Unlike histiocytic sarcoma, which in some forms also consists of highly erythrophagic macrophages, hemophagocytic syndrome is a secondary condition, occurring as a sequela of neoplasia, infection, or other underlying diseases. The macrophage proliferation and hyperactivation is a response to increased production of stimulatory cytokines occurring as part of the primary disease process. Macrophages are found in high numbers in the bone marrow and commonly in other tissues, including lymph nodes, spleen, and liver. Affected animals usually have cytopenias of two or more cell lines. Bone marrow findings reported in animals with hemophagocytic syndrome vary widely, ranging from hypoplasia to hyperplasia of cell lines with peripheral cytopenias, and may also include detection of macrophages containing phagocytosed hematopoietic precursor cells in addition to mature erythrocytes.

DISORDERS OF PLATELETS
IMMUNE-MEDIATED DISORDERS

Immune-mediated thrombocytopenia (IMT)

Immune-mediated thrombocytopenia (IMT) is a condition characterized by immune-mediated destruction of platelets. There are numerous similarities between IMT and IMHA. IMT is a fairly common condition in dogs (it has also been described in horses and cats). It is more common in middle-aged animals, females, and perhaps some breeds of dogs. The disease is usually idiopathic and typically results in severe thrombocytopenia (often <10,000 platelets/µL), although less severe forms of the disease also occur. Affected animals have varying degrees of clinical bleeding tendencies. IMT also sometimes occurs together with IMHA, a condition known as Evans syndrome.

Underlying conditions associated with secondary IMT include infection (e.g., EIAV and ehrlichiosis), drug administration, neoplasia, and other immune-mediated diseases. Many types of infectious agents (viral, bacterial, fungal, protozoal) have been associated with IMT, some of which may also cause thrombocytopenia by other mechanisms. Ehrlichiosis, for example, has been shown to elicit production of antibodies that are cross-reactive with platelet antigens in human beings. Drugs suspected of causing IMT in animals include cephalosporins and sulfonamides.

Neonatal alloimmune thrombocytopenia

A form of immune-mediated thrombocytopenia, known as neonatal alloimmune thrombocytopenia, is recognized in neonatal pigs and foals. The pathogenesis of this disease is virtually identical to that of neonatal isoerythrolysis as a cause of anemia: A neonate inheriting paternal platelet antigens absorbs maternal antibodies against these antigens through the colostrum. In principle, a similar situation may occur following platelet-incompatible transfusion of blood or blood products containing platelets.

INFECTIOUS DISORDERS

This section focuses on infectious agents that specifically affect platelets or platelet precursors. Many other infections may affect platelets indirectly (e.g., via immune-mediated mechanisms).

Anaplasma platys

Anaplasma platys (known until recently as *Ehrlichia platys*) is a rickettsial organism that infects canine platelets, causing recurrent marked thrombocytopenia (the disease is also known as infectious canine cyclic thrombocytopenia). The disease is tick-borne and has been recognized worldwide. Evidence of megakaryocytic hyperplasia and organism-associated antigen within macrophages indicate that thrombocytopenia likely results from increased platelet destruction. Infection is generally considered to be asymptomatic, and morulae within platelets may be detected on blood smears incidentally, but there are rare reports describing more severe clinical signs in infected animals.

Bovine viral diarrhea virus

Thrombocytopenia, often severe, has been reported in association with acute bovine viral diarrhea virus (BVDV) infection in calves and adult cattle. Infection with type II BVDV has been specifically associated with a thrombocytopenic hemorrhagic syndrome. Calves infected with type II BVDV have also been shown to have impaired platelet function. Investigations of the mechanism of BVDV-induced thrombocytopenia have resulted in varying, sometimes conflicting, conclusions. More than one study has shown viral antigen associated both with bone marrow megakaryocytes and with circulating platelets. Evidence of impaired thrombopoiesis (megakaryocyte necrosis, megakaryocyte pyknosis, and degeneration) and increased thrombopoiesis (megakaryocytic hyperplasia, increased numbers of immature megakaryocytes) in the bone marrow has been reported in type II BVDV-infected animals, including concurrent megakaryocyte necrosis and hyperplasia in some experimental subjects. To our knowledge, antibody-mediated destruction of platelets has not been shown.

Feline leukemia virus

As discussed earlier in the section on disorders of erythrocytes, FeLV infects hematopoietic cells and can produce a wide array of hematologic and other disease manifestations. FeLV may be detected in megakaryocytes and platelets in infected cats, and may result in platelet abnormalities, including thrombocytopenia, thrombocytosis, increased platelet size, and decreased function. Proposed mechanisms of FeLV-induced thrombocytopenia include direct cytopathic effects, myelophthisis, and immune-mediated destruction. Platelet life span and function have been shown to be decreased in FeLV-positive cats.

INHERITED PLATELET FUNCTION DISORDERS

Defective platelet function may cause bleeding in individuals that lack other hemostatic abnormalities. Platelet function disorders, also known as thrombopathies or thrombopathias, may be primary or secondary. Box 13-9 shows underlying conditions associated with secondary thrombopathies. Examples of well-characterized primary thrombopathies recognized in

---

Box 13-9

Conditions Associated with Secondary Thrombopathy

- Hyperglobulinemia (as in monoclonal gammopathy due to multiple myeloma, or polyclonal gammopathy due to persistent antigenic stimulation)
- Increased concentrations of fibrinolytic products (because of increased production, as in DIC, or impaired clearance, as in liver insufficiency)
- Uremia
- Immune-mediated thrombocytopenia (antibodies bound to platelets may cause impaired function as well as increased destruction)
- Colloidal plasma expanders (e.g., Hetastarch)
- Infection (BVDV, FeLV)
- NSAIDs—irreversible (aspirin) or reversible inhibition of cyclooxygenase

BVDV, Bovine viral diarrhea virus; *DIC,* disseminated intravascular coagulation; *FeLV,* feline leukemia virus; *NSAIDs,* nonsteroidal antiinflammatory drugs.

---

common domestic animals are discussed in more detail next. Sporadic reports of other thrombopathies in veterinary species have also been reported.

Chédiak-Higashi syndrome

One of the classic features of CHS (discussed earlier in the section on disorders of granulocytes) is a bleeding tendency due to platelet dysfunction. Platelets in individuals with CHS lack the dense granules that normally contain key bioactive molecules involved in hemostasis, including platelet agonists, such as ADP and serotonin, and platelet aggregation in vitro in response to collagen, in particular, is severely impaired.

Simmental hereditary thrombopathy

An inherited platelet function defect resulting in a severe bleeding tendency has been reported in Simmental cattle. The mode of inheritance is apparently not simple mendelian recessive, and the condition may involve mutations of more than one gene. The condition is characterized clinically by spontaneous epistaxis, hematuria, and excessive bleeding in response to minor surgical (e.g., castration) and other (e.g., ear tagging or tattooing) procedures. Platelet aggregation in vitro in response to a number of agonists is markedly impaired. The specific defect has not been identified on the molecular level.

Glanzmann thrombasthenia

Glanzmann thrombasthenia (GT) is an inherited platelet function defect caused by defective expression of the integrin $\alpha_{IIb}\beta_3$ (also known as GPIIb-IIIa). The $\alpha_{IIb}\beta_3$ molecule has a number of functions, but is best known as a fibrinogen receptor that is essential for normal platelet aggregation. Bleeding tendencies vary widely between affected individuals, and bleeding tends to occur mainly on mucosal surfaces. The condition is characterized by an in vitro lack of response to all platelet agonists and severely impaired clot retraction. GT has been recognized in Great Pyrenees and otterhound dogs and in a quarter horse and a thoroughbred horse; a clinically similar condition that does not fulfill molecular criteria of GT has been described in basset hound dogs.

Scott-like syndrome

An inherited thrombopathy resembling Scott syndrome in human beings, in which platelets lack normal procoagulant activity, has been recognized in a family of German shepherd dogs. Affected dogs have a mild to moderate clinical bleeding tendency characterized by epistaxis, hyphema, intramuscular hematoma formation, and increased hemorrhage associated with surgery. The specific defect in these dogs has not been identified on the molecular level, but involves impaired expression of phosphatidylserine on the platelet surface.

von Willebrand disease

von Willebrand disease (vWD) actually refers to a group of inherited conditions characterized by a quantitative or qualitative deficiency of von Willebrand factor (vWF), a soluble multimeric glycoprotein that circulates as a complex with and stabilizes coagulation factor VIII, and mediates binding of platelets to subendothelial collagen (see Fig. 2-18). Although not technically a platelet disorder, vWD is often classified as such because it results in a loss of normal platelet function. vWD is the most common canine heriditary bleeding disorder and has also been described in many other domestic species. Different types of vWD vary in terms of mode of inheritance and severity of clinical disease. Type I vWD is characterized by low plasma vWF concentration but normal multimer proportions and a mild to moderate clinical bleeding tendency; it has been reported in many dog breeds. Type II vWD is characterized by low vWF concentration, absence of large multimers, and a moderate to severe bleeding tendency; it has been reported in German shorthaired pointer and German wirehaired pointer dogs. Type III vWD is characterized by absence of vWF and a severe bleeding tendency; familial and sporadic cases have been reported in numerous dog breeds.

BREED-RELATED PLATELET ABNORMALITIES

Cavalier King Charles spaniels often have a lower than normal concentration of platelets, many of which are abnormally large (a condition known as macrothrombocytopenia). This is likely an autosomal recessive trait. In general, affected dogs are asymptomatic. Cavalier King Charles spaniels have been shown to have abnormal platelet aggregation in vitro in some studies, although the clinical significance of these findings, including a possible causal relationship between platelet abnormalities and mitral valve disease in this breed, is not clear.

Greyhounds tend to have lower concentrations of circulating platelets than other dog breeds (and lower concentrations of erythrocytes and higher MCV and PCV), although this is not of any known clinical significance.

DISORDERS OF LYMPHOCYTES

Disorders of lymphocytes are discussed in the sections on the lymphatic system and in the next section on hematopoietic neoplasia (also see Chapter 6).

HEMATOPOIETIC NEOPLASIA

The term *hematopoietic neoplasia* encompasses a large, diverse group of clonal proliferative disorders of hematopoietic cell types. This section is intended to help the student understand the basic biology (cell type, anatomic distribution, and biologic behavior) and diagnosis of hematopoietic neoplasia in veterinary medicine, with an emphasis on those forms that predominantly affect bone marrow, blood, and lymphoid tissue. Tumors of hematopoietic origin that predominantly affect other tissue, such as skin, will also be mentioned. Before listing specific diseases, it is worthwhile to consider the basic classification of hematopoietic neoplasia and mention some of the emerging diagnostic techniques used in veterinary medicine.

Hematopoietic neoplasia can be broadly classified as lymphoproliferative (lymphoid) or myeloproliferative (myeloid) disease, a distinction based on the fact that the earliest commitment of a pluripotent hematopoietic stem cell is to either a lymphoid or nonlymphoid lineage (Fig. 13-1). Thus clonal proliferations of cells of lymphoid lineage are examples of lymphoid neoplasia, including the various forms of lymphoma (lymphosarcoma), lymphoid (lymphocytic) leukemia, and plasma cell tumors. Clonal proliferations of cells of nonlymphoid hematopoietic lineage (erythroid, granulocytic, monocytic and/or histiocytic, megakaryocytic), are considered myeloid neoplasias, including the various forms of myeloid (or myelogenous) leukemia, myelodysplastic syndrome, and histiocytic neoplasia. Mast cell tumors are not conventionally considered a form of hematopoietic neoplasia, but in a technical sense they are also a form of myeloid neoplasia.

A number of techniques for diagnosing and classifying hematopoietic neoplasia are becoming increasingly available for routine use in veterinary medicine. For example, *immunophenotyping* refers to the use of antibodies recognizing specific molecules expressed on different cell types to determine the identity of a cell population of interest. Immunophenotyping on the basis of these lineage-specific or lineage-associated markers can be performed on histologic sections (immunohistochemistry), air-dried cytology smears (immunocytochemistry), or by laser analysis of cells in suspension in blood or buffer solutions (flow cytometry). Another emerging diagnostic technique is the clonality assay, a PCR test that can help identify neoplastic lymphoid proliferations on the basis of clonal rearrangements of genes encoding lymphocyte antigen receptors. In terms of practical application, the clonality assay is most useful in helping to distinguish lymphoid neoplasia from nonneoplastic lymphoid proliferations mimicking neoplasia.

In the last several decades, as new diagnostic techniques have become available, numerous systems for classifying hematopoietic neoplasia in human beings have been proposed. These systems have been applied to veterinary medicine inconsistently but have helped to demonstrate the diversity of disease subtypes in animals. Some of these systems (the Rappaport and Kiel systems) did not attempt to correlate the classification of the neoplasm based on microscopic features with the clinical course of disease, whereas others (the Working Formulation for classification of lymphomas, sponsored by the National Cancer Institute) attempted to correlate survival data with morphologic criteria but did not take into account the cell of origin (i.e., B lymphocyte or T lymphocyte) of the tumor. The most recent (2002) published system for classifying hematopoietic neoplasia in animals is an adaptation of the 2001 World Health Organization (WHO) system in human beings. An effort is underway to coordinate the classification of hematopoietic neoplasia in human beings and animals in a consistent, clinically relevant manner. This effort, termed the American College of Veterinary Pathology (ACVP) Oncology Initiative, has two main components: a proposal for classification of canine lymphomas and a proposal for classification of myeloid neoplasia in cats and dogs. The ultimate goal of this undertaking is to correlate pathologic findings (cell morphology, immunophenotype, tissue architecture, anatomic location) precisely with clinical behavior of the neoplasm (prognosis, response to therapy).

The next section on hematopoietic neoplasia begins with leukemias (which may be of lymphoid or myeloid origin) and myelodysplastic syndromes, then covers the group of lymphoid malignancies known as lymphomas, and finishes by mentioning some other types of lymphoid and myeloid neoplasia.

LEUKEMIAS AND MYELODYSPLASTIC SYNDROMES

Leukemia is an umbrella term referring to malignant hematopoietic neoplasms that originate in the bone marrow and typically have significant numbers of neoplastic cells in the blood. Hematopoietic neoplasms originating in the spleen, but primarily manifested in the blood, are also considered by some to be forms of primary leukemia. The term *leukemia* is also sometimes used to refer to other forms of hematopoietic neoplasia originating outside of the bone marrow or spleen, such as lymphoma, that may progress to include significant bone marrow and blood involvement. For the purposes of this chapter, cases of secondary bone marrow or blood involvement will not be considered leukemia but rather diseases with a "leukemic phase" of a primary disease other than leukemia. Although primary leukemias usually have high numbers of neoplastic cells in circulation, this is not always the case. Some forms of leukemia (especially acute lymphoid leukemia in cats) have very low numbers of circulating neoplastic cells. This situation is sometimes known as "aleukemic leukemia," although very close examination of blood smears will usually reveal the underlying disease.

Table 13-5   Basic Classification of Leukemias

	Lymphoid	Myeloid
Chronic	CLL	CML
Acute	ALL	AML

ALL, Acute lymphoid leukemia; *AML*, acute myeloid leukemia; *CLL*, chronic lymphoid leukemia; *CML*, chronic myeloid leukemia.

The diagnosis may require confirmation by examination of the bone marrow, which in cases of leukemia contains disproportionately high numbers of neoplastic cells.

Leukemias are conventionally classified into one of four main groups according to cell type (lymphoid or myeloid, with subcategories of both types) and as chronic or acute (Table 13-5). Subcategories exist within each of these groups (e.g., lymphoid leukemias of B- or T-lymphocyte origin, and myeloid leukemias of erythroid, granulocytic, monocytic, or megakaryocytic origin). Chronic and acute leukemias differ both in terms of cell morphology and biologic behavior.

Chronic leukemias are proliferations of well-differentiated cells and are typically indolent, slowly progressive diseases. Often the number of neoplastic cells in circulation is very high. It is not unusual for the concentration to be in the hundreds of thousands per microliter. Mild to moderate nonregenerative anemia is common, but other cytopenias are not usually present. With chronic leukemias, the lineage of the cells is easy to identify by examining a blood or bone marrow smear. The cells look normal, or relatively normal, under the microscope. However, this can pose a diagnostic challenge because it is often not easy to tell whether the cells are a malignant population (i.e., leukemia) or a benign, reactive population (as in the case of marked inflammatory neutrophilia, reactive lymphocytosis, or secondary erythrocytosis), particularly when the concentration of cells in the blood is consistent with either neoplastic or nonneoplastic disease. Diagnosis of chronic leukemia in veterinary species is thus typically one of exclusion. An exception is when the concentration of cells in the blood is so high as to reasonably exclude the possibility of nonneoplastic disease (e.g., the concentration of lymphocytes in cases of chronic lymphocytic leukemia often exceeds 100,000 cells/uL). Necropsy findings are dependent on the stage of disease. In advanced cases with marked organ infiltration with neoplastic cells, there is often uniform splenomegaly, hepatomegaly, and lymphadenopathy. The bone marrow is highly cellular and, histologically, is densely cellular with well-differentiated neoplastic cells. In lymph nodes, there may be follicular lymphoid hyperplasia and neoplastic cells in the sinuses and medullary cords. Similarly the spleen may have follicular lymphoid hyperplasia and accumulation of neoplastic cells in the red pulp. The liver may have accumulations of neoplastic cells in the sinusoids and periportal areas.

Chronic lymphoid leukemias (CLLs) are uncommon in veterinary species. The disease is rarely reported in horses and poorly characterized in cattle. In dogs, CLL is predominantly a disease of middle-aged to older dogs. In the largest study to date, 73% of canine CLL cases were of T-lymphocyte origin. In 54% of the CLL cases, the neoplastic cells were granular T lymphocytes, the vast majority of which expressed CD8 (consistent with cytotoxic T-lymphocyte lineage). Interestingly, most of these cases apparently originated in the spleen, with detectable bone marrow involvement occurring relatively late in the course of disease. There is scant published data regarding CLL in cats, but according to a recent report the majority of cases have a T-helper cell immunophenotype.

Chronic myeloid leukemias (CMLs) are rare in animals, with most reported cases occurring in dogs and cats. Types of CML reported in animals include chronic granulocytic leukemias of neutrophils, eosinophils, and basophils; chronic myelomonocytic leukemia; mast cell leukemia; essential thrombocythemia (CML of platelet lineage); and polycythemia vera (CML of erythrocyte lineage).

In contrast to chronic leukemias, acute leukemias are proliferations of poorly differentiated cells (Fig. 13-34) and typically have a rapid, aggressive clinical course. The distinction between chronic and acute leukemia is not always perfectly clear, either in terms of cell morphology or biologic behavior, and some cases fall "in the middle." Moreover, chronic leukemia may develop into a more acute form (presumably because of additional mutation), a situation sometimes referred to as "blast crisis." Acute leukemia has classically been defined by the presence of greater than 30% blast cells (large, immature cells) in the marrow or blood, although in human beings it has recently been proposed that the threshold be lowered to 20%. In general, the concentration of circulating neoplastic cells in acute leukemias does not tend to be as high as in chronic leukemias. Most animals with acute leukemia have cytopenias of two or more lineages, and pancytopenia is common. With acute leukemias, it is usually obvious from the presence of many large, immature cells in circulation that the patient has hematopoietic neoplasia. However, the cell of origin usually cannot be determined by routine microscopic examination because the cells are poorly differentiated. Identifying the specific cell type is best done by immunophenotyping and/or cytochemical staining. At necropsy, animals with acute leukemia have pale mucous membranes due to anemia, and the bone marrow is highly cellular. Other findings depend on the degree to which neoplastic cells have infiltrated organs. There is often uniform splenomegaly, sometimes with infarcts. Histologically the bone marrow is densely cellular with poorly differentiated neoplastic cells. The splenic red pulp may be extensively infiltrated with neoplastic cells. The lymph nodes may have minor involvement of the medullary cords to diffuse involvement of the entire node.

Myelodysplastic syndrome (MDS) refers to a group of clonal myeloid proliferative disorders characterized by ineffective hematopoiesis. MDS does not meet the traditional definition of acute myeloid leukemia (AML) but is classically diagnosed based on these findings: less than 30% blasts in the bone marrow, cytopenias of more than one cell line, and morphologic evidence of dyshematopoiesis. Studies in people have shown that MDS also differs from AML on the molecular level (MDS is characterized by increased apoptosis compared with AML). MDS may lead to clinical illness and death as a result of the cytopenias and/or from transformation of the neoplasm into AML. MDS is rare in veterinary medicine, occurring most frequently in FeLV-infected cats.

The existing system for classification of AML and MDS in cats and dogs, an adaptation of the French-American-British (FAB) classification system in human beings, was proposed by the Animal Leukemia Study Group (ALSG) in 1991 and has been generally accepted since that time. However, the system does not include immunophenotyping or cytochemical staining characteristics, which have since become key aspects of classifying myeloid neoplasia in people. The ACVP Oncology Initiative group is currently working to develop a new classification system that includes

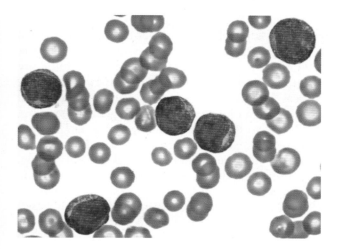

Fig. 13-34   Acute leukemia, canine blood smear. The specific lineage of the large, immature cells cannot be determined reliably based on routine staining. Wright's stain. *(Courtesy Dr. M.M. Fry, College of Veterinary Medicine, University of Tennessee.)*

Box **13-10**

Classification Systems for Acute Myeloid Leukemia

- Classification scheme proposed by Animal Leukemia Study Group in 1991: In Jain NC, Blue JT, Grindem CB et al: Proposed criteria for classification of acute myeloid leukemia in dogs and cats, *Vet Clin Pathol* 20(3):63-82, 1991.
- 2002 WHO Classification of the Myeloid Neoplasms: Vardiman JW, Harris NL, Brunning RD: *Blood* 100 (7):2292-2302, 2002.

---

immunophenotyping and cytochemical staining data. The mission of this group is as follows:

> … to match a classification system (either the original system proposed by the Animal Leukemia Study Group or possibly a system modeled after the recently revised WHO system) with the biologic behavior of myeloid neoplasms. We hope to confirm or challenge the 30% blast cell threshold for distinguishing AML from MDS and associate biological behavior with specific disease subtypes. Similar to the revisions in the human classification system, this project must be done in collaboration with oncology clinics, veterinary institutions, and large diagnostic laboratories.

The existing ALSG system in animals and the 2002 WHO classification system in human beings are referenced in Box 13-10 and in the Suggested Readings list.

Acute lymphoid leukemia (ALL) is rarely recognized in horses and cattle. Cattle with lymphoid neoplasia caused by bovine leukemia virus infection often have high numbers of circulating neoplastic cells, but the disease is generally considered a form of lymphoma and will be discussed next in the section on lymphoma. In a recent immunophenotypic study of 38 cases of acute leukemia in dogs, 6 had B-lymphocyte ALL and 3 had T-lymphocyte ALL of CD8+ granular lymphocytes. Cats with ALL often have low numbers of neoplastic cells in circulation, and examination of the bone marrow may be necessary to make the diagnosis.

AML occurs most often in dogs and cats but has also been reported in other domestic and wild animals. In dogs, the majority of acute leukemias are of myeloid or probable myeloid origin (21 of 38 cases in one recent study). Myelodysplastic syndrome is recognized most often in cats, especially in animals infected with FeLV, but has also been reported in dogs and horses.

LYMPHOMA (LYMPHOSARCOMA)

The term *lymphoma* (also known as lymphosarcoma or malignant lymphoma) encompasses a diverse group of malignancies arising in lymphoid tissue(s) outside the bone marrow. There are many different forms, with notable variability in the following:

- Anatomic location—multicentric, alimentary, mediastinal/thymic, other
- Immunophenotype—B lymphocyte versus T lymphocyte versus non-B/non-T
- Cellular morphology—size, nuclear features, mitotic rate
- Histologic pattern—diffuse versus follicular
- Biologic behavior—from low-grade (indolent) to high-grade (aggressive) tumors

As mentioned previously, there is an ongoing effort within the ACVP to demonstrate the applicability of the new WHO system for classifying hematopoietic neoplasia in people to animals, including a specific project focusing on classification of lymphoma in dogs. The principle underlying this effort is that each category should constitute a distinct, recognized disease entity based on morphology, tissue architecture, immunophenotype, anatomic distribution, signalment data, and full clinical history. A critical component of this effort is to test the consistency (interobserver variability) and reproducibility (intraobserver variability) of interpretation.

Diagnosis and laboratory findings

Lymphoma is often suspected on the basis of organomegaly (e.g., generalized lymph node enlargement) or abnormal ultrasound findings (e.g., thickened intestines with abnormal echogenicity). Initial diagnosis typically is made based on aspiration cytology, biopsy and/or histopathology, or both, of the affected organ(s). In both cytologic and histologic preparations, lymphoma is characterized by a monomorphic population of morphologically atypical lymphocytes. Histologically, lymphoma is also characterized by disruption of normal tissue architecture. In general, lymphomas of small, well-differentiated cells with low mitotic rates are low-grade (indolent, slowly progressive) diseases, whereas lymphomas of large, poorly differentiated cells with high mitotic rates are high-grade (aggressive, rapidly progressive) diseases (Fig. 13-35). The type of tumor and extent of disease may be characterized further by immunophenotyping and clinical staging, respectively. Immunophenotyping is done to determine whether a tumor is of B-lymphocyte or T-lymphocyte origin (this distinction cannot be made reliably based on routine staining). It is not necessarily the case that B-lymphocyte lymphomas have a more favorable prognosis than T-lymphocyte lymphomas because both cell types occur in low-grade and high-grade forms. Clinical staging includes examination of aspirates of bone marrow and other enlarged organs (e.g., spleen, liver, and other lymph nodes).

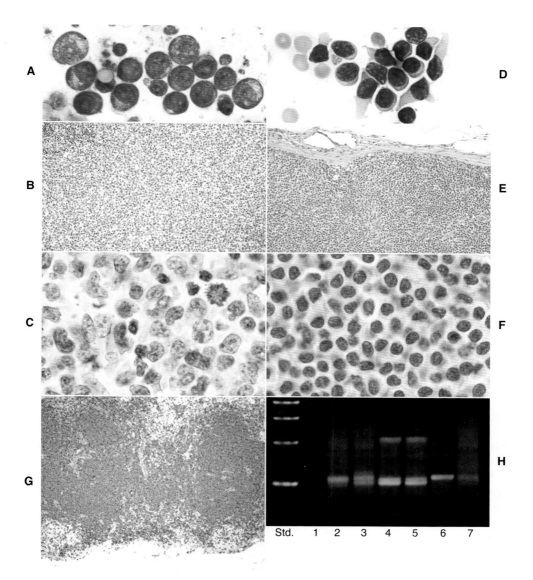

Fig. 13-35   Grading of canine lymphomas, lymph node, dog. Lymphoma (lymphosarcoma): high grade, fine-needle aspirate (**A**), excisional biopsy (**B** and **C**). Neoplastic lymphocytes are large and have large nuclei with dispersed chromatin and prominent nucleoli. Fig. 13-35, *B* and *C* are low- and high-magnification images, respectively, of the same specimen. A mitotic figure is evident at the top right of Fig. 13-35, *C*. Wright's stain (Fig. 13-35, *A*), H&E stain (Fig. 13-35, *B* and *C*). Lymphoma (lymphosarcoma): low grade, fine-needle aspirate (**D**), excisional biopsy (**E** and **F**). Images were taken at the same magnifications as those shown in Fig. 13-35, *A* to *C*. In this sample, neoplastic lymphocytes are of small to intermediate size and have partially condensed chromatin. Wright's stain (Fig. 13-35, *D*), H&E stain (Fig. 13-35, *E* and *F*). Lymphoma (lymphosarcoma): low grade, immunohistochemistry (**G**) and clonality testing (**H**) results for the low-grade lymphoma case shown in Fig. 13-35, *D* to *F*. Fig. 13-35, *G* (from the same area shown in Fig. 13-35, *E*, and taken at the same magnification) shows immunostaining for the T-lymphocyte marker CD3, demonstrating a marked expansion of T lymphocytes. Polymerase chain reaction testing of DNA extracted from the excisional biopsy specimen confirmed that these cells had a clonal T-lymphocyte receptor gene rearrangement, as shown in the gel in Fig. 13-35, *H. Lane 1*, negative control with no DNA; *lanes 2 and 3*, duplicates of a different case of T-lymphocyte lymphoma; *lanes 4 and 5*, duplicates of this case; *lane 6*, positive control; *lane 7*, polyclonal control (i.e., normal). (*A*, Courtesy Dr. M.M. Fry, College of Veterinary Medicine, University of Tennessee. *B, C, E, F,* and *G*, Courtesy Dr. S.J. Newman, College of Veterinary Medicine, University of Tennessee. *D*, Courtesy Dr. D.F. Edwards, College of Veterinary Medicine, University of Tennessee. *H*, Courtesy Dr. W. Vernau, School of Veterinary Medicine, University of California, Davis.)

In cases of advanced disease there may be marked bone marrow and blood involvement, and distinguishing lymphoma from lymphoid leukemia can occasionally be difficult. The distinction can often be made on the basis of immunophenotyping—especially for CD34, which is usually expressed by neoplastic cells in acute leukemias and not in lymphomas. Other laboratory findings with lymphoma are variable. Mild to moderate nonregenerative anemia is probably the most common hematologic abnormality. Lymphopenia is noted more frequently than lymphocytosis, presumably because of abnormal trafficking of normal, nonneoplastic lymphocytes. Hypercalcemia is often associated with lymphoma due to production of parathyroid hormone-related peptide (PTHrP) by the neoplastic cells. Such paraneoplastic hypercalcemia (humoral hypercalcemia of malignancy) may lead to pathologic calcification and related complications (e.g., renal failure).

Necropsy findings in cases of multicentric lymphoma include enlarged lymph nodes that bulge on cut section and are gray-white to light tan or reddish. In advanced cases, the normal architectural distinction between the cortex and medulla is obliterated. Infiltration of spleen and liver can result in diffuse enlargement or nodules. In alimentary lymphoma, affected portions of the gastrointestinal tract are thickened and may be nodular. The lesions may be ulcerated. Enlarged mesenteric nodes may coalesce to form large masses. The gross appearance of thymic lymphoma is a large, gray, soft mass in the cranial mediastinum (Fig. 13-46). Renal lymphoma often affects both kidneys and is evident as bilateral diffuse renomegaly. Central nervous system and bone marrow involvement of lymphoma can be difficult to detect on necropsy because of the similar gross appearance of neoplastic and normal tissue. In any of the various forms of lymphoma, large masses may have areas of central necrosis.

Species differences

Lymphoma is the most common hematopoietic malignancy in animals and has been reported in all the domestic species.

Lymphoma is uncommon in horses, representing 5% or less of all neoplasms. Multicentric lymphoma is the most common form, and alimentary, cutaneous, and other forms may also occur. Most lymphomas in horses are of intermediate or low grade, according to most sources. The multicentric form is characterized by irregular involvement of peripheral lymph nodes with tumor masses in the mediastinum and abdomen. Lymph nodes in different anatomic regions (e.g., superficial, mediastinal, and alimentary) are often similarly affected, and infiltration of liver and spleen is common.

Reports of the frequency of concurrent blood involvement vary from rare to more than 50%. The alimentary form of equine lymphoma is a wasting syndrome, presumably because of involvement of the small intestine, resulting in malabsorption. Cutaneous lymphoma in horses, as in other species, is a chronic disease without blood or internal organ involvement. Equine lymphoma is often of mixed cell type (B lymphocyte and T lymphocyte). B-lymphocyte tumors that also contain many nonneoplastic T lymphocytes (so-called T-lymphocyte–rich B-lymphocyte lymphoma) are especially common as subcutaneous neoplasms.

In cattle, lymphoma is primarily a multicentric B-lymphocyte disease of adult cattle and is strongly associated with BLV infection and BLV-related persistent lymphocytosis. Approximately 30% of cattle infected with BLV develop nonneoplastic persistent lymphocytosis, and of these, less than 5% develop lymphoma. The BLV-induced form of lymphoma is known as bovine enzootic lymphoma. BLV is a retrovirus that persists within lymphocytes for the life of the infected animal. Transmission of the virus is mostly horizontal due to transmission of infected lymphocytes as opposed to free virus in secretions. Blood-sucking arthropods or other mechanical means of transferring small numbers of infected lymphocytes (such as contaminated needles) are the principle means of spread. BLV infection is more common in dairy cattle than in beef cattle, presumably because dairy cattle husbandry favors viral transmission. Incidence of infection varies widely between regions and between herds. Antibodies against viral antigen can be detected by an agarose gel immunodiffusion test, and some herds remain free of BLV by testing and culling infected animals. In addition to lymph nodes, lymphoma in cattle often involves other locations, such as abomasum, vertebral canal, kidney, heart, retro-orbital space, and uterus (Fig. 13-36). Enlargement of superficial lymph nodes is common, and enlarged pelvic and abdominal lymph nodes are often found on rectal palpation. Involvement of the digestive tract and heart may cause vagal indigestion or diarrhea and congestive heart failure, respectively. Lymphoma of the central nervous system is most frequently manifested as posterior paresis or paralysis because of pressure by the extradural mass on the cauda equina or on the lumbar cord. Other sporadic forms of lymphoma not associated with BLV infection also occur in cattle, including thymic, multicentric, and cutaneous forms affecting young animals. The thymic form of sporadic bovine lymphoma is characterized by large cranial thoracic and lower cervical masses, respiratory distress, and weight loss in cattle less than 2 years of age. The sporadic multicentric form is characterized by disseminated disease in calves 3 to 6 months of age. Affected calves frequently have

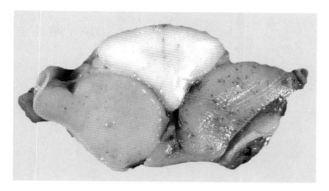

Fig. 13-36   Lymphoma (lymphosarcoma), vertebral canal, epidural space, cow. Bilateral ventrally located soft pink masses compress the spinal cord. In addition to lymph nodes, lymphoma in cattle often involves other locations, such as abomasum, vertebral canal, kidney, heart, retro-orbital space, and uterus. *(Courtesy Dr. J.M. King, College of Veterinary Medicine, Cornell University.)*

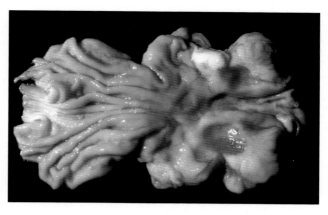

Fig. 13-37   Alimentary lymphoma (lymphosarcoma), stomach, cat. Note the notable thickening of the stomach, which occurred because of infiltration with neoplastic cells. Although uncommon, the mucosal epithelium is focally ulcerated. *(Courtesy Dr. M.D. McGavin, College of Veterinary Medicine, University of Tennessee.)*

widespread lymph node enlargement in addition to hepatic, splenic, and renal involvement. Marked blood and bone marrow involvement may also occur. The cutaneous form is rare, occurs in young cattle, and consists of discrete cutaneous plaques or large scabby lesions.

In dogs, lymphoma is a common form of neoplasia, representing approximately 7% to 9% of all malignancies and the large majority of hematopoietic malignancies. No retroviral or other cause is known. Lymphoma is typically a disease of middle-aged to older dogs. Multicentric lymphoma with generalized lymph node enlargement is the most common form (80% to 85% of all cases of canine lymphoma), and the majority of these (approximately 80%) are intermediate- or high-grade tumors. Other less common forms of canine lymphoma include alimentary, thymic, and cutaneous forms, and sporadically occurring forms in virtually every conceivable location. Approximately 70% to 80% of canine lymphomas are of B-lymphocyte origin. Although the remaining cases are mostly of T-lymphocyte origin, "null" (non-B, non-T, presumably of NK [natural killer] cell origin) lymphomas also occur. Clinical signs may be referable to the specific organ systems affected, but are usually absent or nonspecific when lymphoma is first diagnosed. Approximately 15% of dogs with lymphoma, and approximately 40% of those with mediastinal lymphoma, are hypercalcemic. In the majority of canine lymphoma cases, significant blood or bone marrow involvement is not detected by routine methods upon initial diagnosis, but may be seen with advanced disease. Splenic and hepatic involvement is common in cases of canine multicentric lymphoma.

In cats, lymphoma is among the many hematopoietic abnormalities caused by FeLV, and the epidemiology of feline lymphoma has changed with the development of

routine vaccination and testing for FeLV. Cats infected with FeLV are likely to develop lymphoma at a younger age, and are more likely to develop certain types of lymphoma—especially mediastinal and multicentric T-lymphocyte forms—than FeLV-negative cats. These predispositions still apply, but the percentage of cats infected with FeLV has decreased dramatically. As a result, mediastinal (thymic) and multicentric forms of lymphoma, which used to represent the majority of cases, have become relatively uncommon. At present, approximately 80% to 90% of cats with lymphoma are FeLV-negative, and the majority of lymphoma cases are the alimentary form (Fig. 13-37). Other less common locations in cats include mediastinal, multicentric, renal, and other extranodal sites. FeLV-positive cats with lymphoma still tend to be younger, and their tumors more often of T-lymphocyte origin, than FeLV-negative cats. The large majority (>80%) of cats with mediastinal lymphoma, and approximately one third of cats with multicentric lymphoma, are FeLV-positive. Mediastinal and multicentric forms, although less common now, are still more likely to occur in younger cats, whereas the alimentary form typically develops in older cats (>10 years of age). The neoplastic cell type also tends to vary by anatomic location. Alimentary lymphoma in cats is predominantly a B-lymphocyte disease, whereas mediastinal lymphoma is predominantly a T-lymphocyte disease (consistent with thymic origin). A subtype of intestinal lymphoma in cats, large granular lymphocyte (LGL) lymphoma, is predominantly a T-lymphocyte disease with a highly aggressive biologic behavior. Unlike dogs, cats are usually clinically ill when lymphoma is first diagnosed. In addition to nonspecific signs, such as weight loss, anorexia, and poor grooming habits, cats often have signs referable to the affected organ systems. For example, animals with alimentary lymphoma often have chronic diarrhea and vomiting, and may have palpable abdominal masses, whereas those with mediastinal lymphoma are often dyspneic.

Lymphoma is the most commonly reported malignancy in pigs and may be more likely to affect females than males. Multicentric lymphoma is the most common form of the disease in pigs. Lymph node enlargement is more common in visceral than peripheral nodes. Other commonly affected organs include spleen, liver, kidney, and bone marrow. Lymphoma often affects animals less than 1 year of age, and the mediastinal form of lymphoma tends to affect younger pigs more commonly than the multicentric form. A viral cause (C type viruses) for lymphoma in pigs has been suggested, but transmission studies are lacking. A form of hereditary multicentric lymphoma has also been reported in inbred herds.

OTHER FORMS OF HEMATOPOIETIC NEOPLASIA

In addition to the leukemias and lymphomas, other forms of hematopoietic neoplasia—including lymphoid neoplasms (plasma cell tumors) and myeloid neoplasms (histiocytic, mast cell, and granulocytic tumors)—are also recognized in animals.

Plasma cell neoplasia

There are two main forms of plasma cells tumors recognized in veterinary species: multiple myeloma (MM) and plasmacytoma.

Multiple myeloma. MM is a malignant tumor of plasma cells that arises in the bone marrow and usually secretes large amounts of immunoglobulin (Ig). Blood involvement of the neoplastic cells is not a feature of the disease. MM is a rare disease in animals. Dogs are affected more frequently than other species, but MM has also been reported in horses, cattle, cats, and pigs. The hallmark laboratory finding in patients with MM is hyperglobulinemia, which occurs because of production of large amounts of Ig or Ig subunit by the neoplastic cells. This homogenous protein fraction is often called paraprotein or M protein. Concentrations of other Igs are often decreased.

Diagnosis of MM is based on finding a minimum of two or three (opinions vary) of the following abnormalities:
- Markedly increased numbers of plasma cells in the bone marrow, especially in aggregates (Fig. 13-38, A). A threshold value of plasma cells constituting at least 30% of nucleated cells in the marrow has been proposed as a diagnostic criterion. The neoplastic cells composing the tumor may be well-differentiated plasma cells or poorly differentiated cells with

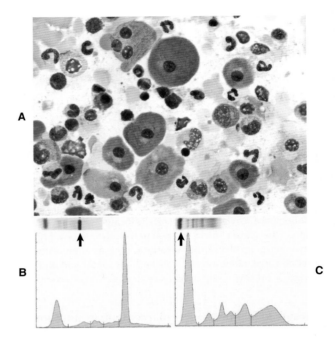

Fig. 13-38 **Multiple myeloma and monoclonal gammopathy. A,** Canine bone marrow aspirate. Many of the neoplastic plasma cells in the bone marrow aspirate have pink-tinged cytoplasm, the result of a high concentration of immunoglobulin. Wright's stain. **B,** Multiple myeloma, cat. Agarose gels and densitometry tracings showing results of serum electrophoresis. The serum has a high concentration of a monoclonal immunoglobulin (*the dark band [arrow] on the right of the gel, corresponding to the tall peak on the right of the tracing*). **C,** Normal cat. Agarose gels and densitometry tracings showing results of serum electrophoresis. The serum has a normal distribution of protein fractions, the most abundant being albumin (*the dark band [arrow] on the left of the gel, corresponding to the tall peak on the left of the tracing*). (**A,** *Courtesy Dr. M.M. Fry, College of Veterinary Medicine, University of Tennessee.* **B** *and* **C,** *Courtesy Dr. S.A. Kania, College of Veterinary Medicine, University of Tennessee.*)

increased anisocytosis and anisokaryosis, visible nucleoli, and multinucleation.
- Monoclonal gammopathy because of clonal production of Ig or Ig fragments by the neoplastic cells. Monoclonality is demonstrated by serum protein electrophoresis (Fig. 13-38, B), and can be characterized further using immunodiagnostic techniques (see later discussion). The term "gammopathy" is used because most Igs migrate in the γ-region of an electrophoresis gel, although some (especially IgA and IgM) may migrate in the β-region. Occasionally biclonal or other atypical electrophoretic patterns may be seen with MM as a result of protein degradation, complex formation, or binding to other proteins, or when the tumor includes more than one clonal population. It is important to note that monoclonal

gammopathy is not specific to MM but has also been reported in cases of B-lymphocyte lymphoma and some nonneoplastic conditions, such as canine ehrlichiosis or leishmaniasis. What appears to be a monoclonal pattern in the γ-region on routine serum electrophoresis may actually be oligoclonal (i.e., may include several Igs with a very similar migration pattern that are increased because of an immunologic response to antigenic stimulation). (This is unlikely to be the case with "spikes" in the β-region, because nonneoplastic conditions typically do not result in high concentrations of IgA or IgM.) Definitively distinguishing monoclonal from oligoclonal patterns in the γ-region requires immunoelectrophoresis or immunofixation using species-specific antibodies recognizing different Ig subclasses and subunits.

- Radiographic evidence of osteolysis. Recent work with human cell cultures has shown that osteoclasts support the growth of myeloma cells, and that direct contact between the two cell types increases the myeloma cell proliferation and promotes osteoclast survival.
- Light chain proteinuria. Free Ig light chains (Bence-Jones proteins) are of low molecular weight and pass through the glomerular filter into the urine. These proteins do not react with urine dipstick protein indicators and are most specifically detected by electrophoresis and immunoprecipitation.

Other pathologic findings in patients with MM may include the following:

- Hypercalcemia, most likely due to increased osteoclast activity
- Lesions associated with marked hyperglobulinemia (hemorrhage caused by secondary platelet dysfunction, renal amyloidosis, and hyperviscosity syndrome)
- Cytopenias due to high numbers of neoplastic cells in the bone marrow

MM typically has a slowly progressive clinical course. Common sites of metastasis include the spleen, liver, lymph nodes, and kidneys.

Plasmacytomas.   Cutaneous plasmacytomas are solid tumors of plasma cell origin that involve the skin or mucous membranes. Masses may be single or multiple. These tumors are usually benign, and excision is usually curative, but more aggressive forms may occur. Cutaneous plasmacytoma is discussed in more detail in Chapter 17. The tumor type known as extramedullary plasmacytoma (EMP) is a malignant solid tissue tumor of plasma cells arising from sites other than the bone marrow. The tumor is rare in animals, occurring most often in dogs and also reported in horses and cats. In one study, there was a disproportionately high percentage of EMP cases in cocker spaniels. The tumors occur most frequently in the gastrointestinal tract but may also occur in the trachea, spleen, kidney, uterus, central

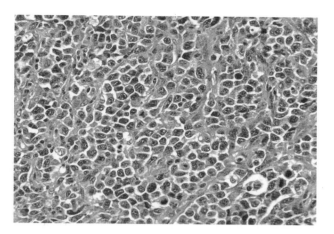

Fig. 13-39   **Plasmacytoma, oral mucosa, dog.** Note the moderately well-differentiated plasma cells arranged in small clusters separated by a fibrovascular stroma. H&E stain. *(Courtesy College of Veterinary Medicine, University of Illinois.)*

nervous system, and elsewhere. Grossly the tumors may be multinodular or cause thickening of the intestinal wall. Metastasis to regional lymph nodes is common. As with MM, the neoplastic cells composing the tumor may be well-differentiated to poorly differentiated (Fig. 13-39). EMPs produce monoclonal immunoglobulins, and monoclonal gammopathy has been reported in some cases of EMP. If there is bone or bone marrow involvement of a malignant plasma cell tumor, it is considered to be MM. Amyloidosis is associated with EMP in many reports and may be useful in distinguishing extramedullary plasmacytoma from other tumors. The distinction between cutaneous plasmacytoma and extramedullary plasmacytoma is not always clear, and benign plasmacytomas of the skin have also been referred to as cutaneous extramedullary plasmacytomas.

Histiocytic neoplasia

Histiocytoma.   Histiocytoma, a benign cutaneous neoplasm of epidermal Langerhans cell origin, is discussed in detail in Chapter 17.

Histiocytic sarcoma.   Histiocytic sarcoma (HS) is an uncommon malignant neoplasm of histiocytic (macrophage or dendritic cell) origin. It occurs most frequently in the dog but has also been reported in the cat. There is a general belief that rottweilers and Bernese mountain dogs are at increased risk for HS, although good epidemiologic data is thus far lacking. Some have called the disseminated form of this disease, with multiple organ involvement, by the name "malignant histiocytosis," reserving the term "histiocytic sarcoma" for cases of single solid tumors, but there is an emerging consensus that the latter term encompasses both forms of the disease. The disseminated form of the disease has a rapid, aggressive clinical course. Sites commonly involved include the spleen, lung, lymph nodes, bone marrow, skin, and subcutis. Liver involvement occurs secondary to disease in the spleen. The solitary form of HS can occur at any of the aforementioned sites, and also in joints (in close association with the subsynovium) or brain. Most cases of HS are of dendritic antigen-presenting cell origin, with a similar immunophenotype to (but dramatically different biologic behavior than) cutaneous histiocytoma. Fewer cases of HS are of macrophage cell origin. These malignant cells have an immunophenotype characteristic of resident macrophages in the splenic red pulp and the bone marrow, and frequently show marked phagocytosis of erythrocytes (hemophagocytosis). Dogs with this form of HS frequently have a hemophagocytic syndrome characterized by severe nonregenerative to mildly regenerative anemia (presumably due largely to destruction of RBCs by the neoplastic cells), splenomegaly, hepatomegaly, and extramedullary hematopoiesis in the spleen and elsewhere. Microscopically, HS tumor cells are large, round to spindloid in shape, and vary from relatively well-differentiated histiocytic morphology to cells with notable features of malignancy (Fig. 13-40).

Cutaneous and systemic histiocytoses. Cutaneous histiocytosis (CH) and systemic histiocytosis (SH) are actually nonneoplastic canine immunoregulatory disorders, rather than hematopoietic neoplasms. They are included in this section because of their clinical similarities with histiocytic neoplasia. CH, a rare disease caused by proliferation of activated dermal dendritic cells, is discussed in more detail in Chapter 17. SH is a familial disorder of Bernese mountain dogs (also found sporadically in other breeds) characterized by large, dense proliferations of activated interstitial dendritic cells in multiple tissues, including skin, peripheral lymph nodes, and ocular and nasal mucosa. The proliferating cells are immunophenotypically identical to those in CH, and the angiocentric skin lesions in SH are histologically identical to those in CH. Lesions of SH in locations other than skin are also angiocentric infiltrates consisting mostly of histiocytes and lymphocytes.

Mast cell neoplasia

Mast cell tumors (MCTs) of the skin and other organs are relatively common in animals, especially in dogs, and are covered in other chapters in this book. Primary leukemia of mast cell origin is a rare form of myeloid leukemia. Mast cells normally are not present in circulation, but the finding of mast cells in the blood (mastocytemia) does not necessarily indicate myeloid neoplasia. In fact, one study found that severity of mastocytemia in dogs was frequently higher in animals without MCTs than those with MCTs, and that random

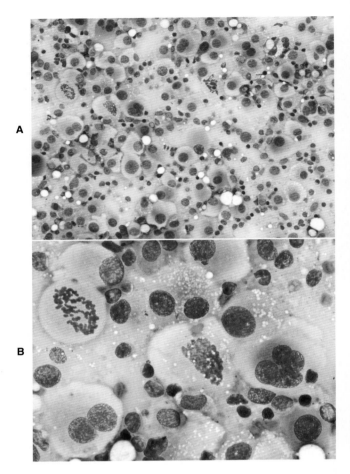

Fig. 13-40 Histiocytic sarcoma, canine mesenteric lymph node. The neoplastic cells are round cells with abundant gray-blue cytoplasm. Note the following features of malignancy: **A,** The low-magnification image shows notable variation in cell and nuclear sizes. **B,** The high-magnification image shows multinucleation, prominent nucleoli, and mitotic figures, as well as a background population of lymphocytes. Wright's stain. (**A** and **B,** *Courtesy Dr. M.M. Fry, College of Veterinary Medicine, University of Tennessee.*)

detection of mast cells in blood smears usually is not due to underlying MCT.

Granulocytic sarcoma

There are rare reports in animals of extramedullary solid tumors of granulocytic origin, known as granulocytic or myeloid sarcomas. These tumors are poorly characterized.

COAGULATION DISORDERS

The section focuses on acquired and inherited primary disorders of coagulation and also includes a secondary condition, disseminated intravascular coagulation (DIC), which is characterized clinically by abnormal hemostasis.

Avitaminosis K

A number of coagulation factors (factors II, VII, IX, and X, as well as the regulatory molecules Protein C and Protein S) must undergo carboxylation to be functional. This posttranslational modification is catalyzed by the enzyme γ-glutamyl carboxylase and requires vitamin K as a cofactor. Vitamin K is oxidized during the carboxylation reaction and is converted back into its active reduced form by the enzyme vitamin K epoxide reductase. The factors requiring this carboxylation step are thus vitamin K dependent, and deficiency or antagonism of vitamin K leads to production of nonfunctional factors and resulting coagulopathy (Fig. 13-41). Conditions associated with avitaminosis K include poisoning with coumarin-related molecules; fat malabsorption (vitamin K is one of the fat-soluble vitamins) due to primary intestinal disease or impaired biliary outflow (uncommon); dietary deficiency (rare); and antibiotics that interfere with vitamin K absorption or usage. Coumarin-related rodenticides, such as warfarin, act by inhibiting vitamin K epoxide reductase, resulting in an absence of vitamin K in its active reduced form. This inhibition lasts until the rodenticide is metabolized and cleared. How long this takes depends on the half-life ($t_{1/2}$) of the rodenticide and dose, but it may take many weeks. Second-generation rodenticides, such as bromadiolone and brodifacoum, are more potent than warfarin, with a longer $t_{1/2}$. Mycotoxins in the same family as anticoagulant rodenticides are associated with mildly sweet clover or sweet vernal grass and cause coagulopathy by the same mechanism. Laboratory findings include prolonged coagulation times (prothrombin time [PT], partial thromboplastin time [PTT], and activated clotting time [ACT]). Early in the course of rodenticide and related toxicoses, PT may be the only one

of these tests that is prolonged, because factor VII has the shortest $t_{1/2}$ of the vitamin K-dependent factors, but the other tests will become prolonged as nonfunctional forms of the other factors accumulate. In uncomplicated cases, patients are not thrombocytopenic. A wide range of hemorrhagic lesions may occur in affected individuals, including ecchymoses, epistaxis, gingival bleeding, hematomas, hemoptysis, melena or hematochezia, hematuria, and other forms of hemorrhage. The treatment for cases of rodenticide and related toxicoses is regular administration of exogenous vitamin K_1 until the toxin is cleared (determined by repeat coagulation testing after withholding treatment).

Disseminated Intravascular Coagulation

DIC is a syndrome characterized by continuous activation of both coagulation and fibrinolytic pathways. Also known as "consumptive coagulopathy," DIC is not a primary disease process, but rather a secondary complication of many types of underlying disease. It is common in critically ill domestic animals. DIC involves an initial hypercoagulable phase, resulting in thrombosis and ischemic tissue damage, and a subsequent hypocoagulable phase as a result of consumption of coagulation factors and platelets, resulting in hemorrhage (Fig. 13-42). The list of underlying conditions associated with DIC includes neoplasia, sepsis, endotoxemia, immune-mediated disease, intravascular hemolysis, shock, heat stroke, and obstetric complications. The pathogenesis of DIC typically involves the release of tissue factor (thromboplastin) and subsequent activation of coagulation pathways and platelets but may also involve defective normal inhibition of coagulation or defective fibrinolysis. Classically, diagnosis of DIC is based on clinical evidence of hemorrhage and/or thromboembolic disease and a triad of laboratory findings: thrombocytopenia, usually moderate (below the lower reference value, but above 50,000/μL); prolonged coagulation times (PT and/or PTT); and decreased fibrinogen, or increased concentration of plasma fibrin degradation products or D-dimer. Milder forms of DIC that do not meet all of the diagnostic criteria also occur. Decreased plasma antithrombin (antithrombin III) concentration and schistocytosis are other laboratory abnormalities often found in patients with DIC.

Inherited Coagulation Disorders
Hemophilia A and B

Hemophilia A refers to an inherited deficiency of functional coagulation factor VIII and has been recognized in horses, cattle, dogs, and cats. *Hemophilia B*, also known as Christmas disease, refers to an inherited deficiency of functional coagulation factor IX and has been recognized in dogs and cats. Both forms of hemophilia have an X-linked recessive mode of inheritance.

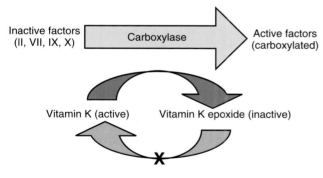

X = Inactivation of vitamin K expoxide reductase, the enzyme that maintains vitamin K in the active form

Fig. 13-41   Schematic diagram of the mechanism of anticoagulant rodenticide toxicity. Anticoagulant rodenticides inhibit the enzyme that converts vitamin K back to its active reduced form.

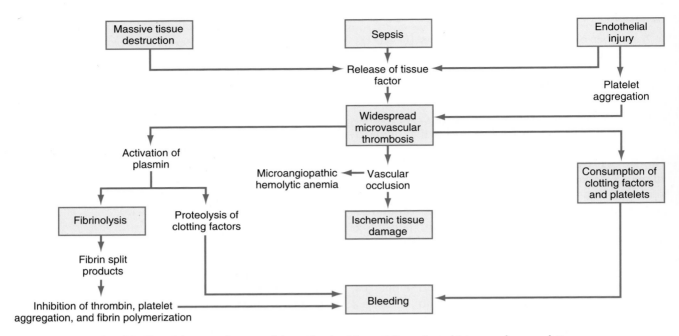

Fig. 13-42   Schematic diagram of the pathophysiology of disseminated intravascular coagulation.
(From Kumar V, Abbas AK, Fausto N: Robbins & Cotran pathologic basis of disease, ed 7, Philadelphia, 2005, Saunders.)

Affected males have variable tendencies to bleed, depending on the severity of the deficiency, exposure to trauma, and size and activity level of the affected individual. Carrier females are usually asymptomatic.

Other inherited factor deficiencies

Factor XI deficiency is the most common inherited coagulopathy in cattle and has also been reported in dogs. The mode of inheritance is probably autosomal recessive. Reports describe excessive bleeding in affected individuals after surgery. The most commonly affected dog breed is the Kerry blue terrier. In these dogs, hemorrhage is often delayed, sometimes developing several days after surgery. Other factor deficiencies also have been reported in animals. These conditions include deficiencies of factor VII (reported in dogs), factor XII (relatively common in cats, also reported in dogs), and prekallikrein (reported in dogs and horses). In most cases, affected individuals are asymptomatic or have only mild clinical bleeding tendencies but may have excessive bleeding following trauma or surgery.

Other inherited coagulopathies

A defect in γ-glutamyl carboxylase, the enzyme required for normal carboxylation of vitamin K–dependent clotting factors, has been recognized as the cause of an inherited coagulopathy in Rambouillet sheep.

LYMPHATIC SYSTEM

DISORDERS OF THE THYMUS

CONGENITAL DISORDERS

Included in this description are the congenital disorders that result in inadequate T-lymphocyte function, and those resulting in B-lymphocyte and plasma cell dysfunction. Many have been described in human beings, and indeed have been invaluable in learning more about mechanisms of immunity and immune regulation. The animal counterparts of immunodeficiency serve as valuable models in comparative immunology research. Combined immunodeficiency disorders (CIDs) are those affecting both humoral and cell-mediated immunity (B and T lymphocytes).

Equine CID is a genetic disorder occurring in Arabian or part-Arabian foals. There is failure of functional B- and T-lymphocyte production, so foals are remarkably susceptible to a variety of microbial agents and usually die before 5 months of age. Adenoviruses that are typically resisted by normal foals are a major cause of death in foals with CID. The viral infection is frequently complicated by various bacterial or protozoal infections that typically result in pneumonia.

Necropsy findings are severe bronchopneumonia in combination with a small thymus, spleen, and lymph nodes. The thymus may be difficult to identify or may consist of a few isolated lobules within the mediastinal fat. Microscopically, it usually consists of a few islands

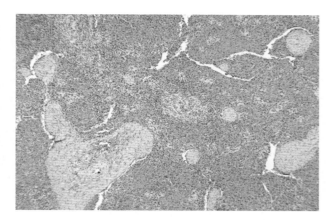

Fig. 13-43   Combined immunodeficiency disease, spleen, foal. The large pale pink areas are splenic trabeculae. Note the almost total absence of white pulp. H&E stain. *(Courtesy Dr. M.D. McGavin, College of Veterinary Medicine, University of Tennessee.)*

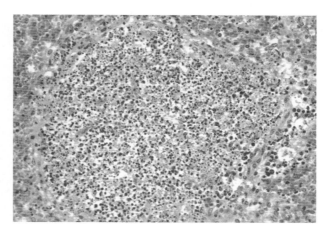

Fig. 13-44   Equine herpesvirus 1, spleen, aborted foal. Most of the splenic follicle is occupied by nuclear debris, the result of lymphocytolysis. The splenic follicle is surrounded by a small rim of red pulp. H&E stain. *(Courtesy College of Veterinary Medicine, University of Illinois.)*

of lymphocyte-like cells and thymic corpuscles. The spleen is smaller than normal because of a marked reduction in the white pulp owing to absence of germinal centers (Fig. 13-43) and periarteriolar lymphoid sheaths. Peripheral lymph nodes and internal lymph nodes may be small and difficult to identify because of the absence of lymphocytes.

X-linked severe combined immunodeficiency (XSCID) has been reported in basset hounds. The affected male pups lack mature functional T lymphocytes. The animals have a normal serum level of IgM but low or undetectable IgG and IgA. The thymus of these dogs is small and often obscured by mediastinal fat. Tonsils, lymph nodes, and Peyer's patches usually cannot be identified at necropsy. Microscopically the thymic tissue consists of small dysplastic lobules with a variable number of Hassall's corpuscles. XSCID has also been described in Jack Russell terrier and Welsh corgi breeds of dogs.

Thymic cysts can be found within the developing and mature thymus and in thymic remnants in the cranial mediastinum. These cysts are often lined by ciliated epithelium and represent developmental remnants of branchial arch epithelium and are usually of no significance.

INFLAMMATORY AND DEGENERATIVE DISORDERS

Thymitis, an infrequent lesion, is seen in porcine circovirus 2 infection (postweaning multisystem wasting syndrome [PMWS]), enzootic bovine abortion (EBA), and salmon poisoning disease of dogs. In PMWS there are multifocal noncaseating granulomas with giant cells, in EBA there is diffuse infiltration of macrophages in both the medulla and septa, and in canine salmon poisoning disease there is infiltration of neutrophils and macrophages into the cortex and medulla of the thymus.

Injury to the thymus resulting in variable degrees of acquired immunodeficiency may be caused by infectious agents (viruses), toxins, chemotherapeutic agents and radiation, malnutrition, aging, and neoplasia.

Viruses damaging the thymus, and often other lymphoid tissues, include canine distemper virus, equine herpesvirus 1 (EHV-1) in aborted foals (Fig. 13-44), feline parvovirus, feline immunodeficiency virus, bovine viral diarrhea virus (BVDV) and hog cholera virus. Lymphocytolysis of the cells of the germinal centers and cortex occurs in feline panleukopenia and in the germinal centers in EHV-1 and BVD infections. In kittens infected with FIV, thymic depletion is an early lesion, and in kittens with progressive FIV infection, ultimately there is complete loss of thymic architecture with only minimal thymic tissue remaining in the connective and adipose tissue.

Environmental toxins such as halogenated aromatic hydrocarbons (e.g., polychlorinated biphenyls and dibenzodioxins, lead, and mercury) have a suppressive effect on the immune system. Fumonisins B_1 and B_2, which are secondary fungal metabolites produced by members of the genus *Fusarium*, cause lymphocytolysis in the thymic cortex. In weaner and grower pigs, aflatoxin causes thymic atrophy because of lymphocyte depletion. In the case of the halogenated aromatic hydrocarbons, there is a genetic basis for susceptibility that is mediated through a complex composed of the aromatic hydrocarbon receptor and the aromatic receptor nuclear transporter. In general, these chemicals cause severe atrophy of the primary and secondary lymphoid organs. Other environmental toxins, such as the metals lead and mercury, cause toxic effects through the interaction of the metal with an enzyme system,

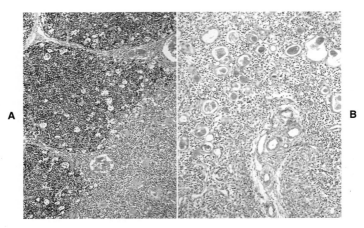

Fig. 13-45   **Effect of ionizing radiation, atrophy of the thymus, cortex and medulla.**
A, Normal thymus. The cortex is heavily populated with numerous thymocytes. The medulla
(bottom right) contains fewer of these cells. H&E stain. **B,** Thymus exposed to ionizing radiation.
Note the depletion of lymphocytes in both cortex and medulla and the preservation of Hassell's
corpuscles (pink, concentric layers). H&E stain. (*A* and *B,* *From Kumar V, Abbas AK, Fausto N: Robbins &
Cotran pathologic basis of disease, ed 7, Philadelphia, 2005, Saunders.*)

cell membrane, or organelle. Similarly, therapeutic agents in general specifically target enzyme systems and cellular components essential for cell replication. Thus they can cause inhibition of a cellular function rather than cause a morphologic change.

Treatments with anticancer drugs, radiomimetic drugs, or ionization radiation can result in immunosuppression. Lymphocytes are very sensitive to these agents. Therapies that cause immunosuppression are best illustrated by the cytotoxic drugs used as chemotherapeutics to treat cancer. In general most cytotoxic drugs inhibit cell division by mechanisms that are centered on the function and activity of nucleic acids. Purine analogs (e.g., azathioprine) compete with purines in the synthesis of nucleic acids, whereas alkylating agents like cyclophosphamide cross-link DNA and inhibit the replication and activation of lymphocytes. Cyclosporin A specifically inhibits the T-lymphocyte signaling pathway by interfering with the transcription of the IL-2 gene. Methotrexate, a folic acid antagonist, blocks the synthesis of thymidine and purine nucleotides. As chemotherapeutics, they have the beneficial effect of targeting cancer cells and the detrimental effect of also targeting noncancerous immune cells—resulting in immunosuppression, the proverbial double-edged sword. Because of the desirable effect of these and other drugs, they are used in the prevention of allograft rejection reactions following transplantation. Corticosteroids are considered to be immunosuppressive, although the degree of suppression is highly variable among species, and, in general, human beings and rodents are corticosteroid sensitive, whereas domestic species are considered corticosteroid resistant.

Ionizing radiation exerts its effects, in part, through lethal mechanisms that target components of DNA and through nonlethal mechanisms related to the generation of highly reactive free radicals. Ionizing radiation can damage lymphoid tissues and cells (Fig. 13-45).

Malnutrition impairs thymic function because it rapidly induces thymic atrophy, with resultant reduction in thymic hormone output. The effect is a reduction in the number of circulating T-lymphocytes in the blood, depletion of T-lymphocytes from the secondary lymphoid organs, and impairment of T-lymphocyte functions. This effect of starvation is mediated by the hormone leptin, whose concentration in the blood is proportional to the mass of fat in the body. Consequently its blood concentration is reduced in starvation, and immunosuppression results.

Aging

With advancing age, all lymphoid organs become reduced in size (atrophic) and have reduced lymphocyte populations. In the case of the thymus, this reduction in size occurs normally after sexual maturity and is more appropriately termed thymic involution. The term *involution* should be reserved for normal physiologic processes in which an organ either returns to normal size after a period of enlargement (e.g., postpartum uterus) or regresses to a more primitive state (e.g., thymic involution) (see previous discussion on gross examination of the thymus). Atrophy, although most commonly used to denote a pathologic decrease in the size of a cell, tissue, or organ, can also be used to indicate a decrease in size of an organ that is dependent on hormonal stimulation. Stated simply, involution should be reserved for nonpathologic physiologic processes, whereas atrophy may or may not imply a pathologic process.

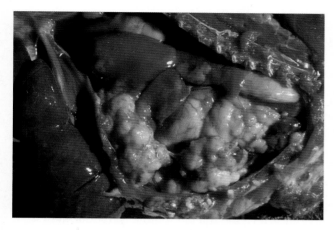

Fig. 13-46   Lymphoma (lymphosarcoma), thymus, dog. The large pale mass in the cranial mediastinum is a thymic lymphosarcoma that has displaced the lungs caudad. *(Courtesy Dr. M.D. McGavin, College of Veterinary Medicine, University of Tennessee.)*

Neoplasia

Because the thymus has both lymphoid and epithelial components, it is possible for either or both to serve as cells of origin of neoplasms. Thymic lymphoma (Fig. 13-46) is a T-lymphocyte neoplasm of young animals, particularly in cats and cattle and less frequently seen in dogs (see Hematopoietic Neoplasia). Clinical findings reflect the presence of a large mass in the cranial mediastinum. This mass can often be forced into the thoracic inlet with gentle compression of the cranial ribs.

Bovine thymic lymphoma most often occurs in beef cattle 6 to 24 months of age and is characterized by massive thymic enlargement. The cause is unknown, and the occurrence of a concurrent leukemia is unusual. The thymus is an important site of lymphoma in cats. The tumors are large white or gray mediastinal masses that result in displacement of adjacent structures and in pleural fluid accumulation. In cats, the fluid is frequently chylous. Microscopically, these diffuse lymphomas are dominated by lymphocytes, which are homogeneous in size, shape, nuclear morphology, and nuclear-cytoplasmic ratio.

Thymomas are usually benign neoplasms that occupy the cranial mediastinum, usually of older animals. They are significantly less common than thymic lymphoma and are only distinguishable microscopically by the presence of neoplastic epithelial cells. Lymphocytes are present within thymomas but are not neoplastic. Thymomas have been associated with myasthenia gravis (which may be accompanied by megaesophagus) and polymyositis (immune-mediated) in dogs. A rare condition, thymic hyperplasia, which results from the formation of B-lymphocyte follicles within the thymus, has also been reported in association with myasthenia gravis in dogs and cats.

Miscellaneous
Thymic hematomas

Thymic hemorrhage and hematomas have been reported in dogs. Many of these die unexpectedly from hypovolemic shock as a result of massive thymic and mediastinal hemorrhage. A variety of causes has been implicated. These include rupture of dissecting aortic aneurysms, trauma from automobile accidents, and ingestion of anticoagulant rodenticides (warfarin, dicumarol, diphacinone, and brodifacoum). In the last type, hemorrhage causes expansion of thymic lobules and interlobular septa and appears to originate in the medulla.

Grossly hemorrhage or hematomas maybe confined to the thymus or extend into the mediastinum. In anticoagulant rodenticide poisoning, hemorrhages may also be at other sites, including the pericardial sac, mesentery, liver, and peritoneum.

DISORDERS OF THE SPLEEN*
Congenital Disorders

Asplenia or the failure of a spleen to develop in utero occurs occasionally in animals. This finding is usually incidental. Because congenital asplenia is so rare, it is not entirely clear whether this affects the resistance of domestic animals to disease. The condition is well known in certain strains of mice, but these are usually maintained under either germ-free or specific pathogen-free (SPF) conditions. However, congenitally asplenic mice have a high mortality rate to experimental plasmodium infection.

Congenital immunodeficiency diseases have been described in Disorders of the Thymus.

Splenomegaly

Although the following conditions have been discussed on the basis of whether or not they cause splenomegaly, it is important to realize that in the early stages, the process involved may not have had sufficient time to cause splenomegaly or splenic nodules.

The diseases and disorders associated with splenomegaly will be discussed using the following categories:
- Uniform splenomegaly with a bloody consistency—bloody spleen (Fig 13-47, *A*)
- Uniform splenomegaly with a firm consistency—meaty spleen (Fig 13-47, *B*)
- Splenic nodules with a bloody consistency
- Splenic nodules with a firm consistency
- Small spleens

Table 13-3 lists the common causes of uniform splenomegaly.

---

*The authors acknowledge Dr. W.L. Spangler for editing this section of the chapter.

A

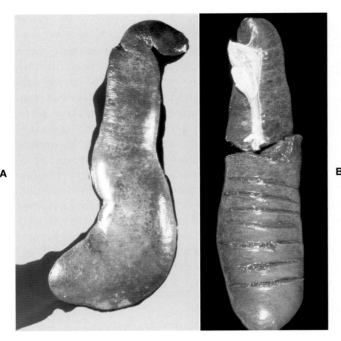

B

Fig. 13-47   Uniform splenomegaly. A, Congested bloody spleen. This condition occurs secondary to compromises in vascular flow into and out of the spleen (e.g., torsion), from intravenous barbiturates (e.g., euthanasia or anesthesia), and from acute hyperemia from septicemia. **B,** Meaty spleen. This condition most commonly results from proliferation of cells, most frequently macrophages in the red pulp and increased splenic phagocytosis in, for example, septicemias and bacteremias. (*A and B, Courtesy College of Veterinary Medicine, University of Illinois.*)

Uniform splenomegaly with a bloody consistency—"bloody" spleen

The common causes of a bloody spleen are congestion (torsion, barbiturate euthanasia, anesthesia), acute hyperemia (inflammation, anthrax), and acute hemolytic anemia.

Congestion

Torsion.   Torsion of the spleen occurs mainly in pigs and dogs, and torsion of the spleen and stomach together occurs in dogs, usually deep-chested ones (see Chapter 7).

In contrast to ruminants, in which the spleen is firmly attached to the rumen, the spleen of dogs and pigs is attached loosely to the stomach by the gastrosplenic ligament. It is the twisting of the spleen on this ligament that results initially in occlusion of the veins, causing splenic congestion, and later in occlusion of the artery, causing splenic infarction.

Grossly the spleen is uniformly and markedly enlarged and blue-black from cyanosis (Fig. 13-47, A). It is often folded back on itself (visceral surface to visceral surface) in the shape of the letter "C." Treatment for this

is splenectomy, but removal of the spleen renders the animal susceptible to certain organisms, such as hemotropic mycoplasma infections (previously known as haemobartonellosis and eperythrozoonosis) in dogs and cattle, and babesiosis and theileriosis in cattle in endemic areas.

Barbiturate euthanasia, anesthesia, or sedation. Acute passive congestion is seen most dramatically at necropsy in horses and dogs that have been euthanized or anesthetized by intravenous injection of barbiturate. When a dog under barbiturate anesthesia and with a markedly congested spleen from the anesthetic was injected with 1 ml of 1:1000 adrenaline into the splenic artery, the splenic volume was reduced by 75%. In past years, when chloral hydrate was used as an anesthetic in cattle, a similar acute splenic congestion was seen at surgery.

Grossly the spleen is extremely enlarged (Fig. 13-48), and the cut surface is notably congested and bulges and oozes blood. The splenic capsule can be fragile and easily ruptured. Histologically, as a result of the distention of the red pulp by blood, the normal architecture of the splenic parenchyma is almost obliterated by masses of blood cells, chiefly erythrocytes (Fig. 13-49). The lymphoid tissues (periarteriolar lymphoid sheaths and splenic follicles) are widely separated and may be absent from the section examined. Because of the splenic distention, trabeculae and the capsule are thin.

Electric stunning of pigs at slaughter is occasionally associated with a large congested spleen.

Acute hyperemia.   In septicemias and bacteremias, microbes are transported to the splenic red pulp, where they are rapidly phagocytosed by the splenic macrophages. Enormous numbers of bacteria injected

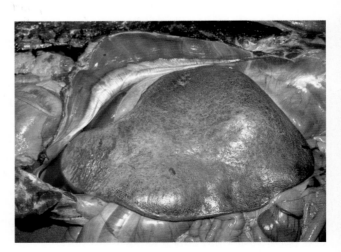

Fig. 13-48   Splenic congestion from barbiturate euthanasia, horse. The spleen is enlarged and congested from storage of blood. (*Courtesy Dr. M.D. McGavin, College of Veterinary Medicine, University of Tennessee.*)

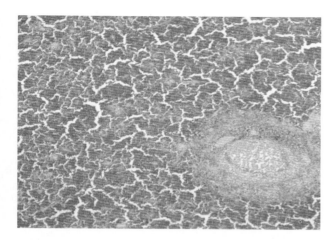

Fig. 13-49   Splenic congestion from barbiturate euthanasia, dog. The red pulp vascular spaces are markedly distended by blood. One focus of white pulp—a splenic follicle with a pale germinal center—is present in the lower right. H&E stain. *(Courtesy Dr. M.D. McGavin, College of Veterinary Medicine, University of Tennessee.)*

intravenously can be cleared from the blood in 20 to 30 minutes. The response of the spleen depends on the duration of the disease. In acutely fatal cases, such as anthrax and fulminating salmonellosis, distension by blood may be the only finding. If there is a longer interval before death, as in swine erysipelas and the less acute forms of salmonellosis, there may be time for neutrophils to accumulate and macrophages in the splenic red pulp to undergo hyperplasia.

In human medicine it has been generally accepted that acute sepsis (septicemia) can cause acute splenitis, loosely defined as splenomegaly, which is the result of acute splenic congestion and neutrophilic infiltrates. A retrospective study in human beings did not support this; in fact, there was little significant change in the spleen. However, in mice injected intraperitoneally with *Burkholderia mallei* (glanders bacillus), there was notable splenomegaly and histologically the spleen was infiltrated initially (within hours) with neutrophils and later (>24 hours) by pyogranulomatous inflammation. Although the Kupffer cells of the liver make up 80% to 90% of the body's macrophages in some animals, in these mice the greatest number of bacilli was present in the spleen.

Grossly in acute septicemias in domestic animals, the spleen is moderately enlarged and red from congestion, and the cut surface oozes blood.

Anthrax.   Anthrax is caused by *Bacillus anthracis* and is primarily a disease of ruminants, especially cattle and sheep. *Bacillus anthracis* is a gram-positive, large rod-shaped, endospore-forming bacterium, which grows in an aerobic to facultative anaerobic environment. Ingested spores replicate locally in the intestinal tract,

spread to regional lymph nodes, and then disseminate systemically, through the blood stream, resulting in septicemia. *Bacillus anthracis* produces exotoxins, which degrade endothelial cell membranes and enzyme systems. The spleen, in a case of anthrax, is uniformly enlarged, is dark red to bluish-black, and contains abundant unclotted blood because of extensive liquefactive necrosis. Impression smears of peripheral blood can contain gram-positive rod-shaped bacteria. Anthrax cases are not normally necropsied, as exposure to air causes the bacteria to sporulate and anthrax spores are extremely resistant and contaminate the environment.

Acute hemolytic anemias.   In hemolytic diseases, such as acute babesiosis, and during the hemolytic crises in equine infectious anemia, because of the need to remove parasitized and altered erythrocytes from the circulation, the spleen is grossly enlarged and congested, and the cut surface oozes blood. If the condition becomes chronic, hyperplasia of the red pulp macrophages takes place, and because of the decreased numbers of parasitized erythrocytes to be phagocytosed, congestion is reduced.

Uniform splenomegaly with a firm consistency—"meaty" spleen

Enlargement and firm consistency of the spleen is due to proliferation of cells, most frequently macrophages in the red pulp (Fig. 13-47, *B*). In fact, splenomegaly from an increased splenic phagocytosis could be considered a response to workload, a sort of "workload hyperplasia" in response to the need to phagocytose organisms in prolonged bacteremias or parasitemias from hemotropic organisms. Other causes are diffuse neoplasia, such as lymphoma, lymphoid hyperplasia, and advanced stages of some storage diseases.

The appearance of the cut surface will vary with the extent of the change in the red and white pulp. In the early stages, red pulp will have its normal color, but it will become paler as lesions become extensive.

The white pulp is not visible in normal spleens, but in cases of marked lymphoid hyperplasia, it may be visible on the cut surface as whitish foci, up to 1 to 2 mm in diameter, scattered through the red pulp. Moderately enlarged, firm spleens with visible white pulp are indicative of "reactive spleens," or lymphoma (lymphosarcoma) (see Lymphoid Hyperplasia).

The common causes of uniform splenomegaly are listed in Table 13-3 and include the following:
1. Bacteremias and low-grade septicemias
2. Chronic infectious diseases, usually granulomatous. A chronic infectious splenitis can be caused by bacteria or fungi. Many of the former produce chronic abscesses, which may be disseminated through the parenchyma or cause a single abscess (see Splenic Nodules).

3. Prolonged hemolytic anemias (such as canine immune-mediated hemolytic anemia)
4. Lymphoid hyperplasia—usually not sufficiently extensive to cause splenomegaly
5. Neoplasms, such as lymphoma (lymphosarcoma)
6. Stored or deposits of material, such as in storage diseases or amyloidosis
7. Extramedullary hematopoiesis as a response to anemia or found in the spleens of aging dogs; but this alone is usually not extensive enough to cause splenomegaly.
8. Splenic myeloid metaplasia, histiocytosis and hypersplenism in dogs

Bacteremias and septicemias. In animals, the most fulminating septicemias (e.g., anthrax) cause splenomegaly with marked congestion (see previous discussion). Less virulent bacteria, which do not result in a quick death but have a longer clinical course, cause hyperplasia of macrophages and accumulations of neutrophils in the spleen. Some of the more common bacteria that cause bacteremia and/or septicemia, include specific serotypes of *Escherichia coli* (septicemic colibacillosis); biotype A and biotype T of *Pasteurella multocida* (septicemic pasteurellosis); *Streptococcus* spp. (neonatal septicemia); *Listeria monocytogenes* (listeric septicemia); *Hemophilus agni* (*Hemophilus* septicemia), *Erysipelothrix rhusiopathiae* (septicemic erysipelas), and *Salmonella* spp. (septicemic salmonellosis).

Chronic infectious diseases. Chronic infectious splenic diseases can cause abscesses (see nodular spleen discussion later), but are commonly associated with uniformly enlarged firm spleens. Firm spleens in these diseases result from one or more of three processes:
1. Macrophage hyperplasia
2. Chronic granulomatosis diseases (granulomatous inflammation)
3. Lymphoid hyperplasia

Macrophage hyperplasia. Macrophage hyperplasia occurs chiefly in the red pulp to phagocytose organisms, bacteria, or parasitized erythrocytes. This process is particularly well exemplified in histoplasmosis and leishmaniasis. *Histoplasma capsulatum* causes a marked proliferation of cells of the monocyte-macrophage system, and the resultant accumulation of macrophages in the spleen may enlarge this organ to several times its normal size (Fig. 13-50). *Leishmania* spp. also cause proliferation of macrophages, and large areas of the spleen may be replaced by macrophages. These cells also infiltrate the bone marrow and portal areas of the liver.

Chronic granulomatosis diseases. These diseases occur: (1) in response to bacteria that are intracellular facultative pathogens of macrophages, which include but are not limited to mycobacteria (*Mycobacterium bovis*, tuberculosis), *Brucella* spp. (brucellosis), and

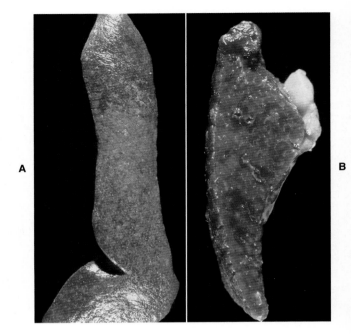

Fig. 13-50 **Histoplasmosis, spleen, dog. A,** There is uniform splenomegaly and the surface of the spleen is mottled from the diffuse granulomatous infiltrate. **B,** Cross section of spleen. The red pulp has been almost completely replaced by diffuse noncaseous granulomatous inflammation. *(A and B, Courtesy Department of Veterinary Biosciences, The Ohio Stare University; and Noah's Arkive, College of Veterinary Medicine, The University of Georgia.)*

Francisella tularensis (tularemia) (see Large Lymph Nodes); (2) in systemic mycoses (see Large Lymph Nodes) such as blastomycosis (*Blastomyces dermatitidis*). Some of these organisms may also produce nodular enlarged spleens from the formation of granulomas (see Splenic Nodules with Firm Consistency).

Lymphoid hyperplasia. Lymphoid hyperplasia, both follicular and of the PALS, are part of the response to blood-borne antigens, which enter the marginal zone and are presented by antigen-presenting cells to T lymphocytes and B lymphocytes, resulting in cell-mediated and humoral immunity. In chronic diseases, the marginal zone may be markedly enlarged.

Prolonged hemolytic anemias. Acute hemolytic anemias cause splenomegaly with congestion (bloody spleens), but if the hemolysis is less severe or more chronic, the spleen is firm and red but not as congested because fewer erythrocytes are being phagocytosed. Proliferation of these macrophages in the red pulp results in an enlarged, firm spleen. Because of extravascular hemolysis of the altered erythrocytes, the red pulp, in addition to being firm, may be red to dark red but does not ooze blood. Splenic enlargement in these diseases may also be partially due to hyperplasia of

T- and B-lymphocyte areas. Acute hemolytic anemias are discussed in more detail earlier in this chapter.

Equine infectious anemia. Equine infectious anemia has cyclical periods of viremia, immunologically mediated damage to erythrocytes and platelets, and phagocytosis to remove altered erythrocytes and platelets. These cycles result in proliferation of red pulp macrophages, hyperplasia of hematopoietic cells (EMH) to replace those lost, and hyperplasia of the T- and B-lymphocyte areas.

Lymphoid hyperplasia. PALSs and splenic follicles become hyperplastic in response to chronic antigenic stimulation (Fig. 13-51). The change in the splenic follicle is similar to that which occurs in the lymphoid follicle. Many of the chronic diseases listed earlier cause lymphoid hyperplasia and proliferation of the macrophages of the red pulp. Lymphoid hyperplasia may also occur focally or regionally, at least in the canine spleen, in the absence of generalized antigenic stimulus. These areas are present grossly as nodular enlargements of the splenic parenchyma generally less than 8 mm in diameter and are often obscured by an associated hematoma. These are discussed in more detail later in the chapter (see Nodular Hyperplasia).

Neoplasia

Primary neoplasms. Primary neoplastic diseases of the spleen arise from cell populations that normally exist in the spleen and include hematopoietic components such as lymphocytes and macrophages and stromal cells such as fibroblasts, smooth muscle, and endothelium. Primary splenic lymphoma, although rare, can produce a uniform splenomegaly (Fig. 13-52, A). Microscopically the normal white pulp follicles are

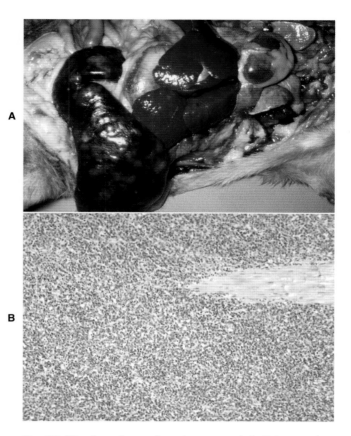

Fig. 13-52 **Lymphoma (lymphosarcoma). A,** Spleen and liver, dog. The spleen is grossly enlarged with pale subcapsular nodules. The mottled appearance of the liver is caused by infiltration of malignant lymphocytes into the portal areas. **B,** Spleen, cow. The pale horizontal band on the upper right is a trabeculum. The remainder of the spleen is diffusely infiltrated by malignant lymphocytes, which have completely obliterated all normal architecture. Note the absence of any normal red or white pulp. H&E stain. (**A,** *Courtesy College of Veterinary Medicine, University of Illinois.* **B,** *Courtesy Dr. M.D. McGavin, College of Veterinary Medicine, University of Tennessee.*)

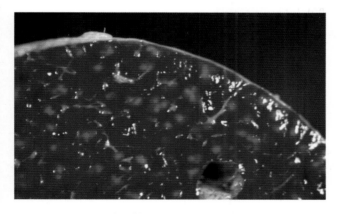

Fig. 13-51 **Lymphoid hyperplasia, cross section of spleen, dog.** Each of the 1- to 3-mm pale foci consists of hyperplastic periarteriolar lymphoid sheaths and splenic follicles. These structures are not visible in the normal spleen but become enlarged and visible from marked lymphoid hyperplasia or from lymphoma. (*Courtesy Dr. S. Wolpert, USDA/FSIS; and Noah's Arkive, College of Veterinary Medicine, The University of Georgia.*)

displaced, and the red pulp is occupied to varying degrees by neoplastic lymphocytes (Fig. 13-52, B). (The different types of lymphoma in domestic animals are discussed under Hematopoietic Neoplasia.) In the advanced stages of disease, acute and chronic leukemias cause uniform splenomegaly. The splenic red pulp appears hypercellular from the extensive infiltration of tumor cells. It should be appreciated that in some cases many of these different types of primary splenic neoplasms will produce nodular lesions discussed later.

Metastatic neoplasms. The spleen is not a common site of metastatic neoplasia, but when it occurs, it generally causes nodules—not uniform splenomegaly. Metastatic neoplasms of the spleen, which cause uniform splenomegaly, can originate from the same hematopoietic cell populations as those that cause primary neoplastic disease, but the neoplastic cells metastasize to the spleen hematogenously. Lymphoma is the most common metastatic neoplasm of the spleen.

Stored deposits of material

Lysosomal storage diseases.   Storage diseases constitute a large heterogeneous group of genetically determined and acquired disorders, which result from the lack of an enzyme required to facilitate the metabolism of a specific substrate. Storage diseases occur in animals less than 1 year of age. In general, these substrates are lipids and/or carbohydrates, which, due to lack of normal processing within lysosomes, accumulate in these cells. Major categories of stored materials include mucopolysaccharides, sphingolipids, lipids, glycoproteins, glycogen, and mucolipids. Macrophages within the spleen are unable to degrade these substrates and essentially serve to store them in an unprocessed form. Ultimately the mass of this undigested substrate results in a uniformly enlarged firm spleen, which may be pale red, depending on the amount of unprocessed lipid or carbohydrate that has accumulated.

Amyloid.   The accumulation of amyloid in the spleen may occur with primary (AL) or secondary (AA) amyloidosis (see Chapters 1 and 5). Rarely can this accumulation be so severe as to cause uniform splenomegaly (Fig. 13-53), in which the spleen is firm, rubbery to waxy, and beige to orange.

Extramedullary hematopoiesis (EMH).   Hormonal or physiologic signaling mechanisms within the spleen initiate the synthesis of progenitor cells from stem cells in an attempt to fulfill the cellular demands of the systemic circulation. However, splenic EMH is often found incidentally, and many consider its presence in the spleen to be within normal limits, at least in dogs. It usually involves cells of the erythroid, myeloid, and megakaryocytes lines, but one type usually predominates. Splenic enlargement from extramedullary hematopoiesis may be minimal, and EMH is often not detectable on gross examination. Extramedullary hematopoiesis may occur in cases of chronic anemia and in conditions such as chronic respiratory disease or chronic cardiovascular disease, in which the circulation is not able to adequately maintain systemic pO_2 concentrations. Extramedullary myelopoiesis may occur in suppurative bacterial diseases such as canine pyometra, in which there is an excessive demand for neutrophils that exceeds the supply from the bone marrow.

EMH is also present in splenic nodular hyperplasia.

Splenic myeloid metaplasia, histiocytosis, and hypersplenism in the dog.   This disease has been described recently and is characterized by severe, diffuse, and persistent splenomegaly, and the splenic capsule may be smooth or have multiple and confluent nodules. There is often random vascular thrombosis, producing grossly visible splenic infarcts. Microscopically, extramedullary hematopoiesis is present with interspersed foci of prominent macrophages (periarteriolar macrophage sheaths [PAMSs]). The process effaces the splenic red pulp and is responsible for the splenic enlargement. This disease may be rather benign, not involving other organs, in which case splenectomy is generally curative. However, EMH may be systemic, involving bone marrow and liver, and this is indicative of a poor prognosis.

Splenic nodules with a bloody consistency

The most common diseases or conditions resulting in nodular splenomegaly with bloody consistency are: (1) hematomas induced by lymphoid hyperplastic nodules; (2) hematomas induced by splenic vascular neoplasms; (3) incompletely contracted areas of the spleen; (4) vascular neoplasms (hemangiomas and hemangiosarcomas); and (5) acute splenic infarcts. The term *nodule* has been applied rather loosely here. In some of these conditions, such as incompletely contracted areas of the spleen, the elevated area of the spleen is not as well defined as the term *nodule* would imply.

Hematomas (induced by lymphoid hyperplastic nodules).   Hematomas in the spleen are usually associated with hyperplastic lymphoid nodules (arising from the PALS of the white pulp) and occur regionally or focally in the splenic parenchyma. These nodules arise idiosyncratically in the canine and (less commonly)

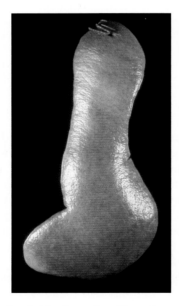

Fig. 13-53   Amyloid spleen, dog. The spleen is pale beige, firm and waxy, and uniformly distended in this advanced case of amyloidosis. *(Courtesy College of Veterinary Medicine, University of Illinois.)*

feline spleens and do not appear to be associated with general antigenic stimulation. Because the circulation in the marginal zone of the white pulp in these two species appears to be "open," the blood exits via open-ended arterial capillaries to percolate among lymphocytes of the marginal zone and reenters through similar open venous capillaries. Distortion of this marginal zone area by hyperplastic lymphocytes disrupts the normal blood flow, resulting in accumulation of pooled blood that is unable to find its way into sinusoids or red pulp vascular spaces (reticular meshwork), thus forming a hematoma that further distorts the splenic architecture.

Hematomas (induced by splenic vascular neoplasms).   Hematomas can also occur secondarily to splenic neoplasms of vascular origin. Bleeding into the red pulp, which is confined by the splenic capsule, produces a red to dark red soft bulging, usually solitary mass of varying size (2 to 15 cm in diameter) (Fig. 13-54). If the capsule over the hematoma ruptures, hemoperitoneum, hypovolemic shock, circulatory failure, and death can ensue. Splenic hematomas progress through a reparative process in which the blood coagulates and, over days, breaks down into a dark red brown soft mass (Fig. 13-55, A). The clotted blood is infiltrated by macrophages, which phagocytose erythrocytes and break down hemoglobin initially with the formation of bilirubin and later hemosiderin (Fig. 13-55, B).

Newly formed capillaries (neovascularization) infiltrate the lesion and fill the site with granulation tissue, which matures to collagen. Collagenous septa divide the clotted blood into distinct "compartments" of varying sizes. The blood eventually liquefies and is

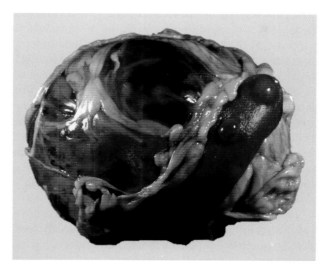

Fig. 13-54   Hematoma, spleen, dog. The ventral extremity of the spleen has a large hematoma on its visceral surface. Note the two nodules of splenic hyperplasia *(dorsal extremity)*, a common site for hematomas to occur **(Fig. 13-59).** *(Courtesy College of Veterinary Medicine, University of Illinois.)*

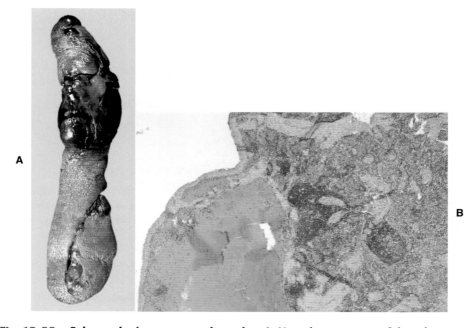

Fig. 13-55   Subcapsular hematoma, spleen, dog. A, Note the separation of the splenic capsule from the underlying parenchyma by a mass of blood. **B,** The yellow material is bilirubin, resulting from the breakdown of erythrocytes in a subcapsular hemorrhage. H&E stain.
*(**A** and **B,** Courtesy Dr. M.D. McGavin, College of Veterinary Medicine, University of Tennessee.)*

phagocytosed and replaced by a scar. In the late stage, histologically the area contains scar tissue and intracellular and extracellular deposits of hemosiderin.

Incompletely contracted areas of the spleen. Acute splenic infarcts can be indistinguishable from areas of incompletely contracted splenic parenchyma. Contraction can occur during circulatory (hypovolemic, cardiogenic, or septic) shock or be a sympathetic response, as in flight or fright situations. Incompletely contracted areas appear as numerous dark red to black, raised, soft, blood-filled areas of various sizes. These are usually at the margins of the spleen, and the intervening areas are depressed and red. The latter areas are normal, contracted splenic red pulp devoid of blood. Incompletely contracted areas were previously confused with splenic infarcts and sometimes hematomas, but they are now recognized to be caused by failure of smooth muscle in some areas to contract, resulting in incomplete splenic evacuation of stored blood.

Vascular neoplasms. The most common cause of nodular splenomegaly associated with a bloody (congested) spleen is neoplasms of vascular endothelial cell origin. Both benign (hemangioma) and malignant (hemangiosarcoma) forms commonly occur.

Grossly, hemangiomas are usually solitary masses, dark red to bluish-purple, friable, and usually covered by a thin shiny serosa. There are no metastases to the liver or peritoneal mesothelium. Hemangiomas are composed of well-differentiated endothelial cells, which differentiate into relatively well-formed vascular spaces. Grossly, hemangiosarcomas can be difficult to differentiate from hemangiomas and hematomas. They are dark red to bluish-purple, friable, and usually covered by a thin serosa (Fig. 13-56), and they commonly occur as numerous large, discrete, and coalescing masses, scattered randomly throughout the spleen and effacing normal splenic architecture. They also may give rise to hepatic, pulmonary, and/or peritoneal metastases, the latter usually occuring by seeding the peritoneal cavity. Hemangiosarcomas are composed of anaplastic endothelial cells, which form haphazardly arranged and poorly defined vascular spaces (Fig. 13-57) that most often contain liquid (nonclotted) blood.

Splenic hemangiosarcomas can occur as primary masses that arise within the spleen or as metastases from distant sites, including skin or right atrium. Primary splenic hemangiosarcomas metastasize to the liver early and frequently; therefore evaluation of the abdomen must include a detailed examination of the entire abdominal cavity for hepatic and peritoneal metastases. Splenic hemangiosarcomas have a poor prognosis.

Acute splenic infarcts. Splenic infarcts occur principally in: (1) the subcapsular areas of the spleen because of poor perfusion and reduced venous return and (2) in areas of acute vascular occlusion or vascultis

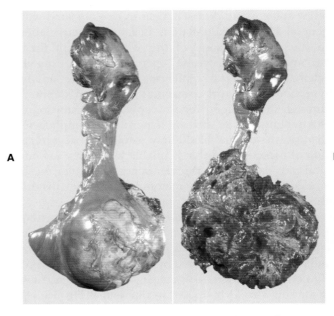

Fig. 13-56 **Hemangiosarcoma, spleen, dog. A,** There are multiple nodules on the dorsal extremity and a large nodule on the ventral extremity of the spleen. **B,** The ventral mass has been incised to reveal the stroma of the hemangiosarcoma. (**A** and **B,** Courtesy Dr. M.D. McGavin, College of Veterinary Medicine, University of Tennessee.)

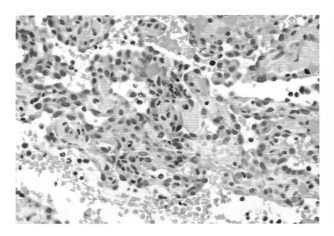

Fig. 13-57 **Hemangiosarcoma, spleen, dog.** Note the haphazardly arranged vascular channels lined by anaplastic endothelial cells. H&E stain. (Courtesy Dr. M.J. Abdy, College of Veterinary Medicine, The University of Georgia; and Noah's Arkive, College of Veterinary Medicine, The University of Georgia.)

induced by infectious agents. Acute splenic infarcts, which are initially hemorrhagic, are not always clearly visible in the early stages but appear as discrete, deeply congested areas with focal capsular distention. As the lesion develops, it becomes somewhat wedge-shaped and gray-white with the base at the splenic capsule (Fig. 13-58).

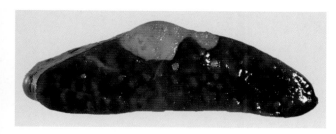

Fig. 13-58   Chronic splenic infarct, spleen, dog. Note the characteristic pale, wedge-shaped area with its base against the capsule of the spleen. *(Courtesy Dr. M.D. McGavin, College of Veterinary Medicine, University of Tennessee.)*

Later a scar forms. Spleens distended with blood are prone to thrombosis and infarction.

Splenic nodules with a firm consistency

The most common diseases or conditions associated with firm-consistency splenic nodules are: (1) nodular hyperplasia, (2) primary neoplasms, (3) metastatic neoplasms, (4) granulomas, and (5) abscesses.

Nodular hyperplasia.   Splenic nodular hyperplasia is most commonly seen in the spleen of older dogs and is often an incidental finding. This lesion has also been called canine nodular splenic hyperplasia and splenoma. Nodules are formed by hyperplastic lymphoid cells or mixed accumulations of hyperplastic erythroid, myeloid, and megakaryocytic cells (EMH) with lymphoid cells. They can appear as single discrete or multiple coalescing firm nodules protruding from the surface but covered by the splenic capsule. The capsular surfaces and cut surfaces often have a mottled red-white pattern because of the intermingling of erythrocytes and hyperplastic leukocytes. Hyperplastic nodules are usually hemispherical and up to 2 cm or larger in diameter (Fig. 13-59). They have no deleterious effect unless they result in a large hematoma, which can rupture and cause hemoperitoneum. Rupture is usually because of trauma or even from a misjudged jump from a couch. These masses must be distinguished from other types of nodules in the spleen, including those of hematoma, hemangioma, hemangiosarcoma, and primary or metastatic neoplasms.

Primary neoplasms.   The primary neoplastic diseases of the spleen that result in nodular enlarged firm spleens include lymphoma, fibroma, fibrosarcoma, osteosarcoma, myxosarcoma, histiocytic sarcoma, myelolipoma, lipoma, liposarcoma, leiomyoma, and leiomyosarcoma. These neoplasms may be solitary or multiple and are locally extensive. They are firm, are raised above the capsular surface but usually confined by the capsular surface, and bulge from the cut surface. Because of the cell of origin (mesenchymal-spindle cells

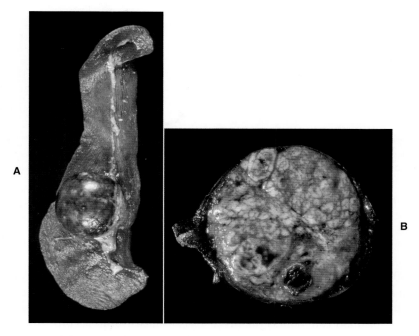

Fig. 13-59   Nodular hyperplasia, spleen, dog. A, A hemispherical 4-cm diameter nodule is protruding from the capsular surface. **B,** Cross section of the nodular mass showing intermixed red and white areas composed of red blood cells and proliferating leukocytes. (**A,** *Courtesy College of Veterinary Medicine, University of Illinois.* **B,** *Courtesy Dr. M.D. McGavin, College of Veterinary Medicine, University of Tennessee.*)

[fibroblasts, myocytes]), the cut surface of these spindle cell neoplasms may have a fibrillar appearance. Myxosarcomas have a distinctively mucinous or slimy character to the cut surface.

Malignant fibrous histiocytomas in canine spleens are considered a continuum of proliferations of fibrous and histiocytic cells (fibrohistiocytic nodule) normally found in the splenic reticular meshwork of the red pulp. They are most often seen as fibrous and histiocytic cellular proliferations in association with hyperplastic lymphoid cells. As the ratio of fibrohistiocytic cells to lymphoid cells increases, the malignant potential of the nodules also increases. Grossly these tumors are often homogeneous, are white, and bulge from the cut surface of the spleen. To our knowledge, there is no evidence that malignant fibrous histiocytoma of the canine spleen is derived from the same cell of origin as the soft-tissue sarcoma of the same name (occasionally called giant cell tumor of soft parts) that occurs in dogs and cats.

Myelolipomas (neoplasms composed of approximately equal quantities of hematopoietic cells and adipose tissue) also may form nodules in the spleen, and these are softer than other mesenchymal-spindle cell neoplasms. Similarly, benign tumors of adipocytes (lipomas) can occur as a single neoplasm and cause splenomegaly.

In cats, the most common neoplasms (primary and secondary) forming nodules in the spleen are, in descending order of frequency, mast cell tumor, lymphoma (lymphosarcoma), myeloid neoplasms, and hemangiosarcomas.

Metastatic neoplasms. Metastatic neoplastic diseases of the spleen that result in enlarged nodular firm spleens can arise from hematopoietic stem cells, from mesenchymal (sarcomas) cell lines, or epithelial (carcinomas) cell lines. These neoplasms may be solitary or multiple and highly invasive and can involve large areas of the spleen. They are firm nodular masses, usually confined by the capsule, and may bulge from the cut surface. Metastatic neoplasms of hematopoietic origin may be lymphoid or myeloid (see Hematopoietic Neoplasia).

Metastatic neoplasms of mesenchymal (sarcomas) origin include fibrosarcomas, leiomyosarcomas, and osteosarcomas. The cut surface of mesenchymal neoplasms may have a fibrillar appearance, which can be difficult to cut if osteoid and/or mineralized bone is present. Metastatic neoplasms of epithelial (carcinomas) origin include most of the common carcinomas (mammary, prostatic, lung) and carcinoids (chemodectomas). The cut surface of epithelial neoplasms may have a lobulated bulging appearance (Fig. 13-60). Malignant melanomas may be black.

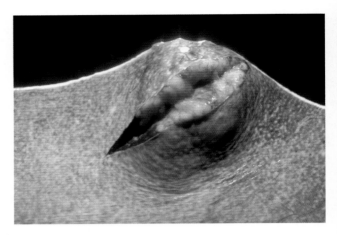

Fig. 13-60   **Metastatic carcinoma, spleen, ox.** The white mass is an undifferentiated carcinoma, which has metastasized to the spleen. Note the lobular texture of the mass and how it bulges from the cut surface. *(Courtesy Dr. M.D. McGavin, College of Veterinary Medicine, University of Tennessee.)*

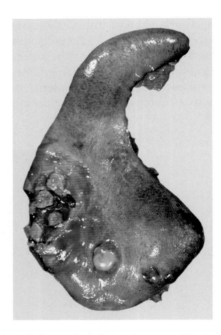

Fig. 13-61   Subcapsular splenic abscesses, *Rhodococcus equi*, spleen, horse. *(Courtesy Dr. P. Carbonell, School of Veterinary Science, University of Melbourne.)*

Granulomas (chronic infectious diseases). Some of the microorganisms listed earlier as causing diffuse granulomatous splenitis and uniform splenomegaly can also cause focal lesions. Others organisms, such as *Brucella abortus* and *Mycobacterium bovis*, cause focal granulomas and nodules in the spleens of pigs. Porcine circovirus 2 causes multifocal noncaseous granulomas with giant cells in the red pulp without splenomegaly.

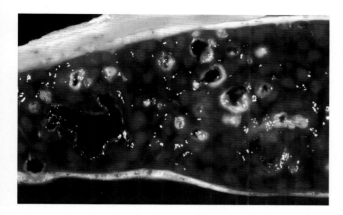

Fig. 13-62   Chronic multifocal suppurative splenitis, splenic abscesses, *Arcanobacterium pyogenes*, spleen, cow. Multiple encapsulated abscesses are present throughout the parenchyma of the spleen, the result of a previous bacteremia. *(Courtesy Department of Veterinary Biosciences, The Ohio State University; and Noah's Arkive, College of Veterinary Medicine, The University of Georgia.)*

Abscesses (acute infectious diseases). Abscesses in the spleen (multifocal chronic suppurative splenitis) are relatively rare but can develop following septicemia and/or bacteremia, usually from pyogenic bacteria such as *Streptococcus* spp., *Rhodococcus equi* (Fig. 13-61), *Arcanobacterium pyogenes* (Fig. 13-62), and *Corynebacterium pseudotuberculosis*. The bacteria are filtered by the monocyte-macrophage system in the spleen but are not killed and replicate within the splenic red pulp to form abscesses of varied sizes, composition, and consistency. Abscesses will bulge from the capsule of the spleen or from cut surfaces. The exudate can vary in texture and color depending on the inciting organism. In most cases, the content is white to yellow-white and moderately thick, and with time becomes encapsulated.

Although there are a large number of diseases and conditions commonly associated with bacteremia, including navel ill, joint ill, chronic respiratory infections, bacterial endocarditis, chronic skin diseases, castration, tail docking, and ear trimming and/or notching, these rarely result in visible splenic abscesses. *Streptococcus equi* ssp. *equi*, the cause of equine strangles, is the prototypical bacterium of acute bacterial infections. The classic lesion of strangles is a nasopharyngitis with lymphadenitis of the regional lymph nodes, usually the mandibular and retropharyngeal. If the organism becomes bacteremic, it commonly causes abscesses in liver, kidney, synovial structures, mesenteric and mediastinal lymph nodes, and occasionally in the spleen. Bastard strangles is the term given to the form of the disease characterized by *Streptococcus equi* ssp. *equi* abscesses anywhere in the body other than the pharyngeal area.

In bovine traumatic reticuloperitonitis, splenic abscesses can result from a direct extension of peritonitis from a penetrating foreign body from the reticulum (see Spleen and Portals of Entry sections). In horses, *Gasterophilus* and *Habronema* spp. can cause gastric ulcers that lead to perforation of the stomach wall and the formation of abscesses in the adjacent spleen.

Small spleens

The most common diseases or conditions associated with small spleens are: (1) developmental anomalies, (2) aging changes, (3) wasting and/or cachectic diseases, and (4) splenic contraction.

Developmental diseases. Immunodeficiency diseases can result in small spleens, as well as small thymuses and lymph nodes. They occur most commonly as primary immunodeficiency diseases of young animals and involve defects in T or B lymphocytes or a combination. Severe combined immunodeficiency (SCID) in Arabian foals is a hereditary disease in which affected foals lack T and B lymphocytes and therefore is characterized by notable lymphoid hypoplasia of primary and secondary lymphoid tissues (Fig. 13-43). Grossly, these spleens are exceptionally small, firm, and pale red. Spleens from affected animals lack lymphoid follicles and PALS, and there are few to no plasma cells. SCID also occurs in the dog, and although the molecular basis is different from that in the horse, the pathologic features of lymphoid tissues are similar. These diseases and their pathologic findings are discussed in Chapter 5.

Accessory spleens can be either congenital or acquired. Congenital accessory spleens are usually small and located in the gastrosplenic ligament. Following rupture of the spleen from injury in dogs, fragments of spleen may be implanted onto peritoneal surfaces. Here they become vascularized and functional. Implanted fragments grossly and histologically resemble normal splenic tissue. They have red and white pulp areas and a thick fibromuscular capsule. These features are important in differentiating accessory spleens from peritoneal implanted fragments (metastases) of hemangiosarcoma, which have a thin shiny serosal covering and a poor prognosis.

Aging changes. The most notable aging change resulting in a small spleen is lymphoid atrophy, the result of loss of T lymphocytes and B lymphocytes.

Grossly the organ is small and the capsule may be wrinkled. Microscopically there is reduction in the white pulp; both PALSs and splenic follicles may be undetectable, and if present, follicles lack germinal centers. Sinuses also lack blood, possibly because of anemia, and are collapsed—resulting in a condensation of their walls, which makes them appear fibrous.

Wasting/cachectic diseases. Any chronic disease, such as starvation, systemic neoplasia, and malabsorption syndrome, may produce cachexia.

Starvation, although having a marked effect on the thymus with resultant atrophy of the T-lymphocyte areas in the spleen and lymph nodes, has little or no effect on the B-lymphoctye areas.

Splenic contraction.   Contraction of the spleen is due to contraction of the smooth muscle in the capsule and trabeculae of storage and intermediate type spleens. It can be induced by the activation of the autonomic system and catecholamine release, which can occur in "fight or flight" situations, and in heart failure and cardiogenic, hypovolemic, and septic shock. It is also present in acute splenic rupture that has resulted in hemorrhage (hemoperitoneum). The contracted spleen is small, its surface is wrinkled, and the cut surface is dry.

MISCELLANEOUS DISORDERS OF THE SPLEEN
Hemosiderosis

Hemosiderin is a form of storage iron derived from the breakdown of erythrocytes, which normally occurs in the spleen. Thus some splenic hemosiderin is to be expected, and the amount varies with the species. It is most extensive in the horse. Excessive amounts of splenic hemosiderin are seen either from a reduced rate of erythropoiesis (less demand for iron) or from rapid destruction of erythrocytes, as in hemolytic anemias (increased stores of iron) such as those caused by immune hemolytic anemias or by hemotropic parasites. Excess hemosiderin may also occur in chronic heart failure and from the injection of iron dextran in pigs. Focal accumulations of hemosiderin in the capsule or parenchyma can be a sequela to hemorrhage, for example from trauma. Intraparenchymal deposits can also be sequelae to hematomas and infarcts. Hemosiderin is also present in siderocalcific plaques (see next section).

Sidero-calcific plaques

Sidero-calcific plaques are also known as Gamna-Gandy bodies. Grossly they are whitish to yellowish, hard, dry encrustations on the capsule. Usually they are most extensive along the margins of the spleen but can be elsewhere on the capsule (Fig. 13-63, A) and sometimes in the parenchyma. Microscopically they are frequently multicolored in an H&E stained section: yellow (bilirubin in early cases), golden brown (hemosiderin), and blue (calcium stained by hematoxylin) (Fig. 13-63, B). As they are often present in older dogs, they have been classified as a senile change, but they may be sequelae to previous hemorrhages.

Splenic rupture

Splenic rupture is not infrequent in dogs and is most commonly from trauma, such as from an automobile accident. Thinning of the capsule can render the spleen more susceptible, and this occurs in splenomegaly at sites of hematomas and infarcts and over tumors such as hemangiomas, hemangiosarcomas, and malignant lymphoma.

On gross examination, in acute cases, the spleen is markedly contracted with a wrinkled surface (Fig. 13-64). The rupture site can be a tear in the capsule, or the spleen can be broken into two or more pieces. Small pieces of splenic parenchyma may be

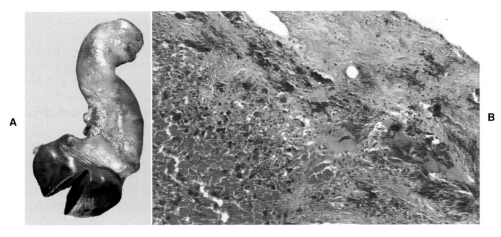

Fig. 13-63   **Sidero-calcific plaque, spleen, dog. A,** Multiple, sometimes confluent raised yellow-white plaquelike foci (sidero-calcific plaques) are present on the capsular surface of the body of the spleen. Note the nodular hyperplasia (incised). **B,** The sidero-calcific plaque lies in the fibrous connective tissue of the capsule and consists chiefly of calcium (blue) and hemosiderin (brown) in fibrous connective tissue. The yellow material is bilirubin, resulting from the breakdown of erythrocytes in a capsular hemorrhage. H&E stain. (**A,** *Courtesy College of Veterinary Medicine, University of Illinois.* **B,** *Courtesy Dr. M.D. McGavin, College of Veterinary Medicine, University of Tennessee.*)

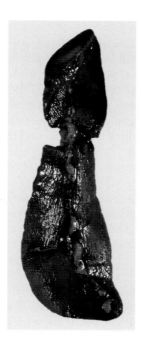

Fig. 13-64   Acute splenic rupture and hemorrhage, spleen, dog. The spleen has been almost transected by trauma. Because of the loss of blood, the spleen has contracted, the surface is crinkled, and the exposed surface of the parenchyma is dry. *(Courtesy Dr. M.D. McGavin, College of Veterinary Medicine, University of Tennessee.)*

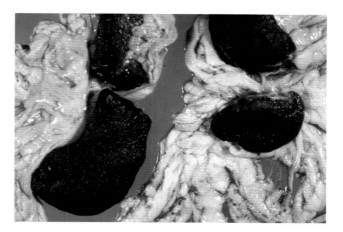

Fig. 13-65   Multiple "spleens," dog. The spleen had been broken into several parts, and the rupture sites have healed. These small pieces of spleen, sometimes referred to as daughter spleens, are functional but not very effective in filtration because of their relatively paltry blood supply. *(Courtesy Dr. H.B. Gelberg, College of Veterinary Medicine, Oregon State University.)*

scattered on the peritoneum (sometimes called "splattered spleen syndrome"). Clotted blood may adhere to the surface at the rupture site. If the rupture is not fatal, the spleen heals by scarring. At necropsy, there may be a capsular scar or two or more separate pieces of spleen adjacent to each other in the gastrosplenic ligament, and/or small accessory "spleens" in the peritoneum (Fig. 13-65). Exactly how functional these "spleens" are is questionable. They have erythrophagocytosis and are presumed to be capable of removing senescent erythrocytes, but as most of them are supplied by small arteries, and thus have limited blood supply, they are not likely to be effective in filtering bacteria out of the body's blood. Also, it is generally considered that at least half of the original splenic mass is required for protection against blood-borne bacterial infections. See previous accessory spleen discussion.

Splenic fissures

Fissures in the splenic capsule are elongated grooves whose axes run parallel to the borders of the spleen. This developmental defect is seen mostly commonly in horses but also occurs in other animals. The surface of the fissure is smooth and covered by the normal splenic capsule.

Chronic splenic infarcts

As in the early stage, chronic splenic infarcts are hemorrhagic and may elevate the capsule. They were discussed previously under Splenic Nodules with a Bloody Consistency. However, as the lesions age, they will diminish in size, become fibrosed, and may be depressed below the level of the adjacent capsule.

Cysts

Occasionally, cystic nodules can be present within the spleen. These cysts are formed by intermediate stages of *Echinococcus granulosa* and *Cysticercus tenuicollis* and are seen most commonly in wild animal species.

DISORDERS OF LYMPH NODES

Many of the inherited immunodeficiency diseases affecting the thymus and spleen cause similar lesions in the lymph nodes—lack of B lymphocytes or T lymphocytes, or both. Congenital hereditary lymphedema has been reported in certain breeds of cattle and dogs. Grossly the most severely affected animals have generalized subcutaneous edema (see Fig. 2-13) and fluid in the serous cavities and are stillborn. Histologically, in severe cases, lymphatics are aplastic, and peripheral and central lymph nodes are hypoplastic. Because at necropsy the pathologist has to evaluate the size of lymph nodes, disorders will be discussed on that basis.

SMALL LYMPH NODES

The most common diseases or conditions associated with small lymph nodes are as follows:
1. Developmental disorders
2. Lack of antigenic stimulation

3. Cachexia and malnutrition
4. Aging
5. Viral infections

Developmental disorders

Hypoplasia, immunodeficiency syndromes. Neonatal animals with primary immunodeficiency diseases of either B lymphocytes or T lymphocytes, or both, often have extremely small to undetectable lymph nodes. In SCID dogs and horses, lymphoid tissues including lymph nodes from affected animals are characterized by an absence of lymphoid follicles and corticomedullary differentiation, and there are few to no lymphocytes and plasma cells.

Lack of antigenic stimulation

Size and components of the lymph node depend on whether it is "resting" or whether it is actively phagocytosing foreign material and/or responding to antigenic stimulation. In specific pathogen-free animals, the lymph nodes are small because they have not been antigenically stimulated. Histologically, there is a small number of primary lymphoid follicles and few or no secondary follicles. This can also be true of peripheral lymph nodes, such as the popliteal, of normal neonatal animals. However, those lymph nodes constantly receiving antigenic material and perhaps bacteria, such as lymph nodes draining the gut, will be large, with active lymphoid follicles containing germinal centers.

It is also important to realize that the immunologic response of a lymph node may be short-lived. After an initial antigenic stimulus, primary lymphoid follicles develop into secondary lymphoid follicles with characteristic germinal centers and produce immunoblasts, which mature into plasma cells and migrate to the medullary cords. Continued stimulation will result in the formation of more primary and secondary lymphoid follicles (follicular hyperplasia). When active, their germinal centers will have many cells undergoing mitosis. Later, as the antigenic response wanes or as the result of long continued stimulation, germinal centers will become depleted of lymphocytes and mitotic figures will be absent. This appearance is described as "depleted germinal centers" or as "reactive depleted lymphoid follicles." Thus lymph nodes may be small because they have never been stimulated (e.g., a peripheral lymph node, such as the popliteal, in a neonatal animal) or because the lymph node has regressed after the cessation of an antigenic stimulus. Thus neither lymphoid follicles, nor germinal centers, are permanent structures. The number of follicles increases or decreases with changes in the intensity of the antigenic stimuli, and the germinal centers go through a cycle of activation, depletion, and rest as described previously.

Cachexia and malnutrition

Any chronic disease such as starvation, systemic neoplasia, and malabsorption syndrome will ultimately produce cachexia. As described under Inflammatory and Degenerative Disorders and Wasting/Cachectic Diseases, starvation mainly reduces the production of T lymphocytes, causing atrophy of the T-lymphocyte areas but having little or no effect on the B-lymphocyte areas.

Aging

Aging results in a depression of the immune system, and as a result, lymph nodes are small. The cortex is reduced, there is a loss of B lymphocytes and T lymphocytes, and lymphoid follicles may be absent.

Viral infections

Many viral infections of human beings and animals target lymphocytes and cause the destruction of lymphoid tissue. In BVD, in the mesenteric lymph nodes, there is a reduction in the number of lymphocytes and necrosis of the germinal centers. Canine distemper virus preferentially infects lymphoid, epithelial, and nervous cells. The distemper virus spreads from the tonsil and tracheobronchial lymph nodes to the spleen, bone marrow, and distant lymph nodes, where it causes lymphoid necrosis. The cortices of lymph nodes of dogs infected with canine distemper are depleted of lymphocytes 6 to 9 days after exposure. This loss of lymphocytes is also reflected hematologically, and affected dogs develop a profound lymphopenia. Although some viruses destroy lymphoid tissue, others can stimulate lymphoid tissue (e.g., Aleutian mink disease virus, maedi-visna virus, and malignant catarrhal fever virus) or cause neoplasia (e.g., feline leukemia virus, bovine leukemia virus, and Marek's disease). Inclusion bodies, typical of porcine inclusion body rhinitis, are found in other epithelia and in lymph nodes, presumably as the result of a viremia.

LARGE LYMPH NODES

Causes of enlarged lymph nodes are as follows:
1. Follicular (B-lymphocyte) and diffuse (T-lymphocyte) lymphoid hyperplasia
2. Lymphadenitis—acute
3. Lymphadenitis—chronic, including encapsulated abscesses; granulomatous inflammation; diffuse or focal
4. Primary neoplasms
5. Metastatic neoplasms
6. Hyperplasia of the monocyte-macrophage system

Lymphoid hyperplasia

Follicular lymphoid hyperplasia can involve large numbers of lymph nodes, as in a systemic disease, or can be localized to a regional lymph node draining an inflamed area. It is thus a common response, provided the animal survives for several days or longer. Follicular lymphoid hyperplasia can be present in the initial stages of a disease, but this may be followed by loss of lymphocytes from the follicles from lymphocytolysis as in many viral diseases (e.g., EHV-1). With time, the lymph follicles become "exhausted," and active proliferation in the germinal centers ceases.

Follicular lymphoid hyperplasia is evident in any regional lymph node draining an area in which there are inflammatory products or antigens (e.g., tuberculin from a tuberculin test or an injected vaccine). It is also particularly notable in lymph nodes draining areas of chronic inflammation (e.g., mammary lymph nodes in chronic bovine mastitis). Follicular lymphoid hyperplasia is characterized by proliferation of lymphoid follicles (Fig. 13-66), which have active germinal centers to produce plasma cells to secrete antibody and an increase in T lymphocytes in the paracortical areas. In acute inflammation, these changes commence after several days.

Grossly, when there is notable lymphoid hyperplasia, lymph nodes will be enlarged, the capsule may be tense, and on incision the parenchyma will bulge. The cortex may be increased in width.

Microscopically, lymph nodes are enlarged chiefly because of the expansion of the cortex by increased numbers of lymphoid follicles (follicular lymphoid hyperplasia), most of which will have active germinal centers with numerous mitotic figures. Plasma cells precursors are generated here and then migrate to the medullary cords where they develop into antibody secreting plasma cells. After about 10 days or more, secondary lymphoid follicles can become depleted of mitotically active cells and lymphocytes. The result is pale germinal centers consisting primarily of stromal and precursor cells. Medullary cords originally densely packed with plasma cells also become depleted, approximately a couple of weeks after the antigenic stimulus ceases.

Acute lymphadenitis

Acute lymphadenitis is usually the result of a regional lymph node draining an inflammatory site and becoming infected (e.g., the medial retropharyngeal lymph nodes in acute rhinitis, tracheobronchial lymph nodes in pneumonia [Fig. 13-67], and the supramammary [mammary] lymph node in mastitis). In some instances, lymphadenitis may be accompanied by inflammation of the afferent lymphatics (lymphangitis). The material draining to the regional lymph node may be bacteria, inflammatory products including mediators, or a sterile irritant. Examination of these lymph nodes should include culturing for bacteria, examination of smears, and histologic sections for bacteria and fungi.

Grossly, lymph nodes are enlarged and may be soft or firm, depending on the amount of exudate. The cut surface may be reddened both from local hyperemia and from blood draining from an inflammatory site. When incised, the parenchyma may bulge, and the surface may be wet with blood, lymph, or pus.

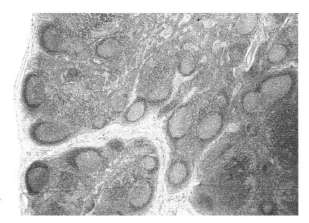

Fig. 13-66   Follicular lymphoid hyperplasia, chronic demodicosis, caudal cervical (prescapular) lymph node, dog. The number of lymphoid follicles has increased (hyperplasia), and all of these have germinal centers (secondary follicles) indicating active proliferation of B lymphocytes to form plasma cells in response to an antigenic stimulus. H&E stain. *(Courtesy Dr. M.D. McGavin, College of Veterinary Medicine, University of Tennessee.)*

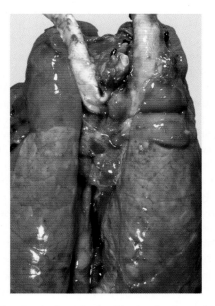

Fig. 13-67   Acute lymphadenitis, tracheobronchial lymph nodes, pig. The nodes are enlarged and reddened from draining the pneumonic cranial lung lobes. Note the red consolidation of the dorsal portion of the cranial lung lobes. *(Courtesy Dr. M.D. McGavin, College of Veterinary Medicine, University of Tennessee.)*

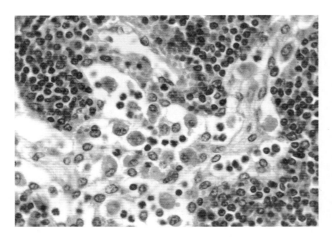

Fig. 13-68   Acute lymphadenitis (early), medulla of lymph node, dog. Medullary sinus with adjacent medullary cords. The lumen of the medullary sinus contains numerous macrophages (large cells, sinus histiocytosis) and a few neutrophils. This is the type of early response seen when a lymph node drains an inflamed area. The medullary cords are packed with lymphocytes and some plasma cells. H&E stain. *(Courtesy Dr. M.D. McGavin, College of Veterinary Medicine, University of Tennessee.)*

Suppuration is usually the result of pyogenic bacteria (*Streptococcus equi* ssp. *equi*, horses; *Streptococcus porcinus*, pig; and *Arcanobacterium pyogenes* in cattle and sheep). Microscopically the lymph node is hyperemic. In the initial stages, neutrophils and usually erythrocytes are present in the sinuses, which are distended with lymph or exudate. After the passage of a day or so, numerous macrophages enter the sinuses (sinus histiocytosis), particularly the medullary sinuses (Fig. 13-68).

In equine strangles caused by *Streptococcus equi* ssp. *equi* and in porcine jowl abscess caused by *Streptococcus porcinus* (Fig. 13-69), the mandibular lymph nodes may rupture and discharge the pus to the surface of the skin. The pathogenesis is similar in both cases. In jowl abscess, *Streptococcus porcinus* colonizes the oral cavity, which results in infection of the tonsils and the regional lymph nodes. The mandibular lymph nodes are the most often affected, but the retropharyngeal and parotid lymph nodes may be involved. Multiple abscesses 1 to 10 cm in diameter may be present in the lymph nodes.

In equine strangles, the etiologic agent *Streptococcus equi* ssp. *equi* causes inflammation of the upper respiratory tract, which results in abscesses in the regional lymph nodes; usually the mandibular and retropharyngeal lymph nodes are most severely affected (Fig. 13-70). Ultimately the abscess may rupture and discharge the pus through a sinus to the surface.

Toxoplasmosis and salmonellosis both cause focal areas of necrosis in infected lymph nodes.

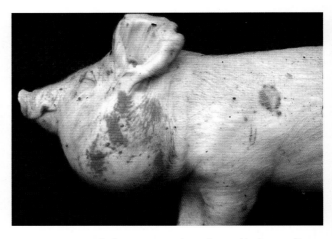

Fig. 13-69   Jowl abscess, pig. The submandibular swelling is caused by marked enlargement of the mandibular lymph nodes from a suppurative lymphadenitis caused by *Streptococcus porcinus.* *(Courtesy Dr. J.M. King, College of Veterinary Medicine, Cornell University.)*

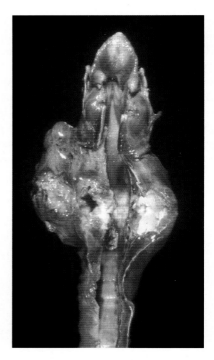

Fig. 13-70   Acute suppurative lymphadenitis, equine strangles (*Streptococcus equi* ssp. *equi*), dorsal view of larynx, left and right retropharyngeal lymph nodes, horse. The lymph nodes are grossly distended with pus. *(Courtesy College of Veterinary Medicine, University of Illinois.)*

If inflammation in the lymph node continues for several days or longer, it will also be enlarged by the response of the immune system, which includes follicular hyperplasia, active germinal centers, and plasma cells in the medullary cords.

Chronic lymphadenitis

Chronic lymphadenitis may be a chronic suppurative (active) lymphadenitis with abscess formation, as in ovine caseous lymphadenitis; granulomatous; diffuse or focal; or a mixture of follicular lymphoid hyperplasia, plasmacytosis, fibrosis, sinus histiocytosis, and microabscesses. In the initial stages, the lymph node may not be notably enlarged. With chronic suppurative inflammation, abscesses range in size from small—causing no increase in the size of the lymph node—to large, even large enough to occupy the whole lymph node.

Granulomatous lymphadenitis may be focal as in tuberculosis, focal coalescing as in blastomycosis and cryptococcosis, or diffuse as in histoplasmosis.

Chronic suppurative lymphadenitis. (encapsulated abscesses).   The classic example of chronic suppurative lymphadenitis is caseous lymphadenitis, a disease of sheep and goats caused by *Corynebacterium pseudotuberculosis*. It is also the cause of ulcerative lymphangitis in cattle and horses and pectoral abscesses in horses. In sheep, the bacterium enters the skin through wounds, such as shearing cuts, and then drains to the regional lymph node. This is usually either the superficial cervical (prescapular) or the subiliac (prefemoral) lymph node because the cuts are frequently on the legs. Here a suppurative lymphadenitis develops. Initially there are multiple microabscesses with numerous eosinophils in the sinuses on the cortex. These coalesce and caseate and become encapsulated by fibrous tissue. However, they continue to enlarge, a process that results in the characteristic concentric lamellae, which can often be seen on a cross section of an old abscess. On gross examination, the pus in the abscess is initially greenish (because of the eosinophils) and semifluid (Fig. 13-71), but it becomes caseous with age (Fig. 13-72), loses its green color, and becomes inspissated. Old abscesses can reach a diameter of 4 to 5 cm. Similar abscesses may be found in the lungs, especially in older sheep. The abscesses in goats are usually more numerous and frequently involve lymph nodes of the head and neck.

Granulomatous lymphadenitis

Focal granulomatous lymphadenitis.   The classic example of focal granulomatous lymphadenitis is tuberculosis caused by *Mycobacterium bovis*, but the more pathogenic members of the *Mycobacterium avium-intercellulare* complex can cause similar lesions in cattle and pigs. Initially, lesions in the lymphatic system are in the regional lymph nodes (e.g., the tracheobronchial lymph nodes in the case of pulmonary tuberculosis), but once tuberculosis is disseminated, lymph nodes throughout the body will have lesions. *Mycobacterium bovis* lesions in lymph nodes are characterized by the formation of caseating granulomas. These are often multiple

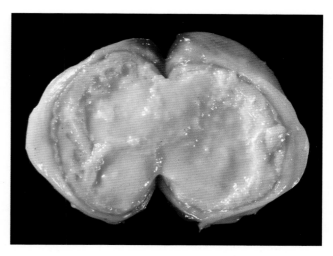

Fig. 13-71   **Caseous lymphadenitis,** *Corynebacterium pseudotuberculosis*, **lymph node, sheep.** The whole lymph node has been replaced by an abscess containing mostly semifluid yellowish pus. This is an early stage of caseous lymphadenitis, before the pus has become inspissated and caseous. *(Courtesy Dr. K. Read, College of Veterinary Medicine, Texas A&M University; and Noah's Arkive, College of Veterinary Medicine, The University of Georgia.)*

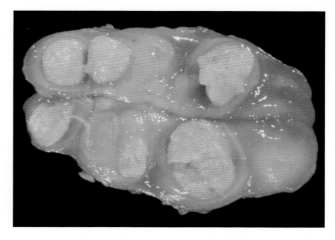

Fig. 13-72   **Chronic caseous lymphadenitis,** *Corynebacterium pseudotuberculosis*, **lymph node, sheep.** The lymph node has been sliced longitudinally exposing three chronic abscesses enclosed by thick fibrous capsules and containing yellowish caseous pus. *(Courtesy Dr. W. Crowell, College of Veterinary Medicine, The University of Georgia; and Noah's Arkive, College of Veterinary Medicine, The University of Georgia.)*

(Fig. 13-73) but can become confluent and occupy the whole lymph node. Grossly the lesions are pale, caseous, and often mineralized in cattle. Microscopically the granulomas have central necrotic debris surrounded by a layer of epithelioid macrophages interspersed

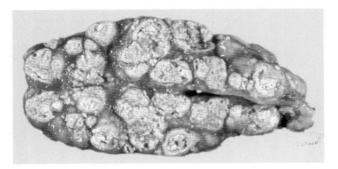

Fig. 13-73 Tuberculosis (*Mycobacterium bovis*), lymph node, ox. The normal architecture of the lymph node has been completely obliterated by multiple caseating granulomas, typical of *Mycobacterium bovis* lesions. *(Courtesy Dr. M. Domingo, Autonomous University of Barcelona; and Noah's Arkive, College of Veterinary Medicine, University of Georgia.)*

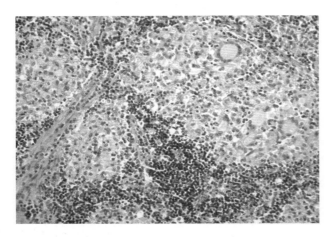

Fig. 13-74 Johne's disease (*Mycobacterium avium* ssp. *pseudotuberculosis*), lymph node, ox. Several noncaseating granulomas *(pale areas)* have replaced the normal lymphoid tissue *(blue)*. Note the Langhans' giant cell *(upper right)*. H&E stain. *(Courtesy College of Veterinary Medicine, University of Illinois.)*

with scattered Langhans' giant cells and lymphocytes. Peripheral to this is a layer of lymphocytes, and in old lesions the granuloma may be surrounded by a fibrous capsule. Pigs ingesting one of the mycobacteria of the *Mycobacterium avium-intercellulare* complex may have caseous lesions confined to the retropharyngeal lymph nodes, and these lesions are self-limiting. In bovine Johne's disease, the mesenteric lymph nodes draining the infected intestine can have noncaseous granulomas (Fig. 13-74).

Focal coalescing granulomatous lymphadenitis. Blastomycosis and cryptococcosis are examples of focal coalescing granulomatous lymphadenitis. Both of these frequently involve a regional lymph node draining an affected area (e.g., the tracheobronchial lymph nodes in

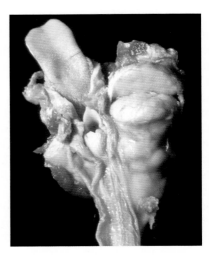

Fig. 13-75 Cryptococcosis (*Cryptococcus neoformans*), right mandibular lymph node, cat. The lymph node is grossly enlarged and the incised surface is bulging and pale, and its normal architecture has been completely effaced. *(Courtesy Dr. M.D. McGavin, College of Veterinary Medicine, University of Tennessee.)*

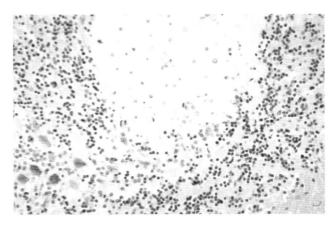

Fig. 13-76 Cryptococcosis, right lymph node, cat. The pale area in the upper center is occupied by *Cryptococcus neoformans*. In H&E stained sections, the capsule of the organism, which is thick, does not stain. The mass of cryptococci is bordered by the diffuse lymphoid tissue of the paracortex. Note the complete absence of any inflammation (usually granulomatous), which frequently occurs in feline cryptococcosis. H&E stain. *(Courtesy Dr. M.D. McGavin, College of Veterinary Medicine, University of Tennessee.)*

the case of pulmonary infections). In advanced cases, the lymph node may be enlarged, the cut surface pale, and its normal architecture totally or almost completely obliterated (Fig. 13-75). In cryptococcosis in cats, there may be little or no inflammatory response (Fig. 13-76), and the enlargement of the lymph node is due mainly to a large mass of organisms (*Cryptococcus neoformans*).

An unusual example of a focal granuloma is the foreign body granuloma that develops around *Demodex* that have drained to a regional lymph node from an area of skin affected with chronic demodicosis.

Diffuse granulomatous lymphadenitis. Diffuse granulomatous lymphadenitis is usually caused by dimorphous fungi. Both *Histoplasma capsulatum* and *Blastomyces dermatitidis* can cause this type of diffuse lesion, but in the early stages the lesions will be microscopic foci that later expand and coalesce to involve most of the lymph node.

Histoplasmosis caused by *Histoplasma capsulatum* is a diffuse disease of the monocyte-macrophage system and causes a marked proliferation of macrophages in a wide variety of tissues including spleen, lymph nodes, liver, lungs, and intestine. The dimorphic fungus *Histoplasma capsulatum* grows as a mold in soil and as a yeast in animal tissue. The fungus is distributed throughout the world, in major river valleys, and in temperate and tropical climates; *Histoplasma capsulatum* grows especially well in soil enriched by bird feces. The greatest incidence of disease is in dogs; the incidence is lower in cats.

In most animals, the organism is inhaled and results in mild self-limiting infections. These are self-limiting but cause enlargement of tracheobronchial lymph nodes. Dogs and cats are usually asymptomatic. Because the fungus is confined to monocytes and macrophages, its spread beyond the respiratory tract is assumed to occur by hematogenous and lymphogenous dissemination of infected cells. Disseminated histoplasmosis in dogs and cats results in gastrointestinal or hepatic disease of long duration.

Disseminated histoplasmosis is characterized by neutrophilia and monocytosis in some animals. Nonregenerative anemia is common because of the chronic inflammation. Nonspecific changes as a result of the damage to the liver are elevated serum alkaline phosphatase activity and hyperbilirubinemia. The total serum protein may be low, normal, or increased, depending upon factors such as extent and duration of the diarrhea and emaciation.

Cytology is useful for the diagnosis of histoplasmosis. The least invasive procedures include examination of cells of body fluids, tracheal wash preparations, and aspirates of bone marrow and lymph nodes. The organisms are visible in macrophages (Fig. 13-77).

Dogs dying of this disease are emaciated. The large bowel is thickened with mucosal corrugations caused by infiltration of the submucosa and lamina propria by macrophages, lymphocytes, and plasma cells. Lymph nodes are uniformly enlarged, and normal architecture may be obscured. In contrast to lymphoma, the nodes are firm when incised.

Histologically in the lymph nodes, coalescing granulomas replace the normal cortical lymphoid tissue.

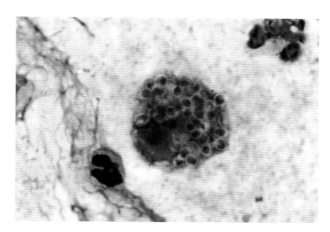

Fig. 13-77   Histoplasmosis, feline transtracheal wash. A macrophage is laden with small, oval, encapsulated yeast forms. **Wright's stain.** *(Courtesy Dr. M.M. Fry, College of Veterinary Medicine, University of Tennessee.)*

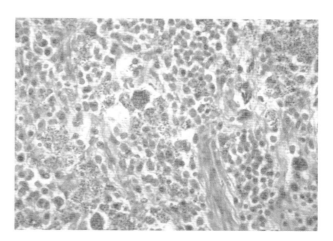

Fig. 13-78   Histoplasmosis, lymph node, dog. Diffuse granulomatous lymphadenitis. Most of the field is occupied by macrophages, many of which have phagocytosed *Histoplasma capsulatum*. **H&E stain.** *(Courtesy Dr. M.D. McGavin, College of Veterinary Medicine, University of Tennessee.)*

Typical yeast organisms, which are 2- to 4-μm-wide hematoxylinophilic dots surrounded by a clear halo, are present in variable numbers in epithelioid macrophages (Fig. 13-78). The spleen and liver are enlarged and firm, and the liver is diffusely gray. Affected organs can be imprinted on glass slides for cytologic evaluation.

Leishmaniasis is a disease of the monocyte-macrophage system caused by protozoa of the genus *Leishmania*. It occurs in human beings, dogs, and other animals and is confined to endemic areas, including parts of Europe, the Mediterranean, the Middle East, Africa, and Central and South America. It may be seen in any part of the world in dogs that have resided in endemic areas. The protozoa proliferate by binary fission in the gut of the sand fly and become flagellated organisms, which are introduced into mammals by insect bites; they then assume a nonflagellated form in macrophages.

Lesions are of two types: cutaneous and/or visceral. The cutaneous lesions in dogs are ulcers at the site of insect bites. These ulcers are directly attributable to proliferation of the organism within macrophages; the accumulation of neutrophils, lymphocytes, and plasma cells; and focal disruption of the dermis and epidermis. In the visceral form of the disease, dogs are emaciated and have general enlargement of abdominal lymph nodes. Dogs have a nonregenerative anemia and a polyclonal hypergammaglobulinemia with total protein concentrations that may exceed 100 g/L (10 g/dL).

At necropsy, dogs with visceral leishmaniasis are emaciated and have an enlarged liver, spleen, and lymph nodes. Histologically the lymph node sinuses are filled with macrophages (sinuses histiocytosis), which are filled with intracytoplasmic organisms. Lymph node aspirates contain macrophages, in which there are organisms. Imprints made of these enlarged organs have macrophages containing numerous round organisms approximately 2 μm in diameter. They have a vesicular nucleus and a small kinetoplast, which aids in distinguishing them from *Histoplasma capsulatum* (Fig. 13-79). The bone marrow is usually hyperplastic. Late in the disease there is usually atrophy of the lymph nodes and spleen.

Mixed inflammatory response. A mixed inflammatory response in the lymph node occurs in reaction to continued drainage from an inflammatory site, such as a joint with chronic erysipelas arthritis (pig) or chronic mastitis (bovine). The lymph node is enlarged because of follicular lymphoid hyperplasia, plasmacytosis (immune response), fibrosis, sinus histiocytosis, and microabscesses. Also there may be hemosiderosis.

Primary neoplasms

The most common primary neoplasm is lymphoma (lymphosarcoma). Many forms of this cause notable enlargement of lymph nodes (Figs. 13-80 and 13-81), and on cross section the normal architecture (cortex and the medulla) may be obliterated by the malignant cells. The cut surface is pale, is often homogeneous, and bulges (see Hematopoietic Neoplasms).

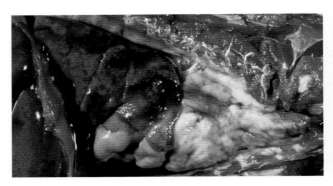

Fig. 13-80 **Lymphoma (lymphosarcoma), cranial mediastinal lymph nodes, cat.** The cranial mediastinal lymph nodes are grossly enlarged, fill the cranial thoracic cavity, and have displaced the lungs and heart caudad. *(Courtesy Dr. M.D. McGavin, College of Veterinary Medicine, University of Tennessee.)*

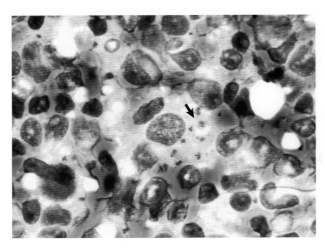

Fig. 13-79 **Leishmaniasis, *Leishmania* spp., canine popliteal lymph node aspirate.** A macrophage contains multiple amastigotes with oval nuclei and smaller bar-shaped kinetoplasts (*arrow*). **Wright's stain.** *(Courtesy Dr. M.M. Fry, College of Veterinary Medicine, University of Tennessee.)*

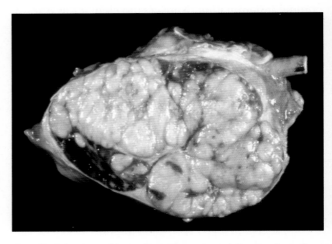

Fig. 13-81 **Lymphoma (lymphosarcoma), bovine lymph node.** Normal architecture of lymph node has been completely obliterated by proliferating lobules of neoplastic tissue composed of malignant lymphocytes. *(Courtesy College of Veterinary Medicine, University of Illinois.)*

Metastatic neoplasms

Carcinomas typically metastasize to the regional lymph node, at least initially. The hematogenous route is typical of metastasis of sarcomas but is often seen with carcinomas. Thus metastatic carcinomas in regional lymph nodes are a common finding, and these lymph nodes may, at least temporarily, prevent further dissemination of the neoplasm. An incomplete list includes squamous cell carcinoma, mammary carcinoma, gastric carcinoma, pulmonary carcinoma, osteogenic sarcoma, malignant melanoma, and malignant mast cell tumor.

If the tumor has induced an inflammatory response at its primary site (e.g., from ulceration such as that caused by an ulcerating squamous cell carcinoma or a perforating gastric carcinoma), this will cause an acute lymphadenitis in the regional lymph node.

Histologically, single cells or clusters of neoplastic cells travel via the afferent lymphatics and are deposited in a sinus, usually the subcapsular sinus. Here the cells proliferate and can ultimately occupy the whole lymph node. They can also send more malignant cells to the next lymph node in the chain.

Lymphoma can be primary or metastatic and both appear grossly similar. The different types of lymphoma are discussed in the section on hematopoietic neoplasia.

PIGMENT IN LYMPH NODES

Lymph nodes may have the following discolorations:
- Red—This may be due to erythrocytes draining from a hemorrhagic or acutely inflamed area, or from hyperemia of the lymph node in acute lymphadenitis. Because of the peculiar anatomy of the porcine lymph node, with large sinuses under the capsule, blood in these nodes is very obvious. It is frequently seen in acute septicemias, in which endotoxin-induced vasculitis or DIC have caused hemorrhages. Histologically, initially there are erythrocytes in the sinuses, and these rapidly undergo erythrophagocytosis by sinus histiocytes, which rapidly increase in number (sinus histiocytosis). If the animal lives, hemosiderin deposits are present within 7 to 10 days in the perisinusoidal macrophages.
- Black—Carbon from pulmonary anthracosis drains to the tracheobronchial lymph nodes and from skin tattoos draining to the regional lymph node.
- Melanin—In chronic dermatitis, melanocytes may be destroyed and their melanin released into the dermis (so-called pigmentary incontinence), and the pigment is then transported in macrophages to the regional lymph node. Also, lymph nodes draining areas of congenital melanosis, such as in porcine lungs, may have melanin deposits. Malignant melanomas, metastasizing to the regional lymph node, may also be black.

- Parasitic hematin—This pigment produced by *Fascioloides magna* in the livers of cattle and *Fasciola hepatica* in the livers of sheep is transported to the hepatic (portal) lymph nodes.
- Brown—Hemosiderin imparts a brown coloration to lymph nodes. This can be due to a breakdown of erythrocytes arriving in the afferent lymph from a congested (e.g., chronic passive congestion of the lungs), hemorrhagic or inflamed area or from the phagocytosis of altered or parasitized erythrocytes in hemolytic anemias. Another cause is drainage of iron dextran to the lymph node from an intramuscular injection site.

The lymph nodes of cattle and sheep are often normally discolored by a brown to blackish pigment.

MISCELLANEOUS LYMPH NODE DISORDERS
Inclusion bodies

Many viruses produce inclusion bodies, and some of these have inclusions in lymph nodes. These include cytomegalic virus in inclusion body rhinitis of pigs, EHV-1 in horses, parvovirus in feline panleukopenia, and the virus of pseudorabies in pigs.

Emphysema

Emphysema in lymph nodes is a consequence of emphysema in their drainage fields and is seen most frequently in the tracheobronchial lymph nodes in bovine interstitial emphysema and in the porcine mesenteric lymph nodes in intestinal emphysema. The appearance of the lymph node varies with the extent of the emphysema. In severe cases, the lymph node is light, puffy, and filled with discrete gas bubbles, and the cut surface may be spongy. Histologically, the sinuses are distended with gas and their walls are lined by macrophages and giant cells. This change has been considered a foreign body reaction to the gas bubbles. Similar lesions are seen in afferent lymphatics.

SUGGESTED READINGS

Alexandre-Pires G: Intermediary spleen microvasculature in canis familiaris—morphological evidence of a closed and open type, *Anat Histol Embryol* 32(5):263-270, 2003.

Avery PR, Avery AC: Molecular methods to distinguish reactive and neoplastic lymphocyte expansions and their importance in transitional neoplastic states, *Vet Clin Pathol* 33(4):196-207, 2004.

Beutler E, Lichtman MA, Coller BS et al, editors: *Williams hematology*, ed 6, New York, 2001, McGraw-Hill.

Boudreaux MK, Lipscomb DL: Clinical, biochemical, and molecular aspects of Glanzmann's thrombasthenia in humans and dogs, *Vet Pathol* 38(3):249-260, 2001.

Chaplin DD: Lymphoid tissues and organs. In Paul WE, editor: *Fundamental immunology*, ed 5, Philadelphia, 2003, Lippincott Williams & Wilkins.

Charles JA: Lymph nodes and thymus, In Sims LD, Glastonbury JRW, editors: *Pathology of the pig: a diagnostic guide*, Victoria, Australia, 1996, Barton, A.C.T.: Pig Research and Development Corp.

Feldman BF, Zinkl JG, Jain NC, editors: *Schalm's veterinary hematology*, ed 5, Philadelphia, 2000, Lippincott Williams & Wilkins.

Ganz T: Hepcidin: a key regulator of iron metabolism and mediator of anemia of inflammation, *Blood* 102(3):783-788, 2003.

Harvey JW: *Atlas of veterinary hematology: blood and bone marrow of domestic animals*, Philadelphia, 2001, Saunders.

Harvey JW: The erythrocyte: physiology, metabolism, and biochemical disorders. In Kaneko JJ, Harvey JW, Bruss ML, editors: *Clinical biochemistry of domestic animals*, ed 5, San Diego, 1997, Academic Press.

Hoover EA, Mullins JI: Feline leukemia virus infection and diseases, *J Am Vet Med Assoc* 199(10):1287-1297, 1991.

Jacobs RM, Messick JB, Valli VE: Tumors of the hemolymphatic system. In: *Tumors in domestic animals*, ed 4, Ames, 2002, Iowa State Press.

Jain NC, Blue JT, Grindem CB et al: Proposed criteria for classification of acute myeloid leukemia in dogs and cats, *Vet Clin Pathol* 20(3):63-82, 1991.

Janeway CA, Travers P, Walport M et al: *Immunobiology: the immune system in health and disease*, ed 5, New York, 2001, Garland Publishing.

Kierszenbaum AL: *Histology and cell biology: an introduction to pathology*, St Louis, 2002, Mosby.

Kumar V, Abbas AK, Fausto N: *Robbins & Cotran pathologic basis of disease*, ed 7, Philadelphia, 2005, Saunders.

Latimer KS, Mahaffey EA, Prasse KW, editors: *Duncan & Prasse's veterinary laboratory medicine: clinical pathology*, ed 4, Ames, 2003, Iowa State Press.

McGill L: *The canine lymphoma classification project: a clinico-pathologic evaluation of the WHO classification system on canine nodal and extranodal lymphoma*, American College of Veterinary Pathologists/American Society for Veterinary Clinical Pathology 2004 Conference Proceedings.

McManus PM: Classification of myeloid neoplasms: a comparative review, *Vet Clin Pathol* 34(3):189-212, 2005.

McManus PM: *Myeloid neoplasms: construction and validation of a classification scheme applicable to animals*, American College of Veterinary Pathologists/American Society for Veterinary Clinical Pathology 2004 Conference Proceedings.

McOrist S, Sims LD: The spleen. In Sims LD, Glastonbury JRW, editors: *Pathology of the pig: a diagnostic guide*, Victoria, Australia, 1996, Barton, A.C.T.: Pig Research and Development Corp.

McQuiston JH, McCall CL, Nicholson WL: Ehrlichiosis and related infections, *J Am Vet Med Assoc* 223(12):1750-1756, 2003.

Messick JB: Hemotropic mycoplasmas (hemoplasmas): a review and new insights into pathogenic potential, *Vet Clin Pathol* 33(1):2-13, 2004.

Raskin RE, Meyer DJ, editors: *Atlas of canine and feline cytology*, Philadelphia, 2001, Saunders.

Sellon DC, Fuller FJ, McGuire TC: The immunopathogenesis of equine infectious anemia virus, *Virus Res* 32(2):111-138, 1994.

Shelton GH, Linenberger ML: Hematologic abnormalities associated with retroviral infections in the cat, *Semin Vet Med Surg (Small Anim)* 10(4):220-233, 1995.

Sims LD, Glastonbury JRW, editors: *Pathology of the pig: a diagnostic guide*, Victoria, Australia, 1996, Barton, A.C.T.: Pig Research and Development Corp.

Spangler WL, Kass PH: Pathologic and prognostic characteristics of splenomegaly in dogs due to fibrohistiocytic nodules: 98 cases, *Vet Path* 35(6):488-498, 1998.

Spangler WL, Kass PH: Splenic myeloid metaplasia, histiocytosis, and hypersplenism in the dog (65 cases), *Vet Pathol* 36(6): 583-593, 1999.

Stockham SL, Scott MA: *Fundamentals of veterinary clinical pathology*, Ames, 2002, Iowa State Press.

Valli VE, Jacobs RM, Parodi AL et al: Histologic classification of hematopoietic tumors of domestic animals. In: *World Health Organization international histological classification of tumors in domestic animals, second series*, vol 2, Washington, DC, 2002, Armed Forces Institute of Pathology.

Valli VEO: Lymphoreticular tissues. In Jubb KVF, Kennedy PC, Palmer H, editors: *Pathology of domestic animals*, ed 4, San Diego, 1993, Academic Press.

Vardiman JW, Harris NL, Brunning RD: The World Health Organization (WHO) classification of the myeloid neoplasms, *Blood* 100 (7):2292-2302, 2002.

Wardrop KJ: The Coombs' test in veterinary medicine: past, present, future, *Vet Clin Pathol* 34(4):325-334, 2005.

Workman HC, Vernau W: Chronic lymphocytic leukemia in dogs and cats: the veterinary perspective, *Vet Clin North Am Small Anim Pract* 33(6):1379-1399, 2003.

APPENDIX **13-1**

TESTS TO EVALUATE PLATELET FUNCTION OR IMMUNE-MEDIATED THROMBOCYTOPENIA

- *Bleeding time (template bleeding time, buccal mucosal bleeding time)*. This assay assesses primary hemostasis (platelet plug formation) by measuring the time interval between inflicting of standardized wound and cessation of bleeding. Sedation may be required. In small animals, the test is usually performed on the buccal mucosa; in large animals, it may be performed on the distal limb. Prolonged bleeding time may be because of a platelet function defect, von Willebrand disease, or a vascular defect. The test is of low sensitivity; reference intervals are species- and site-dependent (can perform test on a normal animal as a control). This test is contraindicated in cases of thrombocytopenia because significant thrombocytopenia can cause a prolonged bleeding time (invalidates interpretation of test results).

- *Clot retraction test.* This assay assesses retraction of a clot, in which platelets play an essential role. This is a crude test that is rarely performed. Different protocols are described. Significant thrombocytopenia invalidates interpretation of test results.
- Tests to characterize platelet function abnormalities more specifically are available through specialized laboratories
  - *Aggregometry*–to assess platelet aggregation in response to different physiologic agonists
  - *Adhesion assays*–to assess the ability of platelets to adhere to a substrate (e.g., collagen)
  - *Flow cytometry*–to assay for expression of surface molecules
  - *PFA-100*–an instrument that simulates a damaged blood vessel, by measuring time for a platelet plug to occlude an aperture; to date, this instrument has mainly been used in research applications
- Tests for immune-mediated thrombocytopenia (IMT)
  - *Flow cytometry*–to detect immunoglobulin bound to the platelet surface, using a fluorescent-labeled antibody
  - *Bone marrow immunofluorescent antibody (IFA) test*–to detect bound immunoglobulin. Sometimes referred to as the "antimegakaryocyte antibody test," this assay actually detects the presence of immunoglobulin nonspecifically: A smear of a bone marrow aspirate is incubated with a fluorescent-labeled antibody to species-specific immunoglobulin.

TESTS FOR EVALUATING THE COAGULATION SYSTEM

- Activated partial thromboplastin time (aPTT or PTT)
  - Required sample: citrated plasma
  - Measures time for fibrin clot formation after addition of a contact activator, calcium, and a substitute for platelet phospholipid
  - Deficiencies/dysfunction in intrinsic and/or common coagulation pathway (all factors except for VII and XIII) will cause prolongation of PTT.
  - Insensitive test–prolongation requires 70% deficiency
  - Other causes of prolongation include polycythemia (less plasma per unit volume, so excess amount of citrate is available to chelate calcium) and heparin therapy.
- Activated clotting time (ACT)
  - Required sample: nonanticoagulated whole blood in special ACT tube (diatomaceous earth as contact activator)
  - Used in practice setting–performed by warming sample to body temperature, monitoring for clot formation; normal clotting times are within 60 to 90 seconds in dogs, 165 seconds in cats

- Less sensitive version of PTT–prolongation requires 95% deficiency
- Severe thrombocytopenia may cause prolongation
- One stage prothrombin time (OSPT or PT)
  - Required sample: citrated plasma
  - Measures time for fibrin clot formation after addition of tissue factor (TF, thromboplastin), calcium, and a substitute for platelet phospholipid
  - Deficiencies/dysfunction in extrinsic (factor VII) and/or common coagulation pathway will cause prolongation of PT
  - Insensitive test–prolongation requires 70% deficiency
- PIVKA (*proteins induced by vitamin K antagonism or absence*) test
  - Required sample: citrated plasma
  - Essentially, a version of the PT using an especially sensitive thromboplastin reagent
  - PIVKA are inactive (uncarboxylated) vitamin K-dependent factors; an increase in PIVKA is not specific for vitamin-K antagonism but may be an earlier and more sensitive detector than PT or PTT.
- Thrombin time (TT)
  - Required sample: citrated plasma
  - Measures time for fibrin clot formation after thrombin (factor IIa) is added
  - Defects directly involving formation and/or polymerization of fibrin will prolong this test (i.e., if the lesion is upstream of the conversion of fibrinogen to fibrin, the TT will be normal). Hypofibrinogenemia or dysfibrinogenemia will cause prolongation of the TT.
- Fibrinogen
  - Required sample: citrated plasma
  - Fibrinogen concentration measured based on time to clot formation after addition of thrombin; this is essentially the same as the thrombin time mentioned earlier and is a more accurate method than the heat precipitation method.
  - Decreased fibrinogen may be because of increased consumption (disseminated intravascular coagulation [DIC]) or decreased production (liver disease).
  - Increased fibrinogen is associated with inflammation, renal disease, and dehydration.
- Fibrin degradation products (FDPs)
  - Required sample: special FDP tube
  - Used in the practice setting
  - Performed by adding blood to a special tube containing thrombin and a trypsin inhibitor (sample clots almost instantly in normal dogs and cats) and incubating two dilutions of serum (1:5 and 1:20) with polystyrene latex particles coated with sheep anti-FDP antibodies (should be negative in normal dogs and cats, but positives have been reported in normal cats)

- D-dimer
  - Required sample: citrated plasma
  - Latex agglutination test
  - To date, only validated in dogs and horses
  - Assay detects a specific type of FDP resulting from *breakdown of cross-linked fibrin*; concentration of plasma D-dimer indicates the degree of fibrinolysis; often used as part of a DIC panel; can be used as a negative predictor to rule out pathologic thrombosis (e.g., pulmonary thromboembolism); will also be increased when there is appropriate clotting.

- Antithrombin (a.k.a. antithrombin III, ATIII)
  - Required sample: citrated plasma
  - Decreased because of decreased production (liver disease), loss (protein-losing nephropathy or enteropathy), consumption (DIC), chronic heparin therapy
- Specific factor assays
  - Required sample: citrated plasma
  - Performed at specialized laboratories

14

Nervous System*

JAMES F. ZACHARY

Central Nervous System

INTRODUCTION

ORGANIZATION OF THE CENTRAL NERVOUS SYSTEM

The central nervous system (CNS) consists of neurons, glia, ependyma, endothelial cells and pericytes of blood vessels, and the meninges (Fig. 14-1, Box 14-1). Neurons vary in size, shape, and function, and their cell bodies are organized into functional groups, such as nuclei, gray columns, and cerebral lamina. Neuronal processes called axons and dendrites traverse through the brain and spinal cord, the former often as organized bundles (tracts, fasciculi) forming synapses on cell bodies, dendrites, and axons of other functionally related neurons. It is estimated that there are 1×10^{11} neurons in the human brain. Each neuron makes approximately 10,000 synapses with other neurons; therefore there are about 1×10^{15} synapses in the human brain.

Exactly which cells are classified as glia has varied over the last few decades. Originally, histologists included astrocytes (astroglia), oligodendrocytes (oligodendroglia), ependymal cells (ependymocytes), and microglia as glial cells; however, they currently recognize astrocytes, oligodendrocytes, and microglia as glial cells. Some classification schemes list astrocytes and oligodendrocytes as macroglia. Astrocytes, oligodendrocytes, and ependymal cells are derived from neuroectoderm; whereas microglia, part of the monocyte-macrophage system, are derived from mesoderm (bone marrow). In the mammalian CNS, glia outnumber neurons 10 to 1. Ependymal cells line the ventricular system, whereas choroid plexus epithelial cells form the outer covering of the choroid plexuses.

The CNS is arranged to form two basic parts: the gray and white matter (Figs. 14-2 and 14-3). In the CNS, gray matter is found in the cerebral cortex, in the cerebellar cortex and cerebellar roof nuclei, around the base of the cerebral hemispheres (basal nuclei [often called basal ganglia]: caudate nucleus, lentiform nucleus [putamen, globus pallidus], amygdaloid nucleus, claustrum), and throughout the brain stem often in nuclei. The gray matter is typified by numerous neuronal cell bodies plus a feltwork of intermingled thinly myelinated axons and dendrites, their synaptic junctions, and processes of oligodendroglia, astrocytes, and microglia. This network of processes and synapses in the gray matter is referred to as the neuropil. The white matter consists of well-myelinated axons that arise from neuronal cell bodies in the gray matter and terminate distally in synapses or myoneural junctions, plus oligodendroglia, astrocytes, and microglia. In the cerebral hemispheres, white matter is located centrally; whereas in the brain stem, white matter is intermingled with gray matter (nuclei). In the spinal cord, white matter is located peripherally surrounding the gray matter.

The exterior of the CNS is covered by the meninges. The meninges consist of three layers named from outermost to inner most layers as the dura mater, arachnoid, and pia mater. The arachnoid and pia enclose the subarachnoid space.

CELLS OF THE CENTRAL NERVOUS SYSTEM

NEURONS

The structure and basic cellular biology of neurons is similar to that of other cells (Fig. 14-4); however, there are, as discussed later, some notable differences. The neuron consists of three structural components: dendrites, a cell body, and a single axon. The length of

---

*Portions of this chapter are from the third edition and were written by Dr. R.W. Storts, College of Veterinary Medicine, Texas A&M University and Dr. D.L. Montgomery, Wyoming State Veterinary Laboratory.

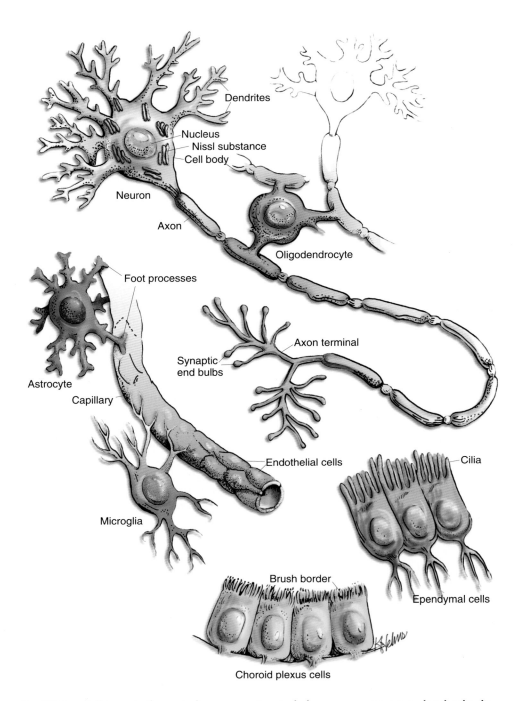

Fig. 14-1 Cell types in the central nervous system include neurons, astrocytes, oligodendroglia, microglia, ependymal cells, choroid plexus epithelial cells, and vascular endothelial cells. *(Courtesy Dr. J.F. Zachary, College of Veterinary Medicine, University of Illinois.)*

the axon varies depending on the function of the neuron. The length of axons of motor or sensory neurons can be 10,000 to 15,000 times the diameter of the neuronal cell body, which results in these axons being several meters in length. The axon terminates in synaptic processes or neuromuscular junctions.

Neuronal cell bodies vary considerably in size and shape, from the large neurons of the lateral vestibular nucleus, Purkinje cell layer of the cerebellum, and the ventral gray matter of the spinal cord to the very small lymphocyte-like granule cells of the cerebellar cortex (Fig. 14-5). Neuronal nuclei tend to be vesicular to

Box **14-1**

Cells of the Central Nervous System and Their Principal Functions

NEURONS

Transmission of electric and chemical impulses
Spatial and temporal interpretation of impulses
Inhibitory and stimulatory regulation of impulses

ASTROGLIA (PROTOPLASMIC [TYPE I] AND FIBROUS [TYPE II])

Regulation of extracellular neurotransmitter concentrations and fluid/electrolyte imbalances
Repair of injury by proliferation of astrocytic cellular processes
Support and bundling of functionally related axons traversing through the central nervous system (CNS)
Participation in barrier systems
   Glia limitans
   Blood-brain barrier

OLIGODENDROGLIA

Myelination of axons within the CNS
Proposed neuronal cell body homeostasis within the CNS

EPENDYMA AND CHOROID PLEXUS EPITHELIAL CELLS

Movement of cerebrospinal fluid (CSF) through the ventricular system
As choroid plexus epithelial cells
   Secretion of CSF
   Barrier function (blood-CSF barrier)

MICROGLIA

Immunosurveillance, immunoregulation, phagocytosis
Monocyte-macrophage system

MENINGES

Arachnoid-CSF barrier
Subarachnoid CSF cushioning of head trauma

ENDOTHELIA

Barrier function (blood-brain barrier)
Selective molecule transport systems

spherical in shape, tend to be usually centrally located, and often, particularly in large neurons, tend to contain a prominent central nucleolus. Neurons contain focal arrays of rough endoplasmic reticulum and polysomes termed Nissl substance that are responsible for the synthesis of proteins involved in many of the neuron's vital cellular processes such as axonal transport. Nissl substance is present in all neurons, regardless of the size of the cell body, but tends to be more prominent in those cells with voluminous cytoplasm such as motor neurons.

AXONAL TRANSPORT

In most cells of the body, proteins and other molecules are distributed throughout the cell by simple diffusion. In neurons, simple diffusion alone is inefficient because synapses are a considerable distance away from the cell body of the neuron and molecules cannot diffuse the length of the axon. In addition, there are no systems in axons or synapses to catabolize molecules resulting from normal metabolic processes. Thus these molecules need to be returned to the cell body for processing.

As a result of these structural differences between neurons and other cells, neurons have developed axonal transport systems to efficiently move molecules and cellular organelles from the cell body through the axon to the synapses and their degradation products back to the cell body (Fig. 14-6). Axons can be longer than a meter in length, especially in an animal such as a giraffe. Lower motor neurons, whose cell bodies lie in the ventral gray horn of the spinal cord, and lumbar dorsal root ganglia, whose axons extend to the distal limb and to the caudal medulla, have the longest axons in the body. The neuron expends considerable energy and materials to move biologic materials up and down the axon. Alterations in the function of these transport systems can lead to neuronal dysfunction.

These transport systems are divided into "fast axonal transport" and "slow axonal transport." The fast axonal transport system has an anterograde component (toward the synapse) and a retrograde component (toward the cell body). The slow axonal transport system has only an anterograde component (toward the synapse).

Fast anterograde axonal transport (up to 400 mm per day) moves materials not intended for use in the cytoplasm of the neuron cell body. These materials formed from the Golgi apparatus are principally membrane-bound vesicles. They include mitochondria and membranous vesicles that contain peptide neurotransmitters, small transmitter molecules, and the enzymes necessary for their activation. These materials are moved down the axon on microtubules by specialized protein motors composed of kinesin and kinesin-related proteins using adenosine triphosphate (ATP) as an energy source.

Fast retrograde axonal transport (200 to 300 mm per day) returns endosomes, mitochondria, and catabolized proteins to the cell body of the neuron for degradation in lysosomes and reuse. This transported material is returned on microtubules, by dynein and microtubule-associated adenosine triphosphatase (ATPase) in the axon. This system will also transport certain toxins, such as tetanus toxin, and viruses, such as rabies virus, from the periphery via the peripheral nervous system (PNS) into the CNS.

Slow anterograde axonal transport (0.2 to 5 mm per day) transfers throughout the axon via microtubules,

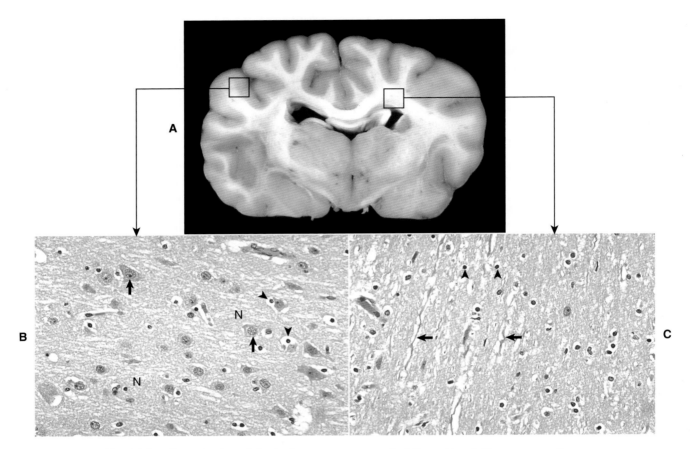

Fig. 14-2 **Organization of the brain, gray matter, and white matter. A,** Transverse section at the level of the thalamus, dog. Gray matter *(darker areas)* of the cerebral cortex lie beneath the leptomeninges on the external surface of the brain, whereas in the thalamus there tends to be a mixture of gray and white matter. Major white matter areas *(light areas)* include corona radiata, centrum semiovale, and corpus callosum of the cerebrum, and internal capsule and optic tracts bordering the lateral and ventral surfaces of the thalamus, respectively. **B,** Gray matter consist primarily of the cell bodies of neurons *(arrows)* and a network of intermingled thinly myelinated axons, dendrites, and glial cell processes. This network is referred to as the neuropil *(N)*. Other components include oligodendroglia (perineuronal satellite cells) *(arrowheads)*, protoplasmic astrocytes, and microglia. H&E stain. **C,** White matter primarily consists of well-myelinated axons *(arrows)* plus oligodendroglia *(arrowheads)* and fibrous astrocytes. The clear spaces surrounding large axons are artifacts formed when the lipid components of myelin lamellae are dissolved away by solvents in the preparation of paraffin embedded sections. H&E stain. *(A, B,* and *C, Courtesy Dr. J.F. Zachary, College of Veterinary Medicine, University of Illinois.)*

the major cytoskeletal proteins, such as microtubule and neurofilament proteins, that are necessary to maintain the structural integrity and transport systems within the axon.

Diseases of the axon that result directly or indirectly from alterations in axonal transport systems are discussed later. The character of the histologic lesions affecting injured nerve fibers can often be related to alterations in specific transport systems. Neurofilament proteins

are synthesized in the neuronal cell body and are assembled and transported into axons. If neurofilaments accumulate in neuronal cell bodies and proximal axons, this lesion is called an axonopathy and is characterized by alterations in slow transport systems, which results in axonal swelling or atrophy and perikaryal neurofibrillary accumulations. Axonal injury and alterations in neurofilament transport can also cause secondary demyelination.

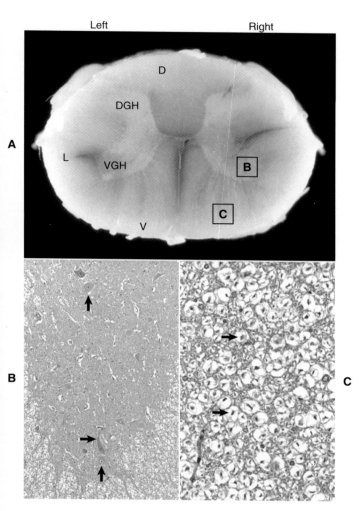

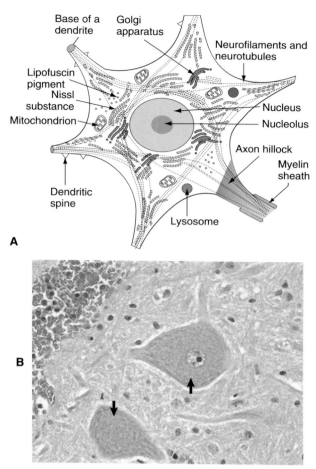

Fig. 14-3   Organization of the spinal cord, gray matter, and white matter. A, White matter in the spinal cord is located peripherally and divided into dorsal, lateral and ventral funiculi. As a general rule, dorsal funiculi (*D*) consist of ascending sensory axons, lateral funiculi (*L*) have a mixture of sensory and motor axons, and ventral funiculi consist of descending motor axons (*V*). *DGH,* Dorsal gray horn; *VGH,* ventral gray horn. Histologically, the right side is a mirror image of the left side. **B,** Transverse section of spinal cord, ventral gray horn, horse. The cell bodies of large motor neurons (*arrows*) are those of lower motor neurons and their axons extend in peripheral nerves to myoneural junctions that innervate skeletal muscle. **C,** Transverse section of spinal cord, ventral funiculus, horse. Because most axons course up and down the length of the spinal cord, in a transverse section, axons (*arrows*) are cut in cross section. They are surrounded by myelin sheaths whose lipid components are dissolved out during the preparation of paraffin embedded sections, resulting in clear spaces that are an artifact. H&E stain. (*A, B,* and *C, Courtesy Dr. J.F. Zachary, College of Veterinary Medicine, University of Illinois.*)

Fig. 14-4   Neuron structure. A, Basic cell biology and structure of neurons are similar to other cells in the body. Additionally, neurons have dendritic arborizations and an axon, specializations for the initiation, propagation, and transmission of impulses that underlie the basic function of these cells. **B,** The cytoplasm of the neuronal cell body has blue (basophilic [H&E stain]) granular material (rough endoplasmic reticulum) called Nissl substance (*arrows*). Nissl substance synthesizes proteins, including precursor neurotransmitter proteins and the structural proteins, (neurofilaments) active in maintaining the integrity (length and diameter) of the axon. H&E stain. (*A, Modified from Kierszenbaum AL: Histology and cell biology, St Louis, 2002, Mosby. B, Courtesy Dr. J.F. Zachary, College of Veterinary Medicine, University of Illinois.*)

MEMBRANE POTENTIALS AND TRANSMITTER/RECEPTOR SYSTEMS

A fundamental activity of neurons is to modulate and effectively transmit chemical and electric signals from one neuron to another via synapses in the CNS or from one neuron to a muscle cell via junctional complexes, myoneural junctions, or motor end plates in the PNS. The process of nerve impulse conduction is made

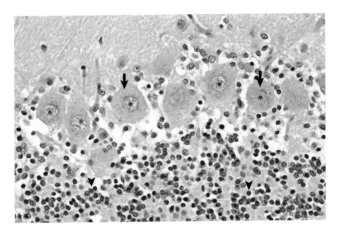

Fig. 14-5   Variations in neuronal morphology, cerebellum, granule cells, and Purkinje neurons, normal animal. The granule cell neurons of the cerebellar cortex (*arrowheads*) are very small lymphocyte-like cells that have relatively little demonstrable Nissl substance when compared with Purkinje neurons (*arrows*) and large motor neurons (depicted in Fig. 14-3, *B*). H&E stain. (*Courtesy Dr. J.F. Zachary, College of Veterinary Medicine, University of Illinois.*)

possible by the establishment and maintenance of an electric potential across the cell membrane of the neuron/axon. Membrane potential is the difference in voltage between the inside and outside of the neuronal/axonal cell membrane and is called the resting potential. This potential is established and maintained by a membrane sodium-potassium ATPase pump. The pump keeps the concentration of sodium ions outside the cell approximately 10 times greater than inside the cell, and the concentration of potassium ions inside the cell 20 times greater than outside the cell. The differences in concentrations of sodium ions outside and potassium ions inside of the cell membrane keep the membrane resting potential at approximately −70 mV. Thus the inside of the neuron/axon is 70 mV less than the outside. Sodium and potassium ions will leak across the cell membrane, and therefore concentration gradients are maintained by the sodium-potassium ATPase pump in the cell membrane. This established equilibrium and the membrane potential places the neuron in a "resting" condition, ready to generate an action potential.

An action potential arises when a neuron transmits information down an axon, away from the neuronal cell body. An action potential is initiated by an event that

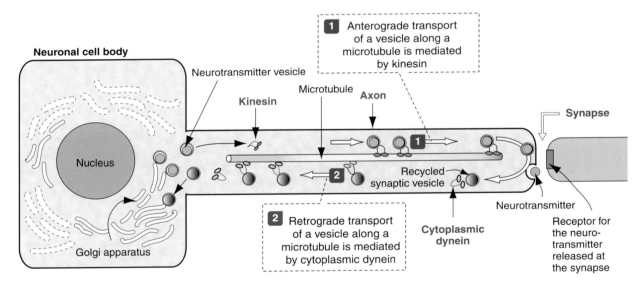

Fig. 14-6   Axonal transport systems. Neurotransmitter vesicles and neurofilament proteins, synthesized in the rough endoplasmic reticulum and packaged in the Golgi apparatus are transported through the length of the axon and to synapses by kinesin. Kinesin is a microtubule motor protein that uses chemical energy from adenosine triphosphate hydrolysis to generate mechanical force and thus bind to and move attached to microtubules. Used vesicles and effete neurofilament proteins are returned along a microtubule (recycled) to the neuron cell body by cytoplasmic dynein, another microtubule motor protein. These transport systems are used by some pathogens (rabies virus, *Listeria monocytogenes*) to enter and spread within the central nervous system. (*Modified from Kierszenbaum AL: Histology and cell biology, St Louis, 2002, Mosby.*)

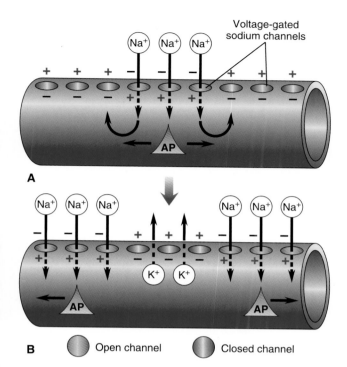

Voltage-gated sodium channels

A

B Open channel Closed channel

Fig. 14-7 Resting and action potentials. Nerve impulse conduction is made possible by the establishment and maintenance of an electric potential across the cell membrane of the neuron/axon. Resting membrane potential is established and maintained by differences in concentrations of potassium ions inside and sodium outside of the cell membrane. Sodium and potassium ions will leak across the cell membrane, and therefore concentration gradients are maintained by a sodium-potassium pump in the cell membrane. When an event depolarizes the cell membrane to a threshold level of approximately −50 mV, an action potential will occur. **A,** An action potential is initiated by an event that opens sodium channels, and the action potential is propagated along the cell membrane by the sequential opening of voltage-gated sodium channels in adjacent sections of the membrane. *AP,* Action potential. **B,** The action potential is regenerated in adjacent sections of the cell membrane as additional sodium channels open. Depolarized segments repolarize as sodium channels close and potassium ions move out of the cell. *AP,* Action potential. (*A and B, From Copstead LC, Banasik JL: Pathophysiology: biological and behavioral perspectives, ed 2, Philadelphia, 2000, Saunders.*)

depolarizes the cell membrane and causes the resting potential to move toward 0 mV. When depolarization reaches a threshold level of approximately −50 mV, an action potential will occur. Once initiated, the strength of an action potential is always the same because the action potential is an intrinsic property of the neuron cell body and its axon.

Action potentials are caused by the movement of sodium and potassium ions across the neuron cell body/axon cell membrane. With an initiating event, sodium

channels are first to open, and large concentrations of sodium ions enter the intracellular microenvironment (Fig. 14-7). Because sodium ions are positively charged, the polarity becomes more positive (−70 mV to −50 mV) and the neuron/axon becomes depolarized. Potassium channels open later in the depolarization process, concurrently with the closing of sodium channels. Potassium ions leave the cell and enter the extracellular fluid. These events cause repolarization of the neuron/axon and a return to a resting potential (−70 mV) via the membrane sodium-potassium ATPase pump. Alterations in these ion channels have been correlated with epilepsy in human beings and will likely be discovered in animals.

Action potentials are most commonly initiated by neurotransmitters such as acetylcholine acting through synapses, but they also occur as a result of mechanical stimuli, such as stretching and sound waves. There are two main classes of synapses: inhibitory and excitatory. Stimulation of inhibitory synapses results in inhibitory postsynaptic potentials that cause hyperpolarization of dendrites and cell bodies. Hyperpolarization decreases the membrane potential (more negative, −80 mV), thus making the neuron less likely to reach the threshold for an action potential. Inhibitory neurotransmitters include γ-aminobutyric acid (GABA), glycine, dopamine, serotonin, norepinephrine (in the CNS), and acetylcholine (in heart muscle).

Stimulation of excitatory synapses results in excitatory postsynaptic potentials that cause depolarization of the dendrites and cell bodies. Depolarization increases the membrane potential (more positive, −50 mV), thus making the neuron more likely to reach the threshold for an action potential. Excitatory neurotransmitters include glutamate, norepinephrine in the PNS, and acetylcholine in skeletal muscle.

The generation of an action potential is a complicated process requiring depolarization of the cell membrane (−50 mV). Inhibitory and excitatory synapses and their inhibitory and excitatory postsynaptic potentials, respectively, are "summed" through processes termed spatial and temporal summation occurring in the dendritic network of the neuron. Spatial summation reflects additive input from different parts of the dendritic network, whereas temporal summation reflects additive input from stimuli that occur closely in time. This summation process is a graded potential and ultimately determines if the threshold for an action potential will occur.

The action potential is a flow of depolarization that travels down the axon to synapses at the distal axon. When the axon lacks myelin, the flow of depolarization down the axon is called continuous conduction. When the axon is myelinated, the speed of conduction is determined by the degree of myelination of the axon

Normal axons (spread of action potential down an axon)

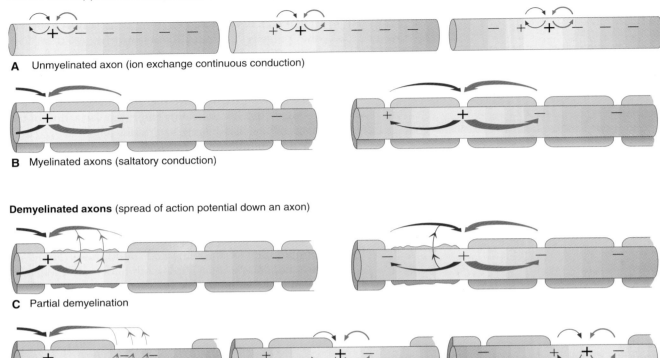

A Unmyelinated axon (ion exchange continuous conduction)

B Myelinated axons (saltatory conduction)

Demyelinated axons (spread of action potential down an axon)

C Partial demyelination

D Complete demyelination

Fig. 14-8 **Axonal action potential conduction and the effect of demyelination.** The speed of the conduction process is determined by the diameter of the axon and the degree of myelination. As axons increase in diameter, the resistance to ion flow decreases, allowing the action potential to flow faster. In addition, the degree of myelination is directly proportional to the diameter of the axon. Thus the concept that the more myelin the faster the speed of the impulse is true up to the point in which the myelin is normal in thickness. For an axon whose myelin is reduced, conduction of the action potential is slower. Under normal conditions, locomotion is a well-coordinated event that requires precise timing (speed) of impulse conduction to get coordinated movements. If the speed of the action potential is altered by disease, especially demyelination, then the conduction of the action potential will be delayed and what are normally coordinated movements become uncoordinated. **A,** In unmyelinated axons, action potentials are conducted at a relatively "slower" velocity by the process of ion exchange continuous conduction (Fig. 14-7). **B,** In myelinated axons, action potentials are conducted at a relatively "faster" velocity by a mechanism called saltatory conduction. Optimal function of saltatory conduction is dependent on having the proper degree of myelination of the axon (as determined by axonal diameter) throughout the full length of the axon. **C,** In axons that have lost some but not all of their myelin lamellae from one or more internodes so that there is a "thinner" covering of myelin, the speed of saltatory conduction is reduced because of leakage of the action potential across this thinner myelin sheath, resulting in clinical dysfunction of the nervous system. **D,** In axons that have lost all of their myelin from one or more internodes (complete primary demyelination of the internode), the speed of saltatory conduction is reduced because of the conversion from saltatory conduction to ion exchange continuous conduction in the areas where internodes have lost their myelin. Thus the speed and timing of the action potential is substantially reduced, leading to clinical dysfunction of the nervous system. (**A** through **D,** *Courtesy Dr. J.F. Zachary, College of Veterinary Medicine, University of Illinois.*)

and is called saltatory conduction. The diameter of unmyelinated axons can range from 0.2 to 1 μm with action potential velocities ranging from 0.2 to 2 m/sec, whereas the diameter of myelinated axons can range from 2 to 20 μm with action potential velocities ranging from 12 to 120 m/sec. The greater the degree of myelination, the faster the speed of impulse conduction down the axon. In unmyelinated axons, action potentials are conducted at a relatively "slower" velocity by the process of ion exchange (continuous conduction). In myelinated axons, action potentials are conducted at a relatively "faster" velocity by a mechanism called saltatory conduction. In this process, action potentials move down the myelinated axon using cable properties, like electric current flow in insulated copper wires. This method is fast, efficient, and requires less energy than ion exchange. However, the action potential would decay if axons were myelinated continuously along their length and likely would not reach synapses at full strength or at all. This decay is caused by loss of current across the cell membrane and capacitance properties of the cell membrane as the action potential travels down the axon. To minimize the decay of action potentials, axons are myelinated in segments called internodes. A gap, called the node of Ranvier, is formed between consecutive internodes and measures between 0.2 and 2 mm in length. At this gap, the action potential is restored to full strength by ion exchange. The node of Ranvier is highly enriched in sodium channels, and these channels are essential for impulse propagation via rapid action potential current restoration. Disease processes that disrupt myelination of axons will interfere with saltatory conduction, slow the action potential, and result in clinical dysfunction of the nervous system (Fig. 14-8).

The axon can be a very long extension of the neuron cell body extending, for example, up to 2 m from the lumbar dorsal root ganglion in a giraffe. At its distal end, the axon splits into several branches that end as specialized structures called axon terminals/terminal buttons/synaptic bulbs. Synapses present at these axon terminals are functional, and structural points of contact between "networked" neurons and these synapses convert the action potential into chemical signals that stimulate the next neuron in the conduction pathway. The cell membrane that releases chemical neurotransmitters is called the presynaptic membrane, and the cell membrane that has neurotransmitter receptors for the chemical neurotransmitters is called the postsynaptic membrane. These membranes are found on dendrites and cell bodies of the next neuron in the neural conduction pathway. The gap between the presynaptic and postsynaptic membranes that chemical neurotransmitters must cross is called the synaptic cleft. The mechanism of diseases, such as tetanus and botulism,

is manifested through presynaptic and postsynaptic membrane receptors.

When an action potential reaches the axon terminal, it causes the release of chemical neurotransmitters from the presynaptic membrane by opening voltage-gated calcium channels, leading to membrane depolarization. The amount of chemical neurotransmitter released into the synaptic cleft is determined by the number of action potentials that reach the axon terminal over time. Chemical neurotransmitters traverse the synaptic cleft and bind to neurotransmitter receptors on dendrites and cell bodies of a new neuron in the neural conduction pathway.

There are two types of chemical neurotransmitter receptors, ionotropic and metabotropic, on the membrane of postsynaptic neurons. Functionally, these receptor types differ in latency and duration of action. Ionotropic receptors have a fast response and short duration of effect, whereas metabotropic receptors have a slower response and a longer duration of effect. In addition, ionotropic receptors are localized to specific sites on the postsynaptic membrane, whereas metabotropic receptors are distributed diffusely and at random.

Chemical neurotransmitter stimulation of ionotropic receptors results in the opening of ion gates or channels, resulting in depolarization of the postsynaptic membrane. Excitatory neurotransmitters, such as glutamate, open postsynaptic membrane sodium channels. Inhibitory neurotransmitters, such as GABA, open postsynaptic membrane chloride channels.

Chemical neurotransmitter stimulation of metabotropic receptors results in the generation of a second messenger such as in the cyclic adenosine monophosphate (cAMP) pathway, which initiates a sequence of metabolic changes in the neuron. Metabotropic receptors are composed of protein subunits that span the postsynaptic cell membrane. An extracellular component of this protein has a high affinity for neurotransmitters and functions as a binding site. Following binding of the neurotransmitter, the receptor undergoes a configurational change that directly or indirectly activates a cell membrane enzyme, such as intracellular G proteins, leading to the formation of the second messenger. cAMP can activate protein kinase A–induced phosphorylation, leading to functional changes in ion channels and protein transcription. Dopamine is an example of a chemical neurotransmitter that uses metabotropic receptor pathways.

ASTROCYTES

The functions of astrocytes in the CNS are regulation, repair, and support, as depicted in Fig. 14-9. Mature astrocytes differentiate from pluripotential progenitor cells during the development of the CNS. Astrocytes are

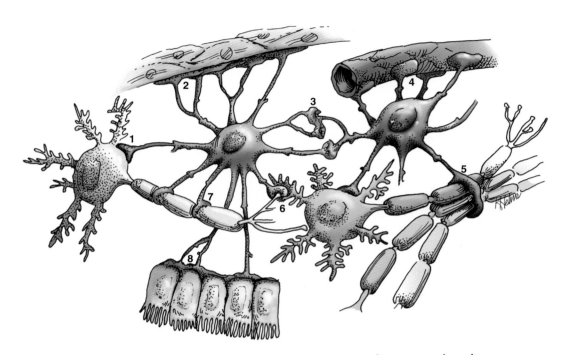

Fig. 14-9   **Functions of astrocytes.** Astrocytes provide structural integrity and regulatory oversight, as depicted in this diagram. They: *1*, monitor and regulate fluid and electrolyte balances within neurons and surrounding extracellular space; *2*, form the glial limitans at the base of the pia mater; *3*, interconnect with other astrocytes to provide a system to monitor and regulate fluid and electrolyte balances throughout the central nervous system (CNS); *4*, possibly participate in the formation and functions of the blood-brain barrier; *5*, participate in the support of axon tracts of functionally related neurons; *6*, monitor for and remove excessive release of neurotransmitters in synapses; *7*, protect and insulate nodes of Ranvier; and *8*, participate in the cerebrospinal fluid-brain barrier. In addition, astrocytes are a reparative (healing) cell following CNS injury with loss of tissue because nervous tissue, per se, is devoid of fibroblasts. Fibroblasts exist in the pia mater and other meninges. Everywhere else, healing is dependent on the astrocyte, which will respond by increased length, branching, and complexity of cellular processes (astrogliosis). The astrocyte has many functions in the nervous system; one of them is to act in healing to produce a scar in attempts to isolate cavities and abscesses. Fibroblasts may also contribute to the formation of a scar, if this cell type is present, as it is in the leptomeninges. *(Courtesy Dr. J.F. Zachary, College of Veterinary Medicine, University of Illinois.)*

the most numerous cell type in the CNS and have traditionally been classified into two types based on morphology. Protoplasmic astrocytes are located primarily in gray matter, whereas fibrous astrocytes occur chiefly in white matter. Microscopically, astrocytes have relatively large vesicular nuclei, indistinct or inapparent nucleoli, and no discernible cytoplasm with routine hematoxylin and eosin (H&E) staining (Fig. 14-10). With suitable histochemical stains, metallic impregnation, or immunohistochemical staining for glial fibrillary acidic protein (GFAP [the major intermediate filament in astrocytes]), the cell body and the extensive arborization and interconnections of astrocytic processes can be demonstrated. Processes vary from short and brushlike to long branching processes in protoplasmic and fibrous astrocytes, respectively (Fig. 14-11). These morphologic

features and their corresponding histochemical and immunohistochemical staining reactions serve as important criteria for the classification of tumors of astrocyte origin.

FUNCTIONS OF ASTROCYTES
Regulation of the microenvironment

The microenvironment of the CNS must be under strict control to maintain normal function. Astrocytes are involved in homeostasis of the CNS and regulate ionic and water balance, antioxidant concentrations, uptake and metabolism of neurotransmitters, and metabolism or sequestration of potential neurotoxins, including ammonia, heavy metals, and excitatory amino acid neurotransmitters such as glutamate and aspartate. Interactions between astrocytes, microglia,

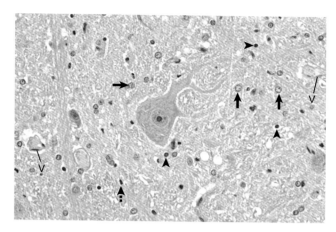

Fig. 14-10   Histologic features of glial cells, ventral gray horn, spinal cord, horse. A neuronal cell body and its processes are in the center of the illustration. To the inexperienced, identifying specific types of glial cells in H&E stained histologic sections can be challenging. Astrocytes (*arrows*) have larger vesicular nuclei (dispersed chromatin) and the cell membrane and cytoplasm are rarely seen in nondiseased conditions. Thus these nuclei just seem to "sit" in the midst of the neuropil. The majority of nuclei in the neuropil here are astrocytic. Oligodendroglial cells (*arrowheads*) have smaller and dense round nuclei (condensed chromatin) often surrounded by a clear zone indicative of cell cytoplasm and a cell membrane. Oligodendroglial cells in gray matter are called perineuronal satellite cells; those in white matter are called interfascicular oligodendrocytes. Microglial cells are difficult to identify in H&E stained sections of the central nervous system, but they often appear as "rod cells," which have small, dense elongated nuclei (*dashed arrow*). The light pink homogenous tissue distributed in large quantities between these cell types is the neuropil. V, Blood vessels. H&E stain. *(Courtesy Dr. J.F. Zachary, College of Veterinary Medicine, University of Illinois.)*

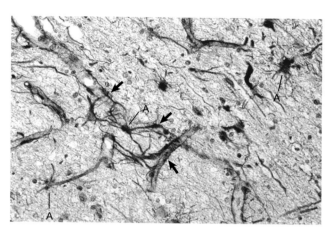

Fig. 14-11   Astrocytic processes, brain, cerebral cortex, normal animal. Processes of astrocytes arborize extensively throughout the central nervous system (structures stained purple). Note that some of the processes are on the outside of blood capillaries (end feet) (*arrows*). A, Cell body of astrocyte. Holzer's stain. *(Courtesy Dr. M.D. McGavin, College of Veterinary Medicine, University of Tennessee.)*

and neurons orchestrate immune reactions in the brain. In this regard, astrocytes can express major histocompatibility complex (MHC) class I and II antigens, a variety of cytokines and chemokines, and adhesion molecules that modulate inflammatory events in the CNS. Astrocytes also secrete growth factors and extracellular matrix molecules that play a role not only in development but also in repair of the CNS.

Repair of injured nervous tissue

In the CNS, reparative processes that occur after injury, such as inflammation and necrosis, are chiefly the responsibility of astrocytes. In these reparative processes, astrocytes are analogous to fibroblasts in the rest of the body. Astrocytes do not synthesize collagen fibers, as do fibroblasts. Instead, repair is accomplished by astrocytic swelling and division, and abundant proliferation of astrocytic cell processes containing intermediate filaments

composed of GFAP, a process called astrogliosis. As an example, neuronal necrosis occurs in some viral diseases of the CNS. When neurons die, the spaces left by the loss of the neuronal cell bodies are filled and such spaces (<1 mm in diameter) are filled by processes of astrocytes. Larger spaces that form following injury, such as an infarct, are often too large to be filled and therefore exist in the CNS as fluid-filled spaces (cysts) surrounded by a capsule of astrocytic processes. Astrocytes will also attempt to wall off abscesses, but they are not as effective as fibroblasts and the capsule can be incomplete or weak (Fig. 14-12). In the case of direct extension of bacteria from the meninges or meningeal blood vessels, which contain or are surrounded by fibroblasts, respectively, fibroblasts will play a larger role in isolating the inflammatory process.

Structural support of the central nervous system

Structurally, astrocytic processes provide support for other cellular elements and ensheathe and insulate synapses. Astrocytes also provide guidance and support of neuronal migration during development; thus, tracts and fasciculi of axons with similar functions are arranged and structurally supported by astrocytic processes. Processes of astrocytes (foot processes) also terminate on blood vessels throughout the CNS, forming a component of the blood-brain barrier. Astrocytes influence the induction of tight junctions between endothelial cells that serve as the structural basis for the blood-brain barrier. A dense meshwork of astrocytic processes also forms the glia limitans beneath the

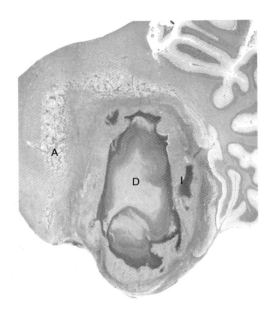

Fig. 14-12 Astrocytic repair, bacterial abscess, brain stem, sheep. The abscess has a central core of necrotic debris (*D*) surrounded by a layer of inflammatory cells (*I*) and a less dense pink-staining zone representing an attempt by astrocytes and fibroblasts to form a capsule (*A*). This capsule is formed by fibrous tissue on the ventral and right sides, those sides closest to the pia, which contains fibroblasts. A fibrous capsule is absent from the dorsal and left sides of the abscess, adjacent to brain parenchyma. Here, there is no population of resident fibroblasts and the capsule is formed by astrocytes and their processes, which are often delicate and do not form an effective capsule (*A*). H&E stain. (*Courtesy Dr. J.F. Zachary, College of Veterinary Medicine, University of Illinois.*)

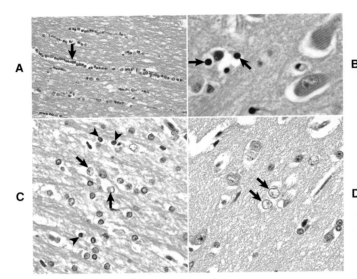

Fig. 14-13 Responses of glial cells to injury in H&E stained central nervous system (CNS) sections. A, White matter. In nondiseased states, oligodendroglia in white matter are often arranged linearly (fascicular oligodendroglia) (*arrow*) and are responsible for the formation of myelin around axons. In gray matter (not shown; see Fig. 14-10), oligodendroglia are dispersed as individual cells around neuronal cell bodies as perineuronal satellite cells (Fig. 14-13, *B*). H&E stain. **B,** Gray matter. When neurons are injured or there exists some pertubation of the perineuronal microenvironment, a long-held belief was that oligodendroglia around neurons hypertrophy and proliferate in a process referred to as satellitosis. Currently, there is no uniform agreement that these cells respond to neuronal injury in this manner. Perineuronal satellite oligodendroglia (*arrows*) surround a small degenerate neuron with condensed chromatin and little cytoplasm. H&E stain. **C,** White matter. Astrocytes (*arrows*) and oligodendroglia (*arrowheads*) have a limited repertoire of responses to injury in the CNS. Astrocytic proliferation can occur but is very difficult to determine in sections stained with H&E. Here, astrocyte nuclei are somewhat enlarged and appear more numerous than expected. H&E stain. **D,** Gray matter. Astrocytes respond to injury in hyperammonemia, such as occurs with hepatic encephalopathy, by forming astrocytes with enlarged, markedly vesicular ("watery"), often elongated nuclei called Alzheimer's type II astrocytes (*arrows*). This type of astrocyte may occur in pairs that are surrounded by a clear space indicative of cellular swelling. H&E stain. (*A, and B, Courtesy Dr. M.D. McGavin, College of Veterinary Medicine, University of Tennessee. C, Courtesy Dr. J.F. Zachary, College of Veterinary Medicine, University of Illinois. D, Courtesy Dr. D. Gould, College of Veterinary Medicine, Colorado State University.*)

pia mater and is variably prominent in subependymal areas. During CNS development, cells termed radial glia provide a scaffold and guidance for migrating neurons. When development is completed, radial glia mature into astrocytes.

OLIGODENDROGLIA

There are two types of oligodendroglia: (1) interfascicular oligodendrocytes and (2) satellite oligodendrocytes (satellite cells). The function of interfascicular oligodendroglia is myelination of axons, whereas the function of satellite oligodendroglia is thought to be regulation of the perineuronal microenvironment. Oligodendroglia have been compared with neurons with regard to their total cell size in that their processes occupy much more space than the cell body. Neurons have very long axons, which account for their size; oligodendroglia have extensive myelin sheaths, which account for their size. In H&E stained sections, oligodendroglia are often confused with lymphocytes because of the similarity of the morphology of their

nuclei and cytoplasmic volume. Interfascicular oligodendroglia and perineuronal satellite oligodendroglia are located primarily in white and gray matter of the CNS, respectively (Fig. 14-13); however, interfascicular oligodendroglia can also be found along axons that

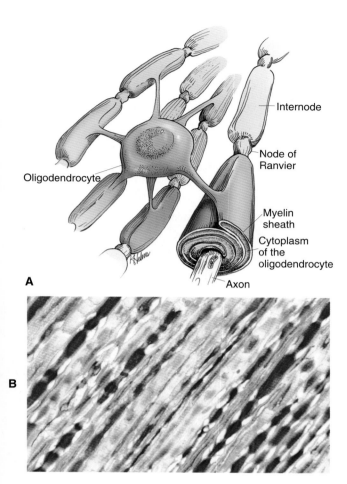

include metallic (silver) impregnation and immunohistochemical methods.

Most interfascicular oligodendroglia (Fig. 14-13) are aligned in rows parallel to myelinated axons and are responsible for the formation and maintenance of segments (internodes) of myelin sheaths. One oligodendroglial cell can form as many as 50 different internodes of myelin, each of which can be located on many different axons (Fig. 14-14). Altered function of oligodendroglial cells, as occurs in infectious canine distemper virus (CDV) infection, can cause primary demyelination of these segments resulting in severe neurologic dysfunction. Oligodendroglia also influence maturation and maintenance of axons, and inhibit regeneration of established myelinated axons.

Perineuronal satellite oligodendroglia (Fig. 14-13) are adjacent to neuronal cell bodies and are also located around blood vessels in the gray matter. They are thought by some investigators to regulate the perineuronal microenvironment and respond to pertubation by proliferation. When the perineuronal microenvironment is altered or neuron cells bodies are injured, perineuronal satellite oligodendroglia in an attempt to regulate the environmental perturbation hypertrophy and proliferate in a process referred to as satellitosis. Similarly, alterations in the microenvironment of gray and white matter away from areas surrounding neuron cell bodies results in hypertrophy of oligodendroglia (Fig. 14-13). Finally, satellitosis can be quite prominent in normal CNS in various areas of the gray matter.

MICROGLIA

The basic functions of microglia are immunosurveillance, immunoregulation, and reparative (phagocytic) activities following neural cell injury and death. The origin of microglia in the CNS has been debated for years. The current consensus is that the cells originate from circulating monocytes (mesoderm-derived) that enter and populate the CNS during embryonic development and early postnatal life, analogous to the formation of the monocyte-macrophage system in other organs. After entry into the CNS, the cells become amoeboid microglia, phagocytosing dead cells and cellular debris during remodeling and maturation of the CNS. Amoeboid cells then enter a quiescent stage and transform into ramified microglia. Ramified microglia constitute up to 20% of the glial cells and are present throughout the mature CNS, serving as sentinels of brain injury. Ramified microglia, also called resting cells, are most numerous in perineuronal and perivascular areas and in interfascicular locations in white matter. Evidence of pinocytosis in ramified cells suggests some role in maintaining the neural microenvironment. The principal function of microglia is phagocytosis, the initiation of and participation in the

Fig. 14-14   Central nervous system (CNS) myelin. Oligodendroglia myelinate axons within the CNS (also see Fig. 14-1). **A,** As depicted in this illustration, each oligodendrocyte sends out numerous cytoplasmic processes that repetitively encircle (myelinate) the portion of an axon between two nodes of Ranvier (internode) on the same and several different axons. Direct or indirect injury to an oligodendrocyte can result in "demyelination" of those internodes myelinated by that oligodendrocyte. This injury will slow the rate of conduction of an action potential, and depending on the site of the lesion may lead to clinical signs of neural dysfunction (ataxia, proprioception deficits). **B,** CNS nerves, longitudinal section. Axons and their neurofilaments (brown stain) and myelin (red stain) are well demonstrated by this immunohistochemical stain for neurofilaments and myelin basic protein. (*A* and *B, Courtesy Dr. J.F. Zachary, College of Veterinary Medicine, University of Illinois.*)

traverse through the gray matter. The mature, small oligodendrocyte has a spherical, hyperchromatic nucleus (Figs. 14-10 and 14-13). As with astrocytes, the cell body and processes of this cell do not stain with conventional H&E staining methods and can only be demonstrated following special procedures that innate and adaptive immune responses, and in degenerative and inflammatory diseases of the CNS.

Microscopically, ramified microglia have small, hyperchromatic ovoid-, rod-, or comma-shaped nuclei and no appreciable cytoplasm with routine H&E staining, hence the term "rod cell" sometimes used to describe them (Fig. 14-10). With special labeling techniques or metallic impregnation, ramified cells have a few delicate branching processes. The small hyperchromatic nuclei and nuclear shape distinguish microglia from astrocytes and oligodendroglia. However, microglia are often difficult to identify in H&E stained sections without some expertise in neuropathology.

Activated microglial cells are not the major source of active macrophages in inflammation of the CNS. Blood monocytes recruited from the circulation account for up to 70% of the macrophages in inflammatory and degenerative diseases of the CNS. These macrophages differentiate from blood monocytes involved in normal "leukocytic trafficking" through the CNS and can be involved in immunologic and phagocytic responses (gitter cells) to disease processes and infectious organisms. They are found mainly in the leptomeninges, choroid plexus, and perivascular areas.

EPENDYMA (INCLUDING CHOROID PLEXUS EPITHELIAL CELLS)

The basic functions of ependymal cells, which line the ventricular system, are to move cerebrospinal fluid (CSF) through the ventricular system via movement of their cilia and to regulate the flow of materials between the CNS and the CSF. The ependyma is a single-layered, cuboidal to columnar, epithelium that lines the ventricles and mesencephalic aqueduct of the brain, and central canal of the spinal cord (Fig. 14-15). This layer of cells is therefore situated between the CSF and nervous tissue. Ependymal cells have cilia that project into the CSF and beat in a coordinated manner in the direction of CSF flow. Other structures, referred to as circumventricular organs, which include the choroid plexuses, are covered by highly specialized ependymal cells. The surface of ependymal cells that form the choroid plexus have microvilli (microvillus border) and cilia that occur singly or more often in groups of three or more. The choroid plexus epithelial cells also have specialized tight junctions (zonulae occludentes) that are a functional part of the blood-CSF barrier. In contrast to the choroid plexus, junctions between the conventional ependymal cells include gap junctions (transmembrane proteins form a pore allowing communication between adjacent cells), and zonulae and fasciae adherentes, which permit movement of materials such as proteins from the CSF into the extracellular space of the brain. This cellular lining, however, is not a static membrane in

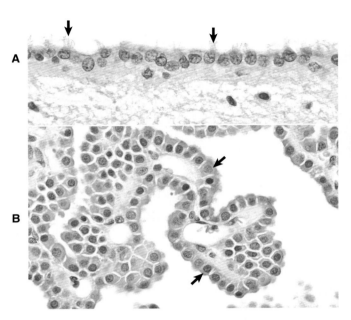

Fig. 14-15 **Ependymal and choroid plexus epithelial cells. A,** Ependymal cells are ciliated (*arrows*) and assist with the flow of cerebrospinal fluid (CSF) through the ventricular system. H&E stain. **B,** Choroid plexus epithelial cells (*arrows*) secrete CSF from a brush-border (microvilli) on the luminal surface. The surface of the choroid plexus also has cilia that occur singly or more often in groups of three or more on a single cell. H&E stain. (*A and B, Courtesy Dr. J.F. Zachary, College of Veterinary Medicine, University of Illinois.*)

that it regulates several processes that involve interaction between the CSF and brain. The functions include regulation of fluid homeostasis between the ventricular cavities and the brain, secretion and absorption of CSF, endocytosis, phagocytosis, and metabolism of substances such as iron resulting from the lysis of erythrocytes following hemorrhage into the ventricular system. Finally, ependymal cells have the structural and enzymatic characteristics necessary for scavenging and detoxifying a wide variety of substances in the CSF.

During embryonic development, the medial wall of the lateral ventricle (choroid fissure), the roof of the third ventricle, and the rostral part of the roof of the fourth ventricle consist of a single layer of neuroectoderm that is adherent on its outer surface to the pia mater. This neuroectoderm-pia union forms the tela choroidea, providing an anchor for the choroid plexuses, which is formed by an invagination of this bilayer membrane into the ventricular spaces.

Choroid plexus epithelial cells are modified ependymal cells. The choroid plexus epithelium is a single-layered, cuboidal to columnar, epithelium with a microvillus border (Fig. 14-15). CSF is secreted from the microvillus border. Choroid plexus epithelial cells, along with capillaries and the pia mater, form the choroid plexuses that project into the lateral, third, and fourth ventricles. The basic function of choroid plexuses is to produce the CSF that fills the ventricular system and the subarachnoid space. CSF has two important functions: (1) to act as a "shock absorber" to mitigate the effects of trauma to the brain and spinal cord and (2) to deliver nutrients to and remove wastes from the CNS.

The normal flow pattern of CSF is regulated by an intraventricular biologic pressure gradient in which the pressure created by secretion of CSF exceeds the pressure created by its absorption in arachnoid villi (arachnoid granulations). Arachnoid villi are focal extensions of the arachnoid and subarachnoid space that extend into the dorsal sagittal venous sinus of the brain. CSF is secreted by the choroid plexuses in the lateral, third, and fourth ventricles. It should be noted, however, that fluid from other sources, such as secretion by the ependyma, interstitial fluid of the brain, and ultrafiltrate of the blood, has also been reported to contribute to the formation of CSF. It moves from the lateral ventricles into the third ventricle, from the third ventricle through the mesencephalic aqueduct (aqueduct of Sylvius in human beings), and then to the fourth ventricle. Once in the fourth ventricle, the CSF exits through the two lateral apertures of the fourth ventricle to enter the subarachnoid space. Lateral apertures are the two openings in the caudal medullary velum that forms the roof of the fourth ventricle into the subarachnoid space, one at each side of the cerebellopontine angle. Although the central canal of the spinal cord is connected to the ventricular system at the caudal end of the fourth ventricle, there apparently is little active movement of CSF within the central canal. CSF in the subarachnoid space is reabsorbed by the arachnoid villi in the brain. Recent evidence indicates that other routes of CSF drainage, in addition to arachnoid granulations, also exist and vary in different species. Venous sinuses, lymphatic drainage, and the cribriform plate appear to play important roles in CSF drainage and the maintenance of normal interventricular CSF pressure. In fact, experimental evidence suggests that the cribriform plate route may be the most important of the four. In human beings, the entire volume of CSF is circulated approximately four times a day; however, with aging, the entire volume of CSF circulates less than two times a day.

MENINGES

The meninges, which enclose the CNS, consist of three layers: the dura mater (outermost layer [pachymeninges]), the arachnoid membrane (mater), and the pia mater (innermost layer) (Fig. 14-16). Together the arachnoid membrane and pia mater are frequently referred to as the leptomeninges, pia-arachnoid layer, or pia-arachnoid. The arachnoid membrane and pia mater are held together by bands of fibrous tissue called arachnoid trabeculae. This arrangement forms a compartment called the subarachnoid space in which CSF flows and which also contains blood vessels and nerves. There is also limited evidence based on studies in human beings with neuro–acquired immunodeficiency syndrome that the brain has a primitive lymphatic system. The leptomeninges form a protective covering for the CNS and provide an external envelope filled with CSF that provides additional protection.

The dura mater, once referred to as the pachymeninx (thick meninges), is a strong and dense collagenous membrane (Fig. 14-17). In the cranium, the dura consists of two layers that are fused with each other. The outer layer serves as the periosteum of the cranial bone, except in the areas of the venous sinuses (surrounded by dura) and falx cerebri, which is the longitudinal layer that extends ventrally between the two cerebral hemispheres. At the level of the foramen magnum, the two layers become separated; the outer layer continues to function as the periosteum of the vertebral (spinal) canal, and the inner layer forms the free dural membrane that surrounds the spinal cord. The inner aspect of dura mater is lined by elongated, flattened mesothelial-like cells. Except in neonates, there is no epidural (extradural) space in the cranial vault as there is in the spinal cord. There can be a "potential" epidural or extradural space in mature animals from hemorrhage caused by trauma.

The arachnoid consists of both the multilayered membrane composed of cells that overlap one another, and the trabeculae that join it to the pia. The arachnoid has tight junctions between its cells, although other junctions have also been described. It contains no blood vessels and has an outer smooth surface formed by mesothelial-like cells that abut similar cells in the dura mater. The mesothelium-like surfaces of the dura and arachnoid oppose and slide over each other, analogous to the parietal and visceral surfaces of other serous membranes.

The pia mater is closely adherent to the surface of the brain and spinal cord and is penetrated by a large number of blood vessels that supply the underlying nervous tissue (Fig. 14-18). The pia mater consists of flat, thin, overlapping connective tissue cells (fibroblasts) that are separated from the underlying neural tissue by variable amounts of loose collagen fibers and the glia limitans. In many areas the pia, which lacks a basal lamina, is only one-cell-layer thick and has fenestrations, so that the glia limitans is exposed directly to the subarachnoid space. Pial and arachnoid cells also ensheathe blood vessels, collagen bundles, and nerves

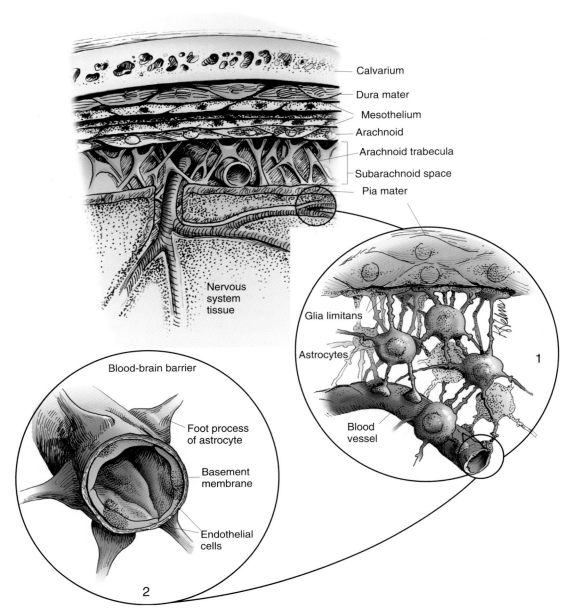

Fig. 14-16   Organization of the meninges. The meninges, from outside to inside, are the dura mater, arachnoid mater, and pia mater as illustrated in the diagram. The arachnoid mater and the pia mater form the leptomeninges. These two layers of the leptomeninges also enclose the subarachnoid space, which contains the arteries, veins, and nerves and is filled with cerebrospinal fluid. The pia mater is attached to the surface of the central nervous system. Astrocytes and their foot processes underlie the pia mater and form the glia limitans (*inset 1*) and surround the endothelial cells that form the blood-brain barrier. As arterioles penetrate the cortex to supply the tissue with blood, they carry the pia and glia limitans with them for 1 to 3 mm until the arteriole structurally becomes a capillary. At this transition site within the cortex, the capillary penetrates the pia and is surrounded by the glia limitans, and the end feet of the astrocytes become part of the blood-brain barrier (*inset 2*). Components of the blood-brain barrier are capillary endothelial cells, basement membrane, and astrocytic foot processes, but the barrier is formed structurally by tight junctions between endothelial cells and functionally by specialized transport systems in these cells. *(Courtesy Dr. J.F. Zachary, College of Veterinary Medicine, University of Illinois.)*

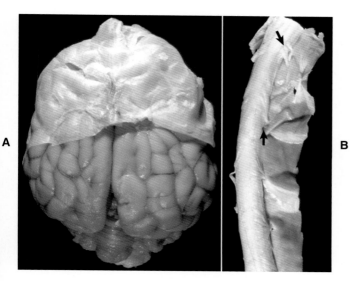

A

B

Fig. 14-17   Layers of the meninges. A, Brain, dog. The dura matter is a thick opaque layer. Here it covers the rostral (cranial) half of the brain and has been dissected away from the caudal half of the brain to expose the underlying leptomeninges. In old animals, the dura mater often fuses with the periosteum of the calvarium, and at necropsy to expose the brain, it is usually removed attached to the calvarium. The leptomeninges are present, but because they are so transparent, in this photograph they are barely visible on the surface of the caudal half of the brain between gyri. **B,** Spinal cord, horse. The dura matter is the thick opaque layer dissected from and lying to the right of the spinal cord. The leptomeninges (pia-arachnoid layer) are present (but not readily visible in this photograph) on the exposed surface of the spinal cord. Arrows indicate spinal nerve roots. (**A** and **B,** *Courtesy Dr. J.F. Zachary, College of Veterinary Medicine, University of Illinois.*)

that are within or cross the subarachnoid space and also are around arteries that penetrate into the CNS up to 1 to 2 mm in depth. Macrophages also are present throughout the leptomeninges.

ENDOTHELIUM

The basic functions of endothelium in the CNS are to line luminal surfaces of blood vessels; form the blood-brain barrier; regulate thrombosis, thrombolysis, and platelet adherence; and maintain a nonthrombogenic boundary between coagulation cascade molecules and luminal surfaces of endothelial cells. Additionally, endothelial cells function as regulatory barriers to small and large molecules crossing the endothelium, and they control the adherence of leukocytes to their luminal surfaces. The endothelial cells of the blood-brain barrier actively transport those molecules that the brain consumes rapidly and in large quantities, such as glucose, amino acids, lactate, and ribonucleosides.

GROUND RULES FOR UNDERSTANDING INJURY IN THE CENTRAL NERVOUS SYSTEM

Before the responses of the CNS to injury are discussed, some fundamental concepts are reviewed in Box 14-2.

RESPONSES OF NEURONS TO INJURY

Neurons are the most vulnerable cells in the nervous system and probably within the body. They have large requirements for energy to maintain normal metabolism, transport systems, and the formation of cytoskeleton proteins in the axon, which can extend over long distances (>1 m), but neurons lack adequate intracellular glucose reserves. Therefore they are completely dependent for survival on an adequate blood supply to provide glucose. Additionally, neurons are vulnerable to free radical oxidative stresses and have a limited ability to buffer shifts of calcium ions into the cell, which can interfere with oxidative phosphorylation and ATP production, such as occurs with ischemia.

Neurons are especially sensitive to excessive stimulation with excitatory amino acid neurotransmitters called excitotoxins, such as glutamate and aspartate. These neurotransmitters are also released in a wide variety of neuronal injuries, especially in neuronal ischemia. Under normal conditions, astrocytic processes surrounding synapses have efficient uptake systems to remove excitotoxins, and neurons are not injured. In excessive quantities, persistent binding of excitotoxins to receptors can lead to neuronal degeneration and death.

The microscopic appearance of the neuronal cell body can vary according to the injury. Characteristic changes of the neuronal cell body are reviewed in Box 14-3.

NEURONAL CELL DEATH

Neurons can die following injury as a result of one of two mechanisms: apoptotic cell death and necrotic cell death. These mechanisms are summarized next and discussed in greater detail in Chapter 1. Both apoptotic and necrotic neuronal cell death can occur concurrently or in temporal or spatial sequences within the nervous system. Although apoptotic and necrotic neuronal death represent different responses of neurons to injury, identical receptors, messenger systems, and mechanisms of cytotoxicity are likely involved in both apoptotic and necrotic cell death. Factors that determine whether the apoptotic or necrotic pathway is activated are unclear but appear to depend on the character on the initiating ligand or injury, type of cell membrane receptors activated, and caspases expressed in response to injury.

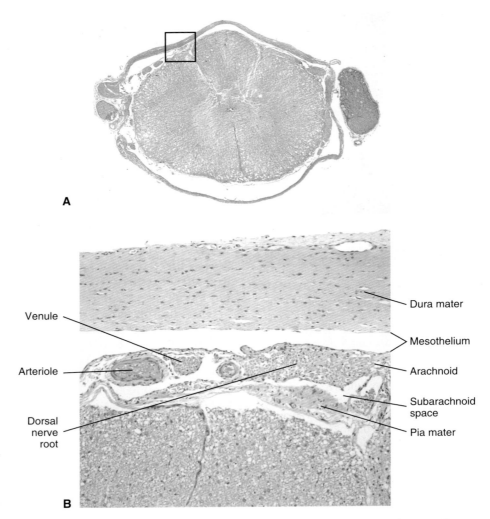

A

Venule

Dura mater

Mesothelium

Arteriole

Arachnoid

Dorsal
nerve
root

Subarachnoid
space

Pia mater

B

Fig. 14-18   **Histologic section of spinal cord and meninges. A,** Low magnification of a
cross section of the spinal cord and meninges with spinal nerve rootlets and a dorsal root
ganglion from which Fig. 14-18, *B* was selected *(box)*. H&E stain. **B,** The inner surface of the
dura mater and the outer surface of the arachnoid mater are covered with mesothelial cells,
and the space between them is the subdural space. Blood vessels and nerves of the dorsal
and ventral roots traverse in the subarachnoid space. H&E stain. (*A and B, Courtesy Dr. J.F. Zachary,
College of Veterinary Medicine, University of Illinois.*)

APOPTOTIC CELL DEATH (PROGRAMMED CELL DEATH)

Apoptosis is a single cell-initiated, gene-directed cellular, self-destructive regulatory mechanism that leads
to "programmed" cell death. This mechanism is used:
(1) during the development of the nervous system to
ensure proper migration and orientation of cell layers
and removal of excess embryonic cells; (2) to remove
"aged" cells (i.e., cell turnover) in organs; and (3) to
maintain cell number homeostasis in organ systems
that have regenerative capacity (endocrine glands).

Apoptotic neuronal death is characterized by a
sequence of cellular degenerative steps that can be

identified biochemically and morphologically. Following
appropriate signals recognized and interpreted by cell
membrane receptors (Fas, tumor necrosis factor [TNF]
receptor-1, TNF-related apoptosis-inducing ligand
receptors), a family of proteins known as caspases are
activated. Caspases cleave cellular substrates that are
required for cellular function and include cytoskeleton
proteins and nuclear proteins, such as DNA repair
enzymes. Caspases also activate other degradative
enzymes such as DNAases, which cleave nuclear DNA.

The role of apoptotic neuronal death in specific neurologic diseases will be discussed in greater detail in subsequent sections. As examples, some viral infections

Box **14-2**

Concepts in Understanding Responses of the Central Nervous System to Injury

1. The cells of the central nervous system (CNS) vary in their susceptibility to injury (neurons > oligodendroglia > astrocytes > microglia > blood vessels). Neurons are the most sensitive to injury, whereas glial and other cells are more resistant to injury.
2. Neurons have only small energy stores; therefore they are dependent on an intact blood flow to supply oxygen and nutrients, particularly glucose. Neurons with the highest metabolic rate, such as some neurons in the cerebral cortex, will die 6 to 10 minutes after the cessation of blood flow after cardiac arrest.
3. There is no regeneration of neurons. The neurons you have now are the ones you were born with; however, their metabolism is dynamic, and metabolites are continually turned over and replaced.
4. If nerve fibers in the CNS are cut by transection of the cord, no or little regeneration of nerve fibers results. Therefore if sufficient motor nerve fibers are cut, there is paralysis; if not, there is a neurologic deficit.
5. If fibers in the peripheral nervous system are cut, they can regenerate under certain circumstances. This outcome depends on axoplasmic flow, alignment of the proximal and distal portions of the nerve, and the preservation and alignment of the proximal and distal portions of the endoneural tube (the structure in which the axon lies).
6. Healing in the CNS is different than in the rest of the body. There are few fibroblasts in the CNS and they are principally found only in the leptomeninges and in the outer few millimeters of the CNS, where they are pulled into the cerebral cortex with blood vessels. Therefore wounds deep in the CNS heal by proliferation of astrocyte processes. Astrocytic processes fill small dead spaces of less than a few millimeters and encapsulate large dead spaces and abscesses. Superficial wounds or wounds that extend through the leptomeninges heal by synthesis and deposition of collagen by fibroblasts (fibrous connective tissue) and by proliferation of astrocytic processes. However, in contrast to the fibroblast, astrocytic processes produce a very poor capsule, which can break down easily.
7. The cranial cavity is nearly filled by the brain, its coverings, and fluids. Therefore many lesions, such as tumors, abscesses, hemorrhages, and hydrocephalus in the brain, produce clinical signs because they are space-occupying lesions, which in neuropathology implies that they cause atrophy or displacement of portions of the brain or cord, depending on the duration of the injury.
8. The blood-brain barrier can exert control over drugs and antibodies from entering the intact brain. It is also a barrier to infection and is formed by the tight junctions of the endothelial cells, aided by basement membrane, and the end feet of the astrocytes, which lie on the outside of the capillary.
9. Although the CNS has the ability to resist infection and injury, once the CNS is infected, it has a low degree of resistance when compared with other tissues of the body. Microbes, such as *Cryptococcus neoformans*, which normally would be relatively nonpathogenic in other organs, may produce death if the CNS is infected. This outcome in part is attributable to the complexity of the CNS and the fact that it is the most vital organ in the body. Any disease process will often cause catastrophic results in the CNS, as opposed to tissues such as in the lung, liver, and kidney.

Box **14-3**

Microscopic Changes That Can Occur in the Neuronal Cell Body

1. Central chromatolysis following axonal injury
2. Ischemic cell change
3. Enlargement of the cell body in lysosomal storage diseases
4. Accumulation of lipofuscin pigment in aging
5. Accumulation of neurofilaments in certain neuronal degenerative diseases
6. Inclusion body formation in certain viral diseases
7. Cytoplasmic vacuolation in spongiform encephalopathies

that occur in utero produce developmental anomalies by initiating apoptosis that leads to faulty differentiation of embryonic granule and Purkinje cell layers, such as occurs in experimental Borna disease. Mild ischemia, excitotoxins, hormones, corticosteroids, and proinflammatory cytokines can induce apoptotic cell death. Rabies virus has been linked experimentally to apoptotic neuronal death.

Apoptosis results in characteristic morphologic changes in cells such as shrinkage, cytoplasmic condensation and blebbing, and chromatin clumping and fragmentation (see Figs. 1-30 through 1-34 in Chapter 1). As cells continue to shrink, nuclear chromatin is cleaved into smaller units and along with condensed cytoplasm is packaged for removal by macrophages. Inflammation is not induced by apoptotic cell death.

NECROTIC CELL DEATH

Necrosis is a process that usually affects groups of cells in contrast to single isolated cells as observed in apoptosis. Necrosis is characterized by the following sequence: hydropic degeneration, swelling of mitochondria, pyknosis and fragmentation of the nucleus, and eventual cell lysis caused by cell membrane damage and the inability of the plasma membrane to control ion and fluid gradients (see Figs 1-11 through 1-17 in Chapter 1).

Cellular debris associated with necrotic neuronal death will illicit an inflammatory response in contrast to apoptotic neuronal death.

Acute neuronal necrosis (ischemic cell change)

Acute neuronal necrosis is a common response to a variety of CNS injuries, such as cerebral ischemia caused by blood loss and hypovolemic shock, vascular thrombosis, and cardiac failure; inflammatory mediators; bacterial toxins; thermal injury; heavy metals; nutritional deficiencies, such as thiamine deficiency; and trauma. Additionally, conditions that reduce ATP generation through oxidative phosphorylation will also lead to neuronal degeneration and death. Such conditions include: (1) interference with cytochrome oxidase activity in mitochondria caused by cyanide poisoning; (2) competitive inhibition of oxygen uptake in carbon monoxide poisoning; and (3) inadequate availability of glucose for neuronal metabolism in hypoglycemia.

The susceptibility of cells and tissue structures of the CNS to ischemia, in decreasing order of susceptibility, are neurons, oligodendroglia, astrocytes, microglia, and blood vessels. However, within groups of neurons, some neurons are more sensitive to injury than others. This phenomenon is called selective neuronal vulnerability. Purkinje cells, some striatal neurons, neurons of the third, fifth, and sixth cerebral cortical lamina, and hippocampal pyramidal cells have the highest vulnerability. A regional vulnerability of neurons has also been reported (cerebral cortex and striatum > thalamus > brain stem > spinal cord). It is hypothesized that the most vulnerable neurons likely produce the most excitotoxins, such as glutamate, and are the most sensitive to them. Because of the microanatomic arrangement of the cerebral cortex, ischemic neurons often occur in a laminar pattern within the cerebrocortical gray matter. This microanatomic pattern accounts for the laminar lesions observed in thiamine deficiency–induced polioencephalomalacia in ruminants and in other diseases, such as salt poisoning in pigs and lead poisoning in ruminants.

Following the various types of CNS injury, there is an early increase in ATP-dependent release of normally sequestered intracellular calcium ions from altered mitochondria and endoplasmic reticulum. Also during this time, neuronal depolarization potentiates the release of the neuroexcitatory neurotransmitter glutamate. Persistent activation of glutamate receptors of target cells results in a disturbance referred to as excitotoxicity. This altered activity leads to a notable influx of extracellular calcium into cells, causing further impairment of mitochondrial function and the generation of reactive oxygen species, such as superoxide, hydrogen peroxide, hydroxyl radicals, and nitric oxide.

These reactive oxygen species, exerting their effects especially on lipid-rich cell membranes, can enhance the existing excitotoxicity, cause further influx of calcium into cells as a result of membrane damage, and ultimately result in neuronal dysfunction and death. Additionally, reperfusion of ischemic tissue after the initial ischemic injury can enhance the generation of reactive oxygen metabolites, thus amplifying the tissue damage. Other influencing factors include the temperature of the brain at the time of ischemia, with lower temperatures (as little as $2°$ C decrease) having a sparing effect and elevated temperatures having an enhanced effect on neuronal injury following ischemia.

Neurons are dependent on a continuous supply of oxygen to remain viable and if the supply is interrupted for several minutes, the vulnerable neurons as described previously will degenerate. Ischemic cell change can also result from metabolic disturbances other than ischemia, such as in thiamine deficiency and cyanide toxicosis, which interferes with oxygen use. In H&E stained sections, the cytoplasm of the neuronal cell body is shrunken, deeply eosinophilic, and frequently sharply angular to triangular in shape (Fig. 14-19). The nucleus is reduced in size, is often triangular, and is pyknotic. The nucleolus and Nissl substance are usually not detectable. Ischemia neurons die and are removed either by a process called neuronophagia, which is phagocytosis by microglial cells and macrophages or by lysis (Fig. 14-19). Following neuronal necrosis, there is swelling of perineuronal and perivascular astrocytic processes.

CHRONIC NEURONAL NECROSIS (BRAIN ATROPHY)

Neuronal death and loss of neurons can occur as a result of progressive disease processes of long duration in the CNS. This loss, termed simple neuronal atrophy, is seen with slowly progressive neurologic diseases, such as cerebral cortical atrophy of aging, ceroid-lipofuscinosis, and primary and multisystem and cerebellar neuronal degeneration. Gross lesions are usually not visible, but when cerebrocortical neurons die, there can be atrophy of cerebral gyri, which results in widening of the sulci (Fig. 14-20). Microscopic lesions indicative of an earlier loss of neurons are diminished numbers of neurons and astrogliosis and atrophy and loss of neurons in functionally related systems. Loss of neurons over time results in progressively worsening neurologic dysfunction.

WALLERIAN DEGENERATION AND CENTRAL CHROMATOLYSIS

Injury to axons of the CNS and PNS can result from a variety of causes such as: (1) traumatic transection leading to Wallerian degeneration; (2) compression

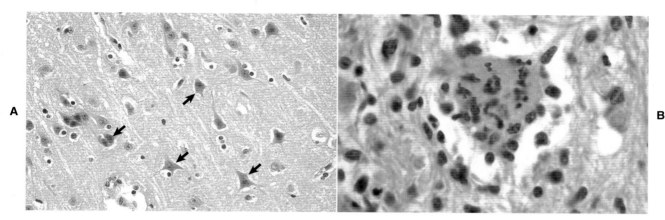

Fig. 14-19   Neuronal necrosis (acute), so-called ischemic cell change, cerebrum, dog.
A, Neuronal ischemia. Neuronal cell bodies of cerebral cortical laminae are red, angular, and
shrunken *(arrows)* and their nuclei are contracted and dense. This lesion can be caused by
neuronal ischemia. H&E stain. **B,** Neuronophagia. This necrotic neuron cell body is surrounded
by macrophages that will phagocytose the cell debris. H&E stain. *(**A,** Courtesy Dr. J. F. Zachary,
College of Veterinary Medicine, University of Illinois. **B,** Courtesy Dr. M.D. McGavin, College of Veterinary Medicine,
University of Tennessee.)*

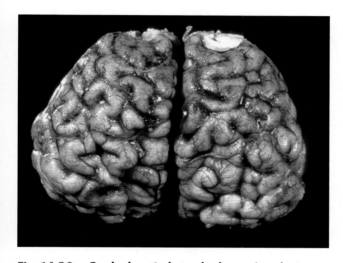

Fig. 14-20   Cerebral cortical atrophy, horse. Atrophy is seen
with a variety of slowly progressive neurological diseases in
which there is a progressive loss of neurons. These diseases
include cerebral cortical atrophy of aging and ceroid-
lipofuscinosis. The characteristic gross lesions are narrowing
of the cerebral gyri with a consequent widening of the sulci.
(Courtesy the Department of Veterinary Biosciences, The Ohio State University.)

and crushing; (3) therapeutic neurectomies; (4) nerve
stretching injury; and (4) intoxication.

WALLERIAN DEGENERATION

In 1850 Dr. Augustus Volney Waller described the
pattern of microscopic lesions (necrosis) in axons and
myelin sheaths following transection. These changes
are characteristic of Wallerian degeneration (Fig. 14-21).
Although Waller described this process in peripheral
nerves, the term *Wallerian degeneration* is also used
to describe necrosis that occurs in nerve fibers in the
CNS after axons are injured (compressed or severed).
The reactions of axon and myelin distal to the site of
injury are to swell and break, and the rate is proportional to the diameter of the fiber. Thus the larger the
diameter of the axon, the faster the rate of Wallerian
degeneration.

Wallerian degeneration in the CNS follows the
same sequence of events as in peripheral nerve fibers,
but the speed of degeneration and phagocytosis is
slower and there is little or no regeneration. In addition, an axon of the PNS has the advantage of: (1) efficient phagocytosis with removal of debris, (2) Schwann
cells to remyelinate the regenerated axon, and (3) an
endoneurial tube to guide the axon as it extends into
the distal segment. On the other hand, an axon of the
CNS has: (1) few microglia (sparse in the white matter)
to remove myelin debris and (2) oligodendrocytes with
a more limited capability to remyelinate axons. In the
CNS, severed axons have a very limited ability to regenerate and successfully reinnervate their appropriate
sensory or motor structures. In the PNS, if the severed
nerves have a large distance between the cut ends,
fibrous tissue scarring can prevent the axons from the
proximal segment entering the distal endoneural tubes
and thus prevent the reparative response, resulting in
the formation of a neuroma. If the severed ends
of nerves are sewn together but the endoneural tubes
are malaligned, which usually occurs, the sensory and

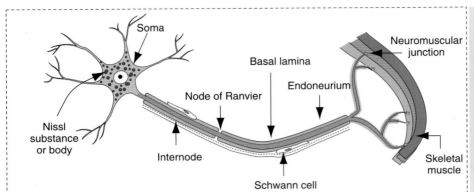

An intact motor neuron is shown with an axon ending in a neuromuscular junction. The axon is surrounded by a myelin sheath and a basal lamina —produced by Schwann cells—and the endoneurium.

The soma of the neuron contains abundant Nissl substance (aggregates of ribosomes attached to the endoplasmic reticulum and free polyribosomes).

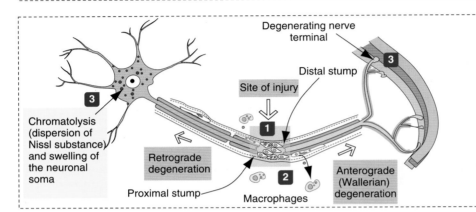

1 An injury damages the nerve fiber. Schwann cells undergo mitotic division and bridge the gap between the proximal and distal axonal stumps.
2 Schwann cells phagocytose myelin. Myelin droplets are extruded from Schwann cells and subsequently are phagocytosed by tissue macrophages.
3 Chromatolysis and degeneration of the axon terminals are seen. The distal and proximal segments of the axon degenerate (anterograde and retrograde degeneration, respectively).

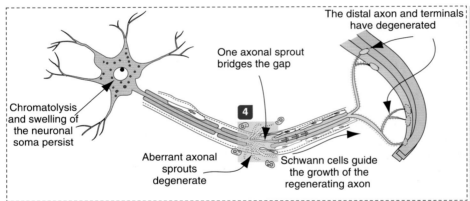

4 The proximal axonal stump generates multiple sprouts advancing between Schwann cells. One sprout persists and grows distally (~1.5 mm per day) to reinnervate the muscle. The remaining sprouts degenerate. In the central nervous system, degeneration of the axon and myelin is similar and microglial cells remove debris by phagocytosis.
The regeneration process starts but is aborted by the absence of endoneurium and lack of proliferation of oligodendrocytes.

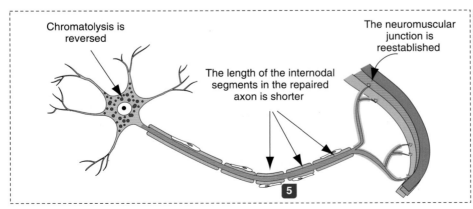

5 Once the regenerated axon reaches the end organ (several months), Schwann cells start the production of myelin. The internodal segments are shorter.

The regenerated axon has a reduced diameter (80% of the original diameter), and therefore the conduction velocity of the nerve impulse is slower.

Fig. 14-21 Peripheral nerve degeneration and regeneration (also applicable to neurons within the central nervous system). *(Modified from Kierszenbaum AL: Histology and cell biology, St Louis, 2002, Mosby.)*

motor nerves will regenerate but reinnervate inappropriate sensory and motor structures.

The sequence of Wallerian degeneration in the PNS (similar in CNS except for significant regeneration; see previously) includes the following:

1. Degeneration and fragmentation of axon and myelin within several days. Proximal segment degenerates back to the next node of Ranvier, but all the distal segment dies.
2. Removal of axonal and myelin debris by phagocytosis. Some phagocytes are from the blood and some phagocytosis is by Schwann cells. All of the debris is cleared out of the endoneural tube within a few weeks.
3. Regeneration of axon if the endoneurium is intact to allow the axon of the proximal segment to enter and slide down the tube.
4. Remyelinization by Schwann cells.

Microscopically, another early lesion in Wallerian degeneration is central chromatolysis, characterized by swelling of the neuronal cell body, dispersion of centrally located Nissl substance, and peripheral displacement of the nucleus (Fig. 14-22). The time of onset depends on how much of the axon has been lost, and thus on how close to the neuronal cell body the axon has been transected. Onset can begin within 24 to 48 hours and reach its maximum in about 18 days following axonal injury. The dispersal of Nissl substance (chromatolysis) is indicative of enhanced synthesis of transport and structural proteins required for regeneration of the axon and reestablishment of fast and slow axonal transport systems. The extent to which chromatolysis develops is related to the degree and location of axonal injury. It is more prominent and can even be followed by neuronal death, the more severe the loss of the volume of the axon and the closer the axonal injury is to the cell body. The time required for recovery of cell bodies can be several months and in most cases will vary from 3 to 6 months, depending on the severity of the axonal injury and the length of axon regenerated.

The change in the axon distal to the point of injury is first evident within 24 hours of injury. Wallerian degeneration is initially characterized by irregularity of the axonal diameter, which is followed after 48 to 72 hours by fragmentation of the axon and myelin along its length (Fig. 14-23). This axonal alteration is followed by disintegration, and usually there is no evidence of the axon remaining by the second week after the injury.

Changes in the myelin sheath surrounding myelinated axons are evident by 28 to 96 hours after injury when axonal disintegration is well advanced. Initially, there are irregularities in the sheath accompanied by folding, lamellar splitting, fracturing, and fragmentation (secondary demyelination). The fragmented myelin can form droplets (termed ellipsoids), which

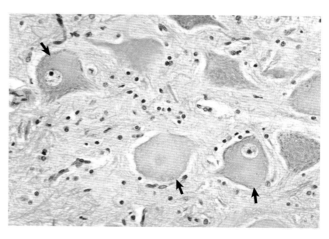

Fig. 14-22   Central chromatolysis, neuron cell body, dog. Compare with Figs. 14-4, *B* and 14-10. Affected neurons have eccentric nuclei and pale central cytoplasm with dispersed Nissl substance (*arrows*). *(Courtesy Dr. M.D. McGavin, College of Veterinary Medicine, University of Tennessee.)*

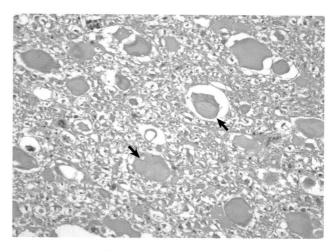

Fig. 14-23   Wallerian degeneration, transverse section of spinal cord, dog. Laceration and/or severe compression of myelinated nerves cause a specific sequence of structural and functional changes in the axon and the myelin (distal from the point of injury), referred to as Wallerian degeneration (Fig. 14-21). Axons are initially swollen (*arrows*) and are eventually removed by phagocytosis to leave clear spaces, which were once the sites of nerve fibers. The cell bodies of affected neurons usually have central chromatolysis, but are metabolically active in an attempt to regenerate the lost portion of the axon (not shown; see Fig. 14-22). *(Courtesy Dr. J.F. Zachary, College of Veterinary Medicine, University of Illinois.)*

surround and enclose isolated fragments and debris of the former axon. Both axonal and myelin debris are then removed by macrophages through phagocytosis. Degeneration of myelin is usually completed by the end of the second week, although evidence of myelin debris can be detected up to 1 to 3 months after axonal injury (the time required for macrophages in the PNS to phagocytose and clear the debris). Myelin debris can be detected in the CNS (when compared with the PNS) for a much longer time after injury.

If the neuronal cell body survives the injury to its axon, regeneration from the proximal stump in the PNS can occur. The degree of axonal regeneration depends on the status of the endoneurial tube (sheath) distal to the original point of injury (Fig. 14-21). The normal endoneurial tube (sheath) and its contents consist (from outside inward) of (1) a connective tissue investment referred to as the endoneurium, (2) the basement membrane that surrounds the Schwann cells plus the Schwann cell cytoplasm, (3) the myelin sheath of myelinated axons, and (4) the axon. Approximately 24 to 72 hours after axonal injury, the endoneurial tube (sheath), formed by persisting basement membrane and endoneurium, contains degenerating remnants of the previously existing axon along with Schwann cells. Schwann cells begin to proliferate and eventually form a longitudinal column of cells referred to as the bands of Büngner.

If the endoneurial tube (sheath) remains intact, as can occur following a compression injury to a peripheral nerve, neural regeneration through the formation of axonal sprouts can occur. A regenerating sprout from the proximal axonal stump can enter the column of Schwann cells and regenerate uninterrupted along its original pathway to the periphery, reestablishing innervation with an end organ (skeletal muscle). Such axons then become remyelinated and regain their physiologic function of impulse transmission. Because of axoplasmic flow, a regenerating neuron lengthens at a rate of approximately 1 to 4 mm/day. Although the time required for axonal regeneration can vary depending on the length of axon to be regenerated, examples of times required for morphologic and functional recovery following crush injury of a peripheral nerve are 250 to 300 and 456 to 486 days, respectively. If, however, the integrity of the endoneurial tube (sheath) is destroyed, as would occur after complete severance of a peripheral nerve, regeneration might not occur, because the proximal axonal stump might be prevented from reaching the distal endoneurial tube (sheath) by proliferated fibrous connective tissue (scar formation) at the site of axonal severance. Regenerating axons may also enter inappropriate endoneurial tubes (sheaths), resulting in improper impulse transmission, such as a sensory neuron axonal sprout entering an endoneurial tube intended for a nerve innervating a muscle.

The microscopic lesions for Wallerian degeneration within the CNS are similar to those described for the PNS, except that in the CNS, degenerated axons and myelin sheaths can remain for months to years before complete removal. With injury to the CNS, some cell bodies have central chromatolysis; others initially have central chromatolysis followed by atrophy and death. Affected axons and their myelin sheaths undergo a rather characteristic series of changes as they degenerate. Initially, axons form linear and bulbous swellings at, and some distance from, the site of injury. These enlargements are termed axonal spheroids. Spheroids consist of neurofilaments, microtubules, and cellular organelles. Because injury to the axon results in dysfunction of axoplasmic flow, any disruption of anterograde and retrograde axonal transport results in the accumulation of neurofilaments, microtubules, cellular organelles, and recycled molecules at or near the point of injury. This process occurs in peripheral nerves as well.

The axonal enlargements can be seen as early as a few hours at the site of injury and remain prominent, particularly for the first week or so (Fig. 14-23). The surrounding myelin sheath is usually distended to create a space between the sheath and the axonal swelling. Progressively, such affected axons and myelin sheaths fragment along their length, forming ellipsoids as in the PNS. Eventually ellipsoids are removed through degeneration and phagocytosis, leaving an empty space, or one still containing myelin debris and macrophages (gitter cells). The latter is termed a "digestion chamber." With time and continued lysis and phagocytosis of the debris, most of the lesion will consist of enlarged empty spaces. The absence of swollen axons in such dilated spaces, especially in the early stages after CNS trauma, does not necessarily mean that the entire axon has degenerated and been removed, which can require several months. It might instead be the site of separation of an enlarged axon from the adjacent axon at the level of the section being examined.

RESPONSES OF MACROGLIA TO INJURY
ASTROCYTES

Common astrocytic reactions in CNS injury are swelling, hypertrophy, division, and the laying down of intermediate filaments in cell processes. The term *astrocytosis* means that astrocytes have increased in size and number in response to injury, whereas the term *astrogliosis* (somewhat synonymous with hypertrophy) implies synthesis of intermediate filaments and an increased length, complexity, and branching of the astrocytic processes. The recognition of these differences is based on histopathologic evaluation.

Swelling is an acute response and is reversible, or it may progress with time to hypertrophy. Swollen astrocytes have clear-staining or vacuolated cytoplasm. Astrocytes swell following ischemia because of the increased uptake of sodium, chloride, and potassium ions and water in an effort to maintain homeostasis in the extracellular microenvironment. It is important to remember that such swelling depends on the astrocyte being viable and still having a semipermeable plasma membrane, even though its function may be altered. With progression, and if the degree and duration of ischemia are sufficiently severe to result in cell death, the plasma membrane becomes fully permeable, and the cell does not swell but becomes shriveled or shrunken and undergoes disintegration, as described for the ischemic cell change of neurons.

If injury is severe, astrocytic processes fragment and disappear followed by lysis of the cell body. Hypertrophied astrocytes often referred to as "reactive," represent a response to a milder and more protracted injury to the CNS. Because of increases in intermediate filaments, mainly GFAP, the cytoplasm becomes apparent along with increased length and branching of the processes with H&E staining. The increase of intermediate filaments and consequently the intensity of GFAP immunohistochemical staining in these cells are so dramatic that some have defined reactive astrocytes on the basis of this change. In protracted degenerative conditions, astrocytes termed gemistocytes can be observed (Fig. 14-24). These cells have eccentric nuclei and abundant pink homogeneous cytoplasm, in contrast to the lack of visible cytoplasm in normal astrocytes, with routine H&E staining. Animals with hepatic encephalopathy can have a unique microscopic lesion in the brain affecting astrocytes of the cerebral cortices. Astrocytic nuclei tend to be in pairs occasionally with prominent central nucleoli and surrounded by a clear space which is the edematous cytoplasm. They are called Alzheimer's type II astrocytes (Fig. 14-13, *D*).

Astrocytic proliferation can occur in CNS injury, but in most instances proliferative capacity is limited. When it occurs, the most dramatic examples are associated with attempts by reactive astrocytes (astrogliosis) to "wall off" abscesses and neoplasms or to fill in cavitated areas that result following lysis of necrotic neurons with the processes of astrocytes. This laying down of glial fibers is referred to as a glial scar. It is formed by a network of interlaced astrocytic processes and provides a loose barrier that separates the injured brain from the more normal adjacent tissue. This astroglia-fibroblast interface in injured CNS attempts to reform the glia limitans, restore the blood-brain barrier, and reestablish fluid and electrolyte balances.

OLIGODENDROCYTES

Oligodendroglia react to injury by cell swelling, hypertrophy, and degeneration. Both perineuronal and interfascicular oligodendroglia can swell, hypertrophy, and degenerate; however, only oligodendroglia precursor cells can proliferate to replace degenerate cells. The role that perineuronal or satellite oligodendroglia play in

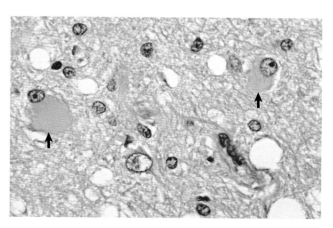

Fig. 14-24   Gemistocytes (gemistocytic astrocytes), cerebrum, dog. When astrocytes react to injury, initially by hypertrophy and later by the synthesis of increased glial filaments (astrogliosis), the nuclei enlarge and often the cell body, which is not normally visible in H&E stained sections, will become visible. These astrocytes are called gemistocytes (plump astrocytes) *(arrows)*. They occur in diseases in which there is alteration of intracellular and extracellular fluid balances or injury to the parenchyma, where healing will be by glial scarring (astrogliosis, e.g., to encapsulate a deep abscess or fill in a small area of dead space). H&E stain. *(Courtesy Dr. J.F. Zachary, College of Veterinary Medicine, University of Illinois.)*

normal neuronal function and neuronal injury has not been definitively clarified. Microscopically, these cells swell and hypertrophy around injured neurons, and this response to injury has been called satellitosis (Fig. 14-13).

Degeneration of interfascicular oligodendroglia caused by ischemia, certain viruses, lead toxicity, and autoimmunity can result in selective degeneration of myelin sheaths referred to as primary demyelination. Primary demyelination is the loss of myelin around an intact axon. Mechanisms of primary demyelination are summarized in Box 14-4. Protracted or repetitive injury to myelinating cells and their myelin sheaths can lead to irreversible neuronal atrophy. Oligodendroglia precursor cells located in the subventricular zone of the CNS can mature into interfascicular oligodendroglia and can also proliferate in response to noncytocidal injury and become involved in remyelination following primary demyelination.

CNS or PNS injury can also lead to loss of myelin secondary to injury of the axon and its cell body or to death of the neuron. When axons are injured, myelin lamellae forming the internodes are retracted and removed by phagocytosis. In some instances oligodendroglia or Schwann cells, the myelin-forming cells in the PNS, also degenerate. This form of myelin degeneration is termed secondary demyelination and is secondary to axon degeneration or loss (resembles Wallerian degeneration).

Box 14-4

Mechanisms of Primary Demyelination

1. Inherited enzyme defects resulting in formation of abnormal myelin
   Leukodystrophies in man and animals
2. Impairment of myelin synthesis and maintenance
   Infection
   Mouse hepatitis virus in mice and progressive multifocal leukoencephalopathy in humans; in both cases oligodendrocytes are selectively destroyed by viral agents and myelin cannot be maintained.
   Nutritional
   Lack of maintenance of myelin are due to copper deficiency, malnutrition, vitamin B_{12} deficiency.
   Toxins
   Cyanide poisoning
   Cuprizone toxicity
3. Loss of myelin as a consequence of cytotoxic edema (status spongiosis)
   Hexachlorophene poisoning, usually prolonged edema
4. Destruction of myelin by detergent-like metabolites
   Lysolecithin, a metabolite of phospholipase A (normally present in the nervous system) may destroy myelin.
5. Immunological destruction of myelin
   Cell mediated
   Experimental allergic encephalitis (EAE)
   Landry-Guillain-Barré (human beings)
   Coonhound paralysis
   Marek's disease (chickens)
   Various stages of multiple sclerosis in human beings
   Various stages of canine distemper

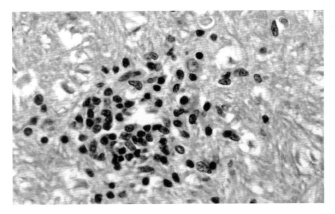

Fig. 14-25   Glial nodule, brain stem, dog. These nodules (*center*), formed by reactive microglial cells and macrophages, occur most frequently in viral encephalitides. H&E stain. (*Courtesy Dr. M.D. McGavin, College of Veterinary Medicine, University of Tennessee.*)

EPENDYMAL CELLS

Ependymal and choroid plexus epithelial cell responses to injury include atrophy, degeneration, and necrosis. Atrophy usually occurs in response to enlargement of the ventricles as occurs with hydrocephalus. The cilia and microvilli of affected cells are reduced in number, and there is also a reduction in their cellular organelles, such as endoplasmic reticulum and mitochondria. An additional lesion that accompanies ventricular enlargement is stretching and tearing of the ependymal lining. In such instances the resulting areas of ependymal discontinuity result in the subependymal CNS being directly exposed to the CSF. Unfortunately, mammalian ependymal cells do not regenerate and therefore do not repair the denuded areas. After 1 to 2 weeks, astrogliosis, which varies greatly in degree and uniformity, occurs in the exposed areas. Astrogliosis can extend into the ventricular space or be minimal in extent and confined to the periventricular area. Periventricular interstitial edema, myelin loss, and axon loss can ensue.

Inflammation of the ependyma, called ependymitis, can also occur, with infection being the most common cause. Microbes most commonly gain entrance to the ependyma via the circulation by lodging in the choroid plexuses, by direct contamination from a rupture of a cerebral abscess into the ventricular system, and by retrograde reflux through the lateral apertures of infected CSF from the subarachnoid space in cases of leptomeningitis. In the case of bacterial infection, the suppurative exudate that forms in the CSF can cause obstructive hydrocephalus, although the development of hydrocephalus cannot always be explained on the basis of obstruction.

RESPONSES OF MICROGLIA TO INJURY

Microglia are often the first cells in the CNS to react to injury, and the magnitude of the response is graded to correlate with the severity of damage. The responses of microglia to injury include hypertrophy, hyperplasia, phagocytosis of cellular and myelin debris, and neuronophagia, the removal of dead neuron cell bodies. After injury, microglia progress through a stage of activation, becoming fully immunocompetent reactive cells. These reactive cells readily proliferate, either focally, forming glial nodules (Fig. 14-25), or more diffusely, depending on the nature of the injury. As mentioned, in concert with astrocytes and neurons, microglia help coordinate inflammatory events in the CNS. Resident microglia and blood-derived macrophages express MHC class I and II antigens, serve as antigen-presenting cells, and possess a broad armament of adhesion molecules, cytokines, and chemokines. Once activated, these cells can also produce nitric oxide, reactive oxygen

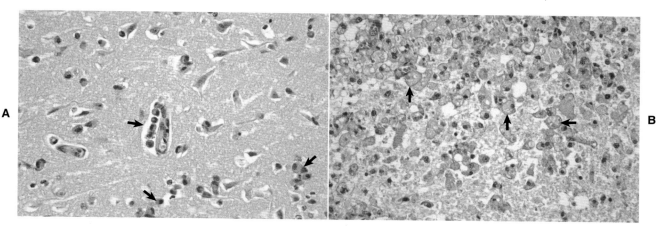

Fig. 14-26   **Gitter cells, cerebrum. A,** Early polioencephalomalacia, cow. Note the angular, eosinophilic neurons with pyknotic nuclei (ischemic cell change). Monocytes (*arrows*) in the perivascular space have been recruited from the vasculature. These cells will become macrophages and phagocytose cellular debris from the necrotic neurons and the myelin from the nerve fibers undergoing degeneration following the death of their neurons. Microglia also participate in this phagocytic response. Macrophages, which have ingested degenerate myelin or other cellular debris, have foamy cytoplasm and are termed gitter cells. H&E stain. **B,** Old necrotic area, dog. The normal brain parenchyma has liquefied and the debris has been ingested by macrophages (*arrows*), which has resulted in the cytoplasm of these cells becoming foamy. They are now designated as gitter cells or simply, foamy macrophages. (**A** *and* **B,** *Courtesy Dr. J.F. Zachary, College of Veterinary Medicine, University of Illinois.*)

intermediates, and other chemical mediators of inflammation that can damage the CNS if not under strict control. When tissue necrosis occurs, macrophages derived from blood monocytes phagocytose the lipid-laden debris of dead neurons and glia, and they become foamy macrophages termed "gitter cells" (Fig. 14-26) and accumulate in the damaged CNS.

RESPONSES OF THE MENINGES TO INJURY

Pathologic processes that initially involve the meninges, most commonly the leptomeninges, can secondarily invade the CNS because of the close apposition between the two tissues. Conversely, processes that primarily affect the CNS can secondarily affect the meninges, most commonly the leptomeninges.

Meningitis refers to inflammation of the meninges. In common usage, the term generally refers to inflammation of the leptomeninges in contrast to inflammation of the dura mater, which is referred to as pachymeningitis. Leptomeningitis can be acute, subacute, or chronic and, depending on the cause, suppurative, nonsuppurative, or granulomatous, and the exudate and inflammatory cells are chiefly in the subarachnoid space. Besides retrograde axonal transport, as occurs with, for example, *Listeria monocytogenes*, infectious agents spread to the meninges hematogenously by direct extension or by leukocytic trafficking.

Other meningeal lesions include: (1) inflammation of the external periosteal dura following osteomyelitis, formation of extradural abscesses, and skull fracture and involve the inner dura as an extension of leptomeningitis; and (2) proliferation of the inner dural mesothelial cells, arachnoid cells, fibroblasts, and cells of the pia mater in response to irritation. Additional lesions likely related to aging or degeneration include formation of cellular nests of mesothelial-like cells on the outer surface of the arachnoid membrane, mineralization of the arachnoid membrane in human beings, and mineralization plus ossification of the dura mater of the spinal cord in both human beings and dogs. Dural ossification in the dog, which tends to affect the ventral, cervical, and lumbar dura mater, is most commonly encountered in large breeds, although smaller breeds can be affected. The clinical significance of this lesion has been debated but not decided.

RESPONSES OF THE CIRCULATORY SYSTEM TO INJURY

ENDOTHELIAL CELL (AND BLOOD VESSEL) RESPONSES TO INJURY

Because many of the infectious and neoplastic disease processes demonstrated in this book are spread through the body via the circulatory system, endothelial cells lining blood vessels, especially capillaries, are subject to a variety of injuries. Bacterial hematogenous CNS diseases occur at the interface between the white and gray matter in the cerebral hemispheres. This phenomenon is thought to result from abrupt changes in vascular flow or luminal diameter of vessels at the interface. These changes may make endothelial cells more susceptible to injury, vasculitis, and thrombosis or predispose the vessels for entrapment of tumor or bacterial emboli.

Endothelial injury can be reversible or nonreversible resulting in necrosis. Injury resulting in endothelial dysfunction can include the activation and release of vasoactive mediators, such as histamine, leading to local and/or systemic changes in vascular flow, pressure, and permeability. Bacterial products and elicited inflammatory cytokines can directly or indirectly cause vascular inflammation (vasculitis) leading to thrombosis and disseminated intravascular coagulation. Thrombotic meningoencephalitis of cattle caused by the bacterium *Histophilus somni* (formerly *Haemophilus somnus*) is an example of this type of injury (Fig. 14-27). Certain herpesviruses and protozoa can also infect endothelial cells and cause endothelial necrosis with vasculitis, hemorrhage, and thrombosis. Finally, some pathogens, such as angioinvasive *Mucor* spp., directly invade blood vessels, resulting in necrosis of the endothelium. Vasculitis resulting in thrombosis can cause tissue ischemia, infarction, and vasogenic edema of the affected area of the CNS. A review of endothelial injury can be found in Chapter 2.

INFARCTION

Infarction means necrosis of a tissue following obstruction (ischemia) of its arterial blood supply. The rate at which ischemia occurs in the CNS determines the degree of injury that follows. The more rapid the onset of ischemia, the more severe the lesion. However, if the obstruction is sudden, as caused by an embolus, many of the neurons can die within minutes and other components within hours. This outcome also applies to compressive injuries to the CNS that produce a sudden reduction in blood flow, such as can happen with sudden compression in rapidly occurring Hansen type I disk herniation in the dog. If the blood flow through an artery is gradually reduced, for example because of arteriosclerosis, there is often sufficient time for anastomotic vessels to dilate and compensate. Anastomoses of the arteries that penetrate from the ventral and cortical surfaces of the brain are insufficient to prevent infarction following sudden occlusion of one or more of these arteries. If the compression is slow—such as is caused by a slowly developing Hansen type II disk herniation in a dog or by a slowly growing neoplasm from the exterior, such as meningioma in a cat—adjacent neural tissue will atrophy to accommodate the mass.

Cerebral necrosis, comparable to infarction following vascular occlusion, can also result from other causes, including cessation of cerebral circulation caused by cardiac arrest, sudden hypotension caused by reduced cardiac output, and reduced or absent oxygen in inspired air. Additional causes include altered function of hemoglobin as a result of carbon monoxide poisoning, inhibition of tissue respiration following cyanide poisoning, toxic substances and poisons, and nutritional deficiencies.

When an artery supplying the CNS is suddenly occluded, blood supply to cells at the center of the infarcted area is rapidly stopped, and if maintained for a sufficient period, all cells die. Neurons at the border of this area continue to receive some blood from nonobstructed vessels. It is proposed that the axonal terminals of degenerated ischemic neurons in the center of the infarct release excessive amounts of the neurotransmitter glutamate, causing injury to still-viable neurons in the borders, which increases the extent of the infarct. This process begins following the binding of the neurotransmitter glutamate to receptors on viable neurons in the borders, inducing an abnormal movement of calcium ions into the recipient cells followed by an increase in intracellular calcium ion concentration. This buildup of calcium ions contributes to a multifunctional cascade that leads to neuronal death. When there is

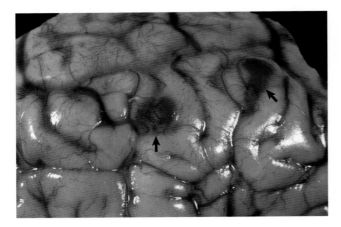

Fig. 14-27 **Vascular thrombosis, thrombotic meningoencephalitis (TEM) (previously called thromboembolic meningoencephalitis [TEME]), cerebrum, cow.** Several red-brown foci (*arrows*) are areas of hemorrhage and/or ischemic necrosis secondary to vasculitis and thrombosis caused by *Histophilus somni* (formerly *Haemophilus somnus*), which reaches the brain hematogenously. *(Courtesy Dr. H. Leipold, College of Veterinary Medicine, Kansas State University.)*

hemorrhage with the infarct, the mechanical injury from the pressure, plus tissue displacement by the hemorrhage, can cause additional damage. See Table 14-1 for the reparative responses associated with the resolution of infarcts.

Areas of cerebral infarction differ somewhat in gross appearance from infarcts in other tissues (Fig. 14-28). The abundance of lipids and enzymes, plus the relative lack of fibrous connective tissue stroma in the brain and spinal cord, results in the affected areas eventually becoming soft because of liquefaction necrosis. The gross appearance of infarction may also differ according to location. Lesions affecting the gray matter tend to be hemorrhagic, whereas infarction of the white matter is often pale. This difference is probably due in part to the less dense capillary meshwork in the white matter, and in part to the fact that the vessels supplying the white matter have fewer anastomoses than those of the gray matter. Infarcted tissue goes through a characteristic sequence of changes that can permit a relatively accurate determination of the age of the infarct. An outline of the chronologic events that occur after an ischemic episode that lasts more than 5 to 6 minutes and is followed by resuscitation of an animal is given in Table 14-1. As can be seen, the tissue changes listed in Table 14-1 take different periods of time to develop in the living resuscitated animal after ischemia occurs. Variation in the times that specific lesions occur depends on the extent and duration of the initial ischemic event. Following removal of cellular and myelin debris, the infarct is repaired by astrocytes. If the infarct is small (<1 mm), it is filled via astrogliosis; if the infarct is larger, it is encapsulated to form a cyst.

Table **14-1** Chronologic Sequence of Changes within Infarcted Tissue (in the Living Animal) following an Ischemic Event

Ischemic Event	TIME FOLLOWING
	Tissue Change
Immediate (seconds)	Cessation of blood flow (ischemia) and accumulation of waste products
Few minutes	Cellular injury and death; coagulation necrosis and edema; hemorrhage (especially in gray matter)
20 min	First microscopic evidence of neuronal injury (perfusion-fixation)
1-2 hr	First microscopic evidence of neuronal injury (immersion fixation)
2 hr	Pale staining of infarct microscopically (white matter); swelling of capillary endothelium; increase in size of astrocytic nuclei
3-5 hr	Ischemic cell change in most neurons; swelling of oligodendroglia and astroglia; beginning clasmatodendrosis of astrocytes
6-24 hr	Beginning neutrophilic infiltration; alteration of myelin (pale staining), 8-24 hours; degeneration and decrease of oligodendroglia, 8-24 hours; astrocytic swelling and retraction and fragmentation of processes (clasmatodendrosis), and degeneration*; cytoplasm of astrocytes visible, 8-24 hours*; vascular degeneration and fibrin deposition, 8-24 hours; thrombosis†, 6-24 hours; beginning endothelial proliferation at margin of infarct, 9 hours
8-24 (up to 48) hr	Initial gross detection of infarct unless hemorrhagic; infarct edematous (swollen), soft, pale, or hemorrhagic and demarcated
1-2 days	Swelling of axons and myelin sheaths; prominent neutrophilic infiltration
2 days	Prominent loss of neuroectodermal cells; continued proliferation of endothelial cells; reduced number of neutrophils; beginning increase in mononuclear cells (gitter cells)
3-5 days	Prominent number of mononuclear cells (gitter cells); disappearance of neutrophils; continued endothelial cell proliferation; number of capillaries appear increased; beginning of astrocytic proliferation (often at margin of infarct)
5-7 days	Grossly, swelling of infarct reaches maximum
8-10 days	Reduction in gross swelling of infarct; liquefaction necrosis; prominent number of mononuclear cells (gitter cells); continued endothelial cell proliferation; beginning fibroblastic activity with collagen formation, variable but most prominent in central nervous system tissue adjacent to the meninges; beginning increase of astroglial fiber production, 5-13 days
3 wk-6 mo	Mononuclear cells decreased; astroglial fiber density increased (especially at margin); astrocytic proliferation reduced; astrocytes return to original appearance; cystic stage of infarct, 2-4 months; vascular network may be present within cyst; endothelial cell proliferation reduced

*The degree of astrocytic injury will depend on location (e.g., central or peripheral) of the cells within the infarct.
†Obviously, thrombosis may occur earlier than 6 hours. This is the time when it may initially be prominent.

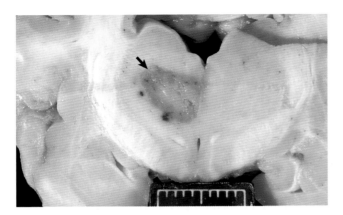

Fig. 14-28   Central nervous system infarct, brain, thalamus, dog. A focal, sharply demarcated area of yellow discoloration and malacia (softening) *(arrow)* in the left central thalamus is most likely an infarct. Scale bar = 2 cm. *(Courtesy Dr. R. Storts, College of Veterinary Medicine, Texas A&M University.)*

CENTRAL NERVOUS SYSTEM SWELLING AND EDEMA

CONGESTIVE BRAIN SWELLING

Congestive brain swelling, as distinguished from cerebral edema, is thought to represent, at least in part, an unregulated vasodilation following trauma, and it can cause serious brain damage (even more severe than the primary injury) if not properly controlled. This lesion therefore represents an enlargement of the brain resulting in elevated intracranial pressure caused by the increased diameter of the blood-containing vasculature, whereas edema results in an increased pressure following accumulation of fluid in the interstitium or intracellularly outside the circulation. Acute brain swelling can be localized (usually of lesser significance) when associated with focal lesions or generalized (often serious) when caused by diffuse brain injury. Although rarely seen in domestic animals, one exception to the importance of focal lesions is extracerebral hemorrhage (acute subdural hematoma in human beings), which—though principally involving the surface of one hemisphere—can cause more mass effect (brain swelling) in the underlying cerebral hemisphere than the hematoma itself. In such circumstances (acute subdural hematoma) the small amount of blood in the subarachnoid space is not the sole reason for the patient's neurologic state. If the hematoma is removed, the acute brain swelling can progress so rapidly that the brain protrudes (herniates) through the craniotomy site.

The more serious forms of diffuse brain injury are associated with generalized acute brain swelling. It is sometimes difficult to determine the relative importance of swelling in affected individuals because initial acute swelling (detectable as soon as 30 minutes after

injury in human beings) can be followed after several hours to days by true cerebral edema (as a result of increased vascular permeability), which can be the actual deleterious lesion. Peroxidative injury to blood vessels has been one proposed cause of pathologic vasodilation in the posttraumatic CNS.

CEREBRAL EDEMA

The basis of our current understanding of cerebral edema was advanced by Klatzo in 1967 when he proposed two distinct types: (1) cytotoxic edema or cell swelling caused by increased intracellular fluid with normal vascular permeability and (2) vasogenic edema or tissue swelling caused by increased extracellular fluid resulting from increased vascular permeability (Fig. 14-29). Other types of cerebral edema have been identified as hydrostatic (or interstitial) edema associated with increased hydrostatic pressure of the CSF (resulting from obstructive internal hydrocephalus) and hypo-osmotic edema, which is dependent on development of an abnormal osmotic gradient between the blood and nervous tissue. The types of edema in the CNS are summarized in Table 14-2. It should be emphasized that, depending on the nature of the injury, multiple mechanisms can contribute to edema in the CNS and these distinctions are not always clearly defined or distinct. For continuity, spongiform change and status spongiosis will also be discussed in this section.

Vᴀꜱᴏɢᴇɴɪᴄ Eᴅᴇᴍᴀ

In animals, vasogenic edema is the most common type of edema in the CNS. It occurs following vascular injury often adjacent to inflammatory foci, hematomas, contusions, infarcts, cerebral hypertension, and neoplasms. The underlying mechanism of vasogenic cerebral edema is a breakdown of the blood-brain barrier that results in movement of plasma constituents, such as water, ions, and organic osmolytes, and proteins into the perivascular extracellular space, particularly that of the white matter (Fig. 14-30, *A*). In addition to extracellular accumulation of fluid, vasogenic edema can also be accompanied by some cellular swelling involving astrocytes. Vasogenic edema with the resulting accumulation of extracellular fluid can cause an increase in intracranial pressure within the CNS. This pressure can also be so severe as to cause neurologic dysfunction and caudal displacement of brain structures, such as the parahippocampal gyri and cerebellar vermis (Figs. 14-86 and 14-87).

Cʏᴛᴏᴛᴏxɪᴄ Eᴅᴇᴍᴀ

Cytotoxic edema is characterized by the accumulation of fluid intracellularly in neurons, astrocytes, oligodendroglia, and endothelial cells (called hydropic degeneration in other cells of the body) as a result

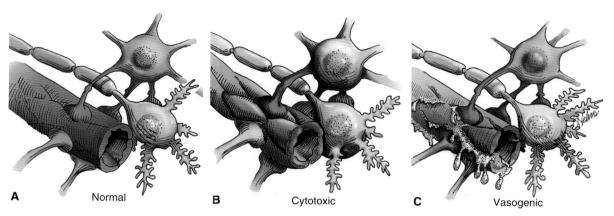

Fig. 14-29   Types of cerebral edema. A, Normal blood-brain barrier. Endothelial cells are red; astrocytes are beige; neurons are light yellow. **B,** Cytotoxic edema. Cytotoxic edema is characterized by the accumulation of fluid intracellularly (in neurons, astrocytes, oligodendroglia, and endothelial cells) as a result of altered cellular metabolism, often caused by ischemia. The gray and white matter are both affected. The fluid taken up by swollen cells is primarily derived from the extracellular space, which becomes reduced in size and has an increased concentration of extracellular solutes. **C,** Vasogenic edema. This type of edema is seen in acute inflammation, and its basic mechanism is an increase in vascular permeability from the breakdown of the blood-brain barrier. This breakdown allows movement of plasma constituents such as water, ions, and plasma proteins into the extracellular space, particularly that of the white matter. (**A, B,** and **C,** *Courtesy Dr. J.F. Zachary, College of Veterinary Medicine, University of Illinois. Based on an illustration from Leech RW, Shuman RM: Neuropathology: a summary for students, Philadelphia, 1982, Harper & Row.*)

Table **14-2**   **Types of Edema in the Central Nervous System**

Type of Edema	Cause	Outcome
Cytotoxic	Altered cellular metabolism (often due to ischemia)	Intracellular accumulation of fluid (neurons, glial cells, endothelial cells)
Vasogenic	Vascular injury with breakdown of the blood-brain barrier	Extracellular accumulation of fluid (cerebrocortical white matter)
Hydrostatic (interstitial)	Elevated ventricular hydrostatic pressure (hydrocephalus)	Extracellular accumulation of fluid (periventricular white matter)
Hypo-osmotic	Osmotic imbalances (blood plasma vs. extracellular and intracellular microenvironments of the central nervous system)	Extracellular and intracellular accumulation of fluid (cerebrocortical gray and white matter)

of altered cellular metabolism, often due to ischemia. Although not all of the cells listed previously may be involved in all cases of cytotoxic edema, affected cells swell within seconds of injury. The mechanism is thought to involve an energy deficit that interferes with normal function of the cell's ATP-dependent sodium-potassium pump. Thus the cell cannot maintain homeostasis, which requires the secretion of intracellular sodium, and the elevated concentration of intracellular sodium and presumably other ions as well as organic osmolytes are followed by an increased influx of water. The gray and white matter of the brain are both affected,

the brain swells, and the sulci and gyri become indistinct and flattened (Fig. 14-31), respectively. The fluid taken up by the swollen cells is primarily derived from the extracellular space, which becomes reduced in size and has an increased concentration of extracellular solutes.

However, for this lesion to be described accurately as cerebral edema, there must be additional fluid movement into the brain and not merely a change of existing fluid from extracellular to intracellular compartments. In practical terms, this is not always the case and can be difficult to determine. The term *cytotoxic edema* has been used rather loosely to refer simply to

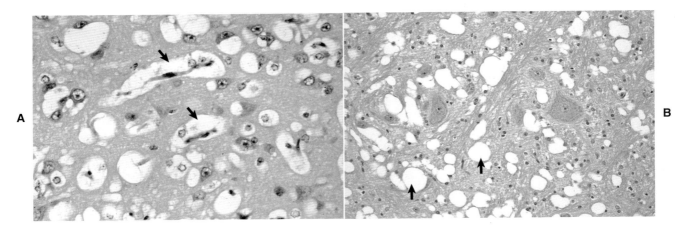

Fig. 14-30   Edema. A, Vasogenic edema. The perivascular spaces are wide as a result of fluid leakage through the blood-brain barrier (*arrows*) (Fig. 14-29). A similar change can be seen around neurons. These fluid-filled spaces are often very difficult to differentiate from artifactual spaces caused by shrinkage from fixation and dehydration in the preparation of the paraffin-embedded sections. H&E stain. **B,** Edema (spongy change, status spongiosis), hepatic encephalopathy, dog. This lesion is characterized by variably sized fluid-filled spaces within the white matter (*arrows*). It can develop by several different mechanisms, which include splitting of myelin sheaths, accumulation of extracellular fluid, and swelling of astrocytic and neuronal cellular processes. Such changes can reflect osmotic imbalances as well as a direct toxic effect on cells (cytotoxic edema). H&E stain. (*A and B, Courtesy Dr. J.F. Zachary, College of Veterinary Medicine, University of Illinois.*)

cellular swelling in many cases. Additional fluid may originate from the circulation by way of the transcapillary fluid exchange or possibly from the CSF, which has extensive diffusional communication with the extracellular fluid of the brain. The blood-brain barrier remains intact during development of this type of edema, so fluid does not enter the brain by a disturbance in vascular permeability. Specific causes of this lesion include hypoxia-ischemia, particularly in the early stages; intoxication with metabolic inhibitors, such as 2,4,dinitrophenol, 6-aminonicatinamide, and ouabain; and severe hypothermia.

INTERSTITIAL (HYDROSTATIC) EDEMA

Interstitial edema is characterized by the accumulation of fluid in the extracellular space of the brain because of elevated ventricular hydrostatic pressure that accompanies hydrocephalus. Fluid moves across the ependyma of the ventricular wall and accumulates extracellularly in the periventricular white matter. Unlike the other forms of cerebral edema that cause swelling of affected CNS tissue, hydrostatic edema causes variable degeneration and loss of the periventricular white matter mostly through primary demyelination accompanied by loss of axons. As the periventricular white matter is reduced in volume, the ventricle expands to fill the void by displacement, thereby exacerbating the hydrocephalus. The blood-brain barrier remains intact in hydrostatic edema.

HYPO-OSMOTIC EDEMA

Hypo-osmotic edema occurs following overconsumption of water (water intoxication) leading to dilution of the osmolality of the plasma. Under normal conditions the osmolality of CSF and extracellular fluid in the CNS is slightly greater than that of plasma. When the osmolality of plasma is further decreased, water moves from the vasculature into the brain following the osmotic gradient resulting in osmotic edema. This form of edema accounts for the clinical signs and lesions in osmotic demyelination syndrome and salt poisoning, as discussed later.

SPONGIFORM CHANGE AND STATUS SPONGIOSUS

Spongiform change is a phrase whose exact meaning varies in different scientific disciplines and experimental situations. In this chapter, wherever possible, spongiform change will be used to describe morphologic changes in H&E stained sections that occur primarily in gray matter. These changes are characterized by small clear vacuoles of varied sizes that form in the cytoplasm of neuron cell bodies and proximal dendrites in diseases such as the transmissible spongiform encephalopathies (TSEs) and rabies encephalitis and in the processes of astrocytes that are spatially related to the affected neurons.

Status spongiosus (spongy degeneration) is also a phrase whose exact meaning varies. It is defined as

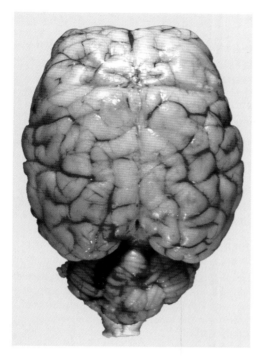

Fig. 14-31   Cerebral edema, polioencephalomalacia, sheep. On the dorsal surface, gyri are swollen and flattened and sulci have become less distinct. Accumulation of extracellular fluid has caused the brain to swell, and because space within the cranial vault is limited, the brain has been pressed against the calvarium. In extreme cases, notable brain swelling can cause caudal displacement of the vermis of the cerebellum and the parahippocampal gyri (Figs. 14-86 and 14-87). Faint yellow discoloration indicates areas of necrosis. *(Courtesy College of Veterinary Medicine, University of Illinois.)*

multiple fluid-filled clear spaces in the white matter of H&E stained sections of the CNS and may be extracellular or intracellular (Fig. 14-30, *B*). This lesion results from the accumulation of edema fluid in the white matter secondary to a variety of causes, including cytotoxic edema, vasogenic edema, intramyelinic edema, Wallerian degeneration, and other hypoxic, toxic, and metabolic diseases.

In some instances the term *spongy degeneration* or *spongy change* has been used in the veterinary literature to describe microscopic lesions in a group of diseases of young dogs, cats, and cows characterized by fluid accumulation in white matter. These diseases will be discussed in later sections.

BARRIER SYSTEMS OF THE CENTRAL NERVOUS SYSTEM

The CNS has several unique structural and functional barrier systems that serve to protect it from diseases affecting the vascular and ventricular systems and to

actively facilitate transfer of necessary molecules, such as glucose, to cells within the CNS.

BLOOD-BRAIN BARRIER

The blood-brain barrier, formed by vascular endothelial cells, endothelial-derived basement membrane, and foot processes of astrocytes, exists in the capillaries of the CNS (Fig. 14-16). The most important structural component of the blood-brain barrier is the tight junctions between endothelial cells of cerebral capillaries. By means of the blood-brain barrier, the CNS can selectively regulate its extracellular compartment and isolate itself from sudden biochemical changes that may occur in the systemic circulation. In the majority of the CNS, endothelial cells are nonfenestrated and are held together by intercellular tight junctions. These tight junctions actively prevent the movement of protein, hydrophilic molecules, and ions from capillary lumina into the intercellular compartment of the CNS. Endothelial cells also have a transmembrane lipophilic pathway for the diffusion of small lipid molecules and numerous highly selective polarized receptor-mediated transport systems for molecules such as insulin, transferrin, glucose, purines, and amino acids. Finally, endothelial cells express a net negative charge on their abluminal side and at the basement membrane, providing an additional selective mechanism that impedes movement of anionic molecules such as chloride ions across the barrier. Foot processes of astrocytes cover more than 90% percent of the abluminal surface of capillary endothelial cells. Experimental evidence suggests that secretion of growth factors from astrocytes promotes the formation and maintenance of the blood-brain barrier.

Capillaries in the area postrema, median eminence, neurohypophysis, pineal body, subfornical organ, commissural organ, and supraoptic crest lack tight junctions and are fenestrated; thus the blood-brain barrier is absent at these sites.

GLIA LIMITANS

The CNS is separated from the subarachnoid CSF by the pia mater and the glia limitans (Fig. 14-16). The glia limitans, which covers the outer surface of the brain and spinal cord and is situated immediately subjacent to the pia mater, consists of astrocytic fibers with many foot processes that form a distinct layer that lies subjacent to the pia mater. In many areas the pia is only one-cell-layer thick and has fenestrations, so that the glia limitans is exposed directly to the subarachnoid space. As arterioles penetrate the cerebral cortex to supply the CNS with blood, they carry the pia mater and surrounding glia limitans with them until the arteriole structurally and functionally becomes a capillary. At the capillary level, the pia mater disappears but the layer of pericapillary astrocytic foot processes remains and serves as a component of the blood-brain barrier. This transition zone occurs at a depth approximately 1 to 3 mm within the cerebral cortex.

BLOOD-CEREBROSPINAL FLUID BARRIER

The blood-CSF barrier is formed by the choroid plexus and the arachnoid. This barrier is formed by tight junctions between apposing surfaces of choroid plexus epithelial cells that cover the choroid plexuses. As noted previously, blood vessels of the choroid plexus are fenestrated. The barrier formed by tight junctions between choroid plexus epithelial cells restricts the movement of molecules that leak from fenestrated capillaries into the extracellular compartment of the choroid plexus and then into the CSF. Similarly, the arachnoid membrane also has tight junctions that prevent the movement of molecules from the blood into the CSF. The arachnoid membrane is generally impermeable to hydrophilic molecules but lacks specialized transport systems, and its role in forming the blood-CSF barrier is largely passive.

CEREBROSPINAL FLUID-BRAIN BARRIER (EPENDYMAL BARRIER)

The CNS is separated from ventricular CSF by ependymal epithelial cells and foot processes of astrocytes. Although the ependymal lining does form a cellular barrier of sorts, materials within the ventricular system can without too much difficulty penetrate into the brain. The CSF-brain barrier is far more permeable than the blood-brain barrier.

DEFENSE MECHANISMS OF THE CENTRAL NERVOUS SYSTEM

Although infectious agents have developed unique approaches to gain entry into the CNS, the body has also evolved a strong suite of defense mechanisms to protect the CNS against infectious pathogens and disease processes. The skin and mucous membranes of the alimentary, respiratory, and urinary systems provide structural and functional barriers against disease. The inflammatory response, immune system, and monocyte-macrophage system provide a strong local and systemic defense against pathogen replication and disease spread. Finally, barrier systems in the CNS, reviewed in an earlier section, represent structural and functional protection against a wide range of pathogens and toxic injuries. These defense mechanisms are summarized in Box 14-5.

INFLAMMATION OF THE CENTRAL NERVOUS SYSTEM

Inflammation of the CNS is different from inflammation in other organs because of the presence of the blood-brain barrier. Under normal conditions, this

---

Box 14-5

Defense Mechanisms against Injury and Infectious Agents in the Central Nervous System

SKIN
Structural and functional (secretions) barrier

CALVARIUM, VERTEBRAE
Structural barrier

MENINGES, CEREBROSPINAL FLUID
Structural and functional (continuous flow of cerebrospinal fluid [CSF]) barrier

BARRIER SYSTEMS
Blood-brain barrier
Structural and functional barrier formed by vascular endothelium, basement membrane, and astrocytic foot processes. This barrier regulates the movement of agents from the blood to the central nervous system (CNS).

Blood-CSF barrier
Structural and functional barrier formed by choroid plexuses cells and the arachnoid membrane. This barrier regulates movement of agents from the blood to the CSF.

GLIA LIMITANS
Formed by astrocytic foot processes immediately subjacent to the pia mater. This structure may have some barrier function in preventing movement of microbes from CSF into the CNS through the pia mater.

MICROGLIA, TRAFFICKING MACROPHAGES
Resident and migrating cells that are part of the monocyte-macrophage system.

IMMUNOLOGIC RESPONSES
Innate and adaptive immunologic responses that form the body's overall immune system.

---

barrier provides limited isolation of the CNS from circulating cellular and humoral elements of the immune system. Macrophages (monocytes) and T lymphocytes can penetrate an intact blood-brain barrier and enter the perivascular and subarachnoid spaces, transit these spaces, and return to the circulation in a role of protective immunologic surveillance of the CNS.

It is important to remember that inflammation in the CNS is regulated by a complex system of recognition and adhesion molecules, cytokines, chemokines, and their corresponding receptors (review Chapters 3 and 4). In particular within the CNS, chemokines and their receptors regulate physiologic and pathologic leukocyte trafficking and cellular migration events.

When pathogens use one of the four portals of entry to gain access to the CNS, the inflammatory process that ensues disrupts the blood-brain barrier. Thus in addition to inflammation, edema and hemorrhage can result. Selectins and integrins in cooperation with chemokines are active in initiating and regulating the acute inflammatory response and the movement of neutrophils across the blood-brain barrier in response to a variety of pathogens. Migration of inflammatory cells within the CNS is poorly understood. Chemotactic gradients are likely established by chemokines that diffuse from sites of production within foci of inflammation. Activated glial cells, including astrocytes and resident microglia, form chemokine networks in areas of inflammation in response to cytokines produced by T lymphocytes that recognize foreign antigens.

Depending on the type of antigen and the pathogenicity of the infectious agent, the inflammatory response will resolve (heal) or progress to a chronic or granulomatous phase with attempts at resolution and clearance of the infectious agent. In the CNS, the type of inflammatory response can vary with the cause. A rather simplistic guideline, to which there are always exceptions, that compares the type of inflammation with different causal agents is as follows:

1. Serous to suppurative or purulent responses can be due to several species of bacteria.
2. Eosinophil responses occur in salt poisoning of pigs and with parasitic larval migration.
3. Lymphocytic, monocytic/macrophage, nonsuppurative, lymphomonocytic, and lymphohistiocytic responses can be due to viruses and certain protozoa.
4. Granulomatous response can be due to fungi, certain protozoa, and some higher-order bacteria, such as the *Mycobacterium* spp.

PORTALS OF ENTRY INTO THE CENTRAL NERVOUS SYSTEM

Disease processes of the CNS enter the brain and spinal cord through one of four principal portals (Box 14-6). These portals include: (1) direct extension, (2) hematogenous entry, (3) leukocytic trafficking, and (4) retrograde axonal transport.

DIRECT EXTENSION

Direct extension is a common portal of entry and includes a wide range of disease processes. Penetrating trauma through the calvarium or vertebrae as a result of a gunshot wound or other forms of trauma can provide a direct portal into the CNS. Disease processes can also extend into the brain and/or spinal cord as a result of: (1) a middle and/or inner ear infection (Fig. 14-32),

---

Box 14-6

Portals of Entry into the Central Nervous System

DIRECT EXTENSION

Penetrating trauma through the calvarium or vertebral bodies

Extension of middle and/or inner ear infection

Extension of a nasal cavity/sinus infection through the cribriform plate or calvarium

Extension from osteomyelitis

HEMATOGENOUS

Localization within capillary beds of the meninges and parenchyma of the central nervous system (CNS)

Localization within capillary beds of the choroid plexuses and extension into the cerebrospinal fluid

LEUKOCYTIC TRAFFICKING

Macrophages or lymphocytes (containing microbes) during their migration through the CNS

RETROGRADE AXONAL TRANSPORT

Transported from the periphery into the CNS by neuronal retrograde axoplasmic flow

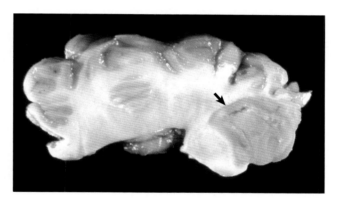

Fig. 14-32   Chronic bacterial abscess, leptomeninges of the cerebellum, sheep. The abscess (*arrow*) resulted from direct extension of infection from an inner ear infection and compresses and distorts the cerebellum. It is walled off from the adjacent cerebellum by a distinct fibrous capsule synthesized by fibroblasts from the adjacent leptomeninges. This abscess likely arose in the leptomeninges of the cerebellum and grew to compress adjacent cerebellum. (*Courtesy College of Veterinary Medicine, University of Illinois.*)

(2) nasal cavity/sinus infection or neoplasia through the cribriform plate or calvarium (Fig. 14-33), or (3) bacterial osteomyelitis or neoplasia of vertebral bodies with extension through the vertebrae into the vertebral canal.

Benign growths of the calvarium and vertebrae, such as osteomas, chondromas, and osteochondromas, often

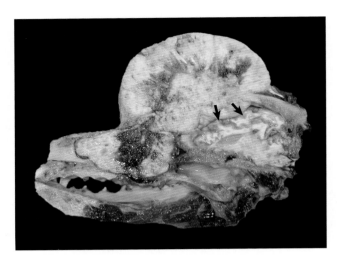

Fig. 14-33   Osteochondrosarcoma, calvarium, dog. The neoplasm has destroyed and penetrated the calvarium and compressed the cerebral hemispheres *(arrows)*. There is also invasion of frontal or nasal sinuses and nasal cavity. *(Courtesy Dr. K. Bailey, College of Veterinary Medicine, University of Illinois.)*

extend into and compress the brain and spinal cord. One specific neoplasm, the multilobular osteoma, has been described as originating from the periosteum of the canine skull. Also, malignant neoplasms adjacent to the cranium or spinal column can cause injury by direct invasion. Some examples include extracranial osteosarcoma and fibrosarcoma in the dog. Also, malignant melanoma of the soft palate in the dog and melanoma involving the paravertebral lymph nodes in the horse can invade adjacent CNS tissue. Other examples of direct extension include lymphosarcoma affecting the spinal cord in the bovine species and less frequently involving the spinal cord or brain in the dog and cat and carcinomas of the ethmoidal area and nasal cavity.

HEMATOGENOUS ENTRY

The most common portal of entry into the CNS is the blood stream. In neonates, infectious agents such as *Escherichia coli* can enter the blood through the umbilical vein or through the venous system following surgical procedures, such as castration. A CNS disease in cows called thrombotic meningoencephalitis is caused by *Histophilus somni* (formerly *Haemophilus somnus*) bacteremia with localization of bacteria in blood vessels of the brain, which leads to vasculitis, hemorrhage, and thrombosis (Fig. 14-27). In adult animals, sites of chronic inflammation, such as abscesses, bacterial skin disease, and ear infections, can also serve as sustained sources of bacteria, which can enter the venous system and spread to distant sites through the blood stream hematogenously.

Capillary beds of the meninges, neuropil, and choroid plexuses are common sites for localization of

specific infectious agents. Such localization patterns may be attributable to receptor-mediated phenomena or vascular flow patterns related to the size of the infectious pathogen. Additionally the blood stream is also a portal of entry into the CNS for metastasizing tumors, such as hemangiosarcoma and a variety of carcinomas.

LEUKOCYTIC TRAFFICKING

As part of the systemic immunologic surveillance system, macrophages (monocytes) and lymphoid cells continually move in and out of capillary beds in the CNS and thus serve as sentinel cells monitoring for the presence of disease processes within the brain and spinal cord. As examples, retroviruses, such as feline leukemia virus, and mycotic agents, such as *Blastomyces dermatitidis*, have stages of their life cycles within the cytoplasm of lymphocytes or macrophages. During the movement of lymphocytes and macrophages in and out of the CNS, cells infected with such agents are activated to release their infectious contents and infect cells of the CNS.

RETROGRADE AXONAL TRANSPORT

Retrograde axonal transport provides a unique portal of entry for viruses such as rabies and the bacterium *Listeria monocytogenes*. These pathogens replicate in tissues richly innervated with receptors and motor end plates from sensory and motor neurons, respectively, which provide a connection between peripheral infection and the CNS. Retrograde axoplasmic flow is then used to gain entry into the CNS (Fig. 14-6).

DISEASES

MALFORMATIONS

NEURAL TUBE CLOSURE DEFECTS (DYSRAPHIA)

Dysraphia literally means an abnormal seam, and these anomalies appear to result from defective interaction of neuroepithelium with adjacent notochordal and mesenchymal cells during closure of the neural tube in the early stages of development. Neuroepithelium is the progenitor cell for neurons and astrocytes, oligodendrocytes, and ependymal cells.

Experimental studies of closure of the neural tube show that it occurs at four distinct locations called closure initiation sites in the embryo, and disruption of this process at these sites leads to site-specific dysraphic anomalies. Closure site I contributes to the posterior neuropore (the opening at the posterior end of the embryonic neural canal), whereas closure sites II to IV contribute to the anterior neuropore (the opening at the anterior end of the embryonic neural canal). Anencephaly is caused by a failure of closure sites II or IV; spina bifida is caused by a failure of closure site I. Genes possibly involved in neural tube closure defects include those of the folate metabolic pathway and folate transport.

Dysraphic anomalies, also called neural tube closure defects, in animals are typified by anencephaly and prosencephalic hypoplasia, cranium bifidum, and spina bifida.

ANENCEPHALY AND PROSENCEPHALIC HYPOPLASIA

Anencephaly literally means an absence of the brain, but in many instances of so-called anencephaly only the rostral part of the brain (cerebral hemispheres) is absent, or very rudimentary, and to varying degrees the brain stem is preserved. Thus this abnormality is best-designated prosencephalic hypoplasia. Such anomalies result from an abnormal development of the rostral aspect of the neural tube. Although the cause for these anomalies is largely unknown, anencephaly has been reported to be associated with anomalies in other body systems in calves. Additionally, anencephaly—following initial cranium bifidum and exencephaly (protrusion of brain not covered by skin or meninges)—has been reported to occur in rat fetuses after exposure of the pregnant dam to excessive concentrations of vitamin A and cyclophosphamide.

MENINGOENCEPHALOCELE AND CRANIUM BIFIDUM

Cranium bifidum is characterized by a dorsal midline cranial defect through which meningeal and brain tissue can protrude. The protruded material, which forms a sac (-cele), is covered by skin and can be lined by meninges (meningocele) or meninges accompanied by a part of the brain (meningoencephalocele) (Fig. 14-34). These malformations are hereditary in pigs and cats and are also caused by griseofulvin treatment in pregnant cats during the first week of gestation.

MENINGOMYELOCELE AND SPINA BIFIDA

Spina bifida is the vertebral counterpart of cranium bifidum. This lesion, which frequently tends to affect the caudal spine, is characterized by a dorsal defect in the closure of one to several vertebral arches that form the dorsal spinal column covering the spinal cord. The lesion results from a failure of the neural tube and developing vertebral arches to close properly, which may result in herniation of either meninges (meningocele) or meninges and spinal cord (meningomyelocele) through the defect, forming a sac covered with skin. In some cases there is no herniation of the meninges or spinal cord through the defect, and this variation is termed spina bifidum occulta (Fig. 14-35). In this variation, there is an absence of skin over the affected vertebral arches, vertebral musculature is visible, and the dura mater and spinal cord can be seen in the spinal canal.

Spina bifida has been reported in several species, including horses, calves, sheep, dogs (especially

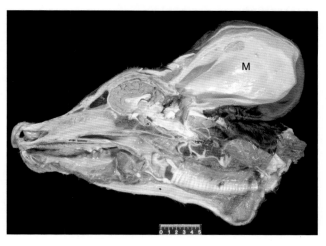

Fig. 14-34   Meningocele (M), brain, calf. A defect in the caudodorsal portion of the skull has allowed the meninges to herniate into a large external pouch covered by skin. The pouch contains fluid and is lined by arachnoid and dura, which are continuous with those surrounding the brain. The cerebellum is small and the occipital cortex truncated. Scale bar = 5 cm. *(Courtesy Dr. R. Storts, College of Veterinary Medicine, Texas A&M University.)*

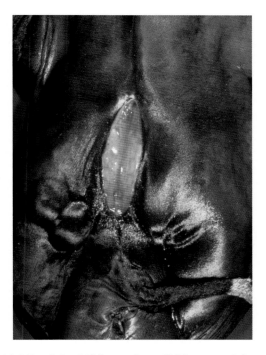

Fig. 14-35   Spina bifida occulta, calf. There is a cleft in several vertebrae of the dorsal spinal column resulting from defective closure of the neural tube. Although not always the case, note the lack of herniation of the meninges or spinal cord through the defect. The spinal cord is not visible (i.e., occulta) because it is located in the vertebral canal at the deepest ventral extent of the cleft and is covered by edematous muscle. *(Courtesy Dr. M.D. McGavin, College of Veterinary Medicine, University of Tennessee.)*

English bulldogs), and cats, particularly the Manx breed, in which it is inherited as an autosomal dominant trait. An additional lesion, myeloschisis, is similar to spina bifida except in its severe form it results from failure of the entire spinal neural tube to close. This lesion is therefore characterized by lack of development of the entire dorsal vertebral column.

HYDROMYELIA

Congenital hydromyelia is an abnormal dilatation of the central canal of the spinal cord (Fig. 14-36) that leads to the formation of a cavity in which CSF may accumulate. In animals, this disorder likely results from infectious or genetic injury that results in damage to ependymal cells lining the canal and the subsequent disruption of the normal flow of CSF and the formation of abnormal CSF pressure gradients within the central canal. As CSF accumulates in the enlarging space, the increased pericanalicular pressure placed on the spinal cord compresses the white and gray matter, leading to loss of white matter and possibly neurons in gray matter. Acquired hydromyelia is rare and is caused by obstruction of the central canal CSF flow. Causes of obstruction include infection, inflammation, and neoplasia.

Clinical signs in young animals with congenital hydromyelia vary depending on the location and size of the dilatation of the central canal in the spinal cord. Signs may include ataxia, urinary incontinence, respiratory difficulty, muscle weakness in front and/or hind limbs, and abnormal proprioceptive reflexes.

NEURONAL MIGRATION DISORDERS
LISSENCEPHALY

Lissencephaly (agyria) and a similar change called pachygyria (large gyri) are developmental anomalies that result in a part or the entire cerebrum having smooth surfaces lacking normal gyri and sulci (Fig. 14-37). The cortex is thicker than normal on a transverse section, and the normal laminar pattern of neurons is disrupted.

This lesion is thought to have a genetic basis and results from an arrest of or defect in neuronal migration during development. Recent experimental studies suggest that this migrational disorder is linked to mutations and/or deletions in the doublecortin, filamin-1, LIS1, and reelin genes. These genes control the spatial and temporal expression of proteins in the extracellular microenvironment that subsequently bind to receptors on migrating cells. Patterns of cell membrane binding signals are interpreted by migrating cells and are reflected in their movements by changes in intracellular cytoskeletal reorganization. This process allows cells to migrate to their final destinations within the CNS. Thus alterations in signaling pathways lead to abnormal neuronal migration and CNS anomalies.

The brains of some laboratory animals, such as rabbits, rats, and mice, lack gyri and sulci; therefore agyria is normal in these species and has no functional significance.

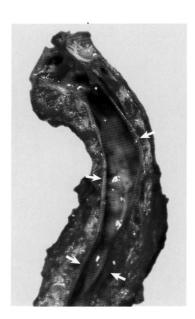

Fig. 14-36   End-stage hydromyelia, spinal cord, dog. The white and gray matter of the spinal cord are missing as a result of compression atrophy from a space-occupying, fluid-filled central canal. The only recognizable remnants of nervous tissue is the dura *(arrows)*. In less severely affected animals, there would be variable dilatation of the central canal of the spinal cord with much less severe compression atrophy. *(Courtesy College of Veterinary Medicine, University of Tennessee.)*

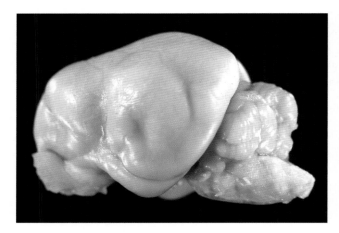

Fig. 14-37   Lissencephaly, brain, dog. Note the smooth surfaces of the cerebral hemispheres, which are without gyri and sulci. Gyri and sulci fail to form, possibly from failure of neuronal development and migration. Lissencephaly is an abnormality in domestic animals, but is normal in mice, rats, rabbits, and birds. *(Courtesy Dr. L. Roth, College of Veterinary Medicine, Cornell University.)*

ENCEPHALOCLASTIC DEFECTS
PORENCEPHALY AND HYDRANENCEPHALY

The formation of fluid-filled cavities in the brain, termed porencephaly (small cavities) and hydranencephaly (large cavities), usually occurs in utero during gestation. *Porencephaly* refers to a cleft or cyst in the wall of the cerebral hemisphere that typically communicates with the subarachnoid space, but it can also communicate with a lateral ventricle. The cavitation results from destruction of immature neuroblasts whose loss prevents normal development as a result of faulty or aberrant neuroblast migration. Hydranencephaly is considered a severe form of porencephaly and is characterized by cavitation in areas normally occupied by the white matter of the cerebral hemispheres and results from improper development of this part of the cerebrum. Hydranencephaly is often quite severe, with very little tissue present between the dilated lateral ventricles and the leptomeninges.

Type I and type II porencephaly have been described in human infants, and cases of porencephaly reported in animals can also be categorized using this scheme. Type I porencephaly is caused by vascular injury or vasculitis. Injury, resulting in infarction in the area of the subependymal germinal matrix, results in the formation of a cyst within the focus of dead cells and effete erythrocytes. The germinal matrix is very sensitive to ischemia because of sparse stroma, delicate vasculature, and high metabolism. The initial focus of hemorrhage can grow by centripetal expansion, depending on the severity of hemorrhage and hypoxia, into a cyst of considerable size. Type II porencephaly is caused by injury of neuroblasts in the germinal matrix and the failure of these neuroblasts to migrate within the matrix to form the cerebral cortex. A cyst results from the expansion of the subarachnoid space into the void left by the absence of the cortex.

Type II porencephaly appears to be the form of porencephaly that occurs in domestic animals. Viruses, such as those that cause Akabane disease, bovine virus diarrhea, blue tongue, border disease, Rift Valley fever, and Wesselsbron disease infect and destroy differentiating neuroblasts and neuroglial cells in the developing fetus in utero. Although neuroblasts appear to be the primary target for viral infection in these diseases, additional experimental studies need to be conducted to clarify whether endothelial cells are also infected.

Grossly, porencephaly/hydranencephaly appears as thin-walled fluid-filled cysts of varied sizes in the cerebral hemispheres. Because of the lack of brain substance, the ventricles expand into this space (hydrocephalus ex vacuo), and the ependymal lining remains relatively preserved or may have scattered defects characterized by absent ependyma. The cranium and meninges are generally unaltered. In some cases, cerebellar hypoplasia (all or part of the cerebellum) and hypoplasia of the spinal cord may also occur. Microscopically, necrosis of undifferentiated cells, including potential neuroblasts and neuroglia, surrounding a fluid-filled cavity is present in the subventricular zone of the cerebral hemispheres. Degeneration and loss of motor neurons of the ventral horns of the spinal cord may also be observed. This lesion may result in denervation atrophy of limb muscles with a resultant lack of joint movement and arthrogryposis, a persistent congenital flexure or contraction of a joint. Nonsuppurative encephalitis, typified by the accumulation of macrophages, lymphocytes, and plasma cells, also occurs.

MALFORMATIONS OF THE CEREBELLUM
CEREBELLAR HYPOPLASIA

In animals the most common causes of cerebellar hypoplasia are parvoviruses (kittens [panleukopenia virus {Fig. 14-38}], puppies [canine parvovirus]), and pestiviruses (calves [bovine virus diarrhea virus {Fig. 14-39}], piglets [classical swine fever virus]). These viruses infect

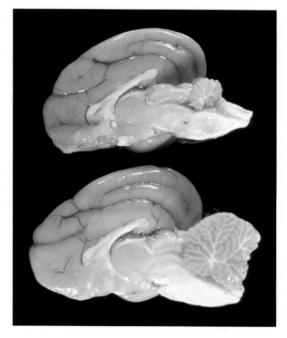

Fig. 14-38   Cerebellar hypoplasia, brain, cat. In the cat, cerebellar hypoplasia (cerebellar hypoplasia, top specimen; normal cat, bottom specimen) most commonly is the result of in utero infection with feline panleukopenia virus (parvovirus). The virus infects and causes lysis of dividing cells in the external granular layer (on the outside of the cerebellum in the fetus). Because these cells are no longer available to migrate to form the (internal) granular layer, the cerebellum remains small. *(Courtesy Dr. Y. Niyo, College of Veterinary Medicine, Iowa State University; and Noah's Arkive, College of Veterinary Medicine, The University of Georgia.)*

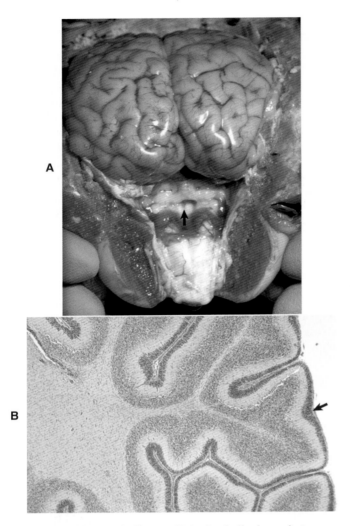

Fig. 14-39   Cerebellum, calf. A, Cerebellar hypoplasia *(arrow)*. In utero infection with bovine viral diarrhea virus (pestivirus) results in cytolysis of dividing germinal cells of the external granular layer (Fig. 14-39, B) and vascular impairment secondary to vasculitis of the cerebellum during organogenesis. The severity of the lesion involving the granule cells is at its greatest if dividing cells are infected during the earliest stages of cellular differentiation, and occurs between 100 to 180 days of gestation. **B,** Normal neonatal calf, external granular layer of the cerebellum *(arrow)*. Although many of these cells migrate to form the (internal) granular layer, some are still present at the time of birth in many domestic animals. Bovine viral diarrhea virus infects and kills mitotic cells of the external granular layer of the cerebellum. These cells are still dividing during the late gestational and early neonatal periods in the cat and between 100 to 180 days of gestation in the calf. Necrosis of these cells means they are not available to migrate to form the internal granular layer, and thus the cerebellum does not obtain full size. Depending on the stage of gestation, injury can also alter development of cells in others ways including altered patterns of migration, resulting in various other lesions termed dysplasia. H&E stain. (**A** and **B,** Courtesy Dr. M.D. McGavin, College of Veterinary Medicine, University of Tennessee.)

and destroy mitotic cells, primarily the cells of the external granular layer of the cerebellum that are still dividing during the late gestational and early neonatal periods. Necrosis of these cells means they are not available to migrate to form the internal granular layer, and thus the cerebellum is hypoplastic. In calves the cerebellar lesion (cerebellar hypoplasia/atrophy), which follows infection at 150 days of gestation (mid trimester), is considered to involve two processes. One process is typified by early necrosis of the undifferentiated cells in the external granular layer. A second process involves viral-induced vasculitis and ischemia of cerebellar folial white matter.

Grossly the size of the cerebellum is reduced; the reduction in size varies in severity depending on the age and developmental stage of the brain when the fetus or neonate is infected.

Microscopically there is necrosis and loss of the external granular layer and degeneration and loss of Purkinje cells that are postmitotic but immature. Reasons for degeneration of Purkinje cells might include infection by the virus or lack of normal development of the cerebellar cortex. The Purkinje cells can also be malpositioned and located in the molecular layer as a result of the viral-induced alteration in development of the cerebellar cortex. In calves, edema of the folial white matter with focal hemorrhage in the cortex, followed by focal cavitation of the white matter and atrophy, may also be present. These latter lesions are due to ischemia resulting from vasculitis. Leptomeningitis, characterized by accumulation of lymphocytes and plasma cells and occasionally fibroplasia, may cause adhesions between adjacent cerebellar folia and focal obliteration of the subarachnoid space.

MALFORMATIONS OF THE SPINAL CORD
SYRINGOMYELIA

Syringomyelia (congenital and acquired forms) is a disorder in which a cyst forms in the spinal cord. The cyst, a tubular cavitation called a syrinx, is not lined by ependyma and is separate from the central canal. The syrinx can extend over several spinal cord segments. The lesion is well known in human beings and has also been described in the dog (Weimaraner breed) and calves. The syrinx can communicate with the central canal but should not be confused with hydromyelia, which means dilatation of the central canal. The cavity contains fluid and is unlined, except for varying degrees of mural astrocytosis, which is usually very mild in the Weimaraner. Proposed causes include presence of an anomalous vascular pattern that results in low-grade ischemia, leading to infarction or failure of cells destined for this area to develop in utero trauma in human beings or an infection that causes degeneration and cavitation. A rare acquired form of syringomyelia is similar to congenital syringomyelia; however, it occurs in older animals. Proposed causes include injury following trauma to the central canal or its vascular supply caused by trauma, infection, or neoplasia that result in degeneration and cavitation of the spinal cord.

Although the central canal of the spinal cord is connected to the ventricular system via the fourth ventricle, there apparently is little active movement of CSF within the central canal. Recently it has been hypothesized that there may be alteration of "normal" CSF flow (see Ependyma, under Cells of the Central Nervous System) with redirection of the flow along a pressure gradient into the central canal and into the syrinx. It has also been suggested that pressure differences in the vertebral column cause CSF to continually move into the cyst, resulting in enlargement of the syrinx and additional compressive damage to the spinal cord.

Clinical signs in young dogs and calves with syringomyelia vary depending on the location and size of the cyst in the spinal cord. Signs may include ataxia, urinary incontinence, respiratory difficulty, muscle weakness in front and/or hind limbs, and abnormal proprioceptive reflexes.

HYDROCEPHALUS

The most common congenital malformations and developmental anomalies in veterinary medicine affecting cells that form the ependyma and choroid plexuses are hydrocephalus, hydromyelia, and syringomyelia. These anomalies will be covered in greater detail later. Of these anomalies, hydrocephalus is the anomaly most likely to be caused by in utero injury following viral infection of the developing fetus. However, in some breeds (brachycephalic breeds), these disorders may have a genetic predisposition, but this mechanism of injury has not been as clearly established in domestic animals as it has in human beings.

In laboratory animals, several neonatal in utero viral infections, including mumps virus, reovirus type I, and parainfluenza virus types I and II, can induce congenital hydrocephalus. Parainfluenza virus can also cause the lesion in the dog. Although there are some differences among the different viral infections, the basic lesion is stenosis of the mesencephalic duct (aqueduct of Sylvius in human beings, mesencephalic aqueduct) that results in the development of noncommunicating hydrocephalus. In the dog, closure of the mesencephalic duct can be incomplete. The virus grows in and causes destruction of ependymal cells lining the ventricular system. The infection is initially accompanied by an inflammation that resolves within 2 weeks.

The notable lesion resulting from this injury to the ependyma of the mesencephalic duct is its occlusion. This end-stage lesion is not the result of an astroglial response or due to the presence of viral antigen.

Instead, the original ependyma-lined aqueduct is replaced by focal aggregates of remaining ependymal cells that have separated from the adjacent tissue, which appears normal. The appearance of the final lesion is therefore more suggestive of an agenesis than a viral infection. Infection of adult laboratory animals (mice with influenza viral infection) also can induce mesencephalic duct stenosis resulting in hydrocephalus, but in contrast to neonatal infection, there is a persistent astroglial response in the area of stenosis.

CONGENITAL HYDROCEPHALUS

CSF can accumulate in the ventricular system, the subarachnoid space, or both. The type of hydrocephalus that develops depends on the site of blockage that disrupts normal flow of CSF.

Exactly which portions of the ventricular system will be dilatated in hydrocephalus depends on the site of the blockage:
1. Blockage of the interventricular foramen between a lateral and third ventricular leads to unilateral dilatation of that lateral ventricle.
2. Blockage of both interventricular foramina leads to bilateral dilatation of both lateral ventricles.
3. Blockage of the mesencephalic duct leads to bilateral dilatation of both lateral ventricles, the third ventricle, and the segment of the mesencephalic duct proximal to the blockage.
4. Blockage of the lateral apertures of the fourth ventricle leads to bilateral dilatation of lateral ventricles, the third ventricle, the mesencephalic duct, and the fourth ventricle.
5. Blockage of reabsorption leads to bilateral dilatation of lateral ventricles, the third ventricle, the mesencephalic duct, the fourth ventricle, and the subarachnoid space.

As an example, following blockage of the interventricular foramina, the pressure in the lateral ventricles increases; the ventricles dilate; the ependyma becomes atrophied and focally discontinuous; and because of the pressure gradient, CSF is forced into the periventricular white matter leading to hydrostatic edema. Hydrostatic edema results in degeneration and atrophy of myelin and axons, and this loss of tissue results in further expansion of the ventricles.

The forms of hydrocephalus are communicating and noncommunicating hydrocephalus. Communicating hydrocephalus, the least common of the two forms, occurs when there is communication of ventricular CSF with the subarachnoid space where the CSF can be in excess. Noncommunicating hydrocephalus results from obstruction within the ventricular system at, or rostral to, the lateral apertures of the fourth ventricle. An area of great vulnerability for obstruction is the mesencephalic aqueduct. Noncommunicating hydrocephalus can also occur without any evidence of obstruction to CSF flow as a result of failure of the reabsorption of CSF.

A recent hypothesis proposes that communicating hydrocephalus is caused by a decreased expansion of intracranial arteries during systole as a result of reduced compliance involving the arterial walls, or the subarachnoid space, and is referred to as "restricted arterial pulsation hydrocephalus." Because the intracranial arteries cannot fully expand, a pressure gradient develops in which there is greater pressure within the brain tissue and the ventricles than outside the brain. Several causes have been advanced, including arteritis, subarachnoid hemorrhage, and meningitis.

A third type of hydrocephalus, referred to as hydrocephalus ex vacuo (or compensating hydrocephalus), is not usually a congenital abnormality but occurs secondary to absence or loss of cerebral tissue. This type of hydrocephalus can occur in utero from destruction and loss of cerebral tissue surrounding the lateral ventricles (e.g., in hydranencephaly). Hydrocephalus ex vacuo is discussed further under Acquired Hydrocephalus.

In domestic animals, congenital hydrocephalus can be caused by in utero viral infections leading to aqueductal stenosis (incomplete closure) in the dog that results in the development of noncommunicating hydrocephalus; however, a genetically programmed predisposition may occur in very small and brachycephalic breeds of dogs.

Gross lesions associated with communicating and noncommunicating congenital hydrocephalus include enlargement (doming) of the cranium if obstruction occurs before the sutures have fused (Fig. 14-40).

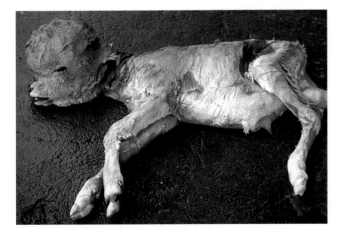

Fig. 14-40   Congenital hydrocephalus, brain, calf. Note the symmetrically enlarged and dome-shaped calvarium. The bone of the calvarium is thinned and distorted from pressure from the expanding brain during gestation. *(Courtesy Dr. J. King, College of Veterinary Medicine, Cornell University.)*

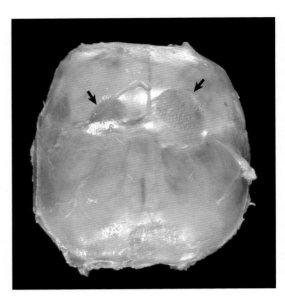

Fig. 14-41   Calvarium, view of the dorsal surface, congenital hydrocephalus, dog. The bone of the calvarium is thin and the fontanelles *(arrows)* are enlarged. The translucent membrane covering the fontanelles is periosteum. *(Courtesy Drs. J. Wright and D. Duncan, College of Veterinary Medicine, North Carolina State University; and Noah's Arkive, College of Veterinary Medicine, The University of Georgia.)*

The bones of the calvarium are extremely thin and the fontanelles are prominent (Fig. 14-41). In the brain there is prominent enlargement of the ventricular system proximal to the point of obstruction (Fig. 14-42). White matter adjacent to the dilated lateral ventricles is reduced in thickness, although the gray matter can retain a relatively normal appearance. As the hydrocephalus progresses, atrophy with fenestration of the interventricular septum (septum pellucidum), atrophy of the hippocampus in the floor of the lateral ventricles, and flattening of cortical gyri can occur. If the obstruction is abrupt and pressure builds rapidly, the cerebral hemispheres can be displaced caudally, causing herniation of the parahippocampal gyri under the tentorium cerebelli and of the vermis of the cerebellum through the foramen magnum. The resulting coning of the cerebellum can be accompanied by necrosis of cells in the cerebellar folia as a result of ischemia and infarction. Microscopically the ependyma can become atrophied and focally discontinuous, and there is loss of cells and cell processes in adjacent white matter and variably in the gray matter.

Clinically, congenital hydrocephalus occurs most frequently in brachycephalic or toy breeds such as the Chihuahua, Lhasa apso, and toy poodle. Clinical signs occur within the first year of life, often before 3 months of age. Behavioral changes are the most common and

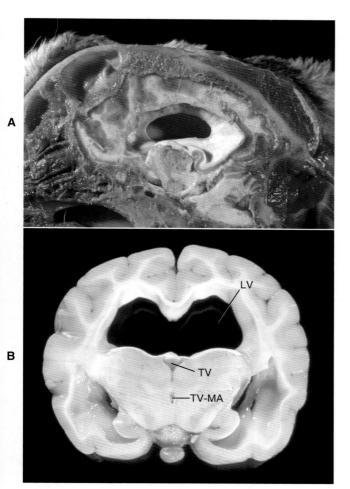

Fig. 14-42 Hydrocephalus, brain, dog. A, Midsagittal section of the head, third ventricle. Note the dilated third and lateral ventricles and the absence of most of the septum pellucidum between the left and right lateral ventricles. **B,** Junction between parietal and occipital lobes, level of thalamus. Bilateral dilation of lateral ventricles dorsally (*LV*), and ventrolaterally. The fornix has separated and lies on the flattened floor of the ventricle. Note that the third ventricle (*TV*) and junctional area between the third ventricle and mesencephalic aqueduct (*TV-MA*) are not enlarged and are possibly even reduced in size, suggesting that the obstruction may be at, or rostral, to this plane of section. (**A,** *Courtesy Dr. M.D. McGavin, College of Veterinary Medicine, University of Tennessee.* **B,** *Courtesy Dr. R. Storts, College of Veterinary Medicine, Texas A&M University.*)

include poor motor skill development; delay in learned behavior, such as house training; somnolence; dullness; episodic confusion; circling; periodic aggression; and seizures.

ACQUIRED HYDROCEPHALUS

Noncommunicating acquired hydrocephalus has been associated with injury of the ependyma, resulting in obstruction of any of the following: the lateral apertures of the fourth ventricle, the cerebral aqueduct, or the interventricular foramen. Causes of obstruction include compression by cerebral abscesses and neoplasms, and blockages by infectious/inflammatory disease resulting in a ventriculitis and, uncommonly, by cholesteatomas in the choroid plexus of the lateral ventricles of the horse. Because the calvarium has now ceased to grow, unlike congenital hydrocephalus, it is of normal size and shape, and its bone is of normal thickness.

A second type of acquired hydrocephalus, referred to as hydrocephalus ex vacuo (or compensating hydrocephalus), usually occurs in the cerebral hemispheres secondary to loss of neural tissue. If there is loss of neurons in the cerebral cortex, as in bovine polioencephalomalacia or other types of laminar cortical necrosis, the axons of these neurons, which normally traverse the white matter of the cerebral hemispheres, will disappear by Wallerian degeneration, and there will be atrophy of the cortex from the loss of neuronal cell bodies and of the white matter from the loss of axons. The lateral ventricles will expand into the space once occupied by white matter. This dilatation of the lateral ventricles may be bilateral when there has been a loss of white and gray matter from both cerebral hemispheres, or it may be unilateral. If the loss of cortex is localized, as in an infarct, then dilatation of the lateral ventricle will not uniformly involve the whole lateral ventricle. Examples of disorders in which hydrocephalus ex vacuo occur include some storage diseases (ceroid-lipofuscinosis in sheep), aging, and postradiation exposure, all of which are associated with cerebral atrophy. There is no evidence of obstruction of the normal flow of CSF in this type of hydrocephalus.

DISEASES CAUSED BY MICROBES
BACTERIA
BRAIN ABSCESSES

Cerebral abscesses in animals are relatively uncommon but arise following entry of bacteria into the CNS. This may occur either from direct extension or hematogenously. With direct extension, abscesses occur following penetrating wounds, such as calvarial fractures, or from spread of infection from adjacent tissues, such as the leptomeninges, paranasal sinuses, and internal ear, and through the cribriform plate of the ethmoid (Fig. 14-12). Diseases that cause bacteremia or septicemia result in infectious agents being trapped in vascular beds within the CNS and meninges. Abscesses usually arise within gray matter because it receives a disproportionate share of blood flow in the CNS, usually at the gray-white (cortex-subcortical white matter) junction. They exert effects in the CNS by disruption and destruction of tissue and by displacement as space-occupying lesions.

If the abscess grows quickly, tissue is more likely to be disrupted and destroyed and in the worst case penetrate the wall of the lateral ventricle and cause a ventriculitis. Bacteria in the CSF may be carried into the subarachnoid space and cause a leptomeningitis. On the other hand, if growth is slow, tissue is more likely to be displaced. Chronic abscesses become encapsulated by either fibrous tissue if they are close to the leptomeninges or by astrocytes away from the meninges. The mechanism of tissue injury is likely a secondary bystander effect related to the actions of the mediators of inflammation and the toxins and other products elaborated from bacteria. Bacteria appear to localize in specific areas of the CNS based on receptor-mediated attachment or because of vascular flow patterns unique to the gray matter–white matter interface of the CNS that allows bacteria to attach to and move through the blood-brain barrier. This latter flow mechanism likely occurs because small blood vessels supplying the cerebrum fail to continue into the white matter and end with their horizontal branches running parallel to the surface of the gyrus within the gray matter at the interface with the white matter. Once within the CNS or meninges, bacteria replicate and elicit an inflammatory response. Lytic enzymes released from lysosomes of neutrophils and other inflammatory cytokines secreted by lymphocytes and macrophages destroy neurons and their processes and disrupt synapses, thus affecting neurotransmission.

Grossly, brain abscesses can be single or multiple, be discrete or coalescing, and have varied sizes (Fig. 14-43). Early in the process, abscesses consist of a white to gray to yellow, thick to granular exudate. The color of the exudate can be influenced by the exuberance of the pyogenic response elicited by the inciting bacteria and by any pigments produced by the bacteria. *Streptococcus* spp., *Staphylococcus* spp., and *Corynebacterium* spp. may produce a pale-yellow to yellow, watery to creamy exudate. Coliforms, such as *Escherichia coli* and *Klebsiella* spp., may produce a white to gray, watery to creamy exudate. *Pseudomonas* spp. may produce a green to bluish-green exudate. The borders of abscesses are often surrounded by a red zone of active hyperemia induced by inflammatory mediators acting on capillary beds. With chronicity, abscesses may be walled off by processes of astrocytes and fibrous connective tissue from the pia mater, especially when the abscess results from a penetrating wound.

Brain abscesses can arise in some food animal species from an extension of otitis interna (Figs. 14-12 and 14-32). These animals often display evidence of facial nerve paralysis, such as a drooping ear. The cerebellopontine angle and adjacent structures are the common locations for such abscesses. In horses, *Streptococcus equi* (strangles) can cause brain abscesses via hematogenous spread from lymphoid tissues (Fig. 14-44). Direct penetration may also occur in small ruminants that lack frontal sinuses because of improper dehorning procedures. Brain abscesses are space-occupying lesions and

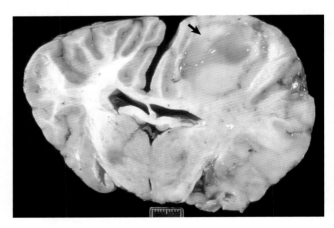

Fig. 14-44 Abscess, right cerebral hemisphere, horse. The cerebral cortex contains an abscess *(arrow)* caused by *Streptococcus equi* entering the central nervous system via the blood (strangles). A fibrous capsule is present on the lateral, medial, and dorsal sides of the abscess (most obvious on the lateral side as a gray band). There is no obvious capsule present on the ventral side (i.e., toward the right lateral ventricle). Microscopically, there would be a thin glial capsule (astrogliosis). Note also the increased size of the right hemisphere with blurring of the distinction between gray and white matter, an indication of edema. Scale bar = 2 cm. *(Courtesy Dr. K. Read, College of Veterinary Medicine, Texas A&M University; and Noah's Arkive, College of Veterinary Medicine, The University of Georgia.)*

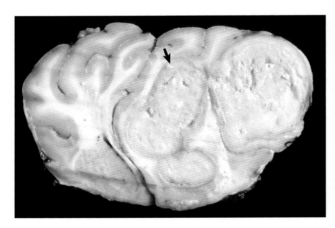

Fig. 14-43 Chronic cerebral abscesses, sheep. Abscesses with caseous centers *(arrow)* have replaced most of the right cerebral hemisphere, enlarged it, and displaced the midline to the left. The abscesses are encapsulated by a thick fibrous capsule generated by fibroblasts of the pia and perivascular spaces of the outer cortex. *(Courtesy Dr. M.D. McGavin, College of Veterinary Medicine, University of Tennessee.)*

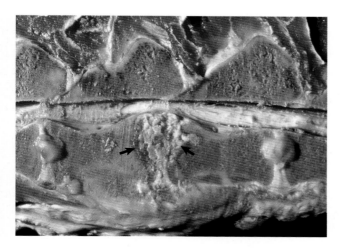

Fig. 14-45   Diskospondylitis, thoracic spinal cord, pig.
This type of abscess *(arrows)* is commonly caused by bacterial emboli that lodge in intervertebral disks or in the body of vertebrae causing osteomyelitis, which can extend into intervertebral disks. Large intervertebral abscesses can compress the spinal cord and cause Wallerian degeneration of nerves, mainly in the ventral funiculi but also in other funiculi. In this case, remodeling and proliferation of the vertebral bone secondary to the infection also contributed to the narrowing of the spinal canal and compression of the spinal cord. *(Courtesy Dr. M.D. McGavin, College of Veterinary Medicine, University of Tennessee.)*

as such can have a devastating effect on brain function. Depending on size and location, compression via mass effect (increased intracranial pressure) of vital structures (nuclei that regulate cardiac and respiratory rhythms) and brain displacements (cerebellar vermis, parahippocampal gyri) are two common sequelae to acute abscesses. Abscesses can occur in the spinal cord as a result of direct extension of bacterial vertebral osteomyelitis through the dura (Fig. 14-45), following tail docking in lambs, and occasionally from hematogenous spread.

Clinically, animals with brain abscesses can show abnormal mental behaviors, ataxia, head tilt, circling, and loss of vision.

DIFFUSE ENCEPHALITIS

Common bacteria have the potential to produce disease in the CNS by hematogenous spread and vasculitis. Also see Neonatal Septicemia.

EPENDYMITIS AND CHOROID PLEXITIS

Infectious agents, especially pus-forming bacteria, such as the coliform and *Streptococcus* spp., can enter the CNS hematogenously or via direct extension, invade the choroid plexuses, and be released into the CSF, gaining access to ependymal cells lining the

ventricular system. Inflammation of the ependyma is called ependymitis, whereas inflammation of the choroid plexus is called choroid plexitis. Gross lesions usually consist of gray-white to yellow-green thick to gelatinous CSF within the ventricular system and choroid plexuses that are granular and gray-white, with areas of active hyperemia and hemorrhage. If the bacteria traverses through the lateral apertures of the fourth ventricle, they can enter and spread throughout the subarachnoid space. possibly inducing suppurative bacterial leptomeningitis. The exudate can also obstruct CSF flow, leading to noncommunicating hydrocephalus. Microscopically, inflammatory cells, especially neutrophils, mixed with fibrin, hemorrhage, and bacteria, can be seen in the exudate.

LISTERIOSIS

Listeriosis, a bacterial disease with particular affinity for the CNS, is seen mainly in domestic ruminants. There is compelling evidence that *Listeria monocytogenes*, a facultative intracellular gram-positive bacterium, invades through the mucosa of the oral cavity and into sensory and motor branches of the trigeminal nerve. Other cranial nerve branches that innervate the oral cavity and pharynx may also be involved. The bacteria migrate via sensory axons using retrograde axonal transport to the trigeminal ganglion and then into the brain (medulla) or via motor axons directly to the midbrain and medulla (motor neurons–nucleus of cranial nerve V). The infection can then spread rostrally and caudally to other areas of the brain stem. Lesions are occasionally found in the cerebellum and cranial cervical spinal cord. These sites are likely the result of direct extension of infection because *Listeria monocytogenes* is a motile bacterium that spreads from cell to cell in its replicative phase.

The mechanism of tissue injury is not completely defined; however, injury to neurons and axons is likely a secondary bystander effect related to inflammation. A correlation between the degree of cell-mediated immunity and severity of brain damage suggests that immunologic injury may occur. Recent studies in a murine model, however, indicate the T lymphocyte response is only slight in early stages of fatal listeriosis. Immunization before experimental infection enhances CD4+ and CD8+ T-lymphocyte responses and provides greater survivability. Other studies have shown increased production of tumor necrosis factor-α (TNF-α) and interleukin (IL)-10 in fatal murine infections. The former is capable of causing brain damage (apoptotic cell death) and augmenting other CNS immune responses; the latter has a suppressive effect on neuroimmunologic reactions. The organism also produces a hemolysin (listeriolysin) that is a virulence factor required for intracellular multiplication.

Once bacteria enter the CNS, recent experimental studies suggest that *Listeria monocytogenes* can directly infect neurons, microglia, choroid plexus epithelial cells, and macrophages recruited in the inflammatory exudate. The bacteria spread from cell to cell using a secreted phospholipase that cleaves a variety of phospholipids, including sphingomyelin (a component of myelin) and phospholipids in cell membranes. Axonal injury and neuronal death are likely attributable to inflammatory processes, especially to the action of listeriolysin and lipases.

Gross lesions are usually absent, but leptomeningeal opacity, foci of yellow-brown discoloration (0.1 to 0.2 mm in diameter in the area of the nuclei of cranial nerves V and VIII), hemorrhage, necrosis in the terminal brain stem, and cloudy CSF have been noted. Microscopically a meningoencephalitis centered about the pons and medulla and involving both gray and white matter is characteristic (Fig. 14-46). The lesions, however, can extend from the diencephalon to the caudal medulla or cranial cervical spinal cord. Small, early lesions consist of loose clusters of microglial cells. With time, these lesions enlarge and contain variable numbers of neutrophils (Fig. 14-46, *B*) and later neutrophils dominate (microabscesses), but in some foci, macrophages can be the principal cell type. Necrosis and accumulation of gitter cells can be prominent in some cases. Numerous gram-positive bacilli can be detected in some lesions (Fig. 14-46, *C*). Leptomeningitis is regularly present and is often severe, and the exudate is composed of macrophages, lymphocytes, plasma cells, and fewer neutrophils. Cranial ganglioneuritis involving the trigeminal nerve and ganglion is often present.

Listeriosis presents in three disease forms: meningoencephalitis, abortion and stillbirth, and septicemia. The last commonly develops in young animals, possibly from an in utero infection. The encephalitic and genital forms of the disease rarely occur together in an individual animal or in the same flock or herd. Infections in human beings also occur. Clinical signs in meningoencephalitic listeriosis are related to lesions in the brain stem and include dullness, torticollis, circling, unilateral facial paralysis, and drooling caused by pharyngeal paralysis. Signs of cranial nerve dysfunction occur because of inflammation in the medulla and pons. Death usually occurs within a few days after the initial signs and is preceded by recumbency and paddling of the limbs. Silage is the most common source of infection. If silage is contaminated with soil containing *Listeria monocytogenes* and is improperly prepared and stored (pH > 5.4), the organism can multiply.

MENINGITIS

Meningitis refers to inflammation of the meninges (Fig. 14-47). In animals, meningitis is most commonly

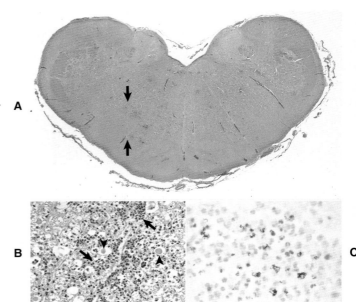

Fig. 14-46   Listeriosis, medulla, cow. A, Microabscesses. Note the areas of faint blue discoloration in this subgross magnification of the medulla *(arrows).* The less well-defined blue areas are aggregates of neutrophils (microabscesses), and the blue linear lesions are perivascular cuffs. *Listeria monocytogenes,* the causative agent, uses retrograde axonal transport via the cranial nerves to enter the central nervous system and localize in the medulla (brain stem) and proximal cervical spinal cord. The lesion is rarely visible on gross observation. H&E stain. **B,** Early microabscesses *(arrows)* and inflammation are the result of inflammatory mediators that have injured axons *(arrowheads)* and will lead to Wallerian degeneration, seen here at the stage of swollen eosinophilic axons. H&E stain. **C,** *Listeria monocytogenes. Listeria monocytogenes,* which is gram-positive *(blue),* can sometimes be detected in microabscesses in a histologic section stained with a Gram stain. Gram stain. *(A, B, and C, Courtesy Dr. M.D. McGavin, College of Veterinary Medicine, University of Tennessee.)*

caused by bacteria such as *Escherichia coli* and *Streptococcus* spp. that traverse to the leptomeninges and subarachnoid space hematogenously. Bacteria can also spread to the meninges by direct extension and leukocytic trafficking. In common usage, the term *meningitis* generally refers to inflammation of the leptomeninges (the pia mater, subarachnoid space, and adjacent arachnoid mater) in contrast to inflammation of the dura mater, which is referred to as pachymeningitis. Leptomeningitis can be acute, subacute, or chronic and, depending on the cause, suppurative, eosinophilic, nonsuppurative, or granulomatous. Inflammation of specific parts of the dura mater of the cranial cavity can occur in the external periosteal dura following osteomyelitis, formation of extradural abscesses and pituitary abscesses, and skull

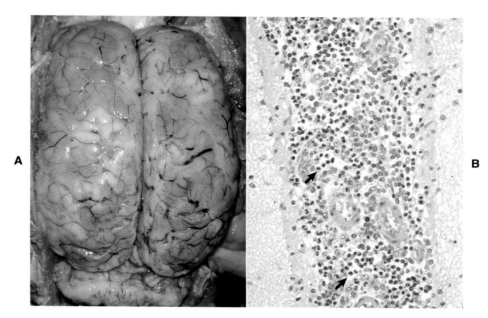

Fig. 14-47   **Suppurative bacterial meningitis, cerebral hemispheres, horse. A,** Pale yellow thick exudate composed principally of neutrophils admixed with bacteria, cellular debris, edema fluid, and fibrin is present in the subarachnoid space on the dorsal surface and also in the sulci. Overall the gyri are flattened, indicating brain swelling and compression. **B,** The arachnoid space of the leptomeninges in this sulcus contains a mixture of neutrophils *(arrows)*, other mononuclear inflammatory cells, cellular debris, edema fluid, and fibrin. H&E stain. (**A,** *Courtesy Drs. C. Lichtensteiger and A. Paulman, College of Veterinary Medicine, University of Illinois.* **B,** *Courtesy Dr. J.F. Zachary, College of Veterinary Medicine, University of Illinois.*)

fracture and involve the inner dura in association with leptomeningitis. Abscesses of the pituitary fossa occur with some frequency in cattle. Bacteria isolated from the cases include *Pasteurella multocida* and *Actinomyces pyogenes.* The abscess can result from spread of infection arising in the caudal nasal cavity or sinuses, possibly through direct extension or through the venous circulation. Incision of the pituitary fossa releases a thick viscous opaque tan to yellow exudate, which can elevate the dura mater surrounding the fossa. Infection can extend via the infundibular recess of the third ventricle into the ventricular system, resulting in ventriculitis, ependymitis, and empyema. Systemic bacterial infections in neonates are a common cause of acute meningitis (leptomeningitis), which are suppurative and fibrinous. In animals, leptomeningitis secondary to a selective viral infection only of the leptomeninges is very rare and is usually seen in combination with viral-induced encephalitides.

NEONATAL SEPTICEMIA

Neonatal septicemia typically involves *Escherichia coli, Streptococcus* spp., *Salmonella* spp., *Pasteurella* spp.,

and *Haemophilus* spp. The release of endotoxins and bacterial cell wall components, such as lipopolysaccharide (LPS), teichoic acid, and proteoglycans, in the CNS vasculature leads to the secretion of cytokines (TNF, IL, platelet-activating factor, prostaglandins, thromboxane, leukotrienes) from the endothelium and trafficking CNS macrophages, followed by adhesion of neutrophils, injury to the endothelium and blood-brain barrier, and vasculitis resulting initially in brain swelling and brain edema and increased intracranial pressure.

Although there are differences in the diseases caused by these organisms, they tend to produce fibrinopurulent inflammation of membranous tissues (serosal surfaces) of the body. Leptomeninges, choroid plexus, and ependyma of the CNS—sites often preferentially involved in hematogenous spread of bacteria, synovium, uvea, and the serosal lining of body cavities—can be affected in various combinations. Infections are often acquired perinatally, and onset is usually within a few days of birth up to 2 weeks (Table 14-3). The initial portal of entry can be oral, intrauterine, umbilical, surgical, via postsurgical procedures such as castration and ear notching, or via the

Table **14-3** Central Nervous System Bacterial Infections in Young Animals

CALF

Escherichia coli–leptomeningitis, choroiditis, ependymitis and ventriculitis, synovitis, ophthalmitis and perioptic neuritis
Pasteurella/Mannheimia spp.–leptomeningitis, ependymitis and ventriculitis
Streptococcus spp.–leptomeningitis, synovitis, ophthalmitis

FOAL

Escherichia coli–leptomeningitis, ventriculitis, polyserositis, synovitis
Streptococcus spp.–leptomeningitis, polyserositis, synovitis
Salmonella typhimurium–leptomeningitis, ependymitis and ventriculitis, choroiditis, synovitis

LAMB

Escherichia coli–leptomeningitis, ependymitis and ventriculitis, peritonitis, synovitis
Pasteurella/Mannheimia spp.–leptomeningitis

PIG

Escherichia coli–leptomeningitis, ophthalmitis
Haemophilus parasuis–leptomeningitis, polyserositis, synovitis
Streptococcus suis type I and II–leptomeningitis, choroiditis, ependymitis, cranial neuritis, myelitis
Salmonella choleraesuis–leptomeningitis, ophthalmitis

respiratory system, but the bacteria eventually spread to the CNS hematogenously.

Gross CNS lesions are commonly present and include congestion, hemorrhage, and diffuse to focal cloudiness or opacity in the leptomeninges, resulting in a leptomeningitis due to accumulation of exudates (Fig. 14-47). The ventricles contain fibrin, usually as a thin layer on the ependymal surface or as a pale coagulum in the CSF of the ventricular lumen, secondary to a choroid plexitis and/or ependymitis.

Microscopic lesions vary according to the organism. With the exception of *Salmonella* spp., the lesions consist of deposits of fibrin and an infiltration of mainly neutrophils in and around the blood vessels and capillaries of the leptomeninges, choroid plexus, and ependymal or subependymal areas of the brain. The epithelium of the choroid plexus and ependymal lining of the ventricles can be disrupted by cellular degeneration, disorganization, and necrosis, and this inflammation can extend into the adjacent CNS. A vasculitis with thrombosis and hemorrhage can be associated with lesions caused by *Escherichia coli*. Lesions caused by *Salmonella* spp. are not limited to the perinatal period. CNS involvement in salmonellosis is generally limited to foals and pigs and in contrast to the above infections,

the leukocytic response tends to have a greater proportion of macrophages and lymphocytes, often to the extent that the inflammation is designated histiocytic or granulomatous. This difference presumably reflects the fact that *Salmonella* spp. can be facultative pathogens of the monocyte-macrophage system. As is true in other tissues, vasculitis, thrombosis, necrosis, and hemorrhage often accompany *Salmonella* infections of the CNS. *Haemophilus parasuis*, which causes Glasser's disease, is also a frequent cause of leptomeningitis, polyserositis, and polyarthritis in 8- to 16-week-old pigs. Again, lesions are as previously noted with fibrinopurulent inflammation involving the leptomeninges, serosal linings of body cavities, and joints.

Bacterial infection with CNS and visceral involvement occurs in neonatal pigs and through the weaning period. These diseases are deserving of special mention because of the incidence and stereotyped nature of the infections. Several strains of *Streptococcus suis* are capable of causing disease. Type 1 strains generally cause disease in suckling pigs ranging in age from 1 to 6 weeks, whereas type 2 strains affect older pigs 6 to 14 weeks old. Type 2 strains are recognized as one of the more important serotypes, causing meningitis not only in pigs but also in human beings, particularly those working with pigs or handling porcine tissues. Other serotypes and untypeable strains can also cause systemic disease that results in leptomeningitis, choroid plexitis, and ependymitis. Extension to involve cranial nerve roots or the central canal of the cervical spinal cord also occurs. The character of the inflammation is fibrinopurulent, and necrotic foci can be found in brain stem, cerebellum, and anterior spinal cord.

Clinically, affected animals are initially ataxic, and then become laterally recumbent with rhythmic paddling of the limbs. As the disease progresses, they may become comatose and die.

THROMBOTIC MENINGOENCEPHALITIS

Histophilus somni (formerly *Haemophilus somnus*), a small gram-negative bacillus, causes a septicemic infection in cattle with variable clinical presentations, including pneumonia, polyarthritis, myocarditis, abortion, and meningoencephalitis. The disease is most prevalent in feedlot cattle but can occur in other situations. All manifestations, particularly meningoencephalitis, tend to be sporadic with single to multiple animals in a herd affected. The CNS form of the disease has been termed thrombotic meningoencephalitis (TME), previously referred to as thromboembolic meningoencephalitis (TEME). Mural thrombi from local vascular injury rather than thromboemboli from distal sites of vascular injury, such as the lungs, are the major type of thrombus in this disease.

The pathogenesis of *Histophilus somni* (formerly *Haemophilus somnus*) infection is not completely understood. Many cattle harbor the organism in the upper digestive tract without evidence of disease, but under some circumstances it invades to cause severe clinical infection. The mechanism(s) of invasion into the blood stream is not definitely known, but the respiratory tract is the initial site of bacterial replication followed by hematogenous spread to the CNS. Once the bacteria gain access to the circulation (bacterial emboli), emboli lodge at the interface of the gray and white matter in microvessels. Organisms adhere to endothelial cells, presumably via a receptor-mediated interaction, which results in endothelial cell contraction and desquamation. Subendothelial collagen is exposed, initiating a cascade of events culminating in vasculitis, thrombosis, and infarction. The bacteria within the infarct replicate and cause inflammation. Lipooligosaccharide, a toxic factor produced by *Histophilus somni* (formerly *Haemophilus somnus*) might protect the bacteria from host defenses. Bovine neutrophils, blood monocytes, and alveolar macrophages are incapable of killing the organism, allowing the infection to become established.

Gross lesions in the CNS are irregularly sized foci of hemorrhage and necrosis scattered randomly, and visible both externally and on cut surfaces (Fig. 14-48). Lesions are most frequent in the cerebrum, commonly at the cortical gray matter–white matter interface. The location of the lesion may reflect a change in the diameter and flow patterns of blood vessels, allowing bacteria to lodge, adhere, and replicate in these vessels. The spinal cord also has lesions. Other lesions include brain swelling due to edema and leptomeningitis with cloudiness of the CSF.

Microscopic lesions in all organs including the CNS are initially marked vasculitis and vascular necrosis, which are followed by thrombosis and infarction. Septic vasculitis, the initial event, is followed by edema and an influx of neutrophils and macrophages in and around vessel walls and adjacent parenchyma. Colonies of small gram-negative bacilli are frequent in thrombi, in and around affected vessels, and in areas of necrosis.

Clinically, affected cows are initially ataxic and circle, head-press, and appear blind. As the disease progresses, they may have convulsions, become comatose, and die.

VIRUSES

The viruses causing CNS disease in domestic animals are listed in Table 14-4.

ARBOVIRUSES

Equine encephalomyelitis

Eastern, western, or Venezuelan equine encephalomyelitis (EEE, WEE, VEE) viruses are members of the

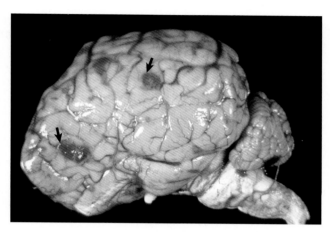

Fig. 14-48   **Thrombotic meningoencephalitis (previously referred to as thromboembolic meningoencephalitis), cerebrum, steer.** On the surface of the cerebral cortex (*arrows*) are several red-brown lesions. These lesions are areas of necrosis, hemorrhage, and inflammation secondary to vasculitis and thrombosis caused by *Histophilus somni* (formerly *Haemophilus somnus*). Such septic infarcts are distributed randomly (hematogenous portal of entry) throughout the central nervous system, including the spinal cord. The lesions depicted here are unusually severe. (*Courtesy Dr. H. Leipold, College of Veterinary Medicine, Kansas State University.*)

family Togaviridae, genus *Alphavirus*. The primary target cell for infection and injury is the neuron; however, these viruses can cause vasculitis followed by thrombosis. Following inoculation (by mosquito), the hematogenously circulating virus initially infects several tissues, including bone marrow, lymphoreticular tissue, muscle, and connective tissue. In lymphoid tissue and bone marrow, this infection may cause cellular depletion, necrosis, or both. A second viremia results in hematogenous infection of the CNS. Experimental evidence suggests that the virus replicates in endothelial cells before entering the nervous system and infecting neurons, for which it has an affinity. There is also evidence that viruses of this group (VEE virus) can cause alterations in the metabolism of neurotransmitters in the CNS and that these alterations are responsible for some of the clinical signs.

Recent experimental evidence from in vivo and in vitro models of VEE suggests that the virus causes upregulation of multiple proinflammatory genes including inducible nitric oxide synthase (iNOS) and TNF-α. This upregulation, occurring principally in astrocytes, affected other glial cells and influenced neuronal survival. In addition to these mediators of innate immune responses, apoptotic cell death was also described as contributing to neurodegeneration following virus infection.

In the CNS, all three viruses induce a polioencephalomyelitis that has similar characteristics, but there are

Table **14-4**   **Viruses Causing Central Nervous System Disease in Domestic Animals**

Virus Group	Disease	Type of Injury
Arboviruses	Equine encephalomyelitis	Encephalitis/myelitis/meningitis/vasculitis
	Japanese encephalitis	Encephalitis/myelitis/meningitis
	Louping ill	Encephalitis/myelitis/meningitis
	West Nile viral encephalomyelitis	Encephalitis/myelitis
	Wesselbron virus	Malformations
Bunyaviruses	Akabane disease	Malformations/encephalitis
	Arthrogryposis hydranencephaly complex (Cache Valley fever)	Malformations/encephalitis
	Rift Valley fever	Malformations/encephalitis
Coronaviruses	Feline infectious peritonitis	Vasculitis/encephalitis/myelitis/meningitis
	Hemagglutinating encephalomyelitis	Encephalitis/myelitis/meningitis/ganglioneuritis
Enteroviruses	Enterovirus-induced porcine polioencephalomyelitis	Encephalitis/myelitis
Herpesviruses	Equine herpesvirus 1 myeloencephalopathy	Encephalitis/myelitis/meningitis/vasculitis
	Bovine malignant catarrhal fever	Encephalitis/myelitis/meningitis/vasculitis
	Infectious bovine rhinotracheitis	Encephalitis
	Pseudorabies	Encephalitis/myelitis/meningitis
Lentiviruses	Visna	Encephalitis/myelitis/demyelination
	Caprine leukoencephalomyelitis-arthritis	Encephalitis/myelitis/demyelination
Orbiviruses	Blue tongue	Malformations/encephalitis
Paramyxoviruses	Canine distemper	Demyelination/encephalitis/myelitis
	Old-dog encephalitis	Encephalitis/demyelination/meningitis/vasculitis
Parvovirus	Feline panleukopenia virus	Malformations/meningitis
Pestiviruses	Classical swine fever	Malformations/hypomyelination/encephalitis/meningitis/vasculitis
	Bovine viral diarrhea	Malformations/meningitis/dysmyelination
	Border disease	Malformations/hypomyelination
Polyomaviruses	Progressive multifocal leukoencephalopathy	Demyelination
Rhabdoviruses	Rabies	Encephalitis/myelitis/meningitis/vasculitis/ganglioneuritis
Unassigned viruses	Borna disease	Encephalitis/myelitis

some differences. Overall, gross lesions include cerebral hyperemia, edema, petechiation, focal necrosis, and increased CSF in the subarachnoid space. Gross lesions are usually found in gray matter as appreciated best in the spinal cord (Fig. 14-49). Microscopic lesions are most prominent in the gray matter of the brain and spinal cord and are characterized by perivascular cuffing with lymphocytes, macrophages, and neutrophils, variable neutrophilic infiltration of the gray matter, microgliosis, neuronal degeneration, focal cerebrocortical necrosis, perivascular edema and hemorrhage, necrotizing vasculitis, thrombosis, choroiditis, and leptomeningitis. Neutrophils are detectable during the early stages (2 days) of clinical EEE and VEE. Vasculitis, thrombosis, and cerebrocortical necrosis are particularly evident in VEE but also in EEE. No lesions are detected in the trigeminal ganglion.

Infection of horses with EEE, WEE, and VEE viruses produces a range of progressive clinical maladies, including fever, rapid heart rate, anorexia, depression, muscle weakness, and behavioral changes such as dementia, aggression, head pressing, wall leaning, circling, blindness, and paralysis of facial muscles. Eastern encephalomyelitis has also been reported in cattle and pigs.

Japanese encephalitis

See Appendix 14-1.

Louping ill

See Appendix 14-1.

West Nile viral encephalomyelitis

West Nile virus, a mosquito-borne virus (family Flaviviridae, genus *Flavivirus*) that causes acute polioencephalomyelitis primarily in human beings, birds, and horses, is most commonly transmitted via a bird-mosquito cycle. In 2002, West Nile virus infection was diagnosed in 47,000 horses in 40 U.S. states and it was estimated that more than 4500 horses died following infection.

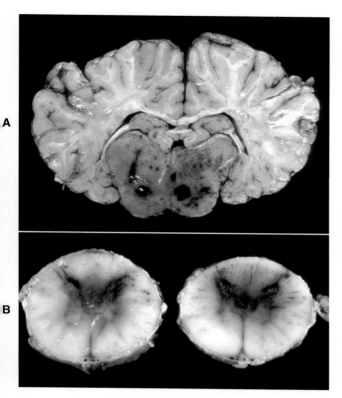

Fig. 14-49 **Neuronal necrosis and vasculitis, eastern equine polioencephalomyelitis, brain stem and spinal cord, horse. A,** Brain, transverse section at the level of the hippocampus, horse. The gray matter of the brain stem has dark red to black discoloration as a result of congestion and hemorrhage. The lesion is the result of viral infection, which has an affinity for neurons; this virus also causes vascular necrosis followed by thrombosis, but this is not common. **B,** Spinal cord, horse. Note the red to brown discoloration of the gray matter in the dorsal and ventral horns (due to congestion and hemorrhage). The lesion is the result of viral infection that has an affinity for neurons; however, this virus can also cause vascular necrosis followed by thrombosis. (**A** and **B,** *Courtesy College of Veterinary Medicine, University of Florida; and Noah's Arkive, College of Veterinary Medicine, The University of Georgia.*)

The pathogenesis of West Nile virus encephalomyelitis remains to be elucidated; however, it is likely to be similar to the mechanism described previously for equine encephalomyelitis viruses. The primary target cell for infection and injury appears to be the neuron; microglial cells are also affected. Experimental studies suggest that viral-induced apoptotic cell death is a mechanism possibly responsible for neuronal injury in experimental West Nile viral infections. Gross lesions of West Nile viral infection in horses usually involve the gray matter and include hyperemia and petechiation to prominent hemorrhage with prevalent involvement of the lower brain stem and ventral horns of the thoracolumbar spinal cord. Microscopic lesions in

birds and horses that have died of the disease are characterized by a nonsuppurative (lymphocytic/histiocytic) polioencephalomyelitis and hemorrhage of the CNS that can vary in degree of severity. Clinical signs of the equine West Nile viral infection include variable fever, depression, ataxia, weakness to paralysis of the hind limbs, tetraplegia, convulsions, coma, and death.

CORONAVIRUSES
Feline infectious peritonitis

Feline infectious peritonitis (FIP), which is caused by a coronavirus and has a worldwide distribution, is mainly a disease of domestic cats, although wild Felidae can be affected. There are two recognized feline coronaviruses (FCoV): feline enteric coronavirus (FECV) and feline infectious peritonitis virus (FIPV), which cause FECV and FIP infections, respectively. The viruses for each infection are antigenically and morphologically indistinguishable and are currently considered to represent avirulent (FECV) and virulent (FIPV) strains of the same basic FCoV virus. Following ingestion, FECV infects and replicates in epithelial cells of the intestine and usually is an insignificant infection, although severe intestinal disease can occur. It has been proposed that when FECV gains the ability (by mutation) to replicate in macrophages, then FIP can occur.

The FIP virus (FIPV) enters the susceptible cat primarily by ingestion of contaminated saliva or feces, although transmission by direct inoculation (cat bites, licking open wounds, etc.) and in utero (rarely) have been reported. Following infection, the virus replicates in macrophages that spread the virus to the liver, visceral peritoneum and pleura, uvea, and the meninges and ependyma of the brain and spinal cord.

Following dissemination of the virus in the body, the development of disease depends on the type and degree of immunity that develops. Virus containment with resistance to disease occurs following development of a strong cell-mediated immunity. Humoral immunity by itself is not protective and can actually enhance development of the effusive form of FIP (wet form) by two proposed mechanisms. The first involves the development of virus-antibody-complement complexes that particularly accumulate in the same areas as infected macrophages around small blood vessels, resulting in inflammation and subsequent vascular injury (type III hypersensitivity) accompanied by effusion of large amounts of fluid. The second mechanism involves a process referred to as antibody-dependent enhancement (demonstrated to occur experimentally), which involves uptake of virus-antibody-complement complexes by macrophages followed by significant viral replication. The heavily infected macrophages, frequently perivascularly orientated, release cytokines that result in alteration of endothelial junctional complexes that leads to leakage of substantial amounts of fluid.

Noneffusive FIP (i.e., dry form), in comparison, is thought to occur when partial cell-mediated immunity (type IV hypersensitivity) develops and represents an intermediate stage between nonprotective humoral immunity alone and protective cellular immunity. Support for this mechanism is the fact that cats that develop the noneffusive form of FIP following experimental infection usually have a preceding and transient bout of effusive-type disease. In addition, there is evidence to support the theory that cats recovered from FIP are immune by a process of "infection immunity" or "premunition." Once these cats no longer retain such infections, they seem to also lose protective (cell-mediated) immunity and are, in fact, more sensitive to a subsequent challenge exposure because of the presence of humoral antibody.

The basic lesion in effusive and noneffusive FIP is a pyogranulomatous inflammation, leading to vasculitis followed by an inconsistent vascular necrosis resulting in infarction. The effusive form is typified by serositis, accumulation of fluid in the abdominal and thoracic cavities, with varying degrees of severity of inflammation. Lesions of the noneffusive form more frequently result in leptomeningitis, chorioependymitis, focal encephalomyelitis, and ophthalmitis, although involvement of the kidneys, hepatic and mesenteric lymph nodes, and less frequently, serosa and other abdominal viscera can occur. In the CNS, pyogranulomatous vasculitis tends to affect blood vessels of (1) the leptomeninges, especially in sulci and near their entrance into subjacent CNS tissue and around the circle of Willis (Fig. 14-50) and (2) the periventricular white matter, especially around the fourth ventricle (Fig 14-51). The uvea, retina, and optic nerve sheath are also commonly involved in FIP.

FIP generally occurs sporadically in cats of all ages, but it is most common in younger cats between the ages of 3 months and 3 years and can be clinically significant because it can result in death. The disease manifests itself in effusive (wet) or noneffusive (dry) forms. Clinical signs caused by involvement of blood vessels in the CNS can include behavioral changes, dullness, coma, paresis, ataxia, paralysis, and seizures.

Hemagglutinating encephalomyelitis

See Appendix 14-1.

ENTEROVIRUSES
Enterovirus-induced porcine polioencephalomyelitis

See Appendix 14-1.

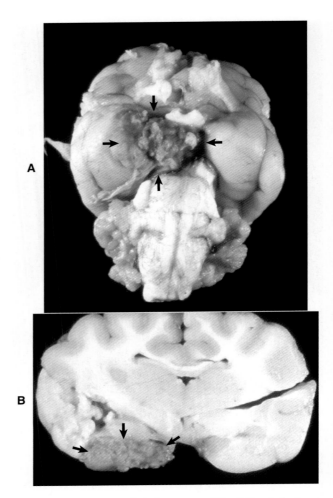

Fig. 14-50   **Pyogranulomatous vasculitis, feline infectious peritonitis, cat. A,** Ventral brain, cerebral vasculature of the circle of Willis. A white-yellow pyogranulomatous inflammation distorts and obscures the blood vessels. Lesions are attributed to deposition of immune complexes (type III hypersensitivity), and in some cases possibly with a cell-mediated component, in the vessel walls that results in inflammation (*arrows*). The character of the inflammatory response can vary from an exudate with accumulation of serous fluid and fibrin mixed with neutrophils and histiocytes to a reaction that is more pyogranulomatous, and in which commonly there are lymphocytes and plasma cells. The severity and magnitude of the lesion depicted here is much more dramatic than usual. **B,** A cross-sectional view of Fig. 14-50, A. The pyogranuloma (*arrows*) is principally in the subarachnoid space and has compressed the adjacent cerebral cortex. (*A and B, Courtesy Dr. J. Sundberg, College of Veterinary Medicine, University of Illinois.*)

HERPESVIRUSES

Encephalitic herpes viruses, members of the subfamilies Alphaherpesvirinae and Gammaherpesvirinae, cause cell injury through: (1) necrosis of infected neurons and glial cells, (2) necrosis of infected endothelial cells, and (3) secondary effects of inflammation, cytokines, and chemokines.

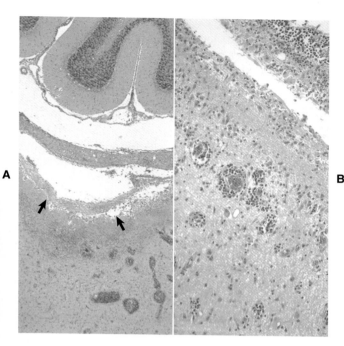

Fig. 14-51 **Pyogranulomatous vasculitis, feline infectious peritonitis (FIP), cat. A,** Periventricular white matter (*arrows*) beneath the fourth ventricle (between the medullary velum and medulla). The type III hypersensitivity and pyogranulomatous inflammation that occur with FIP cause vascular and perivascular injury, vasogenic edema, and parenchymal disruption. H&E stain. **B,** A higher magnification of Fig. 14-51, A. Ventriculitis and ependymitis are evident. Note the prominent perivascular cuffs of small mononuclear cells and macrophages. H&E stain. (**A** *and* **B,** *Courtesy Dr. J.F. Zachary, College of Veterinary Medicine, University of Illinois.*)

Although necrosis appears to be the principal mechanism for cell injury, recent studies indicate that bovine herpesvirus–induced apoptotic cell death can occur.

Neurotropic herpes viruses enter the CNS principally by retrograde axonal transport; however, entry by hematogenous spread via viremia and leukocytic trafficking may occur. These viruses also have a unique survival mechanism that allows them to hide in a latent form in nervous tissue, for example, in trigeminal ganglion of pigs infected with pseudorabies virus. Stress or other factors can activate latent virus resulting in encephalitis.

Bovine malignant catarrhal fever

Malignant catarrhal fever is usually a sporadic highly fatal disease of cattle and other ruminants, including deer, buffalo, and antelope, and can involve several animals in a herd. The disease has a worldwide distribution, and the clinicopathologic features do not differ significantly from one part of the world to another. The primary target tissues are the vasculature and lymphoid organs and epithelial tissue (particularly the respiratory and gastrointestinal tracts), but the kidneys, liver, eyes, joints, and CNS are also affected in some cattle. The virus appears to be transferred between lymphoid tissue/cells and endothelial cells via leukocytic trafficking in T lymphocytes. Two general types of the disease occur, the sheep-associated and wildebeest-derived forms. The causative agents involved belong to the herpesvirus subfamily Gammaherpesvirinae. The disease occurring outside Africa, caused by ovine herpesvirus 2 (OHV-2), often involves close contact of presumed "carrier" sheep with susceptible ruminants. The disease has recently been reported in muskox (*Ovibos moschatus*), Nubian ibex (*Capra nubiana*), and gemsbok (*Oryx gazella*). In Africa, and occasionally in wildlife facilities outside the continent, the source of the infection (designated alcelaphine herpesvirus 1 or AHV-1) is the wildebeest. Two other antigenically related viruses, which apparently do not cause natural disease, include alcelaphine herpesvirus 2 (AHV-2) and hippotragine herpesvirus 1 (HiHV-1), which have been isolated from African hartebeest and roan antelope, respectively. It is generally accepted that cattle and other susceptible ruminants contract the disease in nature following respiratory or oral infection during association with carrier sheep (presumed) and wildebeest, particularly at the time of parturition. A cell-mediated and cytotoxic lymphocytic process has been proposed to be involved in the development of the necrotizing vasculitis.

Gross lesions of the CNS include active hyperemia and cloudiness of the leptomeninges due to nonsuppurative meningoencephalomyelitis and vasculitis. Lymphocytic perivascular cuffing and varying degrees of necrotizing vasculitis occur in the leptomeninges and in all parts of the brain and occasionally in the spinal cord, with the white matter most consistently involved. Other lesions in the affected CNS include variable neuronal degeneration, microgliosis, choroiditis, necrosis of ependymal cells, and ganglioneuritis. Clinical signs referable to CNS infection may include trembling, shivering, ataxia, and nystagmus.

Infectious bovine rhinotracheitis

Although bovine herpesvirus 1 (BHV-1) occasionally causes a nonsuppurative meningoencephalitis, primarily in young cattle, two variants of BHV-1 isolated in Argentina and Australia (referred to as BHV-1, subtypes 3a and 3b, respectively) and recently BHV-5 (isolated in South America, mainly Argentina and Brazil) have a particular tropism for the CNS. Recent evidence suggests that BHV-5 uses an intranasal route to infect and replicate in the nasal mucosa and then enters the CNS by retrograde axonal transport using the trigeminal and olfactory nerves.

Gross lesions are nonspecific and include meningeal congestion and petechiation in ventral areas of the brain. Microscopic lesions consist of lymphomonocytic meningoencephalitis (nonsuppurative) with the occasional presence of neutrophils. Other changes include neuronal degeneration, vasculitis, focal malacia, and presence of intranuclear acidophilic inclusions in neurons and astrocytes.

Clinically, outbreaks of disease occur in young cattle ranging in age from 5 to 18 months. Lesions can also involve the eyes (conjunctivitis) and tissues of the reproductive, alimentary, and integumentary systems in addition to the nervous system.

Pseudorabies

Pseudorabies virus (porcine herpesvirus 1), an alpha-herpesvirus, causes encephalitis primarily in pigs; several species of domestic and wild animals are also susceptible. The disease is also known as Aujeszky's disease and "mad itch." Pseudorabies is not related to rabies but was named because its clinical signs sometimes resemble those seen with rabies.

The route of natural infection in pigs is intranasal, pharyngeal, tonsillar, or pulmonary by direct contact or aerosolization, followed by reproduction of virus in epithelial cells of the upper respiratory tract. The virus then travels to the tonsil and local lymph nodes by way of the lymph vessels. Following replication in the nasopharynx, virus invades sensory nerve endings and is then transported in axoplasm via the trigeminal ganglion and olfactory bulb to the brain. The virus has also been reported to be capable of spreading transsynaptically. Recent studies have additionally shown that some strains produce lesions in the gastrointestinal tract and myenteric plexuses, suggesting that infection might spread from the intestinal mucosa to the CNS via autonomic nerves. In latently infected pigs, the oronasal epithelium can be recurrently infected by virus spreading from the nervous system, followed by its excretion in oronasal fluid. The mechanisms that allow for latency and recrudescence are unclear, but neuronal apoptosis may play a role. The virus can also spread hematogenously, although in low titer, to other tissues of the body. Cellular attachment, entry, and cell-to-cell spread of the virus are mediated by glycoprotein projections that extend from the surface of the viral particle.

Gross lesions in pigs occur in several nonneural tissues including organs of the respiratory system, lymphoid system, digestive tract, and reproductive tract. Focal tissue necrosis also occurs in the liver, spleen, and adrenal glands, particularly in young suckling pigs, and mortality can be high. The CNS is free of gross lesions except for leptomeningeal congestion. Microscopic lesions in pigs are characterized by a nonsuppurative meningoencephalomyelitis with trigeminal ganglioneuritis.

Injury to CNS tissue can be marked, with neuronal degeneration and necrosis. Intranuclear eosinophilic inclusion bodies are not commonly detected in pigs but can be present in neurons, astrocytes, oligodendroglia, and endothelial cells. In cattle, sheep, dogs, and cats, the pathogenesis involving axonal spread to the CNS is comparable to that of pigs, with lesions that include nonsuppurative encephalomyelitis accompanied by ganglioneuritis. Intranuclear inclusion bodies, either eosinophilic or basophilic in their staining characteristics, have been described in neurons of the brain.

The disease in susceptible species other than pigs is generally fatal. Although pigs—particularly young, suckling piglets—can die from infection, most mature pigs remain persistently infected and act as latent carriers. Infection of secondary hosts, such as cattle, sheep, dogs, and cats, regularly involves direct or indirect contact with pigs. Secondary hosts acquire the virus through ingestion, inhalation, and wound infection. Dogs and cats often acquire the virus by ingesting organs from pigs that contain the pseudorabies virus.

Equine herpesvirus 1 myeloencephalopathy

Equine herpesvirus 1 (EHV-1) (an alpha-herpesvirus) is an important cause of equine abortion and perinatal foal infection and death, in addition to myeloencephalitis. EHV-1 can also cause rhinopneumonitis. EHV-1 does not appear to be neuronotropic, which is in contrast to some herpesvirus encephalitides of other species in which the virus replicates in neurons (herpes simplex viral infection in the human, infectious bovine rhinotracheitis viral infection in calves, and pseudorabies viral infection in pigs). In addition to vasculitis being the principal lesion, the infection in the horse also differs somewhat from most other herpetic infections of the CNS in being primarily a disease of the adult, although young animals can be affected.

Equine herpesvirus myeloencephalopathy begins with inhalation of the EHV-1. The virus infects epithelial cells of the nasopharynx and spreads to local lymphoreticular tissue, where it infects lymphocytes and macrophages (monocytes). Through leukocytic trafficking by macrophages (monocytes), EHV-1 is transferred to endothelial cells of the CNS.

The neurologic disease has been experimentally reproduced by intranasal inoculation of the virus (EHV-1, subtype 1), which can replicate in the epithelium of the respiratory or intestinal tracts following infection. Intranuclear inclusions occur in the nasal mucosa. Infection of mononuclear leukocytes (predominantly, but not exclusively, T lymphocytes and macrophages) then occurs and is followed by a cell-associated viremia. The virus, which is endotheliotropic, even though infection of neurons and astrocytes can occur, localizes in small arteries and capillaries of the CNS and some other tissues following direct spread from the circulating infected cells. Inflammation of endothelial cells then results in vasculitis leading to thrombosis and infarction of the neural tissue supplied by the thrombosed vessel. Latent infection of the trigeminal ganglion and lymphoid tissues can also occur.

The characteristic lesion in the CNS caused by EHV-1 infection is a vasculitis affecting endothelial cells of small blood vessels with thrombosis and resulting in focal CNS necrosis (infarction). Lesions occur in both the gray and white matter of the spinal cord, medulla oblongata, mesencephalon, diencephalon, and cerebral cortex (Fig. 14-52, A). The endothelium appears to

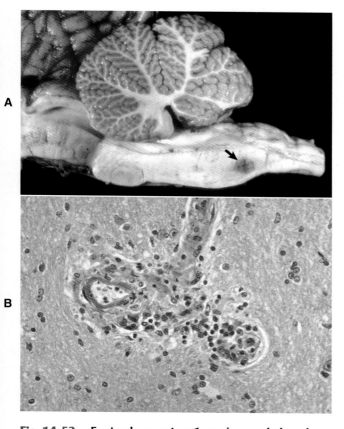

Fig. 14-52   Equine herpesvirus 1 myeloencephalopathy, brain, midsagittal section. A, Hemorrhage, brain stem, horse. Focal or multifocal areas of hemorrhage and/or necrosis *(arrow)* are characteristic of equine herpes virus encephalitis, but also occurs in equine arteritis virus encephalitis, cerebrospinal nematodiasis, and equine protozoal encephalomyelitis *(Sarcocystis neurona)*. **B,** Vasculitis and hemorrhage, brain stem, horse. Vasculitis is the principal lesion. The virus localizes in small arteries, venules, and capillaries of the central nervous system, resulting in vasculitis and fibrinoid necrosis which at times leads to thrombosis and focal infarction of the brain and spinal cord. **(A,** *Courtesy College of Veterinary Medicine, University of Illinois.* **B,** *Courtesy Dr. J. Simon, College of Veterinary Medicine, University of Illinois.)*

be the initial site of involvement (Fig. 14-52, *B*), with the subsequent intimal and medial degeneration resulting in hemorrhage, thrombosis, extravasation of plasma proteins into the perivascular space, axonal swelling with ballooning of the myelin sheath and degeneration of the cell body, and variable mononuclear cellular cuffing. Other lesions include cerebrospinal ganglioneuritis and vasculitis in nonneural tissues, including the endometrium, nasal cavity, lungs, uvea of the eye, hypophysis, and skeletal muscle. Inclusion bodies are apparently not observed in CNS lesions.

The neurologic form of EHV-1 infection has a worldwide distribution and affects other Equidae, including zebras in addition to the horse, but appears to be relatively uncommon when compared with the incidence of abortion and upper respiratory tract disease caused by EHV-1. The neurologic disease may accompany or follow outbreaks of respiratory disease or abortion. An outbreak of epizootic acute encephalitis in Thomson's gazelle (*Gazella thomsoni*) was reported in 1997 from a zoological garden in Japan. That disease resembled equine herpesvirus encephalitis, and the virus, named gazelle herpesvirus 1 (GHV-1), was serologically related to EHV-1 and had a strong tropism for endothelium.

PESTIVIRUSES
Classical swine fever (hog cholera)

See Appendix 14-1.

RHABDOVIRUSES
Rabies encephalitis

Rabies virus (family Rhabdoviridae) is one of the most neurotropic of all viruses infecting mammals. It is generally transmitted by a bite from an infected animal; however, respiratory infection has also been uncommonly reported following exposure to virus in bat caves, accidental human laboratory exposure, and corneal transplants.

The proposed mechanism for spread of rabies virus from the inoculation site to the CNS is illustrated in Fig. 14-53. Rabies virus may first replicate locally at the site of inoculation. Infection of and replication in local skeletal muscle myocytes may be an important initiating event. The virus then enters peripheral nerve terminals by binding to nicotinic acetylcholine receptors at the neuromuscular junction. The probability is greater that the virus will be taken up by both axon terminals and myocytes following a large inoculation dose. If the virus directly enters peripheral nerve terminals, the incubation period will more likely be short regardless of whether muscle cells are infected. With progressively lower doses of virus, however, there is a greater possibility that the virus will enter either nerve terminals or myocytes, but not both. This situation can result in a short

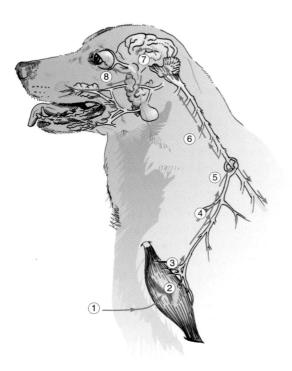

Fig. 14-53 **Rabies pathogenesis.** Following a bite wound, 1, the rabies virus initially replicates in muscle (can enter peripheral nerves directly), 2, enters, 3, and ascends (retrograde axonal transport) the peripheral nerve 4, to the dorsal root ganglion, 5, enters the spinal cord 6, and ascends 7, to the brain via ascending and descending nerve fiber tracts, infects brain cells, spreads to salivary glands 8, and the eye and is excreted in saliva. *(Courtesy Dr. J.F. Zachary, College of Veterinary Medicine, University of Illinois. Based on an illustration from Robinson PA: Rabies virus. In Belshe RB, editor: Textbook of human virology, ed 2, St Louis, 1991, Mosby.)*

incubation period if the virus directly enters nerve terminals as described previously or could result in a more prolonged incubation period if there was initial infection and retention of virus in myocytes before its release and uptake by nerve terminals.

The virus moves from the periphery to the CNS by fast retrograde axoplasmic transport, apparently via sensory or motor nerves, at a rate of 12 to 100 mm per day. Experimental data suggest that rabies virus phosphoprotein interacts with dynein LC8, a microtubule motor protein used in retrograde axonal transport. With sensory axons, the first cell bodies to be encountered following inoculation of a rear leg would be those of spinal ganglia, whose neuronal processes extend to the dorsal horn of the spinal cord. For motor axons, the cell bodies of the lower motor neurons in ventral horn gray matter, or neuronal cell bodies of the autonomic ganglia, are the ones initially infected. It is not known whether viral infection and replication in neurons of dorsal root

ganglia are essential for infection of the CNS. The virus then moves into the spinal cord and ascends to the brain using both anterograde and retrograde axoplasmic flow. During the spread of the virus between neurons within the CNS, there is also simultaneous centrifugal movement via anterograde axonal transport of the virus peripherally from the CNS to axons of cranial nerves. This process results in infection of various tissues, including the oral cavity and salivary glands, permitting transmission of the disease in the saliva. An additionally important feature of rabies is that infection of nervous and nonnervous tissue, such as the salivary glands, occur at the same time, which permits affected animals to have the required aggressive behavior plus passage of the virus into the saliva to facilitate the transmission of the disease.

The results of recent experimental studies have helped clarify the mechanism by which the virus spreads within the CNS. Following axoplasmic spread of the virus from an inoculated rear leg to neurons of the associated segments of the spinal cord, rapid spread of infection to the brain occurs via long ascending and descending fiber tracts, bypassing the gray matter of the rostral spinal cord. This early spread of the virus has been suggested to explain how induction of behavioral changes occurs before there is sufficiently severe injury to cause paralysis and allows dissemination of infection before there is time for a notable immune response. Spread of infection within neurons of the CNS recently has been proposed to occur via both anterograde and retrograde axoplasmic flow, with corresponding neuron-to-neuron spread by axosomatic-axodendritic and somatoaxonal-dendroaxonal transfer of virus. Transsynaptic spread can occur by budding of developing virions from the neuronal cytoplasm (cell body or dendrite) into a synapsing axon or in the form of bare viral nucleocapsid (ribonucleoprotein-transcriptase complexes) in the absence of a complete virion.

In vivo experimental studies using a laboratory strain of rabies virus showed that the virus caused a downregulation of about 90% of genes in the brain at more than fourfold lower levels. Affected genes were those involved in regulation of cell metabolism, protein synthesis, and growth and differentiation. Other experimental studies have shown increased quantities of nitric oxide in brains of rabies-infected animals, suggesting that nitric oxide neurotoxicity may mediate neuronal dysfunction. Finally, the rabies virus has been shown to induce apoptotic cell death of brain neurons in mouse models. The exact mechanism of rabies virus–induced neuronal injury in domestic and wildlife species remains to be fully determined.

Gross lesions of the infected central nervous tissue are often absent. Microscopic lesions of the CNS are typically lymphomonocytic (nonsuppurative) and include

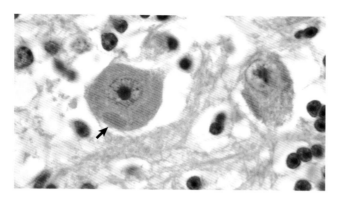

Fig. 14-54   Rabies, Negri body, cerebellum, Purkinje cell, cow. A large pale red (eosinophilic) inclusion (Negri body) is present in the cytoplasm of the neuron cell body *(arrow)*. In the cow, Negri bodies are seen in Purkinje cells and in other neurons, such as those of the red nucleus and cerebral cortex. H&E stain. *(Courtesy Dr. M.D. McGavin, College of Veterinary Medicine, University of Tennessee.)*

a variable leptomeningitis and perivascular cuffing with lymphocytes, macrophages, and plasma cells; microgliosis which sometimes is prominent; variable, but often not severe, neuronal degeneration; and ganglioneuritis. Occasional and slight infection can also involve the leptomeninges, ependyma, oligodendroglia, and astrocytes. Emphasis should be given to the fact that infected neurons often are minimally altered morphologically. Neurons can also contain intracytoplasmic acidophilic (pale red to red) inclusions called Negri bodies (Fig. 14-54). Also, dogs are reported to have a tendency to develop a more severe inflammatory reaction than other species, such as the cow, in which little if any inflammation might occur. Nonneural lesions include variable nonsuppurative sialitis accompanied by necrosis and presence of Negri bodies in canine salivary epithelial cells.

Negri bodies, formed within neurons of the CNS and even in the cranial trigemina, spinal, and autonomic ganglia, have long been the hallmark of rabies infection, although they are not present in all cases. The inclusions are intracytoplasmic and initially develop as an aggregation of strands of viral nucleocapsid, which rather quickly transforms into an ill-defined granular matrix. Mature rabies virions, which bud from the nearby endoplasmic reticulum, can also be located around the periphery of the matrix. With time, the Negri body becomes larger and detectable by light microscopy. Classically, in H&E stained sections, the Negri body, which is eosinophilic, has one or more small, light clear areas called inner bodies that form as a result of invagination of cytoplasmic components (that include virions) in the matrix of the inclusion. Inclusions that do not possess "inner bodies" have been referred to as Lyssa bodies, but they are actually Negri bodies without cytoplasmic indentation. It should also be noted that both fixed viruses (adapted

to the CNS by passage) and street viruses (that produce the naturally occurring disease) produce the same ultrastructural features, but fixed viral strains generally cause severe neuronal degeneration that precludes the development, and thus the detection, of Negri bodies. Negri bodies also tend to occur more frequently in large neurons, such as the pyramidal neurons of the hippocampus, neurons of the medulla oblongata, and Purkinje cells of the cerebellum. Also, inclusions are frequently present in neurons not located in areas of inflammation. Therefore the preferred tissue for rabies examination by light microscopy and by florescent antibody technique for virus include hippocampus, cerebellum, medulla, and the trigeminal ganglion.

A spongiform lesion, indistinguishable qualitatively from the lesion characteristic for several of the spongiform encephalopathies, was described for the first time in 1984 by Charlton. This lesion was initially detected in experimental rabies in skunks and foxes, and later in the naturally occurring disease in the skunk, fox, horse, cow, cat, and sheep. The lesion occurs in the neuropil of the gray matter, especially of the thalamus and cerebral cortex, initially as intracytoplasmic membrane-bound vacuoles in neuronal dendrites and less commonly in axons and astrocytes. The vacuoles enlarge, compress surrounding tissue, and ultimately rupture forming a tissue space. Although the mechanism responsible for the development of this lesion has not been determined, it is thought to result from an indirect effect of the rabies virus on neural tissue (possibly involving an alteration of neurotransmitter metabolism).

The clinical signs in domestic animals are similar with some differences between species. The clinical disease in the dog has been divided into three phases: prodromal, excitatory, and paralytic. In the prodromal phase, which lasts 2 to 3 days, the animal can have a subtle change in temperament. The term *furious rabies* refers to animals in which the excitatory phase is predominant, and dumb rabies refers to animals in which the excitatory phase is extremely short or absent and the disease progresses quickly to the paralytic phase. Cattle and carnivores generally have the furious form of rabies, and affected animals are restless and aggressive. Other somewhat unique signs of cattle with rabies include bellowing, general straining, tenesmus, and signs of sexual excitement followed by paralysis and death. Mules, sheep, and pigs usually have the excitatory form of rabies. Horses can have early signs that are atypical for a neurologic disease but terminally tend to have the excitatory form.

When conducting a necropsy on an animal suspected of having rabies, it is important to remember: (1) to provide additional protection (double-gloves, mask, eye protection, and proper ventilation) for the prosector above those used for routine postmortem examination and (2) to collect the appropriate CNS tissues (hippo-campus, cerebellum, and medulla, and optionally the spinal cord) for examination by immunofluorescence and sometimes mouse inoculation. The remainder of the brain should be fixed by immersion in 10% neutral buffered formalin for histopathologic examination.

UNASSIGNED VIRUSES
Borna disease

See Appendix 14-1.

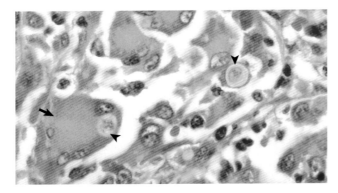

Fig. 14-55   Granulomatous encephalitis, blastomycosis, brain, dog. This inflammatory response, consisting of a mixture of macrophages, multinucleated giant cells (*arrow*), lymphocytes, varying numbers of neutrophils, and occasional plasma cells, is typical of central nervous system infections by fungi and algae. *Blastomyces dermatitidis* organisms are present in the exudate and within macrophages and giant cells (*arrowheads*). H&E stain. *(Courtesy Dr. J.F. Zachary, College of Veterinary Medicine, University of Illinois.)*

FUNGI AND ALGAE

Infection of the CNS by a variety of fungi and algae has been reported in domestic animals. Most reported cases are isolated occurrences and often represent opportunistic infection in immunocompromised individuals. Rare infections have involved genera such as *Aspergillus, Candida, Mucor,* dematiaceous fungi, and the blue-green algae *Prototheca*. These infections do not have a predilection for the nervous system. Of the systemic fungi, CNS infections have occurred with *Coccidioides immitis, Blastomyces dermatitidis, Histoplasma capsulatum,* and *Cryptococcus neoformans,* but only *Cryptococcus neoformans* has a particular affinity for the CNS and will be covered in a separate section later. These agents reach the CNS by leukocytic trafficking and hematogenous spread from primary sites of infection located in other areas (lung) of the body.

This group of pathogens usually elicits, as characterized by *Blastomyces dermatitidis,* a granulomatous to pyogranulomatous inflammatory response (Fig. 14-55). This response can be locally extensive or distinct granulomas can form in the CNS and meninges. Grossly, CNS lesions consist of moderately well demarcated expansile yellow-brown foci that displace and disrupt normal tissue (Fig. 14-56). Microscopically the exudate consists of neutrophils, macrophages (epithelioid type), and multinucleated giant cells. The latter two cell types may contain organisms in their cytoplasm. *Blastomyces dermatitidis* organisms are broad-based budding spherical yeastlike organisms 8 to 25 μm in diameter (Fig. 14-57). The inflammatory response, including cells (granulomatous inflammatory cells) and cytokines, leads to the

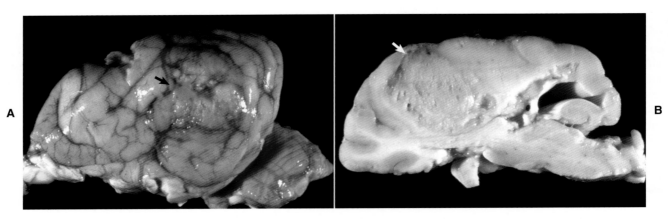

Fig. 14-56   Blastomycosis, cerebrum, dog. A, The subarachnoid space (leptomeninges) of the left cerebral hemisphere (parietal-temporal lobes) contains a locally extensive focus of granulomatous inflammation caused by *Blastomyces dermatitidis* (*arrow*) with extension into subjacent cortex. **B,** A parasagittal section of a similar lesion from another dog shows a moderately well-demarcated granuloma in the white matter of the frontoparietal cortex (*arrow*).
*(**A** and **B,** Courtesy College of Veterinary Medicine, University of Illinois.)*

and the capsule can be stained with mucicarmine and alcian blue (Fig. 14-59, *B*).

Clinically, cryptococcosis with CNS infection occurs in cats, dogs, horses, and cattle. The character of neurologic signs varies with the location of the lesions but can include depression, ataxia, seizures, paresis, and blindness.

OPPORTUNISTIC FUNGI

Opportunistic fungi—including those fungi in the zygomycetes group, such as *Absidia corymbifera*, *Rhizomucor pusillus*, and *Rhizopus arrhizus*, and those fungi in the genus *Aspergillus*, such as *Aspergillus niger*—can invade blood vessels (angiotropic) and cause vascular thrombosis and infarcts in the CNS (Fig. 14-60). It must be noted that the term *opportunistic* implies that some form of tissue damage precedes fungal invasion. As an example, necrotizing enterocolitis caused by *Salmonella* spp. in the horse can provide an "open" vascular bed in the lamina propria of the intestinal mucosa that may be invaded by such fungi. Affected animals are often immunocompromised.

PROTOZOA
EQUINE PROTOZOAL ENCEPHALOMYELITIS (SARCOCYSTOSIS)

Equine protozoal encephalomyelitis is a disease in horses caused by *Sarcocystis neurona*. The organism enters the body through ingestion of sporocysts, but how the parasite enters the CNS is unclear. Experimental studies suggest that ingested sporocysts multiply in visceral tissue, perhaps the intestine, and

then are transported to the CNS probably cytic trafficking. In the CNS, the typical seque events in the pathogenesis of the characteristic lesio thought to be: (1) leukocytic trafficking with focal parasitic activation and replication, (2) marked inflammation, (3) edema, and (4) pronounced tissue destruction affecting both white and gray matter.

Gross lesions can occur throughout the neuraxis but are more common in the spinal cord, particularly the cervical and lumbar intumescences, than in the brain. In the brain, lesions are most commonly seen in the brain stem. When gross lesions are present, they consist of discolored necrotic foci, often with hemorrhage of varied sizes (Fig. 14-61).

Microscopic lesions occur in both the white and gray matter and include necrosis, hemorrhage, and accumulations of lymphocytes, macrophages, neutrophils,

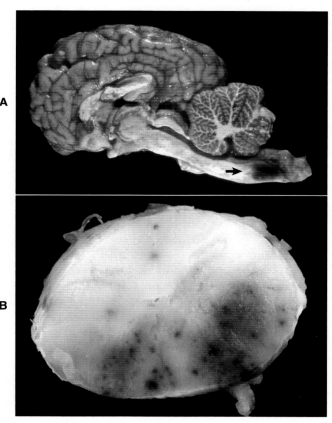

Fig. 14-61   Protozoal encephalomyelitis, brain, saggital section, horse. A, Note the large focus of hemorrhage and necrosis (*arrow*) in the caudal medulla caused by *Sarcocystis neurona*. **B,** Lumbar spinal cord, transverse section. Myelitis due to *Sarcocystis neurona* infection. Prominent focal hemorrhage and necrosis are present in the right lateral funiculus and in the right and left ventral funiculi. (**A,** *Courtesy College of Veterinary Medicine, University of Illinois.* **B,** *Courtesy Dr. R. Storts, College of Veterinary Medicine, Texas A&M University.*)

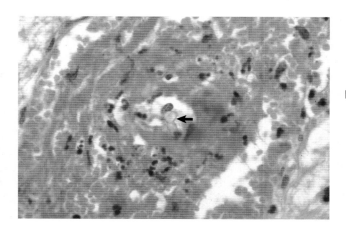

Fig. 14-60   Opportunistic angioinvasive fungi. Fungi such as *Absidia corymbifera, Rhizomucor pusillus,* and *Rhizopus arrhizus* and fungi in the genus *Aspergillus,* such as *Aspergillus niger,* can invade blood vessels (angiotropic) and cause vascular necrosis and infarcts in the central nervous system. Note the vasculitis, hemorrhage, and disruption of the vessel and the fungal hyphae in the lumen (*arrow*). H&E stain. (*Courtesy Dr. J.F. Zachary, College of Veterinary Medicine, University of Illinois.*)

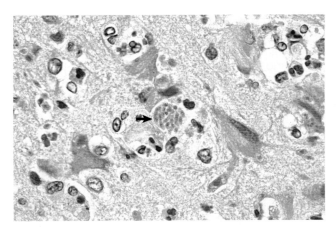

Fig. 14-62 *Sarcocystis neurona*, **brain, horse.** *Sarcocystis neurona* is a small, crescent-shaped to round protozoal organism found in neurons, endothelial cells, and microglial cells. They can be arranged in nonencysted aggregates (*arrow*) or rosettes intracellularly and in central nervous system tissue often with a mixed leukocytic cellular inflammatory response of varied severity. Organisms can be difficult to detect in histologic sections. H&E stain. (*Courtesy Dr. J. Simon, College of Veterinary Medicine, University of Illinois.*)

eosinophils, and a few multinucleated giant cells in perivascular areas and the neuropil, or less commonly, the leptomeninges and the axonal swelling. Gemistocytic astrocytosis can be prominent. In lesions, *Sarcocystis neurona* is small and crescent-shaped to round, has a well-defined nucleus, and is often arranged in aggregates or rosettes (Fig. 14-62). Organisms can be difficult to detect but occur intracellularly in neurons, giant cells, neutrophils, or macrophages or occur extracellularly in cysts within the neuropil. *Sarcocystis neurona* is not typically seen in vascular endothelial cells, a common site for other members of this genus.

Sarcocystis neurona can be propagated in tissue culture where it develops in the host cell cytoplasm. It divides by endopolygeny, with development of schizonts containing merozoites arranged in rosettes around a prominent residual body. The schizont stage of the organism differs from those of the genera *Toxoplasma, Isospora, Eimeria, Besnoitia, Hammondia,* and *Neospora* because the merozoites lack rhoptries but resemble the schizont stage of other genera such as *Sarcocystis* spp. and *Frenkelia*. It is proposed that an opossum coccidian, *Sarcocystis falcatula,* and *Sarcocystis neurona* are synonymous. Studies have suggested that the opossum represents the definitive host and avian species the intermediate host, providing a reservoir for infection of the horse.

Sarcocystis spp. infection in nonequine species involves organisms similar to *Sarcocystis neurona*. Such organisms have been associated with encephalomyelitis in cattle, sheep, and dogs as well as raccoons, but such infections are sporadic. Lesions and organisms have additionally been seen in the CNS of infected bovine fetuses.

Clinical infection typically occurs in young adult horses, and signs are dependent on the area of the CNS parasitized. Signs can include depression, behavioral changes, seizures, gait abnormalities, ataxia, facial nerve paralysis, head tilt, paralysis of the tongue, urinary incontinence, dysphagia, atrophy of masseter and/or temporal muscles, and atrophy of the quadriceps and/or gluteal muscles.

NEOSPOROSIS

Neosporosis, a naturally occurring or experimental disease caused by *Neospora caninum* or a Neospora-like coccidian, has been recognized in a variety of animals, including the dog, cat, cattle, sheep, and horse (*Neospora hughesi*) as well as laboratory rodents. First described in 1988 as a multisystemic infection in the dog, the organism has an affinity for the nervous system. The dog has recently been identified as the definitive host for the organism, but other hosts may exist. Some of the features of the organism similar to those of *Toxoplasma gondii,* include division of tachyzoites by endodyogeny and having both proliferative (tachyzoites) and tissue cyst phases. However, *Neospora caninum* does not develop within a parasitophorous vacuole of a host cell, as does *Toxoplasma gondii*. This latter feature is evident only with the use of transmission electron microscopy.

Although there are morphologic differences between the organisms (*Neospora caninum* has a thicker cyst wall), differentiation by light microscopy is unreliable, and electron microscopic examination or immunohistochemistry is required. Apart from transplacental transmission proposed for a variety of species, the mechanism of infection is unknown. *Neospora caninum* can infect a variety of cell types, but outside of the CNS it appears to have an affinity for cells of the monocyte-macrophage system. The most likely method of spread to the CNS is via leukocytic trafficking.

In the CNS, neurons and ependymal cells, mononuclear cells in the CSF, and cells of blood vessels including endothelium, intimal connective tissue, and tunica media smooth muscle cells can harbor organisms. Organisms have also been detected in spinal nerves. In all animals studied to date, the cyst form of *Neospora caninum* has been seen only in the CNS, whereas tachyzoites have been found in a variety of other tissue. Overall the morphologic pattern and character of lesions caused by *Neospora* spp. in the CNS are most consistent with endothelial tropism, vascular swelling and injury, tissue ischemia, and multifocal infarction.

Neurologic disease can be divided into two categories; that occurring during postnatal life and that associated with midterm to late-term abortions, the latter a notable problem in dairy cattle. Postnatal syndromes have been observed mainly in young and adult dogs, but horses are also affected. In young dogs, clinical signs are due to an ascending polyradiculoneuritis and polymyositis. In adult dogs, clinical signs are more referable to CNS lesions complicated by polymyositis, myocarditis, and dermatitis.

In horses the pathogen causing neosporosis is *Neospora hughesi.* Clinical signs resemble those of protozoal myeloencephalitis caused by *Sarcocystis neurona.* Lesions in horses include meningoencephalomyelitis, variable vasculitis and necrosis with microgliosis, and perivascular cuffing by macrophages, multinucleated giant cells, lymphocytes, plasma cells, or neutrophils, most commonly in the gray and white matter of the spinal cord but also in the pons and medulla.

Gross lesions can involve the white and/or gray matter. Peracute gross lesions may include foci of hemorrhage and necrosis distributed in a vascular pattern. Acute lesions have the same pattern of distribution but are, on cut surface, granular in texture and yellow-brown to gray. In some cases the periventricular white matter may be more affected. Chronic lesions have larger areas of granular yellow-brown to gray discoloration, which often makes white matter indistinguishable from gray matter. Microscopically the lesions and their temporal occurrence are similar to those described for *Toxoplasma gondii* including brain lesions that occur in aborted animals. *Neospora caninum* or *Neospora*-like organisms in lesions can be identified in tissue sections by H&E stain and immunohistochemical staining methods. Clinical signs are similar to those described for encephalitides induced by *Toxoplasma gondii.*

TOXOPLASMOSIS

Toxoplasmosis is a disease in cats and other mammalian species caused by the obligate intracellular protozoan, *Toxoplasma gondii.* Domestic, feral, and wild cats are the definitive hosts of *Toxoplasma gondii.* Cats acquire *Toxoplasma gondii* by ingesting infective cysts, oocysts, or tachyzoites when eating infected prey, such as rodents or birds. Ingestion of one of these stages initiates the intraintestinal life cycle, which occurs only in members of the cat family. *Toxoplasma gondii* replicates and multiplies within epithelial cells of the small intestine and produces oocysts. Oocysts are released into the feces in large numbers for 2 to 3 weeks following initial ingestion of cysts, oocysts, or tachyzoites. When oocysts sporulate, usually within 5 days after passage in the feces, they become infectious for intermediate hosts. Sporulated oocysts are highly resistant and can survive in moist shaded soil or sand for months. Cats are unique in the biology of the organism, serving as both definitive (intraintestinal life cycle) and intermediate (extraintestinal life cycle) hosts.

Toxoplasma gondii can infect a wide variety of animals as intermediate hosts (extraintestinal life cycle) including fish, amphibians, reptiles, birds, human beings, and many other mammals. New World monkeys and Australian marsupials are the most susceptible, whereas Old World monkeys, rats, cattle, and horses seem highly resistant.

Toxoplasma gondii can also parasitize a wide variety of cell types in the intermediate host and can cause lesions in such tissues as the lungs, lymphoid system, liver, heart, skeletal muscle, pancreas, intestine, eyes, and nervous system. Following ingestion, bradyzoites from tissue cysts or sporozoites from oocysts enter intestinal epithelia and multiply. Evidence suggests active penetration of plasma membranes by organism-secreted lytic products, allowing a portal of entry rather than by uptake via phagocytosis. *Toxoplasma gondii* can then spread locally, free in lymph or intracellularly in lymphocytes, macrophages, or granulocytes to Peyer's patches and regional lymph nodes. Intracellularly, organisms multiply as tachyzoites within a parasitophorous vacuole by repeated cycles of endodyogeny during the early acute stages of infection. Dissemination to distant organs is via lymph and blood, either as free organisms or intracellularly in lymphocytes, macrophages, or granulocytes via leukocytic trafficking.

With chronicity and an increasing antibody response by the host, tachyzoites of *Toxoplasma gondii* transform into slow-growing bradyzoites that replicate in cysts within muscle. Infection of the CNS occurs hematogenously; neurons and astrocytes are the eventual target cells. The typical sequence of events in the pathogenesis of the characteristic lesion is similar to that in *Sarcocystis neurona* infection. In utero infections in animals and human beings can result in CNS infection. In fetal brains, foci of necrosis are most common in the brain stem and induce the formation of microglial nodules. Additionally, foci of necrosis and mineralization occur in the cerebrocortical white matter and are caused by fetal hypoxia and ischemia resulting from severe placentitis, fetal myocardial damage, or initiation of a systemic inflammatory reaction in the fetus. In older more mature individuals, *Toxoplasma gondii* infections have been associated with immunosuppression, such as occurs in concurrent CDV infection and toxoplasmosis. In some cases this could represent activation of latent inactive *Toxoplasma gondii* cysts [bradyzoites] in neural tissues.

Immune-mediated mechanisms have been proposed to explain the vascular injury (type III hypersensitivity) and cellular or tissue necrosis (type IV hypersensitivity). Lysis of infected cells by primed cytotoxic, CD8+ T lymphocytes also could potentially contribute to the tissue damage through the production of cytokines, such as INF-γ, which can activate microglia and astrocytes to inhibit parasite replication and induce cytotoxic T lymphocytes to kill infected cells. This exuberant inflammatory response and the cytokine cascade that ensues to kill the organism also causes severe damage to cells in the area of inflammation, especially axons and neurons. Intracellular growth of tachyzoites also has been advanced as a cause of cellular necrosis. The organism does not produce a cytotoxin.

The blood-brain barrier of the CNS is breached when free organisms or those located intracellularly (leukocytic trafficking) infect endothelial cells of the CNS vasculature, especially capillaries. Gross lesions can involve any area of the CNS without predilection for gray or white matter, may also involve nerve rootlets, and may initially include foci of hemorrhage and necrosis and, later, by granular, yellow-brown to gray foci. Peracute lesions initially include endothelial cell swelling due to infection by tachyzoites and vasculitis with hemorrhagic infarcts followed by vasogenic edema. If the edema is of sufficient severity to cause increased brain volume, the edema can lead to brain displacement and herniation.

Early microscopic lesions include infection of and proliferation within endothelial cells by *Toxoplasma gondii* tachyzoites. Endothelial injury results in endothelial cell swelling, endothelial cell degeneration, hemorrhage, capillary occlusion, ischemic necrosis, and edema of adjacent tissue. Subsequently, tachyzoites invade the CNS, inducing a prominent acute inflammatory response leading to necrosis and hemorrhage often striking in severity. With time, the inflammatory response consists of perivascular cuffing of blood vessels within the CNS and leptomeninges by lymphocytes and macrophages. CNS responses to injury consist of microgliosis and astrogliosis; however, these responses are often insufficient to replace the loss of tissue in the cerebral hemispheres, resulting in dilatation of the lateral ventricles (hydrocephalus ex vacuo) and the formation of persistent cysts in the tissue. With chronicity and increasing inflammatory and immunologic responses by the host, tachyzoites change to slow-growing bradyzoites that replicate in and form tissue cysts. Organisms in lesions can often be identified with an H&E stain, but immunohistochemistry facilitates their detection and identification. As the infection is systemic, lesions can occur in several other tissues.

Occasionally, cysts (bradyzoites) can be observed in "normal" CNS tissue without an inflammatory or tissue lesion. These cysts are likely the result of a previous infection with *Toxoplasma gondii* that was successfully resolved. Experimental studies have confirmed that administration of corticosteroids, and hence immunosuppression, increases susceptibility or exacerbates the infection with *Toxoplasma gondii* or both or may contribute to the reactivation of tissue cysts.

Clinical signs can vary depending on the age of the animal, species infected, and areas of the CNS involved and may include depression, weakness, incoordination, tremors, circling, paresis, and blindness.

CHLAMYDIA
Sᴘᴏʀᴀᴅɪᴄ Bᴏᴠɪɴᴇ Eɴᴄᴇᴘʜᴀʟᴏᴍʏᴇʟɪᴛɪs

See Appendix 14-1.

PARASITES

As a general concept, lesions resulting from parasitic infestation of the CNS vary in degree of severity and distribution depending on the parasite and the host response to infection. Gross lesions of hemorrhage and malacia in parasite migratory tracts or space-occupying cysts occur with the various parasitic stages. Microscopically, there is necrosis, hemorrhage, and a leukocytic response, typically with a significant infiltrate of eosinophils. The extent of the host response is often dictated by the degree of trauma and disruption created by the parasite and the level of sensitivity of the host for parasite antigens. This section is not intended to be an extensive review of veterinary parasitology but will cover those parasites most commonly seen in veterinary practice.

Iɴsᴇᴄᴛ Lᴀʀᴠᴀᴇ

Among the most common larvae are those of *Oestrus ovis* and *Hypoderma bovis*. The larvae of *Oestrus ovis* develop in the nasal cavity of sheep but can penetrate into the cranial vault through the ethmoid bone. Larvae of *Hypoderma bovis* can enter the spinal canal during their migration in the subcutis from the hoof to the dorsal midline in cattle and rarely as an aberrant parasite in the brain of horses. Damage in the CNS due to *Hypoderma bovis* in cattle is typically the result of inflammation directed at the degenerating parasites following anthelmintic treatment. Larvae of *Cuterebra* spp., usually a parasite of rabbits and rodents, can invade the CNS of dogs and cats (see Feline Ischemic Encephalopathy).

Cᴇsᴛᴏᴅᴇs

Coenurus cerebralis, the larval form of the dog tapeworm *Multiceps multiceps*, most commonly infests sheep and occasionally other ruminants. The larval forms presumably reach the CNS hematogenously and then cause damage during migration and encystation, forming space-occupying lesions. Another parasite for which human beings are the definitive host is *Taenia solium*, with pigs being the intermediate host. The larval stage, *Cysticercus cellulosae*, generally develops in muscle of the pig but can also occur in the meninges and brain, resulting in a disease called "cysticercosis." Involvement of the CNS has been termed "neurocysticercosis."

Initially, viable cysticerci become "trapped" within capillaries of the CNS, but they do not apparently elicit an inflammatory response. At some point, the host responds immunologically and the cyst becomes denser, collapses inwardly, and disintegrates to eventually become calcified debris in a focus of inflammation. The inflammatory response has humoral and cellular components. Antibodies of the IgG family are directed against the cyst; however, cysts are likely killed by mediators released from eosinophils, which are attracted to the site by mediators released from lymphoid cells in the inflammatory exudate. For undetermined reasons, in "susceptible" animals viable cysts can become established and grow slowly for years. Viable cysticerci can cause asymptomatic infection by actively evading and suppressing the immune response of the host. These cysts cause vasogenic edema and increased intracranial pressure related to behavior as "space-occupying" masses.

Gross lesions are usually seen in the cerebral hemispheres, commonly at the interface of gray and white matter in a hematogenous pattern. Cysts can also be found in the cerebellum, medulla, ventricles, subarachnoid space, and the spinal cord. There are usually no gross changes in the CNS surrounding the cysts. Cysts are round to oval and of varied sizes and number, many of which can be large and visible up to centimeters in diameter. They have a translucent cyst wall and contain a thick, clear fluid. Within the fluid is a scolex, visible as a small 2- to 3-mm nodule. Microscopically, there is little or no inflammation or tissue injury surrounding the cysts, except for compression and edema.

NEMATODES (CEREBROSPINAL NEMATODIASIS)

Aberrant migration of larval stages of nematode parasites into and through the CNS is called cerebrospinal nematodiasis. They gain access to the CNS hematogenously and actively enter the CNS by crossing the blood vessel wall through their locomotive processes. Nematodes cause damage in the cerebromedullary area of the brain and/or spinal cord either from aberrant migration in the definitive host or migration in an aberrant host (Table 14-5; Fig. 14-63). Larval stages of *Strongylus* spp. and *Baylisascaris procyonis*, for example, are typically involved, the exception being *Dirofilaria immitis*, where the adult parasite is found. Greater CNS damage is often created by the migration of the parasites in an aberrant host.

Macroscopic lesions of nematode larval migration often appear as linear or serpentine tracts of necrosis and/or hemorrhage in the tissue. Migration results in endothelial injury, vasculitis, and thrombosis, which may result in vascular occlusion and infarction. Larvae can often be found in histologic sections, and they induce a mononuclear cell inflammatory exudate, including abundant eosinophils (Fig. 14-64).

Table 14-5   **Nematodes Causing Central Nervous System Disease in Domestic Animals**

Parasite	Normal Host	Aberrant Host
NEMATODE MIGRATION IN ABERRANT HOST		
Angiostrongylus cantonensis	Rat	Dog
Baylisascaris procyonis	Raccoon	Dog
Elaphostrongylus rangiferi	Reindeer	Sheep, goat
Parelaphostrongylus tenuis	Deer	Sheep, goat
Setaria digitata	Cattle	Sheep, goat, horse
ABERRANT NEMATODE MIGRATION IN NORMAL HOST		
Angiostrongylus vasorum	Dog (coyote)	
Dirofilaria immitis	Dog (cat)	
Stephanurus dentatus	Pig	
Strongylus spp.	Horse	

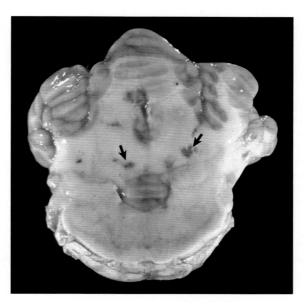

Fig. 14-63   **Cerebrospinal nematodiasis, brain, cerebellum, and medulla at the level of the pons, horse.** *Strongylus vulgaris* migration. Several small foci of hemorrhage and necrosis in the cerebellar white matter are sites of larval migration *(arrows)*. *(Courtesy Dr. R. Storts, College of Veterinary Medicine, Texas A&M University.)*

Halicephalobus (Micronema) deletrix is a free-living rhabditiform nematode that can infest the nasal cavity, CNS, and kidneys of the horse. The life cycle, pathogenesis, and route of infection of *Halicephalobus deletrix* are poorly understood. It has been proposed that the CNS is infected hematogenously in a manner similar to that described for cerebrospinal nematodiasis and that larvae penetrate skin and mucous membranes in recumbent horses with subsequent invasion of sinuses and/or blood vessels. In the CNS, microscopic lesions are prominently associated with blood vessels along which the parasite apparently migrates.

PRIONS

TRANSMISSIBLE SPONGIFORM ENCEPHALOPATHIES

Ovine spongiform encephalopathy (scrapie), bovine spongiform encephalopathy (BSE), and human spongiform encephalopathies are classified within a group

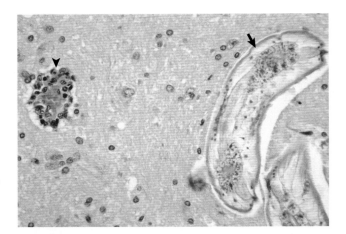

Fig. 14-64 Cerebrospinal nematodiasis, central nervous system (CNS), horse. Migration of *Strongylus vulgaris* larvae *(arrow)* in the CNS elicits a perivascular lymphomonocytic inflammatory response mixed with eosinophils *(arrowhead)* and results in direct injury to blood vessels, axons, and dendrites. *(Courtesy Dr. J.F. Zachary, College of Veterinary Medicine, University of Illinois.)*

of diseases called transmissible spongiform encephalopathies (TSEs). Table 14-6 lists the known TSEs in animals and human beings. These diseases are caused by proteinaceous infectious particles (prions) that: (1) are composed of an abnormal isoform of a normal cellular protein, the prion protein (PrP^c [a 27- to 30-kilodalton polypeptide]), designated PrP^{Sc} and (2) resist inactivation by procedures that degrade nucleic acids and proteins (i.e., heat, ultraviolet irradiation, and strong enzymes). PrP^c is expressed throughout the body and is the product of a highly conserved gene found in organisms as diverse as fruit flies and human beings. The "Sc" superscript is derived from the word "scrapie" because scrapie is the prototype prion disease.

Although the mechanism by which PrP^{Sc} forms has not been completely explained, a posttranslational modification of PrP^c has been proposed (Fig. 14-65). This mechanism proposes that PrP^{Sc} acts as a template on which PrP^c undergoes a conformational change (is refolded) by a process facilitated by another protein (referred as protein X), whereby the α-helical content of PrP^c diminishes and the amount of β-sheet increases, resulting in the formation of PrP^{Sc}. The features of a specific PrP^{Sc} is determined by the animal in which it is formed. When PrP^{Sc} of one species is inoculated into a different species, the recipient is less readily infected and generally has a prolonged incubation period. This resistance to infection is referred to as the "species barrier." A review of prion biology and diseases can be found in Prusiner (2004) in the suggested readings. Dr. Prusiner was awarded the Nobel Prize in Medicine in 1997 for his work on prion diseases.

Table **14-6** Transmissible Spongiform Encephalopathies (i.e., Prion Diseases)

Disease	Natural Host(s)	Prion	Pathogenic PrP Isoform
ANIMALS			
Ovine spongiform encephalopathy (scrapie)	Sheep, goats	Scrapie prion	OvPrP^{Sc}
Bovine spongiform encephalopathy (BSE)	Cows	BSE prion	BoPrP^{Sc}
Feline spongiform encephalopathy (FSE)	Cats	FSE prion	FePrP^{Sc}
Chronic wasting disease (CWD)	Mule deer, elk, black	CWD prion	MdePrP^{Sc}
Transmissible mink encephalopathy (TME)	tailed deer, white tailed deer mink	TME prion	MkPrP^{Sc}
Exotic ungulate encephalopathy (EUE)	Nyala, greater kudu, oryx	EUE prion	UngPrP^{Sc}
HUMAN BEINGS			
Kuru	Human beings	Kuru prion	HuPrP^{Sc}
Creutzfeldt-Jakob disease (CJD)	Human beings	CJD prion	HuPrP^{Sc}
Variant Creutzfeldt-Jakob disease (VCJD)	Human beings	VCJD prion	HuPrP^{Sc}
Gerstmann-Sträussler-Scheinker syndrome (GSS)	Human beings	GSS prion	HuPrP^{Sc}
Fatal familial insomnia (FFI)	Human beings	FFI prion	HuPrP^{Sc}

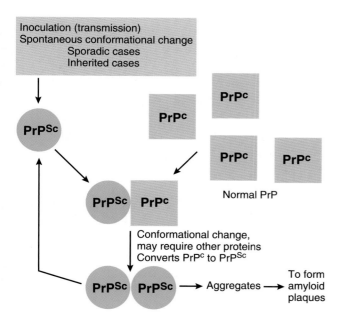

Fig. 14-65   Prion protein. In prion diseases (spongiform encephalopathies), PrP (*PrPc*), a normal neuronal protein, is converted to an abnormal β-pleated sheet isoform (*PrPSc*) through the interaction of PrPSc with PrPc. *(Modified from Cotran RS, Kumar V, Collins T, Robbins SL: Robbins pathologic basis of disease, ed 6, Philadelphia, 1999, Saunders.)*

Spongiform encephalopathies occur through horizontal transmission (scrapie-infected sheep offal* fed to cows [BSE] has been proposed) and through an inherited mutation of the normal human prion gene (parent to child), resulting in the spontaneous formation of PrPSc. In animals the primary route of infection appears to be through horizontal transmission. It has been proposed that prions ingested in infective feedstuffs enter the body through the intestine. The role of the rendering process in the pathogenesis of prion infectivity is also unclear. Prions are thought to cross the intestinal wall at Peyer's patches and are phagocytosed and transported to other lymph nodes by leukocytic trafficking. Prions replicate in lymphocytes and macrophages of the lymphoid system. Because these tissues are innervated, prions have been proposed to be transported by retrograde axonal transport to the brain; however, hematogenous spread via leukocytic trafficking may also be involved. In this example, scrapie infective ovine prions (OvPrPSc) accumulate in neurons and somehow result in the conversion of normal bovine prion proteins (BoPrPc) in neurons to the disease-causing form, BoPrPSc through a process in which a portion of the α-helical and coil structure of PrPc is refolded

into β-sheets (PrPSc). When neurons accumulate sufficient PrPSc to alter the normal function of neurons (it can take years), neurologic signs are observed.

Prion diseases are fatal. The adaptive immune system does not recognize prions as foreign; therefore no immunologic protection develops. How the accumulation of PrPSc causes neurodegeneration and neuron loss in prion diseases is not clear; however, astrocyte and microglial cell activation and apoptosis appear to be likely components of the pathway leading to neuronal injury.

No gross lesions of the nervous system are detectable in animals with spongiform encephalopathies. Microscopic lesions in scrapie-infected sheep and goats are limited to the CNS and are most commonly present in the diencephalon, brain stem, and cerebellum (cortex and deep nuclei), with variable lesions in the corpus striatum and spinal cord. Except for some minor changes, the cerebral cortex is essentially unaffected.

The type of neuronal degeneration can vary and commonly is characterized by shrinkage with increased basophilia and cytoplasmic vacuolation (Fig. 14-66, *A*), although other changes such as central chromatolysis and ischemic cell change variably occur. Astrocytosis in affected areas of the brain, including the cerebellar cortex, can be severe (Fig. 14-66, *B*). There has been speculation whether the astrocytic reaction is a primary or a secondary response. An abnormal protein (prion amyloid protein) first accumulates in astroglial cells in the brain during scrapie infection, which could mean that this cell is the primary site of replication. The spongiform change tends to affect the gray matter, and greater severity of this lesion has been associated with long incubation periods. The lesion in the gray matter is the result of dilation of neuronal processes, but vacuolation of neuronal and astroglial perikarya, swelling of astrocytic processes, dilation of the periaxonal space, and splitting of myelin sheaths have also been reported. Finally, the disease is not accompanied by any notable inflammation within the CNS.

Ovine spongiform encephalopathy (scrapie)

Scrapie is best known as a degenerative disease that affects the CNS of sheep and was first recognized in Great Britain and other countries of Western Europe more than 250 years ago. The disease, which is currently reported throughout the world except for Australia and New Zealand, also occurs naturally in the domestic goat. The name is derived from the characteristic clinical signs of pruritus, which often results in loss of wool in sheep. The disease progresses inexorably with early signs of subtle change in behavior or temperament followed by scratching and rubbing against fixed objects because of the pruritus. Additional signs include incoordination, weight loss (despite retention of appetite), biting of the feet and limbs, lip smacking, gait abnormalities,

---

*Viscera and trimmings of butchered animals considered inedible by human beings.

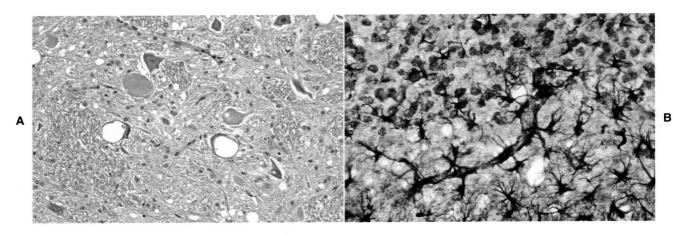

Fig. 14-66 **Spongiform encephalopathy (scrapie), brain, motor neurons, sheep.**
A, Neuronal cell bodies contain one or more discrete and/or coalescing clear vacuoles. There are no inflammatory cells in this disease. Similar spongiosis is evident in the neuropil. H&E stain.
B, Scrapie, experimental, brain, cerebellum, mouse. The cerebellar granule cells are at the top of the figure. There is notable hypertrophy and proliferation (astrocytosis) of astrocytes and their fibers (astrogliosis) *(black branching fibers).* Some of the processes (running diagonally across the illustration) end, as is normal for astrocytes on the walls of capillaries. Cajal's gold sublimate stain for astrocytes. (**A,** *Courtesy Dr. D. Gould, College of Veterinary Medicine; and Biomedical Sciences, Colorado State University; and Dr. M. McAllister, College of Veterinary Medicine, University of Illinois.* **B,** *Courtesy Dr. W.J. Hadlow.*)

trembling (when suddenly stressed), recumbency, and eventually death after 1 to 6 months or longer.

Much of our current understanding of the pathogenesis of the natural infection of scrapie in Suffolk sheep has been advanced by Dr. William Hadlow and coworkers. It should be noted that Dr. Hadlow is a veterinary pathologist and diplomate of the American College of Veterinary Pathologists, who first recognized and reported the similarity between scrapie and kuru of human beings. This important contribution led to the current understanding of the TSEs and a Nobel Prize for the medical scientist (Dr. D. Gajdusek), who originally investigated kuru in the South Pacific.

Bovine spongiform encephalopathy

BSE (mad cow disease) was originally identified in the United Kingdom in 1986 but likely existed there as early as April 1985. Through the end of 2003, more than 183,000 cows from more than 35,000 herds were reported with BSE. With regard to the origins of BSE, epidemiologic evidence strongly suggests that this disease was caused initially (during the early 1980s) by the feeding of rations containing meat and bone meal supplements that were contaminated with the scrapie agent. Countries that have reported cases of BSE or are considered to have a substantial risk to have animals with BSE include: Albania, Austria, Belgium, Bosnia-Herzegovina, Bulgaria, Canada (confirmed May 2003), Croatia, Czech Republic, Denmark, Federal Republic of Yugoslavia, Finland, France, Germany, Greece,

Hungary, Ireland, Israel, Italy, Liechtenstein, Luxembourg, Former Yugoslavia Republic of Macedonia, The Netherlands, Norway, Oman, Poland, Portugal, Romania, Slovak Republic, Slovenia, Spain, Sweden, Switzerland, Japan, and United Kingdom (Great Britain including Northern Ireland and the Falkland Islands).

In December 2003, BSE was confirmed in a single dairy cow from a herd in Washington state. This cow was apparently imported into the United States 2 to 3 years earlier from a farm in northern Alberta, Canada, which was the source of the positive BSE case in Canada confirmed in May 2003. In 2004, additional cases of BSE likely linked to a common source were reported in Washington state, Oregon, and Canada, and in June 2005 a cow tested positive for BSE in Texas.

Signs that accompany BSE include changes in behavior, such as nervousness or aggressiveness, abnormal posture, abnormal gait, incoordination, difficulty in rising, decreased milk production, and loss of body weight despite continued appetite. Clinically affected cattle deteriorate until they either die or require euthanasia. This clinical period usually ranges from 2 weeks to 6 months. All cases of the disease in cattle have occurred in adult animals, with an age range of 3 to 11 years, but most animals have clinical signs develop between 3 and 5 years of age.

The National Veterinary Services Laboratory (APHIS–Animal and Plant Health Inspection Service) of the United States Department of Agriculture has developed and implemented through local and regional veterinary diagnostic laboratories procedures for sampling, preparing, and submitting brains for BSE analysis. Space limitations prevent describing these procedures. They can be obtained through APHIS or a diagnostic laboratory. Dead or sick animals that display neurologic signs and are suspected of being potential BSE candidates are tested using immunohistochemical analysis, Western blot analysis, or enzyme-linked immunosorbent assay to identify PrPSc in brain tissue. Genetically valuable animals that may be exported or have their embryos or DNA saved for future use and are from TSE risk groups can be tested for PrPSc. Immunohistochemical analysis for PrPSc of samples obtained (i.e., under anesthesia) from biopsies of tonsil and lymph follicles of the third eyelid from at-risk groups show promise as diagnostic tools.

DEGENERATIVE DISEASES

METABOLIC

AGING-RELATED DEGENERATIVE MYELOPATHY (GERMAN SHEPHERD MYELOPATHY)

A degenerative myelopathy is most commonly seen in the German shepherd, but a similar condition has been described in other large canine breeds (Belgium shepherd, Old English sheepdog, Rhodesian ridgeback, Weimaraner, great pyrenees). Based on its prevalence in German shepherds, it has been suggested that there is a genetic "aging" predisposition in this breed. Altered suppressor lymphocyte activity has been noted in affected dogs, but the relevance to the CNS disease is unknown. Some investigators have reported low vitamin E concentrations and suggested oxidative stress injury; others have found elevated concentrations of acetylcholinesterase in CSF. The cause of this disorder remains to be discovered.

Gross lesions in the CNS are not present in dogs with age-related degenerative myelopathy; however, atrophy of caudal axial and appendicular muscles occurs. Microscopic lesions are most notable in the thoracic spinal cord and can be diffuse or multifocal. Dorsal aspects of the lateral and ventromedial areas of ventral funiculi can be more severely affected, but lesions can be diffuse in all funiculi. Lesions consist predominately of ballooning and degeneration of myelin sheaths and less prominently of axonal degeneration and loss. Degeneration of dorsal nerve rootlets and peripheral nerves and loss of neuron cell bodies in spinal gray matter occur as well.

Clinically, affected dogs are usually older than 8 years, but the disease has occurred as early as 5 years of age. They have progressive ataxia referable to the thoracolumbar spinal cord and muscle weakness.

AMINOACIDOPATHIES

Two diseases characterized by errors of amino acid metabolism have been described in neonatal calves. One disease, designated maple syrup urine disease (MSUD), occurs in young polled Hereford and Hereford calves. The second disease, bovine citrullinemia, which was originally described in Australia, occurs in neonatal Friesian calves.

MSUD is caused by an inherited defect in branched chain keto-acid dehydrogenase enzyme complex necessary to metabolize the branched-chain amino acids leucine, isoleucine, and valine. These amino acids are essential and must be obtained from protein in the diet. Following consumption, proteins are digested and the amino acids are released to be used to generate energy and for other metabolic processes. In MSUD there is a mutation in one or more of the genes that regulate this degradation process; therefore abnormal metabolites and ketoacids accumulate to toxic levels and cause disease. Urine has a sweet odor attributable to a derivative of isoleucine resembling maple syrup. In human infants the disease is confirmed biochemically by finding elevated concentrations of leucine, isoleucine, and valine in the blood.

Gross lesions are not typically present. Microscopically, marked spongiosis, due to vacuolation of myelin sheaths, is present throughout the neuraxis. The spongiosis affects both gray and white matter. Lesions are often most notable in areas such as the brain stem, where there is an intermingling of gray and white matter.

Affected calves may be normal at birth. Within a few days depression, dullness, and weakness progress to recumbency and opisthotonus.

Bovine citrullinemia is a rare inborn error of metabolism of the urea cycle that results in a pronounced accumulation of citrulline and ammonia in the body fluids because of a failure of the normal synthesis of arginosuccinic acid by the enzyme arginosuccinate synthetase. In human infants the disease is confirmed biochemically by finding elevated concentrations of citrulline in the blood. The cerebral lesions have also been suspected to result from the hyperammonemia or possibly some defect in excitatory neurotransmitter metabolism. However, the pathogenesis of the disease in calves remains unsettled.

Grossly, brains appear normal and have normal weights. Livers are pale yellow. Microscopically, there is fatty change in the liver. Lesions in the brain are characterized by mild to moderate diffuse astroglial swelling in the cerebral cortex.

Calves are normal at birth. Within a few days a severe generalized CNS disorder develops characterized by apparent blindness, depression, and tremors that rapidly progress to seizures, coma, and death within a few hours.

CEREBRAL CORTICAL ATROPHY

Brain atrophy caused by the loss of neurons in the cerebral cortex can occur in animal species but is observed most commonly in sheep with lipofuscinosis. Lipofuscin pigment, a "wear and tear" pigment associated with low-grade chronic membrane damage via lipid peroxidation, is often found in affected neurons. The cause of this lesion is unknown but thought to be related to long-term "wear and tear" on the CNS. Atrophy most frequently involves the cerebral hemispheres, especially the cortex. The cerebral hemispheres are increased in firmness often have a tan color (lipofuscin), and gyri are thinned and the sulci widened. Microscopically, there is loss of neuron cell bodies in cortical laminae without inflammation. Astrogliosis in response to neuronal loss is also observed, as is an increased prominence of the adventitial layer of blood vessels.

CHANNELOPATHIES

Channelopathies are a newly emerging group of inherited neuromuscular diseases of human beings that affect the excitability of membranes of neurons and skeletal myocytes. These diseases result from mutations in genes encoding ion channel proteins that regulate calcium, sodium, and chloride channels and acetylcholine receptors. In human beings, neurologic diseases—such as epilepsy and migraine headaches—have been attributed to channelopathies. In veterinary neurology, channelopathies will likely be shown, in the future, to be the underlying mechanism for epilepsy and other primary neuronal degenerations.

DEGENERATIVE LEUKOMYELOPATHIES

Degenerative leukomyelopathies are a heterogeneous group of familial, likely inherited, and acquired diseases that have been described in dogs, cows, and horses. Although there is not universal agreement, the degenerative leukomyelopathies described here are best characterized as axonal degenerations with spheroid formation predominantly within spinal cord white matter and secondary changes in myelin sheaths and myelin loss. In dogs, familial or inherited diseases include degenerative axonopathy of Ibizan hounds, axonopathy in Labrador retrievers, and axonopathy in Jack Russell and smooth fox terriers. A disease in rottweilers (covered under Primary Cerebellar Neuronal Degenerations in Dogs and Cats) is another disorder with spinal cord white matter involvement that is familial and possibly inherited. An acquired disease, hound ataxia, has been described in the United Kingdom and Ireland in harrier, beagle, and foxhounds. Hound ataxia may represent a nutritional disorder in hunting dogs fed paunch (tripe). Degenerative leukomyelopathies in cattle can be inherited as an autosomal recessive trait or have a familial predisposition. Leukomyelopathies have been reported in Murray Grey, Holstein-Friesian, and in certain lines of Brown Swiss cattle. In horses, a degenerative

leukomyelopathy, covered separately next, is recognized that does not seem to have a well-defined familial or hereditary basis.

Gross lesions are usually not observed. Microscopically, lesions in the white matter of the spinal cord are bilaterally symmetrical and consist of axonal degeneration with formation of spheroids, loss of axons, and secondary myelin degradation. Depending on the species or breed affected, lesions can involve any of the funiculi. Spinocerebellar tracts in the dorsolateral aspects of the lateral and septomarginal areas of ventral funiculi are commonly affected, as is the fasciculus gracilis in the dorsal funiculus. Severe involvement of the dorsal spinocerebellar tracts can extend into the caudal brain stem and via caudal cerebellar peduncles to the cerebellar cortex and Purkinje cells. In some species and breeds, there can also be involvement of additional specific brain stem structures.

Age of onset varies with the familial or inherited disorders. Paresis, ataxia, and dysmetria are the predominant clinical signs.

EQUINE DEGENERATIVE MYELOENCEPHALOPATHY

Equine degenerative myeloencephalopathy has been reported in a variety of pure and mixed breed horses. A similar disease has been reported in zebras. The specific cause of this disorder is unknown. Although a firm relationship does not currently exist, there is some evidence to suggest that vitamin E deficiency could play a role in this disease as well as in a disorder in Morgan and Haflinger breeds termed neuraxonal dystrophy. Investigators have found low vitamin E levels in some horses and that vitamin E supplementation has resulted in clinical improvement or reduced the occurrence of the disease on some premises with a high incidence of degenerative myeloencephalopathy.

Vitamin E functions as an antioxidant, protecting cells from free radical-mediated injury. Vitamin E deficiency associated with abetalipoproteinemia and various fat malabsorption syndromes in human beings, as well as experimentally induced deficiency, result in neurologic disorders with similarities to the equine diseases. A hereditary predisposition for equine degenerative myeloencephalopathy has not been excluded, but a specific mechanism has so far been elusive. Although this disease might be multifactorial or even represent entirely different syndromes with overlapping clinical presentations and lesions, they are grouped here because of similarities in clinical presentation and lesions.

In horses with degenerative myeloencephalopathy, lesions are microscopic. Axonal degeneration in the spinal cord is the most notable lesion, is bilateral, and can affect all funiculi, but the dorsal funiculus is least affected. Dorsal spinocerebellar tracts in lateral funiculi

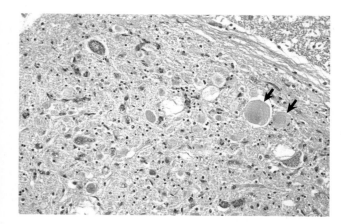

Fig. 14-67   Axonal spheroids and dystrophic axons, degenerative myeloencephalopathy, spinal cord, dorsal gray horn, horse. Axons of the thoracic nucleus are swollen, rounded, and pale pink (axonal spheroids, which are accumulations of neurofilaments and effete organelles) *(arrows).* Although attributed to vitamin E deficiency, its role in central nervous system disease is not firmly established. Vitamin E functions as an antioxidant, protecting cells from free radical–mediated injury. H&E stain. *(Courtesy Dr. J.F. Zachary, College of Veterinary Medicine, University of Illinois.)*

and septomarginal areas of the ventral funiculus are often severely affected. Myelin loss occurs secondary to the axonal degeneration. Depending on duration of clinical illness, astrogliosis occurs. Another, less dramatic, lesion in affected horses is the formation of eosinophilic spheroids (Fig. 14-67). In horses, spheroids have been described in the nucleus gracilis, medial and lateral cuneate nuclei of the terminal brain stem, and thoracic nucleus of the spinal cord. Spheroids represent a focal eosinophilic swelling in the course of an axon that can be somewhat homogeneous, laminated, or granular. The swellings are filled with amorphous debris, membranous profiles, and effete organelles.

A clinically similar syndrome occurs in Morgan and Haflinger horses; changes are termed neuraxonal dystrophy. Lesions consist of eosinophilic spheroids in brain stem nuclei as previously noted, but the severe axonal degeneration does not occur in the spinal cord. The cause of axonal spheroids and dystrophic axons in equine degenerative myeloencephalopathy and neuraxonal dystrophy is unclear; however, alteration of axoplasmic flow is suspected. Immunohistochemical analyses have shown that spheroids and dystrophic axons contain elevated quantities of proteins involved in movement, docking, and fusion of synaptic vesicles to plasma membranes. These findings suggest that disruption of axoplasmic flow plays a role in the pathogenesis of dystrophic axons in equine degenerative myeloencephalopathy and neuraxonal dystrophy.

Clinically, equine degenerative myeloencephalopathy and neuroaxonal dystrophies typically occur in young horses. The onset is insidious and clinical signs are symmetric with spasticity, ataxia, and paresis of the limbs.

EPILEPTIC BRAIN DAMAGE

Brain damage due to prolonged (usually >30 minutes) convulsive seizures (status epilepticus) is not widely recognized or its occurrence even accepted in domestic animals. In human beings and experimental animals, brain damage resulting from status epilepticus is well documented. One study reported a relatively high incidence of brain lesions in dogs caused by status epilepticus. In this study, acute brain damage was widespread and corresponded well with areas of the brain prone to hypoxic-ischemic injury, such as the cerebral cortex, pyriform cortex, basal nuclei, and hippocampus.

The cause of neuronal injury with prolonged convulsive seizures is debatable. It remains unclear if necrosis, apoptosis, or a combination of these two mechanisms cause neuronal injury in status epilepticus. During seizures, there is an increased metabolic demand for glucose and oxygen by neurons; however, cerebral blood flow increases during seizures, so that the amount of glucose and oxygen available for neurons to generate energy remains adequate, at least during earlier stages. Acute neuronal necrosis still occurs even when cerebral blood flow, oxygenation, body temperature, and other metabolic parameters are maintained within normal limits in experimental animals with status epilepticus.

Excitotoxic injury due to accumulation of neurotoxic amino acid neurotransmitters, such as glutamate during the extreme neuronal activity occurring in status epilepticus, is an attractive explanation for neuronal necrosis. Excitotoxicity would account for both the selective vulnerability of certain brain areas and the character of the lesions. Status epilepticus induced experimentally with kainic acid, an excitatory amino acid receptor agonist, in rats has been shown to cause primarily neuronal necrosis and some characteristics of apoptosis. Other experimental studies have suggested that astrocytes produce clusterin during status epilepticus. Clusterin (dimeric acidic glycoprotein), a sulfated glycoprotein, when expressed in cells in elevated concentrations initiates apoptosis. It is proposed that clusterin secreted by astrocytes during status epilepticus is actively endocytosed by hippocampal neurons, and these neurons die by an apoptotic mechanism. The exact mechanism of neuronal injury remains to be proven. There is some evidence that the mature brain is more prone to injury induced by status epilepticus than the immature brain.

Gross lesions, if present, usually consist of widened and flattened gyri and narrow indistinct sulci caused by cerebral edema. Acute neuronal ischemic cell change and astrocytic swelling are observed microscopically. In experimental animals with status epilepticus, neuronal degeneration is observed within 30 minutes and neuronal necrosis within 60 minutes.

Hepatic Encephalopathy

Acute and chronic liver failure, as well as hepatic atrophy associated with congenital or acquired vascular shunts, often results in hepatic encephalopathy and disordered neurotransmission because of the accumulation of toxic substances, principally ammonia, in the systemic circulation and thus the CNS. Ammonia is formed in the gastrointestinal tract by bacterial degradation of amines, amino acids, purines, and urea from proteins consumed in the diet. In healthy animals, ammonia is detoxified in the liver by conversion to urea by the ornithine citrulline arginine urea cycle. Urea is far less toxic than ammonia and is excreted in the urine. Ammonia has several neurotoxic effects such as: (1) changing the transit of amino acids, water, and electrolytes across the neuronal cell membranes and (2) inhibiting the generation of both excitatory and inhibitory postsynaptic potentials in neurons. Ammonia and other toxic metabolites also appear to (1) cause increased permeability of the blood-brain barrier leading to vasogenic edema and (2) alter osmoregulation within the CNS. These mechanisms likely led to the spongy change (status spongiosus) characteristic of the disease microscopically. Because astrocytes play an important role in regulating fluid and electrolyte balances in the CNS and are the primary cell type having lesions (Alzheimer's type II astrocytes) in hepatic encephalopathy, it is not surprising that alterations in osmoregulation are a component of the pathogenesis of the disease. Ammonia and other toxic metabolites likely also affect oligodendroglia. Finally, it has been proposed that alterations in the blood-brain barrier may facilitate passage of neurotoxins, such as short-chain fatty acids, mercaptans, false (pseudo-) neurotransmitters (tyramine, octopamine, and β-phenylethanolamine), ammonia, and GABA into the CNS leading to neuronal dysfunction. A similar condition, termed renal encephalopathy, has been described in dogs, a horse, and a cow with renal failure. It is likely related to high concentrations of ammonia or ammonia-metabolites in the circulation because of inadequate renal clearance caused by severe glomerular or tubular injury.

In all species except the horse, lesions of hepatic encephalopathy are of two types: spongy change and formation of Alzheimer's type II astrocytes (Fig. 14-13, *D*). Spongy change can be present throughout the neuraxis but typically involves areas of confluence or intermingling of gray and white. These areas include the deep cerebrocortical gray-white matter interface, basal nuclei and adjacent internal capsule, reticular areas throughout the brain stem, and deep cerebellar nuclei. The spongy change is due to intramyelinic edema, causing splitting and vacuolation of myelin sheaths. Spongy change can be produced experimentally by ammonia infusion and is reversible. Alzheimer's type II astrocytic change is a subtle alteration but has been reported in all domestic animals and is the only CNS change observed in horses with hepatic failure. Alzheimer's type II astrocytes are found in gray matter and have enlarged vesicular nuclei with peripheral chromatin, glycogen deposits, and demonstrable nucleoli or nucleolar-type bodies. Immunocytochemical staining for GFAP is typically weak or absent, possibly indicating a toxic effect on astrocytes.

Clinically, affected animals show CNS signs such as seizures, ataxia, depressed mentation, walking aimlessly, and head pressing.

Mitochondrial Encephalopathies

In human beings, various encephalopathic and myopathic syndromes due to point mutations in mitochondrial DNA affecting tRNA genes are grouped under the acronyms MELAS (mitochondrial encephalopathy, lactic acidosis, strokelike episodes) and MERRF (myoclonus epilepsy, ragged red fibers). The various human syndromes include Leigh's disease (subacute necrotizing encephalomyelopathy), Kearns-Sayre syndrome, and Leber's hereditary optic atrophy.

Diseases that might be classified as mitochondrial encephalopathies are not well characterized in animals. Despite this caveat, the diseases reported in the Alaskan husky, Australian cattle dogs, English springer spaniel dogs, and a Jack Russell terrier, as well as in Limousin and Simmental cattle and New Zealand South Hampshire sheep, could represent mitochondrial disorders. Table 14-7 summarizes the salient features of the diseases. Characteristics of these diseases in both human beings and animals are symmetric bilateral involvement of the neuraxis and lesions typified by status spongiosus (edema of cerebral white matter) with variable progression to cavitation or necrosis. The CNS is highly dependent on oxidative metabolism and is therefore the most severely affected organ in mitochondrial disorders. Mitochondria isolated from affected human patients have impaired oxygen consumption and reduced respiratory chain enzyme complex activity. Recently, although quite controversial, it has been suggested that alterations in the function of genes in endothelial cells cause dysfunction of the blood-brain and CSF-blood barriers, which may play an important role in the underlying pathogenesis of mitochondrial encephalopathies.

Primary Neuronal Degeneration

The term *primary neuronal degeneration* encompasses three groups of diseases affecting specific regions of the

Table **14-7**   Possible Mitochondrial Encephalopathies in Animals

Animal	Age of Onset	Clinical Signs	Principal Lesions
Alaskan husky	6 to 9 mo	Ataxia, other motor disturbances, anxiety, blindness, hypalgesia	Spongiosis and cavitation in thalamus caudal to medulla
Cattle dog	5 to 12 mo	Seizures, behavioral abnormalities followed by locomotor signs	Spongiosis and cavitation in cerebellum, brain stem nuclei, and spinal gray matter
English springer spaniel	15 to 16 mo	Ataxia, disorientation, visual deficits	Status spongiosis in accessory olivary nucleus; axon loss and gliosis in optic nerve and tracts
Jack Russell terrier (Parson)	2.5 mo	Ataxia, hypermetria, and deafness	Neuronal degeneration and mineralization of the medulla oblongata, vestibulocochlear nerve, choroid plexus, and granule cell layer of the cerebellum
Limousin cattle	1 to 4 mo	Locomotor signs, aggressive behavior, blindness	Spongiosis, cavitation in cerebral and cerebellar white matter, brain stem nuclei, optic chiasm
Simmental cattle	5 to 12 mo	Ataxia, behavioral changes	Spongiosis and necrosis in internal capsule, caudate nucleus, putamen, brain stem nuclei, spinal gray matter

CNS in a temporally and spatially stereotyped manner and are characterized by degeneration, necrosis, and loss of specific populations of functionally linked neurons. Table 14-8 gives an overview of these diseases. The first group includes the multisystem neuronal degenerations, diseases that affect populations of functionally related neurons in the basal ganglia, brain stem, and cerebellum. The second group includes the primary cerebellar neuronal degenerations, diseases that affect populations of neurons restricted to the cerebellum and cerebellar roof nuclei. The third group includes primary spinal cord degenerations, diseases associated with axonal swellings (axonal spheroids) in the neuraxis termed neuraxonal dystrophies. Another term used to denote some of these diseases in the biomedical literature and veterinary textbooks is "abiotrophy" introduced by Gowers in 1902. The term literally means lack of ("a") a vital ("bios") nutrition ("trophy") required to sustain the life of a tissue.

MULTISYSTEM NEURONAL DEGENERATION
Progressive neuronal abiotrophy of Kerry blue terriers

Progressive neuronal abiotrophy of Kerry blue terriers (cerebellar cortical and extrapyramidal nuclear abiotrophy of Kerry blue terriers, abiotrophy of Kerry blue terriers, or hereditary striatonigral and cerebello-olivary degeneration of Kerry blue terriers) is a well-characterized example of a disease with multisystem neuronal degeneration. The disease is inherited and affects connected neural systems, including basal nuclei and the substantia nigra (i.e., striatonigral), and the cerebellar cortex and caudal olivary nucleus (cerebello-olivary).

Table **14-8**   Multisystem Neuronal Degenerations and Brain Stem/Spinal Syndromes in Domestic Animals

MULTISYSTEM NEURONAL DEGENERATIONS

Canine—Kerry blue terrier, red-haired cocker spaniel, Cairn terrier

PRIMARY CEREBELLAR DEGENERATION

Neonatal syndromes

Canine—beagle, Samoyed, Irish setter
Ovine—Welsh mountain, Corriedale
Bovine—Hereford, Hereford cross, Ayrshire

Postnatal syndromes

Canine—Airedale, German shepherd, Gordon setter, rough-coated collie, border collie, Finnish terrier, Bernese mountain dog, Bern running dog, Labrador retriever, golden retriever, cocker spaniel, Cairn terrier, Great Dane
Bovine—Holstein-Friesian, Hereford cross, Angus
Equine—Arabian, Arabian cross, Gotland pony
Ovine—Merino
Porcine—Yorkshire

MITOCHONDRIAL ENCEPHALOPATHY (ENCEPHALOMYOPATHY)

Canine—English springer spaniel, Alaskan husky, Australian cattle dog, English setter dog, Jack Russell terrier
Bovine—Simmental, Limousin
Sheep—New Zealand South Hampshire

(Continued)

Table **14-8** **Multisystem Neuronal Degenerations and Brain Stem/Spinal Syndromes in Domestic Animals—Cont'd**

SPONGY DEGENERATION

Canine—Labrador retriever, Saluki, silky terrier, Samoyed
Bovine—Jersey, shorthorn, Angus-shorthorn, Hereford
Feline—Egyptian mau

BRAIN STEM AND SPINAL SYNDROMES

Neuroaxonal dystrophy

Canine—border collie, Chihuahua, rottweiler
Feline—domestic
Equine—Morgan
Ovine—Suffolk

Motor neuron disease—spinal cord

Canine—Brittany spaniel, Swedish Lapland, English pointer, rottweiler, German shepherd, sheepdog, collie, pug, dachshund, fox terrier
Feline—Siamese
Bovine—Brown Swiss, Hereford (shaker calf syndrome)
Equine—Various breeds (not believed hereditary)
Porcine—Hampshire, Yorkshire

Degenerative leukomyelopathies (spinal cord—white matter)

Canine—German shepherd, Afghan hound, Kooiker, Labrador retriever, Ibizan hound, harrier, beagle, foxhound, rottweiler, smooth fox terrier, Jack Russell terrier
Bovine—Brown Swiss, Holstein-Friesian, Murray gray
Equine—Various breeds (see vitamin E deficiency)

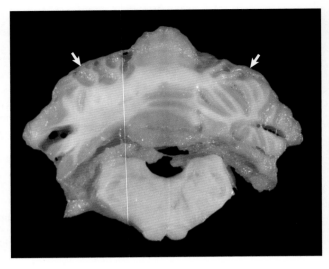

Fig. 14-68 **Striatonigral and cerebello-olivary degeneration, brain, cerebellum, Kerry blue terrier.** Marked atrophy and thinning of folia of dorsal cerebellum (*arrows*) has resulted in increased width of sulci. (*Courtesy Drs. D. Montgomery and R. Storts, College of Veterinary Medicine, Texas A&M University.*)

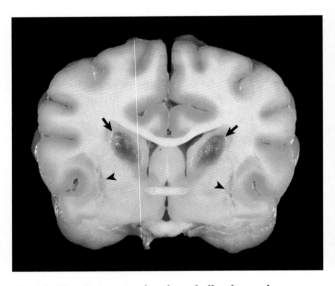

Fig. 14-69 **Striatonigral and cerebello-olivary degeneration, brain, rostral parietal lobe, at level of optic chiasma, Kerry blue terrier.** Note malacia (softening), microscopically due to microcavitation and loss of neurons, in caudate nuclei (*arrows*) and putamen (*arrowheads*). (*Courtesy Drs. D. Montgomery and R. Storts, College of Veterinary Medicine, Texas A&M University; and Vet Pathol 20:143-159, 1983.*)

The pathogenesis is unknown, but an excitotoxic mechanism associated with abnormalities in the glutaminergic cortico-striatal and in the granule-Purkinje cell neurotransmitter systems is proposed. The caudate nucleus and cerebellar cortex are believed to be the primary sites of involvement, whereas lesions in the olivary nucleus and substantia nigra represent transsynaptic degeneration.

Gross lesions are a slight reduction in size of the cerebellum and narrowing of cerebellar folia (Fig. 14-68). In more advanced stages, small foci of softening and discoloration occur in the caudal olivary nucleus and substantia nigra (Fig. 14-69). Lesions in the caudate nucleus initially consist of a vague area of pallor in the body of the nucleus that progresses to marked malacia and ultimately cavitation. There can be similar involvement of the putamen at this advanced stage. Microscopic lesions in chronologic order are degeneration and loss of cerebellar Purkinje and granule cells, followed by neuronal loss in the caudal olivary nucleus, caudate nucleus, putamen, and substantia nigra. Astrogliosis occurs in later stages and is especially prominent in the cerebellar molecular layer. The caudate nucleus and putamen are eventually reduced to microcystic cavities bisected by a few nerve and glial fibers.

In Kerry blue terriers this hereditary disease, with onset from 5 weeks to $5\frac{1}{2}$ months of age, is characterized clinically by rear limb ataxia, intention tremors, hypermetria of front and rear limbs, and atrophy of appendicular and epaxial muscles, presumably from disuse.

Multisystem neuronal degeneration of the red-coated English cocker spaniel

Multisystem neuronal degeneration of the red-coated English cocker spaniel is suspected of being inherited. The pathogenesis is unknown. Bilaterally symmetric diffuse nerve cell loss, astrogliosis, and axonal swellings occur in several nuclei, including septal nuclei, globus pallidus, subthalamic nuclei, substantia nigra, tectum, medial geniculate bodies, and cerebellar and vestibular nuclei. Central cerebellar white matter, corpus callosum, thalamic striae, and subcortical (particularly subcallosal gyri) white matter involvement also are noted. White matter lesions consist of axonal spheroids, intense astrogliosis, subtle myelin loss, and perivascular accumulation of macrophages. Clinical signs occur during the first year of life and consist of progressive ataxia and mental deterioration.

Multisystemic neuronal degeneration of the Cairn terrier

Multisystemic neuronal degeneration of the Cairn terrier has features of an inherited disorder. The pathogenesis is unknown. Widespread neuronal chromatolysis affecting multiple neuronal systems is observed in the CNS and PNS. Affected areas include brain stem sensory and motor nuclei, cerebellar roof nuclei, ventral and dorsal gray columns of the spinal cord, and spinal and autonomic ganglia. Other lesions include degeneration in lateral and ventral spinal funiculi, necrosis of substantia gelatinosa and adjacent white matter most notable in caudal thoracic and cranial lumbar segments, and degeneration in dorsal and ventral spinal nerve rootlets and peripheral nerves. Clinical signs occur between $2\frac{1}{2}$ and 5 months of age, and there is onset of progressive cerebellar ataxia, spastic paresis, and collapse.

PRIMARY CEREBELLAR NEURONAL DEGENERATION

Depending on the degree of maturation of the cerebellum and related systems at the time of birth in the various species, clinical signs in animals with the neonatal syndromes can be manifest in the immediate postnatal period (bovine, ovine) or can be delayed until the time of ambulation (canine). Hereditary transmission is known or suspected in some instances. Lesions vary among affected species and breeds but overall include degeneration or absence of Purkinje cells, proximal swelling of Purkinje cell axons, variable loss of granule cells, cortical astrogliosis, and degeneration of nuclei in the cerebellar medulla.

Animals with postnatal cerebellar syndromes are normal at birth or at the time of ambulation. Onset of ataxia with various other clinical signs referable to cerebellar disease begins weeks or months after a period of apparently normal development. Initial clinical signs are often subtle. Progression of the signs can be slow or rapid, relentless, or with static periods. Some individuals reach a stage without further progression of signs, but this is not typical of the syndrome in most animals.

Grossly the cerebellum can be normal or reduced in size and atrophic. Microscopically, lesions are analogous to those that occur in the neonatal syndromes with loss of Purkinje cells, variable neuronal depletion in the granular layer, and astrogliosis in the molecular layer. Fusiform swellings of proximal Purkinje cell axons are found in the rough-coated collie and the Yorkshire pig. In the rough-coated collie and Merino sheep, lesions occur in other areas of the neuraxis. In these syndromes, degeneration and loss of neurons in the deep cerebellar and other nuclei are accompanied by axonal degeneration in the cerebellum, brain stem, and spinal cord. Loss of spinal ventral horn motor neurons has been noted in the rough-coated collie. An autosomal recessive mode of inheritance is suspected or documented in several of the diseases.

Primary cerebellar neuronal degeneration in dogs and cats

Primary cerebellar neuronal degenerations, as described previously, have been reported to occur in many breeds of dogs and cats, such as American Staffordshire terriers, Australian kelpie dogs, Italian hounds, border collies, Brittany dogs, beagle dogs, Portuguese podengo dogs, Scottish terriers, and domestic shorthair cats. This list is not inclusive and serves only to provide a few common examples. Although most common in young animals of the breeds listed, cerebellar degeneration in Brittany dogs occurs between 7 and 14 years of age. An autosomal recessive mode of inheritance is suspected or documented in several of the diseases. Grossly, the cerebellum can be normal or reduced in size and atrophic. Microscopically, the distribution and characteristics of lesions will vary depending on the breed and species of animal affected. A detailed discussion of the microscopic lesions for each breed and species is outside the scope of this chapter; however, lesions may include a combination of the following changes: loss of Purkinje cells and neurons of the granular layer, astrogliosis, fusiform swelling of proximal Purkinje cell axons, and axonal degeneration in the cerebellum, brain stem, and spinal cord.

Recently, neuronal vacuolation and spinocerebellar degeneration has been reported in young rottweiler dogs. This breed variant of primary cerebellar neuronal degeneration raised biomedical concerns because of the similarities between the vacuolar lesions in neurons of this disease and those of the TSEs (scrapie, BSE). Analyses for protease-resistant scrapie prion protein were performed and were negative. The cause of this disease has not been determined but appears to have a hereditary basis. Apoptotic cell death is apparently not involved in neuronal degeneration. No gross lesions are observed in the brain, but atrophy of the dorsal cricoarytenoid muscles of the larynx has been reported. Microscopic lesions are characterized by spongiform change affecting neuron cell bodies and the neuropil. The cytoplasm of neurons of the cerebellar roof nuclei and nuclei of the extrapyramidal system contain one or more clear vacuoles (1 to 45 μm in diameter). Similar vacuoles are found in neurons in both dorsal nerve root ganglia, myenteric plexus, and other ganglia of the autonomic nervous system. Purkinje cells are also vacuolated, and in terminal stages of the disease there is degeneration with segmental Purkinje cell loss.

Clinical signs, seen as early as 6 weeks (commonly between 3 and 8 months of age in both sexes), include generalized weakness, ataxia, proprioceptive deficits, and paresis that progress in severity over the course of the disease.

Primary cerebellar neuronal degeneration in livestock

Primary cerebellar neuronal degeneration has also been reported to occur in Yorkshire piglets, Merino and Charollais lambs, Holstein Friesian calves, Angus calves, and a moose. An autosomal recessive mode of inheritance is suspected or documented in several of the diseases, but the mechanism of injury is unclear. Grossly the cerebellum can be normal or reduced in size and atrophic. Microscopically, lesions may include loss of Purkinje cells, variable neuronal depletion in the granular layer, fusiform swellings of proximal Purkinje cell axons, and astrogliosis in the molecular layer.

Animals with postnatal primary cerebellar neuronal degeneration are normal at birth or at the time of ambulation. Onset of ataxia with various other clinical signs referable to cerebellar disease begins weeks or months after a period of apparently normal development. Initial clinical signs are often subtle. Progression of the signs can be slow or rapid, relentless, or with static periods. Some individuals reach a stage without further progression of signs, but this is not typical of the syndrome in most animals.

Primary cerebellar neuronal degeneration in horses

Equine cerebellar abiotrophy, a primary cerebellar neuronal degeneration, occurs in Arabian or part-Arabian foals and Swedish Gotland ponies. An autosomal recessive mode of inheritance is suspected, but the mecha-

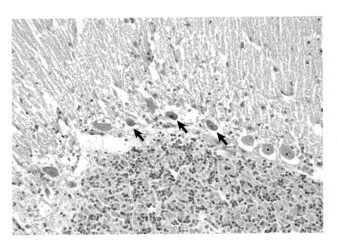

Fig. 14-70   **Equine cerebellar degeneration, cerebellum, horse.** Purkinje cells in the cerebellum show changes consistent with necrosis, such as shrunken cell bodies and nuclear pyknosis (*arrows*). H&E stain. (*Courtesy Dr. J.F. Zachary, College of Veterinary Medicine, University of Illinois.*)

nism of injury is unclear. Although grossly the cerebellum may be slightly reduced in size, microscopically Purkinje cells and their proximal axons are swollen (Fig. 14-70). With time, there may be loss of Purkinje cells and neurons of the granular layer. Clinical signs appear between the time of birth and 9 months of age and include head tremors, ataxia, and spasticity.

Neuraxonal dystrophy

Diseases associated with axonal swellings (axonal spheroids) have been termed neuraxonal dystrophy. Diseases include those putatively associated with vitamin E deficiency or that have been interpreted as an aging change (also see Degenerative Leukomyelopathies and Vitamin E Deficiency). Included here are diseases with a species and breed association and onset relatively early in life, generally before 1 year of age but varying between 4 weeks and 3 years. A hereditary basis is often suspected or proven. Neuraxonal dystrophies have been described in dogs, cats, horses, and sheep. Dystrophy is defined as a disorder arising from defective or faulty nutrition of a cell, tissue, or organ, and the term is most commonly applied to muscle diseases. In this usage it applies to neurons and their axons (neuraxonal). Lesions differ in severity and distribution but are characterized by prominent axonal swellings in various nuclei (often sensory) in the brain stem, cerebellum, and spinal cord. Loss of cerebellar Purkinje and granule cells have been reported in rottweilers and cats and loss of brain stem neurons in cats. In the Morgan horse the axonal swellings are associated with vacuolation.

Neuroaxonal dystrophies are often characterized clinically by severe and often profound muscular weakness and widespread muscle atrophy. Sporadic cases in older adult animals also occur of unknown cause or suspected extraneous influence. Clinical signs vary but include gait abnormalities, dysmetria or hypermetria, proprioceptive disturbance, ataxia, or other cerebellar signs.

Motor neuron diseases

Motor neuron diseases have been described in dogs, cats, cows, horses, and pigs. Degeneration and loss of motor neurons in the ventral horns of the spinal cord and variable axonal degeneration in the ventral spinal nerve rootlets and peripheral nerves characterize the lesions in motor neuron diseases. In some of the motor neuron diseases, there is prominent swelling of ventral horn neuronal cells bodies or axons, or both, associated with marked accumulation of neurofilaments. This accumulation is presumably due to posttranslational protein modification and impairment of neurofilament protein transport. Degeneration in some diseases is not strictly limited to motor neurons of the spinal cord or to motor neurons in general. Other sites of involvement are motor or sensory nuclei, or both, in the brain stem and white matter tracts in the spinal cord.

In horses, lesions in motor neurons are analogous to those already described. The disease affects various breeds, no definitive familial association or age predilections are known, and an inherited basis is not suspected. Generalized weakness, muscle atrophy, and weight loss progress over 1 to several months.

In calves, a disease known as shaker calf syndrome in horned Hereford calves can only be loosely termed a motor neuron disease. There is marked accumulation of neurofilaments within neurons of the central, peripheral, and autonomic nervous systems. All segments of the spinal cord are severely affected. Neurons and neuronal processes in ventral horns, intermediolateral nucleus, Clarke's column, and substantia gelatinosa are swollen and distended. Wallerian degeneration occurs in ventral nerve rootlets and white matter of the spinal cord. Brain stem lesions are less prominent. Swollen cerebellar Purkinje cells and neuronal degeneration in the lateral geniculate body and frontal cortex are reported. The disorder occurs in newborn calves and is characterized clinically by tremulous shaking of the head, body, and tail.

NUTRITIONAL
COPPER

Swayback and enzootic ataxia are diseases caused by copper deficiency in lambs and kid goats. *Swayback* refers to the congenital form of the disease, whereas in enzootic ataxia, onset is delayed for up to 6 months after birth. Although copper deficiency is involved, the pathogenesis is poorly understood. Lesions occur in the cerebrum, brain stem, and spinal cord in the congenital form, but only in the brain stem and spinal cord in cases with a postnatal onset.

Additionally, deficiency of copper can affect wool, hair growth, and pigmentation; musculoskeletal development; and integrity of connective tissue. Copper deficiency can be primarily due to copper-deficient soils and inadequate intake from forage or secondary from defective absorption because of interactions between copper, molybdenum, zinc, cadmium, or inorganic sulfates. Copper is a component of several enzyme systems—including cytochrome and lysyl oxidases such as mitochondrial cytochrome-c oxidase, dopamine β-monoxygenase, peptidyl α-amidating monooxygenase, tyrosinase, and superoxide dismutase—and the protein ceruloplasmin. These enzyme systems are essential for energy generation by mitochondria in the brain, regulating oxidative stress, catecholamine synthesis, and the modification of peptide neurotransmitters.

The pathogenesis of the lesions that occur in swayback and enzootic ataxia is poorly understood. It has been suggested that cerebral lesions result from loss of embryonic cells at the same stage of brain development as occurs in porencephaly and hydranencephaly following in utero viral infection or dysgenesis caused by a biochemical disturbance. Biochemical disturbances could also account for the axonal/neuronal degeneration in the brain stem and spinal cord. Altered function of the mitochondrial enzyme cytochrome oxidase leading to energy failure could play a role in cerebral dysgenesis and axonal and ultimately neuronal degeneration.

More intriguing is the possible involvement of the enzyme copper-zinc superoxide dismutase. A mutation in this enzyme is present in approximately 20% of human beings with familial amyotrophic lateral sclerosis (ALS) and in some individuals with the sporadic form of the disease. This human disorder, which is classified as a motor neuron disease, has a much later onset, and the mutation results in a "gain of function" of the enzyme rather than lack of function as might be present in copper deficiency. Neurofilament accumulation in brain stem and spinal ventral horn neurons and fiber tract degeneration (corticospinal in human beings versus spinocerebellar in lambs and kids with copper deficiency) are similar. Drawing a relevant association between these diseases of human beings and abnormal function of superoxide dismutase in swayback and enzootic ataxia in animals is premature at this time, however. It is also possible that the cortical white matter degeneration and brain stem or spinal lesions arise from different mechanisms.

Grossly, approximately 50% of congenitally affected lambs and rarely kids have bilateral cerebrocortical lesions.

Externally the cerebral cortex can be focally soft and fluctuant or collapsed. These foci correspond to areas of rarefaction, which have either a gelatinous consistency or cystic cavities filled with clear serous fluid, in the white matter of the corona radiate and centrum semiovale. Microscopically a variable astrogliosis is associated with the degeneration of white matter, but the cavities lack a capsule of glial fibers. Myelin degradation and an influx of macrophages are minimal. Delicate neuronal and astroglial processes traverse the cavities. Neuronal necrosis in cortical gray matter overlying these white matter lesions is sometimes observed.

Microscopic lesions in the brain stem and spinal cord in both the congenital (swayback) and delayed-onset (enzootic ataxia) forms of copper deficiency are similar in lambs and kids, and they affect both gray and white matter. Large multipolar neurons of the brain stem reticular formation, certain brain stem nuclei—such as the red and vestibular nuclei—and the ventral, lateral, and, less commonly, dorsal horns of the spinal cord are affected. Neuronal cell bodies lack stainable Nissl's substance (chromatolysis). The cytoplasm is variably dense, pink, and homogeneous to fibrillar as a result of the accumulation of neurofilaments, and nuclei are often displaced to an eccentric position against the cell membrane. The extent of neuronal necrosis varies. Lesions in the white matter of the spinal cord consist of bilateral areas of pallor in the dorsolateral aspects of the lateral funiculi (corresponding roughly to the spinocerebellar tracts) and also in the ventral funiculi adjacent to the ventral median fissure. The pallor of the white matter is due to degeneration of myelinated axons. Involvement of the medial (septomarginal) aspect of the dorsal funiculi is infrequent. In the terminal brain stem, lesions are similar but have a somewhat scattered distribution. The spinocerebellar tracts extending into the middle cerebellar peduncles are affected. Astrogliosis is usually mild. Definitive microscopic lesions in the cerebellum and ventral spinal nerve rootlets and peripheral nerves are usually lacking in lambs, but can be frequent in kids. Changes in Purkinje cells are analogous to those already noted in neurons in other areas. Additionally, ectopic Purkinje cells and thinning of the granular cell layer occur. Bergmann's glial cell processes in the molecular layer hypertrophy. Lesions in ventral spinal nerve rootlets and peripheral nerve are caused by axonal degeneration secondary to injury of motor neurons in the ventral gray horns.

Clinically, CNS disease due to copper deficiency in animals is mainly a disorder of sheep and goats and can be present at birth (swayback in lambs, rarely kids), or onset can be delayed up to 6 months (enzootic ataxia in lambs and kids). Swayback occurs in newborn lambs from ewes with inadequate dietary copper intake. Affected lambs can be born dead, weak, or unable to stand. If mobile, they are ataxic. Enzootic ataxia is characterized by ataxia.

VITAMIN B$_1$ (THIAMINE) DEFICIENCY

Thiamine diphosphate is the active form of thiamine. It is a critical cofactor for several thiamine-dependent enzymes involved in carbohydrate metabolism, and brain damage is thought to be related to a decline in thiamine-dependent enzymes, energy deprivation, and oxidative stress with the abnormal metabolism of free radicals in neurons. These enzymes are also important in the synthesis of several cell constituents, including neurotransmitters. Thiamine deficiency has been associated with neurologic disease in carnivores (Chastek paralysis), human beings (Wernicke's encephalopathy), and ruminants.

Thiamine deficiency in carnivores

In monogastric carnivores and human beings, the relationship between neurologic disease and thiamine deficiency per se is firmly established, and lesions in these species are similar. In carnivores (dog, cat, mink, fox) there is an absolute dietary requirement for vitamin B$_1$. Dietary factors such as the ingestion of fish containing thiaminase, deficient diets, or diets in which the vitamin has been destroyed by other means such as heating, can all lead to thiamine deficiency.

Gross and microscopic lesions are bilaterally symmetric and commonly involve brain stem nuclei, especially caudal colliculi and periventricular nuclei, but the cerebral cortex and cerebellum have also been affected (Fig. 14-71). Lesions consist of neuronal degeneration, neuronal necrosis, status spongiosus, myelin degeneration, and a secondary vascular endothelial and perithelial cell hypertrophy and hyperplasia. Necrotic neurons are those in the caudal colliculi (auditory nerves) that project via axons to the medial geniculate nucleus and those whose cell bodies are located in the periventricular nuclei of the hypothalamus that regulate the release of endocrine hormones from the anterior pituitary. Hemorrhage and an influx of macrophages also occurs in some cases.

Clinical signs in carnivores may include a combination of the following: anorexia, vomiting, depression, wide-based stance, ataxia, spastic paresis, circling, seizures, muscle weakness, recumbency, opisthotonus, coma, or death.

Thiamine deficiency in ruminants

The disease in cattle, sheep, and less commonly, goats, has been termed polioencephalomalacia or cerebrocortical necrosis. Rumen microbes are able to synthesize thiamine, and conclusive evidence of an

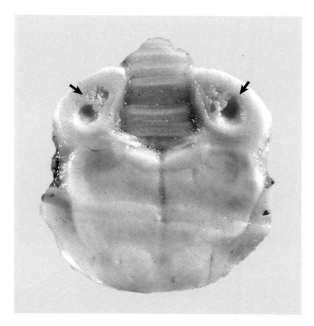

Fig. 14-71   **Thiamine deficiency encephalopathy, midbrain, caudal colliculi, dog.** In the dog, lesions of thiamine deficiency encephalopathy are generally restricted to the brain stem. Note the symmetrically cavitated (malacic) lesions in the caudal colliculi *(arrows)* resulting from neuronal necrosis. *(Courtesy Dr. J. Edwards, College of Veterinary Medicine, Texas A&M University; and Dr. J. King, College of Veterinary Medicine, Cornell University.)*

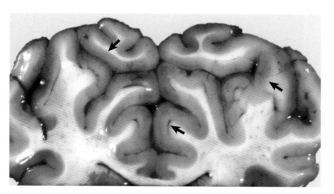

Fig. 14-72   **Acute polioencephalomalacia, cerebral cortex, cross-sectional view, cow.** Cerebral cortical gyri are yellow and swollen *(arrows)*. The cause of this yellow color is unknown, but has been shown experimentally not to be caused by ceroid-lipofuscin pigments. Changes involving the sulci and gyri in acute polioencephalomalacia are shown in Fig. 14-31. *(Courtesy Dr. L. Roth, College of Veterinary Medicine, Cornell University.)*

absolute thiamine deficiency as the sole cause of polioencephalomalacia in ruminants has been elusive. Evidence or theories linking thiamine with the ruminant disorder include the following:

1. Clinical response to thiamine injection in some individuals
2. Decreases in ruminal thiamine, or overgrowth of thiaminase-producing microbes, such as *Bacillus thiaminolyticus*
3. Ingestion of thiaminase-containing plants, such as bracken fern
4. Production of inactive thiamine analogs
5. Decreased absorption or increased fecal excretion of thiamine

Gross lesions, if present, are limited primarily to the cerebral cortex. Initially, 2 days after onset, the surface of the brain can be swollen (cerebral edema) as indicated by flattening of cerebrocortical gyri and narrow sulci. In rare cases with more severe brain swelling, brain displacement with herniation of the parahippocampal gyri beneath the tentorium cerebelli and the vermis of the cerebellum into the foramen magnum can occur. By 4 days after onset, yellow discoloration of the cerebrocortical gray matter occurs (Fig. 14-72), and it is at this time that autofluorescence (see later for

more detail) is seen when the brain is examined under 375 nm ultraviolet light (Fig. 14-73). Eight to 10 days after onset, edematous separation and necrosis involving the middle to deeper lamina or gray-white matter interface may be appreciable (Fig. 14-74). In advanced cases with prolonged survival, areas of marked atrophy of cerebral gyri with an attenuated or absent gray matter zone are covered by meninges (Fig. 14-75).

Microscopically the earliest lesions are laminar cortical necrosis and astrocytic swelling. Laminar cortical necrosis is characterized by neuronal necrosis (ischemic change), with a laminar pattern of edema in the cerebral cortex. Neurons in the middle to deep lamina of the parieto-occipital lobes of the cerebral cortex are preferentially affected. In the early stages or in mild cases, lesions can be limited to the depths of cerebrocortical sulci, but generally there is involvement of entire gyri that may be confluent over extensive areas of the cortex. After 4 to 5 days, neuronal necrosis and edema are more severe, and there is an early influx of blood monocytes that mature into tissue macrophages and become gitter cells as they phagocytose necrotic debris. Macrophages and gitter cells are observed most commonly in perivascular and perineuronal spaces and in the pia arachnoid (Fig. 14-26, A). After 8 to 10 days, necrosis and edema have resulted in laminar separation (at the gray matter–white matter interface) in which there are prominent accumulations of macrophages (Fig. 14-76). Lesions that accompany the necrosis include vascular prominence caused by endothelial cell and perithelial cell hypertrophy and hyperplasia, congestion, and a minimal, if any, influx of neutrophils. Bilaterally symmetric focal lesions, similar

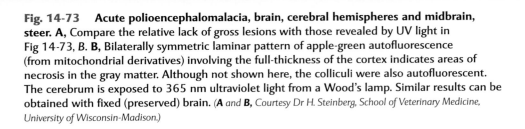

Fig. 14-73   Acute polioencephalomalacia, brain, cerebral hemispheres and midbrain, steer. A, Compare the relative lack of gross lesions with those revealed by UV light in Fig 14-73, *B.* **B,** Bilaterally symmetric laminar pattern of apple-green autofluorescence (from mitochondrial derivatives) involving the full-thickness of the cortex indicates areas of necrosis in the gray matter. Although not shown here, the colliculi were also autofluorescent. The cerebrum is exposed to 365 nm ultraviolet light from a Wood's lamp. Similar results can be obtained with fixed (preserved) brain. *(A and B, Courtesy Dr H. Steinberg, School of Veterinary Medicine, University of Wisconsin-Madison.)*

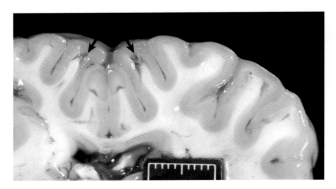

Fig. 14-74   Acute cerebrocortical polioencephalomalacia, thiamine deficiency, brain, parietal lobe, level of thalamus, goat. Note the liquefactive necrosis with varying degrees of tissue separation *(arrows)* in the deep cortex. Scale bar = 2 cm. *(Courtesy Dr. R. Storts, College of Veterinary Medicine, Texas A&M University.)*

to those seen in carnivores, occur in the thalamus and midbrain or colliculi and rarely in other brain stem structures. Animals that survive can have cerebral atrophy and develop hydrocephalus ex vacuo and have been known to live 1 to 2 years. It should be noted that laminar cortical necrosis can be caused by a variety of metabolic abnormalities. In ruminants, in addition to thiamine deficiency, water deprivation-sodium ion toxicosis, lead poisoning, and high sulfur intake can cause polioencephalomalacia and laminar cortical necrosis.

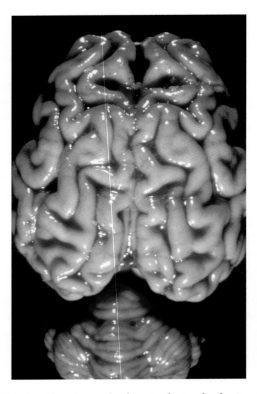

Fig. 14-75   Chronic cerebral cortical atrophy, brain, cow. Cerebral cortical gyri are atrophic. Gyri are narrow, and as a result the sulci are widened. In this case, the loss of cerebral cortex was caused by thiamine deficiency several years previously. *(Courtesy College of Veterinary Medicine, University of Illinois.)*

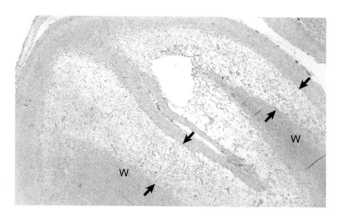

Fig. 14-76   Chronic polioencephalomalacia, cerebral cortex, cow. Areas of microcavitation in the deep cortical laminae next to the subcortical white matter are poorly stained (*area between arrows*) when compared with those of the normal superficial cortex (*left*). *W,* White matter. H&E stain. (*Courtesy Dr. J.F. Zachary, College of Veterinary Medicine, University of Illinois.*)

Although autofluorescence at 365 nm ultraviolet light has been historically attributed to the accumulation of ceroid-lipofuscin in lipophages resulting from lipid degeneration in injured neuronal cell membranes, this supposition has recently been questioned. A recent study of cerebrocortical necrosis reported that autofluorescent substances in degenerating neurons occurred in structures resembling mitochondria and that ceroid-lipofuscin pigments were not demonstrated microscopically in damaged CNS. An association between mitochondria and autofluorescence has also been shown in the neuronal ceroid lipofuscinoses (Batten disease, ceroid-lipofuscin storage diseases). These diseases are characterized by the accumulation of an autofluorescent (365 nm ultraviolet light), intracytoplasmic storage material in CNS neurons composed mostly of subunit c of mitochondrial ATP synthase.

Clinically the disease is seen most commonly in cattle 6 to 18 months of age fed concentrated rations. In sheep, most cases occur in younger age groups (2 to 7 months). Clinical signs in cattle and small ruminants may include depression, stupor, ataxia, head pressing, apparent cortical blindness, opisthotonos, convulsions, and recumbency with paddling, and death. If animals survive or respond to therapy, clinical signs can persist.

Polioencephalomalacia commonly occurs in cattle fed rations rich in carbohydrates with little roughage and is also associated with clinical or subclinical acidosis that may precipitate changes in rumen microflora. The disorder also occurs in association with other dietary factors including cobalt deficiency, molasses- and urea-based diets, and with diets high in elemental sulfur and sulfates

and sulfides, some of which are not specifically associated with thiamine deficiency.

Recently, there has been considerable interest in the relationship of high dietary sulfur to polioencephalomalacia. All sources of sulfur, including formulated rations, plants rich in sulfur (*Kochia scoparia*), and high concentrations of sulfur in the drinking water, are additive. Total dietary intake should not exceed 0.3% to 0.4%. The exact mechanism to explain sulfur-induced polioencephalomalacia in ruminants has not been proven. Although deficiency or disordered metabolism of thiamine can be involved, it would seem not to be the sole cause or, in some instances, even a major factor in the disorder. Alternatively, polioencephalomalacia could represent a multifactorial metabolic disorder with multiple causes, all culminating in cerebrocortical necrosis. Any unifying hypothesis concerning the mechanism(s) of brain damage would have to reconcile all these variables.

VITAMIN A DEFICIENCY

See Chapter 20.

VITAMIN E DEFICIENCY

See Equine Degenerative Myeloencephalopathy.

TOXICOSES

Space constraints do not allow a comprehensive discussion of all toxicities affecting the nervous system. Table 14-9 is a partial listing of poisons with potential to cause neurologic illness and CNS injury. Some of these, such as mercury, have in the past caused high morbidity and mortality in isolated outbreaks. An example is the Minamata Bay incident in Japan (in 1956) of human beings eating fish containing high

Table **14-9**   **Other Toxicities Involving the Nervous System**

CHEMICALS

Heavy metals: cadmium, manganese, mercury, tin (trimethyltin), zinc
Hexacarbons: n-hexane, others
Pesticides: carbaryl, bromethalin, chlorinated hydrocarbons
Drugs: nitrofurazones, ivermectin, levamisole, metronidazole

PLANTS

Cycads, *Chrysocoma tenuifolia*, *Helichrysum* spp., *Solanum* spp. (*dimidiatum, fastigium, kwebense*), sorghum, *Stypandra* spp.

MYCOTOXINS

Acremonium, Aspergillus, Claviceps, Fumonisin, Penicillium

concentrations of methylmercury. Methylmercury accumulates in the aquatic food chain, and thus the highest concentrations exist in predatory fish at the top of the food chain. In human beings and animals with methylmercury toxicosis, neuronal cell bodies of the cerebral cortex and cerebellum die through a mechanism suggested to be apoptosis; however, microtubule dysfunction, oxidative stress, alterations of calcium homeostasis, and the potentiation of glutaminergic excitotoxicity may be involved. The potential remains for serious neurologic illnesses and death from these intoxications, and the interested reader is referred to more comprehensive reference sources. In this chapter, discussion of toxicities will be limited to those conditions most likely to be encountered in veterinary practice.

CHEMICALS

Chemically induced distal axonopathies have been classified by functional alterations affecting motor or sensory neurons, location of injury within the nerve (distal, proximal), or by the type of nerve affected (cranial or spinal). Because of the large number and wide use of chemicals in commerce, there exists an extensive list of experimental studies describing toxic axonopathies and neuropathies. Their complete discussion is outside the scope of this chapter.

Chemicals used in agricultural, industrial, and pharmaceutical commerce can injure nerves by interfering with axoplasmic flow. Such chemicals include: acrylamide (polymerizing agent to strengthen paper), carbon disulfide (fat solvent, used for extraction of oil from oil-bearing fruit such as olives), triorthocresyl phosphate (high-performance lubricants in airplane engines), halomethane (refrigerants), methylene chloride (extraction agents, paint solvents, degreasing agents), carbon tetrachloride (solvents), and butane (fuel source).

Acrylamide causes a unique distal axonopathy (dying-back axonopathy) primarily affecting axons of the PNS (less commonly the CNS) in which there is accumulation of neurofilaments within affected axons. Axonal spheroids are thought to be related to alteration of axonal transport resulting from phosphorylation of neurofilaments and their abnormal rearrangement within the axon. This "dying-back" axonopathy is microscopically characterized by degeneration of axons starting at or near synapses and proceeding toward the neuronal cell body. The most distal axonal projections are furthest from the cell body and thus cannot be maintained. Thus they are most vulnerable to functional alterations; however, it is unclear whether this degeneration is caused by energy deficits, lack of antioxidants, or physical obstruction of axoplasmic flow. Axonal degeneration is followed by secondary demyelination.

Certain types of toxic and biochemical injury to axons result in a stereotypic pattern of morphologic change that affects either distal or proximal segments of the axon and results in the formation of segmental axonal spheroids. Based on the location of the spheroids, such diseases are divided into one of two groups, either diseases affecting axons a distance away from their cell bodies (distal axonopathies) or diseases affecting axons near their cell bodies (proximal axonopathies).

It is hypothesized that axonal spheroid formation and subsequent axonal degeneration are caused by alterations in axoplasmic flow, by alterations of anterograde or retrograde flow depending on the nature of the injury resulting in the accumulation and/or rearrangement of cytoskeletal proteins. The histologic lesion common to these two types of axonopathies is the formation of axonal spheroids with subsequent degeneration of the axon and secondary demyelination, a process that in many ways resembles the lesions described for Wallerian degeneration. Axonal spheroids are common to a variety of neuronal derangements; therefore distal and proximal axonopathies must be differentiated from other diseases that cause spheroids, such as the compressive axonopathies.

Distal and proximal axonopathies have been further subdivided by some scientific disciplines into groups based on whether initial axonal lesions progress in an anterograde or retrograde direction. The terminology and classification schemes, although useful to some, are outside the scope of this chapter and are often confusing. The occurrence of secondary anterograde or retrograde lesions will be discussed in the context of some of the diseases presented next.

Organophosphates

Organophosphates are divided into two groups according to their use, mode of action, and type of toxicity. The first group, organophosphate esters, used as pesticides (parathion, malathion, diazinon, carbaryl, aldicarb), fungicides, herbicides, or rodenticides, cause acute toxicity by inhibiting cholinesterase either directly or indirectly, allowing acetylcholine to accumulate at synaptic (nerve-nerve junctions) or myoneural junctions (nerve-muscle junctions), resulting in persistent depolarization. In acute organophosphate toxicosis, clinical effects vary but are manifested in the following:

1. Parasympathetic nervous system, leading to salivation, lacrimation, urination, defecation, bradycardia, and pupillary constriction
2. Skeletal muscular system, resulting in muscle fasciculations followed by weakness and muscle paralysis (i.e., death is due primarily to respiratory failure)
3. Central nervous system, leading to anxiety, restlessness, hyperactivity, anorexia, and generalized seizures (i.e., observed in dogs and cats, but are uncommon in cattle)

Gross and microscopic lesions in the nervous system are absent, and those in other tissues are nonspecific.

The second group causes chronic toxicosis and is the most common cause of chemically induced distal axonopathy in veterinary medicine. This group of organophosphates includes the cresyl and related compounds, such as triorthocresyl phosphate used in hydraulic fluids, lubricants, flame-retardants, and plasticizers. The triaryl phosphate group of compounds used as high-temperature lubricants is toxic for several species of animals and human beings.

Chronic exposure (delayed neuropathy) to certain organophosphate pesticides and herbicides (trichlorphon, merphos, triorthocresyl phosphate, leptophos, parathion, malathion, diazinon) causes delayed neurotoxicity unrelated to cholinesterase inhibition as seen in acute organophosphate toxicosis. The type of axonal injury caused by these chemicals follows the stereotypic process of morphologic changes described previously and occurs approximately 10 to 14 days following exposure. Organophosphorus compounds causing delayed neurotoxicity inhibit the activity of an enzyme referred to as neuropathy target esterase. The function of the enzyme in the PNS and CNS is not fully understood.

Phosphorylation of the enzyme by the toxic compound is proposed to interfere with its normal function, resulting in axonal injury. Other studies have shown that organophosphates causing delayed neurotoxicity interact with Ca^{2+} or calmodulin kinase II, an enzyme responsible for phosphorylation of cytoskeletal proteins, such as microtubules, neurofilaments, and microtubule-associated protein-2, resulting in disassembly and accumulation of these proteins in the distal portions of axons, producing axonal swelling and degeneration.

No specific gross lesions are present in chemically induced distal axonopathies. Microscopically, there is retrograde degeneration beginning in the distal part of axons, especially those with a larger diameter. Affected areas in the spinal cord include dorsal funiculi, spinocerebellar tracts in lateral funiculi, and ventromedial aspects of the ventral funiculi. Central chromatolysis of cell bodies of affected nerves has occurred.

Clinically, signs of toxicity are usually delayed 1 to 2 weeks after exposure. Young animals, because of their ability to compensate for the neurologic deficits, tend to be less seriously affected, whereas recovery is slow and incomplete in adults. Susceptible animals include cats, domestic and exotic ruminants, chickens, pheasants, and ducks. Small laboratory animals, dogs, and some nonhuman primates are less sensitive. Clinical signs are those of combined sensory and motor neuropathy and spinal cord damage, such as proprioceptive deficits expected by damage to the spinocerebellar nucleus and tract as well as the fasciculus gracilis.

Selenium

An acute paralytic syndrome termed bilateral poliomyelomalacia has been observed in feeder pigs associated with the inadvertent inclusion of toxic amounts of selenium (selenium-enriched yeast, sodium selenite, or sodium selenate) in pig rations. The pathogenesis of the lesions is not proven but could involve an induced nicotinamide or niacin deficiency. Experimentally, 6-aminonicotinamide, a gliotoxin and antagonist of the vitamin, causes lesions analogous to those seen in the natural porcine disease.

Grossly, bilateral (symmetric) areas of softening and yellow discoloration occur in the ventral spinal gray matter of the cervical and lumbar intumescences. Microscopically, acute lesions consist progressively of neuronal chromatolysis, neuronal necrosis, neuronal loss, microcavitation, and glial necrosis. As would be expected, these changes are subsequently followed by astrogliosis and the accumulation of gitter cells. Prominent capillaries are typical. Wallerian degeneration occurs in ventral spinal nerve rootlets of those cord segments whose ventral gray horn motor neurons have been destroyed. Identical lesions have been observed in the brain stem.

Clinically, affected pigs are alert, rest in sternal recumbency, and squeal loudly when disturbed. They eventually progress to quadriplegia with flaccid paralysis of the rear limbs. Cutaneous manifestations of the toxicity also occur and include rough hair coats, partial alopecia, and separation and sloughing of the hoofs. Historically, a similar ovine bilateral symmetric poliomyelomalacia has been reported from Africa, but an association with selenium toxicity was not made.

Sodium chloride

Sodium chloride toxicity, also known as sodium ion toxicosis, water deprivation syndrome, or salt poisoning, occurs primarily in pigs, poultry, and occasionally in ruminants, dogs, horses, and sheep. The disease occurs following over-consumption of sodium chloride in rations or supplements and can be complicated by limited availability of drinking water, resulting in severe dehydration. A similar sequence of events can occur with simple water restriction of sufficient duration to allow compensation by the brain's adaptive response to chronic hypernatremia (hyperosmolarity). Sodium chloride toxicity is due to hyperosmolarity (hypernatremia) caused by excessive intake of sodium salts or severe dehydration followed by rehydration and a "rapid" hypernatremic to normonatremic or hyponatremic shift.

During the initial hypernatremic phase, the brain "shrinks" because of the osmotic loss of water. An influx of sodium, potassium, and chloride ions into the brain, beginning within minutes after the osmotic loss of water, is an acute adaptive response to equalize the sodium imbalance. Maintenance of a normal ionic balance in the brain is critical, however, for normal function and, although a new ionic equilibrium is established, this acute response alone cannot compensate for severe or prolonged hypernatremia.

A second, more delayed adaptive response of the brain is an influx or endogenous production of organic osmolytes, such as certain amino acids, polyols, and methylamines, to equalize the osmotic imbalance created by hypernatremia. This response requires hours or days to establish a new osmotic equilibrium. When animals are given free access to fresh water, an acute hypernatremic to hyponatremic shift occurs. Within minutes, the brain attempts to offset this osmotic imbalance by eliminating sodium, potassium, and chloride ions by actively transporting these ions into the vasculature. This early response cannot, however, offset the osmotic stress created by the increased organic osmolytes in the brain. As a result of the osmotic gradient created by the elevated organic osmolytes, water enters the brain with subsequent brain swelling.

Grossly, lesions are inconsistent but include cerebral and leptomeningeal congestion and edema. Zones of cerebrocortical laminar necrosis can be detected in transverse slices of fixed brain. Microscopically, cerebrocortical neuronal necrosis, often laminar, is accompanied by astrocytic swelling. In pigs, leptomeninges and perivascular spaces can have an infiltrate of eosinophils and, with longer survival, an influx of macrophages occurs depending on the extent of necrosis. The leptomeningeal and perivascular infiltrate of eosinophils is an inconsistent finding. Pallor of subcortical white matter is indicative of edema, and prominence of small cortical blood vessels is due to congestion and swelling of endothelial cell nuclei. In ruminants, arteriolar degeneration with a transmural neutrophilic infiltrate, cerebellar Purkinje cell necrosis, and edema of basal nuclei, thalamus, and midbrain have been observed.

Clinical signs include inappetence and dehydration early followed by heading pressing, incoordination, blindness, circling, paddling, and convulsions. Animals are often found dead in their pasture or pen.

METALS
Arsenic

Toxicity due to ingestion or cutaneous absorption can occur with inorganic and organic arsenicals and can affect multiple organs including the nervous system. Inorganic compounds are predominantly herbicides or pesticides, whereas organic arsenicals (arsanilic acid, 3-nitro-4-phenylarsonic acid) have been used as feed additives in the pig and poultry industries as growth promoters and to control enteric diseases.

Poisoning with inorganic arsenicals is an acute enteric disease with hepatic and renal manifestations, but neurologic signs can occur. Probably because of the nature of the organic compounds and the manner of their use, there is greater potential for neurotoxicity. Arsanilic acid has a greater tendency to cause peripheral and optic nerve and tract damage, whereas 3-nitro compounds tend to affect the spinal cord more severely.

Gross lesions are not present. Microscopically, lesions in cranial and peripheral nerves and spinal cord consist of axonal degeneration and fragmentation of myelin sheaths. In the spinal cord following 3-nitro poisoning, lesions are found chronologically in the cervical and thoracic cord followed by lesions in the lumbar cord. Spinocerebellar tracts and dorsal funiculi are predominantly affected. The distribution of lesions suggests that the distal segments of long ascending fiber tracts can be preferentially injured. Inorganic arsenicals inhibit sulfhydryl enzyme systems and disrupt cellular metabolism. The exact mode of action of organic arsenicals is unknown.

In pigs, clinical signs include blindness resulting from damage to optic nerves and tracts and incoordination, paresis, and paralysis related to spinal cord and peripheral nerve lesions.

Lead

Lead poisoning has occurred in a variety of animals, but with the increased awareness of the potential for toxicity and environmental contamination and current regulations, such as reduced concentrations in paint and unleaded gasoline, poisoning is uncommon and if it occurs is most common in cattle. Potential sources include discarded car batteries and old flaking or peeling lead paint in barns and farm buildings.

Depending on the quantity absorbed, poisoning can be peracute with no gross or microscopic lesions, acute, subacute, or chronic. In peracute or acute cases, contents of the upper digestive tract, such as fragments of battery plates or flakes of paint, could indicate the possibility of lead poisoning. Lead poisoning can affect many tissues and organs, including CNS, PNS, liver, kidneys, gastrointestinal tract, bone marrow, blood vessels, and organs of the reproductive and endocrine systems. In horses grazing lead-contaminated pastures, a cranial neuropathy with laryngeal and facial paralysis has been described.

Lead poisoning in cattle and other species is via the oral route or, less commonly, via the respiratory system or skin (inorganic lead). Lead can damage the brain through a variety of mechanisms. Direct toxic effects on neurons, astrocytes, and cerebral endothelial cells occur by disrupting metabolic pathways and altering the function of dopaminergic, cholinergic, and glutamatergic neurotransmitter systems. Lead crosses the blood-brain barrier rapidly using a cationic transporter, concentrates in the brain because of its ability to substitute for calcium ions in the pump, and enters astrocytes and neurons by voltage-sensitive cell membrane calcium channels. Lead disrupts calcium homeostasis, causing the accumulation of calcium in lead-exposed cells, and induces mitochondrial release of calcium, leading to apoptotic cell death. Astrocytes contain metallothionein and can sequester potentially toxic metals in the CNS, thus protecting more vulnerable neurons from the toxic effects of lead. However, astrocytes may also be sensitive to the toxic effects of lead, leading to functional deficits such as in the uptake, transport, and metabolism of neurotransmitters. Transplacental (human beings and sheep) and neonatal lead exposure can result in delayed brain maturation and biochemical abnormalities.

Gross lesions in the CNS are usually absent. When present, they can resemble those present in polioencephalomalacia of cattle, but this is uncommon. In general, gross lesions, if present, are distributed in a laminar pattern and include meningeal and cerebrovascular congestion, brain swelling with flattening of gyri, or hemorrhage. With longer survival times, there may be foci of cerebrocortical malacia (softening), cavitation, and laminar necrosis followed by cerebral cortical atrophy, widened sulci, narrowed gyri, and loss of white matter.

Microscopically, lesions in peracute cases are absent. In acute cases, congestion, astrocytic swelling, status spongiosis, and microvascular prominence caused by endothelial hypertrophy are present, and often ischemic neuronal cell change is characteristically confined to the tips of cerebrocortical gyri. For most cases in cattle, only a few necrotic neurons at gyral tips and minimal astrocytic swelling, vascular prominence, and congestion can be found. With longer survival times, cerebrocortical lesions progress to laminar necrosis, accumulations of macrophages, or liquefactive necrosis, the last being rare. Because of their similarities, lesions of lead encephalopathy in ruminants must be differentiated from those of thiamine deficiency-induced polioencephalomalacia and sulfur-related polioencephalomalacia.

Lesions in dogs resemble those in cattle, but vascular damage is more obvious and consistent. Vascular lesions can progress to mural hyalinization, necrosis, and thrombosis. Other lesions include neuronal necrosis in the cerebral cortex, hippocampus, and cerebellum (Purkinje cells), myelin destruction in cerebrocortical white matter, and a peripheral neuropathy.

Clinically, affected cows are often found down or dead in the pasture. If clinical signs are present, they range initially from depression, inappetence, and diarrhea to teeth grinding (bruxism), circling, head pressing, incoordination, and blindness later. In small animals, especially dogs, clinical signs include ataxia, tremors, clonic-tonic seizures, blindness, and deafness.

Organotins

Excessive exposure to organotins such as triethyltin (stabilizer, catalyst, wood and textile preservative, fungicide, bactericide, and insecticide) causes cytotoxic edema principally affecting myelin sheaths of oligodendroglial cells in the white matter. Experimental studies have shown that triethyltin selectively damages myelin sheaths and causes a decrease in potassium concentrations in the white matter with a concurrent increase in intracellular water content. The blood-brain barrier is not affected. The mechanism of injury is thought to be uncoupling of oxidative phosphorylation and inhibition of mitochondrial ATPase activity within cell membranes. Loss of Na/K-dependent ATPase activity in cell membranes of myelin lamellae leads to the formation of intramyelinic edema.

Gross lesions, if present, consist of an enlarged brain and spinal cord. Because of compression against the cranium, an affected brain has flattened gyri and shallow indistinct sulci. Microscopically, fluid accumulates between myelin layers and leads to splitting of the myelin lamellae and the formation of intramyelinic spaces.

MICROBIAL TOXINS
Botulism

See Peripheral Nervous System.

Clostridium perfringens type D encephalopathy (pulpy kidney disease, overeating disease)

Clostridium perfringens type D enterotoxemia, associated with epsilon toxin production, is a disease of sheep, goats, and cattle, but only sheep commonly exhibit the neurologic manifestations of the disease. Brain damage is due to vascular injury and breakdown of the blood-brain barrier. Binding of epsilon toxin to endothelial cell surface receptors results in opening of tight junctions, disturbed transport processes, increased vascular permeability that results in vasogenic edema, swelling of astrocytic foot processes, and ultimately necrosis caused by hypoxic-ischemic mechanisms. Some of the effects of epsilon toxin can be mediated by an adenyl cyclase–cAMP system.

Gross lesions are absent in some peracute cases but, when present, consist initially of bilaterally symmetric foci of malacia, leading to yellow-gray to red foci with malacia and cavitation (Fig. 14-77). Lesions can be found in the internal capsule, basal nuclei, thalamus,

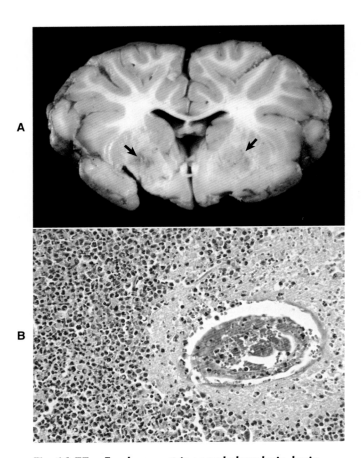

Fig. 14-77   Focal symmetric encephalomalacia, brain, transverse section at the level of the basal nuclei and rostral thalamus, sheep. A, There are bilateral discoloration and malacia (*arrows*) in a portion of the basal nuclei. These lesions are caused by an enterotoxin produced by *Clostridium perfringens* type D. **B,** Microscopically the walls of arterioles can be hyalinized, and endothelial cell nuclei swollen and vesicular (not shown here) with perivascular laking of proteinaceous fluid. Pericapillary hemorrhage and acute necrosis of neurons and macroglia can occur. With longer survival, as seen here, lesions include destruction of neuropil, accumulation of neutrophils and foamy macrophages (*gitter cells—left half of the figure*), and lymphocytic perivascular cuffing. In this case, the inflammatory response is pronounced and would not be considered typical of this disease. H&E stain. (**A,** *Courtesy Dr. D. Cho, College of Veterinary Medicine, Louisiana State University; and Noah's Arkive, College of Veterinary Medicine, The University of Georgia.* **B,** *Courtesy Dr. J. Simon, College of Veterinary Medicine, University of Illinois.*)

hippocampus, rostral colliculus and substantia nigra, pons, corona radiata of frontal cortex, and cerebellar peduncles, especially the middle peduncle. Lesions in other tissue consist of pulmonary congestion and edema, serous pericardial effusion, petechiation, and soft (pulpy) kidneys.

Microscopically the CNS lesion in acute cases is vasogenic edema secondary to vascular injury. The fluid in perivascular spaces is frequently protein rich and eosinophilic. Walls of arterioles can be hyalinized, and endothelial cell nuclei swollen and vesicular. Vasogenic edema, which is interstitial in location, gives a light or pink-staining, spongy appearance to the CNS parenchyma. Both gray matter and white matter are affected. Pericapillary hemorrhage and acute necrosis of neurons and macroglia occur. Other changes occur with longer survival and include axonal swelling, accumulation of neutrophils and foamy macrophages, vascular prominence caused by perithelial-endothelial nuclear enlargement or swelling, lymphocytic perivascular cuffing, and liquefactive necrosis.

Sheep of all ages, except newborns, are susceptible; incidence peaks between 3 and 10 weeks of age and in feeder lambs shortly after arrival at a feedlot. Resistance of newborns can be related to lack in the gut of pancreatic proteolytic enzymes necessary for activation of the epsilon toxin, and to trypsin inhibitors in colostrum. Lambs are typically in good condition and are found dead.

Edema disease (enterotoxemic colibacillosis)

Edema disease is a disorder of rapidly growing, healthy feeder pigs being fed a high-energy ration. The disease is caused by strains of *Escherichia coli* producing a Shiga-like toxin, which is similar to toxins produced by *Shigella dysenteriae* and is designated Shiga-like toxin type IIe (SLT-IIe). This toxin causes necrosis of smooth muscle cells in small arteries and arterioles and a reduction focally in the degree of circulation to the CNS parenchyma, leading to infarction manifested grossly as malacia in the CNS. Glycolipid cell surface receptors on endothelial cells, globotriaosylceramide or globotetraosylceramide, are binding sites for the toxin, and their presence confers susceptibility to the disease. Binding of the toxin to these receptors can initiate a chain of inflammatory and immunologic reactions that lead to vascular damage.

The basic lesion is an angiopathy that leads to edematous and hypoxic-ischemic injury in a variety of tissue, including the brain. Grossly, edema is present in the subcutis often prominent in the palpebrae, cardiac region of the gastric submucosa, gallbladder, colonic mesentery, mesenteric lymph nodes, larynx, and lungs, and serous effusions occur in the thoracic cavity and pericardial sac. Congestion, and sometimes hemorrhage, also occur. The characteristic gross lesions in the brain are usually bilaterally symmetric foci of necrosis in the caudal medulla, but they can extend rostrally as far as the basal nuclei. The lesions are yellow-gray, soft, and slightly depressed.

The primary microscopic lesion, a degenerative angiopathy/vasculitis, is noted most frequently and is most severe in the caudal medulla to the diencephalon and in cerebral and cerebellar meninges. Cerebral, cerebellar, and spinal blood vessels are also affected. Initially, perivascular edema results from early vascular injury. Edema is followed by necrosis of medial smooth muscle cells, deposition of fibrinoid material, and accumulation of macrophages and lymphocytes in the adventitia. Although endothelial cells and their nuclei become swollen and vesicular, this layer generally remains intact, and consequently thrombosis is not a feature. Lesions associated with the angiopathy include pallor and spongiosis of the CNS parenchyma caused by vasogenic edema and necrosis of neurons and glia. An influx of macrophages into the necrotic lesions can be observed with longer survival times.

Pigs are usually 4 to 8 weeks of age, but younger and older pigs can be affected. Clinically, affected animals are initially ataxic and then become laterally recumbent with rhythmic paddling of the limbs. As the disease progresses, they may become comatose and die. Most pigs die within 24 hours; however, pigs that survive for several days typically develop CNS lesions (see chronologic sequence of infarction, Table 14-1).

Leukoencephalomalacia

Ingestion of moldy feed, mainly corn or corn by-products, contaminated with the fungus *Fusarium verticillioides* (formerly called *Fusarium moniliforme*) causes an acute fatal neurologic disease in horses called leukoencephalomalacia. The primary toxin isolated from *Fusarium verticillioides* has been named fumonisin B_1, although other fumonisins have been extracted. The exact mechanism of injury has not been fully defined. Based on the character and progression of lesions, vascular damage has been inferred as the primary injury. Although unproven, the gross lesion is thought to be an infarct by some pathologists. Fumonisins disrupt cellular membranes, are associated with lipid peroxidation of cells and cellular membranes, inhibit synthesis of macromolecules and DNA, and may enhance production of TNF-α by macrophages. Also, fumonisins inhibit the enzyme ceramide synthase, interfering with the synthesis of sphingolipids. Sphingolipids are bioactive compounds that participate in the regulation of cell growth, cell differentiation, cell metabolic functions, and apoptotic cell death.

Gross lesions involve the white matter of the frontal and parietal lobes of the cerebral hemispheres most commonly, but cases with involvement of major white matter tracts in the brain stem and deep cerebellar white matter have occurred (Fig. 14-78). As a result of the white matter damage, including edema, brain swelling is marked with flattening of cerebrocortical gyri. The lesions are often bilateral but not symmetric, are unequal in severity, and can be quite extensive. The characteristic gross lesion at the time of death is yellow gelatinous malacia and liquefaction of the affected white matter due predominately to the breakdown of lipids accompanied by hemorrhage. The reason white matter, including subcortical white matter, is principally involved—whereas the cerebral cortical gray matter is spared—is thought to be related to a unique vulnerability of the blood vessels in the white matter. The mechanism for this selective vulnerability is unknown.

Microscopically the affected white matter is coagulated or liquefied, and the neuropil is disrupted by accumulation of pink-staining proteinaceous fluid with scattered neutrophils and macrophages. The border of the lesion is surrounded by diffuse or perivascular edema, perivascular hemorrhage, and blood vessels with small leukocytic cuffs. Blood vessel walls are degenerate or necrotic, and some are infiltrated with neutrophils, plasma cells, and eosinophils. Although not often detected, thrombosis occurs. Less characteristic changes include edema and perivascular cuffing in the leptomeninges and neuronal necrosis in deeper layers or the entire width of the overlying gray matter. Similar lesions have been reported in the spinal cord where gray matter is preferentially affected.

Leukoencephalomalacia can also be associated with hepatotoxicity, or hepatotoxicity can be the sole manifestation. Additionally, other animals including pigs, ducks, and chickens are susceptible, but clinical disease and lesions generally reflect pulmonary, hepatic, or renal injury. Clinical signs can include depression, somnolence, head pressing, aimless wandering, blindness, or seizures. Rapid progression of these clinical signs followed by death is typical ranging from 1 to 10 days after onset.

Tetanus

Tetanus is a spastic paralytic disease caused by the neurotoxin called tetanospasmin produced by *Clostridium tetani*. Similar to *Clostridium botulinum*, the bacterium is a ubiquitous gram-positive spore-forming anaerobe commonly found in soil. Tetanospasmin is synthesized in anaerobic wounds and first binds at myoneural junctions and/or sensory receptors. It is transported via retrograde axoplasmic flow within the axon and across synaptic junctions until it reaches the CNS. In the CNS, the toxin is transferred across synapses until it becomes fixed to gangliosides in the presynaptic inhibitory motor neuron. Tetanospasmin blocks the release of inhibitory neurotransmitters, such as glycine and GABA. Inhibitory neurotransmitters act to dampen the actions of excitatory nerve impulses from upper motor neurons that are imposed on lower motor neurons. If these impulses cannot be dampened by normal inhibitory mechanisms, the generalized muscular spasms characteristic of tetanus ensue. Tetanospasmin appears to act by selective cleavage of a protein component of synaptic vesicles, thus preventing

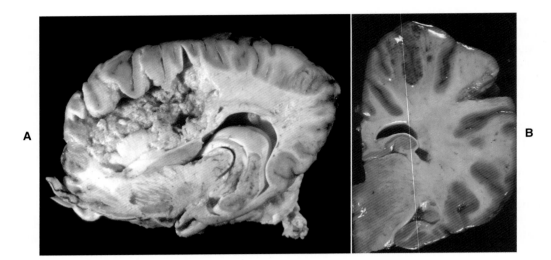

Fig. 14-78   Leukoencephalomalacia, horse, brain. A, Sagittal section. The white matter of the frontal and parietal lobes is necrotic (malacia). The gray matter is not affected. This disease is caused by the toxin fumonisin B_1 produced by the fungus *Fusarium moniliforme* that grows in damaged feed grains. Note that this case demonstrates the extent and distribution of liquefactive necrosis in the white matter in this disease. A more typical presentation is shown in Fig, 14-78, *B*. **B,** Transverse section. The white matter of the three cerebral gyri located at the top of the illustration has areas of yellow gelatinous softening and hemorrhage. Because of the absence of cavitation (liquefactive necrosis), the age of this lesion is likely less than the lesion depicted in Fig. 14-78, A. (**A,** *Courtesy Dr. J. Simon, College of Veterinary Medicine, University of Illinois. **B,** Courtesy Dr. W. Crowell, College of Veterinary Medicine, University of Georgia; and Noah's Arkive, College of Veterinary Medicine, The University of Georgia.*)

the release of neurotransmitters by the cells. Once toxin is bound to synapses, the administration of antitoxin is useless.

This disease is most common in horses but may also occur in lambs castrated in areas contaminated with spores of *Clostridium tetani*. Tetanus also has been reported in cows, pigs, dogs, and cats. Except for the anaerobic wound, there are no macroscopic and microscopic tissue lesions in tetanus. Infected horses initially show signs of colic and muscle stiffness involving muscle groups of the lips, nostrils, ears, jaw (lockjaw), and tail. Horses are hyperesthetic and rapidly have a spastic and tetanic paralytic syndrome develop.

Plant Toxins
Astragalus, Oxytropis, and *Swainsona* poisoning

Astragalus, Oxytropis, and *Swainsona* represent three genera of plants with species that are toxic to livestock. As many as 300 species of *Astragalus* grow in North America, and the genus is the largest of any legume family in this part of the world. Three categories of toxicity can be observed with *Astragalus*, depending on the

mechanism or manner of toxicity: nitro-containing, selenium-accumulating, and poisoning of the locoweed type. Only the last is discussed here. Locoweed poisoning, or locoism, is associated with ingestion of certain species of *Astragalus* and *Oxytropis* in North America and *Swainsona* in Australia. The toxic principles have been termed locoine and swainsonine, respectively.

The mechanism of toxicity has been clarified by the isolation of the indolizidine alkaloids swainsonine and swainsonine N-oxide from *Astragalus lentiginosus*. Both compounds inhibit lysosomal α-mannosidase, thus inducing an acquired α-mannosidosis that mimics the inherited storage disease mannosidosis. Mannosidases are glycoside-hydrolyzing enzymes that are found in the Golgi, lysosomes, and cytoplasm of all mammalian cells. Analyses of tissue from animals poisoned with swainsonine have shown that swainsonine is present in all tissue; however, neurons, epithelial cells in organ systems such as the liver, and macrophages of the monocyte-macrophage system of the spleen and lymph nodes are commonly affected. Therefore, just like in the inherited storage disease (like mannosidosis), acquired swainsonine-induced storage diseases affect similar cells throughout the body. Additionally, swainsonine interferes with normal synthesis of glycoproteins containing asparagine-linked complex oligosaccharides. Swainsonine also inhibits Golgi mannosidase II, an effect not recognized in the inherited disorder.

There are no specific gross lesions in acquired swainsonine-induced storage diseases. Microscopically, lesions involve neuronal cell bodies throughout the neuraxis and autonomic ganglia and are analogous to the inherited lysosomal storage diseases.

Microscopically, neuron cell bodies are swollen and nuclei are sometimes displaced to the periphery of the cell body. The cytoplasm appears foamy or finely vacuolated. The material that accumulates in the cytoplasm does not stain for lipid. Irregular fusiform enlargements, called meganeurites, occur in the proximal axon segment and aberrant synapses form. With time, lesions include distal axonal degeneration and neuronal necrosis with mineralization. The presence of cytoplasmic lesions in other cells of the CNS, such as astrocytes, is dependent on the degree to which α-mannosidase is expressed in individual cell populations. Astrocytes are hydropic or swollen, but their appearance is less dramatic and diagnostic when compared with changes in neurons. Macrophages recruited from the blood stream to phagocytose debris and mannose released from dead neurons also are affected by swainsonine. Microgliosis and neuronophagia are present but inconspicuous.

Similar to the swelling and vacuolation of neurons, this process also occurs in cells throughout the body, including hepatocytes, exocrine pancreatic cells, renal tubular epithelium, endocrine organs (thyroid, parathyroid, and adrenal glands), circulating leukocytes, and cells of the monocyte-macrophage system in liver, spleen, and lymph nodes. Ingestion of the plants of these species by females during gestation can also result in abortion or birth of weak neonates that have similar lesions.

Cattle, sheep, and horses are generally affected. Toxicity is usually insidious, and clinical signs are not observed until after the plants have been grazed on for 14 to 60 days. Clinical signs include poor condition, depression, head pressing, incoordination, circling, blindness, recumbency, and paddling.

Centaurea spp. poisoning

Horses grazing *Centaurea solstitialis* (yellow star thistle) or *Centaurea repens* (Russian knapweed) have a disorder develop known as nigropallidal encephalomalacia. This disease is similar to Parkinson's disease in human beings and has been proposed as a model for experimental studies. The specific cause of the syndrome is not proven. A sesquiterpene lactone isolated from *Centaurea repens* termed repin could provide a basis for the neurotoxicity. Cytotoxicity in cell culture was associated with depletion

of glutathione (a major antioxidant), an increase in reactive oxygen species, and evidence of membrane damage in PC12 cells (a pheochromocytoma cell line) and mouse astrocytes. High concentrations of monoamine oxidase involved in dopamine metabolism normally found in the dopaminergic striatonigral tract (i.e., striatum and substantia nigra [regulate balance and movement]) could render these areas of the brain more susceptible to oxidative damage caused by repin. The mechanism by which repin might cause an increased oxidative state with glutathione depletion, free radical production, and damage to cellular membranes is unknown. Repin is also reported to inhibit dopamine release in the rat striatum, potentially contributing to the clinical manifestations of the disorder. Other potential toxins isolated from *Centaurea solstitialis* include the excitotoxic amino acids aspartate and glutamate. It is unlikely that these amino acids are involved in the naturally occurring disease.

Gross brain lesions are sharply demarcated foci of yellow discoloration and malacia in the globus pallidus (pallidal) and substantia nigra (nigro) (Fig. 14-79). Lesions are usually bilateral and vary in severity; however, unilateral lesions also occur. Microscopically, necrosis with loss of neurons is the primary lesion; however, axons, glia, and blood vessels also are necrotic. The debris is phagocytosed by macrophages (monocytes) recruited into the lesion from the blood stream.

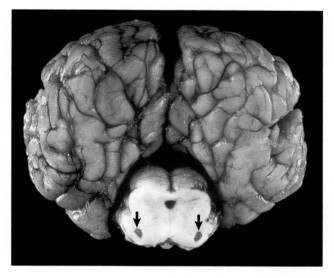

Fig. 14-79   **Equine nigropallidal encephalomalacia, brain, transverse section through the midbrain at the level of the rostral colliculi, horse.** This lesion is caused by yellow star thistle poisoning. Note the symmetrically cavitated (malacia) lesions in the substantia nigra *(arrows)*, resulting from necrosis and phagocytosis by gitter cells. *(Courtesy Dr. L. Lowenstine, School of Veterinary Medicine, University of California-Davis; and Noah's Arkive, College of Veterinary Medicine, The University of Georgia.)*

Grazing the plants for 1 month or longer during the hot summer months when other forage is dried and unpalatable can cause clinical disease. Affected horses are somnolent, have persistent chewing movements, and have difficulty in prehension of feed and drinking water. Death generally is due to emaciation and starvation.

MISCELLANEOUS
CHOLESTEATOMAS

Cholesteatomas, also called cholesterol granulomas, form in choroid plexuses of the ventricles in horses as an aging change. These masses are usually incidental, but reports suggest that if they grow large enough and occlude the flow of CSF, acquired hydrocephalus can result. Cholesteatomas are tan to yellow-brown firm masses with a smooth to, in some cases, papilliform surface (Fig. 14-80). Occasionally the masses are mineralized. This lesion is thought to result from edema and minor but repeated hemorrhages within the choroid plexuses, which result in cholesterol deposits. These deposits elicit a foreign body inflammatory reaction (foreign body granuloma) in the choroid plexus.

DURAL OSSIFICATION

Dural ossification (ossifying pachymeningitis and dural metaplasia) is a metaplastic aging change in dogs, particularly the large breeds. The dura of the cervical and lumbar enlargements of the spinal cord, usually on the ventral and ventrolateral aspects, have well-differentiated bone that can form bone marrow, giving this bone a red color (Fig. 14-81). Thoracolumbar pain in affected dogs is thought to arise

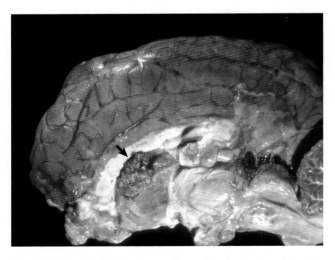

Fig. 14-80   Cholesterol granuloma (cholesteatoma), brain, sagittal section, horse. The choroid plexus of the lateral ventricle contains an expansile mass consisting chiefly of cholesterol and a granulomatous inflammatory response (***arrow***). *(Courtesy College of Veterinary Medicine, University of Illinois.)*

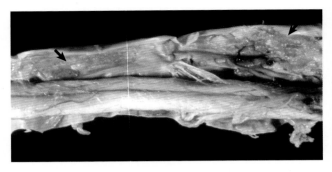

Fig. 14-81   Osseous metaplasia, dura mater, dog. Also called ossifying pachymeningitis and dural ossification, the dura mater contains well-differentiated bone and bone marrow (***arrows***). With movement of the vertebrae, the metaplastic bone can impinge on nerve roots and cause pain in large breed dogs. *(Courtesy College of Veterinary Medicine, University of Illinois.)*

following flexion/extension of the spinal column as a result of compression of spinal roots as they penetrate the metaplastic dura.

INHERITED NECROTIZING MYELOPATHY OF AFGHAN HOUNDS

Inherited necrotizing myelopathy of Afghan hounds seems to have an autosomal recessive inheritance. The lesions are similar to subacute combined degeneration of the spinal cord due to vitamin B$_{12}$ deficiency in human beings and primates, but B vitamin status in affected dogs is considered normal. A similar disease has been reported in Dutch Kooiker dogs, but the relative degrees of axonal degeneration versus demyelination have not been adequately described.

Topographically, gross lesions in the cervical cord are in ventral and less commonly dorsal funiculi, all funiculi in the thoracic cord, and ventral funiculi in lumbar areas. In well-developed lesions, there is severe destruction of the spinal white matter, with an influx of macrophages and myelin degradation that progresses to microcavitation. Neuronal cell bodies in spinal gray matter and ventral nerve rootlets are unaffected. Necrosis, perivascular accumulations of macrophages, and astrogliosis in the dorsal nucleus of the trapezoid body are variable.

Clinical signs begin between 3 and 13 months of age and progress rapidly to paraplegia or tetraplegia within 1 to 3 weeks.

LEPTOMENINGEAL FIBROSIS

Aging dogs will have varying degrees of leptomeningeal fibrosis involving the recesses of the cerebral sulci (Fig. 14-82). This lesion is not present in the

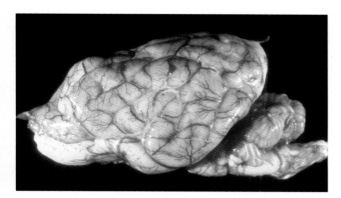

Fig. 14-82 Meningeal fibrosis, leptomeninges (pia-arachnoid mater), dog. In old dogs, the leptomeninges can have areas of fibrosis *(white areas)* particularly in the sulci. This lesion must not be confused with acute leptomeningitis and accumulation of exudate in the leptomeninges and subarachnoid space. In the latter, the exudate extends into the sulci and also covers the gyri (see Fig. 14-47, A). *(Courtesy College of Veterinary Medicine, University of Illinois.)*

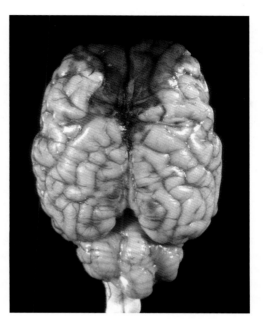

Fig. 14-83 Melanosis, leptomeninges (pia-arachnoid mater), sheep. Note the black pigmentation of the leptomeninges overlying the olfactory poles and dorsal aspect of the frontal lobe. Meningeal melanosis is a normal finding in black-faced sheep and other animals with heavily pigmented skin. *(Courtesy Dr. D. Morton, College of Veterinary Medicine, University of Illinois.)*

leptomeninges covering the outermost surfaces of the gyri. This latter feature can be useful in differentiating meningeal fibrosis from suppurative meningitis. Except for mild meningitis, exudates will also accumulate within the leptomeninges on the outermost surfaces of the gyri.

MENINGEAL MELANOSIS (CONGENITAL)

The leptomeninges of animals and human beings with heavily pigmented skin, especially black-faced sheep and black-skinned pigs, can have melanin (Fig. 14-83). The extent and degree of pigment deposition varies dramatically from animal to animal. Similar pigment deposits can be found in other areas of the body, including the lung, uterine caruncles, liver, and respiratory and alimentary systems' mucous membranes. Congenital meningeal melanosis produces no clinical impairment in affected animals.

RETICULOSIS/GRANULOMATOUS MENINGOENCEPHALITIS

Reticulosis has been reported to occur in several species but is most common in the dog. The term *reticulosis*, at best a somewhat imprecise designation, is used here to give a historical perspective. The spectrum of lesions originally included three disease processes: inflammatory (granulomatous meningoencephalitis) reticulosis, neoplastic reticulosis, and microgliomatosis (proliferation of microglia). Some pathologists have considered the inflammatory and neoplastic forms of reticulosis to represent two opposing ends of a spectrum, with intermediate or transitional forms falling in between. Microgliomatosis is considered to be distinct from the other two types. Recently an additional designation, granulomatous meningoencephalomyelitis, has been used to describe a process that is considered to be analogous, at least in some instances, to the inflammatory form of reticulosis. Ophthalmic lesions also accompany this form and involve the optic nerve, optic disk, and retina.

When present, gross lesions of the three forms are rarely discrete. They frequently are gray-white to red, expansive areas within the brain, which result in a loss of structure (Fig. 14-84). However, lesions can have irregular, well-defined margins, have a gelatinous or rubbery consistency, or appear granular. Microscopically the inflammatory form of reticulosis is characterized by perivascular accumulation of well-differentiated lymphocytes, monocytes, plasma cells, and epithelioid cells with occasional occurrence of neutrophils and giant cells, plus reticulin fibers and collagen. Not infrequently, cells will be predominantly epithelioid. The inflammatory lesion has recently been characterized as consisting primarily of CD3+ T lymphocytes and activated macrophages with strong MHC class II expression, which led to the suggestion that the underlying mechanism of the disease process was a T lymphocyte–mediated delayed-type hypersensitivity of an organ-specific autoimmune disease.

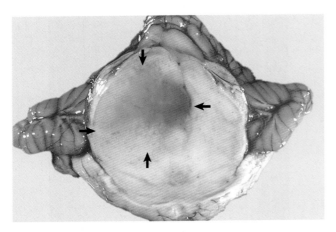

Fig. 14-84   Granulomatous meningoencephalitis (GME, also termed inflammatory reticulosis), transverse section of midbrain just rostral to the pons, dog. The mesencephalon is swollen, discolored, markedly distorted, and soft due to extensive granulomatous inflammation *(arrows)*, which has displaced the midline to the right. The mesencephalic aqueduct is also compressed and distorted. *(Courtesy Dr. J. Edwards, College of Veterinary Medicine, Texas A&M University; and Dr. J. King, College of Veterinary Medicine, Cornell University.)*

With the neoplastic form of reticulosis, cells are arranged around vessels and are also usually present in the tissue. The cells are less differentiated than in the inflammatory form of the disease, and mitotic figures are common. Also, prominent concentrically arranged reticulin fibers are present around vessels and around neurons and glial cells in the tissue.

Reticulosis, with clinical signs of ataxia and proprioceptive deficits, appears to occur more commonly in small breeds such as poodles and terriers. Age of affected dogs is variable and ranges from 9 months to 10 years. In three separate studies involving a total of 85 dogs with reticulosis (including all three forms), the sex distribution was 56 females and 29 males.

CIRCULATORY DISTURBANCES

Many diseases of the CNS in veterinary medicine result from injury to the circulatory system and vascular endothelium. Vascular diseases of the CNS can result from inflammation/infection, either as a component of a systemic disease process or from extension of inflammatory meningeal or cerebral disease. The incidence of cerebrovascular diseases analogous to those in human beings, including trauma, is low in animals, and neurologic manifestations associated with these diseases are uncommon. Arteriosclerosis ("hardening" of arteries) can be categorized as lipid (atherosclerosis) or nonlipid arteriosclerosis; the latter includes arterial

fibrosis, mineralization, and amyloid deposition (see Chapter 10).

ATHEROSCLEROSIS

Atherosclerosis is reported in a variety of animals including nonhuman primates, pigs, dogs, and several avian species. Older pigs are most commonly and severely affected. Occasional older dogs with chronic hypothyroidism or diabetes mellitus can have severe atherosclerosis. The pathogenesis of atherosclerosis and atherosclerotic plaque formation is most well understood in human beings, and the results of experimental studies may have some application to understanding atherosclerosis in domestic animals.

Atherosclerotic plaques arise from a complex and partially understood interaction among endothelium, smooth muscle cells, platelets, T lymphocytes, and monocytes. Endothelial injury induced by oxidized low-density lipoprotein [LDL] cholesterol results in vascular inflammation of the tunica intima. Monocytes migrate into the intima of the vessel wall to phagocytose LDL cholesterol. This process results in the formation of foam cells characteristic of early atherosclerosis (fatty streak). In addition, activated macrophages produce factors that also injure the endothelium. LDL cholesterol concentrations in foam cells and smooth muscle cells often exceed the antioxidant properties of normal endothelium. Oxidized LDL leads to additional metabolic changes that foster a procoagulant microenvironment and enhanced platelet-mediated thrombus formation, as well as initiates a cascade of events leading to the lesions associated with the development of mature atherosclerotic plaques (fibrous plaques with a cap [lipid-laden macrophages walled-off by connective tissue]). The location of atherosclerotic plaques in the circulatory system is dependent on fluid shear stresses and their interaction with injured vascular endothelium. Atherosclerotic plaques characteristically occur in areas of vessel branching or areas where blood undergoes a sudden change in velocity and/or direction of flow.

Although atherosclerotic plaques can reach sizes large enough to significantly reduce blood flow to regions of the brain, the stability of the plaques determines the seriousness of the disease. A stable plaque is characterized by an excess of smooth muscle cells with few lipid-containing macrophages. An unstable plaque is characterized by a large lipid-rich core with abundant lipid-containing macrophages, thin fibrous cap, and inflammation. Rupture of unstable plaques can lead to vascular thrombosis or thromboembolism and infarction of areas supplied by these vessels in the CNS.

Grossly, vessels that can be involved include the aorta and its major branches, extramural coronary arteries, renal arteries, and cerebral arteries. Affected arteries

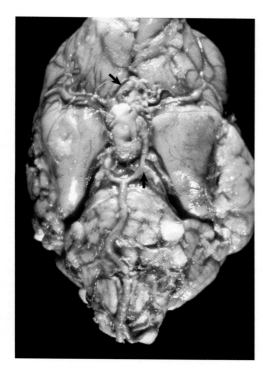

Fig. 14-85   Atherosclerosis, cerebral arteries, brain, ventral surface, dog. The basilar artery, the arteries of the circle of Willis, and the cerebral arteries are segmentally yellow, thickened, and beaded in appearance from atheroma *(arrows)*. This dog had long-standing hypothyroidism. *(Courtesy Dr. J.F. Zachary, College of Veterinary Medicine, University of Illinois.)*

are rigid, irregularly thickened, and white to yellow-white (atheromatous plaques) (Fig. 14-85). Arterial lumina are narrowed or almost obliterated, but there is usually no appreciable ulceration, thrombosis, or hemorrhage. Intimal thickening in intracranial arteries contain less lipid and have a greater tendency for fibrosclerosis than other vessels. In arteries within the brain, there is collagenous adventitial or transmural thickening. The arterial lesions can be associated with hemorrhage or infarcts involving basal nuclei, fornix, internal and external capsules, hippocampus, and thalamus.

In the dog, lesions involve cerebral, coronary, and renal arteries and vessels elsewhere in the body and are most severe in the intima and media. Hemorrhage, ischemia, and infarction of the cerebral cortex are uncommon but can occur.

CEREBRAL EDEMA (PERMEABILITY CHANGES)

The causes and mechanisms of cerebral edema are presented in the section on vasogenic, cytotoxic, and interstitial edema. Cerebral edema has also been associated with "water intoxication," which can result from an increased body hydration caused by (1) excessive, faulty intravenous hydration; (2) compulsive drinking caused

by abnormal mental function; or (3) altered antidiuretic hormone secretion. The increased body hydration produces a hypotonic (hypo-osmolar) plasma, with subsequent development of an osmotic gradient between the hypotonic plasma and the relatively hypertonic state of the normal cerebral tissue. Fluid moves from the plasma into the brain. In this type of edema, the blood-brain barrier remains intact. If it did not, the change in plasma osmolarity would soon be transmitted to the brain tissue (through vascular leakage) and would abolish the necessary osmotic gradient. Fluid accumulation occurs primarily intracellularly, but can also be present extracellularly. In addition, typically a pronounced increase occurs in the rate of formation of CSF originating from the choroid plexus and the extracellular fluid of the brain.

The gross lesions that accompany cerebral edema are the result of enlargement of an organ in an enclosed, limited space; the degree of swelling obviously determines the type and extent of lesions that develop. In evaluating lesions, it is particularly important initially to examine the brain and spinal cord in the fresh state and in situ.

Microscopically, in contrast to some other tissues, such as the lungs, the extracellular fluid associated with vasogenic edema fluid is often not detectable, except in instances of marked vascular injury. When the extracellular space-occupying fluid cannot be identified, only its effects (separation of the cells and their processes causing reduced staining intensity) can be recognized. Additionally, following prolonged vasogenic edema, the lesions include hypertrophy and hyperplasia of astrocytes, activation of microglia, and demyelination. Cytotoxic edema is characterized by cellular swelling, including swelling of astrocytes.

Because of compression against the cranium, an affected brain has flattened gyri and shallow sulci, and it can shift in position. If the edema is confined to one side, the displacement is unilateral, which can be associated with herniation of the cingulated gyrus under the falx cerebri; the extent of the unilateral intracerebral enlargement can be best appreciated following the examination of transverse sections. Diffuse swelling usually causes a caudal shifting that can result in herniation of the brain (parahippocampal gyri of temporal lobes) beneath the tentorium cerebelli (Fig. 14-86) or herniation of the cerebellar vermis through the foramen magnum, resulting in "coning" of the vermis (Fig. 14-87). On a cut surface, the white matter is most often affected (frequently with the vasogenic type of edema, which is the most common). It is swollen and soft, has a damp appearance, and is light yellow in the fresh, unfixed state.

FELINE ISCHEMIC ENCEPHALOPATHY

The cause of feline ischemic encephalopathy has not been definitively established. Although specific vascular lesions (thrombosis or vasculitis) have been found in only a few cases, an ischemic mechanism is suspected and is consistent with the character of the brain damage. Recent evidence strongly supports an aberrant cerebrospinal migration of *Cuterebra* larva following entry into the brain via the nasal cavity. A vascular-mediated vasospasm of the middle cerebral artery,

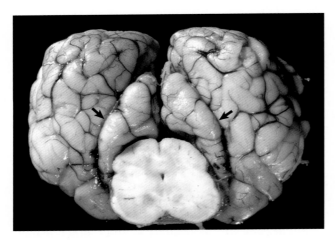

Fig. 14-86   Gyral herniation, parahippocampal gyri, brain, transverse section, caudal face, at level of the rostral colliculi and crus cerebri, horse. The caudal displacement of the parahippocampal gyri (*arrows*) was caused by a sudden swelling of the brain (increase in intracranial pressure) from severe cerebral blunt force trauma to the head. The other cerebral gyri are swollen and flattened and sulci are indistinct **(cerebral edema).** *(Courtesy Dr. M.D. McGavin, College of Veterinary Medicine, University of Tennessee.)*

resulting from hemorrhage or a toxin elaborated by the parasite, has also been proposed. Possible excitotoxic effects of a parasitic toxin have also been suggested.

The gross lesions are unilateral or, uncommonly, bilateral necrosis (but not symmetric) of the white and gray matter of the cerebral hemispheres, usually in the area supplied by the middle cerebral artery (Fig. 14-88). The necrosis can be multifocal or involve up to two thirds of one hemisphere. Hemorrhages can occur in the CNS or leptomeninges. In chronic cases, cerebral atrophy, most severe adjacent to the middle cerebral artery of the affected hemisphere, can occur. Microscopically, lesions include vasculitis, thrombosis, ischemia, and infarction, and the cerebral cortical lesions follow the sequence of changes in infarction listed in Table 14-1.

Feline ischemic encephalopathy has a peracute to acute onset and affects cats of any age. Clinical signs usually reflect unilateral cerebral involvement. The disease most often occurs in the summer months and is accompanied by signs that can include depression, mild ataxia, seizures, behavioral changes, and blindness.

ISCHEMIC MYELOPATHY (FIBROCARTILAGINOUS EMBOLUS FORMATION)

Ischemic myelopathy (necrotizing myelopathy) has been described in the dog, cat, horse, pig, lamb, and turkey. Herniation of degenerative disk material into the vasculature, forming occlusive emboli, is commonly accepted, but the route taken by fibrocartilaginous

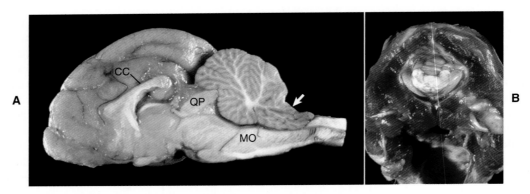

Fig. 14-87   Coning of the cerebellar vermis, brain, cat. A, Sagittal section. Coning of the cerebellum. The caudal cerebellar vermis has been displaced caudally through the foramen magnum, note the notch on the dorsal surface (*arrow*). This result has compressed the medulla oblongata (*MO*), which can cause death from compression of the respiratory center. Note the elevation of the corpus callosum (*CC*) and focal compression of the rostral cerebellar vermis by the tectum (quadrigeminal plate) (*QP*). **B,** Coning of the cerebellum through the foramen magnum, caudal view through the foramen magnum. Note that in this case not only has the cerebellar vermis (upper) been displaced caudally but also the medulla. The caudal cerebellar peduncles have been displaced caudally as far as the foramen magnum. (**A,** *Courtesy Dr. D. Cho, College of Veterinary Medicine, Louisiana State University; and Noah's Arkive, College of Veterinary Medicine, The University of Georgia.* **B,** *Courtesy College of Veterinary Medicine, University of Illinois.*)

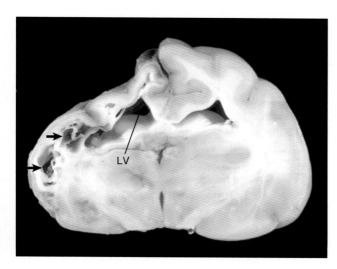

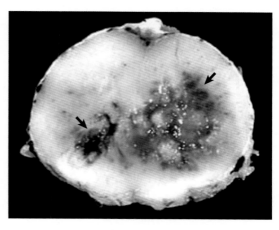

Fig. 14-88 Feline ischemic encephalopathy, brain, transverse section at the junction between the left parietal and occipital lobes, level of thalamus, cat. Chronic feline ischemic encephalopathy with unilateral cerebral degeneration-atrophy. The dorsolateral aspect of the left cerebral hemisphere has undergone necrosis, followed by cyst formation and collapse after phagocytic removal of the necrotic debris. Cysts (*arrows*) have placed the previously existing parenchyma and the left lateral ventricle (*LV*) has expanded into the area of lost tissue (hydrocephalus ex vacuo). *(Courtesy Dr. R. Storts, College of Veterinary Medicine, Texas A&M University.)*

Fig. 14-89 Spinal cord infarction (ischemic necrosis), dog. The yellow-brown region of necrosis (*arrows*) in the right lateral and ventral funiculi was the result of fibrocartilaginous emboli that occluded branches of the ventral spinal artery and obstructed blood flow. *(Courtesy Dr. J. Edwards, College of Veterinary Medicine, Texas A&M University; and Dr. J. King, College of Veterinary Medicine, Cornell University.)*

material into the spinal (or cerebral) vessels is unproven. It has been suggested that trauma to a metaplastic nucleus pulposus causes it to fragment and that the pressure of trauma forces small fragments into damaged veins, venous plexuses, or small arterioles.

The gross lesion is an acute focal infarct involving cervical or lumbar spinal cord most commonly, but any portion can be affected (Fig. 14-89). Microscopically, emboli histochemically identical to the fibrocartilage of the nucleus pulposus of intervertebral disks occlude meningeal or CNS arteries, or veins, or both in affected areas (Fig. 14-90). Clinically, there is a sudden onset of spinal cord deficits, sometimes with cerebral involvement, in certain species. In dogs, larger breeds are more commonly affected. The disease occurs in young and old animals. One study reported that 60% of confirmed cases of canine ischemic myelopathy had a history of trauma or exercise.

NONLIPID ARTERIOSCLEROSIS

Arterial fibrosis occurs more frequently in older animals and has been described in dogs and horses. In the dog, fibrosis of the intima, media, or adventitia occurs with some frequency in cerebrospinal vessels of all types and caliber. Fibrous thickening of the adventitia of small meningeal and CNS arteries can be accompanied

by variable degree of extension of fibrosis into other layers of the vessel wall. A preferential site is the choroid plexus. In old horses, a similar pattern of fibrosis occurs in vessels, and the adventitia may be preferentially affected. Amyloid deposits in meningeal and cerebral vessels are reported in older dogs and other animals. Mineralization (deposition of calcium or iron salts) of cerebral blood vessels occurs in the brains of several species, but is especially common in adult horses. Vessels of the internal capsule, globus pallidus, cerebellar dentate nucleus, and infrequently the hippocampus are preferentially affected in horses, cattle, and less commonly, dogs. Meningeal vessels in old cats, old horses, and cattle, and vessels of the choroid plexus in old cats are other sites of vascular mineralization. Overt ischemic damage is rarely associated with these nonlipomatous vascular lesions in any species; therefore clinical signs are not seen with this lesion.

PERIPARTUM ASPHYXIA SYNDROME

Peripartum asphyxia syndrome (dummy foal, neonatal maladjustment syndrome, or barker foal) is attributed to impairment of normal umbilical blood flow between the mare and foal during parturition, resulting in decreased vascular flow to the brain. Causes usually are those related to interruption of umbilical blood flow, such as a twisted or pinched umbilical cord as occurs in a dystocia or premature separation of the placenta, possibly caused by endophyte fescue toxicity.

Gross lesions are laminar cortical necrosis and look similar to those described for bovine polioencephalomalacia. In the early stages of the disease, the cerebral

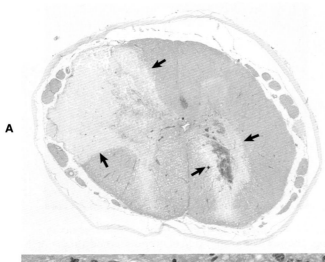

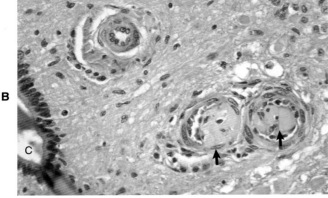

Fig. 14-90   Fibrocartilaginous embolus, spinal cord, dog.
A, Vascular occlusion and infraction. Fibrocartilaginous emboli have obstructed the dorso-lateral artery *(top left)* and branches of the ventral spinal artery to the right ventral gray horn and adjacent white matter, causing infarction *(arrows).* H&E stain. **B,** Fibrocartilaginous emboli in arterioles *(arrows).* **C,** Central canal. H&E stain. (**A,** *Courtesy Dr. M.D. McGavin, College of Veterinary Medicine, University of Tennessee.* **B,** *Courtesy Dr. J. Van Vleet, College of Veterinary Medicine, Purdue University.*)

gyri are edematous and swollen. The cortex may have a yellow-gray discoloration distributed in a laminar pattern several days after onset of the disease. If the animal survives for a longer period of time, there is cerebrocortical atrophy. Microscopically, initial lesions consist of laminar cortical edema and neuronal necrosis, followed by gitter cell accumulation and phagocytosis of cellular debris.

Clinical signs in foals with peripartum asphyxia syndrome include barking like dogs, seizures, aimless wandering, absence of a suckling reflex, and loss of affinity for the mare. Affected foals are usually normal for the first 12 to 24 hours and then decline rapidly as neuronal necrosis ensues.

LYSOSOMAL STORAGE DISEASES

Dysfunction of lysosome-mediated degradation of products (substrates) of normal cellular metabolism results in diseases referred to as lysosomal storage diseases. These substrates cannot be degraded by lysosomes and the accumulated substrate eventually results in death of the affected cells.

Cell death is the end point of a chronic and progressive process of substrate accumulation that interferes with cellular biochemical processes and transport systems. When neurons or myelinating cells die, they release their accumulated substrate into adjacent tissue. Macrophages are recruited from the blood stream as monocytes and they phagocytose cellular debris and unprocessed substrate released from dead cells. Macrophages, however, have the same genetic defect and thus also accumulate substrate in their lysosomes. Although less vulnerable to the effects of substrate accumulation, macrophages eventually die and their released substrate is phagocytosed by additional macrophages recruited from the blood.

Lipid storage diseases, such as globoid cell leukodystrophy, are covered in more detail later. Features of some selected lysosomal storage diseases of animals are provided in Table 14-10. For a comprehensive overview, the reader is referred to a review by Jolly and Walkley (1997).

Lysosomal storage diseases were originally thought to develop exclusively because of mutations that result in a reduction in lysosomal enzyme synthesis. More recently, however, it has become clear that there are other defects such as the following:
1. Synthesis of catalytically inactive proteins that resemble normal active enzymes
2. Defects in posttranslational processing (glycosylation, phosphorylation, addition of fatty acids in the Golgi) of the enzyme, which results in it being misdirected to sites (extracellular) other than to lysosomes
3. Lack of enzyme activator (an enzyme that normally increases the rate of a an enzyme-catalyzed reaction) or protector protein (facilitate repair and refolding of stress-damaged proteins)
4. Lack of substrate activator protein required to assist with the hydrolysis of substrate
5. Lack of transport protein required for elimination of digested material from lysosomes

Characterization of lysosomal disorders has therefore been broadened to include involvement of any protein that is essential for normal lysosomal function.

The best-known diseases are characterized by accumulation of the substrate or substrate precursors and sometimes even by the absence of a critical metabolic product for normal lysosomal function. As a general principle, cell swelling and cytoplasmic vacuolation

Table 14-10   **Classification of Selected Lysosomal Storage Diseases That Involve the Central Nervous System of Animals**

Disease	Storage Product	Deficient Enzyme	Species	Breed
GM$_1$ gangliosidosis	GM$_1$ ganglioside	β-Galactosidase	Bovine	Holstein-Friesian
			Canine	Beagle, English springer spaniel, Portuguese water dog, Alaskan huskies
			Feline	Siamese, domestic shorthair
			Ovine	Suffolk, Coopworth-Romney
GM$_2$ gangliosidosis	GM$_2$ ganglioside	β-Hexosaminidase	Canine	German shorthair pointer, Japanese spaniel
			Feline	Domestic shorthair, Korat
			Porcine	Yorkshire
Globoid-cell leukodystrophy (Krabbe's-like disease)	Galactosylceramide (galactocerebroside) and galactosylsphingosine (psychosine)	Galactosylceramidase (galactocerebroside β-galactosidase)	Canine	West Highland terrier
				Cairn terrier, miniature poodle, blue tick hound, beagle, Pomeranian
			Feline	Domestic shorthair, domestic longhair
			Ovine	Polled Dorset
α-Mannosidosis	Mannose-containing oligosaccharide	α-Mannosidase	Bovine	Angus, Murray gray, Galloway
			Feline	Persian, domestic shorthair
β-Mannosidosis	Mannose-containing oligosaccharide	β-Mannosidase	Caprine	Nubian
			Bovine	Salers
Mucopoly-saccharidosis	Different glycosamino-glycans	Several different enzyme deficiencies	Canine	Plott hound (type I, Hurler's disease), miniature pinscher (type VI, Maroteaux-Lamy disease)
				Breed? (type VII, Sly disease)
			Feline	Domestic shorthair (type I, Hurler's disease)
				Breed? (type VI, Maroteaux-Lamy disease)
				Domestic shorthair (type VII, Sly disease)
			Caprine	Nubian (type III, Sanfilippo's disease)
Ceroid-lipofuscinosis	Subunit *c* of mitochondrial ATPase	Prelysosomal defect?	Canine	English setter, border collie, Tibetan terrier
			Ovine	South Hampshire
			Bovine	Devon
	Sphingolipid Activating proteins A and D	Palmitoyl protein thioesterase	Canine	Miniature schnauzer
			Ovine	Swedish Landrace
	Unknown	Unknown	Canine	Chihuahua, cocker spaniel, Saluki, terrier-cross, blue heeler, Yugoslavian shepherd, Dalmatian, Australian cattle dog, golden retriever, dachshund, corgi
			Ovine	Rambouillet
			Bovine	Beefmaster
			Feline	Siamese, domestic shorthair
Niemann-Pick type c disease	Primarily ganglioside in neurons	Unknown	Feline	Breed?
			Canine	Boxer

?, Unknown; ATPase, adenosine triphosphatase.

occur because of the accumulation of unprocessed substrate in the lysosomes; therefore differences in the size and appearance of cells (neurons versus hepatocytes) depend on the availability of the substrate (carbohydrate or lipid) in the organ system. Many lipids and glycolipids are unique to the nervous system and thus, when there is a lysosomal defect, neural cells often accumulate the substrate.

Examples of lysosomal storage diseases that affect human beings and animals are the gangliosidoses.

With few exceptions, these diseases are inherited in an autosomal recessive pattern. They are also often gene-dose dependent, and correspondingly, recessive homozygotes manifest the disease, whereas heterozygotes are phenotypically and functionally normal, but the effected enzyme's activity is reduced by approximately 50% of normal. The age of onset of clinical signs and the severity of the disease process can vary among the different diseases because the deficiency of the involved enzyme is not always the same. If the gene defect is such that the mutant enzyme is not synthesized at all, there is an early onset of a severe disease. Conversely, if there is some residual synthesis of the deficient enzyme, later onset and a milder form of the disease result because partial catabolism of the accumulated substrate permits a longer period of time before the lysosomes are so distended with substrate that they cause loss of cell function.

Gross lesions of the CNS vary among the different types of lysosomal storage diseases. Brain atrophy occurs with globoid leukodystrophy in latter stages of the diseases because of the loss of myelin. Brain atrophy can also be seen with ceroid-lipofuscinosis but is not prominent in other lysosomal storage diseases, although brains of animals with gangliosidoses can have a firm, rubbery consistency. Microscopically, affected neurons often have a foamy, finely vacuolated, or granular cytoplasm, which is a reflection of the degree to which the stored material is removed during histologic processing (Fig. 14-91). The specific features of the stored material can be best appreciated by ultrastructural examination.

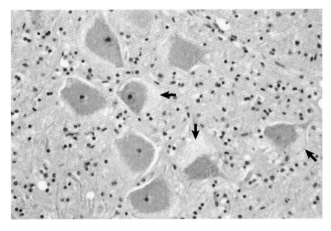

Fig. 14-91 Lysosomal storage disease, brain stem, neuron cell bodies, cat. Note the enlargement of the neuron cell bodies, displacement of nuclei, and accumulation of unprocessed substrate in the cytoplasm of the neuronal cell bodies (*arrows*) giving the appearance of "foamy" cytoplasm. **H&E stain.** (*Courtesy Dr. J.F. Zachary, College of Veterinary Medicine, University of Illinois.*)

Ceroid-lipofuscinosis is a lysosomal storage disease characterized by abnormal sphingolipid (lipopigments) metabolism that occurs in cats, dogs, cattle, and sheep. Its lysosomal dysfunction has not been clearly identified, but experimental studies have shown alterations in the activity of palmitoyl-protein thioesterase and concentration of acid protease. The disease resembles other lysosomal storage diseases in that it can have a recessive mode of inheritance, but it is dissimilar in that it has no gene-dose effect. Brain atrophy occurs with ceroid-lipofuscinosis in later stages of the diseases (in sheep) (Fig. 14-20). The atrophy, which most frequently involves the cerebral cortex but also sometimes the cerebellum, can result in a 50% reduction in brain weight. The cerebral hemispheres are increased in firmness and often have a tan color, whereas the gyri are thinned and the sulci widened, a clear indication of cerebrocortical atrophy. Microscopically the cytoplasm of affected neurons has an eosinophilic granular material (with H&E staining) and a decrease in the number of neurons. Reactive astrogliosis is prominent, and microgliosis may also be observed.

DISEASE PROCESSES AFFECTING MYELIN FORMATION AND MAINTENANCE
HYPOMYELINATION AND DYSMYELINATION

Disorders of myelin formation include hypomyelinogenesis (hypomyelination) and dysmyelination. Hypomyelinogenesis is a process in which there is underdevelopment of myelin. *Dysmyelination* refers to the formation of biochemically defective myelin. Hypomyelinogenesis and dysmyelination most often occur in the early postnatal period and have similar clinical and pathologic features. There are some differences in the lesions and the mechanisms by which they develop. Some of these diseases in domestic animals are outlined in Table 14-11.

HYPOMYELINOGENESIS
Diseases caused by viruses

Classical swine fever (hog cholera) virus, a pestivirus, can be teratogenic in the porcine fetus. The best-known neural defects resulting from fetal infection are hypomyelinogenesis and cerebellar hypoplasia, although other lesions of the CNS, such as microencephaly and nonneural tissue, have been reported. The mechanism of lesion development has not been definitively determined, but a persistent infection that results in inhibition of cell division and function of selected tissues has been proposed.

Border disease viral infection (also a pestiviral infection) is capable of inducing maldevelopment in the CNS and nonneural tissues (skeleton) of lambs and goats after natural infection of the dam during pregnancy.

Table **14-11**   Hypomyelinogenesis and Dysmyelination in Animals

Species	Breed	Disease Designation	Genetic Cause	Infectious Cause	Metabolic Cause
Canine	Dalmatian	Hypomyelinogenesis			
	Chow Chow	Dysmyelination	Suspected		
	Springer spaniel	Shaking pups (hypomyelination)	Sex-linked recessive		
	Samoyed	Tremor (hypomyelination)	Suspected		
	Lurcher	Tremor syndrome (hypomyelination)			
	Weimaraner	Hypomyelination	Suspected		
Bovine	All breeds	Bovine virus diarrhea (dysmyelination)		Bovine virus diarrhea (pestivirus)	
	Charolais	Progressive ataxia	Suspected		
Porcine	Landrace	Congenital tremor (myelin agenesis)	Sex-linked recessive		
	Saddleback	Congenital tremor	Autosomal recessive		
	Chester-white	Myoclonia congenita	Autosomal recessive	Suspected	
	All breeds	Congenital tremor (dysmyelinogenesis and cerebellar hypoplasia)		Classical swine fever (pestivirus)	
	All breeds	Congenital tremor (dysmyelinogenesis)		Unknown virus suspected	
	All breeds	Congenital ataxia and tremor (hypomyelinogenesis and cerebellar hypoplasia)			Trichlorfon (acaricide)
Ovine	All breeds	Border disease (hypomyelinogenesis-dysmyelination)		Border disease virus (pestivirus)	

One of the characteristic lesions in the CNS is hypomyelinogenesis, primarily affecting the white matter of the cerebrum and cerebellum. Grossly, it may be difficult to distinguish between white and gray matter in transverse sections of cerebrum and cerebellum. The brain and spinal cords from affected lambs may be smaller when compared with unaffected lambs. The PNS is unaffected. Hypomyelinogenesis may be related to a viral-induced decrease of myelin-associated glycoprotein, myelin basic protein, and activity of nucleotide phosphodiesterase in oligodendroglia. Other lesions detected in lambs include early inflammation, porencephaly-hydranencephaly, cerebellar malformation including hypoplasia, microencephaly, and reduction in diameter of the spinal cord.

GLOBOID CELL LEUKODYSTROPHY

As discussed previously, *lysosomal storage* generally refers to a cellular alteration in which an increased amount of substrate material, which normally is degraded, accumulates within lysosomes, often eventually resulting in cell death. These diseases have a hereditary basis,

occur in young animals, and are transmitted in an autosomal recessive pattern. Features of some selected lysosomal storage diseases of animals are given in Table 14-10.

Globoid cell leukodystrophy, a sphingolipidosis, is a lysosomal storage disease with its principal lesion being primary demyelination involving oligodendrocytes of the CNS and Schwann cells of the PNS. The disease, which has an autosomal recessive inheritance in the Cairn and West Highland white terrier, is generally seen in younger animals, often younger than 1 year old. It has also been described in beagles, miniature poodles, basset hounds, pomeranians, blue tick hounds, and in domestic shorthaired and longhaired cats.

Mechanistically the proposed sequence of events in this disease includes: (1) early "normal" myelination that progresses up to a certain stage; (2) disruption of normal myelin turnover because of deficient galactosylceramidase activity; (3) degeneration and necrosis of myelinating cells because of the accumulation of psychosine; (4) primary demyelination following degeneration of these cells; (5) recruitment of phagocytes, both resident microglia and trafficking blood monocytes; and (6) infiltration of macrophages, which become globoid cells after phagocytosing myelin byproducts into the nervous tissue. The last-named changes occur in response to the demyelination and unmetabolized galactocerebroside.

Affected oligodendroglia and Schwann cells are deficient in the lysosomal hydrolase, galactosylceramide β-galactosidase (GALC), which is responsible for degradation of galactosylsphingosine (psychosine) and galactosylceramide (galactocerebroside). Psychosine is highly toxic and because it is not degraded, it has been hypothesized that it accumulates during the disease and causes direct injury to oligodendrocytes and Schwann cells, possibly through an apoptotic mechanism of cell death, in part, mediated by psychosine-induced production of cytokines and iNOS.

In globoid cell leukodystrophy, the composition of myelin is not qualitatively abnormal. Galactosylceramide is highly concentrated in myelin but is nearly absent in systemic organs except for the kidney. Peak synthesis and turnover of galactosylceramide coincides with the peak period of myelin formation and turnover during the first year of life. GALC activity also increases in relation to the galactosylceramide peak. Myelination continues at a slower rate as animals mature, and in an adult myelin formation is stable with minimal turnover.

A deficiency in GALC activity results in the accumulation of galactosylceramide, especially during the early phase of myelin maturation and turnover, and results in the formation of globoid cells discussed later. Psychosine also accumulates leading to rapid and massive degeneration of oligodendroglia and Schwann cells, extensive myelinolysis, and reduction in myelination.

Gross lesions of the CNS are characterized by a gray discoloration of the white matter, especially of the centrum semiovale of the cerebral hemispheres and white matter of the spinal cord (Fig. 14-92). The lesion in the spinal cord tends to start in the peripheral white matter and spread inward. Microscopically, such areas have pronounced loss of myelin (Fig. 14-93) and prominent "globoid" cells containing galactocerebroside that can be demonstrated with a periodic acid–Schiff stain (Fig. 14-94). Peripheral nerves are also affected and lesions are typified by primary demyelination and secondary axonal degeneration. Small sensory branches of peripheral nerves are useful sites to take biopsies to make diagnoses (Fig. 14-115).

Clinically, affected animals are ataxic and have limb weakness and tremors that progress to paralysis and muscular atrophy. Poor vision or blindness may also occur.

Spongy Degeneration (Status Spongiosis)

Spongy degeneration is a group of diseases of young animals characterized by a spongy lesion (referred to

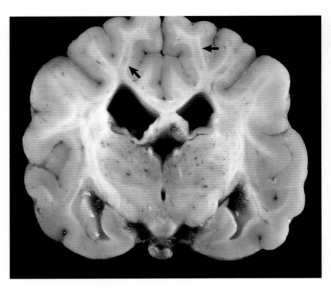

Fig. 14-92   Globoid cell leukodystrophy, brain, transverse section at the level of the mammillary body, dog. The white matter, especially of the gyri, has an off-white appearance (*arrows*). Macrophages (globoid cells) derived from blood monocytes (also enzymatically deficient in β-galactocerebrosidase) accumulate in white matter to phagocytose galactocerebroside and oligodendroglial debris secondary to the toxic effects of galactosylsphingosine (psychosine) on oligodendroglia (and in the peripheral nervous system Schwann cells). There is also bilateral hydrocephalus of the lateral ventricles, presumably hydrocephalus ex vacuo, as a result of the loss of myelin sheaths around axons. *(Courtesy Dr. H.B. Gelberg, College of Veterinary Medicine, Oregon State University.)*

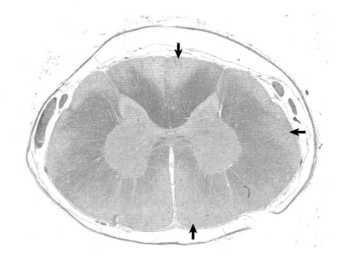

Fig. 14-93   Globoid cell leukodystrophy, spinal cord, dog. This section of spinal cord has been stained with Luxol fast blue, a histochemical reaction that stains myelin blue. Note the loss of myelin from the periphery of the cord (*arrows*), the first area to be affected. Luxol fast blue stain with a nuclear fast red counterstain. *(Courtesy Dr. M.D. McGavin, College of Veterinary Medicine, University of Tennessee.)*

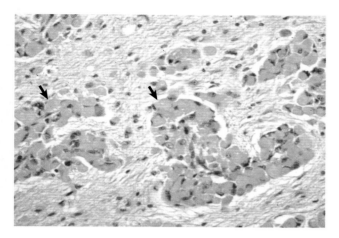

Fig. 14-94   Globoid cell leukodystrophy, cerebrum, dog.
Globoid cells deficient in β-galactocerebrosidase *(arrows)*,
usually located in the perivascular space, increase in size and
number because they are unable to degrade galactocerebroside to a less complex substrate. H&E stain. *(Courtesy*
Dr. M.D. McGavin, College of Veterinary Medicine, University of Tennessee.)

here as status spongiosus) that primarily occurs in the
white matter of the CNS but also extends into the gray
matter. Status spongiosus is a somewhat nonspecific
term and can develop by several different mechanisms.
It includes a variety of lesions, such as splitting of
lamella forming myelin sheaths (characteristic of the
diseases discussed here), accumulation of extracellular
fluid (extracellular cerebral edema), swelling of cellular
processes (astrocytic, neuronal), and Wallerian degeneration at a later stage when the necrotic myelin and
axons have been phagocytosed and the spaces once
occupied by these structures are empty.

Gross brain lesions reported for spongy degeneration range from no gross lesions to swelling, edema,
and pallor of the white matter, and dilation of the ventricles. Microscopically the lesion is characterized by
variably sized empty spaces within the white matter.
Ultrastructurally, with spongy degeneration and some
other disease processes characterized by status spongiosus, there is splitting or separation of the myelin
sheath at the intraperiod line with the formation of large
intramyelinic spaces. In some cases myelin formation
is deficient.

Some species and breeds affected with spongy
degeneration include the canine (Labrador retriever,
Saluki, silky terrier, Samoyed), feline (Egyptian mau),
and bovine (Jersey, shorthorn, Angus shorthorn,
Hereford), and an autosomal recessive mode of transmission has been proposed for some forms of this disorder. A unique form of the spongy degeneration also
occurs in a group of metabolic inherited diseases called
aminoacidopathies.

Not to be confused with spongy degeneration is the
term *spongiform change*. Spongiform change is characterized by small clear vacuoles of varied sizes that form
in the cytoplasm of neuron cell bodies and proximal
dendrites in diseases such as the TSEs and rabies
encephalitis and in the processes of astrocytes that are
spatially related to the affected neurons.

DEMYELINATION

Demyelination, which means degeneration and loss
of myelin already formed, can be divided into primary
and secondary types. *Primary demyelination* refers to a
disease process in which the myelin sheath is selectively affected, with the axon remaining essentially
intact. *Secondary demyelination*, a designation criticized
by some, refers to "secondary" degeneration of myelin
following "primary" injury to and loss of the axon, as in
Wallerian degeneration, and is not a selective injury of
the myelin sheath.

Injury to oligodendroglia that results in myelin
sheath breakdown or direct injury to myelin sheaths
cause the release of lipids and other myelin components into the extracellular space. These materials
readily activate microglial cells and attract blood
monocytes, which phagocytose myelin debris.

METABOLIC CAUSES
Osmotic demyelination syndrome

In human beings this syndrome is termed central
or extrapontine myelinolysis. The disorder was first
reported in 1959, and the majority of cases were in
severely malnourished alcoholics. Since then, the
disorder has been observed in a variety of clinical disease states. A major risk factor is chronic hyponatremia
treated in hospitals by the administration of intravenous saline solution. The disease has been experimentally reproduced in dogs and laboratory rodents by
inducing hyponatremia, allowing a period of stabilization (3 to 4 days is sufficient), and then administering
saline-containing fluids.

Two cases of osmotic demyelination syndrome have
been reported in the veterinary literature, and one
of the authors has observed a case. In all three, there
has been a clinical diagnosis of Addison's disease.
Treatment consisted of intravenous administration
of fluids containing normal saline solution to correct
the hyponatremia typical of hypoadrenocorticism.
The reported rates of correction have been 22 mmol/L
in 24 hours and 16.4 mmol/L in 24 hours. In the
author's case, serum sodium increased by 42 mmol/L
in 4 days. All these rates of correction exceed the limits
established for human beings and are consistent with
human cases of the syndrome.

The pathogenesis of osmotic demyelination syndrome
is thought to be opposite to that occurring with salt

poisoning (i.e., a hyponatremic to hypernatremic shift following saline administration). Lesions occur in areas of the brain where there is a confluence or intermingling of gray and white matter. Rapid (within 24 to 48 hours) correction of chronic hyponatremia from an established equilibrium exceeds the adaptive responses of the brain, resulting in myelin destruction. The exact mechanism of demyelination is not known. It is proposed that osmotic imbalance and water shifts induce osmotic stress in the CNS that result in myelin destruction.

In contrast to human beings, gross lesions in dogs are either not apparent or subtle. Slight softening and discoloration has been observed in affected brain regions. Microscopically, lesions can be limited to the reticular formation at the level of the pons or can be extensive, affecting cerebellar folia, midbrain, thalamus, basal nuclei, and at the interface of the corona radiata and cerebrocortical gray matter. In affected areas, the white matter is pale in routine H&E stained sections and is heavily infiltrated with foamy macrophages. Special stains (Luxol fast blue for myelin), confirm acute myelin destruction and accumulation of myelin debris in macrophages. As is typical of strictly demyelinating lesions, axons are well preserved.

CIRCULATORY AND PHYSICAL DISTURBANCES

Physical compression of CNS tissue that results from various causes usually chronic in nature can also induce demyelination. Some possible mechanisms include compression of myelin sheaths and oligodendroglia, interference with circulation resulting in CNS ischemia, and disease processes resulting in the accumulation of extracellular fluid.

It is well known that vasogenic and hydrostatic edema caused by inflammation, neoplasms, trauma, and obstructive hydrocephalus can cause degeneration of myelin sheaths. The underlying mechanisms for this injury are multiple and include creation of a hypoxic-anoxic environment, degeneration of oligodendroglia, and alteration in stability of the myelin sheath, permitting entrance of injurious proteolytic enzymes from the surrounding environment.

DISEASES CAUSED BY MICROBES
Viruses

Canine distemper.   Canine distemper is one of the most important diseases of the canine species. It is caused by a morbillivirus (family Paramyxoviridae) and has a worldwide distribution. Morbilliviruses other than CDV include measles virus, rinderpest virus, peste des petits ruminants virus, phocine distemper virus of seals, equine morbillivirus. and dolphin and porpoise morbilliviruses. The virus is pantropic and has a particular affinity for lymphoid and epithelial tissues (lung, gastrointestinal tract, urinary tract, skin) and the CNS (including the optic nerve) and eye. In the CNS, there is demyelination without any substantial amount of inflammation.

Dr. Brian Summers (Cornell University, College of Veterinary Medicine) has commented on the sequence of events in CDV infection based on his studies of its pathogenesis. CDV is spread between dogs by aerosol transmission. The virus is trapped in the mucosa of the nasal turbinates (centrifugal turbulence), infects local macrophages, and is spread by macrophages (leukocytic trafficking) to regional lymph nodes (retropharyngeal). CDV replicates in these regional lymph nodes and replication is followed by a primary viremia that infects systemic lymph nodes, spleen, and the thymus approximately 48 hours after exposure. With infection of the lymphoid system, immunosuppression can occur resulting in secondary bacterial infections, such as conjunctivitis, rhinitis, and bronchopneumonia, which are commonly seen in CDV infections.

Four to 6 days after the primary viremia, a secondary viremia occurs largely via leukocytic trafficking. CDV spreads from cells of the lymphoid system to infect the CNS and epithelial cells of the respiratory mucosa, urinary bladder mucosa, and gastrointestinal tract. In the CNS, trafficking leukocytes form perivascular cuffs, and from these cells CDV is disseminated throughout the CNS. It should be noted that the degree of inflammation in the CNS at this stage is minimal.

Under laboratory conditions, the severity of the disease and the cell populations and areas infected in the CNS depend on the (1) age of the dog, (2) strain of CDV, and (3) kinetics of the antiviral immune response. Virtually all cells of the CNS including the meninges, choroid plexus, neurons, and glia are susceptible to infection, but oligodendrocytes are novel in that the infection in these cells is usually defective (incomplete). In dogs infected experimentally with the A75-17 strain of CDV, isolated from a dog with CDV in 1975, approximately a third of the dogs died from encephalomyelitis and the effects attributable to severe immunosuppression. A third of infected dogs developed a timely systemic immune response, and the CNS disease was quickly resolved and they recovered. Finally, a third of the dogs infected with CDV developed a subacute to chronic inflammatory/demyelinating disease of the white matter with some gray matter involvement because of a delayed and deficient immune response.

The encephalomyelitis of canine distemper is initiated following viral entry into the CNS, perhaps 1 week after exposure to CDV. Leukocytic trafficking spreads CDV to the gray and white matter of the CNS and to epithelial cells and macrophages of the choroid plexuses. The virus is shed from choroid plexus epithelial and ependymal cells into the CSF in infected macrophages. It is disseminated throughout the ventricular system, infects ependymal cells lining the ventricular system, and then spreads locally to infect astrocytes and microglia. Periventricular white matter lesions, especially those surrounding the fourth ventricle, are the result of this sequence of events.

By 25 days after exposure, CDV-infected leukocytes in the perivascular cuffs have disappeared; however, lesions in the white matter consist of periventricular foci of myelin degeneration and swollen astrocytes. CDV infects astrocytes, microglia, and other cells. Microglia and recruited blood monocytes phagocytose myelin fragments.

Inflammatory mediators released from lymphocytes, microglial cells, and trafficking macrophages result in expansion of the initial lesions. These inflammatory mediators may cause necrosis of cells and cell processes in the focus but do not result in a "selective" demyelinating process affecting axons. The characteristic white matter vacuolation (intramyelinic edema) seen in H&E stained sections of CDV-infected CNS is apparently caused by a direct effect of the virus on oligodendrocytes, as it appears in the earliest white matter lesions before they have acquired an "inflammatory" character—a dense infiltrate of lymphocytes, monocytes, and plasma cells.

Gross lesions characteristically occur in the cerebellum (medullary area, folial white matter, and subpial white matter) and cerebellar peduncles (with both white matter and sometimes gray matter involvement of the pons). Lesions also occur in medulla oblongata (particularly in the subependymal area of the fourth ventricle), rostral medullary vellum, cerebrum (both white matter and gray matter), optic nerves, optic tracts, spinal cord, and meninges.

Microscopically, in addition to demyelination there is status spongiosus, astrocytic hypertrophy and hyperplasia with focal and variable syncytial cell formation, reduced numbers of oligodendroglia, and variable neuronal degeneration. Inclusion bodies (cytoplasmic, nuclear, or both) are detectable, particularly in astrocytes, which are important target cells for the distemper virus, but also in ependymal cells and occasionally in neurons (Fig. 14-95). The earliest evidence of myelin injury is a ballooning change resulting from a split in the myelin sheath, or more degenerative changes including axonal swelling. This lesion is also variably associated with astroglial and microglial proliferation. This initial injury of the myelin sheath, which has been suggested to be a result of perturbed astrocytic function following viral infection, is followed by a progressive removal of compact myelin sheaths by phagocytic microglial cells that infiltrate the myelin lamellae and variable axonal necrosis.

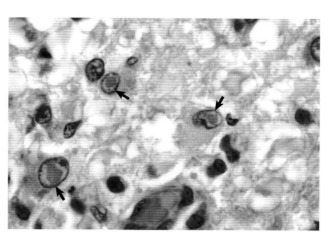

Fig. 14-95   Canine distemper inclusion bodies, brain, midbrain periventricular white matter, dog. Distinct acidophilic (*red*) intranuclear inclusion bodies (*arrows*) are present in astrocytes and some gemistocytes. Similar inclusions can be observed in the cytoplasm of epithelial cells throughout the body (bladder epithelium, respiratory epithelium, gastric epithelium). H&E stain. (*Courtesy Dr. M.D. McGavin, College of Veterinary Medicine, University of Tennessee.*)

A late stage of demyelination, which is a reflection of an affected animal's improved immune status, is more pronounced and is characterized by nonsuppurative inflammation (perivascular cuffing, leptomeningitis, and choroiditis) and also can be accompanied by tissue degeneration and accumulation of gitter cells.

In addition to the dog, animals of the families Ailuridae (red panda), Canidae (fox, wolf), Hyaenidae (hyena), Mustelidae (ferret, mink), Procyonidae (raccoon, panda), Ursidae (bear), Viverridae (civet, mongoose), and Felidae (exotic felids including lions, tigers, and leopards) are also reported to be susceptible to canine distemper viral infection. Additionally, canine distemper has recently been reported in javelinas (collared peccaries) of the family Tayassuidae in the United States.

Neurologic signs in all affected species include convulsions, myoclonus, tremor, disturbances in voluntary movement, circling, hyperesthesia, paralysis, and blindness.

Old-dog encephalitis.   Old-dog encephalitis is thought to arise from long-term persistent infection of the CNS with a defective form of CDV. This pathogenesis has been demonstrated in experimental infections with the CDV. Although the virus has the same general polypeptide composition and contains all of the major viral proteins as the one causing conventional distemper, some differences among peptides have been reported. The mechanisms involved in development of lesions are not known; however, they result in a proliferation of nonsuppurative inflammatory cells.

Lesions are primarily in the cerebral hemispheres and brain stem. Microscopic lesions are characterized primarily by demyelination with a disseminated, nonsuppurative encephalitis with variable, sometimes prominent, lymphoplasmacytic perivascular cuffing, microgliosis, astrogliosis, and variable leptomeningitis and neuronal degeneration. Nuclear and cytoplasmic inclusions, positive for distemper viral antigen, have been detected in neurons and astrocytes in the cerebral cortex, thalamus, and brain stem, but in contrast to distemper, not in the cerebellum.

Old-dog encephalitis is a rare condition occurring in mature adult dogs. Clinical signs include depression, circling, head pressing, visual deficits, seizures, and muscle fasciculations.

Visna.   Visna, which means wasting, is a slowly progressive, transmissible disease of sheep. The disease is caused by a strain of the ovine maedi-visna virus (MVV) complex, one of the eight basic lenti (slow) viruses (family Retroviridae). A different strain of the same virus causes a lymphocytic interstitial pneumonia referred to as maedi.

In recent years, the understanding of the factors associated with infection, including the mechanism of lesion development, has improved. Visna is a persistent viral disease that probably results from the ability of the virus to form provirus and integrate into the host genome. The virus can also change its antigenic characteristics (antigenic drift), which enables it to escape the effects of the host's immune response. Although the visna virus and other lentiviruses can infect promonocytes and monocytes in the bone marrow and blood, viral replication is restricted in these cells, where it remains as provirus DNA until maturation and differentiation to macrophages. Primary viral replication occurs in cells of monocyte-macrophage-microglial lineage. Thus visna virus enters the CNS by way of leukocytic trafficking of virus-infected macrophages. Visna virus can also be present in oligodendrocytes and astrocytes located in foci of demyelination. It has been suggested that the virus gains access to these cells via close contact with infected monocytes. Recent studies suggest the virus can also infect and productively replicate in endothelial cells. This mechanism may provide an additional route for viral entry into the CNS and the potential for alterations of the blood-brain barrier.

Although gross lesions are not frequently observed, they may occur in areas of prominent inflammation where they appear as yellow-tan areas. Early microscopic lesions primarily affect the gray and white matter subjacent to the ependyma of the ventricular system of the brain and central canal of the spinal cord. These lesions are characterized by a nonsuppurative encephalomyelitis accompanied by pleocytosis, variable edema, CNS necrosis, astrocytosis, choroiditis, and nonsuppurative leptomeningitis. The inflammatory response is thought to be caused by the upregulation of expression of major histocompatibility complex class II genes that occurs in virus-infected macrophages. Degeneration of myelin sheaths also occurs at this time but is often accompanied by axonal degeneration, suggesting that it could be a secondary lesion, such as in Wallerian degeneration. Oligodendroglial and neuron injury and necrotic cell death are attributable to cytokines and other toxic factors secreted by inflammatory cells and glial cells. Recent in vitro studies suggest that caspase activation leading to apoptotic cell death may play a role in visna.

Neuronal cell bodies and oligodendroglia are normal (except in areas of necrosis) during this stage of the disease. The latter cells can become infected, however, which leads to later development of demyelination. Primary demyelination, particularly in the spinal cord, has been described in animals infected for prolonged periods (months to years). Such animals also have periventricular inflammation.

The primary demyelination that occurs during the late stages of the disease process (6 months to 8 years after infection) has been proposed to result from oligodendroglial cell infection. The main sources of excreted virus are the udder and lungs (as mainly cell-associated virus), and transmission occurs most readily between the dam and lamb via the milk and between confined individuals, probably via respiratory secretions. The MVV has also been detected in semen of infected rams. It is important to emphasize that no profound immune deficiency occurs with MVV infections, as is the case for immunodeficiency lentiviral infections that infect CD4+ T lymphocytes. Nonetheless, secondary infections can still significantly accompany MVV infection.

In addition to pneumonia, MVVs can also cause mastitis, arthritis (uncommonly of the carpus or hind limb joints), and a mesangial glomerulitis. Irrespective of the target organ, the lesions are to be regarded as chronic and lymphoproliferative, in contrast to the well-known immunodeficiency infections caused by HIV-1, simian immunodeficiency virus (SIV), and feline immunodeficiency virus (FIV).

Viral strain differences and breed of sheep can influence the lesions that develop. For example, the visna form of the disease does not commonly occur in ovine breeds of North America, although some degree of visnalike lesions can be seen with maedi. Visna originally was described in Iceland, but sheep with similar lesions of the CNS have been detected in The Netherlands, Kenya, the United States, and Canada. CNS signs include an abnormal hindlimb gait that progresses to incoordination and rear limb paresis over a period of weeks or months.

Caprine leukoencephalomyelitis-arthritis. Caprine leukoencephalomyelitis-arthritis was first described in the United States and has since been recognized in other parts of the world. The infection can be readily transmitted by colostrum and milk following birth, or by direct contact. A close relationship exists between the MVVs of sheep and the caprine arthritis encephalitis (CAE) virus, but genomic differences between them can be demonstrated. As with MVV infection of sheep, CAE viral infection is also a lymphoproliferative disease with a tropism for the macrophage, which acts as a carrier for the virus.

Gross lesions in the nervous system include tan- to salmon-colored foci of necrosis and inflammation that can occasionally be detected in the brain (Fig. 14-96) and most prominently in the spinal cord. Microscopic lesions of the nervous system are similar to those of visna (nonsuppurative encephalomyelitis) but can be more severe with CAE. Nonneural lesions include interstitial pneumonia of moderate severity in some affected kids. Such lungs fail to collapse completely and are mottled red or blue. As discussed under visna, the mechanism of infection and cell death appear similar.

The pattern of disease in CAE is age dependent. Neurologic manifestations are usually seen in young kids 2 to 4 months of age, but unlike visna in sheep, there is a more rapid progression and signs progressing to quadriplegia develop within weeks to months. As with visna, affected goats have pleocytosis. In adult goats the primary target tissue is the synovium of the joints, and animals that survive the initial infection have lymphoproliferative synovitis and arthritis develop. Pneumonia, lymphocytic mastitis, and encephalomyelitis also occur in adult animals.

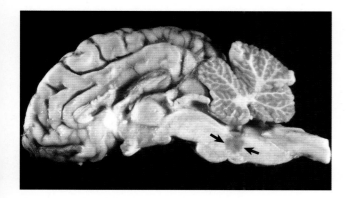

Fig. 14-96   Leukoencephalitis, caprine retrovirus-induced encephalitis, brain stem, goat. A focal area of the brain stem *(arrows)* is yellow-brown and was found, microscopically, to be infiltrated by lymphocytes, plasma cells, and histiocytes. A similar lesion commonly occurs in the spinal cord.
(Courtesy Dr. H.E. Whiteley, College of Veterinary Medicine, University of Illinois.)

Progressive multifocal leukoencephalopathy

See Appendix 14-1.

IMMUNE-MEDIATED DISEASES

In veterinary medicine, naturally occurring immune-mediated demyelination in domestic animals is rare, and other than for canine polyradiculoneuritis (coonhound paralysis), it is usually only suspected rather than proven. These diseases are best known to occur in human beings as sequelae to postinfectious and postvaccinal events. They result in primary demyelination of the CNS. Autoimmune diseases of the CNS are mechanistically either a type II hypersensitivity (antibody-mediated) or a type IV (cell-mediated) hypersensitivity, and T lymphocytes and macrophage-derived cytokines play contributory roles.

Autoimmune injury to oligodendroglia in the CNS arising from aberrant cellular and/or humoral immune responses can result from one of the following four proposed mechanisms:

1. Molecular mimicry: The CNS has antigens that are similar or identical to those expressed by certain pathogens (virus or bacterium). The normal inflammatory and immunologic responses to these pathogens result in the expression of antibodies that cross-react with "antigens" normally expressed by CNS cells.

2. Abrogation of immune tolerance: The CNS is an "immune privileged" organ (like the eye). The immune system therefore does not recognize CNS antigens as innate antigens, and if they are exposed to the immune system following inflammation or trauma, an autoimmune response can ensue. Injury, physical or otherwise, to blood vessels within the CNS can cause the release of "sequestered antigens" into the blood stream leading to an autoimmune response.

3. Genetic factors: Functions of the immune system that are strictly regulated genetically may be under the control of abnormal inherited genes or altered normal genes that regulate immune responses to CNS antigens and thus increase the susceptibility to autoimmune diseases.

4. Stress factors: Environmental stresses mediated through the CNS can depress the functions of the immune system, leading to the formation of autoantibodies.

The mechanism of myelin breakdown in immune-mediated demyelination is not clearly understood. The initial step is thought to be exposure of antigens in myelin basic protein of the major dense line of myelin lamellae following injury. Myelin proteins are substrates for calpain, a calcium-activated neutral proteinase. Calpain has been implicated in several autoimmune diseases and may play an important role in CNS demyelination. Exposed antigens are then recognized by the immune system, and experimental studies suggest that lesions result from a complex interaction between inflammatory cells and their mediators and lamellae of myelinating cells. T lymphocytes, some B lymphocytes, and activated macrophages (recruited monocytes) and microglia cells, adhesion molecules, cytokines, chemokines, and their receptors have been demonstrated in the lesions. This interaction results in primary demyelination.

Gross lesions are usually not present but can include a gray to yellow discoloration of white matter. Microscopically, lesions are best observed in white matter and are characterized by vacuolation of myelin and the presence of lymphocytes, macrophages, and plasma cells. Myelin sheaths degenerate from injury caused by: (1) inflammatory mediators and (2) direct actions of macrophages on lamellae. Myelin lamellae separate as a result of intramyelinic edema, fragment, and are phagocytosed by macrophages.

The best-known model of immune-mediated demyelination is an experimental model referred to as experimental allergic encephalomyelitis (EAE). EAE is produced by inducing a hypersensitivity to myelin or, more specifically, to myelin basic protein. If appropriate laboratory animals are inoculated with white matter or myelin basic protein (suspended in complete Freund's adjuvant), they become paralyzed after 2 to 3 weeks. Lesions are characterized by perivascular (perivenular) demyelination accompanied by accumulation of lymphocytes and macrophages.

A similar process, referred to as postvaccinal encephalomyelitis, occurred occasionally in human beings when human rabies vaccine contained CNS tissue. The incidence decreased after 1957 when duck embryo rabies vaccine came into use. In some cases with mild clinical signs, recovery was complete and axons were remyelinated following immune-mediated demyelination.

A third situation in which this type of demyelination occurs follows infection with certain viruses in human beings (rubeola virus) and animals (e.g., influenza virus). These diseases, which are rare and designated as postinfectious encephalomyelitis, are also characterized by development of lesions in the CNS comparable to those of EAE.

TRAUMATIC INJURY

Traumatic injury of the CNS is caused by physical insults such as compression, stretching, and/or laceration of neurons/axons. When the brain and spinal cord collide with the bony ridges lining the cranial vault and the bony wall of the vertebral canal, respectively, or when axial, rotational, and angular forces (Fig. 14-97)

are applied to neurons and axons during trauma, the force of impact and sudden acceleration of neurons and axons, both within the CNS and in the adjacent cranial and spinal nerves, can cause them to compress, twist, stretch, and tear. Concurrently the same type of forces can injure blood vessels in the CNS and leptomeninges and may result in small hemorrhages or hematomas within the parenchyma of the brain and in the leptomeninges (subarachnoid space) (Fig. 14-98).

Diffuse brain injury (often present in concussion) is caused by acceleration/deceleration forces applied to many areas of the CNS rather than in one specific location. Diffuse brain injury involves neuronal processes, cell bodies, transmitter mechanisms, and macroglial cells and blood vessels. The most severe injury to axons appears to be at the gray matter–white matter junction. A variant of diffuse brain injury is diffuse axonal injury in which axons of large myelinated nerve fibers are injured by shearing forces. In diffuse brain and axonal injury, mechanical deformation results in physical disruption of cell membranes and cytoskeleton and increased membrane permeability, resulting in major ionic fluxes in and out of the cell. Such changes can lead to excessive release of glutamate, excitotoxicity and cell death, free radical formation, apoptosis, and delayed inflammatory responses. The end result can be Wallerian degeneration.

In general, trauma of the CNS in animals occurs less frequently than in human beings. Animals are not exposed as frequently to potentially trauma-causing situations (e.g., automobile travel) as are human beings, and there are anatomic differences (see later), including a quadruped posture, which increases stability and helps protect the brains of animals.

Among animals, trauma to the brain is probably most frequently caused in dogs as a result of automobile-induced injury and in cats from falls from significant heights (high-rise apartment buildings, balconies, and roofs). Even after falling from considerable heights, cats often have remarkably minor injury to the CNS. Other examples include fracture of the spinal column or cranium of jumping horses and fractious animals, such as horses and ruminants, during excitement and restraint.

Predisposition to cerebral trauma is also influenced by anatomic differences. The percentage of brain mass in relation to skull size is much less in domestic animals than in primates, and in the bovine and porcine species the cranial cavity is additionally protected dorsally by prominent frontal sinuses. Birth trauma, which can be important in human beings, is essentially insignificant in animals because in the latter the shoulders, and particularly the pelvis, rather than the head are likely to be compressed in the birth canal. Exceptions to this generalization include brachycephalic

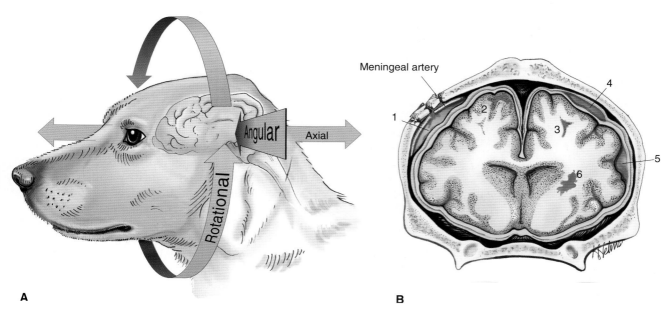

Fig. 14-97   Traumatic central nervous system injury and hemorrhage. A, Axial, rotational, and angular energy applied to the brain during trauma determine the severity of shear, tensile, and compressive forces that cause neuronal and vascular injury. **B,** Locations of hemorrhage, dog, brain. *(1)* Epidural hemorrhage with laceration of meningeal artery; *(2)* cortical hemorrhage; *(3)* hemorrhage in subcortical white matter; *(4)* subdural hemorrhage secondary to laceration of a bridging vein; *(5)* subarachnoid hemorrhage; *(6)* deep intracerebral hemorrhage. (**A,** *Courtesy Dr. J.F. Zachary, College of Veterinary Medicine, University of Illinois.* **B,** *Courtesy Dr. J.F. Zachary, College of Veterinary Medicine, University of Illinois. Redrawn and modified from Leech RW, Shuman RM: Neuropathology: a summary for students, Philadelphia, 1982, Harper & Row.)*

breeds of dogs. Several factors also influence the susceptibility of the spinal cord to trauma. The amount of space between the spinal cord and the wall of the vertebral canal is very important in determining the degree of injury following edema or compression with disk herniation. This space is greater in the cervical area of the dog then at the thoracolumbar level. Thus disk herniation at the latter area is more likely to result in severe spinal cord injury.

Functional factors also play an important role in brain injury. The brain of a freely movable head is much more susceptible to injury than one that is fixed in place. The increased susceptibility of the former has been attributed to the ability of the cranium (the bone) and its contents (the brain) to impact upon each other following nonpenetrating trauma. This interaction occurs because the brain does not completely fill the cranial cavity, thus resulting in a very short distance (or space) between brain and bone.

The type and location of the lesion (contusion and/or hemorrhage) will depend on the location of the point of contact and the direction of the blow, relative to the head. If the blow is directly on the back or front of the head, the head and brain will move straightforward

or backward, respectively (Fig 14-97, axial). If the blow is horizontal to the top of the head or horizontal to the rostral portion, the head will rotate on the atlanto-occipital axis (angularly and rotationally, respectively). In the case of an axial blow to the back of the head (an animal falling onto the back of its head), the head and thus the cranial vault will accelerate faster than the brain, which will lag behind, and the caudal aspect of the vault may move forward and contact the caudal aspect of the cerebral hemispheres, usually the occipital cortex. In the case of an animal falling onto the back of its head, the head will accelerate abruptly and the momentum will carry the brain caudally, where it may strike the inside of the caudal brain in the cranial vault. A vertical blow delivered directly down onto the dorsal surface of the head will have the same type of result on the dorsal aspect of the cerebral hemispheres as the blow to the back of the head. It is more common, from the same blows described previously, to see hemorrhage, usually subarachnoid, on the opposite side of the point of impact with the brain. For example, a vertical blow to the top of the head causes hemorrhage of the ventral surface of the medulla and cerebral hemispheres. Thus, following an

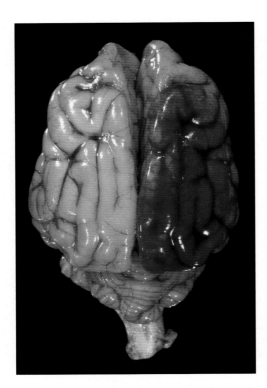

Fig. 14-98 Leptomeningeal (subarachnoid) hemorrhage, brain, right cerebral hemisphere, dog. *(Courtesy Dr. R. Storts, College of Veterinary Medicine, Texas A&M University.)*

impact upon a stationary freely movable head, the bone of the cranial vault will move upon the stationary brain and injure it (coup injury), and on the opposite side the nerves and blood vessels will be stretched, possibly resulting in nerve damage and hemorrhage (contrecoup injury). In addition, the mass and velocity of the object striking the head are important. Trauma following impact of a relatively large blunt object can create notable head movement and a large-impact injury, whereas a small object such as a bullet moving at a high rate of speed can cause less head movement and a smaller but deeper area of direct tissue damage. In summary, the basic concept is the transfer of kinetic energy by the striking object to the head. A large blunt object will cause the head to accelerate without deforming it; a smaller object, such as a bullet, will penetrate.

Factors involved in the protection of the brain include the rigidity of the cranium (dependent on age), the round shape of the dorsum of the skull, the structure of the parietal, occipital, and temporal cranial bones (two layers of compact bone separated by spongy bone referred to as diploë), cranial sutures, sinuses, ridges in the floor of the cranial cavity, meninges, and CSF. The spinal cord is enclosed and protected by the vertebral column, which is surrounded by soft adipose tissue and muscle. Other structures that help protect the spinal cord by absorbing shock are the intervertebral disks and the cancellous bone of the vertebrae. Vertebral ligaments maintain the alignment of the vertebral column; denticulate ligaments support the spinal cord in the middle of the vertebral canal and the meninges, and particularly the CSF cushions trauma.

Clinically, animals with CNS trauma have signs referable to the area injured, brain, or spinal cord. With brain trauma, signs can vary widely and range from unconsciousness lasting a few seconds followed by complete recovery and return to normal function to depression, abnormal behaviors, such as disorientation and irritability, semiconsciousness with responsiveness only to noxious stimuli, and unconsciousness with no response to any stimulus. With spinal cord trauma, signs vary depending on the severity of the injury and the rate of onset. Paralysis results from severance of the cord or ruptured disks. Paresis and ataxia result from less severe injury.

CONCUSSION

Concussion is often thought of as a clinical designation of temporary loss of consciousness with recovery following head injury. As in the human being, a movable head is much more susceptible to trauma than a fixed, supported one. Application of an appropriate concussive trauma to the mobile head of an animal results in a reversible cerebral dysfunction that lasts for a matter of seconds or, at most, a few minutes and is usually reversible, with stronger blows causing more severe injury and even death.

Concussive injuries of the diffuse type also occur in animals, but there are some differences between animals and human beings. For example, it is difficult to produce severe concussion in animals because the margin between the force of a stunning blow and one causing fatal injury is very small. The smaller the brain, the less vulnerable it is to rotational forces and the larger are the forces necessary to cause concussion. It should be noted, however, that concussion, particularly when there is rapid recovery from unconsciousness, can occur more frequently than appreciated in animals because the clinical signs may not be recognized.

Diffuse brain injury does not usually cause gross lesions. Microscopic lesions detected in animals include diffuse axonal injury characterized by axonal degeneration, and this may be followed by Wallerian degeneration. Damage to neurons ranges from central chromatolysis to death and neuronal loss. The more severe forms of diffuse brain injury can also have generalized acute brain swelling caused by unregulated vasodilation, which can be followed after some time by cerebral edema.

Spinal concussion is the term applied to the immediate and temporary loss of function that sometimes follows severe direct blows to the spinal column. Loss of function usually affects the long tracts/bundles of nerve fibers (funiculi), but usually there is no demonstrable external change in the vertebrae or spinal cord. As with cerebral concussion, there is often only a temporary functional disability of the cord after injury, but if the trauma is more severe, permanent neurologic deficits can result.

CONTUSION

Contusion means bruising, which is generally associated with rupture of blood vessels, and in the cerebrum this injury results in grossly detectable lesions such as hemorrhage and can, like concussion, result in unconsciousness and even death. The factors that cause concussion and contusion can occur together in the same animal. Lesions can be superficial (cerebral gyri) or more central (brain stem), and there can be concurrent skull fractures.

Although hemorrhage is the most common lesion, contusion of the brain can also result in tearing of CNS tissue. Tearing results in tissue necrosis and neuronal loss. Two designations are used to identify the location of contusive injury. A coup contusion is located at the impact site, and a contrecoup contusion at a location on the opposite side of the brain. When the two lesions occur together (coup-contrecoup or contrecoup-coup), the first term indicates the site of most severe injury (see Box 14-7 for a summary of the pathogenesis of coup-contrecoup contusion).

Box **14-7**

Pathogenesis of Coup-Contrecoup Contusion

CONDITIONS INVOLVED IN COUP-CONTRECOUP CONTUSION

1. Head freely movable.
2. Head accelerated rapidly (by being struck by a broad object, such as an automobile) or decelerated rapidly (head strikes pavement after a fall from a standing position).
3. Because the brain does not fill the cranial vault, it may lag behind the movement of the cranium when the head is accelerated or decelerated rapidly.
4. As a result, the inside of the cranial vault may strike the stationary brain at the point of impact (coup injury), or the lesion may occur on the opposite side (contrecoup), either from the stretching and tearing of vessels at that site or by the brain being struck by the inside of the cranial vault on the opposite side when there is reduced amount of cerebrospinal fluid buffer present.

Many investigations have been made to determine the mechanisms involved in the development of contusive lesions, and the kinetics are complicated and still not completely resolved. Factors that have been considered to be significant include the ability of the head to move freely, the occurrence of a rotational movement of the brain over rough surfaces on the inside of the cranial vault, and the development within the cranial cavity of positive and negative pressures and gravitational forces. The basic results of the different types of blows to the heads of animals have been discussed previously, and it is interesting to compare these with the lesions in humans. Several neuropathologic principles have been generally accepted regarding craniocerebral contusive trauma in human beings:

1. A blow to the stationary (but freely movable) head produces a cerebrocortical coup contusion beneath the point of cranial impact, but with rare exceptions causes no cerebrocortical contrecoup contusion opposite the point of cranial impact. This outcome is not always true of animals, in which a blow to the dorsum of the head from a flat object, such as a spade, causes marked subarachnoid hemorrhage on the ventral surface (contrecoup).
2. An impact of a moving head (moving before impact, as in a fall from a standing position) against a firm or unyielding surface causes a cerebrocortical contrecoup contusion opposite the point of cranial collision (often at the poles and inferior surfaces of the frontal and temporal lobes), but with rare exceptions there is no contusion beneath the point of impact. In contrast, horses that fall backward and land on their backs and strike the occiput often have subarachnoid hemorrhage over the occipital poles of the cerebral hemispheres.
3. Falls from great heights, and crushing of the head between a strong external force and unyielding surface, are generally not associated with the occurrence of contrecoup lesions.

Dawson and co-workers proposed a mechanism for both contrecoup and coup injury of the human brain that also addressed the specific deficiencies of mechanisms that have been advanced by others. An example explaining the mechanism of contrecoup injury states that when a person falls backward from a standing position because of loss of balance, the gravitational torque acting on the body causes downward acceleration of the head in excess of the acceleration as a result of gravity. Under these circumstances the brain lags toward the trailing anterior surface of the cranium before impact (causing displacement of the protective CSF layer between the brain and skull) and permits compressive stress to develop at this site, although impact occurs at the opposite side of the head. Because dissipation of the CSF at the anterior (contrecoup) site allows compressive stress to be focal at this contrecoup site and because of the shearing stress that is generated, injury occurs. In addition, a relative rotational gliding motion between the brain and skull is produced when the impact suddenly stops the skull's motion and rotation, thus creating an additive shearing stress because the fluid lubrication necessary to facilitate gliding of the brain over the cranial surface is reduced. The concentration of this rotational shearing stress is likely to occur beneath the frontal and temporal lobes because of the rough surface of the skull that exists in this location. In contrast to contrecoup injury, coup contusions occur infrequently in this type of fall. In such situations, the brain lags away from the impact site, which results in a thickening of the protective CSF layer between the brain and skull immediately beneath the point of impact, which helps explain the absence of coup injury in primates and human beings in typical moving head trauma.

Coup injury in human beings can occur when a stationary but freely movable head is impacted. In this type of trauma, there is neither brain lag nor disproportionate distribution of CSF before impact, which accounts for the typical absence of contrecoup contusions. With regard to falls from great heights, the dynamics involving rotation of the body about a fixed point of ground contact associated with a fall from a standing position do not occur. Because gravity produces no torque on a freely falling object, no angular acceleration of the body is produced, and therefore such a fall is a true free-fall state that is associated with an absence of brain lag. For this reason, contrecoup lesions occur infrequently with this type of trauma. One point should be emphasized with regard to the evaluation of coup and contrecoup cortical contusions just described. Displacement of bone associated with skull fracture can contuse the subjacent brain, regardless of the resting or moving status of the head, and such fracture-contusions have nothing to do with the coup-contrecoup mechanisms described. Also, even though the basic mechanisms discussed earlier apply to human beings, they should also be considered when evaluating cerebral contusions of domestic animals, but the situation in human brains is made far more complex because of the numerous wide bony ridges that project into the cranial vault.

Evaluation of spinal cord trauma should include examination not only of the spinal cord but also of the vertebral column and spinal nerve roots. Injuries to the spinal cord can involve concussion, contusion, hemorrhage, laceration, transection, and compression secondary to vertebral trauma and fracture. Contusion in the spinal cord is characterized by vascular tears, hemorrhage, and necrosis. Tears are generally focal and grossly visible. Contusion can occur without fracture of the vertebral column, with fracture, and with fracture

---

Box 14-8

Common Causes of Hemorrhage in Animal Brains

Vasculitis
 (Such as *Histophilus somni* [formerly *Haemophilus somnus*] infection)
Damage to endothelium lining blood vessels
 (By the virus of canine infectious hepatitis, by septicemia or endotoxemia, by immune complexes, or by parasite larval migration)
Trauma
 Contusion
 • Coup lesion
 • Contrecoup lesion
Penetrating wounds

---

plus dislocation of the spinal column. The last-named combination can result in tearing and transection of the spinal cord.

CENTRAL NERVOUS SYSTEM HEMORRHAGE

Although hemorrhage and hematomas in animal brains can be caused by a wide variety of injuries, trauma to the head is the most common cause. (see Box 14-8 for common causes of brain hemorrhage).

Following trauma to the head, hemorrhages can develop in the epidural, subdural, and subarachnoid space, under the pia mater (subpial), and in the brain (Fig. 14-97, *B*). Hemorrhage can be diffuse (Fig. 14-98) or focal (e.g., hematomas) (Fig. 14-99 and 14-100). Such hemorrhages can result from sliding of the brain over bony ridges (jugae) within the cranium with resultant stretching and tearing of blood vessels and tissue, and following the cutting and penetration of bone fragments from skull fracture. Cerebral epidural hemorrhage, which is not commonly described in animals, has been reported in the horse, especially jumpers, resulting from falls while working. Epidural hemorrhage does not usually occur because the dura is tightly adhered to the inner surface of the calvarium and there is no epidural space. In trauma causing skull fractures, bleeding from local blood vessels can separate the dura from the calvarium, forming a hematoma in the epidural space.

Subdural hemorrhage, which is an extravasation of blood between the dura mater and arachnoid membrane, occurs in dogs and cats. It is rare and is usually diffuse and does not form hematomas as seen in human beings, where they can be life threatening from compression and herniation of the brain. Subarachnoid and intracerebral hemorrhage are most common in all

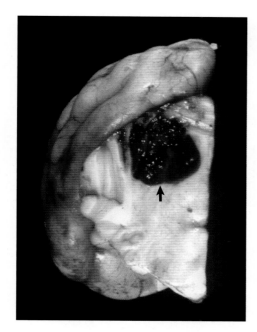

Fig. 14-99   Hematoma (*arrow*), cerebellum, transverse section, dog. Traumatic injury to the head resulted in hemorrhage and the formation of a hematoma from shear, tensile, compressive axial, rotational, and angular forces. *(Courtesy Dr. H.B. Gelberg, College of Veterinary Medicine, Oregon State University.)*

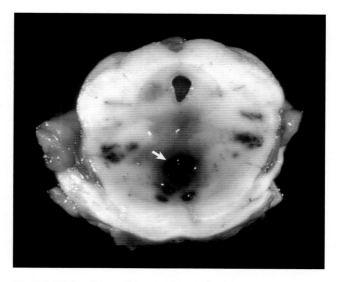

Fig. 14-100   "Duret" hemorrhages, brain stem, transverse section at the level of the pons. Note the multiple hemorrhages in the periventricular white matter *(arrow)*. These hemorrhages are the result of twisting of the brain stem on a longitudinal axis from rotational and axial forces. *(Courtesy Dr. M.D. McGavin, College of Veterinary Medicine, University of Tennessee.)*

species following head injury. Hemorrhage can result from injury to the brain with or without a fractured cranium by the mechanisms given previously and also from penetrating objects (bullets and stab wounds).

The same types of hemorrhage that affect the brain (epidural [rare], subdural [rare], leptomeningeal, and parenchymal) also occur in the spinal cord and its meninges. Causes are similar to those for the brain.

HEMATOMYELIA (HEMORRHAGIC MYELOMALACIA)

Traumatic injury to the spinal cord can cause stretching and tearing of blood vessels, usually arterioles, within the gray matter, resulting in hematomyelia. Hematomyelia is also particularly associated with severe type I disk herniation. If larger vessels are torn, blood pressure can force blood into the gray matter. This outcome results in the formation of a dissecting blood-filled cavity ascending and/or descending initially within the gray matter of the spinal cord. This lesion, which is characterized by a softening to semiliquefaction (myelomalacia) and hemorrhage of the tissue, can develop within 12 to 24 hours after injury and can progress both cranially and caudally from the original site of trauma. As the cavity extends cranially, the hemorrhage at the original site also extends into the white matter and can transect the spinal cord. If this lesion extends to the fifth cervical cord segment, the phrenic

nerves to the diaphragm will be denervated and respiratory paralysis will result. Bleeding continues until pressure in the blood-filled cavity is equal to the vascular pressure or until bleeding ceases because of hemostasis in the vessel. Hemorrhage can also result from bleeding in arteriovenous malformations within the spinal cord. Hematomyelia is characterized by neurologic deficits consistent with a sudden onset of ascending or descending flaccid paralysis and sensory abnormalities.

COMPRESSIVE INJURY

Diseases resulting in compressive injury can affect the brain, spinal cord, or both concurrently. In the brain, diseases such as neoplasia, reticulosis, canine granulomatous meningoencephalitis, and chronic cerebral abscesses can compress adjacent nervous tissue. In the spinal cord, compression can be intramedullary (within the spinal cord) or extramedullary (outside the spinal cord). Causes of intramedullary compression include hemorrhages, neoplasms such as nephroblastoma of the young dog, and chronic expansile inflammatory diseases. Extramedullary compression can be caused by intervertebral disk herniation in the dog, cervical stenotic myelopathy (wobbler syndrome) in the horse and dog, vertebral fracture and dislocation, and neoplasms of the meninges, such as the meningioma; nerve rootlets, such as nerve sheath tumors; or tumor metastasis, such as lymphosarcoma. Finally, developmental

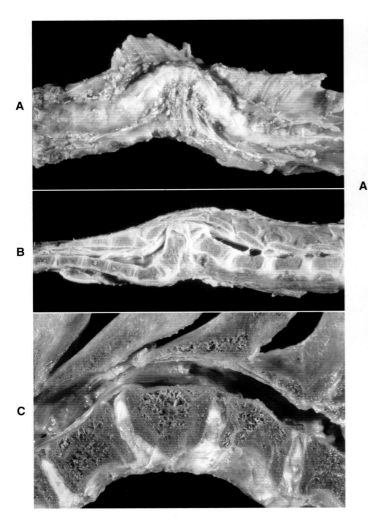

Fig. 14-101   Vertebral abnormalities, vertebral column.
A, Scoliosis, thoracic vertebrae, ventro-dorsal view, sheep. Lateral
deviation of the spinal column. **B,** Kyphosis, thoraco-lumbar
vertebrae, lateral view, sheep. Dorsal deviation of several
vertebrae and a wedge-shaped vertebra (hemivertebra;
Fig. 14-101, C) have resulted in compression of the spinal
cord. **C,** Hemivertebra, lumbar vertebrae, dog. Note that the
cranio-dorsal portion of the body of the hemivertebra has
protruded into the vertebral canal. (*A* and *B,* Courtesy College of
Veterinary Medicine, University of Illinois. *C,* Courtesy Department of
Veterinary Biosciences, The Ohio State University.)

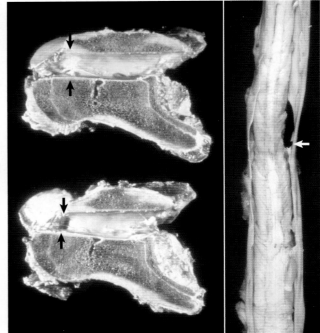

Fig. 14-102   Cervical stenotic myelopathy. A, Cervical
static stenosis, vertebral column, saggital section, sixth
cervical vertebra, horse. The vertebra on the bottom is
stenotic (*arrows*) and will compress the spinal cord. The
vertebra on the top is normal (*arrows*). **B,** Cervical vertebral
instability, spinal cord, fifth cervical segment, dog. Note the
narrowing of the spinal cord at the site of compression (*arrow*).
(*A* and *B,* Courtesy College of Veterinary Medicine, University of Illinois.)

anomalies of bone, such as atlanto-occipital malformation and vertebral deformities with hemivertebrae,
such as scoliosis, lordosis, and kyphosis (Fig. 14-101),
can result in compression of the spinal cord.

Compression of CNS tissue causes neuronal dysfunction by impeding normal anterograde and retrograde
axoplasmic flow in axons (Fig. 14-6). In addition, compression of nerves may result in reduced blood flow to
nerves and thus also contribute to neuronal dysfunction.

Mild compression can result in partial blockage of slow
axoplasmic flow and gradual accumulation of neurofilaments and microtubules, which results in mild
enlargement of the axon proximal to the compression
site, and atrophy of the axon distal to the compression.
Eventually, with a long period of time of complete blockage, the distal axon is lost.

BRAIN DISPLACEMENTS

See Cerebral Edema (Permeability Changes).

CERVICAL STENOTIC MYELOPATHY

Cervical stenotic myelopathy, or wobbler syndrome,
is characterized by stenosis of the cervical vertebral
canal, which causes compressive trauma to the cervical
spinal cord (Fig. 14-102). This disease occurs primarily
in young rapidly growing large breeds of horses and
dogs. Reports indicate that the disease is not caused by
a straightforward mechanism but apparently involves
several factors (multifactorial disease). For example,
stallions that have a genetic predisposition for rapid
growth and large body size are reported to be at greater

risk of developing the disease. Oversupplementation with protein, vitamins, and minerals used to promote rapid growth may also be another environmental factor in developing cervical stenotic myelopathy.

Gross and microscopic lesions of the CNS in cervical stenotic myelopathy are similar to the lesions in intervertebral disk herniation. The severity depends on the speed and degree to which the compression is applied and the specific area of the cord that is involved. Central nervous tissue can tolerate a considerable degree of compression if it is applied slowly. Rapid compression can lead to quickly developing hypoxia-ischemia, necrosis, and direct damage to compressed axons. Lesions detected include a spectrum of changes characterized by axonal injury and disruption of myelin sheaths resulting in Wallerian degeneration and necrosis of the gray or white matter or of both. Lesions can be visible grossly from the exterior but are more commonly seen on cross section of the spinal cord.

Microscopically, particularly at the site of injury, there is initial swelling of axons followed after several days by loss of architecture of the CNS as a result of necrosis and a beginning accumulation of gitter cells that have phagocytosed the lipid-rich tissue debris. Eventually the necrotic area is cleared and a cystic space is formed, which is surrounded by varying degrees of astrocytosis and astrogliosis, although not usually prominent unless there is severe destruction. Rostral and caudal to this location, the lesion is primarily one of Wallerian degeneration in the white matter, and the pattern of lesion development seen depends on the level of the spinal cord that is examined relative to the site of compression. At the site of injury, all parts of the white and gray matter of the spinal cord are affected and often necrotic, if the compressive force is sufficient. Rostral to this site, white matter degeneration is generally limited to the ascending tracts in the dorsal funiculi and the superficial portions of the dorsolateral part of the lateral funiculi. Caudal to the area of injury, degeneration is limited to the descending tracts in the ventral funiculi, and the more central portions of the lateral funiculi. It should also be noted that: (1) a lesion may occur at the point of compression because of ischemia, but a lesion can also occur on the opposite side of the compression also because of ischemia that results from compression of the tissue against bone on that side, and (2) Wallerian degeneration can be observed in distal segments of affected axons far from the point of compression within the spinal cord. In the former case, compressive forces can be transferred through the spinal cord to axons and blood vessels away from the contact point, whereas in the latter example degeneration of the distal axon segments can extend for a length of centimeters to meters away from the point of contact.

Cervical stenotic myelopathy has been known for many years to affect horses and more recently has been recognized in the large dog breeds. The disease in the horse has been referred to by several designations: the wobbler syndrome, wobbles, equine incoordination, and more recently, cervical stenotic myelopathy. The disease has been described in many horse breeds.

Cervical stenotic myelopathy in the horse has been divided into two syndromes, referred to as cervical static stenosis and cervical vertebral instability (dynamic stenosis). Cervical static stenosis commonly affects horses 1 to 4 years of age. The spinal cord is compressed at C5 through C7 as the result of an acquired dorsal or dorsolateral narrowing of the spinal canal (Fig. 14-102). The stenosis is due to formation of bone that requires time to develop. The compressive effect with this type of stenosis is present regardless of head position. The second form of cervical stenotic myelopathy (cervical vertebral instability–dynamic stenosis) occurs in horses ranging in age from 8 to 18 months and is characterized by a narrowing of the spinal canal during flexion of the neck, primarily at C3 through C5 vertebrae.

A disease process with many similarities to that in the horse also affects the dog. It has been known as wobbler syndrome, vertebral instability, vertebral subluxation, and cervical spondylolisthesis. The disease has been most frequently described in the Great Dane and Doberman pinscher breeds but has also been reported in the Saint Bernard, Irish setter, fox terrier, basset hound, Rhodesian ridgeback, and Old English sheepdog. Dogs can have signs develop between 8 months and 1 year of age, with a range of 1 month to 9 years. Great Danes tend to have lesions develop at a young age (8 months to 1 year), whereas Doberman pinschers are generally older, often more than 1 year of age. The vertebral and associated spinal cord lesions in the dog have been reported to most often involve the caudal cervical area from C5 through C7 vertebrae. An exception is the basset hound in which C3 is affected.

INTERVERTEBRAL DISK DISEASE

Although the anatomy of vertebrae and intervertebral disks is similar in dogs and human beings, there are notable differences in the anatomy of the spinal cord and spinal nerve roots that result in differences between the two species in clinical signs caused by herniated disks. Disk herniations in human beings commonly occur laterally, rather than dorsally as in dogs, contributing to the differences in clinical presentations (i.e., lateral herniations compress spinal nerve rootlets, whereas dorsal compression in dogs impinges on the spinal cord directly). In human beings the spinal cord terminates at the level of the second lumbar vertebra. Spinal nerve roots forming the cauda equina traverse in the remaining lumbar and sacral vertebrae before they exit the spinal canal to innervate structures. In dogs the spinal cord terminates at the level of the sixth lumbar vertebra, and nerve roots forming the cauda equina traverse in the remaining lumbar, sacral, and coccygeal vertebrae before they exit the spinal canal to innervate structures. Therefore in human beings, disk disease involving the caudal lumbar vertebrae (caudal to L2) results in compression of spinal nerve roots that innervate limbs and are reflected clinically in a condition know as "sciatica" and defined as referred pain in the sciatic nerve. In dogs, herniated disks in the lumbar vertebra primarily compress the spinal cord and under certain circumstances spinal nerves. Dogs thus present clinically with different neurologic signs.

Differences in clinical signs between dogs and human beings caused by herniated disks arise not only from anatomic differences discussed previously but also from postural differences and the application of shear and stress forces applied to the vertebrae and intervertebral disks. Human beings, with bipedal locomotion and erect posture, dissipate the forces of walking (also running) by transferring these forces from the legs up the vertebral column to the lumbar vertebrae (i.e., first in line to absorb and dissipate forces). In addition, lumbar vertebrae are not stabilized by the rib cage, and thus lumbar vertebrae must also absorb rotational forces (i.e., twisting forces) of motion. Therefore lumbar vertebrae are the primary sites for disk herniation in human beings; however, because of the anatomy discussed earlier, herniated disks compress nerve roots and not the spinal cord. This arrangement results in pain but rarely leg paralysis.

Dogs, having quadrupedal locomotion and horizontal posture, normally dissipate the forces of walking by transferring these forces up the limbs at right angles to the vertebral column and spinal cord. However, when a dog jumps with downward motion, as an example, from a chair to the floor, the force is directed down the vertebral column and results in greater "end on" compression of disks and increased likelihood of herniation. Additionally, thoracic vertebrae are fixed in place by the ribs, and lumbar vertebrae can rotate freely around the axial skeleton. This arrangement directs the impact of stress and shear forces to the thoracolumbar vertebrae and is a primary site of disk herniation and spinal cord compression. In dogs, because the spinal cord is compressed, paralysis of the rear limbs results.

Intervertebral disk disease occurs in the canine species, particularly dogs of the chondrodystrophic breeds typified by the dachshund and Pekingese (Fig. 14-103). Contiguous vertebrae are held together by the annulus fibrosis of intervertebral disks and dorsal and ventral longitudinal ligaments. This anatomic arrangement results in the spinal canal being properly aligned in an

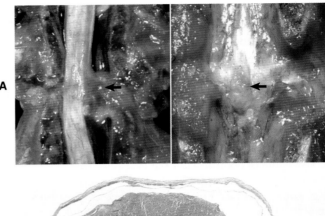

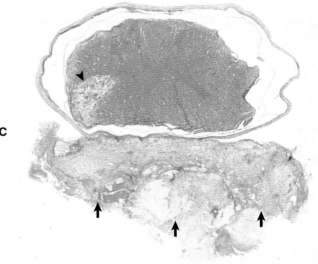

Fig. 14-103   Intervertebral disk disease, dog. A, Disk rupture (herniated intervertebral disk), spinal cord compression. Disk material compresses the spinal cord *(arrow)* resulting in Wallerian degeneration. **B,** Vertebral column, lumbar vertebrae. Herniated intervertebral disk *(arrow)* protrudes into the vertebral canal. **C,** Herniated intervertebral disk, spinal cord. The disk material *(arrows)* lies in the epidural space, touches the dura mater, and compresses the overlying spinal cord. An area of necrosis, possibly caused by infarction is present in the ventral area of the left lateral funiculus *(arrowhead)*. The multiple small holes in all funiculi are the sites of lost nerves as the result of spinal cord compression, which caused Wallerian degeneration. *(A, B, and C, Courtesy Dr. M.D. McGavin, College of Veterinary Medicine, University of Tennessee.)*

axial plane, so the spinal cord can traverse through the space without compression. Extradural space surrounding the cervical, cranial thoracic, and caudal lumbar spinal cord is sufficient to allow for the accumulation of herniated disk material without substantial compression of the spinal cord. In contrast, there is little extradural space surrounding the thoracolumbar spinal cord and it is the site most likely to have clinically significant disk herniation. As a result in dogs, thoracolumbar disk herniation is often more debilitating then cervical disk herniation.

Degeneration of intervertebral disks in chondrodystrophic breeds of dogs is a genetically programmed metaplastic change of the nucleus pulposus, resulting in peripheral to central replacement of the nucleus pulposus with cartilage. It begins as early as 6 months of age, progresses rapidly, and results in the loss of elasticity of the nucleus pulposus. The loss of elasticity places additional mechanical stress forces on the annulus fibrosus, which itself is experiencing degenerative changes similar to those occurring in the nucleus pulposus. The annulus fibrosus is thinnest and thus weakest at its point of contact with the spinal canal. If the annulus fibrosus is ruptured following stress forces placed on the disk by movement, such as jumping downward from a chair, fragments of the nucleus pulposus can be released into the spinal canal (Hansen type I herniation). If the annulus fibrosus ruptures dorsally, fragments compress the ventral funiculi of the spinal cord. If the annulus fibrosus ruptures dorsolaterally to laterally, fragments compress the ventral funiculi, lateral funiculi, and/or spinal nerve roots. Degeneration of intervertebral disks in nonchondrodystrophic breeds of dogs is an aging change of the nucleus pulposus resulting from fibrous metaplasia. This change causes a gradual loss of elasticity of the nucleus pulposus, which may be noticed clinically by 8 to 10 years of age. The gradual loss of elasticity places mechanical stress forces on the annulus fibrosus and results in its protrusion into and compression of the spinal canal (Hansen type II herniation).

Disk herniation causes injury to the CNS by several mechanisms. As discussed previously, the primary injury is caused by the physical trauma of compression and the resulting Wallerian degeneration of affected axons. Additionally, disk material can compress the vascular supply to a spinal cord segment resulting in ischemia, neuronal excitotoxicity, and necrosis. Type I herniation causes the most severe spinal cord damage because there is insufficient time for the spinal cord to compensate and for collateral circulation to develop, as may occur in type II herniation.

TUMORS

In the brain, diseases such as neoplasia cause compression of adjacent nervous tissue. Compression of CNS tissue causes neuronal dysfunction by impeding normal anterograde and retrograde axoplasmic flow in axons. See later discussion of specific types of CNS tumors.

LEPTOMENINGEAL HEMORRHAGE

Physical trauma to the CNS will compress, twist, and stretch blood vessels until they are torn. Such injury results in bleeding and leptomeningeal (subarachnoid) hemorrhage (Fig. 14-98). In the spinal cord, laceration of a large artery or vein can result in prolonged bleeding that ascends or descends the leptomeninges, causing neurologic dysfunction on examination compatible with ascending or descending neurologic deficits in spinal nerve roots.

TUMORS

Neoplasms of the CNS of animals are not as rare as was once believed. In fact, neoplasms occur with a frequency and variety, at least in the dog, similar to those in human beings. The majority of the neoplasms described have been in the dog and cat, and a large portion of these tumors occur in the older population. The intention in discussing CNS neoplasms in this chapter is to present the reader with a brief overview of the more common or better-known neoplasms that occur in animals and is not meant to be all inclusive. The location and characteristics of the primary and common secondary (metastatic) tumors of the nervous system are summarized in Table 14-12.

EMBRYONAL OR PRIMITIVE NEOPLASMS

Considering the complexities of brain development and the fact that astrocytes and oligodendrocytes arise from common stem cells early in development, it should not be surprising that some neoplasms arising in the CNS have multiple lines of differentiation as indicated by immunohistochemistry. One such neoplasm is the rare primitive neuroectodermal tumor. This neoplasm has recently been recognized by two of the authors in a young calf. An additional report in a primate has been made. Peripheral neuroectodermal tumors are tumors composed of poorly differentiated embryonal cells, tend to occur in young age groups, and are aggressive. Immunohistochemical staining for specific markers confirms multiple lines of differentiation such as neuronal, astrocytic, and oligodendroglial. Typically, one cell type dominates, most commonly neuronal.

Another neoplasm of uncertain histogenesis is the rhabdoid tumor. In human beings this neoplasm most commonly arises in the kidneys and brain and is believed to develop from embryonal stem cells. As is true of other embryonal neoplasms, young individuals are commonly affected. A novel concept is the proposal that these neoplasms arise from primordial stem cells that adopt the phenotypic characteristics of cells in the tissue of origin.

Rhabdoid tumors arising in the brain have cell markers of neuronal or glial differentiation. Neoplasms in the kidneys typically lack these markers. Despite their primary location, cell morphology is similar. The cells are large and round to polyhedral, and cytoplasm

Table **14-12**   **Primary Tumors of the Nervous System**

		CENTRAL NERVOUS SYSTEM		
Cell of Origin	Tumor Type	Location	Species Affected	Gross Appearance
Neuron	Medulloblastoma	Cerebellum (WM&GM)	Dog, cow, cat, pig (young animals)	Well-circumscribed, soft, gray to pink expansile mass (usually does not have hemorrhage, cysts, or necrosis)
Oligodendroglia	Oligodendroglioma	Cerebrum, brain stem, interventricular septum (WM&GM)	Dog, cat, cow	Well-demarcated, gray to pink-red, soft or gelatinous expansile mass, usually with areas of hemorrhage
Astroglia	Astrocytoma	Pyriform lobe, cerebral hemispheres, thalamus-hypothalamus, midbrain, cerebellum, spinal cord (WM&GM)	Dog, cat, cow	Poorly demarcated, firm, gray-white when well differentiated; anaplastic neoplasms are moderately to well demarcated, soft and friable, (usually with areas of necrosis, hemorrhage, edema, and cavitation)
Ependyma	Ependymoma	Ventricular system (lateral; less commonly, third and fourth), central canal of the spinal cord	Dog, cat, cow, horse	Poorly, to moderately, to well-demarcated, soft and gray-white, invasive, destructive gelatinous expansile mass (usually with areas of hemorrhage and cavitation)
Choroid plexus epithelium	Choroid plexus tumor	Ventricular system (fourth; less commonly, third and lateral)	Dog, horse, cow	Well-demarcated, granular to papillary, gray-white to red, expansile mass
Microglia	Microgliomatosis (reticulosis)	Cerebrum, brain stem	Dog	Poorly demarcated, gray-white, infiltrative mass (may have perivascular pattern)
Endothelium	Hemangiosarcoma	Cerebrum, brain stem	Dog	Well-demarcated, invasive red to dark red, expansile mass
Mesothelium (fibroblasts)	Meningioma	Meningeal surface of the CNS (basal cow, sheep areas, convexity and lateral surfaces of cerebral hemispheres, cerebellum-tentorium, falx cerebri, surface of the spinal cord)	Cat, dog, horse, cow, sheep	Well-demarcated, variable shapes, firm, encapsulated, and gray-white to soft, red-brown or gray, expansile masses (usually with areas of hemorrhage and necrosis)

		PERIPHERAL NERVOUS SYSTEM		
Cell of Origin	Tumor Type	Location	Species Affected	Gross Appearance
Schwann cells (other supportive cells)	Peripheral nerve sheath tumor*	Cranial nerves, spinal nerves (brachial plexus)	Dog, cow, cat	Firm or soft (gelatinous), white or gray, nodular masses

WM&GM, White matter and gray matter.
*Other names for this tumor type include: schwannoma, neurofibroma, and neurilemmoma.

is eosinophilic and abundant and contains large inclusions composed of skeins of intermediate filaments. A rhabdoid tumor has been reported in the brain of an 18-month-old dog. Immunohistochemical staining demonstrated that cells distributed throughout the tumor stained for vimentin; however, only scattered cells stained for neuron-specific enolase and GFAP. No cells in the tumor stained for S-100.

MEDULLOBLASTOMA

This neoplasm has characteristics similar to the less frequently occurring neuroblastoma, and both are considered to arise from cells of the neuronal lineage. The cell of origin for the medulloblastoma has not been definitely determined, but it has been proposed that the neoplasm can arise from primitive cells originating in the neuroepithelial roof of the fourth ventricle and that give rise to the external granular cell layer.

In animals, medulloblastomas have been reported in dogs, cats, cows, and pigs. There is a predilection for these tumors in young animals. The neoplasm chiefly occurs in the cerebellum of puppies and calves and sometimes also in adult dogs. The neoplasm is well circumscribed, soft, gray to pink, and usually does not have hemorrhages, cysts, or necrosis. The growth can compress the fourth ventricle and cause an obstructive hydrocephalus and can infiltrate adjacent structures including the leptomeninges. It can metastasize through the CSF in the ventricles or subarachnoid space. Microscopically the neoplasm is highly cellular and consists of round to elongated nuclei that have prominent chromatin in an ill-defined cytoplasm. The cells are arranged in sheets or broad bands and also can form pseudorosettes. Mitoses can be numerous.

ASTROCYTOMAS

Astrocytomas have been morphologically classified based on their degree of differentiation (histologic features in H&E stained sections) and include the following three types: diffuse astrocytomas, anaplastic astrocytomas, and glioblastoma multiforme. The degree of differentiation refers to how closely astrocytes forming the tumor resemble normal astrocytes within the CNS. Diffuse astrocytomas tend to have the most well-differentiated astrocytes, whereas glioblastoma multiforme has the most poorly differentiated astrocytes. All of these tumors are malignant; however, the degree of malignancy is often inversely related to the degree of differentiation.

Astrocytomas have been reported in dogs, cats, and cattle but are most frequently diagnosed in dogs (10% incidence) and uncommon in the cat. Brachycephalic breeds such as Boston terriers and boxers and dogs 5 to 11 years of age are most commonly affected. Common sites include the cerebral hemispheres, especially the temporal and pyriform lobes, thalamus-hypothalamus, midbrain, and less frequently, the cerebellum and spinal cord.

Astrocytomas will often displace normal tissue; however, their gross appearance often depends on their rate of growth and degree of differentiation (Fig. 14-104). Slow-growing, well-differentiated astrocytomas (less malignant) are usually difficult to distinguish from normal tissue and are rather solid or firm and gray-white. Rapidly growing, poorly differentiated astrocytomas are more malignant and are easier to discern because they have areas of necrosis, hemorrhage, cavitation, and edema.

Microscopically the more well-differentiated diffuse astrocytomas consist of a rather uniform cell type loosely organized. Cell size varies, and distinct ramifying cytoplasmic processes can be observed. Nuclei vary

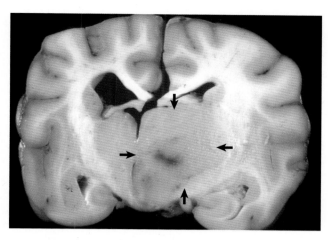

Fig. 14-104   Astrocytoma, brain, transverse section at the level of the thalamus, dog. The deep ventromedial area (thalamus/hypothalamus) of the right hemisphere *(arrows)* contains a poorly demarcated, nonencapsulated, expansile mass, which is a space-occupying lesion that has displaced the midline to the left and compressed the right lateral ventricle. The left lateral ventricle is mildly dilated, most likely from compression of the interventricular foramen. *(Courtesy Dr. M.D. McGavin, College of Veterinary Medicine, University of Tennessee.)*

in size and shape and contain more chromatin than normal astrocytes. Cells tend to be arranged around and along blood vessels. The boundary between neoplastic and normal tissue is indistinct. Anaplastic astrocytomas and glioblastoma multiforme have extreme cellular pleomorphism often with giant cell formation.

Increasing usage of immunohistochemical markers for glial cells and indicators of cellular proliferation will undoubtedly enhance the specificity and prognostic significance of the diagnosis of different glial cell neoplasms in animals. The most reliable marker for astrocytomas is GFAP, although vimentin has proved useful in some cases.

Clinical signs in animals with astrocytomas vary depending on the location of the tumor in the CNS but can include behavioral changes, ataxia, tetraparesis, seizures, circling, and abnormal cranial nerve and proprioceptive reflexes.

CHOROID PLEXUS PAPILLOMAS AND CARCINOMAS

Choroid plexus papilloma occurs most commonly in the dog but has been reported in the horse and in cattle. There is no breed predilection in dogs. In the dog, the neoplasm occurs most frequently in the fourth ventricle, but it also can be located in the third and lateral ventricles.

Grossly the neoplasm is a well-defined, expansive, granular to papillary growth located within the ventricular system that is gray-white to red and compresses

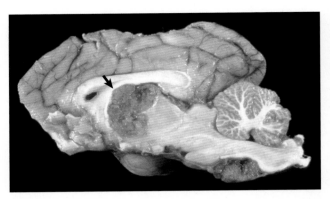

Fig. 14-105   Choroid plexus tumor (carcinoma), brain, sagittal section, dog. The third ventricle contains an expansile mass *(arrow)* that has invaded the normal tissue ventral to it. The mass ventral to the medulla *(right)* may be a metastasis arising from tumor cells that entered the third ventricle and then spread in the cerebrospinal fluid caudally, through the mesencephalic duct, into the fourth ventricle, and out through a lateral aperture into the subarachnoid space. *(Courtesy Dr. Y. Niyo, College of Veterinary Medicine, Iowa State University; and Noah's Arkive, College of Veterinary Medicine, The University of Georgia.)*

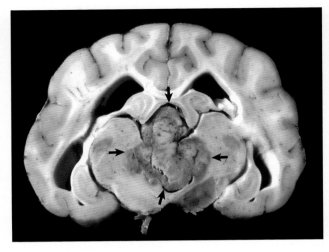

Fig. 14-106   Ependymoma, brain, transverse section at the level of the hippocampus, dog. The third ventricle contains a moderately well-demarcated expansile mass *(arrows)* that has invaded normal tissue ventral to it. Moderate hydrocephalus is present in both lateral ventricles from blockage of the third ventricle. *(Courtesy Dr. M.D. McGavin, College of Veterinary Medicine, University of Tennessee.)*

the adjacent nervous tissue (Fig. 14-105). Noncommunicating hydrocephalus may result from obstruction of CSF flow within the ventricular system. Microscopically these neoplasms generally resemble the choroid plexus and are characterized by an arborizing vascular connective tissue stroma that is covered with a cuboidal to columnar epithelial layer. Mitoses are not present in the benign form. A more malignant variety, choroid plexus carcinoma, is characterized by invasiveness, presence of mitoses, additional occurrence of solid tumor growth, and a tendency to metastasize within the ventricular system, or into the subarachnoid space (through the lateral apertures), where implantation in the ependyma or meninges, respectively, occurs. Currently there are no reliable immunohistochemical markers for these tumors.

The age range of dogs with choroid plexus tumors in one study was 5 to 13 years, except for one dog that was 2 years of age. Clinical signs in animals with choroid plexus tumors vary depending on the location of the tumor in the CNS but can include behavioral changes, ataxia, paresis, seizures, circling, and abnormal cranial nerve and proprioceptive reflexes.

EPENDYMOMAS

Ependymomas are one of the less frequently occurring neoplasms in dogs, cats, cattle, and horses. Some reports on the dog indicate a higher frequency in brachycephalic breeds. Ependymomas usually involve the lateral or, less commonly, third and fourth ventricles. They also occur in the central canal of the

spinal cord. The neoplasm can be observed within the ventricular system and subarachnoid space, likely attributable to local metastasis via the CSF. Noncommunicating hydrocephalus may result from obstruction of CSF flow within the ventricular system.

Grossly, ependymomas are usually large expansile intraventricular masses with generally well-demarcated margins (Fig. 14-106). The neoplasm is soft and gray-white to red depending on blood content and has a smooth cut surface in dogs. In cats the cut surface can be granular in texture. In some ependymomas the cut surface may have gelatinous consistency and be cavitated. More aggressive tumors show invasion into the normal tissue at its margins. Microscopically, ependymomas are highly cellular and well vascularized. Cells have hyperchromic, round to oval nuclei with scant or undetectable cytoplasm. Cells form perivascular rosettes (pseudorosettes) with nuclear polarity away from the vessel wall. Cells are also arranged in sheets and bands. The mitotic rate is variable. Hemorrhage, mucinous and cystic degeneration, and capillary proliferation occur. Malignancy is indicated by invasive growth, frequent mitoses, and anaplasia. Currently there are no reliable immunohistochemical markers for ependymomas.

The average age of affected dogs ranges from 6 to 12 years. Occurrences in a cat as young as 18 months old and in a calf 5 months old have been reported. Clinical signs in animals with ependymomas vary depending on the location of the tumor in the CNS but can include behavioral changes, ataxia, paresis, seizures, circling, and abnormal cranial nerve and proprioceptive reflexes.

OLIGODENDROGLIOMAS

Neoplasms composed of oligodendrocytes occur most commonly in the dog, but cases have been reported in cats and cattle. The reported incidence varies; some reports indicate oligodendrogliomas as the most common neuroectodermal neoplasm (5% to 12% incidence), whereas others place it second to astroglial neoplasms. As with astrocytomas in dogs, there is a predilection for brachycephalic breeds (Boston terriers, boxers, and bulldogs), and the age range is the same as for astrocytomas (5 to 11 years of age). Neoplasms occur in all areas of the white matter of the cerebrum, brain stem, and interventricular septum (Fig. 14-107). Neoplasms tend to extend to meningeal and ventricular surfaces, but dissemination in the CSF is uncommon.

Grossly, most oligodendrogliomas can be relatively well demarcated from surrounding tissue or their margins can be indistinct and blend in with adjacent normal white matter. The neoplasms vary in size, can grow quite large, are gray to pink-red, and are soft or gelatinous with areas of hemorrhage. In larger tumors the central area may be cystic. Microscopically the neoplasms are composed of densely packed cells. Nuclei are centrally located, hyperchromic, and surrounded by pale or nonstaining cytoplasm creating a perinuclear halo. Other patterns include cells arranged in rows, especially peripherally, or in semicircles. Mitoses are generally infrequent. Regressive changes include mucoid degeneration, edema, cavitation, and rarely mineralization. Extensive necrosis is uncommon. Currently there are no reliable immunohistochemical markers for oligodendrogliomas.

MENINGIOMAS

Meningioma is the most common mesodermal neoplasm of the CNS of animals, especially in cats. Sites of occurrence in the dog include the basal area of the brain, the area over the convexity of the cerebral hemispheres, the cerebellum-tentorium area, the lateral surface of the brain, the falx cerebri, and the surface of the spinal cord. Retrobulbar involvement (originating from the optic nerve sheath) also occurs. In the cat, the neoplasm uniquely occurs in the tela choroidea of the third ventricle but also occurs over the cerebral hemispheres, along the falx cerebri, over the cerebellum and tentorium, and rarely at the base of the brain. Occurrence in the meninges of the spinal cord is not common. Meningiomas have been reported to arise from arachnoid "cap cells," which are on the external surface of the arachnoid membrane. These cells cover the surface of the arachnoid layer that oppose the surface layer of the dura mater, and thus these tumors project into the subdural space and often into the CNS parenchyma.

Grossly, neoplasms in the dog are solitary and vary in size. The neoplasms are well defined, spherical, lobulated, lenticular, or plaquelike in shape; firm; encapsulated; and gray-white (Fig. 14-108). Sometimes on the cut surface there are soft, red, brown, or gray areas of hemorrhage and necrosis. Because these neoplasms grow slowly, they cause pressure atrophy of the adjacent nervous tissue. Meningiomas can be invasive, and sometimes there is hyperostosis of the overlying bone. In the cat, meningiomas vary in size from barely detectable to 2 cm in diameter. Cats, and occasionally cattle, can have more than one neoplasm. Other characteristics are comparable with those described in the dog.

Microscopically, several patterns of neoplastic cells can occur, and more than one can be present in a given neoplasm. Based on their cytomorphologic features, these tumors are grouped into one of six categories: (1) epithelioid/meningotheliomatous; (2) fibroblastic; (3) transitional (features of both epithelioid and fibroblastic); (4) psammomatous; (5) angioblastic; and (6) anaplastic/malignant. Cytomorphologic features are beyond the scope of this chapter; however, the more common pattern is characterized by the formation of nests, islands, or laminated whorls of cells. The cells have large cell bodies with abundant cytoplasm, ill-defined

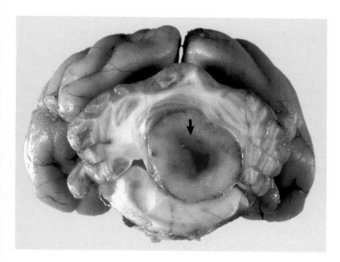

Fig. 14-107   Oligodendroglioma, brain, cerebellum, transverse section caudal to the pons, dog. The tumor is relatively well demarcated from the surrounding cerebellum. Oligodendrogliomas may be well demarcated or merge with adjacent normal brain. They vary in size, are gray to pink-red, and are soft or gelatinous with areas of hemorrhage (*arrow*).
(Courtesy Dr. W. Crowell, College of Veterinary Medicine, University of Georgia; and Noah's Arkive, College of Veterinary Medicine, The University of Georgia.)

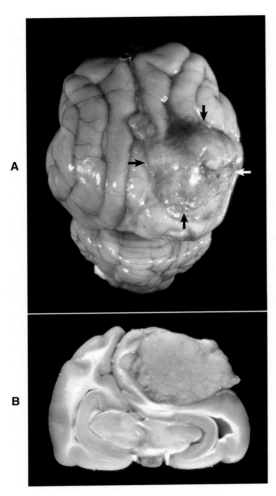

Fig. 14-108   Meningioma, cat, brain. A, On the surface of the right parietal cortex is a mass *(arrows)* that has compressed and distorted the adjacent parenchyma. It is a space-occupying lesion that has displaced the midline (cerebral longitudinal fissure) to the left. **B,** Transverse section at the level of the hippocampus of the brain depicted in Fig. 14-108, A. The tumor has compressed the right cerebral hemisphere and this has resulted in the midline being displaced to the left with compression of the left cerebral hemisphere. The meningioma does not invade the brain and can be "shelled" out at necropsy or surgery. *(A and B, Courtesy College of Veterinary Medicine, University of Illinois.)*

cell boundaries, and elongated, oval, open nuclei with peripherally located chromatin. The number of cells making up a whorl can vary from a few to many, and in the center of such structures can be mineralized material (referred to as psammoma bodies). A second pattern is characterized by strands or streams of elongated cells with a rather irregular or parallel orientation. Regressive changes include hemorrhage and cavernous vascular formations. Invasive growth occurs but is less common

than growth by expansion. Currently vimentin and pancytokeratin may be useful immunohistochemical markers for these tumors.

Meningiomas occur most frequently in the dog and cat but have been reported in other species of domestic animals including horses, cattle, and sheep. In the dog, this neoplasm occurs in several breeds, with dolichocephalic animals being frequently represented. The majority of meningiomas are in dogs between 7 and 14 years of age and in cats 10 years old or older.

Other benign neoplasms of mesenchymal origin, such as neurofibromas of spinal cord nerve roots, occur in the meninges. Spindle cell sarcomas, such as neurofibrosarcomas and dural osteosarcomas, have also been reported in the meninges.

MICROGLIOMATOSIS

Microgliomatosis, which has been classified as a proliferative neoplastic disease, has some features that are quite distinct from the inflammatory and neoplastic forms of reticulosis described in an earlier section (see Reticulosis/Granulomatous Meningoencephalitis). Gross lesions are usually not present. The cells, which infiltrate the CNS without topographic perivascular arrangement, resemble microglia in that their nuclei, which vary in size and shape and have prominent chromatin, are the only visible cellular component following conventional staining. Also, mitoses can be common, and there is no accompanying reticulin fiber formation such as occurs in the inflammatory and neoplastic reticuloses. Microgliomatosis occurs in older dogs.

HEMANGIOSARCOMA

Primary hemangiosarcoma of the CNS is a rare neoplasm arising from endothelial cells. The disease is most common in dogs but can occur in all domestic species. The neoplasm is a solitary expansile red to dark red mass within the cerebral cortex. Its color and bloody consistency are helpful in differentiating it from a primary or metastatic melanoma. Most hemangiosarcomas found in the CNS are from metastases.

METASTATIC TUMORS

Hematogenously metastasizing neoplasms occur and affect the brain more often than the spinal cord. The species in which metastasis has been most commonly reported is the dog; the next most frequent is the cat. Of the metastasizing carcinomas, mammary gland carcinoma in the dog has been reported to occur most frequently, although others have been described. Hemangiosarcoma of the heart, liver, and spleen is one of the most common metastasizing sarcomas in the dog; others are the mesenchymal component of the malignant mixed mammary gland tumor, lymphosarcoma, fibrosarcoma, and malignant melanoma. In the CNS,

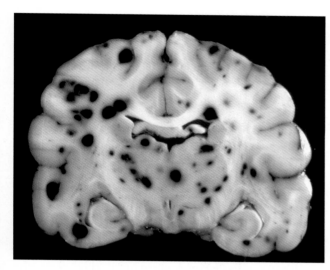

Fig. 14-109   Hemangiosarcoma, metastatic, brain, formalin-fixed, transverse section at the level of the thalamus, dog. Note the prominent hematogenous metastases, which appear as black nodules of various sizes distributed throughout the brain, sometimes at the gray matter–white matter interface. In an unfixed (fresh) specimen, the nodules would be red to dark red from erythrocytes. Black nodules in a fresh specimen would be consistent with metastatic melanoma. *(Courtesy Dr. M.D. McGavin, College of Veterinary Medicine, University of Tennessee.)*

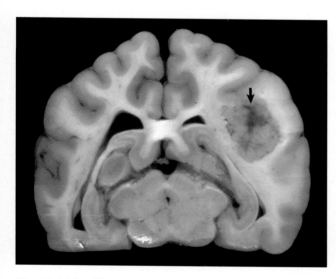

Fig. 14-110   Mammary carcinoma, metastatic, brain, transverse section at the level of the hippocampus, dog. The right cerebral hemisphere contains a well-demarcated mass *(arrow)*, which has caused enlargement of the right cerebral hemisphere and compression of the right lateral ventricle. The left lateral ventricle is slightly dilated, probably because of pressure on the interventricular foramen. *(Courtesy Drs. F. Moore and J. Carpenter, Angell Memorial Animal Hospital; and Noah's Arkive, College of Veterinary Medicine, The University of Georgia.)*

metastatic hemangiosarcomas appear to have predilection for the gray matter–white matter interface (Fig. 14-109). In the cat, the neoplasms that metastasize to the CNS include the mammary gland carcinoma (Fig. 14-110) and lymphosarcoma. Primary CNS lymphomas have been reported.

Peripheral Nervous System

INTRODUCTION

ORGANIZATION

During the last few years, there have been important changes in the approach and terminology used to categorize diseases that involve that portion of the nervous system outside of the CNS. The traditional approach divided these diseases into those of the PNS and the autonomic nervous system (ANS). Advances in neuroscience have resulted in the PNS being divided into three divisions: the sensorimotor division (formerly the PNS), the autonomic division (formerly the ANS), and the enteric division (a newly labeled system). The sensorimotor division is formed by sensory neurons (afferent components of cranial and spinal nerves, sensory receptors, and cranial and spinal ganglia) and motor neurons (efferent components of cranial and spinal nerves, and lower motor neurons) that innervate skeletal muscle via myoneural junctions (Fig. 14-111). The autonomic and enteric divisions consist of networks of afferent and efferent nerves and their ganglia (Meissner's [submucosal] and Auerbach's [myenteric] plexuses) that regulate, as examples, the contractility and relaxation of smooth muscle of the vascular and alimentary (peristalsis) systems and glandular secretions via sympathetic and parasympathetic fibers. Afferent and efferent nerve fibers of the autonomic and enteric divisions are carried in the afferent and efferent branches of the sensorimotor division (cranial and spinal nerves).

Peripheral nerves are composed of groups of axons, both myelinated and nonmyelinated, and of varying caliber (Fig. 14-112). As with the CNS, conspicuous components of axons are neurofilaments and microtubules. Neurofilaments provide structural support; microtubules are intimately involved in bidirectional axoplasmic flow of structural components, nutrients, and trophic factors to and from the cell body required for maintenance of the axons and neuronal integrity. Transport from the neuron cell body to the distal axon (anterograde flow) occurs at fast (400 mm per day or about 0.25 mm per minute) and slow (1 to 4 mm per day) rates. Retrograde transport from the distal axon to the cell body progresses at a rate of 200 mm per day (about 0.125 mm per minute).

Supporting cells in the PNS include Schwann cells and fibroblasts of the endoneurium and the satellite cells (Schwann cell–like cells) of the dorsal root ganglion. Schwann cells surround both myelinated and nonmyelinated axons and are responsible for formation of the myelin sheaths (Fig. 14-112). In contrast to the CNS, where one oligodendroglial cell can send out numerous processes to myelinate many different axonal internodes of several different axons, one Schwann cell myelinates one internode of one axon. As a result, the entire length of an axon in the PNS is myelinated by many individual Schwann cells.

Although Schwann cells do not appear to play a role in axon guidance during formation of the PNS, these cells are necessary for maintenance of axons and secrete neurotrophic factors that play a role in regeneration. Axons are grouped into fascicles along with surrounding loosely organized tissue fibrils and specialized endoneurial fibroblastic cells with phagocytic capabilities (Fig. 14-112). When an axon is damaged so badly as to cause Wallerian degeneration, removal of the debris is by these putative endogenous phagocytic cells, augmented by an influx of blood monocytes. Mast cells and small blood vessels also are present among the nerve fibers.

Depending on species and anatomic location, endothelial cells of endoneurial blood vessels can be joined by tight junctions preventing free passage of some macromolecules and providing an incomplete blood-nerve barrier. Collagen bundles and modified fibroblastic cells, termed perineurial cells, form the perineurium that ensheathes individual nerve fascicles. The perineurium contributes some barrier properties by preventing the free diffusion of macromolecules into the nerve fascicles. The fibrous epineurium is continuous with the dura mater as a peripheral nerve joins the CNS and encloses groups of nerve fascicles. The epineurium contains fibroblasts, mast cells, and adipocytes, the latter probably providing some protection to the nerve. Satellite cells are found in dorsal root ganglia within the matrix formed by the endoneurium that envelops cell bodies of peripheral nerves. They function in a supportive, nonmyelinating role, much like perineuronal oligodendroglia in the CNS.

The autonomic and enteric divisions of the PNS function primarily to transmit impulses from the CNS to peripheral organs (efferent nerves) that regulate (involuntary control) the function of these organ systems

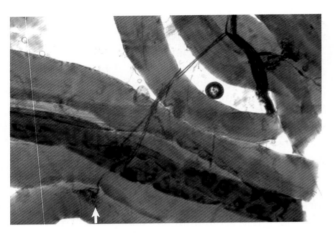

Fig. 14-111   Myoneural junctions. Peripheral nerve with terminal axons ending at myoneural junctions on muscle fibers (*arrow*). Dissected and glycerol-mounted muscle fibers. *(Courtesy Dr. M.D. McGavin, College of Veterinary Medicine, University of Tennessee.)*

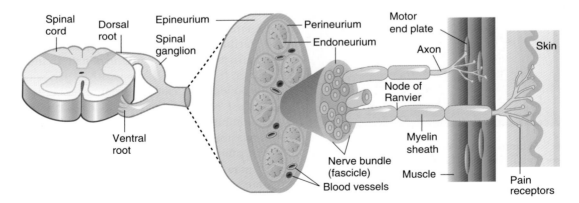

Fig. 14-112   Organization of a peripheral nerve, sensory, and motor branches and their coverings. In human (bipeds) neuroanatomy, spinal nerve rootlets are termed anterior and posterior rather than ventral and dorsal, respectively, in animals. *(From McCance KL, Huether SE: Pathophysiology: the biologic basis for disease in adults & children, ed 4, St Louis, 2002, Mosby.)*

(heart, vascular system, visceral smooth muscle, and exocrine and endocrine glands). These effects include but are not limited to the rate and force of contraction and relaxation in smooth (visceral organs and blood vessels) and striated muscle (heart). Afferent nerves, which transmit from the periphery to the CNS, mediate visceral sensation and vasomotor and respiratory reflexes through baroreceptors and chemoreceptors in the carotid sinus and aortic arch. Autonomic and enteric functions are regulated in the medulla, pons, and hypothalamus of the CNS.

The autonomic division has two structural and functional components: the sympathetic and parasympathetic systems. These systems usually have opposing effects on innervated organ systems. The parasympathetic system acts, as examples, to lessen the effects of increased vasoconstriction (smooth muscle) and contractility (heart rate) exerted by the sympathetic system.

The enteric division of the PNS system exerts effects on digestive processes such as motility, secretion and absorption, and blood flow. The main components of the enteric nervous system are myenteric plexuses (Auerbach's plexuses), located between the longitudinal and circular layers of muscle, and submucosal plexuses (Meissner's plexuses) that innervate esophageal and intestinal smooth muscle. Injury to these plexuses can lead to dysautonomias, which are discussed in a later section.

BARRIER SYSTEMS
BLOOD-NERVE BARRIER

The blood-nerve barrier regulates the free movement of certain substances from the blood to the endoneurium of peripheral nerves. Barrier properties are conferred by tight junctions between endothelial cells of the capillaries of the endoneurium and perineurium, and by selective transport systems in the endothelial cells.

RESPONSES OF THE AXON TO INJURY

See under Central Nervous System: Responses of Neurons to Injury and Wallerian Degeneration and Central Chromatolysis.

DISEASES

PERIPHERAL NEURONOPATHIES AND MYELINOPATHIES

Many disorders affecting the CNS are also manifested in lesions in the PNS, either: (1) because of damage to neuron cell bodies of lower motor neurons residing in the CNS or (2) because the PNS is equally vulnerable

to the disease. As an example in the first case, in lysosomal storage diseases substrate accumulates in cell bodies of lower motor neurons. Cell death and axonal degeneration of the PNS are the end points of a chronic and progressive process of substrate accumulation that interferes with cellular biochemical processes and transport systems. In the second case, substrate will also accumulate in cell bodies of sensory neurons located in the dorsal root ganglion of the PNS, resulting in cell death and axonal degeneration. Despite this caveat, there are certain diseases that primarily affect the PNS. Depending on whether the lesion is in a sensory or motor nerve or both, diseases of the PNS can manifest clinically as motor disturbance, sensory deprivation, or a combination of motor and sensory alterations. Space constraints do not allow an exhaustive coverage of disorders of the PNS. Many of the reported disorders seem to represent isolated occurrences in a specific breed. This section will cover the major types of PNS diseases with reference to specific disorders for illustrative purposes.

CONGENTIAL/HEREDITARY/FAMILIAL DISEASES

Primary sensory neuropathies Included here are the hereditary, familial, and breed- or species-associated syndromes reported in a variety of domestic animals that result in degeneration of PNS sensory neurons (dorsal root ganglion) or axons innervating the limbs. Two examples of primary sensory neuropathies have been described in English pointers and long-haired dachshunds. In pointer dogs, the onset is 2 to 12 months of age with signs of self-mutilation and insensitivity to pain resulting in neuropododermatitis or acral mutilation syndrome (Fig. 14-113). Additional signs can include ataxia, loss of conscious proprioception, and patellar hyporeflexia. In dachshunds, a sensory neuropathy is manifested shortly after birth by ataxia and alterations in the function of the autonomic division of the PNS, such as urinary incontinence and digestive disturbances. Lesions in pointer dogs consist of small dorsal root ganglia with neuronal loss and replacement by satellite cells (nodules of Nageotte) and mild reduction in size of dorsal nerve rootlets, because of degeneration and loss of myelinated and nonmyelinated axons with the presence of cell bands of Büngner (indicative of attempts at remyelination). In dachshunds, lesions are a distal axonopathy with loss of large myelinated and unmyelinated axons. Lesions can occur in the vagus nerve.

Other degenerative distal axonopathies of the PNS have also been reported in Birman cats and in dog breeds, including Bouvier des Flandres, Siberian huskies and crossbreeds, Boxer dogs (sensory axonopathy), rottweilers (sensory axonopathy), dachshunds (sensory axonopathy), Dobermans (dancing Doberman disease—thought to

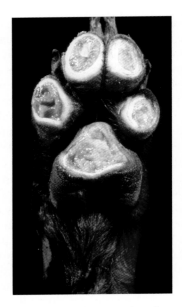

Fig. 14-113   Neuropododermatitis (acral mutilation syndrome), dog. This disorder, a primary sensory peripheral neuronopathy with self-mutilation and insensitivity to pain, is caused by the absence of (or small) dorsal root ganglia, reduction in size of dorsal nerve rootlets, and degeneration and loss of myelinated and nonmyelinated sensory axons. This dog wore off its footpads when placed on a concrete run. Satellite cell proliferation is commonly present in other large autonomic ganglia, (i.e., celiac ganglion). *(Courtesy College of Veterinary Medicine, University of Illinois.)*

be a primary myopathy), German shepherds (giant axonal neuropathy), and Dalmatians. They may have a genetic basis and be inherited.

Gross lesions in the PNS are inapparent; however, microscopically, depending on the breed involved, spheroids can be found in cranial and spinal nerves and brain stem nuclei. Affected animals are usually young (birth to 15 months of age) and show signs of ataxia, muscle weakness (paresis and tetraparesis) followed by muscle atrophy, proprioceptive deficits, urinary incontinence, and digestive disturbances (enteric division involvement).

COLONIC AGANGLIOSIS

Colonic agangliosis (lethal white foal syndrome) is a disorder involving development of the enteric division of the PNS and is analogous to Hirschsprung's disease in infants. This disease occurs most commonly in foals of American Paint Horses with Overo markings. Affected foals have white or nearly white skin color. Specific information on these skin marking patterns can be obtained from the American Paint Horse Association. The gene, which results in the "colonic agangliosis" phenotype being expressed, is inherited as a homozygous dominant.

Recently, mutations in the endothelin-B receptor gene have been detected in affected horses and in

some patients with Hirschsprung's disease. Both glial-derived neurotrophic factor (GDNF) and endothelin-3 (ET-3) are required for normal development of the enteric nervous system and enteric ganglia. It is proposed that GDNF is required for proliferation and differentiation of neuronal precursor cells destined to populate the gut. ET-3 might modulate these effects by inhibiting differentiation, thus allowing sufficient time for precursor cells to migrate and populate the intestinal wall in a cranial to caudal progression before they differentiate to form enteric ganglia.

There are no gross lesions in the intestine related to the enteric division of the PNS. Microscopically the myenteric and submucosal enteric ganglia are absent and the areas affected vary but can extend anywhere between the ileum and distal large colon. Affected foals die soon after birth from functional blockage of the ileum and/or colon because of the lack of innervation and thus normal gut motility.

HYPOMYELINATION/DYSMYELINATION DISEASES

In contrast to the CNS, congenital and postnatal disorders of myelin formation are rare in the PNS but have been described in dogs, calves, and a cat. These disorders are thought to have a genetic predisposition and to be inherited. In dogs, hypomyelination has been described in golden retrievers with onset at approximately 7 weeks of age. Clinical signs include a peculiar hopping gait, depressed spinal reflexes, and circumduction of the limbs while walking. Lesions in peripheral nerves include thin myelin sheaths, increased numbers of Schwann cells, neurolemma cells with abnormally increased cytoplasmic volume, and no evidence of active demyelination or effective remyelination. The lesions are believed to involve a defect in Schwann cells or an abnormal axon–Schwann cell interaction.

In calves a myelinopathic peripheral neuropathy has been described in Santa Gertrudis-Brahman crossbreeds. Microscopically, lesions were present in the vagus nerves, somatic peripheral nerves of the brachial plexuses, and the sciatic nerves. Dorsal and ventral spinal nerve roots also had similar lesions. There was "sausage-shaped" thickening of the myelin sheaths as a result of excess myelin arranged about the axons or as irregularly folded myelin sheaths not surrounding axons. Onset of clinical signs was at 6 to 10 months of age. Clinical signs were dysphagia, abnormal rumination with bloat, and a weak shuffling gait. Congenital hypomyelination has also been described in a 2-month-old Dorsett lamb with tremors and incoordination.

DEMYELINATION DISEASES

A variety of injuries similar to those described in the CNS can cause primary demyelination in the PNS.

Specific demyelinating diseases are covered in the following section. In response to injury, Schwann cells can proliferate to restore the myelin sheaths, often forming longitudinal columns along the course of a degenerated axon termed cell bands of Büngner. Remyelination results in internodes that are shorter than the internodes of adjacent normal myelinated axons, and this change is used microscopically to detect areas of remyelination in peripheral nerves. Another lesion that occurs with repeated episodes of demyelination is proliferation of Schwann cell processes forming concentric whirls, called onion bulbs, that surround the axon.

ACUTE IDIOPATHIC POLYNEURITIS

Acute idiopathic polyneuritis (coonhound paralysis) is an acute, fulminating polyradiculoneuritis with ascending paralysis that occurs in dogs after the bite or scratch of a raccoon. By definition, *polyradiculitis* refers to disease or injury involving multiple cranial or spinal nerve roots, whereas *polyradiculoneuritis* refers to disease or injury involving multiple cranial or spinal nerve roots and their corresponding peripheral nerves.

Coonhound paralysis has been compared with Guillain-Barré syndrome. This human syndrome typically follows a viral illness, vaccination, or some other antecedent disease that results in an autoimmune response resulting in primary demyelination of cranial and spinal rootlets and nerves and delayed conduction of action potentials down the axon. Humoral and cell-mediated components are suspected to be involved in the autoimmune response.

Coonhound paralysis, like Guillain-Barré syndrome, is believed to represent an autoimmune primary demyelination. Despite the lack of close association of macrophages with the degenerating myelin and axons early in the development of the lesions, secretion of TNF-α by these cells could explain both the demyelination and axonal degeneration.

Acute idiopathic polyneuritis has been reported in dogs without an association with raccoons and also occurs rarely in cats, suggesting multiple factors might be involved in this type of nerve damage. Lesions in coonhound paralysis are most severe in ventral spinal nerve rootlets and progressively diminish distally in the peripheral nerve. Involvement of dorsal spinal nerve rootlets and ganglia is not constant and relatively minor. Lesions in the ventral nerve rootlets consist of segmental demyelination with a variable influx of neutrophils, depending on the acuteness and severity of clinical signs, along with lymphocytes, plasma cells, and macrophages (Fig. 14-114). Axonal degeneration is a common sequela. Evidence of remyelination with cell bands of Büngner and axonal sprouting occur during the recovery phase, but the effectiveness of the latter to

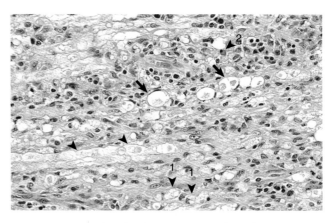

Fig. 14-114   Polyradiculoneuritis, coonhound paralysis, peripheral nerve, dog. This disease is thought to result from an autoimmune response leading to primary demyelination of cranial and spinal rootlets and nerves. Myelin sheaths in this peripheral nerve are distended and fragmented along their length (*arrowheads*) and have been infiltrated by a mixed population of inflammatory cells consisting of lymphocytes, macrophages (*1*), and plasma cells (*2*). Enlarged spaces in the myelin sheath, termed digestion chambers (*arrows*), which form in response to inflammatory and degradative processes, contain myelin debris and macrophages (not shown in this example). Axonal degeneration can occur secondary to primary demyelination. H&E stain. (*Courtesy Drs. R.M. Doty, J.J. Andrews, and J.F. Zachary, College of Veterinary Medicine, University of Illinois.*)

establish continuity of the nerve rootlet and thus reinnervation of muscle is limited.

A chronic polyradiculoneuritis with infiltrations of lymphocytes, plasma cells, or macrophages; demyelination; and variable axonal degeneration in cranial and spinal nerve rootlets and cranial nerves is also reported in dogs and cats. With repeated episodes of demyelination, onion bulbs can be apparent. Both sensory and motor nerves can be involved with sensory disturbances and muscle atrophy.

Clinically, affected dogs have signs of coonhound paralysis develop 1 to 2 weeks after exposure to raccoon saliva. Initial signs of hyperesthesia, weakness, and ataxia are replaced in 1 to 2 days by tetraparesis and/or tetraparalysis that may last from weeks to months. Dogs can die from respiratory paralysis. Recovery is common, but can be prolonged in dogs with extensive muscular atrophy.

CANINE INHERITED HYPERTROPHIC POLYNEUROPATHY

Canine inherited hypertrophic polyneuropathy is a familial disorder in Tibetan mastiffs. The primary defect is in the Schwann cells, but the pathogenesis is undetermined. There are no gross lesions in the PNS. Microscopic lesions consist of demyelination with onion bulb formation. The Schwann cell's cytoplasm is distended by accumulations of actin filaments. Axonal degeneration occurs but is mild. Clinical signs in canine inherited hypertrophic polyneuropathy begin at 7 to 10 weeks of age. They include pelvic limb muscle weakness, depressed spinal reflexes, and muscle atrophy that later progress to involve forelimbs and eventually cause recumbency. Neuropathies with primary developmental demyelination have also been reported in Alaskan malamutes and in beagle-basset hound crosses. A hypertrophic polyneuropathy has rarely been reported in unrelated domestic cats with onset at approximately 1 year of age.

COYOTILLOSIS

Another cause of primary demyelination is the shrub coyotillo (*Karwinskia humboldtiana*) affecting mainly small ruminants in the semidesert areas of the southwest United States. Seeds in the fruit contain polyphenolic compounds that when ingested are toxic. Four toxic compounds have been isolated, including a substance called karwinol A that induces primary demyelination of peripheral nerves.

DYSAUTONOMIAS
HEREDITARY DYSAUTONOMIAS

Dysautonomia is a degeneration of neurons in the ganglia of the enteric division of the PNS that has been reported in dogs, cats (Key-Gaskell syndrome), a llama, sheep, and horses. The cause is unknown, and a hereditary basis is suspected in some cases. A toxic cause has been postulated in the cat. Lesions recently reported in sheep with abomasal emptying defect resemble those reported in dysautonomic diseases of humans and other animals.

Lesions are observed in peripheral and enteric (autonomic) ganglia and vary from neuronal chromatolysis and nuclear pyknosis in more acute cases to loss of neurons and proliferation of satellite cells in cases with longer duration (Fig. 14-115). Minimal to mild leukocytic infiltrates occur, but the lesions are not overtly inflammatory in nature. In cats and dogs, clinical signs are varied and include gastrointestinal disturbances, urinary incontinence, mydriasis, unresponsive pupils, bradycardia, and other signs associated with autonomic dysfunction.

ACQUIRED DYSAUTONOMIAS
Equine grass sickness (equine dysautonomia)

Equine dysautonomia has been suggested to be caused by ingestion of botulinum toxin–contaminated feeds principally affecting postganglionic sympathetic and parasympathetic neurons. Brain stem cranial nerve nuclei have neuronal chromatolysis followed by degeneration and loss of lower motor neurons of the

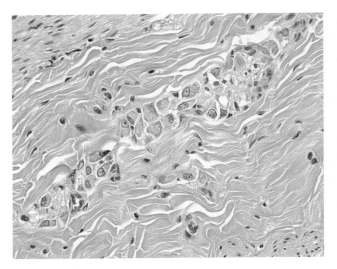

Fig. 14-115 Dysautonomia, submucosal (Auerbach's) plexus, dog. Neuronal central chromatolysis, nuclear pyknosis, and loss of neurons are the characteristic histologic features of enteric dysautonomia reported in dogs, cats, a llama, and horses. *(Courtesy Drs. J.F. Zachary and K. Bailey, College of Veterinary Medicine, University of Illinois.)*

general visceral efferent nuclei of cranial nerves III and X and the general somatic efferent nuclei of cranial nerves III, V, VII, and XII. It has been suggested that equine dysautonomia should be classified as a multisystem disease. Clinically, injury of neurons results in dysphagia and gut stasis (colic).

Although the cause is unknown, oxidative stress, excitotoxicity, fungal toxins, and changes in weather have been proposed. Pasture grasses stressed by rapid growth or sudden cold weather can have reduced concentrations of antioxidants and increased concentrations of glutamate and aspartate (excitotoxic amino acids) and the neurotoxin malonate. It has been proposed that ingestion of high concentrations of these compounds either directly (excitotoxicity-apoptotic cell death) or indirectly (nitric oxide toxicity) induces neuronal injury within the ANS, resulting in alimentary system dysfunction. Because mycotoxins were suspected as a cause of equine grass sickness, studies conducted to investigate this hypothesis demonstrated six species of fungi in pastures from confirmed cases of grass sickness. The significance of these fungi in the pathogenesis of grass sickness is unclear. The similarity between neural lesions induced by *Clostridium botulinum* group III toxins and those in equine dysautonomia has been noted, but the role of such toxins in the disease remains unproven. A recent case report suggests that equine dysautonomia is caused by ingesting grass blades contaminated with botulinum neurotoxin; thus clinically, equine grass sickness has been referred to as a form of botulism.

There are no gross lesions in the PNS, except potentially for lesions related to paralytic ileus; however, microscopically and principally in the small intestine (ileum), the cell bodies of neurons in ganglia of the autonomic and enteric divisions of the PNS are chromatolytic, have displaced and pyknotic of nuclei, are swollen and vacuolated, and with time there is neuronal loss and satellite cell proliferation in affected ganglia. Equine dysautonomia affects horses, ponies, and donkeys primarily between the ages of 2 and 7 years old. The disorder occurs principally between the months of April and July. Injury to enteric neurons results clinically in acute to chronic dysphagia and gut stasis (colic). The only way to diagnose equine grass sickness antemortem is by taking a biopsy of the small intestine during surgery.

Peritonitis-induced dysautonomias

Degeneration of autonomic neurons in the myenteric and submucosal ganglion (plexuses) can occur in animals with peritonitis. The degree of neuronal degeneration appears to be related to the severity and type of inflammatory response in the peritoneal cavity and the ability of inflammatory mediators and other potentially toxic molecules to reach the ganglia by diffusion or hematogenously. Degeneration does not appear to progress to neuronal cell death if the peritonitis is resolved. Affected neurons have vesicular nuclei that are 2 to 3 times normal size (Fig. 14-115). Nissl substance is also displaced (central chromatolysis). Nerve fiber bundles are edematous, and supporting cells can be remarkably hyperplastic and compress adjacent supporting stroma.

This lesion is thought to arise from inflammatory cytokine-mediated injury to autonomic neurons, and this may cause alterations of intestinal motility. It appears that the morphologic changes observed in autonomic and enteric neuron cell bodies are reversible with resolution of the peritonitis. Whether the neuronal lesion results from diffusion, hematogenous, or retrograde axonal transport of cytokines to the ganglion from the site of inflammation remains to be proven.

This lesion is likely the cause of paralytic ileus seen with peritonitis.

ENDOCRINE DISEASES

Of the endocrine disorders, hypothyroidism, hyperadrenocorticism, and diabetes mellitus can affect the PNS. The lesions of these neuropathies are not well characterized and can include evidence of primary demyelination, remyelination, and axonal degeneration. Distal portions of the axon are commonly affected. The extent to which demyelination or axonal degeneration is the primary lesion remains to be determined. From a clinical standpoint, it may be difficult to distinguish neurologic signs from those signs attributed to hormonal-influenced injury of myofibers. Clinical signs can be caused by sensory and motor deficits.

NUTRITIONAL DISEASES
VITAMIN A, VITAMIN D, AND RIBOFLAVIN DEFICIENCIES

Nutritional axonopathies are relatively uncommon and are chiefly caused by vitamin A and some of the B vitamin deficiencies. Vitamin A deficiency results indirectly in peripheral neuropathy by affecting bone growth and remodeling. In neonatal calves, the neuropathy is due to narrowing of the optic foramina caused by continued bone deposition with decreased resorption resulting in compression of the optic nerves, Wallerian degeneration, and blindness. B vitamin deficiencies are primarily diseases of pigs and poultry. In pigs, deficiency of pantothenic acid (B-complex vitamin, vitamin B_5) causes a sensory neuropathy with axonal degeneration, demyelination, and chromatolysis and neuron loss in the dorsal root ganglia, resulting in proprioceptive deficits, goose stepping, and dysmetria. The exact sequence of events in pantothenic acid–deficiency neuropathy is controversial because one study in pigs described initial lesions in the axon; whereas a second study described initial lesions in the cell body. Riboflavin deficiency in poultry, named curly toe paralysis, is primarily a demyelinating neuropathy. Peripheral nerves are swollen because of endoneurial edema, and there is subsequent demyelination with mild axonal degeneration.

VITAMIN E DEFICIENCY
Equine motor neuron disease

Equine motor neuron disease (EMND) resembles amyotrophic lateral sclerosis (ALS) in human beings. Because vitamin E concentrations are very low in affected horses, this and other dietary antioxidant deficiencies have been suggested as a possible factor in the mechanism of equine motor neuron disease. Thus dietary factors, especially the long-term absence (>1 year) of green feeds with high vitamin E concentrations, have been implicated in the pathogenesis of the disease. Vitamin E supplementation may be useful in treating this disease if detected and treated early in its course.

Neural injury in EMND involves the cell bodies and axons of lower motor neurons (ventral horn cells, cranial nerves). Microscopically, cell bodies are swollen, have chromatolysis, and contain spheroids. As the disease progresses, the cell bodies become shrunken and degenerate and are removed by neuronophagia. When the cell bodies are lost, the resulting empty neuronal space can be replaced by astrogliosis. The axons of affected lower motor neurons have lesions consistent with Wallerian degeneration.

The injury in lower motor neurons has been attributed to an oxidative stress mechanism because vitamin E is an antioxidant that offsets the harmful effects of free radicals and reactive oxygen species that can cause membrane lipid peroxidation. However, it is not linked to a mutation in the equine Cu/Zn superoxide dismutase gene. This gene regulates the production of the enzyme superoxide dismutase whose function is to convert free radicals and reactive oxygen species (highly toxic to cells) to hydrogen peroxide (much less toxic to cells). The enzyme catalase is used to convert hydrogen peroxide to water and oxygen molecules. The muscle lesion in EMND is atrophy of type I myofibers secondary to loss of type 1 lower motor neurons.

Clinically, EMND is characterized by progressive degeneration and loss of lower motor neurons resulting in muscle atrophy, weight loss, difficulty standing, and muscle fasciculation.

TOXIC DISEASES
CHEMICALS

These diseases are discussed in greater detail in the CNS. Examples of chemical toxins causing distal axonal degeneration are the vinca alkaloids, vincristine and colchicine, both causing disassembly of microtubules and inhibiting axoplasmic flow. Of interest, taxol—an alkaloid from the western yew (Taxus brevifolia)—promotes the assembly of and stabilizes microtubules but also causes an axonopathy. An outbreak of distal polyneuropathy has been reported in cats fed commercial diets contaminated with the ionophore salinomycin, used as a coccidiostatic drug in poultry and growth promoter in cows. There was acute onset of lameness and paralysis affecting the hindlimbs that progressed to the forelimbs. Demyelination of peripheral nerves followed the axonal degeneration. Some toxins seem to cause different patterns of injury in the CNS and PNS. For instance, in the CNS, lead is noted to cause neuronal necrosis, whereas in the PNS, demyelination, preferentially affecting Schwann cells, is prominent in some species.

OTHER TOXIC NEUROPATHIES

A number of toxins can affect the PNS, with or without damage in the CNS. The initial toxic effects can be at the level of the neuron cell body, the axon, or the myelin sheaths. Examples of toxins targeting neuronal cell bodies are organomercurial compounds such as methylmercury and the cancer chemotherapeutic agent doxorubicin. Methylmercury is particularly toxic because it directly alters biochemical reactions. Although methylmercury poisoning can result from ingestion of water or forage contaminated with industrial discharge, in animals the consumption of fish containing excessive concentrations of methylmercury is the most likely source of the toxin. Fish accumulate methylmercury in their muscle as a result of a "normal" environmental process called biomethylation. Biomethylation converts elemental mercury to methylmercury, which is ingested in the diet of fish. In mercury poisoning, sensory neuron cell bodies of the dorsal root ganglion are preferentially involved and the motor neurons are spared; whereas with doxorubicin, both dorsal root ganglion and autonomic cell bodies are affected. Experimental studies suggest that neuronal cell death is caused by apoptosis of neuronal cell bodies resulting in axonal and Wallerian degeneration.

NEUROMUSCULAR JUNCTION DISEASES
MYASTHENIA GRAVIS

Myasthenia gravis is a disorder of neuromuscular impulse transmission at myoneural junctions and results in flaccid paralysis of skeletal muscle. The disease can be caused by an autoimmune mechanism (acquired) or result from inherited genetic abnormalities (congenital). In autoimmune myasthenia gravis, the antibody binds to acetylcholine receptors (type II hypersensitivity) on postsynaptic muscle membranes. This interaction results in distortion of receptors and blocks binding of the receptors with acetylcholine. Acquired myasthenia gravis often occurs concurrently with thymic abnormalities, such as thymoma and thymic hyperplasia. Because the thymus is responsible for immunologic self-tolerance, thymic abnormalities leading to induced alterations in tolerance have been suggested as the mechanism for developing an antibody response against acetylcholine receptors.

Congenital myasthenia gravis is caused by a genetically determined deficiency in the number of acetylcholine receptors expressed in motor end plates.

There are no gross or microscopic lesions in the PNS or CNS caused by myasthenia gravis. Clinical signs and lesions are due to impairment of skeletal and esophageal muscles, and muscle weakness followed by muscle atrophy.

DISEASES CAUSED BY MICROBES
BACTERIA
BOTULISM

Botulism is characterized by a flaccid paralysis caused by the neurotoxin of Clostridium botulinum type A, B, or C in North America and D in South Africa. The bacterium is a ubiquitous gram-positive spore-forming anaerobe commonly found in soil. This disease most commonly occurs in horses in North America and cows in South Africa. Different forms of botulism affect foals and adult horses. Toxicoinfectious botulism occurs in foals. Foals contract the disease by ingesting soil contaminated with clostridial spores. In past years, spores were thought to vegetate, replicate, and produce toxin in gastric or duodenal ulcers induced by stress or steroids and nonsteroidal antiinflammatory drugs passed in mares' milk. However, recent retrospective studies suggest that gastric or duodenal ulcers are not involved in the pathogenesis of toxicoinfectious botulism in foals. Currently the site of bacterial colonization and toxicoinfection in foals is unknown. In human infants the large intestine is thought to be the site of colonization and toxicoinfection.

In adult horses, poisoning following ingestion of toxin-contaminated forage and less commonly wound botulism occur. Adult horses contract the disease principally through the ingestion of preformed toxin in contaminated feeds, usually haylage that is prepared and stored improperly. Less commonly, adult horses contract the disease through tissue injury and an anaerobic environment, such as hoof abscesses and skin wounds. Spores of *Clostridium botulinum* are either carried into wounds by nails or other contaminated foreign objects or into gastric ulcers by ingestion of contaminated soil. In either case the spores will germinate only in necrotic tissue that has an anaerobic environment. The bacteria replicate and produce exotoxin, which is absorbed through the capillary endothelium and enters the blood stream. In adult horses that ingest contaminated feeds, the toxin is absorbed from the alimentary system and enters the blood stream.

Other than the wound where the bacteria replicates, the toxin of *Clostridium botulinum* causes no macroscopic and microscopic tissue lesions. Once botulinum toxin is in the blood stream, it enters myoneural junctions and binds to receptors on presynaptic terminals of peripheral cholinergic synapses. The toxin is then internalized into vesicles, translocated to the cytosol, and then mediates the proteolysis of components of the calcium-induced exocytosis apparatus, thus interfering with acetylcholine release. Inhibition (blockage) of the release of acetylcholine results in flaccid paralysis of muscles innervated by cholinergic cranial and spinal nerves, but there is no impairment of adrenergic or sensory nerves.

Clinically, affected horses have progressive paralysis of the muscles of the limbs, mandible, larynx/pharynx, upper eyelid, tongue, and tail. Death is usually caused by flaccid paralysis of the diaphragm resulting in respiratory failure. Blockage of acetylcholine release at presynaptic cholinergic terminals is permanent. Improvement occurs only when axons develop (sprout) new terminals to replace those damaged by botulinum toxin.

VIRUSES AND PROTOZOA

Inflammation of the PNS can occur in conjunction with viruses, such as herpesvirus and rabies. Neuritis of the cauda equine in horses and dogs is primarily an inflammatory disorder with secondary demyelination.

This neuritis could have an immune-mediated basis, and adenovirus type 1 has been isolated from affected horses, suggesting a previous viral infection. Polyradiculoneuritis and to a lesser extent ganglionitis occur in toxoplasmosis and neosporosis. The vomiting in pigs infected with hemagglutinating encephalomyelitis virus of pigs is presumed to result from altered function of the vagal nucleus and its ganglion and gastric intramural autonomic plexuses.

LYSOSOMAL STORAGE DISEASES
GLOBOID CELL LEUKODYSTROPHY

Peripheral nerves are also affected in globoid cell leukodystrophy and lesions are typified by primary demyelination followed by axonal degeneration. Small sensory branches of peripheral nerves are useful sites for biopsies to make the diagnoses (Fig. 14-116). Gross lesions are not evident; however, microscopically, such areas have pronounced loss of myelin and abundant globoid cells (activated blood monocytes).

TRAUMATIC INJURY

Trauma to peripheral nerves (lower motor or sensory) is relatively common in animals and can result from lacerations, violent stretching and tearing, or compression or contusion. Reaction patterns following PNS injury are analogous to those in the CNS, but peripheral nerves have a greater capacity for repair.

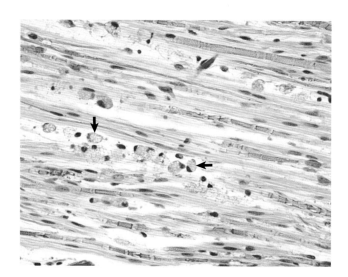

Fig. 14-116   Globoid cell leukodystrophy, small branch of a peripheral sensory nerve, dog. Primary demyelination, secondary axonal degeneration, and globoid cells *(arrows)* between the nerve fibers. Also see Figs. 14-92 through 14-94. **H&E stain.** *(Courtesy Dr. J.F. Zachary, College of Veterinary Medicine, University of Illinois.)*

Three patterns of lesions in the PNS have been described. Mild injury that leaves the axon intact (neuropraxia) can result in temporary conduction block, but total recovery of function is possible. More severe damage that destroys the axon but leaves the connective tissue framework intact (axonotmesis) results in Wallerian degeneration distal to the point of injury, but the potential for regeneration and reinnervation is good. Finally, severance of the nerve with destruction of the supporting framework (neurotmesis) results in Wallerian degeneration distal to the injury with the potential for regeneration but little chance of normal reinnervation. Destruction of the supporting framework results in fibrosis between the proximal and distal ends of the nerve and this gap may be large depending on the severity of the injury. Fibrous tissue can obstruct the regenerating proximal axon from reaching the distal supporting framework of the axon. If the regenerative response is exuberant but unproductive, a "potentially" palpable bulbouslike growth can form at the severed stump of the proximal axon called a "neuroma." The pattern of Wallerian degeneration and the reaction of the neuronal cell body to damage of its axon have been described in an earlier section.

RECURRENT LARYNGEAL NERVE PARALYSIS

Laryngeal paralysis (roarer syndrome) is caused by axonal injury to the left recurrent laryngeal nerve, which results in atrophy of the left dorsal, lateral, and transverse cricoarytenoid muscles and consequently dysfunction of the larynx and laryngeal folds. The cricoarytenoid dorsalis muscle is the main abductor muscle of the larynx, which keeps the arytenoid cartilages in a lateral position. The cause of this axonopathy is unknown, and there may be different causes for different age groups of animals and different forms of the disease. Known causes include: (1) transection of the axon by extension of inflammation from the guttural pouches because the nerve runs through the pouch within a connective tissue fold and (2) other trauma to the nerve. There is also some evidence that laryngeal paralysis may be inherited in younger horses. Currently a genetic age-onset abnormality of axoplasmic flow appears to be the most likely cause in horses in which trauma and inflammation can be excluded as causes.

Affected horses have disabilities of performance and a characteristic and diagnostic "roaring" sound with inspiration. Laryngeal hemiplegia can affect the right or left dorsal cricoarytenoid muscles; however, 95% of cases involve the left side. The cause of this specificity is unclear. Some have suggested it is related to the long course of the left recurrent laryngeal, which extends down into the chest and loops under the arch of the aorta to return to the larynx, but this hypothesis is weakened by the fact that the axonal injury is distal to where the nerve innervates the larynx.

Gross lesions can vary from being recognizable to being inapparent. Microscopically the lesion is Wallerian degeneration. Laryngeal hemiparesis is primarily a disease of large horse breeds between the ages 2 and 7 years old.

NEUROGENIC CARDIOMYOPATHY (BRAIN-HEART SYNDROME)

Neurogenic cardiomyopathy is a syndrome in dogs characterized by unexpected death 5 to 10 days after diffuse CNS injury (usually hit by car). Affected dogs die of cardiac arrhythmias caused by myocardial degeneration. Grossly the myocardium has numerous discrete and coalescing pale white streaks and/or poorly defined areas of necrosis. Neurogenic cardiomyopathy is thought to be caused by overstimulation of the heart by autonomic neurotransmitters and systemic catecholamines released at the time of trauma. It is unknown why there is a 5- to 10-day delay in the development of myocardial necrosis.

NEUROGENIC SHOCK

Neurogenic shock is caused by an alteration in the function of the ANS and its regulation of muscle tone in systemic blood vascular beds (Fig. 14-117). The onset of neurogenic shock usually coincides with traumatic injury to the CNS; however, the factors that determine whether it occurs are poorly understood. It is thought to be caused by massive discharge of the ANS. Following trauma, there is immediate vasoconstriction of vascular smooth muscle. Vasoconstriction is shortly followed by vasodilatation, expanded circulatory volume, and a reduction in blood pressure leading to shock. Brain-heart syndrome in veterinary medicine is likely a manifestation of neurogenic shock and vasoconstriction of arterioles leading to myocardial necrosis.

TUMORS

The objective of this section is to not be all encompassing regarding neoplasms of the peripheral nervous system, but to review one of the best-known examples of how neoplasia can involve this system. Terminology used for neoplasms considered to be of nerve origin in animals is quite confusing. For example, the terms *schwannoma*, *neurofibroma*, and *neurilemmoma* have all been used at various times by different pathologists to identify the same neoplasm. More recently, it has been accepted that the classification of such tumors in veterinary pathology is somewhat arbitrary; therefore these tumors have been simply grouped as benign or malignant peripheral nerve sheath tumors. Malignant tumors show more anaplastic cytoarchitectural features

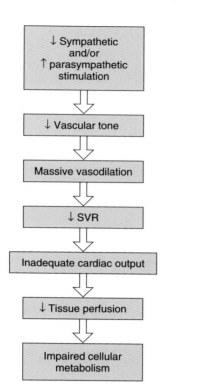

Fig. 14-117   Pathophysiologic mechanism of neurogenic shock. SVR, Systemic vascular resistance. *(From Huether SE, McCance KL: Understanding pathophysiology, ed 2, St Louis, 2000, Mosby.)*

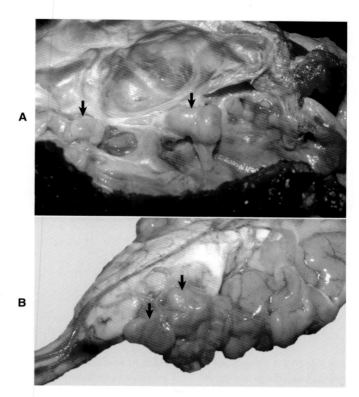

Fig. 14-118   Peripheral nerve sheath tumors. A, Inner surface of the cranial vault, cranial nerves, dog. These tumors are usually lobulated, well-defined, tan, solitary to multiple masses that arise from the coverings of a cranial or spinal nerve *(arrows).* In the central nervous system, the trigeminal nerve is usually affected, and the masseter and temporalis muscles innervated by them may atrophy. Tumors compress the nerves causing Wallerian degeneration. **B,** Brain from dog in Fig. 14-118, A. Peripheral nerve sheath tumors *(arrows).* *(**A** and **B,** Courtesy Dr. J.F. Zachary, College of Veterinary Medicine, University of Illinois.)*

and aggressive growth into adjacent normal tissue. Peripheral nerve sheath tumors occur in both cranial (Fig. 14-118) and spinal nerves (Fig. 14-119) of the PNS. Currently, there are no reliable immunohistochemical markers for these tumors.

Schwannomas of animals have been best recognized in the canine and bovine species, and less commonly in the cat. In the dog, the neoplasm most commonly affects the cranial (fifth) or spinal nerve roots (posterior cervical-anterior thoracic roots of the brachial plexus and their extensions and roots at the thoracic and lumbar levels). Although schwannomas of the skin have been reported, there should always be careful consideration of other neoplasms, such as hemangiopericytoma and fibromas, that can have similar morphologic features. The bovine neoplasm occurs most commonly in mature animals, although the lesion has also been reported in young calves and involves the cranial eighth nerve, brachial plexus, and intercostal nerves. Additionally, autonomic nerves of the liver, heart, mediastinum, and thorax can be affected. The skin can be infrequently involved.

Grossly, schwannomas are nodular or varicose thickenings along nerve trunks, or nerve roots. They can be firm or soft (gelatinous) and white or gray.

Schwannomas of the spinal cord nerve roots can remain inside the dura mater or extend through the vertebral foramina to the exterior.

The main microscopic characteristics described for the human being are also applicable for schwannomas of animals. In human beings, the schwannoma is characterized by having two morphologic features, known as Antoni A and B tissue, and occurs in variable proportions within the neoplasm. Antoni A tissue is cellular and consists of monomorphic spindle-shaped Schwann cells. These cells have poorly defined eosinophilic cytoplasm and pointed basophilic nuclei, and are present in a collagenous stroma of variable extent. The nuclei of these cells are commonly arranged in rows, between which are parallel arrays (stacks) of their cytoplasmic processes, and this arrangement is called a Verocay body. Antoni B areas

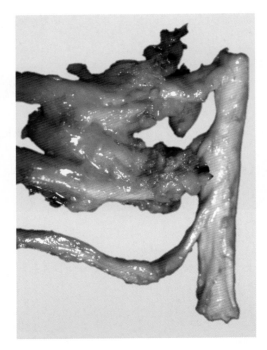

Fig. 14-119   Peripheral nerve sheath tumor, spinal nerve, cow. These tumors are similar to those described in Fig. 14-118 and occur most commonly in cows and dogs. The terms schwannoma, neurofibroma, and neurilemmoma have been used by different pathologists to identify the same neoplasm. Although schwannoma has been proposed as the best term to classify these tumors, the term *peripheral nerve sheath tumor* groups all morphologic diagnoses under a common umbrella. *(Courtesy College of Veterinary Medicine, University of Illinois.)*

are also composed of Schwann cells, but their cytoplasm is inconspicuous and their nuclei appear to be suspended in a copious myxoid, often microcystic, matrix. Also, Schwannomas do not typically contain nerve fibers.

Schwannomas are differentiated from neurofibromas, which consist of Schwann cells, perineurial cells, and fibroblasts. Some microscopic features of the neurofibroma include elongated spindle cells with poorly defined pale eosinophilic, tapering wavy or buckled nuclei, and numerous small nerve fibers (that are not present in schwannomas). Presence of mast cells is also reported. These neoplastic components are situated in a variably prominent fibromyxoid to myxoid matrix (myxoid neurofibroma), although another variant of the neoplasm contains prominent collagen (collagenous neurofibroma).

SUGGESTED READINGS

Appel MJG, Summers BA: Pathogenicity of morbilliviruses for terrestrial carnivores, *Vet Microbiol* 44:187-191, 1995.

Barron KD: Microglia: history, cytology, and reactions, *J Neurol Sci* 207:98, 2003.

Chen Y, Swanson RA: Astrocytes and brain injury, *J Cereb Blood Flow Metab* 23:137-149, 2003.

Cottrell DF, McGorum BC, Pearson GT: The neurology and enterology of equine grass sickness: a review of basic mechanisms, *Neurogastroenterol Motil* 11:79-92, 1999.

Dubey JP, Lindsay DS, Saville WJ et al: A review of *Sarcocystis neurona* and equine protozoal myeloencephalitis (EPM), *Vet Parasitol* 95:89-131, 2001.

Fenner F, Gibbs EP, Murphy FA et al: *Veterinary virology*, New York, 1993, Academic Press.

Gurgo RD, Bedi KS, Nurcombe V: Current concepts in central nervous system regeneration, *J Clin Neurosci* 9:613-617, 2002.

Hadlow WJ, Kennedy RC, Race RE: Natural infection of Suffolk sheep with scrapie virus, *J Infect Dis* 146:657-664, 1982.

Hanisch UK: Microglia as a source and target of cytokines, *Glia* 40:140-155, 2002.

Harkin KR, Andrews GA, Nietfeld JC: Dysautonomia in dogs: 65 cases (1993-2000), *J Am Vet Med Assoc* 220:633-639, 2002.

Jackson AC: Rabies pathogenesis, *J Neurovirol* 8:267-269, 2002.

Jolly RD, Walkley SU: Lysosomal storage diseases of animals: an essay in comparative pathology, *Vet Pathol* 34:527-548, 1997.

Kandel ER, Schwartz JH, Jessell TM, editors: *Principles of neural science*, New York, 2000, McGraw-Hill.

Kierszenbaum AL: *Histology and cell biology: an introduction to pathology*, St Louis, 2002, Mosby.

Lacbawan FL, Muenke M: Central nervous system embryogenesis and its failures, *Pediatr Dev Pathol* 5:425-447, 2002.

Meuten DJ: *Tumors in domestic animals*, ed 4, Ames, 2002, Iowa State Press.

Montgomery DL: Astrocytes: form, functions, and roles in disease, *Vet Pathol* 31:145-167, 1994.

Montgomery DL, Storts RW: Hereditary striatonigral and cerebello-olivary degeneration of the Kerry blue terrier. I. Gross and light microscopic central nervous system lesions, *Vet Pathol* 20:143-159, 1983.

Nelson PT, Soma LA, Lavi E: Microglia in diseases of the central nervous system, *Ann Med* 34:491-500, 2002.

Oliver JE, Lorenz MD, Kornegay JN: *Handbook of veterinary neurology*, ed 3, Philadelphia, 1997, Saunders.

Parent A: *Carpenter's human neuroanatomy*, Baltimore, 1996, Williams & Wilkins.

Prusiner SB: *Prion biology and diseases*, ed 2, Cold Spring Harbor, NY, 2004, Cold Spring Harbor Laboratory Press.

Spencer PS, Schaumburg HH, Ludolph AC: *Experimental and clinical neurotoxicology*, ed 2, New York, 2000, Oxford University Press.

Squire LR, Bloom FE, McConnell SK et al: *Fundamental neuroscience*, ed 2, San Diego, 2003, Academic Press.

Summers BA, Cummings JF, de Lahunta A: *Veterinary neuropathology*, St Louis, 1995, Mosby.

Young B, Stevens A, Lowe JS: *Wheater's basic histopathology: a colour atlas and text*, ed 4, Edinburgh, 2002, Churchill Livingstone.

APPENDIX **14-1**

Necropsy

DIFFICULTIES IN THE EXAMINATION OF THE CENTRAL NERVOUS SYSTEM

There are inherent difficulties in performing a satisfactory examination of the central nervous system (CNS) in all animal species, including rapid autolysis and the fact that removal of the brain and spinal cord is very hard work in older, large animals whose bones are very hard. The gross examination of the CNS requires time (30 to 60 minutes) and a reasonable degree of physical strength.

NECROPSY PROCEDURES

The brain can be removed from the calvarium without great difficulty, but experience gained in veterinary school (diagnostic necropsy rotations) does make the process more efficient and helps to preserve the anatomic integrity of the brain. In the cow and other mammals with large frontal sinuses (pig), the task is more difficult. The bone of the calvarium is cut and removed using a handsaw, hatchet, or Stryker saw (electrically powered saw) with a large blade in large animals or a small handsaw, Stryker saw with a small blade, bone rongeurs, or bone cutting forceps in smaller animals. The equipment used is dependent on the thickness of the bone and the experience of the prosector.

The head is usually disarticulated from the body at the occipitoatlantal joint before examination. A midline incision should be cut through the skin over the calvarium from the occipito-atlantal joint to a point midway between the eyes. The skin is reflected laterally to expose the entire calvarium and the masseter, temporalis, and other muscles. These muscles should be dissected free from the calvarium. The bone of the calvarium is cut in a plane extending from the foramen magnum to a point just behind the eye on each lateral side of the calvarium. A single cut is then made in the calvarial bone behind the eyes at right angles to the initial two cuts. This approach results in connecting the planes of all these cuts through the foramen magnum. If the cuts are complete and connected, the calvarium can be pulled free from the head by pulling in a rostral to caudal direction. In animals with frontal sinuses, the same process is essentially repeated twice to expose the brain.

Once the calvarium is removed, the dura mater, if not removed with the calvarium, should be cut along the midline and reflected laterally to expose the surface of the brain. The falx cerebri and tentorium cerebelli must be cut and removed before attempting to remove the brain; otherwise the brain can be torn during removal. The head is turned upside down and, at the foramen magnum, the cranial nerve roots severed in descending numerical order to release the brain from the cranial vault. The force of gravity will pull the brain out of the cavity onto the necropsy table.

The spinal cord can be removed from small and large animals, but the process is labor intensive; without experience and proper equipment, the process is prone to spinal cord damage and risk to the prosector. The vertebral column must be separated from the limbs, ribs, and visceral and thoracic organs. In large animals, the vertebral column is cut transversely into cervical, thoracic, and lumbar segments. Each segment is then cut in a lateral to medial direction on a saggital plane to the depth of the spinal cord on a heavy-duty band saw. When the vertebral canal is reached, the dura mater is longitudinally cut the length of the cord, the spinal nerves are severed, and the spinal cord removed. A similar method can be used in large dogs, but in smaller animals a complete dorsal laminectomy can be performed, and then the above procedure is followed. The anatomic orientation of the spinal cord needs to be maintained for subsequent histopathologic evaluation.

Even light compression of the spinal cord during necropsy will fracture the gray matter. Heavier pressure will squeeze it out like toothpaste. The CNS is very delicate and must be handled carefully. Bone dust from saws can cause confusion in interpretation of the histological sections.

GROSS EXAMINATION BEFORE FIXATION

Once the CNS has been removed from the calvarium and vertebral canal, and before placing the brain and spinal cord in a fixative, they should be carefully examined for any gross abnormalities. The CNS is a symmetric organ with the right and left sides mirroring each other in structural and functional features across an imaginary midline. These sides should be compared for any alterations in size, symmetry, or color. The sulci, gyri, and the meninges should be examined for inflammation and for any changes suggestive of edema. It is not advisable to section an unfixed specimen of brain or spinal cord unless absolutely necessary.

It is also at this time that a decision must be made regarding the saving of specimens for ancillary testing, such as for bacteriology, virology, and toxicology.

The necessity for these tests will be based on the history, findings of the postmortem examination, and probability of a specific disease occurring in the animal. Fresh CNS tissue should be provided for these ancillary tests in quantities sufficient and satisfactory for the requested analysis, but not in a manner that interferes with further macroscopic and microscopic evaluation of the CNS after fixation. Contact your regional diagnostic laboratory for specific information regarding proper sample selection for these ancillary tests and for evaluation of tissues for rabies virus.

FIXATION PROCEDURES

The CNS should be fixed by immersion in 10% neutral-buffered formalin for histopathologic evaluation. Once the CNS is fixed, it should be sliced like a "loaf of bread" from the olfactory bulbs to the cauda equina in approximately 1-cm-thick sections. The cut surfaces of each section should be carefully examined for changes in size, shape, color, and symmetry when compared with the opposite side. Specimens for microscopic evaluation should be taken from any areas that have visible changes and from areas of the CNS that likely would have lesions for diseases listed in the list of differential diagnoses. In addition, all routine microscopic evaluations of the CNS, in which gross lesions are or are not detected should include specimens from the cerebral cortices (two areas), thalamus/hypothalamus, hippocampus, cerebellum and roof nuclei, brain stem (two areas), and the cervicothoracic and thoracolumbar enlargements of the spinal cord.

The spinal cord and peripheral nerve can be fixed by immersion in formalin. Fetal and neonatal brains should be fixed in 20% neutral-buffered formalin. It is best to fix the entire brain without prior sectioning by submerging it in 10% neutral-buffered formalin and then adding 37% formalin until the brain floats in the solution. The brain should not be randomly sliced in the hope of better tissue fixation. These procedures may vary based on the academic institution.

DISEASES CAUSED BY MICROBES

VIRUSES

BORNA DISEASE

Borna disease is an encephalomyelitis caused by an unusual enveloped RNA virus that replicates in the nucleus of neurons, has no cytopathic effect, and until 1997 its virions had not been visualized ultrastructurally. The disease has been recognized in Central Europe for more than 250 years. Borna disease virus has been classified as the prototype of a new virus family, Bornaviridae.

Experimental evidence indicates that infection of the CNS via olfactory nerves can follow intranasal viral exposure. The virus is highly neurotropic, similar to rabies virus, and is transported by retrograde axonal transport from the periphery to the CNS. Infection of astrocytes, oligodendroglia, ependyma, choroid plexus epithelial cells, and Schwann cells occurs by direct extension when these cells are in close proximity to virus-infected neurons. The virus can also infect the retina by retrograde axonal transport via the optic nerve and cause blindness under experimental conditions. After reaching the CNS, the virus spreads intraaxonally and transsynaptically (proposed) as described for rabies virus. The virus can then also spread centrifugally via the peripheral nervous system (PNS), resulting in infection of various nonneural tissues, including the lacrimal and salivary glands, endocrine tissues, such as the pituitary and adrenal glands, and other tissues. It has also been determined that peripheral blood monocytes can be infected. Experimentally the specific lesions that develop in the CNS appear to depend on a viral-induced, cell-mediated immune mechanism. Antibody to Borna disease virus does not appear to play any significant role in the disease process.

There are no major gross lesions in the CNS. Microscopic lesions, which are limited to the nervous system, consist of a nonsuppurative encephalomyelitis with neuronal degeneration. Lesions are confined largely to the gray matter and are most severe in the midbrain, midbrain-diencephalon junction, hypothalamus, and hippocampus. Inflammation of the meninges and spinal cord is generally mild. Small, round to oval, eosinophilic intranuclear inclusions occur in neurons of the brain stem, hippocampus, and cerebrospinal ganglia. In the PNS, inflammation occurs in the cranial, spinal, and autonomic ganglia and in the peripheral nerves.

The natural infection, which tends to occur more frequently in the spring and summer, has a broad host range, having been reported in horses and sheep (the most frequently cited species), but also in cattle, goats, domestic cats (staggering disease in Sweden and Austria), dogs, rodents, rabbits, deer, alpacas, llamas, pygmy hippopotami, sloths, ostriches, nonhuman primates, and human beings. Borna disease virus infection in horses was originally considered to result in a high mortality, up to 80% to 100% following 1 to 3 weeks of clinical illness. More recent evidence indicates that the majority of infected animals are either asymptomatic or have mild clinical disease that can be accompanied by behavioral changes, followed by recovery. The clinically severe disease in the horse is still largely confined to certain regions in Germany and Switzerland; the asymptomatic infection, which probably also occurs in other species including human beings, is considered to have a worldwide distribution.

Proposed peripheral spread of virus by axonal transport in the autonomic and enteric divisions of the PNS has led to the suggestion that infection of these neurons might cause lesions responsible for colic and other gastroenteric dysfunctions in horses.

Borna disease might also be the first infectious agent recognized to be causally significant in human biologic psychiatry. It is known that behavioral alterations can accompany Borna disease infection in animals (e.g., horses, sheep, domestic cats, and nonhuman primates), especially during the early stages, and also in human beings (schizophrenia, unipolar, and bipolar psychiatric disorders particularly). A proposed mechanism for behavioral alterations involves viral protein interference with neurotransmitter function of infected neurons, particularly those located in the limbic lobe of the brain.

CLASSICAL SWINE FEVER

Classical swine fever (hog cholera) of pigs is caused by a pestivirus. It has a worldwide distribution, except for several countries, including the United States, from which it has been successfully eradicated. Infection under natural conditions occurs by the oronasal route. The virus initially infects epithelial cells of the tonsillar crypts and surrounding lymphoid tissue and then spreads to submandibular and pharyngeal lymph nodes where it replicates. The virus disseminates via leukocytic trafficking to the spleen, bone marrow, visceral lymph nodes, and lymphoid tissue of the intestine where high titers of virus are attained. Target cells for virus replication include endothelial cells, lymphoid cells and macrophages, and epithelial cells. Hematogenous spread of the virus via leukocytic trafficking to endothelial cells throughout the infected pig is usually completed in 5 to 6 days. Infected animals die of disseminated intravascular coagulation.

Lesions of the acute disease, which primarily result from a tropism of the virus for vascular endothelium with subsequent hemorrhage, are present in many organs, including the kidneys, intestinal serosa, lymph nodes, spleen, liver, bone marrow, lungs, skin, heart, stomach, gallbladder, and CNS. Grossly, cerebral edema may be observed. Microscopic lesions of the CNS occur in both gray and white matter and tend to be most prominent in the medulla oblongata, pons, colliculi, and thalamus, but also occur in the cerebrum, cerebellum, and spinal cord. Lesions are characterized by swelling, proliferation, and necrosis of endothelium; perivascular lymphocytic cuffing; hemorrhage and thrombosis; microgliosis; and neuronal degeneration. Choroiditis and leptomeningitis also occur. Special histochemical stains may be required to satisfactorily identify elementary bodies in mononuclear inflammatory cells. Clinical signs resulting from involvement of the CNS include ataxia, paresis, and convulsions.

ENTEROVIRUS-INDUCED PORCINE POLIOENCEPHALOMYELITIS

Teschen disease and Talfan disease, the enterovirus encephalomyelitides of pigs, are caused by porcine enteroviruses (family Picornaviridae) are characterized by polioencephalomyelitis. Teschen disease is caused by porcine enterovirus, possibly by serotypes 2 and 3. Natural infection occurs by the oral route and is followed by viral localization and replication in the tonsil, Peyer's patches, and the intestinal tract (primarily ileum, large intestine, and cervical and mesenteric lymph nodes). These viruses then enter the blood stream and spread hematogenously through the blood-brain barrier to the CNS, where they target motor neurons.

No gross lesions are detectable. Cerebral, cerebellar, and spinal cord involvement vary with the different viruses causing the polioencephalomyelitis. All forms of the disease are characterized microscopically by a nonsuppurative polioencephalomyelitis, which targets motor neurons of the ventral gray horns and craniospinal ganglia. These viruses cause degeneration of neurons with acute swelling, central chromatolysis, necrosis, neuronophagia, microgliosis, and axonal degeneration. Neuronal necrosis is accompanied by lymphocytic perivascular cuffs, especially in the spinal cord. Astrocytosis, and particularly astrogliosis, also occur. Ganglioneuritis, particularly of dorsal root ganglia of the spinal cord, and variable leptomeningitis of varying severity also occur.

Clinical signs include ataxia, excessive squealing, altered or lost vocalization, irritability, muscular tremors/rigidity, grinding of the teeth, and convulsions. In the different diseases, severity varies from notable and associated with death of affected animals (Teschen disease occurring sporadically in Europe and Africa) to less severe disease with signs that include fever, diarrhea, and paralysis, sometimes most severe in the hind legs, in pigs in North America and some other regions of the world.

HEMAGGLUTINATING ENCEPHALOMYELITIS VIRAL INFECTION OF PIGS

In 1958 a disease of nursing pigs characterized by high morbidity, vomiting, anorexia, constipation, and severe progressive emaciation was reported in Ontario, Canada. The causal agent was found to be a coronavirus. Infection by the oronasal route, which has been demonstrated experimentally, is followed by viral replication in epithelial cells of the nasal mucosa, tonsils, lungs, and small intestine. After local replication, the virus spreads to the CNS by retrograde axonal transport in the peripheral nerves, which include the trigeminal and olfactory nerves, vagus, and extensions from intestinal plexuses to the spinal cord. Neurons of craniospinal ganglia also are infected. The vomiting associated with the disease is presumed to result from altered function of neurons (in the vagal nucleus and its ganglion, and gastric intramural plexuses in the enteric division of the PNS) secondary to viral infection.

Gross lesions of the CNS are not present. Microscopic lesions occur in the respiratory tract, stomach, and central and peripheral nervous systems. Similar to enterovirus encephalomyelitis, lesions in the CNS are most pronounced in the gray matter and are characterized by a nonsuppurative meningoencephalomyelitis with neuronal degeneration, lymphocytic perivascular cuffs, and microglial nodules. The caudal brain stem, particularly the medulla and pons, and spinal cord are affected. In the peripheral ganglia, the lesions are nonsuppurative inflammation and neuronal degeneration.

Clinically affected animals may show vomiting caused by neuronal lesions in enteric plexuses, depression, hyperaesthesia, trembling, ataxia, convulsions and paddling of the limbs if laterally recumbent.

JAPANESE ENCEPHALITIS

Japanese encephalitis is a particularly important disease in human beings, but infection also occurs in horses, pigs, cattle, and sheep. The causative virus is classified as a member of the family Flaviviridae (closely related to St. Louis encephalitis and West Nile virus) and is transmitted by mosquitoes, mainly *Culex tritaeniorhychnus*. In nature, infection is maintained in a cycle involving vector mosquitoes, birds, and pigs. Although young susceptible pigs can have signs, detectable illness is not a feature of viral infection in adult or pregnant pigs. However, transplacental fetal infection during pregnancy can result in mummification and stillbirth of fetuses, or the birth of weak live pigs with nervous signs accompanied by nonsuppurative encephalitis and neuronal degeneration.

Factors involved in the pathogenesis of this viral infection include the recent finding that in rats the ability of the virus to infect neurons is closely associated with neuronal immaturity. Such an age-dependent susceptibility of brain to viral infection has also been noted with other flaviviruses, including St. Louis encephalitis virus and yellow fever virus. The fact that fetal and neonatal pigs and young horses appear to be more susceptible than adult animals suggests that such a correlation could also exist in naturally occurring infections of animals.

Grossly, CNS lesions include mild leptomeningeal congestion and hyperemia and occasional hemorrhages within the brain and spinal cord. Microscopically, neurons in the CNS are the target cell. Lesions are characterized by an early leptomeningitis and encephalitis in which neutrophils predominate followed by nonsuppurative encephalomyelitis. This virus also causes degeneration of neurons, especially Purkinje cells of the cerebellum, with necrosis, neuronophagia, microgliosis,

and axonal degeneration. Neuronal necrosis is accompanied by lymphocytic perivascular cuffs. There are no inclusion bodies. The lesions are distributed diffusely throughout the nervous system, but affect the gray matter more than the white matter. Well-documented outbreaks of meningoencephalomyelitis caused by Japanese encephalitis virus in horses have been reported. Young or immature horses are more susceptible to infection than older animals. Its geographic distribution includes India, China, and southeastern Asia.

LOUPING ILL

Louping ill, a tick-transmitted sheep encephalomyelitis, has been recognized in the British Isles for at least 200 years. It is primarily a disease of sheep but also affects cattle, horses, pigs, goats, red deer, dogs, human beings, and the red grouse. It is caused by a flavivirus (family Flaviviridae) and occurs in the British Isles and Norway. A similar disease of sheep occurs in Turkey, Greece, Bulgaria, and Spain. Some cases have been determined to be caused by similar flaviviruses but are distinct from each other and from louping ill virus. The disease occurs in the spring and summer when ticks are alive.

Following infection caused by the tick Ixodes ricinus, the virus replicates in lymph nodes and spleen and reenters the blood stream to cause a high-titered viremia, which is the probable route of infection of neurons. Excretion of the virus in milk of infected ewes and goats has also been reported, with the suggestion that transmission by ingestion is of possible significance in suckling kids.

No major gross lesions are present. Microscopic lesions are characterized by a meningoencephalomyelitis, which is primarily nonsuppurative, although occasional neutrophils can be present. Specific changes also include neuronal degeneration, necrosis, and neuronophagia, most consistently occurring in Purkinje cells of the cerebellar cortex but also affecting neurons of the medulla oblongata, pons, and spinal cord. Lesions in Purkinje cells have been proposed to be at least partially responsible for the unique clinical signs of a peculiar leaping gait displayed by affected animals. No inflammation of spinal ganglia occurs, but inflammation has been detected in sciatic nerves.

CHLAMYDIA-INDUCED VASCULOPATHIES
SPORADIC BOVINE ENCEPHALOMYELITIS

Sporadic bovine encephalomyelitis (chlamydial encephalomyelitis) is uncommon and is caused by *Chlamydophila psittaci* (formally named *Chlamydia psittaci*). The disease was first described in the United States, but cases have since occurred in other countries. Chlamydiae are obligate intracellular organisms now classified as bacteria. *Chlamydophila psittaci* is inhaled or ingested via an oronasal route and infects epithelial cells of oronasal mucous membranes and lungs, endothelial cells, and monocytes and lymphocytes. It appears to spread systemically to infect endothelial cells within the CNS via leukocytic trafficking in monocytes and lymphocytes. Lesions are nonsuppurative meningoencephalomyelitis and serofibrinous polyserositis, arthritis, and tenosynovitis. Gross changes in the CNS, when present, are limited to active hyperemia and edema of the leptomeninges. Microscopic lesions extend throughout the neuraxis and consist of leptomeningeal and perivascular infiltrates of lymphocytes, plasma cells, and a few neutrophils. The basilar leptomeninges are most severely affected. Leukocytes extend into the adventitia of blood vessels accompanied by endothelial swelling and necrosis leading to vasculitis, thrombosis, and ischemia. Additional lesions include neuronal degeneration and parenchymal necrosis with microgliosis. Immune-mediated mechanisms have been suggested as the cause of the vasculitis. Calves younger than 6 to 12 months of age are most susceptible. Affected animals initially are ataxic but terminally may become recumbent and opisthotonos develops.

GLOSSARY OF TERMS

Astrocytosis: increased numbers of astrocytes.

Astrogliosis: reactive astrocytic response with increased number (variable), length, and complexity of cell processes. In the CNS, reparative processes following injury, such as inflammation and necrosis, are facilitated by astrogliosis.

Axonopathy, distal, of the PNS: a neuropathy with degeneration of the terminal and preterminal axon of peripheral nerves.

Axonopathy, distal of the CNS and PNS: degeneration of axons involving distal portions of peripheral nerves, and distal portions of long axons in the CNS (spinal cord).

Axonotmesis: axonal injury of a peripheral nerve in which there is degeneration of the part distal to the site of trauma, leaving the supporting framework intact and allowing for improved potential for regeneration and effective reinnervation.

Blood-brain barrier of the CNS: a barrier to free movement of certain substances from cerebral capillaries into CNS tissue. Relies on tight junctions between capillary endothelial cells and selective transport systems in these cells. Endothelial cell basement membrane and foot processes of astrocytes abutting the basement membrane may play role in barrier function.

Blood-CSF barrier of the CNS: a barrier that consists of tight junctions located between epithelial cells of the choroid plexus and the cells of the arachnoid membrane that respectively separate fenestrated blood vessels of the choroid plexus stroma and dura mater from the CSF.

Blood-nerve barrier: a barrier to free movement of certain substances from the blood to the endoneurium of peripheral nerves. Barrier properties are conferred by tight junctions between capillary endothelial cells of the endoneurium and between perineurial cells and selective transport systems in the endothelial cells.

Brain edema: increase in tissue water within the brain that results in an increase in brain volume. The fluid may be present in the intracellular or extracellular compartments or both. The term also is used to include the accumulation of plasma, especially in association with severe injury to the vasculature.

Brain swelling: marked, rapidly developing, sometimes unexplained, increase in cerebral blood volume and brain volume because of relaxation (dilation) of the arterioles that occurs after brain injury.

Büngner, cell bands of: a column of proliferating Schwann cells that forms within the space previously occupied by an axon following Wallerian degeneration. The proliferating column of cells is surrounded by the persisting basement membrane of the original Schwann cells.

Central chromatolysis: dissolution of cytoplasmic Nissl substance (arrays of rough endoplasmic reticulum and polysomes) in the central part of the neuronal cell body that results from injury to the neuron (often involving the axon). The cell body is swollen, and the nucleus frequently is displaced peripherally to the cell membrane. These structural changes functionally represent a response to injury that can be found (if the cell survives) by axonal regeneration with protein synthesis to produce components of the axon required for fast and slow axonal transport.

Cranium bifidum: a dorsal midline cranial defect through which meninges alone or meninges and brain tissue may protrude into a sac (-cele), covered by skin.

Demyelination: a disease process in which demyelination (destruction of the myelin sheath) is the primary lesion, although some degree of axonal injury may occur. Primary demyelination is caused by injury to myelin sheaths and/or myelinating cells and their cell processes. Secondary demyelination occurs with axonal injury, as in Wallerian degeneration.

Dysraphism: dysraphia, which literally means an abnormal seam, refers to a defective closure of the neural tube during development. This defect, which may occur at any point along the neural tube, is exemplified by anencephaly, prosencephalic hypoplasia, cranium bifidum, spina bifida, and myeloschisis.

Encephalitis: inflammation of the brain.

Encephalo-: a combining form that refers to the brain.

Encephalopathy: a degenerative disease process of the brain.

Ganglionitis: Inflammation of peripheral (sensory or autonomic or both) ganglia.

Gemistocyte: reactive, hypertrophied astrocyte that develops in response to injury of the CNS. The cell body and processes of gemistocytes become visible with conventional staining (e.g., H&E stain). The cell bodies and processes of normal astrocytes are not visible with H&E staining.

Gitter cell: macrophage that accumulates in areas of necrosis of CNS tissue. The cytoplasm is typically distended, with abundant lipid-containing material derived from the lipid-rich nervous tissue. Gitter cell nuclei are often displaced peripherally to the cell membrane. These cells are often referred to as "foamy" macrophages.

Hydranencephaly: a large, fluid-filled cavity in the area normally occupied by CNS tissue of the cerebral hemispheres resulting from abnormal development. The nervous tissue may be so reduced in thickness that the meninges form the outer part of a thin-walled sac. The lateral ventricles are variably enlarged because of their expansion into the area normally occupied by tissue.

Hydrocephalus: accumulation of excess CSF resulting from obstruction within the ventricular system (noncommunicating form) associated with enlargement of any or all of the following: lateral ventricles, third ventricle, mesencephalic aqueduct, and fourth ventricle. Hydrocephalus can also occur with communication of the CSF between the ventricular system and the subarachnoid space (communicating form). Hydrocephalus ex vacuo (compensatory hydrocephalus) is characterized by an expansion of the lateral ventricle (or ventricles) that follows loss of brain tissue.

Leuko-: combining form referring to white matter of the brain or spinal cord.

Leukoencephalitis: inflammation of the white matter of the brain.

Macroglia: a collective term referring to astrocytes and oligodendrocytes. Has also been variously used to refer solely to astrocytes or to astrocytes, oligodendrocytes, and ependymal cells of the CNS, and Müller cells of the retina.

Malacia: grossly detectable (macroscopic lesion) softening of CNS tissue, usually the result of necrosis.

Meningo-: combining form referring to meninges.

Meningomyelocele: a form of spina bifida in which meninges and spinal cord herniate through a defect in the vertebral column into a sac (-cele) covered by skin.

Microglia: resident cells of the CNS believed to arise from monocytes that populate the brain during embryonic development.

Motor neuron, lower: large multipolar neurons in the brain stem and ventral horns of the spinal cord with axons extending into the PNS.

Motor neuron, upper: motor neurons with axons residing solely in the CNS that control lower motor neurons.

Myelitis: inflammation of the spinal cord.

Myelo-: combining form referring to spinal cord.

Myelopathy: a degenerative disease process of the spinal cord.

Myeloschisis: similar to spina bifida, except in its severe form is characterized by complete failure of the spinal neural tube to close and, therefore, a lack of development of the entire dorsal vertebral column.

Neuroglial cells: astrocytes, oligodendroglia, ependymal cells, and microglia of the CNS.

Neuronophagia: accumulation of microglial cells around a dead neuron.

Neuropil: the gray matter feltwork that consists of intermingled and interconnected processes of neurons (axons and dendrites) and their synaptic junctions, plus processes of oligodendroglia, astrocytes, and microglia.

Neuropraxia: traumatic injury to a peripheral nerve with temporary conduction block but with no permanent axonal damage.

Neurotmesis: complete transection of a nerve and supporting framework with little potential for normal reinnervation.

Onion bulb: concentric arrays of Schwann cell cytoplasm around an axon signifying multiple episodes of demyelination and remyelination.

Polio-: combining form referring to gray matter of the CNS.

Polioencephalomalacia: softening (usually the result of necrosis) of the gray matter of the brain.

Polioencephalomyelitis: inflammation of the gray matter of the brain and spinal cord.

Poliomyelomalacia: softening (usually the result of necrosis) of the gray matter of the spinal cord.

Porencephaly: a cleft or cystic defect in the cerebral hemisphere that communicates with the subarachnoid space and also may communicate with the ventricular system. The defect may contain CSF.

Radiculoneuritis (polyradiculoneuritis): inflammation of a spinal nerve rootlet (or rootlets).

Rarefaction: reduction in density of CNS tissue that may result from edema, necrosis, etc. This lesion is usually observed microscopically.

Satellitosis: an accumulation of oligodendroglia around neuronal cell bodies. Although this feature can be seen in normal brains, some consider that it may also be associated with neuronal injury.

Sclerosis: literally means induration or hardening and, when used in describing lesions of the CNS, often refers to induration or hardening of the brain or spinal cord resulting from astrogliosis (astrocytic scar formation).

Spina bifida: a dorsal midline defect involving one to several vertebrae of the spinal column caused by failure of the neural tube to close, permitting exposure of the underlying meninges and spinal cord. The lesion may be associated with herniation of meninges alone or meninges and spinal cord tissue into a sac (-cele) covered by skin, or there may be no herniation (spina bifida occulta).

Status spongiosus: an encompassing term meaning the presence of small focal, ovoid to round "clear (unstained or poorly stained [H&E stain])" spaces in the CNS. The lesion can result from several different tissue alterations, which include splitting of the myelin sheath, accumulation of extracellular fluid, swelling of cellular (e.g., astrocytic and neuronal) processes, and axonal injury (Wallerian degeneration) when swollen axons are no longer detectable within distended spaces.

Syringomyelia: a tubular cavitation (syrinx) in the spinal cord that is not lined by ependyma and may extend over several segments.

Wallerian degeneration: degeneration of the distal component of an injured (compressed or severed) axon. Although the term originally referred to injury of axons in the PNS, current usage also includes the CNS. This process also results in functional and structural alterations in the cell body (central chromatolysis) and proximal internode segment of the axon, and in secondary demyelination.

15

Skeletal Muscle

BETH A. VALENTINE • M. DONALD MCGAVIN

INTRODUCTION

Skeletal muscle has many functions in the body. Some obvious and major functions are maintenance of posture and enabling movement, including locomotion. The rhythmic contraction of the respiratory muscles (the intercostal muscles and the diaphragm) is essential for life. In addition, muscles play a major role in whole body homeostasis and are involved in glucose metabolism and maintenance of body temperature. On a purely esthetic level, muscle contributes to pleasing body contours.

The function of skeletal muscle is intimately related to the function of the peripheral nervous system. The physiologic attributes of a muscle fiber—its rate of contraction and type of metabolism (oxidative, anaerobic, or mixed)—are determined not by the muscle cell itself but by the neuron responsible for its innervation, the ventral horn or the brain stem motor neurons (Fig. 15-1). This fact is significant in evaluating histologic changes in muscle fibers. It is possible to divide changes in muscle fibers into two major classes: neuropathic and myopathic.

Neuropathic changes are those that are determined by the effect or the absence of the nerve supply (e.g., atrophy after denervation). The term "myopathy" should be reserved for those muscle diseases in which the primary change takes place in the muscle cell, not in the interstitial tissue and not secondary to effects from the nerve supply. The term "neuromuscular disease" encompasses disorders involving lower motor neurons, peripheral nerves, neuromuscular junctions, and muscles.

NORMAL SKELETAL MUSCLE

Understanding the normal structure and function of muscle, including gross, histologic, biochemical, physiologic, electrophysiologic, and ultrastructural features, is critical to understanding of muscle disease.

STRUCTURE OF MYOFIBERS

Structural and physiologic features of skeletal muscle determine much of its response to injury. Although muscle cells are frequently called muscle fibers or

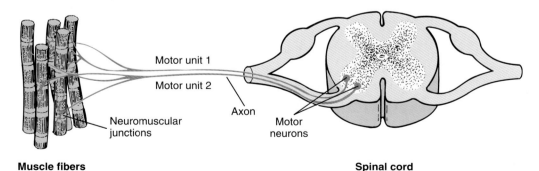

Fig. 15-1 **Schematic diagram of motor units of a muscle.** Each motor unit consists of a motor neuron within the central nervous system and all the myofibers (muscle cells) supplied by the neuron and its axon branches. *(From Huether SE, McCance KL: Understanding pathophysiology, ed 3, St Louis, 2004, Mosby.)*

myofibers, they are in fact multinucleated cells of considerable length, which in some animals may approach 1 meter. Myonuclei are located peripherally in the cylindrical myofiber (Fig. 15-2) and direct the physiologic processes of the cellular constituents in their area through a process known as nuclear domains. This anatomic arrangement allows segments of the cell to react independently of other portions of the cell. Myonuclei are considered terminally differentiated, with little or no capacity for mitosis and thus for regeneration.

Associated with myofibers are the satellite cells, also known as resting myoblasts (Fig. 15-3). These cells are distributed along the length of the myofiber, between the plasma membrane (sarcolemma) and the basal lamina. Satellite cells in skeletal muscle are very different from cells of the same name found within the peripheral

nervous system. Muscle satellite cells are fully capable of dividing, fusing, and reforming mature myofibers. Thus, under favorable conditions, muscle cells (myofibers) are able to fully restore themselves following damage. It is of interest to note that recent studies have found that pluripotent cells derived from bone marrow can also contribute to skeletal muscle repair, albeit only to a very small degree.

Each myofiber is surrounded by a basal lamina and outside of this by the endomysium, a thin layer of connective tissue containing capillaries. Myofibers are organized into fascicles surrounded by the perimysium, a slightly more robust layer of connective tissue (Fig. 15-4). Entire muscles are encased in the epimysium, a protective fascia that merges with the muscle tendon. This connective tissue framework is not inert, but in fact forms an integral part of the contractile function of muscle by storing and relaying force generated by myofiber contraction.

Ultrastructural examination reveals that skeletal muscle is a highly and rigidly organized tissue, with what are perhaps the most highly structured cells in the body. Each myofiber is composed of many closely packed myofibrils containing actin and myosin filaments. The striations visible with light microscopy (Fig. 15-5) represent the sarcomeric arrangement of muscle cells, in which actin and myosin filaments attached to transverse Z bands form the framework, and other organelles and intracytoplasmic materials are interspersed within this framework (Fig. 15-6). The endoplasmic reticulum of myofibers is called the sarcoplasmic reticulum and is modified to contain terminal cisternae that sequester the calcium ions necessary to initiate actin and myosin interaction and thus contraction. Sarcolemmal invaginations that traverse the cell, the T (for transverse)

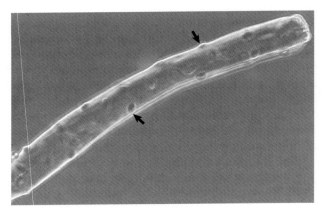

Fig. 15-2   Skeletal muscle, isolated intact myofiber. Note the multiple peripherally located nuclei *(arrows).* Phase contrast microscopy. *(Courtesy Dr. B.A. Valentine, College of Veterinary Medicine, Oregon State University.)*

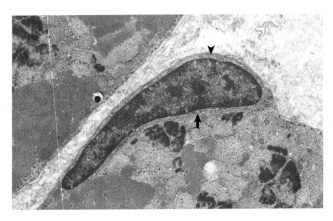

Fig. 15-3   Skeletal muscle myofibers, transverse section. Note the satellite cell (resting myoblast) located between the sarcolemma *(arrow)* and the basal lamina *(arrowhead).* TEM. Uranyl acetate and lead citrate stain. *(Courtesy Dr. B.A. Valentine, College of Veterinary Medicine, Oregon State University.)*

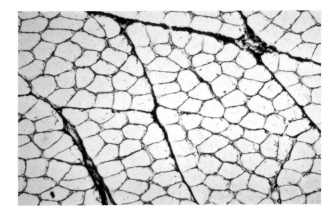

Fig. 15-4   Skeletal muscle, transverse section, normal mammalian muscle. Each myofiber is surrounded by an endomysium of fine collagenous connective tissue. Myofibers are organized into fascicles, which are surrounded by a slightly thicker perimysium. Frozen section, reticulin stain. *(Courtesy Dr. B.A. Valentine, College of Veterinary Medicine, Oregon State University.)*

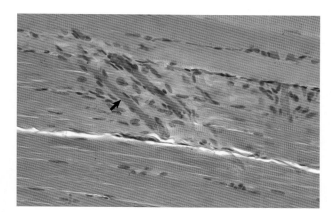

Fig. 15-5   Skeletal muscle, longitudinal section, normal mammalian muscle, cytoarchitectural characteristics. Note the peripherally located myofiber nuclei and cross striations on the muscle fibers. The cross striations correspond to the A bands (*dark lines*) and I bands (*light lines*) in the transmission electron micrograph of Fig. 15-6, *B.* Myofibers are surrounded by an extensive capillary network (*arrow*). Formalin fixation, H&E stain. (*Courtesy Dr. M.D. McGavin, College of Veterinary Medicine, University of Tennessee.*)

tubules, allow for rapid dispersion of a sarcolemmal action potential to all portions of the myofiber. The terminal cisternae of two adjacent sarcomeres and the T tubule form what is called the triad (Fig. 15-6, *A*).

Neuromuscular junctions can only be visualized using electron microscopy or other specialized procedures (Fig. 15-7). Neuromuscular junctions occur only in specific zones within the muscle, usually forming an irregular "band" midway between myofiber origin and insertion.

TYPES OF MYOFIBERS

Mammalian muscles are composed of muscle fibers of different contractile properties. A common classification of these fibers is based on three major physiologic features: (1) rates of contraction (fast or slow), (2) rates of fatigue (fast or slow), and (3) types of metabolism (oxidative, glycolytic, or mixed). These physiologic differences form the basis of histochemical methods that demonstrate fiber types. There are several fiber-type classifications. Classification of fibers into type 1, type 2A, and type 2B (Table 15-1) has proven to have practical application in muscle pathology. It is the classification used in this text. Type 1 fibers are rich in mitochondria, rely heavily on oxidative metabolism, and are slow-contracting and slow-fatiguing. Type 2 fibers have fewer mitochondria and are glycolytic, fast-contracting, and more easily fatigable. In most species, type 2 fibers can be subdivided into type 2A and type 2B. Type 2B fibers are the fast-contracting, fast-fatiguing, glycolytic fibers that depend on glycogen for their

energy supply. Type 2A fibers are mixed oxidative-glycolytic and therefore, although fast-contracting, are also slow-fatiguing. Thus type 2A fibers are "intermediate" in the concentration of mitochondria, fat, and glycogen between type 1 and type 2B.

Most muscles contain both type 1 and type 2 fibers, and these are conveniently demonstrated by the myosin adenosine triphosphatase (ATPase) reaction (Fig. 15-8, *A*). Notice that the different fiber types are normally intermingled, forming what is called a mosaic pattern of fiber types. In most mature muscles, the staining pattern of the ATPase reaction reverses when sections are preincubated in an acid rather than an alkaline solution. There are examples of both patterns in the illustrations in this section. Acid preincubation can also be used to distinguish type 2A and type 2B fibers (Fig. 15-8, *B*). Regenerating fibers, classified as type 2C fibers, stain darkly in both acid and alkaline preparations, which is a distinguishing feature. In most species, oxidative enzyme reactions to demonstrate mitochondria will also demonstrate fiber types to some degree (Fig. 15-9, *A*).

The percentage of each fiber type varies from muscle to muscle (Fig. 15-10). Type 1 fibers (slow-contracting, slow-fatiguing, oxidative) are plentiful in those muscles in which the main function is slow, prolonged activity, such as those that maintain posture. Type 1 predominant postural muscles are most often located deep in the limb. Within the same muscle, the percentage of type 1 fibers often increases in the deeper portions. Muscles that contract quickly and for short periods of time, such as those designed for sprinting, contain more type 2B fibers. Only rarely are muscles composed of only one fiber type (e.g., the ovine vastus intermedius is type 1). Athletic training causes some type 2B fibers to be converted to 2A. There are also variations within breeds and differences in the same muscle in different species. For example, the dog has no type 2B fibers; all canine fibers have strong oxidative capacity (Fig. 15-9, *B*).

INNERVATION AND MOTOR UNITS

The axons of the peripheral nerve trunks contain terminal branches that innervate multiple myofibers. The terminal branches form synapses with the myofibers at the neuromuscular junction. The myofibers innervated by a single axon form a motor unit, all fibers of which will contract simultaneously following stimulation. Different muscles have different sized motor units that relate to their function. For example, extraocular muscle function does not call for forceful contraction, but rather for many fine movements to smoothly move the globe. Therefore, these muscles have very small motor units, with only a small number of myofibers (1 to 4) innervated by each axon. In contrast, the quadriceps muscle is designed, not for fine movement, but for generation of force, and therefore motor units are quite large, with

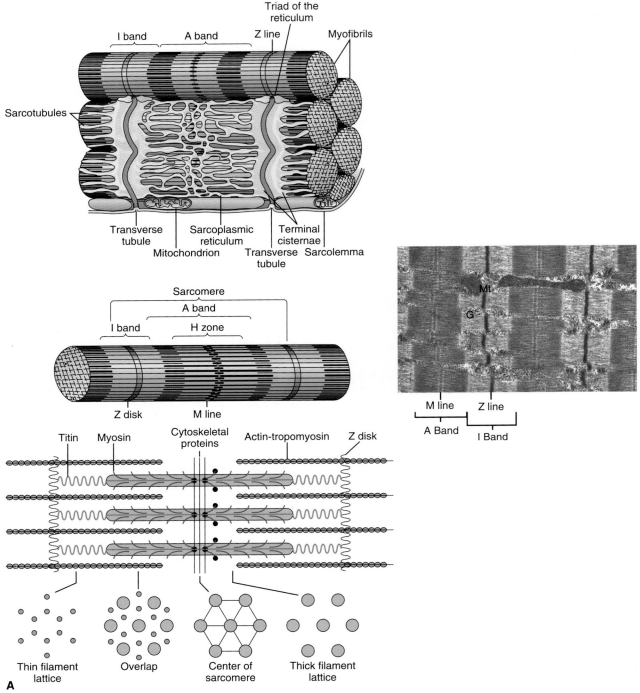

Fig. 15-6 **Myofiber structure. A,** Schematic representation of myofiber orientation, secondary organelles, and ultrastructural arrangement of cytoskeletal proteins within sarcomeres. **B,** Skeletal muscle, longitudinal section, normal mammalian skeletal muscle. Sarcomeres are defined by Z lines, A bands composed of thick myosin filaments, and I bands composed of thin actin filaments. Dense M lines with adjacent clear H zones occur in the center of the A band. Mitochondria *(Mt)* and glycogen *(G)* are interspersed between the myofibrils. TEM. Uranyl acetate and lead citrate stain. (*A,* *From Copstead-Kirkhorn LE, Banasik JL: Pathophysiology: biological and behavioral perspective, ed 3, St Louis, 2005, Saunders. B, Courtesy Dr. B.A. Valentine, College of Veterinary Medicine, Oregon State University.*)

Box **15-1**

Clinical Signs of Muscle Disease

Muscle atrophy
Muscle hypertrophy
Muscle swelling
Weakness
Muscle spasm
Abnormal gait
Esophageal dysfunction (dogs, camelids)

atrophy in a draft horse breed will be more difficult to detect than in a light horse breed.

Weakness can be obvious, as in an animal that is unable to rise or prefers to remain recumbent, or can be manifested primarily as exercise intolerance. Special attention should be paid to gait analysis. The gait of an animal with generalized weakness due to muscle or peripheral nerve dysfunction will have a short stride and often be stiff, and all four legs are often positioned well under the body for support while standing. The abnormal gait of an animal with neuromuscular disease must be distinguished from a similar gait that can occur because of musculoskeletal disease (which is a misnomer, as these disorders affect bone and joint, not muscle). Muscle or peripheral nerve dysfunction in the horse, with this species' unique biomechanics of the pelvic limb, can result in mechanical lameness that can be mistaken for neurologic disease. Odd equine hindlimb gaits designated with such terms as shivers, stringhalt, and fibrotic myopathy are caused by muscle or peripheral nerve disorders. A fibrotic myopathy-like condition also occurs less commonly in the dog and can involve the forelimb. Severe denervating or progressive myopathic conditions that begin in utero or at an early age can cause joint contractures and limb deviation (Fig. 15-48).

Animals with myotonia often exhibit a stiff gait and develop episodic muscle spasms that can lead to collapse. Percussion of muscle groups can cause a persistent muscle contraction known as "dimpling."

In dogs, horses, and ruminants, the esophagus contains a large percentage of skeletal muscle. In dogs and camelids, myopathic, neuropathic, and neuromuscular junction disorders can involve these muscles, causing esophageal dysfunction and megaesophagus. Denervation can also contribute to esophageal dysfunction in cattle with vagal indigestion.

As far as can be determined by clinical evaluation and extrapolation from similar conditions in other species, most neuromuscular disorders in animals are not associated with pain. Muscle cramps, due either to primary myopathy or partial denervation, and muscle swelling are exceptions to this rule.

CLINICOPATHOLOGIC FINDINGS

If the plasma membrane of the myofiber is damaged or a segment of the myofiber becomes necrotic, some of the contents of the muscle cell will "leak out" and be taken up into the blood. The concentrations of some of these components in serum are used as an index of the extent of myofiber damage. The most commonly used is creatine kinase (CK), formerly called creatine phosphokinase (CPK). Aspartate aminotransferase (AST), formerly known as serum glutamic-oxaloacetic transaminase (SGOT), and lactic dehydrogenase (LDH) are also released but are not as specific an indicator of muscle damage because they are also present in other tissues. Because CK has a low renal threshold, it is quickly excreted in the urine. The half-life of circulating CK varies somewhat between species but is generally about 6 to 12 hours. The half-life of AST and LDH in the serum is much longer, and serum AST and LDH concentrations remain elevated for several days following muscle injury. Serum concentration of alanine aminotransferase (ALT) will also increase in all species from severe muscle cell necrosis. Other serum indicators of skeletal muscle injury include carbonic anhydrase III and fatty acid binding protein, but these latter proteins are not part of a routine serum chemistry panel. It has been speculated that the sarcolemma can become "leaky," leading to release of CK and other enzymes, without the affected segment becoming overtly necrotic. This possibility is very hard to prove or disprove.

Although the laboratory testing for CK and AST is relatively standardized, laboratory normal ranges may vary considerably. Determining the normal range of blood values for animals is a difficult task. Normal serum CK concentration in animals is generally less than 500 U/L. Normal serum concentrations of AST, ALT, and LDH vary greatly between species. Tests included in chemistry panels also vary. Some laboratories do not include CK in small animal chemistry panels, which can result in a misdiagnosis of hepatic disease in a dog or cat with a persistent increase in serum AST and ALT concentrations because of degenerative muscle disease. For the purposes of discussion in this chapter, a mild increase in CK or AST is considered to be up to 2 to 3 times normal, a moderate increase is 4 to 10 times normal, and a severe increase is 10 times normal or more.

It should be emphasized that myofibers can be dysfunctional without undergoing necrosis. Myopathic and neuropathic conditions resulting in atrophy, weakness, spasm, stiffness, or myotonia rarely result in significant increase in serum muscle enzyme concentrations. At this time there is no biochemical parameter that will assess muscle fiber function; only muscle fiber integrity can be assessed.

ELECTROMYOGRAPHY

Electromyopathy (EMG) can be a valuable tool when evaluating patients with suspected neuromuscular disease. Concentric needle EMG studies look for abnormal spontaneous activity generated by myofibers. In contrast to other electrodiagnostic studies, a flat line generated by a noncontracting muscle indicates a healthy muscle. Abnormal spontaneous activity includes wave forms designated as positive sharp waves, fibrillations, and myotonic bursts. These abnormal spontaneous electrical events are associated with characteristic sounds emitted by the EMG machine. Abnormal spontaneous activity, typically dense and sustained fibrillations and sharp waves, is generated in denervated muscle because of alteration in sodium channel activity in the membrane of denervated fibers. Spontaneous activity in degenerative myopathies, usually scattered fibrillations, positive sharp waves, and myotonic bursts, is likely related to ionic disturbances associated with fiber degeneration and regeneration; functional denervation following segmental necrosis of the segment containing the neuromuscular junction is also possible. Myotonic conditions result in notably abnormal ionic fluxes leading to waxing and waning of spontaneous potentials with a characteristic "dive bomber" sound. Severe denervating and degenerative disorders, and canine cushingoid myotonia, can be accompanied by myotonic bursts that start and stop abruptly, characteristic of pseudomyotonia.

Nerve conduction velocity studies evaluate the integrity and function of the peripheral nervous system. Primary demyelinating disorders will result in severe reduction of nerve conduction velocity, but axons are intact and muscles are still technically innervated; therefore spontaneous activity does not occur. Repetitive nerve stimulation tests the function of the neuromuscular junctions.

METHODS OF EXAMINATION OF MUSCLE

A variety of examination techniques are often necessary to best appreciate changes occurring in muscle.

GROSS PATHOLOGY AND MUSCLE SAMPLING

Gross examination includes evaluation of changes in size (atrophied, hypertrophied, or normal), color, and texture. The gross pathologic appearance of skeletal muscle can be quite deceiving. What appear to be mild changes in muscle on gross examination often can be severe on microscopic examination, and what appear to be severe changes on gross examination can turn out to be artifact. Subjective evaluation of size can be highly unreliable unless control muscles (e.g., from normal animals or from the opposite sides) are available for weighing and measuring.

Color changes are common. The intensity of the red color of muscle varies depending on the type of muscle, the age and species of animal, and the extent of blood perfusion. Pale muscle can indicate necrosis (Fig. 15-11, A and B; Figs. 15-30, 15-38, A, 15-40, A, and 15-44) or denervation (Fig. 15-11, C; Fig. 15-41), but is also common in young animals and anemic animals. Pale streaking of muscle most often reflects myofiber necrosis and mineralization (Fig. 15-11 A and B) or infiltration by collagen or fat (Fig. 15-11, C and D), and is one of the more reliable indicators of gross pathologic changes. Muscle parasites can be grossly visible as discrete, round to oval, pale and slightly firm zones (Figs. 15-45 and 15-46, A). Dark red mottling of skeletal muscle can indicate congestion, hemorrhage, hemorrhagic necrosis (Figs. 15-36, A and 15-42), inflammation, or myoglobin staining following massive muscle damage (Fig. 15-40, A) or can simply reflect vascular stasis (hypostatic congestion) following death. Hemorrhagic streaks within the diaphragm often accompany death caused by acute exsanguination. A green discoloration can indicate either eosinophilic inflammation (Fig. 15-12) or severe putrefaction. Lipofuscin accumulation in old animals, especially cattle, can cause a tan-brown discoloration of muscle. Black discoloration of the fascia occurs in calves with melanosis as an incidental finding and in older gray horses with metastasis of dermal melanoma to muscle fascia.

Evaluation of texture is also important. Severely thickened and often calcified fascia occurs in cats with fibrodysplasia ossificans progressiva. Fat infiltration or necrosis can result in abnormally soft muscle. Decreased or increased muscle tone can be the result of denervation. Decreased tone can also occur as a result of a lack of muscle conditioning or to postmortem autolysis.

Careful microscopic examination of multiple muscles is often required to detect lesions. In cases of suspected neuromuscular disease, multiple muscle samples should include active muscle (tongue, diaphragm, intercostals, masticatory muscles), proximal muscle (lateral triceps, biceps femoris, semimembranosus, semitendinosus, gluteal), and distal muscle (extensor carpi radialis, cranial tibial). For purposes of a biopsy, certain muscles (e.g., lateral triceps, biceps femoris, cranial tibial, semimembranosus, and semitendinosus) are easier to sample because of their parallel myofiber orientation. The ideal samples will also vary depending on the suspected disorder, such as a type 1 predominant postural muscle for diagnosis of equine motor neuron disease, a type 2 predominant locomotory muscle for diagnosis of equine polysaccharide storage myopathy, and temporal or masseter muscle for diagnosis of masticatory myositis in dogs and masseter myopathy in horses. For physiologic studies in which intact muscle fibers are necessary, and for studies of neuromuscular junction zones, short fibers such as those in the intercostal muscle are preferred.

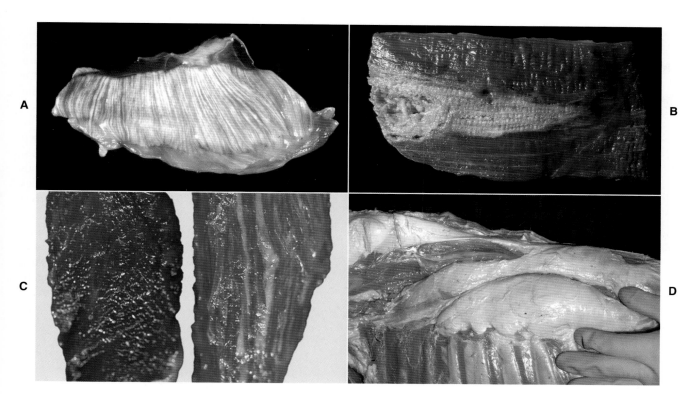

Fig. 15-11   Pathologic changes resulting in pale skeletal muscle. A, Pale streaks, necrosis and mineralization, degenerative myopathy, canine X-linked muscular dystrophy, diaphragm (*left side*), dog. **B,** Localized pallor, necrosis, injection site of an irritant substance, semitendinosus muscle, cow. The irritant was injected just under the perimysium and caused necrosis and disruption of the myofibers. Some irritant seeped down between the fascicles to cause necrosis, but the fascicles of myofibers are still in place. **C,** Overall pale muscle with pale streaks from collagen and fat infiltration, denervation atrophy, equine motor neuron disease, horse. Equine motor neuron disease muscle (*right*) compared with normal muscle (*left*). **D,** Enlargement and pallor, steatosis, longissimus muscles, neonatal calf. The majority of the muscles have been replaced by fat. (**A,** *Courtesy Dr. B.A. Valentine, College of Veterinary Medicine, Oregon State University. For histopathologic findings, see Fig. 15-49.* **B** *and* **D,** *Courtesy Dr. M.D. McGavin, College of Veterinary Medicine, University of Tennessee. For histopathologic findings, see Fig. 15-29.* **C,** *Courtesy Dr. A. de Lahunta, College of Veterinary Medicine, Cornell University. For histopathologic findings, see Figs. 15-23 and 15-41.*)

To ensure proper fixation and orientation of sections prepared from fixed specimens, the sample should be a strip of muscle no more than 1 cm in diameter, with myofibers running lengthwise. Muscle maintains the ability to contract for some time after death, with the time varying depending on the physiologic state of the muscle at the time of death and on the postmortem interval. Contraction of muscle following contact with fixative is the most common cause of an artifact—called contraction band artifact. Contraction can be prevented or at least minimized by use of a specially designed muscle clamp (Fig. 15-13, *A*) or by placing the sample on a rigid surface, such as a portion of a tongue depressor, and fixing the ends with sutures, staples, or clamps before submersion in the fixative (Fig. 15-13, *B*).

MICROSCOPIC EXAMINATION

Frequently, lesions in muscles can be detected and evaluated only by microscopic examination. Proper microscopic examination requires evaluation of both transverse and longitudinal sections. Myofiber diameters, cytoarchitectural changes, and the percentage of abnormal myofibers are most reliably evaluated in transverse sections. Longitudinal sections reveal the length of changes, such as segmental necrosis or regeneration or deposition of storage material. Improperly oriented samples, which result in sections that have obliquely oriented myofibers and thus neither longitudinal or transverse myofibers, are difficult to evaluate. Use of a magnifying glass or dissecting microscope can aid in determining the orientation of myofibers during

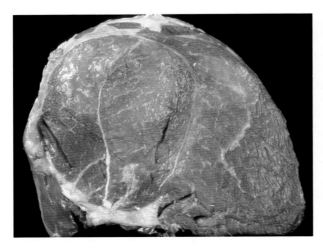

Fig. 15-12   Bovine eosinophilic myositis, gluteal muscles, cow. Green discoloration of the muscle is due to inflammation that has abundant eosinophils. The inflammation is attributed to degenerating *Sarcocystis* spp. *(Courtesy Dr. M.D. McGavin, College of Veterinary Medicine, University of Tennessee. For histopathologic findings, see Fig. 15-43.)*

trimming of muscle before sectioning. Routine stains, such as hematoxylin and eosin (H&E), run the risk of offering the pathologist a "vast pink wasteland" for evaluation (Fig. 15-14, *A*) and are often inadequate for detecting subtle myopathic changes, lesions within intramuscular nerves, or presence of abnormal stored material. Various special stains, including reticulin, Masson trichrome, von Kossa, lipid (performed on frozen sections of fixed samples), and periodic acid–Schiff (PAS) for glycogen, are often invaluable in evaluation of routinely processed skeletal muscle (Table 15-2). Examples of many of these can be found in this section. Other valuable stains and reactions can only be performed on frozen sections of unfixed muscle samples (Table 15-2).

For many decades, myofiber typing could be done only on frozen sections using the myosin ATPase reaction. Recently, immunohistochemical staining of myosin has been developed for demonstration of

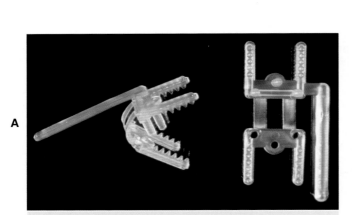

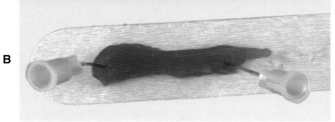

Fig. 15-13   Techniques for collection of a muscle sample for histologic examination. A, Commercially available clamps are used to prevent contraction of a fresh muscle specimen when immersed in 10% neutral-buffered formalin. **B,** Pinning strips of muscle onto a rigid surface, such as a piece of tongue depressor before immersion in 10% neutral-buffered formalin, will also minimize fixation artifacts but is not as effective as the clamps shown above. *(**A**, Courtesy Dr. L. Fuhrer, Clinic Veterinaire de St. Avertin, France. **B**, Courtesy Dr. B.A. Valentine, College of Veterinary Medicine, Oregon State University.)*

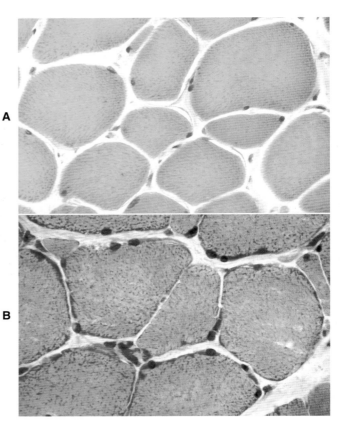

Fig. 15-14   Visibility of mitochondria, formalin-fixed vs. frozen sections, transverse sections of skeletal muscle. A, Formalin fixed, paraffin-embedded sample. Mitochondria stain faintly, and the myofibers lack detail when compared with Fig. 15-14, *B*. H&E stain. **B,** Frozen section. Note the increased detail visible. Blue stained mitochondria are seen throughout the cytoplasm and concentrated at the periphery of the myofibers. H&E stain. *(**A** and **B**, Courtesy Dr. B.A. Valentine, College of Veterinary Medicine, Oregon State University.)*

Table **15-2**   **Useful Special Stains and Enzyme Reactions**

	Stain	**Use**
Routine sections	Masson trichrome	Differentiates collagen (blue) from muscle (red); highlight nerves; differentiate myelin (red) from collagen (blue)
	Reticulin	Identifies reticular fibers of the muscle interstitium; outline individual fibers
	PTAH	Stains cross striations in muscle
	von Kossa	Identifies carbonates and phosphates linked with calcium in mineralized fibers
	Alizarin red S	Identifies calcium in necrotic and mineralized fibers
	PAS	Identifies glycogen and proteoglycans; also stains protozoal cysts
	PAS with amylase (diastase)	Differentiates proteoglycans (amylase resistant) from glycogen (amylase sensitive)
Frozen sections	Modified Gomori's trichrome	Identifies mitochondria (red), nemaline rods (red), collagen (green); differentiates myelin (red) from collagen (green) in nerves
	NADH, SDH, cytochrome oxidase	Identifies mitochondrial enzyme activity
	ATPase	Differentiates fiber types
	Acid phosphatase	Detects macrophages and denervated fibers
	Nonspecific esterase	Detects macrophages and denervated fibers; identifies neuromuscular junctions
	Oil red O; Sudan black	Identifies lipid
	von Kossa, alizarin red S, PAS with and without amylase (diastase)	Same as in routine sections

ATPase, Adenosine triphosphatase; *NADH*, nicotinamide adenine dinucleotide dehydrogenase; *PAS*, periodic acid-Schiff; *PTAH*, phosphotungstic acid hematoxylin; *SDH*, succinate dehydrogenase.

myofiber types in formalin-fixed muscle. This is a major advantage because fiber-type staining is often essential for the complete evaluation of muscle. It is most useful in demonstrating preferential involvement of a fiber type and alteration of the fiber-type pattern because of denervation and reinnervation.

Enzyme histochemistry and immunohistochemistry

There is no question that frozen section histochemistry of unfixed muscle samples is the "gold standard" of muscle pathology. Skeletal muscle may be the one tissue in which the morphology of cells and cellular components is best appreciated in frozen sections (Fig. 15-14, *B*). Routine frozen section histochemistry on muscle includes a battery of stains applied to serial sections. Examples of many of these are provided in this section. Stains applied include H&E, modified Gomori's trichrome, ATPase for fiber typing, nicotinamide adenine dinucleotide dehydrogenase (NADH), succinate dehydrogenase (SDH), cytochrome oxidase, and other mitochondrial enzyme stains, PAS for glycogen, alizarin red S for calcium, alkaline phosphatase and nonspecific esterase for macrophages and denervated fibers, and lipid stains. When indicated, frozen sections also allow for immunostaining for cytoskeletal proteins, such as dystrophin (Fig. 15-50) and the dystrophin-associated proteins.

Certain abnormal structures—such as nemaline rods formed by expansion of Z bands, as seen in nemaline rod myopathy—are not visible in routine sections, but are readily identified in frozen sections stained with modified Gomori's trichrome.

The major disadvantage of frozen section histochemistry is that, unless a neuromuscular disease laboratory is readily available to immediately process unfixed muscle samples, careful preparation for overnight shipping, on ice, in a moist but not overly wet environment, is necessary. Any delay in shipment, or overwetting or overheating of the sample, will result in nondiagnostic samples. In addition, preparation of frozen sections is time and labor intensive, and in most cases only a single transverse section approximately 1 cm in diameter will be examined. This can create a significant sampling error when evaluating a small sample of a large muscle in which lesions may not be evenly distributed.

Complete evaluation to include morphometric examination and calculation of the percentage and mean diameter of each fiber type will detect changes in the percentage of each fiber type and fiber atrophy or hypertrophy. But at this time, morphometric analysis is not routinely performed on samples submitted for diagnostic purposes.

Frozen section histochemistry will always be a powerful tool for evaluation of muscle disease. But in many disorders, it is possible to obtain diagnostic sections from routinely processed muscle samples when appropriate sample selection, handling, and processing are performed, and sections are examined by a pathologist familiar with muscle pathology.

Electron microscopy

Although much of what used to be determined by electron microscopy has been supplanted by newer immunohistochemical procedures, electron microscopic evaluation of muscle is still important. Various structural alterations, such as abnormalities of neuromuscular junctions, mitochondria, sarcomeric disarray, sarcotubular dilation, Z-line streaming, and cytoplasmic inclusions may be best visualized, and in some cases only visualized, by this method. Sampling and handling methods to minimize contraction and other artifacts and to allow for precise transverse and longitudinal sections are imperative.

OTHER METHODS OF EVALUATION

Physiologic testing of isolated intact myofibers in vitro forms the basis for diagnosis of malignant hyperthermia. Short fibers, such as from samples of intercostal muscle, are preferred. While maintained in a physiologic solution, myofiber bundles are exposed to various agents, such as caffeine and halothane, to detect abnormal contractural sensitivity. Biochemical and molecular biologic analysis of muscle samples can evaluate levels of muscle enzymes and other proteins, and genetic analysis can be performed to detect specific gene defects. These latter tests require fresh muscle samples snap-frozen in liquid nitrogen and maintained at −70° C until analysis.

PORTALS OF ENTRY

Portals of entry are summarized in Box 15-2. Injury to muscle can occur secondary to trauma or infection. Muscle lying superficially can be damaged by penetrating wounds, including those created by intramuscular injections (Figs. 15-11, B and 15-15), which can also allow entry of infectious agents. Muscles located deeply are often injured following bone fracture. Crush injuries from external forces will cause extensive muscle damage, and excessive tension can cause muscle tearing. Muscles are endowed with an extensive vascular network that can allow entry of blood-borne pathogens, immune complexes, antibodies and toxins, and inflammatory cells.

Other routes by which muscle can become dysfunctional are summarized in Box 15-3. Some muscular disorders are genetically determined. Inherited or acquired

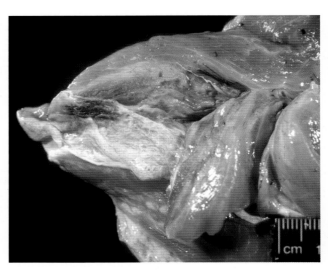

Fig. 15-15   **Inflammation and myofiber necrosis, injection site, muscles, lateral thigh, cow.** Necrotic muscle has been stained green by the injected material, which has spread distally down the fascial plane between the two muscles from the original injection site (**top right**). (*Courtesy Dr. M.D. McGavin, College of Veterinary Medicine, University of Tennessee.*)

Box 15-2

Portals of Entry into the Muscular System

DIRECT

Penetrating wounds
Intramuscular injections
Bone fracture
External pressure causing crush injury

HEMATOGENOUS

Blood-borne pathogens, toxins, autoantibodies, and
    immune complexes
Cytotoxic lymphocytes causing immune-mediated
    damage
Other inflammatory cells

Box 15-3

Other Causes of Muscle Dysfunction

PHYSIOLOGIC

Excessive tension causing muscle rupture
Exercise-induced damage to myofibers
Loss of innervation or blood supply
Endocrine and electrolyte abnormalities

GENETIC

Inborn errors of metabolism
Genetic defects of myofiber structural components
Developmental defects

NUTRITIONAL/TOXIC

Deficiency of selenium and/or vitamin E
Toxic plants or plant products
Feed additives (ionophores)

dysfunction of motor neurons or nerves will cause muscle injury in the form of atrophy. Toxins or an altered endocrine or electrolyte status can affect muscle, and physiologic damage can be caused by exhaustive or overexuberant exercise.

DEFENSE MECHANISMS

Defense mechanisms are summarized in Box 15-4. The thick encircling fascia (epimysium) of many muscles provides some protection from penetrating injuries and from extension of adjacent infection. This fascia can, however, also contribute to injury under circumstances that lead to increased intramuscular pressure causing hypoxia (compartment syndrome). Tissue macrophages are not typically found in normal muscle, but are recruited rapidly from circulating monocytes in the vasculature. Macrophages can cross even an intact basal lamina and effectively clear debris from damaged portions of myofibers, allowing for rapid restoration of the myocyte through satellite cell activation. Neutrophils and other inflammatory cells are also recruited from the blood stream in response to injury or infection. The extensive vascular network of muscle includes extensive collateral circulatory pathways that render muscle relatively resistant to ischemic damage caused by thrombosis or thromboembolism. Despite the high vascular density of muscle, metastasis of neoplasms to muscle is quite rare. There is some evidence to suggest that the capillary endothelium of skeletal muscle is inherently resistant to neoplastic cell adhesion and invasion.

Box 15-4

Defense Mechanisms of Skeletal Muscle

SKIN, SUBCUTIS, AND FASCIA
Form structural barriers to protect against external injury

VASCULATURE
Collateral circulation to protect against ischemia
Recruitment of monocytes that become tissue macrophages
Recruitment of neutrophils and other inflammatory cells
Capillary endothelium resistant to tumor metastasis

IMMUNOLOGIC RESPONSES
Innate humoral and cellular immunologic responses

OTHER
Adequate tissue antioxidant concentrations
Physiologic adaptation
Regenerative capacity

RESPONSE OF MUSCLE TO INJURY

It is often said that the range of response of muscle to injury is limited, consisting primarily of necrosis and regeneration. Actually, muscle is a remarkably adaptive tissue, with a wide range of response to physiologic and pathologic conditions. Myofibers can add or delete sarcomeres to cause elongation or shortening of the entire muscle. In addition to necrosis and regeneration, myofibers can atrophy and hypertrophy, they can split, they can undergo a variety of cytoarchitectural alterations, and they can completely alter their physiologic functions when undergoing fiber-type conversion. To describe muscle response to injury as stereotypical does not do justice to this inherent plasticity. What is true, though, is that it is frequently not possible to determine the cause of muscle injury based on gross or histologic lesions alone. Supplementary tests and clinical histories are often essential.

NECROSIS AND REGENERATION

Myofiber necrosis can accompany a variety of disorders. Because of their multinucleate nature, myofibers often undergo segmental necrosis, with involvement of only one or several contiguous segments within the cell. More than 100 years ago, Zenker described segmental hyaline degeneration (Zenker's necrosis) in the muscles of human patients dying of typhoid, and this term may still be found in some of the older literature. Global necrosis of the entire length of the myofiber occurs only under severe duress, such as extreme pressure to the entire muscle causing crush injury, or widespread ischemia because of pressure on, or thromboembolism of, a large artery.

Necrotic portions of myofibers have several different histologic appearances. The earliest change is often segmental hypercontraction, resulting in segments of slightly larger diameter that are slightly darker staining ("large dark fibers") that are best seen on transverse sections (Fig. 15-16, A). On longitudinal sections, "twisting" or "curling" of affected fibers is often seen. But similar changes occur as an artifactual change in improperly handled samples. The cytoplasm of fully necrotic portions of the fiber is often homogeneously eosinophilic and pale (hyaline degeneration), with loss of the normal cytoplasmic striations and the adjacent muscle nucleus. The affected cytoplasm then becomes floccular or granular as that portion of the myofiber starts to fragment (Fig. 15-16, B; Fig. 15-18, B).

Increased intracellular calcium is a common trigger of necrosis in all cells, and myofibers contain a high level of calcium ions stored in the sarcoplasmic reticulum. Therefore myofibers may be particularly sensitive to calcium-induced necrosis either as a result of damage to the sarcolemma, causing influx of extracellular calcium, or

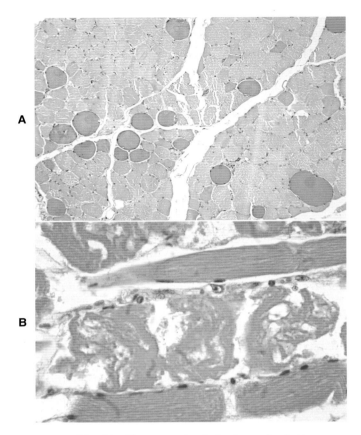

Fig. 15-16　**Myofiber necrosis, skeletal muscle. A,** Hypercontraction, transverse section. Large, deeply stained fibers ("large dark fibers") are hypercontracted segments of a myofiber, the initial stage of necrosis. Note the rounded outline of these myofibers compared with the polygonal outlines of normal myofibers. Formalin fixation, H&E stain. **B,** Segmental necrosis, monensin toxicosis, longitudinal section, horse. Segments of the myofibers have undergone hypercontraction, and the remaining cytoplasm is fragmented. Formalin fixation, H&E stain. (*A* and *B,* Courtesy Dr. M.D. McGavin, College of Veterinary Medicine, University of Tennessee.)

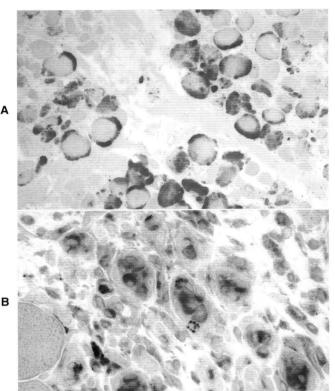

Fig. 15-17　**Myofiber necrosis, skeletal muscle, transverse section. A,** There has been a massive influx of calcium (*stained orange*) into acutely necrotic fibers. Frozen section, alizarin red S stain. **B,** Macrophages with red-brown staining cytoplasm invading necrotic myofibers. Portions of intact fibers are in the lower left. Frozen section, nonspecific esterase stain. (*A,* Courtesy Dr. B.A. Valentine, College of Veterinary Medicine, Oregon State University. *B,* Courtesy Dr. B.J. Cooper, College of Veterinary Medicine, Oregon State University.)

from damage to the sarcoplasmic reticulum, releasing intracellular stores of calcium. Small wonder then that necrotic myofibers are often prone to overt mineralization. Overtly mineralized myofibers appear as chalky white streaks on gross examination (Fig. 15-11, *A*) and as basophilic granular to crystalline material within myofibers on histologic examination. Large deposits of mineral can induce a foreign body granulomatous response. Although the presence or absence of myofiber mineralization has sometimes been used as a diagnostic aid, the circumstances under which a necrotic myofiber segment can become mineralized are so diverse that myofiber mineralization must be considered a nonspecific response, indicative only of myofiber necrosis. Myofiber mineralization can be confirmed with histochemical stains, such as alizarin red S and von Kossa. Histochemical staining for calcium in frozen sections will also detect increased intracytoplasmic

calcium in damaged myofibers that are not overtly necrotic or mineralized (Fig. 15-17, *A*).

Provided there is still an adequate blood supply, macrophages derived from transformation of blood monocytes will rapidly infiltrate areas of myofiber necrosis (Fig. 15-17, *B*). Macrophages are able to traverse the basal lamina and rapidly clear cytoplasmic debris (Fig. 15-18, *A*). Other leukocytes, including neutrophils, eosinophils, and lymphocytes, can also be recruited to sites of extensive myonecrosis, presumably because of various cytokines released from damaged muscle. The infiltration of macrophages and other cells into areas of damaged muscle to clear away necrotic myofibers does not in any way constitute a form of myositis.

Because myonuclei are unable to divide, regeneration of muscle relies on satellite cell activation. Muscle satellite cells are resistant to many of the insults that result in myofiber necrosis, and activation of satellite cells is triggered by necrosis of adjacent myofiber segments. Therefore, as macrophages are clearing cytoplasmic

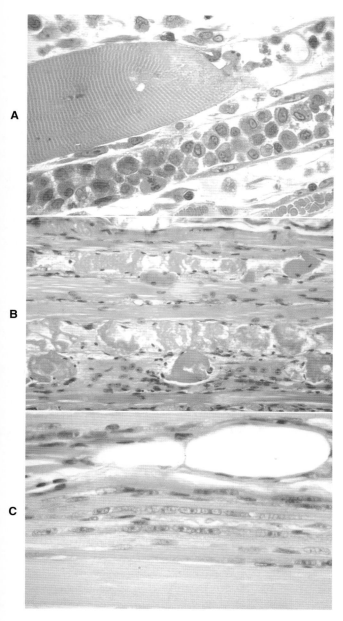

Fig. 15-18, Cont'd   consists of myotubes, which have small diameters, with slightly basophilic cytoplasm and internal rows of large euchromatic nuclei. Formalin fixation, H&E stain. (**A,** *Courtesy Dr. A. Kelly, University of Pennsylvania.* **B,** *Courtesy Dr. B.A. Valentine, College of Veterinary Medicine, Oregon State University.* **C,** *Courtesy Dr. B.J. Cooper, College of Veterinary Medicine, Oregon State University.*)

Fig. 15-18   **Segmental necrosis and regeneration. A,** Monophasic segmental coagulation necrosis, skeletal muscle, longitudinal section of two myofibers. A segment of the upper fiber (*right*) and all the visible portion of the lower fiber have undergone necrosis, and macrophages have invaded through the intact basal lamina and cleared the cytoplasmic debris. Satellite cells on the inner surface of the basal lamina of the lower fiber are activated, and one (*lower left side*) is in mitosis. One μm plastic-embedded section, H&E stain. **B,** Polyphasic injury, segmental coagulation necrosis and regeneration of myofibers, muscle, longitudinal section. Between each of the foci of coagulation necrosis in the lowest myofiber is a segment of small-diameter faintly basophilic cytoplasm lacking cross striations, in which there is an internal chain of euchromatic nuclei. This is a late stage of regeneration. Formalin fixation, H&E stain. **C,** Monophasic injury, late stage regeneration, skeletal muscle, longitudinal section. The regenerating segment of the myofiber

(Continued)

debris, satellite cells are becoming activated and begin to divide in preparation for regeneration of the affected myofiber segment. If the myofiber basal lamina is still intact, it will leave an empty cylindrical space known as a "sarcolemmal tube." This name is clearly a misnomer, dating from the days when the term "sarcolemma" was applied to the tube formed by the basal lamina that remains after segmental myofiber necrosis. Clearly what is now termed the sarcolemma (plasmalemma) of necrotic fiber segments is lost, but this is a misnomer that is firmly entrenched. The important concept to remember is that, if intact, the basal lamina will form a cylindrical scaffold to guide proliferating myoblasts and to keep fibroblasts out. Satellite cells may be seen undergoing mitosis, at which stage they are known as activated myoblasts, on the inner surface of this tube (Fig. 15-18, A). Within hours, proliferating myoblasts will fuse end-to-end to form myotubes (Fig. 15-18, B and C), and within days the myotube will produce thick and thin filaments and undergo maturation to a myofiber and will reestablish myofiber integrity. If the basal lamina is ruptured, myotubes are said to be able to bridge gaps of 2 to 4 mm, but any larger ones heal by fibrosis (see later discussion). The process of myofiber regeneration recapitulates embryologic development of skeletal muscle and is depicted schematically in Fig. 15-19. A percentage of dividing satellite cells will not fuse with the forming myotube, but will instead become new satellite cells capable of future regeneration.

In summary, the success of muscle regeneration depends on (1) the presence of an intact basal lamina and (2) the availability of viable satellite cells. The stages of successful muscle regeneration are summarized in Box 15-5.

Thus myofibers undergoing segmental necrosis in which the basal lamina is preserved, as in metabolic, nutritional, and toxic myopathies, will regenerate very successfully. However, when large areas of satellite cells are killed (e.g., by heat, intense inflammation, or infarction), the situation is very different. In this case, a return to normal is not possible, and healing is chiefly by fibrosis.

If the insult to the muscle is sufficient to disrupt the myofiber basal lamina but not enough to damage the satellite cells, regeneration attempts are ineffective. Because the basal lamina is not intact, there is no tube to guide the myoblasts proliferating from each end. Myoblast proliferation under these conditions results in formation of so-called muscle giant cells (Fig. 15-20). Thus the presence of muscle giant cells indicates that

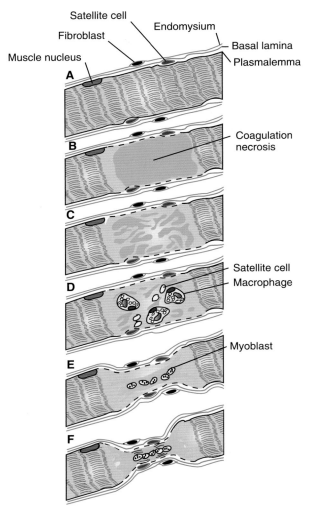

Fig. 15-19   Schematic diagram of segmental myofiber necrosis and regeneration. A, Myofiber, longitudinal section. **B,** Segmental coagulation necrosis. **C,** The necrotic segment of the myofiber has become floccular and detached from the adjacent viable portion of the myofiber. The satellite cells are enlarging. **D,** The necrotic segment of the myofiber has been invaded by macrophages, and satellite cells are migrating to the center. The latter will develop into myoblasts. The plasmalemma of the necrotic segment has disappeared. **E,** Myoblasts have formed a myotube, which has produced sarcoplasm. This extends out to meet the viable ends of the myofiber. The integrity of the myofiber is maintained by the sarcolemmal tube formed by the basal lamina and endomysium. **F,** Regenerating myofiber. There is a reduction in myofiber diameter with central rowing of nuclei. There is early formation of sarcomeres (cross striations), and the plasmalemma has re-formed. Such fibers stain basophilically with H&E. *(A through F, Redrawn with permission from Dr. M.D. McGavin, College of Veterinary Medicine, University of Tennessee.)*

Box 15-5

Stages of Muscle Regeneration under Optimal Conditions

1. Muscle nuclei disappear from the necrotic segment and the sarcoplasm becomes hyalinized (eosinophilic, amorphous, and homogeneous) because of the loss of normal myofibrillar structure (Fig. 15-19, *B*). The necrotic portion may separate from the adjacent viable myofiber (Fig. 15-16, *B*, Fig. 15-18, *A* and *B*, Fig. 15-19, *C*).
2. Within 24 to 48 hours, monocytes emigrate from capillaries, become macrophages, and enter the necrotic portion of the myofiber (Fig. 15-17, *B*, Fig. 15-18, *A*, Fig. 15-19, *D*). Concurrently, the satellite cells, located between the basal lamina and the sarcolemma, begin to enlarge (Fig. 15-18, *A*, Fig. 15-19, *C* and *D*), become vesicular with prominent nucleoli, and then undergo mitosis to become myoblasts.
3. Myoblasts migrate from the periphery to the center of the sarcolemmal tube, among the macrophages (Fig. 15-19, *D*).
4. Macrophages lyse and phagocytose necrotic debris and form a clear space in the sarcolemmal tube, and the shape of the sarcolemmal tube is maintained by the basal lamina (Fig. 15-18, *A*).
5. Myoblasts fuse with one another to form myotubes, which are thin, elongated muscle cells with a row of central, closely spaced nuclei. Developing myotubes send out cytoplasmic processes in both directions within the sarcolemmal tube (Fig. 15-19, *E*). When the processes contact each other or a viable portion of the original muscle fiber, they fuse. The regenerating fiber is characterized by (1) basophilia as a result of increased RNA content, (2) internal nuclei, often in rows, that have differentiated to myonuclei, (3) a lack of striations, and (4) a smaller than normal diameter (Fig. 15-18, *B* and *C*, Fig. 15-19, *F*).
6. The fiber grows and differentiates. Its diameter increases, the sarcoplasm loses its basophilia, and longitudinal and cross striations appear, indicating the formation of sarcomeres.
7. In most species, within several days, the muscle nuclei of regenerating fibers move to their normal position at the periphery of the fiber, just under the sarcolemma.

conditions for regeneration have not been optimal, and occurs following destructive lesions, such as those caused by trauma that transects myofibers, infarction, and intramuscular bacterial infection or injection of irritants. Muscle giant cells are often accompanied by fibrosis, which will unite the ends of the damaged myofibers. This also occurs in muscle damaged by invasive or metastatic sclerosing carcinomas. Cytokines released from damaged muscle fibers contribute to the signaling pathways that initiate macrophage infiltration and regeneration, but they also contribute to interstitial

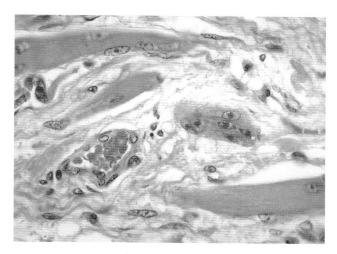

Fig. 15-20   Ineffectual regeneration. Large, bizarre multinucleate muscle giant cells are indicative of regeneration in an area in which the myofiber's basal lamina has been damaged. Because the wall of the "myotube" of basal lamina is not intact, regenerating sarcoplasm exudes through the defect and in cross section this appears as a "muscle giant cell." Formalin fixation, H&E stain. *(Courtesy Dr. M.D. McGavin, College of Veterinary Medicine, University of Tennessee; and Noah's Arkive, College of Veterinary Medicine, The University of Georgia.)*

fibroblast activation. Collagen is inelastic, and thus large areas of fibrosis inevitably reduce the ability of the muscle to contract and to stretch. Fibrosis within locomotory muscles often results in obvious alteration of the gait.

Because segmental necrosis and regeneration are such a common result of a wide variety of insults (e.g., overexertion, selenium deficiency, and toxic injury), a histologic diagnosis of "segmental necrosis" is often not helpful in determining the cause of the disease. Pathologic classification of lesions according to distribution (i.e., focal, multifocal, locally extensive, and diffuse) and duration (i.e., acute, subacute, chronic) has proven to be extremely useful in determining the possible causes of segmental muscle necrosis. Pathologic classification of degenerative myopathies has been further enhanced by Dr. Byron Kakulas, who introduced the terms *monophasic necrosis* and *polyphasic necrosis*. Monophasic lesions are of the same duration, indicative of a single insult. Polyphasic lesions indicate an ongoing degenerative process. Thus a focal monophasic lesion could be the result of a single traumatic incident, such as an intramuscular injection (Fig. 15-11, *B*). A multifocal monophasic lesion could represent a single episode of overly strenuous exercise (exertional myopathy) or a toxin being fed on one occasion (e.g., a horse eating one dose of monensin; Figs. 15-16, *B* and Fig. 15-38, *B*). However, if the insult is repeated or ongoing, such as occurs in muscular dystrophy (Fig. 15-49), selenium deficiency, or continuous feeding of a toxin, then new lesions (segmental necrosis) will form at the same time that regeneration is

taking place; in other words, it will be a multifocal and polyphasic disease (Fig. 15-18, *B*). Using this approach, it is sometimes possible to rule out a diagnosis (e.g., muscular dystrophy and selenium deficiency myopathy are typically polyphasic), but this is not an invariable rule. For example, in livestock with borderline concentrations of selenium, a sudden stress can cause a monophasic necrosis.

The term "rhabdomyolysis" is often encountered, particularly in the clinical arena, and especially in association with exercise-induced muscle injury (exertional rhabdomyolysis) in human beings, horses, and dogs. Technically, *rhabdomyolysis* simply means necrosis (lysis) of striated muscle. This term was coined years ago to replace the term *myoglobinuria* as a description for the clinical entity of severe muscle injury associated with myoglobin release causing dark red discoloration of the urine. Thus rhabdomyolysis generally indicates the presence of a severe degenerative myopathy with a large degree of myofiber necrosis (Fig. 15-40). In horses, the term *exertional rhabdomyolysis* has become firmly entrenched as a clinical entity in which exercise-induced muscle injury is the presenting sign. The term *recurrent exertional rhabdomyolysis* is often employed in cases in which repeated bouts of exercise-induced muscle damage have been documented.

ALTERATION IN MYOFIBER SIZE

The normal myofiber diameter will vary depending on fiber type, the muscle examined, the species, and the age of the animal. In some species (e.g., horse, cat, and human beings), there are three distinct populations based on diameter: Type 1 fibers are the smallest, type 2B fibers the largest, and type 2A fibers are intermediate in size. Differing diameters in part reflect the oxidative needs of the fibers; oxygen diffuses more readily into the interior of small-diameter fibers. In the dog, all fiber types are oxidative, and fiber-type diameter is much more uniform. A histogram generated from morphometric analysis of fiber diameters will reveal the characteristics of individual muscles in various species. Not surprisingly, this type of detailed information is more readily available for human patients than for animals. Even without morphometric analysis, however, a pathologist experienced in examination of muscle can often determine whether there is a normal fiber-size distribution (based on fiber diameter in transverse section), or whether there is an increase in fiber-size variation. The finding of increased fiber-size variation suggests that something is wrong but in itself does not give any indication of cause. Increased fiber-size variation can be a result of fiber atrophy, fiber hypertrophy, or both, and is considered part of the spectrum of changes included in the term "chronic myopathic change" (Box 15-6).

Box **15-6**

Findings Associated with Chronic Myopathic Change

Excessive fiber-size variation
Internal nuclei
Fiber splitting
Other cytoarchitectural changes
Fibrosis
Fat infiltration

Box **15-7**

Fiber Types and Muscle Atrophy

1. Denervation: Type 1 and type 2 fibers; reinnervation leads to altered fiber-type patterns (fiber-type grouping)
2. Disuse: Predominantly type 2 fibers; may vary depending on the species and cause
3. Endocrine disease: Predominantly type 2 fibers; associated with hypothyroidism and hypercortisolism
4. Malnutrition, cachexia, and senility: Predominantly type 2 fibers
5. Congenital myopathy: Often predominantly type 1 fibers

ATROPHY

The term "atrophy" is used to imply either a reduction in the volume of the muscle as a whole or in the diameter of a myofiber. In the early stages of atrophy, it may be difficult or impossible to detect loss of muscle mass by gross observation, and morphometric evaluation of myofiber diameters may be required. Several cellular physiologic processes can be activated to result in muscle atrophy. These include induction of lysosomal action to result in autophagy of cytoplasmic components, apoptosis (programmed cell death), and activation of the cytoplasmic ubiquitin-proteosomal machinery. Lysosomal activation is prominent in denervation atrophy and is the basis for the positive reaction of denervated fibers in alkaline phosphatase and nonspecific esterase preparations. The causes of muscle fiber atrophy include physiologic and metabolic processes, and denervation. In most instances, muscle atrophy is reversible provided the cause is corrected. The type of fiber undergoing atrophy varies depending on the cause, therefore fiber typing is often required for a definitive diagnosis. Interestingly, type 2 fibers are the most likely to atrophy under a variety of circumstances (Box 15-7).

Physiologic muscle atrophy

Decrease in myofiber diameter, and therefore in the overall muscle mass, is a physiologic response to lack of use (disuse atrophy), cachexia, and aging. Type 2 fibers are preferentially affected (Fig. 15-21). Disuse atrophy occurs relatively slowly, and only in muscles not undergoing normal contraction, such as that caused by severe lameness or in muscles of a limb that is splinted or enclosed in a cast. The degree of disuse atrophy will be variable but typically is not as severe as the atrophy of cachexia or denervation (see later discussion). Disuse atrophy is often asymmetric. Muscle atrophy due to cachexia can be profound, especially in cases of cancer cachexia in which increased circulating levels of tumor necrosis factor alter the muscle metabolism, favoring catabolic processes rather than anabolic processes.

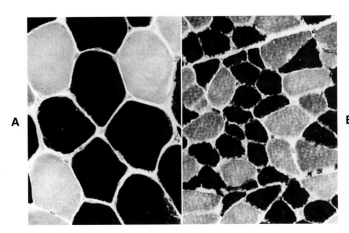

Fig. 15-21   Disuse atrophy, dog. A, Transverse section of normal biceps femoris muscle. **B,** Same muscle, same magnification, 60 days after disuse. Both type 1 *(light)* and type 2 *(dark)* fibers are atrophic, but type 2 fibers are more severely affected. Frozen section, ATPase pH 9.8. (*A and B, Courtesy Dr. M.D. McGavin, College of Veterinary Medicine, University of Tennessee.*)

Cachexia also develops relatively slowly, and causes symmetric muscle atrophy. Muscle atrophy due to aging can be considered a milder form of cachexia. Starvation, malnutrition, and chronic renal and cardiac diseases can also result in cachexia.

Atrophy due to endocrine disease

Preferential atrophy of type 2 fibers causing symmetric muscle atrophy also occurs because of various endocrine disorders. The most common are hypothyroidism and hypercortisolism in dogs. Aging horses with pituitary dysfunction or tumors (leading to equine Cushing's syndrome) often develop muscle atrophy, presumably predominantly of type 2 fibers. The exact mechanisms by which these disorders cause myofiber atrophy are not clear, but myofibers contain a high concentration of surface receptors for several hormones.

Atrophy due to endocrine disease likely reflects the intimate interrelationship between the endocrine and the muscular systems.

Denervation atrophy

This atrophy, also known by the misnomer "neurogenic atrophy," is not uncommon in veterinary medicine. Maintenance of normal myofiber diameter is dependent on trophic factors generated by an intact associated nerve. Loss of neural input results in rapid muscle atrophy, and more than half the muscle mass of a completely denervated muscle can be lost in a few weeks. This trophic effect is not dependent on contractile activity because denervation atrophy is not a feature of neuromuscular junction disorders such as botulism and myasthenia gravis. In these disorders, there is a failure of neuromuscular transmission, but the nerve to the muscle is intact; therefore the muscle is technically still innervated. Generalized neuropathies or neuronopathies, such as equine motor neuron disease, will result in widespread and symmetric muscle atrophy. More commonly, however, only select nerve damage is present, resulting in asymmetric muscle atrophy. One example is equine laryngeal hemiplegia (roaring) secondary to damage to the left recurrent laryngeal nerve (Fig. 15-22). It should

be pointed out that purely demyelinating disorders of peripheral nerves can cause profound neuromuscular dysfunction, but axons are still intact. Associated myofibers are not technically denervated and therefore do not undergo denervation atrophy.

Following denervation, fibers become progressively smaller in diameter as peripheral myofibrils disintegrate. If an atrophic fiber is surrounded by normal fibers, it will be pressed into an angular shape, called an angular atrophied fiber. The angular atrophied fibers of denervation atrophy most often occur either singly or in small contiguous groups (small group atrophy) (Fig. 15-23, A). In more severe denervating conditions, in which many fibers within muscle fascicles are undergoing denervation

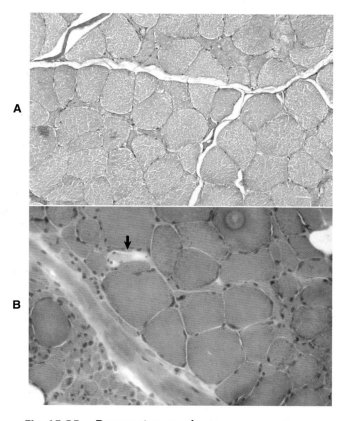

Fig. 15-23   Denervation atrophy, transverse sections. Both sections are from horses with equine motor neuron disease. **A,** In relatively mild denervation, severely atrophied and angular fibers form small contiguous clusters indicative of small group atrophy. Formalin fixation, Masson trichrome stain. **B,** In severe denervation, entire fascicles of fibers undergo rounded atrophy characteristic of large group atrophy (*lower left*). Small group atrophy and admixed fiber hypertrophy are also present. A single pale stained fiber (*arrow*) is undergoing acute necrosis. There is also mild endomysial and perimysial fibrosis and mild fat infiltration (*empty vacuoles in the upper right and lower left*). Frozen section, modified Gomori's trichrome stain. (*A and B, Courtesy Dr. B.A. Valentine, College of Veterinary Medicine, Oregon State University.*)

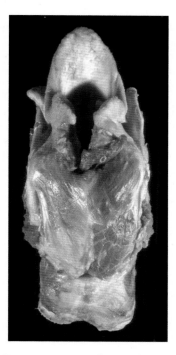

Fig. 15-22   Denervation muscle atrophy, left cricoarytenoideus dorsalis muscle, larynx, dorsal surface, horse. Note the unilateral (*left side*) atrophy and pale gray to white discoloration of the muscle. This horse had a peripheral neuropathy, which had led to laryngeal hemiplegia. *(Courtesy College of Veterinary Medicine, University of Illinois.)*

atrophy, there are no normal fibers to cause compression and angularity, and affected fibers occur as larger groups of small diameter rounded fibers (large group atrophy; Fig. 15-23, *B*). Although myofibrils disappear rapidly, muscle nuclei do not do so at the same rate, and therefore denervation atrophy is often associated with a notably increased concentration of myonuclei. The breakdown of glycogen in the myofiber is an early change in denervation atrophy, and therefore denervated fibers stain faintly, or not at all, with the PAS reaction.

A histologic diagnosis of denervation atrophy may be suspected, based on the characteristic features of routinely processed muscles, but is most reliably documented with histochemistry or immunohistochemistry to detect fiber types. The loss of a nerve fiber to a muscle results in atrophy of all myofibers innervated by that nerve. Because of the intermingling of motor units forming a mosaic pattern of fiber types, myofibers undergoing denervation atrophy are scattered in a section of muscle. Because the motor neuron determines the histochemical myofiber type, and because denervating diseases typically involve both type 1 and type 2 neurons or nerves, atrophy of both type 1 and type 2 myofibers in muscle fasciculi is the hallmark of denervation atrophy (Fig. 15-24, *A*).

In denervation atrophy, histologic examination of the intramuscular nerves is warranted because it may reveal axonal degeneration or loss of myelinated fibers. Masson trichrome stain can be useful here because it will differentiate myelin (red) from collagen (blue). If the nerve damage does not incapacitate the animal and the muscle can still be used (e.g., in locomotion), the remaining innervated myofibers often undergo notable hypertrophy because of increased workload. Often the hypertrophied fibers in chronic denervation are type 1. Even without fiber typing, a pattern of severe small or large group atrophy (Fig. 15-23, *A*), especially if associated with notable fiber hypertrophy (Fig. 15-23, *B*), is strongly suggestive of denervation atrophy. A finding of associated peripheral nerve damage will be definitive.

Under many circumstances, denervated muscle fibers can be reinnervated by subterminal sprouting of axons from adjacent normal nerves. Reinnervation results in return to normal myofiber diameter, but reinnervation will often be from sprouts of a different type of nerve. Because muscle fiber type is a function of the motor neuron, the newly innervated myofiber will take on the fiber type determined by that neuron. This process results in a loss of the normal arrangement of type 1 and 2 myofibers and the formation of groups of the same fiber type adjacent to each other, called fiber-type grouping (Fig. 15-24). Thus fiber-type grouping is the hallmark of denervation followed by reinnervation. What appears to be fiber-type grouping can also occur because

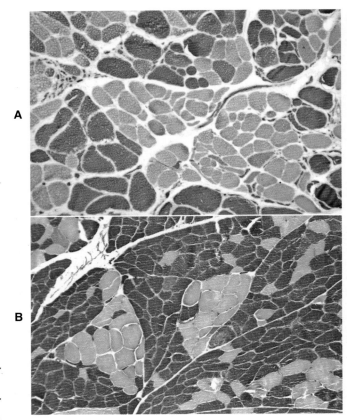

Fig. 15-24 **Denervation atrophy and reinnervation, skeletal muscle, transverse sections. A,** Fiber typing reveals angular atrophy of both type 1 (*light*) and type 2 (*dark*) fibers, characteristic of denervation atrophy. In this case, there is also a loss of the normal mosaic pattern of fiber types, with groups of type 1 and of type 2 fibers indicative of reinnervation. This section is from a horse with laryngeal hemiplegia. Frozen section, ATPase pH 10.0. **B,** Fiber-type grouping in a dog indicative of denervation and reinnervation secondary to corticosteroid therapy. There is a loss of the normal mosaic pattern of fiber types, with grouping of type 1 (*light*) and type 2 (*dark*) fibers. The lack of angular atrophied fibers indicates that active denervation is not occurring at this time. Frozen section, ATPase pH 9.8. (*A, Courtesy Dr. B.A. Valentine, College of Veterinary Medicine, Oregon State University. B, Courtesy Dr. M.D. McGavin, College of Veterinary Medicine, University of Tennessee.*)

of fiber-type conversion (most often to type 1 fibers) in chronic myopathic conditions. Careful evaluation of the peripheral nervous system structure and function will help to distinguish neuropathic from myopathic changes. If previously reinnervated fibers are denervated again, the pattern will include large groups of atrophied fibers of a single fiber type, a process known as type-specific group atrophy. Type-specific group atrophy is far less

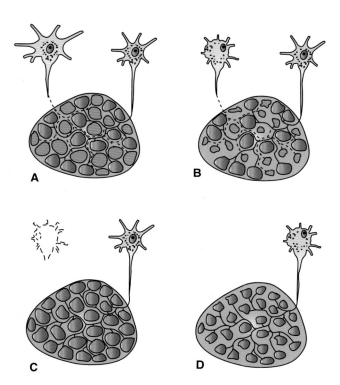

Fig. 15-25 **Schematic diagram of motor units undergoing denervation and reinnervation. A,** Terminal axon branches innervate multiple myofibers, and myofiber type is determined by the electrical activity of the type of neuron innervating the myofiber. Normally the terminal axons of the motor units are intermingled, with the result that the differently stained myofiber types form a mosaic pattern. **B,** If a neuron (or axon) is damaged, the axon will undergo Wallerian degeneration, and the myofibers in that motor unit will undergo denervation atrophy. Small group atrophy is illustrated here. **C,** Axonal sprouts from a healthy neuron can reinnervate affected fibers and cause restoration of their normal diameter. The myofibers will assume the fiber type of the new motor unit, which often causes fiber-type conversion, leading to fiber-type grouping. **D,** If neuronal (or axonal) damage is progressive, denervation atrophy of large groups of fibers of a single type can occur, known as type-specific group atrophy. This type of atrophy is less common in animals than in human beings. (**A** *through* **D,** *Redrawn with permission from Dr. B.A. Valentine, College of Veterinary Medicine, Oregon State University.*)

Atrophy due to congenital myopathy

Congenital myopathy in children is often associated with selective type 1 fiber atrophy. This finding is less common in congenital myopathies identified thus far in animals. Selective type 1 atrophy is, however, a feature

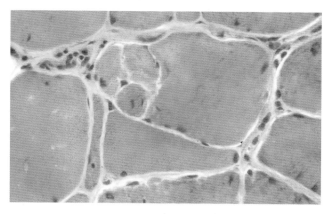

Fig. 15-26 **Fiber type splitting of hypertrophied myofibers, nemaline myopathy, skeletal muscle, transverse section, cat.** Sarcolemmal ingrowth into the myofiber has resulted in multiple partitions with the formation of four myofibers; however, all myofibers are enclosed by one basal lamina. Frozen section, modified Gomori's trichrome stain. (*Courtesy Dr. B.A. Valentine, College of Veterinary Medicine, Oregon State University.*)

of feline nemaline myopathy, an animal model of congenital nemaline myopathy in children.

HYPERTROPHY

Myofibers are increased in diameter by the addition of myofilaments. Physiologic hypertrophy is the normal process of myofiber enlargement that occurs with exercise conditioning. Compensatory hypertrophy occurs because of pathologic conditions that (1) decrease the number of functional myofibers or (2) interfere with normal cellular metabolic or other physiologic processes. Compensatory myofiber hypertrophy is therefore considered a relatively nonspecific response to a variety of insults. Fibers undergoing compensatory hypertrophy can enlarge to more than 100 μm in diameter (normal is less than approximately 60 to 70 μm). Fiber hypertrophy often accompanies fiber atrophy, which contributes to increased fiber-size variation in various myopathic and neuropathic conditions.

Compensatory hypertrophy can occur because of a decrease in the number of functional myofibers. Thus, in a partially denervated muscle, the remaining innervated fibers hypertrophy (Fig. 15-23, *B*), presumably as a result of increased workload. Pathologically hypertrophied fibers will have less oxygen diffusion from interstitial capillaries to internal portions of the myofiber, which can lead to myofiber damage. Mechanical overloading of hypertrophied muscle fibers is also possible. Overloading of hypertrophied fibers can result in segmental necrosis (Fig. 15-23, *B*), or fibers can undergo longitudinal fiber splitting to generate one or more smaller-diameter fragments, all contained within the same basal lamina (Fig. 15-26). Serial sections of areas of fiber splitting

common in animals than in human beings. Fiber-type grouping and type-specific group atrophy can only be detected by methods that distinguish fiber types. Changes occurring as a result of denervation and reinnervation are illustrated in Fig. 15-25.

generally reveals that splits do not extend the entire length of the myofiber. Fiber splitting is considered a form of cytoarchitectural alteration (see later discussion).

CYTOARCHITECTURAL CHANGES

In addition to fiber splitting, a variety of other cytoarchitectural changes can occur within myofibers. Some are degenerative, reflecting an insult that is damaging to the myofiber but that does not culminate in necrosis. Others reflect underlying ultrastructural alterations that may be either pathologic or compensatory in nature. The functional significance of many of the myofiber cytoarchitectural changes is not known.

VACUOLAR CHANGE

Vacuolar change is a common cytoplasmic alteration. In routinely processed muscle samples, or in any sample subjected to less than ideal handling, true vacuolar change can be very difficult to distinguish from artifact. Vacuoles can be an early manifestation of processes leading to necrosis, they can reflect underlying sarcotubular dilation, as occurs in many myotonic conditions (see later discussion), they can be caused by abnormal storage of carbohydrate or lipid, or they can reflect underlying myofibrillar abnormalities. Additional studies are often necessary to determine the cause of vacuolar change. When severe, such as in glycogen storage diseases, the term "vacuolar myopathy" is often employed.

INTERNAL NUCLEI

Myonuclei of mature myofibers are found peripherally, just below the sarcolemma. Nuclei located one nuclear diameter or more from the sarcolemma are known as internal nuclei. (Note: The term "central nuclei" is considered incorrect because few abnormally placed nuclei are exactly centrally located.) Internal nuclei are rare in normal mammalian muscle, but a small percentage can be found normally in avian and reptilian species. Rows of internal nuclei in small-diameter, slightly basophilic myofibers are characteristic of the myotubular stage of regeneration (Fig. 15-18, *B* and *C*). In most species, peripheralization of myonuclei occurs early in regeneration, within days of myotube formation. Rodents are the exception. In rodents, internal nuclei are retained following regeneration, which provides a handy marker for fibers that have undergone necrosis and regeneration in studies using these species. In other mammalian species, the presence of internal nuclei in normal or hypertrophied fibers is a nonspecific finding indicative of chronic myopathic change (Fig. 15-27; Box 15-6). In hypertrophied fibers, the migration of myonuclei to the internal portion of the myofiber can precede the sarcolemmal infolding that creates fiber splitting.

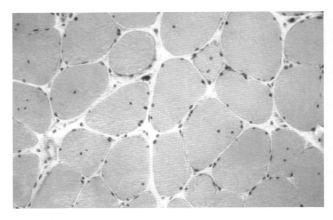

Fig. 15-27   Chronic myopathic change, medial triceps muscle, horse. The variation in myofiber diameter and the presence of one or more internal nuclei in most myofibers are indicative of a chronic myopathic change. Frozen section, H&E stain. *(Courtesy Dr. B.A. Valentine, College of Veterinary Medicine, Oregon State University.)*

WHORLED AND RING FIBERS

The cytoarchitectural rearrangements resulting in whorled and ring fibers are best appreciated on transverse sections. Whorled fibers contain spirals of cytoplasm with internally located nuclei. Whorled fibers can be seen in areas of chronic denervation, and also in areas in which myofiber necrosis with incomplete regeneration has occurred. Ring fibers (also known as "ringbinden") contain a peripheral rim of sarcomeres oriented perpendicular to their normal orientation, resulting in peripheral radiating striations. Ring fibers are visible with many stains, both in frozen sections and in routinely processed sections. In either frozen or routine sections, they are best visualized in sections stained with PAS (Fig. 15-28, *A*). In human beings, ring fibers are common in a specific form of inherited muscular dystrophy known as myotonic dystrophy, but they are also seen in other myopathic and in neuropathic conditions and therefore are not specific for myotonic dystrophy. Similarly, there is no animal disorder in which ring fibers are specific, and these fibers can be seen in a variety of myopathic and neuropathic conditions. The presence of ring fibers can only be considered a chronic myopathic change. For example, in muscle studied from a horse with long-standing, non–weight-bearing foreleg lameness, numerous ring fibers were found in muscle from the weight-bearing limb.

OTHER CYTOARCHITECTURAL CHANGES

Many other cytoarchitectural changes reflect alterations in mitochondrial density or integrity and are best appreciated on examination of frozen sections, in which mitochondria can be visualized, or on ultrastructural examination. The presence of peripheral aggregates of mitochondria that stain red with modified Gomori's trichrome stain form the basis of what are called "ragged red" fibers. Ragged red fibers are a hallmark of mitochondrial myopathy in human beings. In animals, however, ragged red fibers are common in various myopathic conditions, and fibers that would be considered to be ragged red fibers occur in normal dog and horse muscle. Mitochondrial abnormalities are also detected with oxidative enzyme reactions, such as NADH (Fig. 15-28, *B*) and SDH. Nemaline rods, formed by expansions of the Z-line material, stain purple to red with modified Gomori's trichrome stain on frozen sections. These rods can also be seen in animals with other myopathic conditions. Moth-eaten fibers contain multiple pale zones because of loss of mitochondrial oxidative enzyme activity on frozen sections, and occur in denervating disorders and in myopathic conditions (Fig. 15-28, *C*). Sarcoplasmic masses are pale-staining zones at the periphery of myofibers. These can be seen in routinely stained muscle sections. Ultrastructurally, they often contain disarrayed myofilaments with or without degenerate mitochondria. Other less commonly encountered alterations in animal muscle are pale central cores visible with mitochondrial stains, tubular aggregates composed of sarcotubular membranes, and target fibers in which mitochondrial oxidative enzyme reactions reveal central clear zones surrounded by a thin rim of highly reactive cytoplasm.

CHRONIC MYOPATHIC CHANGE

Evaluation of abnormal skeletal muscle often reveals what is known as chronic myopathic change, which includes alterations in fiber size, cytoarchitectural alterations, fibrosis, and fat infiltration (Box 15-6). Chronic myopathic change will accompany a variety of myopathic and neuropathic conditions. In some cases, particularly severe cases, a definitive cause cannot be identified. Chronic inflammation or denervation and chronic degenerative myopathy resulting in repeated bouts of myonecrosis and regeneration often cause diffuse endomysial and perimysial fibrosis (Figs. 15-23, *B* and 15-52, *B*). Interstitial infiltration of muscle by mature adipocytes is less common than fibrosis and occurs most commonly in chronically denervated muscle (Fig. 15-23, *B*), particularly neonatal muscle that lacks appropriate innervation (Fig. 15-29). Fat infiltration can also occur because of severe chronic degenerative myopathy. A chronically damaged or denervated muscle that develops profound fibrosis and/or fat infiltration can be grossly enlarged despite atrophy or loss of myofibers—a condition known as pseudohypertrophy (Fig. 15-11, *D*).

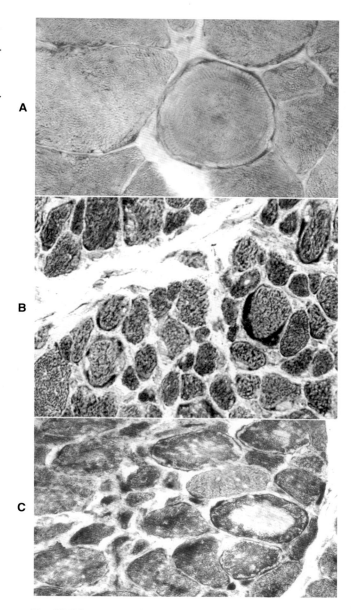

Fig. 15-28   Cytoarchitectural changes, skeletal muscle, transverse sections. A, Ring fiber, extensor carpi radialis muscle, horse. A ring fiber is characterized by a peripheral rim of sarcomeres, arranged circumferentially around a myofiber and with their length at right angles to the long axis of the myofiber. Frozen section, PAS reaction. **B,** Irregular mitochondrial distribution with peripheral aggregates of mitochondria, Labrador myopathy, temporalis muscle, dog. Frozen section, NADH reaction. **C,** Irregularity of mitochondrial distribution and "moth-eaten" fibers, polyneuropathy, dog. Fibers containing pale zones are characteristic of moth-eaten fibers. Frozen section, NADH reaction. (*A, B, and C, Courtesy Dr. B.A. Valentine, College of Veterinary Medicine, Oregon State University.*)

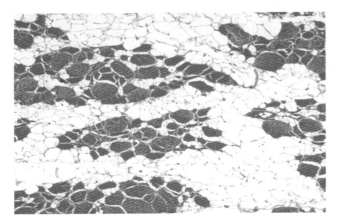

Fig. 15-29   Lipomatosis (steatosis), calf. Lost myocytes have been replaced by mature adipocytes. Islands of remaining myofibers have groups of angular atrophied fibers admixed with hypertrophied fibers, suggestive of denervation atrophy. Formalin fixation, H&E stain. *(Courtesy Dr. M.D. McGavin, College of Veterinary Medicine, University of Tennessee.)*

DISEASES OF MUSCLE

TYPES OF MUSCLE DISEASE

Classification of muscle diseases based on lesions alone is not very satisfactory, and many classifications are based on cause (e.g., toxic myopathy or nutritional myopathy). An example of such a classification is given in Table 15-3. Myopathic conditions can be inherited or acquired. Inherited disorders can affect muscle metabolism or myofiber structure. Acquired muscle disease in livestock is often associated with nutritional deficiency or to ingestion of myotoxins, whereas acquired muscle disease in the dog is most often caused by immune-mediated inflammatory conditions. Other causes of acquired myopathies include ischemia, infectious agents, hormonal or electrolyte abnormalities, and trauma. There are also many neuropathic conditions that result in denervation atrophy (see peripheral nerve discussion). More information on most of the disorders described in this section can also be found under the appropriate species heading or in Appendix 15-1.

DEGENERATIVE

Degenerative myopathies are those resulting in segmental or global myofiber necrosis in which inflammatory cells are not the cause of the myofiber damage.

DISTURBANCE OF CIRCULATION

Given the numerous capillary anastomosis and rich collateral circulation of skeletal muscle, only disorders that result in occlusion of a major artery or that cause widespread intramuscular vascular damage will result in myofiber necrosis (Box 15-8). Vascular occlusion of a major artery, most often aortoiliac thrombosis, occurs

Table **15-3**   **Classification of Muscle Disease**

Classification	Cause or Type of Disorder
Degenerative	Ischemia
	Nutritional
	Toxic
	Exertional
	Traumatic
Inflammatory	Bacterial
	Viral
	Parasitic
	Immune-mediated
Congenital and/or inherited	Anatomic defects
	Muscular dystrophy
	Congenital myopathy
	Myotonia
	Metabolic
	Malignant hyperthermia
Endocrine	Hypothyroidism
	Hypercortisolism
Electrolyte	Hypokalemia
	Hypernatremia
	Other electrolyte imbalances
Neuropathic	Peripheral neuropathy
	Motor neuronopathy
Neuromuscular junction disorders	Myasthenia gravis
	Botulism
	Tick paralysis
Neoplasia	Primary tumors (rhabdomyoma, rhabdomyosarcoma)
	Secondary tumors (hemangiosarcoma, fibrosarcoma, infiltrative lipoma, other tumor phenotypes)
	Metastatic tumors

most commonly in cats (thromboembolism) and horses (mural thrombosis). Intramuscular vascular damage occurs in many species, and there are a variety of causes.

The basic factor in determining the effect of ischemia on muscle is the differential susceptibility of the various cells forming the muscle as a whole. Myofibers are the most sensitive, satellite cells less sensitive, and fibroblasts the least sensitive to anoxia. Thus obstruction of the blood supply to an area of muscle leads first to myofiber necrosis, then to death of satellite cells, and finally to the death of all cells, including the

Box **15-8**

Causes of Muscle Ischemia

1. Occlusion of a major blood vessel
2. External pressure on a muscle
3. Swelling of a muscle in a nonexpandible compartment ("compartment syndrome")
4. Vasculitis/vasculopathy

stromal cells. The size of skeletal muscle infarcts depends on the size of the vessel obstructed and the duration of blockage. Blockage of capillaries causes segmental necrosis, which is usually multifocal and, if the cause is ongoing, polyphasic. However, when larger arteries are blocked, whole areas of muscle, including the satellite cells, are killed, resulting in a monophasic necrosis and healing by fibrosis. Ischemia can also cause peripheral nerve damage and neuropathy, leading to denervation atrophy of intact fibers.

Increased intramuscular pressure can occur in a recumbent animal of sufficient weight after a prolonged period of recumbency, either because of disease or general anesthesia. Myofiber necrosis due to recumbency can occur because of (1) decreased blood flow as a result of compression of major arteries, (2) reperfusion injury causing massive calcium influx into muscle cells when the animal moves or is moved and the compression relieved, (3) increased intramuscular pressure causing compartment syndrome, or (4) any combination of these factors. Localized myonecrosis due to recumbency is common in horses, cattle, and pigs; occurs only in large breeds of dogs; and is virtually unheard of in cats. In downer cows, the weight of the body of the animal in sternal recumbency can cause ischemia of the pectoral muscles and of any muscles of the forelimbs or hindlimbs that are tucked under the body. Ewes in advanced pregnancy with twins or triplets can develop an ischemic necrosis of the internal abdominal oblique muscle, which can lead to muscle rupture. Plaster casts or bandages that are too tight can put external pressure on muscles, leading to ischemia. The duration of ischemia determines the severity of necrosis and the success of regeneration (see Necrosis and Regeneration). Postanesthesic myopathy is a monophasic, multifocal necrosis. In the downer cow, the lesions are multifocal to locally extensive (Fig. 15-30) and, depending on the duration, can be either monophasic or polyphasic.

Any severe insult, whether it be ischemia caused by recumbency or another myodegenerative disorder, that causes myonecrosis within a muscle that is covered by a tight and nonexpansible fascia can result in ischemic injury because early in the necrosis there is increased intramuscular pressure. The resulting compromise of blood circulation leads to ischemic myodegeneration, known as compartment syndrome. The phenomenon of compartment syndrome is best illustrated in the anterior tibial muscle of human beings following strenuous exercise. This condition is believed to be a consequence of swelling of the anterior tibial muscle, which is surrounded anteriorly by the inelastic anterior fascial sheath and posteriorly by the tibia. Swelling impedes blood supply, resulting in ischemia. A similar phenomenon occurs in muscles surrounded by tight fascia in animals, particularly horses. Horses that are recumbent because of general anesthesia can develop

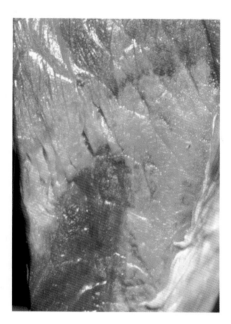

Fig. 15-30   Ischemic necrosis, downer cow syndrome, pectoral muscle, cow. Increased intramuscular pressure during prolonged periods of recumbency has resulted in localized muscle pallor from myofiber necrosis secondary to decreased blood flow caused by compression of arteries. *(Courtesy Dr. M.D. McGavin, College of Veterinary Medicine, University of Tennessee.)*

compartment syndrome affecting gluteal or lateral triceps muscles. Horses can also develop compartment syndrome in gluteal muscles because of exertional rhabdomyolysis, and in temporal and masseter muscles because of selenium deficiency. Compartment syndrome is also possible in the temporal and masseter muscles of dogs with masticatory myositis.

Damage to intramuscular blood vessels will also cause myofiber necrosis. Vasculitis can cause areas of muscle damage (e.g., in horses with immune-mediated purpura hemorrhagica because of *Streptococcus equi* infection [Fig. 15-37] and in pigs with erysipelas). Viral diseases that target blood vessels of many organs, such as bluetongue, can also affect muscle. Exotoxins produced by clostridial organisms cause myositis and severe localized vascular damage, leading to hemorrhage and myofiber necrosis (Table 15-4). The familial myopathy of Gelbvieh cattle is characterized by fibrinoid necrosis of intramuscular blood vessels and associated myonecrosis.

NUTRITIONAL DEFICIENCY

Myofibers are particularly sensitive to nutritional deficiencies that result in loss of antioxidant defense mechanisms. Nutritional myopathies are most common in livestock, including cattle, horses, sheep, and goats (Table 15-5). Although nutritional myopathy of livestock is often referred to as selenium/vitamin E deficiency, in the vast majority of cases it is deficiency

Table **15-4**   **Clostridial Toxins Causing Muscle Damage**

Toxin	Type	Action
α-Toxin	Calcium-dependent phospholipase	Hydrolyzes membrane phospholipids
θ-Toxin	Oxygen-labile cytotoxin (perfringolysin-O)	RBC and WBC lysis
		Induces platelet-activating factor leading to leukostasis and decreased tissue perfusion
κ-Toxin	Collagenase	Contributes to tissue lysis
μ-Toxin, γ- toxin	Hyaluronidases	Disruption of muscle integrity
ε-Toxin	Lipase	Lipid membrane lysis

RBC, Red blood cell; *WBC,* white blood cell.

of selenium that is the cause of myofiber degeneration. The trace mineral selenium is a vital component of the glutathione peroxidase system, which helps to protect cells from oxidative injury. The high oxygen requirement combined with contractile activity makes striated muscle, both skeletal and cardiac, particularly sensitive to oxidative injury. Neonatal animals, which rely on stores of selenium accumulated during gestation, are most often affected. Affected muscle is pale as a result of necrosis (Fig. 15-44); hence the common name white muscle disease. As should be evident from the previous discussion, a gross observation of pale muscle is not specific for necrosis caused by nutritional deficiency; therefore the term nutritional myopathy is much preferred.

TOXIC MYOPATHIES

Here again, livestock are the animals most prone to develop a degenerative myopathy from the ingestion of a toxin (Table 15-5). Myotoxins can be present in plants in pastures or hay, and in plants or plant products in processed feed. Examples of toxic plants and plant products include *Cassia* (coffee senna), *Karwinskia*

(coyotillo), *Eupatorium* (white snakeroot), *Thermopsis* spp., and gossypol present in cottonseed. Clinical signs are weakness, often leading to recumbency, and are accompanied by a moderate to severe increase in serum muscle enzyme concentrations. Gross and histologic findings of multifocal necrosis that can be either monophasic or polyphasic are typical. Diagnosis is based on identification of causative plants within feed, pasture, or stomach contents or, when available, detection of toxic compounds in stomach content or liver.

Ionophore antibiotics such as monensin, lasalocid, maduramicin, and narasin are often added to ruminant feeds to enhance growth. Ionophores form lipid soluble dipolar reversible complexes with cations and allow movement of cations across cell membranes, often against the concentration gradient. This causes a disruption of ionic equilibrium that can be detrimental, especially to excitable tissue such as the nervous system, heart, and skeletal muscle. Ionophore toxicity results in calcium overload and death of skeletal (Figs. 15-16, *B* and 15-38) and cardiac muscle. Most domestic ruminants are quite tolerant of moderate ionophore levels, but toxicity occurs at very high levels. Most cases of ionophore toxicity involve monensin. The LD_{50} (the dose at which 50% of animals die) of monensin in cattle is 50 to 80 mg/kg and for sheep and goats is 12 to 24 mg/kg. Horses are exquisitely sensitive to ionophores and even very low levels are toxic, with an LD_{50} for monensin of only 2 to 3 mg/kg of body weight.

EXERTIONAL MYOPATHIES

The ionic and physical events associated with myofiber contraction can, under certain circumstances, predispose a myofiber to necrosis. Exercise-induced myonecrosis, which can be massive, can occur because of simple overexertion. This outcome is well known in the capture and restraint of nondomesticated species, a syndrome known as capture myopathy. More often, however, exercise-induced myofiber damage occurs in animals with preexisting conditions such as selenium deficiency, muscular dystrophy, severe electrolyte depletion, or glycogen storage disease. The term "exertional

Table **15-5**   **Nutritional and Toxic Myopathies**

Disorder	Species Affected	Cause
Nutritional myopathy	Horses, cattle, sheep, goats, camelids, pigs	Selenium or (less commonly) vitamin E deficiency
Ionophore toxicity	Horses, cattle, sheep, goats, pigs	Monensin, other ionophores used as feed additives
Plant toxicity	Horses, cattle, sheep, goats, pigs	*Cassia occidentalis,* other toxic plants; gossypol in cottonseed products
Pasture-associated myopathy (United Kingdom)	Horses	Unknown

rhabdomyolysis" (also known as exertional myopathy, azoturia, setfast, blackwater, Monday morning disease, and tying up) has long been applied to a syndrome recognized in horses (Fig. 15-40). Only recently have underlying myopathic conditions been identified as the most common predisposing cause of equine exertional rhabdomyolysis (see Muscular Disorders of the Horse). A similar disorder affects working dogs, such as racing sled dogs and greyhounds, the cause of which is still unclear.

TRAUMA

External trauma to muscle includes crush injury, lacerations and surgical incisions, tearing due to excessive stretching or exercise, burns, gunshot and arrow wounds, and certain injections. Some of these result in complete or partial rupture of large muscles. The diaphragm is the most common muscle to rupture and in dogs and cats is most often due to sudden increase in intraabdominal pressure, such as from being hit by a car. In horses, diaphragmatic rupture is thought to occur most often during falls in which the pressure of the abdominal viscera causes diaphragmatic damage. A partial rupture of a muscle results in a tear in the fascial sheath, through which the muscle can herniate during contraction. In racing greyhounds, spontaneous rupture of muscles, such as the longissimus, quadriceps, biceps femoris, gracilis, triceps brachii, and gastrocnemius can occur during strenuous exercise. In horses, damage to the origin of the gastrocnemius muscle has been linked to overexertion during exercise or while struggling to rise. Tearing of muscle fibers occurs in the adductor muscles of cattle doing the "splits" on a slippery floor. Because there is often extensive disruption of the myofibers' basal laminae, most of the healing is accomplished by fibrosis. If muscle trauma is accompanied by fractures of bones, and the animal moves the limb, this can result in further trauma because of laceration by sharp bone fragments.

An abnormal response to localized muscle trauma is thought to be a possible underlying cause of two uncommon reactions of muscle: myositis ossificans and musculoaponeurotic fibromatosis. The term *myositis ossificans* is a misnomer, as the lesion does not involve inflammation, but it has attained the status of acceptance by common usage. Myositis ossificans is a focal lesion usually confined to a single muscle and has been seen in horses, dogs, and human beings. The lesion is essentially a focal zone of fibrosis with osseous metaplasia, often with a zonal pattern. The central zone contains proliferating undifferentiated cells and fibroblasts; the middle one, osteoblast depositing osteoid and immature bone; and the outer one, trabecular bone, which may be being remodeled by osteoclasts. These lesions can cause pain and lameness but are often cured by surgical excision. A connective tissue

disorder in cats, fibrodysplasia ossificans progressiva, has been inappropriately called myositis ossificans. Musculoaponeurotic fibromatosis has so far been described only in horses and human beings. It is a progressive intramuscular fibromatosis that has also been called a desmoid tumor. Musculoaponeurotic fibromatosis is not, however, considered to be a true neoplastic process. Progressive dissecting intramuscular fibrosis accompanied by myofiber atrophy are the characteristic features. In most cases, the extent of intramuscular involvement makes surgical excision impossible, although wide excision of early lesions has proven to be curative.

INFLAMMATORY MYOPATHIES (MYOSITIS, MYOSITIDES [PLURAL])

In addition to the misnomer "myositis ossificans," the term "myositis" has been inappropriately applied to various other veterinary disorders, such as exertional and nutritional myopathy in the horse. These two disorders are degenerative myopathies, not inflammatory myopathies. It is vitally important to distinguish between a true myositis and a degenerative myopathy in which there is a secondary inflammatory response. In the normal response to the necrosis, the necrotic segment is infiltrated by macrophages recruited from the circulating monocyte population (Figs. 15-17, *B* and 15-18, *A*), which phagocytose the cellular debris. Severe acute necrotizing myopathy can also be accompanied by a certain degree of infiltrating lymphocytes, plasma cells, neutrophils, and eosinophils. Cytokines released from damaged muscle fibers are likely to recruit a variety of inflammatory cells under various circumstances, but these cells are not involved in the muscle cell damage. True myositis occurs only when inflammatory cells are directly responsible for initiating and maintaining myofiber injury, and when inflammation is directed at the myofibers and not at the stroma. In some cases, it may take careful evaluation of the overall tissue changes, an understanding of the probable underlying cause, and years of experience with muscle pathology to distinguish a florid cellular response with macrophages on a "clean-up" mission from true inflammation. Lymphocytic myositis must also be distinguished from lymphoma involving skeletal muscle (see Neoplasia).

BACTERIAL

Bacterial infections of muscle are not uncommon, particularly in livestock. Bacteria can cause suppurative and necrotizing, suppurative and fibrosing, hemorrhagic, or granulomatous lesions (Table 15-6). Bacterial infection can be introduced by direct penetration (wounds or injections), hematogenously, or by spread from an adjacent cellulitis, fasciitis, tendonitis, arthritis, or osteomyelitis (see Portals of Entry).

Table **15-6**   **Bacterial Myopathies**

Infectious Agent	Species Affected
Clostridium spp. causing myositis	Horses, cattle, sheep, goats, pigs
Clostridium botulinum	Horses, cattle, sheep, goats, dogs
Pyogenic bacteria	Horses, cattle, sheep, goats, pigs, cats
Agents causing fibrosing and granulomatous lesions	Cattle, sheep, goats, pigs

Table **15-7**   **Viral Myopathies**

	RNA VIRUSES	
Disease	**Family**	**Causal Agent**
Porcine encephalomyelitis	Picornaviridae	Enterovirus
Foot-and-mouth disease	Picornaviridae	Aphthovirus
Bluetongue	Reoviridae	Orbivirus
Akabane disease	Bunyaviridae	Akabane virus

Various clostridial species, particularly *Clostridium perfringens*, *Clostridium chauvoei*, *Clostridium septicum*, and *Clostridium novyi*, can elaborate toxins (Table 15-4) that damage myofibers and intramuscular vasculature, resulting in hemorrhagic myonecrosis (Figs. 15-36 and 15-42). Toxemia is typical and is often lethal. Clostridial myositis is most common in cattle and horses. Clostridial myositis has also been called gas gangrene and malignant edema in horses and blackleg in cattle.

Pyogenic bacteria introduced into a muscle usually cause localized suppuration and myofiber necrosis. This may resolve completely or become localized to form an abscess. In some cases, the infection can spread down the fascial planes (Fig. 15-15). For example, a nonsterile intramuscular injection into the gluteal muscles of cattle can cause an infection that extends down the fascial planes of the muscles of the femur and tibia and erupts to the surface through a sinus proximal to the tarsus. Although the majority of inflammation involves fascial planes, some bacteria extend into and cause necrosis of adjacent muscle fasciculi. *Streptococcus zooepidemicus* (horses), *Arcanobacterium pyogenes* (cattle and sheep), and *Corynebacterium pseudotuberculosis* (horses, sheep, and goats) are common causes of muscle abscesses. After bite wounds, cats can develop cellulitis caused by *Pasteurella multocida* that extends into the adjacent muscle.

Bacteria causing single or multiple granulomas (focal or multifocal granulomatous myositis) are relatively uncommon. Most such lesions are caused by *Mycobacterium bovis* (tuberculosis), usually in cattle and pigs, but this is rare in North America.

Chronic fibrosing nodular myositis of the tongue musculature in cattle is the result of infection with *Actinobacillus lignieresii* (wooden tongue) or *Actinomyces bovis* (the agent causing lumpy jaw). A similar lesion caused by *Staphylococcus aureus* and known as botryomycosis is most commonly seen in horses and pigs. It is most often wound related and can occur at a variety of sites. Histologically, actinobacillosis, actinomycosis, and botryomycosis are similar in that the lesions are encapsulated inflammatory lesions containing a central focus of "radiating clubs" of amorphous eosinophilic material associated with bacteria and neutrophils (Splendore-Hoeppli reaction). Neutrophils admixed with macrophages (pyogranulomatous inflammation) can also be seen. Gram stained tissue can differentiate the clusters of gram-positive cocci in *Staphylococcus* infection, the gram-positive bacilli causing actinomycosis (*Actinomyces bovis*), and the gram-negative bacilli causing actinobacillosis (*Actinobacillus lignieresii*).

VIRAL

Relatively few of these are recognized in veterinary medicine. Spontaneous ones are listed in Table 15-7. Gross lesions may or may not be visible and, if present, are small, poorly defined foci or streaks. Muscle lesions induced by viruses are either infarcts secondary to a vasculitis, as seen in bluetongue in sheep, or multifocal necrosis, presumably because of a direct effect of the virus on the myofibers.

PARASITIC

Parasitic infections of the skeletal muscles of domestic animals are not uncommon and include protozoal organisms and nematodes. The most important ones are listed in Table 15-8 and are discussed under the appropriate species heading. Most parasitic diseases are of little pathologic or economic importance, with the exception of *Neospora caninum*, *Hepatozoon americanus*, and *Trypanosoma cruzi* in dogs, and *Trichinella spiralis* in pigs.

Table **15-8**   **Parasitic Myopathies**

Infectious Agent	Species Affected
Sarcocystis spp.	Horses, cattle, sheep, goats, camelids, pigs
Trichinella spiralis	Pigs
Neospora caninum	Dogs, fetal cattle
Trypanosoma cruzi	Dogs
Cysticercus spp.	Cattle, sheep, goats, pigs
Nematode larval migrans	Dogs
Hepatozoon americanum	Dogs

As the name *Sarcocystis* suggests, intramyofiber protozoal cysts caused by *Sarcocystis* spp. are a common finding. This protozoal organism is a stage of an intestinal coccidium of carnivores that uses birds, reptiles, rodents, pigs, and herbivores as an intermediate host. Ingestion of oocysts by an intermediate host releases sporozoites that invade tissue, including muscle. This parasite rarely causes clinical disease and is therefore most often considered an incidental finding. *Sarcocystis* infection of muscle is seen most often in horses, cattle, and small ruminants and occasionally in cats. Because they are intracellular, cysts are protected from the host's defense mechanisms; thus there is no inflammatory response (Fig. 15-31).

IMMUNE-MEDIATED

Immunologically induced myositis, not associated with vascular injury, has to-date been recognized primarily in the dog. Rarely, immune-mediated myositis occurs in cats and horses. Infiltrating lymphocytes, most often cytotoxic T lymphocytes, are the cause of myofiber injury. Although cytotoxic T lymphocytes are the effector cells causing myofiber damage, the inflammatory infiltrate will be a mixture of lymphocyte types. The characteristic histologic pattern of immune-mediated myositis is an interstitial and perivascular lymphocytic infiltration (Fig. 15-32, *A*; Fig. 15-52), often with invasion of intact myofibers by lymphocytes (Fig. 15-32, *B*). A variety of forms of immune-mediated myositis occur in the dog and can be localized to specific muscles because of proven or suspected unique myosin isoforms within those muscles. These are listed in Table 15-9. Acquired myasthenia gravis is also an immune-mediated disease included in this table for

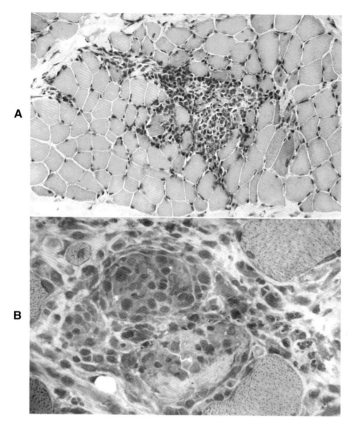

Fig. 15-32   Immune-mediated myositis, canine polymyositis, skeletal muscle, transverse sections, dog. A, There is a dense interstitial infiltrate of primarily mononuclear inflammatory cells. Formalin fixation, H&E stain. **B,** Note the interstitial infiltrate of mononuclear inflammatory cells and mononuclear cells that have invaded an intact myofibers causing myofiber necrosis. Frozen section, modified Gomori's trichrome stain. (**A,** *Courtesy Dr. M.D. McGavin, College of Veterinary Medicine, University of Tennessee.* **B,** *Courtesy Dr. B.J. Cooper, College of Veterinary Medicine, Oregon State University.*)

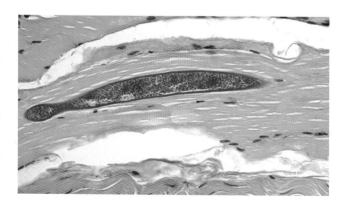

Fig. 15-31   Sarcocystosis, skeletal muscle, longitudinal section, cow. The elongate encysted intramyofiber protozoan is characteristic of *Sarcocystis* spp. There is no associated inflammation. These parasites are common in the muscles of many species of domestic animals and are usually an incidental finding. Formalin fixation, H&E stain. (*Courtesy Dr. M.D. McGavin, College of Veterinary Medicine, University of Tennessee.*)

completeness, but this is a disorder causing damage to the neuromuscular junction rather than to myofibers. In cats, feline immunodeficiency virus infection is a cause of immune-mediated myositis. In horses, lesions consistent with immune-mediated myositis are occasionally found following exposure to *Streptococcus equi* ssp. *equi*

Table **15-9   Immune-Mediated Muscle Disorders**

Disorder	Species Affected
Purpura hemorrhagica	Horses
Viral-associated	Horses, cats
Polymyositis	Dogs
Masticatory myositis	Dogs
Extraocular muscle myositis	Dogs
Acquired myasthenia gravis	Dogs, cats

or infection with equine influenza virus. It should be pointed out that small perivascular and interstitial infiltrates of lymphocytes, with no apparent myofiber damage, are a frequent incidental finding in equine muscle.

Immune-mediated vasculitis resulting in muscle injury occurs in horses and is known as purpura hemorrhagica. Purpura hemorrhagica has been classically associated with *Streptococcus equi* ssp. *equi*, but other bacteria such as *Corynebacterium pseudotuberculosis* can also cause purpura hemorrhagica.

CONGENITAL AND INHERITED DISORDERS

Muscle is subject to numerous hereditary, congenital, and neonatal defects (Table 15-10). Muscular disorders that are apparent at birth are congenital, but they may or may not be inherited. Inherited disorders can manifest at birth or soon thereafter, or they may not be apparent for many years. Molecular biologic studies and development of molecular genetic tests have greatly enhanced our understanding of several muscular disorders of animals and the ability to detect affected and carrier animals.

ANATOMIC DEFECTS

Anatomic defects in skeletal muscle are apparent at birth or soon thereafter. These defects can be either genetic or acquired and result from either abnormal muscle development or abnormal innervation.

Innervation defects

Congenital defects in the lower motor neuron system, involving motor neurons or peripheral nerves, will result in severe alteration of myofiber development. Denervation occurring in fetal and neonatal animals can result in very complex muscle lesions because of the importance of innervation in myofiber development and maturation. Depending on the nature of the nervous system defect, muscular lesions can reflect failure of innervation, denervation of previously innervated fibers, or a combination of both. The most common example of this is arthrogryposis in cattle and sheep in which in utero infection or toxin ingestion causes central and/or peripheral nervous system lesions leading to failure of innervation or to denervation of skeletal muscle. Failure of innervation or severe denervation injury in utero most often result in failure of the myofibers to develop and their subsequent replacement by adipose tissue (fatty infiltration). This outcome can be severe in affected muscle and may be the basis for some cases of congenital muscular steatosis in livestock (Figs. 15-11, *D* and 15-29).

Table **15-10**   **Confirmed or Suspected Inherited Myopathies in Animals**

Disorder	Species Affected	Inheritance
Muscular hyperplasia	Cattle	Autosomal recessive
Myotonia	Horses	Unknown
	Goats	Autosomal dominant
	Dogs	Autosomal recessive
	Cats	Unknown
HYPP	Horses	Autosomal dominant?
Glycogenoses	Horses	Autosomal recessive (glycogen brancher enzyme defect)
		Autosomal dominant (polysaccharide storage myopathy)
	Cattle	Autosomal recessive
	Sheep	Autosomal recessive
	Dogs	Autosomal recessive
	Cats	Autosomal recessive
Mitochondrial myopathy	Horses, dogs	Unknown
Duchenne's type muscular dystrophy	Dogs, cats	X-linked
Inherited myopathy ("muscular dystrophy")	Cattle, sheep	Autosomal recessive
Sarcoglycans deficient muscular dystrophy	Dogs	Autosomal recessive?
Malignant hyperthermia	Horses	Unknown
	Pigs	Autosomal recessive
	Dogs	Autosomal dominant
Labrador myopathy	Dogs	Autosomal recessive
Congenital myasthenia gravis	Dogs	Autosomal recessive
	Cats	Autosomal recessive?

HYPP, Hyperkalemic periodic paralysis.
Question marks denote that inheritance pattern is suspected but not proven.

Genetic defects

The only genetic defect recognized as causing congenital anatomic defects in animals is congenital muscular hyperplasia (double muscling) in cattle. It is possible that with continued selective breeding and advancement in molecular biologic techniques, other defects may occur or be recognized.

Failure of normal development

In addition to failure of myofiber maturation due to innervation defects, inherent myofibrillar developmental defects can occur. This is exemplified by myofibrillar hypoplasia causing splayleg in neonatal pigs. A similar condition has been reported in a calf.

Congenital defects in the diaphragmatic muscle (diaphragmatic hernia) can occur in all species but are most well documented in dogs and rabbits. A genetic basis with a multifactor inheritance is suspected. Clinical signs of respiratory distress due to herniation of abdominal viscera into the thoracic cavity generally occur at or shortly after birth. Defects in the left dorsolateral and central portions of the diaphragm because of failure of closure of the left pleuroperitoneal canal are most common.

MUSCULAR DYSTROPHY

The term "muscular dystrophy" has been grossly misused in the veterinary literature. In the 1930s, the term "nutritional muscular dystrophy" was applied to a disease more appropriately classified as nutritional myopathy, and the misuse of this term has been a source of confusion for years as to exactly what is meant by muscular dystrophy. Following the definition applied to human beings, muscular dystrophy is an inherited, progressive, degenerative primary disease of the myofiber characterized histologically by ongoing myofiber necrosis and regeneration (polyphasic necrosis). Several types of muscular dystrophy occur in human beings and animals. The enormous recent advances in genetic and molecular characterization of muscle diseases have resulted in defining their exact genetic defects, such as those in the dystrophin gene responsible for Duchenne's muscular dystrophy and trinucleotide repeat sequences in myotonic dystrophy, and in the reclassification of others. Similarly, reevaluation of some inherited disorders previously classified as muscular dystrophy, such as muscular dystrophy in sheep and cattle, suggests that they would be better classified as progressive congenital myopathies.

CONGENITAL MYOPATHIES

Those inherited disorders of muscle that do not qualify as anatomic defects, muscular dystrophy, myotonia, or metabolic myopathy (see later discussion) are classified as congenital myopathies. These include structural defects leading to abnormal myofiber cytoarchitecture. In some cases, a specific gene defect is known, whereas the cause of others remains undetermined.

MYOTONIA (CHANNELOPATHIES)

Myotonia is defined as the inability of skeletal muscle fibers to relax, resulting in spasmodic contraction. Various inherited myotonic conditions have been recognized in human beings and animals for many years. Only recently has the basis for many of these myopathies been determined. Most have been found to relate to inherited defects resulting in abnormal ion channel function. Maintenance of ionic equilibrium and control of the ionic fluxes associated with excitable tissue such as muscle are critical to normal muscle functioning. A variety of sarcolemmal ion channels exist that control fluxes of ions such as sodium, potassium, chloride, and calcium. Defective sodium or chloride channels most often result in myotonia.

METABOLIC MYOPATHIES

Inherited disorders of muscle metabolism (Table 15-10) are characterized by reduced muscle cell energy production. Clinical signs include exercise intolerance, exercise-induced muscle cramps, and rhabdomyolysis. Metabolic defects can involve glycogen metabolism, fatty acid metabolism, or mitochondrial function. Metabolic disorders often cause increased blood lactate after exercise. Inheritance patterns vary. Glycolytic, glycogenolytic, and nonmitochondrial DNA–encoded enzyme defects are generally inherited in an autosomal recessive manner. Defects involving mitochondrial DNA–encoded enzymes are inherited through maternal inheritance, because all mitochondria are contributed from the oocyte.

The pathways of glycolysis and glycogenolysis are complex, involving a cascade of enzymatic reactions. Deficiency of a glycolytic or glycogenolytic enzyme leads to accumulation of glycogen and in some cases glycogen-related proteoglycans. There are several different types of glycogen storage diseases depending on which enzyme is deficient. Several types of glycogenoses are recognized in human beings, and five (types II, III, IV, V and VII) cause glycogen accumulation in muscle. Of the glycogenoses affecting muscle, only types II (acid maltase deficiency), IV (glycogen branching enzyme deficiency), V (myophosphorylase deficiency), and VII (phosphofructokinase deficiency) have so far been recognized in animals. Storage diseases in which glycogen accumulates in muscle have been described in horses, cattle, sheep, dogs, and cats.

Inherited lipid storage myopathies have not yet been described in animals, although dogs appear to have a predilection for development of neuromuscular weakness because of acquired lipid storage myopathy with concurrent reduction in skeletal muscle carnitine activity. Mitochondrial myopathies are rarely recognized in animals, perhaps because of the difficulty in documentation of mitochondrial defects. A few such disorders have been described in dogs, and a mitochondrial myopathy has been reported in one Arabian horse. Mitochondrial disorders may affect only muscle, or muscle involvement may be part of an encephalomyopathic condition.

MALIGNANT HYPERTHERMIA

Malignant hyperthermia is a condition characterized by unregulated release of calcium from the sarcoplasmic reticulum, leading to excessive myofiber contraction that causes a severe increase in body temperature. Malignant hyperthermia is often fatal. In human beings, pigs, horses, and dogs a congenital defect in the sarcoplasmic reticulum calcium-release channel, the ryanodine receptor, causes dysregulation of excitation-contraction coupling leading to malignant hyperthermia. Episodes in affected individuals can be triggered by general anesthetic agents, especially halothane, or by stress—hence the name *porcine stress syndrome* for the disorder in pigs (Fig. 15-47).

A malignant hyperthermia-like condition can also occur because of other myopathic conditions, especially those that result in uncoupling of mitochondrial oxidative phosphorylation from the electron transport chain. Inherently uncoupled mitochondria within brown fat are the physiologic basis for production of heat during breakdown of this fat in neonates, and pathologically uncoupled or loosely coupled mitochondria in muscle as a result of an underlying myopathy will also release energy as heat.

Gross and microscopic lesions are described in the section covering the disorder in pigs.

ENDOCRINE AND ELECTROLYTE ABNORMALITIES

Various endocrinologic abnormalities can result in myopathic conditions (Table 15-11). The most common are hypercortisolism and hypothyroidism in dogs.

Table **15-11** **Myopathies Due to Endocrine and Electrolyte Abnormalities**

Disorder	Species Affected
Hypothyroidism	Dogs
Hypercortisolism	Dogs
Hypokalemia	Cattle, cats
Hypophosphatemia	Cattle
Hypernatremia	Cats
Hypocalcemia	Cattle
Hypothalamic/pituitary dysfunction	Horses

In horses, pituitary hyperfunction resulting in Cushing's disease is also associated with muscle disease. In most cases of endocrine myopathy, the end result is myofiber atrophy, particularly of type 2 fibers. A unique syndrome of muscle hypertrophy and pseudomyotonia occurs in dogs associated with hypercortisolism. Endocrine myopathies can also be complicated by pathologic changes in peripheral nerves, leading to a mixture of myopathic (type 2 fiber atrophy) and neuropathic changes (denervation atrophy and alteration in fiber-type pattern) within muscle. Denervation followed by reinnervation leading to fiber-type grouping can be seen in dogs with chronic hypercortisolism (Fig. 15-24, B) and hypothyroidism.

Normal electrolyte status is vital to normal skeletal muscle function. Hypocalcemia, hypokalemia, hypernatremia, and hypophosphatemia can cause profound skeletal muscle weakness, sometimes associated with myofiber necrosis, in various species.

NEUROPATHIC AND NEUROMUSCULAR JUNCTION DISORDERS

Dysfunction of the lower motor neurons, peripheral nerves, or neuromuscular junction can have profound effects on muscle function.

NEUROPATHIC DISORDERS

There are many peripheral nerve disorders, and fewer motor neuron disorders, that can lead to denervation atrophy of muscle in animals. These can be inherited or acquired. Long nerves such as the sciatic and left recurrent laryngeal nerves appear to be particularly sensitive to development of acquired neuropathy. Many of the peripheral nerve disorders of animals are discussed in Chapter 14. Characteristic features of denervation atrophy are described in this chapter under Response of Muscle to Injury.

NEUROMUSCULAR JUNCTION DISORDERS

The neuromuscular junction is a modification of the postsynaptic myofiber membrane. At the neuromuscular junction, the membrane is folded to increase surface area and is studded with specialized ion channels known as acetylcholine receptors. Following arrival of an action potential at the distal end of a motor nerve, the terminal axons release acetylcholine, which diffuses across the synaptic space to bind to the acetylcholine receptors. Binding opens these channels, leading to sodium influx, which initiates the skeletal muscle action potential that culminates in muscle contraction. Acetylcholine is rapidly degraded by acetylcholinesterase released from the postsynaptic membrane, which prevents continued stimulation of the muscle fiber.

Disorders that impair the ability of nerve impulses to travel across the neuromuscular junction have profound effects on skeletal muscle function. Technically, however, the myofibers are still innervated, so denervation atrophy does not occur, and no light microscopic abnormalities in the muscle or nerve are present. Various neurotoxins (i.e., in snake and spider venom) and drugs can affect the neuromuscular junction, but the most common neuromuscular junction disorders affecting animals are myasthenia gravis, botulism, and tick paralysis.

Myasthenia gravis

Myasthenia gravis can be either acquired or congenital. Acquired myasthenia gravis is an immune-mediated disorder caused by circulating autoantibodies against skeletal muscle acetylcholine receptors (Fig. 15-33). Binding of these antibodies to the acetylcholine receptor on the postsynaptic membrane leads to a severe decrease in the number of functional receptors. The mechanisms by which antibodies damage these receptors are (1) direct damage to the neuromuscular junction, which may be visible with electron microscopy as simplification of the membrane, and (2) formation of cross-linked antibodies leading to receptor internalization. Sufficient functional acetylcholine receptors are present to allow initially normal neuromuscular transmission, but the decrease in the number of available receptors leads to progressive weakness and collapse. Therefore acquired myasthenia gravis results in episodic collapse, and repetitive nerve stimulation causes a characteristic rapid decrease in amplitude of the muscle compound motor action potential. Diagnosis of myasthenia gravis can also be made following intravenous injection of cholinesterase inhibitors such as edrophonium chloride (Tensilon, ICN Pharmaceuticals, Costa Mesa, Calif) to collapsed animals. The reduction in cholinesterase activity leads to more available active acetylcholine within the synapse and rapid, although transient, restoration of skeletal muscle activity. Detection of circulating autoantibodies to acetylcholine receptors confirms the diagnosis.

The origin of the autoantibodies causing myasthenia gravis is not always known, but there is a strong link between thymic abnormalities and development of myasthenia gravis in both human beings and animals. Specialized cells within the thymic medulla, known as myoid cells, express skeletal muscle proteins, including those of the acetylcholine receptor. It is thought that these cells participate in development of self-tolerance. Abnormalities of the thymus, most commonly thymoma in animals and thymic follicular hyperplasia in human beings, can lead to loss of self-tolerance to acetylcholine receptors. In such cases, removal of the abnormal thymus can result in restoration of normal neuromuscular junction activity. When thymic abnormalities are not present, treatment with long-acting anticholinesterase agents and in some cases immunosuppressive agents, such as corticosteroids, is necessary.

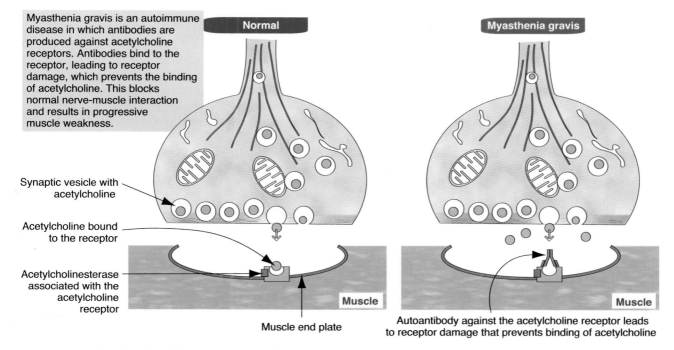

Fig. 15-33   Schematic diagram of the pathogenesis of acquired (autoimmune) myasthenia gravis.
(Modified from Kierszenbaum AL: Histology and cell biology: an introduction to pathology, St Louis, 2002, Mosby.)

Congenital myasthenia gravis is an inherited disorder that is much less common than acquired myasthenia gravis. To date it has been described only in human beings, dogs, and cats. Animals with congenital myasthenia gravis are born with defective neuromuscular junctions that often have a decreased membrane surface area, best visualized with electron microscopy, and inherently reduced acetylcholine receptor density. Such animals may be normal at birth because there are sufficient functional acetylcholine receptors to support muscle contraction in a neonate. But with rapid postnatal growth, clinical signs of profound, sustained, and progressive weakness occur as a consequence of insufficient functional receptors to support the function of growing muscles.

Botulism

Botulism is a neuromuscular disorder caused by the exotoxin of the bacterium *Clostridium botulinum*. Botulinum toxin is considered one of the deadliest of the known toxins. Botulism is characterized by profound generalized flaccid paralysis. Seven serologically distinct but structurally similar forms of botulinum toxin are designated A, B, C, D, E, F, and G. Sensitivity to these toxin types varies among different species. Dogs are most sensitive to type C toxin, ruminants to types C and D, and horses to types B and C.

Botulinum toxin occurs as a light chain and a heavy chain linked by a disulfide bond. Binding of botulinum toxin to receptors on the presynaptic terminals of peripheral nerves leads to toxin endocytosis. Within the endocytotic vesicle of the terminal nerve, the disulfide bond is cleaved, and the released light chain is translocated into the axonal cytoplasm. Botulinum toxin light chains are metalloproteinases. Numerous proteins are involved in the release of acetylcholine from presynaptic vesicles, and botulinum toxin blocks release of acetylcholine by irreversible enzymatic cleavage of one or more of these proteins. Different forms of botulinum toxin affect different proteins, but the end result is the same. Active neuromuscular junctions are the most sensitive, which has lead to use of low levels of injected botulinum toxin as a treatment for localized muscular disorders resulting in spasm.

Clostridium botulinum spores are commonly present in the gastrointestinal tract of animals and in the soil. Under favorable anaerobic and alkalinic conditions, these spores become active, with resultant toxin production. Botulism can occur because of ingestion of preformed toxin, such as in feed contaminated by dead rodents or soil-borne organisms, or from toxin produced by *Clostridium botulinum* organisms within the gastrointestinal tract or superficial wounds (Box 15-9). Dogs and cats, species that are most likely to ingest dead rodents containing botulinum toxin, are quite resistant

Box **15-9**

Portals of Entry—Equine Botulism

Gastrointestinal colonization: Foals up to 6 months of age
Ingestion of preformed toxin: Adults, usually from rodent carcasses in hay or concentrated feed, or environmental contamination
Wound contamination: Adults, deep wounds, uncommon

to developing botulism. In veterinary medicine, horses are the most sensitive to botulinum toxin. Death of horses, most often due to respiratory muscle paralysis, can result from exposure to only very small amounts of botulinum toxin. The damage to presynaptic axon terminals is irreversible, and recovery from botulism occurs only following terminal axon sprouting and reestablishment of new functioning synapses.

Tick paralysis

Dermacentor and *Ixodes* ticks can elaborate a toxin that also blocks release of acetylcholine from axon terminals. Tick paralysis is seen most often in dogs and children. Recovery following tick removal can be rapid (within 24 to 48 hours), indicating that the mechanism of toxin action in tick paralysis does not result in irreversible presynaptic damage and thus is different from that of botulinum toxin.

NEOPLASIA

Neoplasms involving skeletal muscle are most often those that arise within the muscle or its supporting structures or that invade muscle from adjacent tissue.

PRIMARY MUSCLE TUMORS

Tumors with striated muscle differentiation are thought to arise from intramuscular pluripotential stem cells rather than from satellite cells. These tumors are uncommon and are either benign (rhabdomyoma) or malignant (rhabdomyosarcoma). Primary intramuscular tumors can also arise from fibrous tissue, vasculature, or neural elements. The most common tumor to arise from muscle-supporting structures is hemangiosarcoma.

Rhabdomyoma and rhabdomyosarcoma

Tumors of striated muscle that occur at sites other than within muscle are rhabdomyomas of the heart or lung and botryoid rhabdomyosarcomas of the urinary bladder; these are not discussed in this section. Rhabdomyoma and rhabdomyosarcoma arising within skeletal muscle are most common in the dog, followed by the horse and cat. Morphologic variants include round cell, spindle cell, and mixed round and spindle cell, reflecting the developmental stages of skeletal muscle. Historically, diagnosis of tumors of skeletal muscle has relied on identification of cross striations indicative of sarcomeric differentiation. Cross striations are most often seen in elongated multinucleate cells known as "strap cells" (Fig. 34, C) and in ovoid cells known as "racquet cells." They are most easily recognized following staining with phosphotungstic acid hematoxylin (PTAH) stain, but the search for cross striations can be extremely frustrating and unrewarding. These days the diagnosis of tumors of skeletal muscle origin relies primarily on results of immunohistochemical examination using antibodies for muscle-specific proteins. Muscle actin and desmin are expressed by smooth and skeletal muscle tumors, but myoglobin and sarcomeric actin are specific for skeletal muscle. Evidence of muscle differentiation, such as primitive myofilaments and Z-band structures, can also be seen by electron microscopy.

Rhabdomyoma is most often a round cell tumor and occurs most commonly in the larynx of adult dogs. The youngest reported age is 2 years. Tumors are generally smooth and nodular, pink, and unencapsulated. Histologic features are closely packed plump round cells that have central euchromatic nuclei, generally with a single prominent nucleus, and abundant vacuolated to granular eosinophilic cytoplasm. A small number of multinucleate and elongate strap cells can also be seen. Mitoses are rare, and evidence of invasion is uncommon.

Similar to the situation in human beings, rhabdomyosarcomas in animals most often occur at a young age and are most common in the neck or oral cavity, especially in the tongue. These tumors are pink and fleshy, and they often exhibit prominent local invasion. The most common and most distinctive form of rhabdomyosarcoma in animals is embryonal rhabdomyosarcoma, composed of primitive round cells with prominent euchromatic nuclei, a single prominent nucleolus, and either indistinct or prominent eosinophilic cytoplasm ("rhabdomyoblasts"; Fig. 15-34, A and B). Rhabdomyosarcoma can also contain elongate multinucleate strap cells (Fig. 15-34, C) and ovoid racquet cells. Cellular and nuclear pleomorphism is common, as is mitotic activity. These tumors are locally invasive and frequently metastasize, although too few cases have been studied to document any pattern of metastasis.

Hemangiosarcoma

Malignant vascular neoplasms (hemangiosarcoma) arising within muscle are most common in the horse and dog (Fig. 15-35). Clinical signs include swelling within muscle, often with associated lameness. Cytologic preparations frequently reveal only peripheral blood, suggestive of a hematoma. Pathologic diagnosis can be difficult if multiple sites within the lesion are not sampled, as the amount of hemorrhage often far exceeds the area composed of proliferating neoplastic endothelial cells. Intramuscular hemangiosarcoma has a high incidence of metastasis, often to the lungs.

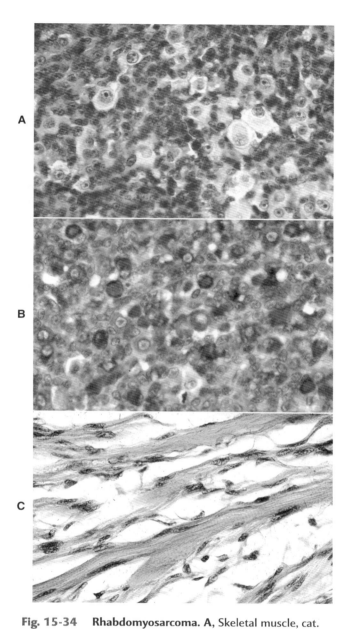

Fig. 15-34   Rhabdomyosarcoma. A, Skeletal muscle, cat. An admixture of small round basophilic cells with a lesser number of larger round cells with prominent eosinophilic cytoplasm is characteristic of embryonal rhabdomyosarcoma. Nuclei are central and euchromatic, most often with a single large nucleolus. H&E stain. **B,** Immunostaining reaction of the same rhabdomyosarcoma as depicted in Fig. 15-34, A showing intense cytoplasmic expression of desmin in many tumor cells, indicative of muscle origin (skeletal, cardiac, or smooth). These cells also express myoglobin and sarcomeric actin (not shown), which differentiates skeletal muscle tumors from smooth muscle tumors. Immunoperoxidase reaction for desmin. **C,** Botryoid rhabdomyosarcoma, urinary bladder, large breed dog. Cross striations, characteristic of a well-differentiated rhabdomyosarcoma, are present in the elongated multinucleate tumor cells. H&E stain. (*A and B, Courtesy College of Veterinary Medicine, Cornell University. C, Courtesy Dr. B.A. Valentine, College of Veterinary Medicine, Oregon State University.*)

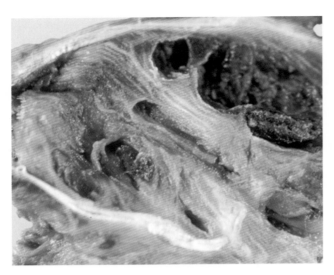

Fig. 15-35   Intramuscular hemangiosarcoma, cervical skeletal muscle, horse. Multiple irregular zones of cavitated (*upper right*) to solid tumor with hemorrhage have replaced normal muscle. Formalin fixed specimen. (*Courtesy Dr. A. de Lahunta, College of Veterinary Medicine, Cornell University.*)

OTHER TUMORS INVOLVING SKELETAL MUSCLE

A variant of lipoma, known as infiltrative lipoma, often involves skeletal muscle. Characteristic gross pathologic and histopathologic findings are mature adipocytes invading skeletal muscle. This tumor is most common in the dog but has also been reported in young horses. Wide excision is the treatment of choice because this tumor will recur as a result of local invasion, but it does not metastasize.

Infiltration of skeletal muscle by neoplastic lymphocytes is not uncommon. Neoplastic lymphocytic infiltrates surround myofibers and can cause myofiber atrophy. These cells do not invade myofibers, however, and myonecrosis is rare. This helps to distinguish intramuscular lymphoma from lymphocytic myositis. Careful examination of infiltrating neoplastic cells typically reveals a relatively monomorphic population of lymphocytes, which may be atypical in appearance. Immunohistochemistry to confirm a single infiltrating cell type is also useful.

Vaccine-associated sarcoma in the muscle of the cat can arise within an intramuscular vaccination site or extend into underlying skeletal muscle from a subcutaneous injection site. Occasionally, mast cell tumors and carcinomas will exhibit prominent skeletal muscle invasion. Melanoma arising in the skin of older gray horses often metastasizes to muscle fascia and may exhibit some extension into the muscle itself. Intramuscular metastasis of tumors is rare (see Defense Mechanisms). Intramuscular metastasis of carcinoma, particularly prostatic, can occur in dogs. When carcinomas associated with sclerosis involve muscle, either by extension or by metastasis, the muscle basement membrane is typically destroyed, often resulting in bizarre multinucleate cells representing attempts at muscle regeneration (Fig. 15-20). These bizarre cells should not be misidentified as tumor cells.

MUSCULAR DISORDERS OF DOMESTIC ANIMALS

Adequate muscle function is essential for the survival of any species. Many domestic animals have been selectively bred for improved musculature for meat production, performance, or appearance. Therefore muscle disease in animals can have a significant economic impact. In some cases, it is selection pressure imposed by human beings that has resulted in development and perpetuation of various myopathic conditions in animals. It is likely that continued selection pressures will lead to new mutations in the future.

It is interesting to compare the effects of muscular disorders that affect human beings and animals. The four-footed stance of animals allows for greater stability, which can allow an animal to remain ambulatory for some time, whereas a similarly affected person would be confined to a wheelchair. However, disorders that result in recumbency, even if it is transitory, can be devastating in livestock. It is much more difficult to nurse a large animal through a period of recumbency than it would be for a hospitalized human being or small animal patient.

The most common and important muscle disorders of animals are discussed by species because this is the way diseases are considered clinically. The same disease may occur in different species. Details of less common muscle disorders are presented in Appendix 15-1.

MUSCULAR DISORDERS OF THE HORSE

There is perhaps no other domestic animal species for which optimal muscle development and function is so critical as the horse. Selective breeding for better muscling has occurred in virtually all horse and pony breeds. The ability of such selection pressure to result in equine muscle mutations is exemplified by the relatively recent occurrence of hyperkalemic periodic paralysis (HYPP), in which a muscle mutation results in visually appealing increased muscle bulk and definition. Unfortunately, as you will see in the discussion of HYPP later, such mutations do not often result in improved muscle function.

BACTERIAL AND PARASITIC MYOPATHIES

Infection by various bacterial organisms and clostridial toxins can cause myopathy in the horse. Protozoa (*Sarcocystis* spp.) are common incidental findings in equine muscle, but protozoal myopathy is rare.

Clostridial myositis (malignant edema; gas gangrene)

Clostridial myositis in the horse is an often fatal disorder caused by infection by various toxin-producing clostridial species, which are large gram-positive anaerobic bacilli. *Clostridium septicum* is the most common cause of clostridial myositis in horses, but *Clostridium perfringens* types A to E, *Clostridium chauvoei*, *Clostridium novyi*, and *Clostridium fallax* can also cause infection. Infection can involve more than one clostridial species. *Clostridium* spp. are ubiquitous organisms that form spores within the soil and within the gastrointestinal tract. Unlike cattle, in which nonpenetrating trauma causes muscle bruising and anaerobic conditions that activate clostridial spores already in the muscle, clostridial myositis in horses is virtually always secondary to a penetrating wound. Most often this is an injection site of a nonantibiotic substance, but infection of sites of puncture wounds and perivascular leakage of irritants in intravenously administered compounds are also possible. It is also possible that clostridial bacteria from the gastrointestinal tract can colonize damaged muscle. This is one possible explanation for the frequent occurrence of signs of colic before development of clostridial myositis at sites of injection of medications such as flunixin meglumine. Under anaerobic conditions, clostridia proliferate and produce toxins that damage blood vessels, resulting in hemorrhage and edema, and cause necrosis of adjacent muscle fibers (Table 15-4).

Clinical signs are acute onset of heat, swelling, and pain within a muscle group and adjacent fascia, with concurrent fever, depression, dehydration, and anorexia. If sufficient muscle necrosis is present, serum CK and AST concentrations may be mildly to moderately increased. Death from toxemia and/or septicemia often occurs within 48 hours. Affected muscle and adjacent fascia are swollen and often hemorrhagic, with edema, suppurative inflammation, and necrosis; gas may also be present (Fig. 15-36). Vasculitis is not seen. Gram-positive bacilli characteristic of *Clostridium* spp. are generally demonstrable within affected tissue.

The diagnosis can be made with reasonable certainty based on typical historical, gross pathologic, cytologic, and histopathologic findings. *Clostridium* spp. can also be identified by culture under anaerobic conditions or by a fluorescent antibody test. Treatment must be initiated rapidly and includes surgical incisions into affected muscle to allow drainage and oxygenation, antibiotic therapy, and supportive care.

Botulism

Technically this disease is a neuromuscular junction disorder and is included in this section for convenience. Botulism is caused by *Clostridium botulinum* toxin

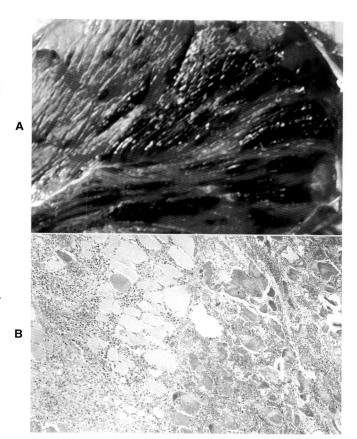

Fig. 15-36 **Clostridial myositis, malignant edema, horse.** **A,** *Clostridium septicum* is the most common cause of clostridial myositis in horses. Affected muscle (*shown here*) and adjacent fascia (*not shown here*) are swollen and often hemorrhagic. **B,** Interstitial edema, hemorrhage, and inflammatory cells surround numerous swollen and fragmented necrotic myofibers. Formalin fixation, H&E stain. (**A,** *Courtesy College of Veterinary Medicine, Cornell University.* **B,** *Courtesy Dr. B.A. Valentine, College of Veterinary Medicine, Oregon State University.*)

and is often not associated with *Clostridium botulinum* infection. The portals of entry of botulinum toxin in horses are summarized in Box 15-9. *Clostridium botulinum* bacteria are found as spores within the gastrointestinal tract of many mammals, and spores are common in the soil. Preformed toxin within contaminated feed or soil is the most common cause of botulism in adult horses. However, in foals, usually between 1 week and 6 months of age, ingestion of *Clostridium botulinum* spores can lead to proliferation of toxin-producing *Clostridium botulinum* within the intestinal tract, resulting in toxicoinfectious botulism (shaker foals). Wound infection is an uncommon cause of botulism in horses.

The pathogenesis of botulism has been previously discussed (see Neuropathic and Neuromuscular Junction Disorders). Irreversible binding of toxin to presynaptic nerve terminals and blockage of acetylcholine release lead to the profound generalized flaccid paralysis that is the hallmark of botulism. Clinical signs are acute and progress rapidly, generally resulting in recumbency. Dysphagia and tongue weakness are common findings that help to distinguish botulism from other neuromuscular diseases causing recumbency. Serum concentrations of CK and AST are within normal limits (indicating the absence of damage to myofibers) or are possibly slightly increased as a result of ischemic myopathy secondary to recumbency (see later discussion).

No specific gross or histopathologic lesions are present in horses dying with botulism, although aspiration pneumonia caused by dysphagia can occur. Muscle fibers are intact unless recumbency has compromised their blood supply, causing ischemia and localized myofiber necrosis.

Evaluation of stomach contents or contaminated feed may reveal the presence of toxin. However, horses are exquisitely sensitive to botulinum toxin, and as only a small concentration of the toxin may be present in an affected horse, available tests may not detect such a low concentration of toxin. In most equine cases, the diagnosis is made based on the clinical history after elimination of other possible causes of profound muscular weakness. Affected animals should be treated with polyvalent botulinum antitoxin to prevent further binding of toxin. Recovery occurs following terminal axon sprouting and reestablishment of functional neuromuscular junctions. Vaccination with botulinum toxoid is an effective preventive measure.

Corynebacterium pseudotuberculosis (pigeon fever)

Intramuscular abscesses due to *Corynebacterium pseudotuberculosis* occur almost exclusively in horses in arid regions of the Western United States and Brazil. *Corynebacterium pseudotuberculosis* is a gram-positive pleomorphic facultative anaerobic bacillus present within the soil. It can enter muscle via penetrating wounds, including injection sites. The biotype most common in horses is different from that which affects sheep and goats as it is unable to reduce nitrates to nitrites. The high lipid content of the bacterial cell wall contributes to survival within macrophages, and bacterial exotoxins, such as phospholipase D, contribute to vascular damage and inhibition of neutrophil function. Equine infections occur most frequently during the fall and early winter, and a higher incidence of the disease is often seen following rainy winters. Infections are most common in the pectoral muscles, but other locations are possible. Affected muscles are swollen and edematous, and contain variably sized zones of localized suppurative inflammation. Fever is common. The causative agent is readily isolated from affected tissue and can be seen in aspirates from intramuscular abscesses. Treatment is generally curative and includes

antibiotic therapy and establishment of drainage of abscesses. Rarely, infection with *Corynebacterium pseudotuberculosis* in horses leads to immune-mediated vasculitis (purpura hemorrhagica; see next discussion).

Streptococcal-associated myopathies

Two distinct degenerative myopathies are associated with infection or exposure of the horse to *Streptococcus equi* ssp. *equi.* One, known as purpura hemorrhagica, has been recognized for many years. The other, known as streptococcal-associated rhabdomyolysis and muscle atrophy, has only recently been recognized.

Purpura hemorrhagica.   In this disease, muscle damage is not caused by the direct infection of the muscles but rather by an immune response to the bacterial pathogen. *Streptococcus equi* is the most common cause of purpura hemorrhagic in horses, but other bacteria can also be involved. In cases caused by *Streptococcus equi*, circulating immune complexes composed of immunoglobulin A (IgA) antibodies and streptococcal M antigen deposit in small vessels. This leads to vasculitis and vascular wall necrosis (Fig. 15-37), with resultant hemorrhage and infarction of myofibers. It is also possible that antibodies to streptococcal M protein cross-react with skeletal and cardiac muscle myosins to cause direct injury.

Signs of myopathy often accompany systemic signs of poststreptococcal purpura in horses (i.e., depression, fever, dependent edema, petechiae or ecchymoses, leukocytosis, increased serum fibrinogen, and anemia), but myopathy can also be the primary presenting disease process. Affected horses are weak, may have a short-strided gait, and can become recumbent. Myoglobinuria and very

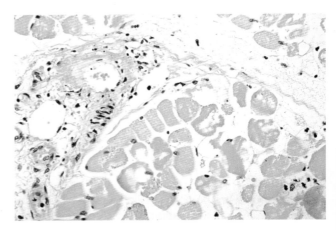

Fig. 15-37   Intramuscular vasculitis, purpura hemorrhagica, skeletal muscle, transverse section, horse. In the wall of the blood vessel (*upper left*) is a band of circumferential fibrinoid necrosis containing nuclear debris. Many of the adjacent myofibers are necrotic. Some of these myofibers are fragmented, and a small number contain fine basophilic deposits of mineral. Formalin fixation, H&E stain. (*Courtesy Dr. B.A. Valentine, College of Veterinary Medicine, Oregon State University.*)

high increases in serum concentrations of CK and AST are common.

Multiple muscles are involved (as opposed to the locally extensive lesion of clostridial myositis), and affected muscles contain multifocal to locally extensive hemorrhage and edema that dissects between necrotic muscle fibers. Gross pathologic findings are similar to those seen in clostridial myositis (Fig. 15-36, A), but lesions do not contain gas bubbles. Vasculitis (Fig. 15-37) is present on microscopic examination and is the diagnostic feature.

Diagnosis is based on a history of exposure of the horse to *Streptococcus equi* and typical clinical, clinicopathologic, and histopathologic findings. Because this is an immune-complex disorder, histopathology, cytology, and bacterial cultures of affected muscle do not reveal *S. equi*. This organism or other causative organisms may be cultured from other affected tissues, especially lymph nodes or guttural pouch. A high serum titer to *Streptococcus equi* M protein is strongly supportive of streptococcal-associated purpura hemorrhagica. Treatment includes corticosteroid therapy and supportive care, but horses frequently succumb to other manifestations of systemic vasculitis, such as gastrointestinal infarcts.

Streptococcal-associated rhabdomyolysis and muscle atrophy. A syndrome of severe acute rhabdomyolysis and profound rapidly progressive generalized muscle atrophy has also been seen in horses infected or even just exposed to *Streptococcus equi*. This syndrome occurs most frequently in young to young adult quarter horses, but young horses of other breeds can also be affected. Clinically recognized muscle atrophy is often most evident in paraspinal and gluteal muscles. Some cases have microscopic evidence of concurrent polysaccharide storage myopathy (see Inherited or Congenital Myopathies), which may be a predisposing factor. In others, nonsuppurative perivascular and interstitial inflammation has been detected, and immune-mediated damage caused by cross reaction of streptococcal antibodies with muscle proteins has been proposed. Affected horses do not show typical signs of purpura hemorrhagica but often have very high serum concentrations of CK and AST. Affected horses may respond to corticosteroid therapy. Most will recover, but recurrence following subsequent *Streptococcus equi* exposure is possible.

Protozoal myopathy

Protozoa (*Sarcocystis* spp.) are common incidental findings in equine skeletal and cardiac muscle. As the protozoa are in cysts within the myofiber itself and thus are protected from the body's surveillance, there is no inflammatory response. Massive infection by *Sarcocystis fayeri* is suspected of causing a degenerative myopathy in horses, but this is rare. Rarely, localized thickening of the tongue has been found in horses with granulomatous myositis, the result of sarcocystis organisms within tongue musculature.

Ear tick–associated muscle spasms

Episodic muscle spasms can occur in horses with ear ticks (*Otobius megnini*). The mechanism is not known. Dimpling of affected muscles following percussion can be seen, but myotonic discharges are not found with electromyography. Treatment for ear ticks results in rapid recovery.

NUTRITIONAL AND TOXIC MYOPATHIES

Nutritional deficiency, most often of selenium, and various toxins are relatively common causes of degenerative myopathy in the horse.

Nutritional myopathy

Foals (most commonly up to 2 weeks of age) and young adult horses are most susceptible to nutritional myopathy because of a deficiency of the antioxidants selenium or (less commonly) vitamin E. In severely selenium-deficient areas, such as the Pacific Northwest, selenium deficiency myopathy can occur in horses of any age. Selenium present in the soil is taken up by growing plants. In many areas, the soil is selenium deficient, and selenium supplements to the animal's ration must be provided. Vitamin E deficiency occurs in horses that eat marginal- to poor-quality grass hay and have little or no access to pasture and no supplemental vitamin E. Oxidative injury to actively contracting muscle fibers occurs as a result of a lack of antioxidant activity.

Affected foals are most likely to be those born to selenium-deficient mares. Foals have generalized weakness, which may be present at birth or become apparent soon after birth. Affected foals may become recumbent but are generally bright and alert. They often continue to suckle if bottle fed, but weakness of the tongue and pharyngeal muscles can lead to weak suckling.

Affected adult horses are most often stabled horses fed only selenium-deficient hay, with clinical disease being seen most commonly in the late winter or early spring. In the Pacific Northwest, selenium deficiency myopathy can occur in adult horses fed only pasture or hay, and it can occur at any time of year. Affected adult horses often show preferential involvement of the temporal and masseter muscles (sometimes inappropriately termed maxillary myositis or masseter myositis) with swelling and stiffness of these muscles and impaired mastication. Involvement of pharyngeal muscle results in dysphagia, which can be mistaken for botulism. In more chronic cases, bilaterally symmetric atrophy of the masseter muscles may be evident, which can be mistaken for atrophy secondary to protozoal myeloencephalitis. Careful examination of these horses often reveals generalized weakness, evident as a stiff, short-strided gait.

Severely affected horses can have an acute onset of recumbency that mimics neurologic disease.

Serum concentrations of CK and AST are generally mildly to moderately increased, although extremely high concentrations can be seen in severely affected foals and horses. Concentric needle electromyography of affected muscles results in abnormal spontaneous activity (positive sharp waves, fibrillations, and myotonic bursts).

Muscles of affected horses appear pale (hence the common name *white muscle disease*), often in a patchy distribution (Fig. 15-44). The most severely affected muscles are those that have the highest workload (e.g., cervical muscles, proximal limb muscles, tongue, and masticatory muscles). The gross appearance depends on the extent of the necrosis and the stage. In early stages, yellow and white streaks are present, and later pale, chalk white streaks often appear. Horses with impaired swallowing can have cranioventral aspiration pneumonia. Severely selenium-deficient foals and horses will also have pale areas of necrosis within the myocardium, especially the left ventricular wall and septum. The stage of the necrosis depends on the age of the lesions. In foals with severe, acute myopathy leading to death or euthanasia, lesions are at the stage of massive muscle necrosis and mineralization with minimal macrophage infiltration (monophasic). In animals that have lived longer (i.e., subacute cases), the lesions are polyphasic, and active necrosis, macrophage infiltration, and regeneration are present. Although type 1 fibers may be more likely to develop necrosis because of nutritional myopathy, in severely affected muscles almost all fiber types are affected. In cases with myocardial involvement, myocardiocyte necrosis and mineralization are present. If the animal survives, the necrotic myocardiocytes are replaced by fibrovascular connective tissue that forms a scar.

Diagnosis of nutritional myopathy is based on typical history, increases in serum concentrations of CK and AST, deficient blood concentrations of selenium or vitamin E, and characteristic gross and histopathologic findings. If horses live long enough, myofiber regeneration can restore the muscles to normal. This disorder in foals can be prevented by supplementing the ration of mares with selenium during gestation. Foals born in selenium-deficient areas can also be given injectable vitamin E and selenium soon after birth. Young adult horses should be given sufficient dietary vitamin E and selenium. Treatment with selenium and vitamin E after the onset of clinical signs is far less effective than prevention.

Ionophore toxicity

The pathogenesis of ionophore toxicity is discussed in the section titled Toxic Myopathies. Horses are exquisitely sensitive to ionophores and will succumb to very small doses. Ionophores may be present as contaminants within horse feed, or the horse may be accidentally fed ionophore-containing feeds intended for other domestic animals.

Most of the available literature relates to monensin toxicity, but the effects of other ionophores should be similar. In acute monensin toxicity, death occurs because of shock and cardiovascular collapse, and no specific lesions are seen on postmortem examination within the first 48 hours. If the horse survives 3 to 4 days, cardiac muscle necrosis and segmental necrosis of skeletal muscle occurs (Fig. 15-38, *B*, Fig. 15-16, *B*), with concurrent increases in serum concentrations of CK and AST, which may be severe. Affected skeletal and cardiac muscles will often contain pale streaks (Fig. 15-38, *A*). Given the profound sensitivity of horses to ionophores, ionophore toxicity in horses is typically the result of a single dose and thus the lesion is a monophasic multifocal process. This helps to differentiate ionophore toxicity from nutritional myopathy, which is often polyphasic. Both type 1 and type 2 fibers are affected. If the horse survives, necrosis is followed by myofiber regeneration, which can restore the muscles to normal. Necrotic myocardiocytes will be replaced by fibrosis because of the lack of significant regeneration of the myocardium. Horses dying at 14 days postionophore exposure often have normal skeletal muscles and extensive myocardial fibrosis. Acute cardiac failure and death because of myocardial scarring can occur months to years following apparent recovery from ionophore exposure.

Diagnosis is based on a history that includes both ingestion of ionophores and the presence of the characteristic gross or histopathologic findings. Analysis of feed or stomach contents for ionophores is definitive. Treatment for ionophore-intoxicated horses is supportive, as there is no specific therapy.

Plant toxicities

A number of toxic plants are known to cause muscle necrosis in horses (see also Toxic Myopathies). These include *Cassia occidentalis* (coffee senna) and *Thermopsis* spp. Most plant-associated toxicities in horses are associated with plants growing in pastures or baled into hay. Necrosis is most often polyphasic. Cardiac myonecrosis may or may not also be present. In the United Kingdom, a syndrome of pasture-associated myonecrosis has been documented in horses for which the cause is as yet unknown.

INHERITED OR CONGENITAL MYOPATHIES AND MYOTONIC DISORDERS

Hyperkalemic periodic paralysis (HYPP)

This myotonic disorder affects horses whose ancestry traces back to a quarter horse stallion named Impressive. Affected horses generally have remarkably well-defined

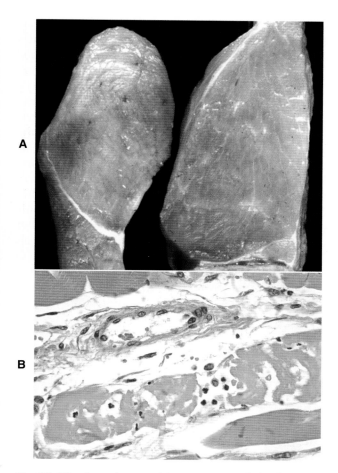

Fig. 15-38 **Ionophore toxicity, monensin, skeletal muscle.** **A,** Necrosis. The pale white to gray foci are areas of necrotic myofibers. Myocardium will often contain similar lesions. **B,** Segmental myofiber necrosis (2 days old), longitudinal section, horse. The segment of myofiber visible here is necrotic, fragmented, and infiltrated by macrophages and neutrophils. Note the intact basal lamina and endomysium on both sides of the myofiber, which will contain the regenerating myofiber and thus facilitate resolution. Ionophore toxicity results in calcium overload and death of skeletal (also cardiac) myocytes. Formalin fixation, H&E stain. (**A,** *Courtesy Dr. J. Wright, College of Veterinary Medicine, North Carolina State University; and Noah's Arkive, College of Veterinary Medicine, The University of Georgia.* **B,** *Courtesy Dr. M.D. McGavin, College of Veterinary Medicine, University of Tennessee.*)

muscle groups, which has lead to their popularity for showing in halter. The disease is inherited as an autosomal dominant disease. Therefore affected horses can be either heterozygotes or homozygotes. Homozygous foals often have a distinctive laryngeal muscle dysfunction that results in laryngospasm and labored breathing, and most homozygous horses are considered nonviable.

The underlying defect in HYPP is a point mutation in the gene encoding the α subunit of the skeletal muscle sodium channel. This defect causes abnormal (delayed) inactivation of sodium channel activity, resulting in membrane instability and continuous muscle fiber electrical activity, which is reflected in EMG findings (see later discussion). The pathogenesis of clinical signs of HYPP is complex and not entirely understood, either in horses or in human beings with a similar disorder. Affected heterozygotes have a mosaic of abnormal and normal sodium channels, and resting muscle membrane potentials are typically lower than normal. This leads to an increased likelihood of electrical generation of a prolonged muscle action potential, resulting in transient myotonia. When abnormal sodium channels are activated, the response to the abnormally increased intracellular sodium is release of potassium to the extracellular space and blood stream, resulting in hyperkalemia. Hyperkalemia is not, however, a consistent finding. Feeding of high potassium feeds, such as alfalfa products or feeds with added molasses, can precipitate clinical signs of HYPP, possibly by activating abnormal sodium channels. Another potential consequence of prolonged activation of abnormal sodium channels is inactivation of normal sodium channels, resulting in flaccid paralysis and collapse. This result would explain the typical signs seen during episodes, which include transient muscle spasm (myotonia), with protrusion of the third eyelid, followed by flaccid paralysis. Decreased muscle temperature, as can occur as a result of a chilling rain, can precipitate episodic collapse in HYPP horses, possibly by decreasing the activity of the muscle sodium-potassium exchanger (the Na-K ATPase), an important means by which affected muscle compensates for abnormal sodium channel activity. Postanesthetic recumbency and anesthesia-associated hyperthermia have also been seen in HYPP horses. Affected horses can appear normal for many years, can have multiple episodes of collapse, or can die acutely. Serum concentrations of CK and AST are generally normal. Abnormal ionic fluxes occur at all times in affected horses, and concentric needle electromyography between paralytic episodes reveals characteristic persistent myotonic bursts.

There are no gross pathologic findings in HYPP horses other than prominent muscling. Affected skeletal muscle is generally histologically normal, although scattered intracytoplasmic vacuoles (vacuolar myopathy) can be present in type 2 fibers. The characteristic pathologic finding of HYPP is only evident at the ultrastructural level, where dilated terminal cisternae of the sarcoplasmic reticulum are found.

Diagnosis can be made with reasonable certainty based on characteristic clinical signs and clinicopathologic findings in a horse of Impressive line breeding. Myotonic bursts with concentric needle electromyography are also diagnostic. The simplest and most reliable test, however, is a DNA-based test performed on peripheral white blood cells or, more recently, on cells obtained from the base of pulled mane or tail hairs. Treatment consists of feeding a low-potassium diet, which means avoiding alfalfa products and molasses. A low-potassium diet can be successful in controlling signs in many cases. More severe cases can be treated with the diuretic acetazolamide, which causes increased urinary excretion of potassium. Acute episodes can be treated by intravenous dextrose or insulin or with oral sugar solutions such as sugar syrup. Administration of glucose to stimulate insulin secretion, or of insulin itself, will aid in alleviating signs by helping to drive intracellular movement of potassium along with glucose.

Polysaccharide storage myopathy

This myopathy, designated with the acronyms EPSM, PSSM, or EPSSM, is most commonly recognized in quarter horse, warm blood, Arabian, Morgan, pony of the Americas, and draft-related breeds. It also occurs in many other horse and pony breeds, including miniature horses. Survey examination of equine muscle samples has revealed an astonishing incidence of approximately 66% in all draft-related horses and approximately 30% in all light horses. Not all affected horses exhibit obvious clinical signs of muscle dysfunction. This disorder is thought to be inherited as an autosomal dominant trait, although the exact mode of inheritance is not clear at this time.

In contrast to other glycogenoses affecting skeletal muscle, to-date no abnormality in the glycolytic or glycogenolytic pathways in skeletal muscle has been identified, making this equine disorder unique, but an underlying carbohydrate metabolic disorder is still suspected. Affected horses appear to have a more rapid intramuscular uptake of blood glucose than controls, although the exact mechanism for this phenomenon is still unknown. Abnormal accumulation of intracytoplasmic glycogen (confirmed by being PAS-positive, amylase-sensitive) within type 2 fibers is the histologic finding. In severe cases, aggregates of abnormal glycogen are eventually ubiquitinated, resulting in amylase-resistant inclusions composed of glycogen and filamentous protein. Certain breeds, such as quarter horse and draft-related breeds, seem to be most prone to the development of amylase-resistant inclusions, whereas glycogen aggregates are more common in other breeds. The explanation for this difference is as yet unknown.

Clinical signs are variable, and all are thought to be caused by insufficient energy production by affected muscle fibers. Abnormal myofiber function due to architectural alteration secondary to deposition of complex polysaccharide is also possible, although the excellent response to therapy even in horses with severe intramyofiber inclusion accumulation suggests that this is

less significant than is altered energy metabolism. Recurrent exertional rhabdomyolysis (see later discussion) is a commonly recognized sign, but unexplained pelvic limb lameness is even more common than clinical rhabdomyolysis. Affected horses can also have a stiff gait, symmetric muscle atrophy, back soreness, muscle cramping resulting in abnormal hindlimb flexion characteristic of shivers, and bilateral pelvic limb or generalized weakness. In draft horses, sudden onset of spontaneous recumbency or postanesthetic recumbency because of myopathy can occur. Serum concentrations of CK and AST are markedly increased after episodes of exertional rhabdomyolysis but may be only mildly to moderately increased in affected horses after exercise or onset of recumbency. Normal serum levels of CK and AST in affected horses are thought to indicate that the muscle dysfunction is not associated with overt myonecrosis. Concentric needle electromyography may reveal abnormal spontaneous activity (scattered positive sharp waves and fibrillations).

In severe cases, in which horses have died or been euthanatized because of rhabdomyolysis or recumbency, muscles may be pale pink or diffusely red-tinged, which can be mistaken for autolysis. Multifocal pale zones may be present (Fig. 15-40, A). In draft horses, chronic myopathy can result in overall reduction in muscle mass. Muscles in severely affected draft horses can also be of normal size but may contain pale streaks where myofibers have been replaced by fat. The most severely affected muscles are those of the proximal thigh and epaxial muscles of the back (e.g., longissimus), although any of the large "power" muscle groups, including pectoral and shoulder girdle muscles, can be affected. Swollen, dark kidneys (pigmentary nephrosis) caused by myoglobinuria can be seen in horses dying with severe rhabdomyolysis. The extent of overt myofiber necrosis is extremely variable; massive necrosis or regeneration can be seen after severe rhabdomyolysis, whereas only minimal scattered fiber necrosis may be seen in recumbent horses. Lesions are monophasic if there has been only a single bout of exertional rhabdomyolysis, or polyphasic if there have been repeated bouts of less severe exercise-induced injury. Fiber necrosis is uncommon in muscle biopsy samples taken from affected horses while they are clinically normal.

The characteristic histologic finding is aggregates of intracytoplasmic material that stain positively with PAS reaction for glycogen (Fig. 15-39, A). In severe cases, multiple pale intracytoplasmic inclusions will also be seen with H&E stain (Fig. 15-39, B). These inclusions are PAS-positive (Fig. 15-39, C) and resist digestion by amylase and are thus not glycogen. Terms used to describe this amylase-resistant material include amylopectin, polyglucosan, and complex polysaccharide. In chronic cases, myofibers also exhibit chronic myopathic

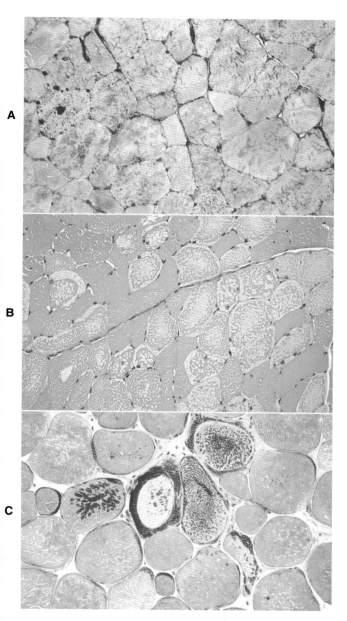

Fig. 15-39 Equine polysaccharide storage myopathy, semimembranosus muscle, transverse sections, horse.
A, Note the increased amount of and irregularly distributed dark-pink staining glycogen. Abnormal aggregates are present both beneath the sarcolemma and within the cytoplasm. Formalin fixation, PAS reaction. **B,** Severe form. Numerous myofibers contain multiple pale (*very light pink*) subsarcolemmal and intracytoplasmic inclusions of stored polysaccharide. Formalin fixation, H&E stain. **C,** These inclusions shown in Fig. 15-39, *B* stain intensely with PAS but are not digested by amylase (not shown) and are characteristic of what is called complex polysaccharide, amylopectin, or polyglucosan. Formalin fixation, PAS reaction. (*A, B, and C, Courtesy Dr. B.J. Cooper, College of Veterinary Medicine, Oregon State University.*)

change (atrophy, hypertrophy, internal nuclei), and fat replacement of myofibers can occur in severe cases.

At this time, the diagnosis of polysaccharide storage myopathy depends on finding characteristic histopathologic changes in muscle samples of horses with appropriate clinical signs. Gluteal, semimembranosus, or semitendinosus muscle samples are preferred, although changes in longissimus muscle are also found, especially in horses with back pain. A presumptive diagnosis of polysaccharide storage myopathy can be made based on characteristic clinical findings in a predisposed breed. Treatment has relied on altering the diet to minimize starch and sugar intake (less than 15% of total daily calories) and maximize fat intake (at least 20% to 25% of total daily calories from fat). Grains and sweet feeds are replaced by high-fiber, low-starch, low-sugar feeds, with added fat in the form of vegetable oil, powdered fat, or high-fat rice bran supplements. Provision of as much time in a pasture or paddock and regular exercise as possible are also important. Treatment is very successful in most cases.

Glycogen brancher enzyme deficiency (glycogenosis type IV)

This disorder is due to a congenital lack of a glycogenic enzyme, glycogen brancher enzyme (GBE), and is an emerging disease in quarter horses and American paint horses. This disorder is inherited as an autosomal recessive trait. Affected foals may be aborted, stillborn, or weak at birth or can have contracted tendons, rhabdomyolysis, or cardiac failure at an early age. The consequence of GBE deficiency is the accumulation of long unbranched chains of glucose within cells that leads to abnormal glycogen formation and deposition. These molecules would normally be converted into glycogen in the presence of GBE in the final step in the formation of glycogen. There are no specific gross pathologic findings. Pulmonary edema may be found in foals that die from cardiac failure. Characteristic histologic findings are round hyaline inclusions resembling amylopectin (polyglucosan bodies) within skeletal and cardiac myocytes, especially Purkinje fibers, and to a lesser degree within hepatocytes. Inclusions are also common in the brain and spinal cord and, unlike glycogen, are PAS-positive and resistant to amylase digestion. As with other carbohydrate metabolic defects, a lack of energy production by affected fibers is thought to underlie cellular dysfunction. Disruption of cytoarchitecture due to amylopectin deposition may also contribute. Analysis of peripheral blood or skeletal muscle for GBE activity will identify affected animals with severely reduced GBE activity and carriers in which GBE activity is moderately reduced. A DNA test using pulled mane or tail hairs is now available to detect carriers and affected horses. There is no treatment for this disorder.

Myotonia and mitochondrial myopathy

A myotonic disorder occurs occasionally in horses, and a mitochondrial myopathy has been described in an Arabian horse. These disorders are discussed in more detail in Appendix 15-1.

OTHER EQUINE MYOPATHIES
Exertional rhabdomyolysis

Equine exertional rhabdomyolysis (tying up, azoturia, Monday morning disease, setfast, blackwater) is characterized clinically by sudden onset of stiff gait, reluctance to move, swelling of affected muscle groups (especially gluteal), sweating, and other signs of pain and discomfort. Serum concentration of CK and AST are often markedly increased. Signs may appear during or immediately after exercise, but only rarely is exertional rhabdomyolysis associated with exhaustive exercise. In severely affected horses, even minimal exercise such as walking out of a stall can cause clinical signs. An association with high grain feeding and lack of regular exercise has been recognized for many years. Previous theories regarding the pathogenesis of equine exertional rhabdomyolysis include development of muscle lactic acidosis, vitamin E and/or selenium deficiency, hypothyroidism, and electrolyte abnormalities. It is only recently that studies have concluded that lactic acidosis is not a finding in horses with exertional rhabdomyolysis, that hypothyroid horses show no signs of degenerative myopathy, and that electrolyte abnormalities as a primary cause of equine exertional rhabdomyolysis are rare. It is still thought that vitamin E or selenium deficiency can exacerbate signs of exertional rhabdomyolysis in predisposed horses, but neither vitamin E nor selenium deficiency is considered a primary cause. Recent studies have found that affected horses typically have an underlying myopathy, most often polysaccharide storage myopathy. There is some evidence to suggest that recurrent exertional rhabdomyolysis in thoroughbreds is because of abnormal calcium homeostasis within skeletal muscle, although other affected thoroughbreds have been found to have polysaccharide storage myopathy. As muscle necrosis per se is neither painful, nor does it cause muscle swelling, it is suspected that other factors play a role in this disorder in the horse. These factors include oxidative injury to muscle membranes occurring secondary to segmental necrosis and release of reactive compounds from damaged membranes, which may explain the perceived benefit of supplemental vitamin E and selenium to affected horses, and vascular injury, which results in ischemia (i.e., compartment syndrome).

Gross findings are similar to those described for polysaccharide storage myopathy (Fig. 15-40, A). Histologic findings are localized or widespread muscle fiber necrosis (Fig. 15-40, B) followed by the usual

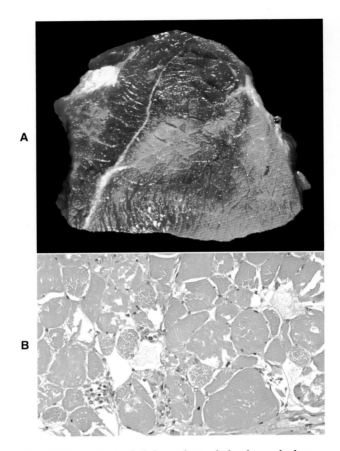

Fig. 15-40   Acute rhabdomyolysis, skeletal muscle, horse. A, Affected muscles may be pale pink or diffusely red-tinged, which can be mistaken for autolysis. Multifocal pale zones may also be present. **B,** Segmental myofiber necrosis, semitendinosus muscle, transverse section. Most of the myocytes are necrotic and at the stage of coagulation necrosis. In a few myofibers, necrosis is at a later stage and the necrotic sarcoplasm has lysed, leaving empty sarcolemmal tubes. A couple of necrotic myofibers are at an even later stage and contain a small number of macrophages. Formalin fixation, H&E stain. (**A,** *Courtesy Dr. W. Crowell, College of Veterinary Medicine, University of Georgia; and Noah's Arkive, College of Veterinary Medicine, The University of Georgia.* **B,** *Courtesy Dr. B.J. Cooper, College of Veterinary Medicine, Oregon State University.*)

sequence of events, macrophage infiltration and regeneration. Affected fibers are primarily type 2 fibers. Lesions can be either monophasic or polyphasic.

Diagnosis is based on typical clinical signs and clinicopathologic evidence of muscle injury (increased activity of CK or AST). Treatment for an acute episode includes nonsteroidal antiinflammatory agents, acepromazine, and rest. Careful evaluation of the patient for evidence of renal damage ([pigmentary] myoglobinuric nephrosis) because of myoglobin released from damaged muscle is indicated. Long-term treatment and prevention include correction of any concurrent electrolyte, mineral, or vitamin deficiencies and most importantly a change in diet to one that is high in fat and fiber and low in starch and sugar, as described for horses with polysaccharide storage myopathy (see Inherited or Congenital Myopathies). Thoroughbreds with recurrent exertional rhabdomyolysis due to suspected underlying calcium handling abnormalities also respond well to this type of diet.

Hyperthermia

Malignant hyperthermia occurring during general anesthesia and development of postanesthetic hyperthermia (sometimes called hypermetabolism to distinguish it from true malignant hyperthermia) occurs in horses. A genetic defect in the skeletal muscle ryanodine receptor, similar to malignant hyperthermia in human beings, dogs, and pigs, has been identified in some horses with malignant hyperthermia triggered by anesthetic agents. Some affected horses with a hyperthermia-like syndrome occurring during anesthesia or with hyperthermia occurring during recovery from anesthesia have HYPP or polysaccharide storage myopathy, but in some cases the exact cause of these conditions is not clear. It is likely that, similar to hyperthermia in human beings, a variety of underlying myopathies, especially those that result in uncoupling of mitochondria within skeletal myocytes (see Malignant Hyperthermia), can predispose animals to anesthesia-associated hyperthermia. Studies of muscle from horses with exertional rhabdomyolysis have detected loosely coupled mitochondria, which could predispose them to malignant hyperthermia–like episodes. The extent of overt muscle fiber necrosis due to hyperthermia varies but is often severe.

Ischemic myopathy

In addition to vascular damage due to clostridial toxins or immune-mediated vasculitis, ischemic myopathy of pectoral and limb muscle can be seen in recumbent horses as the result of pressure interfering with vascular perfusion. Once the horse is moved or is standing, reperfusion injury can occur. Development of compartment syndrome can contribute to ischemic injury (see Disturbance of Circulation). Ischemic myopathy of the abdominal muscles can be seen after prolonged lifting of a horse with a sling. In these cases, affected muscles generally show degenerative or regenerative changes that are all at about the same stage (monophasic necrosis). Concurrent necrosis and regeneration (polyphasic necrosis) can also be seen in horses that are in a sling or recumbent for an extended period of time. Recovery will depend on the extent of injury and the ability to regenerate (i.e., depending on whether the basal lamina is intact and the extent of satellite cell injury and necrosis).

Transient pelvic limb muscle ischemia due to aortoiliac mural thrombosis occurs in horses. The cause of the thrombosis is unknown, although it has been attributed to migration of strongyle larvae. Typically the thrombus is not occlusive, and clinical signs of pelvic limb dysfunction occur only during or after strenuous exercise, such as racing. A short-strided gait and a decreased surface temperature of the distal portion of the affected limb during episodes are characteristic. Because the ischemia is transient, pathologic studies are few. But overt myofiber necrosis is thought to be minimal, and recovery is typically rapid.

Postanesthetic myopathy

Degenerative myopathy can occur in horses undergoing prolonged recumbency during general anesthesia. In some cases, muscle damage may be due to ischemia from systemic hypotension leading to muscle hypoxia or from pressure caused by the weight of large muscle masses during recumbency, especially when adequate padding has not been provided. Underlying myopathy of various types will also predispose to postanesthetic myopathy. In ischemic damage, the location of the lesions depends on the position of the horse during anesthesia. In dorsal recumbency, the gluteal and the longissimus muscles are ischemic; in lateral recumbency, the triceps brachii, pectoralis, deltoideus, and brachiocephalicus muscles of the leg under the body become ischemic. The basic mechanism is that the pressure in the muscle exceeds the perfusion pressure in the capillaries. The use of adequate padding under the recumbent horse and the maintenance of normal blood pressure during anesthesia have greatly reduced the incidence of postanesthetic myopathy from muscle ischemia in horses. These days, underlying myopathy, particularly polysaccharide storage myopathy, appears to be the most common cause of postanesthetic myopathy in horses.

Endocrine myopathies

Although hypothyroidism is often suggested to be a cause of muscle dysfunction in the horse, studies of experimentally thyroidectomized horses have failed to support hypothyroidism as a cause of equine myopathy. Pituitary hyperfunction due to adenoma or hyperplasia in older horses, causing equine Cushing's disease, is the most common equine endocrine disorder causing muscle atrophy and weakness. The characteristic pot-bellied appearance of affected horses is thought to be secondary to abdominal muscle weakness.

DENERVATING DISEASES

Localized or generalized muscle dysfunction can be caused by disorders affecting motor neurons or peripheral nerves. Several syndromes of peripheral nerve dysfunction are recognized in the horse.

Peripheral neuropathy

Injury to the motor nerves in a peripheral nerve results in localized muscle atrophy and dysfunction of those myofibers innervated by those nerves. Damage to the suprascapular nerve results in unilateral scapular muscle (supraspinatus and infraspinatus) atrophy, and the clinical condition is known as sweeney. In working draft horses, this nerve can be compressed by a poorly fitted harness collar. In nonharness horses, trauma is the most common cause. Traumatic injury to the radial nerve or axillary plexus is also relatively common in horses.

Sporadic pelvic limb neuropathy causing an exaggerated flexion of one or both limbs is known as stringhalt. It can be caused by trauma to the hind leg, ingestion of plant toxins, or can be of unknown cause. Outbreaks of stringhalt in pastured horses in Australia and New Zealand are the result of ingestion of *Hypochoeris radicata* and related species, also known as flatweed, false dandelion, and hairy cat's ear. Lesions of denervation atrophy are found in the distal lateral digital extensor muscle, and surgical removal of this muscle is one method of correction. Laryngeal hemiplegia due to denervation can also occur in affected horses (see later discussion). *Hypochoeris radicata* grows prolifically in the Pacific Northwest and a similar syndrome of plant-induced stringhalt is said to occur there, but evidence to support this hypothesis has been hard to find, and feeding trials at Oregon State University have failed to reproduce the syndrome.

In addition to hamstring (semitendinosus, semimembranosus, and biceps femoris) muscle trauma, pelvic limb neuropathy as a result of trauma or unknown causes can cause the characteristic abnormal gait known as fibrotic myopathy, in which the forward swing of the affected pelvic limb is restricted. Affected muscle shows characteristic microscopic lesions of denervation atrophy.

Laryngeal hemiplegia is a well-documented condition in horses in which degenerative lesions within the left recurrent laryngeal nerve result in unilateral laryngeal muscle denervation atrophy (Fig. 15-22) and laryngeal dysfunction. Affected horses often make a characteristic respiratory noise during exercise, hence the name *roaring*. There are many possible causes of injury to the left recurrent laryngeal nerve, including extension of infections from the gutteral puches or tumors in that area, lead toxicity, and direct trauma. Most cases, however, are considered idiopathic. Although the exact cause of idiopathic laryngeal hemiplegia in horses is not known, the fact that it occurs only in tall, long-necked horses, and virtually never in ponies, suggests that whatever the mechanism of injury, very long nerves are predisposed.

Lead intoxication can also cause generalized peripheral neuropathy, muscle atrophy, and weakness mimicking equine motor neuron disease (see later discussion). Polyneuritis equi (neuritis of the cauda equina) and peripheral nerve lymphoma also cause denervation atrophy in horses. Polyneuritis equi most often involves the caudal nerve roots and facial nerves, and lymphoma has been found affecting multiple nerve roots or selectively involving the facial nerve.

Motor neuronopathy

Damage to motor neurons in the brain stem or ventral horns of the spinal cord will result in degeneration of peripheral nerves. In the horse, protozoal myeloencephalitis due to *Sarcocystis neurona* is a common cause of unilateral denervation atrophy, usually of facial or gluteal musculature. Affected horses often also exhibit ataxia and proprioceptive deficits indicative of upper motor neuron and general proprioceptive pathway dysfunction (see Chapter 14).

Equine motor neuron disease occurs as the result of severe and prolonged vitamin E deficiency, which leads to motor neuron degeneration. Clinical signs are sudden onset of rapid muscle wasting, weakness, trembling, and increased time spent in recumbency. Type 1 motor neurons and muscles are preferentially affected, supporting the proposed pathogenesis of oxidative injury to motor neurons secondary to vitamin E deficiency. The severe denervation atrophy occurring in

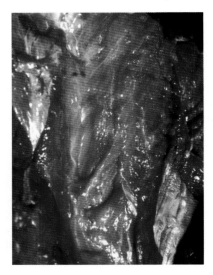

Fig. 15-41   Denervation atrophy, equine motor neuron disease, medial triceps muscle, horse. The medial triceps muscle, a type 1 predominant postural muscle deep in the foreleg, is diffusely pale tan and gelatinous in appearance because of severe denervation atrophy. The adjacent muscles *(left and right)* have a normal appearance. *(Courtesy College of Veterinary Medicine, Cornell University. For histopathologic findings, see Fig. 15-23.)*

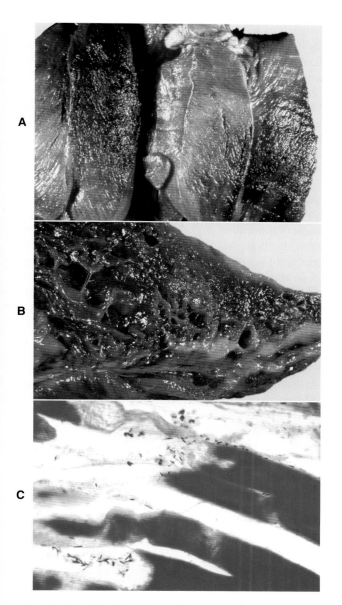

Fig. 15-42   Blackleg, hemorrhagic-necrotizing myositis (*Clostridium chauvoei*), thigh muscle, cow. A, The dark red areas are caused by hemorrhagic necrosis of the underlying muscle. These lesions are characteristic of blackleg. **B,** *Clostridium chauvoei* can also produce substantial quantities of gas within infected tissues as shown here by the numerous ("pseudocystic") spaces within hemorrhagic and necrotic muscle. **C,** Gram-positive bacilli are present in the serous exudate. Formalin fixation, Gram stain. (*A, Courtesy College of Veterinary Medicine, Cornell University. B and C, Courtesy Dr. M.D. McGavin, College of Veterinary Medicine, University of Tennessee.*)

postural muscles (medial head of the triceps, vastus intermedius, sacrocaudalis dorsalis medialis) in horses with motor neuron disease often results in a remarkable pale yellow-tan color (Fig. 15-41, Fig. 15-11, C) and gelatinous texture of the affected muscle. Severely

affected horses may become persistently recumbent, leading to death or euthanasia. In some cases, high-dose vitamin E supplementation (10,000 IU or more per day) can halt the progression of the disorder, and affected horses on vitamin E therapy can even develop some compensatory muscle hypertrophy and regain muscle mass. There is little or no evidence of reinnervation in this disorder, and affected horses are considered disabled for life.

MUSCULAR DISORDERS OF CATTLE

Although cattle have not been selected for muscle performance, many breeds have been selected for meat quality. This has lead to selection for at least one genetic disorder. Disorders affecting muscle can have a profound economic effect on the cattle industry.

BACTERIAL AND PARASITIC MYOPATHIES
Clostridial myositis (blackleg)

This disease, due to *Clostridium chauvoei*, is economically an extremely important disease that is most common in beef cattle. It can also occur in dairy cattle, especially those housed in free-stall barns. *Clostridium chauvoei* is a spore-forming, gram-positive anaerobic bacillus. Its spores are ubiquitous in the soil and following ingestion are capable of crossing the intestinal mucosa, entering the blood stream, and being carried to skeletal muscles. The spores lie dormant until localized trauma to the muscle, which in cattle is most often due to bruising during handling in a chute or from trauma in a crowded feedlot, results in muscle damage and localized hypoxia. The resultant anaerobic conditions allow the spores to activate and the bacteria to proliferate and produce toxins (Table 15-4) that cause capillary damage, hemorrhage, edema, and necrosis of adjacent myofibers.

The most common presentation is acute death. Signs before death are referable to toxemia; to the heat, swelling, crepitus, and dysfunction of the affected muscle group; and to fever. Serum concentrations of CK and AST are typically increased. Locally extensive hemorrhage and edema, often with crepitus due to gas bubbles, are seen in affected muscles and in overlying fascia and subcutaneous tissue. Necrotic muscle fibers appear dark red to red-black. Lesions are either wet and exudative (early lesions) or dry (later lesions) (Fig. 15-42, A). Cardiac muscle can also be involved. A characteristic odor of rancid butter due to butyric acid is typical. In other parts of the body, hemorrhages and edema can occur from the toxemia. Affected carcasses autolyze rapidly, likely due to the effects of clostridial toxins on tissue and of high body temperature before death. Histologically, locally extensive areas of muscle fibers undergoing coagulation necrosis and fragmentation, and interstitial edema and hemorrhage are seen. Overt vasculitis is not seen. Gas bubbles are typical.

Gram-positive bacilli whose appearance is compatible with that of *Clostridium chauvoei* may be demonstrable within affected muscle (Fig. 15-42, C).

Isolation of *Clostridium chauvoei* on anaerobic media or visualization by fluorescent antibody techniques are useful for the diagnosis of blackleg, but are confirmatory only if typical gross and histopathologic lesions are present, as dormant spores of *Clostridium chauvoei* can be found in normal muscle. The vaccination history and evaluation of husbandry practices are also important; unvaccinated or poorly vaccinated animals in situations in which muscle trauma is possible are most at risk. There is generally no effective treatment for cattle with blackleg, and death occurs rapidly. Prevention is the best treatment. Vaccination against clostridial toxins and maintenance of a safe environment are critical.

Botulism

Botulism due to ingestion of *Clostridium botulinum* toxin from contaminated feed or soil occurs in cattle, and clinical signs and pathogenesis are similar to those in the adult horse. Cattle are most susceptible to type C and D botulinum toxins, and herd outbreaks are possible. Cattle, however, are much more resistant to botulism than are horses. Botulinum toxin within silage, haylage, or hay is the most common cause of outbreaks of botulism in cattle. Abnormal eating habits (pica) can result in ingestion of *Clostridium botulinum* toxin from the soil or carrion. Botulism in cattle is usually fatal.

Pyogenic bacteria

Cattle are prone to develop abscesses caused by pyogenic bacteria, most commonly *Arcanobacterium pyogenes*. Abscesses in muscle occur most commonly in the hind leg. Swelling and lameness of the affected limb because of widespread necrotizing cellulitis and myositis are seen.

Arcanobacterium pyogenes is a ubiquitous bacterium that can infect muscle by two routes: by direct contamination of wounds and injection sites and hematogenously. The bacterium can be found within the reproductive tract of cows and within the rumen wall, and it has been speculated that *Arcanobacterium pyogenes* from a transient bacteremia after parturition or from disruption of the rumen wall can result in colonization of damaged muscle. Lesions vary depending on the virulence of the bacteria and the age of the lesions. They vary in extent from encapsulated intramuscular abscesses adjacent to the site of injection to a diffuse purulent cellulitis extending down the tissue and fascial planes. The cellulitis may be so severe as to involve much of the musculature of the affected limb. Grossly, encapsulated abscesses are filled with thick, yellow-green, foul-smelling pus. In cases of cellulitis, pus dissects along fascial planes outside the muscle and between perimysial sheaths within muscles. Inflammation extends into the adjacent myofibers, resulting in myonecrosis and subsequent replacement by fibrous tissue. The greenish color of the exudate is distinctive, and small gram-positive pleomorphic bacteria are often seen within tissue sections or cytologic preparations. *Arcanobacterium pyogenes* is readily isolated on aerobic culture.

Actinobacillus lignieresii (wooden tongue)

Infection of oral tissue, particularly of the tongue musculature, by *Actinobacillus lignieresii* results in a severe chronic suppurative and fibrosing myositis. Infection occurs through oral wounds or by penetrating plant fragments. Affected cattle have difficulty prehending and swallowing, and often have excessive salivation. Histologic features are of marked fibrosis with microabscesses containing eosinophilic material ("radiating clubs") and characteristic gram-negative bacilli. Aggressive antibiotic therapy can be curative.

Actinomyces bovis (lumpy jaw)

Actinomyces bovis frequently involves bones of the jaw, causing chronic suppurative and fibrosing osteomyelitis. Occasionally *Actinomyces bovis* involves the musculature of the tongue, causing gross and histologic lesions similar to those caused by *Actinobacillus lignieresii*. Gram stain reveals gram-positive bacilli, which distinguishes this lesion from the gram-negative *Actinobacillus lignieresii* infection.

Protozoal myopathies

Intracytoplasmic protozoal cysts of *Sarcocystis* spp. are common incidental findings in skeletal and cardiac myofibers of cattle (Fig. 15-31). Massive exposure may result in fever, anorexia, and progressive wasting, but this is uncommon. More often, *Sarcocystis* infection is diagnosed as an incidental finding at necropsy or during meat inspection at slaughter. If the cyst wall breaks down, a focus of myofiber necrosis and later granuloma formation results.

Eosinophilic myositis is a disease of cattle thought to be a relatively uncommon manifestation of *Sarcocystis* infection that may involve hypersensitivity. There is overt green discoloration (Fig. 15-12) of affected muscles caused by the massive infiltration of eosinophils (Fig. 15-43, A and B). This is accompanied by myofiber necrosis and, in chronic cases, fibrosis. Fragments of degenerating intralesional protozoa can sometimes be found (Fig. 15-43, C).

Cattle can also be infected with *Neospora caninum*. Adults have no clinical disease, but infection of the fetus can cause nonsuppurative inflammation of skeletal muscle and of heart and brain.

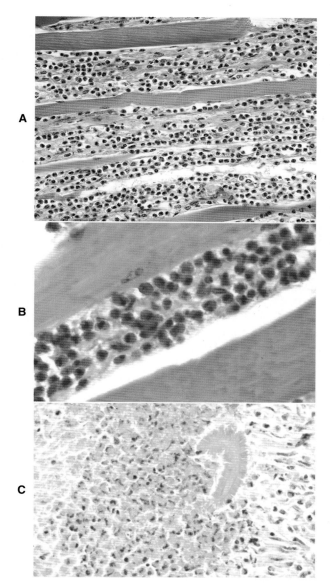

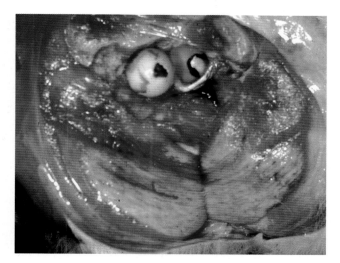

Fig. 15-44   Nutritional myopathy (white muscle disease), skeletal muscles of the caudal thigh, sagittal section, calf. In this early stage, affected muscles have yellow and white streaks, often in a patchy distribution. These streaks are areas of necrotic myofibers. Later as the necrotic myofibers calcify, white streaks (chalky texture, mineralization) are visible grossly. *(Courtesy Dr. G. K. Saunders, Virginia-Maryland Regional College of Veterinary Medicine; and Noah's Arkive, College of Veterinary Medicine, The University of Georgia.)*

Fig. 15-43   Bovine eosinophilic myositis, skeletal muscle, longitudinal section, cow. A, A dense interstitial infiltrate of eosinophils has separated the muscle fibers, some of which are atrophic. Formalin fixation, H&E stain. **B,** Higher magnification demonstrating the large population of eosinophils in the inflammatory exudate. Formalin fixation, H&E stain. **C,** Degenerate *Sarcocystis* organism surrounded by degenerate eosinophils. Formalin fixation, H&E stain. **(A,** *Courtesy Dr. M.D. McGavin, College of Veterinary Medicine, University of Tennessee; and Noah's Arkive, College of Veterinary Medicine, The University of Georgia.* **B,** *Courtesy Dr. M.D. McGavin, College of Veterinary Medicine, University of Tennessee.* **C,** *Courtesy Dr. R. Bildfell, College of Veterinary Medicine, Oregon State University.)*

NUTRITIONAL AND TOXIC MYOPATHIES
Nutritional myopathy

Similar to horses, calves and young cattle are susceptible to nutritional myopathy because of selenium or (less commonly) vitamin E deficiency. But the profound involvement of temporal and masseter muscles ("maxillary myositis") that can occur in horses is not seen in cattle. In the latter species, the postural muscles and muscles of locomotion are most commonly affected. Muscles of affected calves appear pale pink to white, often in a patchy distribution. The gross appearance depends on the extent of the necrosis and the stage of the lesion. In early stages, yellow and white streaks are present, and later pale, chalk white streaks often appear, thus the common name *white muscle disease* (Fig. 15-44).

Plant toxicities

Cassia occidentalis (coffee senna, coffee weed) is the most common cause of degenerative myopathy in cattle due to plant toxicity in cattle. This plant grows throughout the southeastern United States. Pale areas within skeletal muscle, with lesser involvement of cardiac muscle, are due to fiber necrosis, generally with minimal to no mineralization. Other plant toxicities are discussed in the toxic myopathies section.

Ionophore toxicity

The pathogenesis of ionophore toxicity is discussed in the toxic myopathy section. Ionophore toxicity in cattle is seen only with overdoses because of improper feed mixing. Anorexia, diarrhea, and weakness are the primary clinical signs. Serum concentrations of CK and AST are often extremely high. Pale areas within skeletal and cardiac muscle are due to myofiber necrosis. In animals that survive, regeneration will restore the skeletal muscle integrity, but cardiac lesions heal by fibrosis.

CONGENITAL OR INHERITED DISORDERS
Steatosis

This disease in cattle, sometimes called lipomatosis, is most often recognized as an incidental finding at necropsy or at slaughter. This disorder is thought to be the result of defective muscle development, in which large areas of myofibers are replaced by adipocytes. An inherited basis has not been established. Lesions can be symmetric or asymmetric, with the most severely affected muscles being those of the back and loin (longissimus muscles; Fig. 15-11, *D*). Severely affected muscles are composed entirely of fat, whereas less severely affected muscles appear streaked because of partial replacement by fat. Histologically the space normally occupied by myofibers is filled with mature adipocytes. In utero denervation or failure of innervation will result in a similar muscle lesion (Fig. 15-29), and careful evaluation of the peripheral nerves and spinal cord is indicated.

Diagnosis is readily made on gross examination and can be confirmed by histologic examination, specifically in sections stained with oil-red-O or Sudan black for fat. As this condition is usually not diagnosed during life and the loss of myofibers is irreversible, treatment is neither necessary nor possible.

Other bovine congenital or inherited myopathies and neuronopathies

Congenital muscular hyperplasia ("double muscling") due to defects in the myostatin gene occurs in a variety of cattle breeds. An unusual multisystemic disease with characteristic necrotizing vasculopathy occurs in young Gelbvieh cattle. Glycogenosis type II (acid maltase deficiency) has been recognized in shorthorn and Brahman cattle, and glycogenosis type V (myophosphorylase deficiency) occurs in Charolais cattle. An inherited motor neuron degenerative disease occurs in Brown Swiss cattle. These disorders are discussed in more detail in Appendix 15-1.

ELECTROLYTE ABNORMALITIES
Hypokalemic myopathy

Decreased potassium interferes with normal muscle cell function and can lead to muscle weakness and myofiber necrosis. Type 2 fibers are preferentially affected. The pathogenesis of hypokalemic myopathy is not clear, but myofiber necrosis may be the end result of either decreased myofiber energy production or of focal ischemia secondary to vasoconstriction. Hypokalemia can also interfere with normal cardiac conduction, and atrial fibrillation is common. Hypokalemia in cattle can be due to anorexia. A history of ketosis

occurring within a month of parturition is common. Glucocorticoids with high mineralocorticoid activities, such as isoflupredone acetate used to treat ketosis, are a recognized cause of hypokalemic myopathy in cattle. Activation of glucose transport into cells by intravenously administered glucose or insulin will also cause intracellular movement of potassium and can result in hypokalemia. No specific findings are present at postmortem examination, although ischemic necrosis secondary to recumbency can be seen in muscles of the hindlimbs (see later discussion). Examination of muscles not involved in weight-bearing reveals multifocal polyphasic myofiber necrosis and vacuolated myofibers (vacuolar degeneration), indicative of myodegeneration as a direct effect of hypokalemia.

Affected cows are profoundly weak and become recumbent and unable to support the weight of their heads. Serum concentration of potassium is below normal (<2.3 mEq/L), and CK and AST levels are moderately high. The diagnosis is based on typical historical and clinical findings and a low serum potassium concentration. Intravenous and oral supplementation with potassium salts and supportive therapy may result in recovery in some cases, but this disorder is often fatal.

Other electrolyte abnormalities

Both hypocalcemia and hypophosphatemia can result in profound muscle weakness and recumbency in cattle. In hypocalcemia, weakness is primarily due to disruption of neuromuscular transmission. Significant changes are not seen in affected muscles, although ischemic necrosis can occur secondary to recumbency (see later discussion). Diagnosis relies on clinical findings and identification of abnormal serum electrolyte concentrations. Treatment includes correction of the electrolyte defect by intravenous administration of the appropriate electrolyte-containing fluids, supportive care, and correction of any dietary abnormalities that may predispose to electrolyte problems.

ISCHEMIC MYOPATHY

Ischemic muscle necrosis due to recumbency is common in cattle. The muscular lesion is similar to that seen in other species, but in cattle prolonged sternal recumbency is more common than lateral recumbency, and pectoral muscles and muscles of limbs tucked under the body or splayed out limbs will be most prone to injury (Fig. 15-30).

MUSCULAR DISORDERS OF SMALL RUMINANTS

Selection pressures and economic consequences of muscle disorders similar to those in beef cattle exist in small ruminants raised for meat. In goats, selection for an interesting mutant has resulted in perpetuation of myotonia.

BACTERIAL AND PARASITIC MYOPATHIES
Clostridial myositis (blackleg)

This disorder occurs occasionally in sheep and goats and is similar to the disease in cattle.

Botulism

Botulism can occur in small ruminants, but, as in cattle, it is rare.

Protozoal myopathy

Intracytoplasmic cysts of *Sarcocystis* spp. are commonly found within skeletal and cardiac muscle fibers of sheep and goats as an incidental finding, similar to cattle. Eosinophilic myositis due to sarcocystosis is rare in sheep and is not recognized in goats. In camelids, massive infection with *Sarcocystis* can occur (Fig. 15-45), especially in animals imported from South America where sarcocystosis is common. In rare cases, *Sarcocystis* infection in camelids is associated with widespread eosinophilic myositis.

NUTRITIONAL AND TOXIC MYOPATHIES

Degenerative myopathy due to nutritional deficiency or toxin ingestion is relatively common in many small ruminant species. The eating habits of goats make them particularly likely to ingest poisonous plants.

Nutritional myopathy

Young goats and sheep are susceptible to degenerative myopathy associated with selenium or, less commonly, vitamin E deficiency. A similar disorder occurs rarely in young camelids. The disease in these species is similar to the disease in young cattle.

Toxic myopathies

Sheep and goats are susceptible to plant and ionophore toxicities similar to those in cattle. In goats, ingestion of honey mesquite (*Prosopis glandulosa*) causes degeneration of the motor nucleus of the trigeminal nerve, resulting in denervation atrophy of the muscles of mastication, and consequent inability to adequately chew feed, leading to progressive emaciation.

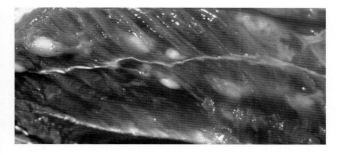

Fig. 15-45   Sarcocystosis, skeletal muscle, alpaca. Multiple pale nodules within the muscle indicate the location of *Sarcocystis* cysts. *(Courtesy College of Veterinary Medicine, Cornell University.)*

CONGENITAL OR INHERITED MYOPATHIES
Myotonia in goats

Myotonia in the goat is inherited as an autosomal dominant trait, and the variable clinical severity is attributable to increased severity in homozygotes compared with heterozygotes. The genetic defect affects the skeletal muscle chloride channel, resulting in decreased chloride conductance and associated ionic instability of the sarcolemma. Affected goats develop severe muscle spasms in response to sudden voluntary effort, for example when startled by the blowing of a locomotive horn, starting at about 2 weeks of age. Episodes of myotonia can last from 5 to 20 seconds and are characterized by generalized stiffness and adoption of a "sawhorse" stance. Goats often fall over. Sustained muscle dimpling occurs after percussion. Serum concentrations of CK and AST are normal. Concentric needle electromyography reveals the characteristic waxing and waning ("dive bomber") spontaneous activity of myotonia. There are no gross pathologic findings. Histologically, muscle fibers in affected goats may show moderate hypertrophy. But characteristic abnormalities are revealed only with ultrastructural examination in which dilated and proliferated T tubules and terminal cisternae of sarcoplasmic reticulum are seen. Diagnosis is based on characteristic clinical signs and EMG findings. There is no treatment for this disorder, and it is rarely fatal. Affected animals are actually prized by collectors of so-called fainting goats. If nothing else, housing for these animals is simplified, as fencing need not be nearly as high as that required for normal goats.

Other inherited myopathies

An inherited myopathy (ovine muscular dystrophy) in Merino sheep and an inherited glycogen storage myopathy have been identified in sheep in Australia. These disorders are discussed in more detail in Appendix 15-1.

MEGAESOPHAGUS IN CAMELIDS

The esophagus of camelids contains a large amount of skeletal muscle, and adult llamas and alpacas are prone to develop abnormal motility and dilation of the esophagus (megaesophagus). Affected animals often lose body condition and exhibit abnormal rumination of feed boluses. Histopathologic findings of angular atrophy of type 1 and type 2 fibers suggest that this disorder is an acquired denervating disease, but further studies are necessary.

MUSCULAR DISORDERS OF PIGS

The economic impact of muscle disease in pigs is profound. The high percentage of pigs with the genetic defect that predisposes to malignant hyperthermia is another example of selection pressure leading to skeletal muscle genetic mutations.

BACTERIAL AND PARASITIC MYOPATHIES
Clostridial myositis (malignant edema)

Pigs occasionally develop clostridial myositis (*Clostridium* spp.) particularly at sites of intramuscular injection. The resulting disease is similar to that seen in cattle, sheep, and goats, although heart involvement appears to be rare.

Pyogenic bacteria

Abscesses within muscles and their fascia as a result of infection by pyogenic bacteria, such as *Arcanobacterium pyogenes*, are common in pigs and are similar to those in cattle.

Trichinosis

Infection of pigs by the nematode parasite *Trichinella spiralis* is of major economic importance to the porcine industry and poses a serious health hazard to human beings. Pigs infected with *Trichinella spiralis* show no clinical signs.

The adult nematode resides in the mucosa of the small intestine. Larvae penetrate the intestinal mucosa and enter the blood stream, through which they gain access to the muscle. Larvae invade and encyst within myocytes. Encysted larvae are typically not visible on gross examination, although dead larvae can calcify and be visible as 0.5- to 1-mm white nodules (Fig. 15-46, *A*). Active muscles such as the tongue, masseter, diaphragm, and intercostal, laryngeal, and extraocular muscles are preferentially affected. Focal inflammation consisting of eosinophils, neutrophils, and lymphocytes occurs associated with invasion of the muscle by *Trichinella* larvae. After cyst formation, the larvae are protected from the host's immune response, and inflammation is minimal to absent (Fig. 15-46, *B*).

Diagnosis is based on identification of the characteristic nematode larvae encysted within muscle fibers. In those cases in which the larvae have died and calcified, a presumptive diagnosis of trichinosis can still be made.

Protozoal myopathies

Intracytoplasmic cysts of *Sarcocystis* spp. are not common in pigs but can occasionally be found in the skeletal and cardiac muscle fibers as an incidental finding. Eosinophilic myocarditis has been reported following experimental infection.

NUTRITIONAL AND TOXIC MYOPATHIES
Nutritional myopathy

Young pigs are susceptible to degenerative myopathy because of selenium or vitamin E deficiency, and the pathologic changes are similar to those seen in calves. A distinctive clinical disorder seen in very young Vietnamese pot-bellied pigs, in which affected piglets

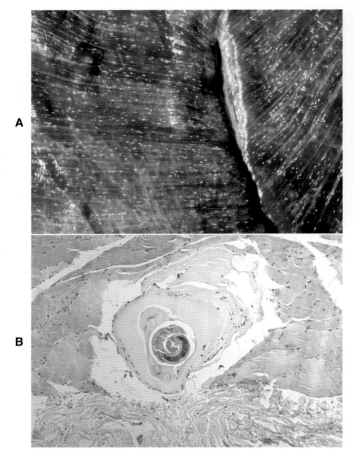

Fig. 15-46   Trichinosis, encysted larvae, diaphragm, bear. A, Encysted larvae of *Trichinella spiralis* appear as pale elongated foci in the muscle. **B,** Encysted larvae of *Trichinella spiralis* incite minimal inflammation until they die. Formalin fixation, H&E stain. (*A* and *B*, *Courtesy Dr. M.D. McGavin, College of Veterinary Medicine, University of Tennessee.*)

have a short, stilted gait and tend to stand on their toes, is thought to be related to selenium or vitamin E deficiency. Histologically, there is a multifocal polyphasic degenerative myopathy. Affected piglets appear to recover spontaneously.

Toxic myopathies

Pigs are susceptible to poisoning by *Cassia occidentalis* and develop segmental necrosis of myofibers, especially in the diaphragm. Monensin toxicity results in segmental necrosis of skeletal muscle and necrosis of cardiac muscle, particularly atria. The pathogenesis of ionophore toxicity is discussed in the section on Toxic Myopathies. Gossypol present in cottonseed products is toxic to pigs when these products are fed at 10% or more of the ration and causes skeletal and cardiac muscle necrosis as well as lesions in the liver and lung.

CONGENITAL AND INHERITED MYOPATHIES
Myofibrillar hypoplasia (splayleg)

This congenital disorder affects young piglets and results in splaying of the limbs to the side (abduction). Affected animals propel themselves by pushing against the ground with the pelvic limbs. This posture results in progressive flattening of the sternum. Although delayed myofibril development has been suggested, the histopathologic findings are inconclusive because similarly poorly developed myofibers can be seen in normal littermates. Affected piglets can recover with treatment, which includes the use of a harness that partially supports their bodies, holds their legs under their bodies, and encourages locomotion. Providing affected pigs with a nonslip floor is also important.

Steatosis

Pigs can have large areas of muscle replaced by mature adipose tissue, similar to that described in cattle.

Malignant hyperthermia (porcine stress syndrome; pale soft exudative pork)

This disorder affects several strains of pigs, most commonly those with unpigmented hair coats. A similar syndrome occurs in Vietnamese pot-bellied pigs. Incidence varies, but can be very high within certain herds. The disease in pigs is an accurate animal model of the disease in human beings and is an important cause of economic losses in the pig industry. Susceptibility to malignant hyperthermia is inherited as an autosomal recessive trait. The genetic defect results in abnormal activity of the skeletal muscle ryanodine receptor. The ryanodine receptor is a calcium release channel located in the sarcoplasmic reticulum terminal cisternal membrane that links the T tubule to the sarcoplasmic reticulum during excitation-contraction coupling. Uncontrolled intracytoplasmic calcium release because of abnormal ryanodine receptor activity leads to excessive contraction and heat production. Clinical disease occurs only in pigs homozygous for the defect, although human heterozygotes can also be susceptible to hyperthermic episodes following halothane anesthesia. It is suspected that this defect originated years ago in a foundation animal and resulted in offspring with increased muscling and reduced body fat. Affected pigs are clinically normal until an episode of hyperthermia is triggered by a precipitating factor, such as halothane anesthesia or stress. Episodes consist of severe muscle rigidity and dramatically increased body temperature. Severe cases progress rapidly to death. Serum concentrations of CK and AST are markedly increased during episodes.

In animals dying during a hyperthermic episode, affected muscles are pale, moist, and swollen and appear "cooked" (Fig. 15-47), hence the common name "pale,

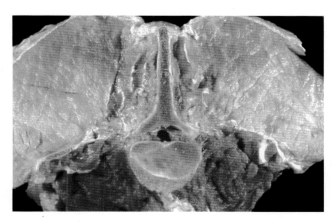

Fig. 15-47   Malignant hyperthermia, (porcine stress syndrome; pale soft exudative pork), lumbar epispinal muscles, transverse section, pig. The affected muscles are pale pink, moist, and swollen and have a "cooked" pork appearance ("parboiled"). *(Courtesy Dr. J. Wright, College of Veterinary Medicine, North Carolina State University; and Noah's Arkive, College of Veterinary Medicine, The University of Georgia.)*

soft, exudative pork." Muscles of the shoulder, back, and thigh are preferentially affected. Affected fibers are either hypercontracted or, if the animal has survived for some hours, undergoing coagulation necrosis. Histopathologic findings in susceptible pigs sampled during clinically normal periods include chronic myopathic change (fiber-size variation, internal nuclei) and rare necrotic fibers.

This disorder is most commonly diagnosed in pigs dying acutely and is made based on the clinical history of a precipitating stress and on the characteristic gross and histopathologic findings. Given that the precise defect is known, genetic testing allows for identification of carrier and affected animals. Avoidance of precipitating stress factors in susceptible pigs and removal of carrier and affected animals from the breeding stock will reduce the incidence of this disorder.

ISCHEMIC MYOPATHY

Large pigs are susceptible to ischemic myopathy secondary to recumbency, resulting in ischemic necrosis similar to that seen in horses and cattle. The proximal limb muscles are most susceptible.

MUSCULAR DISORDERS OF THE DOG

Selection pressures for a certain type of muscular development are far less frequent in dogs than in livestock. A few disorders, such as myotonia, have been suggested to occur more often in dogs originally bred for meat, but this is pure speculation. The canine genome may have genes prone to new mutations, similar to human beings, leading to genetic disorders, such as X-linked muscular dystrophy. In general, the impact of muscular disorders in dogs is much less than in livestock. Dogs with muscular weakness can still make good house pets.

PARASITIC MYOPATHIES
Protozoal myopathy

The parasitic diseases affecting skeletal muscle in the dog are primarily caused by protozoal organisms, of which *Neospora caninum* is the most important. It is now suspected that early reports of myositis and radiculoneuritis caused by *Toxoplasma gondii* in young dogs were actually *Neospora caninum* infections. *Neospora caninum* is often transmitted in utero, and evidence suggests that affected bitches are chronic carriers of the organism. Both the peripheral nervous system and the skeletal muscle are invaded by organisms. Ventral spinal roots are preferentially involved, and damage results in denervation atrophy of muscles. Signs of progressive neuromuscular weakness, most profound in the pelvic limbs, begin in affected pups several weeks of age. Marked muscle atrophy of the pelvic limb muscles occurs rapidly, and fixation of pelvic limb joints occurs as a result of denervation of muscle in an actively growing limb. Serum concentrations of CK and AST may be slightly increased. Concentric needle electromyography reveals dense, sustained spontaneous activity (fibrillations and positive sharp waves) consistent with denervation.

Pelvic limb muscles are severly atrophied, firm, and pale. Fixation of the pelvic limb joints persists after anesthesia or death. Scattered foci of mixed inflammation with associated segmental myofiber necrosis are often seen within skeletal muscle, and characteristic intracytoplasmic protozoal cysts may be present.

Neospora caninum infection should be suspected based on characteristic progressive neuromuscular dysfunction in a young growing pup. Infection of older dogs is also possible but is uncommon. The finding of a mixed inflammatory-neuropathic lesion within affected skeletal muscle should prompt a search for protozoa, although these are often present in small numbers and may not be seen. Serologic tests can detect antibodies to *Neospora caninum*, and antibodies are available for immunohistochemical studies of paraffin-embedded, formalin-fixed tissue. Antiprotozoal treatment may kill the organisms, but denervation atrophy and pelvic limb fixation will persist.

Hepatozoon americanum and *Trypanosoma cruzi* are other protozoal organisms that can affect canine skeletal muscle. These parasitic diseases are discussed in more detail in Appendix 15-1.

Other parasites

Rarely, cysts of *Trichinella spiralis* are found as an incidental finding in canine muscle.

CONGENITAL OR INHERITED MYOPATHIES
X-linked muscular dystrophy (Duchenne's type)

This disorder has been confirmed or suspected in several breeds of dogs, including Irish terrier, golden retriever, Labrador retriever, miniature schnauzer, rottweiler, Dalmatian, Shetland sheepdog, Samoyed, Pembroke Welsh corgi, Japanese spitz, and Alaskan malamute. This canine disorder is homologous to Duchenne's muscular dystrophy of human beings and involves defects in the dystrophin gene, which codes for a membrane-associated cytoskeletal protein present in skeletal and cardiac muscle. The absence of dystrophin renders skeletal muscle fibers susceptible to repeated bouts of necrosis and regeneration. Necrosis of cardiac myocytes also occurs and is followed by replacement with connective tissue, resulting in a progressive cardiomyopathy. This disorder is inherited as an X-linked recessive trait, affecting approximately 50% of males born to a female carrier. Experimentally, affected females have been produced from breeding of an affected male to a carrier female. It is suspected that new mutations in the canine dystrophin gene may be relatively common, as is the case in human beings. Therefore this disorder could occur in any breed, including crossbreeds. There is variable severity of clinical disease even within littermates, and small breed dogs are often less severely affected than are large breed dogs.

Severely affected pups develop a rapidly progressive weakness and die within the first few days of life. In less severely affected dogs, clinical signs are a stiff, short-strided gait and exercise intolerance beginning at 8 to 12 weeks of age, followed by progressive weakness and muscle atrophy. Development of a degree of joint contracture and splaying of the distal limbs is typical (Fig. 15-48). Weakness of the tongue, jaw, and pharyngeal muscles results in difficulty with prehension and swallowing of food, and affected dogs often drool excessively. Involvement of skeletal muscle within the esophagus can result in megaesophagus, regurgitation, and aspiration pneumonia. Markedly increased concentrations of serum CK, AST, and alanine aminotransferase (ALT) are characteristic, even before the onset of obvious clinical disease. Concentric needle electromyography reveals remarkable spontaneous activity in the form of pseudomyotonic bursts. Muscles do not dimple with percussion.

In pups dying within the first few days of life, the thin superficial muscles of the shoulder, neck, and pelvic limbs (trapezius, brachiocephalicus, deltoid, and sartorius), and the diaphragm have pale yellow-to-white streaks throughout (Fig. 15-11, *A*). Death in these cases is thought to be caused by respiratory failure related to severe diaphragmatic myonecrosis. In animals with clinical disease beginning at 8 to 12 weeks, pale streaks within muscle are much less evident, although affected

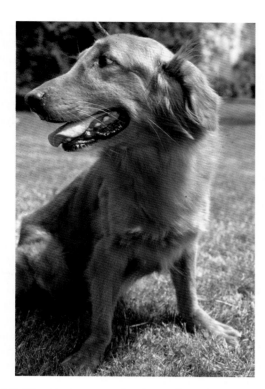

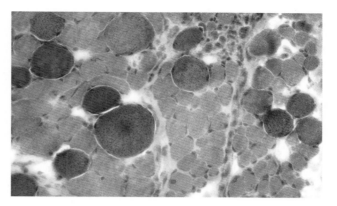

Fig. 15-49   Canine muscular dystrophy, X-linked muscular dystrophy, biceps femoris muscle, transverse section, dog. The numerous large dark fibers (*left*) are undergoing acute necrosis, and the cluster of small-diameter fibers with large prominent nuclei (*top right*) are regenerating. The presence of both necrotic and regenerating fibers is indicative of polyphasic necrosis. Frozen section, modified Gomori's trichrome stain. (*Courtesy Dr. B.A. Valentine, College of Veterinary Medicine, Oregon State University.*)

Fig. 15-48   Canine muscular dystrophy, X-linked muscular dystrophy, adult golden retriever. Note the diffuse muscle wasting and splaying (outward rotation) of the forelimbs. (*Courtesy Dr. B.A. Valentine, College of Veterinary Medicine, Oregon State University.*)

muscles often appear diffusely pale and may be fibrotic. All skeletal muscles, with the exception of the extraocular muscles, appear to be affected to varying degrees. Overt myofiber necrosis is most severe in earlier stages of the disorder and typically affects small clusters of contiguous fibers. Scattered large, darkly stained fibers ("large dark fibers") in the early stages of hypercontraction and necrosis are common (Fig. 15-16, *A*) Regeneration of affected segments occurs rapidly, and characteristically both myofiber necrosis and fiber regeneration are present within the same section (i.e., the lesion is a multifocal polyphasic necrosis) (Fig. 15-49). Scattered mineralized fibers can also be found. With time, ongoing necrosis and regeneration are less common, and endomysial fibrosis occurs. Chronically affected muscles can have remarkable fibrosis, infiltration by adipocytes, and other chronic myopathic changes. Fiber-type conversion can also be seen as a chronic myopathic change.

In all dogs 6 months of age or older, multifocal pale yellow–to–white zones will be present within the heart, predominantly involving the subepicardial region of the left ventricular wall, the papillary muscles, and the ventricular septum. Histologically, necrosis, mineralization, and progressive dissecting myocardial fibrosis

are found. Death in older animals is due either to aspiration pneumonia secondary to dysphagia or to progressive cardiac failure, although affected dogs may survive for many years.

The diagnosis should be suspected based on characteristic clinical findings in a young male dog but must be confirmed by muscle biopsy and analysis of muscle for dystrophin. The absence of dystrophin in muscle fibers of affected dogs can be confirmed using immunohistochemical staining on frozen sections (Fig. 15-50) or by Western blot analysis. There is no treatment for this disorder.

Carrier females show no clinical signs, but scattered necrotic and regenerating fibers and moderate increases in serum CK and AST are common in young carriers. At birth, dystrophin in carriers is expressed in a mosaic pattern in both cardiac and skeletal muscle (Fig. 15-50, *C*). Because they are multinucleate, skeletal myofibers are able to eventually up-regulate and translocate dystrophin to restore this protein within the entire myofiber. Fiber necrosis is therefore rare in older carriers. Cardiac muscle, however, remains mosaic for life. Foci of necrosis and development of fibrosis occurs in the cardiac muscle of carrier females, but to-date none have developed overt cardiac failure. Any female dog producing affected pups is a carrier, and approximately half of all of her female offspring will also be carriers. Carrier females can also be identified either by dystrophin or DNA analysis and should be spayed.

Other canine muscular dystrophies

Dystrophin has been found to be associated with a series of dystrophin-associated proteins, forming a

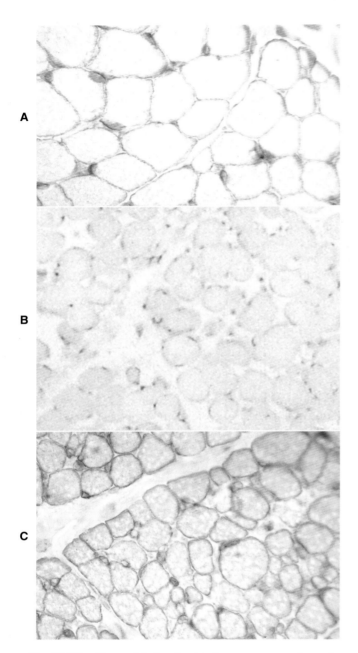

Fig. 15-50 **Dystrophin localization in transverse sections of canine muscle, immunostain for dystrophin, skeletal muscle. A,** Normal dog. Note that the dystrophin is localized at the sarcolemma. Frozen section, immunoperoxidase reaction for dystrophin. **B,** X-linked muscular dystrophy, dog. Dystrophin is completely absent. Frozen section, immunoperoxidase reaction for dystrophin. **C,** X-linked muscular dystrophy carrier, young carrier female dog. Note the mosaic pattern in which some fibers contain normal dystrophin and others completely lack dystrophin. Frozen section, immunoperoxidase reaction for dystrophin.

(*A, B,* and *C, Courtesy Dr. B.J. Cooper, College of Veterinary Medicine, Oregon State University.*)

membrane complex. The genes for many of these proteins are autosomally inherited; therefore not all canine muscular dystrophies are X-linked disorders. Autosomal recessive inheritance of dystrophin-associated gene defects leading to muscular dystrophy is common in human beings, and defects in dystrophin complex proteins leading to non-Duchenne's type muscular dystrophy have also been identified in various breeds of dogs. These are discussed in more detail in Appendix 15-1.

Labrador retriever myopathy

This disorder is inherited as an autosomal recessive trait. Affected dogs occur within the working or sporting breed lines rather than the show dog lines. Despite extensive study, the underlying defect is not known. Recent studies suggest similarity to inherited centronuclear myopathy of human beings. Affected Labrador retrievers develop signs of neuromuscular weakness within the first 6 months of life. Exercise intolerance leads to collapse during prolonged exercise, and episodes of collapse can also be elicited by exposure to cold. Loss of triceps and patellar reflexes is characteristic. Affected dogs usually do not develop normal musculature. Concentric needle electromyography reveals intense and abnormal spontaneous activity with normal motor nerve conduction velocities. Serum concentrations of CK and AST are often normal, although they can be mildly to moderately increased. Megaesophagus can be present.

The only specific abnormalities seen at necropsy are poor muscling and possibly megaesophagus. On histologic examination, affected dogs have remarkable myopathic changes characterized by clusters of atrophic myofibers, myofiber hypertrophy, and internal nuclei (Fig. 15-51). Abnormal mitochondrial distribution, often with peripheral mitochondrial aggregates (identified as ragged red fibers in frozen sections stained with Gomori's modified trichrome stain), can also be seen (Fig. 15-28, *B*). A primary defect of the myofiber is suspected, but segmental necrosis and regeneration are rare. Therefore this disorder does not qualify as a muscular dystrophy. Although the initial reports described this disorder as a type 2 deficiency myopathy, further studies have shown that fiber-type proportions vary remarkably between muscles and between dogs, although an increase in type 1 fibers (type 1 fiber predominance) is often seen. Alteration of the normal mosaic pattern of myofiber types is also seen. There is fiber-type grouping, usually considered a neuropathic change, despite the absence of peripheral nerve lesions. These changes are thought to reflect fiber-type conversion unassociated with denervation.

Based on the clinical findings, the diagnosis may be suspected but should be confirmed by a muscle biopsy. There is no treatment for the disorder, although the

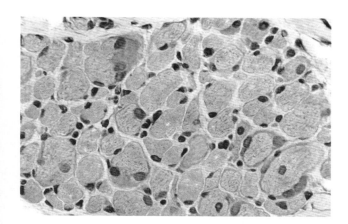

Fig. 15-51   Labrador myopathy, skeletal muscle, transverse section, Labrador dog. There is excessive fiber-size variation, and some fibers contain one or rarely two internal nuclei. Nuclei are abnormally large. Frozen section, H&E stain. *(Courtesy Dr. B.A. Valentine, College of Veterinary Medicine, Oregon State University.)*

disease is nonprogressive after 6 months to 1 year of age, and affected animals can still be kept as pets. Dogs producing affected pups should not be rebred.

Congenital myotonia

Myotonia is seen most commonly in the Chow chow dog, miniature schnauzer, and Staffordshire terrier. Autosomal recessive inheritance has been confirmed in the miniature schnauzer, and available evidence supports similar inheritance in the Chow chow. The underlying cellular defect in miniature schnauzers is decreased chloride conduction, and a similar defect is suspected in Chow chow dogs. Affected pups can begin to show signs of a stiff gait as early as 6 weeks of age. The signs progress for several months, and then stabilize with variable severity. Affected dogs move with splayed, stiff thoracic limbs and often "bunny hop" in the pelvic limbs. Signs are most severe on initiation of movement and improve with continued exercise. But affected dogs are never clinically normal. During severe episodes, dogs can fall over, and laryngospasm can result in transient dyspnea and even cyanosis. The musculature becomes remarkably hypertrophied, and sustained muscle dimpling occurs after percussion. Characteristic waxing and waning ("dive bomber") myotonic bursts are found with concentric needle EMG. Serum concentrations of CK and AST are normal or mildly increased.

Overall muscle hypertrophy, with prominently defined muscle groups, is the only finding on postmortem examination. In early stages of the disease, muscle appears relatively normal on histologic examination. With time, myofiber hypertrophy and myofiber

atrophy of both type 1 and type 2 fibers, and rare scattered segmental necrosis or regeneration, are seen. Fibrosis is mild to inapparent.

Diagnosis is based on clinical signs and can be confirmed by concentric needle electromyography or by examination of a muscle biopsy. Molecular testing is available to detect carrier and affected miniature schnauzers. Therapeutic agents that act to stabilize excitable cell membranes, such as quinidine, procainamide, and phenytoin, can relieve some of the signs of myotonia.

Swimmer pups

These puppies are clinically similar to piglets with splayleg. Affected pups cannot adduct the limbs beneath their bodies, and develop a characteristic "swimming" gait, and progressive flattening of the sternum. Although this syndrome can occur in pups with neuromuscular disease of any sort that leads to weakness, it is more commonly associated with overfeeding leading to excess body weight. Affected overfed pups often recover after reduction in total daily milk intake, provision of a nonslippery floor surface, and development of harnesses and physical therapy to encourage them to bring their legs underneath their bodies and walk. Sternal flattening and abnormal lateral deviation of the limbs are consistent findings. Histopathologic abnormalities in muscle will vary depending on the cause and will be absent in pups in which this disorder simply reflects overfeeding.

ENDOCRINE MYOPATHIES
Hypothyroidism

Because of its role in muscle metabolism, decreased thyroid hormone often results in skeletal myofiber weakness and atrophy. Hypothyroidism can also cause a peripheral neuropathy, and damage to motor nerves can cause denervation atrophy and contribute to the neuromuscular weakness. Signs of neuromuscular dysfunction due to hypothyroidism are extremely varied and include generalized weakness, muscle atrophy, laryngeal paralysis, and megaesophagus. Electromyographic studies are often normal; abnormal spontaneous activity and decreased motor nerve conduction velocities can be found if there is concurrent peripheral neuropathy. Serum concentrations of CK and AST are generally normal. Other systemic manifestations of hypothyroidism may or may not be present.

At necropsy, overall muscle atrophy can be seen. Thyroid glands are often bilaterally atrophied, and megaesophagus can be present. Symmetric alopecia (endocrine dermatopathy) can also be seen. Type 2 myofibers are preferentially atrophied. Axonal degeneration can occur in peripheral nerves and can lead to angular atrophy of both type I and type II fibers because of denervation, and to fiber-type grouping as a result of reinnervation.

Diagnosis is suspected on the basis of clinical findings and selective type 2 atrophy or evidence of denervation or reinnervation in affected muscles but should be confirmed by evaluation of thyroid function. In many cases, replacement thyroid hormone will improve the signs of neuromuscular weakness.

Hypercortisolism

This disorder can occur because of either increased adrenocortical cortisol production or administration of exogenous corticosteroids. Clinical findings of neuromuscular weakness can be very similar to those in hypothyroidism. A unique manifestation of hypercortisolism in some dogs is development of a remarkably stiff, stilted pelvic limb gait, with increased bulk and tone of proximal thigh muscles (Cushingoid pseudomyotonia). The cause of Cushingoid pseudomyotonia is not known, although induction of sarcolemmal ionic instability is postulated. Concentric needle electromyography of these muscles reveals myotonic bursts that do not wax and wane (pseudomyotonic activity). Muscles do not dimple after percussion. Other systemic signs of hypercortisolism such as symmetric muscle atrophy and alopecia can also be present. Serum concentrations of CK and AST are normal. Adrenal glands have bilateral cortical atrophy due to exogenous corticosteroid administration or bilateral hypertrophy due to stimulation secondary to pituitary neoplasia. Adrenal cortical neoplasia causes enlargement of the affected gland and atrophy of the contralateral gland. Findings in affected muscle and peripheral nerves are similar to those seen in hypothyroid myopathy (i.e., selective type 2 fiber atrophy) and evidence of axonal degeneration in peripheral nerves, type 1 and type 2 fiber atrophy indicative of denervation atrophy, and fiber-type grouping reflecting reinnervation are possible (Fig. 15-24, B).

Diagnosis is suspected on the basis of clinical and histopathologic findings but should be confirmed by evaluation of adrenocortical function and total serum cortisol. Cessation of exogenous corticosteroids, removal of adrenal neoplasia, or chemical destruction of hyperplastic adrenal cortical tissue results in improvement in muscle mass and strength, although signs of pseudomyotonia may persist.

IMMUNE-MEDIATED MYOPATHIES (LISTED IN TABLE 15-9)
Polymyositis

Polymyositis is due to immune-mediated inflammation that attacks components of the skeletal myofibers and results in myofiber necrosis (Fig. 15-32). The immunologic injury can be directed against skeletal muscle only or can be part of a more generalized immune-mediated disease, such as systemic lupus erythematosus. Polymyositis can also occur in dogs with thymoma. This generalized inflammatory myopathy can have an acute and rapidly progressive course or an insidious onset of muscle atrophy and generalized weakness. Temporal and masseter muscle atrophy may be most obvious, mimicking the appearance of dogs with masticatory myositis (see later discussion). Esophageal muscle involvement can lead to esophageal fibrosis and esophageal dysfunction, including megaesophagus. Respiratory muscle involvement can occur and, if severe, will cause respiratory distress. Pain on palpation of muscles is rare. Serum concentrations of CK, AST, and ALT can be increased, but in chronic cases these concentrations can also be within normal limits. Concentric needle electromyography often reveals scattered foci of abnormal spontaneous activity, and motor nerve conduction velocities are normal.

At necropsy, overall muscle atrophy may be the only finding. Aspiration pneumonia can occur secondary to megaesophagus. Histologic findings within affected muscles are extremely variable. In acute, fulminating cases, the muscle sections are filled with inflammatory cells, predominantly lymphocytes and plasma cells (Fig. 15-52, A), although eosinophils and neutrophils can also be present. The degree of myofiber necrosis is variable. Necrotic fibers in early stages will have a rim of lymphocytes that can be seen to invade intact myofibers (Fig. 15-32, B). Necrosis is followed by regeneration, but basal lamina damage is common and will result in some degree of healing by fibrosis. In more chronic and insidious cases, the only lesion consists of scattered lymphocytes adjacent to myofibers, with a variable degree of fibrosis and chronic myopathic change (Fig. 15-52, B). Sampling multiple muscles for histopathologic examination is recommended.

Polymyositis should be suspected based on the clinical findings, but identification of characteristic changes within muscle sections is often necessary to confirm the diagnosis. A positive circulating antinuclear antibody titer (ANA) is useful but is not always found. Treatment with immunosuppressive drugs such as corticosteroids can be curative, but affected animals may require lifelong therapy.

Masticatory myositis (eosinophilic myositis; atrophic myositis)

The type 2 myofibers in the masticatory muscles of the dog contain a unique myosin isoform (type 2M myosin). On occasions, antibodies to this myosin form, and the result is an inflammatory myopathy confined to the temporalis and masseter muscles. Severe, acute cases display bilaterally symmetric swelling of and pain in those muscles and an inability to fully open the jaw. Affected dogs can have difficulty prehending food. More chronic or insidious cases have bilaterally symmetric atrophy of the temporal and masseter muscles

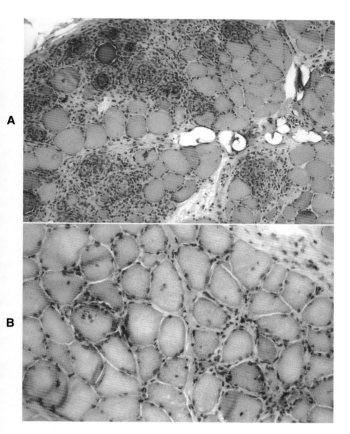

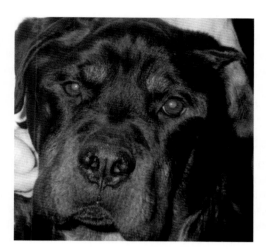

Fig. 15-53   Chronic masticatory myositis, skeletal muscle, dog. Note the severe atrophy of the temporalis and masseter muscles. *(Courtesy Dr. W. Hornbuckle, College of Veterinary Medicine, Cornell University.)*

Fig. 15-52   Canine polymyositis, skeletal muscle, transverse section, dog. A, Acute polymyositis. Dense interstitial and intramyofiber mononuclear inflammatory cell infiltrates are associated with myofiber necrosis. Frozen section, H&E stain. **B,** Chronic polymyositis. At this stage, there are only scattered interstitial mononuclear inflammatory cell infiltrates, scattered degenerate fibers, and chronic myopathic change (excessive fiber-size variation, internal nuclei, endomysial fibrosis). Frozen section, H&E stain. (**A,** *Courtesy Dr. L. Fuhrer, Clinic Veterinaire de St. Avertin, France.* **B,** *Courtesy Dr. B.A. Valentine, College of Veterinary Medicine, Oregon State University.*)

The presence of fibrosis is an important prognostic indicator because fibrosis is an irreversible change.

The diagnosis is suggested on the basis of characteristic clinical findings. Masticatory myositis must be differentiated from polymyositis, which can also have severe involvement of the temporal and masseter muscles. Serologic testing to detect anti–type 2M myosin antibodies specific to masticatory muscle myositis is available, and serum from affected dogs will bind to type 2M fibers (Fig. 15-54). Electromyography and histopathologic evaluation of multiple muscles can also

(Fig. 15-53) and decreased jaw mobility. Pain may or may not be evident at this stage. Concentric needle EMG often reveals foci of spontaneous activity in active cases, but can be normal in more chronic cases. Serum concentrations of CK and AST are normal or only mildly increased.

Severely atrophied muscles often contain pale streaks. The degree and nature of the inflammation are variable. In acute cases, infiltrates of lymphocytes and plasma cells, similar to those in polymyositis, are present. There can also be numerous eosinophils, and eosinophils can be the predominant cell type. Neutrophils are much less common. Inflammation is associated with myofiber necrosis. Regeneration can restore myofibers, but because the basal lamina is often damaged, development of fibrosis is common.

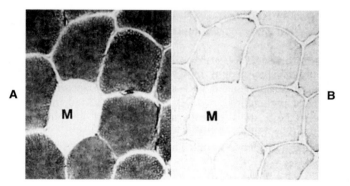

Fig. 15-54   Canine masticatory myositis, skeletal muscle, temporalis muscle, transverse sections, normal dog. A, A single type 1 fiber *(light staining, M)* surrounded by type 2 fibers *(dark staining).* Frozen section, ATPase pH 9.8. **B,** After incubation with serum from a dog with masticatory myositis, type 2 fibers stain positively because of binding of anti–type 2M myosin antibodies from the affected dog. Notice that the type 1 fiber *(M)* is unstained. Frozen section, staphylococcal protein A-peroxidase. (**A** and **B,** *Courtesy Dr. G. D. Shelton, University of California, San Diego.*)

help to differentiate these two disorders. Treatment with immunosuppressive doses of corticosteroids generally alleviates pain and results in increased mobility of the jaw and increase in muscle mass. Some degree of atrophy and loss of complete jaw mobility can persist. A single course of corticosteroids can be curative; however, some cases require extended therapy.

Extraocular muscle myositis

An immune-mediated attack directed specifically at extraocular muscles is the suspected cause of this disorder. Acute onset of bilateral exophthalmos is seen. Affected dogs are usually less than 2 years of age, and golden retriever dogs appear to be predisposed. Serum concentrations of CK and AST are generally normal.

The extraocular muscles, with the exception of the retractor bulbi muscle, are swollen and pale yellow. A predominantly lymphocytic inflammation resulting in myofiber necrosis and regeneration is seen. Because it is difficult to obtain a biospy sample of the extraocular muscles, diagnosis is generally based on typical clinical findings. Corticosteroid therapy is effective, but episodes can recur.

DISORDERS OF THE NEUROMUSCULAR JUNCTION
Myasthenia gravis

The pathogenesis of myasthenia gravis is discussed in the section on neuropathic and neuromuscular junction disorders (Fig. 15-33). In most cases, myasthenia gravis is an acquired disease, with circulating antibodies directed at the acetylcholine receptors of the neuromuscular junction. An inherited predisposition to development of acquired myasthenia gravis has been reported in Newfoundland dogs. In some cases, onset of myasthenia gravis occurs because of thymoma or, less commonly, thymic hyperplasia. Congenital myasthenia gravis is due to abnormal development of the neuromuscular junction and is inherited as an autosomal recessive trait in Jack Russell terriers, smooth fox terriers, and Springer spaniels. Congenital myasthenia gravis also occurs in smooth-haired miniature dachshunds. Typical signs of acquired disease are episodic collapse in an adult dog, with normal gait and strength after rest. Clinical signs can, however, be variable. The canine esophagus contains a large percentage of skeletal muscle in its wall; therefore megaesophagus is common in dogs with myasthenia gravis and may be the only presenting sign. In some cases, mild weakness persists between episodes. Clinical signs of congenital myasthenia gravis appear at an early age (6 to 8 weeks of age) and in most affected breeds are progressive and typically quite severe. Affected dachshunds, however, appear to recover by 6 months of age. Repetitive motor nerve stimulation reveals an initial sharp decremental response, followed by relatively uniform amplitude potentials. Serum concentrations of CK and AST are normal.

No findings are evident at postmortem examination unless megaesophagus or thymic abnormalities are present, and no abnormalities in muscle are seen on light microscopic examination. Ultrastructural abnormalities of the neuromuscular junctions (simplification of the postsynaptic membrane) can be seen.

Diagnosis is suspected on the basis of typical clinical findings and results of repetitive nerve stimulation. In patients with acquired myasthenia gravis, dramatic transient improvement in muscle strength following administration of intravenous acetylcholinesterase inhibitors such as edrophonium (Tensilon) will be seen, and the diagnosis is confirmed by identification of circulating antibodies to skeletal muscle acetylcholine receptors. In cases of acquired myasthenia gravis, the presence of thymic abnormalities should be determined, as removal of a thymoma or of a hyperplastic thymus results in resolution of clinical signs. In other cases, long-acting acetylcholinesterase inhibitor therapy, sometimes combined with corticosteroid therapy, is often beneficial. There is no effective treatment for congenital myasthenia gravis.

Tick paralysis

In a dog with flaccid tetraparesis, a diagnosis of tick paralysis should be considered along with polyradiculoneuritis (coonhound paralysis; See Disorders of Peripheral Nerves) and botulism. Clinical signs of tick paralysis appear 5 to 7 days following infestation with causative *Dermacentor* or *Ixodes* ticks. Initial clinical signs are of pelvic limb weakness, with progression to recumbency within 48 to 72 hours. Cranial nerve function is normal. Clinical signs of tick paralysis are very similar to those of coonhound paralysis (see peripheral nerve discussion). Treatment for tick infestation can result in recovery within a few days, although death due to respiratory muscle paralysis is still possible.

Botulism

Botulism occurs in dogs, resulting in rapid onset of flaccid tetraparesis, but is rare. Reported cases of canine botulism are most often due to types C and D of *Clostridium botulinum* neurotoxins. Diagnosis is often presumptive, based on a failure to identify other causes of diffuse neuromuscular weakness and, with luck, a history of consumption of a rotted carcass. Recovery has been reported in dogs with botulism, although many cases are fatal.

OTHER CANINE MYOPATHIES
Exertional rhabdomyolysis

Massive acute rhabdomyolysis associated with exertion occurs in racing greyhounds and sled dogs.

Muscles of the back (longissimus) and thigh (gluteal) are most often affected and may be severely swollen. Predisposing factors are not clear, but in sled dogs a change to a very high-fat diet has resulted in decreased exercise-induced muscle injury.

Malignant hyperthermia

Malignant hyperthermia occurs sporadically in dogs, and breeding studies indicate an autosomal dominant inheritance. The cause has been determined to be a genetic defect in the muscle ryanodine receptor, which is also the cause of malignant hyperthermia in pigs and human beings. Malignant hyperthermia-like episodes can also occur in any dog following ingestion of hops used for brewing beer.

Other breed-specific myopathies

A number of breed-specific myopathies have been reported in the dog, including dermatomyositis in collies and Shetland sheepdogs, mitochondrial myopathy in Old English sheepdogs and other breeds, and myopathy of Bouvier des Flandres dogs, English Springer spaniels, and rottweilers. Myoclonus and intramuscular La Fora-like bodies occur in wirehaired miniature dachshunds. These are discussed in more detail in Appendix 15-1.

IDIOPATHIC MASTICATORY MUSCLE ATROPHY

Dogs can develop a progressive atrophy of temporal and masseter muscles that is not associated with pain or difficulty opening the jaw or prehending food. Examination of affected muscle from these dogs reveals mild generalized atrophy of myofibers, but there is no evidence of inflammation, degeneration, fibrosis, or denervation. The cause is not known, and there is no treatment.

DENERVATING DISEASES

There are numerous causes of inherited and acquired peripheral nerve disorders causing axonal damage and resultant denervation in dogs (see Disorders of the Peripheral Nervous System). Motor neuron disease is most often inherited, such as in the Brittany spaniel and rottweiler. Such disorders cause symmetric atrophy of affected muscle. Neoplasms arising in peripheral nerves (nerve sheath neoplasms) cause compression of the nerve and axonal degeneration and loss, leading to progressive gait abnormalities and ultimately denervation atrophy of muscles of the affected limb.

MUSCULAR DISORDERS OF THE CAT

Relatively few muscular disorders have thus far been identified in cats. This may, in part, be due to the low performance expectations of the average house cat. It is entirely possible that there are many cats lying around with muscular disorders that have, as yet, gone unrecognized.

INHERITED OR CONGENITAL MYOPATHIES
X-linked muscular dystrophy (Duchenne's type)

Dystrophic cats lack the muscle cytoskeletal protein dystrophin, which is also the cause of Duchenne's dystrophy in boys and X-linked muscle dystrophy in the dog. Affected cats develop a progressive, persistent, stiff gait associated with marked muscular hypertrophy. The cause of the remarkable muscular hypertrophy seen in affected cats, as opposed to the muscle atrophy seen in the dog and in human beings, and the pseudo-hypertrophy as a result of fat infiltration that can occur in human beings, is not known. Age of onset is from a few months to 21 months of age. Affected cats have difficulty grooming, jumping, and lying down. Concentric needle EMG reveals dense and sustained abnormal spontaneous activity, similar to findings in the dystrophic dog. Serum concentrations of CK, AST, and ALT are elevated, typically to very high levels. Affected cats can die under anesthesia or following restraint or sedation because of a malignant hyperthermia-like syndrome.

At necropsy, all muscles are severely hypertrophied and may contain pale areas. Focal pale or chalky areas within the myocardium are typically found. Histologically, muscles show a range of changes. Concurrent segmental myonecrosis and myofiber regeneration (polyphasic necrosis) are characteristic. Chronic myopathic changes, found in older animals, include severe myofiber hypertrophy, myofiber atrophy, internal nuclei, and mild to moderate endomysial fibrosis. Myocardial lesions consist of multifocal necrosis and mineralization of cardiac myofibers and fibrosis, primarily in the left ventricular free wall, papillary muscles, and septum. Affected cats may have a relatively normal life span, although unexpected death during anesthesia or forced restraint is common. The exact cause of this is unclear.

The diagnosis is suspected on the basis of characteristic clinical, clinicopathologic, and histopathologic findings in a young male cat. Confirmation relies on assay of muscle samples for dystrophin or on immunohistochemical staining for dystrophin in frozen sections.

Other feline inherited or congenital myopathies

Glycogenosis type IV (glycogen branching enzyme defect) affecting skeletal muscle is seen as an inherited disorder in Norwegian Forest cats. A histologically similar condition occurs occasionally in other breeds. Feline nemaline myopathy is a rare congenital myopathy in the cat. A poorly understood condition that may be myopathic occurs in Devon Rex cats. These disorders are discussed in more detail in Appendix 15-1.

MYOPATHIES DUE TO ELECTROLYTE ABNORMALITIES (HYPOKALEMIA AND HYPERNATREMIA)

Similar to cattle, cats with severe electrolyte abnormalities can show signs of neuromuscular weakness that can cause a degenerative myopathy. Although degenerative myopathy has been reported secondary to increased blood sodium concentrations (hypernatremia), hypokalemic myopathy occurs far more frequently.

The cause of the weakness and myofiber necrosis associated with electrolyte abnormalities is complex and involves abnormal skeletal muscle energy metabolism and possible ischemia because of vasoconstriction. Hypokalemia (potassium less than 3.5 mEq/L) can occur because of decreased dietary intake or increased urinary excretion of potassium. In cats, hypokalemia is often a consequence of chronic renal disease. It can also occur secondary to gastrointestinal disease or inappropriate fluid therapy. Hyperthyroidism has been associated with development of hypokalemic myopathy in cats. Hypernatremic myopathy is less common, but has been reported in a 7-month-old cat with hydrocephalus and transient hypopituitarism.

Affected cats show severe generalized weakness, with notable ventroflexion of the neck. Concentric needle EMG often demonstrates foci of abnormal spontaneous activity. Serum concentrations of CK, AST, and ALT are often increased, sometimes severely. Blood concentrations of potassium are low in hypokalemia, and blood concentrations of sodium are high in hypernatremia.

No specific gross pathologic findings are present except in cats with hypokalemia as a result of chronic renal disease, in which the kidneys are small and fibrotic. In hypokalemic myopathy, myofiber necrosis and regeneration of variable severity are present concurrently (polyphasic necrosis). If renal disease is present, chronic interstitial nephritis is most commonly seen. No abnormalities were detected in a muscle biopsy from the cat with hypernatremic myopathy, although the mildly increased serum concentration of creatine kinase and abnormal EMG suggest mild and perhaps transient myofiber necrosis and regeneration.

Diagnosis is based on characteristic clinical findings of weakness and concurrent hypokalemia or hypernatremia. Treatment of affected cats has been very successful. Immediate fluid therapy is used to correct the electrolyte abnormality, followed by diet change to maintain normal electrolyte concentrations. If there is an underlying hyperthyroidism, this should also be treated.

IMMUNE-MEDIATED DISORDERS

An immune-mediated myositis has been described in cats infected with feline immunodeficiency virus.

Serum concentration of CK is moderately increased, but clinical signs of muscle dysfunction are not apparent. Infiltration of muscle by CD8+ lymphocytes, similar to HIV-associated polymyositis in human beings, is characteristic.

DISORDERS OF THE NEUROMUSCULAR JUNCTION
Myasthenia gravis

Feline acquired and congenital myasthenia gravis are similar to these disorders in the dog but occur less commonly.

Botulism

Although theoretically possible, we are not aware of any confirmed or highly suspicious cases of botulism in cats. This likely reflects both inherent resistance to botulinum toxin and the typical feline fastidious appetite.

DENERVATING DISEASES

Disorders affecting peripheral motor nerves are much less common in cats as compared with dogs. A chronic relapsing polyneuritis primarily affecting ventral spinal roots has been seen in young adult cats, which can cause denervation atrophy in affected muscles. Diabetes mellitus can also result in peripheral neuropathy in cats.

■ SUGGESTED READINGS

Beech J: Equine muscle disorders 2, *Eq Vet Educ* 20(4):208-213, 2000.

Blot S: Disorders of the skeletal muscles. In Ettinger SJ, Feldman EC, editors: *Textbook of veterinary internal medicine,* ed 5, Philadelphia, 2000, Saunders.

Bradley R, Fell BF: Myopathies in animals. In Walton J, editor: *Disorders of voluntary muscle,* ed 4, Edinburgh, 1981, Churchill Livingstone.

Cooper BJ: Animal models of human disease. In Karpati G, Hilton-Jones D, Griggs RC, editors: *Disorders of voluntary muscle,* ed 7, Cambridge, UK, 2001, Cambridge University Press.

Cooper BJ, Valentine BA: Tumors of muscle. In Meuten DJ, editor: *Tumors in domestic animals,* ed 4, Ames, 2002, Iowa State Press.

de Lahunta A: Lower motor neuron-general somatic efferent system. In: *Veterinary neuroanatomy and clinical neurology,* ed 2, Philadelphia, 1983, Saunders.

Dubowitz V: *Muscle biopsy: a practical approach,* ed 2, London, 1985, Baillière.

Evans J, Levesque D, Shelton GD: Canine inflammatory myopathies: a clinicopathologic review of 200 cases, *J Vet Intern Med* 18(5):679-691, 2004.

Kakulas BA, Cooper BJ: Experimental and animal models of human neuromuscular disease. In Walton J, Karpati G, Hilton-Jones D, editors: *Disorders of voluntary muscle,* ed 6, New York, 1994, Churchill Livingstone.

Podell M: Inflammatory myopathies, *Vet Clin North Am Small Anim Pract* 32(1):147-167, 2002.

Shelton GD: Myasthenia gravis and disorders of neuromuscular transmission, *Vet Clin North Am Small Anim Pract* 32(1):189-206, 2002.

Shelton GD, Cardinet GH III: Pathophysiologic basis of canine muscle disorders, *J Vet Intern Med* 1(1):36-44, 1987.

Taylor SM: Selected disorders of muscle and the neuromuscular junction, *Vet Clin North Am Small Anim Pract* 30(1):59-75, 2000.

Valentine BA: Postoperative complications—myopathy/neuropathy. In Mair T, Divers T, Ducharme N, editors: *Manual of equine gastroenterology,* Philadelphia, 2002, Saunders.

Valentine BA: Mechanical lameness in the hindlimb. In Ross MW, Dyson SJ, editors: *Diagnosis and management of lameness in horses,* St Louis, 2003, Saunders.

Van Vleet JF, Ferrans VJ, Herman E: Cardiovascular and skeletal muscle system. In Haschek-Hock WM, Rousseaux CG, editors: *Handbook of toxicologic pathology,* Orlando, Fla, 1991, Academic Press.

Van Vleet J, Valentine BA: Muscle and tendon. In Jubb KVF, Kennedy PC, Palmer N, editors: *Pathology of domestic animals,* ed 5, New York, Academic Press (in press).

APPENDIX **15-1**

VIRAL CAUSES OF MYOSITIS

Porcine encephalomyelitis is caused by a coronavirus of the *Enterovirus* genus. Besides the destruction of the neurons, which results in paralysis, the virus can also cause multifocal necrosis of myofibers, accompanied by a focal interstitial and perivascular infiltrate of lymphocytes, macrophages, and a few neutrophils.

The major lesions of foot and mouth disease virus in ruminants and pigs are vesicles in the skin and mucous membranes. In addition, the heart and skeletal muscles can have yellow streaks and pale foci, which microscopically are areas of segmental myofiber necrosis accompanied by an intense lymphocytic and neutrophilic infiltration.

Akabane virus (Bunyaviridae family) can produce a nonsuppurative myositis in the bovine fetus.

Bluetongue, caused by a virus of the family Reoviridae, is a noncontagious, insect-borne viral disease of sheep that causes vasculitis in a wide array of tissue, particularly the oral mucosa. Gross lesions in muscles are foci of necrosis (infarctions) and hemorrhage. Depending on the age of the lesions, necrosis, calcification, or regeneration may be present. Because of the size of the infarcts, regeneration is usually not possible, and healing is by fibrosis.

PARASITIC MYOSITIDES

The larval forms of *Ancylostoma caninum* migrate somatically, primarily in human beings. After entering the muscles of paratenic hosts, development is arrested. The larvae cause inflammation and myonecrosis. As they continue to migrate, they leave a trail of inflammation and segmental myofiber necrosis.

Toxocara canis larvae migrate through numerous tissues of the dog (visceral larval migrans). Some larvae are arrested, and granulomas form around them. These have been found in a wide array of tissue, including kidney, liver, lung, myocardium, and skeletal muscle.

The lesion in muscle is a focal granulomatous myositis, with the larvae and granulomas lying between myofibers.

Dirofilaria immitis, a nematode normally found in the hearts of dogs and cats, can occasionally involve the external and internal iliac arteries and their branches. Thromboemboli from debris and parasites can cause multiple infarcts in the muscles of the hindlimbs (see Disturbance of Circulation).

Cysticercus is a larva with a solid caudal portion and a bladderlike proximal portion. It is the intermediate stage in the life cycle of several tapeworms. *Taenia solium* and *Taenia saginata,* both tapeworms of human beings, have a cysticercus stage in the pig (*Cysticercus cellulosae*) and cattle (*Cysticercus bovis*). These cysticerci preferentially lodge in the most active muscles, especially the heart, masseter, diaphragm, and tongue, where they appear as small white or gray cysts. Histologically, there is displacement of myofibers by the cyst, but little myositis; there may be a few lymphocytes, macrophages, and eosinophils around the cyst, which lies in the interstitial tissue, not within the myofiber. With time, the immunologic system of the host kills the cysticercus. *Cysticercus cellulosae* in pigs can become calcified. *Cysticercus ovis* in the heart and shoulder muscles of sheep and goats is the intermediate stage of *Taenia ovis,* a tapeworm of dogs.

Hepatozoon americanum is a protozoal organism, previously classified as *Hepatozoon canis,* that infects multiple tissues, including the skeletal muscle of dogs. It is most common in South Africa and the Middle East, but also occurs in areas of the United States (primarily Oklahoma and the Gulf Coast area). Young dogs, up to 6 months of age, are most susceptible to infection. The organism is transmitted by ingestion of an infected tick, such as *Rhipicephalus sanguineus.* Sporozoites invade through the intestinal wall and travel to multiple tissues, particularly liver and skeletal muscle, where they undergo schizogony. Suppurative to granulomatous inflammation occurs following rupture of schizonts within tissue. Encysted stages, however, do not elicit an inflammatory response. Clinical signs include fever, anorexia, weight loss, body pain, and gait abnormalities. Respiratory signs can also occur. Serum CK activity is often mildly increased. Radiographs often reveal a characteristic periosteal proliferation of long bones similar to that of hypertrophic osteopathy. Diagnosis is made by identification of the organism either within peripheral neutrophils or within affected tissue.

In dogs, infection by *Trypanosoma cruzi* (Chagas' disease) causes myocarditis with lesser involvement of skeletal muscle. Inflammation consists of lymphocytes admixed with macrophages. Protozoal organisms are typically readily identified in affected tissues.

CONGENITAL AND INHERITED MYOPATHIES

CONGENITAL MUSCULAR HYPERPLASIA (DOUBLE MUSCLING) IN CATTLE

This disorder is seen in several beef breeds, including Charolais, Angus, Belgian blue, Belgian white, South Devon, Santa Gertrudis, and Piedmontese cattle. This disorder is inherited as an autosomal recessive trait with incomplete penetrance. The genetic defect is inactivation of the myostatin gene, which regulates the number of myofibers. Affected calves have large, bulky muscles, especially of the shoulder and rump, because of an increased number of otherwise normal fibers. This increased muscle bulk predisposes to dystocia. Body fat deposits and intramuscular fat are reduced to about 60% of normal, which is considered desirable in a meat-producing animal. The diagnosis of this disorder is readily made based on typical clinical findings. There is no treatment.

MUSCULAR DYSTROPHY

BOVINE DIAPHRAGMATIC DYSTROPHY

A muscular dystrophy affecting diaphragm and respiratory muscles has been recognized in Meuse-Rhine-Yssel cattle in Europe and Holstein cattle in Japan. This disorder appears to be inherited as an autosomal recessive trait. The most common clinical sign is recurrent bloat. Clinical signs appear in adults 2 years of age or older and include loss of condition, decreased rumen activity, and recurrent bloat. Serum activity of muscle enzymes is normal. The diaphragm is found to be thickened and pale. Examination of affected muscle indicates a progressive myopathy with severe cytoarchitectural alterations and other chronic myopathic changes, including fibrosis. Scattered necrotic fibers can be found, but this myopathy does not have the characteristic ongoing progressive myofiber necrosis and regeneration of muscular dystrophy. Central corelike lesions are prominent and have been found to contain actin and ubiquitin with immunohistochemical studies. This disorder would be best defined as a progressive inherited myopathy, possibly a myofibrillar myopathy. There is no treatment, and animals producing affected offspring should not be rebred.

OVINE MUSCULAR DYSTROPHY

A progressive disorder known as ovine muscular dystrophy is recognized in Merino sheep in Australia. The underlying defect is not known. The disease is inherited as an autosomal recessive trait. Clinical signs of neuromuscular weakness occur as early as 1 month of age and are characterized by a stiff gait and exercise intolerance. Serum concentrations of CK and AST are increased. Because the disease affects only type 1 myofibers, gross lesions are most easily seen in muscles that consist primarily or only of type 1 myofibers (e.g., vastus intermedius). The appearance depends on the age of the animal. Initially the muscle is pale and lacks tone but is close to normal size. In the next few years, the muscle becomes firm, more atrophic, and pale gray to almost white as the space formerly occupied by the myofibers is filled with adipocytes and fibrosis. There is atrophy and hypertrophy of the myofibers, along with myopathic features, such as internal nuclei and subsarcolemmal masses. Lesions do not have the characteristic ongoing progressive myofiber necrosis and regeneration of muscular dystrophy, and this disorder may be best defined as a progressive inherited myopathy. Diagnosis is based on characteristic clinical and histopathologic findings. There is no treatment for this progressive disorder, and animals producing affected lambs should not be rebred.

OTHER CANINE MUSCULAR DYSTROPHIES

Defects in sarcoglycan, a protein that is part of the sarcolemmal dystrophin glycoprotein complex, have been found in both male and female dogs of various breeds. Affected dogs exhibit signs of neuromuscular disease by 1 year of age. Serum activities of CK, AST, and ALT are increased. Electromyography detects abnormal spontaneous activity, including myotonic bursts, and histopathologic findings of multifocal polyphasic necrosis are consistent with muscular dystrophy.

OTHER MUSCULAR DISORDERS OF CATTLE

MYOPATHY OF GELBVIEH CATTLE

A necrotizing myopathy of juvenile Gelbvieh cattle has been recognized. An inherited basis is suspected.

Clinical signs include neuromuscular weakness. The characteristic histopathologic change in affected muscles is necrotizing vasculitis that results in myofiber necrosis. The pathogenesis of this disorder is not known; both vitamin E deficiency and immune-mediated disease have been suggested. Pathologic changes are also found in the kidney, dorsal spinal tracts of the spinal cord, and in peripheral nerves. Cardiac lesions can occur but are uncommon. Treatment with vitamin E may be of some benefit.

BROWN SWISS CATTLE NEURONOPATHY

An inherited neuronal degenerative disease designated as a form of spinal muscular atrophy occurs in brown Swiss cattle. Clinical signs of a progressive lower motor neuron weakness appear by 2 to 6 weeks of age. Neuronal degeneration within the ventral gray matter of the spinal cord leads to axonal degeneration of peripheral nerves and denervation atrophy of muscle. The disorder is inherited as an autosomal recessive trait, and pedigree analysis has identified a common ancestor thought to be the founder animal. Animals producing affected calves should not be rebred.

OTHER BREED-ASSOCIATED DISORDERS OF DOGS

CANINE DERMATOMYOSITIS

A condition involving skin and muscle has been described in collies and Shetland sheepdogs, and has been compared with dermatomyositis of human beings. In human beings, characteristic skin lesions and immune-mediated damage to muscle capillaries occur. In dogs, the dermatopathologic changes are distinctive, but muscle involvement is much less common, and the muscle lesions seen are not always convincingly vascular in nature. In cases studied by one of the authors, occasional muscle inflammation appeared to reflect extension of inflammation from overlying ulcerated skin.

MYOPATHY OF BOUVIER DES FLANDRES DOGS

A progressive degenerative myopathy affecting males and females is recognized in Bouvier des Flandres dogs. Onset of clinical signs of neuromuscular weakness varies from about 2 months to 2 years of age. Esophageal and pharyngeal muscles are often most severely affected. Generalized muscle atrophy, weakness, and abnormal gait are typical. Serum activities of CK and AST are often moderately increased. Electromyography reveals abnormal spontaneous activity (myotonic bursts). Generalized muscle atrophy and megaesophagus are common

necropsy findings. Histopathologic changes are generally severe chronic myopathic change with notable cytoarchitectural changes. Multifocal fiber necrosis and regeneration occurs but is not common. Cardiac necrosis and fibrosis can also be seen.

DISTAL MYOPATHY OF ROTTWEILER DOGS

Both males and females are affected. Clinical signs of progressive muscle weakness and development of a plantigrade and palmigrade stance are apparent by about 2 months of age. This disorder is characterized histologically by severe fiber atrophy and fat infiltration, primarily of distal limb musculature. Myonecrosis and fibrosis are mild. Serum activities of CK and AST can be normal or slightly increased. Electromyography reveals rare spontaneous activity (fibrillations and positive sharp waves). Decreased serum and muscle carnitine concentrations suggest that this may be a lipid metabolic disorder.

MYOPATHY OF ENGLISH SPRINGER SPANIELS

A myopathy with involvement of esophageal muscle occurs in English springer spaniel dogs. Affected dogs also have dyserythropoiesis and cardiomegaly. Histologic findings are of chronic myopathic change with central linear or granular inclusions within myofibers.

MYOCLONUS IN WIREHAIRED MINIATURE DACHSHUNDS

A syndrome of sustained muscle contraction (myoclonus), seizures, and early dementia is recognized in related wirehaired miniature dachshunds. Inclusions of PAS-positive, amylase-resistant polyglucosan bodies similar to La Fora bodies described in human beings occur in skeletal muscle and central nervous tissue.

OTHER BREED-ASSOCIATED DISORDERS OF CATS

Feline nemaline myopathy is a congenital disorder described in domestic short-haired cats. Affected cats develop a characteristic progressive gait abnormality and muscle atrophy at an early age. The characteristic pathologic finding of expanded Z-line material (nemaline rods) within skeletal muscle fibers is only apparent in frozen sections or ultrastructurally. The mode of inheritance is not known.

A congenital disorder resulting in spasticity has also been described in Devon Rex cats. At this time it is not known if this is truly a myopathic disorder, nor has the mode of inheritance been determined.

MYOTONIA

EQUINE SPECIES

Congenital or early-onset myotonia is seen in thoroughbreds, standardbreds, and quarter horses. Various similar disorders, designated as myotonic dystrophy-like or muscular dystrophy-like, are likely to be the same or similar disorders. As with all congenital myotonias, an underlying abnormal ion channel leading to continuous abnormal muscle activity is suspected. But to-date the defect and potential for inheritance have not been defined. Affected horses have remarkable exercise intolerance, with stiffness of posture and gait apparent at birth or soon thereafter, and often, remarkably well-defined to hypertrophied muscle groups. Clinical signs of stiffness are most apparent when the animals first begin to move, with some decrease in stiffness with exercise. Serum concentrations of CK and AST are generally normal to only slightly increased. Muscles often show prolonged dimpling after percussion. Concentric needle electromyography demonstrates characteristic waxing and waning ("dive bomber") myotonic bursts.

No specific gross lesions are present, other than prominent muscling. On histologic examination, affected muscle fibers vary tremendously in size and shape, with numerous internal nuclei, altered cytoplasmic areas beneath the sarcolemma (sarcoplasmic masses), and other cytoarchitectural alterations, such as ring fibers. Scattered fiber necrosis and regeneration may be seen, but is not a prominent feature. In chronic cases, affected muscles can develop a variable degree of replacement of myofibers by fat, indicating a previous loss of myofibers.

The diagnosis of myotonia is based on characteristic clinical signs in a young horse and can be confirmed by electromyography or muscle biopsy. No specific treatment is known at this time.

FELINE SPECIES

The pathogenesis of feline congenital myotonia is not known at this time, although a skeletal muscle ion channel defect is suspected. Cats with congenital myotonia have signs similar to those of cats with X-linked muscular dystrophy, but the muscular hypertrophy is less remarkable. A stiff gait is the most obvious sign. Serum concentrations of CK and AST are normal or only slightly increased. Concentric needle electromyography reveals waxing and waning ("dive bomber") potentials characteristic of myotonia.

Other than mild muscular hypertrophy, there are no findings at necropsy. Significant myofiber hypertrophy and increased variation in myofiber diameter are the only histopathologic findings. Dilation of sarcotubular elements is the characteristic ultrastructural finding. The diagnosis of congenital feline myotonia is based on characteristic clinical findings. At this time, no type of treatment has been attempted.

METABOLIC MYOPATHIES

ACID MALTASE DEFICIENCY (GLYCOGENOSIS TYPE II; POMPE'S DISEASE)

This defect has been described in shorthorn and Brahman cattle and is inherited as an autosomal recessive trait. The enzyme defect results in blockage of the glycolytic metabolic pathway and in cellular dysfunction, which is most evident in skeletal muscle, Purkinje cells of the heart, and neurons. Myofiber necrosis is thought to be a result of a cellular "energy crisis" (i.e., energy deprivation).

Affected shorthorn cattle often show clinical signs of weakness by 3 to 7 months of age and die as a result of respiratory and cardiac failure. Affected shorthorn cattle may also develop relatively normally until 1 to $1^1/_2$ years of age, at which time weakness and neurologic deficits are evident. Affected Brahman cattle grow poorly and have muscular weakness and neurologic disease. Electrocardiographic studies reveal abnormalities of cardiac conduction. Serum concentrations of CK and AST can be increased, with notable increases evident in severely weak animals before death.

There may be no obvious changes within the skeletal and cardiac muscle at necropsy, although pale streaks may be evident in those animals undergoing myofiber necrosis before death. No gross pathologic lesions are evident in the nervous system. On histopathologic examination, affected myofibers, cardiac myocytes, and neurons are filled with vacuoles containing glycogen (vacuolar myopathy and neuronopathy), which can be demonstrated by PAS reaction. Glycogen accumulation in skeletal myofibers is segmental, whereas in neurons it is diffuse. Both degeneration and regeneration of skeletal muscle fibers and chronic myopathic change (fiber atrophy, hypertrophy, and internal nuclei) are present.

Diagnosis of a glycogenosis can be made based on characteristic clinical and histopathologic findings. Assay of affected tissue for glycolytic enzyme activities is necessary to determine the specific enzyme defect. There is no effective treatment for this disorder, and cattle known to produce affected calves should not be rebred.

MYOPHOSPHORYLASE DEFICIENCY (GLYCOGENOSIS TYPE V; McARDLE DISEASE)

This disorder has been identified in Charolais cattle. Myophosphorylase deficiency is an autosomal recessive disorder with glycogen storage similar to acid maltase deficiency, but with only skeletal muscle involvement. Clinical signs of exercise intolerance and inability to keep up with herd mates are recognized at a relatively early age. If forced to exercise, affected cattle become recumbent for up to 10 minutes. Serum concentrations of CK and AST are often mildly to markedly increased. No specific findings are evident at necropsy. Histopathologic findings in skeletal muscle are similar to those of acid maltase deficiency. Diagnosis can be based on characteristic clinical and histopathologic findings. Affected animals and carriers can be detected after analysis of peripheral blood leukocyte DNA by polymerase chain reaction assay. There is no treatment, and carrier animals should not be used for breeding.

A glycogen storage myopathy due to myophosphorylase deficiency has been identified in sheep in Australia and is similar to the disease in cattle.

PHOSPHOFRUCTOKINASE DEFICIENCY (GLYCOGENOSIS TYPE VII)

This is an autosomal recessive disorder in dogs caused by a point mutation in the muscle isoenzyme of phosphofructokinase, an important enzyme in the glycolytic pathway. This disorder has been recognized in English springer spaniels and American cocker spaniels. Muscles from older affected dogs can have myopathic changes and inclusions of a PAS-positive, amylase-resistant substance classified as complex polysaccharide. Clinical signs of neuromuscular dysfunction do not occur, however, because skeletal muscle up-regulates expression of the liver isoenzyme of phosphofructokinase. Absence of erythrocyte phosphofructokinase results in hemolysis during periods of increased respiratory activity (panting) and resultant mild respiratory alkalosis.

FELINE GLYCOGENOSES

Glycogenosis type IV occurs in Norwegian Forest cats because of decreased activity of glycogen branching enzyme (GBE), resulting in defective carbohydrate metabolism and a generalized glycogen storage disease. The disorder is inherited as an autosomal recessive trait. Affected cats may be stillborn or die within a few hours of birth. Those that survive lack energy and develop muscle tremors and a bunny-hopping pelvic limb gait at about 5 months of age. The disease is progressive, resulting in severe generalized muscle atrophy and tetraplegia. Concentric needle EMG reveals abnormal spontaneous activity with normal motor nerve conduction velocities. Serum concentrations of CK and AST are mildly to moderately increased. Muscle atrophy and fibrosis are evident in affected pelvic limb muscles of cats surviving 1 year or longer. Storage of PAS-positive, amylase-resistant material forming "lakes" within skeletal muscle fibers is the characteristic histopathologic finding. Myofiber atrophy is also prominent, and myofiber necrosis and regeneration can be seen. Cardiac myocytes have similar inclusions and undergo necrosis and replacement by fibrosis. Abnormal glycogen storage is also seen within smooth muscle and neurons in the central nervous system. Diagnosis can be suspected on the basis of characteristic clinical and histopathologic findings. Confirmation is based on assay of GBE concentration in blood leukocytes. There is no treatment for this disorder.

Similar intramyofiber inclusions of PAS-positive, amylase-resistant inclusions resulting in clinical signs of neuromuscular weakness are found rarely in older cats of mixed breeding, suggesting that there is more than one cause for this finding in cats.

EQUINE MITOCHONDRIAL MYOPATHY

A single case of mitochondrial myopathy in a 3-year-old Arabian filly has been reported. Deficiency of mitochondrial respiratory chain complex I was detected. Clinical signs were stiff gait and profound exercise intolerance. Lactic acidosis developed with minimal exercise. Skeletal muscle samples exhibited increased muscle mitochondrial content with bizarre cristae formation on ultrastructural examination.

CANINE MITOCHONDRIAL MYOPATHIES

A mitochondrial myopathy has been recognized in Old English sheepdogs. Clinical signs are exercise intolerance leading to episodic weakness and exercise-induced lactic acidosis. A suspected mitochondrial myopathy occurs in Welsh terrier dogs. Involvement of skeletal muscle occurs in Alaskan husky and Australian cattle dogs as part of a mitochondrial encephalomyopathy syndrome.

OTHER CANINE METABOLIC MYOPATHIES

Pyruvate dehydrogenase deficiency occurs in Clumber and Sussex spaniels in the United States and Belgium. Clinical signs are profound exercise intolerance with exercise-induced lactic acidosis. No gross or histopathologic lesions are found in muscle.

16

Bone and Joints

STEVEN E. WEISBRODE

INTRODUCTION

The skeleton consists of bones and joints and is responsible for supporting and protecting the body and enabling movement initiated by the nervous system and moved by muscles. The skeleton can be divided into axial skeleton (head, vertebrae, ribs, and sternum) and appendicular skeleton (thoracic and pelvic limbs). The postmortem examination and evaluation of the skeleton is presented in the appendix at the end of the chapter (Appendix 16-1).

NORMAL STRUCTURE AND FUNCTION OF BONE

BONE AT THE CELLULAR LEVEL

Structure and function can be discussed at the organ, tissue, and cellular levels. In this section, normal structure and function are briefly reviewed beginning at the cellular level and include bone matrix and mineral. Cells directly involved with the structural integrity of bone include osteoblasts, osteocytes, and osteoclasts (Box 16-1).

Osteoblasts are cells on any bone surface (periosteal, endosteal, trabecular, intracortical) that produce bone matrix (osteoid), initiate the mineralization of this matrix (deposition of hydroxyapatite), and seemingly paradoxically initiate the resorption of this matrix by osteoclasts. Osteoblasts are derived from mesenchymal stem cells. Active osteoblasts are plump (Fig. 16-1), with abundant basophilic cytoplasm rich in rough endoplasmic reticulum, prominent Golgi apparatus, and numerous mitochondria (Fig. 16-2). Inactive osteoblasts are disk-shaped with little cytoplasm because of the reduction in organelles needed for matrix synthesis and secretion (Figs. 16-3 and 16-4). Osteoblasts likely interact with osteocytes to assist in fine control of calcium homeostasis and detection of mechanical use and microscopic

damage to bone as discussed later. An indirect measurement of osteoblast activity is reflected in blood concentrations of the enzyme alkaline phosphatase and the noncollagenous protein osteocalcin. Alkaline phosphatase is an enzyme on the osteoblasts' surface whose function is uncertain, but it is suspected to play a role in mineralization and in pumping calcium across cellular membranes. Osteocalcin is a protein of uncertain function secreted by osteoblasts and found in bone matrix. Blood concentrations of osteocalcin and the bone isoenzyme of alkaline phosphatase correlate well with osteoblast synthetic activity.

Osteocytes are osteoblasts that have been surrounded by mineralized bone matrix (Fig. 16-5). They occupy small spaces in the bone called lacunae (singular: lacuna) and make contact with osteoblasts and other osteocytes by means of long cytoplasmic processes that pass through thin tunnels in the bone called canaliculi (singular: canaliculus). Under conditions of extreme stress to calcium homeostasis, osteocytes might have the ability

---

Box **16-1**

Bone Cell Function

Osteoblasts	Cells on the surface of bone that form bone matrix, initiate bone mineralization, and initiate bone resorption in response to physiologic stimuli
Osteocytes	Cells residing within bone matrix that detect changes in stress (force applied to the bone) and strain (structural deformation in response to the force) in the bone and signal these changes to osteoblasts to either form bone or initiate resorption
Osteoclasts	Cells that resorb bone

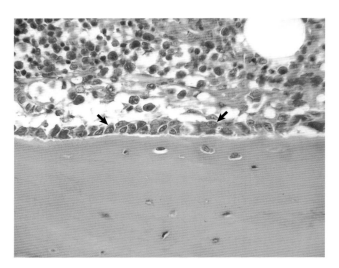

Fig. 16-1   Osteoblasts and osteocytes, long bone, young dog. Prominent cuboidal osteoblasts (*arrows*) line the endosteal surface. Hematopoietic marrow is present. More mature (older) osteocytes are present deeper in the cortex and are recognizable as small elliptical cells. The more recently embedded (younger) osteocytes are closer to the surface, ovoid, and in large lacunae. H&E stain. (*Courtesy Dr. S.E. Weisbrode, College of Veterinary Medicine, The Ohio State University.*)

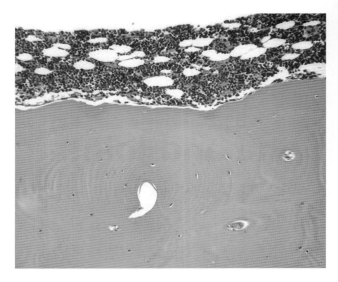

Fig. 16-3   Osteoblasts, vertebra, adult dog. Osteoblasts on the endosteal surface are fusiform with little cytoplasm and form an inconspicuous layer between the cortical bone and active hematopoietic marrow of the adult axial skeleton. H&E stain. (*Courtesy Dr. S.E. Weisbrode, College of Veterinary Medicine, The Ohio State University.*)

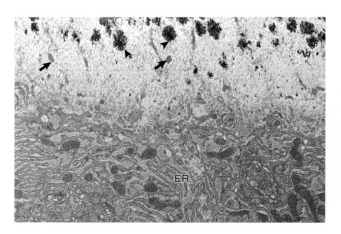

Fig. 16-2   Osteoblasts, bone, tibia, rodent. Osteoblasts with abundant endoplasmic reticulum (*ER*) on an actively mineralizing surface. Cell processes (*arrows*) of the osteoblasts extend out into the osteoid. Mineralization (*black spicules*) is initiated within matrix vesicles (*arrowheads*), then grows onto the adjacent collagen. TEM. Uranyl acetate and lead citrate stain. (*Courtesy Dr. S.E. Weisbrode, College of Veterinary Medicine, The Ohio State University.*)

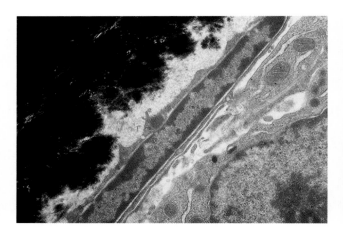

Fig. 16-4   Inactive osteoblast, bone, tibia, rodent. Inactive osteoblast with reduced cytoplasmic volume because of the less-developed or less-active organelles, which are necessary for collagen synthesis. The narrow rim of unmineralized (*white*) bone matrix, the lamina limitans, acts as a protective layer for the underlying mineralized bone. TEM. Uranyl acetate and lead citrate stain. (*Courtesy Dr. S.E. Weisbrode, College of Veterinary Medicine, The Ohio State University.*)

to resorb perilacunar mineral and matrix, thus enlarging the lacuna (osteocytic osteolysis). This process apparently is rare and likely does not contribute significantly to development of osseous lesions. Osteocytes also retain a limited capacity to form bone. Other functions of osteocytes are somewhat speculative and are presented later in osteoblast-osteocyte interactions.

Osteoclasts are multinucleated cells responsible for bone resorption (Fig. 16-6). They are derived from hematopoietic stem cells of the granulocyte-monocyte series. They have abundant eosinophilic cytoplasm and a specialized brush border adjacent to the bone surface that is being resorbed (Fig. 16-7). For osteoclasts to resorb bone, they must gain access to the bone surface that is

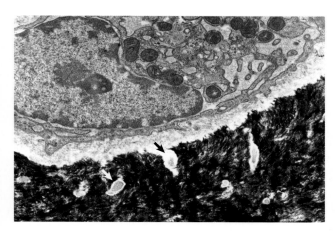

Fig. 16-5   Osteocyte, bone, tibia, rodent. A recently embedded osteocyte still has residual rough endoplasmic reticulum and Golgi apparatus used during its osteoblastic period. Cell processes are extending into the mineralized matrix *(black)* through tunnels called "canaliculi" *(arrows)*. TEM. Uranyl acetate and lead citrate stain. *(Courtesy Dr. S.E. Weisbrode, College of Veterinary Medicine, The Ohio State University.)*

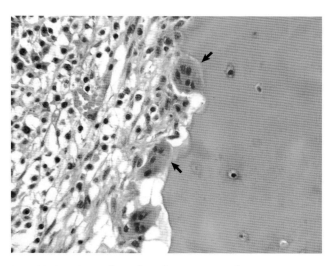

Fig. 16-6   Osteoclasts, long bone, young dog. Several multinucleated cells (osteoclasts) *(arrows)* are resorbing endocortical bone and creating a scalloped appearance of the surface. These scalloped cavities of resorbed bone are called Howship's lacunae. H&E stain. *(Courtesy Dr. S.E. Weisbrode, College of Veterinary Medicine, The Ohio State University.)*

usually covered by osteoblasts, and they must attach to the mineralized surface by transmembrane receptors in their sealing zones. These receptors bind to specific ligands in the matrix, likely residing in noncollagenous proteins. Osteoclasts are not able to bind to unmineralized bone matrix even though it contains these same ligands. Once bound to the matrix, the osteoclast resorbs bone in two stages. First, the mineral is dissolved by secretion of hydrogen ions through a proton pump located in the brush border. These hydrogen ions are derived from carbonic acid produced within the osteoclast from water and carbon dioxide by the enzyme carbonic anhydrase. Second, the collagen of the matrix is cleaved into polypeptide fragments by cysteine and metalloproteinases and cathepsins released from the numerous lysosomes in the osteoclast and secreted through the brush border. The concavity in the bone created by the resorption is called a Howship's lacuna. Physiologically, osteoclast activation is controlled by osteoblasts and bone marrow stromal cells (see later discussion of interactions). Calcitonin is a systemic inhibitor of osteoclasts. Osteoclasts have receptors for calcitonin and respond to this hormone by involuting their brush border and detaching from the bone surface. The activity of osteoclasts can be indirectly measured by determining blood concentrations of collagen degradation products (pyridinoline and deoxypyridinoline cross links).

Osteoblast-osteocyte interactions are apparent from their connections to each other by thin, tortuous, cytoplasmic processes. This network of osteoblasts and osteocytes forms a functional membrane that separates

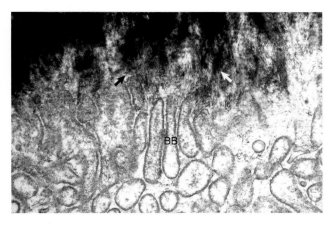

Fig. 16-7   Osteoclasts, brush border, bone, tibia, rodent. Spicules of hydroxyapatite *(arrows)* are apparent between the projections of the brush border *(BB)*. The crystals have been separated from the matrix and are in the process of being dissolved by acid and enzyme secretions across the brush border. TEM. Uranyl acetate and lead citrate stain. *(Courtesy Dr. S.E. Weisbrode, College of Veterinary Medicine, The Ohio State University.)*

the extracellular fluid bathing bone surfaces from the general extracellular fluid and can regulate the flow of calcium and phosphate ions to and from the bone fluid compartment (Fig. 16-8). Because of the large surface area of perilacunar and canalicular bone available for

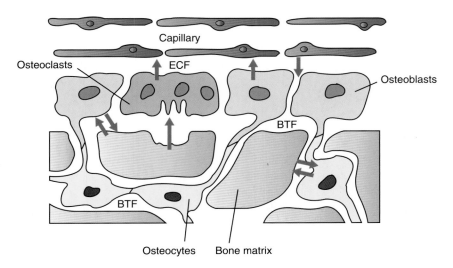

Fig. 16-8   Schematic diagram of the hypothesized intracellular and extracellular movement of calcium (*arrows*) in bone and the relationships of osteoblasts, osteocytes, and osteoclasts to blood vessels, extracellular fluid (*ECF*), and bone tissue fluid (*BTF*) compartment. *(Redrawn from Matthews JL, Vander Wiel C, Talmage RV: Adv Exp Med Biol 103:456, 1978.)*

rapid ion exchange, significant amounts of calcium can be shifted from the bone fluid compartment to the extracellular fluid compartment without structural changes within the bone. In addition, this network allows osteocytes to detect alternations in the fluid flow within the bone extracellular fluid compartment. It is thought such flow contributes to electric currents called streaming potentials. Changes in these streaming potentials caused by altered stress and strain on the bone or disruption of these potentials by microcracks (minuscule fractures within the bone visible only microscopically) might be detected by osteocytes with subsequent signaling to the overlying osteoblasts to initiate bone formation or resorption.

Osteoclast-osteoblast/stromal cell interactions are required for physiologic resorption of bone. The bone surface is protected from osteoclastic resorption by a continuous layer of osteoblasts and also by a very thin layer of unmineralized bone matrix normally present beneath resting osteoblasts (lamina limitans) (Fig. 16-4). Osteoclasts are not able to bind to unmineralized bone matrix). For parathyroid hormone (PTH) to initiate bone resorption, receptors on the osteoblast bind PTH (osteoclasts do not usually express receptors for PTH). The binding of PTH to osteoblasts signals them to retract and secrete collagenases, which erode the unmineralized layer of matrix allowing osteoclasts access to a mineralized bone surface. In addition, osteoblasts and stromal cells activated by binding PTH, and in response to a variety of other bone resorbing stimuli (1,25 dihydroxyvitamin D_3, interleukin [IL]-1 and IL-11, tumor necrosis

factor-α [TNF-α], prostaglandin E_2 [PGE$_2$], and glucocorticoids) will express or secrete osteoclast differentiation factor (ODF), also called rank ligand. ODF binds to receptors on osteoclasts (rank) and activates the resorption process. Osteoblasts and bone marrow stromal cells also can secrete osteoprotegerin (OPG), a protein that blocks ODF. OPG expression can be stimulated by transforming growth factor-β (TGF-β). Therefore osteoblasts and stromal cells have the ability to both up- and down-regulate osteoclastic bone resorption (Fig. 16-9). In conditions of inflammation and necrosis, inflammatory mediators such as IL-1 and TNF-α can stimulate osteoclasts directly, causing bone resorption independent of viable osteoblasts.

BONE AT THE ORGANIC MATRIX AND MINERAL LEVEL

The mineralized matrix of bone, its interstitium, provides the organ's strength. Bone organic matrix consists of type I collagen and "ground substance" (the noncollagenous extracellular matrix: water, proteoglycans, glycosaminoglycans, noncollagenous proteins, and lipids, discussed later). Type I collagen polymers are secreted by osteoblasts and assembled into fibrils that are embedded in the ground substance and then mineralized. The type I collagen molecule is composed of three intertwined amino acid chains. Unique to these chains is the hydroxylated form of the amino acid proline (hydroxyproline). Type I collagen molecules have extensive cross linkages among the amino acid chains within the molecule and between adjacent molecules.

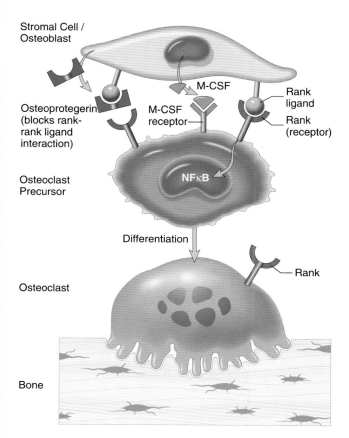

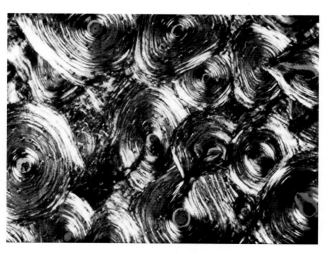

Fig. 16-10   Osteonic remodeling, bone, endocortical surface. Endocortical surface of bone has undergone extensive osteonal remodeling. Collagen fibers are birefringent when viewed in appropriate plane with polarized light. Usually, alternate lamellae polarize when viewed in the same plane. This alternating pattern of birefringence demonstrates the parallel arrangement of collagen layers in lamellar bone. All of the bone present is lamellar. Much of the cortex has been remodeled into osteonal bone (concentric layers with central channel for vessels and nerves), but there are areas of cortex that remain unosteonized (unremodeled). Unstained and fully mineralized. Polarized light micrograph. *(Courtesy Dr. L. P. Krook, College of Veterinary Medicine, Cornell University.)*

Fig. 16-9   Schematic diagram showing interaction between stromal cells/osteoblasts and osteoclast/osteoclast precursors. Stromal cells and osteoblasts produce "rank ligand," which binds to the "rank" receptor on the osteoclast and its precursors; this binding stimulates osteoclasis. Conversely, osteoblasts and stromal cells can inhibit the activation of osteoclasts by secreting osteoprotegerin, which can bind to "rank ligand" and block its binding to "rank receptor." *M-CSF,* Macrophage colony-stimulating factor; *NFκB,* nuclear factor kappa B. *(From Kumar V, Abbas AK, Fausto N: Robbins & Cotran pathologic basis of disease, ed 7, Philadelphia, 2005, Saunders.)*

Collagen molecules are deposited in rows with a gap between each molecule and with the rows staggered so that the molecules overlap by one fourth of their length. This specific packing of the collagen molecules and the cross linkages contribute to the strength and insolubility of the fibrous component of the bone matrix. Other than in rapidly deposited bone (woven bone found in primary trabeculae, bone of early fetal development, and pathologic conditions such as fracture repair), collagen fibers are arranged in parallel lamellae (singular: lamella) and called lamellar bone. The orientation of the collagen fibers in each lamella is slightly different, giving a herringbone-like pattern. In Haversian (osteonal) bone, lamellae are arranged concentrically (Fig. 16-10).

In trabecular bone, the lamellae usually are arranged parallel with the surface. The collagen content of bone and its lamellar arrangement give bone its strength and flexibility. The ground substance of bone, also synthesized by osteoblasts, consists of noncollagenous proteins, proteoglycans, and lipids. Many of the noncollagenous proteins are cytokines capable of influencing bone cell activity. These cytokines, such as TGF-β, may play pivotal roles in controlling the extent of bone formation and resorption in normal remodeling and in disease (Fig. 16-11). Also, among the noncollagenous proteins are enzymes that can function in degradation of collagen (e.g., matrix metalloproteinases) and can destroy inhibitors of mineralization (e.g., pyrophosphatases). Other noncollagenous proteins in the matrix can function as adhesion molecules and help bind cells to cells, cells to matrix, and mineral to matrix. Examples are osteonectin and osteocalcin. The role of proteoglycans in bone matrix is uncertain. They could play a role in inhibiting mineralization and promoting cell matrix interactions. Lipids can assist in binding calcium to cell membranes and in promoting calcification.

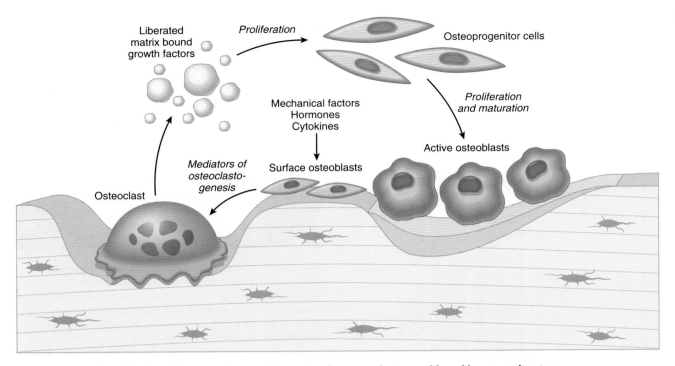

Fig. 16-11   Schematic diagram illustrating that osteoclasts are able to liberate and activate growth factors from the matrix that are stimulatory to osteoblast progenitor cells and "couple" the process of osteoclastic bone lysis with subsequent bone formation. *(From Kumar V, Abbas AK, Fausto N: Robbins & Cotran pathologic basis of disease, ed 7, Philadelphia, 2005, Saunders.)*

Bone mineral is in the form of a crystal called hydroxyapatite. Fully mineralized bone is approximately 65% of the bone by weight and consists in part of calcium, phosphorus, carbonate, magnesium, sodium, manganese, zinc, copper, and fluoride. The mineral content gives bone its hardness. The production of osteoid (unmineralized organic matrix) by osteoblasts is followed by a period of maturation, after which mineral is deposited at the exchange of water. The process of mineralization is initially rapid until the matrix is about half saturated with mineral. Complete saturation of the matrix with mineral takes several months. Mineralization in woven bone is initiated within cytoplasmic blebs (matrix vesicles) of osteoblasts in the osteoid (Fig. 16-2). Initiation of mineralization involves concentrating calcium, phosphorus, and other elements in these matrix vesicles (intracellularly) to a concentration that causes precipitation of the mineral in the vesicle in the form of amorphous (not yet crystalline) hydroxyapatite. These vesicles have phospholipids and enzymes, such as alkaline phosphatase and adenosine triphosphatase in their membranes. It is speculated that these membrane phospholipids attract calcium and phosphorus to the surface of the vesicle, and that the alkaline phosphatase and adenosine triphosphatase enzymes might

function in the pumping of these ions into the cell against a concentration gradient.

Upon reaching a critical mass, the amorphous mineral becomes crystalline. The crystalline hydroxyapatite pierces the lipid membrane of the matrix vesicle and extends to the gaps (holes) between collagen molecules. It is within these holes that the mineral crystals are first deposited in collagen. For the mineralization to spread beyond these gaps between the tropocollagen molecules, it is necessary for naturally occurring inhibitors of mineralization in the matrix to be destroyed. One such inhibitor is inorganic pyrophosphate. Inorganic pyrophosphates are normal by-products of cellular metabolism and are deposited in unmineralized matrix by osteoblasts. The phosphatase enzymes described previously on the matrix vesicles have the ability to cleave these inorganic pyrophosphates and in doing so, destroy these inhibitors. Once the gaps are filled with mineral and inhibitors of mineralization are destroyed, the process continues so that eventually the surfaces of collagen fibers as well as spaces between collagen fibers are mineralized. Initiation of mineralization in lamellar bone might not require matrix vesicles. Glycoproteins, such as sialoprotein and osteonectin, can act as the nidus for the mineralization process.

BONE AS A TISSUE

Bone is organized into osteons or Haversian systems in the compact bone of the cortex and in the bone beneath articular surfaces (subchondral bone) of larger animals. In cortical bone, osteons are cylinders of concentric layers of lamellae that contain centrally located vessels and nerves. These cylinders are oriented parallel to the longitudinal axis of the bone. Haversian or compact bone is made up of numerous osteons (Fig. 16-12 and Fig. 16-10). Bone between the osteons is called interstitial lamellae. Layers of bone oriented parallel to the internal and external circumference of the bone (beneath the endosteal and periosteal surfaces) are called circumferential lamellae. The osteonal system provides channels for the vascular supply to thick bone of the cortex and also acts as tightly bound cables, giving the cortical bone strength yet limited flexibility. This osteonal system also might be important in limiting propagation of microcracks in bone by diverting cracks along cement lines, which are collagen poor, and

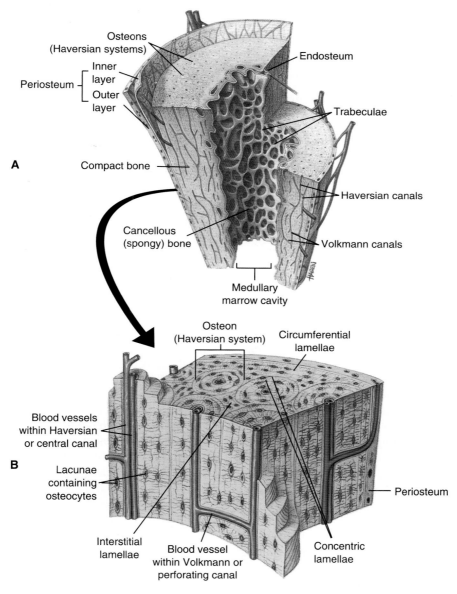

Fig. 16-12   **Schematic diagram of the structure of compact and cancellous bone. A,** Longitudinal section of a long bone showing both cancellous and compact bone. **B,** A magnified view of compact bone.

(Continued)

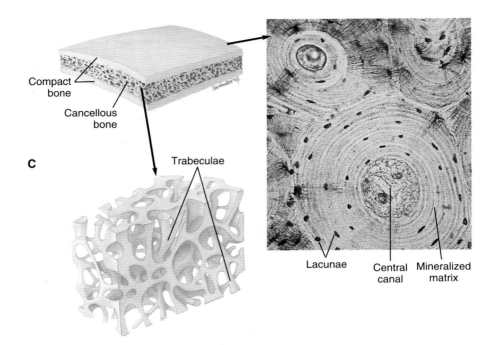

Compact bone

Cancellous bone

C

Trabeculae

Lacunae   Central   Mineralized
             canal   matrix

Fig. 16-12, cont'd   C, Section of a flat bone. Outer layers of compact bone surround cancellous bone. Fine structure of compact and cancellous bone is shown to the right. (**A, B,** and **C,** *From Thibodeau GA, Patton KT:* Anatomy and physiology, *ed 5, St Louis, 2003, Mosby.*)

proteoglycan-rich seams between adjacent remodeling or modeling units (see later discussion). In histologic sections, cement lines appear as basophilic lines in H&E stained sections of decalcified bone.

In contrast to the dense compact bone of the cortex and the subchondral bone plates, the bone in the medullary cavity is in the form of anastomosing plates or rods and is called cancellous, trabecular, or spongy bone (Fig. 16-12). The orientation of the trabeculae usually reflects adaptation (modeling) to mechanical stresses applied to the bone. This is readily apparent when examining the patterns of the trabeculae in the femoral neck. They are in lines and arcs perpendicular to the stress applied and thicker and more numerous on the ventral aspect (side of compression) compared with the dorsal aspect (side of tension). The lamellae within a trabecula usually are arranged parallel to the surface of the trabecula. They are not arranged into tubes or osteons, as in cortical bone.

In most species, bone undergoes a low but constant replacement called remodeling: Old bone is resorbed and replaced by new. The basal level of this remodeling activity (number of sites in the skeleton being remodeled at any one time) is likely "programmed" for each species. The number of these active remodeling sites, however, can be markedly increased or decreased in response to altered mechanical use (see later discussion). This turnover of old bone to new bone allows for the repair of accumulated microscopic injury in the bone (microfractures). In normal bone remodeling, slightly less bone is replaced than removed, leaving a small negative net change in bone mass with each remodeling cycle. This partly explains the reduced bone mass in aged animals. In disease states such as hyperparathyroidism, resorption is often increased and formation decreased, leaving a significant net negative bone balance. Not all species undergo bone remodeling; in small, short-lived animals, such as the mouse and rat, cortical bone is not remodeled. Not all areas of bone in larger species undergo remodeling. It is common to find unremodeled cortical bone in aged small dogs and cats. These unremodeled regions likely have been spared vigorous mechanical use (stress) and did not experience strain (deformation in structure) sufficient to initiate remodeling. The remodeling unit of cortical bone is called the osteon, and for trabecular bone, it is called the basic structural unit. The shape of the osteon is cylindrical. The basic structural unit has the contour of a shallow trench filled with parallel lamellae. The time required from initiation to completion of these remodeling units is estimated to be 3 to 4 months in human beings. At the periphery of these remodeling units are cement lines, which separate the units from each other. Because there are no collagen fibers extending across the cement lines, there can be slight movement of these columns or plates of bone in relation to each other providing flexibility and possibly a means of distributing shearing forces. Cement lines indicating the limit of previous resorptive activity are usually somewhat scalloped, reflecting the Howship's lacunae created by osteoclasts. These lines are called "reversal lines" (where resorption stopped and the process was reversed by formation) (Fig. 16-13). Cement lines also can occur when osteoblast formation ceases and subsequently resumes. The reason for the cessation is usually not obvious. These cement lines are called "resting lines" and are usually smooth and follow the contour of the overlying surface.

The term "modeling" is used to describe change of the shape or contour of a bone in response to normal growth, altered mechanical use, or disease. In modeling, bone surfaces (periosteal, endosteal, intracortical, and trabecular surfaces) can go from resting directly to either formation or resorption depending on the stimulus. This process allows the shape or size of bone to change and enables the medullary cavity to enlarge and the overall shape of the bone to be maintained while the bone is growing. Modeling is in contrast to normal remodeling in which resorption must precede formation to keep bone mass and shape constant.

BONE AS AN ORGAN

Individual bones of the skeleton vary in their manner of formation, growth, structure, and function. Flat bones of the skull develop by the process of intramembranous ossification, in which mesenchymal cells differentiate into osteoblasts and produce bone directly. Cartilage precursors are not involved. Most bones develop from cartilaginous models by the process of endochondral ossification. Cartilaginous models are invaded by vessels, and primary (diaphyseal) and secondary (epiphyseal) centers of ossification develop and provide for further growth and increasing strength.

The long appendicular bones and the vertebral bodies are divided anatomically into epiphyses, metaphyseal growth plates (physes), metaphyses, and diaphyses (Fig. 16-14).

BLOOD SUPPLY TO BONE

Arterial blood from the systemic circulation enters bones through nutrient, metaphyseal, periosteal, and

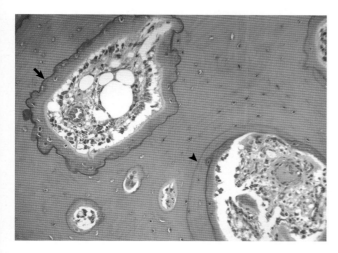

Fig. 16-13   Remodeling in compact subchondral bone adjacent to a joint with bacterial infection, bone, horse. Resting cement appear as basophilic smooth lines indicating where formation has temporarily stopped (*arrowhead*). Reversal lines are scalloped basophilic lines (*arrow*) indicating where in the bone resorption stopped and was followed by formation. H&E stain. (*Courtesy Dr. S.E. Weisbrode, College of Veterinary Medicine, The Ohio State University.*)

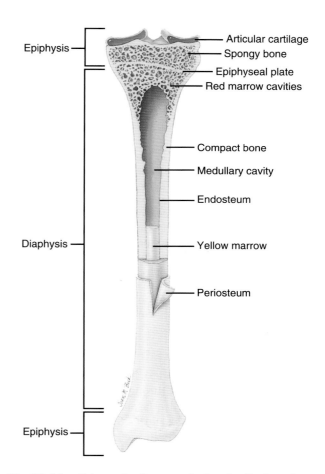

Fig. 16-14   Schematic diagram of a longitudinal section of long bone (tibia) showing spongy (cancellous) and compact bone. The name *epiphyseal plate* in the diagram is commonly used but not preferred for this growth plate. This growth plate elongates the metaphysis and is the metaphyseal growth plate or physis. The growth plate responsible for enlarging the epiphysis is the articular-epiphyseal complex (see **Bone Growth**). (*From Thibodeau GA, Patton KT:* Anatomy and physiology, *ed 5, St Louis, 2003, Mosby.*)

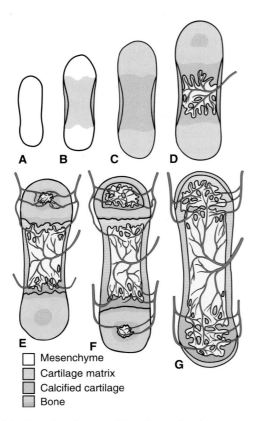

Fig. 16-15 **Correlation of long bone development and vascularization.** The primitive mesenchyme that makes up the skeletal primordia has no blood vessels (**A**). This mesenchyme condenses and undergoes mineralization, and a bony collar forms in the periosteum of the diaphysis (**B** and **C**). The nutrient artery enters the mineralized cartilaginous tissue in the diaphysis, bringing osteogenic and osteoclast precursors enabling endochondral ossification to occur (primary center of ossification) (**D**). Similarly, the epiphyseal arteries bring these cells to the secondary centers of ossification in the epiphyses (**E**). Extensive anastomoses develop as the bone continues to develop and as the growth plates close (**F** and **G**). *(From Banks WJ: Applied veterinary histology, ed 3, St Louis, 1993, Mosby.)*

epiphyseal arteries (Fig. 16-15). Nutrient arteries penetrate the diaphyseal cortex through a nutrient foramen covered by strong, protective fascial attachments; once within the medulla, these arteries divide into proximal and distal intramedullary branches. Other arteries penetrating the cortex are the proximal and distal metaphyseal arteries. These are smaller and more numerous than the nutrient artery. They penetrate the cortex and anastomose with the terminal branches of the nutrient arteries in the medullary cavity. These anastomoses protect against infarction if a nutrient artery is obstructed.

Small periosteal arteries also pass through the diaphyseal cortex at sites of fascial attachment and can supply one quarter to one third of the outer cortex. The remainder

of the cortex is supplied by the nutrient artery and its anastomotic branches. This blood flow is centrifugal (from medulla to periosteum)because of greater pressures in the intramedullary vessels. The chondrocytes of the physis nearest the epiphysis are supplied by epiphyseal arteries. The chondrocytes of the physis nearest the metaphysis are supplied by branches of metaphyseal and nutrient arteries. As capillaries from these vessels approach the metaphyseal side of the physis, they make abrupt turns (loops). These loops are sites predisposed to bacterial embolization in neonatal sepsis.

BONE GROWTH

Bone grows in length by interstitial growth within the cartilage growth plates (Fig. 16-16). The mineralized longitudinal septa of the growth plates serve as struts on which bone is deposited. This process is called endochondral ossification. The metaphyseal growth plate, or physis, is primarily responsible for lengthening the bone. Cartilage of the metaphyseal growth plate is divided into a reserve or resting zone, a proliferative zone, and a hypertrophic zone (Fig. 16-17). The hypertrophic zone is sometimes further subdivided into zones of maturation, degeneration, and calcification. The zone of degeneration is suspected to be a form of apoptosis, but usually there is nuclear and cytoplasmic swelling

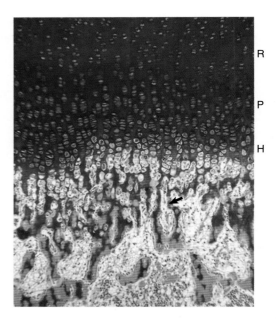

Fig. 16-16 **Growth plate, long bone, dog.** Resting (*R*), proliferating (*P*), and hypertrophic (*H*) zones of the growth plate are visible. Apoptotic chondrocytes are released from their lacunae by invading vessels and chondroclasts leaving only the longitudinal septa (*arrow*) as a base on which bone will be deposited to form a primary trabeculae. H&E stain.
(Courtesy Dr. S.E. Weisbrode, College of Veterinary Medicine, The Ohio State University.)

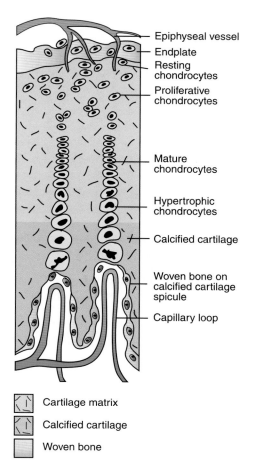

Epiphyseal vessel
Endplate
Resting chondrocytes
Proliferative chondrocytes
Mature chondrocytes
Hypertrophic chondrocytes
Calcified cartilage
Woven bone on calcified cartilage spicule
Capillary loop

Cartilage matrix
Calcified cartilage
Woven bone

Fig. 16-17   **Schematic diagram of the major blood supply to the physis.** Branches of the epiphyseal artery supply the resting zones of the growth plate. Branches of the metaphyseal artery form capillary loops at the metaphyseal end of the physis undergoing endochondral ossification. *(From Banks WJ: Applied veterinary histology, ed 3, St Louis, 1993, Mosby.)*

for the mineralization, a nearby blood supply is necessary, and vascular invasion does not take place in mammalian growth plates unless there is mineralization of the longitudinal septum. Vascular invasion of the growth plate is a critical step in endochondral ossification. Blood vessels from the metaplysis invade into the advancing growth plate, bringing with them osteoblasts that form bone on the cartilage spicules (Fig. 16-17). The chondroosseous junction in the metaphysis is a fragile lattice of bone-covered spicules of calcified cartilage (primary trabeculae). As the growth plate advances and elongates the metaphysis, the more mature trabeculae deeper in the metaphysis become fewer and thicker (secondary and tertiary trabeculae) and often contain residual fragments of cartilage.

Growth of the epiphysis also contributes to the overall length of the bone and is accomplished by endochondral ossification at the articular-epiphyseal (AE) complex. The AE complex is the zone of endochondral ossification beneath the articular cartilage in growing animals (Fig. 16-18). The residue of the AE complex will become the zone of mineralized articular cartilage in the adult.

Growth plates are thickest when growth is most rapid; as growth slows, the plate becomes thin and "closes" (it is entirely replaced by bone) at skeletal maturity (Fig. 16-19). The times for closures of specific growth plates in an individual animal can vary greatly. The AE complex usually closes before the physis. The physes of vertebra will usually remain open longer than the physes of the long bones. Androgens and estrogens play a major role in determining the time of growth plate closure, and early castration in the dog results in delayed growth plate closure with the subsequent increased length of bones.

Bone grows in width by intramembranous bone formation. Except for articular surfaces (including the ends of the vertebral bodies), the surfaces of bones are covered

light microscopically, and this is not typical of apoptosis. The resting or reserve zone serves as a source of cells for the proliferating zone where cells multiply, accumulate glycogen, produce matrix, and become arranged in longitudinal columns. In the hypertrophic zone, chondrocytes secrete macromolecules that modify the matrix to allow capillary invasion and initiate matrix mineralization; eventually these chondrocytes die. The overall lengthening of the bone is due to a combination of the effects of the proliferating zone and hypertrophying zone. Calcification begins in the longitudinal septa of cartilaginous matrix between columns of chondrocytes. Matrix vesicles derived from chondrocytes (analogous to those described previously for mineralization of bone) form in the hypertrophic zone and initiate the mineralization process as previously described for bone. The processes of mineralization and vascular invasion of the growth plate are co-dependent events. To supply salts

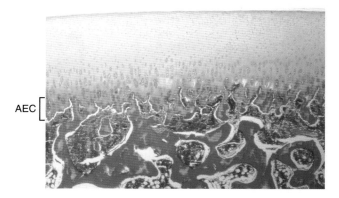

AEC

Fig. 16-18   **Articular-epiphyseal complex (AEC), bone, articular cartilage, young dog.** The AE complex is the growth plate beneath the articular cartilage. Its function and structure are essentially the same as the metaphyseal growth plate (Fig. 16-16). H&E stain. *(Courtesy Dr. S.E. Weisbrode, College of Veterinary Medicine, The Ohio State University.)*

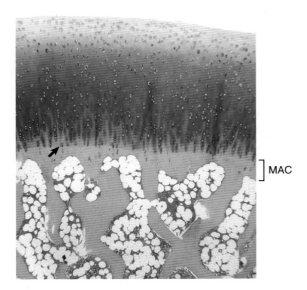

Fig. 16-19   Bone and cartilage, humerus, proximal end, adult dog. Growth of the skeleton, specifically the epiphysis, has ceased, and cartilage that was portion of the articular epiphyseal complex is retained as the mineralized layer of the articular cartilage (*MAC*). The MAC is separated from the unmineralized articular cartilage by a basophilic line called the tidemark (*arrow*). Collagen fibers cross the tidemark and are shared by the MAC and overlying unmineralized articular cartilage. There are no collagen fibers crossing the junction between the subchondral bone and MAC because they are of different collagen types. H&E stain. (*Courtesy Dr. S.E. Weisbrode, College of Veterinary Medicine, The Ohio State University.*)

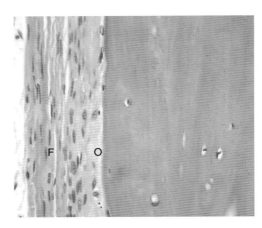

Fig. 16-20   Periosteum, bone, dog. The outer fibrous layer (*F*) and inner osteogenic layer (*O*) line the periosteal surface. The osteogenic layer is able to rapidly deposit woven bone as a nonspecific response to injury. H&E stain. (*Courtesy Dr. S.E. Weisbrode, College of Veterinary Medicine, The Ohio State University.*)

NORMAL STRUCTURE AND FUNCTION OF JOINTS

Joints (articulations) join skeletal structures, provide for movement, and in some cases have shock-absorbing functions. Most of the material in this section is confined to the synovial joints.

Synovial joints occur in both the axial and appendicular skeleton. Such joints allow for a variable degree of movement and, anatomically, are composed of two bone ends joined together by a fibrous capsule and ligaments. The inner surface of the articular capsule is lined by a synovial membrane, and the bone ends are covered by articular cartilage. The joint space contains synovial fluid, and fibrocartilaginous menisci or disks are present at some sites (e.g., femoro-tibial and temporomandibular joints). Synovial joints operate with very low coefficients of friction and are self-lubricating. Articular cartilage serves as the bearing substance and subchondral bone as the supporting material. Articular cartilage functions to minimize friction created by movement to transmit mechanical forces to underlying bone and to maximize the contact area of the joint under load. Joints receive and absorb energy of impact. Both articular cartilage and subchondral bone deform under pressure, but it is the subchondral bone that has the most significant force-attenuating properties.

ARTICULAR CARTILAGE

Articular (hyaline) cartilage is normally a white to blue-white material with a smooth, moist surface. Cartilage thickness is greatest in the young and at sites of maximal weight bearing. Thinning and yellow discoloration occur in old age. At its margins, articular cartilage merges with a periosteal surface that is lined by fibrous tissue

by periosteum. This covering is a thin membrane that is loosely attached to underlying bone except at heavy fascial attachments on bony prominences and at tendon insertions, where its attachments are strong and are associated with large vessels penetrating the underlying bone. Microscopically the periosteum is composed of an outer fibrous layer that provides structural support and an inner osteogenic or cambium layer, capable of forming normal lamellar appositional bone on the cortex of growing bones, and abnormal woven bone formation in response to injury (Fig. 16-20). The periosteum is well supplied with lymph vessels and with fine myelinated and nonmyelinated nerve fibers that explain the intense pain when the periosteum is injured.

The periosteum covering the physis is called the perichondrial ring. The perichondrial ring adds new cartilage to the periphery of the physis, enabling the physis to expand in width as the animal grows. The metaphyseal cortex immediately adjacent to the perichondrial ring is normally very thin in the growing bone because its surfaces are the sites of very active osteoclastic bone resorption. Structurally, this area is the weakest part of the bone.

contiguous with the synovial membrane. Synovial fossae are normal depressions on non–weight-bearing articular cartilage surfaces (Fig. 16-21, *A* and *B*) that develop bilaterally in the larger appendicular joints of the horse, pig, and ruminant. These are not present at birth but are fully formed by skeletal maturity. The function of synovial fossae is not known. They are significant because they can easily be mistaken for lesions. Articular cartilage contains no nerves or blood or lymph vessels, and its nutrients are obtained by diffusion from synovial fluid and to a lesser extent from subchondral vessels. In the immature skeleton, articular cartilage overlies the still growing cartilage of the epiphysis (epiphyseal cartilage). The epiphyseal cartilage contains blood vessels and will undergo endochondral ossification and thereby contribute to the growth of the epiphysis. Defects at the junction of the articular cartilage and epiphyseal cartilage (the articular epiphyseal complex) occur in osteochondrosis. At skeletal maturity, the epiphyseal cartilage has been replaced by a bony subchondral plate. The deeper regions of the articular cartilage mineralize and remain—they are not removed by endochondral ossification. The junction between the unmineralized articular cartilage and the deeper mineralized cartilage is called the tidemark (Fig. 16-19). As animals age, multiple tidemarks can be formed, indicating an advance (thickening) of the mineralized layer of articular cartilage and thinning of the overlying nonmineralized articular cartilage. The mineralized cartilage serves to anchor articular cartilage to subchondral bone and limits the diffusion of substances between bone and cartilage.

Articular cartilage is 70% to 80% water by weight. It is a viscoelastic, hydrated fiber-reinforced gel that contains chondrocytes, collagen fibers (mostly type II), and proteoglycan aggregates. The largest proteoglycan

is aggregin. Aggregin is composed of the immensely long, nonpolysulfated glycosaminoglycan hyaluronon, to which core proteins are attached in a perpendicular arrangement like bristles on a brush. Again, in bottle brushlike fashion, smaller polysulfated glycosaminoglycans (chondroitin sulfate and keratan sulfate) are attached to these core proteins. Aggregin is extremely hygroscopic. By binding water and forming a hydrated gel, proteoglycans provide stiffness to resist compression and impede the outflow of water when cartilage is under load (weight bearing). The lacunae in which chondrocytes reside are different from those in bone. There is no fluid space within a chondrocyte lacuna as in osteocyte lacunae. The space in the chondrocyte lacunae often seen in light microscopy is a shrinkage artifact. In fact, chondrocytes have surface receptors for matrix components (e.g., hyaluronan), so there is direct communication between matrix and cell.

Collagen fibers provide tensile strength and are arranged in arcades so that the tops of the arcades are parallel to the articular surface, and the sides are perpendicular to the surface and parallel with the radial or intermediate zone of chondrocytes. Functionally the superficial zone of articular cartilage (which has significant amounts of type I collagen) resists shearing forces, the middle zone functions in shock absorption, and the mineralized deep zone of cartilage serves to attach articular cartilage to the subchondral bone by their irregular (and therefore interlocking) interfaces. In scanning electron micrographs, the surface of articular cartilage is not smooth but rather has numerous depressions that can serve as reservoirs for synovial fluid.

Chondrocytes are responsible for the production, maintenance, and turnover of intercellular substances. Normal turnover is enzymatic and is balanced by

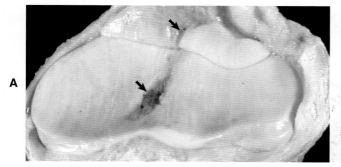

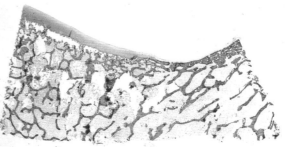

Fig. 16-21 **Synovial fossa, joint, radius and ulna, bone, proximal end, adult horse.** **A,** Synovial fossae are recognized as depressions in the cartilage on the non–weight-bearing surfaces of the sagittal ridge of the radius and in the semilunar notch of the ulna (*arrows*). The parallel linear grooves apparent on the weight-bearing surface (articular cartilage) of the radius are the result of degenerative joint disease. **B,** Histologically, synovial fossae are regions where the endochondral ossification of the epiphyseal cartilage is complete (leaving no articular cartilage), and only a thin fibrous membrane is present on the surface separating the bone from the joint cavity. H&E stain. (**A** and **B,** *Courtesy Dr. S.E. Weisbrode, College of Veterinary Medicine, The Ohio State University.*)

enzyme inhibitors. Disease occurs if there is increased destruction or decreased synthesis of components of the matrix. It is important to remember that compared with bone, which normally renews itself by remodeling, only the proteoglycans turn over in cartilage. The cells and collagen of cartilage are infrequently, if ever, replaced under normal conditions. Chondrocytic mitotic activity is minimal in adult animals, and cellularity of articular cartilage declines with age.

ARTICULAR CAPSULE/SYNOVIUM/SYNOVIAL FLUID

The articular capsule consists of outer fibrous and inner synovial tissue layers. The outer layer is a heavy sheath that contributes to joint stability and at its insertion attaches to bone at the margins of the joint and thereby encloses a segment of bone of variable length within the joint cavity. It is well supplied with blood vessels and nerve endings. The synovial membrane covers all the inner surfaces of the joints except for that of the surface of the articular cartilage. The synovial membrane is normally very thin and barely visible grossly. Tiny surface projections (villi) are normally present and are more prominent in some areas than in others. Synovial intimal or lining cells, one to four cells thick, form a discontinuous surface layer (Fig. 16-22). They are designated as A cells (phagocytic cells that produce hyaluronate); B lymphocytes (fibroblast-like cells, rich in rough endoplasmic reticulum), which may produce glycoprotein; and "intermediate" cells, which have some of the characteristics of both. A cells are of bone marrow origin and are part of the monocyte-macrophage cell system. The synovial subintima can be classified according to the type of predominant tissue (areolar, adipose, or fibrous). It contains blood and lymph vessels that supply and drain the intraarticular structures.

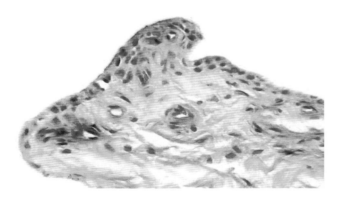

Fig. 16-22   Synovial membrane, joint, dog. The normal synovial membrane consists of an incomplete layer of histiocytes (phagocytic cells) and fibrocytes with subjacent loose fibrous and/or fibrofatty tissue. The joint lumen is at the top. **H&E stain.** *(Courtesy Dr. S.E. Weisbrode, College of Veterinary Medicine, The Ohio State University.)*

Adipose tissue sometimes accumulates in the deep layers of the synovium, forming fat pads that serve as soft cushions in joint cavities (e.g., the infrapatellar fat body of the stifle joint separates the fibrous layer of the articular capsule from the synovium on the anterior aspect of the joint distal to the patella).

Synovial fluid is a dialysate of plasma, supplemented with proteoglycans from the synovial intima that nourishes and lubricates intraarticular structures. Normally, it is a clear, colorless to pale yellow, viscous fluid.

Joint lubrication depends on the microscopic roughness, elasticity, and hydration of articular cartilage and on the presence of mucin (hyaluronate and glycoprotein) in synovial fluid. Lubrication of the synovial membrane itself is hyaluronate-mediated boundary lubrication. Boundary lubrication implies that a substance sticks to the surface and minimizes contact. Lubrication of articular cartilage is accomplished by the complementary action of weeping (squeeze-film) and boundary lubrication. In weeping lubrication, the weight-bearing articular surface is supplied with pressurized fluid that carries most of the load. This fluid is synovial fluid admixed with water released from the underlying cartilage subsequent to pressure of weight bearing. When non–weight-bearing, the water returns to the cartilage because of the hydrophilic properties of proteoglycans. This flushing of water in and out of the articular cartilage enables nutrients to enter cartilage from the synovial fluid and waste products to be removed. Joint stiffness is often due to inability of periarticular soft tissue to lengthen rather than to intraarticular friction.

SUBCHONDRAL BONE

The subchondral bone acts to support the overlying cartilage and dissipate concussive forces to the peripheral cortical bone (Fig. 16-23). The thickness of the subchondral bone plate varies in proportion to the degree of weight bearing. In larger animals, subchondral bone can be compact osteonal bone.

REACTIONS OF BONE TO INJURY

Mechanical forces that can affect bone are both internal and external. Internal forces associated with extremes in work or exercise can influence modeling or remodeling (see previous discussion) and occasionally cause fracture (failure of the bone). External forces (trauma) are more commonly associated with damage to the periosteal surface or fracture of the cortex and/or trabecular bone.

Hormonal agents, particularly calcitriol and parathyroid hormone, enter the bone by the blood stream as described previously.

Infectious agents will be discussed later under Inflammation of Bone.

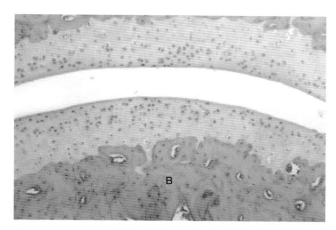

Fig. 16-23   Rat. Compact bone (*B*) supports the articular cartilage in the adult animal when there is no longer endochondral ossification occurring at the articular epiphyseal complex. H&E stain. *(Courtesy Dr. S.E. Weisbrode, College of Veterinary Medicine, The Ohio State University.)*

Defense against mechanical forces include the structure of the bone and the bone's ability to model and remodel to adapt to chronic changes in forces applied to it. The dense bone of the cortex enables the bone to resist most external forces. The formation of osteons and cement lines in the cortex (primary remodeling) facilitates dissipation of microcracks and bending of the bone in response to stress.

Defense against hormonal agents that are capable of resorbing bone include the protective covering on mineralized surfaces by the lamina limitans and osteoblasts. In addition, hormonal signaling to resorb bone is done through the osteoblast, which has the ability to modulate the resorption signal. Defense against infectious agents will be discussed later under Inflammation of Bone.

The hard tissue of bone can be likened to the rings in a tree in leaving clues to its history embedded in its hard structure. Interpreting these clues requires understanding the ways in which bone uniquely responds to injury (Box 16-2).

Box **16-2**

Bone-Specific Reactions to Injury

1. Disruption of endochondral ossification will affect metaphyseal trabeculae.
2. Bone will change its shape to adapt to damage and abnormal use.
3. Bone will alter its mass in response to systemic disease and altered use.
4. Bone deposited rapidly is woven rather than lamellar.
5. Injured periosteum often responds by forming bone.

Disruption of endochondral ossification can alter the appearance of the primary trabeculae. Examples of this are growth retardation lattice and growth arrest lines. Growth arrest lines can be seen in cases of multiple nutrient deficiencies, such as occur in debilitating disease or general malnutrition. The growth plate becomes narrow (growth is impaired), and the metaphyseal face of the plate can be sealed by a layer of bone as a result of transverse trabeculation (trabecular bone forming parallel with the growth plate). If growth resumes, this layer of bone is left in the metaphysis as the physis moves away from the metaphysis (Fig. 16-24, A and B). The bony lines parallel to the growth plate that can be seen grossly and radiographically in such conditions are called growth arrest lines.

A growth retardation lattice results from acquired impairment of osteoclastic activity within the primary

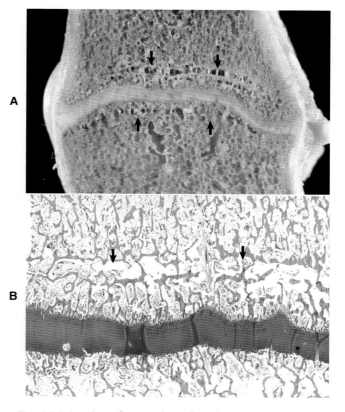

Fig. 16-24   Growth arrest lines, long bone, metaphysis, young zebra. Gross (**A**) and microscopic (**B**) appearance of growth arrest lines. The zebra was ill from a bacterial renal infection and became anorexic. The animal made a brief clinical recovery before euthanasia. The period of inappetence is responsible for the parallel horizontal lines of bone in the metaphysis (*growth arrest lines; arrows*). These lines are due to transverse (horizontal) orientation of the trabeculae during the period of slowed growth. H&E stain. (**A** and **B,** *Courtesy Dr. S.E. Weisbrode, College of Veterinary Medicine, The Ohio State University.)*

trabeculae, which causes retention of primary trabeculae. These trabeculae elongate because of continued production by the growth plate. The retention of the primary trabeculae results in a dense band of vertically oriented trabecular bone beneath the growth plate; this band is called a growth retardation lattice (Fig. 16-25, A and B). The band is apparent because the normal modeling process that resorbs many primary trabeculae completely and molds the remaining ones into progressively fewer but thicker secondary and tertiary trabeculae is impaired. Diseases that cause growth retardation lattices include canine distemper and bovine viral diarrhea. In addition, toxic damage to osteoclasts, such as in lead poisoning, can cause a growth retardation lattice (lead line). The name *growth retardation lattice* is perpetuated here because it is in common use, but it is important to understand that the lesion is in modeling of the trabeculae rather than a reduction in longitudinal growth. Abnormal retention of primary trabeculae also can be seen with congenital defects in the function of osteoclasts (see later discussion of osteopetrosis).

Weakening or destruction of the matrix of the physeal cartilage, as occurs in animals with hypervitaminosis A and with manganese deficiency, can lead to premature closure of growth plates. If the entire plate is affected, no further longitudinal growth is possible. If closure is focal, as can be seen subsequent with localized inflammation or traumatic damage to vessels, there will be uneven growth of the growth plate, which will produce angular deformities.

Osteochondrosis is an important example of diseases caused by disruption of endochondral ossification and will be discussed under disorders of endochondral ossification later.

The ability of bone to change its shape and size (modeling) to accommodate altered mechanical use is called Wolff's Law (Fig. 16-26). Tension and compression are important mechanical factors that affect bone modeling with formation favored at sites of compression and resorption favored at sites of tension. In addition, trabecular bone will align along lines of stress. How bone cells detect altered mechanical use is not precisely known but likely is because of inputs from a variety of signals, including stretch receptors on bone cells, streaming potentials, and piezoelectrical activity. Streaming potentials are electrical currents in bone caused by fluid fluxes through canalicular spaces. These are detected by the osteocytes-osteoblast network. Piezoelectrical activity refers to currents in bone as a result of deformation of collagen fibers and mineral crystals. Electrical currents can affect cell function (bone formation and resorption) and thus influence bone modeling.

Bone mass can be altered to accommodate mechanical use. This is done by the effects of mechanical use on remodeling. Mechanical use is required for maintenance of bone mass. Normal mechanical use suppresses programmed bone resorptive activity. Decreased mechanical use reduces this inhibition (allowing resorption to proceed) as well as suppresses bone formation. The net

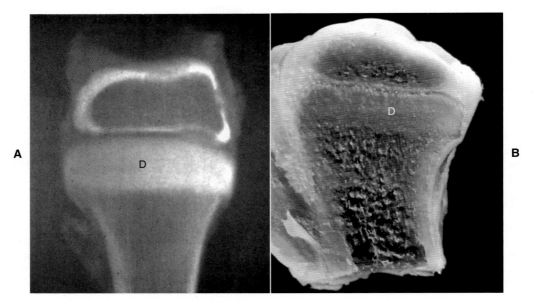

Fig. 16-25   Growth retardation lattice, bone, radius, distal end, dog. Radiograph (**A**) and longitudinal section (**B**) of a growth retardation lattice. The increased bone density (*D*) of the metaphysis represents failure of osteoclasts to resorb unnecessary primary trabeculae. In this case, the failure of osteoclastic resorption was due to canine distemper virus infection of osteoclasts. (*A* and *B,* Courtesy Dr. S.E. Weisbrode, College of Veterinary Medicine, The Ohio State University.)

effect of decreased mechanical use therefore is less bone because of increased resorption and decreased formation (Fig. 16-27). Increased mechanical use will suppress bone resorption and allow bone mass to increase (Fig. 16-28). Chronic suppression of remodeling, however, could lead to accumulated microcracks, which in turn could override the suppression and stimulate remodeling in regions of the microcracks.

Woven bone is the haphazard, hypercellular bone that is deposited in times of repair. Rather than collagen fibers being lamellar, they are irregularly arranged (Fig. 16-29). In woven bone, osteocytes are larger and more numerous per unit area than in lamellar bone, and there is no orientation to their lacunae as seen in lamellar bone in which the alignment of the elliptical lacunae are parallel with the lamellae. When woven bone is formed, the body is responding to a sudden need for more mass and can wait to model and remodel this new bone into lamellar bone once the injury subsides.

The periosteum is programmed to respond to injury by producing woven bone (Fig. 16-29). Usually this is in the form of spicular bone oriented perpendicularly to the long axis of the cortex. If the lesions are nodular, they are called osteophytes. The term enthesiophytes refers

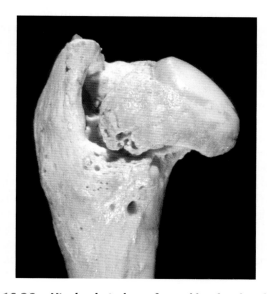

Fig. 16-26   Hip dysplasia, bone, femoral head and neck, dog. The shapes of the femoral head and neck are noticeably abnormal. The head is flattened, and periosteal new bone and coalescing osteophytes have formed a massively thickened femoral neck. Macerated and bleached specimen. (*Courtesy Dr. S.E. Weisbrode, College of Veterinary Medicine, The Ohio State University.*)

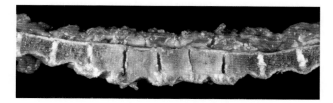

Fig. 16-28   Osteosclerosis, bone, vertebrae, dog. Osteosclerosis (increased bone per unit of area) is evident in the four vertebrae in the center of the vertebral column. The cancellous bone of the medullary cavities has been obliterated by newly formed compact bone. The osteosclerosis is in response to increased mechanical stress in the bodies of the vertebrae as a result of degeneration and loss of the intervertebral disks between these vertebrae. (*Courtesy Dr. S.E. Weisbrode, College of Veterinary Medicine, The Ohio State University.*)

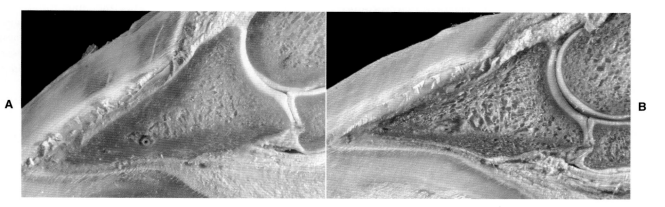

Fig. 16-27   Bone, third phalanx, left rear leg, foal. The leg was in a cast for 2 months to repair an avulsion of gluteal muscles from their insertions and thus could not be used. **A,** Normal right third phalanx. **B,** Left third phalanx. There is pronounced disuse osteopenia (atrophy) compared with the phalanx on the left (**A**). The increase in resorption and decrease in formation associated with disuse has resulted in marked porosity of the cortical and subchondral bone. The cortex now has the appearance of cancellous bone (cancellization of the cortex). (**A** *and* **B,** *Courtesy Dr. S.E. Weisbrode, College of Veterinary Medicine, The Ohio State University.*)

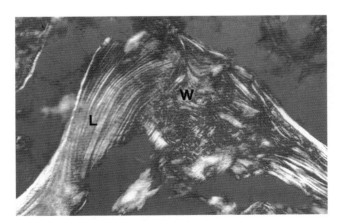

Fig. 16-29   Cancellous and woven bone. A spicule of cancellous bone *(L)* with a sharply demarcated focus of woven bone *(W)*. The woven bone polarizes light, but its collagen fibers are not arranged in uniform parallel layers as in the adjacent normal lamellar bone. This focus of woven bone may represent the site of a healing fracture in this trabecula. Unstained and fully mineralized. Polarized light micrograph. *(From Burkitt HG, Young B, Heath JW: Wheater's functional histology: a text and color atlas, ed 3, New York, 1993, Churchill Livingstone.)*

to osteophytes in regions of insertions of tendons or ligaments. This reactive periosteal woven bone can be admixed with hyaline cartilage. Lesions even can be predominantly cartilage. The extent to which there is cartilage production by the periosteum is thought to be a result of the oxygen available. When oxygen tension is low, cartilage proliferation can predominate. When oxygen is normal, there may be no cartilage present. Cartilage produced in such circumstances can eventually undergo endochondral ossification. Woven bone produced by the periosteum can undergo modeling to lamellar bone or could undergo osteoclastic resorption and be removed. The periosteum certainly is not limited to production of woven bone. Lamellar bone is produced by the periosteum during slower stages of appositional growth of the diaphysis. In addition to bone formation, the periosteal surface can have osteoclastic bone resorption. During growth, the regions of the cut-back zone of the metaphysis, in which the bone is tapered from its diameter at the physis to the narrower diameter of the diaphysis, have marked osteoclastic bone resorption at the periosteal bone surface. Also, infectious inflammation of the periosteum can lead to marked osteoclastic bone resorption at the periosteal bone surface.

REACTION OF JOINTS TO INJURY

ARTICULAR CARTILAGE

Although articular cartilage contains metabolically active cells, it has a limited response to injury and minimal capacity for repair. Superficial cartilage defects (cartilage erosion) that do not penetrate into subchondral bone persist for long periods. Clusters or clones of chondrocytes (evidence of local chondrocyte replication in response to injury) are present but are ineffective in filling a defect. Some flow or spreading of cartilaginous matrix into the defect might also occur. This phenomenon of matrix flow is likely facilitated by load bearing and joint movement. In short, superficial injuries to articular cartilage neither heal nor necessarily progress, although progression can occur when there is stiffened (sclerosis of) subchondral bone. However, if a cartilaginous defect extends into subchondral bone (cartilage ulceration), the defect is quickly filled with vascular fibrous tissue that often undergoes metaplasia to fibrocartilage, but rarely to hyaline cartilage. Formation of fibrocartilage can be hastened in full-thickness cartilaginous defects by exercise or prolonged passive motion. Injury to articular cartilage is not painful unless the synovium or subchondral bone is involved. Having no blood supply, articular cartilage does not participate directly in the inflammatory response but is very much affected by inflammation in the synovium, subchondral bone, or subarticular growth (vascularized) cartilage of the epiphysis in young animals. Given that alternating compression and release of normal weight bearing facilitates the diffusion of fluid with nutrients into the articular cartilage and fluid with metabolic waste products out of articular cartilage, it follows that constant compression or lack of weight bearing leads to atrophy (thinning) of articular cartilage.

Sterile injury to cartilage can be a consequence of trauma, joint instability, or lubrication failure because of changes in synovial fluid, synovial membrane, or incongruity in joint surfaces. Destruction of articular cartilage in response to sterile injury and infectious inflammation is mediated by a combination of enzymatic digestion of matrix and failure of matrix production when chondrocytes become degenerate or necrotic. These changes can be initiated by damage to the cartilage directly, or indirectly, by lesions in the synovium.

Matrix metalloproteinases are enzymes capable of matrix digestion; they are normal constituents of the matrix, but are present in an inactive form. Matrix metalloproteinases can be broadly categorized as gelatinases, collagenases, and stromelysins. Collagenases are most capable of digestion of collagen fibers; gelatinases digest type I collagen and basement membrane collagens but are less effective against type II collagen of cartilage. Stromelysins destroy noncollagenous proteins. Matrix metalloproteinases can be activated by products of degenerating or reactive chondrocytes and inflammatory cells. In addition to acting as a control on the destructive effects of activated metalloproteinases, tissue inhibitors of metalloproteinases (TIMPs) are present in the matrix.

Normal   Fibrillation   Eburnation

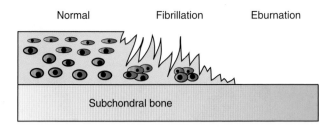

Subchondral bone

Fig. 16-30   Schematic diagram showing the structural changes that characterize fibrillation and eburnation of articular cartilage overlying subchondral bone. In the area of eburnation, the cartilage is missing, and the exposed subchondral bone has increased density.

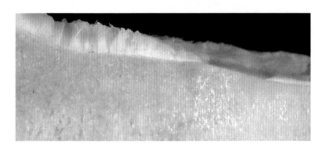

Fig. 16-31   Fibrillation and ulceration, degenerative joint disease, tibia, proximal articular cartilage, sagittal section, bull. To the left, the cartilage is frayed (fibrillation) and its surface has the appearance of a shag rug. To the right of the fibrillated region is an ulcer. Note that the cartilage is missing from the bed of the ulcer in the plane of the section, but the edge of the ulcer with a rim of normal cartilage is visible at its back. The cartilage to the right of the ulcer is very thin, indicating erosion. *(Courtesy Dr. S.E. Weisbrode, College of Veterinary Medicine, The Ohio State University.)*

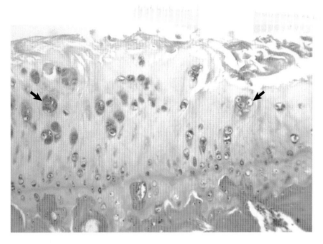

Fig. 16-32   Degenerative joint disease, hip dysplasia, femoral head, articular cartilage, dog. The superficial cartilage is fibrillated and hypocellular (necrosis) with clusters of chondrocytes *(arrows)* representing ineffectual attempts at repair. H&E stain. *(Courtesy Dr. S.E. Weisbrode, College of Veterinary Medicine, The Ohio State University.)*

The loss of proteoglycans from cartilage alters the hydraulic permeability of the cartilage, thereby interfering with joint lubrication and leading to further mechanically induced injury to the cartilage. The loss of proteoglycans, with subsequent inadequate lubrication of the articular surface, leads to disruption of collagen fibers on the surface of articular cartilage. The surfaces of affected areas of cartilage are yellow-brown and have a dull, slightly roughened appearance. As more proteoglycans are lost, the collagen fibers condense and fray (fibrillation) with multiple clefts and/or fissures forming along the vertical axis of the arcades of collagen fibers (Figs. 16-30 to 16-32). The vertical axis of the collagen fibers in these arcades is perpendicular to the plane of movement of the joint. Fibrillation is accompanied by loss of surface cartilage (erosion) and eventual thinning of the articular cartilage. Subsequent to fibrillation and erosion, necrosis of individual chondrocytes occurs in the radial zone, thus making cartilage hypocellular. In response to the fibrillation, erosion, and necrosis of chondrocytes, remaining chondrocytes can undergo regenerative hyperplasia (cluster or clone

formation), but the ability of chondrocytes in the adult to divide is limited and the regenerative attempt is almost always ineffective. Loss of articular cartilage can become complete with exposure of subchondral bone (ulceration) (Fig. 16-33).

ARTICULAR CAPSULE/SYNOVIUM/ SYNOVIAL FLUID

Intraarticular prostaglandins, nitric oxide, TNF-α, IL-1, and neurotransmitters—such as substance P among other cytokines and chemokines—are increased in degenerative and inflammatory joint disease. Prostaglandins and nitric oxide inhibit proteoglycan synthesis in synovium and chondrocytes; this reduction in proteoglycan content can lead to degeneration and loss of the cartilage (see previous discussion). IL-1 and TNF-α are cytokines secreted by activated macrophages (synovial type A cells or subintimal macrophages); they promote secretion of prostaglandins, nitric oxide, and neutral proteases from synovial fibroblasts and chondrocytes. Increasing concentrations of these agents will decrease matrix synthesis and increase matrix destruction. Cytokines and growth factors that can be anabolic to cartilage include IL-6, TGF-β, and insulin-like growth factor.

Lysosomal enzymes (collagenase, cathepsins, elastase, arylsulfatase) and neutral proteases, which are capable of degrading proteoglycans or collagen, can be derived from inflammatory cells, synovial lining cells, and chondrocytes.

The synovial membrane commonly responds to injury by villous hypertrophy and hyperplasia, hypertrophy and hyperplasia of synoviocytes (Fig. 16-34), and pannus

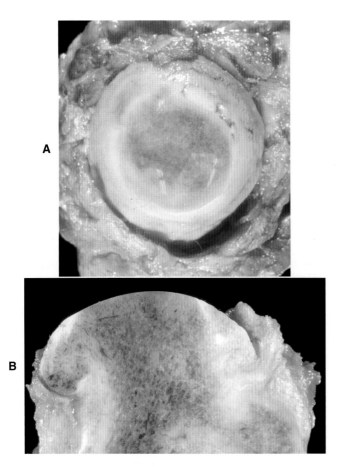

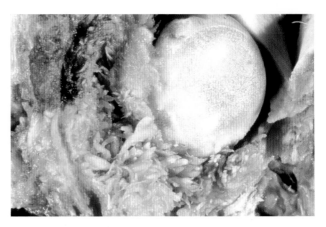

Fig. 16-34   **Synovial villous hyperplasia, hip dysplasia, coxofemoral joint, articular capsule and femoral head, dog.** There is marked villous synovial hyperplasia. The extent of this proliferation is unusually severe for hip dysplasia. Microscopically, this hyperplasia is routinely accompanied by variable lymphoplasmacytic inflammation that is independent of the cause of the articular damage. (*Courtesy Dr. S.E. Weisbrode, College of Veterinary Medicine, The Ohio State University.*)

Fig. 16-33   **Degenerative joint disease, hip dysplasia, bone, femur, head, dog.** The femoral head viewed from the medial aspect (**A**) and sagittal plane (**B**). The head is flattened (modeled) and ulcerated. The ulcerated region appears darker because congestion of blood vessels in the marrow spaces of the subchondral bone is visible through the thinned articular cartilage of the femoral head. The zone of attachment of the round ligament to the head of the femur has been destroyed. (**A** *and* **B,** *Courtesy Dr. S.E. Weisbrode, College of Veterinary Medicine, The Ohio State University.*)

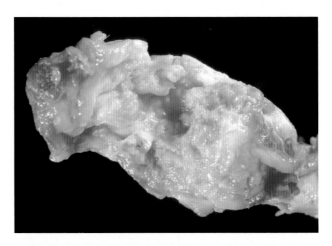

Fig. 16-35   **Pannus, rheumatoid-like arthritis, radius and ulna, proximal end, dog.** Note the fibrovascular tissue (pannus) covering all articular surfaces. (*Courtesy Dr. S.E. Weisbrode, College of Veterinary Medicine, The Ohio State University.*)

formation (see later discussion). Villous hypertrophy occurs with and without synovitis. The proportions of A and B cells in the synovium also can change in various disease processes. Fragments of articular cartilage can adhere to the synovium, where they are surrounded by macrophages and giant cells. Larger pieces of detached cartilage (as in osteochondrosis) can float free and survive as "joint mice" that continue to be nurtured and remain viable by synovial fluid.

Inflammatory cell infiltrates (see later section under Inflammatory Lesions: Infectious and Noninfectious Arthritis) in the synovial membrane can impair fluid drainage from the joint, and joint fluid can lose some of its lubricating properties because hyaluronic acid can

be degraded by the superoxide-generating systems of neutrophils.

Pannus can develop in association with chronic infectious fibrinous synovitis and with some immune-mediated diseases, such as rheumatoid arthritis. Pannus is a fibrovascular and histiocytic tissue that arises from the synovial membrane and spreads over articular cartilage as a velvety membrane (Figs. 16-35 and 16-36). In the pannus, tissue histiocytes and monocytes of bone marrow origin transform into macrophages, and they, along with the collagenases from fibroblasts, cause lysis

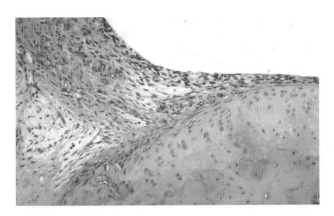

Fig. 16-36   Pannus, rheumatoid-like arthritis (experimentally induced), articular cartilage, tibia, distal end, rat. The experimentally induced rheumatoid-like arthritis was produced by injecting Freund's adjuvant and *Mycobacterium butyricum* into the subcutis at the base of the tail. The pathogenesis of "adjuvant arthritis" is uncertain, other than it appears to be T-lymphocyte mediated. Here, fibrovascular repair tissue (pannus) is seen arising from the synovium (*left*) and growing onto the surface of the articular cartilage. There is not yet any damage to the cartilage beneath the pannus. H&E stain. *(Courtesy Dr. S.E. Weisbrode, College of Veterinary Medicine, The Ohio State University.)*

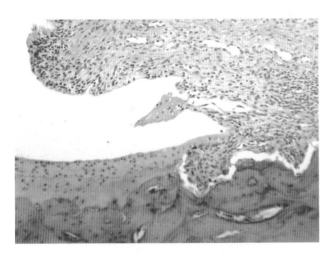

Fig. 16-37   Pannus, rheumatoid-like arthritis (experimentally induced), articular cartilage, tibia, distal end, rat. Pannus originating from the synovium (*right*) is invading and destroying the articular cartilage and bone. H&E stain. *(Courtesy Dr. S.E. Weisbrode, College of Veterinary Medicine, The Ohio State University.)*

of cartilage (Fig. 16-37). As the pannus spreads, the underlying cartilage is destroyed. In time, if both opposing cartilaginous surfaces are involved, the fibrous tissue can unite the surfaces, causing fibrous ankylosis (fusion of the joint). In some cases of immune-mediated arthritis, pannus is present in the subchondral bone marrow as well as in the synovium. Pannus can develop in marrow

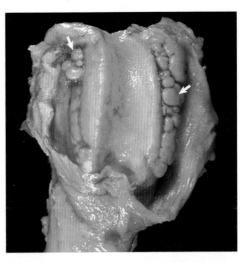

Fig. 16-38   Osteophytes, degenerative joint disease, distal femur, dog. Note the marked formation of osteophytes (*arrows*) at the lateral and medial margins of the trochlear ridges. *(Courtesy Dr. H. Liepold, College of Veterinary Medicine, Kansas State University; and Noah's Arkive, College of Veterinary Medicine, The University of Georgia.)*

from subchondral bone and penetrate into the overlying articular cartilage.

Sterile degenerative changes in articular cartilage are often accompanied by the formation of periarticular osteophytes (Fig. 16-38) and by some degree of secondary synovial inflammation and hyperplasia. The synovitis is characterized by the presence of variable numbers of plasma cells, lymphocytes, and macrophages in the synovial subintima (beneath the layers of synoviocytes) and by hyperplasia and hypertrophy of synovial lining cells. The pathogenesis of this synovitis is not known, but is suspected to be secondary to release of sequestered or altered host antigens by the degenerate cartilage osteophytes that form as multiple bony or cartilaginous outgrowths. They can arise from mesenchymal cells with chondro-osseous potential within the synovial membrane at the junction of the synovial membrane with the perichondrium/periosteum, just peripheral to the articular cartilage or on the surface of the bone where the articular capsule and the periosteum merge. Osteophytes do not grow continuously, but once formed, they persist as multiple periarticular spurs of bone. These spurs can be confined within the joint cavity if they arise from the perichondrium or can be protrusions from the periosteal surface of the bone if they arise from the insertion site of the joint capsule with the periosteum. Osteophytes can result from mechanical instability within the joint causing stretching or tearing of the insertions of the articular capsule or ligaments, or they can form from stimulation by cytokines such as TGF-β released from reactive or degenerating mesenchymal cells within the joint.

Because of their antiinflammatory effect, glucocorticoids are injected into joints. Sometimes this is followed by a rapid progression of degenerative changes within the joint and is designated "steroid arthropathy." These degenerative changes relate to the antianabolic effects of glucocorticoids on chondrocytes. They reduce the synthesis of cartilaginous matrix, lead to proteoglycan depletion, retard repair, and reduce the mechanical strength of cartilage.

SUBCHONDRAL BONE

With loss of proteoglycans, concussive forces are less attenuated by degenerate or thin articular cartilage and a greater component of these forces then is transmitted to the subchondral bone. The bone responds to the increased mechanical use by decreasing resorption and increasing formation resulting in denser (sclerotic) bone. If the cartilage ulcerates to the level of the bone and the joint is still used, the dense bone can become polished and ivory-like (eburnation) (Fig. 16-33, A). There is interest in the possible role subchondral bone might play in initiating cartilage damage in degenerative joint disease. Overweight human beings (and animals) are predisposed to develop degenerative joint disease. In the human knee, the density of the subchondral bone is greater in overweight people presumably in response to increased weight bearing. This change precedes the development of degenerative joint disease. Some believe this dense bone is less effective in dissipating normal concussive forces and causes some of the impact to be deflected back into the articular cartilage causing injury to the chondrocytes.

PORTALS OF ENTRY INTO BONE

Infectious agents can enter bone directly through the periosteum and cortex or by the blood stream. Agents can gain access through the periosteum by means of trauma that may or may not break the bone or by extension from adjacent inflammation, as in periodontal tissue (periodontitis becoming a mandibular or maxillary osteomyelitis) or the middle ear (otitis media extending into the bone to become an osteomyelitis of the tympanic bulla). Blood vessels gain access to the marrow cavity of the diaphysis and metaphysis by the nutrient foramen. The epiphysis in the young animal depends mostly on the epiphyseal artery and small branches of that artery that cross the epiphyseal cortex. Blood-borne bacterial infection of bone in the perinatal animal may originate from the umbilicus or oral-pharyngeal route, with the latter being more likely. In theory, hematogenous osteomyelitis can begin in any capillary bed in bone where bacteria lodge and survive. In practice, it occurs most commonly in young animals and is localized typically at the zone of vascular invasion of the growth plate (either at the physis [Fig. 16-39] or AE complex [Fig. 16-40]) where capillaries make sharp bends to join

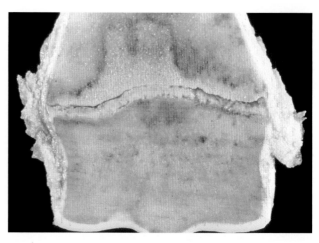

Fig. 16-39   Embolic (suppurative) osteomyelitis and physitis, bone, radius, distal end, foal. The pale region in the metaphysis extending upward to the top middle border of the illustration represents suppurative inflammation and necrosis. It is bordered by a red rim of active hyperemia. A fissure *(the linear and horizontal space on the metaphyseal side of the growth plate)* and the porosity *(darker regions within the growth plate, right)* are the result of bone lysis (primary trabeculae) caused by the physitis. *(Courtesy Dr. S.E. Weisbrode, College of Veterinary Medicine, The Ohio State University.)*

medullary veins (Fig. 16-12). Here, bacterial localization is apparently facilitated by slow flow and turbulence of blood in the larger descending limbs, a lower phagocytic capacity, and discontinuous endothelial cells. No vascular anastomoses are located in this region, and thrombosis of these capillaries results in bone infarction that is a predisposing factor for bacterial localization. It is likely that ligand-receptor binding between bacteria and endothelial cells plays a role. From this nidus at the physis or AE complex, the exudates can extend into other structures. At the AE complex the inflammation can extend into the overlying joint cavity (Fig. 16-40). At the physis, the inflammation can extend into the epiphysis, periosteum, or joint cavity (Figs. 16-41 and 16-42).

PORTALS OF ENTRY INTO JOINTS

Microbial and other agents enter the joints via hematogenous spread and direct extension (Fig. 16-43). Neonatal bacteremia secondary to omphalitis or oral-intestinal entry commonly leads to polyarthritis. Bacteria can also reach the joint by direct inoculation, as in a puncture wound, by direct extension from periarticular soft tissues, or by extension from adjacent bone.

DEFENSE MECHANISMS OF BONE

The defense against infectious agents is no different in bone than in other tissue. However, the consequences

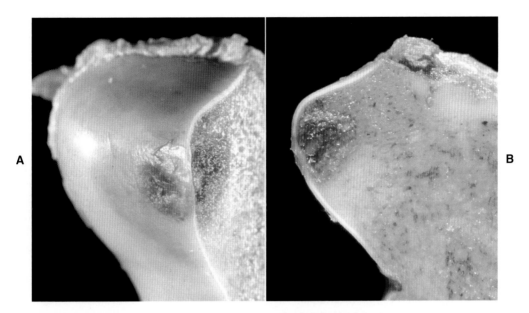

Fig. 16-40   Embolic (suppurative) osteomyelitis, bone, distal femur, medial trochlear ridge, transverse section, horse. A, Oblique view of articular cartilage and transverse section. **B,** The suppurative osteomyelitis has extended from its site of origin in the cancellous bone into the articular epiphyseal complex and then into the overlying articular cartilage, with resulting collapse and fragmentation of the articular cartilage. (*A and **B,** Courtesy Dr. S.E. Weisbrode, College of Veterinary Medicine, The Ohio State University.*)

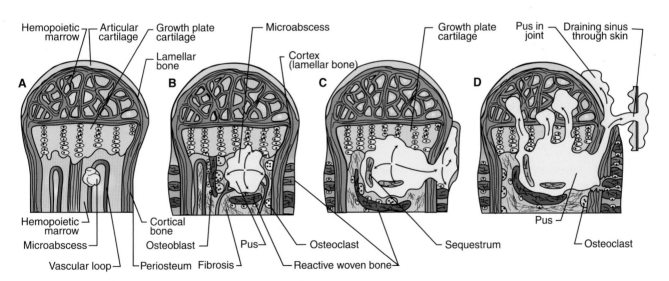

Fig. 16-41   Schematic diagram showing patterns of spread of embolic osteomyelitis from the physis. The septic embolus lodges in capillary loops at the physis (**A**). The inflammation causes lysis of metaphyseal bone and growth plate cartilage. This lysis can cause mechanical instability to which the periosteum responds by producing reactive bone (**B**). The exudates can lyse the cortex at its thinnest point (the metaphyseal cut back zone) and extend into the periosteum (periostitis) or into the joint (arthritis) (**C and D**). (*A through **D,** Redrawn from Rubin E:* Essential pathology, *ed 3, 2001, Lippincott Williams & Wilkins.*)

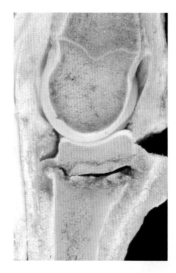

Fig. 16-42 **Embolic bacterial physitis, osteomyelitis, periostitis, proximal first phalanx and arthritis, metacarpal-phalangeal joint, horse.** Bacterial inflammation has destroyed the physis and has extended into the periosteum and joint cavity (*left*). *(Courtesy Dr. S.E. Weisbrode, College of Veterinary Medicine, The Ohio State University.)*

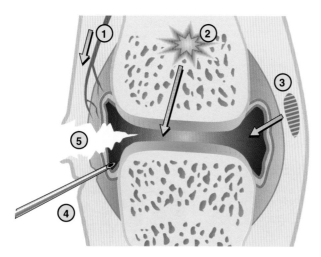

Fig. 16-43 **Schematic diagram of the routes of infection for a joint in an adult.** *1*, The hematogenous route. *2*, Extension from osteomyelitis. *3*, Spread from an adjacent soft tissue infection. *4*, Diagnostic or therapeutic procedures. *5*, Penetrating damage from puncture or cutting. *(From Huether SE, McCance KL: Understanding pathophysiology, ed 2, St Louis, 2000, Mosby.)*

of an inflammatory response can have great effect on the structure and function of bone. Many soluble inflammatory mediators can increase both bone formation and resorption, resulting in varying extent of reactive bone formation and bone lysis. The exudate associated with some acute infections in the medulla can increase

the pressure in the marrow cavity and cause compression of the nutrient artery resulting in ischemic necrosis. If resorbed cortical bone is replaced by scar tissue (fibrous repair tissue), the bone can become unstable.

DEFENSE MECHANISMS OF JOINTS

The cellular and humoral defenses against infectious agents are no different in the joint from those in other tissue. Details are presented previously in response to injury and later in the presentation of lesions in infectious and noninfectious arthritis. However, because articular cartilage has such limited ability to regenerate, the consequences of inflammation that destroy the ability of synovium to provide nutrients and synovial fluid to the cartilage or that destroy areas of the cartilage itself could progress to degenerative joint disease after the inflammation subsides.

DISEASES OF BONE

ABNORMALITIES OF GROWTH AND DEVELOPMENT

DISORDERS OF BONE RESORPTION

Osteopetrosis is an osteosclerotic (increased bone density per unit area) disease that occurs in dogs, sheep, horses, cattle, and several strains of mice and is described by some as a "metaphyseal dysplasia." The basic disorder is due to failure of osteoclasts to resorb bone. The nature of the osteoclast failure has been defined in several strains of mice with spontaneous disease. In addition, knockout mice have been useful in defining possible mechanisms for osteosclerosis, including knockouts for genes that encode for osteoclast differentiation factor and tartrate resistant acid phosphatase (an osteoclast lysosomal enzyme). The specific osteoclast defects are not yet known in domestic animals with osteopetrosis.

Growth plate: There are no primary lesions in the growth plate in osteopetrosis.

Trabecular bone: Osteoclasts are unable to resorb and shape (model) the primary trabeculae (Fig. 16-44). As a result, spicules of bone with central cores of calcified cartilage fill the medullary cavity. This process affects all bones that develop in a cartilaginous model (elongate by endochondral ossification from a growth plate). Affected bones are dense and have no medullary cavity. The rare disease has been reported in a variety of domestic and exotic animals. The defect in Angus cattle is inherited as an autosomal recessive trait. Affected calves are typically stillborn a few weeks premature and also have brachygnathia inferior, impacted molar teeth, and deformed cranial vaults that compress the brain.

Cortical bone: The cortical bone is essentially normal. The cut back zone of the metaphysis, although not as

A   B   C

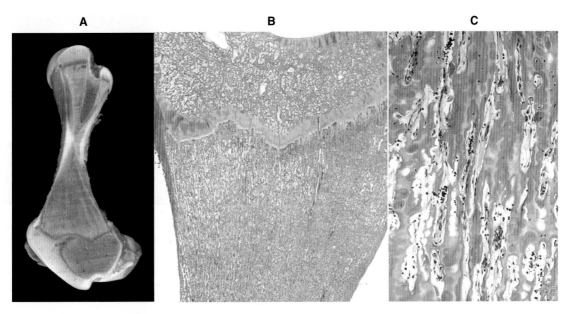

Fig. 16-44   Osteopetrosis, bone, femur, calf (Aberdeen Angus). A, The primary trabeculae are retained and fill the entire medullary cavity. **B** and **C,** Retained straight unremodeled trabeculae with cartilaginous cores fill the medullary (marrow) cavity. H&E stain. (**A,** *Courtesy Dr. H. Leipold, College of Veterinary Medicine, Kansas State University.* **B** and **C,** *Courtesy Dr. S.E. Weisbrode, College of Veterinary Medicine, The Ohio State University.)*

acutely angled as normal, is still present indicating periosteal osteoclast function might be less affected.

DISORDERS OF BONE FORMATION

Osteogenesis imperfecta is an osteopenic (reduced bone mass) disease and has been described in calves, lambs, and puppies; it involves bone, dentin, tendons, and sclera. Clinically, affected animals may have multiple fractures, joint laxity, and defective dentin. The basis of the lesion is a defect in osteoblastic and/or odontoblastic production of type I collagen and in some cases decreased synthesis of certain noncollagenous proteins (i.e., osteonectin). In human beings, and likely in animals, the disease is mostly due to mutations in one or both of the genes that code for type I collagen. In cases in which errors are not found in the collagen genes themselves, alterations should be looked for in genes for enzymes responsible for posttranslational modification of collagen. Mild forms of the disease, because of inactivation of an allele of one the genes, result in normal collagen but in reduced amounts. Mutations that cause substitutions in critical amino acids necessary for collagen helix formation and cross-linking can result in structurally inferior collagen that can be produced in normal amounts. It is interesting that the clinical manifestations of these mutations are usually limited to the bone, teeth, and eyes, even though type I collagen is the major structural collagen in the skin as well.

Growth plate: Growth plates are not affected in osteogenesis imperfecta and would not be expected to be because cartilage collagen is mostly type II.

Trabecular bone: In severe cases, there is much less trabecular bone than normal and without evidence of marked osteoclasis or proliferation of fibrous tissue, as might be expected in severe cases of fibrous osteodystrophy (see later discussion). Osteoblasts can appear normal or small. In some cases, the amount of bone and its microscopic appearance is normal, but there is evidence of fracture disease. Fractures can be present at birth, some with callus formation indicating in utero fractures. Bone fragility in cases with normal bone mass and appearance is likely because of errors in helix formation or cross-linking of tropocollagen molecules. Calves with notable bone fragility (evidence of preparturition and postparturition fractures) can have bone that is normal microscopically and without obvious reduction in bone mass. These calves become osteopenic, possibly secondary to decreased mechanical use because of bone pain from fractures.

Cortical bone: There is a delay in the compaction of cortical bone. Compaction is the term used for the process of completing the formation of cortical bone during development. Depending on the species, varying size and contoured spaces are left between laminae or spicules of woven bone in the developing cortex. The filling of these spaces by bone to solidify the cortex is called compaction. The cortices in osteogenesis imperfecta can be composed of spicules or layers of woven bone with large vascular spaces remaining unfilled by bone. If the animal survives, these vascular spaces may eventually fill in with bone and form compact cortical bone.

Teeth: Because at birth bones can be structurally normal other than the presence of fractures, examination of teeth can be important in reaching a diagnosis of osteogenesis imperfecta morphologically. Grossly, teeth can be pink due to the visibility of the dental pulp through the thin crown. Histologically the dental tubules are short, tortuous, and sometimes absent. The disorganization of the dentin is a qualitative change that allows confirmation of the diagnosis without needing a control animal.

DISORDERS OF BONE MODELING
CONGENITAL CORTICAL HYPEROSTOSIS

Congenital cortical hyperostosis is an autosomal recessive inherited disease of newborn pigs (an example of diaphyseal dysplasia) characterized by the abnormal periosteal bone formation on major long bones. Lesions can be a consequence of disorganization of the perichondral ossification groove (the chondrogenic membrane surrounding the growth plate that enables the growth plate to expand in diameter). One or several limbs can be affected. Piglets are stillborn or die shortly after birth because of other defects. The pathophysiology of the bone lesions is not understood.

Growth plate: Growth plates are not involved.

Trabecular bone: Trabecular bone is not involved.

Cortical bone: Cortical bone only is affected by the production of spicules of woven bone radiating outwards from the periphery of the preexisting cortex. These spicules are oriented perpendicular to the long axis of the cortex and arise from the cambium layer of the periosteum and other than extent of the change, is typical of the nonspecific reaction of the periosteum to injury described previously. The underlying cortex is normal.

CRANIOMANDIBULAR OSTEOPATHY

Craniomandibular osteopathy, also known as "lion jaw," typically occurs as an autosomal recessive condition in West Highland white terriers. Lesions like those in this breed have been reported as isolated occurrences in other breeds and have been associated with a leukocyte adhesion deficiency (suggesting an infectious cause) in a litter of Irish setter pups that also had lesions of hypertrophic osteopathy (see later discussion under noninfectious inflammation of bone). Lesions are bilaterally symmetric, resulting in overall irregular thickening of the mandibles, the occipital and temporal bones, and, occasionally, other bones of the skull (Fig. 16-45).

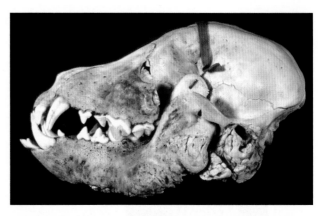

Fig. 16-45   Craniomandibular osteopathy, bone, skull, dog (West Highland white terrier). Extensive periosteal new bone formation on the lateral surfaces of the body and ramus of the mandible, caudolateral maxilla, bulla tympanica, and occipital condyle. Macerated and bleached specimen. *(Courtesy Dr. H. Leipold, College of Veterinary Medicine, Kansas State University.)*

The tympanic bullae are often severely affected. Less commonly the disease can affect the appendicular skeleton. The disease often becomes apparent at 4 to 7 months of age and can regress. For affected dogs, mastication is painful and difficult, and the muscles of the skull become atrophic from disuse. The etiopathogenesis of this disease is unknown. A similar self-limiting disease has recently been reported in the calvaria of young bull mastiffs.

Growth plate: Growth plates are not involved.

Trabecular bone: In the medullary cavities of the bones of the skull and jaw, trabeculae become osteosclerotic (increased bone density per unit area) because of proliferation of woven bone by the osteoblasts of the endosteum with subsequent modeling and remodeling (see next discussion on cortical bone).

Cortical bone: In the skull and jaw, the cortices are thickened because of proliferation of woven bone by the periosteum. Characteristic of the disease is rapid disorganized modeling and remodeling of this bone, causing a mosaic of reversal cement lines with regions of lamellar bone adjacent to regions of woven bone.

DISORDERS OF ENDOCHONDRAL OSSIFICATION
CHONDRODYSTROPHIES

Chondrodystrophies are disorders of bone growth as a result of primary lesions in growth cartilage. Growth cartilage includes the physis, AE complex and epiphyseal cartilage (articular epiphysis yet to undergo endochondral ossification [AE complex] as the secondary center of ossification expands). *Chondrodystrophy* generally implies a widespread abnormality of growth cartilage but could be expressed only in the AE complex selectively affecting the epiphysis (epiphyseal dysplasias such as spider lamb in Suffolk and Hampshire sheep) or only in the physis (metaphyseal dysplasias such as chondrodysplasia in the Alaskan malamute, Norwegian elkhound, and Great Pyrenees breeds). Chondrodystrophies can result in dwarfism. Affected animals usually are short-legged with normal-sized heads because the bones of the calvarium (but not the maxilla and mandible) arise from membranous bone rather than endochondral bone. These are called disproportionate dwarfs. Proportional dwarfism is usually due to underlying endocrine disease (pituitary dwarfism) or malnutrition.

The mechanisms of chondrodysplasias in animals is rarely determined, but defects can be caused by inherited errors in genes that control chondrogenesis. In human beings, the most common dwarfism is called achondroplasia (a misnomer because growth cartilage is present). The condition is inherited as an autosomal dominant trait caused by a single point mutation in the fibroblast growth factor receptor 3 (FGFR3) gene. This mutation results in constant activation of this receptor causing down-regulation of chondrocyte proliferation.

Skeletal dysplasias have also been reported in animals with inherited lysosomal storage diseases, such as mucopolysaccharidosis and gangliosidosis. Chondrocytes can be vacuolated because of retained glycosaminoglycans and lipid.

Growth plate: Growth plates can appear normal or thin depending on the disease. Likewise the arrangements of the chondrocytes can be in normal columns or markedly disorganized. The cartilage matrix can appear normal or rarified.

Trabecular bone: The primary trabeculae can be reduced in amount with the cartilage cores being coarse and misshaped rather than fine regular spicules. This can vary greatly with the type of chondrodysplasia.

Cortical bone: Lesions in cortical bone are greatly variable and mostly due to abnormality in shape or size. Little would be learned from microscopic examination of cortical bone.

OSTEOCHONDROSIS

The osteochondroses consist of a heterogeneous group of lesions in growth cartilage of young animals and are characterized by focal or multifocal failure (or delay) of endochondral ossification. As such, osteochondrosis involves the metaphyseal growth plate and the AE complex. The lesions are common and represent an important orthopedic entity that has a number of different clinical manifestations in pigs, dogs, horses, cattle, poultry, and rats. Many investigators have made the point that the term "osteochondrosis," which implies degeneration of cartilage and bone, is inappropriate because the lesions are initially in the cartilage. The hallmark of the uncomplicated gross lesions of osteochondrosis is focal or multifocal retention of growth cartilage due to its failure to become mineralized and replaced by bone (a failure of endochondral ossification).

The cause of osteochondrosis is unknown. The high incidence of osteochondrosis in species bred and fed to achieve maximal body weight at a young age suggests that it might be a mechanical complication superimposed on minor multifocal defects of endochondral ossification that occur normally. Presumably, uneven patterns of endochondral ossification are common, and most go undetected. Only in animals selected for rapid weight gain might these develop into clinically significant lesions. Little evidence is available to indicate that the lesions of osteochondrosis result from a specific nutritional deficiency. However, copper deficiency, perhaps induced by excess dietary zinc, has produced lysis of the AE complex and formation of thin flaps of cartilage in thoroughbred suckling foals. Also, lesions of cartilage retention are less frequent in foals from mares fed increased dietary copper. Osteochondrosis-like lesions have been reported at greater incidence in growing dogs fed high-calcium diets.

Not only are the causes of osteochondrosis unknown, but the nature of the initial lesion in areas of dysplasia is still under debate. Necrosis of cartilage in the epiphysis of the pig, likely secondary to ischemia from physiologic thrombosis of cartilage vessels, might contribute to lesions of osteochondrosis in the AE complex. Studies examining the role of apoptosis in the development of osteochondrosis in poultry have revealed contradictory findings.

Foci of retained cartilage in the physis or AE complex can be unrelated to osteochondrosis and can be secondary to anything that will interfere with vascular invasion of the cartilage, such as infractions (fractures without affecting the external contour of the bone) of the primary trabeculae or inflammation.

The simplest forms of osteochondrosis have been called dysplasias of the physis and AE complex.

Growth plate: Grossly the dysplasia is usually a well-demarcated wedge of white, firm hyaline cartilage at the AE complex or physis (Fig. 16-46). Variations in this gross appearance might reflect stages of resolution or secondary necrosis. Hemorrhage and mineralized debris can occur at the junction of the dysplastic and adjacent bone. Often small dysplastic areas produce no clinical signs. Such dysplasias are common, especially in the distal femurs of pigs; the distal femur, distal tibia, and vertebral articular facets of horses; the proximal humerus of dogs; and the proximal tibia of rapidly

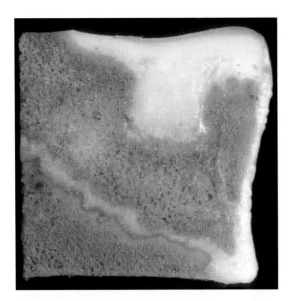

Fig. 16-46   Dysplasia of the articular-epiphyseal complex, bone, distal femur, lateral trochlear ridge, horse. The cartilage extending into the epiphysis is from epiphyseal cartilage that has failed to undergo endochondral ossification and been retained as cartilage, whereas the remainder of the epiphysial cartilage has been converted to bone. *(Courtesy Dr. S.E. Weisbrode, College of Veterinary Medicine, The Ohio State University.)*

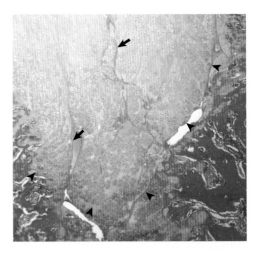

Fig. 16-47   Dysplasia of the articular-epiphyseal complex, bone, distal femur, lateral trochlear ridge, horse. Note the retained cartilage outlined by arrowheads; it has no evidence of vascular invasion. There are numerous eosinophilic streaks (*arrows*), which sometimes contain cavitations. The cause and significance of these streaks and cavities are uncertain. Because the specimen was decalcified for ease of sectioning, it cannot be used to confirm that mineralization is absent. H&E stain. *(Courtesy Dr. S.E. Weisbrode, College of Veterinary Medicine, The Ohio State University.)*

growing birds. Microscopically, these areas are composed of hypertrophic, sometimes poorly aligned chondrocytes without evidence of mineralization or vascular invasion (Fig. 16-47). Particularly in horses, acellular streaks are present within the cartilage. Microscopically, these streaks are eosinophilic due to loss of proteoglycans and condensation of the collagen fibers. Sometimes splitting of the condensed collagen occurs causing fissures within the streaks (Fig. 16-47). These streaks might be sequelae to physiologic necrosis of chondrocytes that can occur when blood vessels that extend across the growth plate undergo normal thrombosis. These streaks are found in normal cartilage, but they can appear exaggerated in some cases of osteochondrosis. Dysplasias can progress, spontaneously resolve by endochondral ossification, or undergo necrosis and cavitation.

Trabecular bone: Immediately subjacent to a dysplastic area, the trabeculae are usually coarse, modeled, and without cartilage cores. Often due to the failure of endochondral ossification, there is some discontinuity between the retained cartilage and the bone; this space is occupied by slight fibrosis. If the dysplastic areas are large and became necrotic, a cystic space filled with serumlike fluid and lined by fibrous tissue can form in the metaphysis.

Cortical bone: Lesions in cortical bone are not expected with dysplasias of osteochondrosis, but dysplasias of the physis can cause angular limb deformities as a result of uneven longitudinal growth. This condition

of angular limb deformity subsequent to lesions in the growth plate or primary trabeculae is sometimes lumped under the term "epiphysitis" in horses. Epiphysitis in horses can be due to true dysplasias of osteochondrosis or can be secondary to trauma or inflammation of the growth plate and/or primary trabeculae.

OSTEOCHONDRITIS DISSECANS

Osteochondritis dissecans (OCD) is the name given to dysplasias at the AE complex that form clefts in the retained cartilage with subsequent fracture of the overlying articular cartilage (Fig. 16-48). The result is a cartilaginous or osteochondral flap, depending on the extent of bone that is associated with the cartilage. Should this flap fracture off and become free in the joint space, it is called a "joint mouse." OCD can be accompanied by pain, joint effusion, and nonspecific secondary lymphoplasmacytic synovitis. Free-floating joint mice occasionally interfere with mechanical movement of the joint. The lesions of OCD develop in various synovial joints, including those of the facets of the vertebral column. Common sites of OCD are the humeral head in the dog, the anterior aspect of the intermediate ridge of the distal tibia in horses, and the medial condyles of the distal femur and distal humerus in pigs. The disease is a significant cause of lameness in young breeding pigs. The articular cartilage defect in OCD might never heal, and such joints are destined to develop some degree of degenerative joint disease.

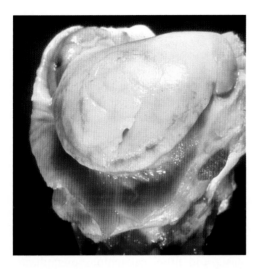

Fig. 16-48   Osteochondritis dissecans (osteochondrosis), bone, articular cartilage, humerus, proximal end, dog. A flap of cartilage with articular-epiphyseal complex dysplasia (not visible from this view of the surface) has detached from the underlying bone. The synovium is hyperemic and hyperplastic. *(Courtesy Dr. S.E. Weisbrode, College of Veterinary Medicine, The Ohio State University.)*

Growth plate: For the development of OCD, clefts must develop in dysplasias at the AE complex (Fig. 16-49). These clefts can be linear and be formed by necrosis of cartilage, possibly induced by pressure or failure of nutrient diffusion, or they may be consequences of eosinophilic streaks as described previously. Cleft formation can cause mechanical instability and lead to separations within cartilage or between cartilage and the underlying bone. Trauma can cause the cleft to extend through the overlying articular cartilage, resulting in the formation of a flap.

Lesions of OCD can develop in horses without predisposing dysplasias (retention of growth cartilage). In these cases, articular cartilage of normal thickness can be peeled from the subjacent bone because of fissuring in the deeper layers of the AE complex. Such lesions have been seen in foals licking fences with zinc-based white paint. The pathogenesis of the lesion is thought to involve copper deficiency induced by the zinc excess. Copper is a required cofactor for enzymes that facilitate cross linkages between tropocollagen molecules, but these foals do not appear to have any generalized

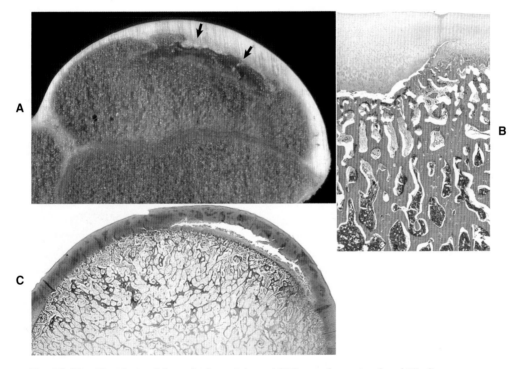

Fig. 16-49   Dysplasia of the articular-epiphyseal (AE) complex, osteochondritis dissecans (osteochondrosis), bone. A, Humerus, pig. The retained cartilage has separated from the subchondral bone (*arrows*) but a fissure has not formed to the articular surface. **B,** AE complex, femur, distal end, horse. A linear fissure between the dysplastic AE complex and underlying (subchondral) bone is extending into adjacent normal (*right*) articular cartilage. H&E stain. **C,** Humerus, horse. Note the fissure within the region of the AE complex. A preexisting dysplasia is not obvious. H&E stain. *(**A** and **B,** Courtesy Dr. S.E. Weisbrode, College of Veterinary Medicine, The Ohio State University. **C,** Courtesy Dr. C. Bridges, College of Veterinary Medicine, Texas A&M University; and Dr. J. King, College of Veterinary Medicine, Cornell University.)*

collagen dysplasia. In addition, a relatively common and often clinically incidental lesion of lysis of the AE complex cartilage without flap formation is seen in articular facets of 1- to 2-year-old horses. In such cases there is coagulation necrosis of the AE complex of inapparent cause and no dysplasia. There is a fissure formed, but the overlying articular cartilage usually does not fracture free to form a flap.

Trabecular bone: Changes in trabecular bone of the epiphysis reflect the extent of the cleft formation and whether the flap detached. Marked fibrosis and formation of reactive woven bone is expected at the base of the flap.

Cortical bone: Lesions in cortical bone are not expected with OCD.

EPIPHYSIOLYSIS

Epiphysiolysis is the separation of the epiphysis from the metaphysis because of fissure formation horizontally through the physis. This is not associated with focal or multifocal dysplasia and because of that is different from the osteochondroses presented previously (other than that seen in foals with zinc toxicity). The condition is most common in pigs and dogs. The femoral head can be involved in market-weight pigs and in young gilts. In young sows, separation of the ischial tuberosity at its growth plate is a common cause of caudal weakness and inability to stand. In dogs, the process of epiphysiolysis can affect the anconeal process of the ulna (ununited anconeal process). Epiphysiolysis is the only form of osteochondrosis found in the cat. In the cat, a diffuse physeal dysplasia with slipped capital femoral epiphysis is described in heavy young adult castrated male cats. The growth plates in these cats appears to remain open longer than expected and might, along with weight, be a predisposing factor for lesion development.

Growth plate: Grossly there is a horizontal fissure/fracture through the physis with complete or partial separation of the epiphysis from the metaphysis. The growth plate may be delayed in closing and have fewer chondrocytes than expected with their arrangement being somewhat disorganized.

Trabecular bone: The response to trabecular bone in epiphysiolysis is that expected from trauma and fracture. There is marrow fibrosis and proliferation of reactive woven bone with variable hemorrhage in the marrow cavity.

Cortical bone: There are no primary changes in cortical bone with this condition, and any lesions that would develop would be secondary to altered mechanical use.

CERVICAL VERTEBRAL MYELOPATHY

Cervical vertebral myelopathy (CVM) is secondary to static or dynamic compression on the spinal cord by abnormal cervical vertebrae. The abnormal vertebrae can cause this compression constantly as a result of an absolute stenosis of the canal or intermittently during movement (usually flexion). It is useful therefore to try to determine clinically if the lesion represents a static compression or dynamic compression. Clinical localization of the lesion by neurologic examination, myelography, or computerized tomography is very helpful to the pathologist. The condition is seen most often in horses and giant breed dogs. In thoroughbred and standard bred horses and in dogs, the static compression is usually due to a grossly appreciable narrowing of the spinal canal from caudal to cranial within a single vertebral body (Fig. 16-50). The pathogenesis of this is not known but is likely developmental. In quarter horses, localized hyperplasia and fibrocartilaginous metaplasia of the ligamentum flavum (the ligament between the dorsal lamina), likely secondary to chronic mechanical irritation and/or trauma, can protrude into the spinal canal and cause static compression of the spinal cord.

The lesions associated with dynamic compression of the cord are more variable and less definitive because often identical lesions can be found in asymptomatic animals. In horses, the most common lesions are those of osteochondrosis (see previous discussion) of the cervical facets. Osteochondrosis can cause abnormal and asymmetric development of the facets or abnormally

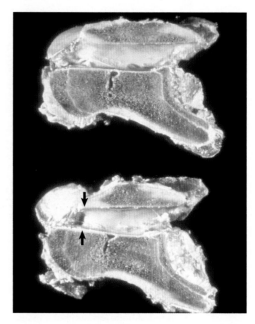

Fig. 16-50 **Static stenosis, bone, cervical vertebra, sagittal section, horse.** Static stenosis (narrowing) of the vertebral canal due to malformation of the vertebra (*bottom vertebra*). Note the smaller diameter of the vertebral canal at the cranial end (*arrows*) of this vertebra. The top vertebra is normal.
(Courtesy College of Veterinary Medicine University of Illinois.)

large cranial epiphyses of the vertebral bodies. With each of these, it is possible that during flexion, the dorsal aspect of the vertebral body compresses the ventral aspect of the cord, causing transient ischemia. Such compression can at first cause functional deficits only without lesions in the spinal cord, but can progress to notable Wallerian degeneration. Horses with clinical signs of dynamic cervical vertebral myelopathy have the same frequency of osteochondrosis in the cervical vertebrae as clinically normal horses, but the severity of the lesions are worse in clinically affected horses. In addition, the diameter of the vertebral canal is smaller in affected horses, suggesting that compression of the cord in these horses would be easier to achieve. The frequency and severity of osteochondrosis lesions in the appendicular skeleton are greater in horses with clinical signs suggesting a systemic condition.

METABOLIC BONE DISEASES

These systemic skeletal diseases are generally of nutritional, endocrine, or toxic origin (Tables 16-1 and 16-2). Structural abnormalities occur in both growing and adult skeletons during normal modeling and remodeling. Metabolic bone diseases are often called osteodystrophies. The term "osteodystrophy" is a general one and implies defective bone formation. The classical metabolic osteodystrophies are osteoporosis, fibrous osteodystrophy, rickets, and osteomalacia. These terms imply specific pathologic changes but do not necessarily imply a specific cause. For example, osteoporosis can be due to a calcium deficiency, glucocorticoid therapy, or physical inactivity. Different osteodystrophies can coexist in the same skeleton. For example, the skeleton of an animal with a severe calcium deficiency accompanied by excess dietary phosphorus might have features of both osteoporosis and fibrous osteodystrophy. In practice, most nutritional deficiencies in domestic animals do not involve a single element; more often, deficiencies are multiple, not severe, and not the "classic" lesions produced under experimental conditions.

OSTEOPOROSIS

Clinically, osteoporosis is the disease of bone pain and fracture secondary to a reduction in bone density or mass (Fig. 16-51). The bone present, although reduced in amount, is normally mineralized. When there is reduced bone mass but no clinical disease, the term *osteopenia* is more appropriate. If the disease progresses and clinical signs appear, the disease is called osteoporosis. Osteopenic bone lacks strength and is more easily fractured. In senile osteoporosis in human beings, in addition to decreased bone density, the turnover rate is reduced, allowing microcracks (small cracks in the

Table **16-1**   **Metabolic Bone Disease**

Disease	Characteristics	Causes
Osteoporosis	Reduced bone mass—porous, thin, and brittle bones	Protein calorie malnutrition, immobilization, dietary calcium deficiency, glucocorticoid excess, menopause in human beings
Osteomalacia (adult animals)	Decreased bone mineralization (accumulation of osteoid)—soft bones	Vitamin D deficiency, phosphorus deficiency
Rickets (growing animals)	Decreased bone mineralization (accumulation of osteoid)—soft bones; thickened growth plates (failure of endochondral ossification)	Vitamin D deficiency, phosphorus deficiency
Fibrous osteodystrophy	Decreased bone mass because of resorption and replacement by fibrous tissue, rubbery bone	Hyperparathyroidism 1. Primary—functional chief cell adenoma of parathyroid gland 2. Paraneoplastic—parathyroid hormonelike-related protein from neoplasia-like adenocarcinoma of apocrine glands of anal sac 3. Secondary nutritional hyperparathyroidism from diets low in calcium and high in phosphorus 4. Secondary renal hyperparathyroidism from failure of the kidney to secrete phosphorus and reduced synthesis of 1,25-dihydroxyvitamin D

Table **16-2** Toxic Osteodystrophies

Principal	Route/Source	Lesions	Mechanism
Vitamin D	Ingestion of plants (e.g., *Solanum malacoxylon*) that contain water-soluble glycosides of the vitamin; ingestion of excess vitamin D added to Feed	Acute high-dose exposure: widespread soft tissue mineralization Chronic lower dose exposure: osteosclerosis with formation of abnormal woven bone matrix with increased basophilia	Acute high dose: increased absorption of calcium from intestines and increased release by osteoclasts from bone Chronic lower dose: suppression of bone resorption by hypercalcemia, which suppresses parathyroid hormone and increases calcitonin secretion Vitamin D also likely has direct stimulatory effect on osteoblasts
Vitamin A	Ingestion of excessive retinoids (not carotenoids) as found in certain plants (sweet potatoes) and meat (liver) or drug toxicity	Growing animals: multifocal premature closures of growth plates with subsequent growth deformity, osteoporosis, and pathologic fractures Adult animals: osteosclerosis, periosteal bone formation, and exostoses	Retinoids cause degeneration and necrosis of chondrocytes and osteoblasts in growing animals and paradoxically are stimulatory to osteoblasts in adult animals
Lead	Ingestion usually from licking lead-based paint	Characteristic lesion is a "lead line," an osteosclerotic band of bone parallel to the growth plate; osteoclasts can have acid-fast lead inclusions; osteoporosis also can be present, but likely secondary to systemic illness of lead toxicity	Lead is stored in bone mineral; part of the sclerosis seen radiographically is a result of the radiodensity of the lead; lead is toxic to osteoclasts; bone mineral with lead is somewhat resistant to osteoclasis
Fluoride	Ingestion of rock phosphates naturally high in fluoride; grazing on pastures with naturally high fluoride soil content or contaminated with fluoride as industrial by product; drinking water with naturally high fluoride content	Chronic low toxic levels cause osteosclerosis; chronic higher toxic levels cause osteopenia and periosteal bone formation	At lower toxic levels fluoride is stimulatory to osteoblasts and its incorporation in the hydroxyapatite make the crystal more resistant to resorption At higher toxic levels the mechanisms are uncertain, but direct toxic injury to osteoblasts is possible, resulting in osteopenia with the periosteal proliferation; begins a reaction to support the mechanically weakened skeleton

bone visible only microscopically) to accumulate. These microcracks superimposed on the reduced bone mass make bones more brittle than would be predicted from the reduced mass alone. In growing animals, osteoporosis is potentially reversible. In adults, however, once trabecular bone is lost, it is very slow to be replaced physiologically. For some locations, such as the femoral neck, trabecular bone contributes much to the bone's strength. In the femoral diaphysis, it is the thickness and density of the cortex that determine strength.

Some of the causes of osteopenia include calcium deficiency, starvation, physical inactivity, and the administration of glucocorticoids. A calcium deficiency can result in hypocalcemia, which is compensated for by increased PTH output and increased bone resorption. It is not clear why calcium deficiency does not result in fibrous osteodystrophy, as described later. Starvation and malnutrition can result in arrested growth and osteoporosis, largely because of reduced bone formation because of deficiencies of protein and mineral.

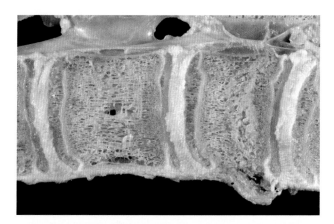

Fig. 16-51   **Osteoporosis, bone, lumbar vertebrae, median section, horse.** Note the markedly thin cortices, particularly the dorsal ones. The thickness of trabeculae has been reduced, but this is difficult to appreciate. The vertebra to the right has a compression fracture, seen as collapsing of the trabeculae into each other, shortening of the length of the body between the growth plates and buckling of the ventral cortex. The marrow has been flushed from the specimen for purposes of illustration of the bone changes. *(Courtesy Dr. S.E. Weisbrode, College of Veterinary Medicine, The Ohio State University.)*

Reduced physical activity (disuse or immobilization osteoporosis) causes increased bone resorption and decreased bone formation. This disuse loss of bone might be mediated through changes in piezoelectrical activity, streaming potentials, and stretch receptors that are able to detect decreased mechanical use of the skeleton. Loss of bone mass associated with long-term paralysis or immobilization is not necessarily progressive; rather, the skeleton stabilizes at a new (reduced) level. Postmenopausal osteoporosis is a common and important disease in women; it often results in vertebral deformity or collapse and pathologic fractures of the femoral neck. Declining concentrations of estrogens, physical inactivity, reduced muscle tone, and inadequate calcium intake are factors that can be responsible for causing osteopenia to progress to osteoporosis. Estrogen generally potentiates bone formation and inhibits bone resorption, likely by altering cytokine production from osteoblasts and monocytes. Estrogens promote secretion of TGF-β (an anabolic cytokine) and decrease production of IL-1, IL-6, and TNF-α (cytokines that promote osteoclasis). The loss of estrogen in menopause will have the opposite effect. IL-6 knockout mice do not get osteopenia following ovariohysterectomy, confirming the critical role of cytokines in this process. Interestingly, ovariohysterectomy in the bitch is not associated with clinical osteoporosis. In experimental studies, a transient osteopenia has been found in ovariectomized dogs; these studies confirm years of veterinary clinical observations that spayed dogs are not at risk to develop osteoporosis. Osteopenia associated with reduced estrogens

from ovarian atrophy or ovariectomy appears to be greatest in animals with estrous cycles that extend throughout the year (e.g., rat, pig, and primate).

Growth plate: Lesions in the growth plate are not expected in osteoporosis unless the disease is related to pituitary dysfunction or protein calorie malnutrition, in which the plate would be thin.

Trabecular bone: Trabeculae become thinner, become fewer in number, and develop perforations within the plates. With time the normal structure of trabecular bone (anastomosing plates) is replaced by strut or rodlike bone. The loss of these anastomoses results in reduced ability of the trabeculae to withstand stress. In most long bones of adults, trabeculae extend from the epiphysis to the metaphyseal-diaphyseal junction. The degree to which the trabeculae do not reach this distance suggests the extent of the osteopenia (Fig. 16-52, A).

Cortical bone: Cortical bone becomes thin because of osteoclastic resorption on the endosteal surface with corresponding enlargement of the medullary cavity. The cortex becomes porous because of increased resorption within the cortical vascular spaces and Haversian systems and/or decreased osteoblastic activity (Fig. 16-52, B). In severe cases, cortices become brittle, and the force required to break them is notably reduced.

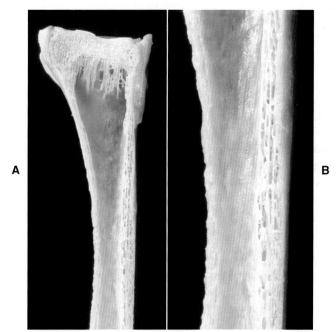

A   B

Fig. 16-52   **Osteopenia, bone, metatarsal, sheep. A,** There is marked reduction in the number and length of trabeculae. **B,** The cranial cortex (*right*) is markedly porous, and the caudal cortex (*left*) is thin. The marrow has been flushed from the specimen for purposes of illustration of the bone changes. *(A and B, Courtesy Dr. S.E. Weisbrode, College of Veterinary Medicine, The Ohio State University.)*

RICKETS AND OSTEOMALACIA

Failure of mineralization with subsequent bone deformities and fractures is called rickets in the growing skeleton and osteomalacia (soft bone) in the adult. In the immature animal, rickets is a disease of bone and cartilage undergoing endochondral ossification. In the adult, osteomalacia is a disease only of bone. Clinically, affected animals have bone pain, pathologic fractures, and deformities such as kyphosis and scoliosis.

The most common causes of rickets and osteomalacia are deficiency of vitamin D or phosphorus. However, failure of mineralization and rickets and/or osteomalacia can occur in chronic renal disease and in chronic fluorosis. Dietary phosphorus deficiency is not common but can occur in herbivores grazing on phosphorus-deficient pastures. Phosphorus-deficient animals often have reduced feed intake, are unthrifty, and have impaired reproductive performance. Vitamin D deficiency is rare today because this vitamin is commonly added to commercial feed, and animals exposed to adequate sunlight should be able to synthesize their own if they have normal kidneys. It is not clear why phosphorus deficiency and vitamin D deficiency cause osteomalacia and calcium deficiency does not. An observation to further complicate the issue is that knockout mice with no receptors for vitamin D get rickets, but this can be corrected by feeding a high-calcium diet. Apparently, in the distal small intestine, calcium absorption is passive and not vitamin D dependent. This suggests that vitamin D deficiency causes rickets as a result of reduced intestinal absorption of calcium and adds to the confusion over why dietary calcium deficiency does not result in rickets. Species variation is important in this matter. In fact, birds will get ricketslike lesions with calcium deficiency, but this is not the case with mammals.

Growth plate: The growth plates in rickets are thickened because of failure of mineralization (Fig. 16-53). The costal-chondral junctions can be prominent and nodular, and historically the lesion has been called "rachitic rosary" because of its resemblance to a string of prayer beads. This thickening is apparent grossly as retained cartilage. Microscopically the columns of chondrocytes in the plate are disorganized. In mammals, there is a marked increase in the number of chondrocytes in the zone of proliferation compared with normal. This is presumably due to the inability of these proliferating chondrocytes to mature. It is uncertain if the disorganization of chondrocytes in vitamin D-deficiency rickets is due to a primary effect of vitamin D metabolites (specifically, 24,25-dihydroxyvitamin D) or a mechanical consequence of the failure of endochondral ossification. Because of the inadequate absorption of calcium in rickets, the growth plate does not undergo mineralization. In mammals, when mineralization of the cartilage matrix does not occur, blood vessels with accompanying

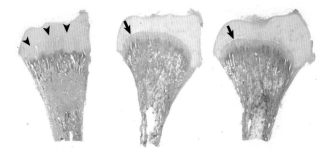

Fig. 16-53   Vitamin D deficiency (experimental), bone, tibia, chicken. Left specimen—rachitic tibia; middle and right specimens—normal chicken and a chicken fed a vitamin D deficient diet supplemented with calcitriol. The latter two specimens appear normal and are indistinguishable from each other. In these normal-appearing bones, notice the tapering of the metaphysis ("cutback" zone) and the thickness of the growth plate. In these normal chickens, the cleft (*arrows*) separating the growth plate from the epiphyseal cartilage is an artifact. There is no ossification center present in the epiphysis, which is normal for young broilers. The growth plate in the rachitic bird is thickened. The arrowheads indicates the junction between the growth plate and the epiphyseal cartilage. The metaphysis has not undergone modeling ("cutback"). H&E stain. *(Courtesy Dr. L. Nagode).*

chondroclasts do not invade the physis. Because the ability of the chondrocytes to proliferate and hypertrophy is at least partially retained in rickets, the growth plate thickens because the rate of its removal by endochondral ossification is reduced.

Trabecular bone: Grossly and radiographically the metaphyses are "flared" in rickets because of failure of bone and cartilage removal in the cutback zones (Fig. 16-53). Poorly mineralized matrixes cannot be resorbed because osteoclasts cannot bind to an unmineralized matrix (see previous discussion). Microscopically the surfaces of trabecular bone in rickets and osteomalacia have excessive amounts of osteoid (unmineralized matrix) (Fig. 16-54). Osteoclasts are not able to adhere to, or resorb, osteoid. Therefore bone modeling and remodeling is impaired. Hypocalcemia can develop in a vitamin D deficiency, and lesions of secondary hyperparathyroidism (fibrous osteodystrophy [see later discussion]) also can develop.

Cortical bone: Grossly cortical bone can be of normal appearance or the softened bone can be deformed by weight bearing. In severe cases, the bones are so soft that they can be cut with a knife. Microscopically, endocortical and trabecular surfaces in the cortex can have numerous wide seams of unmineralized osteoid. Osteomalacic bone is susceptible to accumulation of microcracks because of the impaired remodeling and modeling secondary to osteoid surfaces interfering with osteoclasis.

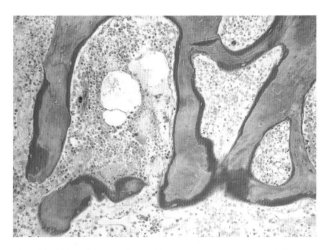

Fig. 16-54   Osteomalacia, bone, cross section, metaphysis, trabeculae, human being. This person had osteomalacia secondary to malabsorption of fat soluble vitamins (including vitamin D) associated with gastrectomy. This section was not demineralized and was stained to show the difference between osteoid (*red*) and fully mineralized bone (*blue-green*). Normally no more than 10% of trabecular surfaces should be covered by osteoid seams, but in this case almost all surfaces are covered by osteoid. Goldner's trichrome stain. (*Courtesy Dr. S.E. Weisbrode, College of Veterinary Medicine, The Ohio State University.*)

FIBROUS OSTEODYSTROPHY

Fibrous osteodystrophy is the name given to the skeletal lesions of increased widespread osteoclastic resorption of bone and replacement by fibrous tissue because of primary, secondary, and pseudohyperparathyroidism. Weakening of bones leads to lameness, pathologic fractures, and deformities. As described previously, osteoblasts—but not osteoclasts—have receptors for parathyroid hormone and respond by up-regulating production of osteoclast differentiation factor and down-regulating secretion of osteoprotegerin. Bone marrow stromal cells also have receptors for parathyroid hormone, and when the hormone is expressed constantly at high levels, these cells differentiate into fibroblasts. Paradoxically, intermittent doses of parathyroid hormone have the opposite effect on bone. Daily injections of parathyroid hormone is, as of this writing, the most potent inducer of new bone formation in women with advanced stages of postmenopausal osteoporosis.

In domestic animals, primary hyperparathyroidism, as in cases of functional parathyroid adenoma, parathyroid carcinoma, or idiopathic bilateral parathyroid hyperplasia, is rare. Secondary hyperparathyroidism is more common and can be either nutritional or renal in origin (nutritional or renal fibrous osteodystrophy). Nutritional hyperparathyroidism is caused by dietary factors that tend to decrease the concentration of serum ionized calcium, to which the parathyroid glands respond by increasing output of PTH. It is most common in young, growing animals that are fed rations deficient in calcium and have a relative excess of phosphorus. Unsupplemented cereal grain rations fed to pigs, all-meat diets fed to dogs and cats, and bran fed to horses are examples of low-calcium, high-phosphorus diets that can cause secondary nutritional hyperparathyroidism and eventually fibrous osteodystrophy. Increased concentrations of dietary phosphorus are important in the evolution of fibrous osteodystrophy, perhaps by interfering with the intestinal absorption of calcium.

Growth plate: No primary lesions are expected in the growth plate or AE complex.

Trabecular bone: Trabeculae are thinned by osteoclastic resorption. Osteoblastic proliferation can be marked but ineffectual in that they produce little osteoid. Proliferation of fibrous tissue in the marrow space is usually marked but in early stages can be subtle and consist of only two or three layers of cells between the bone lining cells and the marrow space (Fig. 16-55). In severe cases, the marrow cavity is obliterated by fibrous tissue.

Cortical bone: Bone resorption and replacement by fibrous tissue can be so extensive that the bone becomes pliable (Fig. 16-56). Clinically and at postmortem examination, in severe cases bones can be bent at a right angle without fracture. Osteoclastic resorption begins on the endocortical bone surface, but any vascular spaces within the wall of the bone can undergo marked enlargement by osteoclastic resorption and replacement by fibrous tissue. In advanced disease, entire cortices can be replaced by reactive woven bone and fibrous tissue. Sometimes the proliferation of fibrous tissue is exuberant and associated with increased external dimension of the bone (Fig. 16-57). This process is

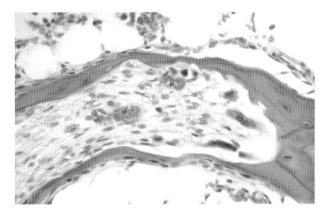

Fig. 16-55   Tunneling resorption (within a trabecula), fibrous osteodystrophy, bone, longitudinal section, dog. Osteoclasts (*right*) have resorbed the central portion of the trabecula, and this space is being replaced by fibrous tissue rather than bone, as in normal remodeling. H&E stain. (*Courtesy Dr. S.E. Weisbrode, College of Veterinary Medicine, The Ohio State University.*)

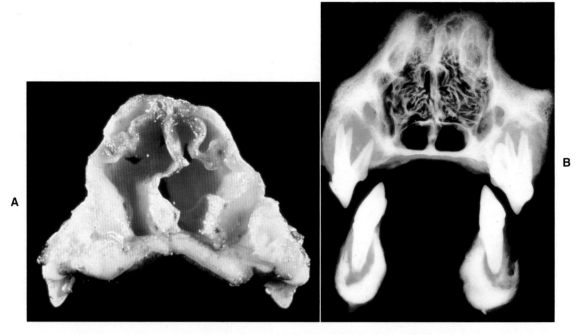

Fig. 16-56   Fibrous osteodystrophy, bone, maxillae and mandible, transverse section, dogs.
A, The pliable nature of the bone can be seen by the collapsed and folded (not fractured)
appearance of the nasal septum and maxilla. **B,** Radiograph. There is marked loss of bone density
around the teeth in both maxillae and mandibles. These changes are detectable only by radiographic
examination. (**A** and **B**, Courtesy Dr. S.E. Weisbrode, College of Veterinary Medicine, The Ohio State University.)

more common in the maxilla and mandible and might reflect the response of the weakened bone to the intense mechanical stress of mastication.

RENAL FIBROUS OSTEODYSTROPHY

Renal fibrous osteodystrophy is a general term that refers to the skeletal lesions that develop secondary to chronic, severe renal disease. Osteomalacia and fibrous osteodystrophy can occur as separate diseases or in combination as a result of chronic renal disease in human beings. Fibrous osteodystrophy, which is sometimes complicated by osteomalacia, occurs in the dog, the animal most commonly affected with renal osteodystrophy. Dogs can have bone pain (lameness) and loss of teeth and deformity of the maxilla or mandible because of the osteoclastic resorption of bone and replacement by fibrous tissue. The pathogenesis of renal osteodystrophy is complex and likely varies depending on the extent and nature of the renal disease and the availability of dietary vitamin D. Loss of glomerular function, inability to excrete phosphate, inadequate production of 1,25-dihydroxyvitamin D by the kidneys, and acidosis are central to the development of renal osteodystrophy. Phosphate retention because of decreased renal excretion leads to hyperphosphatemia. As the calcium and phosphorus product exceeds solubility, calcium is precipitated in soft tissue resulting in hypocalcemia.

This hypocalcemia stimulates PTH output with subsequent fibrous osteodystrophy. The reduced production of 1,25-dihydroxyvitamin D by the diseased kidneys together with impaired mineralization because of the acidosis of uremia explain the development of osteomalacia.

INFLAMMATION OF BONE
INFECTIOUS INFLAMMATION OF BONE

Inflammation of bone is called osteitis, periostitis if the periosteum is involved, and osteomyelitis if the medullary cavity of the bone is involved (Table 16-3). These can be common and sometimes life threatening and require early diagnosis and vigorous treatment. Osteomyelitis is often a chronic, disfiguring process caused by necrosis and removal of bone and by the compensatory production of new bone; the two processes often proceed simultaneously over a prolonged period. Osteitis is often a painful process leading to debilitation of the affected animal. Infectious inflammation of bone in animals is usually caused by bacteria, although viral, fungal, and protozoal agents can be involved. Hematogenous bacterial osteomyelitis is uncommon in dogs and cats, but it is common in neonatal animals used for food and fiber production and foals. A wide range of gram-positive and gram-negative bacteria is responsible

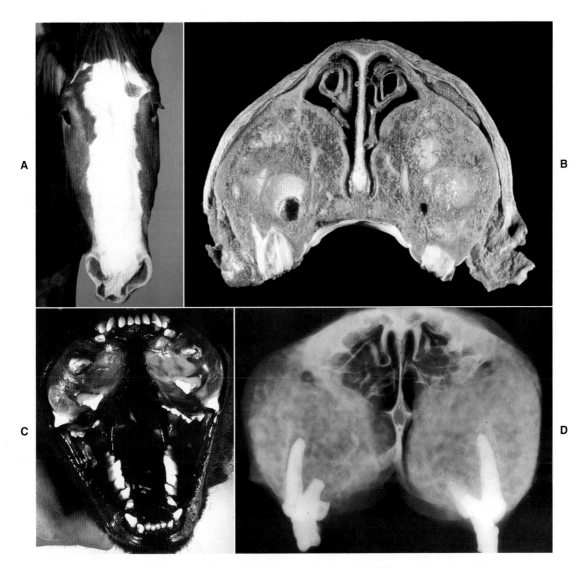

Fig. 16-57   Fibrous osteodystrophy, bone, maxillae and mandibles. A, Nutritional fibrous osteodystrophy, horse. Note the swelling of the facial crest. **B,** Maxillae, transverse section, horse. Proliferating and poorly organized fibroosseous tissue in the maxillae has distorted and extended their contours laterally and compressed the nasal cavity medially. Note the absence of normal bone. **C,** Renal fibrous osteodystrophy, dog. Exuberant poorly mineralized woven bone and fibrous tissue has caused the maxillary bones to expand and distort the positioning of the teeth. Similar changes affect the mandible, and its teeth are also malpositioned. **D,** Radiograph, renal fibrous osteodystrophy, dog. Postmortem transverse slab section demonstrating the reduced bone density (radiodensity) of the proliferated woven bone and fibrous tissue that has replaced the preexisting maxillary bones. Note the absence of normal radiodense bone. (*A* and *D,* Courtesy Dr. S.E. Weisbrode, College of Veterinary Medicine, The Ohio State University. **B,** Courtesy Dr. W. Crowell, College of Veterinary Medicine, The University of Georgia; and Noah's Arkive, College of Veterinary Medicine, The University of Georgia. **C,** Courtesy Department of Veterinary Biosciences, The Ohio State University; and Noah's Arkive, College of Veterinary Medicine, The University of Georgia.)

for hematogenous osteomyelitis in calves and foals. *Arcanobacterium pyogenes* and other pyogenic bacteria (e.g., *Streptococcus* spp., *Staphylococcus* spp.) and *Salmonella* spp., *Escherichia coli*, and other coliforms are among the most common microbes that cause hematogenous osteomyelitis. *Staphylococcus intermedius* is the most common cause of hematogenous osteomyelitis in the dog.

Fungi and viruses also can cause disease in bone. Mycotic agents such as *Coccidioides immitis* and *Blastomyces dermatitidis* are frequently spread hematogenously to bone to produce granulomatous or pyogranulomatous osteomyelitis, with bone lysis and irregular new bone formation. Various viral agents also localize in bone. The viruses of hog cholera and infectious canine

Table **16-3**   Lesions of Inflammatory Joint Disease

	Synovial Fluid	Location Synovial Membrane	Articular Cartilage
TIME/EXUDATE			
Acute suppurative	Reduced viscosity Neutrophils	Hyperemia Edema	No lesions
Subacute suppurative	Reduced viscosity Neutrophils	Hyperplasia Lymphoplasmacytic Inflammation	Usually no lesions
Chronic suppurative	Reduced viscosity Neutrophils	Hyperplasia Lymphoplasmacytic inflammation Fibrosis	Erosion Ulceration
Acute fibrinous	Reduced viscosity Fibrin	Hyperemia Edema	No lesions
Subacute fibrinous	Reduced viscosity Fibrin	Hyperplasia Lymphoplasmacytic Inflammation	Usually no lesions
Chronic fibrinous	Reduced viscosity Fibrin	Hyperemia Lymphoplasmacytic Fibrin Pannus	Erosion Ulceration Pannus

hepatitis can cause endothelial damage, resulting in metaphyseal hemorrhage and necrosis, and acute inflammation. Osseous localization of the distemper virus injures osteoclasts, disrupting metaphyseal modeling and producing a growth retardation lattice as described earlier. A variant of the feline leukemia virus has been associated with myelosclerosis (increased density of medullary bone) in cats. These latter two viruses do not cause an inflammation of bone.

Growth plate: Epiphyseal cartilage (Fig. 16-58) (cartilage of the epiphysis that has yet to undergo endochondral ossification) and physeal cartilage can be eroded by invasion of inflammation from adjacent bone or direct bacterial embolization in the blind-loop vessels at sites of endochondral ossification (see portals of entry section). In contrast to cartilage lysis, it is possible for growth cartilage to appear thickened, secondary to osteomyelitis caused by disruption of endochondral ossification by the inflammatory process and failure to replace cartilage with bone. In growing animals, articular cartilage can be lysed by extension of osteomyelitis from the subjacent AE complex, so what appears to be a primary arthritis actually began in the underlying epiphysis.

Trabecular bone: The composition of the exudates in metaphyseal osteomyelitis is determined by the infectious agent, but in bacterial infection in domestic animals it is typically purulent. Exudate in the medullary cavity increases the intramedullary pressure and can cause compression of vessels resulting in thrombosis and infarction of intramedullary fat, hematopoietic marrow, and bone. Thrombosis of vessels and local tissue infarction are important in the evolution of

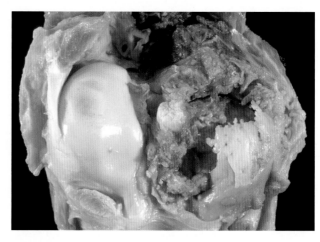

Fig. 16-58   **Emboli (suppurative) epiphysitis, bone, femur, distal end, foal.** Bacterial emboli in the articular-epiphyseal complex have produced suppurative inflammation that has destroyed both the subchondral bone and overlying articular cartilage of the condyle (**right**). (Courtesy Dr. S.E. Weisbrode, College of Veterinary Medicine, The Ohio State University.)

bacterial osteomyelitis. In areas of inflammation, bone resorption is mediated mostly by osteoclasts stimulated by prostaglandins and cytokines released by local tissue and inflammatory cells. Reduced blood flow through large vessels also promotes osteoclastic bone resorption, possibly by altering electrostatic charges in bone. In addition, proteolytic enzymes released by inflammatory cells and activation of matrix metalloproteinases

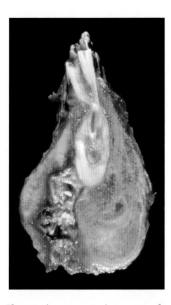

Fig. 16-59   Chronic (suppurative) osteomyelitis, bone, mandible, transverse section, sheep. Chronic suppurative osteomyelitis has caused a fistulous tract that penetrates through the full dorso-ventral thickness of the mandible. This lesion likely began as a periodontal bacterial infection. The ventral progression of the lesion reflects the effects of gravity on the exudate. *(Courtesy Dr. S.E. Weisbrode, College of Veterinary Medicine, The Ohio State University.)*

by the acid environment of inflammation assist in resorbing matrix. Lack of drainage and persistence of the offending agent in areas of necrotic bone account for the chronicity of the process. Bacteria can persist for years in cavities and areas of necrosis in bone. Inflammation in the medullary cavity can penetrate into and through cortical bone and undermine the periosteum, where it can further disrupt the blood supply to the bone at the nutrient foramen and nutrient canal.

Cortical bone: The lesions in cortical bone with infectious osteomyelitis can vary with the route of entry of the organism and the nature of the exudates (Fig. 16-59). With suppurative inflammation, bone lysis is expected. The lysis would be subperiosteal for bacteria induced traumatically by way of the periosteum and endosteal in cases of embolic osteomyelitis. Lysis within the cortex begins within existing vascular channels and can occur with either route of entry. Periostitis can develop by direct inoculation from trauma (e.g., puncture wounds) or by centripetal spread from the marrow cavity and through the cortex. Chronic bacterial periostitis is characterized by multiple spreading pockets of exudates and areas of irregular periosteal new bone formation and cortical lysis (Fig. 16-60). Additional sequelae of osteomyelitis include extension of inflammation to adjacent bone, hematogenous spread to other bones and soft tissue, pathologic fractures, and development of sinus tracts that penetrate cortical bone and drain to the exterior. Occasionally, fragments of dead bone become isolated from their blood supply and surrounded by a pool of

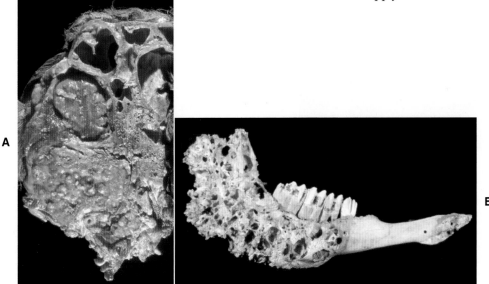

Fig. 16-60   Chronic pyogranulomatous osteomyelitis and sinusitis, actinomycosis (*Actinomyces bovis*), maxillary sinus, cow. A, Transverse section of the maxillae. The nodules apparent within the masses in the sinuses and maxilla represent pockets of pyogranulomatous inflammation that are surrounded by fibrous tissue and woven bone. **B,** Macerated and bleached specimen of the mandible. Note the spicules of woven bone radiating from the mandible. Within the spaces formed by this reactive bone were nodules of pyogranulomatous inflammation and colonies of *Actinomyces bovis*. (**A** *and* **B,** *Courtesy Dr. S.E. Weisbrode, College of Veterinary Medicine, The Ohio State University.*)

exudates (bone sequestrum). Sequestra can form when bone fragments are contaminated at the site of a compound fracture, when the fragments at a fracture site become infected hematogenously, or when fragments of necrotic bone become isolated and thus avascular in osteomyelitis (Fig. 16-61). These isolated fragments of bone (sequestra) and associated exudates can become surrounded by a dense collar of reactive bone (the involucrum). Extracellular matrix is not living tissue. With the death of the cells in the bone and marrow space, there is no way for the bone matrix to be resorbed from within bone (matrix devoid of cells will not liquefy). Therefore relatively large sequestra can persist for long periods and interfere with repair. They often become pale and chalky and lack the glistening appearance of normal bone.

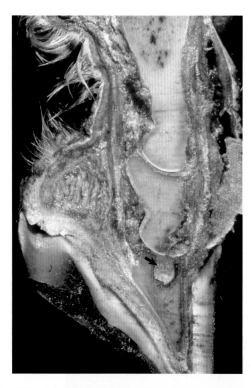

Fig. 16-61   Suppurative periostitis and osteomyelitis, phalanges, horse. Trauma to the dorsal aspect of the hoof inoculated bacteria into the subcutis, causing suppurative cellulitis and periostitis and, subsequently, cortical osteolysis of the dorsal aspect of the distal first phalanx and the entire dorsal surface of the second phalanx. From there, the infection spread to the distal interphalangeal joint and then to the third phalanx, where it caused suppurative osteomyelitis, loss of articular cartilage, and formation of a sequestrum in the proximal portion of the third phalanx (*arrow*). The viable tissue immediately adjacent to the sequestrum is not different from that further away, implying that in this case an involucrum (reactive bone surrounding the exudate around a sequetrum) was not formed. *(Courtesy Dr. S.E. Weisbrode, College of Veterinary Medicine, The Ohio State University.)*

NONINFECTIOUS INFLAMMATION OF BONE
HYPERTROPHIC OSTEODYSTROPHY

Also termed metaphyseal osteopathy, hypertrophic osteodystrophy is a disease of young, growing dogs of the large and giant breeds. These names are unfortunate because they are misleading. The initial lesions are those of a suppurative and fibrinous osteomyelitis of the trabecular bone of the metaphysis. The cause and pathogenesis are unknown; infectious agents have not been isolated. There have been reports of hypertrophic osteopathy in litters of Weimaraners, in which granulocytopathies have been suspected, and in littermates of Irish setters, in which canine leukocyte adhesion deficiency was confirmed. This would suggest infectious agents in that these dogs are susceptible to infections, but the cause of the bone lesions was not determined in these reports. Clinically, hypertrophic osteopathy is characterized by lameness, fever, and swollen, painful metaphyses in multiple long bones.

Growth plate: Lesions in the growth plate are not expected in hypertrophic osteopathy.

Trabecular bone: Lesions are usually bilaterally symmetric. Radiographically, metaphyseal zones of increased lucency and increased density are adjacent and parallel to the physes (Fig. 16-62, A and B). Microscopically the lucent areas represent suppurative and fibrinous inflammation and necrosis of the metaphyseal marrow and bone (Fig. 16-62, C). The death of osteoblasts results in primary trabeculae that are not reinforced by apposition of bone matrix. These trabeculae collapse and fracture without external distortion of the bone (infractions) and appear radiographically as relatively dense regions.

Cortical bone: The inflammation can extend from the medulla through the cutback zone into the periosteum. This periosteal inflammation, along with mechanical instability due to the metaphyseal infractions can cause notable new metaphyseal periosteal bone formation in chronic cases.

EOSINOPHILIC PANOSTEITIS

Eosinophilic panosteitis is another canine bone disease with an unfortunate name. The lesion is neither inflammatory nor eosinophilic. The cause is not known, and the disease is almost always self-limiting. It occurs in growing (usually large-breed) dogs and is painful. Morphologic studies are few because the disease is easily recognized clinically and resolves spontaneously so that biopsy evaluation is rarely necessary. Radiographically the lesions are recognized as increased densities in the medullary cavity in the diaphysis, usually beginning near the nutrient foramen. Increased densities can also be present in the periosteum. These densities are due to proliferation of well-differentiated woven bone and

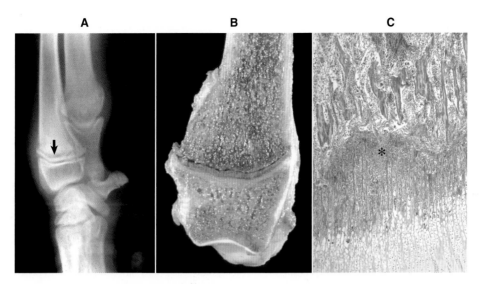

Fig. 16-62   Hypertrophic osteodystrophy, bone, distal radius, dog. A, Radiograph. The radiolucent line (*arrow*), parallel with the level of the primary trabeculae, is characteristic of hypertrophic osteopathy. **B,** Grossly, this line appears to be a fracture within the metaphysis, parallel with the growth plate. The zone of primary trabeculae is more visible in the radiograph than in this gross specimen. **C,** Histologically, this line is a hypercellular band (*) of neutrophils between the primary and secondary trabeculae. (**A, B,** and **C,** *Courtesy Dr. S.E. Weisbrode, College of Veterinary Medicine, The Ohio State University.*)

fibrous tissue. No inflammation is present. The cause of the lameness is presumed to be pressure on nerves by the proliferating woven bone both within the medullary cavity and on the periosteum.

ASEPTIC NECROSIS OF BONE

Aseptic necrosis of bone in human beings occurs in a variety of clinical conditions, including occlusive vascular disease (bone infarction), hyperadrenocorticism, fat embolism, nitrogenous embolism, sickle cell anemia, and intramedullary neoplasms, all of which likely result in arterial or venous infarction of the bone (Table 16-4). In domestic animals, aseptic necrosis of bone has been associated with intramedullary neoplasms and various nonneoplastic lesions. Decreased venous outflow from the bone and increased bone marrow pressure are important factors in the pathogenesis of ischemic or aseptic necrosis of bone. The gross appearance of necrotic bone varies with its extent and the response to it. Microscopically the hallmark of bone necrosis is cell death and loss of osteocytes from their lacunae.

Following an episode of ischemia leading to infarction, the cellular elements of the marrow lose their differential staining, and circular spaces (pooled lipid) develop within a few days. If the region of dead bone remains avascular, the coagulated tissue and mineralized matrix can persist for some time. Dead osteocytes

elicit little reaction; their nuclei become pyknotic, but their disappearance from lacunae is slow and might not be complete for 2 to 4 weeks.

Reaction to and repair of necrotic bone requires revascularization that is associated with infiltration of macrophages and invasion by fibrous tissue that advances from the margins of the lesion. The bone marrow might eventually regenerate entirely, or a scar might form and remain. The necrotic matrix remains fully mineralized and might even "hypermineralize" because of calcification of the dead osteocytes and their lacunae. This mineralization is only possible if there is vascularization that brings additional calcium to the region. Dead bone is slowly removed by osteoclasts. The resorption of necrotic bone with simultaneous replacement by new bone is termed "creeping substitution." The process is slow and often incomplete. Small areas of bone necrosis might not be detected clinically or radiographically.

Growth plate: Ischemic necrosis of metaphyseal bone and bone marrow can result in retained growth cartilage. The metaphyseal necrosis would not affect the zones of proliferating and hypertrophying chondrocytes, and the physeal thickness would increase because its removal by endochondral ossification would be impaired. Ischemic necrosis of the epiphysis could result in premature closure of the growth plate because of death of the proliferating chondrocytes, which are dependent on the epiphyseal blood vessels. Endochondral ossification

Table **16-4** Necrosis of Bone

Cause/Duration of Necrosis	Lesion	Clinical Significance
Acute aseptic (ischemic) necrosis	Death of bone cells and marrow; bone structure intact	Can be clinically silent
Chronic aseptic (ischemic) necrosis	1. If no revascularization, dead bone can remain intact structurally for a long time but will accumulate microcracks 2. If revascularization takes place, dead bone can be resorbed slowly and replaced by new bone 3. If revascularization takes place, dead bone may be resorbed slowly and NOT be replaced by bone but by fibrous tissue	1. Can remain clinically silent, but risk of microcrack progressing to complete clinical fracture increases with time and mechanical use 2. Can remain clinically silent from initiation of lesion to completion of repair 3. Can cause structural failure and collapse of the bone (e.g., chronic idiopathic necrosis of the femoral head)
Acute septic necrosis	Exudate, usually suppurative, will form at junction of dead bone and viable tissue with subsequent bone lysis and reactive bone formation	Pain due to cytokines from the inflammation and pressure in marrow cavity and periosteum
Chronic septic necrosis	1. If the focus of dead bone is relatively small, it can be completely resorbed by the inflammatory process and osteoclastic bone lysis; there can be marked modeling of bone, usually with resorption predominating and replacement by fibrous tissue; in some cases excess formation can occur 2. If the focus of dead bone is relatively large, it can be sequestered (sequestrum) by a peripheral wall of reactive fibrous tissue or reactive bone (involucrum)	Pain due to cytokines and pressure in marrow cavity and periosteum; draining tracts can form; strength of the bone can be weakened because of resorption or its function can be affected by exuberant formation

would continue normally if the metaphyseal blood supply is not affected, and the plate would close because of failure to replenish new chondrocytes.

Trabecular bone: In the femoral heads of young, small, and miniature breed dogs, aseptic necrosis of the femoral head is associated with clinical signs because of the collapse of the articular cartilage as a result of resorption of the necrotic subchondral bone (Legg-Calvé-Perthes disease) that occurs late in the course of the disease. Apparently the initial infarction is asymptomatic (Fig. 16-63). The cause of the infarction is usually not determined but might be caused by venous compression or increased pressure within the articular cavity. This pressure can result in increased intraosseous pressure and bone necrosis. In clinical cases of aseptic necrosis, the dead bone is not replaced by creeping substitution but is ultimately resorbed and replaced by fibrous tissue. The fibrous tissue does not provide adequate support for the articular cartilage, and the femoral head collapses. In stages before complete resorption, it is common in revascularized necrotic medullary bone, for reactive new bone to be deposited on trabeculae of necrotic bone (Fig. 16-64). This sandwich of

central dead bone covered by viable reactive woven bone can persist for months and give (along with osteocyte mineralization described previously) the affected region a radiodense appearance. Ultimately in clinical cases of aseptic necrosis of the femoral head, even these foci of new bone formed on top of dead bone are resorbed and replaced by fibrous tissue. Although the long-term use of steroids in human beings has been associated with necrosis of the femoral head in adults, steroids do not appear to induce osteonecrosis in domestic animals.

Cortical bone: Large areas of necrotic cortical bone have a dry, chalky appearance; the periosteum can be removed easily; and they can remain for years and be subclinical. The formation of sequestra almost always requires inflammation. Sequestra formation in sterile necrosis of bone is unlikely.

PROLIFERATIVE AND NEOPLASTIC LESIONS

Surprisingly, bone, as a tissue, offers little resistance to an expanding or invading neoplasm, and many skeletal

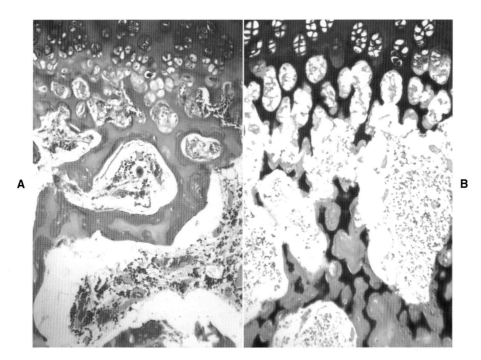

Fig. 16-63   Femoral head, necrosis (experimental), bone, femur, pig. Necrosis was produced experimentally by a ligature placed around the femoral neck. Several days after the procedure, the only difference between the control (**A**) and the infarcted bones (**B**) is the coagulation necrosis of the marrow and bone cells. The hard tissue of the cartilage and bone remains unaffected. H&E stain. (**A** and **B**, *Courtesy Dr. S.E. Weisbrode, College of Veterinary Medicine, The Ohio State University.*)

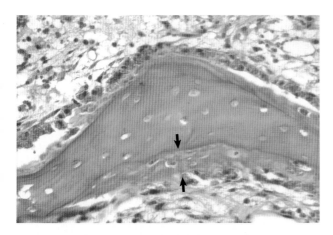

Fig. 16-64   Revascularization, ischemic necrosis (experimentally induced), 1-month duration, femoral head, epiphyseal (cancellous) bone, pig. Reactive woven bone (*between arrows*) has been deposited on the surface of the necrotic bone. Empty lacunae and karyolytic nuclei in the bone indicate that it is necrotic. Fibrovascular repair tissue in the marrow surrounds the bone. H&E stain. (*Courtesy Dr. S.E. Weisbrode, College of Veterinary Medicine, The Ohio State University.*)

neoplasms are accompanied by both bone resorption and new bone formation (Fig. 16-65). Pain, hypercalcemia, increased serum alkaline phosphatase activity, pathologic fracture, and distant metastases are other possible manifestations of a skeletal neoplasm. New bone formation occurs, at least in part, in response to mechanical stress on a weakened cortex and is prominent in neoplasms that have a marked fibrous stroma. Neoplasms with little stroma, such as plasma cell myeloma and lymphosarcoma, have minimal reactive bone formation, even though bone can be weakened by marked bone lysis. Tumor-associated bone destruction is largely accomplished by osteoclasts, but prostaglandins, cytokines, acid metabolic by-products, and lytic enzymes released by inflammatory or neoplastic cells can be responsible for local bone resorption and formation. Hypercalcemia, due in part to bone resorption induced by release of bone-resorbing factors from extraskeletal neoplasms, is well documented (humoral hypercalcemia of malignancy). In animals, the most common example is adenocarcinoma of the apocrine glands of the anal sac in the dog. This neoplasm produces PTH-related protein and it metastasizes widely, but rarely to bone.

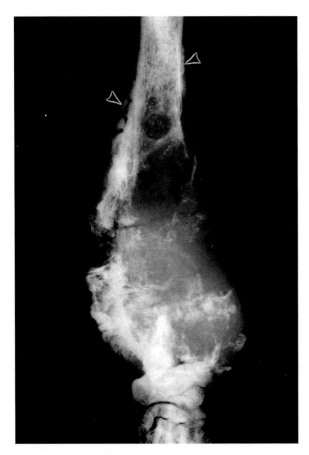

Fig. 16-65   Osteosarcoma, bone, distal radius, dog.
Osteosarcoma with extensive destruction of preexisting bone and some new bone formation on the periosteal surface (*arrowheads*). Radiograph. *(Courtesy Dr. S.E. Weisbrode, College of Veterinary Medicine, The Ohio State University.)*

NONNEOPLASTIC PROLIFERATIVE AND CYSTIC LESIONS

Lesions considered here vary widely in their cause, structure, and ultimate effect on the host. Reactive bone formation, sometimes exuberant, can occur in fracture repair, chronic osteomyelitis, and degenerative joint disease in the form of periarticular osteophytes. An exostosis or osteophyte is a nodular, benign, bony growth projecting outward from the surface of a bone. An enthesophyte is an osteophyte at the insertion of a ligament or tendon. In addition to bone, these proliferations can have variable amounts of cartilage. The bone component can be woven and/or lamellar, depending on rate of growth and duration of lesion. Hyperostosis usually is used to indicate that the diameter of the bone has increased and implies more uniform thickening on the periosteal surface rather than the nodular appearance of an osteophyte. An enostosis is a bony growth within the medullary cavity, usually originating from the cortical-endosteal surface, and can result in obliteration of the

medullary cavity. The above lesions are nonneoplastic proliferative lesions in which growth is seldom continuous. Some exostoses can remodel and some regress. Nonneoplastic proliferative lesions can be mistaken for skeletal neoplasia in some biopsy specimens. Conversely, small superficial biopsies might contain only nonneoplastic reactive bone overlying a malignancy. These statements serve to highlight the problem of making a morphologic diagnosis from a small biopsy specimen, without the benefit of a clinical history, radiographic findings, and other laboratory data. One must also remember that more than one process might be active at any one site (e.g., osteosarcoma might be complicated by fracture repair or by osteomyelitis).

Hypertrophic osteopathy (hypertrophic pulmonary osteopathy) occurs in human beings and in domestic animals, with the dog being the most commonly affected. The disease is characterized by progressive, bilateral, periosteal, new bone formation in the diaphyseal regions of the distal limbs (Fig. 16-66). The word "pulmonary" is included because most cases have intrathoracic neoplasms or inflammation. Other less commonly associated lesions or agents are endocarditis, heartworms, rhabdomyosarcoma of the urinary bladder in young giant-breed dogs, and ovarian neoplasms in the horse. Although the association between the pulmonary lesions and the proliferation of new periosteal bone on the extremities is not clear, it has been postulated that pulmonary lesions lead to reflex vasomotor changes (mediated by the vagus nerve) and to increased blood flow to the extremities. In hypertrophic osteopathy, woven bone is rapidly deposited by the periosteum of the diaphysis of the long bones. Similar periosteal woven deposition can occur in the metaphysis, but in hypertrophic osteopathy the lesions are usually less severe and less frequent in the metaphysis compared with the diaphysis. This periosteal new bone causes notable thickening of the limb bones. The lesions can regress if the primary lesion is removed.

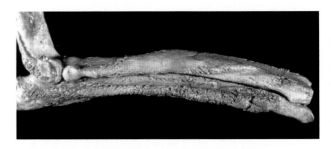

Fig. 16-66   Hypertrophic pulmonary osteopathy, bone, radius and ulna, dog. Marked periosteal proliferation of woven bone has caused a roughened irregular surface, particularly of the ulna. Macerated and bleached specimen. *(Courtesy Dr. S.E. Weisbrode, College of Veterinary Medicine, The Ohio State University.)*

Regression of the bone lesions also occurs after vagotomy. Increased arterial pressure, hyperemia, and edema of the periosteum lead to thickening of the periosteum both by fibrous tissue and later by new bone formation. Lesions similar to hypertrophic osteopathy can be reproduced in dogs by creating shunts that allow blood to bypass the pulmonary circulation, thereby increasing the stroke volume of the left side of the heart and increasing the blood flow to peripheral tissue.

Osteochondromas (multiple cartilaginous exostoses) occur in dogs and horses and reflect a defect in skeletal development rather than a true neoplasm. This condition is inherited and lesions appear shortly after birth. Osteochondromas project from bony surfaces as eccentric masses that are located adjacent to physes. They arise from long bones, ribs, vertebrae, scapulas, and bone of the pelvis and can be numerous (Figs. 16-67 and 16-68). Microscopically, they have an outer cap of hyaline cartilage that undergoes orderly endochondral ossification to give rise to trabecular bone that forms the base of the lesion (Fig. 16-68, C). The medullary cavity of the osteochondroma usually communicates with the medullary cavity of the underlying bone, because the cortex of the underlying bone at this site has not completely developed. Trabecular bone and bone marrow are continuous with those of the adjacent bone. Normally, growth ceases at skeletal maturity when the cartilage cap is replaced by bone. Although the origin of osteochondromas is not clear, some arise secondary to a defect in the perichondral ring as peripheral pieces of physeal cartilage are pinched off and carried away from the growth plate by longitudinal growth. Clinically, their importance is threefold: They might interfere mechanically with the action of tendons or ligaments; they can act as space-occupying masses that protrude into the vertebral canal and cause spinal cord compression; and they can undergo malignant transformation and give rise to chondrosarcomas. Osteochondromas in cats are different in that they develop in mature animals, less commonly affect long bones, do not have orderly endochondral ossification, and might be of viral origin. Osteochondromas in cats, like those in horses and dogs, can undergo malignant neoplastic transformation. The term osteochondroma is sometimes used (but not recommended) for cartilaginous osteophytes that have undergone central endochondral ossification. As will be discussed in callus formation in fracture repair, the osteogenic tissue (cambium layer) of the periosteum can form hyaline cartilage instead of bone when the oxygen tension of the tissue is low.

Fibrous dysplasia is an uncommon focal to multifocal, lytic, intraosseous lesion that has been found at various sites (skull, mandible, and long bones) in young animals. It could be a developmental defect. Typically, preexisting bone is replaced by an expanding mass of fibro-osseous

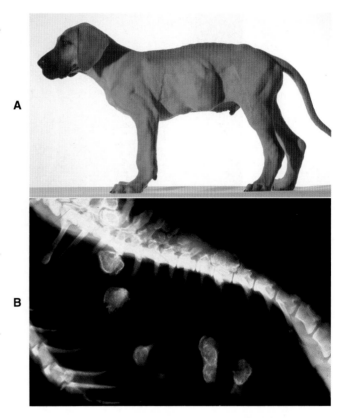

Fig. 16-67   Osteochondromas, young dog. A, Multiple protruding nodules of osteochondromas (cartilaginous exostoses) are present as single and coalescing masses on the ribs. **B,** Radiograph. The cartilaginous exostoses have undergone endochondral ossification and appear in this case as exophytic nodules on the ribs and the dorsal spinous processes of the vertebral bodies. (**A** and **B,** Courtesy Dr. S.E. Weisbrode, College of Veterinary Medicine, The Ohio State University.)

tissue that can weaken the cortex and enlarge the external contour of the bone. The lesion is firm, often has mineralized areas when sectioned, and can have multiple cysts filled with sanguinous fluid. Microscopically, well-differentiated fibrous tissue has relatively regularly spaced and sized trabeculae of woven bone. Osteoblasts are not recognizable on trabecular surfaces, a feature that helps to distinguish this lesion from ossifying fibroma.

Bone cysts are classified as subchondral, simple, or aneurysmal. Radiographically, all appear as lucent areas without evidence of aggressive growth. Subchondral cysts are sequelae to osteochondrosis and degenerative joint disease. Subchondral bone cysts due to osteochondrosis represent failure of endochondral ossification with subsequent necrosis and cavitation of retained growth cartilage. Bone never was present in such lesions. Subchondral cysts secondary to degenerative joint disease represent herniation of synovial fluid into the subchondral bone through fissures in the

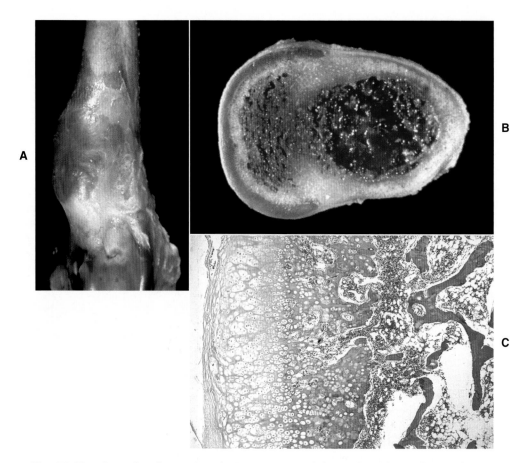

Fig. 16-68 **Osteochondromas (cartilaginous exostoses), bone, distal femoral metaphysis, dog. A,** A plateaulike mass (*left*) protrudes from the metaphyseal cortex. **B,** On cross section, the mass (*left*) has a cartilage cap. **C,** Histologically, the cartilage cap is undergoing endochondral ossification as would be seen in an articular-epiphyseal complex. H&E stain. (**A, B,** and **C,** *Courtesy Dr. S.E. Weisbrode, College of Veterinary Medicine, The Ohio State University.*)

articular cartilage. These herniations become lined by a synovial cell-like membrane. Bone lysis is by osteoclasis secondary to either pressure or cytokines released from the expanding cyst.

Simple bone cysts can contain clear, colorless, serumlike fluid, or the contents can be notably serosanguinous. The wall of the cyst is composed of variably dense fibrous tissue and woven to lamellar bone. Bone peripheral to this has undergone modeling to accommodate the expansile growth of the cyst. The category of simple bone cysts can overlap substantially with that of fibrous dysplasias; a clear distinction between them can be difficult to make.

Aneurysmal bone cysts consist of spaces filled with blood or serosanguinous fluid. Tissue adjacent to the spaces can vary from well-differentiated fibrous or fibroosseous tissue to pronounced proliferation of undifferentiated mesenchymal cells admixed with osteoclast-like multinucleated giant cells. Hemorrhage and hemosiderosis are frequent. An endothelial cell

lining is usually not present. The cause of simple and aneurysmal bone cysts is unknown. They could be consequences of ischemic necrosis, hemorrhage, or congenital or acquired vascular malformations. Caution should be exercised in the interpretation of microscopic lesions in biopsy specimens of cysts, and these lesions should be correlated with the radiographic appearance to rule out cystic cavitation in a neoplasm.

PRIMARY NEOPLASMS OF BONE

The histopathologic diagnosis of skeletal neoplasia in domestic animals often involves evaluation of needle, trephine, or wedge biopsies (Table 16-5). It is important that the pathologist be aware of the radiographic findings to determine if the biopsy is representative of the clinical process. Often biopsies consist only of reactive periosteal tissue, and if the lesion is both lytic and proliferative, the clinician should be told that the biopsy specimen is not likely representative of the entire mass.

Table **16-5**   **Primary Skeletal Neoplasms of the Dog**

Name	Cell of Origin	Incidence	Primary Site	Biologic Behavior
Osteoma	Osteoblast	Rare	Flat bones	Benign
Osteosarcoma	Osteoblast	Common	Predominantly metaphyses of larger appendicular bones	Highly malignant with metastases early in clinical course
Chondroma	Chondroblast/chondrocyte	Rare	Flat bones	Benign
Chondrosarcoma	Chondroblast/chondrocyte	Relatively rare	Ribs, sternum, nasal cavity	Metastases not common and late in clinical course
Fibroma	Fibroblast			Not significantly recognized as a primary tumor of bone
Fibrosarcoma	Fibroblast	Relatively rare	Diaphysis of bones of appendicular skeleton	Metastases relatively late in clinical course

The pathologist must explain any conflicts between the interpretation of the biopsy and radiographic findings. Radiographically aggressive lesions with mass effect usually indicate malignancy or inflammation. If a lesion is radiographically aggressive, the pathologist should not definitively conclude that a process is benign based only on the microscopic findings unless there is an explanation of the aggressive appearance (e.g., secondary infection in a benign neoplasm; pathologic fracture).

Ossifying fibromas are uncommon masses in the maxillae and mandibles of horses and cattle. In their early stages, these are intramedullary neoplasms. Although considered benign, they destroy adjacent cortical and trabecular bone by expansile growth. Microscopically, they are composed of well-differentiated fibrous tissue with scattered spicules of woven bone covered by osteoblasts.

Fibrosarcomas are malignancies of fibroblasts that produce collagenous connective tissue but not bone or cartilage. Microscopically the matrix of fibrosarcomas should not mineralize and entrap cells in lacunae as happens in normal and neoplastic bone and cartilage. Cells can be arranged in a whirling or interlacing pattern. Central fibrosarcomas arise from fibrous tissue within the medullary cavity, whereas periosteal fibrosarcomas arise from periosteal connective tissue. Central fibrosarcomas must be distinguished grossly and microscopically from osteosarcoma. In general, central fibrosarcomas grow more slowly, are accompanied by less formation of reactive new bone, are slower to metastasize, and produce a smaller tissue mass than osteosarcomas. Grossly, fibrosarcomas are gray-white,

fill part of the medullary cavity, and replace cancellous and cortical bone.

Chondromas are benign neoplasms of hyaline cartilage. They are very rare neoplasms of dogs, cats, and sheep and often arise from flat bones. Cartilaginous neoplasms in the skeleton do not arise from articular cartilage, most likely because of its low mitotic potential and avascularity. They are usually in adult animals that do not have growth cartilage, so the cell of origin is presumed to be a stromal cell with chondrogenic potential. Chondromas are multilobulated and have a blue-white cut surface. They tend to enlarge slowly but progressively and can cause thinning of underlying bone. Microscopically, they are composed of multiple lobules of well-differentiated hyaline cartilage. Endochondral ossification of the neoplastic cartilage is possible. They are difficult to distinguish from low-grade, well-differentiated chondrosarcomas. Chondromas that arise in the medullary cavity are called enchondromas.

Chondrosarcomas are malignant neoplasms in which the neoplastic cells produce cartilaginous matrix but not osteoid or bone. They are most common in mature dogs of the large breeds and in sheep. In sheep, they arise from the ribs and sternum; in dogs, the major sites of origin are the nasal bones, ribs, and pelvis. In general, chondrosarcomas most frequently arise in the flat bones of the skeleton (Figs. 16-69 and 16-70). Chondrosarcomas can evolve from multiple cartilaginous exostoses in dogs and in human beings. Most arise in the medullary cavity and destroy preexisting bone. Given time, they become large, lobulated neoplasms with a gray or blue-white cut surface. Some neoplasms

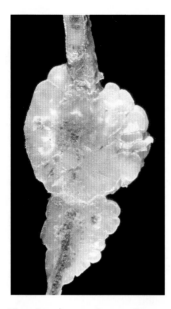

Fig. 16-69   Chondrosarcoma, bone, rib, cat. A chondrosarcoma arising in a rib has destroyed and replaced the medulla and cortices. *(Courtesy Dr. S.E. Weisbrode, College of Veterinary Medicine, The Ohio State University.)*

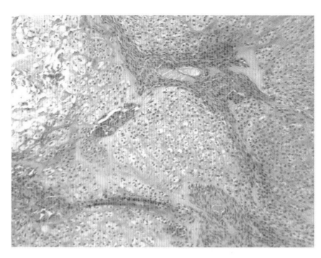

Fig. 16-71   Chondrosarcoma, bone, dog. Chondrocyte lacunae are prominent in well-differentiated regions. Lacunae are not as apparent in the less well-differentiated regions *(lower right)*. Cytological and nuclear atypia is minimal, but this cannot be seen at this magnification. H&E stain. *(Courtesy Dr. S.E. Weisbrode, College of Veterinary Medicine, The Ohio State University.)*

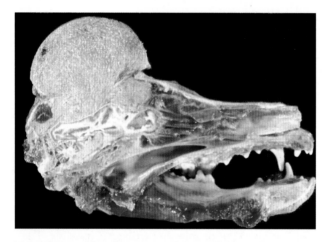

Fig. 16-70   Chondrosarcoma, bone, calvarium, dog. A chondrosarcoma protrudes from the skull, compresses the underlying brain, and has invaded the frontal sinus. The widespread white foci within the mass could represent areas of mineralization of the neoplastic cartilage or nonneoplastic bone formed by endochondral ossification. *(Courtesy Dr. K. Read, College of Veterinary Medicine, Texas A&M University; and Noah's Arkive, College of Veterinary Medicine, The University of Georgia.)*

are gelatinous on sectioning, and some have large areas of hemorrhage and necrosis. Microscopically (Fig. 16-71) the range of differentiation of neoplastic cells is wide: Some neoplasms are well differentiated and are difficult to distinguish from chondroma (conventional chondrosarcomas); some have mostly the appearance of primitive mesenchyma tissue (myxosarcoma-like) with abundant basophilic interstitial mucin and rare foci of chondroid differentiation (mesenchymal chondrosarcoma); other neoplasms are composed of highly anaplastic cells and have only a few areas in which differentiation into chondrocytes and chondroid matrix is apparent. Nonneoplastic bone can be present because of endochondral ossification of the malignant cartilage. Chondrosarcomas have a longer clinical course, grow more slowly, and develop metastases later than osteosarcomas. Metastases are usually to the lung by way of the venous system without metastasis to the regional or bronchial lymph nodes.

Osteomas are uncommon benign neoplasms that usually arise from bones of the head. They occur as a single, dense mass that projects from the surface of the bone (Fig. 16-72). They do not invade or destroy adjacent bone; their growth is slow and progressive but not necessarily continuous. Microscopically, osteomas are covered by periosteum and are composed of cancellous bone that becomes denser with time. Trabeculae are lined by well-differentiated osteoblasts and osteoclasts. The intertrabecular spaces contain delicate fibrous tissue, adipocytes, and hemopoietic tissue.

Osteosarcomas are malignant neoplasms in which neoplastic cells form bone, osteoid, or both. They can be classified as simple (bone formed in a collagenous matrix), compound (both bone and cartilage are present), or pleomorphic (anaplastic, with only small islands of osteoid present). Classification has also been based on cell type and activity (osteoblastic, chondroblastic, or

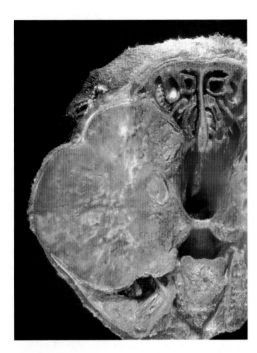

Fig. 16-72   **Osteoma, bone, maxilla and maxillary sinus, sheep.** The osteoma has proliferated and formed a dome-shaped mass above the normal contour of the maxilla and has compressed the maxillary sinus. This mass was hard throughout and composed of closely spaced trabeculae lined by well-differentiated osteoblasts. An *Oestrus ovis* larva is present in the nasal cavity. *(Courtesy Dr. S.E. Weisbrode, College of Veterinary Medicine, The Ohio State University.)*

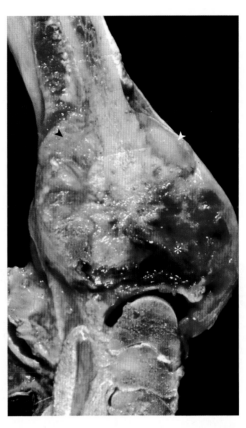

Fig. 16-73   **Osteosarcoma, bone, distal radius, dog.** Osteosarcoma has lysed and replaced normal bone. There is reactive periosteal bone formation *(arrowheads)* and a large area of hemorrhage and necrosis (*). *(Courtesy Department of Veterinary Biosciences, The Ohio State University; and Noah's Arkive, College of Veterinary Medicine, The University of Georgia.)*

fibroblastic), radiographic appearance (lytic, sclerotic, or mixed), or origin (central, juxtacortical, or periosteal). An uncommon form of osteosarcoma is the telangiectatic type that grossly resembles hemangiosarcoma. Microscopically, telangiectatic osteosarcomas are composed of osteoblasts, osteoid, and large cystic, blood-filled cavities lined by malignant osteoblasts. Osteosarcomas are common neoplasms, comprising approximately 80% of all the primary bone neoplasms in the dog. They arise most commonly in the metaphyses (distal radius, distal tibia, and proximal humerus are the most usual sites) (Fig. 16-73). However, osteosarcomas can occur in ribs, vertebrae, bones of the head, and various other parts of the skeleton (Fig. 16-74). Rarely, they arise in soft tissue (extraskeletal osteosarcoma). Typically, these neoplasms occur in mature dogs of the large and giant breeds. Growth of the neoplasm is often rapid and painful. Grossly, central or intraosseous osteosarcomas have a gray-white appearance and contain variable amounts of mineralized bone. Large, pale areas surrounded by zones of hemorrhage (areas of infarction) and irregular areas of hemorrhage are common in rapidly growing intramedullary neoplasms. Neoplastic tissue tends to fill the medullary cavity locally and can extend

proximally and distally, but typically does not penetrate articular cartilage. Therefore osteosarcomas do not invade into the joint space. Cortical bone is usually destroyed, and neoplastic cells penetrate and undermine the periosteum and can extend outwardly as an irregular lobulated mass. Destruction of cortical bone is accompanied by varying amounts of reactive (nonneoplastic) periosteal bone. Microscopically, variable amounts of woven bone or osteoid are produced by the neoplastic osteoblasts (Fig. 16-75). Bone formation by the malignant cells can be abundant and widespread, or it can be minimal, as in anaplastic or fibroblastic osteosarcomas that are composed of sheets of poorly differentiated mesenchymal cells or fibroblastic tissue. Distinguishing between an intramedullary fibrosarcoma, and fibroblastic osteosarcoma can be difficult to impossible, especially in small biopsy samples. It was hoped that immunostaining for the osteoblast-specific protein osteocalcin might be useful in this regard, but it has been reported in human medicine that fibroblastic osteosarcomas commonly no longer express osteocalcin so the applied value of this technique can be low. In terms of biologic behavior, osteosarcomas in the dog are characterized by aggressive local invasion and, except for those arising in the axial skeleton and particularly the head, early hematogenous pulmonary metastasis. Although pulmonary metastasis is common and occurs early, metastasis can be widespread and can involve both soft tissue and other bones.

The previous description relates to central or intraosseous osteosarcomas. Periosteal osteosarcomas also have an aggressive behavior and invade into the medullary cavity from the periphery. As with central or intraosseous osteosarcomas, periosteal osteosarcomas cause bone lysis and reactive bone formation in

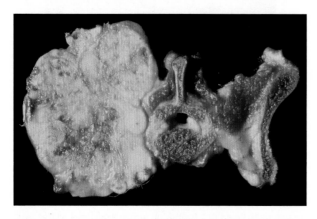

Fig. 16-74   Osteosarcoma, bone, wing of ilium, dog.
Although the mass appears to be growing mostly by expansion into the adjacent soft tissues, it has invaded and lysed the underlying ilium and is focally invading the lumbar vertebra. (*Courtesy Dr. S.E. Weisbrode, College of Veterinary Medicine, The Ohio State University.*)

addition to production of neoplastic bone. At the time of presentation, often it is not possible to determine if the osteosarcoma originated from the periosteum or the medullary cavity. Rarely, osteosarcomas are also juxtacortical (parosteal) in origin. These neoplasms arise within the periosteum and form an expansive mass that adheres to and surrounds, but does not invade, the underlying cortex. Invasion of the shaft and metastasis can occur with parosteal osteosarcomas but is a late event, so early en bloc excision might effect a cure. Although parosteal osteosarcomas are very rare, it is important to distinguish them from periosteal osteosarcomas because parosteal osteosarcomas have a more favorable prognosis.

Multiple skeletal osteosarcomas that occur in human beings and dogs could represent a primary neoplasm that has metastasized to bone. The lesions have a random distribution, and pulmonary metastases are likely to be present. Alternatively, multiple skeletal osteosarcomas could have a multicentric origin. Metastasis of skeletal osteosarcoma to other bones in the dog has been reported to be higher in dogs receiving chemotherapy.

Although the cause of naturally occurring osteosarcomas in human beings and domestic animals is largely unknown, osteosarcomas can develop in association with other diseases. Osteosarcomas have been associated with bone infarctions, previous fractures, and the use of metallic fixation devices in human beings and domestic animals. Osteosarcomas of viral origin are reported in mice.

A unique form of skeletal malignancy occurs in the skull of the dog and is awkwardly called a multilobular tumor of bone (older literature calls this chondroma rodens). These are single, nodular, smooth-contoured,

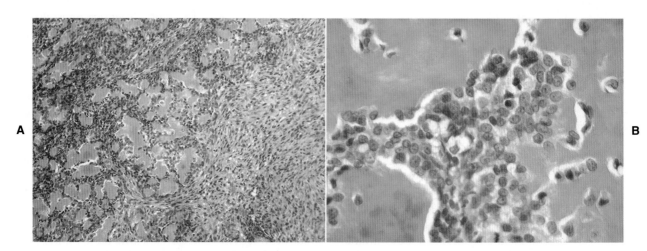

Fig. 16-75   Osteosarcoma, bone, dog. A, Islands of eosinophilic osteoid are being produced by sheets of malignant osteoblasts. **B,** At higher magnification, malignant osteoblasts can be seen becoming embedded (malignant osteocyte formation) in the osteoid. Mineralization is not apparent. H&E stain. (**A** *and* **B,** *Courtesy Dr. J. Sagartz, College of Veterinary Medicine, The Ohio State University; and Noah's Arkive, College of Veterinary Medicine, The University of Georgia.*)

immovable masses on the flat bones of the skull (bones of membranous origin) and the hard palate. Neoplastic tissue is firm and the cut surface is composed of multiple, gray, partially mineralized lobules set in a background of fibrous tissue. These neoplasms are slow growing, are locally invasive, and can compress and invade the brain. They metastasize to the lungs late in the clinical course, and the metastases are frequently small and clinically silent. The microscopic appearance consists of multiple lobules, each having centrally located cartilage or bone surrounded by plump mesenchymal cells that blend into well-differentiated interlobular fibrous tissue.

Various other neoplasms such as liposarcomas, giant cell tumors, and hemangiosarcomas can arise in bone, and neoplasms such as lymphosarcomas and plasma cell myeloma can involve the bone marrow and surrounding bone.

SECONDARY NEOPLASMS OF BONE

At autopsy, 60% of (human) cancer patients have skeletal metastases. These are predominantly in red bone marrow, where the vascular sinusoidal system is apparently predisposed to trap circulating malignant cells. The true incidence of skeletal metastasis in animals is unknown and might be low because early euthanasia shortens the course of the disease. However, bone scanning techniques and detailed necropsies might establish that skeletal metastases are more common than presently estimated. Metastatic neoplasms in bone can be associated with pain, hypercalcemia, lysis of bone, pathologic fracture, and reactive new bone formation. Rib shafts, vertebral bodies, and humeral and femoral metaphyses (proximal appendicular skeleton) are common sites of metastatic neoplasms in dogs. In about 50% of the carcinomas present in the proximal appendicular skeleton in the dog, there is no clinical evidence of a primary carcinoma, and at postmortem, a primary carcinoma is not found. Consideration should be given to these being primary intraosseous carcinomas. In cats, skeletal metastases are rare, but the distal appendicular skeleton appears to be the predisposed sites. In cats, clinically silent pulmonary carcinomas can have a history of sloughing of multiple claws. Histopathologic examination of an amputated affected digit reveals metastatic pulmonary carcinoma with involvement mostly in the third phalanx causing destruction of the nail bed epithelium and sloughing of the claw.

FRACTURE REPAIR

Broken bones are a common occurrence. It is important to understand how and why fractures heal, and more importantly why they do not. Fractures can be classified as traumatic (normal bone broken by excessive force) or pathologic (an abnormal bone broken by minimal trauma or by normal weight bearing). Osteomalacia, osteomyelitis, and bone neoplasms are examples of lesions that can weaken a bone and predispose it to pathologic fracture. Microcracks might predispose to development of fracture with less than expected trauma, but to date this has not been proven.

Growth plate: The Salter-Harris classification of growth plate fractures has been widely accepted and can be readily found in texts on clinical orthopedics. Growth plate fractures that involve only the hypertrophied layers of cartilage and/or the primary trabeculae (Salter-Harris I and II) usually heal with few or any complications. Fractures which cross the growth plate (III and IV) or crush the plate (V and VI) have the potential to heal with secondary growth deformities. Fractures that crush or cross the growth plate could irreversibly injure chondrocytes of the reserve (resting) cell layer of the growth plate or damage the branch of the epiphyseal artery that nourishes these cells. Loss of reserve cells can result in premature closure of the growth plate in these regions.

Trabecular bone: Fractures of trabeculae without external deformation of the cortex are called infractions. These are often associated with inflammation or necrosis of bone as predisposing factors.

Cortical bone: Fractures of cortical bone can be classified in many other ways: closed or simple, if the skin is unbroken; open or compound, if the skin is broken and the bone is exposed to the external environment; comminuted, if the bone has been shattered into several small fragments; avulsed, if the fracture was caused by the pull of a ligament at its insertion into bone; greenstick, if one side of the bone is broken and the other side is only bent so that there is no separation or displacement; and transverse or spiral, depending on the orientation of the fracture line.

Stable fracture repair means that the fracture ends have been immobilized to give relative clinical stability (not necessarily weight-bearing ability), but have not been rigidly fixed by surgery (Table 16-6). The events that normally occur in the healing of a closed stable fracture of cortical bone are summarized later (Fig. 16-76). The reader should understand that this description represents a summary of a complex process that is subject to a great deal of variation. At the time of fracture, the periosteum is torn, the fragments are displaced, soft tissue is traumatized, and bleeding occurs forming a hematoma. Because of impaired blood flow and isolated bone fragments, bone at the broken ends and marrow tissue can undergo necrosis. The hematoma and tissue necrosis can be important in subsequent callus formation. Growth factors are released by macrophages and platelets in the blood clot and the proliferating osteogenic tissue, and even from the dead bone by the lysis and acidification of the matrix. These growth factors (bone morphogenetic proteins, TGF-β, and platelet-derived growth factors among others) are important in stimulating proliferation of repair tissue (woven bone). Undifferentiated mesenchymal cells having osteogenic potential and reactive vascular proliferation begin to penetrate the hematoma from the periphery in 24 to 48 hours. The mesenchymal cells are derived from the periosteum, endosteum, stem cells in the medullary cavity, and possibly from metaplasia of endothelial cells. These mesenchymal cells proliferate in the hematoma to form a loose collagenous tissue. This proliferation of collagen-producing mesenchymal cells and neovascularization has been called "granulation tissue." This is misleading because granulation tissue is committed to becoming fibrous tissue, whereas the mesenchymal cells in the early stages of fracture healing have the potential to

undergo metaplasia to cartilage and bone. Woven bone is visible microscopically as early as 36 hours and regenerating nerve fibers are visible in the hematoma as early as 3 days.

The term "callus" refers to an unorganized meshwork of woven bone that forms after a fracture. It can be external (that formed by the periosteum) or internal (that formed between the ends of the fragments and in the medullary cavity or endosteum). This "primary" callus should bridge the gap, encircle the fracture site, and stabilize the area (Fig. 16-77). In time, woven bone at the fracture site is replaced by stronger, mature lamellar bone (secondary callus). Depending on the mechanical forces acting at the site, the callus can eventually be reduced in size by osteoclasts until the normal shape of the bone is restored. This process, however, might take years to complete.

Callus can contain hyaline cartilage. The amount of cartilage present in the callus reflects the adequacy of the blood supply. Less than optimal oxygen supply promotes mesenchymal stem cells to differentiate into chondroblasts rather than osteoblasts. Cartilage does not provide as strong a callus as woven bone. However, it will eventually undergo endochondral ossification and therefore ultimately contribute to the formation of the bony callus.

Rigid fracture repair is usually due to surgical intervention and application of devices to keep the bone ends in contact or in very close proximity and keep the fracture stable during the repair process. Ideally (but rarely achieved across an entire fracture) contact healing occurs. This is when the fractured ends are touching each other and there is no instability. In such conditions, healing is

Table 16-6   Stable Fracture Repair

Time	Tissue at Repair Site	Stability
Immediate	Hematoma	Unstable
24-48 hr	Undifferentiated mesenchymal cells and neovascularization	Unstable
36 hr	Earliest woven bone	Unstable
4-6 wk	Primary callus of woven bone and possibly hyaline cartilage	Stable
Months to years	Modeling of woven bone into lamellar bone	Stable

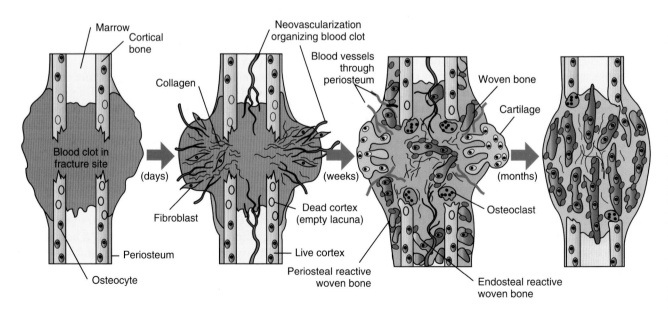

Fig. 16-76 Schematic diagram of the temporal course of callus formation and fracture repair.
(Redrawn from Rubin E: Essential pathology, ed 3, Baltimore, 2001, Lippincott Williams & Wilkins.)

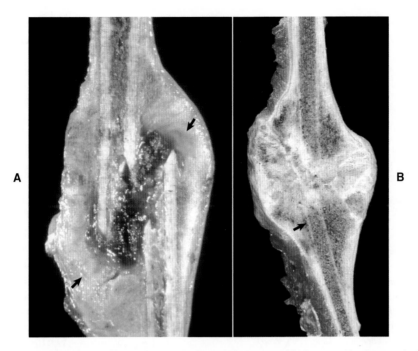

Fig. 16-77   Fractures, stable and unstable, bone, rib. A, Unstable fracture. The fractured edges of the rib are improperly aligned, and there is abundant external callus composed of both cartilage and bone (*arrows*) and fibrous tissue mixed with hemorrhage. Fibrous tissue is produced in regions of tension in an unstable fracture. **B,** Stable fracture. The fractured edges of the rib are adequately aligned, and the fracture is stabilized by abundant cartilaginous callus that is being replaced by new bone. Note the location of the original cortex (*arrow indicates original periosteal surface*). (**A,** *Courtesy College of Veterinary Medicine, University of Illinois.* **B,** *Courtesy Dr. F. A. Leighton, College of Veterinary Medicine, University of Saskatchewan; and Noah's Arkive, College of Veterinary Medicine, The University of Georgia.*)

by direct osteonal bridging of the fracture site (Fig. 16-78). Osteoclasts forming channels for new osteons will "jump" the fracture line and the new osteons will "knit" the bone ends together without formation of a callus. If there is a gap present between the bone ends but it is less than 1 mm, bone cells will migrate from the fracture ends and form lamellar bone at a right angle to the fracture line (Fig. 16-79). This will eventually model into osteonal bone parallel to the long axis of the bone. In rigid fractures with gaps greater than 1 mm, woven bone fills the gap and must be modeled into osteonal bone.

The most common complications of fracture healing are inadequate blood supply, instability, and infection. If the blood supply is less than optimal, then hyaline cartilage will form as described previously. If blood supply is disrupted to the point of anoxia, necrosis will occur. Mechanical tension and compression at the fracture site influence the reparative process. Excessive movement and tension favor the development of fibrous tissue. Mature fibrous tissue is not wanted in the callus because it does not stabilize the fracture and, unlike cartilage, will not act as a template for bone formation. Excessive fibrous tissue between bone ends

in a fracture might result in a nonunion. With time, the bony ends of the nonunion can become smooth and move in a pocket of fibrous tissue and cartilage to form a false joint or pseudoarthrosis. Other factors that can interfere with the normal repair process include malnutrition, bacterial osteomyelitis, and the interposition of large fragments of necrotic bone, muscle, or other soft tissue that might lead to delayed union or nonunion. Fractures heal more slowly in aged animals likely because of decreased presence of red marrow and its stromal stem cells.

There are several complications of fracture repair specifically associated with metallic implants used in fracture stabilization. Metallic devices that are too large deprive the bone of normal mechanical forces (stress shielding) and result in bone loss (disuse atrophy). Intramedullary fixation devices have the potential to damage the blood supply. Implanted material (metal, plastics, and bone cement) often is separated from the surrounding bone by a thin layer of fibrous tissue, sometimes with metaplastic cartilage that forms in response to operative trauma, implant mobility, or corrosion of the implant. In addition, the implant surface

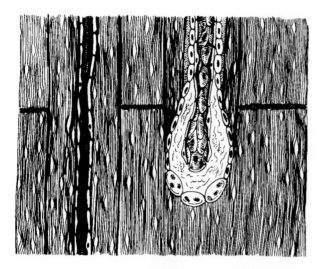

Fig. 16-78　**Schematic diagram of "direct or contact healing" in bone.** The fracture line is represented by a vertical line. In the lower portion of the illustration, a cutting cone is crossing the fracture and subsequently filling in with bone. *(From Olmstead ML: Small animal orthopedics, St Louis, 1995, Mosby.)*

can be a nidus for bacterial growth, and the admixture of bacteria with amorphous host fluid can form a biofilm that is resistant to antibiotics and host inflammatory cells. Microscopic particulate debris from implanted fixation materials ("wear debris") can elicit a macrophage or multinucleated giant cell response. These inflammatory cells can release cytokines and growth factors that result in bone resorption and

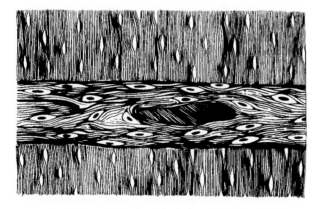

Fig. 16-79　**Schematic diagram of "small gap healing" in bone.** The gap has been filled with lamellar bone deposited in a plane perpendicular (vertical in the illustration) to the fractured ends. *(From Olmstead ML: Small animal orthopedics, St Louis, 1995, Mosby.)*

deterioration at the bone-implant surface, causing loosening and failure of the implant. Neoplasia thought to be induced by metallic fracture fixation devices has been reported rarely in the veterinary literature and is usually secondary to chronic osteomyelitis. The mechanism by which chronic osteomyelitis could be a predisposing factor for development of osteosarcoma is not known for certain. Generally, it is believed that any lesion that causes cell proliferation (as would be expected in chronic osteomyelitis) can increase the chance of cancer-causing spontaneous DNA damage by such things as free radicals and solar radiation. Pulmonary embolization of marrow fat from the trauma of the fracture or from trauma associated with repair of the fracture can cause severe clinical disease in human beings. It appears that the frequency of fat embolization secondary to trauma to the bone marrow is relatively common in human beings and dogs, but that clinical consequences of such embolization are relatively rare. Experimentally, fat embolization can be created readily in dogs by the reaming of the medullary cavity followed by pressurization. Interestingly, fat released from the marrow cavity in dogs by reaming is greater from intact bones than from fractured bones, presumably caused by decompression of the marrow cavity by the fracture in the latter. About 1% of human beings with hip replacement surgery can develop acute right-sided congestive heart failure because of embolization of fat from the surgery site to the lung.

DISEASES OF THE JOINTS

The joints or junctions between the bones can be classified as those that provide for little movement (fibrous joints or synarthrosis [e.g., sutures between the bones of the skull]) or limited movement (cartilaginous joint or amphiarthrosis [e.g., intervertebral joints]) and those that facilitate motion (synovial joint or diarthrosis [e.g., stifle joint]). The postmortem examination and evaluation of the joints is presented in Appendix 16-1.

ABNORMALITIES OF GROWTH AND DEVELOPMENT

ARTHROGRYPOSIS

Arthrogryposis refers to the congenital contracture of a joint. Usually this is bilateral and symmetric. The cause of arthrogryposis is often not established when it occurs sporadically. However, the pathogenesis is well established in outbreaks involving damage to the fetal central nervous system with intrauterine viral infections (Akabane virus and bluetongue virus) in cattle and sheep or ingestion of poisonous plants by the dam (lupine poisoning in cattle and poison hemlock in pigs).

In some cases, the central nervous system lesions are clearly hereditary, with significant numbers of offspring affected after introduction of a new sire. The central nervous system lesions result in degeneration or atrophy of muscle groups with subsequent contraction of the distal limb. Alternatively, maternal intoxication with certain alkaloids (coniine in poison hemlock) and lupine plants (anagyrine) is believed to cause sustained contraction of uterine muscle. It is suspected that such uterine tension causes flexion of the distal limbs and eventually atrophy of the flexure muscles. In all of these situations, there is no primary problem in the joint. Usually upon sectioning the tendons or the articular capsule these contractures can be relieved and the joint straightened. In rare circumstances, there is congenital articular malformation resulting in incongruous joint surfaces.

Articular cartilage: Articular cartilage is usually normal, but subtle malformations can be present.

Articular capsule, synovium, synovial fluid: Articular capsule/synovium/synovial fluid is without gross lesions other than the lack of flexibility.

Subchondral bone: Subchondral bone is usually normal other than subtle malformation.

HIP DYSPLASIA

Hip dysplasia of the dog is a major orthopedic problem and is most common in large and giant breeds. Many different theories regarding the etiopathogenesis have been advanced, but most agree that it is a biomechanical disease in which joint laxity of the hip (instability) is one of the essential early findings, eventually resulting in chronic subluxation and severe secondary degenerative joint disease with marked modeling of the acetabulum and femoral head and neck. Heredity clearly plays a role, and by selective breeding the prevalence of the disease has been significantly reduced. The lesions are not present at birth but can be well advanced by 1 year of age. Weight and overexercise also might contribute to the time of onset of signs and severity of the disease. Dogs on restricted calorie intake have significantly delayed time of onset of both hip dysplasia and degenerative joint disease.

Hip dysplasia, which might be inherited, also occurs in bulls of some beef breeds. Affected animals have shallow acetabula, joint laxity, and instability, which lead to degenerative joint disease early in life.

Articular cartilage: In the advanced disease, there is notable erosion and ulceration of articular cartilage of both the femoral head and acetabulum.

Articular capsule/synovium/synovial fluid: In advanced disease, the articular capsule is stretched and thickened, and areas of osseous and cartilaginous metaplasia can develop within it. The round ligament of the femoral

head can be ruptured. It has been reported that the earliest detectable microscopic lesion in hip dysplasia is a mild lymphoplasmacytic synovitis (see previous discussion in reactions to injury). Although this is likely secondary to undetectable early cartilage breakdown, it is intriguing that this inflammation is the first observable microscopic lesion in any structure of the joint in hip dysplasia.

Subchondral bone: In advanced disease, the dorsal rim of the acetabulum flattens and becomes shallow and wide. Subsequent to ulceration of cartilage of the femoral head there is eburnation of underlying bone and formation of periarticular osteophytes on the femoral neck and acetabulum (Fig. 16-23).

INFLAMMATORY LESIONS

The term *arthritis* implies lesions present in articular cartilage in addition to inflammation of the synovial membrane, whereas the term synovitis is restricted to inflammation of the synovium (Table 16-3). Arthritis is characterized by the presence of inflammatory cells in the synovial membrane, but the nature of the inflammatory process is often reflected best in the volume and character of the exudate in the joint fluid. It is useful to classify joint diseases as inflammatory or noninflammatory. The problem with this classification becomes apparent when striking lymphoplasmacytic and histiocytic synovitis is found in "noninflammatory" diseases, such as hip dysplasia and degenerative joint disease. Arthritis can be classified by cause (bacterial, viral, sterile immune-mediated, or urate deposits of gout), duration (acute, subacute, or chronic), or the nature of the exudate produced (serous, fibrinous, purulent, or lymphoplasmacytic). The term "arthropathy" is all-encompassing and refers to any joint disease. Like osteomyelitis, arthritis can be a serious threat to the well-being of an animal. It is painful and can lead to permanent deformity and crippling. Chronicity can be due to an inability of the animal to remove the causative agent or substance, repeated trauma, persistence of bacterial cell wall material, or ongoing autoimmune-mediated inflammation. If there is irreversible damage to cartilage or synovium, even if the cause of the primary inflammation is cleared, the joint could progress to degenerative joint disease. Injury to intraarticular structure can be due to the offending agent or substance, to the inflammatory process, to proteolytic enzymes released from cells of cartilage or synovial tissues, to activation of latent matrix metalloproteinases, or to failure of degenerating or necrotic chondrocytes to maintain the proteoglycan content of the matrix. Mediators of inflammation that contribute to joint injury include prostaglandins, cytokines, leukotrienes, lysosomal enzymes, free radicals, nitric oxide, neuropeptides, and products of the activated coagulation, kinin, complement, and fibrinolytic systems in synovial fluid.

INFECTIOUS ARTHRITIS

Neonatal bacteremia secondary to omphalitis or oral-intestinal entry commonly leads to polyarthritis in lambs, calves, piglets, and foals. Bacteria can also reach the joint by direct inoculation, as in a puncture wound, by direct extension from periarticular soft tissue, or by extension from adjacent bone. Bacterial osteomyelitis can extend through the cortex at the metaphysis (Fig. 16-45) (especially in young animals in which this cortex is not a completed wall of bone) into the joint, or epiphyseal osteomyelitis can lyse directly through articular cartilage (Fig. 16-46). Bacterial arthritis is not common in dogs or cats. In a retrospective study in a university veterinary hospital, most cases of bacterial arthritis in dogs involved the stifle and were complications from surgery on the stifle joint. Next most frequent in this series was hematogenous arthritis, and in most of these dogs an underlying chronic degenerative arthritis was thought to be the predisposing factor. The mechanisms of this predisposition is uncertain but might be related to the increased blood flow.

Because the lesions of infectious arthritis can be very similar from different inciting agents, lesions will be presented first. Lesions are presented by time and whether the initial exudates is/was mostly neutrophilic (suppurative arthritis) or fibrinous (fibrinous arthritis) (Table 16-3).

Articular cartilage: The response of cartilage to inflammation with time will depend on the nature and severity of the exudates. In acute inflammation independent of the nature of the initial exudate, the articular cartilage is normal grossly and microscopically. In subacute suppurative or fibrinous arthritis, there can be thinning of the cartilage because of lysis and erosion (see previous discussion) of collagen by the enzymes in the exudates, activation of matrix metalloproteinases, and collapse of the cartilage as a result of a loss and failure to replace the water-binding proteoglycans by the degenerate or necrotic chondrocytes. In chronic suppurative arthritis, extensive cartilage erosion and ulceration is expected (Fig. 16-80). In chronic fibrinous arthritis, there can be cartilage ulceration as well, but it as not as consistent as with chronic suppurative arthritis. In addition, in chronic fibrinous arthritis, pannus formation can occur (pannus is unusual with chronic suppurative arthritis). As described previously, cartilage erosion and ulceration is expected subsequent to pannus formation. In chronic infectious arthritis in which there was no acute exudate into the joint, cartilage loss might be quite slow and be secondary to low grade lymphoplasmacytic synovitis (see later discussion).

Articular capsule/synovium/synovial fluid: In acute suppurative and fibrinous arthritis, the synovial fluid is usually reduced in viscosity because of a combination of enzymatic digestion of the glycosaminoglycans and dilution of the synovial fluid with edema. The fluid may be turbid because of the presence of neutrophils and strands of fibrin and possibly reddened because of presence of slight hemorrhage. Exudate in the synovial fluid can be extensive in acute lesions (Fig. 16-81), whereas the synovial membrane can appear only slightly hyperemic and edematous even microscopically. Therefore in acute arthritis, evaluation of synovial fluid is much more informative than evaluation of synovial membrane. Reports in the horse suggest that

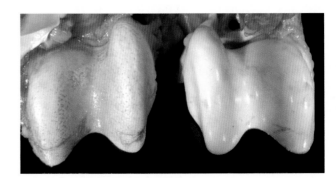

Fig. 16-80   Chronic suppurative (active) arthritis, right tibial-tarsal bone, articular surface, hock, horse. The suppurative inflammation has caused widespread erosions (lysis) of the articular cartilage that appear as darkened pitted areas on the articular surface (*left*). The cartilage erosion has allowed the red appearance (vascularization) of the underlying subchondral bone marrow to be seen. Normal left tibial-tarsal bone is on the right. (*Courtesy Dr. S.E. Weisbrode, College of Veterinary Medicine, The Ohio State University.*)

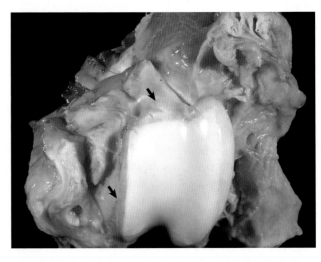

Fig. 16-81   Acute fibrinous arthritis, bone, tibial-tarsal joint (hock), calf. The articular cavity is distended by layers of yellowish-brown fibrin that coat the synovial surface (*arrows*) of the joint capsule. (*Courtesy Dr. C.S. Patton, College of Veterinary Medicine, University of Tennessee.*)

culturing for bacteria in synovial fluid is more sensitive than culturing synovial membrane or looking for bacteria in the synovial membrane with special stains histopathologically. In contrast, in the dog, culturing the synovial membrane has been reported to be more sensitive than the synovial fluid. In acute fibrinous or suppurative bacterial arthritis that has been treated effectively with antibiotics, the lesions can resolve without residual defects.

In subacute suppurative and fibrinous arthritis and in subacute infectious arthritis in which there was no acute exudate into the joint, independent of cause, the synovium is expected to have lymphoplasmacytic inflammation and variable hyperplasia of synovial lining cells (Fig. 16-82). The lymphoplasmacytic inflammation reflects the immunogenicity of the infectious agent. The synovial hyperplasia is a nonspecific response but presumably is an attempt at increasing production of synovial fluid. In subacute (and chronic) suppurative and fibrinous arthritis, it is uncommon to find significant numbers of neutrophils and fibrin deposits, respectively, in the synovial membrane. Rather, the neutrophils and fibrin exude from the membrane and enter the joint space.

In chronic suppurative arthritis, granulation tissue with pronounced lymphoplasmacytic inflammation can replace the synovial membrane and there can be notable fibrosis of the articular capsule. In chronic fibrinous arthritis, if deposits of fibrin are extensive, they can be invaded and replaced by fibrous tissue, leading to restricted articular movement. Chronic fibrinous arthritis (e.g., erysipelas and mycoplasmosis [see later discussion]) of long duration is often accompanied by pronounced villous hypertrophy, lymphoplasmacytic synovial inflammation and pannus formation, and progressive destruction of cartilage (Fig. 16-83). In both chronic fibrinous arthritis and chronic suppurative arthritis, fibrin and pus (suppurative exudate) continue to be produced and are present in the joint space in active (bacteria is still present) lesions. Fibrous ankylosis of joints can occur in extreme cases of either fibrinous or suppurative arthritis.

Subchondral bone: Subchondral bone is affected only secondarily in infectious arthritis. In chronic purulent arthritis, the exudates can erode the articular cartilage and extend into the subchondral bone plate (Fig. 16-84). If there is severe chronic lameness, the subchondral bone can undergo disuse atrophy and appear osteopenic.

BACTERIAL ARTHRITIS

Lesions of infectious arthritis based on the nature of the exudates and duration of the lesion were presented previously. The duration of bacterial arthritis is variable. Some organisms are rapidly removed and synovitis

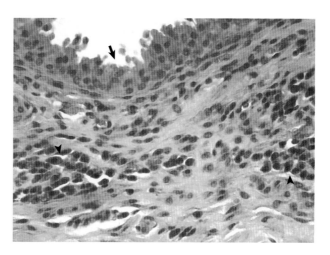

Fig. 16-82   Subacute synovitis, joint capsule, dog. There is marked synovial cell hyperplasia (*arrow*) and infiltration of lymphocytes and plasma cells into the synovial membrane (inner layer of the articular capsule) (*arrowheads*). H&E stain. *(Courtesy Dr. S.E. Weisbrode, College of Veterinary Medicine, The Ohio State University.)*

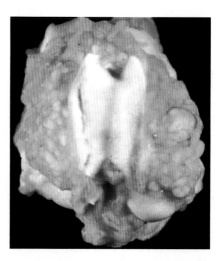

Fig. 16-83   Chronic fibrinous (active) synovitis, erysipelas, stifle joint, pig. A chronic arthritis from *Erysipelothrix rhusiopathiae* has resulted in villous hypertrophy of the synovial membrane. The tips of some villi are hemorrhagic and necrotic. *(Courtesy Dr. D. Harrington, College of Veterinary Medicine, Purdue University; and Noah's Arkive, College of Veterinary Medicine, The University of Georgia.)*

is short-lived. In other instances, bacteria can persist, and the inflammatory process can become chronic but still active. The extent and mechanism of cartilaginous destruction differ somewhat depending on the nature of the exudates. In turn, the nature of the exudates can depend on the infectious agent involved. Generally, fibrinous inflammation is expected more often with gram-negative bacteria, whereas suppurative arthritis

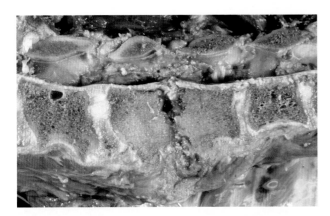

Fig. 16-84 **Suppurative discospondylitis, joint, intervertebral disk, dog.** Chronic marked suppurative discospondylitis (inflammation of the intervertebral disc and adjacent vertebrae) with marked lysis of the disk and cortices, epiphyses, and metaphyses of the adjacent vertebrae. *(Courtesy Dr. S.E. Weisbrode, College of Veterinary Medicine, The Ohio State University.)*

is expected more often with gram-positive bacteria. The exudates in the joint in acute stages of infection with gram-positive bacteria, however, can be mostly fibrinous and become purulent with time. An example of chronic fibrinous arthritis is that caused in pigs by *Erysipelothrix rhusiopathiae* septicemia. This is an exception to the above generality about fibrinous inflammation being due to gram-negative bacteria. *Erysipelothrix rhusiopathiae*, a gram-positive bacteria, causes a fibrinous arthritis that does not become purulent with time. Survivors can have lesions secondary to localization of *Erysipelothrix rhusiopathiae* in the skin, synovial joints, valvular endocardium, or intervertebral disks. Chronic painful polyarthritis is a common sequela. *Arcanobacterium pyogenes* is a common cause of suppurative arthritis in cattle and pigs. Many different infectious agents cause arthritis in animals. For example, *Escherichia coli* (fibrinous) and streptococci (suppurative) initially cause septicemia in neonatal calves and piglets and then localize in joints, meninges, and, sometimes, serosal surfaces. Often synovitis is acutely serofibrinous and becomes more purulent with time. *Haemophilus parasuis* (fibrinous) causes Glasser's disease in pigs 8 to 16 weeks of age. Lesions consist of fibrinous polyserositis, polyarthritis, and meningitis. Acute serofibrinous polyarthritis is seen frequently in cattle dying of thrombotic meningoencephalitis caused by *Haemophilus somnus*.

Borrelia burgdorferi, a spirochete, is the tick-borne cause of Lyme disease (borreliosis). The arthritis in Lyme disease is seen in dogs, cattle, and horses. Single or multiple joints can be affected. In experimental studies in dogs, lameness developed in about half of the infected animals. Time of onset of the lameness was 2 or more months

after infection. In the acute stages of the disease, the exudate is a combination of fibrinous and suppurative (fibrinopurulent) inflammation. In the chronic stages, pannus (usually a sequela to fibrinous arthritis) and chronic suppurative inflammation can be seen.

MYCOPLASMA ARTHRITIS

Generally the nature of the lesions of mycoplasma arthritis are comparable to those described previously for bacteria causing fibrinous arthritis. Usually multiple joints are involved, indicating the hematogenous route of infection. In pigs, *Mycoplasma hyorhinis* and *Mycoplasma hyosynoviae* can be commonly isolated from nasal and pharyngeal regions in asymptomatic pigs. *Mycoplasma hyorhinis* causes fibrinous polyarthritis and polyserositis in weanling pigs. *Mycoplasma hyosynoviae* causes fibrinous polyarthritis in older pigs (more than 3 months old). It is not certain how these mycoplasma gain access to the circulation and ultimately the joints, but it is likely an oral-pharyngeal/pulmonary route secondary to stress or concurrent respiratory disease.

Mycoplasma bovis causes fibrinous to pyogranulomatous polyarthritis in feedlot cattle, and the disease is characterized by lameness and swelling of the large synovial joints of the limbs, which can contain large volumes of serofibrinous to frankly suppurative exudate. *Mycoplasma bovis* likely gains access to joints through the blood stream, possibly secondary to mycoplasma pneumonia or mastitis.

VIRAL ARTHRITIS

The first viral arthritis discovered was the reoviral arthritis in chickens. At the time, there was great hope that idiopathic arthritides (such as rheumatoid arthritis) would also be shown to be viral. However, other than in goats, viral arthritis does not appear to be a significant or even recognized disease in domestic mammals. The caprine arthritis-encephalitis virus (a retrovirus) causes chronic fibrinous arthritis in older goats. The disease is characterized by debilitating lameness, carpal hygromas, and distention of the larger synovial joints. Peculiar to chronic cases of viral arthritis in goats due to caprine arthritis-encephalitis virus, necrosis and mineralization of synovial villi can give the membrane a chalky white appearance. Also present is lymphoplasmacytic synovitis, synovial villous hyperplasia, and pannus formation typical of chronic fibrinous arthritis.

NONINFECTIOUS ARTHRITIS

The causes of inflammatory conditions should be considered in two broad categories: infectious and noninfectious. The infectious causes of arthritis were presented previously. Here we consider specific joint diseases that have inflammation as the initiating event but are known to be sterile. Noninfectious arthritis is often classified as erosive or nonerosive depending on the effect of the disease on articular cartilage. Following are three types of sterile erosive arthritis.

RHEUMATOID ARTHRITIS

Rheumatoid arthritis in the dog is an uncommon, chronic, sterile, erosive polyarthritis that resembles the disease in human beings. In human beings and dogs, the cause is unknown, although it is clear that the process is immune mediated (involves humoral and cell-mediated immunity). Antibodies (rheumatoid factor) of the immunoglobulin (Ig)G or IgM classes are produced in response to an unknown stimulus. Alterations in the stearic configuration of IgG, persistent bacterial cell wall components that cross-react with normal proteoglycans, anticollagen antibodies, and defective suppressor T-lymphocyte activity are factors that may be involved. Neutrophils activated by ingestion of immune complexes release lysosomal enzymes, which sustain the inflammatory reaction and injure intraarticular structures. The pathogenesis of joint destruction in rheumatoid arthritis was described previously in reaction to injury of joints to inflammation. In addition to inflammatory mediators and their effects on synovium and cartilage, rheumatoid arthritis characteristically has exuberant pannus formation (see Fig. 16-35). Fibroblasts in pannus can enzymatically degrade cartilage, and pannus can act as a physical barrier between the synovial fluid and the cartilage preventing nutrition of the chondrocytes. Antibodies against normal and altered collagen from articular cartilage are present in human cases of rheumatoid arthritis and might be important mediators of the ongoing joint inflammation and injury that occur in this disease. In dogs, rheumatoid arthritis is characterized by progressive lameness involving the peripheral joints of the limbs.

REACTIVE ARTHRITIS

Reactive arthritis is the name given to a sterile erosive oligoarthritis of uncertain pathogenesis. This condition is rarely reported in domestic animals and is presented here because it likely is underdiagnosed. It is a known problem in primate research colonies as an arthritis that develops subsequent to diarrheal disease. In the dog, the term *reactive arthritis* is being used for sterile nonerosive arthritis secondary to infectious disease elsewhere in the body (see later section titled Nonerosive Noninfectious Arthritis). This is at odds with the condition recognized in human beings and nonhuman primates. Reactive arthritis is defined clinically as sterile inflammation in joints that occurs subsequent to infectious inflammation in other organ systems—usually intestinal and urogenital in human beings; and usually caused by bacteria such as *Yersinia, Salmonella, Campylobacter,* and *Shigella.* Several hypotheses

have been presented: cross-reactivity (molecular mimicry) between bacterial heat-shock proteins and articular glycosaminoglycans, inexplicable homing of sensitized gut lymphocytes to joints, and inexplicable localization of antigenic bacterial peptidoglycans in joints. These are not mutually exclusive.

POSTINFECTIOUS STERILE ARTHRITIS

Postinfectious sterile arthritis is suspected to represent the immune reaction to antigenic breakdown products of bacterial cell walls that can remain sequestered in a joint after a confirmed bacterial infection within the joint.

Articular cartilage: Rheumatoid arthritis, reactive arthritis and postinfectious arthritis are all erosive, and in some cases, the ulceration can be extensive. Cartilage erosion is not expected until at least the subacute phases of the disease. These diseases can be very chronic, lasting for months because of difficulty in controlling the condition with medication.

Articular capsule/synovium/synovial fluid: Grossly the lesions in advanced cases consist of marked villous hypertrophy of the synovial membrane, pannus formation, formation of periarticular osteophytes, and, when severe, fibrous ankylosis of affected joints. In severe cases, pannus formation can result in a velvetlike layer overlying the subchondral bone. Microscopically the alterations in the joint are hyperplasia of synovial lining cells and infiltration of large numbers of plasma cells and lymphocytes into the synovium. Additionally, necrotic foci, fibrinous exudate, and infiltrating neutrophils can be present in the synovium. Large numbers of neutrophils are present in the synovial fluid.

Subchondral bone: With severe ulceration and pannus formation, rather than sclerosis of subchondral bone, there can be lysis of subchondral bone by the ongoing pannus.

NONEROSIVE NONINFECTIOUS ARTHRITIS

Nonerosive noninfectious arthritis has been best described in the dog. Most are idiopathic symmetric oligoarthritides, but they can be associated with concurrent sterile immune-mediated diseases such as steroid responsive meningitis/arteritis, neoplasia, and infectious inflammation in other organ systems (nonerosive reactive arthritis). Systemic lupus erythematosus (SLE) can be associated with nonerosive arthritis. SLE is a chronic nonerosive oligoarthritis that is recognized in dogs. These dogs can have, in addition, dermatitis, anemia, thrombocytopenia, polymyositis, and glomerulonephritis. It is thought that synoviotrophic immune complexes are the mediators of this inflammation. Why this does not result in articular destruction as in rheumatoid arthritis is not apparent.

Articular cartilage: Articular cartilage lesions are not expected in nonerosive arthritis even when it is chronic.

Articular capsule/synovium/synovial fluid: In these diseases, villous hypertrophy can be minimal to marked with variable neutrophilic and lymphoplasmacytic synovitis. Pannus formation does not occur, and destruction of articular cartilage is not to be expected. The exudate in the synovial fluid in chronic nonerosive arthritis is neutrophilic.

Subchondral bone: Subchondral bone lesions are not expected in nonerosive arthritis.

In sterile inflammatory joint disease, a definitive diagnosis is not often possible. It should be remembered that response to antibiotics does not confirm that a process was a result of infectious agents. Antibiotics that reduce gram-positive bacteria in the intestine may allow coliform overgrowth and increased lipopolysaccharide production. Increased intestinal absorption of lipopolysacchoride is associated with decreased clinical signs in autoimmune arthritis, possibly by the immune system down-regulating or by establishing a more rigorous recognition of self.

CRYSTAL DEPOSITION DISEASE

Crystal deposition disease is characterized by deposits of minerals such as urates, calcium phosphates, and calcium pyrophosphates in articular cartilage and/or the soft tissue of joints. Clinical disease due to crystal deposition is rare in domestic mammals. Crystal-induced synovitis with secondary degeneration of articular cartilage occurs in gout when urate crystals are deposited in and around joints. Gout occurs in species that do not have the enzyme uricase (human beings, birds, and reptiles). Deposits of urate, called tophi, incite an acute to chronic granulomatous inflammation and can appear grossly as white caseous material. Deposition of calcium and phosphorus in different forms (calcium pyrophosphate deposition disease, "pseudogout," and calcium phosphate deposition disease) in the soft tissue of the synovium, articular capsule, and adjacent ligaments has been reported in young dogs. Underlying metabolic diseases are not recognized. Single or multiple joints can be involved. The variable bone and cartilage changes that can be present might be secondary. Perhaps the most common crystal deposition disease, but usually clinically silent, is intraarticular crystal deposition disease. This is usually due to calcium pyrophosphate deposition. In horses and dogs, this can be present in locations subject to increased mechanical use (scapulohumeral joint of racing dogs and metacarpal- and metatarsal-phalangeal joints of horses). The deposition is initiated around the chondrocytes and can be seen grossly as bright white foci. The significance of the deposition is uncertain, but it might play a role in the progression of degenerative joint disease.

DEGENERATIVE JOINT DISEASE

Degenerative joint disease (osteoarthritis, osteoarthrosis), recognized since antiquity, is a destructive disease of articular cartilage of synovial joints that occurs in all animals with a bony skeleton (Table 16-7). It can be monoarticular or polyarticular, can occur in immature or mature animals, and can be symptomatic or clinically silent. Affected animals have variable degrees of joint enlargement and deformity, pain, and articular malfunction. The etiopathogenesis of degenerative

Table **16-7**   **Degenerative Joint Disease**

Name of Stage	Gross Appearance	Microscopic Lesion
Chondromalacia	Softened	Decreased proteoglycan content apparent with histochemical stains for mesenchymal mucins
Erosion	Ranges from matted appearance and normal thickness to grossly apparent thinning	Loss of cartilage layers–ranges from earliest loss only of the surface layer to later stages of loss extending to tangential, radial, and eventually deep (mineralized layer)
Fibrillation	Frayed appearance	Condensation of collagen fibers (because of loss of water at this stage) and splitting of the matrix along the vertical axis of the collagen fibers (perpendicular to the joint surface)
Ulceration/eburnation of subchondral bone	Exposure of the subchondral bone; the bone surface can be polished very smooth by wear	Loss of cartilage to the level of the subchondral bone; vascular and marrow spaces of the bone become smaller as they fill with bone (osteosclerosis) because of increased mechanical use; the surface of the exposed bone can be smooth; this combination of increased density (osteosclerosis) and surface smoothness is termed eburnation

joint disease is incompletely understood, and it is likely that the term encompasses a variety of diseases that have a common end stage. Initial changes can be due to traumatic injury to articular cartilage, inflammation of the synovium, increased stiffness of the subchondral bone, or abnormalities in conformation, joint stability, and congruence of joint surfaces (Fig. 16-85). In addition, age-related degeneration of articular cartilage is common in all species but often is clinically insignificant. Lesions are of greatest importance when they occur at an early age and progress rapidly.

The initial biochemical change in articular cartilage in degenerative joint disease is loss of proteoglycan aggregates. In the early stages of degeneration, this loss of proteoglycans is associated with an increase in water content in the cartilage matrix. This early increase in the water content of the cartilage matrix in early stages of degenerative joint disease, coinciding with a decrease in cartilage matrix proteoglycans, seems contradictory because in normal cartilage, proteoglycans play a critical role in binding water. The explanation for this is not clear, but the increased water in the matrix is not bound normally to the proteoglycans and does not contribute to the normal lubrication and flushing of nutrients and waste products as described previously. Core proteins of proteoglycan aggregates are susceptible to the action of neutral proteoglycanases, which are increased in early degenerative joint disease. In electron micrographs, the findings include focal loss of the amorphous layer

covering the surface of the articular cartilage and fraying of the superficial collagen fibers. Continued proteoglycan loss interferes with joint lubrication and allows collagen fibers to collapse on each other along lines perpendicular to the joint surface because of the loss of the hydrated gel of proteoglycans and water that kept the fibers separated.

Synovitis in degenerative joint disease is secondary to release of inflammatory mediators by injured chondrocytes and from synovial macrophages that have phagocytosed cartilaginous breakdown products.

Articular cartilage: Lesions can be focal to diffuse within a joint. The loss of proteoglycans and improper binding of water (actual increase in water content) causes the articular cartilage to become soft (chondromalacia). In hinge-type joints, linear grooves can often be seen particularly in horses (see Fig. 16-21). Histologically, these grooves are not erosions or ulcers but have all layers intact. They represent linear depressions in the cartilage associated with scattered necrotic chondrocytes and localized loss of proteoglycan. It is presumed that these depressions represent areas of collapse of the collagen fibers because of loss of proteoglycans and water. The pathogenesis of these grooves is uncertain, but they might represent sequelae to jetties of synovial fluid secondary to incongruities of the joint surfaces. Chondromalacia is followed by abnormal wearing of the cartilage and loss of very superficial layers (early erosion) resulting grossly in a matted appearance.

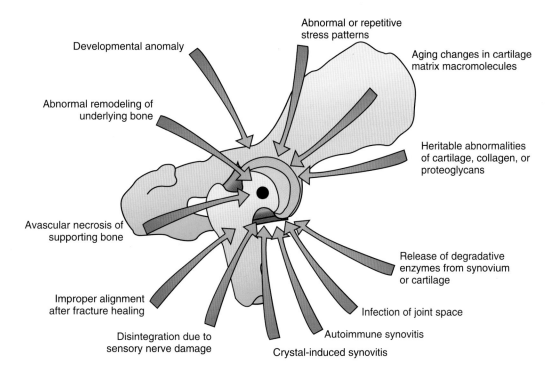

Fig. 16-85   Schematic diagram illustrating degenerative joint disease of the coxofemoral joint. *(From Damjanov I, Linder J: Anderson's pathology, ed 10, vol 2, St Louis, 1996, Mosby.)*

As the lesions progress, erosions becomes deeper (cartilage is thinner) and grossly apparent fraying of collagen fibers along their radial arrangement can be seen (fibrillation) (see Figs. 16-30 to 16-32). Fibrillated cartilage can be yellow to brown. Advanced lesions can have notable loss of cartilage down to the mineralized layer and subchondral bone (ulceration) (see Fig. 16-33).

Articular capsule/synovium/synovial fluid: Synovitis characterized by villous hypertrophy, hyperplasia of synoviocytes, and infiltration of lymphocytes, plasma cells, and macrophages is usually present in chronic cases (see Fig. 16-34). The synovial fluid does not have exudates and is clear and colorless but might have reduced viscosity because of increased plasma filtrate relative to glycosaminoglycans in the synovial fluid, and increased degradation of glycosaminoglycans by enzymes released by the inflamed synovium. Fibrosis of the articular capsule because of instability or release of cytokines such as TGF-β might contribute, along with osteophytosis and joint incongruity, to the joint stiffness and limited range of motion seen in advanced degenerative joint disease.

Subchondral bone: Degenerative joint disease often progresses to sclerosis of subchondral bone, but some investigators consider stiffness (sclerosis) of subchondral bone to be the initial lesion and that this stiffness predisposes the cartilage to mechanical damage. If there is ulceration of cartilage and the joint is still used, the exposed bone can be polished smooth by wear (eburnation). Marginal (periarticular) osteophytes form and there can be pronounced modeling of the epiphyseal and metaphyseal bone because of altered mechanical use (see Fig. 16-38). The joint might fuse because of combination of bony or fibrous bridging (ankylosis) of the joint space (Fig. 16-86). Subchondral bone cysts in degenerative joint disease are cavities in the subchondral bone with a synovial-like lining and peripheral osteoclastic bone lysis and fibrosis. Presumably, they arise secondary to fissures in the overlying cartilage or eburnated bone, allowing synovial fluid to be forced into the subchondral bone. These appear to be more common in human beings than domestic animals, and this might reflect the longer duration of the lesions in human beings. The Hartley guinea pig spontaneously develops degenerative joint disease in the stifles before 1 year of age. Subchondral cysts are present in the proximal tibial articular surface, and in this model they appear to be invaginations of synovial membranes surrounding the cruciate ligaments as they insert into the subchondral bone.

DEGENERATION OF INTERVERTEBRAL DISKS

Degeneration of the intervertebral disks is often an age-related phenomenon in many species. In general, loss of water and proteoglycans, reduced cellularity, and an increase in collagen content of the nucleus pulposus occur, so that the distinction between the nucleus pulposus and the annulus fibrosus is obscured. The central part of the disk is yellow-brown and is composed of friable fibrocartilaginous material (Fig. 16-87). These degenerative changes are likely caused by various metabolic and mechanical insults that lead to a breakdown of proteoglycan aggregates in the nucleus pulposus and to degenerative changes in the annulus fibrosus. Both rotational and compressive types of movement injure the annulus fibrosus. Changes in structure of the nucleus pulposus, together with a weakened annulus,

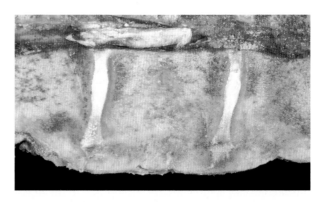

Fig. 16-86   Ankylosing spondylosis, joints, intervertebral, bull. Periosteal new bone formation on the ventral and lateral periosteal surfaces (not visible in this plane of section) of the vertebrae is called spondylosis and can be a result of mechanical instability or excess mechanical stress on the intervertebral discs (joints). The bony proliferation (ventrally) has bridged the joint space between the adjacent vertebrae and caused fusion (ankylosis) or ankylosing spondylosis. *(Courtesy Dr. S.E. Weisbrode, College of Veterinary Medicine, The Ohio State University.)*

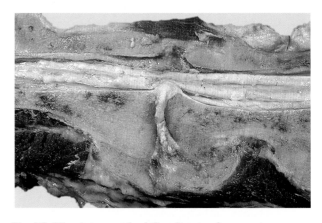

Fig. 16-87   Intervertebral disc disease, degenerate intervertebral disc, prolapsed disc, ankylosing spondylosis, intervertebral joint, dog. Dorsal protrusion of a degenerate nucleus pulposus has compressed the spinal cord. Marked ventral ankylosis (coalescing periarticular osteophyte formation) is secondary to the instability of the joint. *(Courtesy J. King, College of Veterinary Medicine, Cornell University.)*

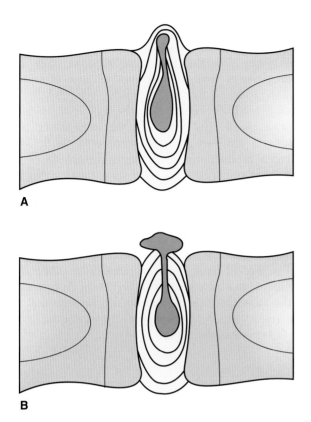

A

B

Fig. 16-88   Schematic diagram illustrating stages of prolapse of the nucleus pulposus in intervertebral disc disease. **A,** Prolapse of the nucleus pulposus may be secondary to partial rupture of the annulus fibrosus. **B,** Complete rupture of the annulus fibrosus allows extrusion of the nucleus pulposus into the vertebral canal.

often lead to concentric and radial tears or fissures in the annulus that allow bulging or herniation of the nucleus pulposus material (Fig. 16-88). Herniation is usually dorsal in domestic animals. In human beings (rarely in domestic animals), disk material can be extruded through the end plate into the vertebral body, producing a lesion known as Schmorl's node.

In chondrodystrophic breeds of dogs, such as the dachshund, chondroid metaplasia of the nucleus pulposus is followed by calcification during the first year of life. These alterations can result in disk prolapse, with total rupture of the annulus fibrosus and extrusion of disk material into the vertebral canal at sites of mechanical stress, such as the cervical and thoracolumbar vertebrae.

Senile degenerative disk disease is independent of breed in the dog and also occurs in human beings, pigs, and horses. These lesions are characterized by progressive dehydration and collagenization of the nucleus pulposus and degeneration of the annulus fibrosus. The lesions develop slowly, and calcification is rare. Prolapse of the disk is secondary to partial rupture of the annulus fibrosus and is characterized by bulging of

the dorsal surface of the disk into the vertebral canal. An important consequence of degeneration of intervertebral disks is prolapse of the disk. Prolapse or herniation can be dorsal (spinal cord compression) or lateral (spinal nerve compression and entrapment). Because each intervertebral joint is a three-joint complex (intervertebral joint and two facet joints), the reduced disk thickness that follows degeneration and dehydration allows overriding of articular facets and some degree of joint instability. These changes contribute to the evolution of degenerative disease and enlargement of articular facets. Enlargement of the facets can cause impingement on spinal nerves and even compression of the spinal canal because the medial aspect of these facets is adjacent to the intervertebral foramen. Degeneration of intervertebral disks and the ensuing intervertebral joint instability can result in the development of osteophytes on the ends of the vertebral bodies around or adjacent to the disk (spondylosis) in many species, such as dogs, cattle, pigs, and horses. Vertebral osteophytes are usually ventral and lateral; if dorsal, they can cause stenosis of the vertebral canal.

NEOPLASMS OF JOINTS

Essentially only malignant tumors are recognized as primary neoplasms within joints, and these arise from the synovial membrane but vary notably in their metastatic potential. These tumors are uncommon in dogs and very rare in other species. Articular cartilage, likely because of the limited ability of chondrocytes to divide, is not known to give rise to neoplasms. Two different malignancies of the synovium are recognized. One is derived from histiocytic cells and is called a histiocytic sarcoma. If the histiocytic malignancy is multicentric (present at multiple sites) the term *malignant histiocytosis* is used. If present as a single focus, it is called a histiocytic sarcoma. When presenting at multiple sites, it cannot be determined if this is a histiocytic sarcoma with metastasis or a truly multicentric malignant histiocytosis. As the name implies, these cells have a histiocytic phenotype; atypia is sometimes extreme with bizarre mitotic figures and pronounced pleomorphism. Histiocytic sarcomas have a high chance of distant metastasis.

Synovial cell sarcoma is the term given to a malignancy of synovial fibrocyte origin (Fig. 16-89). These are more common in joints, but synovia of tendon sheaths can be involved. These malignant cells are negative for histiocytic cell markers, positive for mesenchymal markers (vimentin), and inexplicably, a small percent of the malignant cells with a fibrocytic phenotype are positive for epithelial markers (cytokeratins). Such epithelial cell expression is not found in the synovia of normal joints. In human beings, there is a characteristic gene translocation that occurs in synovial cell sarcomas.

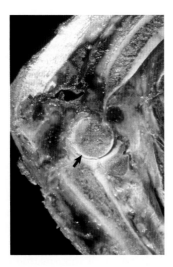

Fig. 16-89   Synovial cell sarcoma, joint, elbow, dog.
Synovial cell sarcoma presenting as a tan and hemorrhagic mass (*left*) within the joint has invaded into the distal humeral condyle (*arrow*) and caused pronounced lysis of the proximal ulna. (*Courtesy Dr. S.E. Weisbrode, College of Veterinary Medicine, The Ohio State University.*)

Synovial cell sarcomas have a moderate to low chance of distant metastasis. Some fibrocytic cell tumors in the synovium have notable myxomatous metaplasia and have been called myxomas and benign because of the absence of distant metastasis. However, because of their ability to invade bone, these should also be considered low-grade malignancies. The lesions described later are for the fibrocytic synovial cell sarcoma and not histiocytic sarcoma.

Articular cartilage: Articular cartilage is usually not affected other than secondarily as a result of a loss of subchondral bone support by the invading malignancy.

Articular capsule/synovium/synovial fluid: Synovium can be markedly and asymmetrically thickened with a gray to tan mass that has variable hemorrhage. The masses can be firm to gelatinous because of myxoid matrix produced by the neoplastic cells. Usually the mass is relatively confined to the region of the joint. Microscopically the mass has the appearance of a moderate- to low-grade fibrosarcoma, with little collagen production. Myxomatous metaplasia of the malignant cells can be seen in some cases giving the tumor a myxosarcoma appearance.

Subchondral bone: Radiographically, there is evidence of invasion into bone, usually on both sides of the joint space. However, this bone invasion can be subtle and often not apparent on gross examination. Subchondral and periosteal bone lysis can range from minimal to extensive but characteristically is present on both sides of the joint space. Sometimes it can be seen that the malignancy invades the epiphysis by way of the canals for the epiphyseal vessels.

SUGGESTED READINGS

Bullough PG: *Atlas of orthopedic pathology with clinical and radiographic correlations*, Philadelphia, 1992, JB Lippincott.

Palmer N: Bones and joints. In Jubb KVF, Kennedy PC, Palmer N, editors: *Pathology of domestic animals*, ed 4, San Diego, 1992, Academic Press.

Pool RR, Thompson KG: Tumors of joints. In Meuten DJ, editor: *Tumors of domestic animals*, ed 4, Ames, 2002, Iowa State Press.

Thompson KG, Pool RR: Tumors of bones. In Meuten DJ, editor: *Tumors of domestic animals*, ed 4, Ames, 2002, Iowa State Press.

Vigorita VJ: *Orthopedic pathology*, Philadelphia, 1999, Lippincott Williams & Wilkins.

Woodard JC: Skeletal system. In Jones TC, Hunt RD, King NW, editors: *Veterinary pathology*, ed 6, Baltimore, 1997, Williams & Wilkins.

APPENDIX **16-1**

POSTMORTEM EXAMINATION AND EVALUATION OF BONES

The entire skeleton is rarely examined at necropsy. Instead, the extent of the examination is dictated by the clinical history. Antemortem clinical and radiographic findings are valuable and should be in hand before the postmortem examination is begun, especially for cases suspected of having relatively small localized lesions. It should be remembered that a lesion responsible for lameness may involve the skeletal, muscular, or nervous systems.

Pathologists should routinely examine certain areas of the skeleton. This procedure provides completeness to the necropsy and leads to familiarity with normal osseous structures. At least one long bone should be cut longitudinally and examined at necropsy. This examination should include an assessment of marrow for fat cell stores and hemopoietic activity, thickness of cortical bone, amount and distribution of cancellous bone, thickness and uniformity of metaphyseal growth plates, articular surfaces, and tendon insertions. In small animals, testing bone strength by breaking a rib can be informative, but because of the marked variation in sizes of small animals, this becomes very relative. More important than the strength required to break a rib is noting the degree to which the rib will bend before breaking. Increased pliability might indicate fibrous osteodystrophy. Bony tissues are more readily seen if bone marrow contents are flushed out with a jet of water. Some lesions can be best visualized radiographically. Postmortem radiographs of slabs of bones or entire bones with much of the soft tissue removed can be very informative. Postmortem autolytic changes do not usually pose major problems in the evaluation of the skeleton at necropsy. Postmortem bacterial invasion is less rapid than in most other tissue, and bone marrow cultures can be useful in detecting bacteremia (e.g., salmonellosis). Bones can be fractured at euthanasia and by postmortem transport and handling. Postmortem fracture of bones will not be associated with hemorrhage in bone or adjacent soft tissue. Fracture of bones during euthanasia could be difficult to distinguish from recent fracture, especially if recent antemortem trauma was reported in the history. However, as in a postmortem bone fracture, less blood from hard and soft tissue is expected in agonal fracturing of bones.

POSTMORTEM EXAMINATION AND EVALUATION OF JOINTS

Several large synovial joints, such as the shoulder and hip, should be opened and examined routinely at necropsy to become familiar with the expected age-related changes in cartilage. Septicemic joint disease may not affect these larger joints, and when suspected, many joints should be examined, including the carpal and tarsal joints. Joints should be disarticulated so that articular surfaces, synovial fluid, and all associated structures are clearly visible. Consideration should be given to aspirating synovial fluid before disarticulation to obtain a sample free of contamination and suitable for culture and analysis that includes viscosity (mucin precipitation), cell count, and cytology. Articular cartilage must be examined as soon as the joint is opened because dehydration of cartilage occurs rapidly on exposure to air. Fine finger-like proliferations of synovium (villous hypertrophy) are best evaluated if the specimen is submerged in water, saline, or formalin. Microscopic examination of synovium might be required to confirm the presence of synovitis.

17

The Integument

ANN M. HARGIS • PAMELA E. GINN

INTRODUCTION

BASIC FUNCTION, STRUCTURE, AND HOST DEFENSE MECHANISMS OF THE INTEGUMENT

FUNCTIONS OF THE SKIN

The skin is not only the largest organ in the body, but one of the most important. Without the skin, terrestrial mammalian life could not exist. The skin has numerous functions, which are listed in Box 17-1. The skin prevents significant loss of fluid and electrolytes (e.g., the stratum corneum barrier), protects against physical and chemical injury (e.g., the stratum corneum barrier, keratin filaments, desmosomal and hemidesmosomal junctions, collagen, and elastic fibers), participates in temperature and blood pressure regulation (e.g., the hair coat, sweat glands, and vascular supply), produces vitamin D (e.g., ultraviolet light photolysis of dehydrocholesterol), serves as a sensory organ (e.g., tactile hairs, Merkel cells, and nerves), and stores fat, water, vitamins, carbohydrates, protein, and other nutrients (e.g., subcutaneous fat). Absorption, although not a primary function, also occurs. In addition, the keratinocyte, a major source of cytokines and antimicrobial peptides, is now considered to be an integral part of the innate and adaptive immune systems protecting against microbial injury and participating in inflammation and tissue repair.

MORPHOLOGY OF THE SKIN

The skin is the largest organ in the body and has haired and hairless portions (Figs. 17-1 and 17-2). The skin consists of epidermis, dermis, subcutis, and adnexa (hair follicles and sebaceous, sweat, and other glands). The histologic structure varies greatly among different sites and among different species of animals. The haired skin is thickest over the dorsal aspect of the body and on the lateral aspect of the limbs, and is thinnest on the ventral aspect of the body and the medial aspect of the thighs. Haired skin has a thinner epidermis, whereas nonhaired skin of the nose and footpads has a thicker epidermis (Figs. 17-1 and 17-2). The skin of large animals is generally thicker than the skin of small animals. The subcutis, consisting of lobules of adipose tissue and fascia, connects the more superficial layers (epidermis and dermis) with the underlying fascia and musculature.

EPIDERMIS

The epidermis is divided into layers based on the morphology of the keratinocyte, the major cell type of the epidermis. The epidermis of haired skin consists of four basic layers (stratum corneum, stratum granulosum, stratum spinosum, and stratum basale) (Fig. 17-3). The epidermis of hairless skin consists of five layers; the fifth layer is the stratum lucidum, which is located between the stratum granulosum and stratum corneum. Keratinocytes originate from germinal cells in the stratum basale of the epidermis, ascend through the layers of the epidermis,

---

Box 17-1

Functions of the Skin

Provides a protective barrier against fluid loss, microbiologic agents, chemicals, and physical injury
Regulates temperature and blood pressure
Produces vitamin D
Acts as sensory organ
Stores nutrients
Absorptive surface
Participates in innate and adaptive immunity and inflammation and repair

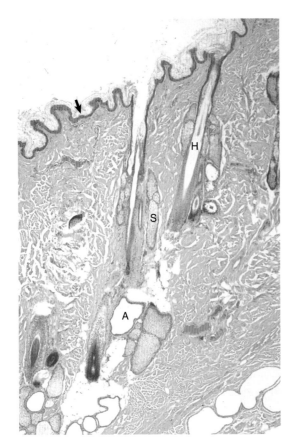

Fig. 17-1   Normal skin, haired, thorax, dog. The epidermis *(arrow)* in haired skin has an undulating surface but lacks rete ridges. The epidermis in haired skin has fewer nucleated cell layers than the epidermis in nonhaired (hairless) skin such as the nose and footpads (Fig. 17-2); thus it is referred to as "thin" skin. Hair follicles *(H)*, apocrine glands *(A)*, and sebaceous glands *(S)* are present. The haired skin is thickest over the dorsal aspect of the body and on the lateral aspect of the limbs, and it is thinnest on the ventral aspect of the body and the medial aspect of the thighs. H&E stain. *(Courtesy Dr. Ann M. Hargis, DermatoDiagnostics.)*

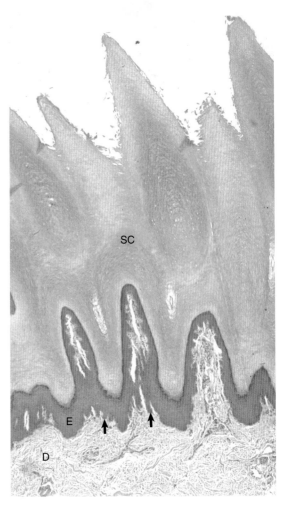

Fig. 17-2   Normal skin, hairless, footpad, dog. The epidermis *(E)* in hairless (nonhaired) skin has more numerous nucleated cell layers and more abundant stratum corneum than the epidermis in haired skin; thus it is referred to as "thick" skin. Note the dense zone of compact stratum corneum *(SC)* over the surface. The epidermis and dermal papillae *(D)* interdigitate to form rete ridges *(arrows)*. The rete ridges strengthen the attachment between the epidermis and dermis. In the dog, the contour of the epidermal surface follows the epidermal ridges and thus is papillated. H&E stain. *(Courtesy Dr. Ann M. Hargis, DermatoDiagnostics.)*

differentiating in each layer until they reach the stratum corneum. Keratinocytes are continuously shed from the stratum corneum. The time of transit for a keratinocyte in the stratum basale to shedding at the stratum corneum is approximately 1 month, although this time can be accelerated in some disorders, such as primary seborrhea characterized clinically by scaling.

The outermost layer of the epidermis is the stratum corneum, which consists of many sheets of flattened, keratinized cells termed corneocytes. Keratin is an intracellular fibrous protein that is in part responsible for the toughness of the epidermis, enabling the epidermis to form a protective barrier. The next layer is the stratum granulosum, which consists of effete cells with basophilic keratohyalin granules. In nonhaired skin,

the stratum corneum and stratum granulosum are separated by an additional layer of compacted, fully keratinized cells, the stratum lucidum, best seen in the footpad. Deep to the stratum granulosum is the stratum spinosum, a layer of polyhedral-shaped cells attached to one another by desmosomes. During fixation and processing for microscopic examination, the cells of the stratum spinosum contract, except for the desmosomal attachments. These attachment sites create the appearance of "spines" or intercellular bridges, leading to the

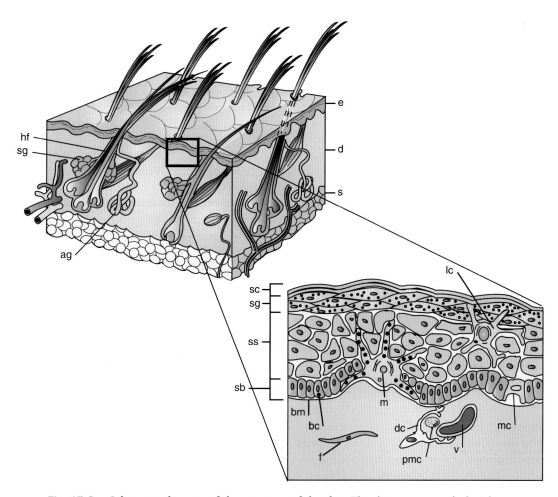

Fig. 17-3   Schematic diagram of the structure of the skin. The skin is composed of epidermis (*e*), dermis (*d*), and subcutis (*s*), with adnexa consisting of hair follicles (*hf*), sebaceous glands (*sg*), and apocrine glands (*ag*). **B,** This projection of the epidermis demonstrates the progressive upward maturation of basal cells (*bc*) in the stratum basale (*sb*) through the stratum spinosum (*ss*), stratum granulosum (*sg*) into the cornified squamous epithelial cells of the stratum corneum (*sc*). Melanocytes (*m*), midepidermal dendritic Langerhans' cells (*lc*), and Merkel cells (*mc*) are also present. The subjacent dermis contains small vessels (*v*), fibroblasts (*f*), perivascular mast cells (*pmc*), and dendrocytes (*dc*), potentially important in dermal immunity and repair. *(Adapted from Cotran RS, Kumar V, Collins T, Robbins SL: Robbins pathologic basis of disease, ed 6, Philadelphia, 1999, Saunders; and Gawkrodger DJ: Dermatology: an illustrated colour text, ed 2, New York, 1997, Churchill Livingstone.)*

name of this layer. The visibility of the intercellular bridges is enhanced when there is intercellular edema of the epidermis. The stratum spinosum in haired areas is thinner in dogs and cats and is thicker in cattle, horses, and pigs. The innermost layer of the epidermis is the germinal layer or stratum basale, which consists of a single layer of cuboidal cells resting on a basement membrane. Intermixed within the basal cell layer are melanocytes, Langerhans' cells, and Merkel cells.

Melanocytes, embryologically derived from neural crest cells, are also present in lower layers of the stratum spinosum and produce melanin pigment, giving skin and hair their color. Melanocytic granules are transferred to and distributed in keratinocytes as a caplike cluster of granules between the nucleus and the external surface of the skin to help protect the nucleus from ultraviolet light–induced injury. Langerhans' cells are bone marrow–derived cells of monocyte-macrophage lineage that process and present antigen to sensitized T lymphocytes, thereby modulating immunologic responses of the skin. Langerhans' cells are present in the basal, spinous, and granular layers of the epidermis but have a preference for a suprabasal position. Merkel cells are neuroendocrine cells located in the basal layer that join with keratinocytes via desmosomal junctions. Merkel cells are located in haired and hairless skin, particularly in regions of the body with high tactile sensitivity (digits and lips), and in the outer portion of hair follicles. In some sites, Merkel cells are present in tylotrich pads where they form a Merkel cell–neurite complex. Merkel cells have granules that contain neurotransmitter-like substances (met-enkephalin, vasoactive intestinal peptide, chromogranin A, acetylcholine, calcitonin gene-related peptide, neuron-specific enolase, and synaptophysin). The specific role these substances play in paracrine or autocrine control of keratinocytes or hair follicle epithelial cells remains speculative. Merkel cells also function as slowly adapting mechanoreceptors.

BASEMENT MEMBRANE ZONE

The epidermis and dermis are separated by a basement membrane. In hairless areas, such as the footpads and nasal planum, this junction is irregular because of epidermal projections that interdigitate with dermal papillae (e.g., rete ridges/a.k.a. rete pegs), thus strengthening the epidermal-dermal attachment by providing resistance to shearing. In densely haired areas, the junction is smoother and has an undulating appearance as the epidermal-dermal attachment is strengthened by the hair follicles. The more sparsely haired skin of pigs has more epidermal-dermal interdigitations (rete ridges) and fewer hair follicles. The basement membrane zone is composed of hemidesmosomes of basal cells (i.e., tonofilaments and attachment plaques), the lamina lucida (plasma membrane, subdesmosomal dense plate, and anchoring filaments), and the lamina densa (i.e., type IV collagen), which also serve to anchor the epidermis to dermis (Fig. 17-4). The importance of the basement membrane in anchoring function is noted in some immune-mediated diseases where antibodies bind to a component in the basement membrane and result in the formation of bullae (see Selected Autoimmune Reactions, Reactions Characterized Grossly by Vesicles or Bullae as the Primary Lesion and Histologically by Vesicles or Bullae within the Basement Membrane [Bullous Dermatoses]). The basement membrane zone also serves as a scaffold for migration of epidermal cells in wound healing and as an initial barrier to invasion of the dermis by neoplastic epidermal cells.

DERMIS

The dermis (corium), consisting of collagen and elastic fibers in a glycosaminoglycan ground substance, supports hair follicles, glands, vessels, and nerves. By convention, the dermis is generally subdivided into superficial and deep layers that blend together without a clear line of demarcation. The superficial dermis conforms to the contour of the epidermis and generally supports the upper portion of the hair follicle and sebaceous glands. It is composed of fine collagen fibers and is wider in the skin of cattle and horses than in the skin of dogs and cats. The deep dermis supports the lower portion of the hair follicle and apocrine glands and is composed of collagen bundles larger than those in the superficial dermis. Smooth muscle fibers of the arrector pili muscle attach the connective tissue sheath of the hair follicle to the epidermis and are responsible for causing the hair to stand erect. Skeletal muscle fibers from the cutaneous muscle extend into the lower dermis and are responsible for voluntary skin movement. Mast cells, lymphocytes, plasma cells, macrophages, and rarely eosinophils and neutrophils can be found in normal dermis. These cells are bone marrow derived-cells and arrive via the blood vascular system; thus they are typically concentrated around small superficial blood vessels.

VESSELS AND NERVES

Cutaneous arteries give rise to three vascular plexuses: deep, middle, and superficial. The deep plexus supplies

Fig. 17-4   **Schematic diagram of basement membrane structure of the skin.** Keratinocytes attach to each other via desmosomes and to the basement membrane via hemidesmosomes. The projection of the basement membrane zone illustrates the multiple, interconnecting layers of this zone. The most superficial layer consists of the basal layer hemidesmosomes (tonofilaments and attachment plaques). The next layer, the lamina lucida, is an electron-lucent zone composed of the plasma membrane (not labeled), subdesmosomal dense plate, and anchoring filaments. The deepest layer is the lamina densa, an electron-dense zone that consists of type IV collagen. Collagen rootlets extend from the lamina densa for a short distance into the papillary dermis, and microfibrils, long delicate elastic fibrils, blend with underlying elastic structure of the dermis. The interconnecting layers of the basement membrane zone provide an important function in epidermal-dermal adherence, are the site of immune reactant deposition in cutaneous disease (Table 17-12), and serve as a barrier to invasion by malignant epidermal tumors. *ag*, Apocrine glands; *d*, dermis; *e*, epidermis; *hf*, hair follicles; *s*, subcutis; *sg*, sebaceous glands. *(Adapted from Cotran RS, Kumar V, Collins T, Robbins SL: Robbins pathologic basis of disease, ed 6, Philadelphia, 1999, Saunders; and Rubin E, Farber JL: Pathology, ed 3, Philadelphia, 1999, Lippincott-Raven.)*

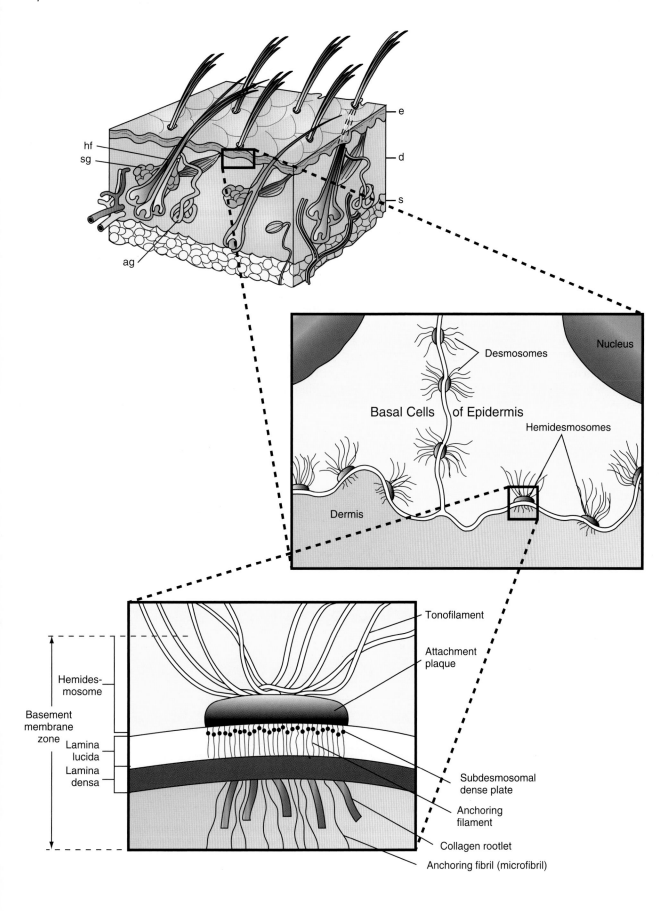

the subcutis and deep portions of follicles and apocrine glands; the middle plexus supplies the sebaceous glands, midportion of follicles, and arrector pili muscles; and the superficial plexus supplies the superficial portions of follicles and epidermis. Lymph capillaries arise in the superficial dermis and connect with a subcutaneous plexus. The lymph vessels then converge to form larger channels that eventually reach peripheral lymph nodes.

The skin is an important sensory organ containing millions of microscopic nerve endings that perceive itch, pain, temperature, pressure, and touch (Fig. 17-5). The nerve endings consist of Meissner's corpuscles, pacinian corpuscles (Pacini's corpuscles), free sensory nerve endings, and mucocutaneous end organs (similar to Meissner's corpuscles but located in mucocutaneous skin). These nerve endings are minute, and the free sensory nerve endings are so delicate that they require special staining techniques, such as silver impregnation, to be visualized microscopically. The sensations of itch, pain, touch, temperature, and displacement of body hair are detected by the free sensory nerve endings. Itching, a form of mild pain that promotes the desire to scratch, is one of the most common reasons animals are presented to veterinarians. The sensations of touch and pressure are detected by Meissner and Pacini's corpuscles.

Sensations detected by free sensory nerve endings and by the corpuscles are transmitted to the spinal cord via the dorsal root ganglia. Sensory fibers to the facial area are supplied by the trigeminal nerve. Motor fibers (adrenergic and cholinergic) are supplied by the sympathetic component of the autonomic nervous system (Fig. 17-5). Adrenergic fibers travel from the spinal cord through postganglionic fibers in peripheral nerves and arborize into plexuses that innervate blood vessels, arrector pili muscles, and apocrine sweat glands. Stimulation by these adrenergic fibers causes vasoconstriction and piloerection (raising of the hair shafts). Cholinergic fibers travel from the spinal cord and arborize into plexuses that innervate the eccrine sweat glands. Stimulation of these fibers in human beings causes widespread eccrine sweating, important in thermoregulation and recognized clinically as "beads of sweat" on the skin. Because the eccrine ducts open directly on the surface of the skin, the secretion is more easily seen clinically. This phenomenon does not occur in dogs or cats because they lack eccrine glands in haired skin. However, cholinergic and to a lesser degree adrenergic fiber stimulation in dogs and cats causes sweating of the eccrine glands of footpads at times of excitement or agitation. Physiologic control of sweating in horses is

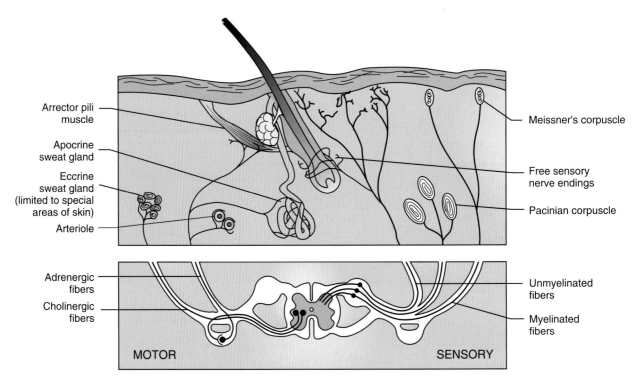

Fig. 17-5   Schematic diagram of cutaneous innervation. Unmyelinated cutaneous nerve endings transmit sensations of touch, pressure, temperature, pain, and itch via dorsal root ganglia to the central nervous system. Motor fibers in skin are supplied by the autonomic nervous system. Adrenergic fibers activate arterioles, arrector pili muscles, and apocrine glands; cholinergic fibers stimulate eccrine glands. *(Adapted from Ackerman AB: Histologic diagnosis of inflammatory skin diseases, Philadelphia, 1978, Lea and Febiger.)*

primarily neural due to adrenergic fiber stimulation of apocrine glands, but a humoral component mediated by adrenergic agonists released from the adrenal medulla into the circulation also plays a role during exercise. Eccrine sweat glands have not been described in the horse. The only other domestic animal in which apocrine gland secretion is thought to play a thermoregulatory role is cattle, but sweating is not typically clinically visible except in horses.

SUBCUTIS (PANNICULUS, HYPODERMIS)

The subcutis attaches the dermis to subjacent muscle or bone and consists of adipose tissue and collagenous and elastic fibers, which provide flexibility. Adipose tissue insulates against temperature variation and, in the case of footpads, serves in shock absorption.

ADNEXA
Hair follicles

The growth of hair occurs within hair follicles in a sequence of stages (Fig. 17-6). These stages include hair genesis, growth, maturation, and loss. In the anagen stage of the hair cycle, mitotic activity and growth occur. The catagen stage is a transitional phase during which cellular proliferation ceases. The follicle then enters a

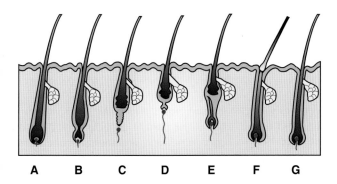

A   B   C   D   E   F   G

Fig. 17-6 **Schematic diagram of the hair cycle. A,** Anagen. During this growing stage, hair is produced by mitosis in epithelial cells covering the apex of the follicular papilla (dermal papilla), which is enveloped by hair matrix cells at the hair bulb. **B,** Early catagen. In this transitional stage, a constriction occurs at the hair bulb, and the hair shaft above this becomes a "club hair." **C,** Catagen. The distal follicle becomes thick and corrugated and pushes the hair outward. **D,** Telogen. This is the resting stage in which the dermal (follicular) papilla separates and an epithelial strand shortens to form a secondary germ. **E,** Early anagen. The secondary germ grows down to enclose the dermal (follicular) papilla, and a new hair bulb forms. **F,** Exogen. This refers to the shedding of the old hair shaft. **G,** Anagen. The hair elongates as growth continues. Note that the anagen hair bulbs are located deeper in the dermis than the catagen and telogen hair bulbs. (**A** through **G,** *From Scott DW, Miller WH Jr, Griffin CE: Muller and Kirk's small animal dermatology, ed 6, Philadelphia, 2001, Saunders.*)

resting stage, telogen, after which mitotic activity and new hair production resumes. The exogen stage is the phase in which the old hair is shed. In many animals hair follicle growth occurs in cycles, resulting in periodic loss or shedding of the hair coat. The reason the hair growth occurs in cycles is not clear. Some hypotheses include that the cycle provides the ability: (1) to shed fur to cleanse the body surface, (2) to adapt and change body cover in response to changing environment (winter to summer) or social conditions, or (3) to protect against malignant transformation that might occur in a rapidly dividing tissue. The regulation of hair cycling is exceedingly complex and incompletely understood. Factors that play a role include genetics, photoperiod, temperature, nutrition, hormones, health status, and neural mechanisms. Genetic factors determine the hair shaft length (e.g., short-haired versus long-haired breeds of dogs). The exact signals that control the hair cycle have not been identified; however, growth factors, such as epidermal growth factor, fibroblast growth factor, hepatocyte growth factor, platelet-derived growth factor, transforming growth factor-β (TGF-β), and insulin-like growth factor, have been localized to the skin and hair follicles. These growth factors probably play a crucial role in regulation of the hair cycle and follicle growth.

Photoperiod acts via the hypothalamus, pituitary, and pineal glands, which secrete tropic hormones, such as melatonin and gonadal, thyroid, and adrenal hormones, that also influence hair growth. Some hormones, such as thyroid and growth hormone, stimulate hair growth, whereas excessive levels of estrogen or glucocorticoids suppress hair growth. The cells in the follicular papilla (sometimes called dermal papilla) regulate epithelial growth and are probably the target of the tropic hormones. Nutrition and health status have a significant influence on hair growth and quality. Hair is largely composed of protein. Thus diets low in protein or disease states associated with severe protein loss result in poor quality hair coat. Animals in poor health have larger numbers of hair follicles in telogen, and because telogen hairs are more easily shed than anagen hairs, animals in poor health tend to shed more heavily than healthy animals. Also, in disease states, cuticle formation can be defective, resulting in a dull or dry hair coat. It is also thought that the hair cycle is influenced by the nervous system. Evidence of such is implied by the abundant nerve supply of the hair follicle, the high density of Merkel cells in the hair follicle epithelium, and facts that keratinocytes express several neurotransmitter and neuropeptide receptors whose stimulation can alter keratinocyte proliferation and differentiation. Indirect influence by autonomic nerves could also be mediated by alteration of hair follicle blood flow and thus of oxygen and nutrient supply.

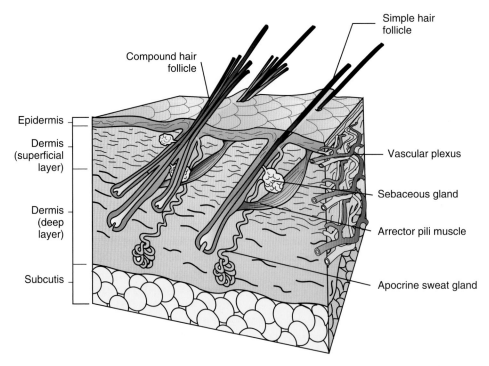

Fig. 17-7 **Schematic diagram of the skin and simple and compound hair follicles.** For the purpose of simplification, the vascular supply is illustrated on one face only. Note the simple hair follicle *(right)* and the compound hair follicle *(left)*. Simple follicles consist of one large primary follicle with the hair bulb in the dermis or subcutis (depth varies with species), and with sebaceous and apocrine glands, and arrector pili muscles. Compound follicles consist of a large primary follicle and smaller secondary follicles. The hair bulbs of secondary follicles are located more superficially in the dermis than the hair bulbs of primary follicles. Secondary follicles may have sebaceous glands but lack apocrine glands and arrector pili muscles. *(From Dellman DH, Brown EM: Textbook of veterinary histology, ed 3, Philadelphia, 1987, Lea and Febiger.)*

Forms of hair follicles vary in different animals (Fig. 17-7). Cattle and horses have evenly distributed simple follicles with one large (i.e., primary) follicle, usually with sebaceous and apocrine glands and arrector pili muscles. Pigs have simple follicles grouped in clusters. Goats, dogs, and cats have compound follicles that consist of primary follicles and smaller secondary follicles. Sheep have simple follicles in hair-growing areas and compound follicles in wool-growing areas. Primary follicles have the hair bulb rooted more deeply in the dermis than secondary follicles. The depth of the hair bulbs varies with species. In dogs and cats, the anagen hair bulbs of primary follicles are at the dermal-subcutaneous junction, whereas in horses and cattle the anagen hair bulbs are in the mid dermis. In all species, the bases of telogen follicles are more superficially located than the bases of anagen follicles. Typically, primary and secondary hair shafts emerge through a common follicular opening. Tactile hairs include sinus and tylotrich hairs. Sinus hairs, also termed vibrissae, arise in simple follicles with a blood-filled sinus located between the inner and outer layers of the dermal sheath. Sinus hairs

generally occur on the nose, above the eyes, on the lips and throat, and on the palmar aspect of the carpus of cats. Sinus hairs function as mechanoreceptors (i.e., touch receptors). Tylotrich hairs also function as mechanoreceptors and are scattered among the regular body hairs. The arrector pili muscles extend from the connective tissue sheath of the hair follicles at the junction of the middle and inferior portion of the follicle and attach to the superficial dermis. The arrector pili smooth muscles are oriented almost perpendicularly to the wall of the follicle, and are well developed on the back of animals, especially dogs. Muscle contraction causes erection of hairs and expression of the contents of sebaceous glands.

Sweat glands

There are two basic types of sweat glands: apocrine glands and eccrine glands. Apocrine glands are located throughout haired areas of skin in domestic animals and are tubular- or saccular-coiled glands. The ducts of the apocrine glands open in the superficial portion of the hair follicle; thus these glands are also called "epitrichial glands." The glands are lined by secretory cuboidal to low columnar epithelium surrounded by contractile myoepithelial cells. Other apocrine glands include the interdigital glands of small ruminants, glands of the external ear canal and eyelids of domestic animals, anal sac glands of dogs and cats, and the mental organ of pigs. Eccrine glands are merocrine in secretion and, in contrast to ducts of apocrine glands, the ducts open directly onto the surface of the epidermis. Thus eccrine glands are also called "atrichial glands." They are tubular glands lined by cuboidal epithelium surrounded by myoepithelium and are confined mainly to footpads of dogs and cats, frog region of ungulates, carpus of pigs, and nasolabial region of ruminants and pigs.

Sebaceous glands

Sebaceous glands are simple, branched, or compound alveolar glands that undergo holocrine secretion, with ducts opening into hair follicles except at some mucocutaneous junctions where the glands open on the surface of the skin (e.g., meibomian gland/a.k.a. tarsal gland). Well-developed sebaceous glands are found in the supracaudal gland of dogs and cats; infraorbital, inguinal, and interdigital regions of sheep; the base of the horn of goats; the anal sac glands of cats; the preputial glands of horses; and the submental organ of cats.

Specialized structures

Anal sacs are specialized cutaneous structures that are especially prone to develop lesions. Anal sacs are bilateral diverticula located between internal and external anal sphincter muscles in dogs and cats, and have ducts that open onto the anus at the level of the anocutaneous junction. Ducts and sacs are lined by stratified squamous epithelium. In cats, the sac wall has sebaceous and apocrine glands, but in dogs the wall has only apocrine glands. The anal sacs can become distended with secretory products, rupture following trauma, and cause bacterial infection and chronic inflammation (foreign body reaction) in contiguous tissues.

Hepatoid (i.e., circumanal or perianal) glands occur most commonly in the skin around the anus and are also present in skin near the prepuce, tail, flank, and groin. These glands have nonpatent ducts and are composed of peripheral reserve cells that surround lobules of differentiated cells resembling hepatocytes, resulting in the name "hepatoid" glands.

The claws of dogs and cats shield the third phalanx and consist of a wall (i.e., dorsal and lateral sides) and sole (i.e., ventral side), both of which are stratified squamous keratinizing epithelium. The wall consists of hard keratin and the sole of softer keratin. The dermis of the claw consists of dense collagen, elastic tissue, and blood vessels that can bleed profusely if the claw is trimmed too short. The claw fold is a fold of skin that covers the wall laterally and dorsally for a short distance. Hooves consist of the wall, sole, and frog in solipeds; and a wall, sole, and prominent bulb in ruminants and pigs. The hoof wall comprises three structurally distinct layers (i.e., stratum externum, stratum medium, and stratum internum), which are formed by the proliferation and downward movement of epidermal cells arising from a specialized junction of the epidermis and dermis, a region known as the coronary band. The stratum internum interdigitates with the dermal collagen, thereby anchoring the hoof to the dermis. In general, the deeper portion of the dermis blends with the periosteum of the third phalanx.

The digital pads of dogs and cats have a thick epidermis composed of all layers, including the stratum lucidum. The surface is covered by compacted layers of stratum corneum and is smooth in the cat; however, in the dog, the surface is covered by conical papillae that conform to the outline of the epidermal surface (Fig 17-2). The epidermis and dermis interdigitate via rete ridges and dermal papillae, thus providing resistance to shear forces. Eccrine (atrichial) glands are present in the dermis and the adipose tissue. Lobules of adipose tissue that act as a cushion are subdivided by collagenous stroma and elastic tissue.

The chestnuts and ergots of the horse are considered to be vestiges of the first, second, and fourth digits. Chestnuts are located in the supracarpal and tarsal area on the medial surface of the limbs, and the ergot is located at the flexion of the fetlocks (metacarpophalangeal articulation). Chestnuts and ergots are histologically similar, and consist of compact stratum corneum covering thick cellular layers of the epidermis. The rete ridges are long and interdigitate with long dermal papillae.

PORTALS OF ENTRY INTO THE SKIN

Normal intact skin has many natural defenses and barriers that render it impenetrable to most organisms and protect the body from a variety of other types of insults that include pressure, friction, mild mechanical trauma, temperature extremes, ultraviolet light exposure, and chemical absorption.

The route by which an infectious agent gains entry into the body is called the portal of entry (Box 17-2). Many pathogens can only cause disease when entering the body via their specific portal of entry. A few pathogens, such as hookworm larvae, are able to penetrate intact normally functioning skin. Dermatophytes are able to colonize the cornified structures (hair, claws) and the stratum corneum, and cause disease without ever entering living tissue. Clinical disease in a dermatophyte infection is the result of the host's reaction to the organism and its byproducts. The skin only becomes an

Box **17-2**

Portals of Entry into the Skin

EPIDERMIS

Absorption through stratum corneum and epidermis
Penetrating trauma, including injection from exterior
Penetration of ultraviolet or γ-radiation
Direct contact with heat, cold, irritants, caustic
    substances, and microbiologic agents

ADNEXA

Penetration through follicular openings
Rupture of follicle, gland, or other structure (anal sac)

DERMIS AND PANNICULUS

Vessels (Hematogenous)

Drugs or toxins
Localization within capillary beds
Embolism
Leukocyte trafficking

Nerves

Migration from ganglion along sensory nerves via
    axonal flow to epithelial cells

SUPPORT STRUCTURES

Penetrating trauma from bone fracture
Extension of tumor or infection from adjacent lymph
    node, gland, muscle, or bone

efficient portal of entry for microorganisms when the barrier is damaged by trauma, excessive moisture, heat or cold, or by disruption of the normal flora of the integument. A number of microorganisms (e.g., *Staphylococcus intermedius, Streptococcus* sp., *Corynebacterium pseudotuberculosis, Pasteurella* sp., *Proteus* sp., *Pseudomonas* sp., and *Escherichia coli*) gain entrance to the body by either entering through natural pores, such as hair follicles or glands with ducts that traverse the epidermis, or by the parenteral route, which includes all types of breaks in the skin including injections, insect bites, and other types of wounds. Organisms that are able to inhabit hair follicles, such as mites or bacteria, gain entry to the body when the wall of the follicle is ruptured, leading to emptying of follicular contents into the dermis. Similarly, rupture of glands or ducts can lead to entry of microorganisms. From here, infectious agents can stimulate a robust host immune response or possibly spread to other areas of the body by gaining entry to the blood stream or traveling to regional and distant lymph nodes via lymph flow.

Intact skin with its waterproof barrier provides some protection against weak acids and alkali substances and water-soluble compounds, but certain lipid-soluble compounds can be absorbed directly through intact skin as can some artificially engineered gases developed for chemical warfare. Ultraviolet radiation can damage the skin by direct exposure if the body's natural defenses, such as the hair coat and melanin pigments, are not present or are inadequate. The lesions of actinic dermatitis (see Disorders of Physical, Radiation, or Chemical Injury; Solar Dermatosis, Keratosis, and Neoplasia) typify the effects of chronic exposure to ultraviolet radiation. In addition to actinic dermatitis, squamous cell carcinomas, hemangiomas, and hemangiosarcomas have an increased tendency to develop in skin chronically damaged by ultraviolet radiation.

The dermal capillaries can be a portal of entry to the skin via the hematogenous route. Embolization of infectious agents, such as bacteria (*Erysipelothrix rhusiopathiae* [diamond skin disease]) or fungi (systemic infection with *Blastomyces dermatitidis*) can damage the skin via this route during hematogenous dissemination. Tumor cells (hemangiosarcoma) can also embolize to the skin and lead to metastatic tumor foci or possible cutaneous infarction. The hematogenous route is also most often the delivery system for drugs (adverse cutaneous reactions to the administration of trimethoprim-potentiated sulfonamides; photosensitization dermatitis that occurs with phenothiazine ingestion) and toxins (gangrenous ergotism caused by the mycotoxin of *Claviceps purpurea*) to reach the skin.

Rarely an infectious agent that is neurotropic can migrate from a ganglion along sensory nerves via axonal flow to the skin (reactivation of feline herpesvirus 1 infection in cats resulting in ulcerative facial dermatitis). The skin can also be secondarily infected or traumatized or damaged by extension of pathologic processes affecting adjacent support structures such as bone, muscle, lymph nodes, or glands (locally invasive mammary gland carcinoma resulting in cutaneous ulceration).

HOST DEFENSE MECHANISMS AGAINST INJURY

The skin is a complex organ composed of many integrated components structurally and functionally designed to protect the host. Host defenses against injury principally consist of three broad mechanisms: (1) physical defense, (2) immunologic defense, and (3) repair mechanisms. The most critical defense is the barrier derived from the more superficial layers of the skin, which include the stratum corneum, epidermis, basement membrane, and superficial dermis. Without these outer layers of the skin, animals cannot survive (consider, for example, the deleterious effects of extensive burns and immune-mediated diseases, such as pemphigus vulgaris). One of the most important cells in the skin is the keratinocyte. The keratinocytes terminally differentiate to form the stratum corneum, the outermost barrier of the skin. The keratinocytes produce keratin filaments, desmosomes, and hemidesmosomes, providing structural integrity to the cytoplasm and an interconnecting network that anchors the keratinocytes to each other and the basement membrane. Keratinocytes produce cytokines (interleukin-1 [IL-1], IL-6, IL-8, IL-3, tumor necrosis factor-α [TNF-α], colony-stimulating factors) and growth factors (TGF-α, TGF-β, platelet-derived growth factor [PDGF], fibroblast growth factor [FGF]), thus participating in innate and adaptive immunity and in the communication between the two. Keratinocytes also dissolve desmosomes and hemidesmosomes and form actin filaments so they can migrate to cover skin wounds and then proliferate to regenerate the wounded skin. Keratinocytes thus not only orchestrate the activities of the skin but also serve as many members of the orchestra.

PHYSICAL DEFENSE MECHANISMS
BARRIER FUNCTIONS

Barriers of the skin against physical injury are listed in Box 17-3. The hair coat, particularly the long dense hair coat of some dogs and cats, serves as a physical barrier to temperature extremes, ultraviolet radiation, and minor trauma. The hair coat also sheds water as a result of the lipids provided by sebaceous gland secretion. Vibrissae, or tactile hairs, and sensory neurons provide awareness of the physical environment, allowing the animal to make appropriate reactions for survival, such as reflex responses to heat and other noxious stimuli. Claws, especially on cats, serve as a quite effective barrier against predators by providing traction for climbing and serve as weapons to be used against aggressors. Horns of cattle, sheep, and goats also provide some physical defense capabilities.

The stratum corneum is an exceedingly important component of the barrier, imparting protection from the exterior and preventing water loss from the interior. The stratum corneum is the "bricks and mortar" of the barrier. The bricks are the flattened, cornified cells that are eventually shed from the surface through daily frictional trauma and that are continually renewed by regeneration of basal cell keratinocytes. The mortar consists of intercorneocyte lipids derived from lipid membranes extruded from the lamellar granules of keratinocytes in the outer granular layer. About 90% of the corneocyte is tightly packed keratin filaments arranged parallel to the skin surface; the remaining 10% is the cornified cell envelope, a resilient protein-lipid polymer. The strength of the protein component is the result of cross-linking of structural proteins (e.g., keratin intermediate filaments, desmosomal proteins, and others) by disulfide and isopeptide bonds.

Box **17-3**

Host Defense Mechanisms against Injury: Physical Defense Mechanisms

BARRIER FUNCTIONS

Hair follicles: Physical and thermal
Tactile hairs and neurons: Sensory
Claws and horns: Physical defense
Stratum corneum: Barrier function
Adnexal glandular secretions: Barrier function
Apocrine glands horses and cattle: Defense against excessive heat
Melanin: Defense against ultraviolet radiation
Basement membrane zone: Filter to macromolecules, and barrier to invasion of neoplastic epidermal cells
Panniculus: Barrier against temperature extremes

RESISTANCE TO MECHANICAL FORCES

Hair follicles and epidermal-dermal interdigitations: Anchor epidermis to dermis
Stratum corneum: Corneocyte, corneocyte envelope, and intercellular lipid adhesion
Desmosomes and hemidesmosomes: Intercellular and basement membrane adhesion
Basement membrane: Anchors epidermis to dermis
Collagen and elastic tissue: Resilience, strength, and support of adnexa
Panniculus: Shock absorption, facilitates movement, anchors dermis to fascia

---

The lipid component surrounds the protein component to which it is covalently bound and provides adhesion of the cornified cells (i.e., bricks) to the intercellular lipids (i.e., mortar). Layers of the corneocytes and their corneocyte envelope (i.e., bricks), and intercellular lipids (i.e., mortar) form a tough and resilient protective barrier. The waterproofing and repellency of the stratum corneum is in part provided by the keratinocyte and sebum-derived lipids. Secretion from apocrine glands in cattle and horses provides defense against excessive heat.

Other barrier functions of the skin include defense against antioxidant injury provided by vitamin E in sebaceous gland secretion, and defense against ultraviolet light provided by the hair coat and also by melanin pigment in keratinocytes. The cap of melanin pigment over the nucleus helps protect the nucleus (and its nucleic acid) against ultraviolet light–induced injury by scattering and absorbing ultraviolet light rays. The basement membrane zone serves as an initial barrier to invasion of the dermis by neoplastic epidermal cells. The panniculus through its insulating properties serves as a barrier against cold temperatures.

RESISTANCE TO MECHANICAL FORCES

Anatomic features of the skin that provide resistance to physical injury are listed in Box 17-3. Hair follicles help anchor the epidermis to the dermis, as do epidermal-dermal interdigitations, thus these interdigitations are most numerous in nasal planum and footpad where hair follicles are absent and resistance to shearing force is necessary. Host defense against mechanical injury is also provided by the resilience of the cornified envelope due in part to cross-linked peptides, such as keratin intermediate filaments, and adhesion of cornified envelope and intercellular lipids. The keratinocytes contain keratin filaments and form desmosomal junctions with adjacent cells (Fig 17-4). The keratin filaments perform a structural role (i.e., cytoskeletal) in the cells, and the desmosomes promote adhesion of epidermal cells and resistance to mechanical stresses. The desmosomes in the outermost stratum corneum undergo proteolytic degradation allowing individual corneocytes to shed. The basement membrane anchors the epidermis to the dermis providing structural integrity against trauma. Collagen and elastic tissue provide resilience and strength to the skin and support for the vessels, nerves, and adnexa. The panniculus protects against surface trauma by providing some shock absorption (e.g., footpads), by facilitating movement, and by anchoring the dermis to fascia. Thus the various components of the epidermis, dermis, adnexa, and panniculus provide a flexible interconnecting framework to protect the host against mechanical injury.

IMMUNOLOGIC DEFENSE MECHANISMS
INNATE IMMUNITY

Innate immunity is a primitive, highly conserved response that quickly detects and impairs pathogens and harmful environmental stimuli encountered daily in life and does not require antigen-specific receptors. Innate immunity protects the host during the first 7 days of exposure to a pathogen before development of an adaptive immune response, and also initiates and assists the adaptive immune response (Table 17-1). The diversity of microorganisms requires equal diversity in host defense responses. The first phase of innate host defense consists of the barrier of the stratum corneum, which prevents pathogen adherence and provides an antimicrobial surface consisting of antimicrobial peptides and fatty acids. The antimicrobial peptides (e.g., β-defensins and cathelicidins) are effective against many organisms including viruses, bacteria, protozoa, and insects, and probably kill some of these pathogens by damaging their lipid membranes. The surface barrier also includes normal flora of nonpathogenic bacteria that competes with pathogenic microorganisms for nutrients and for attachment sites on cells. The normal flora also produces antimicrobial substances that prevent pathogen colonization. Because the dry cornified surface is such an effective barrier to pathogens, a wound or abrasion is usually necessary for a pathogen to gain entrance. If the epidermis sustains injury or if a microorganism otherwise penetrates the surface barrier, it is met by the second phase of innate host defense, namely tissue macrophages and other immune cells that by cell surface receptors contact and bind many types of pathogens. A significant challenge to the innate immune system is for the host to differentiate large numbers of pathogen antigens from self-antigens with the use of a limited number of receptors. It is now known that pathogen recognition is mediated by pattern-recognition receptors, which recognize molecular structures (i.e., pathogen-associated molecular patterns) common to broad

---

Table 17-1   Innate Immunity Host Defense Mechanisms

Stratum corneum barrier	Prevents pathogen adherence and provides antimicrobial surface
Macrophages (dendritic cells) with pattern-recognition receptors	Recognize broad classes of pathogens, differentiate pathogen antigens from self-antigens, initiate Toll signaling pathway, and secrete cytokines, facilitating inflammation and innate immunity
Toll signaling pathway	Promotes expression of large numbers of genes, resulting in production of cytokines, chemokines, and adhesion molecules important in inflammation and innate immunity
Macrophages and neutrophils	Recognize, ingest, and destroy pathogens
Endothelial cells	Express adhesion molecules and trigger kinin and coagulation systems, facilitating influx of plasma proteins and migration of leukocytes (cell trafficking) necessary to control infection
Coagulation system	Forms blood clot in case of injury to control blood loss and prevents microorganisms from entering the blood stream
Complement enzyme cascade	Recruits inflammatory cells, opsonizes pathogens, and kills some pathogens
Lipid mediators	Increase vascular permeability and induce influx and activation of leukocytes sustaining inflammatory responses

Innate immunity protects the host in the first 7 days of exposure and does not require antigen-specific receptors but does not provide protection to later reexposure.

classes of pathogens and that efficiently differentiate pathogen antigens from self-antigens.

A few examples of pathogen-associated molecular patterns include lipopolysaccharide (most gram-negative bacteria), lipoproteins (non-spore-forming, anaerobic, gram-positive rods), peptidoglycan (gram-positive bacteria); CpG motifs (mostly bacterial pathogens), lipoarabinomannan (mycobacteria), mannans and zymosan (yeast), and heat shock proteins (bacteria, fungi, algae, protozoa). Most pattern-recognition receptors act by stimulating signaling pathways, such as the Toll signaling pathway. The Toll signaling pathway is a phylogenetically ancient signaling pathway conserved in plants, insects, and mammals, which translates injury mediated by microorganisms or trauma into biochemical signals that rapidly optimize host defense. This signaling pathway is initiated when pathogen-associated molecular patterns are expressed by microorganisms, initiating a cascade of cytokine and chemokine release. These patterns are recognized by pattern-recognition receptors on the surface of macrophages and dendritic cells. Once triggered, the pathogen-receptor complex recruits an important adaptor molecule, called MyD88, which through a series of less well-understood intracellular signaling steps eventually frees a crucial molecule in host defense, known as NF kappa B, from its sequestered cytoplasmic location in the activated cell to migrate to the nucleus, where it acts as a transcription factor promoting the expression of large numbers of genes resulting in production of cytokines, chemokines, and adhesion molecules important in inflammation and the innate immune response. Thus the important outcome of pathogen-receptor binding is activation of macrophages and dendritic cells and others responsible for host defense, such as lymphocytes, to release cytokines and chemokines (e.g., IL-8 and IL-1), to recruit neutrophils and monocytes to the site of infection, and to activate the arachidonate cascade. Both macrophages and neutrophils play a key role in innate immunity by recognizing, ingesting, and destroying pathogens without the aid of the adaptive immune response.

The complement enzyme cascade, activated rapidly in response to many types of injury, also facilitates the elimination of pathogens by producing proteins (C3b and C4b) that opsonize the surface of pathogens. Opsonization enhances phagocytosis, the recruitment of additional phagocytes, and the killing of some pathogens. After phagocytosis, macrophages and neutrophils kill pathogens via lysosomal enzymes, toxic oxygen-derived products, toxic nitrogen oxides, and antimicrobial peptides, enzymes, and competitors. Cytokines (IL-1, IL-6, and TNF-α) also produced by macrophages cause fever, synthesis of acute-phase response proteins, and leukocytosis in the acute inflammatory response. Fever is beneficial to host defense because most pathogens grow better at temperatures lower than those associated with fever, and host cells are protected from harmful effects of some cytokines at temperatures elevated above normal body temperature (i.e., above 37° C). The acute-phase response proteins can opsonize a broad range of pathogens and can also activate the complement cascade, making pathogens more susceptible to phagocytosis and killing by macrophages and neutrophils. Finally, cytokines cause leukocytosis by increasing the number of circulating neutrophils available to migrate to the site of the pathogen and participate in phagocytosis.

Cytokines and other mediators released by activated immunocytes induce an acute inflammatory response (see Chapter 3) resulting in the five cardinal signs of inflammation—heat, pain, redness, swelling, and loss of function. The acute inflammatory response is characterized by changes in local blood vessels including: (1) vasodilation of arterioles, which causes increased blood flow at reduced velocity to capillary beds and postcapillary venules, (2) activation of endothelial cells to express adhesion molecules to bind circulating leukocytes so they can stop circulating, attach to the endothelium, and then migrate to the site of inflammation, and (3) increased vascular permeability that enhances the accumulation of plasma proteins (e.g., fibrinogen, complement) at the site of inflammation.

Activated endothelial cells can also trigger activation of the kinin and coagulation systems. The kinin system causes pain via production of bradykinin and substance P (i.e., activation of sensory nerve fibers) and enhances the acute inflammatory response by increasing vascular permeability. The coagulation cascade promotes blood clotting, thus preventing the spread of pathogens via the vasculature. Once initiated, the innate immune response helps to start the antigen-specific immune response (i.e., adaptive immunity). Innate immunity is crucial to protecting the host in the early days of infection; however, pathogens can evade innate immunity, and innate immunity does not lead to immunologic memory characteristic of adaptive immunity.

THE INTERACTION BETWEEN INNATE AND ADAPTIVE IMMUNITY

The link between innate and adaptive immunity is complex; however, IL-1 is proposed to be particularly important. If the epidermis sustains injury or if a microorganism penetrates the surface barrier, it is quickly met by an arsenal of stored IL-1α within the keratinocytes and stratum corneum. IL-1α induces the expression of more than 90 genes regulating adhesion molecules, chemokines, cytokines, proteolytic enzymes, and matrix proteins in various cell types, including keratinocytes, endothelial cells, and fibroblasts. The induction of gene expression of this magnitude is done through the activation of the Toll signaling pathway. Other signaling pathways are also activated by the binding of IL-1 to its receptor, further amplifying the inflammatory events associated with IL-1 activation. These events include: (1) stimulation of keratinocyte synthesis of cytokines and chemokines, (2) Langerhans' (i.e., dendritic) cell migration from epidermis to dermis and eventually to skin-associated lymph nodes, and (3) the expression of endothelial adhesion molecules (i.e., E-selectin, intercellular adhesion molecule-1 [ICAM-1], and vascular cell adhesion molecule-1 [VCAM-1]). These events recruit a subpopulation of memory T lymphocytes bearing cutaneous lymphocyte antigen (CLA) on the cell surface, and this molecule mediates passage of lymphocytes out of postcapillary venules. Thus IL-1 participates in both the innate and adaptive immune system.

ACQUIRED (ADAPTIVE) IMMUNITY

Whereas innate immunity works immediately to detect and destroy microorganisms, acquired or adaptive immunity develops later because the lymphocytes that contribute to adaptive immunity specific for the invading pathogen must increase in number by clonal expansion. The major components of the cutaneous adaptive immune system include keratinocytes, dendritic antigen-presenting cells (Langerhans' cells and dermal dendritic cells), lymphocytes, and endothelial cells (Table 17-2). The adaptive-immune response is initiated by a stimulus (e.g., microbial invasion, contact with environmental allergens, injury, or tumor growth), at which time the bone-marrow derived antigen-processing and antigen-presenting cells (Langerhans' cells in the epidermis and dendritic cells in the perivascular dermis) ingest and process the antigen. The major

function of Langerhans' cells and dermal dendritic cells is antigen processing and presentation; thus these cells are referred to as "professional antigen processing and presenting cells." Langerhans' and dermal dendritic cells reexpress the ingested and processed antigen on their cell surfaces, and migrate via afferent lymphatics to the paracortical areas of skin-associated lymph nodes, where they arrive as mature and powerful antigen-presenting cells. These skin-derived dendritic cells then initiate a pathogen-specific protective immune response by presenting antigen to the naïve T lymphocytes. Langerhans' cells also produce cytokines (e.g., IL-1 and TNF-α), thus participating in up-regulation of inflammatory and immune responses in the skin.

The T lymphocytes activated by antigen presentation in the skin-associated lymph nodes then express skin-associated homing receptors (e.g., cutaneous lymphocyte antigen/CLA) that interact with adhesion molecules (E-selectin, P-selectin, VCAM-1, and ICAM-1) on cytokine-activated endothelial cells in the dermal vessels at the site of initial injury, thus providing a way for the activated lymphocytes to find their way back to the site of the pathogen. Once in the skin and after receipt of a renewed antigenic stimulus by the professional antigen-presenting cells, the sensitized T lymphocytes undergo clonal expansion, resulting in the generation of protective effector mechanisms. Most of the lymphocytes in the skin are T-helper lymphocytes, but various types of T lymphocytes and B lymphocytes contribute to adaptive immunity. Lymphocytes recognize pathogens (i.e., antigens) via cell surface receptors. The B lymphocytes have immunoglobulin molecules as the receptors for antigen, and upon activation,

Table **17-2** **Adaptive Immunity Host Defense Mechanisms**

Langerhans' cells in epidermis and dendritic cells in dermis	Ingest and process antigen; present antigen to naïve T lymphocytes in lymph nodes; present antigen to sensitized T lymphocytes at site of injury; and produce cytokines that up-regulate inflammation and immune responses
T lymphocytes	After stimulation by antigen-presenting cells in lymph node, migrate back to the site of injury
CD8 (cytotoxic lymphocytes)	Recognize antigen expressed on the cell surface and kill the cell (cytotoxic lymphocytes); responsible for killing neoplastic cells, some bacteria and parasites, and all viruses that replicate inside cells
CD4 $T_H 1$	Activate macrophages, helping to control infection by intracellular bacteria
CD4 $T_H 2$	Activate B lymphocytes, helping eliminate extracellular pathogens
B lymphocytes	Secrete immunoglobulin, providing defense against pathogens (often bacteria) in extracellular spaces
Endothelial cells	Express adhesion molecules and bind to stimulated T lymphocytes
Keratinocytes	Produce cytokines and growth factors up-regulating or down-regulating inflammation and immune responses
Cytokines, chemokines, and adhesion molecules	Contribute as in innate immune response

Adaptive (acquired) immunity develops after innate immunity because the lymphocytes that contribute to adaptive immunity specific for the invading pathogen must increase in number by clonal expansion and provides protection upon later reexposure to pathogen.

B lymphocytes secrete immunoglobulin, which provides defense against pathogens (often bacteria) in the extracellular spaces. In contrast, T lymphocytes have receptors that recognize foreign antigens expressed as peptide fragments bound to major histocompatibility complex (MHC) proteins (see Chapter 5 for a review). One class of T lymphocyte expresses the CD8 molecule on the surface (i.e., CD8 T lymphocytes) and is responsible for cell-mediated immune responses. These CD8 T lymphocytes recognize peptide fragments (viral antigens and others) bound to MHC I. CD8 T lymphocytes kill some bacteria and parasites, and all viruses that replicate inside cells. These CD8 T lymphocytes recognize the antigen expressed on the cell surface, then kill the cell, and thus are also called "cytotoxic" T lymphocytes.

Another class of T lymphocytes express the CD4 molecule on their surface. This class of T lymphocyte is divided into two subclasses. One CD4 T-cell subset (T_H1) recognizes peptide fragments (e.g., microbial antigen) bound to MHC II and activates macrophages, thus helping to control infection by intracellular bacteria, such as *Mycobacteria* spp. Upon phagocytosis, the lipoprotein on the surface of mycobacterial organisms binds surface receptors (including Toll-like receptors) on macrophages. This binding further stimulates macrophages, resulting in the secretion of macrophage IL-2, and production of nitric oxide within macrophages. Nitric oxide is toxic to the bacteria, and facilitates their killing. IL-2 stimulates CD4 T lymphocytes to release cytokines (interferon-γ [IFN-γ] and TNF-α), which activate and recruit more macrophages to the site of infection. The accumulating macrophages phagocytose and kill mycobacterial organisms and form granulomas. The other CD4 T-lymphocyte subset (T_H2 [T-helper] cells) recognizes peptide bound to MHC II and activates B lymphocytes to secret immunoglobulin, thus helping eliminate extracellular pathogens. Most antigens require an accompanying signal from helper T lymphocytes before they can stimulate B lymphocytes to proliferate and differentiate into plasma cells secreting antibody. Thus T lymphocytes are crucial to adaptive immunity by destroying pathogen-infected cells, by activating macrophages, and by activating B lymphocytes.

Down-regulation (i.e., a decrease in the number of or affinity for receptors on the cell surface) of the immune response has been less well studied. Typically the elimination of the stimulus results in resolution of the inflammatory or immune response. Also, some growth factors, particularly TGF-β, and other cell products, such as prostaglandin E_2, can have immunosuppressive functions leading to down-regulation of inflammatory and immune responses. Thus complex interactions between host cells, pathogens or other antigens, and inflammatory mediators of the adaptive immune system typically result in appropriate host defenses, the

removal of the inciting pathogen, and the generation of differentiated memory lymphocytes through clonal expansion, allowing faster specific immune responses in future encounters with the offending antigen. However, impaired function of the adaptive immune system can lead to increased susceptibility to infection and to development of neoplasia. Similarly, uncontrolled inflammatory responses also can lead to chronic inflammation or autoreactive disorders, such as contact hypersensitivity, atopic dermatitis, or lupus erythematosus.

REGENERATION AND REPAIR

Regeneration and repair also constitute a host defense mechanism to injury (Box 17-4). The details of

---

Box 17-4

Host Defense Mechanisms against Injury: Regeneration and Repair

BLOOD CLOTTING AND INFLAMMATION

Clot forms in vessel and wound space, provides matrix for cell migration, and dries to form scab over wound

Platelets and coagulation and complement cascade recruit inflammatory cells

Neutrophils and macrophages phagocytize pathogens and foreign debris

Macrophages secrete collagenase, facilitating tissue débridement, and transition between inflammation and repair

REEPITHELIZATION, FIBROPLASIA, AND ANGIOGENESIS

Reepithelization

Epithelial cells produce proteases to dissect between viable and nonviable tissue, migrate and proliferate to cover wound, and reestablish basement membrane

Fibroplasia

Fibroblasts produce proteolytic enzymes to provide path for migration, migrate and proliferate in wound site, and produce extracellular matrix to form connective tissue

Angiogenesis

Endothelial cells form tubular structures that become blood vessels and reestablish blood flow

WOUND CONTRACTION AND COLLAGEN PRODUCTION

Fibroblasts produce collagen and contractile microfilaments that link to matrix

Newly formed collagen bundles link to each other and to collagen bundles at wound edge to contract the wound

Inflammation, edema, and vascularity gradually disappear

tissue regeneration and repair are covered in Chapter 4, whereas the basic mechanisms involved in healing of cutaneous wounds will be summarized here. Two common types of cutaneous wounds will be used as examples, and these include wounds with opposed edges, such as surgical incisions, and larger wounds in which the edges cannot be opposed, such as broad ulcers, necrosis associated with deep burns, or large areas of trauma where portions of the skin have been lost (Fig. 17-8). Recall that regeneration and repair are

a dynamic process involving multiple and overlapping stages. These stages include: (1) blood clotting and inflammation (12 to 24 hours after injury), (2) reepithelization, fibroplasia, and angiogenesis (3 to 7 days after injury), and (3) wound contraction and collagen production (1 to 2 weeks after injury).

HEALING OF WOUNDS WITH OPPOSED EDGES

The simplest healing involves the clean, uninfected, surgical incision in which the edges of the wound are

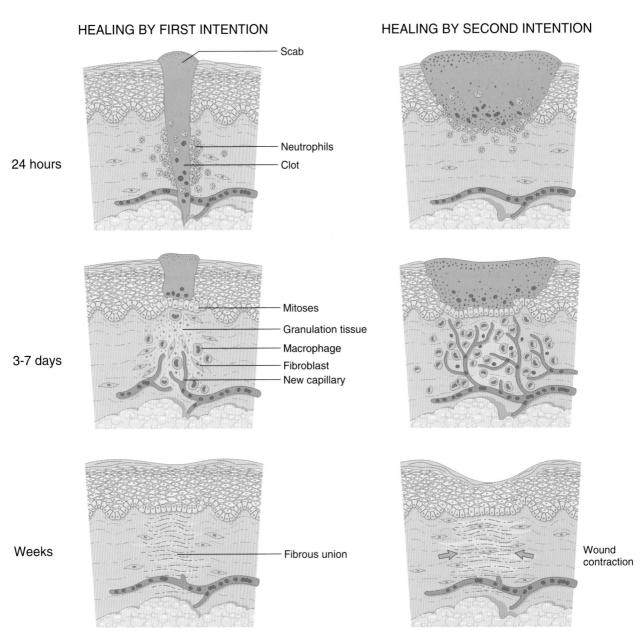

Fig. 17-8   Schematic diagram of the steps in wound healing by first intention (*left*) and second intention (*right*). Note large amounts of granulation tissue and wound contraction in healing by second intention. *(From Kumar V, Abbas A, Fausto N: Robbins & Cotran pathologic basis of disease, ed 7, Philadelphia, 2005, Saunders.)*

closely opposed by sutures so the wound space is narrow (Fig. 17-8). Healing of these wounds is called primary union or healing by first intention. These wounds cause minimal necrosis of cells of the epidermis, dermis, and adnexa and minimal disruption of the basement membrane. Thus they heal quickly without significant architectural change, although a thin scar remains and the adnexa destroyed by the incision are permanently lost.

The first stage of wound healing is blood clotting and inflammation and begins within the first 12 to 24 hours of injury. The process begins with blood vessel disruption, platelet aggregation, blood coagulation, and clot formation in the vessel and wound space. Dehydration of the surface of the clot forms the scab that covers the wound. The clot in the wound space provides the matrix for migration of inflammatory cells, endothelial cells, and fibroblasts. Platelet-derived factors and factors associated with the coagulation and complement cascades facilitate recruitment of inflammatory cells such as neutrophils and macrophages to phagocytose pathogens, foreign particles, and debris. Many of the cytokines and chemokines that govern inflammation in regeneration and repair are the same as those participating in inflammatory processes of other causes. Neutrophils, the first cells to arrive at the margins of the incision, phagocytose pathogens and debris, then either slough with desiccated tissue, are phagocytosed by macrophages, or undergo apoptosis. Macrophages replace neutrophils, secrete collagenase (facilitates tissue débridement), and release growth factors initiating the formation of granulation tissue.

The second stage of wound healing consists of reepithelialization, fibroplasia, and angiogenesis and is maximal between 3 and 7 days of injury. The process of reepithelialization begins within hours of injury from basal cell keratinocytes adjacent to the incision. In order for the basal cells to become mobile, they retract intercellular tonofilaments, dissolve desmosomes and hemidesmosomes, and form cytoplasmic actin filaments. In addition to mobility, within 24 to 48 hours from injury, there is mitosis of basal cells at the edges of the wound. The mitosis is induced by growth factors from epidermal cells, macrophages, and dermal parenchymal cells. Basal cells from both sides of the wound migrate along the cut edges of the dermis separating nonviable tissue from viable tissue by using the expression of various surface integrin receptors on viable cells and through the production of collagenase, which débrides dead tissue. The basal cells join at the midline of the wound, and as reepithelialization develops, the nonviable tissue above this newly united epidermis, is sloughed. Basal cells also produce extracellular matrix, such as fibronectin, to facilitate reestablishment of the basement membrane. The basal cells revert to a nonmigratory normal phenotype, form hemidesmosomes, and firmly reattach to the newly formed basement membrane, thus beginning the reestablishment of the epidermis over the wounded skin.

Fibroplasia and angiogenesis begin with the formation of granulation tissue, the term applied to a specialized type of tissue composed of proliferative fibroblasts and vascular endothelial cells produced in healing of soft tissue injury. Granulation tissue is the hallmark of healing and is named for its clinical appearance of soft pink to tan tissue with minute red foci consisting of capillaries (granules). However, it is the histologic appearance that is diagnostic, a lattice-work array of proliferative capillaries (angiogenesis) oriented perpendicular to proliferative fibroblasts (fibroplasia). The fibroblasts produce extracellular matrix, which is remodeled, ultimately resulting in scar formation (i.e., cicatrix formation).

The process of forming granulation tissue begins about 3 days after injury. Fibroplasia (fibrosis) is induced when cytokines (IL-1, TNF-α) and growth factors (TGF-β, PDGF, endothelial growth factor [EGF], FGF) from inflammatory cells (especially macrophages), platelets, and endothelial cells stimulate fibroblasts to proliferate, migrate, and ultimately produce extracellular matrix. As in reepithelialization, the ability of fibroblasts to migrate into the clot or provisional matrix requires alteration in expression of surface receptors and production of proteolytic enzymes to provide a path for migration. When fibroblasts have migrated into and filled the wound space, growth factors and cytokines (TGF-β, PDGF, FGF, IL-1, IL-13) direct fibroblasts to switch from migration to protein (collagen) production, providing the structural protein that eventually contributes to wound strength. Collagen production begins by days 3 to 5 and persists for several weeks, depending on the size of the wound.

Concurrent with fibroblast migration into the wound space, angiogenesis, the formation of new blood vessels in an area of tissue injury, is also occurring (see Chapter 2). Angiogenesis develops from preexisting vessels and also from endothelial precursor cells (angioblast-like cells) from the bone marrow. Many growth factors play a role in angiogenesis, but vascular endothelial growth factor (VEGF) is considered to be the most important. In angiogenesis from preexisting vessels, macrophages and injured cells in the wound site release cytokines (such as FGF and VEGF), causing endothelial cells to release proteinases (e.g., procollagenase). The proteinases degrade components of the endothelial cell basement membrane. The disruption of the endothelial cell basement membrane removes the barrier otherwise confining endothelial cells, thereby permitting endothelial cells to migrate into the injured site in response to cytokines and growth factors released from injured or stimulated cells (e.g., FGF from macrophages, VEGF from keratinocytes, and heparin from mast cells). The migratory endothelial cells form tubes that express $\alpha_v\beta_3$ integrin, facilitating endothelial cell adhesion and migration. The endothelial cells deposit provisional matrix of fibronectin and proteoglycans, and eventually form new basement membrane.

The growth factors continue to stimulate endothelial cell proliferation, ensuring a supply of endothelial cells for the extension of capillary tubes so that blood flow to the area of soft tissue injury can be reestablished. In angiogenesis from endothelial precursor cells, VEGF stimulates the mobilization of endothelial cell precursors from the bone marrow, and proliferation and differentiation of these cells at the site of injury; however, the mechanism whereby these cells are directed to the site of injury is unclear. Once at the site of injury, these endothelial cell precursors form a delicate capillary plexus that eventually links to existing capillaries, facilitating formation of a capillary network. The newly formed vessels, whether produced by sprouting from preexisting capillaries or from endothelial precursor cells, are provided structural support by pericytes (recruited by angiopoietin 1 interacting with Tie 2, an endothelial cell receptor) and smooth muscle cells (recruited by PDGF), and by production of extracellular matrix proteins (stimulated by TGF-β).

Angiogenesis is a well-regulated process. More than 20 molecules present in tissue act as angiogenesis inhibitors and modulate the reparative process. By the end of the second stage of wound healing, the incision is filled with granulation tissue, neovascularization is maximal, collagen fibrils bridge the incision, and reepithelialization has been completed. By day 7, the usual time to remove sutures, the tensile strength of the incision site is about 10% that of unwounded skin.

The third and final phase of wound repair involves collagen production and wound contraction. However, wound contraction principally affects large wounds that heal by second intention and is described later. Production of collagen and proliferation of fibroblasts (directed by cytokines, such as TGF-β) progress fairly rapidly in this phase of wound repair. In contrast, inflammation, edema, and increased vascularity disappear. The proliferation and maturation of endothelial cells, fibroblasts, and inflammatory cells that contribute to wound repair are dependent on complex feedback control mechanisms between cells, cytokines, enzymes, and the extracellular matrix microenvironment. This complex interaction has been called "dynamic reciprocity." As the wound space is bridged by granulation tissue and fibroblasts produce collagen, the endothelial cells undergo apoptosis, thus reducing capillary numbers. Similarly, fibroblasts and macrophages also undergo apoptosis. The reduction of endothelial cells, fibroblasts, and inflammatory cells leads to formation of an acellular scar. By the third week of wound repair, the wound has about 20% the tensile strength of normal skin. Over the ensuing months, collagen production is reduced, but there is continued slow remodeling of the extracellular matrix leading to a healed wound that at maximum strength is only 70% to 80% that of unwounded skin.

HEALING OF WOUNDS WITH SEPARATED EDGES

Healing of wounds with separated edges (healing by second intention) occurs when there is more extensive loss of skin tissue. Healing by this process is more difficult and time consuming, and larger scars result and replace the cutaneous architecture. The principal differences between healing by primary intention and healing by second intention include: (1) in healing by second intention, inflammation is usually more extensive because there is more tissue damage that must be removed and secondary infection is more likely; (2) granulation tissue is more extensive because the wound has wider edges so there is a larger gap to fill; and (3) wound contraction occurs, reducing the size of the wound to a fraction of the original size (experimentally, it has been shown that large wounds in rabbits are reduced to 5% to 10% of their original size in about 6 weeks).

Wound contraction begins during the second week of healing when fibroblasts develop phenotypic characteristics of smooth muscle cells. These consist of cytoplasmic bundles of actin-containing microfilaments, and formation of cell-cell and cell-matrix linkages. Fibroblasts link to the extracellular fibronectin matrix and collagen matrix by fibronectin (e.g., $\alpha_5\beta_1$) and collagen (e.g., $\alpha_1\beta_1$, $\alpha_2\beta_1$) receptors and to each other through direct adherens junctions. Also, newly synthesized collagen bundles form covalent cross-links with themselves and with collagen bundles at the wound edge. These linkages thus provide a conduit across the wound space so that the traction of fibroblasts on the matrix can contract the wound, substantially reducing its size and facilitating healing by second intention.

THE RESPONSES OF THE SKIN TO INJURY (A PRIMER TO HISTOLOGIC PATTERNS)

A number of "new" terms commonly used to classify diseases of the skin are used throughout this chapter. For convenience and to provide quick reference, these terms are listed at the end of this chapter in a glossary. Although there are many new terms to learn, it should be realized that the system of forming of these terms is similar to that used for other anatomic systems. Basically, prefixes and suffixes are added to word roots to create specific terms that define the pathology of the skin. For example, the prefix "epi" (meaning upon or above) combined with the word root "dermat(o)" (referring to skin) creates the word "epidermis," which simply means the portion of the skin above the dermis. Likewise, the term *hypodermis* refers to the portion of the skin below the dermis, also called the subcutis or panniculus. Suffixes are used in the same way. For example, the suffix "itis" (meaning inflammation) combined with the word root "dermat(o)" forms the word "dermatitis," which simply means inflammation of the skin. Similarly, terms referring to inflammation predominantly within the epidermis, follicles, or the panniculus are epidermitis, folliculitis, and panniculitis, respectively. The suffix "osis" refers to a disease process, often noninflammatory. Thus combining dermat(o) and osis forms the word "dermatosis," which means any disease of the skin, especially one not characterized by inflammation. Dermatoses is the plural of dermatosis and thus means noninflammatory skin diseases.

Numerous endogenous and exogenous factors can potentially cause injury of the skin (Fig. 17-9). Determining a definitive diagnosis of a skin disorder depends on obtaining a complete history, including age, breed, and sex of the animal; conducting a thorough physical examination, paying particular attention to the distribution of skin lesions; and performing additional diagnostic tests, such as a complete blood count, serum chemistry panel, skin biopsy sampling, and microbiologic cultures. Results from cutaneous biopsy sampling are often useful and can be necessary to establish a definitive diagnosis for skin diseases. Although the skin has a limited range of responses to injury, the distribution and types of inflammatory cells in the lesion often represent a recognizable pattern that can be used to: (1) formulate a list of specific etiologic agents that could cause the lesion or (2) suggest categories of disease with similar lesions and a common pathogenesis. Algorithms (i.e., a set of directions for accomplishing some task that has a recognizable end point) have been developed for the recognition of histopathologic patterns in veterinary dermatopathology (Table 17-3). Recognition of patterns, both clinically and histologically, can facilitate differential diagnoses of skin disease (Table 17-4).

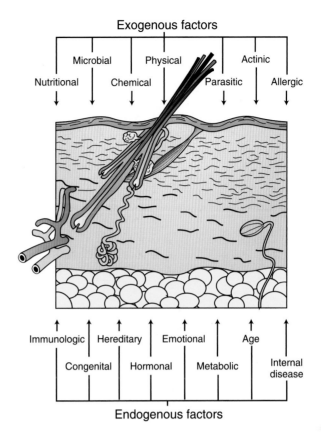

Fig. 17-9   Schematic diagram of the exogenous and endogenous factors that influence the skin. A myriad of exogenous and endogenous factors influence the gross and microscopic appearance of the skin. Because the skin can respond to these factors in a limited number of ways, different skin disorders may have a similar appearance. Identification of the cause of a skin disorder therefore often requires not only histopathologic evaluation but also clinical history, including clinical lesion distribution and appearance.
(Courtesy Dr. Ann M. Hargis, DermatoDiagnostics.)

Table **17-3**   **Examples of Pattern Diagnosis in the Skin**

Component of Skin	Reaction to Injury	Pattern	Disease Examples
Epidermis	Prominent hyperkeratosis	Hyperkeratotic diseases of the epidermis	Primary seborrhea Ichthyosis Vitamin A deficiency Callus
Dermis	Interface inflammation	Interface dermatitis	Lupus erythematosus Erythema multiforme
Follicle	Inflammation of the follicular lumen	Luminal folliculitis	Infection with staphylococci, dermatophytes, Demodex sp.
Panniculus	Predominantly neutrophilic inflammation	Neutrophilic panniculitis	Abscess Feline pansteatitis (early)

A pattern consists of two parts: a component of the skin (e.g., epidermis) + a histologic reaction of that component to injury (e.g., hyperkeratosis) = pattern (hyperkeratotic diseases of the epidermis).

Table **17-4** Differential Diagnoses of Selected Patterns That Can Be Recognized Clinically and Histologically

Pattern	Pustules Crusts (epidermal)	Vesicles Bullae (epidermal) to subepidermal)	Necrosis or ulceration (epidermal)	Scaling or other hyperkeratotic lesions* (epidermal)	Nodules ± draining tracts (dermal and pannicular)	Alopecia (adnexal)	Hypopigmentation or depigmentation (epidermal)
Disorders	Superficial bacterial infection	Pemphigus vulgaris	Vasculitis/ infarction	Primary seborrhea	Masses caused by deep infections with bacteria, fungi, algae, Pythium, migratory parasites (e.g., actinomycosis, feline leprosy, mycetoma, blastomycosis, pythiosis, habronemiasis abscesses)	Folliculitis: Infectious Noninfectious	Vitiligo
	Pemphigus foliaceus and panepidermal pustular pemphigus	Paraneoplastic pemphigus	Chemical and thermal burns	Ichthyosis		Postinflammatory and posttraumatic	Uveodermatologic syndrome
	Dermatophilosis	Lupus erythematosus	Superficial necrolytic dermatitis	Zinc responsive dermatosis		Endocrine alopecia	Lupus erythematosus
	Exudative epidermitis	Dermatomyositis	Erythema multiforme	Sebaceous adenitis		Idiopathic flank alopecia	Copper deficiency
	Subcorneal pustular dermatosis	Subepidermal bullous dermatoses	Stevens-Johnson syndrome	Ear margin seborrhea		Telogen effluvium	Alopecia areata (healing stage)
	Foot pads*	Drug reactions	Toxic epidermal necrolysis	Vitamin A responsive dermatosis		Anagen defluxion	Inherited disorders (Chédiak-Higashi syndrome, Maltese and other coat color dilutions)
	Pemphigus foliaceus	Chemical and thermal burns	Ergot/fescue grass toxicity	Feline exfoliative dermatosis	"Sterile" nodular inflammation (e.g., foreign body reactions, histiocytosis, sterile pyogranuloma, xanthoma, venomous bites, injection site reactions, eosinophilic granulomas)	Post clipping alopecia	Waardenburg-like syndrome
	Superficial necrolytic dermatitis	Photosensitization	Frostbite	Feline paraneoplastic dermatosis and thymoma		Follicular dysplasia	Piebaldism
	Lupus erythematosus	Viral diseases	Feline indolent ulcer	Callus		Congenital alopecia and hypotrichosis	Albinism
			Feline ulcerative dermatosis	Cutaneous horn		Feline psychogenic alopecia	Cyclic hematopoiesis
			Vesicular cutaneous lupus erythematosus	Actinic dermatitis		Poor nutrition with protein deficiency	Contact with rubber
			Self-trauma		Panniculitis/ steatitis	Feline paraneoplastic alopecia	
			Epitheliogenesis imperfecta		Neoplasms		

Some of these disorders could be placed in different patterns. For instance, disorders characterized by vesicles or bullae may develop into an ulcerative pattern after the vesicles or bullae rupture.
*Hyperkeratotic disorders may also affect the nasal planum and footpads; see Box 17-12.

Patterns of responses to injury are illustrated by changes in the epidermis, dermis, adnexa, and panniculus and are discussed in the following sections.

RESPONSES OF THE EPIDERMIS TO INJURY
ALTERATIONS IN EPIDERMAL GROWTH OR DIFFERENTIATION

The basal cells (i.e., basal keratinocytes) in their postmitotic state migrate outward from the basal layer, eventually forming the cornified layers (stratum corneum) of the epidermis. In the normal epidermis, balance is established between the rate of proliferation of the basal cells (germinal cells) and the rate of loss of differentiated cells (squamous epithelial cells) from the surface, resulting in the constant thickness of the epidermis and each of the layers. The orderly proliferation, differentiation, and cornification of epidermal cells is regulated by cytokines (e.g., epidermal growth factor, fibroblast growth factors, insulin-like growth factors, interleukins, and tumor necrosis factor), hormones (e.g., cortisol and vitamin D_3), and nutritional factors, such as protein, zinc, copper, fatty acids, and vitamin A and the B vitamins. The cytokines that regulate keratinocyte growth and differentiation are produced by a variety of cell types in the skin, including endothelial cells, leukocytes, fibroblasts, and keratinocytes. Thus keratinocytes also have a self-regulatory role (i.e., autocrine) in their growth and differentiation, and inflammatory cells, among others, can influence keratinocyte growth and differentiation.

Disorders of cornification

Disorders of cornification (i.e., alterations in the formation of the stratum corneum) can be primary, such as in primary seborrhea, but more often are secondary to a variety of factors, such as inflammation, trauma, or metabolic or nutritional disorders. A disorder of cornification called hyperkeratosis is characterized by an increase in the thickness of the stratum corneum and occurs in two forms: orthokeratotic and parakeratotic hyperkeratosis. In orthokeratotic hyperkeratosis (also referred to as hyperkeratosis), squamous epithelial cells are anuclear, and in parakeratotic hyperkeratosis (also referred to as parakeratosis), the squamous epithelial cells have nuclei. Subtypes of hyperkeratosis include basket weave (exaggerated undulating pattern of layers the normal stratum corneum), compact (compacted layers of basket weave stratum corneum), and laminated (layers of stratum corneum that are more linear and less undulating). Both parakeratosis and hyperkeratosis are common nonspecific responses to chronic stimuli (e.g., superficial trauma, inflammation, or sun exposure) and also occur as primary lesions. For example, hyperkeratosis is a feature of the primary cornification disorder of the cocker spaniel (Fig. 17-10), ichthyosis, and vitamin A deficiency. Diffuse parakeratosis is a feature of zinc-responsive dermatosis and superficial necrolytic dermatopathy (hepatocutaneous syndrome) (Fig. 17-11). Hyperkeratosis and parakeratosis can be accompanied by alterations in the thickness of the granular cell layer (stratum granulosum). Generally, hyperkeratosis is associated with an increased thickness of the granular cell layer (hypergranulosis), and parakeratosis is associated with a decreased thickness of the granular cell layer (hypogranulosis).

Epidermal hyperplasia

Epidermal hyperplasia is an alteration in epidermal growth or differentiation characterized by an increase

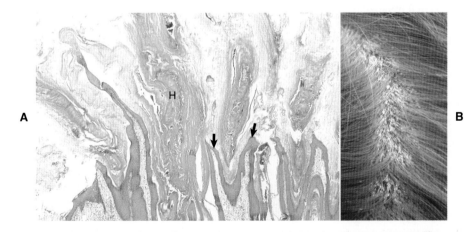

Fig. 17-10   Idiopathic seborrhea, skin, haired, dog. A, Note the marked orthokeratotic hyperkeratosis *(H)*. The stratum corneum within the hair follicles is increased in quantity, extends through the follicular opening to the external skin surface, and distends follicular openings *(arrows)*, creating a papillomatous appearance in the epidermis. H&E stain. **B,** Hair is parted to reveal excessive scaling, the result of orthokeratotic hyperkeratosis. *(A and B, Courtesy Dr. Ann M. Hargis, DermatoDiagnostics.)*

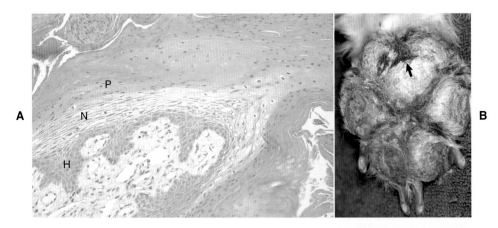

Fig. 17-11   **Superficial necrolytic dermatitis, skin, dog. A,** Nuclei of the the thickened stratum corneum have been retained (parakeratotic hyperkeratosis [parakeratosis]). The epidermis has a trilaminar pattern created by three layers: (1) parakeratotic layer *(P)*, (2) subparakeratotic edema/necrolytic layer *(N)*, and (3) deep epidermal hyperplasic layer *(H)*. The pathogenesis of superficial necrolytic dermatitis is not completely understood but is speculated that in most cases it is the result of an underlying systemic disease (such as severe liver disease or diabetes mellitus) that interferes with the normal nutrient metabolism needed to form a healthy epidermis. H&E stain. **B,** Footpad. Note the fissure *(arrow)* and crusts. The crusting is due largely to the parakeratosis. Secondary infections by bacteria, yeast, and fungi can also contribute to the formation of crusts by causing fluid, leukocytes, and other cellular debris to accumulate on the surface. (**A** and **B,** *Courtesy Dr. Ann M. Hargis, DermatoDiagnostics.*)

in the number of cells within the epidermis, most often within the stratum spinosum, and is also referred to as acanthosis. Hyperplasia is a response common to a variety of stimuli, often chronic, and occurs in a variety of types including regular, irregular, papillated, and pseudocarcinomatous (pseudoepitheliomatous) (Fig. 17-12). Some forms of epidermal hyperplasia (regular, irregular, and pseudocarcinomatous) can develop in sequence. In early stages of epidermal hyperplasia, the epidermal dermal interface is mildly undulating, but as the hyperplasia progresses, there often is an elongation of the rete ridges (ridges that extend into the dermis and interdigitate with dermal papillae) that can be regular or irregular. In regular epidermal hyperplasia, the rete ridges are approximately evenly sized and shaped, whereas in irregular epidermal hyperplasia, the rete ridges are less uniform. Pseudocarcinomatous hyperplasia is a chronic and late stage of epidermal hyperplasia that develops after milder forms (regular or irregular). It refers to marked hyperplasia of the epidermis, resulting in many branching and anastomosing epidermal ridges that deeply interdigitate with dermal collagen fibers. Mitotic figures can be numerous in proliferating basal cells, but in contrast to squamous cell carcinoma, the keratinocytes maintain normal polarity, are not atypical, and do not penetrate the basement membrane. Pseudocarcinomatous hyperplasia develops after chronic injury, as seen in skin damaged by long-term actinic radiation (i.e., repeated

exposure to ultraviolet light) or at the edges of persistent, nonhealing ulcers. Psoriasiform epidermal hyperplasia is an exaggerated type of regular epidermal hyperplasia in which the epidermis forms elongated rete ridges that are of similar length and width and that interdigitate with similarly elongated dermal papillae. This type of hyperplasia has very regular or uniform histologic appearance and is a feature of certain disease syndromes, such as psoriasiform lichenoid dermatitis of the springer spaniel and porcine juvenile pustular psoriasiform dermatitis (pityriasis rosea). Papillated epidermal hyperplasia is a unique form of epidermal hyperplasia in which fingerlike (papillary) projections of epidermis develop above the skin surface; it is a feature of some papillomas, hamartomas, and calluses.

Dyskeratosis

Dyskeratosis is an alteration in epidermal differentiation characterized by premature keratinization of cells in the viable layers of the epidermis. Dyskeratotic keratinocytes are shrunken, are separated from adjacent keratinocytes, and have a pyknotic nucleus and brightly eosinophilic cytoplasm because of the accumulation of keratin filaments. Dyskeratosis occurs when epidermal maturation is deranged, such as in zinc-responsive dermatosis. Dyskeratosis is also a feature of epidermal dysplasia, which is a premalignant change in actinic keratoses.

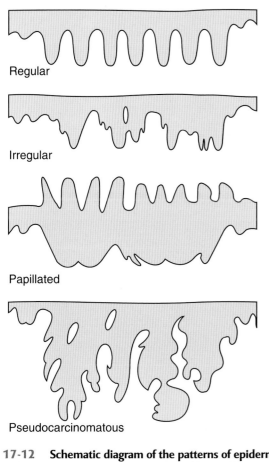

Fig. 17-12   **Schematic diagram of the patterns of epidermal hyperplasia.** Exaggerated regular epidermal hyperplasia is also called "psoriasiform" epidermal hyperplasia, named after the human condition of "psoriasis," which is characterized by this type of epidermal hyperplasia. *(Adapted from Ackerman AB, Boer A, Bennin B et al, editors:* Histologic diagnosis of inflammatory skin diseases, *ed 3, New York, 2005, Ardor Scribendi.)*

Apoptosis

Apoptosis refers to programmed cell death. Apoptotic keratinocytes have the morphologic features of dyskeratotic cells. However, in apoptosis, the cytoplasmic eosinophilia is due to condensation of cytoplasmic organelles. Apoptotic cells are phagocytosed by adjacent keratinocytes. Phagocytosis before cellular disintegration prevents the development of an acute inflammatory response that would be elicited by the liberated cellular constituents. Thus the process of apoptosis is significantly different from that of necrosis, in which cell lysis releases cellular contents into the extracellular space and causes an inflammatory response. Apoptosis is seen with diseases such as lupus erythematosus and erythema multiforme (Fig. 17-13).

Necrosis

Necrosis refers to the death of cells and is characterized by nuclear pyknosis (shrunken and dense nucleus),

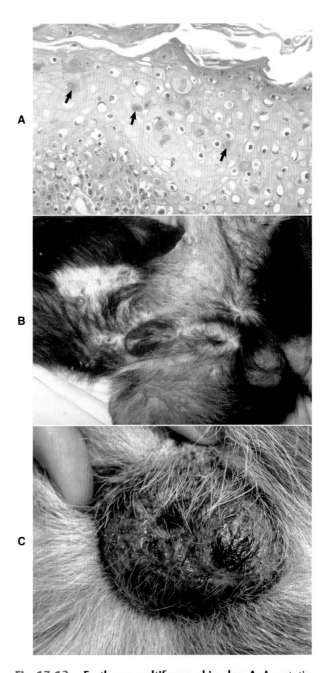

Fig. 17-13   **Erythema multiforme, skin, dog. A,** Apoptotic keratinocytes *(arrows)* are present in the cellular layers of the epidermis. The increased staining intensity of apoptotic keratinocytes is a result of condensation of cytoplasmic organelles and nuclei. H&E stain. **B,** Skin of abdomen, inguinal region, and scrotum. Note the circular and linear erosions. The clinical lesions resulting from apoptotic keratinocytes depend on the prevalence and location of the apoptotic cells in the epidermal strata. Numerous deeply located apoptotic keratinocytes can lead to loss of part of the epidermis, resulting in erosions that develop into ulcers. **C,** Scrotum erythema, ulceration, and crusting are present. Crusts form because the ulceration (injury) results in release of inflammatory mediators leading to the accumulation of fluid and cellular exudate that cover and dry on the ulcerated surface. (**A,** *Courtesy Dr. Ann M. Hargis, DermatoDiagnostics.* **B,** *Courtesy Clinical Dermatology Service, College of Veterinary Medicine, University of Florida.* **C,** *Courtesy Dr. Alexander Werner, Valley Veterinary Specialty Service.)*

karyorrhexis (nuclear membrane rupture with fragmentation and release of contents), or karyolysis (complete dissolution of the nucleus with loss of chromatin material), organelle swelling, plasma membrane rupture, and release of cytoplasmic elements into the extracellular space accompanied by an acute inflammatory response. Causes of epidermal necrosis include physical injury (lacerations, thermal burns), chemical injury (irritant contact dermatitis), and injury as a result of ischemia and infarction (vasculitis, thromboembolism). Necrosis of the epidermis can result in erosion (loss of a superficial portion of the epidermis) or ulceration (loss of an area of the entire epidermis and portion of the dermis).

Dysplasia

Dysplasia is defined as abnormal development. Classically, it refers to alteration in size, shape, and organization of adult cells (keratinocytes). Dysplasia is a stage of abnormal development that precedes the formation of a noninvasive (in situ) carcinoma. This is the stage of carcinoma that occurs before the abnormal epidermal cells penetrate the basement membrane. The histologic features include irregular stratification of keratinocytes, variation in cell and nuclear size, increase in number of mitoses, and large hyperchromatic nuclei.

Atrophy

Atrophy is a decrease in the number and size of the cells within the epidermis and occurs as a consequence of sublethal cell injury. Cutaneous atrophy occurs in response to hormonal imbalances, such as hyperadrenocorticism in dogs and cats, partial ischemia, and in severe malnutrition.

ALTERATIONS IN EPIDERMAL FLUID BALANCE AND CELLULAR ADHESION

Edema and intracellular fluid accumulation

Edema refers to fluid accumulation between cells. Intercellular edema of the epidermis is called spongiosis because as the intercellular space expands with fluid, the epidermis develops a "spongy" appearance (Fig. 17-14). The term "spongiosis" is used in other chapters of this book to describe responses to injury that are unique to other tissues or organ systems, and in those circumstances the term "spongiosis" will have different meanings. Severe intercellular edema of the epidermis results in the formation of spongiotic vesicles, which are variably sized vesicular spaces in the epidermis. The spongiotic vesicles often blend with intercellular spaces that are also widened, but to a lesser degree; thus intercellular bridges are often prominent between keratinocytes bordering spongiotic vesicles. Spongiosis is common in epidermal inflammation (epidermitis) caused by staphylococci or *Malassezia* sp.

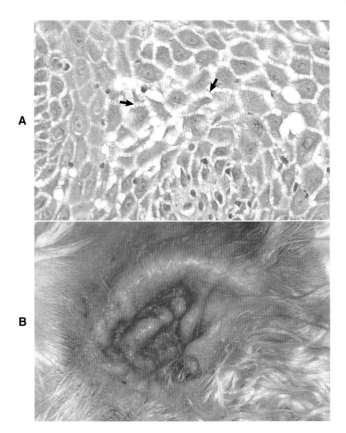

Fig. 17-14   **Edema, skin, dog. A,** Intercellular epidermal edema. Note the appearance of "spines" between keratinocytes (*arrows*) caused by widening of the intercellular spaces by edema. The keratinocytes remain connected to each other via desmosomal attachment sites (Fig. 17-4). H&E stain. **B,** Acute allergic otitis, ear. Note erythema from dermal congeston (hyperemia) and the moist glistening surface of the skin from dermal and epidermal edema. (**A,** *Courtesy Dr. Ann M. Hargis, Dermato Diagnostics.* **B,** *Courtesy Dr. David Duclos, Animal Skin and Allergy Clinic.*)

Intracellular fluid accumulation results in cytoplasmic swelling of keratinocytes, and if the swelling is severe, the swollen keratinocytes can burst, forming microvesicles supported by the walls of the ruptured cells. This type of epidermal damage is termed "reticular degeneration." Intracellular fluid accumulation limited to the basal layer of the epidermis is termed hydropic or vacuolar degeneration and can result in the formation of intrabasilar vesicles. Hydropic degeneration is a consequence of damage to basal keratinocytes when the basal keratinocytes cannot maintain normal homeostasis, and fluid accumulates within the cells (Fig. 17-15). Examples of diseases commonly resulting in hydropic degeneration include lupus erythematosus, dermatomyositis, and drug eruptions. Ballooning degeneration, a form of intracellular fluid accumulation of keratinocytes in more superficial layers of the

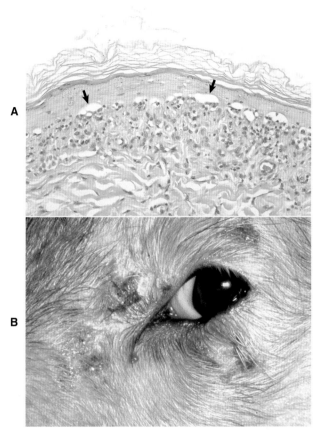

Fig. 17-15 Hydropic degeneration, skin, dog. A, Note vacuolization of the cells of the basal layer. In this photomicrograph, the vacuolated basal cells resemble clefts *(arrows)* between the epidermis and dermis. Lymphocytes are also present in the superficial dermis and lower layers of the epidermis, obscuring the junction between the epidermis and dermis. H&E stain. **B,** Dermatomyositis, periocular. Erythema, depigmentation, erosion, and crusting are the result of injury to basal cells. The vacuolar degeneration of basal cells weakens the epidermal dermal attachment and results in formation of vesicles, erosions, and ulcers. In addition, inflammatory mediators are released, resulting in fluid and cellular exudate, which dry on the surface and form crusts. *(A and B, Courtesy Dr. Ann M. Hargis, DermatoDiagnostics.)*

epidermis, such as the stratum spinosum, is characterized by swollen cells losing their intercellular attachments. This type of degeneration can result in the formation of a fluid-filled vesicle. Viruses that infect cells of the epidermis, such as the pox and parapox viruses, can cause lysis of cytoplasmic keratin and a buildup of excessive fluid, resulting in ballooning degeneration (see Pathologic Reactions of the Entire Cutaneous Unit).

Acantholysis

Acantholysis is the disruption of intercellular junctions (desmosomes) between keratinocytes of the epidermis.

The process is initiated by damage to transmembrane glycoproteins belonging to the cadherin family of adhesion molecules, and leads to splitting of the extracellular core of the desmosomes. Subsequently the desmosomal plaques dissolve and intermediate filaments retract to the perinuclear region of the keratinocytes. Acantholysis occurs with immune-mediated injury, as seen in pemphigus (type II cytotoxic hypersensitivity) or with neutrophilic enzymatic destruction, as seen in superficial pyoderma or uncommonly with some *Trichophyton* sp. infections. The microscopic lesions vary with the location of acantholysis within the various layers of the epidermis. In pemphigus foliaceus, acantholysis occurs in the subcorneal epidermis, resulting in release of free-floating keratinocytes in subcorneal vesicles and pustules (Fig. 17-16). In pemphigus vulgaris, acantholysis occurs in the epidermis, just above the basal layer, resulting in the separation of the upper epidermis from the basal cells (which are often referred to as "a row of tombstones") attached to the basal lamina (Fig. 17-17). Fluid accumulating between the separated layers of the epidermis forms vesicles of varied sizes and shapes.

Vesicles

Vesicles are fluid-filled cavities within or beneath the epidermis (Fig. 17-18). If the cavity is less than 1 cm in diameter, it is called a vesicle; if it is greater than 1 cm in diameter, it is called a bulla (pl. bullae). Vesicles can develop in any layer of the epidermis or beneath the epidermis and can form as the result of acantholysis, epidermal or dermal edema, degeneration of basal cells and keratinocytes, or other processes, such as frictional trauma and burns that cause a lack of cohesion between the epidermal cells or between the epidermis and dermis, resulting in the accumulation of fluid within a cavity. The location of vesicles or bullae within the layers of the epidermis is suggestive of certain diseases. For instance, intraepidermal vesicles can occur in viral infections, subcorneal vesicles in pemphigus foliaceus, suprabasilar vesicles in pemphigus vulgaris (Fig. 17-17), and subepidermal vesicles in bullous pemphigoid or thermal burns (Fig. 17-19).

INFLAMMATORY LESIONS OF THE EPIDERMIS

Acute inflammation of the epidermis actually begins in the dermis with active hyperemia, edema, and migration of leukocytes, often neutrophils (see inflammatory disorders of the dermis section). The edema fluid arises from dilated venules and can move intercellularly through the epidermis, widening the intercellular spaces and causing spongiosis. In thermal burns of the skin, larger quantities of fluid accumulate within or below the epidermis forming vesicles; the fluid reaching the epidermal surface dries to form a

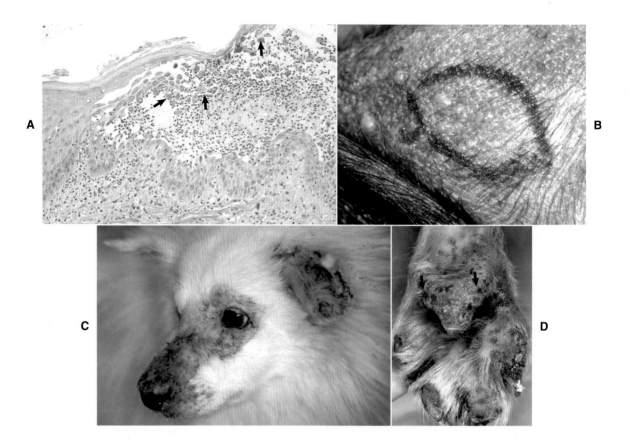

Fig. 17-16 **Pemphigus foliaceus, skin. A,** Horse. The subcorneal pustule contains neutrophils and acantholytic cells (*arrows*), which are epidermal cells separated from each other as a result of the loss of desmosomal attachments. In pemphigus foliaceus, the pustule is located in the superficial epidermis, resulting in clinical lesions that are superficial (pustules that can rupture to form erosions and crusts). The roof of the pustule is the stratum corneum, and the base of the pustule is the stratum spinosum. Forceful clipping or scrubbing the surface of the pustule can lead to rupture and thus can make the sample nondiagnostic. H&E stain. **B,** Inguinal region, dog. Multiple pustules (circumscribed accumulations of pus in the epidermis visible as irregularly ovoid, slightly elevated tan areas) are present in the sparsely haired skin of the inguinal region. The skin within the circle has been injected with local anesthetic in preparation for biopsy sampling. **C,** Face, dog. Erythema, alopecia, focal erosion, crusting, and depigmentation are present on medial surface of the pinnae, periocular skin, and dorsum of the muzzle and the nasal planum. Crusts develop as the result of upward growth of the epidermis and disruption of pustules. Erosions develop as the result of loss of stratum corneum and pustular exudate, which exposes the stratum spinosum. Depigmentation can result from inflammation and damage to pigment containing epidermal cells. **D,** Foot pad, dog (same dog as in Fig. 17-16, C). Erosions (*arrows*), depigmentation, and crusts are present. (*A,* Courtesy Dr. Pamela E. Ginn, College of Veterinary Medicine, University of Florida. *B,* Courtesy Dr. David Duclos, Animal Skin and Allergy Clinic. *C* and *D,* Courtesy Dr. Ann M. Hargis, DermatoDiagnostics.)

largely acellular crust. The leukocytes (often neutrophils in acute inflammation) migrate from the superficial dermal vessels, through the superficial dermis, and into the intercellular spaces of the deep and then superficial layers of the epidermis. The aggregation of migrating leukocytes in the epidermis is termed "exocytosis." Exocytosis of leukocytes is common in inflammation and is usually accompanied by spongiosis. If the inflammation progresses, the migrating leukocytes form pustules within the epidermis or the stratum corneum. Pustules usually dry rapidly and become crusts (Fig. 17-20). The type of leukocyte recruited into the epidermis is influenced by complex interactions of cytokines involved in the pathogenesis of the disease and can be useful in

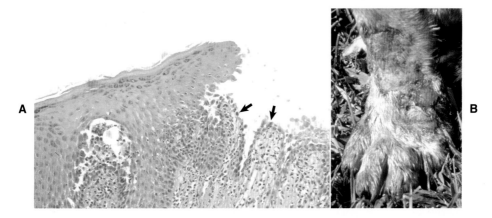

Fig. 17-17   Pemphigus vulgaris, skin, dog. A, Suprabasilar clefting has left a row of basal cells *(arrows)* attached to the dermis. The single row of basal cells is fragile and easily damaged leading to formation of ulcers, with subsequent fluid loss and secondary bacterial infection. H&E stain. **B,** Leg. Note the erythema and large confluent areas of ulceration. In contrast to pemphigus foliaceus (more commonly characterized by erosions and crusts), pemphigus vulgaris is characterized by ulcers because the acantholysis in pemphigus vulgaris occurs deeper in the epidermis (in the cells of the lower epidermis). Vesicles are not frequently seen as they rapidly progress to ulcers, the more common clinical lesion. **(A,** *Courtesy Dr. Ann M. Hargis, DermatoDiagnostics.* **B,** *Courtesy Dr. Alan Mundell, Animal Dermatology Service.)*

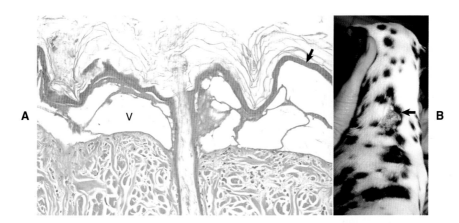

Fig. 17-18   Thermal burn, full thickness (third degree) skin, dog. A, There is necrosis of the epidermis *(arrow)*, follicular epithelium, and dermis. Because of increased capillary permeability, fluid has accumulated between the dermis and epidermis, forming vesicles *(V)*. H&E stain. **B,** The dry necrotic skin is the site of the burn *(arrow)*. *(A and B, Courtesy Blackwell Publishing.)*

classifying and ultimately diagnosing the disease. For instance, intraepidermal eosinophils can be seen in association with ectoparasite bites. Lymphocytic infiltrates into the epidermis are often seen with immune-mediated diseases such as lupus erythematosus. Malignant lymphoma affecting the epidermis is also characterized by intraepidermal lymphocytes. Erythrocytes can also be present in the epidermis, usually associated with trauma, or circulatory disturbances, such as marked vasodilation and vasculitis.

Pustules

Pustules (microabscesses) are accumulations of inflammatory cells (pus) within the epidermis (Fig. 17-16). Epidermal pustules vary in inflammatory cell content and location in the epidermis, depending on the pathogenesis of the disease. The pustules of superficial bacterial infections generally contain degenerate neutrophils and coccoid bacteria and are often located beneath the stratum corneum (subcorneal). In ectoparasitic hypersensitivity, pemphigus foliaceus, and feline eosinophilic

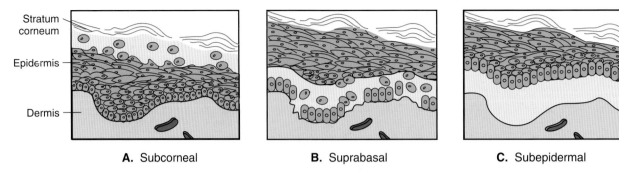

A. Subcorneal   **B.** Suprabasal   **C.** Subepidermal

Fig. 17-19   Schematic diagram of the sites of vesicle formation in the skin. A, In a subcorneal vesicle, the stratum corneum forms the roof of the vesicle (as in impetigo or pemphigus foliaceus). **B,** In a suprabasal vesicle, a portion of the epidermis (stratum spinosum) forms the roof (as in pemphigus vulgaris). **C,** In a subepidermal vesicle, the entire epidermis separates from the dermis and forms the roof (as in bullous pemphigoid). (*A, B,* and *C, From Cotran RS, Kumar V, Collins T, Robbins SL: Robbins pathologic basis of disease, ed 6, Philadelphia, 1999, Saunders.*)

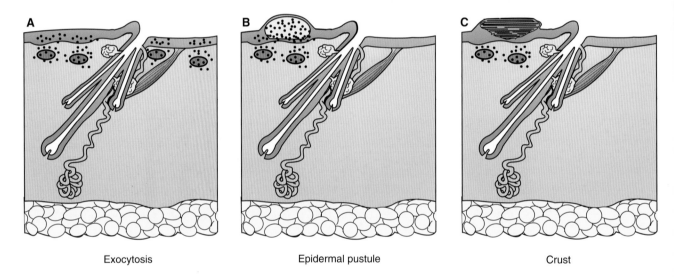

Exocytosis   Epidermal pustule   Crust

Fig. 17-20   Schematic diagram of the inflammatory patterns of the epidermis. A, Leukocytes (*black dots*) migrate from the perivascular dermis into the epidermis, a process called exocytosis. **B,** Leukocytes migrate into the epidermis and accumulate to form a pustule. **C,** The pustule dries to form a crust. (*A, B,* and *C, Courtesy Dr. Ann M. Hargis, DermatoDiagnostics; and Dr. Pamela E. Ginn, College of Veterinary Medicine, University of Florida.*)

plaque, the pustules can be filled with eosinophils. Small pustules containing neoplastic lymphocytes (Pautrier's microabscesses) are present in epitheliotropic lymphoma.

Crusts

Crusts are composed of dried fluid and cellular debris (i.e., dried exudates) located on the epidermal surface; thus crusts are indicative of a previous exudative process. Crusts are not specifically diagnostic but can hold the key to diagnosis in some diseases. For example, in dermatophilosis, the most diagnostic portion of the skin is the crust, which is multilaminated and contains the gram-positive, branching coccoid organism *Dermatophilus congolensis.* Similarly, crusts formed through aging of pustules in pemphigus foliaceus are multilaminated and frequently contain numerous acantholytic cells. Crusts can also contain hair shafts infected with spores and hyphae of dermatophytes.

ALTERATIONS IN EPIDERMAL PIGMENTATION

Pigmentary alterations include hyperpigmentation, hypopigmentation, and pigmentary incontinence. Melanin is produced by melanocytes located in the basal and lower spinous layers of the epidermis, in the external root sheath and hair matrix of follicles, and perivascularly in the dermis. Melanocytes have surface receptors for hormones, such as melanocyte-stimulating hormone, and these hormones regulate melanogenesis. Other factors that influence the amount of melanin pigment in skin and hair are genes, age, temperature, and inflammation.

Hyperpigmentation

Hyperpigmentation results from an increased production of melanin from existing melanocytes or an increase in the number of melanocytes. An example of hyperpigmentation due to an increased number of melanocytes is a lentigo, a rare localized nonneoplastic proliferation of melanocytes confined to the epidermis and resulting in formation of a black macular circumscribed lesion that is usually less than 1 cm in diameter. Most hyperpigmentation of the epidermis results from increased production of melanin from existing melanocytes. Possible mechanisms of increased melanin production include increases in the rate of production of melanosomes (i.e., granules within melanocytes that contain tyrosinase and synthesize melanin), in melanosome size, in rates of melanosome transfer to keratinocytes and increased survival of melanosomes in keratinocytes. Examples of epidermal hyperpigmentation by increased production of melanin include chronic inflammatory diseases (most common cause), such as chronic allergic dermatitis, and endocrine dermatoses, such as hyperadrenocorticism. Hyperpigmentation secondary to inflammation is thought to result from release of melanocyte-stimulating factors from keratinocytes. It is thought that these factors are present in normal epidermis, but that their level or activity is increased in response to stimulation or keratinocyte stress.

Hypopigmentation

Hypopigmentation can be congenital or hereditary and develops because of a lack of melanocytes, failure of melanocytes to produce melanin, or failure of transfer of melanin to epidermal cells. Hypopigmentation can also be acquired via a loss of existing melanin or melanocytes (depigmentation). Because copper is a component of tyrosinase, production of melanin pigment is dependent on copper, and copper deficiency can result in reduced pigmentation.

Pigmentary incontinence

Pigmentary incontinence refers to the loss of melanin pigment from the basal layer of the epidermis caused by damage to the cells of the basal layer and the accumulation of the pigment in macrophages in the upper dermis. Pigmentary incontinence can be a nonspecific lesion associated with inflammation; however, it is also seen with diseases that specifically damage basal cells or melanocytes, such as lupus erythematosus or vitiligo. Leukotrichia (Fig. 17-21) and leukoderma

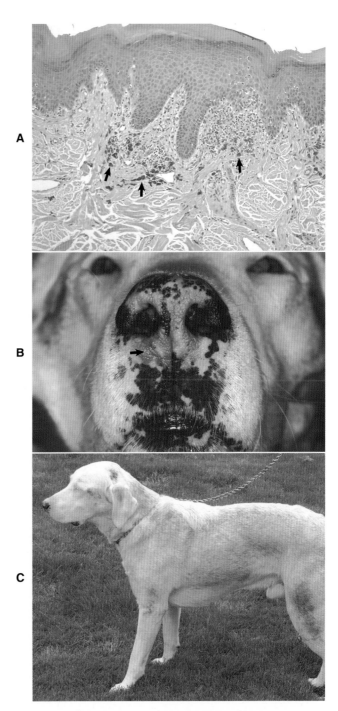

Fig. 17-21   **Leukoderma, skin, dog. A,** Injury to the epidermal pigment containing cells (predominantly melanocytes) has caused loss of melanin pigment in the epidermis (leukoderma). The pigment from the damaged melanocytes has been phagocytosed by dermal macrophages (pigmentary incontinence) *(arrows)*. Mild to moderate lymphocytic inflammation is present along the epidermal dermal interface. H&E stain. **B,** Nose and lips. Areas of the normally black skin of the planum nasale and lips have been partially *(bluish-gray)* or totally *(pink)* depigmented. The bluish-gray areas are in the process of becoming depigmented. Biopsy samples should be collected from the bluish-gray areas *(arrow)* to identify active inflammation and diagnostic lesions.

(Continued)

Fig. 17-21, cont'd Biopsy samples from black skin or from already totally depigmented skin will likely only show normal appearing black or nonpigmented skin, respectively, with no evidence of inflammation. **C,** Leukotrichia, body. This dog is the same one depicted in Fig. 17-21, *B.* He is a black Labrador retriever mix. More than 90% of the black hair coat became white (leukotrichia). Biopsy samples from white-haired areas may be normal because the inflammatory event that caused the pigment loss is likely gone by the time nonpigmented hair shafts emerge from the hair follicles. (*A, Courtesy Dr. Ann M. Hargis, DermatoDiagnostics. B and C, Courtesy Dr. David Duclos, Animal Skin and Allergy Clinic.*)

refer to decreased pigmentation of hair and skin, respectively.

RESPONSES OF THE DERMIS TO INJURY
ALTERATIONS IN GROWTH, DEVELOPMENT, OR TISSUE MAINTENANCE

Dermal atrophy

Dermal atrophy results from a decrease in the quantity of collagen fibrils and fibroblasts in the dermis and leads to a decrease in the thickness of the dermis noted clinically by thin, translucent skin with more

visible vasculature. The principal causes of dermal atrophy in domestic animals are catabolic diseases associated with protein degradation, such as hyperadrenocorticism (particularly in dogs and cats), and starvation. In cats with hyperadrenocorticism, collagen loss is sufficient to increase fragility of the skin, which tears with normal handling. Severe dermal atrophy can also be caused by repeated topical application of glucocorticoids.

Fibrosis

Fibrosis (fibroplasia) develops in response to various injuries, particularly ulceration of the epidermis. It consists of proliferation of fibroblasts and newly formed collagen fibrils (extracellular matrix). In the early stage of fibroplasia called "granulation tissue," the long axis of the fibroblasts and collagen fibrils are parallel to the surface of the skin and are oriented perpendicular to vertically aligned proliferative vessels. Clinically the capillaries are seen on the surface as minute red dots that create a "granular" appearance, thus the name "granulation tissue." Microscopically the orientation pattern provides a "lattice-work" appearance to the tissue (Fig. 17-22). Fibrosis refers to the gradual deposition and maturation of collagen to form a scar. During fibrosis, collagen production increases and fibroblast and capillary numbers decrease, resulting in less

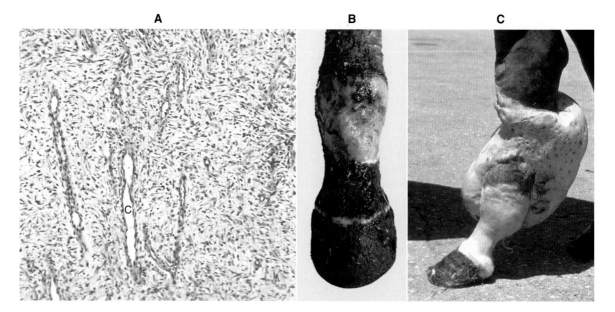

Fig. 17-22 **Granulation tissue, skin, horse. A,** Note vertically oriented capillaries (C) and horizontally oriented fibroblasts and a few collagen fibers providing a "lattice-work" appearance to the granulation tissue. **B,** Leg. Note ulcerated area filled with granulation tissue. **C,** Exuberant granulation tissue, leg. Granulation tissue is a normal component of wound healing. However, excessive or exuberant granulation tissue can develop as a pathologic process. This condition occurs especially in horses, when an ulcer fails to become reepithelialized. Although this process is commonly called "exuberant granulation tissue," at the stage depicted in this photograph, most of the granulation tissue has been converted to fibrous connective tissue. (*A, B, and C, Courtesy Dr, M.D. McGavin, College of Veterinary Medicine, University of Tennessee.*)

cellular dense collagen oriented in thick hyaline bundles in parallel arrangement (e.g., a scar), which grossly appear white and glistening.

Collagen dysplasia

Collagen dysplasia is generally an inherited abnormality of collagen that results in decreased tensile strength and an increased ability of the skin to stretch beyond normal limits. Because the tensile strength is reduced, even minor trauma can cause the skin to tear. Healing results in formation of scars. Microscopic features vary among the different types of collagen dysplasia disorders, and in some the skin has no microscopic alterations. Collagen bundles can vary in size and shape and consist of tangled fibers with an abnormal organizational pattern.

Solar elastosis

Solar elastosis is caused by chronic exposure of the skin to the ultraviolet spectrum of sunlight. Sunlight consists of visible, ultraviolet (UV), and infrared light rays. The portion of the UV light most damaging to the skin is ultraviolet B (UVB) and is in the range of 290 to 320 nm. The amount of light reaching the skin is dependent on a variety of environmental and host factors that can greatly influence the geographic incidence and anatomic locations of solar damage. Environmental factors include quantity of ozone, smog, and cloud cover that tend to absorb and scatter some of the UV rays. Altitude and latitude are also very important. The atmosphere at high altitude is thinner, so there is less oxygen and particulate matter to absorb and scatter the UV rays. Latitude is also critically important. It has been estimated that the incidence of sunlight-induced cancer in human beings doubles for every 265 miles closer to the equator that human beings reside. At high latitudes, the path of sunlight through the ozone layer is longer than at lower latitudes, so more of the harmful UV light is absorbed by the ozone. The path of sunlight through the ozone layer is also one of the reasons that sunlight has more damaging UV rays in summer months and at midday. Increased wind velocity has also been shown to have an enhancing influence on damaging effects of UV light on the skin. Local environmental factors can influence the quantity of UV light reaching an animal's skin. Such factors include availability of shelter from sunlight in the form of trees, shade panels, or indoor housing, and color of the ground material (lightly colored sand) that can increase exposure to UV light through reflection. Host factors include quantity of hair, degree of pigmentation, thickness of stratum corneum, and other difficult to define genetic factors. Therefore solar damage is more prevalent in high altitude, low latitude parts of the world and in animals residing outside for long periods of time. Lesions generally develop in poorly haired and lightly pigmented sites. Solar elastosis consists of increased numbers of thick, interwoven, basophilic elastic fibers in the superficial dermis. In the nonpigmented abdominal skin of dogs, solar elastosis may develop intermixed with or below a linear band of scarring parallel to the epidermal surface. In human beings, studies have revealed that the solar-damaged elastic tissue is newly formed as a result of altered function of fibroblasts, not a degeneration product of preexisting elastic fibers. Solar elastosis is less prominent in the skin of domestic animals than in human beings but is often prominent in lightly pigmented, poorly haired sun-exposed skin and eyelids of horses and in the lower eyelids of Hereford cattle residing in sunny locations.

DEGENERATIVE COLLAGEN DISORDERS OF THE DERMIS

The term "collagen degeneration" has been used to refer to an altered histologic appearance of collagen fibers in hematoxylin and eosin (H&E) stained sections, whereby there is brightly eosinophilic granular to amorphous material bordering the fibers and somewhat obscuring the fiber detail. The collagen fibers and bordering eosinophilic material have also been referred to as "flame figures" due in part to the irregular, sometimes radiating, edges and brightly eosinophilic staining intensity. Electron microscopic studies in cats and human beings indicate that the collagen fibers can be disrupted, but they are not "degenerate." Instead, the brightly eosinophilic granular and amorphous material consists of aggregates of many eosinophils and eosinophil granules that border slightly disrupted but otherwise normal collagen fibers. These flame figures are seen in conditions in which eosinophils are prominent, including in reactions to insect bites, mast cell tumors, and eosinophilic granulomas (collagenolytic granulomas) (Fig. 17-23). Collagen lysis refers to dissolution of collagen fibrils morphologically consisting of amorphous, lightly eosinophilic material lacking fibrillar detail. Collagen lysis is likely a secondary event caused by proteolytic enzymes released by a variety of cells, including eosinophils (collagenase) and neutrophils (collagenolytic proteinase, collagenase).

DISORDERS CHARACTERIZED BY ABNORMAL DEPOSITS IN THE DERMIS

Amyloid

Amyloid is an abnormal proteinaceous substance that can be deposited in the skin as a result of a primary abnormality of immunocytes (primary amyloidosis), in which case the amyloid is derived from components of immunoglobulin light chains (AL amyloid), or as a result of chronic inflammatory conditions (secondary amyloidosis), in which case the amyloid is derived from serum amyloid-associated protein (SAA protein), an acute phase reactant produced by the body in response

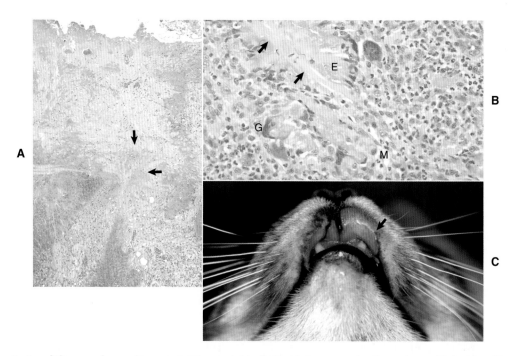

Fig. 17-23 **Eosinophilic granuloma, skin, cat. A,** Ulcerated skin *(left)* with fragmented collagen *(arrows)* is bordered by degranulated eosinophils. H&E stain. **B,** Fragmented collagen *(arrows)* is bordered by a row of macrophages *(M),* multinucleated giant cells *(G),* and degranulated eosinophils *(E),* somewhat resembling a flame ("flame figure"). H&E stain. **C,** Upper lip. Bilateral ulcers are present on the upper lips, but the ulcer on the right side of the photograph is more extensive *(arrow).* *(**A,** **B,** and **C,** Courtesy Dr. Ann M. Hargis, DermatoDiagnostics.)*

to inflammation. Cutaneous deposition of amyloid is rare but is seen in dogs and horses. Cutaneous deposition of amyloid in dogs can be triggered by a monoclonal gammopathy or plasma cell tumors (AL amyloid) or by dermatomyositis (SAA protein). Clinical lesions reflect the triggering disease. In horses, cutaneous amyloidosis is most often due to deposits of amyloid derived from SAA protein, but underlying inflammatory conditions are not usually identified. Clinical lesions vary from papules and plaques to nodules that usually are covered by a normal hair coat. Similar nodules can also develop in the respiratory mucosa and regional lymph nodes. Histologic lesions include nodular to diffuse granulomatous dermatitis and panniculitis with deposition of amyloid, an eosinophilic hyaline material.

Mucin

Mucin (glycosaminoglycan [GAG]), a normal component of the ground substance of the dermis, consists of protein bound to hyaluronic acid and can be deposited in increased quantity in focal areas or diffusely. Because hyaluronic acid has a great affinity for binding water, the skin in cases of mucin deposition (mucinosis) has a thick, puffy appearance. In cases of severe mucinosis, the skin, when pricked with a needle, can exude mucin (a stringy fluid material). In histologic sections, much of the water is lost and mucin appears as fine amphophilic granules or fibrils that separate dermal collagen. Examples of disorders with dermal

mucin deposition are termed myxedema in hypothyroidism and mucinosis in the Chinese Shar-Pei dog.

Calcium deposits

Calcium deposits are deposits of insoluble calcium salts within cutaneous tissue and are referred to as mineralization or calcification. Mineralization can occur in three basic forms: (1) dystrophic, (2) metastatic, and (3) idiopathic. Dystrophic mineralization occurs as a result of injury or degeneration of skin components. Mechanisms leading to calcium deposition in dystrophic mineralization are complex and involve reduced pH of injured tissue, mitochondrial concentration of calcium and phosphorus, and the influx of calcium into injured cells. Examples include deposition of mineral in granulomas and calcinosis cutis seen in some cases of hyperadrenocorticism. In metastatic mineralization, the calcium deposits develop in association with abnormal metabolism of calcium, phosphorus, and vitamin D. Mechanisms thought to participate in mineral deposition are loss of mineralization inhibitors, changing of ions into a solid phase, and phosphate ion initiation of crystal formation. Examples include deposition of calcium salts in soft tissues in chronic renal disease and in poisoning with cholecalciferol (vitamin D_3). The causes of idiopathic mineralization are not known. Mineralization can affect individual or groups of collagen fibers, resulting in increased basophilia and fragmentation of fibers in H&E stained sections. Calcium can also be deposited as amorphous nodular aggregates (calcinosis circumscripta). Calcium deposits can elicit a granulomatous inflammatory response, a foreign-body reaction to the deposits.

INFLAMMATORY DISORDERS OF THE DERMIS

Dermatitis is inflammation of the dermis. Acute dermatitis begins with active hyperemia (increased blood flow), edema, and migration of leukocytes and results from release of cytokines and other mediators of acute inflammation (see Chapter 3). Active hyperemia is due to vasodilation of arterioles, which causes increased blood flow at reduced velocity to capillary beds and postcapillary venules. Edema is due to increased vascular permeability. Fluid leaves vessels mostly through widened interendothelial cell junctions. With a mild increase in vascular permeability, the edema fluid is clear (serous) because there are very few plasma proteins in the fluid. With increasing vascular permeability or endothelial cell injury, larger protein molecules such as fibrinogen escape from vessels, and the edema fluid becomes more eosinophilic and amorphous to fibrillar (fibrinous). The next step in acute dermatitis is migration of leukocytes from vessels into the perivascular dermis. The slowing of the blood flow and the endothelial cell expression of adhesion molecules that bind circulating leukocytes permit the migration of leukocytes in acute inflammation. The slowing of the blood flow allows leukocytes to move from the center of the vessel, where blood flow is fastest, to the margin, where they contact and attach to the activated endothelial cells.

After attaching to activated endothelial cells, leukocytes migrate between the endothelial cells into the perivascular dermis. The type of leukocyte that migrates and the sequence of cellular influx depend on activation of different adhesion molecules and chemotactic factors in the different phases of inflammation. In many types of acute inflammation, neutrophils are one of the first cells to arrive. Neutrophils predominate in the first 6 to 24 hours of injury and are generally replaced by macrophages in 24 to 48 hours. There are exceptions to this sequence of cellular exudation. For instance, in reactions mediated by immunoglobulin E (IgE) cross-linking, such as type I hypersensitivity responses, mast cells (located in the perivascular dermis) are stimulated to release contents of granules (occurs in seconds), and synthesize and release inflammatory mediators (prostaglandins, leukotrienes, cytokines) resulting in the influx of eosinophils, basophils, CD4-T_H2 lymphocytes, and macrophages. Mast cell degranulation and T_H2 lymphocyte activation cause eosinophils to accumulate in large numbers. Thus eosinophils often comprise the majority of leukocytes in inflammatory reactions against parasites and other allergic reactions. Also in type IV hypersensitivity reactions mediated by sensitized T lymphocytes (delayed-type

hypersensitivity), CD4 lymphocytes (T_H2 [helper]) are present first and constitute a majority of the perivascular inflammatory cells in fully developed lesions.

Acute dermatitis typically results in one of four outcomes. First, there can be complete resolution, which occurs when the inciting stimulus has short duration and there is little tissue damage that is completely repaired. Second, an abscess can form, which occurs with pus-producing (pyogenic) bacterial infections. Third, healing occurs by replacement of the injured area by fibrous connective tissue (e.g., scarring), which occurs when there is significant tissue destruction (such as a deep burn) in which the parenchymal tissues are lost and thus cannot regenerate. Fourth, there is progression of acute dermatitis to chronic dermatitis.

Chronic dermatitis is inflammation of the skin that lasts weeks or months. Histologic features of chronic dermatitis include: accumulation of macrophages, lymphocytes, and plasma cells; tissue destruction in part caused by the inflammatory cells; and a reparative host response of fibrosis and angiogenesis. Chronic dermatitis is usually caused by persistent infections often associated with delayed hypersensitivity and the formation of granulomas (e.g., *Mycobacteria* sp.), presence of foreign material in the skin (e.g., embedded suture), or autoimmune reactions in which self-antigens provoke an ongoing immunologic inflammatory response against host tissue (e.g., lupus erythematosus). Macrophages are a key cell in chronic dermatitis. They arise from monocytes in the peripheral blood and mature to macrophages whose primary function is phagocytosis. Macrophages also become activated by a variety of chemical mediators, including the cytokine IFN-γ secreted by sensitized T lymphocytes. When activated, macrophages also secrete many mediators of tissue injury (toxic oxygen metabolites, proteases, coagulation factors) and fibrosis (growth factors, angiogenesis factors, collagenases) that contribute to chronic inflammation. The presence of lymphocytes and plasma cells in chronic inflammation is indicative of a host immune response.

The inflammatory milieu in the progression of acute and chronic dermatitis can be further complicated by other superimposed factors, notably physical injury from self-trauma, secondary bacterial infection of traumatized surface, injury from insect bites attracted by odor or exudate, and moderation by the host immune response or therapy. Thus dermal inflammatory responses to different stimuli often have overlapping histologic features, providing a diagnostic challenge for the dermatopathologist. Even so, the distribution of leukocytes often evolves into recognizable patterns that, when combined with the inflammatory cell type, suggest a group of differential diagnoses or the cause or pathogenesis of a specific disease (Tables 17-3 and 17-4). Dermal patterns of inflammation that have been used in histologic diagnosis include perivascular dermatitis, interface dermatitis (mild inflammation affecting the basilar epidermis and superficial dermis that often obscures the epidermal dermal interface), nodular to diffuse dermatitis with infectious agents, and nodular to diffuse dermatitis without infectious agents (Fig. 17-24). For example, perivascular dermatitis with eosinophils is suggestive of hypersensitivity associated with parasites or other antigens; interface dermatitis with lymphocytes is suggestive of an immune response directed toward epidermal cells, such as lupus erythematosus or erythema multiforme; and nodular dermatitis with macrophages (granulomatous dermatitis) indicates a persistent stimulus, such as infection with acid-fast bacteria or fungi. Thus patterns of inflammation combined with cellular composition of infiltrates are useful in microscopic diagnosis.

RESPONSES OF THE ADNEXA TO INJURY

The term "adnexa" refers to appendages or adjunct parts, which in the skin includes hair follicles and

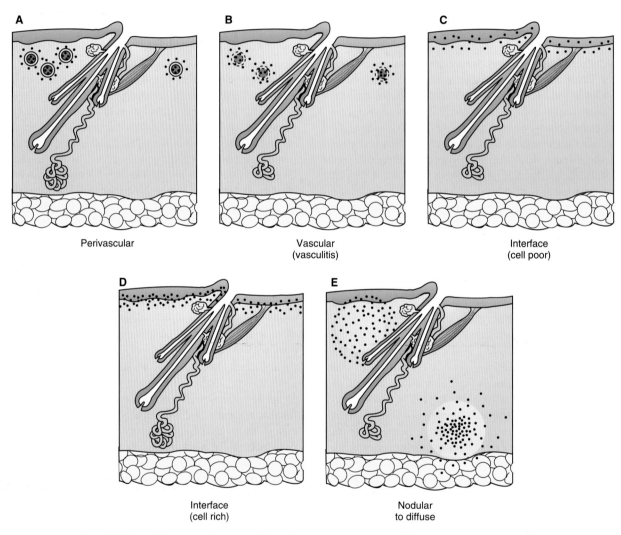

Fig. 17-24 **Schematic diagram of the inflammatory patterns of the dermis. A,** Perivascular: Leukocytes (*black dots*) migrate from the dermal vessels into the perivascular dermis. This is the least specific pattern because all inflammatory patterns are at one stage perivascular. **B,** Vascular (vasculitis): Leukocytes target the vessel wall, resulting in necrosis, inflammation, leakage of fibrin and red blood cells, and if severe, thrombosis and infarction. **C,** Interface, cell poor: Mild, often lymphocytic, inflammation located along the epidermal dermal interface with vacuolar or apoptotic degeneration of basal cells. **D,** Interface, cell rich: Dense band of inflammation along the epidermal dermal interface, obscuring the basilar layer of the epidermis, and with vacuolar or apoptotic degeneration of basal cells. **E,** Nodular to diffuse with or without microorganisms: Inflammation, typically granulomatous to pyogranulomatous, which partially effaces the architecture of the dermis. May be associated with infectious agent or may be sterile. (*A through E, Courtesy Dr. Ann M. Hargis, DermatoDiagnostics; and Dr. Pamela E. Ginn, College of Veterinary Medicine, University of Florida.*)

glands. The major clinical and histologic changes involve the hair follicles, and thus follicular lesions will be emphasized in the following discussion.

ALTERATIONS IN MAINTENANCE, GROWTH, AND DEVELOPMENT

Atrophy

Atrophy refers to gradual reduction (involution) in size and can be physiologic or pathologic. Physiologic atrophy is related to the normal progression of the hair follicle cycle (i.e., the hair cycle stages of growth [anagen], transition [catagen], rest [telogen], and shed [exogen]). Pathologic atrophy occurs when the degree of atrophy is greater than that expected for a given stage of the hair cycle. Causes of follicular atrophy include hormonal abnormalities, nutritional abnormalities, inadequacy of blood supply, inflammation, and general state of health, including stressful events or systemic illness. Some types of pathologic atrophy can be reversed when the underlying cause is corrected. Damage to germinal epithelium can result in destruction or total loss of the adnexa with replacement by a scar. Examples include extensive inflammation and disruption of the follicle (folliculitis and furunculosis) and bordering glands and dermis that destroy a significant portion of the adnexal germinal epithelium, thermal burns sufficiently deep to involve the adnexa and dermal vessels, thrombosis causing infarction (i.e., diamond skin disease in pigs), and severe physical trauma, such as lacerations that remove components of the skin including adnexa.

Hypertrophy

Hypertrophy is an increase in the unit size of a structure or an individual cell. Follicular hypertrophy, follicles that are longer and wider than normal for the site, develops secondary to repeated surface trauma, such as in acral lick dermatitis. Hyperplasia is an increase in the number of cells in a structure. Enlargement of adnexa, a common response to injury, usually involves both hypertrophy and hyperplasia, and is observed in follicles and sebaceous and apocrine glands associated with chronic allergic dermatitis.

Abnormalities of hair cycle stages

Abnormalities of hair cycle stages occur when there is disruption in the normal progression from the anagen, catagen, telogen, and exogen stages of the hair cycle (Fig. 17-6). Clinical and histologic lesions are diverse. Some animals have failure of hair to regrow after clipping (hypothyroidism, post clipping alopecia). Other animals have sudden shedding of hair coat (synchronous change of many follicles from telogen into anagen, resulting in loss of old telogen hair shafts as new hair shafts emerge, termed "telogen effluvium").

Yet other animals have gradual, but progressive, loss of hair shafts associated with endocrine disease, such as hyperadrenocorticism.

Follicular dysplasia

Follicular dysplasia refers to incomplete or abnormal development of follicles and hair shafts. Different types of follicular dysplasia syndromes are described, but most are poorly characterized. Microscopic features vary but include abnormal keratinocytes in the hair matrix or abnormally formed follicles, which produce abnormal hair shafts, resulting clinically in a reduced or absent hair coat. The lesions of follicular dysplasia that are most easily recognized microscopically are color associated and include color mutant alopecia (color dilution follicular dysplasia) and black hair follicular dysplasia (Fig. 17-25) in which melanin pigment abnormalities serve as a marker for the dysplasia. These pigment abnormalities include abnormally clumped melanin pigment granules in melanocytes in the epidermis and follicular hair matrix cells; and irregularly sized, shaped, and distributed melanin pigment clumps in hair shafts; and macrophages containing melanin pigment and located in the perifollicular dermis. The pathogenesis of the abnormal hair coat appears to involve breakage of

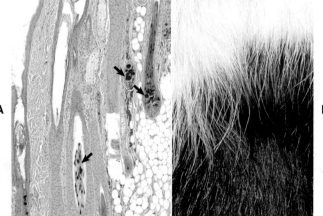

Fig. 17-25   **Black hair follicular dysplasia, skin, dog.** **A,** Large and variably sized and shaped melanin pigment granules are present in hair shafts and hair matrix cells *(arrows).* Macrophages that have phagocytosed melanin pigment are present in the dermis, most prominently near hair bulbs. The melanin presumably comes from damaged hair matrix cells. H&E stain. **B,** Note alopecia in black-haired area and normal hair coat in white-haired area. The skin in the black-haired area is pigmented; thus alopecia is not easily recognized from a distance. (**A,** *Courtesy Dr. Ann M. Hargis, DermatoDiagnostics.* **B,** *Courtesy Blackwell Publishing.)*

hair shafts in areas of large pigment clumps, an abnormality of development of the cuticle, and also possibly an abnormality of hair shaft development caused by damaged hair matrix cells.

ADNEXAL INFLAMMATORY DISORDERS
Folliculitis

Folliculitis is inflammation of a hair follicle. Folliculitis can be histologically classified according to the anatomic segment of the hair follicle affected and the type of leukocytes present in the inflammatory infiltrate (Fig. 17-26). The types of follicular inflammation include perifolliculitis, mural folliculitis, luminal folliculitis, and inflammation of the hair bulb (bulbitis). The inflammation of hair follicles begins in the perifollicular blood vessels with the same hemodynamic, permeability, and leukocytic changes that comprise dermal inflammation. Leukocytes migrate from perifollicular blood vessels to the dermis, resulting in perifolliculitis (inflammation around, but not involving, the hair follicle). Perifolliculitis is not specific for any category of disease but is an initial event in the development

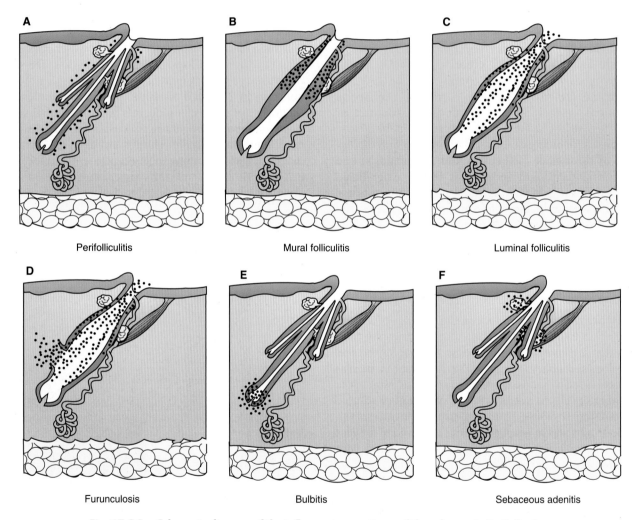

Perifolliculitis   Mural folliculitis   Luminal folliculitis

Furunculosis   Bulbitis   Sebaceous adenitis

Fig. 17-26   Schematic diagram of the inflammatory patterns of the adnexa. A, Perifollicular: Leukocytes *(black dots)* migrate from the dermal vessels near follicles into the perifollicular dermis. **B,** Mural folliculitis: Inflammation targets the follicular wall. There are subtypes of mural folliculitis that vary with level of involvement (superficial versus inferior), type of the inflammation (pustular versus necrotizing), and the degree or severity of penetration into the follicular wall (interface versus infiltrative). **C,** Luminal folliculitis: Inflammatory exudate is present in the follicular lumen, and inflammation also usually involves the wall, often a response to follicular infection. **D,** Furunculosis: Disruption of the follicular wall resulting in release of luminal contents into the bordering dermis. **E,** Bulbitis: Inflammation targeting the inferior segment of the hair follicle, also called the "hair bulb." **F,** Sebaceous adenitis: inflammation targeting the sebaceous glands. (**A** through **F,** *Courtesy Dr. Ann M. Hargis, DermatoDiagnostics; and Dr. Pamela E. Ginn, College of Veterinary Medicine, University of Florida.*)

of folliculitis. Perifolliculitis also often coincides with folliculitis of a variety of causes. The perifollicular inflammatory cells then migrate into the follicular wall, resulting in mural folliculitis (inflammation limited to the wall of the follicle). Depending on the cause of the inflammatory process, the leukocytes can remain localized to the follicular wall or can progress into the follicular lumen.

Mural.   In mural folliculitis, leukocytes remain largely confined to the follicular wall. Mural folliculitis is further subdivided by the location, type, or severity of involvement of the follicular wall, such as interface (outer aspect of the follicular wall), infiltrative (more infiltration into the follicular wall), pustular (presence of pustules in the follicular wall), or necrotizing (necrosis and disruption of the follicular wall). The subtype of mural folliculitis can provide insight into the pathogenesis of folliculitis (e.g., disease process). For example, pustular mural folliculitis is a feature of pemphigus foliaceus, and interface mural folliculitis is a feature of demodicosis (Fig. 17-27).

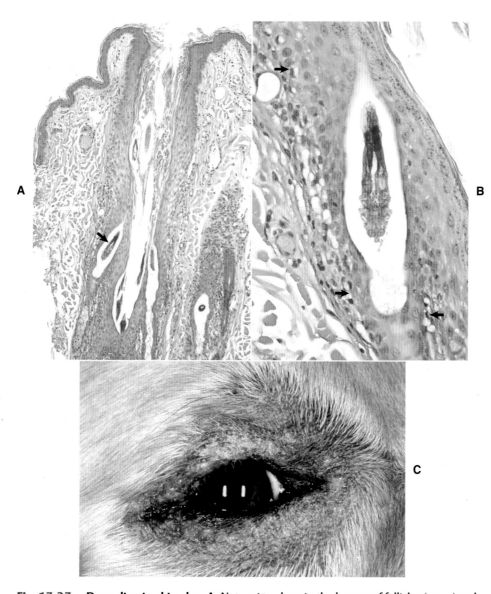

Fig. 17-27   **Demodicosis, skin, dog. A,** Note mites deep in the lumens of follicles (*arrow*) and also inflammation in the outer wall of the follicle (interface mural folliculitis) and in the perifollicular dermis (perifolliculitis). H&E stain. **B,** Note the mite in the follicular lumen. There are a few lymphocytes bordering the follicular wall and mild vacuolar degeneration of basal cells (*arrows*) (lymphocytic interface mural folliculitis) of the follicular wall. H&E stain. **C,** Localized demodicosis, periocular. Skin is alopecic, lichenified, and hyperpigmented. Alopecia is likely due to inflammation, initiated by an immune response to mite infestation and possibly secondary bacterial infection, that results in damage and sometimes disruption of the follicular wall (furunculosis). (*A, B,* and *C,* Courtesy Dr. Ann M. Hargis, DermatoDiagnostics.)

Bulbitis.   Bulbitis refers to inflammation directed at the deepest portion of the follicle, the hair bulb. Alopecia areata is a specific example of bulbitis. It develops in horses, dogs, cats, and cattle; is characterized by lymphocytic infiltrates around and in growing hair bulbs; and results in alopecia. In dogs and horses, antifollicular cell-mediated immunity and humoral immunity participate. Cellular infiltrates of the hair bulb are mostly cytotoxic CD8+ lymphocytes and CD1+ dendritic antigen-presenting cells, whereas CD8+ and CD4+ lymphocytes predominate in the peribulbar infiltrate. Autoantibodies target trichohyalin, hair keratins, and other components of the hair follicle. The damage to hair matrix cells within the hair bulb results in formation of dystrophic (abnormal) hair shafts. Alopecia areata can spontaneously resolve, but the newly growing hairs can be white instead of pigmented, probably as a result of damage to melanocytes in the hair bulb.

Luminal.   Luminal folliculitis refers to inflammation involving the lumen of the follicle and usually the wall of the follicle (Fig. 17-28). Luminal folliculitis develops when the leukocytes in the follicular wall migrate into the lumen, usually as a result of a stimulus in the follicular lumen, such as a follicular infection with bacteria (staphylococci) or dermatophytes (*Microsporum, Trichophyton*), or infestation with parasites (*Demodex, Pelodera*). The inflammation can weaken the follicular wall leading to rupture, known as furunculosis (Fig. 17-29), and release of follicular contents into the dermis. There are other causes of furunculosis, including trauma to the surface of the skin resulting in epidermal hyperplasia at the opening of the follicle, plugging of the follicle by stratum corneum, and accumulation of follicular contents including glandular secretions (comedo formation). The gradual accumulation of this luminal material can cause thinning of the follicular wall, leading to rupture. Regardless of the cause of furunculosis, the presence of hair fragments, keratin proteins, sebum, and possible infectious agents in the dermis leads to a suppurative inflammatory response that progresses to more long-standing chronic pyogranulomatous inflammation and scarring. Perifolliculitis, luminal folliculitis, and furunculosis often follow in sequence (Fig. 17-30). The inflammation can resolve with appropriate therapy, can extend into the deep dermis and panniculus, and/or can form sinuses that drain to the surface of the skin and are difficult to resolve. Severe inflammation can lead to complete destruction of adnexal units and replacement by scar tissue.

Sebaceous adenitis

Sebaceous adenitis is a specific inflammatory reaction that targets sebaceous glands; it occurs in dogs (Fig. 17-31) and rarely in cats. Early lesions are

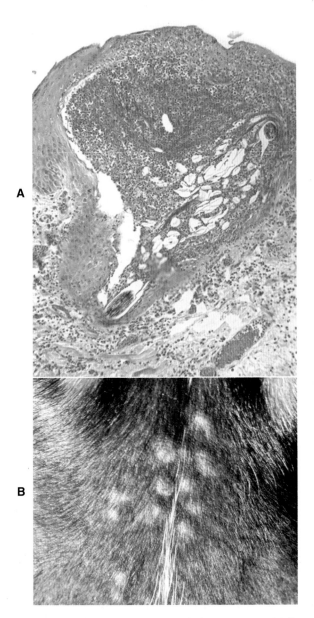

Fig. 17-28   Folliculitis, skin, haired, dog. A, Luminal folliculitis. Note the distention of hair follicle with inflammatory cells (mostly neutrophils). H&E stain. **B,** Multiple alopecic papules are caused by perifollicular inflammation and edema and hair follicles distended with exudate. (*A, Courtesy Dr. M.D. McGavin, College of Veterinary Medicine, University of Tennessee. B, Courtesy Dr. Ann M. Hargis, DermatoDiagnostics.*)

characterized by accumulations of lymphocytes around sebaceous ducts. Fully developed lesions consist of lymphocytes, neutrophils, and macrophages that efface sebaceous glands. Chronic lesions have total loss of sebaceous glands (atrophy), scarring, and epidermal and follicular hyperkeratosis. Sebaceous gland inflammation also can occur secondary to folliculitis, demodicosis, uveodermatologic syndrome, or leishmaniasis, in which

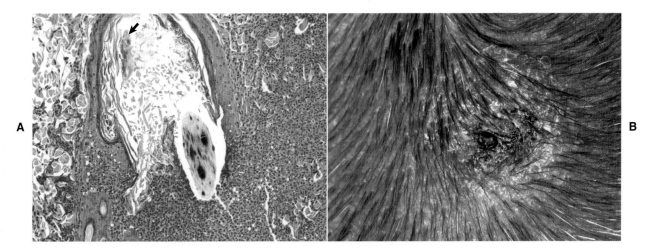

Fig. 17-29   Folliculitis and furunculosis, skin, haired, dog. A, The wall of the follicle has become disrupted, resulting in the release of follicular contents (a hair shaft, stratum corneum of the follicle, and exudate) into the dermis. The follicular lumen also contains numerous coccoid bacteria *(arrow).* The hair shaft has variably sized and shaped melanin pigment granules, indicating that this dog also had coat color dilution. H&E stain. **B,** A circular area of erythema, scaling, and crusting is caused by follicular inflammation and rupture (furunculosis). The inflammation in the perifollicular dermis has extended into the surrounding dermis and formed a draining sinus to the epidermal surface. The exudate on the surface has dried to form a crust. (**A** *and* **B,** *Courtesy Dr. Ann M. Hargis, DermatoDiagnostics.*)

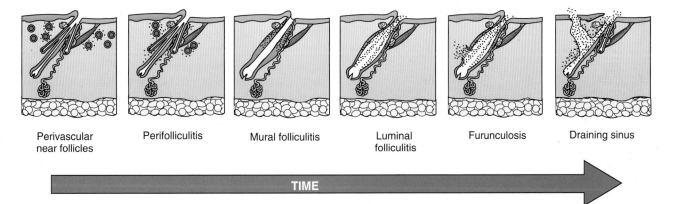

| Perivascular near follicles | Perifolliculitis | Mural folliculitis | Luminal folliculitis | Furunculosis | Draining sinus |

TIME

Fig. 17-30   Schematic diagram of the progression of folliculitis. Inflammation begins with migration of leukocytes *(black dots)* from perifollicular dermal vessels into the perifollicular dermis (perifolliculitis). Inflammation progresses to involve the follicular wall (mural folliculitis) and then the lumen (luminal folliculitis). If the inflammation continues, the follicular wall is weakened, ruptures, and follicular contents are released into the dermis. The inflammation can extend into the deep dermis and panniculus, and/or form sinuses that drain to the surface of the skin. *(Redrawn with permission from Dr. Ann M. Hargis, DermatoDiagnostics; and Dr. Pamela E. Ginn, College of Veterinary Medicine, University of Florida.)*

the inflammation targets other areas of the skin (follicles, epidermal cells, or dermis) and involves the neighboring sebaceous glands because of their proximity to the inflammation.

Hidradenitis

Hidradenitis, inflammation of apocrine glands, has rarely been studied in detail in domestic animals. Suppurative hidradenitis has been described in dogs in which most cases developed in conjunction with staphylococcal folliculitis and furunculosis, either affecting the same or other follicular units. It is speculated, because of the physical connection between the apocrine gland and hair follicle in dogs, that suppurative hidradenitis is most often an extension of hair follicle infection and is due to the bacteria that cause

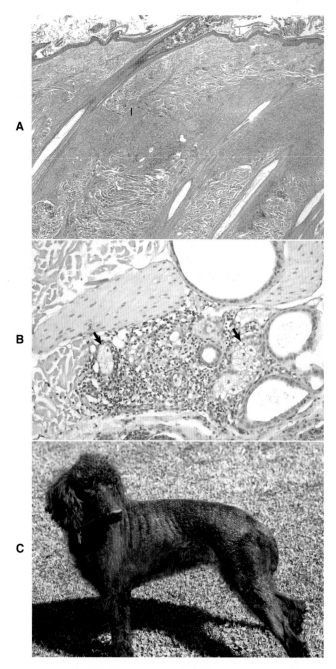

Fig. 17-31   Sebaceous adenitis, skin, haired, dog. A, Note the inflammation (*I*) concentrated in and around sebaceous glands. The inflammation forms a band of inflammatory cells parallel to the epidermis at the level of the sebaceous glands. H&E stain. **B,** Inflammation is beginning to efface the sebaceous glands. A few sebaceous glands (*arrows*) are visible within the area of inflammation. H&E stain. **C,** Alopecia and scaling are evident. The pathogenesis of the alopecia and scaling is incompletely understood. (**A, B,** and **C,** *Courtesy Dr. Ann M. Hargis, DermatoDiagnostics.*)

the folliculitis (usually *Staphylococcus intermedius*). There are no clinical signs that are unique to or suggest the presence of hidradenitis other than the association with follicular bacterial infection. Histologically, dogs with hidradenitis associated with bacterial folliculitis and furunculosis have suppurative inflammation of the apocrine gland and surrounding dermis.

RESPONSES OF THE VESSELS TO INJURY

Vasculitis, inflammation of vessels (Fig. 17-24) in which the vessels are the primary target of injury, can be the result of infection by microbes, immunologic injury, toxins, or disseminated intravascular coagulation or can be idiopathic. The species most commonly presenting with vasculitis are the horse and the dog, and most cases are idiopathic in that a specific cause cannot be determined. Histologic diagnosis of vasculitis is often challenging because it is often difficult to differentiate between vessels taking part in inflammation simply by providing a conduit for inflammatory cells to reach a site of injury in the epidermis or dermis from those vessels that are actually the target of injury. Also, the type of inflammatory cell that participates in the inflammatory process can vary more with the age of the vascular lesion than with the type of disease process. Histologic lesions in vasculitis include damage to the vessel wall, such as the presence of few necrotic cells or foci of fibrinoid necrosis, mural infiltrates of leukocytes, and intramural or perivascular edema, hemorrhage, or fibrin exudation. Vascular injury leads to the clinical lesions of edema and hemorrhage and, if severe, can include ischemic necrosis and infarction. Ulceration with or without sloughing of the skin can occur. Classic examples include immune-complex deposition in vessel walls (systemic lupus erythematosus), infection with an endotheliotropic organism (*Rickettsia rickettsii*), and septicemia with bacterial embolism and infarction in pigs (*Erysipelothrix rhusiopathiae*).

RESPONSES OF THE PANNICULUS TO INJURY
PANNICULITIS

Panniculitis, inflammation of the subcutaneous adipose tissue, can be caused by infectious agents (bacteria, fungi), immune-mediated disorders (systemic lupus erythematosus), physical injury (trauma, injection of irritant material, foreign bodies), nutritional disorders (vitamin E deficiency), or pancreatic disease (pancreatitis, pancreatic carcinoma) or can be of undetermined cause (idiopathic). Panniculitis can be primary or secondary. In primary panniculitis, the subcutaneous adipose tissue is the target of the disease process (Fig. 17-32). An example of primary panniculitis is feline pansteatitis, which occurs in cats fed diets high in polyunsaturated fats and low in antioxidants, such as vitamin E. Lack of vitamin E leads to oxidation of lipids (free radical–induced

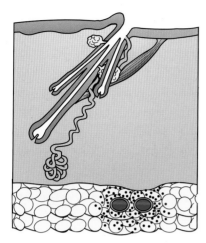

Panniculitis

Fig. 17-32   Schematic diagram of inflammation in the panniculus. Note the leukocytic inflammation *(black dots)* in the subcutaneous adipose tissue (panniculitis). In addition to spreading locally, the inflammation can form a sinus through the dermis and epidermis to the surface. The exudate can have an oily composition due to the fat content of the panniculus. *(Redrawn with permission from Dr. Ann M. Hargis, DermatoDiagnostics; and Dr. Pamela E. Ginn, College of Veterinary Medicine, University of Florida.)*

membrane lipid peroxidation) of the subcutaneous adipose tissue, inciting a pyogranulomatous inflammatory response. In secondary panniculitis, the subcutis is affected by inflammation primarily involving the contiguous dermis; the inflammation extends down into the subcutis. For example, deep bacterial folliculitis with furunculosis can lead to a secondary panniculitis, as can a penetrating wound contaminated with microbial agents or a foreign body. Animals with panniculitis clinically have palpable nodules that can ulcerate and drain an oily or hemorrhagic material. Lesions are most often on the trunk and proximal limbs and can be solitary or multifocal. Solitary lesions may be cured by excision, whereas multiple lesions may resolve with specific therapy or result in scar formation. In animals, panniculitis is subdivided based on cell type and presence or absence of microorganisms into the following basic categories: predominantly neutrophilic, predominantly lymphocytic, predominantly granulomatous to pyogranulomatous with infectious agents, and predominantly granulomatous to pyogranulomatous without infectious agents.

PATHOLOGIC REACTIONS OF THE ENTIRE CUTANEOUS UNIT

Disease processes involving the skin uncommonly affect just one component of the skin (i.e., only the epidermis or only the lumens of hair follicles). More often, multiple components of the skin are involved in the disease process. In addition, lesions evolve through different stages; some lesions can resolve, and there can be secondary lesions, such as self-induced trauma, complicating the initial lesions. Therefore multiple biopsy samples collected from different areas of the skin are often necessary to help illustrate the range of lesions necessary to reach a diagnosis. Multiple biopsy samples provide a more representative picture of the disease process than could a single biopsy sample. Even so, evaluation of multiple biopsy samples does not always lead to a specific diagnosis, but the pattern of lesions identified often suggests categories of disease and rules out other differential diagnoses.

The involvement of the multiple components of the skin in a disease process can be illustrated by a poxvirus infection (Fig. 17-33). When a poxvirus invades the epidermis, the virus replicates in the cells of the stratum spinosum and causes cytoplasmic swelling (ballooning degeneration) and rupture (reticular degeneration) of some of the epidermal cells. Cytoplasmic viral inclusions form in some cells. Cellular constituents released from damaged epidermal cells act as chemical mediators of the acute inflammatory response and are chemotactic for leukocytes. These chemical mediators and chemotactic factors: (1) increase blood flow to the site of viral invasion by dilation of arterioles, (2) cause margination of leukocytes in capillaries and postcapillary venules in the dermis, (3) increase vascular permeability (dermal edema), and (4) cause migration of leukocytes out of vessels into the tissue, creating the formation of macular lesions. The epidermal degeneration, dermal edema, and perivascular inflammation can progress to exudative lesions. Ballooning and reticular degeneration of keratinocytes result in the formation of intraepidermal vesicles. Leukocytes in perivascular sites under the influence of inflammatory mediators from the epidermis migrate to the epidermis and enter the vesicle to form pustules. Some poxviruses also cause epidermal hyperplasia by stimulating host cell DNA synthesis, presumably by a viral gene product similar to epidermal growth factor, resulting in pseudoepitheliomatous hyperplasia. The pustule enlarges and eventually ruptures, releasing the exudates onto the skin surface. The exudates dry and form a crust (scab). The primary lesions of vesicles and pustules are fragile and often transient, lasting only hours, and so are difficult to identify and collect in biopsy samples. The secondary lesions of crusting and scarring are more long-standing. In this way, multiple components of the skin participate in the development of the lesions and are responsible for the clinical stages of macule, papule, vesicle, pustule, crust, and scar.

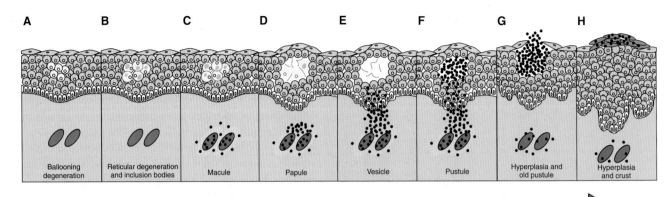

Fig. 17-33 **Schematic diagram of the development of a poxvirus lesion over time.**
A, Ballooning degeneration and **B,** reticular degeneration with inclusion bodies in
keratinocytes are subclinical stages. **C,** Congestion, edema, margination, and migration of leukocytes
(*black dots*) form the macule stage. **D,** Continued epidermal reticular degeneration, epidermal
hyperplasia (acanthosis), dermal edema, and perivascular inflammation form the papule stage.
E, The vesicle stage develops by coalescing of areas of reticular degeneration (disruption of
swollen keratinocytes). **F,** Inflammatory cells migrate from the dermal vessels into the vesicle
and accumulate in the vesicle to form the pustule stage. **G,** The epidermis begins to proliferate
and becomes more acanthotic, and the old pustule is moved toward the epidermal surface.
H, Epidermal hyperplasia progresses with the formation of elongated epidermal dermal
interdigitations, and the old pustule ruptures to form a crust. Larger pustules can be umbilicated, involve the dermis, and result in scarring. (*A* through *H,* Courtesy Dr. Ann M. Hargis, Dermato-
Diagnostics; and Dr. Pamela E. Ginn, College of Veterinary Medicine, University of Florida.)

DEFINITIONS OF CLINICAL TERMS

Knowledge of the clinical appearance of skin lesions,
distribution of lesions, and correlation between the
gross and histologic lesions is often critical in formulating differential and final diagnoses. In skin diseases,
the clinical lesions represent the gross lesions and are
typically examined by a practitioner, not the pathologist; thus the practitioner essentially serves as the eyes
for the pathologist. It is therefore important for the
practitioner to develop the ability to accurately recognize clinical lesion morphology and translate that
information to the pathologist. To facilitate this process,
Table 17-5 is provided to illustrate the morphology of
the various clinical lesions and provide examples of the
disease processes in which those lesions occur.

TECHNIQUES FOR SKIN BIOPSY SAMPLING

Important tips for biopsy sampling of the skin are listed in
Table 17-6. Biopsy do's and don'ts are listed in Boxes 17-5
and 17-6, respectively.

WHEN TO COLLECT BIOPSY SAMPLES

Knowing when to collect biopsy samples helps obtain
the most diagnostic samples; facilitates obtaining samples

early so acute, serious, or neoplastic disorders are diagnosed quickly; and prevents the frustration and economic loss when samples are inappropriately collected,
such as when concurrent therapy might alter diagnostic lesions, when lesions are in a quiescent stage and
might not be diagnostic, and when dermatologic evaluation would have been a better method of achieving
a diagnosis. Biopsy sampling is recommended when:
1. The therapy for the skin disorder is associated with
   significant side effects (to confirm the clinical diagnosis before starting therapy).

Text continued on p. 1155.

Box 17-5

Biopsy Sampling Do's

Be gentle
Biopsy early
Collect multiple samples representative of the range
   of lesions
Include crusts
Biopsy before using antiinflammatory therapy
Use the correct biopsy procedure for the type of lesion
Label samples from different areas
Prevent samples from freezing

Table **17-5**   Definition and Morphology of Primary and Secondary Skin Lesions

Lesion Definition	Drawing	Clinical Photograph
CALLUS* Thick, hard, hairless plaque with increased skin creases Example: Trauma over bony prominence such as elbow or sternum	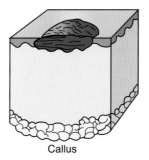 Callus	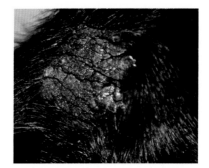
COMEDO Plug of stratum corneum and sebum (*arrows*) within the lumen of a hair follicle Examples: Canine actinic dermatosis, chin acne, Schnauzer comedo syndrome, hyperadrenocorticism	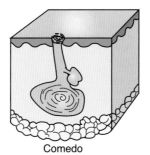 Comedo	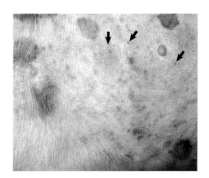
CRUST Dried exudate on the skin surface Example: Chronic stage of pustular disease such as staphylococcal infection or pemphigus foliaceus	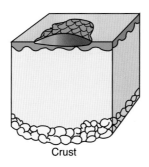 Crust	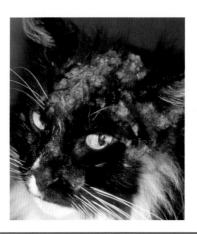

All drawings modified from Copstead LC, Banasik JL: *Pathophysiology: biological and behavioral perspectives*, ed 3, Philadelphia, 2005, Saunders. All clinical photographs courtesy Dr. Ann M. Hargis, DermatoDiagnostics, unless otherwise noted.
*Courtesy Washington Animal Disease Diagnostic Laboratory.

(Continued)

Table **17-5** Definition and Morphology of Primary and Secondary Skin Lesions—Cont'd

Lesion Definition	Drawing	Clinical Photograph
CYST Cavity lined by epithelium and filled with liquid or semisolid material and located in the dermis or subcutis Examples: Follicular cyst, dermoid cyst	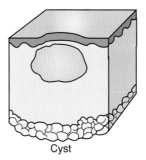 Cyst	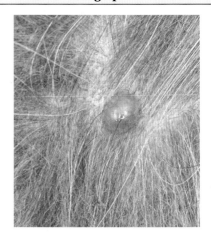
EPIDERMAL COLLARETTE Flat to minimally elevated ring (*arrows*) of scale that enlarges peripherally Examples: Superficial bacterial infection, insect bite, fungal infection	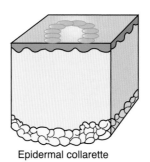 Epidermal collarette	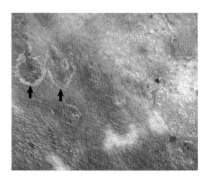
EROSION Loss of part of the epidermis; depressed, moist, glistening (*arrows*) Examples: Secondary to vesicle or pustule rupture or secondary to surface trauma	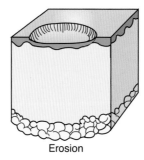 Erosion	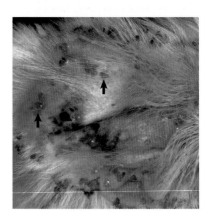

Table **17-5**   **Definition and Morphology of Primary and Secondary Skin Lesions—Cont'd**

Lesion Definition	**Drawing**	**Clinical Photograph**
EXCORIATION* Linear loss of epidermis (*arrows*) Example: Abrasion or scratch	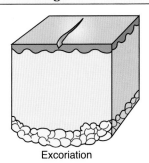 Excoriation	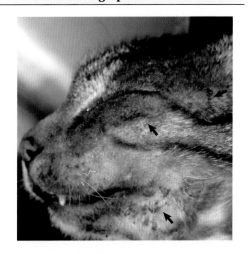
FISSURE Linear crack or break (*arrows*) from the epidermis to the dermis Examples: Footpad fissure seen in pemphigus foliaceus, superficial necrolytic dermatitis, or digital hyperkeratosis	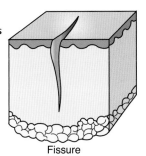 Fissure	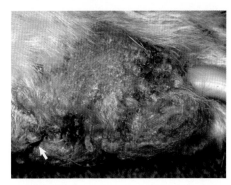
LICHENIFICATION† Rough, thickened epidermis secondary to persistent rubbing, scratching, or irritation Example: Chronic dermatitis	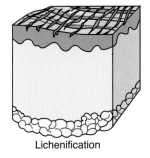 Lichenification	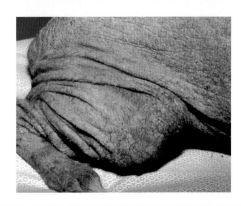

*Courtesy Dr. David Duclos, Animal Skin and Allergy Clinic.
†Courtesy Dr. Helen Power, Dermatology for Animals.

(Continued)

Table **17-5**   **Definition and Morphology of Primary and Secondary Skin Lesions—Cont'd**

Lesion Definition	**Drawing**	**Clinical Photograph**
MACULE Flat, circumscribed area that is a change in the color of the skin, <1 cm in diameter Examples: Hemorrhage, lentigo, vitiligo	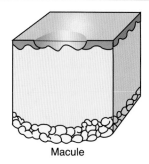 Macule	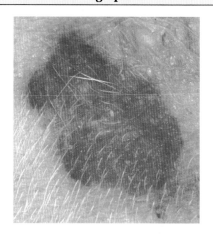
NEOPLASM* "An abnormal mass of tissue, the growth of which exceeds and is uncoordinated with that of normal tissue and persists in the same excessive manner after cessation of the stimuli, which evoked the change"† Examples: Lipoma, mast cell tumor, squamous cell carcinoma	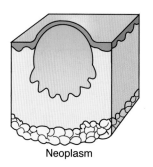 Neoplasm	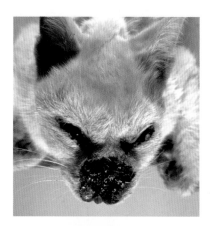
NODULE‡ Elevated, firm, circumscribed lesion 1-2 cm in diameter Examples: Bacterial or fungal infection, infectious or sterile granuloma	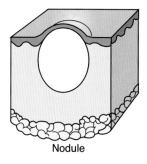 Nodule	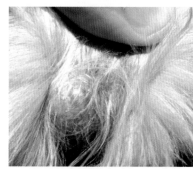
PAPULE Elevated, firm, circumscribed area <1 cm in diameter (*arrows*) Examples: Insect bite, papilloma, superficial folliculitis	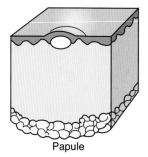 Papule	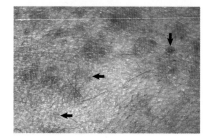

*Courtesy Dr. Donald McGavin.
†From Willis RA: *Pathology of tumors*, Philadelphia, 1948, FA Davis.
‡Courtesy Dr. Alan Mundell, Animal Dermatology Service; and Dr. Ann M. Hargis, DermatoDiagnostics.

Table **17-5**   **Definition and Morphology of Primary and Secondary Skin Lesions—Cont'd**

Lesion Definition	Drawing	Clinical Photograph
PLAQUE Elevated, firm, lesion with a flat top surface >1 cm in diameter Examples: Calcinosis cutis, reactive histiocytosis, eosinophilic plaque	Plaque	
PUSTULE, EPIDERMAL* Elevated superficial accumulation of purulent fluid within the epidermis *(arrow)* Examples: Bacterial infection, pemphigus foliaceus	Pustule	
SCALE Fragmented, keratinized cells, flaky skin, irregular, thick or thin, dry or oily Examples: Cornification disorders, sebaceous adenitis, ichthyosis	Scale	
SCAR Thin to thick fibrous tissue that replaces normal skin following injury or laceration to the dermis Examples: Healed wound, surgical scar	Scar	

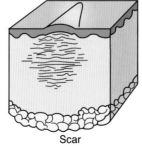
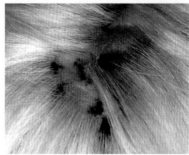

*Courtesy Dr. David Duclos, Animal Skin and Allergy Clinic.

(Continued)

Table **17-5**   Definition and Morphology of Primary and Secondary Skin Lesions—Cont'd

Lesion Definition	Drawing	Clinical Photograph
ULCER[*] Loss of epidermis and basement membrane with exposure of dermis, concave Examples: Ischemic lesions resulting from vasculitis, indolent ulcer, feline herpesvirus infection, feline ulcerative dermatosis syndrome	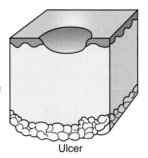 Ulcer	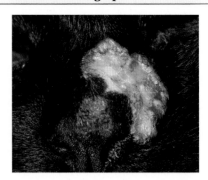
VESICLE AND BULLA[†] Vesicle: Elevated, circumscribed, fluid-filled lesion <1 cm in diameter Bulla: A large vesicular lesion >1 cm in diameter (*arrows*) Examples: Burn, viral infection, immune-mediated diseases such as bullous pemphigoid	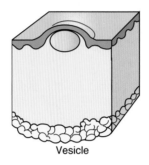 Vesicle	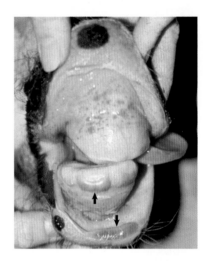
WHEAL[*] Elevated, irregular-shaped area of cutaneous edema; solid, transient (*arrows*) Examples: Insect bites, urticaria, allergic reaction	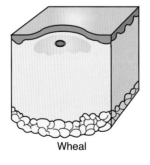 Wheal	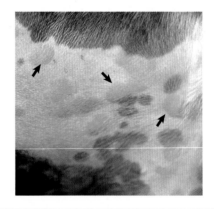

[*]Courtesy Dr. David Duclos, Animal Skin and Allergy Clinic.
[†]Courtesy Dr. Pamela E. Ginn, College of Veterinary Medicine, University of Florida; and Ginn PE, Hillier A, Lester GD: *Vet Dermatol*, 9:249-256, 1998.

Table **17-6**   **Biopsy Sampling Tips**

Preparation	Very gently clip or scissor if necessary
	Do not surgically prepare the site if sampling lesions in epidermis or dermis
	Caveat: Can surgically prepare site for excision of lesions deep in the subcutis or to remove large nodular mass, such as a neoplasm
Lesions	Collect *multiple* samples representative of the range of lesions
	If crusting is significant, collect crust, wrap in lens paper, and place in formalin
	For *alopecic* conditions: Collect samples from the most alopecic areas; draw a line on the sample in the direction of the hair coat
	For *ulcers or depigmenting lesions* (junction important): Use incisional or excisional method or use an 8-mm biopsy punch instrument, and draw a line on the sample perpendicular to the junction between lesion and normal skin
Punch samples	Use 6- or 8-mm punch instruments for haired skin
	Use 4-mm punch for periocular skin, footpads, or nasal planum
Incisional and excisional samples	Use incisional or excisional methods if smaller punch would damage large pustule or vesicle
	Gently place thin incisional or excisional samples, subcutis side down, on a piece of cardboard; let adhere for about 30 seconds, then place in formalin (prevents warping); Note: Do not let sample dehydrate
	For lesions in the panniculus, use incisional or excisional method to ensure that the sample is of sufficient size and depth for diagnosis
Fixation	Fix samples in 10% buffered formalin with 10 times the volume of formalin for the volume of samples
	For diagnosis of autoimmune skin disease or tumors, begin with standard histopathology; selected immunohistochemical stains can usually be done later on the formalin-fixed samples if desired
Important finale	Submit a history with differential diagnoses

---

Box **17-6**

Biopsy Sampling Don'ts

Do not surgically prepare the site if lesions are in the epidermis or dermis

Do not use electrocautery or laser for small biopsy samples

Do not grasp the punch biopsy samples or lesion areas of larger samples with a tissue forceps

Do not use a biopsy instrument that is too small (4 mm is the *minimum* useful diameter)

Do not forget to collect multiple samples

Do not forget to submit a history

---

2. A nodular lesion, ulcer, or nonhealing wound might represent a tumor (so that surgical excision of the tumor can be performed as early as possible).
3. Lesions develop suddenly, are severe, or are unusual (to help identify a serious disease so that therapy can be instituted early).
4. Lesions develop during the course of therapy (to identify a potential adverse reaction to drug therapy).
5. When lesions are active and before use of therapy that might alter the histologic appearance of the lesions, and when there are multiple clinical differential diagnoses and the thorough dermatologic and clinical examinations do not differentiate the conditions (so samples are collected in their early stage, and when other means of diagnosis are insufficient).

6. When a skin disorder fails to respond to apparently appropriate therapy or when the disorder responds to therapy but recurs when therapy is stopped (to establish the correct diagnosis, or evaluate for predisposing factors). Recall that antiinflammatory therapy can alter lesions.

SITE SELECTION

Multiple cutaneous sites representative of the range of lesions should be selected for biopsy. Fully developed nontreated primary lesions, such as macules, papules, pustules, nodules, neoplasms, vesicles, and wheals, are often the most useful for diagnosis (Table 17-5). However, primary lesions may not be present at the time the animal is examined, so secondary lesions, such as scales, crusts, ulcers, comedones, or scars then need to be sampled and evaluated (Table 17-5). These secondary lesions can be diagnostic or contribute substantially to the diagnosis when multiple cutaneous sites are selected for biopsy. One of the most useful secondary lesions is the crust, because acantholytic cells from drying pustules in pemphigus foliaceus and organisms, such as *Dermatophilus congolensis* or dermatophytes, may be identified in crusts, providing the information necessary for diagnosis. Also, the margin of a chronic ulcer may represent a squamous cell carcinoma, or the scale at the edge of an epidermal collarette (i.e., peripherally expanding ring of epidermal scales) may represent superficial spreading pyoderma, thus providing the key to diagnosis.

METHODS

Excisional biopsy samples (entire lesions) are recommended for large pustules or vesicles that can be damaged by use of a smaller punch biopsy instrument. Deeper excisional biopsy samples are generally necessary for diagnosis of lesions, such as panniculitis, that are deep to the epidermis and dermis. Digital amputation can be required, particularly in dogs, for the diagnosis of claw bed lesions. Electrocautery or laser should not be used for small biopsy samples because the samples can be damaged and rendered nondiagnostic. Tissue forceps should grasp, if at all, only one nonaffected margin, preferably in the subcutis.

SITE PREPARATION

Generally the skin at a punch biopsy site should not be surgically prepared because the procedure may remove a diagnostic portion of the sample (Fig. 17-16). Gentle clipping of hair is acceptable, but for an excisional biopsy of lesions deep to the epidermis, surgical preparation of the skin is acceptable. For collection of biopsy samples in areas of alopecia, drawing a line with a fine-tipped permanent marking pen in the direction of the hair coat helps laboratory personnel orient the sample (Fig.17-34, A). In the laboratory, the sample is cut along the line so that the hair follicles are oriented longitudinally (Fig. 17-34, B). If the line is not drawn on the sample, the sample might be cut so that the follicles are in cross or tangential section rather than longitudinal section (Fig. 17-34, C), which reduces histologic value of the sample when evaluating for follicular disease. For collection of ulcers, depigmented lesions, or other lesions where the interface between normal and affected skin is critical to diagnosis, use of incisional or excisional samples collected from affected skin and contiguous normal skin is often preferable. However, a large (8 mm) biopsy punch instrument can be used to collect the junction between normal and affected skin if a line with a fine-tipped permanent marking pen is drawn perpendicular to the junction between the normal and affected tissue before sample collection (Fig. 17-35). The line instructs laboratory

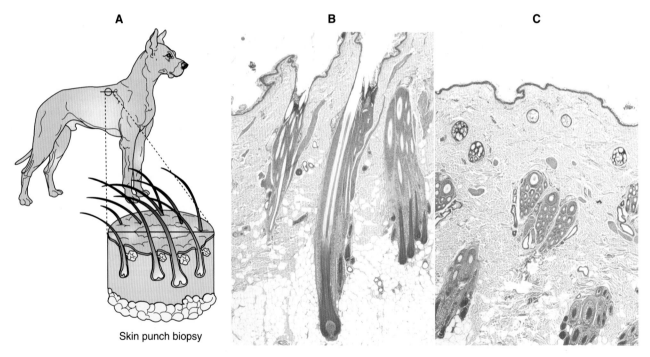

A   **B**   **C**

Skin punch biopsy

Fig. 17-34 **Sampling of the skin for histopathologic evaluation, haired, dog. A,** Schematic diagram of the line drawn (with fine tipped permanent marking pen) on the skin in the direction of the hair coat. The line directs laboratory personnel to cut and embed the sample parallel to the hair follicles. Cutting the sample parallel to the hair follicles allows visualization of the entire length of the follicles during microscopic examination, which facilitates evaluation for causes of alopecia. For simplicity, simple follicles are used in this illustration. **B,** Section of skin trimmed parallel to the hair follicles. Note that the hair follicles are cut longitudinally, and that the full length of the hair follicle is present. H&E stain. **C,** Section of skin trimmed in cross section to the hair follicles. Note that the hair follicles are cut tangentially, and that only portions of each follicle are present for examination, which reduces the ability to evaluate follicular morphology. H&E stain. (*B* and *C, Courtesy Dr. Ann M. Hargis, DermatoDiagnostics.*)

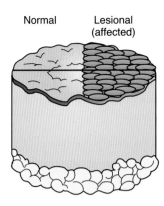

Normal   Lesional
              (affected)

Fig. 17-35   Schematic diagram of collecting the margin of a lesion and normal skin using a large punch biopsy instrument (8 mm). It is necessary to draw a line on the sample from normal into affected skin to direct laboratory personnel to cut and embed the sample so that the interface between the normal and affected skin is present for microscopic examination. Without this line, the sample could be cut at a right angle to the desired line and thus miss the interface between normal and affected skin essential for histologic examination of the area most likely to have diagnostic changes.

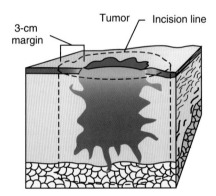

3-cm
margin   Tumor   Incision line

Fig. 17-36   Schematic diagram of excisional sampling. If possible, 3-cm margins should be collected if the nodule is suspected of being an invasive neoplasm. This facilitates examination of the margins for completeness of excision.

personnel how to trim the sample to ensure that the critical areas are present for dermatopathologic evaluation. For lesions suspected of being invasive tumors, complete excision of the mass, including a 3-cm margin of clinically normal skin around all borders, is recommended (Fig. 17-36).

FIXATION

Punch biopsy specimens should be placed in 10 times the volume of 10% neutral buffered formalin (NBF). To prevent warping in the fixative, thin excisional biopsy specimens should be gently attached to a flat object, such as a piece of cardboard or tongue depressor, and permitted to dry for 20 to 30 seconds. Twenty to 30 seconds is all that is necessary for the sample to adhere to the flat object. The specimen and flat object are then immediately immersed in formalin. Care should be taken not to let the sample become dehydrated (i.e., remain unfixed for longer than 20 to 30 seconds), which could damage the morphology of small samples and the lesions. In cold climates during winter months, adding 1 part alcohol to 9 parts 10% NBF reduces the chance of freezing of specimens during transport.

HISTORY

Accurate histopathologic diagnosis and interpretation require knowledge of the gross features of the lesions. Therefore it is essential to include with biopsy samples the following information: (1) age, breed, and sex of the animal; (2) location, gross appearance, and duration of the lesions; (3) presence or absence of lesion symmetry; and (4) presence or absence of pruritus affecting the animal (Box 17-7). Clinical information including results of laboratory evaluations (i.e., hemograms, serum biochemical analyses), results of skin cultures or scrapings, current medications, and response to therapy should be included along with a list of clinical differential diagnoses. History can be critical to reaching a diagnosis. For instance, presence of luminal and mural folliculitis with no apparent follicular infectious agents in H&E stained sections in conjunction with the history of lack of response to appropriate antibiotic therapy would suggest to the pathologist that a fungal stain to evaluate for occult dermatophyte infection should be performed. Without the history of lack of response to appropriate antibiotic therapy, the folliculitis could easily be presumed to be of bacterial origin, and a fungal infection missed.

Box 17-7

What Constitutes a History?

Age, breed, sex
Lesion distribution
Lesion appearance and severity
Lesion duration
Influence of specific therapy and/or recent therapy that could change lesions
Other clinical problems
Laboratory analyte abnormalities
Differential diagnoses (important)

ANCILLARY PROCEDURES

Other diagnostic procedures can supplement information gained from histologic examination of biopsy samples. These procedures include aspiration of pustule contents for cytologic evaluation, performing touch imprints of the cut surface of suspected neoplastic or infectious lesions for cytologic evaluation, aseptically collecting a tissue sample for microbiologic culture, and collecting biopsy samples of suspected immune-mediated diseases or poorly differentiated tumors for immunostaining. Use of immunostaining for identification of cell surface or cytoplasmic proteins (to aid in diagnosis of tumors) or for identification of immunoglobulin, complement, or other antigens (to aid in the diagnosis of immune-mediated skin disease, such as pemphigus) can be helpful in some cases.

Unfortunately, immunostaining techniques can give false-positive or false-negative results; thus they must be done in conjunction with standard histopathology. For autoimmune diseases, if immunofluorescence evaluation is desired, specimens can be fixed in Michel's medium, which preserves immunoglobulin and complement. If immunohistochemistry (immunoperoxidase) staining is desired, formalin-fixed samples are used; however, for best results, samples should not remain in formalin longer than 48 hours. Prolonged fixation in formalin results in cross-linking of proteins and false-negative results. For autoimmune disease, newer techniques that detect more specific antigens, such as desmoglein (transmembrane glycoproteins found in desmosomes that provide physical connections between keratinocytes), use of "salt-split" skin sections (a technique used in immunostaining of the skin where sodium chloride splits the epidermis from the dermis through the lamina lucida, allowing better differentiation of subepidermal bullous diseases), use of better substrates for indirect immunostaining, and use of immunoblotting and enzyme-linked immunosorbent assay (ELISA) techniques will improve diagnostic accuracy of immune-mediated skin diseases in the future. For identification of cell surface or cytoplasmic proteins in poorly differentiated tumors, evaluation of a series (panel) of antibodies is preferred because the pattern of staining with a panel of antibodies is more reliable than staining with one or two antibodies. Formalin-fixed specimens are acceptable for some procedures, but for others, fresh or frozen specimens are better. Discussion with a pathologist is recommended regarding when to use immunostaining procedures.

DISEASES OF THE SKIN

CONGENITAL AND HEREDITARY DISORDERS

The terms "congenital" and "hereditary" are not synonymous. Congenital lesions develop in the fetus (in utero), are present at birth, and have a variety of causes. An example is hypotrichosis in the fetus associated with maternal dietary iodine deficiency. Inherited conditions are transmitted genetically and are not always manifested phenotypically in utero or at birth but may develop later in life. An example is sebaceous adenitis, which may not develop until 1 to 2 years of age or later.

CONGENITAL ALOPECIA AND HYPOTRICHOSIS

Congenital alopecia or atrichia (absence of hair from skin where hair is usually present) and hypotrichosis (less than the normal amount of hair) have been reported in most species of domestic animals. In most instances, congenital hypotrichosis is a hereditary condition due to spontaneous genetic mutations affecting genes responsible for or influencing the normal development and/or maintenance of hair follicles or other components of the skin. In most cases, the exact mutation has not been identified. In some of these animals, the alopecia or hypotrichosis has been recognized as standard for the breed (e.g., Mexican hairless dog, Sphinx cat, and Ulster pig), and the mutation is purposefully propagated. Animals with congenital hereditary hypotrichosis can have defects in other body systems, including brachygnathism (abnormal smallness of the mandible), and dental, thymic, and genital abnormalities. When the condition involves the hair follicles plus adnexal glands and teeth, which all arise from the ectoderm, the condition is also termed "ectodermal dysplasia." In addition to health problems created by oral, dental, or thymic defects (inability to efficiently chew or graze and immune deficiency that can lead to death), animals with hypotrichosis are more susceptible to sunburn, temperature extremes, and bacterial and fungal infections. The degree, location, and age of onset of hairlessness vary. Hair that is present is usually abnormally coarse or fine and easily broken or epilated. Morphologic changes in the skin and hair follicles vary from species to species, most likely representing differences in mutations. A useful example is congenital hypotrichosis with anodontia in German Holstein calves (Fig. 17-37). In this condition, hypotrichosis, lack of most teeth, and complete absence of eccrine nasolabial glands is inherited as a monogenic X-linked recessive trait. Because the condition affects the hair follicles, some adnexal glands, and teeth, it is also classified as an ectodermal dysplasia. The condition varies in severity, with some calves more affected than others. Affected calves have reduced numbers of hairs per surface area in various anatomic locations (especially head, pinnae, neck, back, and tail), and also have reduced length and numbers of eyelashes and vibrissae. The alopecia and hypotrichosis are most severe in newborn calves because the presence of fine hairs increases with age. There are no defects in the horns, endocrine

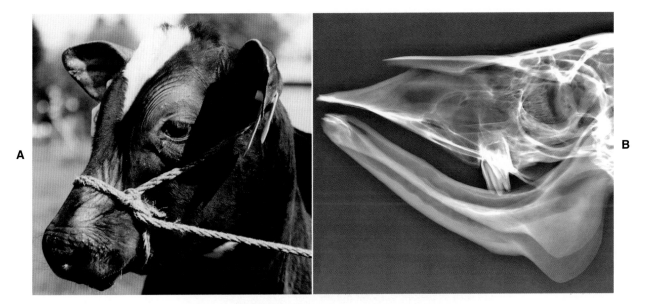

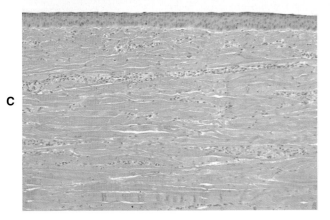

Fig. 17-37   Congenital hypotrichosis with anodontia, calf. A, The hair coat is sparse and short. Eyelashes and tactile hairs are also sparse and very short. The tail switch (not in this photograph) was about one third the normal length. **B,** Radiograph, skull. Note that most of the teeth are missing. When congenital hypotrichosis involves the hair follicles plus adnexal glands and teeth, which all arise from the ectoderm, the condition is also termed "ectodermal dysplasia." **C,** Affected skin. Note the lack of hair follicles. Animals with hypotrichosis are susceptible to extremes of temperature, and the skin is more likely to sustain traumatic injury and secondary infection because of the lack of the protective hair coat. H&E stain. (**A,** *Courtesy Professor Tosso Leeb, Institute of Animal Breeding, School of Veterinary Medicine Hannover; and Drogemuller C, Kuiper H, Peters M et al: Vet Dermatol 13:6;307-313, 2002. **B,** Courtesy Professor Tosso Leeb, Institute of Animal Breeding, School of Veterinary Medicine Hannover; and Tierarztl Prax. **C,** Courtesy Dr. Frank Seeliger, Department of Pathology, Tieraerztliche Hochschule Hannover.*)

glands, genital organs, or other internal organs. Histologically, hair follicles and adnexal glands are absent in the skin on the back of the ears. Hair follicle density is often reduced in other areas. When present, hair bulbs are small and poorly developed. In some areas, the apocrine glands are reduced in quantity, and eccrine nasolabial glands are absent.

Especially for purposes of herd health management and disease prevention, it is important to differentiate the congenital inherited alopecia and hypotrichosis disorders from the nongenetic congenital alopecic disorders. The latter includes congenital hypotrichosis due to maternal iodine deficiency in pigs, calves, lambs, and foals; in utero infection with bovine virus diarrhea or hog cholera virus; and defects in other systems, such as adenohypophyseal hypoplasia in some breeds of cattle (Table 17-7).

It should be realized that there is some overlap between the congenital alopecia and hypotrichosis disorders and the follicular dysplasia disorders. Recall that

Table **17-7**   Categories, Causes, and Age of Onset of Hypotrichosis and Alopecia

Category	Cause	Age of Onset	Species
Congenital hypotrichosis or alopecia	Usually inherited, may be accompanied by odontogenic, thymic, genital, or other defects that influence neonatal viability	Usually present at birth or within the first month of life	Mostly calves; less often piglets, puppies, kittens; rarely foals
	Maternal dietary influences (e.g., iodine deficiency)	Present at birth	Calves, piglets, lambs, foals
	Secondary to other defects (adenohypophyseal hypoplasia)	Present at birth	Guernsey and Jersey calves
	In utero infection with bovine virus diarrhea or hog cholera virus	Present at birth	Calves, pigs
Follicular dysplasia	Usually inherited	Months to years after birth	Dogs, cattle, horses
Endocrine disorders and alopecia X in dogs*	Abnormal function of pituitary, thyroid, adrenal or pineal glands, or gonads; or iatrogenic administration of hormones	Develops in young adults to aged	Predominantly dogs
Hair cycle abnormalities	Nonendocrine factors that influence hair growth such as therapy with antimitotic drugs (anagen defluxion), stress, fever, illness (telogen effluvium), or clipping plush-coated breeds of dogs (post clipping alopecia)	Typically adults	Any species, often dogs
Neoplasia	Paraneoplastic: internal malignancy, often of pancreas or liver	Aged	Cats
	Direct involvement of epidermis, dermis, or adnexa (example: epitheliotropic lymphoma)	Usually adult to aged	Dogs, cats
Inflammatory conditions	Follicular infection	Any age	Any species; dogs most frequently affected with follicular infection and sebaceous adenitis
	Posttraumatic and inflammatory Sebaceous adenitis		
Excessive grooming	Hypersensitivity reactions or psychogenic causes	Any age	Most often affects cats
Nutrition	Severe protein or protein-calorie nutrition	Any age, especially young or pregnant	Any species

*Endocrine:
1. Alopecia X of Nordic breeds of dogs is a group of poorly characterized dermatoses, including castration responsive dermatosis, growth hormone responsive dermatosis, and follicular dysplasia in Siberian huskies or Alaskan malamutes.
2. Clinically manifested endocrine disease in cats is usually caused by hyperadrenocorticism where marked dermal atrophy leads to tearing of the skin with normal handling procedures. Alopecia can be a feature, but skin fragility is a more significant problem.
3. Clinically manifested endocrine disease in horses is usually caused by hyperadrenocorticism and is typified paradoxically by hypertrichosis rather than alopecia (possibly because of production of adrenal androgens, other hormones, or pressure of the pituitary on thermoregulatory areas of the hypothalamus).

follicular dysplasia is usually an inherited abnormality of the hair follicles in which there is failure of hair growth, production of defective hair shafts, or failure to maintain hair within follicles (Fig. 17-25). The principal differentiating features include: (1) animals with follicular dysplasia having hair follicles that are defective or dysplastic, not absent or only reduced in number; (2) animals with follicular dysplasia having alopecia and hypotrichosis, which are not typically congenital, but develop in the months to years after birth; and (3) animals with follicular dysplasia typically not having defects in other organ systems. However, these differentiating features are not absolute. Consider, for example, that animals with congenital hereditary hypotrichosis and alopecia can have areas of the skin with hair, but the hair is abnormally coarse or fine and easily broken or epilated; thus they also technically have follicular dysplasia in some areas of the body.

COLLAGEN DYSPLASIA AND MUCINOSIS

Collagen dysplasia (hyperelastosis cutis, dermatosparaxis, cutaneous asthenia) occurs in most domestic animals and comprises a clinically, genetically, and biochemically heterogeneous group of diseases that are rare. In each, skin tears easily, is hyperextensible, and loose, but the severity of these lesions varies among species. Specific enzyme defects of collagen synthesis or processing are the cause of some collagen dysplasia syndromes. Abnormal synthesis or processing of collagen leads to structurally abnormal dermal collagen that has decreased tensile strength. The causes of other collagen dysplasia syndromes have not been established. Gross lesions consist of cutaneous hyperextensibility and laxity (Fig. 17-38), frequent skin wounds that result even from normal handling and activity, and numerous scars, which are the result of previous tearing of the dermal connective tissues. Microscopic features vary among the different types of collagen dysplasia syndromes, and in some the skin is histologically normal. If microscopic lesions are present, the collagen bundles can vary in size and shape, can be separated by wide spaces, or have a haphazard arrangement. Electron microscopy or biochemical analyses are sometimes required to make a definitive diagnosis.

Mucinosis (mucin deposition in the dermis) occurs normally in some breeds of dogs, such as the Shar-Pei or in association with myxedema of hypothyroidism. The presence of mucin in the Shar-Pei causes the thick, wrinkly skin that typifies this breed. However, in some Shar-Pei dogs, the mucin deposition is excessive and "lakes" or pools of mucin develop. In these areas of mucin accumulation, there is a concomitant reduction in dermal collagen fibers and dilated lymphatic channels. These areas of the skin are fragile, and if traumatized, thick, stringy mucin exudes from the dermis.

EPIDERMOLYSIS BULLOSA (RED FOOT DISEASE)

Epidermolysis bullosa refers to a group of mechanobullous diseases, resulting in development of cutaneous blisters (bullae) in response to minor mechanical trauma. Blisters develop as a result of poor cohesion of the epidermis and dermis as a result of structural defects at the basement membrane zone. The structural defects are the result of mutations in genes responsible for the synthesis of a variety of structural components of this anatomic region of the skin and include abnormalities in keratin intermediate filaments, hemidesmosome-associated proteins, and anchoring fibrils, such as type VII collagen. The diseases vary in mode of inheritance, clinical manifestations, and anatomic location of the blisters. Animals affected with the diseases usually die because of their inability to obtain nourishment, loss of fluid and protein, and secondary infection leading to bacteremia. Epidermolysis bullosa has been reported in some breeds of sheep, horses, cattle, and dogs. Lesions can be present at birth or develop shortly thereafter and are located where epithelial surfaces are subjected

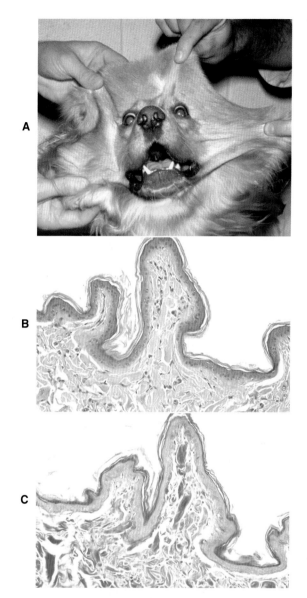

Fig. 17-38   Collagen dysplasia, skin, dog. A, The skin is hyperextensible. In this dog, the skin can be stretched more than the skin of a normal dog. **B,** The collagen bundles are irregular in size and shape and are arranged haphazardly. The abnormally functioning collagen is responsible for the hyperextensibility of the skin, which predisposes to tearing with normal handling and activity. H&E stain. **C,** Deeper level of the sample shown in Fig. 17-38, *B.* Collagen bundles are stained blue. The variation in diameter and shape of the collagen bundles and their haphazard arrangement is accentuated with this stain. Masson's trichrome stain. (**A,** *Courtesy Dr. Ben Baker, Washington State University.* **B** *and* **C,** *Courtesy Dr. Ann M. Hargis, DermatoDiagnostics.*)

to minor mechanical trauma, such as oral mucosa, lips, and extremities, including the coronary band. Shearing forces that normally cause no problem are sufficient to cause injury in these animals. Microscopic lesions are those of an epidermal vesicular disease in which vesicles form in different locations (subepidermal, epidermal-dermal junction, intraepidermal) depending on the specific disease. The vesicles progress to ulcers, or if secondarily infected become pustules. As healing occurs, the reepithelization causes sloughing of the dried exudates over the ulcer, and the pustules dry to form crusts.

EPITHELIOGENESIS IMPERFECTA (APLASIA CUTIS)

Epitheliogenesis imperfecta results from the failure of the stratified squamous epithelium of skin, adnexa, and/or oral mucosa to develop completely. The disease varies in severity and has been reported in most domestic species. It is the result of inherited genetic mutations in some species, but inheritance is not proven in other species. Additional information regarding the pathogenesis is not known. Without the protective covering of the stratified squamous epithelium, the underlying tissue is easily traumatized, can become infected, and bacteremia can develop. Grossly, lesions consist of sharply demarcated areas devoid of the epidermis and adnexa or mucosa, exposing the underlying red, moist dermis or submucosa. Lesions are located most often on the face, extremities, or mucous membranes, and can be small (1 cm) or involve extensive regions, such as the entire distal limb (Fig. 17-39). Small lesions can heal with scarring and not interfere with life. With extensive involvement, the entire skin can be affected, including hooves, ears, lips, and eyelids, and may result in abortion of the affected fetus. Animals born alive with extensive lesions usually die from infection or dehydration and electrolyte abnormalities from extensive fluid loss through nonepithelialized surfaces.

CONGENITAL HYPERTRICHOSIS

Excessive growth of hair can be congenital or hereditary. Abnormally hairy fleece at birth develops in fine- and medium-wooled fetal lambs because of an in utero border disease virus infection. Fetal infection before 90 days of gestation results in an initial phase of retardation of follicular growth followed by an extended period of rapid growth of primary follicles. The altered growth rate of follicles results in production of larger, more heavily medullated primary wool fibers. The exact mechanism controlling the exaggerated growth of primary follicles is unknown. It has been speculated that reduction in number of the later developing secondary fibers could be the result of impaired nutrition because of placentitis. In addition to abnormal fleece, affected sheep have defective myelination of the brain and spinal cord, abnormalities of body conformation, poor growth, and reduced viability. Microscopically, primary follicles and wool fibers are enlarged and the number of the secondary follicles and wool fibers is reduced (see Morphology of the Skin, Hair Follicles and Fig. 17-7). In utero hypertrichosis can develop in lambs secondary to hyperthermia in pregnant ewes living in areas of high environmental temperature.

DERMATOSIS VEGETANS

Dermatosis vegetans is an inherited disorder of young pigs characterized by vegetating skin lesions, hoof malformation, and giant cell pneumonia. The condition is

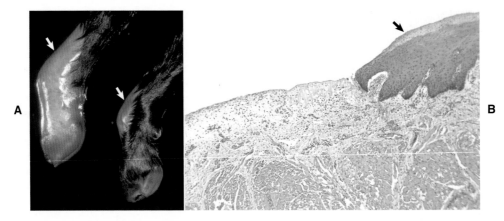

Fig. 17-39   Epitheliogenesis imperfecta, calf. A, Skin. Areas of epidermis over the extremities are missing (*arrows*). This condition is the result of inherited genetic mutations in some species, but inheritance is not proven in other species. **B,** Oral mucosa. Junction of normal and affected mucous membrane. Epithelium is present on the right (normal area) (*arrow*) but is abruptly missing on the left. The lack of germinal epithelium results in the failure of the epidermis, adnexa, or mucosal epithelium to develop completely. Skin, adnexa, and oral mucosa can be affected in this disease. (*A* and *B, Courtesy Dr. M.D. McGavin, College of Veterinary Medicine, University of Tennessee.*)

a simple autosomal recessive trait of Landrace pigs. The pathogenesis of lesion formation is unknown. Skin lesions can be present at birth but might not develop until 2 to 3 months of age. Lesions begin as erythematous papules on the ventral abdomen and medial aspect of the thighs and possibly the sides and back. The papules enlarge peripherally to form plaques with a depressed center filled with gray to brown-black granular brittle material. Each crusty plaque is sharply demarcated from normal skin by a hyperemic raised border. As lesions spread peripherally, they coalesce to form extensive horny, papilloma-like areas covered by black crusts. Foot and hoof lesions, if they occur, are always present at birth. Usually all digits, including accessory digits, on more than one limb are affected. The coronary region is markedly swollen and erythematous, and the skin is covered by a yellow-brown greasy material. The wall of the hoof is thickened by ridges and furrows parallel to the coronary band. Histologically, fully developed cutaneous lesions have marked orthokeratotic and parakeratotic hyperkeratosis, prominent irregular epidermal hyperplasia, intercellular edema, and intraepidermal pustules and microabscesses containing eosinophils and neutrophils. Affected piglets frequently die of secondary infection when skin lesions reach the typical papilloma-like stage (5 to 8 weeks of age) either from entrance of bacteria from skin lesions or a bacterial pneumonia complicating the giant cell pneumonia characteristic of this disease. Skin lesions begin to resolve if the pig survives.

DISORDERS OF PHYSICAL, RADIATION, OR CHEMICAL INJURY
ACTINIC INJURY

Sunlight is composed of visible (400 to 700 nm), ultraviolet (100 to 400 nm), and infrared (700 to 20,000 nm) light rays. The portion of the ultraviolet (UV) light most damaging to the skin is ultraviolet B (UVB) and is in the range of 290- to 320-nm wavelength. However, photodynamic chemicals, if present in the skin, can chemically react with longer wavelengths, thus releasing energy and leading to the formation of reactive oxygen intermediates that initiate a chain of reactions resulting in cutaneous damage (photosensitization, phototoxicity). The amount of light reaching the skin is dependent on a variety of environmental and host factors, such as quantity of ozone, smog, and cloud cover (tend to absorb and scatter some of the UV rays), and the amount of pigment and hair (reflect or otherwise block UV rays from reaching the skin). Solar damage is more prevalent at high altitudes and at latitudes close to the equator, in areas with a high number of cloudless days, and in animals spending most of their time outdoors. The susceptibility of animal skin to actinic injury depends on the density of hair, degree of pigmentation, and thickness of the stratum corneum. Lesions generally develop in poorly haired and lightly pigmented skin.

SOLAR DERMATOSIS, KERATOSIS, AND NEOPLASIA

The damage to skin by UV light can be acute (sunburn) or chronic (solar dermatosis, neoplasia). An early transient erythema may be due to the heating effect of the light rays and possibly to photochemical changes. The later developing erythema is called "sunburn erythema," and the skin is warm, tender, and swollen. The pathogenesis of sunburn erythema may involve diffusion of inflammatory mediators, such as cytokines, from radiation-damaged keratinocytes, or from direct damage to endothelial cells of superficial dermal capillaries by UV light. One of the more influential alterations caused by exposure to UV light rays is the formation of thymidine dimers between pyrimidine bases of DNA. The damage can be easily and accurately repaired before the cell undergoes mitosis by an enzyme system that removes the damaged area and synthesizes a new strand of DNA. However, if the cell undergoes mitosis before the damage is repaired, a gap in the DNA strand is left at the location of the thymidine dimer. The gap is repaired by a postreplication repair method that is thought to be error-prone and may lead to mutations and the development of neoplasms. Factors that irritate the skin and increase the rate of cell division increase the number of cells repaired by the postreplication repair method and therefore can enhance development of neoplasms. UV radiation may also alter immunologic reactivity by inducing suppresser T lymphocytes, which favor growth of neoplastic cells. Preneoplastic and neoplastic lesions are common in chronically solar-damaged skin in domestic animals.

The lesions of sun-induced injury occur in all domestic animals. In cats, gross lesions occur where there is little or no hair and little pigment, particularly on external ear tips, eyelids, nose and lips, and are most severe in white cats. In dogs, lesions develop most commonly in nonpigmented, sparsely haired skin of the ventral abdominal, inguinal, and perianal areas (Fig. 17-40). Lightly pigmented young pigs are also susceptible, and the pinnae and tip of the tail can slough if injury is severe. In horses, lesions occur on the eyelids, nose, and around the prepuce. The eyelids of Hereford cattle are also prone to development of lesions. In lightly colored dairy goats, lesions can develop on the lateral aspects of the udder and teats. Grossly, lesions begin as erythema, scaling, and crusting. After years of exposure, the skin becomes wrinkled and thickened secondary to epidermal hyperplasia, hyperkeratosis, fibrosis, and in some species, elastosis. One or more papular or plaque-like foci covered with thick scale (hyperkeratosis)

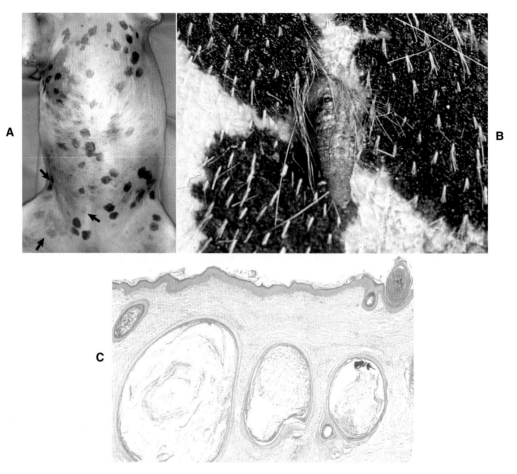

Fig. 17-40   Solar dermatitis, skin, dog. A, Ventral abdomen and thorax. The nonpigmented and sparsely haired skin is erythematous, has comedones and crusts, and is palpably thickened *(arrows)*. The densely pigmented black spots are clinically unaffected, but lightly pigmented spots are affected. Comedones can rupture (furunculosis), releasing follicular contents that cause a foreign body inflammatory response and secondary bacterial infection. Clinically, the inflammation is prominent (erythema and furuncles) and can be misinterpreted as primary. Clinically, the distribution pattern of affected nonpigmented sparsely haired skin and unaffected haired or pigmented skin is supportive of the diagnosis of solar dermatitis. **B,** Ventral abdomen. Solar dermatitis with an actinic keratosis that has formed a cutaneous horn. Cutaneous horns are keratoses formed from multiple layers of compacted stratum corneum. They may arise from benign or malignant lesions in the epidermis (actinic keratosis, squamous cell carcinoma) or adnexa (infundibular keratinizing acanthoma). **C,** The epidermis is thickened by acanthosis, and comedones (follicular hyperkeratosis) are present. If comedones rupture, a large amount of endogenous foreign material (stratum corneum, hair shafts, and sebum) is released into the dermis, causing a foreign-body inflammatory response and bacteria that typically cause a secondary bacterial infection. H&E stain. (**A, B,** *and* **C,** *Courtesy Dr. Ann M. Hargis, DermatoDiagnostics.*)

known as solar keratoses may develop, some of which progress to squamous cell carcinoma. Occasionally the hyperkeratosis is dense and compact, and resembles a "horn" (Fig. 17-40, *B*). Hemangiomas and hemangiosarcomas have developed in the nonpigmented conjunctiva of dogs and horses and in the skin of dogs, cats, and a few goats. The cutaneous hemangiomas and hemangiosarcomas are often seen on the abdomen and flanks of dogs that spend time resting in the sun. The difference in type

of neoplasm can be due in part to thickness of the epidermis, which influences the depth of penetration of the UV rays. UV light may also play a role in the development of melanomas in goats.

Microscopically, in early UV-induced injury, the number of apoptotic cells (sunburn cells) scattered in the epidermis can be so numerous as to form a band of these cells along with intercellular edema, vacuolation of keratinocytes, and loss of granular cell layer. By 72 hours, hyperkeratosis, parakeratosis, and acanthosis are present along with dermal lesions of hyperemia, edema, perivascular mononuclear infiltrates, capillary endothelial cell swelling, and hemorrhage. Hyperkeratosis, parakeratosis, and acanthosis can persist, and pseudocarcinomatous hyperplasia (marked hyperplasia of the epidermis resulting in many branching and anastomosing epidermal ridges reaching down into the dermis) and dermal fibrosis can develop. The thickened epidermis with adherent compact and parakeratotic stratum corneum create the solar keratoses. Comedones (hair follicles dilated with a plug of follicular stratum corneum and sebum) develop in some dogs (Fig. 17-40, C). In some animals and in some anatomic locations, elastic tissue and collagen are damaged by solar radiation.

PHOTOSENSITIZATION

Photosensitization is a disorder caused by long-wavelength UV, or less frequently visible light, absorbed by a photodynamic chemical in the skin, or by a complex of photodynamic molecule and a biologic substrate, which results in a release of energy that produces reactive oxygen molecules, including free radicals. Generation of reactive oxygen molecules leads to mast cell degranulation and the production of inflammatory mediators, which causes damage to cell membranes, nucleic acids, proteins, and organelles. The photodynamic agent usually enters the dermis via the systemic circulation. However, direct contact and absorption of some photodynamic agents can result in localized contact photosensitization.

Photosensitization can occur in several forms. Type I or primary photosensitization, is often due to ingestion of preformed photodynamic substances contained in a variety of plants; thus herbivores are most commonly affected. The plants causing photosensitization usually contain helianthrone or furocoumarin pigments. The helianthrone pigments are red fluorescent pigments such as hypericin (found in *Hypericum perforatum* [St. John's wort]) and fagopyrin (found in *Fagopyrum esculentum* [buckwheat]). Photosensitization caused by furocoumarin pigments is due to the presence of psoralens, photodynamic agents found in a variety of plants including *Cymopterus watsonii* (spring parsley), *Ammi majus* (bishop's weed), and *Thamnosma texana* (Dutchman's breeches). Furocoumarin pigments also form phytoalexins, a group of compounds formed in plants in response to fungal infection or other injury and that inhibit or destroy the invading agent. The phytoalexins formed in fungus-infected parsnips and celery have caused phytophotocontact dermatitis when they are absorbed into the skin and react with UV light.

Primary photosensitization can also occur with the administration of drugs such as phenothiazine, which is converted to a photoreactive metabolite in the intestinal tract. This metabolite is usually converted to a nonphotoreactive compound in the liver by mixed function oxidases, but occasionally either the reactive metabolite bypasses the liver or mixed function oxidase activity in the liver is compromised or insufficient, and the reactive metabolite reaches the skin.

Type II photosensitization develops because of abnormal porphyrin metabolism, leading to the blood and tissue accumulation of photodynamic agents. These diseases usually are inherited as an enzyme deficiency, resulting in abnormal synthesis of photodynamic agents, including uroporphyrin and coproporphyrin. Examples include bovine congenital porphyria and bovine erythropoietic (hematopoietic) protoporphyria. Photosensitization due to abnormal porphyrin metabolism has also been reported in pigs and cats.

Type III or hepatogenous photosensitization is due to impaired capacity of the liver to excrete phylloerythrin, which is formed in the alimentary tract from the breakdown of chlorophyll. This is the most common type of photosensitization and occurs most commonly in herbivores, but any animal with generalized hepatic disease on a chlorophyll rich diet and that is exposed to sufficient solar radiation can develop hepatogenous photosensitization. Hepatogenous photosensitization occurs secondary to primary hepatocellular damage, inherited hepatic defects, or bile duct obstruction. Toxic plants, including but not limited to *Lantana camara* (lantana) and *Tribulis terrestris* (puncture vine), and mycotoxins such as sporidesmin are the most common cause of this type of photoensitization. Other plants that cause hepatic damage (such as those that contain pyrrolizidine alkaloids) can also contribute to the development of hepatogenous photosensitization.

Grossly, in photosensitization, lesions are located on areas of the body with nonpigmented skin and hair, and on parts of the body exposed to the sun, such as the face, nose, and distal extremities in horses. In cattle, lesions occur in white-haired areas and on the teats, udder, perineum, and nose. In sheep with heavy fleeces, lesions occur on the pinnae, eyelids, face, nose, and coronary band, but in shorn sheep, lesions can occur on the back. Sheep can have extensive edema of the head resulting in the synonyms of "swelled head" and "facial eczema." Onset of lesions may take only hours and initially include erythema and edema, followed by blisters, exudation, necrosis, and sloughing of necrotic tissue. The microscopic lesions consist of coagulative necrosis of the epidermis and possibly follicular epithelium, adnexal glands, and superficial dermis. Subepidermal vesiculation can occur. Endothelial cells of the superficial, middle, and deep dermal vessels are swollen and necrotic, and fibrinoid degeneration and thrombosis can result in edema; infarction; sloughing of the epidermis, dermis, and adnexa; and secondary bacterial infection.

PHOTOENHANCED DERMATOSES

Photoenhanced dermatoses are immune-mediated disorders that are aggravated by exposure to UV radiation, and include lupus erythematosus and dermatomyositis. Cytokines liberated from keratinocytes may play a role in photoenhancement. Clinical and histologic lesions are consistent with those of the specific disease process. Photoactivated vasculitis in horses may also represent a photoenhanced dermatosis; however, the cause and pathogenesis of this disorder are unknown. Sun exposure appears to trigger lesion development in some horses, but lesions do not always resolve with removal from sun exposure. Lesions typically develop in the white-haired extremities of horses, but rarely similar lesions occur in legs covered with dark hair. Lesions initially consist of well-demarcated erythematous, moist, crusted areas. More chronic lesions consist of plaques of epidermal acanthosis, hyperkeratosis, and crusting. Microscopically, lesions occur in small, thin-walled vessels of superficial dermal papillae. There is vascular dilation, endothelial degeneration, mild hyalinization of vessel walls, thrombosis, and perivascular edema and mild hemorrhage without significant inflammation.

IONIZING RADIATION INJURY

Advances in the treatment of cancer in companion animals have made the possibility of radiation-induced skin injury more likely. Ionizing radiation consists of electromagnetic radiation (x-rays, γ-rays) and particulate radiation (electrons, neutrons, protons, etc.), and is most damaging to highly proliferative cells, such as those of the anagen hair matrix, but epidermal basal cells and vascular endothelial cells are also affected. Available radiation modalities offer differing degrees of tissue penetration and thus differing potential for tissue injury. Some forms of radiotherapy penetrate deeper tissues while sparing the skin, and others are more concentrated in the superficial tissues or are preferentially absorbed by specific tissues. The type of radiation therapy, source, dose, intensity, and duration of exposure dictate the range of possible side effects. Ionizing photons disrupt chemical bonds in cells, leading to injury or cell death. Some cells are not lethally damaged, but sustain DNA damage to the extent that replication and/or replacement is not possible. The effects of radiation damage can be divided into acute and chronic forms.

Acute radiation injury to the skin is a result of damage to rapidly dividing cells. Damage is self-limiting and recovery is associated with rapid cell turnover. Clinical lesions of radiation dermatitis appear 2 to 4 weeks after exposure. Initially, there is erythema, pain, edema, and heat, followed several weeks later by dry or moist desquamation depending on the degree of injury. Histologically the lesions resemble a second-degree burn, with suprabasilar or subepidermal bullae formation, dermal edema with fibrin exudation, and a marked leukocytic infiltrate. Reepithelialization occurs over a period of 10 to 60 days. The damage sustained to germinal epithelium of hair follicles and sebaceous glands leads to alopecia within 2 to 4 weeks after exposure. Hair regrowth will follow over the next several months, but damage to sebaceous glands is not reversible and leads to permanent scaling manifesting histologically as hyperkeratosis. The chronic lesions of radiation injury are evident months to years after treatment and are primarily due to damage to the microvasculature. Chronic changes include pigmentary alterations (hyperpigmentation with lower doses and hypopigmentation with higher doses), leukotrichia (depigmentation of hair shafts because of loss of follicular melanocytes), dermal scarring, epidermal atrophy, and ulceration. The epidermis is thin, friable, and in some areas hyperplastic and can become neoplastic. Squamous cell carcinomas can develop in some sites of severe radiation damage because of sublethal DNA damage. Chronic nonhealing exudative ulcers can develop, but granulation tissue does not form. The dermis is fibrotic with atypical fibroblasts, telangiectasia, and possibly deep arteriolar changes. Endothelial swelling, necrosis, and thrombosis lead to occlusion and excessive endothelial proliferation, which, when combined with the effects of vascular leakage, leads to vascular collapse. This condition of progressive vessel abnormalities is referred to as obliterative endoarteritis and is known to form a "histohematic" (tissue-blood) barrier to surrounding tissue, leading to continued anoxia and nutrient shortage.

CHEMICAL INJURY

Chemical injuries to the skin can result from local application directly onto the skin or from absorption of chemicals via the gastrointestinal tract and subsequent distribution to the skin. For a chemical to cause injury via local application, it must penetrate the hair and protective epidermal layers. Penetration is enhanced by physical damage to the stratum corneum, especially that caused by excessive moisture. Chemical injuries of the skin include contact irritant dermatitis (local application), systemically distributed chemicals, such as arsenic, mercury, thallium, iodine, and organochlorines and organobromines, and poisonings by fungal-contaminated plants and plants containing selenium, mimosine, and trichothecenes. Externally applied agents that produce irritant contact dermatitis induce cutaneous damage by altering the water-holding capacity of the epidermis or by penetrating the epidermis and directly damaging cells. Systemically absorbed and distributed chemical agents cause lesions by a wide variety of mechanisms, some of which are not known. An example is toxicity due to systemic absorption of some organochlorine and organobromine compounds, such as highly chlorinated napththalenes, which were used as additives in lubricants for farm machinery, such as feed pelleting equipment. As a result, highly chlorinated napththalenes were frequent feed contaminants. Toxicosis occurred most commonly in cattle, the most susceptible species, and was known as X-disease or bovine hyperkeratosis. Fortunately, this toxicosis is largely of historical interest as highly chlorinated napththalenes have not been used in lubricants since the 1950s. Lesions of chlorinated naphthalene toxicity are due to the interference of the conversion of carotene to vitamin A, and result in vitamin A deficiency. Vitamin A is necessary for normal differentiation of stratified squamous epithelium. Clinical lesions consist of alopecia and lichenified, fissured plaques of scale that spare only the legs. Histologic lesions consist of marked hyperkeratosis of the epidermis and follicles. Squamous metaplasia of the epithelial lining of the glands and ducts of the liver, pancreas, kidneys, and reproductive tract also develop.

IRRITANT CONTACT DERMATITIS

There are two forms of contact dermatitis, one is immunologically mediated (see Selected Hypersensitivity Reactions, Allergic Contact Dermatitis), and the other is due to direct damage by irritant substances. Allergic contact dermatitis (immunologically mediated) requires prior sensitization to the offending agent. Most cases of contact dermatitis are nonimmunologic and are caused by direct contact with substances, such as body or wound secretions; application of drugs; or exposure to acids, alkalies, soaps, detergents, or irritant plants. These substances overwhelm the protective mechanisms of the skin and directly injure cells. It is important to realize that the two types of contact dermatitis can produce very similar histologic lesions, thus differentiation between immune-mediated and irritant contact dermatitis is largely dependent upon history, clinical signs, and anatomic distribution of the lesions. In dogs and cats, lesions of irritant contact dermatitis develop on the glabrous (sparsely haired) skin of the abdomen, axillas, flanks, interdigital spaces, perianal area, ventral tail, ventral chest, legs, eyelids, and feet. Horses develop lesions on the nose, ventrum, lower limbs, and where riding tack contacts the body, and on the perineum and caudal aspect of the rear legs. Grossly, erythematous patches, papules, and, rarely, vesicles develop, but self-inflicted trauma can lead to ulcers and crusts. Microscopically, lesions consist of spongiotic dermatitis, neutrophilic vesicopustules, and superficial dermal perivascular neutrophilic inflammation. Chronic lesions consist of epidermal hyperplasia, hyperkeratosis, and superficial perivascular inflammation. Lesions can be obscured by self-inflicted trauma, making histologic diagnosis difficult. Corrosive substances (strong acids or alkalies) can cause epidermal necrosis.

INJECTION SITE REACTIONS

Injections of vaccines or therapeutic drugs into the subcutis can result in granulomatous nodules. Injected materials, such as adjuvant and other vaccine components are highly antigenic, and can incite a local and persistent immunologic response resulting in a palpable subcutaneous nodule. Histologic descriptions of the acute or subacute reactions to similar injected materials are not reported in the literature. Histologic changes represented by the palpable nodules at the site of previous vaccination consist of a localized area of deep dermal or subcutaneous necrosis containing foreign material thought to be adjuvant or vaccine components. The central zone of foreign and necrotic material is bordered by macrophages and multinucleated giant cells with a peripheral zone of lymphocytes and variable numbers of plasma cells and eosinophils (foreign body granuloma). Macrophages usually contain amphophilic granular foreign material. Lymphoid follicular development at the margins of these lesions can be extensive. Although many injection site lesions heal without serious consequences, in cats there is a causal relationship between postvaccination inflammation and development of fibrosarcomas, osteosarcomas, rhabdomyosarcomas, malignant fibrous histiocytomas, and chondrosarcomas. The antigen load and degree of persistent inflammation and eventual fibroblastic proliferation caused by subcutaneous vaccine administration are thought to be important factors predisposing to tumor development in cats. It is speculated that during tissue repair, fibroblasts or myofibroblasts are stimulated by the immunogenic substances in the vaccine reaction site and this, in combination with other factors such as oncogene alterations or unidentified carcinogens, leads to malignant transformation of cells. Tumor development can take months to years, with eventual neoplastic transformation of mesenchymal cells.

In small, often soft-coated, breeds of dogs, especially poodles, injection of killed rabies vaccine can result in localized lymphoplasmacytic panniculitis, subtle vasculitis, and localized ischemia leading to severe follicular atrophy in overlying dermis (Fig. 17-41) that is clinically apparent as a focal area of alopecia and hyperpigmentation. Immunofluorescence staining has identified rabies antigen in the vessels and epithelium of the hair follicles. A low-grade, immune-mediated vasculitis with resultant tissue anoxia leading to the atrophic changes in the adnexa has been suggested as the pathogenesis. Vascular lesions are characterized by hyalinization of the vessel wall, lack of endothelial cells, intramural karyorrhectic debris, and perivascular lymphocytic infiltrates. Rarely, small numbers of

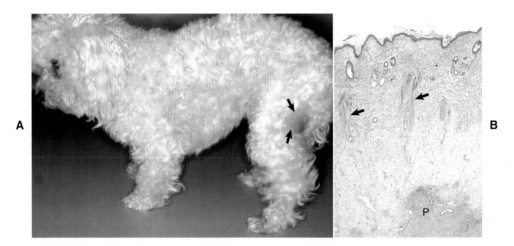

Fig. 17-41 **Rabies vaccine-associated alopecia, skin, haired, dog. A,** This type of alopecia (*arrows*) generally develops 3 to 6 months after vaccination. **B,** Note panniculitis (*P*) with lymphocytes, plasma cells, and histiocytes that has resulted from subcutaneous injection of killed rabies vaccine. Small, atrophic hair follicles (*arrows*) are in the dermis. H&E stain. (**A,** *Courtesy Dr. Lynn Schmeitzel, College of Veterinary Medicine, University of Tennessee.* **B,** *Courtesy Dr. Ann M. Hargis, DermatoDiagnostics.*)

lymphocytes are found within the walls of affected vessels.

Injection site eosinophilic granulomas with necrotic centers have been reported to occur in horses 1 to 3 days after injections of various substances using silicone-coated needles. The reaction is suspected to be a form of delayed hypersensitivity.

SNAKE AND SPIDER BITES (ENVENOMATIONS)

The families Elapidae (coral snake) and Viperidae (rattlesnake, water moccasin, and copperhead) contain the majority of the poisonous snakes in the United States. The genera *Latrodectus* (e.g., black widow) and *Loxosceles* (e.g., brown recluse) are the most common venomous spiders causing cutaneous injury. Effects are dependent upon composition of the venom, individual victim response, anatomic location of the envenomation, and specific characteristics of the offending snake or spider, which can be influenced by season of the year, geographic location, time since last inflicted bite or sting, depth of injury, etc. Different species of animals respond differently to the same venom.

Spider bites occur most often on the face and legs. The brown recluse spider (*Loxosceles reclusa*) is the spider most known to induce dermal necrosis, although there are a number of others. Brown recluse venom contains hyaluronidase and sphingomyelinase-D, which degrade tissue. A blister with a surrounding pale halo and more peripheral erythema characterizes initial reactions documented in human beings and some experimental animals. Necrosis and eschar formation occur within 5 to 7 days. Ulceration can be extensive.

Histologically, there is hemorrhage and edema, neutrophilic vasculitis, and arterial wall necrosis. The epidermis and dermis undergo infarction that can extend into the subcutis and underlying muscle. Panniculitis can be present. Eventually, there is dermal scarring and replacement of the subcutis and muscle by hypocellular connective tissue. Brown recluse spider bites in human beings can also lead to massive hemolysis. Differentials include other venomous bites, vasculitis, slough due to iatrogenic injection of irritating substances, thermal burns, necrotizing fasciitis or other cutaneous infection, septic embolization, or trauma. Some putative spider bites (and possibly wasp and bee stings) in the dog develop as acute, painful, swollen areas on the dorsal or lateral nose that histologically consist of severe eosinophilic folliculitis and furunculosis (see Miscellaneous Skin Disorders, Nasal Eosinophilic Folliculitis and Furunculosis in Dogs) leading to the theory that these lesions are probably caused by hypersensitivity reactions to injected venom.

Snake bites are common in the dog, horse, and to a lesser degree cats and most often are inflicted on the head or legs. Snake venom contains various enzymes, proteins, peptides, and kinins. Of the five genera of venomous snakes in the United States, *crotaline* (rattlesnake, copperhead, cottonmouth, and others) *venom* contains the highest concentration of proteolytic enzymes. Snakebite envenomation produces pain, edema, and erythema that, if severe, are followed by necrosis and sloughing of tissue, and sometimes death of the animal. Variable systemic effects occur, including paralysis, coagulation disturbances, shock, increased capillary permeability, myocardial damage, rhabdomyolysis, and renal failure.

ERGOT

Ergot poisoning is due to the ingestion of toxic alkaloids produced by the fungus *Claviceps purpurea*. This fungus infects the seed heads of grasses and grains. The alkaloids, particularly ergotamine, cause direct stimulation of adrenergic nerves supplying arteriolar smooth muscle, resulting in marked peripheral arteriolar vasoconstriction and damage to capillary endothelium. Arteriolar spasm and damage to capillary endothelium lead to thrombosis and ischemic necrosis (infarction) of tissue. Cold temperatures increase the severity of the lesions. The species most commonly poisoned are cattle fed contaminated grain or cattle grazing pastures infected with the alkaloid-producing fungus. Lesions develop after about 1 week of consumption, and begin as swelling and redness of the extremities, particularly the hind legs. The tips of pinnae and tail are affected with dry gangrene (infarction) and can slough.

TALL FESCUE GRASS

Lesions identical to those of ergot poisoning occur after the ingestion of tall fescue grass, a common pasture plant, infected by the endophytic fungus *Neotyphodium coenophialum* (formerly *Acremonium coenophialum*). Lesions develop about 2 weeks after ingestion of the toxic plant, and consist of necrosis (dry gangrene) of distal extremities. The ergot alkaloids, particularly ergovaline, are responsible for toxicity and act as peripheral vasoconstrictors.

SELENIUM

Selenium poisoning is due to ingestion of plants that have accumulated toxic concentrations of selenium, or to an overdose of a selenium supplement. Some plants selectively accumulate selenium, regardless of soil selenium content. These selective accumulators (obligate accumulators; e.g., *Astragalus, Stanleya*) require selenium for growth, generally are not palatable, and are eaten only when other plants are unavailable. Many other plants (facultative accumulators; e.g., *Aster, Atriplex*) do not require selenium for growth but will accumulate toxic concentrations of selenium if grown in soil with high selenium concentrations. These facultative accumulator plants are commonly eaten by livestock, and more often are the cause of poisoning. The mechanism by which selenium is thought to exert its effects on the integument and appendages is through its competitive replacement of sulfur, which modifies the structure of keratin, a sulfur-containing molecule. Replacement of sulfur by selenium in other molecules can also contribute to toxicity. Acute or chronic selenium poisoning has developed in most domestic animals, although susceptibility to selenium poisoning varies with species, dosage, diet, rate of consumption, chemical form, and other factors. In acute poisonings, signs relate to involvement of multiple organ systems. Chronic selenium toxicity usually develops in livestock (cattle, sheep, and horses) consuming seleniferous forages. It occurs worldwide but is more frequent in Nebraska, Wyoming, and the Dakotas in the United States and in portions of Western Canada. Animals with chronic selenium intoxication are emaciated, have poor-quality hair coat, and have partial alopecia. Horses lose the long hair of the mane and tail, develop hoof deformities, and shed the hooves.

VETCH TOXICOSIS AND VETCHLIKE DISEASES

Vetch toxicosis is most commonly seen as a syndrome characterized by dermatitis, conjunctivitis, diarrhea, and granulomatous inflammation of many organs. It occurs in cattle and to a lesser extent in horses after consumption of vetch-containing pastures. Hairy vetch (*Vicia villosa* Roth) is a cultivated legume used as pasture, hay, and silage in most of the United States and in other countries. Toxicity from vetch seeds is known to be a result of the presence of prussic acid. The cause of the granulomatous inflammation in this syndrome remains unclear. One proposed pathogenesis is that ingestion of vetch or another substance leads to antigen formation in the form of a hapten or a complete antigen that sensitizes lymphocytes and evokes the cell-mediated immune response upon repeat exposure.

Initial lesions in cattle consist of a rough coat with papules and crusts affecting the skin of the udder, teats, escutcheon (back of udder and perineum), and neck, followed by involvement of the trunk, face, and limbs. The skin becomes less pliable, alopecic, and lichenified. Marked pruritus leads to excoriations from self-induced trauma. The dermis has perivascular to diffuse infiltrates of monocytes, lymphocytes, plasma cells, multinucleated giant cells, and eosinophils. There is marked hyperkeratosis, and dermal and epidermal edema.

The clinical syndrome begins 2 or more weeks after consumption and consists of pruritic dermatitis, diarrhea (possibly bloody), and wasting. Morbidity is low and mortality is high. Holstein and Angus cattle, and cattle 3 years or older, are more often affected. Death in cattle occurs approximately 10 to 20 days after illness begins. At necropsy, yellow nodular infiltrates of mononuclear leukocytes are seen that disrupt the architecture of a wide range of organs but are most severe in myocardium, kidney, lymph nodes, thyroid, and adrenal glands. In cattle, other species of *Vicia* and additional compounds are capable of inducing disease indistinguishable from vetch toxicity. These include feed additives, such as diureidoisobutane and citrus pulp.

Hairy vetch toxicosis in horses resembles that in cattle, except for the infrequent finding of eosinophils in the infiltrate and lack of heart involvement. Conditions very similar to vetch toxicosis have been reported in horses with no vetch exposure. These cases have been variably referred to as "idiopathic granulomatous disease involving the skin," "systemic granulomatous disease," "generalized granulomatous disease," or "equine sarcoidosis." Organ involvement is variable. Skin lesions include scaling, crusting, and alopecia on the face or limbs that progress to a generalized exfoliative dermatitis. Histologically the skin has multifocal, sometimes perifollicular to deep dermal nodules of granulomatous inflammation. These idiopathic conditions in the horse are fairly indistinguishable and should be considered "vetchlike disease" until more information is available.

The diagnosis of vetch toxicity or vetchlike disease is a diagnosis by exclusion. It is made after review of the herd history and of character and distribution of the lesions. The combination of lesions is fairly distinctive.

PHYSICAL INJURY
Acral lick dermatitis

Acral lick dermatitis (lick granuloma, neurodermatitis) is a relatively common psychogenic dermatitis usually developing on an extremity (acral = extremity or apex) in dogs, and is caused by persistent licking or chewing. The cause is not known, but a mild sensory polyneuropathy that incites a sensation of pruritus or pain may be associated with lesion development. The constant licking and chewing of the skin is a form of repeated trauma that leads to the gross and histologic changes. Boredom can also play a role. Usually a single lesion develops in carpal, metacarpal, metatarsal, tibial, or radial areas. Grossly, lesions are circumscribed, hairless, and, sometimes, ulcerated (Fig. 17-42). Microscopically, there is compact hyperkeratosis and acanthosis of the epidermis and follicular epithelium. Ulcers are occasionally seen, the result of chronic irritation from licking. The dermis is thickened by fibrosis. Capillaries and some collagen fibers are oriented parallel to hair follicles, called "vertical streaking." Sebaceous glands and hair follicles are hypertrophic, and there is perivascular and periadnexal plasmacytic dermatitis. Some lesions are complicated by secondary bacterial folliculitis and furunculosis.

PYOTRAUMATIC DERMATITIS (ACUTE MOIST DERMATITIS, "HOT SPOTS")

Pyotraumatic dermatitis, especially common in dogs, is secondary to irritation and is principally the result of self-inflicted trauma from biting or scratching because of pain or itching caused by allergies, parasites, matted hair, or irritant chemicals. Dogs with long hair and dense undercoats are predisposed, and lesions develop more commonly in hot humid weather. Flea bite dermatitis is a common predisposing cause, and lesions can coalesce to involve large portions of dorsal lumbar and thigh skin. Type I hypersensitivity reaction to flea bites leads to severe pruritus and self-trauma. Excoriated, moist skin is conducive to bacterial colonization. Grossly the lesions are hairless, red, exude fluid, and have circumscribed edges. Microscopically, affected dogs have either superficial erosive to ulcerative exudative dermatitis or a deeper suppurative folliculitis (pyotraumatic folliculitis,

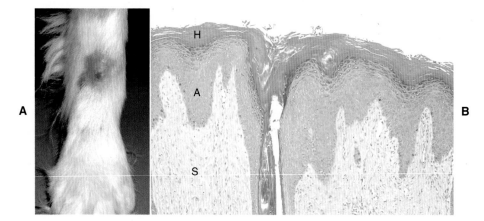

Fig. 17-42   Acral lick dermatitis, skin, leg, dog. A, Chronic licking has resulted in an area of alopecia and a small dark ulcer in the alopecic area. Alopecia can be caused by mechanical removal of the hair or breakage of hair from licking, and in cases with secondary folliculitis, alopecia can also be due to follicular inflammation (folliculitis) and sometimes follicular rupture (furunculosis). Ulceration also can be caused by mechanical trauma to the skin surface. **B,** The epidermis is thickened by compact hyperkeratosis (*H*) and acanthosis (*A*), and the dermis is thickened by granulation tissue and fibrosis (scarring [*S*]). H&E stain. (*A* and **B,** *Courtesy Dr. Ann M. Hargis, DermatoDiagnostics.*)

deep pyoderma). The pyotraumatic folliculitis lesions are considered to represent a deep pyoderma and develop more commonly on the cheek and neck of young golden retrievers, Saint Bernards, Labrador retrievers, and Newfoundland dogs. Biopsy is required to differentiate the more superficial pyotraumatic dermatitis from the deeper suppurative folliculitis.

FELINE ULCERATIVE DERMATITIS SYNDROME

Feline ulcerative dermatitis syndrome is an uncommon disorder that may have more than one underlying cause. Previous injections and hypersensitivity are thought to initiate the syndrome in some, but not all, cats. The pathogenesis is not known, but self-trauma appears to significantly contribute to and perpetuate lesions. Lesions develop most commonly in the skin of the dorsal neck or interscapular regions, and grossly consist of a nonhealing ulcer with serocellular exudate that can mat the adjacent hair. Microscopic lesions consist of an ulcer covered by fibrinonecrotic crust. The dermis subjacent to the ulcer contains components of necrotic epidermis and adnexa intermixed with degenerate neutrophils. Adnexal effacement by fibrosis is seen in severe cases. Inflammation in adjacent and deeper dermis is variable, but often scant, and consists of a few neutrophils, eosinophils, and mixed mononuclear cells. Chronic lesions consist of acanthosis of bordering epidermis with a linear band of fibrosis beneath and parallel to the adjacent intact epidermis. In those cases attributed to previous vaccination, nodular lymphoplasmacytic to histiocytic panniculitis is present.

CALLUS

A callus is a raised, irregular, patch of thickened skin that develops because of friction, usually over pressure points on bony prominences or on the sternum (Table 17-5). Callosities can develop in all domestic animals, but are particularly common in giant breed dogs and in pigs kept on concrete or other hard flooring without adequate bedding. Secondary folliculitis, furunculosis, and ulceration can develop. Microscopically the epidermis and follicular epithelium are thickened by hyperkeratosis and acanthosis. Regular epidermal hyperplasia (rete ridge and dermal papilla interdigitation) also occurs. Comedones are present in some lesions. The follicular openings can be widened by excessive keratin. Dilated follicles can rupture (furunculosis), releasing bacteria, keratin proteins, and sebum, resulting in secondary pyoderma and a foreign body inflammatory response (callus pyoderma).

INTERTRIGO (SKIN FOLD DERMATITIS)

Intertrigo is superficial dermatitis occurring on apposed skin surfaces, such as the facial fold (brachycephalic breeds), lip fold (breeds with large lips such as the Saint Bernard), body fold (Shar-Pei breed), vulvar fold (obese female dogs with a small vulva), and tail fold (dogs with corkscrew tails, such as English bulldogs) (Fig. 17-43). Intertrigo also occurs in cows with large pendulous udders and develops between the udder and the medial thigh (udder-thigh dermatitis). The cause and pathogenesis involve the presence of closely apposed skin surfaces, frictional trauma between the skin surfaces, accumulated moisture (from tears, saliva, cutaneous glandular secretions, or urine), and bacterial infection. The moisture and frictional trauma predispose to bacterial growth and subsequent infection. Early gross lesions of intertriginous dermatitis typically consist initially of erythema and edema. Later, pustules, ulcers, and crusts can develop. Late lesions in cows can be severe, with occasional sloughing of skin and subcutis. Microscopically, in early stages there is congestion and edema with early perivascular inflammation that progresses to a more diffuse band of inflammation in the superficial dermis, parallel to the epidermis, but often sparing the epidermal-dermal junction. Inflammatory cells include plasma cells, fewer lymphocytes, neutrophils, and macrophages. In more severe cases, there can be exocytosis of neutrophils into the epidermis, epidermal pustules, crusts, ulcers, and, in cows, necrosis that leads to sloughing of tissue. If the cause is corrected, early and mild chronic lesions heal without scarring (most cases). However, when there is ulceration or necrosis and sloughing of tissue (minority of cases), lesions heal by second intention with the formation of granulation tissue, wound contraction, and scarring.

TEMPERATURE EXTREMES

Exposure to cold temperatures causes different types of injury depending on the severity of the temperature extreme and length of exposure. The pathogenesis involves both direct freezing and disruption of cells and vascular damage, leading to tissue anoxia. In direct freezing, the initial injury results in the formation of extracellular ice crystals that damage cellular membranes, leading to cell death. As freezing continues, a shift in intracellular water to the extracellular space leads to cellular dehydration and increased intracellular sodium concentration and, eventually, to intracellular ice crystal formation. When intracellular ice crystals form and expand, the cell is mechanically and irreversibly damaged. Lesions are located in the extremities, such as the ear tips of cats, the scrotum of dogs and bulls, and the ear tips, tail, and teats of cattle. Grossly, lesions consist of infarction (dry gangrene) and sloughing of necrotic tissue.

In contrast, slow chilling produces vasoconstriction with endothelial and parenchymal cell damage. Subsequent secondary vasodilation causes increased vascular permeability followed by edema and neutrophilic inflammation.

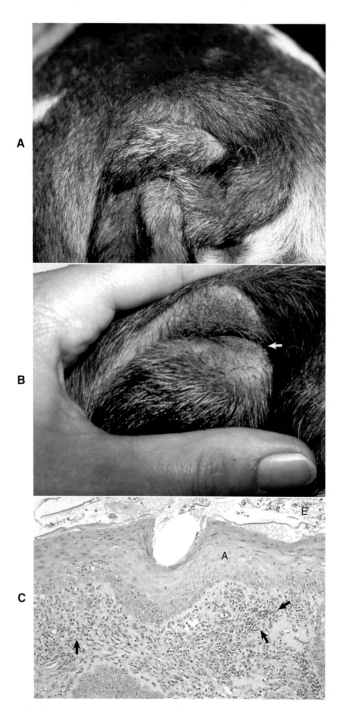

Fig. 17-43   Intertriginous inflammation (screw tail), skin, tail, dog. A, "Screw tail," English bulldog. Excessive skin folds around the tail cause friction and moisture accumulation, predisposing to bacterial growth. **B,** Intertriginous pyoderma, English bulldog. The skin fold *(arrow)* of the dog depicted in Fig. 17-43, A has been opened to expose the erythema, hyperpigmentation, and lichenification. **C,** Intertriginous dermatitis. The epidermis is acanthotic *(A)* and partially covered by fluid and cellular exudate *(E),* and there is inflammation composed of numerous plasma cells and fewer lymphocytes and neutrophils in the dermis *(arrows).* H&E stain. *(A and B, Courtesy Dr. Alexander Werner, Valley Veterinary Specialty Service. C, Courtesy Dr. Ann M. Hargis, DermatoDiagnostics.)*

Exposure to more severe and persistent cold temperatures causes vasoconstriction, necrosis of vessels, increased blood viscosity, and coagulative necrosis of tissue because of anoxia. Cutaneous lesions due to cold temperatures are uncommon in well-nourished healthy animals but can develop in an animal recently moved from a warm to a cold climate or in neonates that are hypoglycemic or inadequately dried at birth.

Thermal burns are caused by exposure to excessive heat. Examples of heat sources include hot liquids, flames, friction, electricity, heating pads, blow dryers, drying cages, and lightning. Burns are categorized as partial (first- or second-degree) or full-thickness (third-degree). Longer exposure to lower temperatures is more damaging than shorter exposure to higher temperatures. Dry heat causes desiccation and carbonization, whereas moist heat causes coagulation of tissue. In less severe burns, damage is due to accelerated cellular metabolism, inactivation of enzymes, and vessel injury. In first-degree burns only the epidermis is affected, whereas in second-degree burns the epidermis and part of the dermis are damaged. In third-degree (full-thickness) burns, there is coagulation of the epidermis and all dermal components including connective tissue, blood vessels, and adnexa. Fourth-degree burns are similar to third-degree burns, but damage extends into the subcutaneous fascia and underlying tissue. Gross lesions of burns vary from erythema and edema due to capillary dilation and increased capillary permeability (first-degree burn) to vesicle formation as a result of fluid accumulation at the dermal-epidermal junction, which produces the "burn blister" (second-degree burn), to desiccation and charring of the epidermis, with underlying amorphous accretion of connective tissue representing the coagulated dermis and adnexa (third-degree burn). Microscopically, partial-thickness burns consist of coagulation necrosis of the epidermis, subepidermal vesicles as a result of accumulation of fluid from superficial capillaries (Fig. 17-18), necrosis of superficial portions of follicles and sebaceous glands, and degeneration of the subepidermal collagen. In partial-thickness burns, there is preservation of part of the epidermis or dermal portions of adnexa from which epithelial regeneration develops. Full-thickness (third-degree) burns are represented by coagulation of all components of the skin accompanied by acute inflammation. Subcutaneous vasculitis can be present. Partial-thickness burns involving the epidermis (first-degree burns) heal completely, as remaining epidermis and epithelium from adnexa reepithelialize the surface, and the dermis and adnexa are intact, so there is no scarring. However, partial-thickness burns that also involve the superficial dermis and superficial adnexa (second-degree burns) can result in superficial dermal scarring, but the adnexa are preserved. In full-thickness burns, over time histiocytes infiltrate the tissue, the necrotic tissue sloughs, and the defect is filled in by granulation tissue. Permanent scarring with loss of adnexa results unless skin grafts are performed, and if much of the body is affected, the lesions are life threatening because of fluid loss and possible sepsis from lack of the skin's protective barrier. In human beings, the prognosis in severe burn injury can be roughly calculated by adding the patient's age plus the percentage of the body with full-thickness burns (third-degree). If the total is 100, the likelihood of survival is low.

Moderate heat dermatosis (erythema ab igne) is an uncommon disorder reported in dogs and cats, and is caused by repeated chronic (weeks to months) exposure to moderate heat, too low to cause a thermal burn. Heat sources that have caused moderate heat dermatosis include heating pads, heated kennel mats, electric blankets, plant warmers, heat registers, and concrete driveways. When the heat source is in direct contact with the skin, conduction probably plays a role in mediating the injury, but the pathomechanism at the cellular level by which conductive heating causes moderate heat dermatitis has not been investigated. In dogs and cats, the cutaneous lesion distribution typically reflects chronic exposure to moderate heat during lateral or sternal recumbency. Clinical lesions consist of irregular areas of erythema, alopecia, and sometimes hyperpigmentation. Histologic lesions include keratinocyte karyomegaly, atypia, and degeneration, mixed dermal mononuclear inflammation, adnexal atrophy, and a variable number of wavy eosinophilic elastic fibers in the dermis. Hyperpigmentation is due to accumulation of melanophages and hemosiderophages in the dermis. Recall that exposure to moderate heat sources (e.g., heating pads on low temperature setting) can also cause thermal burns. Therefore lesions of thermal burns (e.g., coagulation of the epidermis) can coexist with those of moderate heat dermatosis.

MICROBIAL AND PARASITIC DISORDERS

Cutaneous infections develop when there is disruption in the defense mechanisms of the skin (see Host Defense Mechanisms against Injury). Predisposing factors to skin infections involve compromised epidermal barrier integrity caused by friction, trauma, excessive moisture, dirt, matted hair, chemical irritants, freezing or burning, irradiation, and parasitic infestation. Suppressed immune function resulting from inadequate nutrition, therapy with glucocorticoids, and other acquired or inherited immunologic abnormalities can also contribute to increased susceptibility to microbial and parasitic infections. Infectious agents enter the body via their specific portal of entry (see Portals of Entry into the Skin),

which includes traversing the epidermal surface, entering via hair follicles or the ducts of glands, and migrating via nerves or sometimes via the hematogenous route.

VIRAL INFECTIONS
POXVIRUSES

Poxviruses are DNA epitheliotropic viruses that infect most domestic, wild, and laboratory animals and birds (Table 17-8). Dogs and cats are rarely infected with poxviruses, although infection with contagious ecthyma (parapoxvirus) has been reported in dogs, and cutaneous infection caused by a poxvirus of the orthopoxvirus genus (cowpox) has been reported in cats in Europe. There are major differences between different poxviruses and in the range of species they will infect, with some being species-specific and others zoonotic. Many poxviruses of animals, such as the contagious ecthyma parapoxvirus, can cause skin lesions in human beings. Poxviruses induce lesions by a variety of mechanisms. Lesions develop secondary to pox viral invasion of epithelium, by ischemic necrosis caused by vascular injury, and by stimulation of host cell DNA, resulting in epidermal hyperplasia. Hyperplasia may be explained by a gene, present in several poxviruses including molluscum contagiosum, whose product has significant homology with epidermal growth factor. Poxviruses also encode for functions that may counteract host defenses. These include genes related to those encoding the serpins (a superfamily of related proteins important in regulating serine protease enzymes that mediate kinin, complement, fibrinolytic, and coagulation pathways) and genes encoding antiinterferon activities. The severity of poxviral infection varies depending on whether the infection is localized or systemic and whether there are secondary infections. The sequence of the lesions are macule, papule, vesicle (varies in severity), umbilicated pustule, crust, and scar (Fig. 17-33). Histologically, pox lesions begin as epidermal cytoplasmic swelling and vacuolation, usually first affecting the cells of the outer stratum spinosum. Rupture of the damaged keratinocytes produces multiloculated vesicles, so-called reticular degeneration. The early dermal lesions include edema, vascular dilation, a perivascular mononuclear cell infiltrate, and a variable neutrophilic infiltrate. Neutrophils migrate into the epidermis and aggregate in vesicles to form microabscesses. Large intraepidermal pustules can form and sometimes extend into the superficial dermis. There is usually marked epithelial hyperplasia and sometimes pseudocarcinomatous hyperplasia of the adjacent epithelium. This contributes to the raised border of the umbilicated pustule. Rupture or drying of the pustule produces an inflammatory crust, often colonized on its surface by bacteria. Poxvirus lesions often contain characteristic intracytoplasmic eosinophilic

Table **17-8**   **Viral Infections of the Skin**

Virus	Diseases	Species Affected	Distribution
Parapoxvirus	Contagious pustular dermatitis	Sheep, goats, cattle; rarely dogs	Cutaneous
	Papular stomatitis	Cattle	
	Pseudocowpox	Milking cows; zoonotic	
Orthopoxvirus	Cowpox	Some such as cowpox and	Cutaneous
	Vaccinia	vaccinia affect many species;	
	Horsepox*	others are more host specific	
	Equine papular dermatitis†		
Molluscipox	Molluscum contagiosum	Horses, rarely dogs	Cutaneous
Capripoxvirus	Sheeppox	Most species specific	Systemic
	Goatpox		
	Lumpy skin disease	Cattle	
Suipoxvirus	Swine pox	Pigs	Cutaneous
Unclassified poxvirus	Ulcerative dermatosis of sheep	Sheep	Cutaneous
Bovine herpesvirus 2 (dermatotropic)	Bovine ulcerative mammillitis (bovine herpes mammillitis) Pseudo-lumpy skin disease	Cattle	Cutaneous
Bovine herpesvirus 4 (dermatotropic)	Bovine herpes mammary pustular dermatitis	Cattle	Cutaneous
Feline herpesvirus 1	Feline facial dermatitis and stomatitis	Cats	Cutaneous, oral, ocular, upper respiratory
Ovine herpesvirus 2‡ (in United States)	Malignant catarrhal fever	Cattle	Cutaneous, oral, systemic
Papillomavirus	Warts	All species	Cutaneous, oral, mucocutaneous
Papillomavirus	Fibropapilloma	Cattle	Cutaneous, genital
Papillomavirus	Sarcoid (fibropapilloma)	Horse, cat	Cutaneous
Papillomavirus	Bowen's-like disease	Cat, less in dog	Cutaneous
Papillomavirus	Pigmented epidermal plaques	Dog	Cutaneous
Picornavirus	Foot-and-mouth disease	Ruminants, pigs	Oral, cutaneous
Picornavirus	Swine vesicular disease	Pigs	Oral, cutaneous
Rhabdovirus	Vesicular stomatitis	Horses, cattle, pigs	Oral, cutaneous
Calicivirus	Vesicular exanthema	Pigs	Oral, cutaneous
Calicivirus	Feline calicivirus	Cats	Oral, cutaneous, systemic
Parvovirus	Porcine parvovirus	Piglets	Oral, cutaneous
Retrovirus	Feline leukemia virus Feline immunodeficiency virus	Cats	Secondary skin infections; cutaneous horns with feline leukemia virus

*Horsepox may be due to human or cattle orthopoxviruses.
†Virus not fully characterized.
‡Indirect evidence of viral involvement.

inclusion bodies. These are single or multiple and of varying size and duration. Sheeppox and goatpox are the most pathogenic poxviruses, and infection causes significant mortality, especially in young animals as a result of systemic disease. Sheeppox and goatpox do not occur in the United States or Canada.

Contagious ecthyma

Contagious ecthyma (contagious pustular dermatitis, orf, sore mouth) is a common localized infection of young sheep and goats caused by a parapoxvirus with worldwide distribution. Less commonly, human beings, cattle, wild ungulates, and dogs are infected. Morbidity in lambs is usually great and, although mortality is usually low, it can approach 15% in lambs. Lesions are initiated by abrasions from pasture grasses or forage, begin at the commissures of the mouth, and spread to the lips (Fig. 17-44), oral mucosa, eyelids, and feet. Lambs can transfer the virus to the teats of ewes, and the lesions can spread to the skin of the udder. Contagious ecthyma

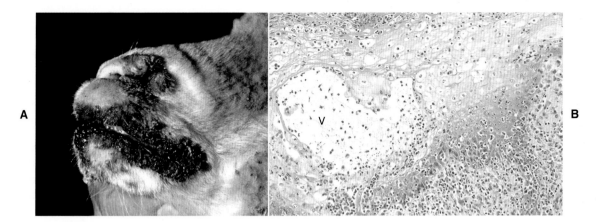

Fig. 17-44   Contagious ecthyma, skin, lamb. A, Note crusts around nose and lips. These lesions are the late stage of the disease, are formed after rupture of vesicles and pustules, and are responsible for the common name "scabby mouth." **B,** Note the epidermal hyperplasia (acanthosis), ballooning degeneration, vesicle (V), and neutrophils accumulating in the vesicle, which will subsequently result in the formation of a pustule. Epidermal hyperplasia, upward movement of the pustule, and rupture of the vesicle or pustule contribute to crust formation as seen in Fig. 17-44, **A.** H&E stain. (**A,** *Courtesy Dr. M.D. McGavin, College of Veterinary Medicine, University of Tennessee.* **B,** *Courtesy Dr. Ann M. Hargis, DermatoDiagnostics.*)

is of economic importance due to weight loss in lambs that are reluctant to eat because of the pain associated with oral and perioral lesions. Pathogenesis of lesion formation and gross and microscopic features are consistent with the typical poxvirus lesions (see previous discussion and Fig. 17-33), except that the vesicle stage is very brief, the ulcer and crust stage persists and is clinically prominent, and the epidermis is markedly hyperplastic. Inclusion bodies are only briefly detectable histologically at the vesicular stage.

Molluscum contagiosum

Equine molluscum contagiosum is a mildly contagious, self-limiting cutaneous infection in the horse caused by a poxvirus from the genera *Molluscipoxvirus* (molluscum contagiosum virus), a virus closely related to the human molluscum contagiosum virus. The equine lesions are small and often incidental and may be localized to the penis, prepuce, axillary and inguinal areas, and nose. The pathogenesis of lesion formation is typical of poxvirus infection (see previous discussion). Commencing as multiple, circular, smooth-surfaced, gray-white papules 1 to 2 mm in diameter, the lesions become umbilicated and develop a central pore from which a caseous plug is extruded. The microscopic lesions of molluscum contagiosum consist of well-demarcated foci of epidermal hyperplasia and hypertrophy that form invaginated lobules of the epidermis in the superficial dermis. Keratinocytes containing inclusions exfoliate through a pore that forms in the stratum corneum

and enlarges into a central crater. The individual keratinocytes are markedly swollen and contain large intracytoplasmic eosinophilic inclusions, known as "molluscum bodies," which can be identified histologically and in cytologic preparations. There is usually no dermal reaction. Rarely, molluscum contagiosum has developed in dogs.

Swinepox

Pox lesions in pigs are caused by the host-specific poxvirus *Suipoxvirus* (swinepox). Normally, swinepox is transmitted by contact, although transplacental infection has not been ruled out. The sucking louse *Haematopinus suis* often acts as a mechanical vector and assists infection by causing skin trauma. The virus persists in dried crusts from infected animals. The pathogenesis of lesion formation and morphology of the gross and histologic lesions are consistent with the typical pox infection. The gross lesions typically affect the ventral and lateral abdomen, lateral thorax, and medial foreleg and thigh. Occasionally, lesions on the dorsum predominate. Lesions can be generalized and rarely involve the oral mucosa, pharynx, esophagus, stomach, trachea, and bronchi. The erythematous papules usually transform into umbilicated pustules without a significant vesicular stage (Fig. 17-45). The inflammatory crust eventually sheds to leave a white scar. The disease occurs worldwide and is endemic to areas of intensive swine production. The disease affects young, growing piglets and is mild with very low mortality.

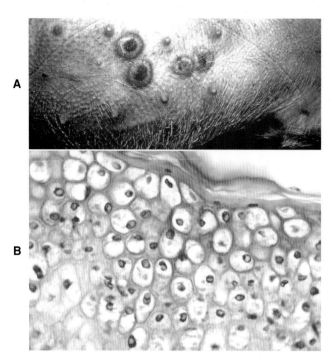

Fig. 17-45   Swine pox, skin, piglet. A, Note the four umbilicated pustules in the abdominal skin. **B,** Note keratinocytes with ballooning degeneration and eosinophilic cytoplasmic inclusion bodies. Ballooning degeneration develops before vesicle formation. H&E stain. (*A* and *B, Courtesy Dr. M.D. McGavin, College of Veterinary Medicine, University of Tennessee.*)

Cowpox

Cowpox virus infections occur rarely in cattle in the United Kingdom and other areas of Europe. There is increasing evidence that small wild rodents (i.e., mice, squirrels, voles) serve as a reservoir for infection, and that cattle, cats, and rarely other mammals become infected through contact with the wild rodents. Cutaneous infections in cattle usually develop on the teats and udder of cows and on the muzzle of suckling calves. Lesions follow the typical sequence of cutaneous pox viral infections. In cats, poxvirus infection is uncommon and usually occurs in outdoor cats living in rural areas, presumably because these cats hunt and have contact with rodents harboring the poxvirus. Primary cutaneous lesions typically develop on the face, neck, or forelegs and consist of an ulcerated or crusted macule or plaque. Lesions can develop into deep ulcers that heal with granulation tissue or less commonly develop into abscesses or cellulitis. Rarely oral or mucocutaneous junctional areas are affected. Additional secondary cutaneous lesions can develop within about two weeks after viremic distribution to other cutaneous sites and less commonly to the upper or lower respiratory tract. The microscopic lesions are

sharply demarcated, often deep ulcers covered by fibrinonecrotic exudate. Intracytoplasmic inclusion bodies in keratinocytes or follicular or sebaceous glandular epithelial cells help establish the diagnosis.

HERPESVIRUSES

Herpesviruses are DNA viruses that only occasionally produce cutaneous lesions (Table 17-8). Cutaneous lesions have rarely been reported in nondermatotropic herpesviruses infections, such as infectious bovine rhinotracheitis (bovine herpesvirus 1) and equine coital exanthema (equine herpesvirus 3), and in cats with feline herpesvirus 1 infection. Two dermatotropic herpesvirus infections with economic importance are bovine herpesvirus 2 and bovine herpesvirus 4. Herpesviruses can be latent, with inactive virus persisting in tissue such as the trigeminal nerve ganglia. It is speculated that up to 80% of adult cats recovered from feline herpesvirus 1 infection as kittens or young cats have latent herpesvirus 1 infections. During times of stress, the virus is reactivated and lesions can recur. Herpesviruses infect epithelial cells and replicate in the nucleus, leading to lysis of nuclear contents. As immature viral particles enter the cytoplasm, there is degeneration of cytoplasmic organelles, accumulation of cytoplasmic lipid, and precipitation of protein. Death of keratinocytes leads to spread of virus to neighboring cells, leading to rapid necrosis of focally extensive areas of the epidermis. Gross lesions consist of vesicles that rupture to form ulcers that are then covered by crusts. Microscopic lesions in herpesvirus infections depend on the stage, but early degenerative changes include ballooning and reticular degeneration, the sequelae of degeneration of epidermal cells and acantholysis. Syncytial cells may be seen. Intranuclear inclusions develop, but because of rapidly developing necrosis may not be found except at the margins of ulcers. The appearance of the viral inclusions varies with the specific herpesvirus. Some herpesviruses produce large, hyaline amphophilic inclusions that fill the nucleus (feline herpesvirus 1), whereas others (bovine herpes mammillitis) produce typical Cowdry type A inclusions, which are also intranuclear but smaller and eosinophilic.

Bovine herpesvirus 2

Bovine herpesvirus 2, a dermatotropic virus (Allerton virus), can cause generalized disease (pseudo-lumpy skin disease) or, as seen in the United States, localized infection of the teat called bovine ulcerative mammilitis (bovine herpes mammillitis). Mammillitis is inflammation of the teat or nipple. Localized infection occurs more commonly in lactating dairy cows but can develop in beef cows, pregnant heifers, and suckling calves. Trauma is implicated in the pathogenesis because normal skin is resistant to viral penetration. The pathogenesis of lesion formation was discussed earlier. Bovine ulcerative mammillitis is of economic importance because of decreased milk production and secondary bacterial mastitis. Lesions develop on the teats and skin of the nearby udder or occasionally the perineum. Suckling calves develop lesions on the muzzle (nose).

Bovine herpesvirus 4

Bovine herpesvirus 4 (bovine herpes mammary pustular dermatitis) causes a similar but milder disease than the localized form of bovine herpesvirus 2.

Feline ulcerative facial dermatitis and stomatitis

Feline herpesvirus 1 is an uncommon cause of ulcerative, often persistent, facial dermatitis or stomatitis in cats of various ages and sexes. Glucocorticoid therapy or stresses, such as overcrowding, are thought to play a role in lesion development. Most lesions develop under circumstances suggesting reactivation of latent herpesvirus infection. The pathogenesis is typical of that described for herpesviruses in the previous section. Gross lesions are ulcerative and crusted (Table 17-5). Histologically, there is extensive necrosis of the epidermal, follicular, and sometimes sebaceous gland epithelium accompanied by prominent mixed dermal inflammation that frequently includes numerous eosinophils. Follicular epithelium can be destroyed, and free keratin in the dermis is associated with eosinophils and foci of eosinophil degranulation bordering collagen fibers and collagen degeneration. Large amphophilic or hyaline intranuclear inclusions are present in the surface and adnexal epithelium. Inclusion bodies are often easily overlooked, variable in number, and sometimes present in small rafts of epithelial cells surrounded by necrotic debris. The lesions are different from those previously reported in domestic cats in that they persist and are limited to the skin of the face or oral mucosa and often have significant eosinophilic inflammation. The inflammation in feline herpesvirus dermatitis overlaps with that of the hypersensitivity reactions, including mosquito bite hypersensitivity, and also with that of eosinophilic ulcers, thus warranting close scrutiny of eosinophilic necrotizing cutaneous lesions for intranuclear inclusion bodies.

PAPILLOMAVIRUSES

Papillomaviruses are typically species- and site-specific pathogens that infect the squamous epithelium and cause benign proliferative masses and less commonly malignant tumors. All domestic animals are affected by one or more papillomaviruses (Table 17-8). Papillomaviruses cause lesions by two different mechanisms. In some cells, infection elicits increased activity, mitosis, and proliferation that lead to the gross and histologic changes of hyperplasia and hyperkeratosis (nonproductive infection). The hyperplastic cells are considered transformed. In other cells, infection leads to degeneration, virion production within the cell nucleus, and eventual cell death (productive infection). The effect the papillomavirus has on the cell (i.e., proliferation or virion production leading to cell death) is dependent on the way the viral genome is inserted into the host cell genome and on the stage of the cell cycle of the host cell at the time of infection. In the epidermis, virion production is limited to cells of the suprabasilar layer. Clinical and histologic lesions are diverse. The most common type of cutaneous papillomavirus infection (papilloma, wart, cutaneous papillomatosis) consists of clinical lesions that are alopecic, flat, or papilliferous benign masses (Fig. 17-46). Histologically, stratified squamous epithelium is covered by thickened orthokeratotic or parakeratotic keratin, is acanthotic, and has elongated epidermal-dermal interdigitations. The epidermis rests on a collagenous core. In some papillomas, keratinocytes, especially of the upper stratum spinosum, are swollen with amphophilic cytoplasm and have an eccentric nucleus and a perinuclear halo; these keratinocytes are termed "koilocytes" (meaning hollow or concave). Keratohyalin granules are irregular. Also, pale basophilic intranuclear inclusion bodies, located in degenerating cells in the outer layers of the stratum spinosum and granulosum in which virion production is taking place, occur in some but not all papillomas. Papillomas spontaneously regress, and in regressing stages, there is reduced epidermal hyperplasia, increased proliferation of fibroblasts, deposition of collagen, and infiltration of T lymphocytes at the epidermal dermal interface.

In cats and horses, papillomavirus infection also causes development of cutaneous fibropapillomas (sarcoids). These are flat, verrucous, or nodular masses in which the proliferation of dermal fibroblasts is the prominent feature, often surpassing that of the epidermal hyperplasia (Fig. 17-47). Equine sarcoids are caused by a nonproductive infection of bovine papillomavirus and are locally aggressive, nonmetastatic fibroblastic skin tumors of horses, mules, and donkeys. They are the most common skin tumor of horses, accounting for up to 30% of tumors, and occur in any breed, sex, or age. Young adult horses 3 to 6 years of age are most commonly affected. Sarcoids frequently develop in areas subjected to trauma or at sites of wounds 6 to 8 months after wound healing, and develop anywhere but are most common on the head, legs, and ventral trunk. They can be single or multiple. The tumors are classified according to their gross appearance as verrucous, fibroblastic, mixed, or occult. The verrucous type is a small wartlike growth, usually measuring less than 6 cm in diameter, with a dry, rough surface and

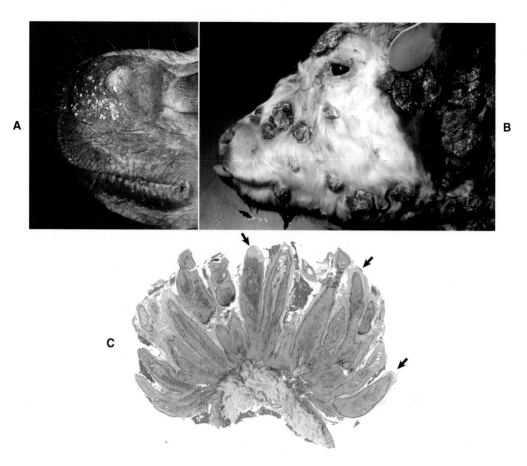

Fig. 17-46   **Cutaneous papillomas, skin. A,** Chin, horse. Note multiple, small, verrucous masses arising in the skin. **B,** Head, cow. Note multiple, irregular, alopecic, verrucous papillomas. **C,** The papillary projections *(arrows),* often called fronds, are composed of hyperkeratotic epidermis covering a collagenous core. H&E stain. (**A,** *Courtesy Dr. David Duclos, Animal Skin and Allergy Clinic.* **B** *and* **C,** *Courtesy Dr. M.D. McGavin, College of Veterinary Medicine, University of Tennessee.)*

variable alopecia. The fibroblastic type of sarcoid is more variable in appearance and can range from a well-circumscribed firm nodule with intact surface to a large mass, greater than 25 cm in diameter, with an ulcerated surface prone to hemorrhage, and resembling exuberant granulation tissue. The mixed type is a transitional form in which a verrucous sarcoid becomes a fibroblastic type as a result of trauma or biopsy. The occult form consists of a slow-growing, slightly thickened area of skin with slight surface roughening and alopecia that remains static for a long period.

Histologically, sarcoids are typically biphasic tumors composed of both epidermal and dermal components; however, the epidermal component may be minimal or absent in some tumors, especially those with extensive ulceration. When the epidermis is intact, hyperkeratosis, parakeratosis, and acanthosis with thin rete pegs extending deep into the dermis are common features. The dermal component consists of fibroblasts and

collagen in various proportions. The fibroblasts have plump nuclei, and nucleoli may be prominent. The mitotic index is usually low. Fibroblasts at the dermal-epidermal junction are frequently oriented perpendicular to the basement membrane in a "picket fence" pattern, which is a distinctive histologic feature seen in most sarcoids. The cells are arranged in whorls, interlacing bundles, or haphazard arrays of variable density. Tumor margins are typically indistinct and adequacy of excision is frequently difficult to determine. Spontaneous remission can occur after several years in up to 30% of cases. The tumors are characterized by a high rate of recurrence, up to 50%, following surgical excision. Bovine papillomavirus DNA has also been identified in feline fibropapillomas (sarcoids).

Papillomavirus infection may also contribute to the development of another syndrome in cats and less often in dogs termed, "multicentric squamous cell carcinoma in situ" (Bowen's-like disease). Although not all the factors

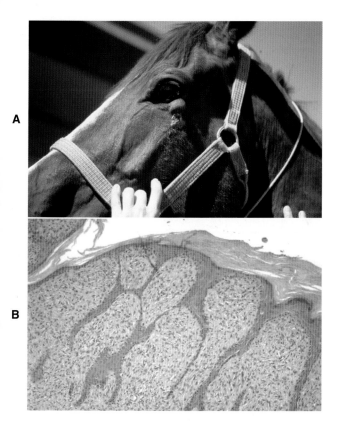

Fig. 17-47 **Sarcoid, skin, horse. A,** Equine sarcoid, face. The irregular multinodular mass is present on the ventrolateral periocular skin. **B,** Sarcoid. The sarcoid consists of an epidermal and dermal component. The hyperplastic epidermis has thin rete pegs that extend into the dermis. The dermis is thickened by proliferating fibroblasts and collagen. H&E stain. (**A,** *Courtesy Dr. Helen Power, Dermatology for Animals.* **B,** *Courtesy Dr. Pamela E. Ginn, College of Veterinary Medicine, University of Florida.*)

contributing to lesion formation have been documented, papillomavirus DNA has been identified in these lesions in cats, suggesting a nonproductive infection promotes the epithelial hyperplasia characteristic of this disease. Multicentric squamous cell carcinoma in situ clinically consists of sharply demarcated single, or more often multiple, scaly verrucous or irregular plaquelike lesions 0.5 to 3.0 cm in diameter. Histologically the epidermis and follicular infundibular epithelium are thickened by proliferation of basal keratinocytes that tend to stream together, providing a "windblown" appearance to the epidermis. Nuclei are often varied in size with hyperchromatic nuclei, large nucleoli, and numerous mitoses, some of which are located above the basal layer. The basement membrane, at the time of histologic examination, is intact. Most lesions remain as "in situ" carcinomas indefinitely, but an occasional lesion has progressed to invasive basal cell carcinoma or invasive squamous cell carcinoma.

Pigmented epidermal plaque (epidermodysplasia verruciformis) is caused by papillomavirus infection in certain breeds of dogs (miniature schnauzers, pugs, and Shar-Peis) or in other breeds of dogs that are immunosuppressed. Clinical lesions occur most commonly on the ventral abdomen, groin, ventral thorax, or neck, and consist of variably irregular, pigmented macules, or plaques. Histologically the lesions are sharply demarcated, hyperkeratotic foci, or plaques with pigmented, acanthotic epidermis, and large keratohyalin granules. These pigmented epidermal plaques do not regress, are slowly progressive, and occasionally develop into a squamous cell carcinoma.

OTHER VIRUSES

Cutaneous lesions are seen with foot-and-mouth disease (picornavirus), vesicular stomatitis (rhabdovirus), swine vesicular disease (picornavirus), vesicular exanthema (calicivirus), and malignant catarrhal fever (herpesvirus) (see Chapter 7) (Table 17-8). Feline leukemia virus (FeLV) can cause the development of lymphoma and fibrosarcoma. A few cats with FeLV infection have developed dermatitis characterized by epidermal and follicular acanthosis with epidermal giant cells, dyskeratosis, necrosis, and ulceration. In addition, a few FeLV-infected cats have also developed one or more localized areas of marked compact hyperkeratosis of the footpads that clinically resemble "horns" (cutaneous horns). In immunoperoxidase-stained sections, the hyperplastic epidermis in cases with epidermal giant cells is strongly positive for FeLV. Both FeLV and feline immunodeficiency virus (FIV), because of their immunosuppressive capabilities, can cause cats to be susceptible to chronic skin infections, including abscesses, paronychia, and demodicosis.

Feline calicivirus, usually the cause of upper respiratory infection and oral ulcers with high morbidity but low mortality, rarely produces cutaneous ulcers. More recently, virulent systemic strains of feline calicivirus with mortality rates between 30% and 60% have been described. These strains cause alopecia, cutaneous ulcers, and subcutaneous edema. The pathogenesis involves lysis of epithelial cells of the epidermis, follicles, oral mucosa, bronchioles, alveoli, and exocrine pancreas, in addition to lysis of endothelial cells. The lysis of epithelial and endothelial cells leads to necrosis, edema, fibrin exudation, and thrombosis from vascular injury, and release of inflammatory mediators from damaged cells. Clinical lesions include ulcers of the nose, lips, pinnae, feet, and oral mucosa, variable alopecia of limbs and ventrum, and subcutaneous edema, especially of the limbs and face. Systemic signs of fever, anorexia, icterus, red and swollen conjunctival mucosa, and nasal or ocular discharge are present. The most consistent microscopic lesions are epithelial necrosis with subsequent ulceration of the skin and oral and nasal mucosa. Vascular injury consists of edema, microthrombosis, and fibrin exudation. Broncho-interstitial pneumonia and necrosis of the liver, pancreas, spleen, and lymph nodes are present in some cats. In contrast to infection with the more common and less virulent field strains of feline calicivirus, the systemic virulent strains cause more severe disease in adult cats than kittens.

BACTERIAL INFECTIONS

The portals for entry of bacteria into the skin include pores (follicular openings), hematogenous spread, or direct entry through damaged skin. Cutaneous bacterial infections vary in location (e.g., epidermis, dermis, subcutis, adnexa, or systemic), morphology (e.g., pyogenic, granulomatous, or necrotizing), distribution (e.g., focal, multifocal, regional, mucocutaneous, haired skin, or interdigital), and severity (e.g., mild and asymptomatic to severe with systemic signs). The variation is due to the specific organism involved, predisposing or coexisting factors, and host-immune response. The so-called superficial and deep bacterial infections are frequently pus-producing infections (pyogenic) and are thus referred to as pyodermas. In contrast, bacterial granulomas are characterized by an abundance of macrophages and are usually caused by traumatic implantation of bacteria that generally are saprophytes of low virulence. Systemic bacterial infections or localized infection with toxin-producing bacteria are often most severe because of vascular damage or the presence of endotoxins or exotoxins that have systemic consequences. The most common bacterial infections of the skin are listed in Box 17-8.

SUPERFICIAL BACTERIAL INFECTIONS (SUPERFICIAL PYODERMAS)

These infections involve the epidermis and the upper infundibulum of hair follicles, usually heal without scarring, and usually do not involve the regional lymph nodes. Gross lesions include erythema, alopecia, papules, pustules, crusts, and peripheral expanding rings of scale also called "epidermal collarettes" (Table 17-5). The early microscopic feature of superficial bacterial infection that involves the epidermis is intraepidermal pustular dermatitis. The intraepidermal pustules are fragile and can rupture, leading to crust and superficial scale formation. The major microscopic feature of superficial bacterial infection that involves the follicles is superficial suppurative luminal folliculitis. The cellular infiltrate in and around hair follicles plus dermal congestion and edema correspond to the clinically evident papules and follicularly oriented pustules. Follicular injury leads to alopecia. Although gram-positive cocci, such as *Staphylococcus* sp., are usually the cause of the superficial bacterial infections, the bacteria are not

---

Box **17-8**

Cutaneous Bacterial Infections

SUPERFICIAL PYODERMAS

Superficial pustular dermatitis (impetigo)
Superficial spreading pyoderma
Mucocutaneous pyoderma
Dermatophilosis
Exudative epidermitis
Ovine fleece rot
Superficial folliculitis (see staphylococcal folliculitis and furunculosis below)

DEEP PYODERMAS

Staphylococcal folliculitis and furunculosis
Abscesses

BACTERIAL GRANULOMATOUS DERMATITIS

Mycobacterial granulomas
Granulomas caused by nonfilamentous bacteria
 Staphylococcus spp.
 Streptococcus spp.
 Pseudomonas aeruginosa
 Actinobacillus lignieresii
 Proteus spp.
Filamentous bacterial granulomas
 Nocardia spp.
 Actinomyces spp.
 Streptomyces spp.
 Actinomadura spp.

SYSTEMIC OR TOXIC REACTIONS

Erysipelothrix rhusiopathiae
Systemic salmonellosis, pasteurellosis, *Escherichia coli* infection
Canine toxic shock syndrome and necrotizing fasciitis due to streptococcal or staphylococcal infection
Clostridial dermatitis
 Clostridium novyi or *Clostridium chauvoei*
Streptococcus equi

BACTERIAL DIGITAL INFECTIONS OF RUMINANTS

Contagious foot rot
Necrobacillosis of the foot
Papillomatous digital dermatitis

---

always microscopically demonstrable. Predisposing factors, such as allergy, seborrhea, immune deficiency, and other causes of follicular inflammation or dysfunction often play a role.

Superficial pustular dermatitis (impetigo)

This infection is observed in dogs, cats, piglets, cows, does, and ewes and is caused by coagulase-positive

Staphylococcus sp. in association with such predisposing factors as cutaneous abrasions, viral infections, increased moisture, and poor nutrition. *Staphylococcus intermedius* is the most frequent cause of the condition. This organism produces proinflammatory mediators, such as protein A, which binds to the Fc receptor of IgG, leading to the activation of complement and the eventual production of substances chemoattractant for leukocytes initiating a chain of events that mediate inflammation and lead to tissue damage. Older dogs with immunosuppression, usually because of hyperadrenocorticism, may develop a bullous impetigo. In cows, does, and ewes, lesions are predominantly on the udder. In kittens, the dorsum of the neck and shoulders are affected because of overzealous "mouthing" by the queen; *Streptococcus* sp. and *Pasteurella* sp. are the more common bacterial isolates as these are part of the oral flora. Gross lesions consist of pustules that develop into crusts, principally in nonhaired skin (except in kittens). The microscopic lesion is a nonfollicular neutrophilic subcorneal pustule. In bullous impetigo, the lesions are more severe with large interfollicular flaccid pustules that when ruptured lead to more extensive loss of the superficial epidermis. Dermal inflammation in impetigo is minimal.

Superficial spreading pyoderma

Superficial spreading pyoderma is a common, often pruritic, superficial bacterial infection in dogs caused by *Staphylococcus intermedius*. The pathogenesis is poorly understood. Initial studies revealed that dogs with the superficial spreading variety of pyoderma more frequently had IgE antibodies directed against staphylococci than dogs with other forms of staphylococcal pyoderma, suggesting that bacterial hypersensitivity might play a role. In addition or alternatively, proinflammatory mediators, including protein A as described earlier for impetigo, might contribute directly. Clinical lesions are most frequently recognized in the glabrous ventral thoracic and abdominal skin, but can affect the haired skin of the dorsal and lateral trunk as well. Early clinical lesions include erythematous macules, papules, and transient pustules. Older clinical lesions include epidermal collarettes, crusts, alopecia, and hyperpigmentation. Early microscopic lesions are superficial, spongiotic epidermal pustules that rapidly crust and form basophilic debris, often with cocci, on the surface of the epidermis. This basophilic debris can dissect peripherally (laterally) between the epidermis and stratum corneum and is thought to form the rim of scale that clinically represents the epidermal collarette. Occasionally, superficial spreading pyoderma can originate from superficial folliculitis where follicular pustular formation is minor and epidermal collarette formation more prominent. Dermal lesions include superficial

perivascular to interstitial accumulations of neutrophils, eosinophils, and mixed mononuclear cells. Some dogs have neutrophilic vasculitis involving superficial venules possibly due to immune-complex deposition, a feature suggesting a hypersensitivity response to bacterial antigens. Dermal congestion and edema are usually present.

Mucocutaneous pyoderma

Mucocutaneous pyoderma is a putative bacterial infection of mucocutaneous junctional skin in dogs. A variety of breeds are affected, but the German shepherd breed is thought to be predisposed. The pathogenesis is unknown. Lesions consist of erythema, depigmentation, crusting, and in severe cases ulceration. Lesions are most common on mucocutaneous skin of the lips, but mucocutaneous skin of prepuce, vulva, and anus can be affected. Histologic lesions include a dense band of lymphoplasmacytic inflammation at the epidermal dermal junction (lichenoid inflammation), typically without basal cell degeneration. Other features include spongiosis and cellular exocytosis into the epidermis, neutrophilic pustular crusts, and folliculitis of adjacent follicles. Over time pigmentary incontinence develops. Although classic cases are said not to have basal cell degeneration, there is interface inflammation obscuring the epidermal-dermal interface of some cases of mucocutaneous pyoderma, preventing definitive differentiation from discoid lupus erythematosus.

Dermatophilosis (streptothricosis)

This infection, caused by *Dermatophilus congolensis*, is characterized by crusty cutaneous lesions (Fig. 17-48), and occurs in cattle, sheep, and horses more often than dogs, cats, pigs, and goats. The bacterium is transmitted by carrier animals and is more common in tropical and subtropical countries and during wet weather. Lesions tend to develop on the dorsum of the back and distal extremities and after epidermal irritation from ectoparasites, trauma, or prolonged wetting of the skin, hair, or wool, which allows penetration of the damaged epidermis by the *Dermatophilus* "zoospore."

The bacterium grows in the outer root sheath of the hair follicle and superficial epidermis and produces gram-positive filamentous branches that subdivide longitudinally and transversely (Fig. 17-48). These bacteria stimulate an acute inflammatory response in which neutrophils migrate from superficial vessels into the dermis and through the epidermis to form intraepidermal microabscesses. The inflammation inhibits further penetration of the bacterium. However, residual bacterial organisms subsequently invade the newly regenerated epidermis. Thus repeated cycles of bacterial growth, inflammation, and epidermal regeneration result in the formation of the multilaminated pustular crusts.

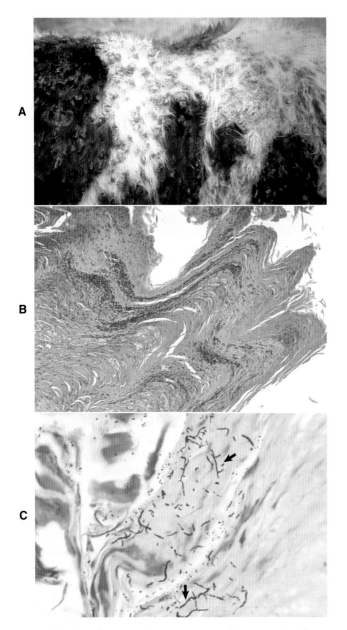

Fig. 17-48 *Dermatophilus congolensis* **infection, skin, haired, cow. A,** The hair is matted by a crust composed of dried exudate, stratum corneum, and bacteria. **B,** Note thick laminated crust formed of alternating layers of hyperkeratotic/parakeratotic cells and degenerate neutrophils. H&E stain. **C,** The stratum corneum contains filamentous bacteria *(arrows)*. These bacteria subdivide longitudinally and transversely and can result in a "railroad track" appearance (not evident here). Brown and Brenn stain. *(A, Courtesy Dr. F. Lozano-Alarcon. B, Courtesy Dr. M.D. McGavin, College of Veterinary Medicine, University of Tennessee. C, Courtesy Dr. Ann M. Hargis, DermatoDiagnostics.)*

Grossly, lesions consist of papules, pustules, and thick crusts that can coalesce and mat the hair or wool (Fig. 17-48). The microscopic lesions consist of hyperplastic superficial perivascular dermatitis with multilaminated crusts of alternating layers of keratin

and neutrophils covering the skin surface. Samples of crusts obtained by biopsy are necessary to identify organisms and make a definitive diagnosis.

Exudative epidermitis of pigs (greasy pig disease)

Exudative epidermitis, caused by *Staphylococcus hyicus (hyos)*, is an acute, often fatal, dermatitis of neonatal piglets but a mild disease in older piglets. Predisposing factors include cutaneous lacerations and poor nutrition. *Staphylococcus hyicus (hyos)* produces an exotoxin, called "exfoliatin," which binds to filaggrin in the keratohyalin granules of the stratum granulosum in the epidermis. This reaction probably causes focal erosion of the stratum corneum. Dermatitis and brownish exudates develop around the eyes, pinnae, snout, chin, and medial legs and spread to the ventral thorax and abdomen, giving the animal an overall "greasy" appearance (Fig. 17-49). The lesions rapidly coalesce and become generalized, resulting in greasy, malodorous exudates covering an erythematous skin. If piglets survive, the exudate hardens, cracks, and forms fissures. Subacute disease develops gradually in older piglets, and lesions are generally localized to the skin of the face, pinnae, and periocular regions. Grossly the epidermis is thickened with scaling. The early histopathologic lesion is subcorneal pustular dermatitis, which extends to the hair follicle, resulting in superficial suppurative folliculitis. In the fully developed lesion, the epidermis is hyperplastic and has thick crusts of keratin, microabscesses, and cocci. The term exudative epidermitis is descriptive of this condition as the inflammatory changes largely involve the epidermis, and there is an accumulation of exudates on the surface. The dermis is congested and edematous. In the early stages, the dermatitis is superficial and perivascular with neutrophils and eosinophils, and in the later stages is perivascular and mononuclear.

Ovine fleece rot

Ovine fleece rot is a superficial bacterial dermatitis usually caused by excessive moisture (usually in the form of rain) that penetrates the fleece (wool), wets the skin, and causes proliferation of *Pseudomonas* spp. Approximately 1 week of continual wetting is usually sufficient to cause marked proliferation of the bacteria on the skin and in the fleece. This is followed by an acute inflammatory response with serum exudation and matting of the fleece. The fleece is also discolored because of production of pigments (chromogens) by the pseudomonas bacteria and has a rotten odor. Microscopic lesions include epidermal pustular dermatitis and superficial folliculitis. Ovine fleece rot is important economically because the malodor attracts flies, predisposing to myiasis (infestation of tissue by

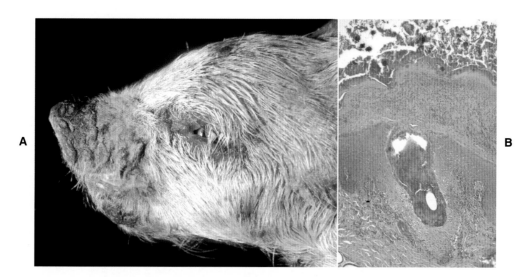

Fig. 17-49   Exudative epidermitis, *Staphylococcus hyicus (hyos)*, skin, piglet. A, Head. Exudative epidermitis is also called greasy pig disease. The skin around the nose and eye in this piglet is lichenified and has fissures. Greasy exudate focally has adhered to the hair and the surface of the skin. **B,** Note the epidermal hyperplasia (acanthosis) and suppurative exudate within the lumen of a hair follicle and on the surface of the epidermis. The exudate has dried to form a crust that is fragmenting superficially. H&E stain. (**A,** *Courtesy Dr. M.D. McGavin, College of Veterinary Medicine, University of Tennessee.* **B,** *Courtesy Dr. Pamela E. Ginn, College of Veterinary Medicine, University of Florida.*)

the larvae of dipterous flies), and the value of the affected wool is reduced.

Superficial bacterial folliculitis

Staphylococcal folliculitis and furunculosis are discussed with deep bacterial infections next.

DEEP BACTERIAL INFECTIONS (DEEP PYODERMAS)

Deep pyodermas are bacterial infections of the hair follicle, dermis, and/or subcutis. They are caused by a variety of bacteria, including *Staphylococcus* sp., *Streptococcus* sp., *Corynebacterium pseudotuberculosis*, *Pasteurella* sp., *Proteus* sp., *Pseudomonas* sp., and *Escherichia coli*. *Staphylococcus intermedius* is the primary pathogen of canine skin. Organisms typically enter the skin via natural pores such as hair follicles or any form of wound, including direct penetration of the skin. Deep bacterial infections of hair follicles often have predisposing causes, such as immune suppression, demodicosis (dogs), or disorders associated with follicular hyperkeratosis (callus or comedo formation), and also originate as a sequela to superficial bacterial folliculitis. Deep bacterial infections are less common than superficial infections and develop most frequently in dogs.

Staphylococcal folliculitis and furunculosis (Table 17-9)

Infection of the hair follicle can be superficial or deep. Superficial infections involve the follicular infundibulum but can spread to involve the deeper portions of the follicle (the infundibulum and below). Mild to moderate folliculitis without furunculosis can resolve completely with appropriate antibiotic therapy. However, untreated or severe folliculitis can progress to involve deeper aspects of the follicle and result in follicular distention with rupture (furunculosis) and release of follicular contents (hair, follicular stratum corneum, bacteria) into the dermis and sometimes subcutis. The bacteria proliferate in the deep dermis and subcutis and can reach draining lymph nodes. Draining tracts often develop as a foreign body response to extruded follicular contents (e.g., hair and follicular stratum corneum). Thus the infection and severe inflammation spread into the surrounding dermis and subcutis, resulting in the need for intensive long-term treatment and increasing the potential for systemic infection and local scarring.

Staphylococcal folliculitis and furunculosis develop most commonly in the dog (Figs. 17-28 and 17-29), frequently affect the horse, goat, sheep, but are uncommon in the cow, cat, and pig. In dogs, lesions are localized or generalized and develop on the dorsal nose, pressure points, interdigital areas, and chin. Other cutaneous areas can also be affected, especially if predisposing conditions (e.g., follicular dysplasia, cornification disorders, or demodicosis) are present. Deep pyoderma of adult German shepherd dogs (German shepherd folliculitis, furunculosis, and cellulitis) is a unique deep pyoderma with an apparent genetic predisposition.

Table 17-9 Bacterial Folliculitis and Furunculosis

Organisms	Predisposing Causes	Portal of Entry	Clinical Lesions	Histologic Lesions	Anatomic Locations	Species
Staphylococcus sp. are most frequently involved Others: Streptococcus sp., Corynebacterium pseudotuberculosis, Pasteurella sp., Proteus sp., Pseudomonas sp., and Escherichia coli	**Superficial folliculitis:** Allergy Seborrhea Parasitic infestations Hormonal factors Local irritants Matted hair coats **Deep folliculitis:** Sequel to superficial bacterial folliculitis Immune suppression Stresses (large animals) Demodicosis (dogs) Follicular hyperkeratosis (callus or comedones) Irritation from tack (horses) Increased environmental temperature and moisture (horse) **Pastern folliculitis (horses):** Excessive moisture, trauma, contact dermatitis, mite infestation	Hair follicle openings	**Superficial folliculitis:** Papules, crusted papules, pustules, epidermal collarettes, and alopecia **Deep folliculitis:** Same as superficial folliculitis plus hemorrhagic bullae, nodules, and draining tracts	**Superficial:** Superficial luminal folliculitis **Deep:** Superficial and deep suppurative luminal folliculitis with follicular distention often in conjunction with furunculosis Pyogranulomatous dermatitis in response to release of follicular contents Tracts that drain to the surface Scarring with loss of adnexa and permanent alopecia localized to affected skin	Dorsal nose, pressure points, interdigital areas, chin, and can be generalized	Dog; common
					Area covered by tack, especially the skin of the saddle area, the tail, or on the caudal aspect of the pastern* or fetlock†	Horse; frequent
					Face, pinnae, distal limbs, and glabrous areas of the udder, ventral abdomen, medial thighs, and perineum	Goat; frequent
					Adult sheep: face, especially around the eyes, ears, base of horns, limbs, or teats Lambs: mild lesions most commonly on the lips and perineum; usually spontaneously regress	Sheep; frequent
					Tail, perineum; less often scrotum and face	Cattle, more in young bulls; uncommon
					Piglets younger than 8 weeks: generalized body hindquarters, abdomen, chest Young growing piglets: facial lesions related to sharp canine teeth	Piglets; uncommon
					Crusted papular eruption indistinguishable from miliary dermatitis; any where, including head and neck	Cat; rare

*Pastern (proximal interphalangeal articulation).
†Fetlock (metacarpophalangeal articulation).

Lesions are located on the dorsal lumbosacral, ventral abdominal, and thigh areas. Hypersensitivity to the bites of fleas or alterations in immune or neutrophil function have been proposed as predisposing causes, but most of these potential causes have been discounted. Deep folliculitis and furunculosis, especially on the cheek area or neck of some large-breed dogs (golden and Labrador retriever, Saint Bernard, and Newfoundland), can clinically resemble superficial pyotraumatic dermatitis (acute moist dermatitis), belying the deep nature of the lesions.

In horses, lesions develop most commonly in association with tack, especially on the skin of the saddle area, the tail, or the caudal aspect of the pastern (proximal interphalangeal articulation) or fetlock (metacarpophalangeal articulation). When the skin of the pastern or fetlock is involved, the condition is called equine pastern folliculitis (a.k.a. grease heel, scratches). Equine pastern folliculitis is a complex disorder in which secondary staphylococcal folliculitis plays a role. Predisposing factors are numerous and include excessive moisture, trauma, and contact dermatitis. Also, many other conditions affect the pastern skin in horses, including immune-mediated diseases (pemphigus foliaceus, vasculitis, photosensitization), other infections (dermatophilosis, dermatophytosis), and mite infestation (*Chorioptes* sp.), necessitating an early thorough clinical evaluation and sometimes microbiologic or histopathologic evaluation to differentiate staphylococcal folliculitis of the skin of the pastern from these other disease processes. In severe chronic lesions, initiating causes may no longer be identifiable.

In goats, the face, pinnae, distal limbs, and glabrous areas of the udder, ventral abdomen, medial thighs, and perineum are most commonly affected. In adult sheep, lesions develop on the face, especially around the eyes, or on the limbs or teats. In otherwise healthy lambs, mild lesions develop most commonly on the lips and perineum, and usually spontaneously regress.

Grossly the lesions of superficial folliculitis include papules, crusted papules, pustules, epidermal collarettes, and alopecia. Deep folliculitis can have similar lesions plus hemorrhagic bullae, nodules, and draining tracts. The microscopic patterns include superficial or deep luminal folliculitis, pyogranulomatous furunculosis, draining sinuses, and occasionally, panniculitis. Microscopic lesions include suppurative luminal folliculitis with follicular distention often in conjunction with furunculosis. Pyogranulomatous dermatitis in response to release of follicular contents is often severe, may efface the dermal architecture, extend into the deep dermis and panniculus, and form tracts that drain to the surface. Scarring can lead to loss of adnexal structures and permanent alopecia localized to affected skin.

Subcutaneous abscesses

Subcutaneous abscesses are localized collections of purulent exudate located within the dermis and subcutis. Abscesses are common in cats because of the frequency of bacterial contamination of puncture wounds. Abscesses also are common in large animals. In addition to puncture wounds, other predisposing causes include foreign bodies, injections, and shearing and clipping wounds. Granulation tissue or mature fibrous connective tissue borders the exudate. Subcutaneous abscesses frequently rupture and drain spontaneously, and heal by scarring. A wide variety of bacteria can cause subcutaneous abscesses. Commonly isolated bacteria include *Pasteurella multocida* (dog and cat bite wounds), *Corynebacterium pseudotuberculosis* (horses, sheep, and goats), and *Arcanobacterium pyogenes* (sheep, goats, cattle, pigs). Other frequently isolated bacteria include β-hemolytic streptococci, *Fusobacterium* sp., *Peptostreptococcus* sp., *Bacteroides* sp., *Staphylococcus* sp., and *Clostridium* sp.

BACTERIAL GRANULOMATOUS DERMATITIS (BACTERIAL GRANULOMAS)

Bacterial granulomatous dermatitis is usually caused by traumatic implantation of bacteria, which are generally saprophytes of low virulence. Causative organisms usually stimulate a strong cell mediated-immune response by persisting as an antigen in the tissue. Grossly, lesions are slowly progressive, nodular or diffuse, and can ulcerate and drain through the surface of the skin via fistulas. Microscopic lesions consist of mixed populations of inflammatory cells, especially macrophages, thus lesions are granulomatous to pyogranulomatous. Multinucleated giant cells and caseous necrosis are present in some lesions. Causal agents can be present in macrophages, exudate, or in clear spaces or fat vacuoles within tissue but are often in such low numbers that they are difficult to identify in histologic sections.

Mycobacterial granulomas

Mycobacterial organisms produce granulomatous to pyogranulomatous dermatitis and panniculitis in many species of animals, particularly cats and less frequently dogs and cattle. The majority of mycobacteria are intracellular pathogens that are able to persist in tissue by entering macrophages. Many are able to survive and replicate within the macrophages by inhibiting fusion with lysosomes. Tissue destruction results from persistence of antigen in the tissue and a cell-mediated inflammatory response. Infection occurs with obligate pathogens that require a vertebrate host to multiply and saprophytes in the environment that occasionally cause opportunistic infections. Infection occurs with the tuberculosis group considered to be obligate pathogens (*Mycobacterium tuberculosis, Mycobacterium bovis*), the leprosy group considered to be obligate pathogens (*Mycobacterium lepraemurium*), and the opportunistic group considered to be saprophytes or facultative pathogens (subdivided based on growth rate and pigment production). Rapid-growing opportunistic organisms (*Mycobacterium fortuitum, Mycobacterium smegmatis, Mycobacterium chelonae, Mycobacterium abscessus,* and *Mycobacterium thermoresistible*) and slow-growing opportunistic organisms (*Mycobacterium avium-intracellulare* complex, *Mycobacterium kansasii, Mycobacterium ulcerans*) are inhabitants of soil, water, and decomposing vegetation, and infection tends to occur via wound contamination or traumatic implantation. To avoid confusion in terminology, by convention, infections caused by *Mycobacterium tuberculosis* and *Mycobacterium bovis* are referred to as "tuberculosis." In contrast, infections caused by other mycobacterial agents are referred to as "mycobacteriosis," which is sometimes further defined by the group of agents involved (e.g., atypical, opportunistic, or avian).

Mycobacterial infection is more common with the rapidly growing opportunistic mycobacteria (also called atypical mycobacteria), and infections are more common in cats, in which lesions are characterized by recurrent nodules, with draining sinuses frequently located in the dermis and subcutis of the inguinal area. The microscopic lesions are characterized by pyogranulomatous inflammation. Organisms are more often found extracellularly in clear spaces sometimes lined by neutrophils (Fig. 17-50). Infections with the slow-growing, opportunistic mycobacteria are more commonly disseminated (not limited to the skin) and resemble those caused by *Mycobacterium tuberculosis.*

In cattle, cutaneous infections with opportunistic mycobacterial organisms, historically called "skin tuberculosis," occur as single or multiple nodules 1 to 8 cm in diameter in the dermis and subcutis, particularly of the lower legs. But lesions can spread to the thighs, forearms, shoulder, and abdomen through skin lymphatics. The skin of the udder is sometimes involved. The lymph nodes are unaffected. The causative organisms are thought to be saprophytic atypical mycobacteria that probably enter through cutaneous abrasions. In most of these infections, the specific mycobacteria have not been identified by culture, but *Mycobacterium kansasii* has been identified in a few cases. A more appropriate name for this condition is bovine cutaneous opportunistic mycobacteriosis. Clinical lesions are either firm or fluctuant nodules connected by thin cords of tissue that represent inflamed lymphatic channels (lymphangitis). The firm nodules consist of pyogranulomatous inflammation with fibrosis and sometimes mineralization. The fluctuant nodules are thick-walled abscesses that can ulcerate, rupture, and drain thick, tan exudate. Small lesions can spontaneously resolve, but larger lesions are persistent. This disease became apparent during the time of intense tuberculosis eradication efforts because infection with these opportunistic mycobacterial

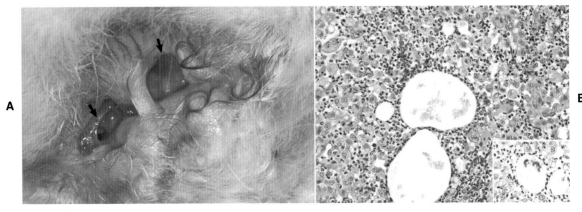

Fig. 17-50 **Atypical mycobacteriosis (opportunistic mycobacterial infection), rapidly growing *Mycobacterium* sp., pyogranulomatous panniculitis, skin, abdomen, cat. A,** Note the draining sinuses (*arrows*) that overlie areas of nodular pyogranulomatous inflammation in the dermis and panniculus. **B,** Note pyogranulomatous inflammation (neutrophils and macrophages) surrounding a vacuole containing bacteria. In atypical *Mycobacterium* sp. infections of this type, the mycobacterial organisms are extracellular. H&E stain. *Inset:* Pyogranulomatous inflammation with a vacuole containing acid-fast bacilli. Fite's method for acid-fast organisms. (**A,** *Courtesy Dr. David Duclos, Animal Skin and Allergy Clinic.* **B** and **Inset,** *Courtesy Dr. Pamela E. Ginn, College of Veterinary Medicine, University of Florida.*)

organisms can cause false-positive reactions to bovine tuberculin tests. Bovine cutaneous opportunistic mycobacteriosis is much less commonly identified in current times, partly because the prevalence of and thus testing for bovine tuberculosis has been reduced.

Feline leprosy, caused by *Mycobacterium lepraemurium* and probably other mycobacterial organisms (see later discussion) develops in cats living in cold, wet areas of the world, including the northwestern United States and Canada. Mode of transmission is not known, but bites of cats or rodents, soil contamination of cutaneous wounds, or possible transmission via biting insect vectors may be involved. *Mycobacterium lepraemurium* does not grow in culture using standard techniques but has been identified by polymerase chain reaction (PCR) with DNA sequencing. These molecular techniques have resulted in the identification of other, potentially causative, mycobacterial agents (i.e., *Mycobacterium visibilis* [*Mycobacterium visibile*]) in cutaneous lesions clinically consistent with feline leprosy. Lesions develop most commonly on the head, neck, and limbs but can occur anywhere (Fig. 17-51). Histologically, two distinct morphologic patterns of inflammation are present. In one, there is diffuse granulomatous inflammation without necrosis and with large numbers of intracellular acid-fast bacilli. In the other pattern, there are granulomas with central necrosis surrounded by a zone of lymphocytes. Few to moderate numbers of acid-fast bacilli are generally limited to the areas of necrosis.

Rarely a nodular granulomatous dermatitis due to acid-fast bacilli develops on the head, dorsal pinnae, or other distal extremities in dogs, often with short-hair coats (canine leproid granuloma syndrome). Saprophytic mycobacterial organisms transmitted via the bites of flies are thought to be the cause of the syndrome. The dogs are healthy otherwise, and cultures are negative.

Cutaneous infections caused by *Mycobacterium tuberculosis* and *Mycobacterium bovis* are rare; alimentary and pulmonary infections are more common, but skin infections can develop alone or in combination with disseminated infection. Tentative diagnosis of mycobacterial infections is made by considering the animal species affected, clinical lesion appearance and location, and cytologic or histopathologic detection of acid-fast bacilli. In the past, culture was required for definitive identification of the organism involved. The acid-fast bacilli can be rare in tissue sections, especially with the saprophytic opportunistic agents, and some organisms, such as those in feline leprosy and canine leproid granuloma syndrome are exceedingly difficult to grow on culture media; thus diagnosis is challenging. Fortunately the need for cultural identification is being reduced by use of immunohistochemistry and PCR techniques that can identify the organisms or their genetic material in tissue and can be completed within a few days.

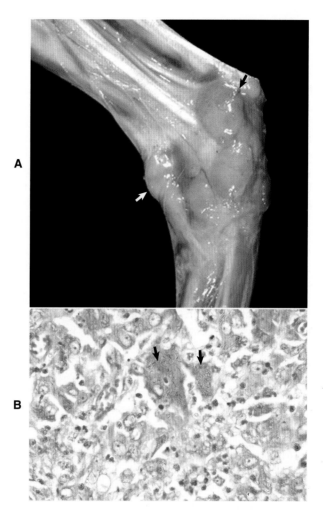

Fig. 17-51   **Feline leprosy syndrome, *Mycobacterium lepraemurium* (and sometimes other *Mycobacterium* sp.), nodular granulomatous panniculitis, subcutis, cat. A,** Leg. Note multiple grouped nodules *(arrows)* consisting of granulomatous inflammation. In feline leprosy, slowly growing nodules are present in the skin or subcutis, especially of the face, forelegs, or trunk. **B,** Macrophages contain numerous mycobacteria *(arrows)*. Ziehl-Neelsen stain. (**A,** *Courtesy Dr. Charles Leathers, Washington State University.* **B,** *Courtesy Dr. Ann M. Hargis, DermatoDiagnostics, Edmonds, Washington.*)

The use of genetic techniques is enhancing studies of mycobacterial diseases in human beings and animals. For example, within the genus *Mycobacterium*, 42 new species have been detected since 1990. It is likely that taxonomy of mycobacterial diseases will be refined based on the use of the genetic techniques.

Bacterial granulomatous dermatitis caused by other bacteria

Botryomycosis is a term for a granulomatous dermatitis caused by nonfilamentous bacteria, typically *Staphylococcus* spp., *Streptococcus* spp., *Pseudomonas aeruginosa, Actinobacillus lignieresii,* and *Proteus* spp. In botryomycosis, these bacteria form small yellow "sulfur" granules, which consist of centrally located bacterial colonies surrounded by radiating club-shaped bodies of homogeneous eosinophilic material termed Splendore-Hoeppli material. This material is considered to be antigen-antibody complexes. Clinically the lesions are progressive nodular masses located in cutaneous or subcutaneous areas and that are composed of granulomatous inflammation with the embedded bacterial colonies bordered by the Splendore-Hoeppli material. Histologic differential diagnoses of botryomycosis include infections with filamentous bacteria that cause similar nodular masses (actinomycotic mycetomas) and nodular masses caused by fungi (eumycotic mycetomas).

Filamentous bacteria also cause bacterial granulomatous dermatitis with granules bordered by Splendore-Hoeppli material and are differentiated from botryomycosis by gram staining and culture. The bacteria are introduced through traumatic injury; are gram-positive, filamentous, and branching; and include various species of *Nocardia* and *Actinomyces*. Other actinomycetes (e.g., *Actinomadura, Streptomyces*) can also contribute. The granules contain mycelial filaments that are 1 μm or less in diameter. *Nocardia* spp. have a limited tendency to clump together; thus they typically do not form granules. The clinical lesions are progressive nodular cutaneous and subcutaneous masses, often with draining sinuses, which can extend into and involve underlying bone. These nodular masses are called "actinomycotic mycetomas." Histologic lesions are nodular areas of granulomatous inflammation with abundant fibrosis and embedded bacterial colonies bordered by Splendore-Hoeppli material. Histologic differential diagnoses include botryomycosis and mycetomas caused by fungi (see Subcutaneous Mycoses, Eumycotic Mycetomas). A classic example of actinomycotic mycetoma in cattle is the so-called "lumpy jaw" wherein the infection begins via traumatic implantation of *Actinomyces bovis* into the mandibular mucosa (rather than skin), which progresses to involve mandibular bone (see Chapter 16).

DERMAL LESIONS SECONDARY TO SYSTEMIC BACTERIAL INFECTIONS OR INFECTION WITH TOXIN PRODUCING BACTERIA

Systemic bacterial infections can cause skin lesions in animals by bacterial embolization to the skin during sepsis, toxin production, direct infection of vascular endothelial cells, or precipitation of immune-complex disease. In some infections, more than one mechanism is involved. Lesions often reflect vascular damage, specifically vasculitis and thrombosis.

Cutaneous lesions caused by *Erysipelothrix rhusiopathiae* (erysipelas) in pigs are a result of bacterial embolization to the skin during sepsis. Lesions consist

of square to rhomboidal, firm, raised, pink to dark purple areas (Fig. 17-52) and are caused by vasculitis, thrombosis, and ischemia (infarction). The rhomboidal shape likely represents the area of skin supplied by the thrombosed vessel.

Septicemic salmonellosis causes cyanosis of the external ears and abdomen because of capillary dilation,

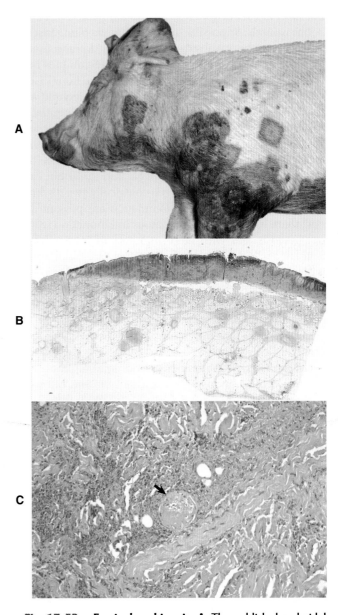

Fig. 17-52   Erysipelas, skin, pig. A, The reddish rhomboidal lesions in the skin are infarcts secondary to thrombosis, from the embolization of septic emboli. **B,** The epidermis and dermis are necrotic from infarction. The only normal dermis and epidermis are at the extreme left. H&E stain. **C,** Note the thrombosis of the vessel *(arrow)*. H&E stain. *(A and B, Courtesy Dr. M.D. McGavin, College of Veterinary Medicine, University of Tennessee. C, Courtesy Dr. Pamela E. Ginn, College of Veterinary Medicine, University of Florida.)*

congestion, and thrombosis. The thrombosis leads to necrosis of distal extremities. The mechanism of vascular damage involves endotoxin-induced venous thrombosis. Systemic infection with *Pasteurella multocida* can cause similar lesions in pigs. *Escherichia coli* production of Shiga-like toxin-II causes edema disease of pigs. The Shiga-like toxin damages the endothelium and tunica media of small arteries and arterioles throughout the body, causing vascular degeneration, necrosis, and edema. Gross lesions of the skin in edema disease consist of accumulation of clear fluid (edema) in the subcutis of the snout, eyelids, submandibular area, ventral abdomen, and inguinal areas. Histologically the subcutis is edematous and sometimes, edema, hemorrhage, smooth muscle necrosis, and hyaline degeneration of the tunica media of vessels may be evident in the skin and other areas of the body.

Recently, conditions that resemble toxic shock syndrome in human beings have been described in dogs. *Streptococcus canis* has been documented as the cause in most dogs; however, other bacteria, especially *Staphylococcus intermedius*, that produce exotoxins—including toxic shock syndrome toxin-1—could potentially play a role. The site of infection can be the skin, as seen with necrotizing fasciitis (inflammation of the subcutaneous fat and fascial planes); however, the primary site of infection in some dogs has been the lung or urinary tract. Initial clinical signs in dogs with necrotizing fasciitis include rapid onset of extreme pain associated with a relatively minor wound or blunt injury to skin. The bacteria are thought to enter through a minor cutaneous wound anywhere on the body and produce exotoxins leading to severe tissue damage initially in the region of the skin injury. However, the portal of entry or initial wound in some cases of necrotizing fasciitis may not be apparent. Clinically, lesions of necrotizing fasciitis are painful, hot, and swollen. The subcutaneous fat, fascia, and overlying skin can become necrotic and can slough. The swelling is due to necrosis of fat and exudate accumulating between the fascial planes (fasciitis and/or cellulitis). Histologic lesions include edema, hemorrhage, necrosis, suppurative inflammation, and thrombosis. Occasionally, vasculitis and colonies of cocci are seen. The condition can rapidly lead to sepsis, multiorgan failure, and death if not treated early and aggressively. In dogs with toxic shock-like syndrome, but without necrotizing fasciitis, clinical skin lesions include multicentric to generalized cutaneous erythema. Some dogs also have edema and vesicles or pustules that progress to ulcers. The ears, extremities, and ventrum are frequently affected, and dogs can be depressed and have fever, anemia, thrombocytopenia, and neutrophilia. Histologically, these dogs have superficial dermatitis with apoptotic keratinocytes bordered by neutrophils. The lesions can progress to full-thickness necrosis and ulceration of the epidermis. As in necrotizing fasciitis, lesions can be fatal without early therapy with appropriate antibiotics. The cause of the skin lesions in the dogs with toxic shock–like syndrome, but without necrotizing fasciitis, has not been determined. In human beings, the pathogenesis of the skin lesion is thought to be a result of nonspecific stimulation of lymphocytes by exotoxins with superantigen activity and the release of cytokines, including TNF-α.

Bacterial infections can also develop from direct extension of bacterial infections of deeper tissue, such as clostridial myositis and cellulitis. *Clostridium novyi* can cause severe cellulitis, toxemia, and death in young rams whose heads have been traumatized by butting during the breeding season. Spores in the soil gain entrance through cutaneous lacerations at the base of the horns, germinate, produce toxins, and result in cellulitis and toxemia. Swelling of the head and neck result in the common term "big head" or "swelled head." *Clostridium chauvoei* is a secondary invader of wounds, where spores can germinate, proliferate, and produce necrotizing and hemolytic exotoxins leading to extensive necrosis of the skin and underlying tissue (gas gangrene).

Rocky Mountain spotted fever, the most important rickettsial disease associated with cutaneous lesions, is caused by *Rickettsia rickettsii*, an organism that infects endothelial cells. This organism is transmitted by ticks, mainly *Dermacentor andersoni* and *Dermacentor variabilis*. The disease is seasonal, corresponding with the increased activity of ticks and contact with ticks. In addition to systemic signs, affected dogs have cutaneous, ocular, genital, and oral erythema with petechiae, edema, necrosis, and ulceration as a result of the direct endothelial cell damage and vasculitis caused by the rickettsia.

In horses, purpura that develops occasionally as a sequela to *Streptococcus equi* are caused by immune-complex vasculitis. Clinically, horses have petechial hemorrhages of the skin and mucous membranes and edema with serum exudation of distal extremities. Microscopic lesions consist of vascular wall disruption by neutrophils (neutrophilic vasculitis), perivascular edema, hemorrhage, and fibrin exudation.

DIGITAL INFECTIONS OF RUMINANTS (BACTERIAL PODODERMATITIS)

Infections of the digits of cattle and sheep are usually mixed bacterial infections sometimes separated into two basic groups, "contagious foot rot" and "necrobacillosis of the foot," based on the contagious nature of the infection and the type of bacteria principally responsible for infection (Table 17-10). Contagious foot rot is caused principally by *Dichelobacter nodosus* (formerly *Bacteroides nodosus*) acting synergistically with *Fusobacterium necrophorum* and other bacteria. Necrobacillosis of the foot is caused principally by *Fusobacterium necrophorum* and other bacteria, including *Bacteroides melaninogenicus* in cattle.

Contagious foot rot

Contagious foot rot in sheep develops when predisposing factors, such as moisture and trauma, damage the interdigital epidermis and allow colonization by a variety of microorganisms, including *Fusobacterium necrophorum* from skin or feces. If the sheep harbors the obligate anaerobic bacteria, *Dichelobacter nodosus* in interdigital skin, foot rot will develop. Contagious foot rot is a synergistic bacterial infection principally involving *Dichelobacter nodosus* (elaborates proteases and growth-enhancing factors, which aid bacterial penetration of the epidermis and bacterial growth) and *Fusobacterium necrophorum* (responsible for most of the necrosis and inflammation). Contagious foot rot in

sheep occurs in virulent and benign forms. The virulent form is due to more virulent *Dichelobacter nodosus* that produces significantly more proteolytic enzymes (proteases including elastase), allowing more bacterial penetration of the epidermis. The proteases in the virulent form also tend to be more heat stable. Virulent foot rot is more persistent (can last for more than 1 year if not treated), affects a high percentage of sheep, affects more than one foot, and can result in death of sheep due to emaciation as a result of severe pain and reluctance to graze. Early lesions of virulent foot rot begin in the interdigital axial (inner) bulbar notch, affect both digits, and consist of red, moist, and swollen eroded skin. The infection spreads around the bulb of the heel to the epidermal matrix of the hoof and results in a malodorous exudate that separates the horn from the interdigital skin. Lesions progress to the bulb and

Table **17-10**   **Digital Infections of Ruminants**

Species	Disorder	Predisposing Factors	Bacteria Involved	Severity	Contagious
Sheep	Contagious foot rot, virulent form	Moisture and trauma	*Dichelobacter nodosus* plus *Fusobacterium necrophorum* and other bacteria	Severe; virulent strains of *Dichelobacter nodosus* produce more proteolytic enzymes	Yes
Sheep	Contagious foot rot, benign form (foot scald)	Moisture and trauma	*Dichelobacter nodosus* *Fusobacterium necrophorum*	Mild; less virulent strains of *Dichelobacter nodosus* produce fewer proteolytic enzymes and are less pathogenic	Yes
Sheep	Necrobacillosis of the foot I. Ovine interdigital dermatitis		*Fusobacterium necrophorum* Other bacteria, but no *Dichelobacter nodosus*	Clinically similar to benign foot rot	No
	II. Foot abscesses A. Heel abscesses (infective bulbar necrosis) B. Toe abscesses (lamellar abscesses)	Wet seasons Heavy adult sheep	*Fusobacterium necrophorum* *Arcanobacterium pyogenes*	Can cause severe lameness with permanent foot deformity	No
Cattle	Foot rot	Trauma and moisture	*Dichelobacter nodosus* *Fusobacterium necrophorum* Other bacteria	Mild; similar to benign foot rot in sheep	Yes
Cattle	Necrobacillosis of the foot (foul-in the-foot)	Trauma	*Fusobacterium necrophorum* *Bacteroides melaninogenicus*	Can be severe with cellulitis involving tendons, joints, and bone	No
Cattle	Papillomatous digital dermatitis (foot warts; hairy heel warts)	Prolonged wet conditions	Probably *Treponema* sp. spirochete	Moderate to severe lameness	Yes

sole, and finally to the axial and abaxial (outer) surfaces of the hoof wall. The germinal epithelium is not destroyed and regeneration is attempted, but the new horn is destroyed. In chronic infections, hooves can become long and misshapen. Benign foot rot (foot scald) is mild, confined to interdigital skin, and can have slight separation of the horn of the heel; also the hoof can overgrow. Foot rot in cattle is similar to benign foot rot in sheep.

Necrobacillosis

Necrobacillosis of the foot in sheep includes ovine interdigital dermatitis and foot abscesses. Ovine interdigital dermatitis is an acute necrotizing dermatitis that clinically is similar to benign foot rot. Ovine interdigital dermatitis is differentiated from foot rot by the failure to demonstrate *Dichelobacter nodosus* in smears or cultures of exudate. Foot abscesses include heel abscesses (infective bulbar necrosis) and toe abscesses (lamellar abscesses). Foot abscesses are more common in wet seasons and in heavy adult sheep. In addition to *Fusobacterium necrophorum*, *Arcanobacterium pyogenes* (*Actinomyces pyogenes*) may be isolated from the lesions.

Necrobacillosis (foul-in-the-foot) of cattle occurs secondary to trauma to the interdigital skin and is caused by *Fusobacterium necrophorum* and *Bacteroides melaninogenicus*. There is lameness with an interdigital dermatitis and cellulitis with fissures and necrosis that may extend into the deeper structures of the foot, such as the distal phalanx, distal sesamoid bone, distal interphalangeal joint, and tendons.

Papillomatous digital dermatitis

Papillomatous digital dermatitis, also known as foot warts or hairy heel warts, is a painful, contagious dermatitis of the feet of cattle (Table 17-10). It occurs worldwide. The cause of papillomatous digital dermatitis is unknown, but spirochetes belonging to the genus *Treponema*, structurally similar to *Borrelia burgdorferi*, are suspected. The condition is also usually associated with management conditions in which the feet of cattle remain wet for prolonged periods. The pathogenesis of lesion formation is not yet known. Papillomatous digital dermatitis most commonly affects the skin proximal and adjacent to the interdigital space at the caudal (plantar) aspect of the hind feet. Early gross lesions are well-circumscribed, round-to-oval, red plaques up to 6 cm in diameter with a moist granular surface prone to bleeding and with a very strong, pungent odor. Lesions are partially to completely alopecic and can be bordered by hypertrophied hairs two to three times longer than normal. Microscopically, this corresponds to areas of mild epidermal hyperplasia with foci of erosion, necrosis, ballooning degeneration, and microabscesses. The dermis contains minimal perivascular inflammation.

Mixed bacteria can be present in the outer necrotic debris, but only spirochetes are present in the deeper viable epidermis. The lesions become progressively more proliferative and less painful with time. Mature lesions are irregular wartlike growths or filamentous papillae that measure 0.5 to 1.0 mm in diameter and 1 mm to 3 cm in length and are pale yellow, gray, or brown. Histologically the older lesions are composed of frondlike projections or plaques of markedly hyperplastic epidermis with parakeratosis and hyperkeratosis. Foci of necrosis and hemorrhage, ballooning degeneration, and aggregates of neutrophils are scattered throughout the hyperplastic epidermis (Fig. 17-53). At this later stage, inflammation is more intense in the dermis and plasma cells can be numerous. Lesions are painful, forcing the animal to shift its weight to the toe of the affected foot, which results in a smooth contour to the toe (clubbing) and atrophy of the bulbs of the heels.

Papillomatous digital dermatitis is economically important because it frequently causes moderate to severe lameness that results in weight loss, decreased milk production, and poor reproductive performance. The vast majority of cases are in dairy cows, but the infection has also been reported in beef cattle. Although the disease occurs in cattle of all ages, the highest incidence appears to be in replacement dairy heifers.

FUNGAL (MYCOTIC) INFECTIONS

Mycotic infections have been classified into four basic categories: superficial, cutaneous, subcutaneous, and systemic (Box 17-9). Ability to mount an inflammatory response is paramount to clearing the infection. Mycotic infections tend to occur more often in animals with compromised resistance because of debilitating systemic diseases—such as diabetes mellitus or neoplasia—or in animals treated with glucocorticoids or other immunosuppressive agents or with long-term, broad-spectrum antibiotics.

SUPERFICIAL MYCOSES

Superficial mycoses are infections restricted to the stratum corneum or hair with minimal or no dermal reaction. Piedra is a rare superficial mycosis caused by *Trichosporon beigelii* and has been reported in horses and dogs. Lesions consist of minute swellings restricted to the extrafollicular portion of the hair shaft.

CUTANEOUS MYCOSES

Cutaneous mycoses (also included as superficial mycoses by some authors) are infections of keratinized tissue, including hair, claws, and epidermis. The fungi are usually restricted to the cornified layers and only very rarely are found in the dermis or subcutis, but tissue destruction and host response can be extensive.

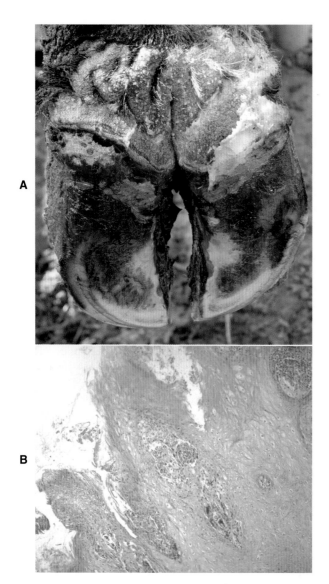

Fig. 17-53 **Papillomatous digital dermatitis, skin, cow.** **A,** Note the moist, irregular, and reddened alopecic areas on the bulbs of the heel. The lesions are of several weeks to a few months duration. **B,** Note the papillated epidermal hyperplasia (see also Fig. 17-12). The epidermis is thickened by hyperkeratosis and acanthosis. Most of the acanthotic cells have ballooning degeneration. The hyperplastic epidermis covers dermal papillae, which contain hyperemic vessels and foci of mixed inflammatory cells. H&E stain. (**A,** *Courtesy Dr. Jan Shearer, College of Veterinary Medicine, University of Florida.* **B,** *Courtesy Dr. Pamela E. Ginn, College of Veterinary Medicine, University of Florida.*)

Infections in animals include dermatophytosis, cutaneous candidiasis, and *Malassezia* dermatitis.

Dermatophytoses

Dermatophytoses are fungal infections of the skin, hair, and claws of animals caused by taxonomically

---

Box **17-9**

Cutaneous Fungal Infections

SUPERFICIAL (LIMITED TO HAIR OR STRATUM CORNEUM)

Piedra
  Trichosporon beigelii

CUTANEOUS (LIMITED TO HAIR, STRATUM CORNEUM, CLAWS)

Dermatophytes
  Microsporum canis
  Microsporum gypseum
  Trichophyton mentagrophytes
Candida spp.
Malassezia spp.

SUBCUTANEOUS (USUALLY LIMITED TO CUTANEOUS AND SUBCUTANEOUS TISSUE, SOMETIMES LYMPHATICS)

Eumycotic mycetoma
  Curvularia geniculata
  Madurella spp.
  Acremonium spp.
  Pseudoallescheria spp.
  Phaeococcus spp.
Dermatophyte pseudomycetoma
Phaeohyphomycosis
Hyalohyphomycosis
Sporotrichosis
Entomophthoromycosis (zygomycosis)
Oomycosis (pythiosis and lagenidiosis)

SYSTEMIC (USUALLY PULMONARY PORTAL OF ENTRY, BUT CAN AFFECT DERMIS AND SUBCUTIS)

Blastomycosis
Coccidioidomycosis
Cryptococcosis
Histoplasmosis

related fungi known as dermatophytes. Pathogenic genera include *Epidermophyton*, *Microsporum*, and *Trichophyton*. Dermatophytosis occurs worldwide, is the most important cutaneous (superficial) mycosis, and is common in human beings and animals, especially cats. Superficial and cutaneous mycoses (dermatophytosis) are acquired by contact with infected animals or by contact with scales shed from infected animals. Dermatophytes are able to colonize the cornified structures (hair, claws) and the stratum corneum and cause disease without ever entering living tissue. Clinical disease in a dermatophyte infection is the result of the host's reaction to the organism and its by-products. Dermatophytes are more contagious than other fungal infections, are more common in hot, humid environments, and young animals are more susceptible than adults. Animals kept in overcrowded, dirty, or damp areas and those with inadequate nutrition are also more susceptible. Species that more commonly infect domestic animals are included in the genera *Microsporum* and *Trichophyton*. *Epidermophyton* is adapted to human beings (anthropophilic) and rarely infects animals. Zoophilic dermatophytes (e.g., *Microsporum canis*) are primary animal pathogens but can infect human beings. *Microsporum canis* is so well adapted, especially in long-haired, purebred cats that inapparent infections occur. Geophilic dermatophytes (e.g., *Microsporum gypseum*) occur in soil as saprophytes, but under favorable conditions can infect human beings and animals if the integrity of the skin is broken or the host immune system is compromised.

Dermatophytes invade cornified tissues (stratum corneum, hair shafts, and claws) by producing proteolytic enzymes, which help them penetrate the surface lipid coat. The fungal hyphae invade the cornified tissue, and the hyphae break into chains of arthrospores. The products elaborated by the dermatophytes cause dermal irritation and damage to the epidermis. The fungal products and cytokines released from damaged keratinocytes result in epidermal hyperplasia (hyperkeratosis, parakeratosis, acanthosis) and dermal inflammation. Inflammatory cells arrive via the superficial vessels (superficial perivascular dermatitis) and, subsequently, migrate through the epidermal layers (exocytosis) to the invaded keratinized layers, forming intracorneal microabscesses. Exocytosis of inflammatory cells into follicular walls and lumens results in mural and luminal folliculitis and, if the follicular wall is destroyed, in furunculosis. Bacterial infection increases the severity of the folliculitis and furunculosis. Gross and microscopic lesions are highly variable and range from an asymptomatic infection to an eruptive nodular mass (kerion), to deep granulomatous nodular dermal and pannicular masses containing distorted fungal hyphae (pseudomycetoma), to discolored, malformed, friable, broken, or sloughed claws (onychomycosis).

Gross lesions in haired skin are often circular or irregularly shaped, scaly to crusty patches of alopecia (Fig. 17-54), which can coalesce to involve large portions of the body. Fungi tend to die in areas of inflammation in the center of lesions but are viable at the periphery, thus giving rise to the peripheral red ring and the term "ringworm." Hair loss is due to breakage of hair shafts and loss of hair shafts from inflamed follicles. Follicular papules and pustules can be present. In animals with severe furunculosis, the inflammation can extend into the deep dermis and subcutis leading to draining tracts. Microscopic patterns include perifolliculitis, luminal folliculitis, or furunculosis, and epidermal hyperplasia with intracorneal microabscesses.

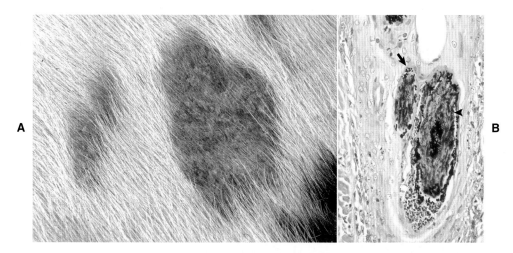

Fig. 17-54 **Dermatophytosis, luminal folliculitis, skin, haired. A,** Dermatophytosis, presumed to be *Trichophyton verrucosum*, cow. Note irregularly ovoid, hairless areas with mild surface crusting. **B,** Dermatophyte infection presumed to be *Microsporum canis* involving hair follicle, dog. Note spores (*arrow*) along periphery and hyphae (*arrowhead*) within hair shaft. The hair loss is due to breakage of hair shafts and mural and luminal folliculitis, which interfere with production of new hairs and cause increased loss of old hairs. Gomori's methenamine silver nitrate-H&E counter stain. (*A, Courtesy Dr. H. Denny Liggitt, University of Washington. B, Courtesy Dr. Ann M. Hargis, DermatoDiagnostics.*)

In many lesions, septate hyphae or spores are present in hair shafts and in the stratum corneum of the epidermis or follicles (Fig. 17-54, *B*).

Candidiasis

Candidiasis is a yeast infection caused by *Candida* sp., normal inhabitants of the skin and gastrointestinal tract. Infection occurs when host resistance is compromised. Infections with *Candida* sp. are rare in domestic animals and usually occur on mucous membranes and at mucocutaneous junctions. Gross lesions consist of exudative and pustular to ulcerative inflammation of the lips (cheilitis), oral mucosa (stomatitis), and external ear canal (otitis externa). Microscopic lesions consist of spongiotic neutrophilic pustular inflammation, parakeratosis, and ulceration with exudation. The yeast organisms are present in the superficial exudates.

Malassezia dermatitis

Malassezia dermatitis is caused by *Malassezia pachydermatis (Pityrosporum canis)*, a yeast isolated from the normal external ear canal and skin. This yeast proliferates and causes clinical disease when the microclimate or host defenses are altered. Lesions can be regional (interdigital, otic, perianal, or intertriginous) or more generalized (Fig. 17-55). Grossly the lesions are erythematous, often hyperpigmented, lichenified, alopecic, and scaly. Microscopic lesions consist of hyperkeratosis, focal parakeratosis, variable spongiotic pustular dermatitis, acanthosis, and the presence of *Malassezia pachydermatis* within the surface keratin. Because *Malassezia*

organisms can be lost during tissue processing, cytology is often a more reliable method of assessing the number of yeast present. Low numbers in histologic sections with lesions compatible with *Malassezia* dermatitis are often considered significant, especially with concurrent characteristic gross lesions. (Fig. 17-55).

SUBCUTANEOUS MYCOSES

Subcutaneous mycoses are caused by fungi that, after traumatic implantation, invade cutaneous and subcutaneous tissue. Some infections remain localized, but others spread to the lymph vessels. Diseases in this category include eumycotic mycetomas, dermatophyte pseudomycetoma, subcutaneous phaeohyphomycosis, subcutaneous hyalohyphomycosis, sporotrichosis, subcutaneous entomophthoromycosis, and oomycosis (pythiosis and lagenidiosis, not true fungi). The gross appearance of subcutaneous mycoses and deep granulomatous infections caused by bacteria are similar, usually one or more ulcerative nodules, sometimes with draining sinuses. Microscopically the lesions of subcutaneous mycoses consist of nodular to coalescing, suppurative, pyogranulomatous, or granulomatous inflammation.

Eumycotic mycetomas

Eumycotic mycetomas develop most often in horses and dogs and are rare fungal infections resulting in progressive cutaneous and subcutaneous nodular enlargements of granulomatous inflammation that can have draining sinuses and that resemble botryomycosis and actinomycotic mycetomas. The portal of entry is through traumatic injury into the dermis or subcutis, and most

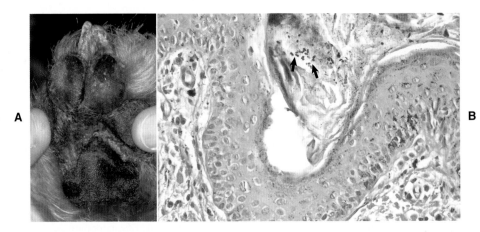

Fig. 17-55 **Interdigital dermatitis (*Malassezia pachydermatis*), skin, dog. A,** In this dog with atopic dermatitis, the interdigital skin is erythematous, moist, and mildly lichenified indicating chronicity. **B,** Haired skin. Stratum corneum contains numerous *Malassezia pachydermatis* yeast (*arrows*), which are bilobed ("peanut"-shaped). The dermis is mildly edematous—note the mild separation of the collagen bundles by nonstaining to lightly amphophilic edema fluid. Gomori's methenamine silver stain-H&E counter stain.
(**A,** *Courtesy Dr. David Duclos, Animal Skin and Allergy Clinic.* **B,** *Courtesy Dr. Ann M. Hargis, DermatoDiagnostics.*)

of the fungi involved in these infections are saprophytes. *Curvularia geniculata* is the most commonly isolated fungus in animals; other fungal genera include *Madurella, Acremonium, Pseudoallescheria,* and *Phaeococcus.* Histologic lesions are nodular masses of granulomatous inflammation with fibrosis and exudate in which there are embedded granules composed of masses of septate, branching fungal hyphae measuring 2 to 4 microns in diameter. The granules vary in size, shape, color, and texture, and are bordered by Splendore-Hoeppli material. Culture identifies the organism involved.

Dermatophytic pseudomycetoma

Dermatophytic pseudomycetoma is a rare, deep dermal and subcutaneous infection usually caused by *Microsporum canis,* and that develops predominantly in Persian cats, suggesting the possibility of a specific genetic deficit in innate or adaptive immunity in this breed. It is presumed that follicles rupture, releasing dermatophytes into the subfollicular dermis. Gross lesions are similar to other subcutaneous mycoses. Microscopic lesions are in the subfollicular dermis or subcutis, and consist of a granulomatous inflammatory response and intermixed aggregates of fungal hyphae with irregular dilations. Hair shafts within adjacent follicles contain *Microsporum* hyphae and spores.

Phaeohyphomycosis

Phaeohyphomycosis is a mycotic infection caused by species of pigmented fungi (dematiaceous) of a variety of genera that have dark-walled, septate hyphae. Genera include *Alternaria, Drechslera,* *Exophiala, Phialophora,* and others. These fungi are plant pathogens, soil saprophytes or, in some instances, normal flora that enter the skin at sites of trauma. Most of these infections remain localized to the skin and subcutaneous tissue, but they can spread to other tissue via lymphatic drainage in immunocompromised hosts. Grossly, lesions consist of alopecic or haired cutaneous nodules that can ulcerate and drain (Fig. 17-56). Microscopically, lesions consist of foci of granulomatous, pyogranulomatous, or lymphocyte-rich granulomatous inflammation containing pigmented fungal organisms. Culture is necessary for specific identification of the fungus involved. Subcutaneous phaeohyphomycosis occurs in cats, cattle, horses, and rarely dogs. Hyalohyphomycosis (paecilomycosis) is similar to phaeohyphomycosis except that the fungal hyphae in tissue are nonpigmented (nondematiaceous). Organisms include *Pseudoallescheria* sp., *Acremonium* sp., *Fusarium* sp., *Paecilomyces* sp., and *Geotrichum* sp.

Sporotrichosis

Sporotrichosis, caused by *Sporothrix schenckii,* is an uncommon mycosis that occurs in cutaneous, cutaneolymphatic, and disseminated forms in horses, mules, cattle, cats, and dogs. *Sporothrix schenckii* is a saprophytic dimorphic fungus found in moist organic debris, and entry into the body is by traumatic implantation. Ulcerated cutaneous nodules and fistulas develop at the site of inoculation and along lymph vessels (lymphangitis), but visceral dissemination is uncommon. Deep dermal to subcutaneous pyogranulomatous inflammation develops. Organisms are ovoid to elongate

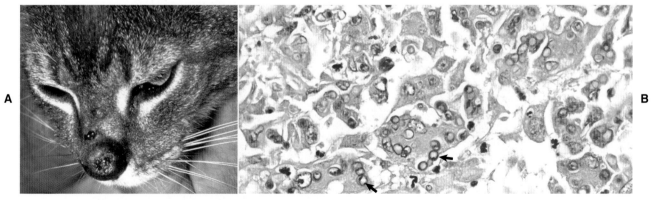

Fig. 17-56   **Cutaneous opportunistic fungal infection, phaeohyphomycosis, granulomatous dermatitis, skin, cat. A,** Infection of nasal planum and dorsum of muzzle. There is nodular ulcerative and granulomatous dermatitis primarily on the planum nasale. An ulcer is on the dorsum of the muzzle. **B,** Granulomatous dermatitis. Note macrophages containing yeastlike pigmented (dematiaceous) fungi (*arrows*). The presence of the pigmented fungi indicate that the condition is phaeohyphomycosis. The specific fungal organism was not cultured. H&E stain. (**A,** *Courtesy Dr. Alexander Werner, Valley Veterinary Specialty Service.* **B,** *Courtesy Dr. Ann M. Hargis, DermatoDiagnostics.*)

(cigar-shaped) bodies, which are often sparsely distributed and difficult to find except in cats, where organisms are numerous. The exudate containing organisms is infectious to human beings if introduced into cutaneous wounds.

Oomycosis (pythiosis and lagenidiosis)

Oomycosis refers to dermal and subcutaneous infection by *Pythium insidiosum* or *Lagenidium* sp., which are both aquatic dimorphic water molds and members of the Oomycetes in the kingdom Protista. Pythiosis most often affects the skin of the limbs and trunk of dogs, cattle, cats, and horses. Lagenidiosis has only been reported in dogs. Many infections develop in conjunction with exposure to freestanding water. Contamination of minor skin wounds is thought to be necessary for infection to occur. Infections are more common in tropical or subtropical climates, including the Gulf Coast of the United States, and are characterized clinically by erythematous, sometimes necrotizing, nodular lesions that ulcerate and drain (Fig. 17-57). There can be extensive tissue destruction by inflammation and necrosis. A unique gross feature of pythiosis is yellow, friable, fragments of necrotic tissue and hyphae, which can be dislodged from the lesions. Pythiosis in the dog is a rapidly progressive, debilitating, and often fatal disease seen most often in young, large-breed dogs. Lagenidiosis in the dog is also a very aggressive disease, and dogs may have lesions in organs other than the skin and lymph nodes.

Histologically, hyphae or hyphal-like structures are in areas of eosinophilic to pyogranulomatous dermal or subcutaneous inflammation. Organisms may not be readily visible in H&E stained sections; thus special stains, such as Gomori's methenamine silver stain, may be required to identify the organisms. Pythiosis, lagenidiosis, and entomophthoromycosis (see next discussion) cannot be reliably differentiated from one another via examination of histologic sections. PCR assays to detect oomycotic DNA and immunoblot analyses are required to differentiate these diseases from one another. Special collection and culture techniques are also necessary.

Entomophthoromycosis (zygomycosis)

Entomophthoromycosis refers to dermal and subcutaneous infections caused by *Basidiobolus* sp. and *Conidiobolus* sp., saprophytic fungi that gain entry to the body by inhalation or traumatic implantation by wounds or insects. Most *Basidiobolus* sp. infections have been seen in the horse. Infections with *Conidiobolus* sp. have been seen in dogs, llamas, sheep, and horses. Systemic dissemination of *Conidiobolus* sp. has developed in the dog and sheep. As in oomycosis, infections are more common in tropical or subtropical climates. Clinical and histologic features are similar to those of oomycosis. Differentiation between entomophthoromycosis and oomycosis requires culture and other techniques, such as PCR assays and immunoblot analyses,

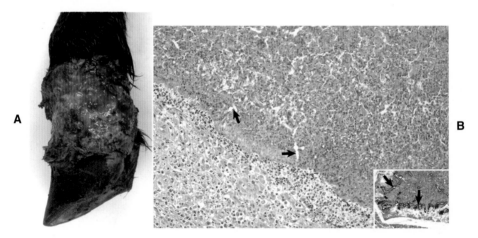

Fig. 17-57   Cutaneous pythiosis, *Pythium insidiosum* skin, horse. A, Distal leg. Note the extensive ulcer with multinodular coalescing granulomatous and exudative dermatitis. Infection with *Pythium insidiosum* results in extensive inflammation and tissue damage. Necrotic tissue and inflammatory debris exude from the ulcerated surface. **B,** Note margin of necrotic debris (*above*) and granulomatous and eosinophilic dermatitis. Hyphal-like structures of *Pythium insidiosum* do not stain well with H&E but may be visible as irregular clear hyphal-like spaces embedded within the necrotic debris (*arrows*). H&E stain. Inset: Numerous *Pythium insidiosum* organisms stained black (*arrows*). Gomori's methenamine silver stain. (**A,** *Courtesy University of Florida Clinical Dermatology Service.* **B** and **Inset,** *Courtesy Dr. Pamela E. Ginn, College of Veterinary Medicine, University of Florida.*)

and is therapeutically important because infections with Zygomycetes (true fungi) can be responsive to antifungal treatment, whereas infections with Oomycetes are not.

SYSTEMIC MYCOSES

The respiratory tract, especially the lung, is almost invariably the primary portal of entry and infection in the systemic mycoses, but cutaneous and subcutaneous infections can occur as part of the disseminated disease or by direct implantation of fungi by trauma. Systemic mycoses include *Blastomyces dermatitidis, Coccidioides immitis, Cryptococcus neoformans,* and *Histoplasma capsulatum.* Infections with these fungi can occur in animals with apparently normal immune function, but are more extensive in immunocompromised animals. Grossly, one or more nodular areas in the skin can ulcerate and have draining sinuses. Histopathologically, there are nodular areas of granulomatous or pyogranulomatous inflammation in the dermis and possibly subcutis. *Cryptococcus neoformans* can cause a granulomatous response, but generally the inflammation is less severe than with the other fungi. The cryptococcal organisms have a mucinous capsule that does not stain with H&E. When inflammation is mild, the capsules of the numerous organisms in a lesion give the tissues a multicystic appearance microscopically. Cytology or microscopy is required for diagnosis. The morphologic features of the organisms (including mucicarmine-positive capsule) are sufficient for diagnosis.

ALGAL INFECTIONS

Protothecosis is a rare infection of animals caused by achloric (colorless) alga of the genus *Prototheca. Prototheca* inhabit sewage, animal waste, and slime flux of trees. They enter the body via ingestion of contaminated water or food (see Chapter 7) or traumatic implantation. The organisms are usually of low pathogenicity, but severe or even disseminated infections occur in immunologically compromised hosts. Cell-mediated immunity is considered vital to control or eliminate the infection. Infection is most often reported in the dog and cat. Grossly the lesions are nodular, and the microscopic pattern is nodular to diffuse granulomatous dermatitis and panniculitis. The organisms can be identified in tissues by the characteristic endospores especially when stained with Gomori's methenamine silver stain or with immunohistochemical techniques. *Prototheca* sp. can also be identified by culture.

PARASITIC INFECTIONS

Ectoparasites include mites and ticks (which have eight legs), and lice, fleas, and flies (which have six legs) (Box 17-10). The presence of these ectoparasites is called an infestation. Endoparasites causing cutaneous lesions include nematodes, trematodes, and protozoa, and their presence is called an infection. Parasites cause a number of untoward effects including damage to hides and predisposition to secondary infection. Arthropod parasites (jointed limbs) also serve as vectors of bacterial, spirochetal, helminthic, rickettsial, protozoal, and viral infections. The cutaneous reaction to parasites varies with parasite number, location, feeding habits, and host immune response. The cutaneous

---

Box **17-10**

Cutaneous Parasitic Infestations

MITES
Demodex sp.
Sarcoptes sp.
Notoedres sp.
Otodectes sp.
Psoroptes sp.
Chorioptes sp.
Cheyletiella sp.
Psorergates sp.
Neotrombicula and *Eutrombicula* spp.

TICKS
Argasid (soft)
Ixodid (hard)

LICE
Mallophaga (biting)
Anoplura (blood sucking)

FLEAS
Ctenocephalides felis and *Ctenocephalides canis*

FLIES
Adult fly bites
    Horn fly, stable fly, horse fly, deer fly, black fly, biting
        gnats, mosquitoes
Myiasis
Calliphorids, sarcophagids, *Cuterebra* sp., *Hypoderma* sp.,
    screwworm, *Dermatobia* sp.

HELMINTHS
Larvae
    Hookworms, *Habronema* sp., *Pelodera* sp., *Necator* sp.,
        Strongyloides sp., *Gnathostoma* sp., *Bunostomum* sp.
Filarial
    Onchocerca sp., *Stephanofilaria* sp., *Elaeophora* sp.,
        Parafilaria sp., *Suifilaria* sp., *Dirofilaria* sp.,
        Acanthocheilonema sp.

PROTOZOA
Leishmania sp.
Rarely other genera

reaction is often mediated in part by immune mechanisms (hypersensitivity).

MITES

Mite infestations can cause serious cutaneous lesions in domestic animals and economic loss in food animals. Sheep in the United States are free of mite infestation except for *Demodex* sp.. Cattle, however, can be infested with a variety of mites, including *Sarcoptes, Psoroptes,* and *Chorioptes* genera, which are reportable diseases. Mite infestations are rare in horses, except for *Chorioptes* sp., which produce dermatitis of distal limbs in heavy breeds. Mite infestations can also cause serious cutaneous diseases in dogs (*Demodex canis, Sarcoptes scabiei, Otodectes cynotis*), cats (*Demodex cati, Demodex gatoi, Otodectes cynotis, Notoedres cati*), and pigs (*Sarcoptes scabiei*). In *Sarcoptes scabiei* infestation, mites can be difficult to find, except for infestation of the skin of the external ears of pigs.

Most species of *Demodex* mites live their entire life cycle in the lumens of hair follicles or sebaceous glands as part of the normal fauna of the skin of most mammals. It is only when the normal equilibrium between the host and the parasite is changed to favor proliferation of the mite that skin lesions of demodectic mange are produced. Thus identification of large numbers of adult mites or an increased number of immature mites in skin scrapings or biopsy samples is required for diagnosis of demodicosis. Demodicosis is caused by host-specific mites; it is a major problem in dogs, but is uncommon in other animals.

Demodicosis

Demodicosis is one of the most common skin disorders of dogs in North America. Canine demodicosis is caused by *Demodex canis* and occurs in two clinical forms, localized and generalized, both of which are more common in juvenile dogs. Transmission from mother to offspring occurs via close skin contact as occurs during suckling. Purebred dogs of many breeds are predisposed to infestation, suggesting an inherited basis for the disease related to a primary deficit in cell-mediated immunity. Research studies suggest the defect is one of T-lymphocyte helper dysfunction resulting in damage by cytotoxic T lymphocytes. Active lesions of demodicosis result in lymphocytic mural folliculitis with lymphocyte-mediated damage to the keratinocytes of the follicular wall. It is speculated that follicular keratinocytes express altered self-antigens or *Demodex* antigens, which leads to immune-mediated destruction of the follicular wall. Secondary immunodeficiency, due to T-lymphocyte suppression, is also associated with demodicosis, particularly if a secondary *Staphylococcus intermedius* infection is present. The secondary immunodeficiency improves as the demodicosis resolves. Results of studies conflict as to whether the secondary immunodeficiency is caused by the accompanying bacterial infection or to the mite infestation. Demodicosis occurs in adult dogs with underlying metabolic disorders (hypothyroidism, hyperadrenocorticism) or that are given drugs (glucocorticoids or cytotoxic drugs) that can compromise the immune system. Idiopathic cases also occur.

Gross lesions of localized demodicosis in the dog consist of one to several small scaly, erythematous, alopecic, areas on the face or forelegs (Fig. 17-27). Canine generalized demodicosis usually involves large areas of the body; lesions consist of larger coalescing patches of erythema, alopecia, comedones, scales, and crusts. The early microscopic lesions include epidermal hyperkeratosis, perifolliculitis, and lymphocytic interface mural folliculitis, including mild degeneration of follicular basal cells, follicular pigmentary incontinence, and intraluminal mites (Fig. 17-27). Follicles can become plugged with large numbers of mites, keratin, and sebum. Secondary bacterial infection leads to neutrophilic folliculitis that in conjunction with mite proliferation and follicular hyperkeratosis, progresses to follicular rupture. Mites, bacteria, keratin, and sebum spill into the dermis, stimulating a granulomatous to pyogranulomatous dermatitis. Perifollicular granulomas with portions of mites are often seen. Gross lesions in dogs with severe secondary bacterial infection include papules, pustules, edema, and draining tracts. In severe demodicosis, inflammation and organisms spread into the subcutis, and lymphadenitis and septicemia can develop. Severe chronic lesions consist of dermal fibrosis with effacement of adnexal structures.

In cats, demodicosis is rare and is caused by two species of mites, one (*Demodex cati*) lives in follicles and sebaceous glands, and the other (*Demodex gatoi*) resides on the skin surface within the stratum corneum. Unless the immune response is compromised, lesions associated with *Demodex cati* are usually localized to the chin, eyelids, head, or neck. When the immune response is compromised, as in feline retroviral infections, generalized lesions of erythema, scaling, alopecia, pustules, and crusts develop. Histologically, cats with *Demodex cati* have epidermal and follicular hyperkeratosis and follicular atrophy. Inflammation is minimal. The most common sign associated with the presence of *Demodex gatoi* is pruritus, resulting in excessive grooming and symmetric alopecia. *Demodex gatoi* is contagious between cats, and there is an asymptomatic carrier state.

Demodicosis in cattle (*Demodex bovis, Demodex tauri,* and *Demodex ghanaensis*) and goats (*Demodex caprae*) is of little clinical significance, but extensive infection can damage hides by development of multifocal nodules in the skin of shoulders, neck, and face, or in a more generalized distribution. Nodules correspond to follicular cysts that are filled with mites and keratinaceous material. Rupture of the cysts leads to severe granulomatous dermatitis and damage to the hide. Similarly, *Demodex phylloides* of pigs causes scale-covered papules progressing to nodules that are filled with keratinaceous debris and mites, and that damage the hide. Lesions develop in the ventral body skin, eyelids, and snout. Sheep have two species of mites. *Demodex ovis* is located in hair follicles or sebaceous glands distributed over the body and can cause alopecia, erythema, scaling, pustules, and matted fleece. Lesions develop on the face, neck, shoulders, and back, but the ears, limbs, and coronary bands can also be affected. *Demodex aries* is located in sebaceous glands of the vulva, prepuce, and nostrils, and can cause papular, rarely pustular, or nodular lesions. Demodectic mange is rare in the horse. *Demodex caballi* is commonly present in pilosebaceous units of eyelids and nose, generally without producing lesions. In contrast, *Demodex equi* is distributed over the body. Clinical lesions are rare, but when present develop on the face, neck, shoulders, or forelimbs, and consist of localized to diffuse alopecia and scaling, or of papules, nodules, and pustules.

Scabies

Scabies is caused by *Sarcoptes scabiei*. This highly contagious mite is the most important ectoparasite of pigs, is common in dogs, and is uncommon to rare in horses, cattle, sheep, goats, and cats. The mites burrow in tunnels in the stratum corneum and cause intense pruritus due principally to hypersensitivity reactions, although irritation from secretions also plays a role. Lesions begin on the external ears, head, and neck, and can become generalized. Early gross lesions include erythematous macules, papules, crusts, and excoriations. Chronic lesions are scaly, lichenified, and hairless (Fig. 17-58). Microscopically, early lesions consist of superficial perivascular dermatitis with eosinophils, mast cells, and lymphocytes. Mild focal spongiosis can be seen. Small parakeratotic crusts can develop as spongiotic lesions age. Chronic lesions are associated with epidermal acanthosis with marked rete ridge formation, compact hyperkeratosis, parakeratosis, crusting, and perivascular dermatitis with eosinophils, mast cells, and lymphocytes. In areas of excoriation, neutrophils—and with time, dermal scarring—may be evident. Mites, mite eggs, or feces may be found in tunnels in the stratum corneum (Fig. 17-58), but are not commonly seen in tissue sections because of small numbers of mites.

Notoedric mites

Notoedric mite infestation is caused by *Notoedres cati*. This mite infests cats, rabbits, and occasionally foxes, dogs, and human beings. It is a rare but highly contagious pruritic disease characterized initially by an erythematous papular rash followed by scales, crusts, and alopecia, and, when chronic, with lichenification. Lesions begin on the neck and pinnae and extend to the head, face, and paw and can become generalized.

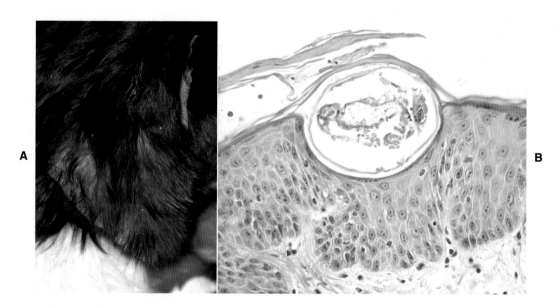

Fig. 17-58   *Sarcoptes scabiei* **infestation, skin, dog. A,** Ear. Note the alopecia, erythema, and scaling along the margin of the ear. **B,** Note the section of a mite in the stratum corneum. The epidermal hyperkeratosis, acanthosis, and rete ridge formation are in response to both the mite itself and also to self-trauma caused by intense pruritus. H&E stain. (**A,** *Courtesy Dr. Ann M. Hargis, DermatoDiagnostics.* **B,** *Courtesy Dr. M.D. McGavin, College of Veterinary Medicine, University of Tennessee.*)

Microscopic lesions consist of a hyperplastic, perivascular eosinophilic dermatitis with mild spongiosis, and crusts. In cats, mites are readily found in the stratum corneum in tissue sections or in skin scrapings.

Otodectic mites

Otodectic mite infestation caused by *Otodectes cynotis* occurs in the external ear canals of dogs and cats and occasionally can be present on other parts of the body. The mite lives on the skin surface and can be seen by direct visualization. Because *Otodectes* can be present in areas of the body other than ears, it is important to differentiate it from *Sarcoptes* and *Notoedres* mites, which can be identified in microscopically examined skin scrapings or sometimes in tissue sections.

Psoroptic mites

Psoroptic mite infestation in sheep, cattle, horses, goats, rabbits, and other animals is caused by several species of host-specific mites. *Psoroptes cuniculi* live on the surface of the skin, feeding on lipids and later on serous and hemorrhagic crusts that exude from the traumatized skin. It infests the external ear canals of rabbits, horses, goats, and sheep. *Psoroptes equi* infests the base of the mane and tail, and skin under the forelock of horses. *Psoroptes ovis* causes serious disease in cattle and sheep, producing parasitic lesions of thickened skin and dry scales and crusts that begin on the withers and spread because of persistent self-inflicted trauma. In sheep, psoroptic mite infestation is called "sheep scab." Lesions develop on the withers and sides. The wooled areas are chiefly involved with crusts that become adherent to the matted fleece and in time expand and coalesce. Damage is due to self-inflicted trauma, resulting from the pruritus associated with irritation and hypersensitivity reactions. The microscopic lesion is a spongiotic, hyperplastic, hyperkeratotic, or exudative superficial perivascular dermatitis with eosinophils. Self-trauma leads to erosions, ulcers, and exudation of serum and leukocytes. No cases of *Psoroptes ovis* have been reported in sheep in the United States since 1970.

Chorioptic mange

Chorioptic mange, caused by *Chorioptes bovis*, affects cattle, horses, goats, and, in some countries, sheep. The mite is not host specific. Mites on the skin surface cause irritation and pruritus leading to self-trauma and the gross lesions of erythematous, papular, crusted, scaly, hairless, thickened skin on the lower hind limbs, scrotum, tail, perineum, udder, and thigh of cattle; lower limbs of horses; scrotum and lower hind limbs of sheep; and lower limbs, hindquarters, and the abdomen of goats. Microscopic lesions are similar to those seen in other surface-dwelling mite infestations.

Cheyletiellosis

Cheyletiellosis, caused by infestation with *Cheyletiella* sp., occurs in dogs, cats, rabbits, wild animals, and human beings. The mite lives on the surface of the skin and induces hyperkeratosis. In dogs and cats, lesions consist of hyperkeratosis manifested as dry, white, scaly dandruff along the dorsal midline of the back. Some infestations are asymptomatic. Cats can have focal, multifocal, to generalized red papules or crusts, characterized microscopically by superficial perivascular dermatitis with eosinophils. The diagnosis requires identification of the mites via skin scrapings, acetate tape, or brush techniques because mites are not usually seen in tissue sections.

Psorergatic mites

Psorergatic mite infestation, caused by *Psorergates ovis*, occurs in sheep in Australia, New Zealand, South Africa, and Argentina. Sheep in the United States have been free of *Psorergates* sp. mites since 1973. Suspected cases of psorergatic mange should be reported to the state veterinarian. The infestation initially results in papules and scales along the trunk. Over time, the fleece becomes ragged as severe pruritus leads to secondary crusts, lichenification, and hyperpigmentation with alopecia.

Trombiculiasis

Trombiculiasis is infestation by larvae of trombiculid (harvest) mites also known as chiggers. *Eutrombicula (Trombicula) alfreddugesi* (North American chigger), and *Eutrombicula (Trombicula) splendens* are some of the species implicated in trombiculiasis in cats, dogs, and horses. *Neotrombicula (Trombicula) autumnalis*, the European harvest mite, attacks most domestic species. *Eutrombicula (Trombicula) sarcina*, an Australian species known as the leg-itch mite, is an important parasite of sheep, although its principal host is the gray kangaroo. The larvae tunnel into the epidermis and inject saliva that gels to form a characteristic stylostome used to obtain digested tissue fluids. Grossly, small red papules or crusts containing several orange to red larvae develop on parts of the skin in close contact with plants or the ground. Lesions are intensely pruritic. The microscopic lesions are a hyperplastic, superficial perivascular dermatitis with eosinophils, mast cells, and intraepidermal mites. Identification of a stylostome microscopically is pathognomonic.

TICKS

Ticks comprise two families, Ixodidae (hard ticks that contain a scutum, a hard chitinous plate on the anterior dorsal surface) and Argasidae (soft ticks that lack the scutum). Most of the pathogenic ticks are in the family Ixodidae. An exception is *Otobius megnini*, the spinose ear tick, which is parasitic to all domestic animals and causes severe otitis externa. Heavy tick infestations, particularly by adult argasid ticks that engorge repeatedly, can cause anemia. As obligate bloodsucking ectoparasites, ticks also serve as vectors for many potentially severe blood-borne diseases, such as *Rickettsia rickettsia* (Rocky Mountain spotted fever), *Borrelia burgdorferi* (Lyme disease), *Anaplasma marginale* (anaplasmosis), and African swine fever. Tick bites also cause direct damage to the skin at the site of attachment, which predisposes to secondary bacterial infection leading to abscesses or septicemia, and to myiasis. Adverse reactions to ticks depend in part on the content of salivary secretions. Tick saliva has been shown to contain factors that are antihemostatic, antiinflammatory, and immunosuppressive; a key factor contributing to these functions is prostaglandin E_2. These factors are thought to facilitate feeding and the transmission of tick-borne diseases. In addition, salivary secretions of several species of ixodid ticks (e.g., *Dermacentor andersoni* and *Dermacentor variabilis* in North America) contain neurotoxins that can cause an acute ascending lower motor neuron paralysis of the host. If the tick is removed, symptoms disappear rapidly.

The severity of local cutaneous reactions varies not only with salivary secretions, but also with host resistance. In experimental studies, it has been shown that in nonsensitized hosts, the inflammatory response to tick mouth parts embedded deeply in the dermis develops in the immediate site of the bite, is composed largely of neutrophils, and is minor even about 2 days after the tick attaches. In contrast, previously sensitized hosts develop more rapid and intense local reactions (as early as 1 hour postattachment). Cutaneous lesions are present a greater distance from the site of attachment, and basophils, eosinophils, and neutrophils are present in the epidermis and dermis. Cutaneous basophil hypersensitivity, a form of delayed-type hypersensitivity, plays an important role in immunity to ticks.

In naturally occurring cases, gross lesions include red papules that progress to circular erythematous areas up to 2 cm in diameter. Lesions progress to foci of necrosis, erosions, ulcers, crusts, and in some animals, nodules. Lesions heal with scarring and alopecia. Histologic lesions include congestion, edema, and sometimes hemorrhage with an intradermal cavity below which the tick mouthparts may be present. Inflammation consists of perivascular to diffuse accumulations of neutrophils, eosinophils, and basophils. Later developing lesions include epidermal and dermal necrosis, the granulocytic leukocytes of more acute lesions plus accumulations of lymphocytes and macrophages at the margin of the necrotic dermis. In a cross section of skin, these lesions can be triangular with the apex at the panniculus. Some lesions comprise granulomas (arthropod bite granulomas) in which the inflammatory cells efface the tissue architecture and lymphoid follicles form.

LICE

Pediculosis is infestation with lice and is caused by two orders of lice: Mallophaga (biting lice) and Anoplura (blood-sucking lice). Infestations are relatively host specific, are spread by direct contact, and are relatively easy to control because the life cycle takes place entirely on the host. Pediculosis occurs more commonly in winter when temperatures are cooler, the wool or hair coat is longer, animals are congregated, and the plane of nutrition is lower. Thus heavy infestations are usually an indication for underlying problems, such as overcrowding, poor sanitation, or poor nutrition. Generally, pediculosis is not a significant threat to the host, and animals with low infestations may not have clinical signs or lesions. Most problems are related to skin irritation and resultant pruritus. However, the Anoplura have piercing mouth parts and suck blood, thus heavy infestations can cause anemia. In addition, *Haematopinus suis*, a sucking louse that parasitizes pigs, is economically important because the lice transmit *Eperythrozoon suis*, and the viruses of swinepox and African swine fever. The Mallophaga cause less severe signs as they feed on epithelial cellular debris. Primary lesions caused by lice are few, and most are secondary to scratching, rubbing, or biting. The cause of the pruritus is not known, but is thought to be a result of more than mechanical irritation alone. Gross lesions consist of papules, crusts, excoriations, and damage to hair, wool, or skin. Lice and eggs are visible on hair or wool. Animals infested with sucking lice can be anemic. Weight loss and reduced production of milk can result from the constant irritation associated with some infestations.

FLEAS

Flea infestation is principally a problem in dogs and cats. *Ctenocephalides felis* is the most common flea causing infestation, and it also transmits *Dipylidium caninum*. Infestation can occur with *Ctenocephalides canis*, and less commonly with fleas that parasitize other mammals and birds. Fleas can cause severe skin irritation because of frequent biting and release of enzymes, anticoagulants, and histamine-like substances, hypersensitivity reactions to saliva, and secondary host-inflicted trauma from scratching and biting. Severe infestations can cause blood loss (anemia), especially in puppies, kittens, or small debilitated adults. Lesions occur over the dorsal lumbosacral region (Fig. 17-59), caudomedial thighs, ventral abdomen, flanks, and, in cats the neck area, and consist of multiple red papules and secondary excoriations (see insect bite hypersensitivity section).

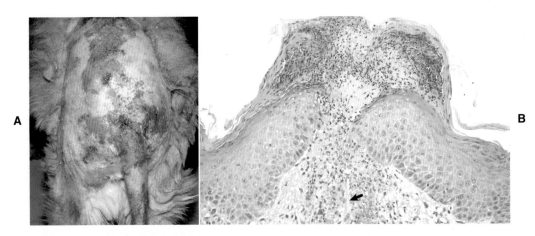

Fig. 17-59 **Insect bite hypersensitivity, skin, acute moist dermatitis (pyotraumatic dermatitis), dog. A,** Flea bite hypersensitivity. The hair has been clipped to allow better visualization of the lesions. Self-inflicted trauma is largely the source of the erosion, moist exudation, and crusting in the skin of this dog with flea bite hypersensitivity. **B,** Insect bite. The serocellular crust on the epidermal surface covers a defect in epidermis, beneath which in the dermis is a vertical zone of necrosis infiltrated by eosinophils *(arrow)*. Hypersensitivity reactions to insect bites can be pruritic and initiate scratching and result in acute moist dermatitis. H&E stain. (**A,** *Courtesy Dr. Ben Baker, Washington State University.* **B,** *Courtesy Dr. Ann M. Hargis, DermatoDiagnostics.*)

FLIES

Cutaneous reactions due to fly bites range from minor to severe, and are due to bites by adult flies and to myiasis by larvae. Reactions to the bites of flies vary and include irritation, anemia, direct toxicity, and hypersensitivity. Biting flies include *Haematobia irritans* (horn fly), *Stomoxys calcitrans* (stable fly), and horse flies, deer flies, black flies, biting gnats, mosquitoes, and the sheep ked (*Melophagus ovinus*), a common wingless fly that sucks blood. Lesions of biting flies are due to local irritation and include wheals and papules centered around a puncture wound that can bleed. Such lesions can persist with hair loss, scales, hemorrhagic crusts, erythema, and secondary excoriations because of self-inflicted trauma, especially if the animals are hypersensitive to the bites. Such hypersensitivity occurs with *Culicoides* sp. in horses (Queensland itch, sweet itch; see Selected Hypersensitivity Reactions, Culicoides Hypersensitivity) and mosquitoes in cats (see Selected Hypersensitivity Reactions, Mosquito Bite Hypersensitivity in Cats). Microscopic lesions associated with fly bites vary depending on the fly involved. Dermal hemorrhage and edema with a central area of epidermal necrosis are early lesions seen with bites of some flies. Hemorrhagic crust covers areas of necrosis, and perivascular neutrophilic, eosinophilic, and mixed mononuclear inflammation can be seen. Intraepidermal eosinophils including eosinophilic pustules are sometimes identified, and eosinophilic folliculitis and furunculosis can be present

in reactions to mosquito bites. Epidermal hyperplasia, hyperkeratosis, parakeratosis, and crusting are associated with self-trauma.

Myiasis is infestation of tissues by the larvae of dipterous flies (flies with two wings or winglike appendages), and is a disease of neglect. Lesions develop in skin kept moist and soiled by urine, feces, or body secretions. Flies are attracted by the odor of such areas. Sheep, largely because of ovine fleece rot (see Superficial Bacterial Infections) are most commonly affected. In myiasis caused by blow flies (calliphorids) and flesh flies (sarcophagids), eggs are deposited in wounds or on soiled hair or wool. Gross lesions consist of matted hair or wool and multiple irregular cutaneous holes or ulcers with an offensive odor. Secretion of proteolytic enzymes by larvae causes lesions to spread. Death can result, and is due to septicemia or toxemia.

In cuterebral myiasis, eggs of *Cuterebra* sp. are deposited on stones or vegetation near the burrows of rabbits and rodents, the natural hosts. Less often cats or dogs become infested. The eggs hatch to first-stage larvae on the vegetation, and when the host contacts the vegetation, larvae attach to the hair coat and move to the skin. Once on the skin, larvae move to natural body openings such as the nares, where they penetrate the mucosa. Other portals of entry are direct penetration of the skin or ingestion by the host during grooming. The larvae migrate to the subcutis, produce a cyst-like subcutaneous nodule in which the larvae mature and cut a hole in the skin for respiration. The larvae feed on tissue debris. Wounds heal slowly after larvae are removed or released, but secondary bacterial infection can develop.

In hypoderma myiasis, larvae of *Hypoderma lineatum* and *Hypoderma bovis* penetrate the skin of the legs of cattle and less frequently horses and migrate proximally in the subcutis of the leg. The larvae can be found in many areas of the body. After weeks to months, first-stage larvae reach the esophagus (*Hypoderma lineatum*) or vertebral canal (*Hypoderma bovis*) where they develop into second-stage larvae. These second-stage larvae then migrate to the subcutis of the back, become established in subcutaneous nodules similar to those of *Cuterebra* sp. with an opening for respiration, and mature to third-stage larvae (Fig. 17-60). Microscopically, these larvae are located in a cavity filled with fibrin and a few eosinophils and bordered by granulation tissue containing clusters of eosinophils.

Screwworm myiasis is caused by two species of Diptera larvae, *Cochliomyia hominivorax* (Coquerel) the New World screwworm, and *Chrysomyia bezziana* (Villeneuve), the Old World screwworm. *Cochliomyia hominivorax* occurs in tropical and semitropical regions of the Western hemisphere including Central and South America and some Caribbean islands. It has been eradicated in the United States and Mexico. *Chrysomyia bezziana* (Villeneuve) is found in tropical and semitropical regions of the Eastern Hemisphere including Africa and Southern Asia. Screwworm flies deposit eggs in wounds or near mucocutaneous junctions of living animals. The eggs develop into first-stage larvae that move into the wound. Larvae have sharp, pointed mouth hooks that tear living tissue. Larvae feed on tissues liquefied by secretions of proteolytic enzymes. Screwworm myiasis is an important disease in domestic and wild animals because screwworm larvae destroy viable tissue. Grossly, malodorous wounds contain larvae, shreds of tissue, and copious amounts of reddish-brown fluid. Once an animal is infested, death is almost inevitable unless the larvae are removed. When it is necessary to differentiate screwworm myiasis from cutaneous myiasis caused by other flies, larvae can be preserved in 70% alcohol and submitted for identification. Screwworm myiasis is a reportable disease in some countries, including the United States.

Larvae of the tropical warble fly, *Dermatobia hominis*, cause cutaneous myiasis in numerous species of mammals, most commonly and importantly in cattle, in South and Central America. Adult *Dermatobia hominis* attaches its eggs to the legs of other insects that then transport the eggs to the mammalian hosts. While the insects feed, the eggs are deposited on the skin, hatch into larvae, and quickly penetrate the skin of the host mammal. The larvae grow in subcutaneous nodules similar to those of *Cuterebra* sp. with an opening on the skin surface for respiration, after which they leave the nodule and drop to the ground to complete their life cycle. *Dermatobia* myiasis is of economic importance because it causes condemnation of hides at slaughter and predisposes the skin to myiasis by other flies.

HELMINTHS

Cutaneous infections with helminths are generally not life threatening but can be unsightly and irritating in companion animals and cause hide damage in food animals. Infections are due to migration of helminth larvae that as adults live in noncutaneous sites, or by filarial infections (filarial dermatitis) in which adults or microfilaria spend some time in the skin or subcutis.

Helminth larval migrans

Hookworm dermatitis.   Hookworm dermatitis is caused by cutaneous migration of the larvae of *Ancylostoma* or *Uncinaria* sp. Red papules that coalesce and develop into lichenified alopecic areas occur on the feet of dogs and, less frequently, on other areas in contact with an unsanitary environment contaminated by hookworm larvae. Footpads can become soft, the keratinized portion can separate, and secondary bacterial dermatitis and paronychia can develop. Hyperplastic spongiotic perivascular dermatitis with eosinophils, serocellular crusts, and migration tracks are the microscopic lesions. Parasitologic evaluation of fresh tissue may allow larval identification.

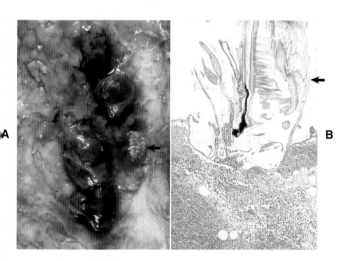

Fig. 17-60   Myiasis, skin, subcutis. A, Hypodermal myiasis, *Hypoderma* sp. larva, cow. Multiple nodules each contain a single larva. One nodule *(right)* has been incised to expose a larva *(arrow).* **B,** Cuterebral myiasis, *Cuterebra* sp. larva, dog. Note a portion of a subcutaneous cystic nodule that contains a segment of a larva *(arrow).* The panniculitis is largely comprised of eosinophils. H&E stain. *(A and B, Courtesy Dr. Ann M. Hargis, DermatoDiagnostics.)*

Cutaneous habronemiasis.   Cutaneous habrone-miasis (summer sores) occurs in horses and is caused by infection with the larvae of *Habronema* sp. or *Draschia* sp. deposited on the skin by house or stable flies. Larval deposition and lesions occur on parts of the body where the skin is either traumatized, such as the legs, or moist and soft, such as the prepuce and medial canthus of the eye (Fig. 17-61). Larvae are unable to pen-etrate normal skin, but fly bites cause sufficient damage to allow larval penetration. Grossly, single or multiple, proliferative, ulcerated red to brown, nodular masses are present that on section have small, yellow to white, gritty foci. The microscopic lesion is a nodular dermatitis with eosinophils, epithelioid macrophages, and, some-times, giant cells bordering larvae or necrotic debris (Fig. 17-61, *B*). Granulation tissue infiltrated by neutro-phils is present on the ulcerated surface.

Other helminth parasites associated with cutaneous larval migration include *Pelodera*, *Necator*, *Strongyloides*, *Gnathostoma*, and *Bunostomum*. Schistosome cercariae, especially of birds, can cause similar lesions.

Filarial dermatitis.   Onchocerciasis is a filarial dermatitis principally affecting horses. Adult parasites are located in nodules in connective tissue and can be asymptomatic. Microfilariae are located in the dermis, particularly of the ventral midline, and are the source of the major lesions. Intermediate hosts, such as the Simuliidae (black flies, gnats) and Ceratopogonidae (biting midges), transmit the microfilariae. Not all horses with microfilariae have clinical signs or lesions. In those horses with cutaneous inflammation attrib-uted to microfilariae, dead or dying microfilariae induce the most intense inflammation, and inflamma-tion can be enhanced by microfilarialcidal therapy. Differences in lesion severity between horses may reflect different degrees of hypersensitivity to microfi-lariae, different degrees of hypersensitivity to the bites of intermediate hosts, or possibly other factors. Recent evidence in human filarial disease has revealed that the acute inflammatory response in two important diseases, elephantiasis and river blindness, may largely be a result of the endosymbiotic bacteria (*Wolbachia*) harbored within the filarial parasites and released into the blood by living parasites or following death or damage of the adults or microfilariae. The inflamma-tory stimulus is thought to be caused by endotoxin-like activity that is dependent on pattern recognition receptors known to contribute to innate immunity. *Wolbachia* have been identified in a number of filarial parasites in animals including *Onchocerca gutturosa*, *Onchocerca lienalis*, and *Onchocerca cervicalis*. However, further research is needed to determine the role, if any, of these bacteria in filarial parasitic diseases in animals. In equine onchocerciasis, clinical lesions related to microfilariae develop on the head, neck, medial

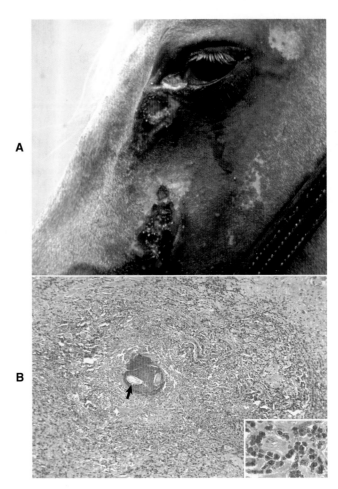

Fig. 17-61   **Cutaneous habronemiasis, *Habronema* sp., skin, horse. A,** Face. Multiple coalescing nodular granuloma-tous and ulcerated areas are present on the skin of the medial canthus, skin immediately ventral to the eye, and the skin of the lateral surface of the face. Lesions of cutaneous habrone-miasis develop in areas of the skin that are traumatized (often the legs) or in soft moist skin (around the genitalia or eyes). In this case, moisture from ocular secretion (tears) may have predisposed to bites of house or stable flies, with subsequent emergence and migration of *Habronema* sp. larvae into the dermis. **B,** Note sections of larvae (*arrow*) within nodule of granulomatous and eosinophilic dermatitis. H&E stain. Inset: The inset illustrates eosinophils in the inflammatory response. H&E stain. (*A*, *Courtesy Dr. Valerie Fadok, College of Veterinary Medicine, University of Florida. **B** and **Inset,** Courtesy Dr. Pamela E. Ginn, College of Veterinary Medicine, University of Florida.*)

forelimbs, ventral thorax, and abdomen, and consist of patchy to diffuse alopecia, erythema, scaling, crusting, and pigmentary changes. Some horses have a charac-teristic, variably pigmented, circular area of dermatitis on the forehead. Keratitis, conjunctivitis, and uveitis are observed in some horses. Microscopic cutaneous lesions vary from none to superficial and deep perivas-cular to interstitial dermatitis with eosinophils, lymphocytes, and microfilariae. Fibrosis is seen in older lesions.

Stephanofilariasis, a filarial dermatitis of cattle, buffalo, and goats, is transmitted by flies and caused by six species of parasites of the genus *Stephanofilaria*. Each species of *Stephanofilaria* causes lesions in a different body location. Cutaneous lesions are caused by a reaction to the parasites free in the dermis, to the bites of the flies serving as the vector, and self-inflicted trauma. *Stephanofilaria stilesi* occurs in cattle in the United States and causes lesions along the ventral midline that consist initially of small (1 cm) circular patches with moist erect hairs, foci of epidermal hemorrhage, and serum exudation. Such foci expand and coalesce into a large area covered by crusts, which upon healing, consist of thickened hairless plaques as large as 25 cm in diameter (Fig. 17-62). Microscopic lesions consist of superficial and deep perivascular dermatitis with eosinophils, epidermal hyperkeratosis, parakeratosis, acanthosis with spongiosis, eosinophilic microabscesses, and crusts. Adult parasites and microfilaria can be seen. Other causes of filarial dermatitis include *Elaeophora* sp., *Parafilaria* sp., *Suifilaria* sp., and rarely *Dirofilaria* sp. or *Acanthocheilonema* sp.

PROTOZOA

In the United States, cutaneous protozoal infections develop as part of systemic infections, principally with members of the genus *Leishmania*. Rarely, cutaneous

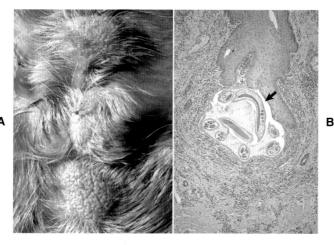

Fig. 17-62   Stephanofilarial dermatitis, *Stephanofilaria stilesi*, skin, cow. A, Ventral abdomen. Note the thickened plaquelike area of alopecia and lichenification. **B,** Note longitudinal and cross sections of adult parasite. The adult parasites usually live in a cystlike space at the base of a hair follicle *(arrow)* and can destroy follicles. Note the marked infiltrate of mixed mononuclear cells around the cystic space and base of the follicle (perifolliculitis). H&E stain. (**A,** *Courtesy Dr. M.D. McGavin, College of Veterinary Medicine, University of Tennessee.* **B,** *Courtesy Dr. Pamela E. Ginn, College of Veterinary Medicine, University of Florida.)*

infection with *Caryospora* sp., *Neospora* sp., *Sarcocystis* sp, or *Toxoplasma* sp. has been reported. Leishmaniasis occurs in human beings, dogs, cats, horses and other mammals. Members of the *Leishmania donovani* complex, an intracellular parasite of the mononuclear-phagocytic system, cause most infections. Sandflies serve as the vector for infection of animals. Dogs, cats, and rodents serve as reservoirs of infection for human beings. Leishmaniasis is endemic in Mediterranean countries and some parts of Africa, India, and Central and South America. The disease, which can occur in cutaneous, mucocutaneous, or visceral forms, is rare in animals in the United States except in endemic areas in Oklahoma, Texas, and Ohio. However, visceral leishmaniasis has been identified recently in about 21 states in the United States and in southern Canada, indicating an increase in the prevalence of this disease. Infections in animals in the United States also have been associated with foreign travel of human beings and their animals.

The skin is one of the main organs affected in systemic leishmaniasis in dogs. Resistance to infection is dependent upon a $CD4^+$ T_H1 lymphocyte immune response, and lesion severity and character vary with host immune response and concurrent disease. Dogs with the alopecic form of the cutaneous disease have fewer organisms and a more robust cellular immune response including larger numbers of antigen-presenting Langerhans' cells, MHC II-positive keratinocytes, and infiltrating T lymphocytes. In contrast, dogs with the nodular form of cutaneous disease have fewer antigen-presenting cells and greater numbers of macrophages and larger numbers of organisms. Therefore it has been suggested that the clinical and histologic lesions can be useful in establishing a prognosis for remission, in that the character of the lesions reflects immune competence. Cutaneous lesions in dogs consist of generalized alopecia with silvery white scales, or more severe lesions of nodules and ulcers. Lesions occur chiefly in anatomic areas where sandflies feed—around the muzzle (nose), ears, and eyes. Paronychia and deformed claws have also been reported. Microscopically, lesions include hyperkeratosis, parakeratosis, crusts, and granulomatous nodules in the dermis including periadnexal regions. Accumulations of macrophages, lymphocytes, and plasma cells can efface sebaceous glands. *Leishmania* sp. are most commonly identified within macrophages, however, they can occasionally be found within other leukocytes, endothelial cells, or fibroblasts. In areas of necrosis, the organisms can be free within the interstitium. *Leishmania* sp. can be distinguished from other protozoa via light microscopy by recognizing the kinetoplast oriented perpendicular to the nucleus. Cytology, immunohistochemistry, PCR, and serologic testing can help confirm the diagnosis.

Mechanisms of Tissue Damage in Hypersensitivity or Autoimmune Diseases

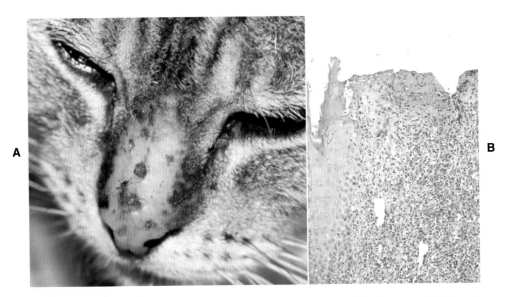

Fig. 17-63   **Resolving mosquito bite hypersensitivity dermatitis, skin, face, cat. A,** Alopecia, erythema, and erosions are present. Note the mosquito that is biting the skin. The two red depressions nearest the mosquito are healing biopsy sites collected previously during a more active stage of the disease. Mosquitoes have been kept away from this cat for one week, allowing the active lesions of hemorrhagic crusting to resolve. **B,** The dermis under the ulcer is heavily infiltrated with eosinophils, lymphocytes, and plasma cells. H&E stain. (**A,** *Courtesy of Dr. Kenneth V. Mason, Animal Allergy and Dermatology Service, Springwood, Queensland, Australia.* **B,** *Courtesy Dr. Ann M. Hargis, DermatoDiagnostics.*)

with foci of degranulated eosinophils (flame figures) and eosinophilic folliculitis and furunculosis. The epidermis is acanthotic with foci of erosion, ulceration, and cellular crusting (Fig. 17-63).

ALLERGIC CONTACT DERMATITIS

Allergic contact dermatitis, an example of a type IV hypersensitivity reaction, is due primarily to contact with chemicals such as aniline dyes in carpets, plant resins, chemicals in shampoo, and historically to plastics in food dishes. These chemical substances contain low molecular weight haptens that require binding to cell-associated proteins before they are recognized by cytotoxic T lymphocytes (CD8+). Lesions develop upon reexposure to the antigen. The lesions are pruritic, result in self-inflicted trauma, vary in severity, and are located in regions in contact with the antigen, typically in areas of glabrous (smooth and bare or hairless) skin unless the antigen is a liquid or aerosol. Grossly, lesions consist of erythema, papules with or without vesicles, and exudates that develop into crusts. Chronic lesions consist of lichenification, hyperpigmentation, and alopecia. Early microscopic lesions are spongiotic superficial perivascular dermatitis with lymphocytes, macrophages, and, usually, infrequent eosinophils. However, some lesions have many perivascular eosinophils and eosinophilic epidermal pustules. More chronic lesions, often those identified in biopsy samples, have acanthosis and foci of parakeratotic cellular crusts. Lesions associated with self-induced trauma can also be seen.

HYPERSENSITIVITY REACTIONS TO DRUGS

Hypersensitivity reactions to drugs are uncommon in dogs and cats, are rare in other domestic animals, and can result from any of the four types of hypersensitivity reactions. The drugs most commonly associated with hypersensitivity reactions include penicillins and trimethoprim-potentiated sulfonamides, but many drugs can cause a hypersensitivity reaction. Gross and microscopic lesions vary greatly. Microscopic lesions have different histopathologic patterns and include perivascular dermatitis, interface dermatitis, epidermal necrosis, vasculitis, vesiculopustular dermatitis, necrotizing dermatitis, perforating folliculitis (i.e., furunculosis), or panniculitis.

SELECTED AUTOIMMUNE REACTIONS
REACTIONS CHARACTERIZED GROSSLY BY VESICLES OR BULLAE AS THE PRIMARY LESION AND HISTOLOGICALLY BY ACANTHOLYSIS

Pemphigus is a group of diseases clinically characterized by transient vesicles or bullae and histologically by acantholysis (Table 17-12). This group of diseases is

Table **17-12**   Immune-Mediated Dermatoses in Which Bullae Form within or below the Epidermis

Disorder	Species	Prevalence	Clinical Distribution	Target	Location of Bullae
Pemphigus foliaceus	Dog Cat Horse Goat	Common	Skin	Desmoglein 1 in human beings and about 6% of affected dogs	
Pemphigus foliaceus subtype (pan-epidermal pustular pemphigus)	Dog	Uncommon	Oral Skin	Undetermined, possibly multiple antigens	
Pemphigus vulgaris	Dog Cat Horse Goat	Rare	Oral Skin	Desmoglein 3	
Paraneoplastic pemphigus	Dog	Rare	Intraepidermal Oral Skin	210 kD envoplakin 190 kD periplakin 170 kD uncharacterized	
Bullous pemphigoid	Dog Cat Horse Pig	Rare	Mucosal epithelium and skin	BP 180 BPAG2 Type XVII collagen (NC16A domain of BPAG2)	
Epidermolysis bullosa acquisita (EBA)	Dog	One of the more common of these bullous dermatoses	Oral Skin, areas of trauma	Type VII collagen, anchoring fibrils in sublamina densa	

BP, Bullous pemphigoid; *BPAG*, bullous pemphigoid antigen; *IgA*, immunoglobulin A; *LAD-1*, leukocyte adhesion deficiency-1; *SLE*, systemic lupus erythematosus.

(Continued)

Table **17-12**   **Immune-Mediated Dermatoses in Which Bullae Form within or below the Epidermis—Cont'd**

Disorder	Species	Prevalence	Clinical Distribution	Target	Location of Bullae
Linear IgA dermatosis	Dog	Rare	Oral Skin	Extracellular portion of BPAG2 after intracellular transmembrane and NC16A domains have been removed by proteolysis; 120 kD linear IgA (LAD-1) in upper lamina lucida	
Mucous membrane pemphigoid	Dog	Rare	Oral Skin	97 kD antigen, possibly C-terminus of BPAG2 and laminin-5 in lower lamina lucida	
Lupus erythematosus* (systemic and cutaneous forms)	Dog Cat Horse	Uncommon	Oral Skin Systemic form	Many membrane and solid antigens including DNA, RNA, nucleoprotein, histone-related antigens, and in bullous SLE subtype, type VII collagen	

*The level of bulla formation depends on subtype of lupus erythematosus and antigen targeted, typically subepidermal with basal cell degeneration. Bullous SLE subtype is similar to EBA.

caused by a type II response and involves autoantibodies produced against proteins responsible for keratinocyte cell-to-cell adhesion (desmosomes). Recall that desmosomes are the sites where cells of the stratum spinosum attach to each other, and during fixation and processing for microscopic examination, the cells of the stratum spinosum contract, except for the desmosomal attachments, which provide the appearance of "spines" or intercellular bridges (see Morphology of the Skin, Epidermis).These desmosomal protein antigens are found in various stratified squamous epithelia including skin, mucocutaneous junctions, oral mucosa, esophagus, and vagina. Damage to desmosomes results in acantholysis, which leads to the formation of vesicles or bullae within varying levels of the epidermis according to the location of the target antigen. The pathogenesis of acantholysis is unknown, but the autoantibodies themselves induce acantholysis and thus are considered pathogenic. In addition, complement activation or activation of the plasminogen-plasmin system independent of complement may play a role. However, studies using plasminogen activator knockout mice suggest that this system may not be necessary for blister formation as once thought. Other mechanisms involved in acantholysis include release of keratinocyte-derived cytokines, including IL-1 and TNF-α. Other autoantibodies may contribute by weakening intercellular adhesion by interfering with desmosomal protein expression or preventing new production of desmosomes. The severity of clinical disease is related to the depth of the formation of the bullae. The more severe signs are caused by separations deep within the epidermis, and the more mild signs are caused by separations in the subcorneal epidermis.

Pemphigus foliaceus

Pemphigus foliaceus (PF) is the most common and milder form of pemphigus and in domestic animals has been reported in the dog, cat, horse, and goat. The disease develops spontaneously and, in dogs and cats, as an adverse reaction to drug therapy. In human beings, PF autoantibodies recognize the desmosomal protein, desmoglein 1, which is expressed predominantly

in the upper layers of the epidermis and in small amounts in the oral mucosa. Thus antibodies targeting desmoglein 1 cause cutaneous, rather than oral lesions, and the acantholytic process occurs at a superficial level in the epidermis, producing clinical lesions that are typically exfoliative (Fig. 17-64). Pemphigus foliaceus in animals is thought to be similar to that in human beings. In fact, autoantibodies to desmoglein 1 have been identified in the serum of a small percentage of dogs with pemphigus foliaceus. However, autoantibodies to other keratinocyte antigens and to the basement membrane were identified in affected dogs, indicating that canine pemphigus foliaceus is an immunologically heterogeneous disease. Autoantibodies involved in the development of pemphigus foliaceus have not been

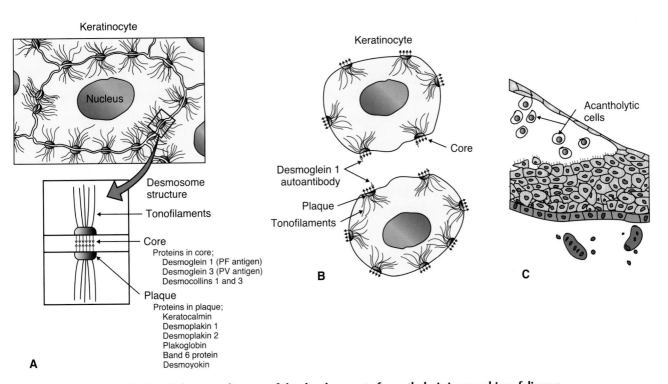

Fig. 17-64   Schematic diagram of the development of acantholysis in pemphigus foliaceus.
In human beings and about 6% of dogs with pemphigus foliaceus, acantholysis develops when autoantibodies bind to desmoglein 1, a glycoprotein within the extracellular core of the desmosome.
A, Desmosomes provide physical connections between keratinocytes and consist of keratinocyte tonofilaments, an intracytoplasmic plaque region where tonofilaments insert, and an extracellular core region. Proteins in the plaque region consist of desmoplakins, plakoglobuin, and others. Proteins in the core region consist of desmogleins 1 and 3 and desmocollins 1 and 3.
B, Autoantibody attaches to desmoglein 1, which is located predominantly in desmosomes of the upper layers of the epidermis. Simple binding of the autoantibody to desmoglein 1 induces keratinocyte detachment, probably by impairing function of desmoglein 1. Keratinocyte-released cytokines or other autoantibodies may contribute by further weakening cell-to-cell attachment.
C, An intraepidermal vesicle containing acantholytic keratinocytes is the result of loss of desmosomes between keratinocytes in the upper layers of the epidermis. *PF,* Pemphigus foliaceus; *PV,* pemphigus vulgaris. (**A, B,** *and* **C,** *Adapted from Rubin E, Farber JL: Pathology, ed 3, Philadelphia, 1999, Lippincott-Raven; and Lin MS, Mascaro JM Jr, Liu Z et al: Clin Exp Immunol 107 suppl 1:9-15, 1997.)*

studied in cats, horses, or goats. The gross lesions are similar in all species. The primary lesions consist of transient vesicles that rapidly become pustules, which can be localized to specific areas of the skin (nose, pinnae, periocular skin, footpads, claw beds, coronary bands), or can be more generalized and symmetric. The pustules are in the superficial epidermis, covered by only a small amount of stratum corneum or a few epidermal cells. Because the pustules are fragile, they quickly rupture from minor mechanical pressure on the surface, and this leads to secondary crusts, scales, alopecia, and superficial erosions (Fig. 17-16). In the dog and cat, lesions tend to appear first on the nose, and then spread to periorbital areas, the ears, neck, and ventral abdomen. Involvement of the feet produces marked papillary hyperkeratosis and crusting of the footpads, and there is a predilection for the claw beds, occasionally leading to sloughing of claws. In cats, lesions are often seen around the nipples in addition to lesions on the face and ears. In horses, lesions often begin on the face or distal extremities, or can be localized to the coronary bands. In any species the lesions can become generalized.

Microscopically, acantholysis results in the formation of very transient "vesicles" (in animals the vesicle stage is not a major clinical feature as it is in human beings because the vesicle stage in animals very rapidly progresses to the pustular stage). Pustules form and progress to crusts. In the horse, subcorneal or intragranular pustules that contain the acantholytic cells are observed, but in the dog pustules often are in the stratum spinosum. Crusts should be included in the biopsy sample, especially if well-developed pustules are no longer present, as laminated crusts with acantholytic cells can help establish the histologic diagnosis. The laminated crusts are composed of multiple layers of dried pustules, one on top of the other. The dermis contains perivascular to interstitial accumulations of mixed inflammatory cells. Eosinophils are the predominant inflammatory cell in about one third of the canine and equine cases. Deposition of IgG at intercellular bridges in all layers of the suprabasilar epidermis or in the superficial epidermis demonstrated by immunofluorescence (IF) or immunohistochemistry (IHC) is a feature of PF, but is not specific for PF. With immunostaining there are frequent false negative results (poor lesion selection or prior glucocorticoid or immunosuppressive therapy) and false positive results (chronic skin lesions with plasma cells and secondary immunoglobulin diffusion into the epidermis), thus immunostaining must be interpreted carefully and in conjunction with clinical and histologic findings.

Pemphigus vulgaris

Pemphigus vulgaris (PV) is a very severe form of pemphigus and has been reported in the dog, cat, horse, and goat (Table 17-12). In the dog, autoantibodies are formed against desmoglein 3, one of the prominent desmosomal proteins involved in adhesion of basal cells of the epidermis and mucosal epithelium, thus lesions in pemphigus vulgaris, in contrast to pemphigus foliaceus, occur deeper in the epidermis and also in the oral mucosa. Microscopic lesions consist of separation of keratinocytes of the lower epidermis owing to loss of intercellular attachments. However, basal cell keratinocytes remain attached to the basement membrane, resulting in a suprabasilar vesicle leaving a row of basal cells attached to the basement membrane ("row of tombstones") (Fig. 17-17). There usually is accompanying superficial perivascular to interface mixed inflammation. Vesicles or secondary erosions and ulcers are found in the oral mucosa, at mucocutaneous junctions, and skin subject to mechanical stress such as in the axilla or groin. Animals can be febrile, depressed, and anorectic and have leukocytosis. Drooling is often a presenting complaint, as involvement of the oral mucosa is almost always present.

Paraneoplastic pemphigus

Paraneoplastic pemphigus (PNP) is an aggressive form of pemphigus associated with solid or hematopoietic neoplasms (Table 17-12). One documented case in the dog could not be demonstrated to be associated with the presence of a neoplasm, so it is possible for this condition to occur without a concurrent malignancy. PNP has been documented in human beings and dogs. Cutaneous lesions can precede detection of the neoplastic process, and are resistant to treatment. Lesions consist of severe mucosal and mucocutaneous blistering and erosions. Histologically, lesions have a pattern of combined erythema multiforme and suprabasilar acantholysis resembling pemphigus vulgaris. One case of PNP-like disease in the horse has been documented, but in the horse there was dermoepidermal separation characteristic of bullous pemphigoid rather than pemphigus vulgaris. Lymphohistiocytic cell–rich interface dermatitis with apoptosis of keratinocytes is present. In addition, lymphocytes border apoptotic keratinocytes (this is often called "lymphocytic satellitosis"). Labeling of intercellular bridges is detected by IHC or IF. In human beings, immunoprecipitation reveals a typical set of five protein bands with molecular weights of 250, 230, 210, 190, and 170 kD. These protein bands have been identified as desmoplakins I and II, bullous pemphigoid antigen 1, envoplakin and periplakin. In one dog, immunoprecipitation revealed the main antigen targets were 210, 190, and 170 kD.

Pemphigus foliaceus subtypes

Pemphigus foliaceus subtypes, called "panepidermal pustular pemphigus" (PPP) by some veterinary dermatopathologists, refers to a form of pemphigus in the dog that has some of the features of PF, pemphigus vegetans, and pemphigus erythematosus. It is considered to be a subtype or variant of PF. It is similar to PF in that lesions develop in the superficial epidermis, but lesions are not restricted to the superficial layers of the epidermis and thus it does not neatly fit the same criteria as PF. Immunological studies have not definitively documented the presence of autoantibodies to desmosomal or hemidesmosomal proteins in PPP, but new studies evaluating autoantibody epidermal binding patterns in dogs with pemphigus foliaceus have identified four main IgG intercellular epidermal patterns. One of the patterns was seen in dogs with autoantibodies against desmoglein 1 (and thus is consistent with pemphigus foliaceus). Other IgG autoantibodies have been detected against intracellular keratinocyte antigens in the stratum basale, spinosum granulosum, and corneum as well as antibasement membrane antibodies. These studies suggest that superficial forms of pemphigus in the dog are heterogeneous immunologically, and these antibody-binding patterns may explain the variation in location of epidermal pustules in canine pemphigus foliaceus. Original designations of pemphigus vegetans and pemphigus erythematosus in animals were based on similarities to the human conditions. Further studies suggest the conditions are not directly comparable. Pemphigus erythematosus was considered to be a variant of PF with a facial or "lupus" lesion distribution occurring in dogs and cats. Criteria for diagnosis and differentiation from PF were dependent upon the immunological demonstration of both a diffuse cell surface IF or IHC pattern typical of the pemphigus group plus a linear band of immunoglobulin, with or without complement, deposited at the basement membrane zone. False-positive and false-negative IF and IHC results occur with such frequency that using these criteria to establish pemphigus erythematosus as a separate disease entity has come under scrutiny. Reported cases of pemphigus vegetans in veterinary patients are very limited and originally were thought to be benign variants of pemphigus vulgaris. The lack of clear clinical or histologic distinction between pemphigus vegetans and pemphigus erythematosus in the dog has led to the new inclusive entity of PPP by some veterinary dermatopathologists; however, this classification is controversial. Features used to differentiate PPP from typical cases of PF are discussed next.

Panepidermal pustular pemphigus is less common than PF. Akitas and Chow chows are predisposed to develop both entities. Although initially the character and distribution of gross lesions are similar and consist of erythematous macules followed by vesiculopustular lesions, over time the lesions of PPP progress to proliferative, scaly and crusted plaques or papules.

Verrucous vegetations studded with small pustules are characteristic. Depigmentation of the nasal planum can develop. The predominant histologic lesions are numerous, large, intraepithelial pustules composed of eosinophils, neutrophils, and a few to large numbers of acantholytic epithelial cells that develop at various levels of the epidermis, including the subcorneal epithelium through and including the suprabasal layers. The pustules also involve the infundibular outer root sheath, and eosinophilic to neutrophilic intrainfundibular mural folliculitis can be present. In mature lesions, there is papillated epidermal hyperplasia. The dermis has perivascular to interstitial mixed cellular infiltrates including eosinophils. Biopsy samples from the mucocutaneous junction or the nasal planum can be intensely plasmacytic with a dense band of inflammation parallel to the epidermal dermal interface. IFA or IHC may demonstrate immunoglobulin at intercellular bridges and/or the basement membrane zone; however results can be variable. Histological differentials include predominantly facial PF, bacterial pustular dermatitis, and dermatophytosis.

REACTIONS CHARACTERIZED GROSSLY BY VESICLES OR BULLAE AS THE PRIMARY LESION AND HISTOLOGICALLY BY VESICLES OR BULLAE WITHIN THE BASEMENT MEMBRANE (BULLOUS DERMATOSES)

Bullous dermatoses are a rare group of disorders caused by autoantibodies directed toward one or more antigens within the basement membrane zone (see Morphology of the Skin, Basement Membrane Zone; and Table 17-12), and characterized clinically and histologically by vesicles and bullae. The disorders include bullous pemphigoid (autoantibodies against bullous pemphigoid antigen 2 [BPAG2; BP180], which is type XVII collagen, a hemidesmosomal transmembrane molecule), epidermolysis bullosa acquisita (autoantibodies against type VII collagen in the anchoring fibrils), linear IgA bullous dermatosis (autoantibodies against the 120-kD linear IgA bullous dermatosis antigen [LAD-1] in the upper lamina lucida), mucous membrane pemphigoid (autoantibodies against a 97-kD antigen in the lower lamina lucida, and laminin-5), and bullous systemic lupus erythematosus (autoantibodies against the noncollagenous amino terminus of type VII collagen) reported in one dog.

Bullous pemphigoid

Bullous pemphigoid (BP) is caused by autoantibodies directed against hemidesmosomal proteins. In human beings the autoantibodies are directed toward bullous pemphigoid antigen 1 (BPAG1, a 230-kD intercellular antigen) and bullous pemphigoid antigen 2 (BPAG2, also called type XVII collagen, a 180-kD hemidesmosomal transmembrane molecule). In animals, only bullous pemphigoid antigen 2 has been identified. The location and character of clinical lesions are similar to those of pemphigus vulgaris (e.g., vesicles that progress to erosions and ulcers in the oral mucosa, mucocutaneous junctional skin, and skin in the axilla or groin). Bullous pemphigoid has been reported in the dog, cat, horse, and pig (Fig. 17-65). Separation of the hemidesmosomes of the basal layer cells from the upper lamina lucida of the basement membrane leads to the microscopic lesions of vesicles and bullae. Direct immunofluorescence staining most commonly reveals IgG and complement linearly distributed at the dermoepidermal junction. Evaluation of salt-split epithelial substrates with indirect immunofluorescence reveals staining on

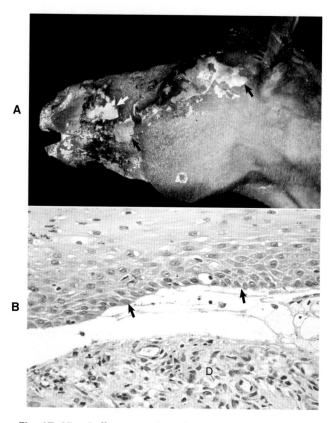

Fig. 17-65   Bullous pemphigoid-like dermatitis, skin. A, Bullous pemphigoid-like dermatitis, face, horse. Severe ulceration and hemorrhage are present in the skin, especially lateral to and above the eye, on the nose, and on the chin. Both cutaneous and mucocutaneous sites of the body lined by stratified squamous epithelium were affected. The epidermis had separated easily from the underlying dermis, leading to the formation of vesicles, bullae, and areas of ulceration *(arrows).* **B,** Subepidermal bullous dermatosis, dog. Note subepidermal vesicle formed when the intact epidermis, including the stratum basale *(arrows)* separated from the dermis *(D).* H&E stain. *(**A,** Courtesy Dr. S. Terrell, College of Veterinary Medicine, University of Florida. **B,** Courtesy Dr. Ann M. Hargis, DermatoDiagnostics.)*

the epithelial side of the artificial split, helping to differentiate bullous pemphigoid from epidermolysis bullosa acquisita and mucous membrane pemphigoid that are located in the sublamina densa or lower lamina lucida, respectively. The presence of eosinophils is considered to be suggestive of bullous pemphigoid. A superficial perivascular to dense band of inflammation parallel to the epidermal dermal interface can also be present, particularly if ulceration has occurred.

REACTIONS CHARACTERIZED GROSSLY BY DEPIGMENTATION, PLEOMORPHIC PAPULAR TO MACULAR ERUPTIONS, OR ULCERATION AND HISTOLOGICALLY BY BASAL CELL OR KERATINOCYTE DEGENERATION OR INTERFACE INFLAMMATION

Lupus erythematosus

Systemic lupus erythematosus (SLE) is a multiorgan disease of dogs and rarely cats and horses. Factors involved in development include genetic predisposition, viral infections, hormones, and UV light. SLE is a disease of immune dysregulation, with abnormalities in both cellular and humoral immunity, including defective T-lymphocyte suppressor function and cytokine dysregulation. The defective T-lymphocyte suppression function may be due to anti–T-lymphocyte antibodies or a primary suppressor T-lymphocyte deficiency. The defective T-lymphocyte suppression function results in B-lymphocyte hyperactivity and in the formation of autoantibodies to a variety of membrane and soluble antigens, including nucleic acids. Antibodies are also directed to organ-specific antigens, clotting factors, and cells (e.g., erythrocytes, leukocytes, platelets). A bullous form of systemic lupus erythematosus caused by autoantibody directed to type VII collagen has been reported in one dog (bullous SLE). Although the autoantibodies can damage tissue, the principal mechanism of injury in SLE occurs via antigen-antibody binding (i.e., immune-complex formation), and deposition of the antigen-antibody complexes in a variety of tissues, including skin. The deposition of these immune complexes, which in the skin occurs at the basement membrane and in the walls of dermal blood vessels, results in a type III hypersensitivity response. Lesions are intensified by exposure to UV light. The enhanced damage may occur via UV-induced expression of nuclear antigens on the keratinocyte surface, autoantibody binding to the newly expressed antigens with resultant keratinocyte damage, and release of keratinocyte cytokines (e.g., Il-1, Il-6, and TNF-α). Ultraviolet light may also act by inducing the expression of adhesion molecules, thus facilitating trafficking of leukocytes to the epidermis. Systemic signs are variable, but can include polyarthritis, fever, anemia, proteinuria (from glomerulonephritis), and thrombocytopenia.

Cutaneous lesions are highly variable, can be localized or generalized, but commonly involve the face, pinnae, and distal extremities. Lesions consist of erythema, depigmentation, alopecia, scaling, crusting, and ulceration. Stomatitis or panniculitis can be present. Microscopic lesions include lymphohistiocytic interface dermatitis with basal cell apoptosis, pigmentary incontinence, and the presence of subepidermal vacuolization. The basal cell degeneration and subepidermal vacuolization can lead to formation of subepidermal vesicles, which can rapidly ulcerate and crust. Basement membrane thickening caused by accumulation of immune complexes, and immune-complex vasculitis of small dermal vessels can also be seen.

Discoid lupus erythematosus (DLE), also called localized cutaneous lupus erythematosus and photosensitive nasal dermatitis, is seen most commonly in the dog but is rare in the cat and horse. Historically, DLE has been considered to be a mild variant of SLE in which there is no involvement of other organ systems and the antinuclear antibody titer is negative. However, with the recent recognition of another disease, "mucocutaneous pyoderma" (see Superficial Bacterial Infections [Superficial Pyodermas], Mucocutaneous Pyoderma), and the clinical and histological overlap between localized cutaneous lupus erythematosus and mucocutaneous pyoderma, the classification of DLE as a distinct entity is being revisited. Investigative studies are needed to better define these two conditions. Clinical lesions of DLE consist of depigmentation, erythema, scaling, erosion, ulceration, and crusting, and generally occur in the skin of the nasal planum, dorsal surface of the nose, and less commonly, the pinnae, lips, and periocular region, and in the oral mucosa. DLE can be exacerbated by sunlight. Microscopic lesions include accumulations of lymphocytes and plasma cells at the epidermal dermal interface. In early cases the infiltrate can be sparse, but in some cases the lymphocytes and plasma cells are arranged in a dense bandlike pattern that obscures the epidermal-dermal interface. In addition, there are apoptotic basal cells resulting in loss of epidermal pigment that is phagocytosed by dermal macrophages (pigmentary incontinence). As with SLE, the basal cell degeneration can, in more severe cases, lead to subepidermal vesicles, loss of the epidermis, and ulceration and crusting. Other forms of lupus erythematosus also uncommonly occur in dogs.

Exfoliative cutaneous lupus erythematosus is formerly known as lupoid dermatosis of the German shorthair pointer. Lesions develop in German shorthair pointers between 3 months and 3 years of age. Clinical lesions consist of scaling and crusting first seen on the face, ears, and back. Lesions then become generalized. The lesions persist, but wax and wane. Fever and lymphadenopathy can be present. Rarely there is a positive antinuclear antibody titer. Histologic lesions consist of lymphocytic interface dermatitis with hydropic degeneration of basal cells and apoptosis of keratinocytes. Interface inflammation also affects the basilar epithelium of follicles and sebaceous glands, resulting in sebaceous gland atrophy.

Vesicular cutaneous lupus erythematosus is a disorder formerly known as ulcerative dermatosis of the collie and Shetland sheepdog. Lesions develop in middle age to older dogs. The Shetland sheepdog and collie appear predisposed to lesion development. Clinical lesions develop in the groin and axillary areas and consist of vesicles and bullae that progress to ulcers. Lesions can be cyclic, and worsen in association with estrus. Histologic lesions include interface lymphocytic dermatitis with hydropic degeneration of basal cells, keratinocyte apoptosis, and extensive vesicles and bullae at the epidermal-dermal junction that progress to ulcers.

Lupus panniculitis is a rare manifestation of lupus erythematosus, and is seen in dogs. Clinical lesions consist of nodules occurring predominantly in the subcutis of the trunk and proximal aspects of the legs. Histologic lesions consist of nodular masses of lymphoplasmacytic and histiocytic inflammation often with fat necrosis. Vasculitis can also be present. In addition, there may be apoptotic basal cell degeneration, pigmentary incontinence, and thickening of the basement membrane.

Erythema multiforme (EM), Stevens-Johnson syndrome (SJS), and toxic epidermal necrolysis (TEN)

These are uncommon to rare diseases affecting the skin and sometimes mucous membranes. The conditions can be the result of adverse drug reactions, secondary to systemic or localized infections or neoplasia, or may be idiopathic. There is considerable overlap in both gross and histological lesions among EM, SJS, and TEN, with clinical forms varying from mild to very severe. Future in-depth studies of these cases scrutinizing the character and extent of clinical and histological lesions in correlation with the clinical history may help determine the likelihood of drug causation. In human beings, studies of this nature have indicated that drugs are the more likely cause in patients with more severe lesions of the epidermis (SJS, TEN), whereas patients with less severe lesions (EM) were more likely to be associated with an underlying infection, particularly with herpesvirus. Results of these studies in animals are not yet available.

EM has been seen in dogs, cats, horses, and cattle and is characterized clinically initially by circular areas of erythema. The erythema disappears from the center of the lesions, producing targetlike lesions that are most common on the trunk and groin. Papules, vesicles, ulcers, erosions, and serpiginous erythematous lesions also can be seen (Fig. 17-13). Histologically, individual keratinocytes in all layers of the epidermis undergo apoptosis (Fig. 17-13) and are surrounded by lymphocytes (lymphocytic satellitosis). Apoptotic keratinocytes can coalesce, leading to the clinically visible erosions and possibly ulcers. Hydropic lymphocytic interface dermatitis of varying severity is also present. Mucous membranes can be involved in the more severe forms of EM (EM major), and some refer to the more severe form of EM as the Stevens-Johnson syndrome. The condition can be self-limiting. Graft-versus-host disease, seen after bone marrow transplantation, is similar histologically to erythema multiforme. TEN is seen principally in dogs and cats, is a more serious condition than EM, and may overlap in the spectrum of gross and histological lesions with the more severe forms of EM and with the SJS. TEN is a life-threatening, severe ulcerative disorder of the skin and oral mucous membranes that begins clinically as widespread erythematous macules that coalesce. Later there is full-thickness epidermal necrosis that results in large subepidermal bullae and widespread ulceration as the necrotic epidermis is sloughed. Lesions are often present on the face, mucocutaneous junctions, and footpads, but can be more widespread. Histologically there is full-thickness coagulative necrosis of the epidermis, with separation of the epidermis from the dermis forming bullae, which detach and leave the dermis denuded. Dermal inflammation in the acute lesions is minimal.

Uveodermatologic syndrome (Vogt-Koyanagi-Harada-like [VKH] syndrome)

This is a rare syndrome of histiocytic interface dermatitis and granulomatous uveitis in dogs, particularly akitas, Chow chows, samoyeds, and Siberian huskies. The pathogenesis is thought to involve an immune-mediated attack against melanin or melanocytes. Ocular lesions usually develop before cutaneous lesions. Clinical lesions consist of symmetrical patchy to diffuse depigmentation of the skin of the nose, lips, eyelids, and footpads. Lesions are occasionally more widespread. Leukotrichia of adjacent hair can be present. Uncommonly lesions are more severe, and consist of erosion, ulceration, and crusting. Fully developed histologic lesions are cell-rich interface inflammation, primarily of histiocytic cells containing melanin pigment (pigmentary incontinence). Basal cell degeneration is uncommon.

REACTIONS CHARACTERIZED GROSSLY BY HEMORRHAGE, EDEMA, NECROSIS, ULCERATION, INFARCTION, OR BY ALOPECIA AND SCARRING AND HISTOLOGICALLY BY VASCULITIS OR THROMBOSIS

In human medicine, two principal mechanisms are thought to contribute to the pathogenesis of vasculitis; these include direct invasion of vessels by infectious agents (e.g., *Rickettsia*, herpesvirus) and immune-mediated mechanisms (immune-complex formation, antineutrophil cytoplasmic antibodies, and antiendothelial cell antibodies). This is likely true for vasculitis in animals. Evidence for the role of immune-complex deposition is derived from experimental studies (Arthus phenomenon and serum sickness), and from identification of immune complexes in serum and tissues in patients with vasculitis caused by infectious agents and hypersensitivity reactions to drugs. Thus infectious agents can contribute to immune complex–mediated vasculitis. The immune complexes can form in the circulation, in the vessel wall, or both. The role for antineutrophil cytoplasmic antibodies in causing cutaneous vasculitis is less clear. Although these antibodies are present in the serum of patients with vasculitis, there is no proof that these antibodies actually play a causative role. It is thought that the antibodies form after an initial stimulus, such as an infection, which causes release of proinflammatory cytokines (TNF) and microbial products (endotoxin). These inflammatory mediators can cause neutrophils to express surface receptors (i.e., proteinase-3 and myeloperoxidase) against which the antibodies develop. It is theorized that the binding of the antibodies to receptors on activated neutrophils causes neutrophil degranulation and damage to tissue, including damage to endothelial cells. Resultant endothelial-cell damage potentially could cause release of "non-self" antigens and stimulation of additional antibody or cell-mediated immune responses, further perpetuating vascular injury.

Dermatomyositis and similar disorders with cutaneous and vascular lesions

Dermatomyositis is an inherited disease with variable expressivity that occurs in juvenile and adult onset forms in collies and Shetland sheepdogs (Fig. 17-66). Other breeds are occasionally affected. The pathogenesis involves vasculitis of skin, muscle, and sometimes other tissues. The vascular lesions are subtle and include mild thickening of the vessel wall, occasionally pyknotic cells in the vessel wall, and occasionally lymphocytes within the wall; these changes are termed "cell-poor" vasculitis. Circulating immune complexes have been identified, and likely play a role. Dermatomyositis develops in puppies as early as 8 weeks of age. Early lesions include vesicular dermatitis of face, lips, and external ears, which progresses to involve the distal extremities,

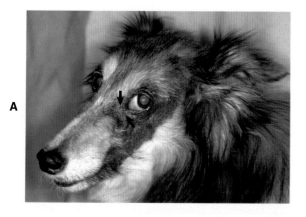

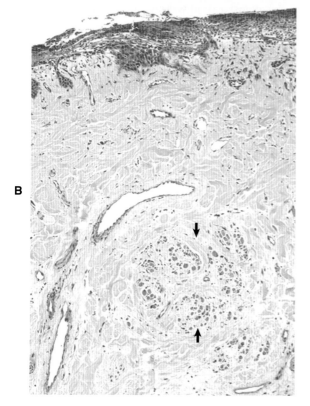

Fig. 17-66   Dermatomyositis, skin, dog. A, Face. Chronic lesions of hair loss, hyperpigmentation, and scarring are present in the skin around the eye and on the lateral side of the face. Interface dermatitis, myositis, and vasculitis have resulted in ischemic follicular atrophy, muscle atrophy, and scarring. The scarring and possibly also some muscle atrophy have contributed to the contraction of the skin of the eyelid and the inability to close the eyelids fully at the medial canthus (*arrows*). **B,** Lip. Erosion is present on the surface of the lip skin at the far right. Atrophy of the dermis and adnexa (adnexa not present here) can predispose to injury of the epidermis and superficial dermis by minor trauma. Muscle atrophy (*arrows*) and scarring around the muscle fibers are present. If muscle is present in skin biopsy samples with features of dermatomyositis, and if muscle atrophy or myositis are seen, the diagnosis of dermatomyositis is strengthened. H&E stain. (*A* and *B,* Courtesy Dr. Ann M. Hargis, DermatoDiagnostics.)

especially over bony prominences and the tip of the tail. Myositis and atrophy of muscles of mastication, distal extremities, and, sometimes, esophagus develop after the dermatitis (Fig. 17-66). The myositis is variably severe and multifocal, but more prevalent in peripheral anatomic locations. The muscle inflammation consists of lymphocytes, plasma cells, histiocytes, and fewer neutrophils or eosinophils. Perifascicular myofiber atrophy (atrophy at the periphery of muscle fascicles) occurs occasionally. The rostral and most superficial portion of the temporalis muscle is the biopsy site of choice to confirm the myositis. Dermatomyositis varies in severity. Mild skin lesions heal without scarring, but moderate skin lesions heal with permanent foci of alopecia, hyperpigmentation, and scarring. Hypopigmentation can also develop from damage to melanin-containing cells in the basal layer of the epidermis. Skin and muscle lesions in dogs with severe disease are progressive and disfiguring, the result of severe scarring of the skin and atrophy of muscle. Microscopic skin lesions include interface dermatitis with basal cell degeneration of the epidermis and follicular wall, variable epidermal vesicles and pustules, follicular atrophy, and dermal scarring. Cell-poor vasculitis, a major feature contributing to the lesions in dermatomyositis, is not always identified in small biopsy samples. The combination of interface dermatitis and mural folliculitis with follicular atrophy and cell-poor vasculitis has been considered to represent ischemic lesions, and is referred to as "ischemic dermatopathy."

Skin and vessel lesions indistinguishable from those in dermatomyositis occur in multifocal rabies vaccine–induced dermatitis in dogs and in the syndrome of cutaneous vasculitis in Jack Russell terriers. In some of the Jack Russell terriers, cutaneous and vascular lesions develop 2 to 3 weeks after vaccination. Rabies vaccine–induced dermatitis develops as a localized form limited to the site of vaccination and as a more widespread form, both developing in the months following rabies vaccination. In the localized form, rabies antigen has been detected in follicular epithelial cells and in vessels in affected skin. In the widespread form, lesions are present at the site of vaccination, ear margins, periocular skin, and skin over bony prominences, tip of tail, and paw pads. Lingual erosions and ulcers also occur. In addition, some dogs develop perifascicular muscle atrophy and perimysial fibrosis, with C5b-9 in the microvasculature. The development of lesions after vaccination and the identification of rabies-virus antigen in the vessels and follicular epithelial cells in dogs with the localized form of rabies vaccine–induced dermatitis has resulted in the speculation that lesions might be a result of an immunological reaction to viral antigen in these sites in genetically predisposed dogs.

Familial vasculopathy of German shepherd dogs appears to have a genetic basis, but the underlying cause and pathogenesis are unknown. Cutaneous and vascular lesions have similarities to ischemic dermatopathy. Puppies, about 1 to 2 months of age are affected, and some puppies develop lesions after vaccination. The major clinical lesion is swelling of footpads, and some puppies develop ulcers on the footpads, ear margins, and tail tip, and nasal planum with depigmentation of the nasal planum or nasal commissures. Histologically, early vessel lesions include neutrophil infiltration of small venules and arterioles, but more commonly vascular lesions are subtle and consist of cell-poor vasculitis (mild thickening of the vessel wall with occasional pyknotic cells and lymphocytes within the wall). In addition, cutaneous lesions consist of mild interface dermatitis with pigmentary incontinence. The nodular lesions in footpads are in the dermis and subcutis, and early lesions consist of focal collagen degeneration bordered by neutrophils and mononuclear cells. Chronic lesions have dermal and subcutaneous fibrosis sometimes accompanied by degeneration and fibrosis of skeletal muscle bundles.

Cutaneous and renal glomerular vasculopathy of the greyhound

Greyhounds with this condition are typically from race track environments. The cause and pathogenesis are unknown; however, there is speculation that the disorder is similar to hemolytic-uremic syndrome in human beings where a verotoxin (Shiga-like toxin) damages vascular endothelium. Most racing greyhounds eat raw meats, which could contain the *Escherichia coli*-producing toxin. Clinical lesions include hemorrhagic macules that progress to deep ulcers of the tarsus, stifle, or inner thigh. Occasionally lesions develop on the front legs, groin, or trunk. Lesions heal slowly (usually over 1 to 2 months) by fibrosis. Histologically, capillaries, venules, and arterioles in the dermis and occasionally the subcutis have degenerate walls with pyknotic or karyorrhectic nuclei, and occasionally fibrinoid necrosis. Fibrin thrombi can result in cutaneous infarction. About 25% of the affected greyhounds also have systemic signs of renal failure because of glomerular arteriolar inflammation, necrosis, and thrombosis.

Cold agglutinin disease

Cold agglutinin disease is an autoimmune disease that has rarely been reported in dogs and cats, and is caused by the presence of autoantibodies directed against erythrocytes. The autoantibodies are active at cool temperatures (0° to 37° C). Clinical lesions include erythema, hemorrhage, cyanosis, necrosis, and ulceration of the extremities. Histologic lesions include edema, hemorrhage, necrosis, ulceration and inflammation associated with secondary infection. Vessels with homogeneous eosinophilic material (cryoglobulin) occasionally are identified.

DIAGNOSIS OF AUTOIMMUNE SKIN DISORDERS

The diagnosis of autoimmune disorders is based on distribution and appearance of gross and microscopic lesions. Other diagnostic tools include the demonstration of immunoglobulin (IgG, IgM, or IgA) with or without complement, via direct immunohistochemistry, in intercellular areas (pemphigus vulgaris and foliaceus), at the basement membrane (BP, SLE, DLE, and linear IgA dermatosis), or in vessels (cutaneous vasculitis), and the results of clinical immunologic tests such as antinuclear antibody titers and Coombs' test. Unfortunately, false negative and false positive results are frequent in direct immunohistochemical staining, limiting the usefulness of this procedure. Newer techniques that detect more specific antigens such as desmoglein, use of "salt-split" skin sections for subepidermal bullous diseases, and use of better substrates for indirect immunostaining improve diagnostic accuracy of immune-mediated skin diseases, but these testing procedures currently are not universally available. The "salt-split" technique uses a 1-molar solution of NaCl to split the skin through the lamina lucida. This allows identification of autoantibodies that bind to the roof (epidermal), floor (dermal), or combined sides of the split and increases accuracy of diagnosis in bullous dermatosis.

DISORDERS WITH ALOPECIA OR HYPOTRICHOSIS

Cutaneous endocrine disorders are due to imbalances in hormones and generally are manifested as nonpruritic, bilaterally symmetric alopecia or hypotrichosis (Box 17-11). The remainder of the hair coat is dull, dry, easily epilated, and fails to regrow after clipping. The epidermis is often hyperpigmented. These lesions are referred to as "endocrine alopecia." In disorders associated with alterations in sex hormones, the alopecia often begins in the perineal and genital areas and can extend cranially. However, it is not uncommon for a cutaneous endocrine disorder to have asymmetric alopecia and epidermal hyperpigmentation along with secondary pyoderma or seborrhea. Microscopically, uncomplicated endocrine disorders of the skin consist of hyperkeratosis of superficial epidermis and of hair follicles; normal, atrophic, or hyperplastic epithelium; dilated follicles from hyperkeratosis; increased numbers of catagen or telogen hair follicles; lack of hair shafts in follicles; and increased epidermal pigmentation. These general features support the diagnosis of an endocrine disease, but often are not sufficiently specific

Box 17-11

Conditions with Prominent Alopecia or Hypotrichosis

ENDOCRINE DISORDERS

Hypothyroidism
Hyperadrenocorticism
Hyperestrogenism
Alopecia X of Nordic breeds*
Hypersomatotropism
Hyposomatotropism
Cyclical flank alopecia (pineal gland)

NONENDOCRINE HAIR CYCLE ABNORMALITIES

Post clipping alopecia
Telogen effluvium
Anagen defluxion

DISORDERS ASSOCIATED WITH EXCESSIVE GROOMING

Feline psychogenic alopecia
Feline hypersensitivity reaction

FOLLICULAR DYSPLASIA SYNDROMES AND CONGENITAL ALOPECIA AND HYPOTRICHOSIS

OTHER CONDITIONS ASSOCIATED WITH ALOPECIA

Sebaceous adenitis
Folliculitis—infectious and noninfectious
Feline paraneoplastic alopecia
Poor nutrition
Postinflammatory and posttraumatic

*Alopecia X of Nordic breeds is a group of poorly characterized dermatoses, including but not limited to castration responsive dermatosis, growth hormone responsive dermatosis, and follicular dysplasia in Siberian huskies or Alaskan malamutes.

to be diagnostic for an individual endocrine disorder. Also, inflammation due to secondary seborrhea or pyoderma frequently complicates the diagnosis. Selected clinical and histologic features of individual endocrine disorders (e.g., clinical evidence of cutaneous and muscle atrophy and histologic evidence of mineral deposition in the case of hyperglucocorticoidism) in conjunction with clinical testing are used to establish a more definitive diagnosis. Cutaneous endocrine disorders are more common in dogs than in cats, food animals, or horses.

CUTANEOUS ENDOCRINE DISORDERS

HYPOTHYROIDISM

Deficiency of thyroid hormone is considered the most common endocrine disorder in dogs and is caused by idiopathic thyroid atrophy and lymphocytic thyroiditis. Thyroid hormones play an essential role in normal growth and development of many organs including the skin, and can result in a variety of systemic and cutaneous signs and lesions. In dogs, the hair follicle is considered to be an important target for thyroid hormones, where the hormones are thought to be necessary for the initiation of the anagen stage of the hair cycle. Clinical lesions of thyroid deficiency consist of a dull, dry, easily epilated hair coat that fails to regrow after clipping. Alopecia of the dorsal surface of the nose is present in some hypothyroid dogs. Symmetrical truncal alopecia is also considered to be a feature of hypothyroidism, but may not be as common as once thought. Microscopically, the primary hair follicles are usually in the telogen stage of the hair cycle, and the old primary hair shafts are retained in follicular lumens. There are increased numbers of secondary hair follicles in the telogen stage of the cycle, but these follicles generally have lost the old secondary hair shafts. Follicular infundibular hyperkeratosis with plugging of the follicular opening is also present. Other histologic changes attributed to hypothyroidism include acanthosis of epidermis and follicular infundibular epithelium, an increase in dermal mucin (myxedema), which results in dermal thickening, and vacuolated or hypertrophic arrector pili muscles. Secondary staphylococcal infection can develop.

Hypothyroidism can also be the result of congenital iodine deficiency. Iodine deficiency develops in fetuses because of maternal ingestion of diets deficient in iodine or containing substances that interfere with production of thyroid hormones (goitrogens). These factors result in insufficient synthesis of thyroxine and reduced blood levels of thyroxine and triiodothyronine. The reduced levels of these hormones are detected by the hypothalamus and pituitary gland, stimulating secretion of thyrotropin and resulting in hyperplasia of the thyroid follicular cells. Regions of North America that are deficient in iodine include the Great Lakes Basin, the Rocky Mountains, the Northern Great Plains, the upper Mississippi Valley, and the Pacific Coast region. Paradoxically, maternal diets high in iodine can also result in congenital hypothyroidism. High blood iodine also interferes with one or more steps of thyroid hormone production, leading to low blood thyroxine levels, hypothalamic and pituitary stimulation, and secretion of thyrotropin. Congenital iodine deficiency can occur in any domestic animal but usually is seen in large animals; it is associated with the birth of dead fetuses or weak neonates. These neonates can have alopecia, and thyroid glands are usually enlarged because of the follicular cell hyperplasia.

HYPERADRENOCORTICISM

Hyperadrenocorticism results in cutaneous lesions principally in dogs and cats, and is usually caused by bilateral adrenal cortical hyperplasia secondary to a pituitary neoplasm, a functional adrenal cortical neoplasm, a functional nodule of cortical hyperplasia, or the administration of exogenous glucocorticoids. In dogs, cutaneous lesions include endocrine alopecia that generally spares the head and extremities, thinning of the skin, comedones, increased bruising, poor wound healing, and increased susceptibility to infection (Fig. 17-67). Dystrophic calcification of the dermis of the back, inguinal, and axillary areas can occur in dogs, particularly in iatrogenic hyperadrenocorticism (calcinosis cutis) (Fig. 17-68). Grossly, lesions of calcinosis cutis are firm, thickened, sometimes gritty, often ulcerated and alopecic, crusted plaques or nodules (Fig. 17-68). In cats, the dermal collagen fibers can be markedly thin and atrophic, resulting in extremely

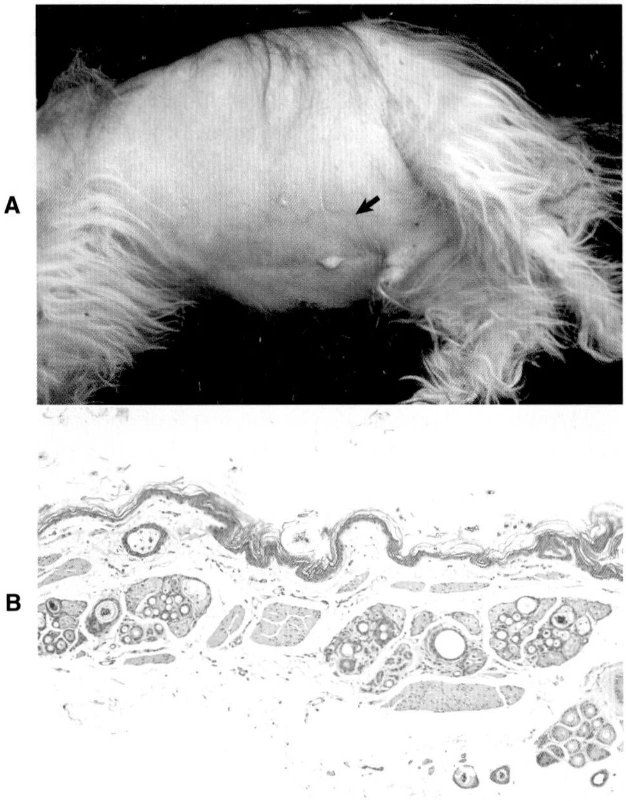

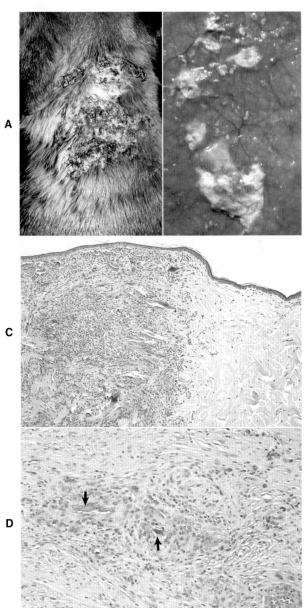

Fig. 17-68   Calcinosis cutis, hyperadrenocorticism, skin, dog. A, Dorsal neck. The skin is partially alopecic, ulcerated, and crusted. It is also palpably thickened. **B,** Subcutis. Mineral deposits are visible as white nodular foci. **C,** Skin at the margin of a plaque is thickened by dermal mineralization and granulomatous inflammation (*left half*). H&E stain. **D,** Higher magnification of dermal mineralization (*arrows*) and granulomatous inflammation. H&E stain. (**A,** *Courtesy Dr. Alan Mundell, Animal Dermatology Service.* **B,** *Courtesy Dr. M.D. McGavin, College of Veterinary Medicine, University of Tennessee.* **C** *and* **D,** *Courtesy Dr. Ann M. Hargis, DermatoDiagnostics.*)

Fig. 17-67   Truncal alopecia, hyperadrenocorticism, skin, dog. A, Note the alopecia, distended abdomen, and thin skin in which blood vessels are faintly visible (*arrow*). The distended abdomen and visibility of blood vessels are a result of protein catabolism and loss of muscle and dermal collagen, respectively. The distended abdomen and thin skin with greater visibility of blood vessels in conjunction with symmetrical alopecia suggest that a catabolic endocrine disease such as hyperadrenocorticism is likely. **B,** Atrophy of dermal collagen fibers is so severe that the collagen has almost disappeared, leaving the adnexa and arrector pili muscles readily visible. Hair follicles are in the telogen (resting) stage of the hair cycle. H&E stain. (**A,** *Courtesy Dr. Alan Mundell, Animal Dermatology Service.* **B,** *Courtesy Dr. Ann M. Hargis, DermatoDiagnostics.*)

fragile skin that can tear with normal handling. Microscopically, the lesions of hyperadrenocorticism include epidermal, dermal, and follicular atrophy (Fig. 17-67), follicular hyperkeratosis, and calcinosis cutis, especially in dogs (Fig. 17-68). A foreign body reaction (granulomatous inflammation) and draining sinuses can develop in association with the calcium deposits.

HYPERESTROGENISM

Hyperestrogenism can develop in male and female dogs. In females, the estrogen originates from ovarian cysts, rarely an ovarian neoplasm, or from estrogen administration. In males, elevated serum concentrations of estrogen are usually derived from a functional testicular Sertoli cell tumor. Iatrogenic estrogen administration has also caused hyperestrogenism in male dogs (Fig. 17-69). In addition to endocrine alopecia, female dogs have an enlarged vulva and abnormalities of the estrus cycle. Male dogs can develop gynecomastia, pendulous prepuce, or an enlarged prostate because of squamous metaplasia of prostatic ducts. Cutaneous microscopic lesions include orthokeratotic hyperkeratosis, follicular hyperkeratosis, and telogen follicles (Fig. 17-69).

ALOPECIA X OF NORDIC BREEDS (ADRENAL SEX HORMONE ALOPECIA, CASTRATION RESPONSIVE DERMATOSIS, GROWTH HORMONE RESPONSIVE DERMATOSIS)

This condition is seen most often in Nordic breeds of dogs (e.g., Pomeranian, Chow chow, Samoyed, Keeshond,

Siberian husky, Alaskan malamute, Norwegian elkhound, Finnish spitz, American Eskimo). Poodles, and sporadically other breeds of dogs, are also affected. Dogs with this condition (or conditions) are grouped together by having in common (1) plush hair coats in the normal state (e.g., when not affected with this condition), (2) alopecia sparing head and distal extremities, (3) normal thyroid and glucocorticoid levels, and (4) skin biopsy samples with telogen follicles and often prominent flame follicles (follicles with prominent tricholemmal keratin that forms spikes into the follicular stratum spinosum). The alopecia often develops at 1 or 2 years of age in otherwise healthy dogs of either sex. The alopecia is symmetric and involves the perineum, caudal thighs, ventral abdomen and thorax, neck, and trunk. The head and distal extremities are spared. Hyperpigmentation is usually present (Fig. 17-70). Thyroid function testing, ACTH (adrenocorticotropic hormone) response test, low-dose dexamethasone suppression test, and serum chemistry results are normal. Abnormalities in a number of hormones have been detected, but most work has involved the evaluation of 21-hydroxylase enzyme and other adrenocortical enzymes necessary for adrenal steroidogenesis. In the Pomeranian dog, partial deficiency of 21-hydroxylase enzyme has been detected and results in dysregulation of adrenal hormone synthesis, decreased cortisol levels, and in hyperprogestinism and hyperandrogenism (similar to late-onset, nonclassic congenital adrenal hyperplasia in human beings). Castration provides a temporary

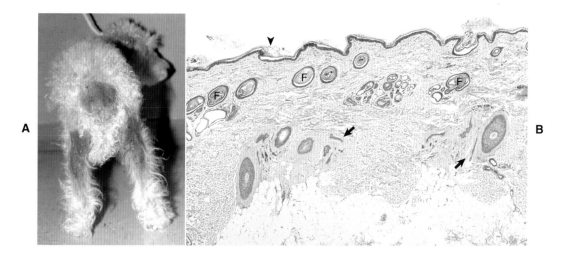

Fig. 17-69   Symmetrical alopecia and hyperpigmentation, hyperestrogenism (iatrogenic from diethylstilbestrol therapy), skin, dog. A, Note the symmetrical alopecia and hyperpigmentation over the caudal dorsal trunk and caudolateral hind legs. In male dogs, the symmetrical alopecia in conjunction with enlargement of nipples, pendulous prepuce, and attraction of other male dogs suggest the possibility of hyperestrogenism. **B,** Note epidermal orthokeratotic hyperkeratosis *(arrowhead),* follicles dilated with keratin *(F),* and small atrophic follicles *(arrows)* in the telogen (resting) stage of the hair cycle. H&E stain. *(A and B, Courtesy Dr. Ann M. Hargis, DermatoDiagnostics.)*

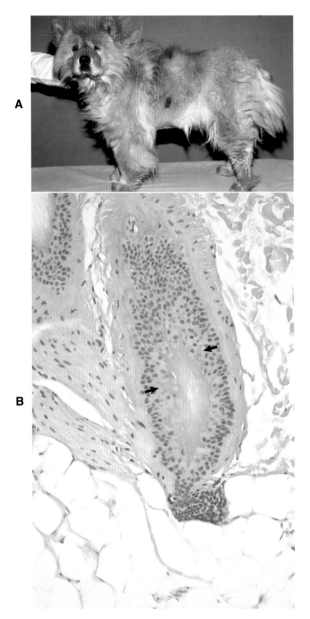

Fig. 17-70   Alopecia X, skin, dog. A, "Alopecia X of Nordic breeds," Chow chow. Note the partial alopecia and hyperpigmentation of trunk. The alopecia is not diagnostic for a specific condition. The breed suggests that alopecia X of Nordic breeds should be considered as one of the differential diagnoses. **B,** Flame follicle, haired skin. The hair follicle has excessive trichilemmal keratinization resembling the spikes *(arrows)* of a flame and consistent with a "flame follicle." H&E stain. (**A,** *Courtesy Dr. Alan Mundell, Animal Dermatology Service.* **B,** *Courtesy Dr. Ann M. Hargis, DermatoDiagnostics.*)

response to the alopecia by eliminating the influence of testicular hormones. Microscopic lesions include follicular inactivity (telogen-stage follicles without hair shafts) and prominent formation of flame follicles (Fig. 17-70, B). Prominent diffuse flame follicle formation is suggestive of alopecia X, but flame follicles can be seen normally, especially in some breeds (Shar-Pei dogs), in other endocrine dermatoses (hyperestrogenism and hyperadrenocorticism, particularly in plush-coated breeds), and in follicular dysplasia of the Siberian husky. Follicles similar to flame follicles but with less exaggerated tricholemmal keratin spikes and with hair shafts retained are seen in normal plush-coated breeds of dogs and in post clipping alopecia. Epidermal hyperpigmentation and dermal atrophy are variable.

HYPERSOMATOTROPISM

This syndrome rarely occurs in adult dogs, and is a result of excess levels of growth hormone (somatotropin). The excess growth hormone can arise from acidophil tumors of the anterior pituitary gland, injection of pituitary gland extracts, administration of progestins, or with the metestrus (luteal) phase of the estrous cycle in intact female dogs. Hypersecretion of growth hormone results in increased production of connective tissue, bone, and viscera. Clinical lesions consist of acromegaly (enlargement of parts of the skeleton, especially distal extremities), and thick, folded myxedematous skin over the head, neck, and extremities. The hair coat can be long and thick, and the claws thick and hard. Histologic lesions include thickened dermis caused by increased production of glycosaminoglycans and collagen by dermal fibroblasts. Myxedema is present in about a third of cases.

HYPOSOMATOTROPISM

Deficiency of growth hormone in dogs younger than 3 months of age is usually due to failure of the normal development of the pituitary gland leading to cyst formation. Deficiencies of thyroid, adrenal, and gonadal hormones are frequent accompanying problems. Pituitary deficiency results in failure to grow, retention of the puppy hair coat, and development of endocrine alopecia. Microscopically, the features are consistent with endocrine alopecia (e.g., hyperkeratosis of superficial epidermis and of hair follicles; normal or atrophic epithelium; follicular dilation from hyperkeratosis; increased numbers of telogen hair follicles; lack of hair shafts in follicles; and increased epidermal pigmentation). The numbers of dermal elastic fibers are reduced in the skin of some dogs.

CYCLICAL FLANK ALOPECIA (SEASONAL FLANK ALOPECIA, IDIOPATHIC FLANK ALOPECIA)

Cyclical flank alopecia develops more commonly in dogs living in northern latitudes. The cause of cyclical flank alopecia is not known, but changes in the photoperiod, and thus melatonin released from the pineal gland, might play a role. Many breeds are affected, but English bulldogs, boxers, and Airedale terriers are among the more commonly affected breeds. Alopecia develops

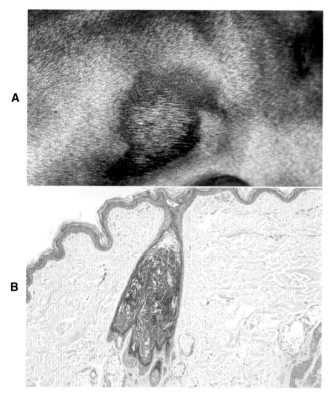

Fig. 17-71   Cyclical flank alopecia (seasonal flank alopecia), skin, dog. A, Alopecia and hyperpigmentation are present in the skin of the flank of a boxer dog. The breed of dog, location of the alopecia, and often cyclic nature of the condition suggest that cyclical flank alopecia is a likely diagnosis. Hair is regrowing in the central area of alopecia (*brown area within hyperpigmented zone*), indicating that lesions are resolving. **B,** Note the distorted follicle with dilations at the base. The follicle resembles an upside-down "footprint." This histologic feature, in conjunction with clinical history of cyclical flank lesions in the predisposed breeds, supports the diagnosis of this condition. H&E stain. (**A,** *Courtesy Dr. David Duclos, Animal Skin and Allergy Clinic.* **B,** *Courtesy Dr. Ann M. Hargis, DermatoDiagnostics.*)

seasonally or cyclically in the skin of the flank, usually bilaterally (Fig. 17-71). Histologically, follicles are in the telogen stage of the hair cycle, and primary follicles are markedly dilated and distorted by follicular hyperkeratosis. The follicular hyperkeratosis also distends the openings of secondary follicles as they enter the primary follicle, giving the follicles the distorted appearance of an upside-down "footprint" (Fig. 17-71, *B*). The condition, as the name suggests, is often transient but can be recurrent.

CUTANEOUS NON-ENDOCRINE DISORDERS ASSOCIATED WITH HAIR CYCLE ABNORMALITIES
POST CLIPPING ALOPECIA

Post clipping alopecia is a failure of the hair to regrow in apparently normal dogs after close clipping.

The condition usually occurs in long-haired or heavily coated (plush-coated) breeds of dogs such as the Chow chow. The cause is not known. It has been speculated that close clipping could cause a change in thermoregulation that may stimulate active follicles to simultaneously enter the telogen (resting) stage of the hair cycle. Alternatively, it is thought that heavily coated breeds of dogs have a prolonged telogen stage of the hair cycle, possibly to conserve energy by avoiding frequent cycles of shedding. Thus clipping when the hair coat is in a prolonged inactive stage of the hair cycle would result in lack of quick regrowth of the hair coat. The hair coat may not regrow until there is another significant growth phase, which may take 6 to 12 months. Most affected dogs regrow hair coat after they go through a cycle of heavy shedding. Histologic lesions consist of normal epidermis, dermis, and sebaceous glands, and hair follicles in the telogen stage of the hair cycle with prominent tricholemmal keratin resembling flame follicles but in which the hair shafts are retained.

TELOGEN EFFLUVIUM

Telogen effluvium develops when an animal is systemically ill or is severely stressed such as occurs with high fever, pregnancy and lactation, or anesthesia and surgery. The illness or stressful event triggers a sudden termination of the growth stage of follicles. This causes a majority of the hair follicles to synchronously enter the catagen and then telogen stages of the hair cycle. Gross lesions do not develop until about 1 to 3 months after the systemic illness or stress resolves, and the telogen (or inactive) follicles synchronously enter into the anagen stage of the hair cycle. When the new anagen hair shafts emerge from the follicle, the old telogen hair shafts are suddenly shed. The alopecia resolves as the new hair shafts emerge from the follicles, and the new hair coat becomes visible. Histologic lesions during the stage of excessive shedding are essentially normal and consist of the majority of follicles in the anagen stage of the hair cycle.

ANAGEN DEFLUXION

Anagen defluxion occurs when there is an insult to the anagen (or growing) hair bulbs. This most commonly occurs in dogs with continuously growing hair coats such as poodles, when given antimitotic drugs that damage the hair matrix cells (keratinocytes) of the anagen hair bulb. Gross lesions consist of alopecia that develops suddenly after the administration of the antimitotic drug. Histologic lesions can be subtle and include degeneration and fragmentation of nuclei in the keratinocytes of the hair matrix of the anagen hair bulbs, and eosinophilic hair shafts within the follicular canal.

DISORDERS ASSOCIATED WITH NORMAL FOLLICLES

Excessive grooming, particularly in cats, can result in symmetrical alopecia or hypotrichosis that clinically resembles endocrine dermatoses. Excessive grooming can be the result of pruritus (usually associated with cutaneous hypersensitivity reactions) or allegedly from psychogenic problems such as boredom or stress (feline psychogenic alopecia). Thus it is important to determine if the alopecia or hypotrichosis is the result of excessive grooming, and if so, what the underlying stimulus is.

FELINE PSYCHOGENIC ALOPECIA

Psychogenic alopecia occurs in cats of the more emotional breeds, including Siamese and Abyssinian, and possibly others. A partial alopecia is due to the breaking of hairs from gentle, but persistent, licking. Linear or symmetric areas of alopecia are found along the caudal dorsal midline or in the perineal, genital, caudomedial thigh, or abdominal areas. Microscopically, the skin is generally normal, but the number of telogen follicles is increased. The principal differential diagnosis is alopecia due to hypersensitivity (see next discussion). Endocrine associated alopecia is rare in the cat.

ALOPECIA DUE TO HYPERSENSITIVITY REACTIONS IN THE CAT

Clinical signs of alopecia due to hypersensitivity reactions are often identical to those of feline psychogenic alopecia. Pruritus typically is due to hypersensitivity reactions of a variety of causes (food allergy, parasitism, atopy). Histologically, there is perivascular dermatitis, usually with eosinophils, mast cells, and lymphocytes. The inflammation helps to distinguish alopecia associated with hypersensitivity from that of feline psychogenic alopecia.

DISORDERS ASSOCIATED WITH DYSPLASTIC FOLLICLES

FOLLICULAR DYSPLASIA SYNDROMES

Follicular dysplasia syndromes, defined as incomplete or abnormal development of follicles and hair shafts, comprise a group of generally poorly characterized disorders recognized most commonly in dogs, but occasionally in horses, cattle, and cats. Clinical lesions are alopecia or hypotrichosis, and consequently, there is clinical resemblance to the endocrine disorders. Some of the more common follicular dysplasia syndromes are associated with coat color dilution (color dilution follicular dysplasia, color mutant alopecia) or occur in black versus white haired areas (black hair follicle dysplasia) (Fig. 17-25). Microscopic features of follicular dysplasia vary with the syndrome. The conditions associated with coat color dilution or those that occur in black-haired areas have densely clumped melanin pigment in the hair bulb, hair shafts, and also in the basal layer of the epidermis (Fig. 17-25). Lesions in other conditions include lipid distention of hair matrix cells, abnormally formed follicles or hair bulbs, and abnormal hair shafts. The microscopic features help to differentiate syndromes of follicular dysplasia from the endocrine dermatosis.

DISORDERS RELATED TO NUTRIENT IMBALANCES, DEFICIENCIES, OR ALTERED METABOLISM

MALNUTRITION

Malnutrition can be primary (dietary deficiency of proteins, fats, carbohydrates, vitamins, minerals, amino acids, or fatty acids) or secondary (diet is adequate, but malnutrition results from nutrient malabsorption, impaired nutrient use, increased nutrient loss, or increased nutrient needs such as pregnancy, neonatal growth, disease states, or cold weather). Inadequate diets can involve imbalances between dietary nutrients (e.g., copper deficiency and molybdenum excess, and vitamin E deficiency and excess dietary fatty acids). Diets inadequate in one nutrient may be inadequate in multiple nutrients, or there may be a greater deficiency in one nutrient relative to the others (e.g., starvation, the diet may be inadequate in protein, fats, and carbohydrates, and vitamins and minerals, or there may be a greater deficiency in protein relative to other nutrients). A variety of nutritional deficiencies result in similar cutaneous lesions. The lesions heal when the animal is fed a balanced diet. Deficiencies affecting the skin include protein-energy malnutrition (starvation), fatty acid deficiency, vitamin deficiencies (A, C, E), and deficiencies of riboflavin, pantothenic acid, biotin, niacin, iodine, cobalt, copper, and zinc. A few selected deficiency conditions are described.

PROTEIN-CALORIE MALNUTRITION

Protein-calorie malnutrition results in a range of clinical syndromes from inadequate dietary intake of protein and calories to meet the needs of the body. Often diets are deficient in multiple components including protein, carbohydrates, and fats, which together are responsible for the total caloric intake. Deficiency of calories per se results in weight loss (adults) or retarded growth (young growing animals) and reduced subcutaneous fat and muscle, producing a thin, emaciated appearance. Increased energy demands such as pregnancy or cold weather can worsen the severity of the malnutrition, leading to ketosis in pregnant sheep, birth of weak neonates or dead fetuses, lack of estrus cycles, and death. A greater deficiency of protein relative to calories also results in malnutrition, referred to herein as "protein deficiency." In early stages, protein deficiency malnutrition resembles that from deficiency of calories, and results in weight loss and reduced production (e.g., milk) in adults and reduced growth in young animals. In addition, prolonged protein deficiency also results in edema caused by the reduction in the concentration of the serum protein, albumin. Because of the requirement of protein for the production of hair coat, the hair coat of malnourished animals (protein-calorie malnutrition and protein deficiency) is thin and dull, with failure to shed or to complete the normal hair cycle. The epidermis, dermis, and adnexa are atrophic with reduced subcutaneous fat and muscle, and surface scales (hyperkeratosis) can be present. In long-standing severe protein deficiency, dermal and subcutaneous edema is present.

ZINC DEFICIENCY

Zinc deficiency occurs chiefly in pigs and dogs and is of less importance in ruminants. It results from diets containing high concentration of phytic acid (binds zinc), low concentration of zinc, or high concentration of calcium (reduces absorption of zinc), or from inherited defective absorption or metabolism.

ZINC DEFICIENCY IN PIGS

Zinc deficiency, although once common in pigs, occurs infrequently today because of dietary supplementation. Gross lesions are generally symmetrical, circumscribed, reddened macules that develop first on the ventral abdomen and medial thighs, and spread to the lower limbs especially over joints, periocular areas, pinnae, snout, scrotum, and tail. The macular lesions progress to papules and plaques that become covered with scales and crust. The crusts thicken, and develop fissures filled with debris including soil and bacteria. The fissures provide a route of entrance for bacteria that can cause infection including the development of subcutaneous abscesses. Microscopically, the lesions are parakeratosis, hypergranulosis, acanthosis, and pseudoepitheliomatous hyperplasia. Secondary bacterial invasion results in epidermal pustular dermatitis and folliculitis. The fissures filled with debris can become infected by mixed populations of bacteria and lead to the development of subcutaneous abscesses.

CANINE ZINC RESPONSIVE DERMATOSIS

This dermatosis occurs in two forms. One form occurs principally in Siberian huskies and Alaskan malamutes, but other large-breed dogs can be affected. Alaskan malamutes have an inherited reduced ability to absorb zinc from the intestine. Scaling and crusting develop in the skin around the mouth, chin, eyes (Fig. 17-72), external ears, pressure points, and footpads. The second form

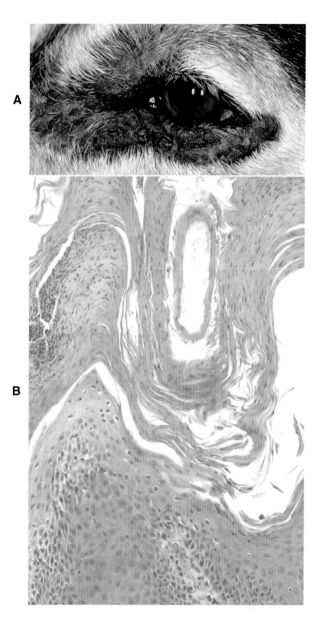

Fig. 17-72   Zinc responsive dermatosis, skin, dog.
A, Siberian husky. Periocular skin is thickened, alopecic, pigmented, and covered by tightly adherent scale. In Siberian huskies and Alaskan malamutes in particular, scaling and crusting develop in the skin around the mouth, chin, eyes, external ears, pressure points, and footpads.
B, Note the papillary epidermal hyperplasia with marked parakeratosis. The parakeratotic hyperkeratosis and acanthosis form the thickened adherent scale. Although epidermal hyperplasia and parakeratosis are features of zinc-responsive dermatosis, they also occur in other conditions (such as superficial necrolytic dermatitis, chronic surface trauma, and nasal parakeratosis). Therefore breed, lesion distribution, and other features in the clinical history or clinical chemistry analysis are important in differential diagnosis. H&E stain. (*A* and **B,** *Courtesy Dr. Ann M. Hargis, DermatoDiagnostics.*)

of zinc deficiency occurs in rapidly growing pups of large-breed dogs fed diets low in zinc or high in calcium or phytates, which can interfere with zinc absorption. Clinically dogs with this form have scaly plaques located on those areas of the skin subjected to repeated trauma (e.g., elbows and hocks), the footpads, and planum nasale. Microscopically, there is marked diffuse parakeratosis (Fig. 17-72, *B*) that extends into the hair follicles, and an accompanying superficial perivascular lymphocytic and sometimes eosinophilic dermatitis. Another disorder, generic dog food dermatosis, a largely historic disease that occurred in the 1980s in dogs fed generic dog foods, has clinical and histologic lesions similar to those of canine zinc responsive dermatosis. However, dogs with generic dog food dermatosis had a more rapid onset of lesions, and also had systemic signs such as fever, depression, lymphadenopathy, and pitting edema of the dependent areas. The acute onset and systemic signs suggested that more than zinc deficiency played a role in generic dog food dermatosis.

LETHAL ACRODERMATITIS OF BULL TERRIERS

Lethal acrodermatitis is an autosomal recessive inherited disease of defective zinc metabolism in white bull terriers. The exact cause or pathogenesis of the disorder is not known. Although defective zinc metabolism and/or absorption are thought to play a role, affected dogs do not respond to oral or parenteral zinc supplementation. The concentrations of serum zinc and copper are low in affected bull terriers compared with those of control dogs, suggesting that copper deficiency might contribute. Lesions generally begin between 6 and 10 weeks of age. Most affected dogs are dead by 15 months of age, usually because of bronchopneumonia. The thymus is small or absent, and T lymphocytes are deficient in lymphoid tissues, likely contributing to immunodeficiency and increasing the potential of infection. Cutaneous lesions begin between the digits and on footpads and progress to involve mucocutaneous areas, especially of the face. Severe interdigital pyoderma, paronychia (inflammation of the skin around the claws), and villous thickening and fissuring of footpad keratin ensue. Exfoliative dermatitis can also develop on pinnae, external nose, elbows, hocks, and, in some dogs, can become more generalized, with crusting, ulceration, and secondary pyoderma. Microscopically, the principal lesions are extensive diffuse parakeratotic hyperkeratosis, responsible for the exfoliative dermatitis, and accompanying acanthosis. Lesions of secondary infection consist of epidermal pustular dermatitis and folliculitis.

DIETARY ZINC DEFICIENCY IN RUMINANTS

Dietary zinc deficiency has been reported in cattle, sheep, and goats. Cutaneous lesions include alopecia, scaling, and crusting of the skin of the face, neck, distal extremities, and mucocutaneous junctions. In uncomplicated cases, microscopic lesions consist of parakeratosis and sometimes hyperkeratosis.

HEREDITARY ZINC DEFICIENCY

Hereditary zinc deficiency (lethal trait A-46, hereditary parakeratosis, hereditary thymic aplasia) is an autosomal recessive inherited form of zinc deficiency that has been reported in young calves (Friesian and Black Pied Danish cattle of Friesian descent in Europe, and shorthorn cattle in the United States). The disease is due to intestinal malabsorption of zinc, and lesions resolve with zinc supplementation. The disease is multisystemic. Skin lesions usually begin at 1 to 2 months of age, and without zinc supplementation, calves usually die within a few months from secondary infections associated with immune dysfunction. Skin lesions begin on the nose and spread to periocular areas, pinnae, intermandibular space, and distal extremities including coronary bands. Ventral abdominal, flank, and perineal skin can also be affected. Lesions consist of erythema, exudation, crusting, scaling, and a rough hair coat that fades to lighter color. The calves have thymic hypoplasia, reduced humoral and cell-mediated immunity, and secondary infections. The major histologic lesion is marked diffuse parakeratotic hyperkeratosis (parakeratosis). There also can be perivascular edema and dermatitis with neutrophilic exocytosis forming crusts colonized by cocci.

COPPER DEFICIENCY

Copper is an essential component of tyrosinase, an enzyme critical in melanogenesis. Animals with copper deficiency or depressed tyrosinase activity have depigmented hair or wool. Copper deficiency can be due to simple deficiency or secondary to excessive dietary sulfate and molybdenum, which interfere with absorption. This pigmentary disorder is seen primarily in cattle and sheep. Affected cattle with normally black coats become rusty-brown and develop "spectacle" lesions of depigmented hair around the eyes. Black sheep develop intermittent bands of light-colored wool corresponding to periods of restricted availability of copper. The deficiency of copper also affects the physical nature of the wool or hair. In sheep, the wool has less crimp, prompting the colloquial name of "string" or "steely" wool. The straightness of the wool is due to inadequate keratinization, probably caused by imperfect oxidation of sulfhydryl groups in prekeratin, a process that involves copper.

VITAMIN E DEFICIENCY

Cats fed diets containing an excess of dietary fatty acids such as canned red tuna can develop inflammation of the subcutaneous and abdominal fat (steatitis). This condition develops when the diet is high in fat and when food processing or oxidation inactivate vitamin E. Vitamin E has a number of functions that contribute to its role as an antioxidant that stabilizes lysosomes. Grossly, the subcutaneous fat contains firm, nodular, yellow to orange masses. Microscopic lesions consist of fat necrosis that stimulates a lobular to diffuse neutrophilia followed by granulomatous inflammatory response. Macrophages and multinucleated giant cells contain ceroid pigment, which is responsible for the yellow to orange color of the affected fat.

VITAMIN A RESPONSIVE DERMATOSIS

Vitamin A responsive dermatosis is a rare disorder primarily occurring in cocker spaniels, although a few other breeds of dogs have been affected. Because lesions respond to vitamin A therapy and relapse when treatment is withdrawn, vitamin A plays a role in the pathogenesis. However, vitamin A deficiency is not the cause of the lesions, as plasma concentrations of vitamin A are within the normal range. Vitamin A might contribute to lesion resolution by influencing epithelial differentiation. Gross lesions consist of generalized scaling, dry hair coat, and hyperkeratotic plaques with large "fronds" of stratum corneum extending from distended follicular openings (large open comedones). The plaques are most prominent in the ventral and lateral thorax and abdominal skin, but can also occur on the face and neck. Microscopic lesions consist of mild orthokeratotic hyperkeratosis, mild irregular epidermal hyperplasia, and follicles markedly distended by hyperkeratosis.

DISORDERS OF EPIDERMAL GROWTH OR DIFFERENTIATION

PREDOMINANT EPIDERMAL HYPERKERATOSIS (SCALE)

PRIMARY IDIOPATHIC SEBORRHEA

Primary idiopathic seborrhea is a disorder of epidermal hyperproliferation that results in increased production of corneocytes and visible scale. It occurs most commonly in dogs and less commonly in horses and cats. Most experimental work has been performed in cocker spaniels. The pathogenesis of the disease involves hyperproliferation of the epidermis, hair follicle infundibulum, and sebaceous glands. The basal cell labeling indices are 3 or 4 times higher in cocker spaniels with seborrhea than in normal dogs. The hyperproliferation results in reduction in the epidermal turnover time to about one third (e.g., from 22 days to 8 days in the cocker spaniel). In the cocker spaniel the disorder appears to be the result of a primary cellular

defect in the keratinocyte, as the epidermal cells remain hyperproliferative when grown in culture and after being grafted onto the dermis of normal dogs. In seborrhea, quantitative studies on sebum production have not been performed, but it is known that there is a relative increase in free fatty acids and a relative decrease in diester waxes on the surface of the seborrheic skin of various breeds. In addition, there is a change from nonpathogenic resident bacteria to pathogenic, coagulase-positive staphylococci. Clinically, two forms of seborrhea have been described, a dry form (seborrhea sicca) with dry skin and white to gray scales that exfoliate (Fig. 17-10), and a greasy form (seborrhea oleosa) with scaling and excessive brown to yellow lipids that adhere to the surface of the skin and hair. An animal can have seborrhea sicca in some areas of the body and seborrhea oleosa in others. Microscopic lesions include marked hyperkeratosis of the epidermis and follicular epithelium. The epidermis has a papillary appearance due to widening of follicular ostia by the follicular hyperkeratosis (Fig. 17-10). Comedones (follicles dilated with a plug of follicular stratum corneum and sebum) are present in some animals. At the edges of follicular ostia, foci of parakeratosis form over a spongiotic epidermis containing a few scattered leukocytes. The superficial dermis is congested and edematous.

ICHTHYOSIS

Ichthyosis is an inherited cutaneous disease seen principally in dogs and cattle. It has also been reported in llamas and pigs. The skin is thickened by marked hyperkeratosis and can crack into plates resembling fish scales, thus the origin of the name. The basic defect is increased adherence of keratinocytes, which prevents normal desquamation. In cattle, two forms of the disease have been described. One (ichthyosis fetalis) is lethal, and most calves are stillborn or die within days of birth. Grossly and microscopically the skin is alopecic and covered by thick cornified plaques separated by fissures. Fissuring of the skin leads to exudation of protein, and secondary bacterial and fungal infections that often lead to death or euthanasia. In the second and less severe form (ichthyosis congenita), lesions in some calves are mild at birth and progress with age. The skin becomes thickened, folded, and covered by scale, and partial alopecia develops. More severe lesions are seen where hair is shorter, particularly on the limbs, abdomen, and nose. In dogs, ichthyosis is rare and usually present at birth. Grossly, there are scales adherent to the epidermis, which shed in sheets attached to hair shafts (Fig. 17-73). There can be marked thickening of nasal planum and digital pads by accumulated stratum corneum forming fronds. Alopecia is sometimes present. In addition to marked

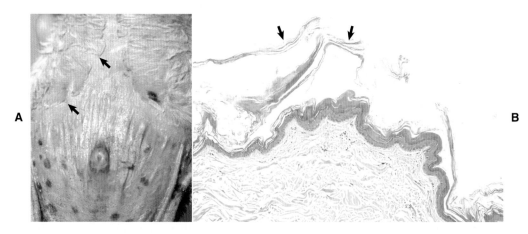

Fig. 17-73   Ichthyosis, skin, dog. A, Abdomen. The skin is covered with adherent plates of scale (*arrows*), and the skin surface is wrinkled. **B,** Compact hyperkeratosis is present. Plates of stratum corneum are separating from each other and are lifting off the surface (*arrows*). H&E stain. (**A,** *Courtesy Dr. Diane Lewis, College of Veterinary Medicine. University of Florida.* **B,** *Courtesy Dr. Ann M. Hargis, DermatoDiagnostics.*)

epidermal and follicular hyperkeratosis, hypergranulosis, keratinocyte vacuolation, and reticular degeneration are seen in the skin of some affected animals.

SEBACEOUS ADENITIS

Sebaceous adenitis, inflammation of sebaceous glands, is probably immune-mediated. Sebaceous adenitis occurs most commonly in dogs. Lesions are diffuse in the longer-haired breeds and multifocal, annular, and serpiginous in shorter-haired breeds. Microscopic lesions include inflammation of the sebaceous glands (Fig. 17-31), and in some dogs, extensive orthokeratotic hyperkeratosis. Chronically affected dogs have no remaining sebaceous glands, but mild residual inflammation and fibrosis are present in the perifollicular dermis near the isthmus (site normally occupied by sebaceous glands).

HYPERKERATOSIS OF NASAL PLANUM OR FOOTPADS IN DOGS

Nasal and/or digital hyperkeratoses have a variety of underlying causes, including infectious disease (e.g., canine distemper [see Chapter 14], leishmaniasis, putative papillomavirus infection), immune-mediated disorders (e.g., pemphigus foliaceus and lupus erythematosus), familial or inherited disorders (e.g., idiopathic seborrhea, familial footpad hyperkeratosis of Irish terriers and Dogue de Bordeaux, ichthyosis, familial nasal hyperkeratosis, nasal parakeratosis of the Labrador retriever), metabolic or nutritional disease (e.g., superficial necrolytic dermatitis, zinc-responsive dermatosis), adverse reaction to drug therapy, and neoplasia (e.g., cutaneous lymphoma) (Box 17-12). In some

---

Box 17-12

Hyperkeratosis of the Nasal Planum or Footpads in Dogs

IMMUNE MEDIATED

Pemphigus foliaceus
Lupus erythematosus
Drug reaction

INFECTIOUS

Canine distemper
Leishmaniasis
Putative papillomavirus infection

METABOLIC

Superficial necrolytic dermatitis
Zinc-responsive dermatosis

INHERITED

Familial footpad hyperkeratosis
Ichthyosis
Familial nasal hyperkeratosis
Nasal parakeratosis of the Labrador retriever

IDIOPATHIC

Idiopathic seborrhea
Idiopathic nasodigital hyperkeratosis

NEOPLASTIC

Cutaneous lymphoma

cases, an underlying cause is not determined, thus the condition is considered to be idiopathic (occurs most commonly in old dogs). Some of the disorders in which nasal or digital hyperkeratosis is a feature also have skin lesions in other sites, and systemic disease can be present. Gross lesions on the footpads or nasal planum include a dry, thick, irregular and rough surface in which crusts, fissures or erosions can develop (Figs. 17-11 and 17-16). The edges of the footpads and non–weight-bearing pads are more severely affected because friction on weight-bearing surfaces wears through some of the excessively thick stratum corneum. Histologic lesions reflect the underlying cause. In the idiopathic nasodigital hyperkeratosis of old dogs, irregular epidermal hyperplasia with marked orthokeratotic to parakeratotic hyperkeratosis is present. In familial nasal parakeratosis, there is variable parakeratotic hyperkeratosis with intraepidermal serum and leukocytic exocytosis. The dermis has perivascular to interface or interstitial mixed inflammation. In familial footpad hyperkeratosis, there is moderate to extensive epidermal acanthosis and marked diffuse orthokeratotic hyperkeratosis in which the surface stratum corneum forms many papillary projections.

PREDOMINANT FOLLICULAR HYPERKERATOSIS (COMEDONES)

Comedones (Table 17-5) occur in numerous skin disorders, including those associated with surface trauma (callus, actinic dermatosis), endocrine dermatosis (especially hyperadrenocorticism), nutritional or inherited disorders of cornification (primary seborrhea, vitamin A responsive dermatosis), and in some disorders associated with follicular infection (especially demodicosis). In addition, comedones are prominent in two conditions wherein the comedones are considered a major feature of the disease.

SCHNAUZER COMEDO SYNDROME

Schnauzer comedo syndrome affects some miniature schnauzers and probably has an inherited basis. Gross lesions develop on the dorsum of the back and consist of comedones, papules and crusts. Histologic lesions consist of follicles distended with a plug of follicular stratum corneum and sebum (comedones). Because the follicular opening is connected to the epidermis, the dilated follicles can contain coccoid bacteria. The dilated follicles can rupture (furunculosis) and release contents into the dermis resulting in a foreign body response and bacterial infection.

ACNE

Feline acne is a disorder of follicular cornification in the skin of the chin, lower lip, and less commonly upper lip. Cats of a variety of ages, sexes, and coat lengths are affected. Gross lesions consist of comedones that can progress to papules, crusts, nodules, and diffuse swelling. Histologic lesions begin as mild follicular hyperkeratosis and progress to comedones, which can become secondarily infected by bacteria, rupture (furunculosis), and cause panniculitis and cellulitis.

Canine acne is a chronic disorder that develops in the skin of the chin and lips of young dogs, usually with short hair coats. The cause of the disorder is not known, but a follicular cornification disorder has not been definitively documented. Early lesions consist of follicular papules and comedones that with time enlarge to nodules that can ulcerate and drain. Histologically early lesions consist of moderate to marked follicular hyperkeratosis (the papules and comedones), and later of folliculitis, furunculosis, and draining sinuses (the nodular, ulcerated, and draining lesions).

PREDOMINANT EPIDERMAL HYPERPLASIA (LICHENIFICATION OR CRUSTS)

SECONDARY SEBORRHEA

Secondary seborrhea is not a primary disorder of cornification; however, it clinically resembles the primary cornification disorders (dry exfoliative or greasy adherent scales) and thus needs to be differentiated from them. Secondary seborrhea is common, and is caused by a variety of unrelated cutaneous disorders such as allergy, ectoparasitism, fungal infection, dietary deficiency, endocrine disease, and internal diseases. The lesions of secondary seborrhea resolve completely if the underlying disease is eliminated. Microscopic changes include epidermal and follicular hyperkeratosis with or without parakeratosis plus the lesions associated with the underlying disease.

PORCINE JUVENILE PUSTULAR PSORIASIFORM DERMATITIS (PITYRIASIS ROSEA)

This disorder develops in suckling and young pigs (3 to 14 weeks of age), usually resolves spontaneously by 4 weeks of onset, and is thought to be inherited. A few piglets in the litter or entire litters can be affected. Lesions are symmetric and develop on the abdomen, groin, and medial thigh and begin as small papules covered by brown crusts. The lesions coalesce and spread, and develop into umbilicated plaques with white centers and erythematous, scaly borders that can progress into mosaic patterns (Fig. 17-74). These clinical lesions resemble those of dermatophytosis, swinepox, and dermatosis vegetans, from which they need to be differentiated, but otherwise the clinical lesions are of no significance. Microscopically, the early histologic lesions are superficial and deep perivascular neutrophilic, eosinophilic, and mixed mononuclear dermatitis. Epidermal spongiosis and leukocytic exocytosis result in spongiform pustules. Later lesions consist of marked

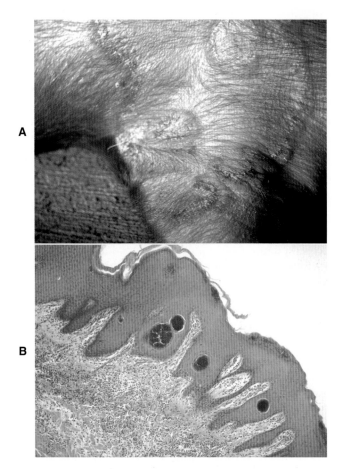

Fig. 17-74   Porcine juvenile pustular psoriasiform dermatitis (pityriasis rosea), skin, pig. A, Abdomen. Note the circular to serpiginous *(wavy)* lesions with distinct raised and reddened border and the adjacent scale. These lesions need to be differentiated from those of dermatophytosis, swinepox, and dermatosis vegetans. **B,** Note the epidermal hyperplasia (acanthosis with elongated rete ridges) and intraepidermal pustules. The dermis contains diffuse accumulations of neutrophils and mixed mononuclear inflammatory cells. The disease receives its name from the juvenile age of onset, the formation of epidermal pustules, and the exaggerated regular epidermal hyperplasia (psoriasiform hyperplasia). H&E stain. *(A, Courtesy Dr. M.D. McGavin, College of Veterinary Medicine, University of Tennessee. B, Courtesy Dr. Pamela E. Ginn, College of Veterinary Medicine, University of Florida.)*

psoriasiform epidermal hyperplasia (regular epidermal hyperplasia with epidermal ridges of uniform length and width) and parakeratotic cellular crust.

EQUINE CORONARY BAND DYSTROPHY

Equine coronary band dystrophy is a condition of unknown etiology and pathogenesis. Clinically, the coronary band (coronary border of hoof) is thickened, crusty, and scaly. Cracks and fissures can lead to lameness. The chestnuts and ergots (cornified protuberances

considered to be vestiges of the first, second, and fourth digits) are similarly affected and can be ulcerated. Usually all four limbs are affected; however, the lesion may not involve the entire coronary band. Histologically, the epidermis of affected areas has marked papillary epidermal hyperplasia (Fig. 17-12) and marked orthohyperkeratosis to parakeratotic hyperkeratosis. In some areas, there is ballooning degeneration of keratinocytes. Dermal inflammation is minimal unless secondary infection is present. The diagnosis is made by ruling out the various differential diagnoses, including pemphigus foliaceus, hepatocutaneous syndrome, bacterial or fungal infection, selenium toxicosis, mite infestation, and eosinophilic exfoliative dermatitis. The condition is chronic and treatment palliative. Although the condition affects adult horses of any breed, draft breeds are considered predisposed.

DISORDERS OF PIGMENTATION

Melanin pigments are responsible for the coloration of the hair, skin and eyes, and also play an important role in photoprotection. Melanin is synthesized by melanocytes, which are dendritic cells originating as melanoblasts in the neural crest. Melanoblasts develop in the neural crest and migrate to peripheral sites including the basal and lower spinous layers of the epidermis, hair follicles, and dermis. Melanoblasts differentiate into melanocytes, and synthesize melanosomes and melanin. Tyrosinase, a copper-containing enzyme, plays a critical role in the synthesis of melanin. Genetic mutations affecting any of the steps in the formation of melanin can lead to hereditary hypopigmentation. Many types of exogenous influences, such as inflammation, UV radiation, endocrinopathies, autoimmune diseases, and nutritional status, can affect melanocytes in the skin, resulting in acquired hypopigmentation or hyperpigmentation. Examples of some of the disorders include Chédiak-Higashi syndrome, color mutant (dilution) alopecia, the Maltese dilution of cats, leukoderma and/or leukotrichia of Doberman pinschers and rottweilers, periocular leukotrichia in Siamese cats, and Arabian fading syndrome. Immune-mediated disorders associated with depigmentation include discoid lupus erythematosus and uveodermatologic syndrome (VKH-like disease).

HYPOPIGMENTATION

Disorders associated with reduced pigment can (1) be inherited or acquired, (2) involve skin or hair, (3) be generalized or localized, or (4) be idiopathic or linked with other diseases. Reduction in pigmentation of the skin is leukoderma, and of the hair is leukotrichia. Leukoderma and leukotrichia can occur independently. They can result from a decrease in melanin (hypomelanosis), a complete absence of melanin (amelanosis), or from a loss of existing melanin (depigmentation). These events result from either an absence of the pigment-synthesizing melanocytes or from a failure of melanocytes to produce normal amounts of melanin or to transfer it to adjacent keratinocytes. Because copper is a component of tyrosinase, production of melanin pigment is dependent on copper, thus copper deficiency can result in reduced pigmentation.

INHERITED HYPOPIGMENTATION

Hereditary hypopigmentation can be divided into melanocytopenic hypomelanosis, characterized by the absence of melanocytes in affected areas, and melanopenic hypomelanosis, in which melanocytes are present but defective. Hypopigmentation can be localized, focally extensive, or generalized.

Syndromes analogous to the human Waardenburg's syndrome have been reported in cats, dogs, and horses. In this melanocytopenic hypomelanosis, there is failure of melanoblasts to migrate from the neural crest into the skin, or failure to survive in the skin. Affected animals typically have white coats and blue or heterochromatic irides, and are deaf. In cats, this has been shown to be a result of an autosomal dominant mutation with complete penetrance for loss of pigmentation and incomplete penetrance for deafness. In dogs, this syndrome has been described in breeds such as the Dalmatian, bull terrier, Sealyham terrier, collie, and Great Dane. A syndrome analogous to human Waardenburg type-4 (Hirschsprung's disease) has been reported in American Paint horses in which white foals from overo mares are born with aganglionic colons. These foals develop colic from greatly distended colons, and die shortly after birth.

Piebaldism is also a form of genetic melanocytopenic hypomelanosis resulting in multifocal white patches in which there is an absence of melanocytes because of either a congenital failure of melanoblasts to migrate from the neural crest to the skin, or by their inability to survive and proliferate in the skin. Piebaldism has been seen in many species including horses, dogs such as the Dalmatian, cats, and cattle.

Vitiligo is a melanocytopenic hypomelanosis of human beings and animals, which is characterized by gradually expanding pale macules that are often symmetrical or segmental in distribution. The immediate cause of vitiligo is the destruction of melanocytes. It is considered to be a genetic amelanosis inherited as an autosomal recessive trait in animals. Theories regarding the pathogenesis of this disease include autoimmune destruction of melanocytes, a neurogenic theory involving release of a neurochemical from peripheral nerves that inhibits melanogenesis, a self-destruction theory that involves failure of protection of melanocytes against the toxic effects of melanin precursors, or a combination of factors. Vitiligo has been described in the dog, cat, horse, and cattle. The condition is best characterized in Belgian tervurens. The depigmentation in this breed occurs chiefly on the pigmented skin and mucous membranes of the face and mouth in young adult dogs. Histologic examination of affected skin shows an epithelium devoid of both pigment granules and DOPA-positive cells. Electron microscopy confirms the lack of melanocytes in the lesions, their place being taken by Langerhans' or indeterminate dendritic cells.

The various forms of albinism are examples of melanopenic hypomelanosis. In albino animals and human beings, melanocytes are present and normally distributed but are defective in function and fail to synthesize melanin. The extent of the biochemical defect varies, so that albinism covers a spectrum from amelanosis, oculocutaneous albinism, through graded pigmentary dilution. Oculocutaneous albinisms and pigment dilutions are inherited as autosomal recessive traits. In albino animals with white hair and skin, and translucent irides, there is a mutation in the tyrosinase gene resulting in no residual enzyme activity.

Chédiak-Higashi syndrome in human beings, Hereford, Brangus, and Japanese Black cattle; Persian cats; and various other animal species is an example of partial albinism and is inherited as an autosomal recessive trait. While melanin is produced, there is a mutation of the beige gene, which plays a major role in generating cellular organelles. This results in a membrane defect leading to the formation of giant melanosomes that are transferred with difficulty to the keratinocytes. The clumping of these giant melanosomes produces the color dilution effect. Chédiak-Higashi syndrome is discussed with the hematopoietic system (see Chapter 13).

Cyclic hematopoiesis (cyclic neutropenia), a lethal hereditary disease of collie dogs, is caused by an autosomal recessive gene with a pleiotropic effect on coat color dilution. Affected dogs are silver-gray. The abnormal hair pigmentation results from the diminished formation of melanin from its precursor tyrosine rather than from pigment clumping. The normal collie coat color is restored in animals receiving bone marrow transplants to correct cyclic hematopoiesis. The hematological aspects of this disease are considered with the hematopoietic system (see Chapter 13).

Coat color dilution has been reported in many species. It occurs in many breeds of dogs, cats, horses, and cattle, but is particularly common in Siamese cats. The pale coat coloration is due to clumping of large melanin granules in hair shafts, hair matrix cells, and sometimes in the epidermis. In cats, dilute coat color is thought to be a result of an autosomal recessive trait (Maltese dilution).

Acquired Hypopigmentation

Acquired hypopigmentation follows damage to the epidermal melanin unit by various insults, including trauma, inflammation, radiation, contactants, endocrinopathies, infections and nutritional deficiencies. In general, the severity of the injury determines whether an insult will result in hypopigmentation or hyperpigmentation. Mild injury results in pigmentary incontinence and epidermal hypopigmentation from death of melanin containing keratinocytes. However, hyperpigmentation can occur, possibly from release of melanocyte-stimulating factors from surviving keratinocytes and subsequent increase in production of melanosomes. It is thought that these factors are preset in normal epidermis, but their level or activity is increased in response to stimulation or keratinocyte stress. In contrast, severe injury results in the death of melanocytes, which do not regenerate, and thus there is no repigmentation.

Cutaneous depigmentation in dogs and horses can result from contact with rubber. The monobenzene ether of hydroquinone, a common ingredient in rubber, inhibits melanogenesis. In horses lesions result from contact with equipment such as rubber bit guards, crupper straps, or with feed buckets (lips, buttocks, face). In dogs lesions result from contact with rubber dishes or toys (lips or nose).

In dogs, hypopigmentation can occur in immune-mediated diseases such as lupus erythematosus, dermatomyositis, and uveodermatologic syndrome (see Selected Autoimmune Reactions). The hypopigmentation develops from injury and subsequent loss of the melanin-containing keratinocytes or melanocytes. Leukotrichia (depigmentation of hair) can be seen in the healing stage of alopecia areata, an immune-mediated condition characterized clinically by alopecia, and microscopically by lymphocytic inflammation of the hair bulb.

HYPERPIGMENTATION
Secondary Hyperpigmentation

Hyperpigmentation can result from inflammation, irritation, and metabolic disorders. Consequently hyperpigmentation is seen in all species with epidermal melanin pigment. Hypermelanosis results from an increased rate of melanosome production, an increase in melanosome size, or an increase in the degree of melanization of the melanosome. It is usually associated with an accelerated melanocyte turnover with an increased number of melanosomes, as occurs following trauma and ultraviolet light exposure.

Acanthosis Nigricans

Primary idiopathic acanthosis nigricans is considered a genodermatosis (genetically determined skin disorder) of young dachshunds. The disease is manifested by bilateral axillary hyperpigmentation, lichenification, and alopecia, which can involve large areas and include secondary seborrhea and pyoderma. Histological examination reveals hyperplastic dermatitis with orthokeratotic and parakeratotic hyperkeratosis, acanthosis and rete ridge formation. All layers of the epidermis are heavily melanized. Spongiosis, neutrophilic exocytosis and serous crusts can also be present. The dermal inflammatory reaction is mild, pleomorphic in cell type, and superficial perivascular in location. The term "acanthosis nigricans" has also been used to encompass a variety of chronic inflammatory and pruritic disorders that in their chronic form are manifested by axillary or more diffuse lichenification, alopecia, and hyperpigmentation. Consequently, the diagnosis of primary acanthosis nigricans requires clinical correlation together with the histologic findings to support the diagnosis in a young dachshund with compatible lesion distribution.

Nonneoplastic Pigmented Macules or Plaques
Lentigines (focal macular plaques)

Lentigines are rare, nonneoplastic, well circumscribed, macular to slightly raised plaques found most often on the mucocutaneous junctions of the mouth, eye, nose, and footpads. Histologically, lentigenes are characterized by irregular epidermal hyperplasia, hyperpigmentation, and increased numbers of pigmented melanocytes. Lentigines are often multifocal and have been described in dogs and cats. The lesions are of no significance except that they can be confused clinically with melanoma or epidermal pigmented plaques.

Pigmented epidermal plaques

See Viral Infections, Papillomaviruses.

MISCELLANEOUS SKIN DISORDERS
DISORDERS CHARACTERIZED BY INFILTRATES OF EOSINOPHILS OR PLASMA CELLS

These diseases are listed in Box 17-13. In addition to the syndromes discussed herein, eosinophils are often a prominent feature of hypersensitivity or parasitic dermatoses, especially in cats and horses, and are also often a feature in feline herpesvirus facial dermatitis.

Eosinophilic Plaques

These common lesions of the skin of cats occur on the abdomen and medial thigh and are thought to be associated with hypersensitivity reactions. Lesions consist of raised, variably sized erythematous, pruritic, and eroded to ulcerated plaques. Microscopically, epidermal

Box **17-13**

Disorders Characterized by Infiltrates of Eosinophils or Plasma Cells

Eosinophilic plaques
Eosinophilic granulomas
Nasal eosinophilic folliculitis and furunculosis in dogs
Hypereosinophil syndromes with systemic signs or lesions
    Multisystemic eosinophilic epitheliotropic disease in the horse
    Feline hypereosinophilic syndrome
    Eosinophilic dermatitis with edema in the dog
Feline plasma cell pododermatitis
Hypersensitivity and parasitic dermatitis (see Mechanisms of Tissue Damage in Hypersensitivity Reactions)
Feline herpesvirus facial dermatitis (see herpesvirus section)

lesions include acanthosis, variable spongiosis, erosion, and ulceration, accompanied by superficial and deep, perivascular to diffuse, predominantly eosinophilic dermatitis.

EOSINOPHILIC GRANULOMAS (COLLAGENOLYTIC GRANULOMAS)

Eosinophilic and granulomatous lesions with brightly eosinophilic, granular to amorphous material bordering collagen fibers and somewhat obscuring the fiber detail (flame figures) occur in cats, dogs, and horses. The causes of these syndromes are poorly understood. The tinctorial change can develop in any lesion with large numbers of eosinophils such as reactions to parasites, foreign bodies (including hair), or in mast cell tumors. Eosinophils congregate and degranulate near collagen bundles causing the tinctorial change. Eosinophil degranulation results in release of a wide range of toxic granule proteins (e.g., major basic protein), enzymes (peroxidase, collagenase), cytokines (IL-3, IL-5, GM-CSF), chemokines (IL-8), and lipid mediators (leukotrienes and platelet-activating factor) augmenting an inflammatory response. Gross lesions include papules, nodules, plaques (sometimes linear), and ulcers in the skin (Fig. 17-23). Nodular or ulcerated lesions can also develop in the oral mucosa of dogs and cats, and footpads of cats. Microscopically, nodular dermatitis (or stomatitis) consists of an inflammatory response with a prominence of eosinophils, flame figures, and macrophages, some of which are multinucleated (Fig. 17-23). Collagen lysis develops in some lesions, likely a secondary event caused by the proteolytic enzymes (e.g., collagenase). Some indolent

ulcers on the upper lip of cats have areas of flame figures and granulomatous inflammation and are considered to be eosinophilic granulomas.

NASAL EOSINOPHILIC FOLLICULITIS AND FURUNCULOSIS IN DOGS

Nasal eosinophilic folliculitis and furunculosis develops primarily on the dorsal and lateral surfaces of the nose of young dogs, and is thought to be a result of arthropod bites (bees, wasps, spiders). Lesions develop acutely, and are often painful swollen areas that rapidly ulcerate and can drain bloody fluid. Lesions can progress to involve the periocular, pinnal, and sometimes the glabrous ventral abdominal skin. Because lesions develop rapidly and appear clinically severe, biopsy samples are typically collected early in the course of the disease. At this time, microscopic lesions consist of ulceration, superficial and deep interstitial eosinophilic to mixed inflammation with eosinophilic folliculitis and furunculosis.

HYPEREOSINOPHILIC SYNDROMES WITH SYSTEMIC SIGNS OR LESIONS

Multisystemic eosinophilic epitheliotropic disease in the horse

This generalized, exfoliative dermatitis of horses is of unknown etiology; however, one case report documents the coexistence of an intestinal T-lymphocyte lymphoma and postulates a role for tumor cell overproduction of IL-5, a powerful eosinophilopoietin. Initial cutaneous lesions include dry scales and serous exudates of the epithelium of the skin of the head, coronary bands, and oral mucosa. The lesions progress to generalized excoriations with ulceration and alopecia. Secondary infections are common. Histologically there is superficial and deep, perivascular to interstitial, eosinophilic lymphoplasmacytic, and sometimes granulomatous dermatitis with irregular epidermal hyperplasia and orthokeratotic and parakeratotic hyperkeratosis. Eosinophils, lymphocytes, and apoptotic keratinocytes can be prominent in the epidermis, and eosinophilic folliculitis, furunculosis, and flame figures are occasionally seen. The dermatitis is accompanied by a similar inflammatory response with fibrosis in other organs including the alimentary tract, pancreas, liver, uterus, and bronchial epithelium. Clinically, the horses lose weight and become progressively debilitated.

Feline hypereosinophilic syndrome

Feline hypereosinophilic syndrome is a rare multisystemic disorder of unknown cause that is associated with moderate to marked peripheral eosinophilia and infiltrates of mature eosinophils in multiple organ systems, sometimes including the skin. Middle-aged female cats are more often affected. Gross lesions of the skin include erythema and excoriations associated with severe pruritus. Histologically, there is superficial and deep, perivascular dermatitis with prominent eosinophils. Clinical signs include anorexia, diarrhea, weight loss, and vomiting.

Eosinophilic dermatitis with edema in the dog

Eosinophilic dermatitis with edema is a newly described condition affecting adult dogs of a variety of breeds, although Labrador retrievers may be overrepresented. The cause is not known, but a hypersensitivity reaction to medications, arthropod bites, or other antigens is suspected. Gross lesions consist of extremely erythematous macules that progress and coalesce into arciform and serpiginous plaques. Facial or generalized pitting edema is often seen. Lesions involve the pinnae, ventral abdomen and thorax, and less often the extremities. Histological lesions consist of diffuse, predominantly eosinophilic dermatitis, vascular dilation, and edema. Eosinophil aggregation and degranulation are seen in some lesions. Depression, hypoproteinemia, and pyrexia are present in some dogs.

PLASMA CELL PODODERMATITIS

Feline plasma cell pododermatitis is an uncommon condition of undetermined pathogenesis. It is characterized clinically by soft, painless swelling of multiple footpads that can lead to collapse of the footpad and ulceration, hemorrhage, and lameness. Histologically, the skin of the footpad is heavily infiltrated by plasma cells with variable numbers of Russell body plasma cells, neutrophils, and lymphocytes. This condition is sometimes accompanied by plasmacytic stomatitis, hypergammaglobulinemia, immune-mediated glomerulonephritis, or renal amyloidosis. A recent study indicated 50% of cases are positive for feline leukemia virus.

NODULAR GRANULOMATOUS INFLAMMATORY DISORDERS WITHOUT MICROORGANISMS

These diseases are listed in Box 17-14. The disorders in this category have traditionally been considered to be sterile because no microorganisms have been identified by microscopic examination, including with special stains for organisms, by electron microscopic examination, by cultures, or by cytologic evaluation for organisms. However, newer techniques, including the PCR that detects minute amounts of DNA, suggest the potential for microbial participation in the pathogenesis of some of these seemingly sterile inflammatory disorders, especially in human beings. It is possible, for instance, for an abnormal immune response to an as yet unidentified microbial antigen to initiate a macrophage-dominated inflammatory response.

> **Box 17-14**
>
> ## Nodular Granulomatous Inflammatory Disorders without Microorganisms
>
> Juvenile sterile granulomatous dermatitis and lymphadenitis
> Sterile pyogranuloma syndrome (idiopathic sterile granuloma and pyogranuloma)
> Canine reactive histiocytosis
> Idiopathic sterile nodular panniculitis
> Xanthoma (xanthogranuloma)
> Equine generalized granulomatous disease (see Vetch Toxicosis and Vetchlike Diseases)
> Feline nutritional pansteatitis (see Vitamin E Deficiency)

Defective down-regulation of the immune response to the organism could lead to a persistent granulomatous inflammatory process. Currently, this issue remains unresolved, but as more of these lesions are probed for microbial agents, a better understanding of these so-called "sterile" inflammatory disorders will hopefully develop.

JUVENILE STERILE GRANULOMATOUS DERMATITIS AND LYMPHADENITIS (JUVENILE CELLULITIS, JUVENILE PYODERMA, PUPPY STRANGLES)

This disorder of unknown cause occurs in pups younger than 4 months (Fig. 17-75), with one or more of the pups of a litter developing pustular and nodular dermatitis and edema of the face, ears, and mucocutaneous junctions. The pustular and nodular lesions tend to rupture, drain, and crust. Microscopically, early lesions consist of multifocal granulomatous or pyogranulomatous perifolliculitis and dermatitis (Fig. 17-75). Early lesions are adjacent to, but do not involve, follicles; however, lesions typically progress to folliculitis, furunculosis, panniculitis, cellulitis, and granulomatous to pyogranulomatous lymphadenitis. The lesions initially are considered to be sterile, but secondary bacterial infections develop and can lead to sepsis if not treated. About half of the puppies are lethargic, and anorexia, fever, and joint pain can also occur.

IDIOPATHIC STERILE GRANULOMA AND PYOGRANULOMA (STERILE PYOGRANULOMA SYNDROME)

These lesions are seen most commonly in dogs and rarely cats and horses, are of unknown cause, and are characterized grossly by single or multifocal papules, plaques, or nodules most commonly in the skin of the head and extremities. Early microscopic lesions include periadnexal to coalescing nodular accumulations of leukocytes predominantly consisting of macrophages (histiocytes), neutrophils, and lymphocytes.

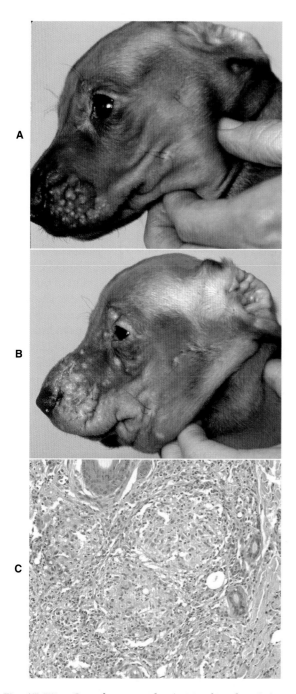

Fig. 17-75   **Granulomatous dermatitis, skin, dog. A,** Juvenile sterile granulomatous dermatitis and lymphadenitis (juvenile pyoderma), dachshund puppy. The pustules on the muzzle are of 1 day duration. The mandibular lymph node *(held between thumb and index finger)* is enlarged. **B,** Juvenile sterile granulomatous dermatitis and lymphadenitis (juvenile pyoderma), dachshund puppy (same as in Fig. 17-75, A). The lesions, of 12 days duration, have progressed to include alopecia, thickening of the skin from edema, and crusting. The mandibular lymph node *(held between thumb and index finger)* has at least doubled in size. **C,** Note the periadnexal mixture of macrophages and fewer lymphocytes, plasma cells, and neutrophils in the dermis. No microorganisms are present. H&E stain. *(A and B, Courtesy Dr. David Prieur, College of Veterinary Medicine, Washington State University. C, Courtesy Dr. Ann M. Hargis, DermatoDiagnostics.)*

Older lesions can efface adnexa and extend into the subcutis. Neither microorganisms nor foreign material are found microscopically, and cultures and cytology for organisms are negative. The lesions must be differentiated from those of the infectious granulomatous disorders and the reactive histiocytic disorders recognized in dogs (reactive histiocytosis).

CANINE REACTIVE HISTIOCYTOSIS

Canine reactive histiocytosis is a poorly understood disorder that occurs in cutaneous and systemic forms in dogs of a variety of ages and breeds. Cultures and special stains fail to reveal causative agents, and the disorder is thought to be the result of immune dysregulation. The disorder typically has a slowly progressive, waxing and waning course but can respond favorably, as least for a time, to immunomodulatory therapy. The lesions require long-term management and often lead to death, particularly if there is systemic involvement. The cutaneous form consists of single or multifocal, nonpainful plaques or nodules composed of histiocytic cells that are immunophenotypically identified as dermal perivascular activated dendritic antigen-presenting cells (CD1+, CD4+, CD11c+, CD11b+, MHC II+, ICAM-1+, and CD90+). Also intermixed with the histiocytic cells are CD3+, CD8+, TCRαβ+ T lymphocytes and CD11b+ neutrophils. The systemic form is identical immunophenotypically, but can also involve the nasal mucosa, eyelids, sclera, lung, spleen, liver, bone marrow, and multiple lymph nodes in addition to the skin. Gross lesions in the cutaneous form are restricted to the skin and subcutis, can be alopecic or haired, and are most often on the head, neck, perineum, scrotum, and extremities. Histologically, there are single or multifocal infiltrates of large, round-to-oval histiocytes mixed with lymphocytes and neutrophils that, in early lesions, are periadnexal to elongate and are oriented vertically. Later the infiltrates coalesce into larger deep dermal and subcutaneous masses. Vessels are often surrounded and invaded by the infiltrates, which can result in thrombosis and infarction.

IDIOPATHIC STERILE NODULAR PANNICULITIS

These lesions develop in dogs, cats, and rarely horses, are of unknown cause, and are characterized grossly by single or multifocal plaques or nodules in the subcutis and occasionally deep dermis of any anatomic site. Lesions can rupture and drain, thus involve the dermis secondarily. Microscopic lesions consist of discrete, coalescing, or diffuse accumulations of macrophages (histiocytes), neutrophils, lymphocytes, and occasionally other leukocytes. The lesions must be differentiated from those of the infectious granulomatous disorders, sterile pyogranuloma syndrome, and the reactive histiocytic disorders recognized in dogs (see section on reactive histiocytosis [cutaneous and systemic histiocytosis]).

XANTHOMAS (XANTHOGRANULOMAS)

Xanthomas are rare, usually multifocal, light tan to yellow papules, plaques, or nodules located in the skin of cats and more rarely dogs and horses. The lesions take their name from the Greek "xanthos" meaning yellow. Some xanthomas are associated with abnormalities in triglyceride or cholesterol metabolism and are thus seen in animals with hereditary defects in lipid metabolism or with metabolic disorders, such as diabetes mellitus, hypothyroidism, or hyperadrenocorticism. Histologically, xanthomas associated with abnormalities in triglyceride or cholesterol metabolism consist of sheets of macrophages filled with foamy cytoplasm, scattered giant cells, and interstitial areas of granular to amorphous lipid material and cholesterol clefts. The lipids in the lesions impart a yellow to tan color to the clinical lesions, which is responsible for the name. Rarely xanthogranulomas also have developed in apparently healthy cats and dogs.

Other syndromes including equine generalized granulomatous disease (see Vetch Toxicosis and Vetch-like Diseases), and nutritional pansteatitis (see Vitamin E Deficiency) are also categorized as sterile granulomatous disorders.

DISORDERS OF THE CLAW BED AND LUPOID ONYCHODYSTROPHY

Onychodystrophy refers to abnormal formation of the claw (nail), onychomadesis to sloughing of claws, and paronychia to inflammation of the skin of the claw fold. These conditions are rare. Onychodystrophy and paronychia of multiple claws on multiple feet have a variety of causes including infections (e.g., bacterial, fungal), immune-mediated disorders (e.g., pemphigus, lupus erythematosus), systemic disease (e.g., hyperadrenocorticism, disseminated intravascular coagulation), and disorders of unknown cause (e.g., lupoid onychodystrophy, idiopathic onychodystrophy). Diagnosis can require amputation of the third phalanx and the adjacent skin proximal to the claw fold for histopathologic evaluation. Lupoid onychodystrophy is probably the most common cause of onychomadesis that leads to onychodystrophy of multiple claws involving multiple feet in dogs. The condition affects many breeds of dogs of varying ages; the dogs are healthy otherwise. History includes sudden loss of claws, eventually involving all claws on all feet. There is partial regrowth of misshapen, friable claws that continue to slough. Paronychia is usually absent. Histologic lesions are more prominent on the dorsal aspect of the claw and claw bed skin and include interface lymphoplasmacytic inflammation with basal cell vacuolation and apoptosis and pigmentary incontinence. Secondary bacterial infection and osteomyelitis can develop.

CUTANEOUS MANIFESTATIONS OF SYSTEMIC DISEASE

LAMINITIS

The term "laminitis" refers to inflammation of the laminar structures of the hoof, but laminitis is a complex disease in which inflammation is only a part of the disease process. Laminitis can be seen in any hoofed animal, but is of greatest importance in horses and cattle. Laminitis occurs in three phases (developmental or preclinical, acute, and chronic). By definition, chronic laminitis (also called "founder") refers to the stage of laminitis associated with radiographic or physical evidence of rotational or vertical displacement of the third phalanx relative to the hoof wall. In severe laminitis, rotation can occur as early as 24 hours after the appearance of lameness. A variety of systemic conditions cause laminitis including, but not limited to, alimentary carbohydrate overload, toxemia, and sepsis. Repeated trauma to the foot can also cause laminitis. The pathogenesis of laminitis is complex, not completely understood, and controversial. There are two basic hypotheses, vascular and toxic-metabolic, that address mechanisms responsible for the systemic causes of laminitis. The vascular hypothesis argues that digital ischemia is the primary event. The toxic-metabolic hypothesis argues that there is direct damage to epithelial cells of the laminae or to the basement membrane, and that the vascular lesions are secondary. Gross findings of the external foot in acute laminitis can be minimal. Swelling or edema of the coronary band can be seen. Extravasation of serum through the skin above the coronary band is indicative of severe laminitis. Chronic lesions are highly variable, ranging from minimal gross changes to a totally gangrenous foot. Common gross lesions include parallel circumferential hoof rings (ridges, founder rings), altered foot shape, separation of the wall from the epidermis at the coronet, depression of coronary band, flattened sole, and, in some cases, penetration of the third phalanx through the sole.

The principal clinical sign of laminitis is pain manifested as lameness, abnormal stance, or reluctance to move. Diagnosis of laminitis is based principally on clinical, radiographic, and gross findings. Histopathology is used to facilitate understanding of the pathogenesis of laminitis. Regardless of whether the initial damage is ischemic or direct injury to the epithelium or basement membrane, the lesions of acute laminitis are degeneration and necrosis of epithelial cells of the laminae, separation of epithelial cells from the basement membrane, and loss of the basement membrane. If the epithelial and basement membrane damage is minor and patchy, regeneration of the damaged cells and basement membrane occurs preserving structural integrity of the epithelial laminae and hoof, and the animal does not enter into the chronic stage of laminitis. If the epithelial and basement membrane damage is more severe and confluent, the stability created by the interdigitating epithelial laminae attaching the hoof wall to the dermis and third phalanx is disrupted and the structural integrity of the foot is weakened. In addition, the epithelial necrosis causes release of inflammatory mediators such as cytokines, which result in congestion, edema, and an influx of a small to moderate number of neutrophils and mixed mononuclear cells. The edema adds to the soft tissue swelling and, in the confines of the rigid hoof wall, further compromises digital perfusion. If the tissue damage is subtotal, remaining epithelial cells regenerate. The hyperplasia and increased cornification of epithelial cells of the primary and secondary laminae cause broadening and fusion of the laminae, which reduces the surface area of the laminae and weakens the structural support of the hoof wall. The weakened structure of the epithelial laminae and basement membrane as a result of degeneration, necrosis, and subsequent epithelial hyperplasia, combined with the weight of the animal on the hoof and pulling force of the digital flexor tendon, contribute to displacement of the third phalanx, the hallmark of chronic laminitis, and to the altered shape of the foot in chronic laminitis (Fig. 17-76). For example, the circumferential hoof rings develop because the heel growth exceeds that of the dorsal wall. The unequal growth rate of the heels compared with the dorsal wall plus the mechanical forces on the wall also lead to abnormal hoof shape such as the concave profile of the dorsal hoof, often accompanied by long under-run heels. Depression of the coronary band and flattened or dropped sole are a result of displacement of the distal phalanx relative to the hoof wall, and thus are an indication that collapse of the foot has occurred.

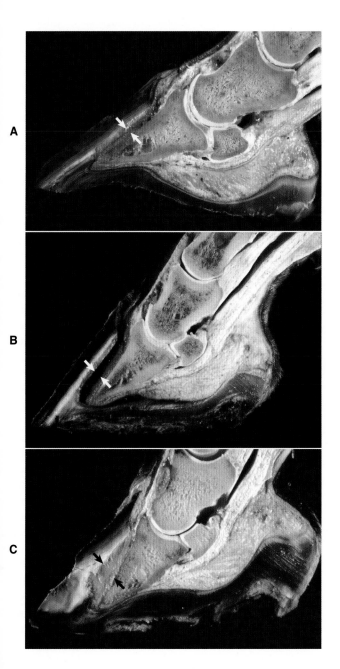

←

Fig. 17-76   Laminitis, hoof, horse. A, Normal hoof, midsagittal section. Note that the dorsal surface of the third phalanx is parallel to the epidermal laminae of the inner surface of the hoof wall *(arrows)*. No space is visible at this junction or at the junction of the ventral surface of the third phalanx and the internal (weight-bearing) surface of the hoof. **B,** Acute laminitis. Note that the dorsal surface of the third phalanx has separated from the epidermal laminae of the inner surface of the hoof wall *(arrows)*, leaving a large gap. The tip of the third phalanx has rotated ventrally slightly, resulting in a space between the ventral aspect of the third phalanx and the internal surface of the horny sole (weight-bearing surface of the hoof). **C,** Severe chronic laminitis. The dorsal surface of the third phalanx is widely separated from the epidermal laminae of the inner surface of the hoof wall, and the tip of the third phalanx has rotated ventrally. This space is filled with proliferated epithelium, connective tissue, and areas of inflammation *(arrows)*. The shape of the entire weight bearing surface of the hoof, the external surface of the horny sole, has been altered, leading to turning up and irregular wear of the toe region and thickening of the heel of the horny sole. (**A,** *Courtesy Dr. Pamela E. Ginn, College of Veterinary Medicine, University of Florida.* **B,** *Courtesy College of Veterinary Medicine, University of Illinois.* **C,** *Courtesy Dr. T. Boosinger, College of Veterinary Medicine, Auburn University; and Noah's Arkive, College of Veterinary Medicine, The University of Georgia.)*

Box **17-15**

Principal Cutaneous Paraneoplastic Syndromes

Paraneoplastic alopecia and internal malignancies in the cat
Exfoliative dermatitis and thymoma
Superficial necrolytic dermatitis
Pancreatic panniculitis (necrotizing panniculitis)
Nodular dermatofibrosis and renal or uterine tumors in dogs
Paraneoplastic pemphigus (see Selected Autoimmune Diseases)

CUTANEOUS PARANEOPLASTIC SYNDROMES

Cutaneous paraneoplastic syndromes are rare dermatoses that occur in association with internal malignancies (Box 17-15). Confirmation of a dermatosis as a paraneoplastic syndrome requires strict adherence to established clinical, histopathologic, and in some instances, immunologic criteria. Conditions meeting these criteria currently recognized in animals include paraneoplastic pemphigus (discussed in the section on autoimmune diseases); paraneoplastic alopecia and internal malignancies in the cat; exfoliative dermatosis and thymoma in the cat, dog, and rabbit; and superficial necrolytic dermatopathy in the dog and cat. Dermatofibrosis in the dog, pancreatic panniculitis, and multisystemic eosinophilic epitheliotropic disease in the horse have also been associated with underlying neoplasia; however, they have not yet been proven to be true paraneoplastic syndromes. This list is exclusive of the endocrine dermatoses associated with functional tumors of endocrine organs. Many other syndromes are documented in human beings, and it is likely more will be documented in animals in the future. The refractory nature of these syndromes and their significance as an indicator of systemic disease underscores the importance of their recognition.

PARANEOPLASTIC ALOPECIA ASSOCIATED WITH INTERNAL MALIGNANCIES IN THE CAT (PANCREATIC PARANEOPLASTIC SYNDROME)

This syndrome is a rapidly progressive, largely ventrally distributed, symmetric alopecia that develops in older cats with metastatic pancreatic or biliary carcinomas. The pathogenesis of this condition is not known. The alopecia typically affects the ventrum, legs, and footpads. The ears and periocular skin are less frequently involved. Alopecic skin is smooth, soft, and often has a shiny or glistening appearance. Histologically, affected skin has small inactive hair follicles with a reduction or absence of the stratum corneum. Some cats groom excessively, and it has been suggested that the smooth shiny appearance of the skin is because of the absence of the stratum corneum. In other areas of the skin there is variable orthokeratotic and parakeratotic hyperkeratosis in which *Malassezia pachydermatis* is sometimes identified. In addition to the alopecia, the cats have systemic signs of anorexia, weight loss, and lethargy.

EXFOLIATIVE DERMATITIS AND THYMOMA

A generalized exfoliative dermatitis has been documented as a paraneoplastic syndrome of older cats with thymomas. More recently, the condition has been recognized in dogs and rabbits. Immune dysregulation probably plays a role in lesion development. Gross lesions begin as scaling and erythema of the head and ears and progress to generalized alopecia with scales, crusts, and ulcers. Histologically, the lesions include basal cell hydropic degeneration, lymphocyte exocytosis, and lymphocyte clustering around apoptotic keratinocytes of the epidermis and outer follicular root sheath. The lesions are compatible with the diagnosis of erythema multiforme or a graft-versus-host-type reaction. Cats with this syndrome often have clinical signs referable to an intrathoracic mass resulting in dyspnea.

SUPERFICIAL NECROLYTIC DERMATITIS (DIABETIC DERMATOPATHY, HEPATOCUTANEOUS SYNDROME, NECROLYTIC MIGRATORY ERYTHEMA, METABOLIC EPIDERMAL NECROSIS)

This is an uncommon disorder reported primarily in older dogs with deranged nutrient metabolism because of diabetes mellitus, hepatic dysfunction, or less commonly with glucagon-secreting pancreatic islet tumors. Anticonvulsant therapy has also preceded the development of superficial necrolytic dermatitis, but it is uncertain if anticonvulsant therapy causes the disease or possibly exacerbates subclinical disease. The disorder is rarely seen in cats; one cat with superficial necrolytic dermatitis had concurrent pancreatic endocrine carcinoma. The pathogenesis of superficial necrolytic dermatitis is not completely understood, and may vary with the underlying defect. When glucagon is elevated, persistent gluconeogenesis is thought to result in a negative nitrogen balance with protein degradation, including proteins in the epidermis. However, when glucagon is not elevated, as occurs in human beings with some types of hepatic or malabsorptive disease and in dogs with diabetes and multinodular vacuolar hepatopathy, it is thought that deficiencies of certain essential fatty acids, zinc, and amino acids play a role. Clinical lesions of scaling, crusting, erythema, and alopecia develop on the face, distal extremities, and genitalia. Footpad lesions consist of crusting and fissuring or ulceration (Fig. 17-11), and result in lameness. Microscopic lesions, when fully developed, are considered diagnostic and consist of trilaminar thickening of the epidermis in which the stratum corneum has marked parakeratosis, the upper stratum spinosum is pale with reticular degeneration, and the lower spinous and basal cell layers are hyperplastic (Fig. 17-11). Secondary infections with bacteria or yeast frequently complicate lesions, and secondary infection with dermatophytes also has been seen.

PANCREATIC PANNICULITIS (NECROTIZING PANNICULITIS)

Pancreatic panniculitis is an acute rare disorder that has developed in dogs with pancreatic neoplasia and pancreatitis. The lesions are thought to be a result of the release of pancreatic enzymes (e.g., lipases) either from damaged pancreatic exocrine cells or from neoplastic exocrine cells. The lipases enter the systemic circulation and subsequently locate in the panniculus. Gross lesions consist of multiple, frequently ulcerated and hemorrhagic nodules within the subcutis. Histologically there is necrosis of adipose tissue (caused by the lipases) with fine basophilic granularity (caused by mineralization of the necrotic fatty tissue). Neutrophilic inflammation occurs at the periphery of the necrotic foci.

NODULAR DERMATOFIBROSIS AND RENAL DISEASE IN THE DOG

In nodular dermatofibrosis, multiple cutaneous nodules composed of excessive collagen coexist with renal cystadenomas, cystadenocarcinomas, hyperplastic epithelial cysts, or uterine smooth muscle tumors. Renal lesions are often bilateral and may not be detectable clinically for months or years after the appearance of the cutaneous nodules. The syndrome has been described in the German shepherd, boxer, golden retriever, and mixed-breed dogs, and is thought have an autosomal dominant mode of inheritance in the German shepherd. Whether the condition is a true paraneoplastic syndrome with the renal neoplasm inducing dermal fibrosis or the simultaneous occurrence of two independent conditions with a common hereditary linkage is undetermined. Gross lesions consist of firm dermal and subcutaneous nodules on legs, head or ears. Histologic lesions consist of nodular dermal and subcutaneous aggregates of poorly cellular, mature dermal collagen bundles that are slightly thickened. In the dermis, the collagen bundles blend often imperceptibly with bordering collagen, but in the subcutis, the nodules are usually circumscribed. Adnexa are normal or hyperplastic. The cutaneous nodules are benign but serve as a marker for the more serious renal lesions.

PARANEOPLASTIC PEMPHIGUS

See Selected Autoimmune Reactions, Paraneoplastic Pemphigus.

CUTANEOUS NEOPLASIA

The skin is a common site of neoplastic growth in most animals; the neoplasms are of ectodermal, mesodermal, and melanocytic origin (Box 17-16). Ectodermal neoplasms of the epidermis and adnexa are most often benign with the exception of the neoplasms of the apocrine sweat glands, apocrine glands of the anal sac, and neoplasms of the surface epithelium (squamous cell carcinomas).

Benign neoplasms do not metastasize or invade adjacent tissue. In general, benign neoplasms are circumscribed, grow by expansion, and are composed of well-differentiated cells that closely resemble the cells or tissue of origin (Box 17-16). Malignant neoplasms are locally invasive and often metastasize. They are more often composed of anaplastic cells with a high mitotic index that no longer resemble the cells of origin. Anaplastic cells are pleomorphic (vary in cell size and shape) and have a large, vesicular nucleus with increased size and number of nucleoli (Box 17-16). Malignant cells develop surface alterations such as altered antigenicity, decreased numbers or altered location of receptors for adjacent cells, and increased receptors for components of the extracellular matrix. Changes such as these allow malignant cells to detach from the primary site of tumor growth, move through tissues, and in some cases escape detection by the host's immune system. A specific example is the loss of E-cadherins (proteins responsible for epithelial cell to cell attachment) by some types of carcinomas. E-cadherins are partially responsible for the "contact inhibition" that leads to density control and inhibits uncontrolled proliferation of epithelial cells.

Neoplasms of the skin develop secondary to the same basic molecular changes, leading to the development of neoplasms of any tissue. The neoplastic transformation of a cell is the end result of a series of events causing damage to the cellular DNA. Most agents that are known to be carcinogenic target and damage DNA. Solar radiation, x-radiation, viral infections, and continued trauma are important contributors to neoplastic transformation of components of the skin. Continued trauma contributes to tumor development by increasing cell turnover, which in turn increases the chance of mutations. Not all factors contributing to the development of cutaneous neoplasms are known.

Four categories of genes encode for a large number of proteins responsible for regulation of cellular proliferation and differentiation. These categories are the tumor suppressor genes, the protooncogenes, genes that

Text continued on p. 1259.

BOX 17-16

Examples of Tumors of the Skin

ECTODERMAL TUMORS
Basal Cell Tumor

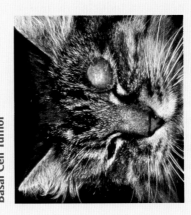

Basal cell tumor, skin, upper eyelid and dorsal to eye, cat. The tumor is circumscribed, raised, and sparsely haired. The tumor and bordering skin can be easily moved from side to side above the deeper tissue because the tumor has not invaded into underling tissue.*

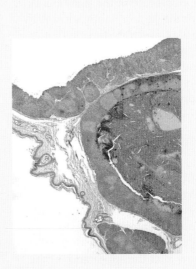

Basal cell tumor of epidermal origin, skin, cat. The dermis is expanded by multiple lobules of neoplastic basal epithelial cells. The centers of some of the lobules have cystic degeneration and contain pigmented debris. Basal cell tumors arise from basal cells of the epidermis and those of hair follicles. H&E stain.†

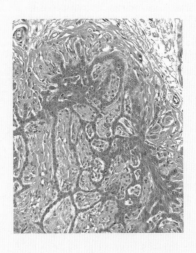

Trichoblastoma (basal cell tumor of follicular origin), skin, dog. Note ribbon (medusoid) pattern produced by the proliferating basal cells. This pattern is one of several patterns (ribbon, trabecular, granular cell, spindle cell) typical of basal cell tumors of follicular origin, also called trichoblastomas. H&E stain.‡

(Continued)

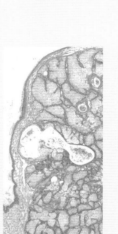

Infundibular keratinizing acanthoma, skin, dog. Higher magnification of wall of the tumor. The lobules border concentric laminations of stratum corneum and are supported by scant mucinous stroma. These tumors resemble squamous cell carcinoma but have a circumscribed, noninvasive border. H&E stain.

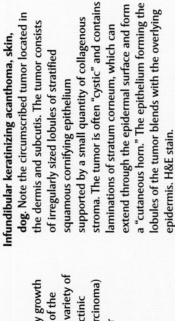

Infundibular keratinizing acanthoma, skin, dog. Note the circumscribed tumor located in the dermis and subcutis. The tumor consists of irregularly sized lobules of stratified squamous cornifying epithelium supported by a small quantity of collagenous stroma. The tumor is often "cystic" and contains laminations of stratum corneum, which can extend through the epidermal surface and form a "cutaneous horn." The epithelium forming the lobules of the tumor blends with the overlying epidermis. H&E stain.

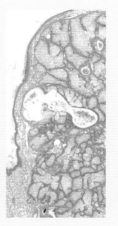

Infundibular Keratinizing Acanthoma

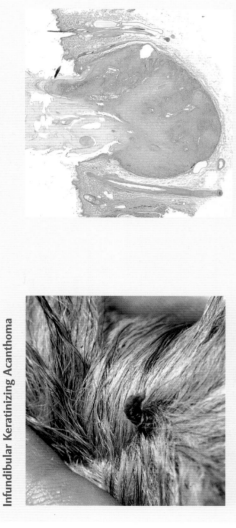

Infundibular keratinizing acanthoma (intracutaneous cornifying epithelioma, keratoacanthoma), skin, dog. Note horny growth (cutaneous horn) projecting from surface of the tumor. Cutaneous horns can arise from a variety of benign or malignant epidermal lesions (actinic keratosis; Fig. 17-40, *B*, squamous cell carcinoma) or adnexal lesions, especially infundibular keratinizing acanthomas.[§]

Sebaceous Gland Adenoma

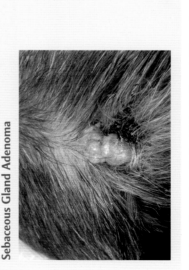

All photographs courtesy Dr. Ann M. Hargis, DermatoDiagnostics, unless otherwise noted.
*Courtesy Dr. Peter Ihrke, College of Veterinary Medicine, University of California-Davis.
†Courtesy Dr. Pamela E. Ginn, College of Veterinary Medicine, University of Florida.
‡Courtesy Dr. M. Donald McGavin, College of Veterinary Medicine, University of Tennessee.
§Courtesy Dr. Helen Power, Dermatology for Animals.

Box 17-16

Examples of Tumors of the Skin—Cont'd

Sebaceous gland adenoma, skin, dog. This common tumor of sebaceous glands often protrudes above the epidermal surface. The tumors are hairless and greasy because of sebaceous gland secretion.

Sebaceous gland adenoma, skin, dog. Lobules of well-differentiated sebaceous glands are present in the dermis and cause polypoid elevation of the overlying epidermis. A duct with sebaceous secretion is also present. Ducts connect via follicular epithelium to the epidermis providing the sebaceous (greasy) secretion to the surface. H&E stain.

Sebaceous gland adenoma, skin, dog. Note the close resemblance of the lobules of tumor cells to those of nonneoplastic sebaceous glands, a feature suggesting benign behavior. H&E stain.

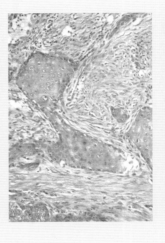

Squamous Cell Carcinoma

Squamous cell carcinomas, skin, abdomen, dog. Note multiple ulcerated squamous cell carcinomas in nonpigmented, sparsely haired abdominal skin. These are solar induced squamous cell carcinomas that developed in a beagle dog living outdoors at a high altitude region where the level of UV light is increased.

Squamous cell carcinoma, skin, dog. The dermis is invaded by neoplastic squamous epithelial cells that have arisen from the basal cells of the epidermis (*above center*) and that have differentiated to form irregular islands of squamous epithelium. H&E stain.[‡]

Squamous cell carcinoma, skin, dog. Islands of neoplastic epithelial cells with squamous differentiation have invaded the dermis and are surrounded by proliferating fibroblasts and collagen (desmoplasia). H&E stain.[‡]

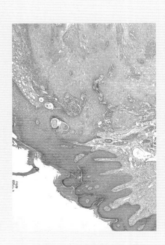

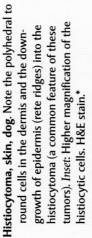

Histiocytoma, skin, dog. Note the polyhedral to round cells in the dermis and the down-growth of epidermis (rete ridges) into the histiocytoma (a common feature of these tumors). *Inset:* Higher magnification of the histiocytic cells. H&E stain.*

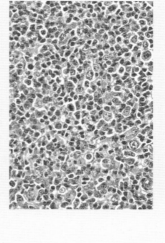

Cutaneous lymphoma, skin, horse. Note the population of different appearing lymphoid cells.

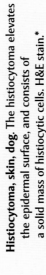

Histiocytoma, skin, dog. The histiocytoma elevates the epidermal surface, and consists of a solid mass of histiocytic cells. H&E stain.*

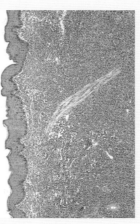

Cutaneous lymphoma, skin, horse. Sheets of neoplastic lymphocytes and infiltrating

MESODERMAL TUMORS
Cutaneous Histiocytoma

Cutaneous histiocytoma, skin, nose, dog. Circular raised alopecic tan nodule is present. Cutaneous histiocytomas frequently spontaneously regress. *Inset:* section of cutaneous histiocytoma illustrating the non encapsulated, solid dermal mass protruding above the epidermal surface.

Cutaneous Lymphoma

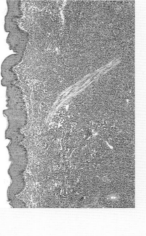

Cutaneous lymphoma, skin, neck and lateral thorax, horse. Note the nodules that are masses of

*Courtesy Dr. M. Donald McGavin, College of Veterinary Medicine, University of Tennessee.

(Continued)

Box 17-16

Examples of Tumors of the Skin—Cont'd

neoplastic lymphocytes and infiltrating nonneoplastic lymphocytes in the dermis, causing elevation of overlying epidermis.*

nonneoplastic lymphocytes have obliterated the normal dermal architecture except for an arrector pili muscle (*center*). The overlying epidermis is normal. H&E stain.

Some resemble normal lymphocytes and are small and well differentiated, whereas others are large and pleomorphic with vesicular nuclei and prominent nucleoli. Immunohistochemical and genetic studies of many cases of cutaneous lymphoma in the horse have demonstrated that the small well-differentiated lymphocytes are nonneoplastic T lymphocytes, whereas the large pleomorphic lymphocytes are neoplastic B lymphocytes. It is speculated that the neoplastic B lymphocytes produce cytokines that lead to infiltrates of nonneoplastic T lymphocytes and sometimes other leukocytes. Cutaneous lymphoma in the horse with this morphology and immunophenotype is referred to as a T-lymphocyte rich B-lymphocyte lymphoma subtype. H&E stain.

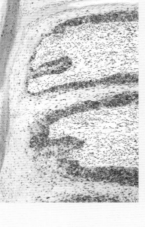

Epitheliotropic Lymphoma

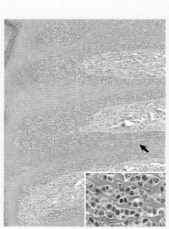

Epitheliotropic lymphoma, skin of lip and oral mucosa, dog. Note swelling, erythema, and depigmentation. Lymphocytes invade the epithelium and can cause depigmentation by displacing and damaging pigment containing epithelial cells and resident melanocytes of the basal region of the epidermis. Because of the involvement of the oral mucosa and mucocutaneous junctions and the presence of depigmentation and sometimes erosions, epitheliotropic lymphoma can be clinically confused with immune-mediated diseases such as systemic lupus erythematosus.

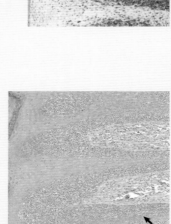

Epitheliotropic lymphoma, skin, dog. Neoplastic lymphocytes are located predominantly in the lower layers of the epidermis (*arrow*). *Inset:* Higher magnification of the neoplastic lymphocytes in the epidermis. Some of the lymphocytes are clustered together, forming microabscesses (Pautrier's microabscesses). H&E stain.[†]

Epitheliotropic lymphoma, skin, dog. Neoplastic lymphocytes are located predominantly in the lower layers of the epidermis and are labeled for CD3, indicating that they are T lymphocytes.

Mast Cell Tumor

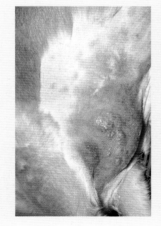

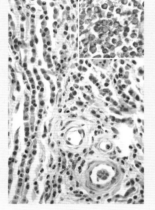

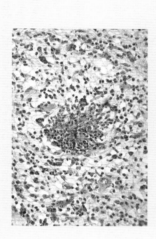

Mast cell tumor, skin, ventral thorax, dog. Note the irregular nodular and erythematous masses. Mast cell tumors in dogs can clinically resemble areas of inflammation because mast cells can degranulate and release inflammatory mediators (e.g., histamine, factors chemotactic for eosinophils and neutrophils, prostaglandins, serine esterases, and tumor necrosis factor-α) causing the inflammatory response.[†]

Mast cell tumor, skin, dog. The dermis is infiltrated by well-differentiated neoplastic mast cells with abundant gray to blue, finely granular cytoplasm and centrally located nuclei. H&E stain. *Inset:* Mast cells stained to illustrate metachromatic granules. In some cases, it can be difficult to differentiate round cell tumors such as histiocytomas, lymphomas, and mast cell tumors from each other. Demonstration of metachromatic cytoplasmic granules is an indicator of the presence of mast cells. *Metachromasia* means that the tissue or cellular component stains a color different from that of the staining dye because of a chemical reaction between the dye and the tissue component. For example, mast cell granules stain purple with the blue dye, toluidine blue. Toluidine blue stain.[‡]

Mast cell tumor, skin, dog. Mast cell tumor with degranulated eosinophils that border a collagen fiber. The collagen fibers and bordering eosinophilic material have been referred to as "flame figures" due in part to their irregular, sometimes radiating, edges and brightly eosinophilic staining intensity. H&E stain.[‡]

(Continued)

*Courtesy Dr. Donald McGavin, University of Tennessee.
[†]Courtesy Dr. Pamela E. Ginn, College of Veterinary Medicine, University of Florida.
[‡]Courtesy Dr. David Duclos, Animal Skin and Allergy Clinic.

Box **17-16**

Examples of Tumors of the Skin—Cont'd

Fibrosarcoma

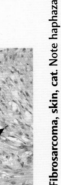

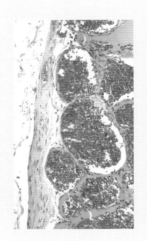

Fibrosarcoma, skin, cat. Note haphazardly arranged intersecting bundles of anaplastic spindle shaped neoplastic cells within a collagenous stroma. Anaplastic cells are pleomorphic in that they vary in cell size and shape and have a large, vesicular nucleus with increased size and number of nucleoli. Numerous mitotic figures are also present (*arrows*). H&E stain.[†]

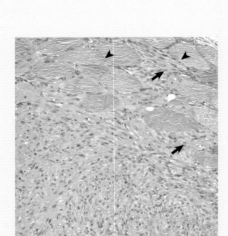

Fibrosarcoma, skin, cat. Cells of the fibrosarcoma (*arrows*) have infiltrated between skeletal muscle fibers (*arrowheads*). H&E stain.

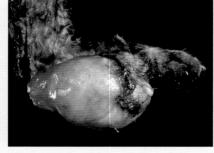

Fibrosarcoma, skin, leg, cat. The tumor has enlarged to such a degree that it has caused ulceration of the epidermis. Fibrosarcomas are locally invasive and difficult to excise completely. Amputation is an option for fibrosarcomas located on distal extremities.

Hemangioma

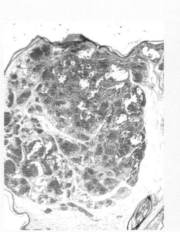

Hemangioma, skin, dog. The dermis is expanded by a circumscribed mass of blood filled vascular channels lined by well-differentiated endothelial cells. Note flattened well-differentiated endothelial cells (*arrows*) that form a single uniform layer. H&E stain.[†]

Hemangioma, skin, dog. Well-defined mass of proliferative, blood-filled, vascular channels in the dermis has elevated the epidermis. H&E stain.

Hemangioma, skin, hind leg, dog. Note raised red to dark red circumscribed mass in nonpigmented and sparsely haired skin.

Hemangiosarcomas

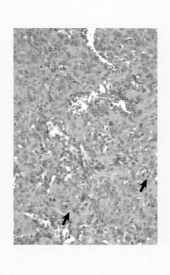

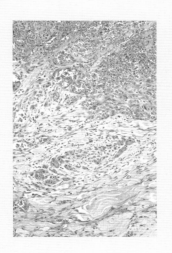

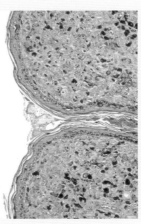

Hemangiosarcoma, skin, dog. Note multiple raised red masses in nonpigmented and sparsely haired skin of whippet.

Hemangiosarcoma, skin, dog. Note poorly demarcated margin between tumor (*mostly on the right*) and normal tissue (*mostly on the left*). H&E stain.

Hemangiosarcoma, skin, dog. The dermis is effaced by highly irregular vascular channels lined by plump, hyperchromatic endothelial cells with numerous mitotic figures (*arrows*). H&E stain.[†]

MELANOCYTIC TUMORS
Melanoma

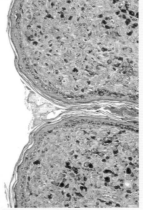

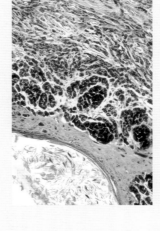

Melanocytoma, skin, dog. Note raised pigmented brown to black hairless mass.*

Melanocytoma, skin, dog. The dermis is diffusely infiltrated by sheets of variably pigmented melanocytes, which have prominent nucleoli and moderate variation in the size of cells and nuclei. H&E stain.[†]

Melanoma, skin, dog. Note clusters of pigmented melanocytes within the epidermis. This is called "junctional activity" and is a feature of melanocytic tumors. H&E stain.[†]

(Continued)

*Courtesy Dr. David Duclos, Animal Skin and Allergy Clinic.
[†]Courtesy Dr. Pamela E. Ginn, College of Veterinary Medicine, University of Florida.

Table 17-13   Selected Cutaneous Neoplastic and Neoplastic-like Lesions of Domestic Animals

Lesion	Cause	Species Age, Breed, Sex	Location	Gross Pathology	Histopathology	Biologic Behavior	Unique Features
Cutaneous papilloma (wart) (verruca) (Fig. 17-46)	Often caused by papillomavirus	Common in horses, cattle Infrequent in dogs, goats, sheep Rare in cats Often young age Congenital in foals	Horse: about the nose, lips, inner aspect of ears (aural plaques) Any location, often the head	Flattened to papillary mass, single or multiple, on narrow or broad base Inverted variety occurs	Papillary projections of epithelium over collagen core Epithelium thickened by hyperkeratosis and acanthosis	Most benign and will regress Occasional transformation to squamous cell carcinoma	May have viral inclusion bodies May have koilocytes (keratinocytes with swollen clear or gray cytoplasm)
Fibroepithelial polyp (skin tag)		Dogs	Any location	Raised smooth polyp	Epidermis covering collagen core	Benign	More collagen than squamous papilloma
Fibropapilloma (also see sarcoid)	Bovine papilloma virus 2	Young bulls, cows	Glans penis of bulls Vulva and vagina cows	Irregular mass attached to glans penis, less papillary than cutaneous papilloma	Proliferative epithelium and whorls and fascicles of fibroblasts and collagen	Look aggressive histologically and may recur after excision, but do not metastasize	Location Viral cause
Cutaneous cysts (Table 17-5, cyst) Follicular Sebaceous duct Dermoid Apocrine Ciliated	Follicular and apocrine (occluded follicles or ducts) Dermoid (genetic) Ciliated (developmental anomaly)	Any species, often dogs and cats	Anywhere on skin Dermoid: dorsal midline of Rhodesian ridgeback Ciliated: neck of cats	Cyst filled with soft, tan, greasy stratum corneum and sebum (follicular and sebaceous); hair (dermoid); or clear fluid (apocrine and ciliated)	Cystic structure with the wall composed of epidermal or adnexal epithelium Ciliated: from thyroglossal duct or respiratory epithelium	Nonneoplastic	Rupture and foreign body inflammation may develop
Cutaneous horn (Box 17-16)	Associated with benign or malignant epithelial tumors FeLV cat footpads Dermatophilus associated Papillomavirus	All domestic species	Any location Footpads of cats Areas of Dermatophilus infection in ruminants	Hard conical hornlike growth Greater height than diameter	Horn consists of laminations of compact stratum corneum Base may be a hyperplastic, neoplastic, or inflammatory lesion	Both neoplastic and nonneoplastic varieties Depends on nature of underlying lesion	Gross appearance

Tumor	Etiology	Species predisposition	Location	Clinical appearance	Histologic features	Biologic behavior	Comments
Hair follicle tumors Trichoepithelioma Tricholemmoma Trichoblastoma Pilomatricoma Trichoblastoma (hair follicle tumor of basal cells)	Genetic (breed predilections) May be multicentric in predisposed breeds	Dogs, occasionally cats Pilomatricoma Kerry blue terrier Trichoepithelioma Basset hound	Any location	Firm and discrete tumors Some cystic Some ulcerate Some mineralize	Variable depending on tumor Resemble portion of follicle from which they arise	Most tumors of follicular origin are benign Malignant varieties of trichoepithelioma and pilomatricoma have been described	May mineralize May result in foreign body response if cystic tumor ruptures
Infundibular keratinizing acanthoma (intracutaneous cornifying epithelioma) (Box 17-16)	Genetic (breed predilection)	Norwegian elkhound, may be multicentric	Often back and tail when multicentric	Dermal or subcutaneous mass, often with pore opening onto skin surface May be covered with cutaneous horn	Invaginated cyst with wall composed of lobules of stratified squamous epithelium	Benign	Resembles squamous cell carcinoma histologically
Malignant trichoepithelioma (matrical carcinoma) Malignant pilomatricoma	Unknown	Dogs	Any location in skin	Large, dermal or subcutaneous mass Poorly circumscribed, invade subcutis	Not usually connected with epidermis Similar to benign, but greater nuclear pleomorphism and mitotic activity	Malignant variety Trichoepithelioma: frequent metastasis to lymph nodes or lungs; recurrence also reported Pilomatricoma: may metastasize	Matrical keratinization Pilomatricoma has no trichohyalin granules; often has calcification or ossification
Benign basal cell tumor* (Box 17-16) Basal cell carcinoma	Unknown	Benign basal cell tumor of epidermal origin (cats) Carcinoma (dogs and cats) Rare in other domestic animals	Often head, neck, and cranial trunk	Generally solitary, firm nodules or plaques, which may ulcerate Carcinoma: may be multicentric	Benign: resemble basal cells Carcinoma: ragged margins; solid, clear cell; and keratinizing types	Benign Carcinoma locally aggressive with low potential for metastasis	Lack intercellular bridges May contain melanin pigment and can be confused with melanoma May be contiguous with epidermis

FeLV, Feline leukemia virus. *FeSV*, feline sarcoma virus; *FIV*, feline immunodeficiency virus.
*Classification and terminology of benign basal cell tumors varies with authors. Differences appear largely related to epidermal versus follicular origin and therefore histologic appearance of the tumors.

(Continued)

Table **17-13**   Selected Cutaneous Neoplastic and Neoplastic-like Lesions of Domestic Animals—Cont'd

Lesion	Cause	Species Age, Breed, Sex	Location	Gross Pathology	Histopathology	Biologic Behavior	Unique Features
Squamous cell carcinoma (Box 17-16) (in situ carcinoma termed Bowen's-like disease develops in cats in haired, often pigmented skin, multicentrically)	Solar radiation Trauma Carcinogens Papillomavirus in Bowen's-like disease Some unknown	All species, especially white cats, Hereford cattle, light-colored horses, white or partly white dogs Less in pigs Adults to aged	Nonpigmented or lightly pigmented and sparsely haired skin Nail bed (dogs, cats) Penis/prepuce (horses)	Variable: nodular, proliferative, crusty, ulcerative Cutaneous horn may be present	Cords and islands of squamous cells Keratin pearls Dyskeratosis Intercellular bridges Basement membrane disrupted	May recur Metastasis to lymph nodes and beyond may develop Those of equine penis and feline nail bed are more aggressive Solar-associated are slow to metastasize	Keratin pearls, intercellular bridges Spindle-cell and pseudoglandular varieties occur
Claw bed tumors Inclusion cyst Papilloma Keratoacan-thoma Squamous cell carcinoma Melanoma	Unknown Trauma	Dogs: large-breed, black-haired, predisposed to multiple squamous cell carcinomas Cats	Claw bed May be multiple	Variable Swelling of claw bed Loss of claw Deformed claw	Depends on type of lesion or tumor	Malignant melanoma of dogs and squamous cell carcinoma of cats can be aggressive	Differentiate from pulmonary carcinoma in cat, which may metastasize to multiple digits
Apocrine adenoma: simple, complex, mixed, and ductal Apocrine adenocarcinoma: simple, complex, mixed, and ductal	Unknown	Older dogs and cats	Any location glands present Older female dogs: bilateral adenocarcino-mas may develop from apocrine glands of anal sacs	Adenoma: small, slow growing, cystic, circumscribed Carcinomas: firm, infiltrative	Benign: variable appearance, resemble glandular or ductal epithelium Mixed type have myoepithelium, cartilage, or bone Carcinomas of anal sac usually solid	Adenomas: benign Carcinomas: aggressive, may metastasize early	Carcinomas may resemble exudative dermatitis Anal sac carcinomas are often associated with hypercalcemia
Sebaceous gland adenoma (Box 17-16) Sebaceous gland epithelioma Sebaceous gland carcinoma	Unknown	Adenoma common in adult dogs: Cocker spaniel, poodle Less common in cats Rare in other animals	Head, neck, anywhere	Adenoma: gray-tan, greasy, lobulated, raised Epithelioma: discrete, firm; may ulcerate Carcinoma: often ulcerated	Adenoma: similar to sebaceous gland Epithelioma: more basal cells and mitoses Carcinoma: less fat in cells, less differentiated	Adenomas: benign Epitheliomas may recur Carcinomas: locally invasive; rarely metastasize	Eyelid meibomian gland tumors are similar Nodular hyperplastic lesions of sebaceous glands also very common

Tumor	Cell of origin	Signalment	Location	Gross appearance	Histology	Biologic behavior	Comments
Perianal gland adenoma (hepatoid gland adenoma) Perianal gland epithelioma Perianal gland carcinoma	Hormonal influence	Older dogs Intact males predisposed	Skin near anus, base of tail, prepuce, vulva; less elsewhere	One or more raised nodules often ulcerated, circumscribed, orangish tan and greasy on cut surface	Adenoma: similar to perianal gland Epithelioma: more basal cells and mitoses Carcinoma: infiltrative, less differentiated, and more mitoses	Most are adenomas, which are benign In males, castration or estrogen therapy may cause regression of adenomas Carcinomas: low grade malignancy	Location and hormonal sensitivity
Canine cutaneous histiocytoma (Box 17-16)	Unknown Langerhans' cell of origin (epidermal dendritic antigen-presenting cell)	Dogs: more than half of the tumors develop before 2 years of age Purebred dogs predisposed	Head, especially distal pinna; distal forelegs; and feet	Usually single Dome-shaped Circumscribed Often ulcerated	Sheets of large round cells (histiocytes) replace adnexa and collagen Frequent mitoses Later necrosis and lymphocytic inflammation	Rapid growth followed by regression Rarely recur No metastasis	Young dogs Rapid growth Regression
Canine reactive histiocytosis (cutaneous and systemic)	Unknown Activated, dermal, perivascular antigen-presenting cell (dendritic cell) origin	Adult dogs Systemic: Bernese mountain dogs and a few other breeds	Cutaneous: multiple cutaneous sites Systemic: skin and other organs	Multiple cutaneous and subcutaneous plaques and nodules ± systemic lesions	Histiocytic cells and variable mix of lymphocytes, plasma cells, and neutrophils	Remissions, relapses Prolonged course Slowly progressive	Recurrent May have nasal lesion or systemic involvement
Histiocytic sarcoma (disseminated) (also known as malignant histiocytosis)	Unknown Nonactivated, dendritic cell (antigen presenting cell) origin	Bernese mountain dog Retriever (golden, Labrador) Rottweiler, others	Skin and subcutis are rarely affected Multisystemic involvement	Multinodular, invasive, destructive	Anaplastic, large, round and/or plump spindle cells, other leukocytes	Aggressive Usually fatal disease	Breed predisposition Multisystemic masses Anaplastic cell populations

(Continued)

Table 17-13   Selected Cutaneous Neoplastic and Neoplastic-like Lesions of Domestic Animals—Cont'd

Lesion	Cause	Species Age, Breed, Sex	Location	Gross Pathology	Histopathology	Biologic Behavior	Unique Features
Cutaneous lymphoma Dermal form (Box 17-16) T-lymphocyte type Epidermal form (mycosis fungoides) (Box 17-16) T-lymphocyte type Angiocentric form (lymphomatoid granulomatosus)	Unknown	Dogs; less common in cats and horses Age variable	Skin or oral Dermis or epidermis	Variable 1. Red scaly skin 2. Mucocutaneous ulceration/ depigmentation 3. Single/multiple cutaneous masses 4. Infiltrative and ulcerative mucosal epithelium ± systemic lesions	Dermal: sheets of lymphocytes in dermis Epidermal: lymphocytes in epidermis and adnexal epithelium Angiocentric: lymphohistiocytic dermal masses with angiocentric pattern	Ultimately terminate fatally Lymphomatoid granulomatosus is aggressive, has angio-centric pattern, and may invade vessels and cause infarction	Epidermal form may mimic dermatitis, autoimmune disease, or stomatitis Equine lymphosarcoma is pleocellular and can be confused with inflammation
Merkel cell tumor	Neuroendocrine origin	Dog, rare tumor	Skin or oral	Nodular mass	Nests of round cells with collagen septa	Usually benign	200-nm granules seen ultrastructurally
Cutaneous plasmacytoma (extramedullary plasmacytoma)	Unknown	Dog, rarely cat Aged adult Both sexes	Ear, lip, digit, and other mucocutaneous and cutaneous sites	Usually solitary, raised, reddish discrete, nodule	Densely cellular; single or multiple variably sized nuclei; many mitoses Resemble plasma cells; may have amyloid	Usually do not recur Subcutaneous or those with amyloid may be aggressive and recurrent Rare association with multiple myeloma	Cytoplasmic immunoglobulin present May have amyloid deposits
Mast cell tumor (mastocytoma) (Box 17-16)	Unknown Genetic influence In cats, FIV associated	Common tumor of dogs, especially boxers, less common in other species Siamese cats have histio-cytic variety Generally adults, less common in neonates	Dog: often legs, trunk Feline: head	Solitary or multiple nodules Poorly circumscribed edematous swellings May ulcerate early	Sheets of large round cells with bluish granular cytoplasm Not encapsulated Many eosinophils, in dogs especially Vasculitis Collagen degeneration	Canine: behavior may correspond to histologic grade May disseminate Feline histiocytic-type may spon-taneously regress Equine generally benign	Metachromatic granules, eosinophils Other lesions: vasculitis, collagen degeneration, gastrointestinal ulceration Prolonged coagulation time

Tumor	Cause	Species	Location	Gross appearance	Histologic features	Biologic behavior	Comments
Melanoma: benign (melanocytoma) junctional dermal compound (Box 17-16) Malignant melanoma	Genetic factors Unknown Ultraviolet light Angora goats	Common: dogs and horses, and some strains of pigs and angora goats Uncommon: cats Rare: other species	Dog: head, eyelids, legs, digits Horse: perineal skin and underside of root of tail Feline: head Angora goat: dorsal ear, face, perineum	Dog and cats: single Horse: multiple Macules to nodules Usually dark brown or black	Epithelioid to spindle-shaped cells containing variable quantity of pigment Nests of these cells bordered by thin collagen septa Malignant; are anaplastic and may be amelanotic	Canine: oral, mucocutaneous, subungual, often malignant; haired skin often benign Gray horses: usually progressive and multicentric; are Malignant Location, size, mitotic index, and cell morphology help predict behavior	Melanin pigment in cytoplasm Common in horses that fade to gray
Fibroma Fibrosarcoma (Box 17-16)	Fibrosarcoma: 1. FeLV and FeSV are associated with development of multiple sarcomas in young cats 2. Vaccination in cats	Adult to aged All domestic animals Fibrosarcomas: common in cats, less common in dogs, rare in other species	Head, legs, and sites of vaccination in cats	Circumscribed (fibroma) Firm to soft Resilient Gray-white	Interlacing bundles of fibroblasts and collagen Fibrosarcoma may have multinucleated giant cells	Fibromas: benign Fibrosarcomas are infiltrative and often recur, but metastasis is uncommon	Fibrosarcomas in cats have been caused by FeLV plus FeSV, and by vaccination
Equine sarcoid Feline sarcoid (Fig. 17-47)	Bovine papillomavirus/equine papillomavirus Probable papillomavirus/feline	Most common skin tumor of horses Donkey, mule Cat	Skin of legs, head, ventral trunk	Types: verrucous fibroblastic flat or occult mixed	Fibroblastic proliferation with pseudoepitheliomatous hyperplasia	Locally invasive Frequently recur Do not metastasize	Autotransplantable Rare spontaneous regression

Table **17-13**   Selected Cutaneous Neoplastic and Neoplastic-like Lesions of Domestic Animals—Cont'd

Lesion	Cause	Species Age, Breed, Sex	Location	Gross Pathology	Histopathology	Biologic Behavior	Unique Features
Myxoma Myxosarcoma	Unknown	Rare in domestic animals Adult to aged	Any location, often limbs	Poorly defined and infiltrative, soft and mucoid Gelatinous	Fusiform and stellate cells within mucinous matrix	Infiltrative Recur frequently Myxosarcomas metastasize uncommonly	Some consider myxomas (sarcomas) to be a type of fibroma (sarcoma)
Hemangiopericytoma (cell of origin is controversial, probably pericyte or possibly neural)	Unknown Some consider this to be a malignant peripheral nerve sheath tumor	Dogs Adult to aged More in females Cats, very rare	Dermis and subcutis of extremities	Gray to pink Lobulated Firm and nodular or more gelatinous	Concentric laminations of spindle cells	Often recur Locally invasive Rarely metastasize	Concentric laminations of spindle cells around vessels
Nerve sheath tumors Neurofibroma Schwannoma	Unknown	Dogs, less others	Cutaneous tumors are uncommon, more common on head of cats, legs of dogs, and eyelids of horses	Nodular Firm to gelatinous White-gray Associated with nerve	Bundles, whorls, and palisades of spindle cells	Dogs and cats: locally invasive, may recur	Cells arranged in palisades Associated with nerves
Lipoma Infiltrative lipoma Liposarcoma	Unknown	Lipoma: common in adult to aged dogs; less common in horse and cow; rare in cat, sheep, pig Infiltrative lipoma: adult dogs Liposarcoma: rare	Legs, thorax, abdomen	Lipoma: circumscribed, greasy, soft, white, slightly translucent; float in formalin Infiltrative lipoma: poorly delineated soft enlargements of muscle or soft tissue Liposarcoma: firmer, nondiscrete, gray to white	Lipoma: mature fat cells Infiltrative lipoma: mature fat cells replacing normal muscle or collagen Liposarcoma: round to spindle-cell tumor, cellular, vacuolated cytoplasm	Lipomas do not recur Infiltrative lipomas are locally invasive and recur but do not metastasize Liposarcomas are locally invasive, may recur, and rarely metastasize	Fatty tumor Float in formalin

Tumor	Cause	Signalment	Location	Gross appearance	Histology	Behavior	Comments
Hemangioma Hemangiosarcoma (Box 17-16)	Unknown Trauma or solar radiation for some types	Adult to aged More common in dogs, less common in cats, horses, cattle, sheep, pigs Foals: congenital hemangiomas	Hemangioma: dermis or subcutis Hemangiosarcoma: primary to skin or metastatic from visceral tumor Seen more in white, poorly haired dermis, especially of dogs	Red, brown to black Circumscribed (hemangioma) Soft Ooze blood on cut surface Dermal may bleed	Interconnecting blood channels lined by endothelium Hemangiosarcoma may resemble fibrosarcoma or have benign appearance (especially if metastatic)	Hemangiomas do not recur Hemangiosarcoma in white cat ear tip and eyelid recur Metastatic potential is high in canine hemangio-sarcomas	Thrombosis frequent in hemangioma Coagulation disorder may be associated with these tumors, especially if tumors are large, malignant, or multifocal
Lymphangioma Lymphangio-sarcoma	Some are believed to be congenital in young animals	Uncommon to rare	Lymphatics associated with skin	Poorly defined Cavernous/spongy Soft May dissect along fascial planes	Interconnecting channels lined by endothelium, usually without erythrocytes	May be difficult to remove due to dissection along fascia, so tumors tend to recur	
Feline ventral abdominal angiosarcoma	Unknown	Adult cats	Ventral abdominal skin	Same as for lymphangioma and sarcoma May be difficult to distinguish benign and malignant types	Cat ventral abdominal angiosarcoma is invasive and recurs.		
Leiomyoma Leiomyosarcoma	Unknown	Very rare	Skin associated with arrector pili muscles, or cutaneous blood vessels	Circumscribed Solitary Firm	Interlacing bundles of smooth muscle fibers tend to intersect at right angles Nuclei have blunt ends	Leiomyoma: benign Leiomyosarcoma is locally invasive	
Cutaneous nodular fasciitis (overlap with fibrous histiocytoma)	Unknown Nonneoplastic	Rare Dog and cat	Usually solitary Subcutaneous fascia	Solitary, firm Nondiscrete Subcutaneous Head, face	Mixtures of fibroblasts, giant cells, and inflammatory cells in vascular stroma Mitoses present	Nonneoplastic but can have clinically aggressive behavior	Similar lesion on cornea/third eyelid, especially in collies, is termed "nodular granulomatous episclerokeratitis"

(Continued)

Table **17-13** Selected Cutaneous Neoplastic and Neoplastic-like Lesions of Domestic Animals—Cont'd

Lesion	Cause	Species Age, Breed, Sex	Location	Gross Pathology	Histopathology	Biologic Behavior	Unique Features
Benign fibrous histiocytoma (overlap with cutaneous nodular fasciitis)	Unknown	Uncommon: dogs, especially collies Rare: cats Younger adult	Multiple Face Dermal	Often multiple Firm Dermal	Mixture of fibroblasts, and histiocytes Lymphocytes and plasma cells at periphery	May recur Neoplastic nature questioned	Similar eye lesions probably represent "nodular granulomatous episclerokeratitis"
Malignant fibrous histiocytoma (extraskeletal giant cell tumor)	Unknown Pleocellular tumor that probably is either of primitive mesenchymal cell origin, or individual tumors may originate from different cell lines, requiring immunohistochemical differentiation	Older ages Cats, dogs, horses Uncommon to rare	Skin of limbs and neck	Firm, solitary Nonencapsulated Variable size and shape	Densely cellular spindle cell tumor with two cell types: fibroblastic and histiocytic Many mitoses Multinucleated cells in cats	Locally aggressive Usually slow to metastasize; however, this can depend on cell of origin	Histiocytic and fibroblastic cells Giant cells, especially in cats

regulate apoptosis, and genes that regulate DNA repair. Damage to these genes results in deranged cellular proliferation by the abnormal expression or function of proteins such as growth factors, growth factor receptors, signal-transducing proteins, cell cycle regulators, and nuclear transcription factors. The majority of malignant neoplasms have evidence of damage (mutation) of multiple genes within these categories. Mutations are often collected by cells in a stepwise manner that imparts increasing degrees of malignant potential. These molecular changes are known to correlate with morphologic changes and the clinical behavior of some neoplasms. For example, it is known that squamous cell carcinomas often develop in a stepwise manner and progress through several recognizable stages: hyperplasia (increased number of cells; no cellular atypia or tissue disorganization) → dysplasia (increased mitoses, cellular atypia, and tissue disorganization consisting of loss of polarity) → carcinoma in situ (increased tissue disorganization, mitoses, anaplastic nuclei, but no invasion of underlying basement membrane) → invasive squamous cell carcinoma (disruption of the basement membrane with dermal invasion by anaplastic carcinoma cells).

The progression of the disease from mere hyperplasia to an invasive carcinoma represents a series of molecular events whereby the population of cells harbors an increasing number of damaged genes belonging to the four categories of genes listed. This series of changes takes place over long periods of time, often years, before a tumor reaches full malignant potential. The process may be halted in the early stages if the agents causing continued genetic damage can be removed (for example, exposure to UV radiation).

Most cutaneous neoplasms are primary, as the skin is an uncommon to rare site for metastasis; however, the skin can be the site of secondary tumor growth. Examples include mammary gland neoplasms that invade into adjacent skin, feline pulmonary bronchogenic carcinomas that metastasize to multiple digits of the feet, and canine visceral hemangiosarcomas that can metastasize to the skin. Table 17-13 gives an abbreviated listing of the salient features of cutaneous neoplasms.

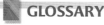 **GLOSSARY**

Acantholysis: loss of cohesion between keratinocytes due to the breakdown of intercellular bridges.

Acanthosis: thickening of the spinous cell layer (stratum spinosum).

Acral: distal parts of the extremities.

Alopecia: hair loss.

Anagen: phase of hair cycle in which hair synthesis takes place.

Anaplasia: lack of cellular differentiation and organization, a feature of neoplastic cells.

Angioedema: vascular reaction involving the deep dermis or subcutis and consisting of edema manifested as giant wheals and caused by dilation and increased permeability of capillaries (deeper version of urticaria).

Apoptosis: programmed cell death.

Atrophy: reduction in size of a cell, tissue, organ, or part.

Ballooning degeneration: marked intracellular fluid accumulation in the cells of the epidermis.

Blister (vesicle or bulla): localized collection of fluid usually in or beneath epidermis.

Bulla: large blister (>1.0 cm).

Catagen: transition phase of the hair cycle between growth and resting phases.

Comedo (plural = comedones): plug of follicular stratum corneum and dried sebum in a hair follicle.

Cornification: production of stratum corneum by terminal epidermal differentiation.

Crust: material formed by drying of exudate or secretion on the skin surface.

Cytokines: small molecular weight protein molecules (generally <30 kD) that are mediators of inflammation and growth.

Dematiaceous: naturally pigmented black or brown mycelium or conidium.

Dermatitis: inflammation of the skin.

Dermatophytosis: infection of the stratum corneum of the epidermis, hair, or claws with fungi of the genera *Microsporum, Epidermophyton,* or *Trichophyton.*

Dermatosis: noninflammatory lesion of the skin.

Dyskeratosis: abnormal, premature, or imperfect keratinization.

Dysplasia: abnormal development.

Effluvium: shedding of hair.

Epidermal collarette: peripheral expanding ring of scale.

Epidermitis: inflammation of the epidermis.

Epidermolysis: separation of the epidermis from the dermis.

Erosion: loss of all or part of the thickness of the epidermis.

Eruption: rapid development of skin lesion associated with redness.

Erythema: redness of skin due to congestion of capillaries.

Excoriation: superficial loss of epithelium due to physical trauma (scratching).

Exfoliation: shedding of layers or scales.

Exogen: the stage of the hair cycle where old hairs are shed.

Exudate: fluid, cells, or debris from blood vessels deposited in or on other tissues.

Fissure: cleft or groove.

Folliculitis: inflammation of a hair follicle.

Furuncle: circumscribed, painful nodule (accumulation of pus) in the dermis secondary to follicular rupture.

Genodermatosis: a genetically determined disorder of the skin.

Glabrous: smooth skin, hairless skin.

Hamartoma: growth of cells in a localized area that surpasses the growth of cells in the surrounding area, and presumed to be of congenital origin.

Hydropic degeneration: intracellular fluid accumulation in cells of the basal epidermis.

Hyperkeratosis: histologic term for thickening of stratum corneum.

Hyperplasia: increase in the number of normal cells.

Hypoplasia: incomplete development.

Hypotrichosis: less hair than normal.

Ichthyosis: congenital skin disorder in which the skin is thickened by scales (hyperkeratosis) that can crack into plates resembling fish scales.

Impetigo: bacterial dermatitis characterized by pustules.

Indolent: slow growing, a term applied to persistent ulcers on the lips of cats, and sometimes incorrectly called "rodent ulcer," a term from the human literature used to refer to ulcerated basal cell carcinoma.

Indurated: Hardened.

Interface: inflammation arranged in a layer close to and often obscuring the epidermal-dermal junction (interface), and with vacuolar and sometimes apoptotic basal cells; the inflammation can be mild (cell poor) or extensive (cell rich).

Intertrigo: dermatitis that develops because of friction between apposing skin surfaces (e.g., adjacent folds).

Keratinocytes: the epidermal cells that synthesize keratin and comprise more than 90% of epidermal cells.

Keratosis (plural = keratoses): an uncommon to rare circumscribed papular, plaquelike, or linear focus of proliferative keratinocytes covered by thick stratum corneum; keratoses can be caused by sun exposure (actinic keratoses) or can be idiopathic (lichenoid, linear, cannon [metatarsal bone] keratoses).

Langerhans' cells: antigen-presenting cells of the skin.

Lichenification: thickening of skin with accentuation of skin creases.

Lichenoid: confusing term that generally refers to a dense zone of dermal inflammation parallel to the epidermis usually without basal cell injury.

Lichenoid dermatoses: uncommon to rare, often idiopathic, single or grouped papules, plaques, or papillomatous foci covered by scale, and histologically composed of epidermal hyperplasia, lichenoid lymphoplasmacytic dermal inflammation, hyperkeratosis and parakeratosis.

Macule: flat, circumscribed lesion of altered skin color.

Melanin: dark, amorphous pigment consisting of dihydroxy indoxylic acid.

Melanophage: macrophage containing ingested melanin.

Merkel cell: a neuroendocrine cell found in the stratum basale.

Mucin: glycosaminoglycan (GAG), a normal component of the ground substance of the dermis, consists of protein bound to hyaluronic acid.

Mycelium: a mass of hyphae.

Mycetoma: a slowly progressive infection of the cutaneous and subcutaneous tissue, fascia, and sometimes underlying bone caused by traumatic implantation of actinomycetes (actinomycotic mycetoma) or fungi (eumycotic mycetoma).

Myxedema: nonpitting edema of the skin because of abnormal deposits of mucin in the dermis.

Nevus: circumscribed malformation of the skin assumed to be of congenital or inherited origin, and consisting of any component of the skin. The term "hamartoma" is preferred to nevus to avoid confusion with the pigmented nevus (mole) that arises in the skin of human beings.

Nodule: a circumscribed, solid elevation of skin (>1 cm).

Onychodystrophy: abnormal formation of the claw.

Onychomadesis: sloughing of claws.

Panniculitis: inflammation of subcutaneous adipose tissue.

Papule: circumscribed, solid elevation of skin (<1 cm).

Parakeratosis: retention of pyknotic nuclei in epidermal cells of the stratum corneum.

Paronychia: inflammation of skin around the claws.

Pemphigus: cutaneous disease associated with blistering.

Phaeohyphomycosis: mycotic disease caused by pigmented fungi (dematiaceous fungi) of a variety of genera and species that do not form sclerotic bodies or granules.

Pigmentary incontinence: melanin pigment within dermal macrophages or free in the dermis developing via injury to pigment containing basal layer cells.

Plaque: a flat-topped, solid elevation in the skin that occupies a relatively large surface area in comparison with its height.

Pruritus: itching.

Pustule: small, circumscribed accumulation of pus within the epidermis or within a hair follicle.

Pyoderma: pyogenic (pus-producing) bacterial infection of the skin.

Rodent ulcer: a term used in human medicine to define an ulcerative basal cell carcinoma; sometimes used inappropriately in veterinary medicine to refer to an indolent ulcer affecting the lip of cats.

Scale: a thin, platelike accumulation of stratum corneum on surface of skin.

Seborrhea: nonspecific term for clinical signs of scaling, crusting, and greasiness. Primary seborrhea is a more specific term applied to inherited cornification disorders.

Sebum: secretion of sebaceous glands.

Spongiosis: intercellular edema which, by widening of the intercellular space and stretching of the "intercellular bridges," creates a spongelike appearance to the epidermis.

Telogen: resting phase of the hair cycle.

Ulcer: loss of epidermis and at least the superficial portion of dermis.

Urticaria: usually transient vascular reaction in the upper dermis consisting of edema manifested clinically as wheals (hives); a more superficial version of angioedema.

Vesicle: small blister within the epidermis or at or below the dermal-epidermal interface (<1.0 cm) (Fig. 17-19).

Vibrissa (plural = vibrissae): (sinus hair, tactile hair) long, coarse hair located about the nose.

Vitiligo: acquired disorder characterized by circumscribed areas of depigmentation in the skin.

Wheal: smooth, circumscribed, slightly elevated area on skin caused by dermal edema.

Yeast: unicellular budding fungus.

SUGGESTED READINGS

Veterinary Dermatology
Mueller RS: *Dermatology for the small animal practitioner*, Jackson, Wyo, 2000, Teton NewMedia.
Scott DW, Miller Jr. WH: *Equine dermatology*, St Louis, 2003, Mosby.
Scott DW, Miller Jr. WH, Griffin CE: *Muller and Kirk's small animal dermatology*, ed 6, Philadelphia, 2001, Saunders.

Veterinary Dermatopathology
Bettenay SV, Hargis AM: *Practical veterinary dermatopathology for the small animal clinician*, Jackson, Wyo, 2006, Teton NewMedia.
Ginn PE, Mansell JEKL, Rakich PM: The skin and appendages. In Maxie MG, Slocombe RF, editors: *Pathology of domestic animals*, ed 5, Oxford, Elsevier Ltd., in press.
Gross TL, Ihrke PJ, Walder EJ et al: *Skin diseases of the dog and cat: clinical and histopathologic diagnosis*, ed 2, Oxford, Blackwell, 2005.
Yager JA, Wilcock BP: *Color atlas and text of surgical pathology of the dog and cat. Dermatopathology and skin tumors*, Spain, 1994, Mosby-Year Book Europe Ltd.

Veterinary Neoplasia
Goldschmidt MH, Dunstan RW, Stannard AA et al: *Histological classification of epithelial and melanocytic tumors of the skin of domestic animals*, second series, vol III, Washington, DC, 1998, Armed Forces Institute of Pathology.
Goldschmidt MH, Hendrick MJ: Tumors of the skin and soft tissues. In Mueten DJ, editor: *Tumors of domestic animals*, ed 4, Ames, 2002, Iowa State University Press.
Goldschmidt MH, Shofer FS: *Skin tumors of the dog and cat*, New York, 1992, Pergamon Press Ltd.
Hendrick MJ, Mahaffey EA, Moore FM et al: *Histological classification of mesenchymal tumors of skin and soft tissues of domestic animals*, second series, vol II, Washington, DC, 1998, Armed Forces Institute of Pathology.

Human Dermatopathology
Ackerman AB: *Histologic diagnosis of inflammatory skin diseases: an algorithmic method based on pattern analysis*, ed 2, Baltimore, 1997, Williams and Wilkins.
Elder D, Elenitsas R, Jaworsky C et al, editors: *Lever's histopathology of the skin*, ed 8, Philadelphia, 1997, Lippincott-Raven.
Hood AF, Kwan TH, Burnes DC et al: *Primer of dermatopathology*, Boston, 1984, Little Brown and Co.

18

Female Reproductive System*

ROBERT A. FOSTER

The reproductive system is arguably the most important in terms of survival of a species. In production animals, reproduction is essential for the continued supply of product, be it meat, fiber, milk, or any of the many other by-products. Diseases of the reproductive system have not changed much in the last few decades, but our understanding of many of the processes has progressed dramatically and many of the accepted "dogmas" have now been challenged and/or modified. In addition, the traditional approach to diseases of the reproductive system has focused on information about specific conditions for which some information is known, rather than taking into consideration the overall significance in a clinical setting. In this chapter, each component or region will be examined in turn; however, the relative importance of specific diseases or processes will be emphasized. The traditional approach also concentrated on bovine and, to a lesser extent, equine reproductive diseases. In this chapter, diseases of all species including companion animals will be undertaken.

INTRODUCTION

ORGANIZATION

FEMALE REPRODUCTIVE SYSTEM

The female reproductive systems of domesticated animals, although diverse in anatomy, share many similarities in structure and function. Whereas the female reproductive tract was thought to be the embryonic default when the male reproductive tract did not form, it is now considered to involve unique actions of various genes and subsequent processes.

Genes initiate the pathways of ovarian differentiation and development. *DAX1* is one such gene that both promotes ovarian development and inhibits testicular development. In development of the ovary, the germ cells undergo meiosis and the supporting cells surround the oocytes to become the cells of the follicles. Steroid-producing cells become the thecal cells. The differentiation of a female phenotype occurs with the development of the paramesonephric (Müllerian) ducts to form the uterine tube, uterus, and upper part of the vagina, and for the genital tubercle to develop into the distal vagina and vulva.

The structural arrangement of the ovary is relatively uniform except in the mare. The ovary itself has an outer layer of epithelium, which is of mesothelial origin. The cortex of the ovary contains follicles, stromal connective tissue, and blood vessels. The medulla has many large blood vessels, lymphatics, nerves, and loosely arranged connective tissue. Remnants of the mesonephric tubules, called the rete ovarii, are present in this region.

The follicles are where the ova develop, and they are named according to their stage of development: primordial, primary, secondary, and tertiary types. Each developing follicle has multiple layers of granulosa cells and more peripheral thecal cells. Ovulation occurs when the follicle ruptures, releasing the ovum and allowing the space to fill with blood and then with luteal cells to form the corpus hemorrhagicum and corpus luteum, respectively. Follicles that do not ovulate become atretic. In addition to these various ovarian structures, cats have interstitial glands that are cells of an endocrine type. The canine ovary has small ingrowths of the ovarian surface that are called subsurface epithelial structures.

Oogenesis is usually completed by birth. In most species, ovulation occurs through the outer surface of the ovary from whence the ovum is collected by the infundibulum.

The ovary of the mare differs from the other species in several ways. Equine fetal gonads undergo hypertrophy wherein interstitial glands expand and produce a

*Chapters on this subject in earlier editions were written or partially written by Dr. H. Acland of the Pennsylvania Veterinary Laboratory, Harrisburg, Pa.

gonad that is extremely large. Stimulation by pregnant mare gonadotropins is believed to induce the large size. These atrophy before birth. The ovary of the mare has a kidney shape with a depression that is called the ovulation fossa. It is from this small depression that the ovum is released. The cortex of the ovary extends into the center of the gonad, and the "medulla" is at the periphery. The follicles in the mare can attain a large size—up to 7 cm. Mares can therefore form a large corpus hemorrhagicum. On occasion, this and the corpus luteum can extend out through the ovulation fossa.

The uterine tube has four regions—the infundibulum, ampulla, isthmus, and uterotubal junction. It is supported by a mesosalpinx. The mesosalpinx of the dog completely surrounds the ovary and has a large amount of fat; a small hole connects the bursa to the abdominal cavity. The infundibulum surrounds the ovary of each species, except in the horse where it only covers the ovulation fossa. The uterine tube is where fertilization occurs, and the conceptus then moves into the uterus.

All species have a bicornuate uterus with uterine horns and a uterine body. In ruminants, each uterine horn contains four rows of protuberances that are the caruncles. These can be pigmented in sheep. The placenta of ruminants is cotyledonary. The uterus of the mare has longitudinal folds. Endometrial cups are formed between 37 and 150 days of gestation and are the site of production of pregnant mare serum gonadotropins (Fig. 18-1). These typically form around the pregnant horn at the bifurcation. Their disappearance is an immune-mediated event. The placenta of the horse is diffuse and microcotyledonary. Dogs and cats have a zonary placenta with a marginal hematoma. The placenta of the pig is diffuse with small villi.

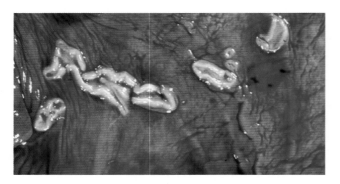

Fig. 18-1   Endometrial cups, uterus, mare. Endometrial cups are plaquelike structures in the endometrium that form when trophoblasts invade the endometrium early in pregnancy. They are present between 37 and 150 days of pregnancy. The chorionic surface opposite each cup is called the chorioallantoic pouch and is avillous. *(Courtesy Dr. K. Read, College of Veterinary Medicine, Texas A&M University; and Noah's Arkive, College of Veterinary Medicine, The University of Georgia.)*

The cervix is the structure that separates the external genitalia from the uterus and is an effective barrier from the external environment. Cervical mucus is viscous except during estrus when it becomes more plentiful and thinner. The cervix in the mare, dog, and cat does not have transverse folds as it does in the ruminants and sows. The cervix of the dog and cat tends to open dorsally.

MAMMARY GLAND
MAMMARY DEVELOPMENT, LACTATION, AND INVOLUTION

Embryologically the mammary glands arise from the mammary ridge that is formed by ventrolateral ectoderm. Mammary buds push into mesenchyme with their number equaling the number of glands. Sprouts form from each bud, and the number determines the number of openings and therefore papillary ducts—1 in cattle, sheep, and goats; 2 in horses and pigs; 3 to 7 in cats, and 8 to 14 in dogs. Glands develop in male embryos, but in domesticated species they only regress fully in the stallion.

As puberty approaches, there is branching of ducts mediated by prolactin, growth hormone and insulin-like growth factors, and many other factors. There is an intimate interaction between the mesenchyme and epithelium, as the ducts branch and alveoli eventually develop. With the onset of lactation, mammary development is at its zenith. Milk flows from the alveoli through the lactiferous ducts to a lactiferous sinus (in large animals) and, with suckling, through the papillary duct or ducts.

There is variation between the species in the amount of regression that occurs when milking ceases. As expected, there is a reduction in the area of secretary epithelium, and a relative increase in the amount of stroma of the gland. When secretion ceases completely, any mammary fluid is resorbed. Bovine mammary glands do not regress as much as in other species, and as such have completed involution in about 2 weeks. Ewes take about 4 weeks to involute. Leukocytes infiltrate the involuting gland; macrophages are most numerous.

FUNCTIONS
FEMALE REPRODUCTIVE SYSTEM

The overall function of the female reproductive tract is to provide a location for the conception, development, and eventual release of viable offspring. One offspring is sufficient for dairy cows, but the largest number possible is required for production animals. Each anatomic site has its own particular function.

The function of the ovary is to develop and release an ovum or ova and to produce hormones, such as estrogen and progesterone, that influence animal behavior and affect other organs and tissue to maintain pregnancy.

The uterine tube acts as a transport system and storage site for spermatozoa. It also collects and transports the ovum or ova and provides a location for fertilization. The conceptus that is formed is nourished and eventually transported to the uterus for subsequent development.

The uterus provides a sterile and inert environment for the development of the conceptus. Exchange of nutrients and trophic factors, immunologic components such as immunoglobulin molecules, and waste products is a major function. This is achieved via placental attachment sites that increase the surface area of the interface between maternal and fetal tissue. At the appropriate time, the muscles of the uterus contribute to the release and birth of the developing individual.

The cervix has a gatekeeper function of holding the products of conception within the uterus until the appointed time. It also provides a seal that prevents entry of organisms and substances from the cranial vagina. Its dilation is an important part of parturition.

The vagina and vulva provide a passageway that allows an internal site for the deposition of semen. This protects the spermatozoa from desiccation and excessive contamination with organisms and materials that would excessively irritate or infect the uterus and uterine tube. The vagina also has a function in reducing contamination of the cervix, especially during pregnancy. It is also a portal for the fetus at parturition.

MAMMARY GLAND

The mammary glands have the basic function of providing immunity and nutrients to neonates. Milk is the source of many defenses, including antimicrobial, antiinflammatory, and immune-modulating molecules and substances. In the immediate neonatal period, passive transfer of immunoglobulin via colostrum is an important means of providing immediate immunity to offspring of all domestic species. Most domestic species rely on colostrum entirely in the first 24 hours as the sole source of serum immunoglobulin. Dogs and cats are exceptions, as there is some transplacental transfer. Components of the cellular immune system, such as lymphocytes and cytokines, are also transferred in milk. After the immediate postnatal period, substances in ingested milk (including immunoglobulin) provide some local protection against intestinal and respiratory pathogens.

The mammary gland of the modern dairy animal is expected to provide much more milk than is necessary for these functions, and the high-producing dairy cow is a special creature, developed to provide a product of good quality with a long shelf life and with modifications to the components of milk to suit consumers. This includes high production with a low somatic cell count.

CELL TYPES
FEMALE REPRODUCTIVE SYSTEM

The cells of the ovary are unique, but those of the rest of the tract are of a type seen in other locations. In general terms, much of the reproductive system has a barrier between the external environment and the internal environment that is based on epithelium and on an active mucosal immune system. Superimposed on this arrangement are the modifications that occur with the estrus cycle and with pregnancy.

The cell types of the ovary include the epithelium (surface epithelium, subsurface epithelial structures of the bitch, and the rete ovarii), the stroma, germ cells, and follicular cells. Lymphoid cells are usually absent. Control of ovarian function is from the hypothalamus and pituitary through release of gonadotropin-releasing hormone (GnRH) as well as follicle-stimulating hormone (FSH) and luteinizing hormone (LH) (see Fig. 12-4).

The uterus is a unique environment that is separated from the external environment by the cervix. Because it is designed to protect and nourish the fetus, there are some unique features of the endometrium. The endometrium has an epithelial lining of columnar and sometimes ciliated cells. There is also a stromal component of the endometrium. Inflammatory and immune cells are present, particularly during estrus, when the uterus is open to the external environment and to spermatozoa or semen (horses and pigs have intrauterine insemination). Mild inflammation is a "normal" part of the estrus cycle.

The "external" component of the female reproductive tract, being the vulva, vagina, and part of the cervix, is lined by a stratified squamous epithelium that varies with the stage of cycle. This is best illustrated in the bitch and queen, in which vaginal cytology is used as a practical guide to determine the stage of cycle. During anestrus, the epithelium is predominantly of a basal type, having a large nucleus and a small amount of cytoplasm. With the progressive approach of estrus (i.e., during proestrus), the epithelium becomes more mature so that at estrus the majority of cells are superficial epithelial cells with either pyknotic nuclei or no nuclei. Lymphoid follicles beneath the epithelium are a normal part of the distal vagina.

Pregnancy brings about a world of change to the reproductive system. The maintenance of pregnancy and the exchange of nutrients between mother and fetus and of other products from fetus to mother depend on the interactions of the trophoblasts with the endometrium. During pregnancy, the trophoblasts are directly opposed and in contact with the endometrial epithelium. In cattle, the maintenance of pregnancy depends on the inhibition of prostaglandin $F_{2\alpha}$ ($PGF_{2\alpha}$) production in the endometrium so luteolysis does not occur. The trophoblast must avoid rejection by the mother and maintain a barrier yet provide a system for the exchange of nutrients and waste products. There is much to be learned about the enigma that is pregnancy.

Some of the cells that we would ordinarily consider "inflammatory" cells have specific and individual functions separate from their usual roles. Thus uterine macrophages, natural killer cells, and, even in some cases, neutrophils have separate and distinct functions. For example, macrophages are important in maintaining the size and shape of bovine caruncles, CD2+ T lymphocytes and natural killer-like cells are important in early pregnancy in pigs, and neutrophils are involved in cervical relaxation at parturition in sheep. Thus the usual function of inflammatory cells can be modified or used by the reproductive tract for specific but otherwise unexpected purposes that result in the maintenance of pregnancy.

MAMMARY GLAND

The mammary gland is sequestered from the outside world by the gatekeeper functions of the sphincter of the mammary papilla (teat) and the papillary duct and, at least in the ruminant, its lining of keratinized squamous epithelium. The lactiferous sinus and ducts are lined by columnar epithelial cells, and the alveoli have the secretory epithelium. Secretion of milk components occurs in the alveoli. Mammary epithelial cells, specifically the alveolar cells, have receptors for immunoglobulin G (IgG); they are present for about 1 week before parturition, but the receptors disappear during lactation. Epithelial cells also allow for the transfer of IgA, which is produced locally in subepithelial plasma cells, into the alveolar lumens.

Lymphoid cells in the normal gland are derived from blood, and there is also homing of lymphocytes from the intestine (the enteromammary link) as part of the common mucosal immune system. Lymphocytes of the cellular immune system are present also, but in low numbers.

RESPONSES TO INJURY
FEMALE REPRODUCTIVE SYSTEM

Little is known about the response of the ovary to infection or insults. Observations of neutrophilic and, in viral infections, lymphocytic inflammation indicates that the ovary is capable of inflammatory and immune responses as one would expect with other parts of the body. Hyperplasia of the surface epithelium is a common response, just as it is with mesothelium elsewhere.

The uterine tube is such a narrow structure that its function is altered readily with edema, inflammation, and scarring. Exocytosis of neutrophils from blood vessels via the interstitium can be rapid. In sufficient numbers, pus is formed. Local immune responses can develop and result in the accumulation of lymphocytes, plasma cells, and, in some instances, lymphoid follicles. Granulation tissue formation in severe inflammatory conditions leads to scarring and subsequent obstruction of the tube is followed by an accumulation of fluid (hydrosalpinx) or pus (pyosalpinx).

Much has been studied about the responses of the uterus to infection. Inflammation varies from mild, in the case of postmating endometritis, to severe in bacterial metritis and pyometra. In mild acute inflammation of the endometrium (endometritis) of species—apart from the dog and cat—neutrophils and macrophages migrate through the epithelium into the lumen, and the stratum compactum is edematous. This becomes more florid with an increased severity. Neutrophils and necrotic debris accumulate in the uterus until pyometra forms. Lymphocytes and plasma cells accumulate in the stroma of the endometrium. With chronicity and in severe situations, the epithelium becomes squamous and so there is squamous metaplasia. Necrosis and erosion of the epithelium will induce the formation of granulation tissue, and varying degrees of fibrosis are commonplace in severe infectious or inflammatory disease.

The canine endometrium in particular, and also the feline endometrium, responds with cystic endometrial hyperplasia. Any injury or insult, be it inert foreign material or pathogenic infectious agents, will stimulate this response. This occurs in diestrus, and the luminal epithelium becomes papillated and can resemble a placental site.

Because of the stratified squamous epithelium of the vulva and vagina, inflammation and infection of the external part of the reproductive tract results in hyperplasia and keratinization. Exocytosis of inflammatory cells does occur, predominantly with neutrophils. These inflammatory cells do so with some difficulty because of the intercellular junctions. The inflammatory response is typically lymphocytic and plasmacytic, and these cells form a thick band of cells beneath the epithelium. Lymphoid follicles often form and give the affected region of the vagina a granular macroscopic appearance.

Reactions of the placenta are stereotyped and rely heavily on the maternal response and, to a lesser extent, the fetal immune systems. There is some species variability that can be related to the types of placenta and the usual route of infection. The response of the fetus and placenta tends to be relatively rudimentary. Trophoblasts are phagocytic, and they will take up debris, blood, and infectious agents. Reactions of fluid exudation and of connective tissue with granulation and fibrosis occur as elsewhere. The reactions of fetal macrophages and neutrophils are less obvious than is seen where maternal leukocytes are readily accessible. Placentitis occurs when there is sufficient time for a response: Fetal loss can be rapid with fetal distress, and there can be insufficient time to mount an effective response. Chronic lesions are much more obvious and are seen in ruminants especially. The cotyledonary placenta means that attachment of the placenta to the endometrium is restricted to a relatively small area in relation to the total placental area. The intercotyledonary area is a potential space that can accumulate a large volume of exudate. Chronic inflammation in ruminants is typified by fibrosis and exudates of suppurative material. Lymphoid follicles and plasma cells are a lesser component of the reaction, but lymphocytes do accumulate beneath the layer of trophoblasts and around blood vessels. The neutrophils are probably mainly of maternal origin. In the equine placenta, placentitis involves a small area, usually around the cervical star. There is no potential space because of the diffuse microcotyledonary type of placenta, so exudates and suppuration are much less prominent, and chronic placentitis is rare. The inflammatory reaction in the pig, dog, and cat is mild and is rarely seen because chronic placentitis is very rare.

MAMMARY GLAND

The mammary gland is usually sterile, but it can respond rapidly to infection or other irritants. The responses are relatively stereotyped, however. The columnar epithelial cells can become hyperplastic, but the cells are not able to withstand injury to the same extent as stratified epithelium, so squamous metaplasia is a frequent occurrence when irritants, such as infection or intramammary preparations, are introduced. Necrosis of the epithelium is common in infectious disease, and granulation and scarring of the lining of the ducts and sinus are frequent.

Although the immune system of the normal mammary gland is quiescent, injury quickly results in recruitment of the various elements. Neutrophils and macrophages are rapidly recruited. Humoral and cellular immunity is typically seen in infectious conditions. The accumulation of large numbers of plasma cells, recruited to the area because of the development of a local immune system, is an invariable component of the immune response in infection. Edema and subsequent fibrosis are part of the reaction to injury. The flow of milk is often halted by injury and exudates, so the normal involutionary processes that result in resorption of secretion (macrophage and epithelial uptake) also operate.

PORTALS OF ENTRY
FEMALE REPRODUCTIVE SYSTEM

It is critical that organisms are excluded from the uterus; otherwise fertility or pregnancy can be jeopardized. Portals of entry are listed in Box 18-1. Organisms that

---

Box 18-1

Portals of Entry into the Female Reproductive System, Especially the Uterus

Ascending infection through cervix
- At insemination
- Excessive vaginal contamination
- Postpartum and with retained fetal membranes

Hematogenous
- Localization in maternofetal interface

Descending from ovary via uterine tube

Transneural with recrudescence of herpesvirus infection

---

cause inflammation of the uterus can enter through the vulva (ascending infection) or can arrive via the blood (hematogenous infection). Reinfection of the external genitalia from nerves is a unique feature of infection with some herpesviruses.

Ascending infections are initiated at estrus, breeding, and parturition. At estrus, the cervix is open to admit spermatozoa. Contamination of the cranial vagina is very important in determining whether infection of the uterus occurs or not. Conformational and structural changes in the vulva and vagina are also important determinants of infection. These will be discussed in more detail later. A subcategory of ascending infection is infection of semen by infectious agents. There are many agents, including bacteria, viruses, protozoa, and *Ureaplasma* and *Mycoplasma*, some of them with a recognized venereal transmission, which can be acquired in this fashion. These will be discussed further in examining diseases of the uterus. Ascending infection is the major portal by which the equine placenta becomes infected with bacteria or fungi. The cervix in the mare is "loose," attains a much larger diameter, and can be readily opened with digital pressure. It is virtually impossible to penetrate the cervix of other species with a probe without creating severe trauma. Infection of the uterus and or placenta by the ascending route with a pure culture of *Streptococcus zooepidemicus* is common in the mare, but most ascending infections in other species includes a mixture of bacteria. This is particularly the case with postpartum infection.

Hematogenous infections are less common and are usually involved in specific infections, such as in brucellosis, salmonellosis, pestiviral and herpesviral infections, and they usually occur during pregnancy. Many of the fungal infections of the placenta occur via the hematogenous route.

There are some instances in which infections appear to descend from the ovary through the uterine tube. Some viral, chlamydial, and *Ureaplasma* infections can be descending.

Box 18-2

Portals of Entry into the Mammary Gland

Ascending ductular route
- Bacteria, fungi, parasites
- Therapeutic agents

Systemic infection and localization
- Systemic fungi, viruses, mycoplasmas, mycobacteria

Lymphatic spread
- Teat lesions

Direct penetration
- Penetrating injury

Box 18-3

Defenses of the Female Reproductive System

Innate defenses
- Vaginal epithelium
- Cervical barrier
- Conformation
- Myometrial tone and contraction
- Drainage of secretions
- Neutrophils
- Macrophages
- Complement
- Cytokines

Adaptive defenses
- Humoral immunity including common mucosal immune system
- Cellular immunity

Transaxonal infection of the distal reproductive tract occurs with some herpesviruses, where stressful events such as parturition cause a recrudescence. Neonates can be exposed and infected via this route, but clinical disease in the mother is unusual.

MAMMARY GLAND

Portals of entry are listed in Box 18-2. Most infectious agents and foreign material (intramammary preparations) enter the gland in an ascending fashion via the papillary duct. Small (bacteria) and large (leeches) pathogens can enter the gland via this route. There are some instances where organisms home to the mammary gland from systemic infection, but their number is small. Viruses such as the retroviruses of caprine arthritis and encephalitis, ovine maedi-visna, and *Mycoplasma* spp. are good examples. Penetrating injury is rare.

DEFENSE MECHANISMS
FEMALE REPRODUCTIVE SYSTEM

Whereas the adaptive immune system has been a focus of attention in defense of the reproductive system, innate, nonimmune, or physical factors are much more important. In many instances, failure of the physical factors, and infection of the tract, is too late for the fetus and infertility and failure of pregnancy occurs. Defense mechanisms are listed in Box 18-3.

INNATE IMMUNITY

The reproductive tract requires much of its defense system, as it must provide a sterile environment for the fetus but allow entry of antigenic and infectious materials (semen). It does this by providing specialized epithelium in the "contaminated" environment of the vulva and vagina, and then has a specialized structure, the cervix, to exclude most agents from the upper "sterile" regions. Vaginal epithelium has intercellular tight junctions that inhibit the transepithelial migration of agents and molecules and is likely to have molecules

that detect pathogen-associated molecular patterns. These molecules, presumably including defensins, exclude or direct actions against many pathogens.

The anatomy and integrity of the cervix is very important in the exclusion of infectious agents from the uterus. Contamination of the cranial vagina is an additional factor, and so conformation of the external genitalia is the physical factor that has received the most attention in relation to uterine infections. In older multiparous mares, the vulva is frequently higher than the floor of the pelvic canal and tends to become horizontal; air and contaminants, including feces, will be sucked in or allowed entry into the vagina or even into the uterus. Urine can pool in the vagina of mares with defective function of the vestibule and vulva muscles. When contamination and pooling of urine occur, the vestibule and vagina become inflamed, and the cervix and uterus become inflamed at the onset either from direct contact with environmental organisms or from local spread of the inflammation.

Muscular contractions of the uterus and gravitational drainage of secretions (mucus, lochia) from the uterus and vagina is a physical factor that can flush out infectious organisms. Congenital malformations and anomalies, such as persistent hymen, can reduce outflow and increase pooling in the vagina and uterus. The altered environment of the vagina in spayed, obese bitches can predispose the vagina and vulva to infection.

Following infection or irritation from semen, changes include hyperemia and edema of the uterine wall and lumen. These have the theoretical effect of diluting infectious or irritant substances. Recruitment of neutrophils from the blood occurs in response to chemotactic substances released by bacteria, complement, and inflammatory mediators from endometrium and leukocytes. Attracted neutrophils infiltrate the endometrium and enter the uterine lumen and contribute additional amounts of inflammatory mediators, providing additional chemotactic stimuli. Complement activation, directly by bacteria via the alternate pathway or by specific antibody via the classical pathway, can eliminate bacteria either by lysis following attack on their membranes or by phagocytosis enhanced by opsonization.

ADAPTIVE IMMUNITY

The reproductive tract is a unique environment because it must respond adequately to challenge from pathogens, yet tolerate the allogeneic spermatozoa and fetus. Adaptive immune responses, be they humoral or cellular, have to be carefully controlled. Control is achieved by differing cytokine expression of epithelial cells and their effects on regulatory T lymphocytes that make "decisions" as to the type and extent of the response. There is likely to be variation in the response, depending on the location. The response in the "sterile" compartments of the uterus and uterine tube will be different than that of the "nonsterile" vagina and ectocervix.

Although the upper reproductive tract is part of the common mucosal immune system, it differs from intestinal and bronchial tissues because it does not have mucosal-associated lymphoid tissue analogous to Peyer's patches. This is no doubt because of the lack of continuous antigenic stimulation. Lymphoid follicles, however, are present in the vulva and distal vagina. The uterus also has the added potential influence of hormones to modify responses.

T lymphocytes are critical in determining whether the appropriate response is predominantly humoral or cell mediated. CD8+ T lymphocytes are the most common lymphocytes of the luminal endometrial epithelium and stroma (stratum compactum especially), although there is variation depending on the location in the uterus. For example, CD4+ lymphocytes are more common in the horns of the uterus of mares, whereas CD8+ lymphocytes are more numerous in the body.

Little is known of the T lymphocyte and cell-mediated immune system of the reproductive tract; much more is known about its humoral immune system. It is generally believed that locally produced antibodies are more important in those diseases that are acquired by ascending infection, for example, *Tritrichomonas foetus* in cattle, whereas systemic immunity is more important in systemically or hematogenously acquired infections, such as *Brucella* sp. infection. The immunoglobulin isotype (IgA or IgG) and subisotype (IgG$_1$ or IgG$_2$) that is found in an individual infection is unique to that infection. The generalization that IgA is the main mucosal antibody is not always the case. The response to specific infectious agents is not uniform, and there are differing responses between species. Protection against *Tritrichomonas foetus* in cattle, for example, is mostly by IgG$_1$. Local transfer of immunoglobulin occurs at all levels of the tract.

Leakage of serum into the uterine lumen from an inflamed endometrium also contributes to the antibody content of the uterine fluid. Opsonization of bacteria by antibodies, especially IgG, promotes more efficient phagocytosis by neutrophils and macrophages; thus they enhance the innate cellular response by phagocytes.

The influence of the estrus cycle on antibodies in the uterus is controversial, but data suggest that concentrations of luminal immunoglobulins and immunoglobulin-containing cells in the endometrium are not influenced by the stage of the estrus cycle.

Locally produced IgA interferes with attachment of bacteria to mucosal surfaces and can activate complement via the alternate pathway. It is not directly bactericidal and neither acts as an opsonin nor as a macrophage activator. Variations occur among species on the position in the tract where the concentration of IgA is greatest, but the sites correspond to the site of semen deposition (uterus in mares, vagina in cows).

HORMONAL INFLUENCES ON INNATE AND ADAPTIVE IMMUNITY

Infections of the uterus are more easily overcome at estrus than at other stages of the cycle. This increased response at estrus is probably due, at least in part, to better drainage through an open cervix. Both estrogen and progesterone affect neutrophil and lymphocyte function, but there is variation in results obtained when the effects of hormones have been studied. In some species, such as the mouse, estrogen induces an influx of neutrophils and macrophages (at estrus). Estrogen can also be involved in the up-regulation of subsets of T lymphocytes. There is variation in the numbers of lymphocytes in the reproductive tract during the estrus cycle. Even so, there is evidence that CD4+ lymphocytes increase in number with increases in estrogen. Progesterone, which dominates during the luteal phase and pregnancy, antagonizes the "proinflammatory" activity of estrogen. Studies in cattle and sheep indicate an up-regulation of T- and B-lymphocyte responses during the follicular phase of the estrus cycle, when estrogen dominates. Major histocompatibility antigen II expression is enhanced at estrus in direct relationship with rising estrogen concentration. The influence of the estrus cycle on antibodies in the uterus is controversial, but data suggest that concentrations of luminal immunoglobulins and immunoglobulin-containing cells in the endometrium are not influenced by the stage of the estrus cycle. Generally the uterus is more susceptible to infection during the progestational or luteal phase of the estrus cycle and during pregnancy. The nonpregnant uterus is highly resistant to infection. The mechanisms involved in the effect of sex hormones on neutrophils is unknown, and receptors for sex hormones have not been demonstrated in them.

Prostaglandins are normally produced by the endometrium. In most species (excluding the dog, cat, and primates), prostaglandins are responsible for lysis of the corpus luteum. In acute inflammation, prostaglandin production by the endometrium is increased, and lysis of the corpus luteum occurs. When chronic inflammation progresses to the stage of epithelial and mucosal surface loss, production of prostaglandins is decreased, and the corpus luteum persists, with the result that the more susceptible environment of a progestational uterine environment is maintained.

MAMMARY GLAND

As with the body in general, the mammary gland has a full range of mechanisms to prevent and control infectious disease. It relies heavily on isolation. The structure and function of the papillary duct of the teat, and the keratin that accumulates there to form a plug, prevents many potential pathogens from entering the gland. Secretions of the gland contain antimicrobial, antiinflammatory, and immune-modulating substances. Within the gland, there also are humoral and cellular defenses. Defense mechanisms are listed in Box 18-4.

INNATE IMMUNITY

Physical factors are very important in the resistance to infection. The teat orifice, with its sphincter, and the papillary duct offer mechanical resistance to the entry of organisms. The keratin and waxy nature of the inner aspect of the papillary duct can be protective by having bactericidal fatty acids, by adsorbing bacteria and desquamating when coated with bacteria, and by desiccating. Delays in the formation of the keratin plug at drying off or cracks in the teat ends increase the risk of intramammary infection. Regular milking of the lactating mammary gland probably is a natural defense mechanism because of the flushing of organisms and products of inflammation from the gland.

Soluble factors are numerous and contribute to resistance to infection. Lactoferrin, the major iron-binding protein of saliva and milk, is a nonspecific natural protective factor in milk. Mammary gland epithelial cells produce the bulk of lactoferrin in milk. Lactoferrin concentration is increased in acute mastitis and in the involuting gland. The binding of iron withholds this essential nutrient from pathogenic bacteria and thus has a bacteriostatic effect. The lactoperoxidase-thiocyanate-H_2O_2 system temporarily inhibits some streptococci and coliforms and *Staphylococcus aureus*. Lactoperoxidase is synthesized by mammary gland epithelium, thiocyanate is derived from certain green feeds, and H_2O_2 is produced by enzymic constituents of milk by streptococci or from an exogenous source. Hypothiocyanite produced by the lactoperoxidase system damages the inner bacterial membrane, killing the bacteria. Lysozyme, synthesized locally or from blood, destroys bacteria by lysis of cell wall peptidoglycan. Complement activated in mastitis by the alternate pathway in response to the presence of bacterial endotoxin can be important in bactericidal activity, opsonization, and promoting inflammation. Normal milk is antiinflammatory. Cytokines have a broad range of immunomodulation. Molecules of this general group include the interleukins (IL-2 especially), colony-stimulating factors, interferons, and tumor necrosis factor.

Cells that are not part of the adaptive or acquired immune system include the macrophages, neutrophils, and natural killer cells. Macrophages are usually the most numerous leukocyte in mammary secretions. They phagocytose bacteria and act as antigen-presenting cells. Macrophages can be found free in the alveoli and the interstitium, as well as in the lamina propria of the lactiferous sinus and interlobular and intralobular lactiferous ducts. In a lactating cow, apparently at least 500,000 phagocytes per milliliter of milk are necessary for defense of the mammary gland against invading bacteria. In an uninfected bovine mammary gland, 50,000 to 200,000 neutrophils and macrophages are found per milliliter of milk, with the macrophages predominating. Lymphocytes represent about 10% of the leukocytes in lactation. Neutrophils are present only in low numbers unless there is bacterial infection or injury, when their influx can be dramatic. Neutrophils play an extremely important role in antibacterial action by phagocytosis and the release of antibacterial substances.

Box 18-4

Innate or Nonspecific Defenses of the Mammary Gland

Physical factors
- Sphincter and keratin of teat orifice
- Flushing action of milk

Soluble factors
- Lactoferrin
- Lysozyme
- Complement
- Cytokines

Cellular factors
- Macrophages
- Neutrophils
- Natural killer cells

Their function is inhibited in the periparturient period. Recruitment of neutrophils from the blood to an infection site is one of the first steps in an inflammatory response. Recruitment can be rapid, so that neutrophils are the dominant cells as early as 2 hours after infection. Cell counts in milk can average 700,000 per milliliter in subclinically infected quarters, and millions of neutrophils per milliliter are common in clinical infections.

In experimental staphylococcal mastitis, the numbers of inflammatory cells (mostly neutrophils) in milk cycle up and down every several days, with a corresponding inverse cycling of the number of viable bacteria. When cell counts are at a peak, bactericidal activity per cell is most efficient, by as much as 10,000-fold, and phagocytosis is optimal. The frequency and periodicity of the cycle, as well as the amplitude of the cell and bacterial counts, are independent for each infected quarter. The likely source of reinfection of the mammary gland are neutrophils that are inefficient at killing phagocytosed bacteria at the time of low cell count. As these cells undergo necrosis and lysis, their previously protected intracellular viable bacteria are released to multiply, and the inverse cycling of neutrophils and bacterial numbers continues.

Although neutrophils recruited from the blood are important in fighting infection in the mammary gland, they do not kill bacteria as well in milk as they do in blood. Milk seems to be a poor medium for the functioning of neutrophils. Some possible reasons include the absence of glucose in milk for the glycolytic metabolism of neutrophils, decreased amounts of glycogen in milk neutrophils, deficiency of opsonins and complement in milk, coating of the surface of neutrophils with casein, loss of neutrophil pseudopodia caused by phagocytosis of fat, and a decrease of hydrolytic enzymes within neutrophils after phagocytosis of casein and fat.

In the first week after parturition, when neutrophils are likely most needed to deal with mammary gland infections, bovine blood neutrophils already are defective before they pass into the mammary gland. They have significantly impaired chemokinesis and decreased superoxide anion production, antibody-dependent cell-mediated cytotoxicity, and phagocytosis of bacteria. The causes are probably some combination of the effects of stress, energy, and protein demands of early lactation and the hormonal fluxes of this stage of the reproductive cycle. In the parturient period, the concentration of glucocorticoids is increased. This means that leukocyte function is less effective, because expression of L-selectin and CD18 on neutrophils are down-regulated by glucocorticoids. This down-regulates adhesion between blood neutrophils and vascular endothelium and transendothelial migration of neutrophils. Neutrophils are also important in creating bystander injury when the products of neutrophil granules, such as superoxide anions and enzymes, are released during phagocytosis and with neutrophil destruction.

Natural killer cells use perforin to kill bacteria in a major histocompatibility complex (MHC) independent way, and so are part of the nonspecific defenses of the gland.

ADAPTIVE IMMUNITY

The humoral immune system operates in the mammary gland in several ways apart from the transfer of immunoglobulin in colostrum and during lactation. Antibody concentration in normal bovine milk is small, about 1 mg per milliliter, and includes IgG_1, IgG_2, IgM, and IgA. Most IgG is serum derived; IgG_1 is selectively transferred into mammary gland secretion and is the major immunoglobulin class in milk obtained from healthy mammary glands. IgG_2 is both serum derived and locally produced by resident plasma cells, especially in inflammation. IgA and IgM are synthesized locally in the stromal tissue of the acini of the mammary gland and may be part of the enteromammary link of the mucosal immune system, whereby lymphocytes from gut-associated lymphoid tissue home to the reproductive tract. Local production is caused by stimulation of subepithelial lymphocytes.

Particulate antigens, such as bacteria, stimulate an antibody response in the mammary gland of the cow, whereas soluble antigens do not. In colostrum and in milk from inflamed mammary glands, antibody concentration approaches 50 mg per milliliter. Early in inflammation, IgG_1 and IgG_2 opsonize bacteria to enhance phagocytosis by macrophages, but later the importance of IgG_2 as an opsonin increases as neutrophils enter the gland. Neutrophils can transport IgG_2 to the mammary gland as they move to the site of inflammation. IgM also functions as an opsonin. IgA does not opsonize but could prevent bacterial adherence to epithelium, inhibit bacterial multiplication, neutralize leukocyte-inhibiting bacterial toxins, and agglutinate bacteria. Concentrations of immunoglobulin are reduced in the periparturient period and may contribute to the increased susceptibility of the gland to infection.

Cell-mediated immunity in the gland is stimulated in infectious disease. Interleukins from mammary gland macrophages stimulate the immune system by activating T and B lymphocytes. Only a few B lymphocytes are present in the normal mammary gland and milk. T lymphocytes in normal mammary gland tissue and milk of cows and pigs are mostly CD8+ α/β-T lymphocytes. The CD4+/CD8+ ratio is <1, which is reversed from the ratio in blood. The mammary gland thus has selective lymphocyte trafficking, favoring CD8+ lymphocytes, which have either cytotoxic or suppressor function. T lymphocytes, which activate B lymphocytes,

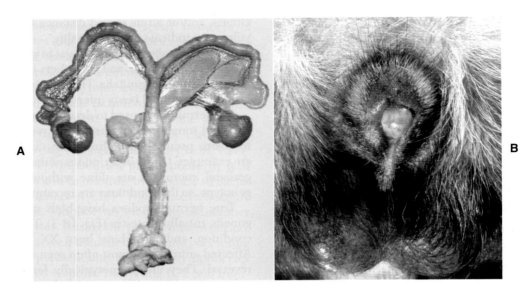

Fig. 18-4   **Male pseudohermaphrodite, reproductive tract. A,** Pig. A testis and epididymis are present on each side. Note the well-developed uterus, cervix, and vagina. No ovarian tissue is present. **B,** Clitoral enlargement, dog. The clitoris protrudes between the labia of the vulva and is visible on the ventral floor of the vulva. Note the formation of a bifid scrotum ventral to the vulva. (**A** and **B,** *Courtesy Dr. K. McEntee, Reproductive Pathology Collection, University of Illinois.*)

an XY genotype, testes, but female tubular elements (Fig. 18-4). Miniature schnauzers with persistent Müllerian ducts have a complete Müllerian system with uterine tube, uterus, and cranial portion of the vagina. They lack Müllerian inhibitory substance or its receptor. Testicular feminization syndrome is a type of male pseudohermaphroditism, as the individuals lack testosterone or its receptors, and as such do not develop a typical male external genitalia. XX pseudohermaphrodites include freemartins and other chimeras.

Chimerism

Animals that are chimeras or mosaics for the sex chromosomes have ambiguous reproductive organs (Fig. 18-5). Chimeras and mosaics have two or more cell types, each with a different chromosomal constitution. The cells of a chimera come from two different sources (such as from male and female members of a set of twins in the bovine freemartin), whereas the cells of a mosaic come from the same source.

The most common chimera in domestic animals is the freemartin calf (Fig. 18-5). Placental vascular anastomoses, which allow exchange of blood between fetuses, are a requirement for the occurrence of a freemartin. These anastomoses occur most often in the bovine species, and less frequently in other ruminants and pigs. The freemartin is the female of a set of male and female twins. The percentage of male cells in freemartins varies widely. Gene products from the cells of the male cause the differentiation of fetal Sertoli

cells and seminiferous cordlike structures in the female twin's ovaries. The ovaries are small, ranging from organs with reduced number of or no germ cells, to organs partially converted to testes, or to organs composed entirely of structures resembling seminiferous tubules. The paramesonephric (Müllerian) duct derivatives vary from almost normal to cordlike structures, but communication is never made with the vagina. The vagina, vestibule, and vulva are hypoplastic. Seminal vesicles are always present; other mesonephric (Wolffian) structures are present to varying degrees. Externally the animal appears female, but the vestibule and vagina are short, the vulva is hypoplastic, and the clitoris is enlarged. The male twin is minimally affected.

Anomalies with normal sexual development

There are many different anomalies found in individuals that have a normal matching of genotypic, gonadal, and phenotypic sex organs. Although there are too many to list, most fit into the categories of failure of the normal maturation, hypoplasia, and aplasia. Because normal development requires such intricate timing of events—including regression of some parts, the joining of tubes and tubules, migration of components from one site to another, the interaction of genes, and hormones and local factors—it is no wonder there are a myriad of anomalies.

Segmental aplasia of the paramesonephric duct system can have a variety of forms. Little is known of

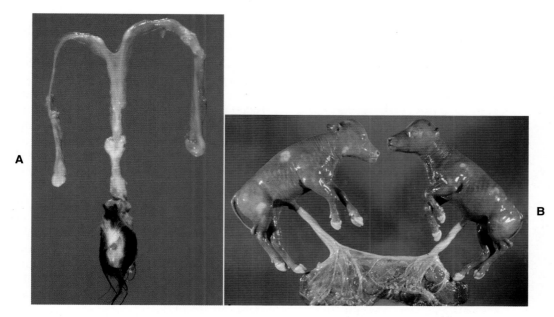

Fig. 18-5   Bovine freemartinism. A, Phenotypically female, reproductive tract, cow. The freemartin is the female of a set of male and female twins. Freemartins are chimeras. There is a vulva and vagina with a prominent clitoris. The internal genitalia consist of bulbourethral and vesicular glands, ductus deferentes, and short incomplete segments of uterus. The gonads are testis with epididymides attached. This major anomaly renders the cow infertile. **B,** Placenta, twin fetuses. Placental vascular anastomoses, which allow exchange of blood between fetuses, are a requirement for the occurrence of a freemartin. These anastomoses occur most often in the bovine species. (*A* and *B,* *Courtesy Dr. R. A. Foster, Ontario Veterinary College, University of Guelph.*)

the pathogenesis of segmental aplasia, apart from studies indicating a genetic basis in some breeds of cattle. Segmental aplasia of the paramesonephric duct system most often occurs in shorthorn cattle, in which it is associated with the recessive gene for white coat color. The simplest form is failure of the paramesonephric duct to make a proper connection with the urogenital sinus, leaving a persistent hymen, a membrane where the two precursor tissues join. A perforated hymen often persists and is of no clinical significance (Fig. 18-6). However, if the hymen is completely imperforated and there is no drainage, the vagina, cervix, and uterus fill with normal secretions. In the more severe forms, one or more segments of the vagina, cervix, uterine body, and uterine horns are absent or rudimentary. Generally the ovaries, uterine tubes, and most cranial parts of the uterine horns are present and normal, except that the horns can be distended by secretion.

Aplasia of a segment of the uterus (Fig. 18-7) can affect cattle. Prostaglandin can be synthesized and released from a uterine horn made blind by the absence of a segment, just as it would be produced by a normally connected uterine horn. In species such as the pig in which systemic transmission of $PGF_{2\alpha}$ from the endometrium to the corpus luteum is important, prostaglandins from the blind uterine horn can have a

lytic effect on the corpora lutea of pregnancy in the contralateral ovary. In species such as the cow, in which the local utero-ovarian pathway is important for luteolysis, the absence of a large segment of the uterus could result in an amount of $PGF_{2\alpha}$ insufficient to cause regression of the corpus luteum. Even a small segment of uterine aplasia can have the same effect if the cranial segment becomes distended with fluid and does not synthesize prostaglandins. In the dog and cat, the uterus does not play a role in the regression of the corpus luteum.

Imperfect fusion of the paired paramesonephric ducts is a common cause of anomalies. Normally the two ducts unite first at the cloacal end to form the vagina and the process moves cranially to form the cervix and the uterine body. A double uterine body, called uterus didelphys, and a double cervix are normal structures at an early stage of development. Malformations due to imperfect fusion are most common in and adjacent to the cervix. They range from a dorsoventral fibrous band in the cranial vagina together with a normal cervix, to failure of fusion of the caudal cervix with bifurcation of the cervical canal, to complete duplication of the cervix and body of the uterus.

Hypoplasia (and its extreme, aplasia) of a portion of the reproductive tract apart from the tubular genitalia comes in many different degrees. Gonadal hypoplasia

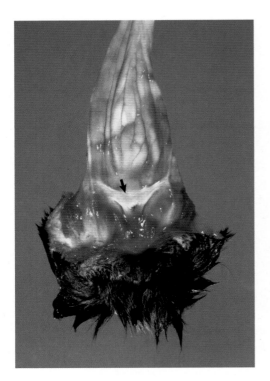

Fig. 18-6 **Persistent hymen, vagina and vulva, bitch.** The membrane *(arrow)* partially separates the vestibule from the vagina and is just cranial to the urethral opening. This minor anomaly is of little consequence and does not interfere with coitus or parturition. *(Courtesy Dr. R. A. Foster, Ontario Veterinary College, University of Guelph.)*

is common, especially in males, and these will be discussed in the relevant sections.

MINOR ANOMALIES

Minor or incidental anomalies are myriad in the reproductive tract. The same factors influencing the development of major anomalies in animals with normal sexual differentiation are at work here too. Minor anomalies are those curiosities that are incidental and are of no clinical significance apart from being mistaken for lesions that do cause infertility, subfertility, or are life threatening. Foremost of these are the numerous cysts and tubular remnants that can be found in many individuals. The so-called paraovarian cysts are extremely common and can be confused with cystic neoplasia. They can be derived from paramesonephric ducts, mesonephric ducts, and mesonephric tubules. Table 18-2 lists the location and names of common incidental cystic anomalies. They will be discussed in more detail later.

Cysts of the reproductive tract not derived from embryonic elements are called inclusion cysts. One of the more common types is the serosal inclusion cyst of the uterus in bitches (Fig. 18-8). It is assumed to arise from small groups of mesothelial cells that get trapped beneath the serosal surface during involution of the uterus. These grapelike clusters of semitransparent thin-walled cysts are found on the serosal surface of the uterus. Subsequent distention and enlargement result in numerous cysts developing.

COMMON SYNDROMES

Many of the commonly seen syndromes of sexual development were mentioned earlier in the relevant sections, but they are combined with those of the male reproductive system and listed in Table 18-1.

OVARY
DEVELOPMENTAL ANOMALIES

Occasionally, agenesis from unknown cause involves one or both ovaries. The reproductive tract can be absent as part of the defect. In cases of bilateral agenesis, the tubular genitalia remain infantile. Duplication of an ovary is a rare anomaly, arising by two different mechanisms: originating separately or splitting from an already developing ovary. The latter type, an accessory ovary, is close to the normally located organ and is usually connected to it. This anomaly is an uncommon cause of ovarian remnant syndrome. Ovarian remnant syndrome is a syndrome that develops in previously spayed cats and dogs that come into heat (estrus) again. Failure of complete surgical removal at the time of spaying is the usual cause.

Hypoplasia of the ovaries occurs most commonly in cows and to a lesser extent in other species. It is usually bilateral but nonsymmetric. The affected ovaries are small and lack follicles or surface scars from ovulation. Microscopically, cortical stroma and ova are absent or poorly developed. The tract remains infantile after puberty. Other causes of an infantile reproductive tract are malnutrition or other forms of debility. Ovaries in these animals, however, have numerous primordial follicles and can respond to gonadotropic hormones after removal of the debilitating factor.

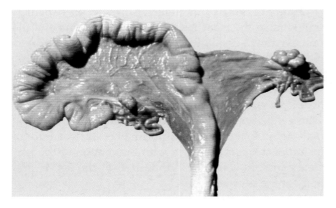

Fig. 18-7 **Segmental aplasia of a uterine horn, uterus, pig.** The right uterine horn is completely missing. *(Courtesy Dr. K. McEntee, Reproductive Pathology Collection, University of Illinois.)*

Table 18-2   Cysts of the Female Reproductive Tract by Location

Cyst		Origin	Species
Intraovarian	Cystic rete ovarii	Mesonephric tubule	Dog and cat
	Inclusion cyst	Ovarian epithelium	Mare
	Subsurface epithelial structure	Normal invagination of ovarian epithelium	Dog
	Cystic follicles	Graafian follicle	Cow, sow
	Anovulatory cyst	Graafian follicle	Mare
	Luteal cyst	Graafian follicle	Cow, sow
	Cystic corpus luteum	Graafian follicle	Cow
	Cystadenoma, cystadenocarcinoma	Rete ovarii, subsurface epithelial structure, surface epithelium	Dog and cat
Paraovarian	Accessory uterine tube (hydatid of Morgagni)	Paramesonephric duct	Mare
	Fimbrial cyst	Paramesonephric duct	
	Bursal cyst	Ovarian bursa	Cow
	Mesonephric duct cysts	Mesonephric ducts	Dog
	Hydrosalpinx	Obstruction of uterine tube	
Uterine	Serosal inclusion cyst	Serosal mesothelium	Dog
	Adenomyosis	Endometrium	Dog and cat
	Cystic endometrial hyperplasia	Endometrium/endometritis	Dog and cat
Vaginal	Mesonephric (Gartner's) ducts	Mesonephric duct remnants	Cow
Vestibular	Cystic vestibular (Bartholin's) gland	Inflammation of vestibular glands	Cow

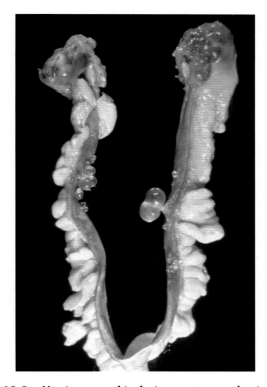

Fig. 18-8   Uterine serosal inclusion cysts, reproductive tract, bitch. The cysts projecting from the serosal surface of the uterus are believed to arise from mesothelial cells trapped within serosal connective tissue. These cysts are an incidental finding at ovariohysterectomy. Note that there are also multiple thin-walled cysts around the right ovary. These cysts are remnants of embryonal ducts and are called paraovarian cysts. *(Courtesy Dr. K. McEntee, Reproductive Pathology Collection, University of Illinois.)*

Hypoplasia caused by genetic and chromosomal abnormalities has been reported. Ovarian hypoplasia occurs in Swedish Highland cattle as an autosomal recessive trait with incomplete penetrance. The ovarian defect is either unilateral or bilateral. The number of primordial follicles and the proportion of Graafian follicles are less then normal. Luteinization tends to occur without ovulation. Ovarian hypoplasia has been associated with cytogenetic anomalies such as XXX chromosomes in the mare and cow and XO chromosomes in the mare. The latter type is similar to the XO disease in human females, called Turner's syndrome, with such features as small stature, lack of uterine cyclic activity, and underdevelopment of the endometrium. The fetal gonad is normal, but the adult ovary has no follicles.

Vascular hamartomas of the ovary are incidental findings in the cow, sow, and mare. They occur as a dark red mass on the surface of the ovary and consist of connective tissue and vascular channels lined by mature endothelial cells.

Cysts in and around the ovary are common findings in many species, particularly in dogs and cats during ovariohysterectomy (Table 18-2). They are of two types: those within the ovary and those outside the ovary. The latter cysts are grouped as paraovarian cysts, and they arise from either paramesonephric ducts or the mesonephric tubules and ducts. Location of the cyst is the most reliable method of differentiating them. Sometimes, histologic similarities with a normal uterus allows identification of those cysts that are of paramesonephric ductal origin.

Cystic remnants of the paramesonephric ducts include the fimbrial cyst and the cystic accessory tube.

This latter cyst is common in the mare and is called the hydatid of Morgagni (Fig. 18-9). They can be several centimeters in diameter. There are many cysts that arise from mesonephric remnants, and some develop in and around the ovary from mesonephric tubules. One of the most common in the dog and cat is the cystic rete ovarii (Fig. 18-10). They can reach several centimeters in diameter. Cystic rete ovarii expand into the ovarian stroma, as they are located in the ovarian hilus. They are lined by ciliated columnar to flattened epithelium.

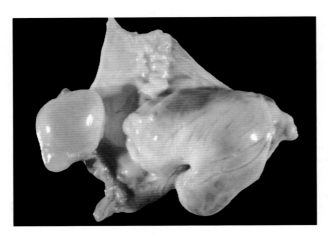

Fig. 18-9 Hydatid of Morgagni, ovary, mare. This cystic structure is located in the fimbria, adjacent to the ovary. They are very common in mares and are cystic remnants of paramesonephric ducts. *(Courtesy Ontario Veterinary College, University of Guelph.)*

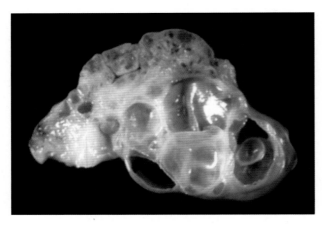

Fig. 18-10   Multiple cystic rete ovarii, ovary, bitch. Note the multiple cysts within the ovary at the hilus. They are incidental findings in bitches and are of little consequence. They develop from the rete (mesonephric tubules) of the ovary and become cystically distended. In cats, they can be unilocular and very large and cause pressure atrophy of the ovary. They must be differentiated from cystadenomas and cystadenocarcinomas, histologicallly. *(Courtesy Dr. R. A. Foster, Ontario Veterinary College, University of Guelph.)*

Cystic ovarian neoplasms are an important differential diagnosis of cysts of or near the ovary. Histologic examination may be required to differentiate them. They are described under Neoplasms. Other cysts of the ovary are derived from the ovarian surface or from the Graafian follicle and will be described under Lesions of the Ovarian Follicles.

ACQUIRED OVARIAN LESIONS

Oophoritis, or inflammation of the ovary, is rare in domestic animals. Experimentally, infectious bovine rhinotracheitis virus (bovine herpesvirus 1[BHV-1]) can induce necrotizing oophoritis in the postestrus cow subsequent to viremia. The corpus luteum is hemorrhagic, and thick, cloudy fibrinous fluid fills some follicles. Microscopically the lesions in the corpus luteum range from focal necrosis and infiltration of mononuclear cells to diffuse hemorrhage and necrosis. Most affected ovaries also have necrotic follicles and diffuse mononuclear cell infiltrates in the stroma. Bovine viral diarrhea (BVD) virus, a vertically and horizontally transmitted virus responsible for mild to fatal enteric disease and reproductive failure, can localize in bovine oocytes and cumulus cells and cause chronic oophoritis. Infection of ovarian oocytes with BVD virus is one of several possible routes of transmission of the virus from cow to fetus. Bacterial oophoritis occasionally is found in cats and dogs. In cats, it must be differentiated from feline infectious peritonitis. The inflammation is around the ovary and within the uterine tube, suggesting that the causative bacteria ascended from the uterus.

Ovarian bursal adhesions vary from thin bands to large sheets of fibrous tissue binding the walls together or crossing the cavity of the ovarian bursa, a peritoneal pouch formed around the ovary by the broad ligament and the mesosalpinx. The lesion is often bilateral in cows and could result from an ascending uterine infection that follows a retained placenta after parturition. Physical trauma from manipulations of the ovary is another possible cause; bursal adhesions are common in beef heifers. Adhesions can obstruct or cause retention of fluids in the bursa and result in a cystic bursa.

Epithelial inclusion cysts are common in mares, in which they can be a cause of infertility (Table 18-2). It is believed that epithelium from the surface of the ovary becomes pinched off and embedded in the stroma during ovulation. This epithelium produces a fluid that causes the structure to enlarge and eventually reach several centimeters in diameter. They are identical in appearance to large follicles, and they do not appear and disappear as follicles should; histologic assessment is necessary for accurate diagnosis. Their size and number may block ovulation. Similar cysts in other species and cysts of the subsurface epithelial structures of the bitch are usually small and incidental.

LESIONS OF THE OVARIAN FOLLICLES

Hemorrhage into follicles is sometimes present in calves, and hemorrhages into cystic follicles happen occasionally in the bitch. A small amount of hemorrhage is normal at the time of ovulation in all species. The mare is an exception because normally much blood is present in the cavity of the follicle, forming the corpus hemorrhagicum. In rare cases, the hemorrhage can be extensive enough to form an ovarian hematoma or even hemoperitoneum can occur. If it extends through the ovulation fossa, the corpus luteum can be external to the ovarian capsule. In the mare and cow, a focal area of serositis is detectable at the point of ovulation. Progression through a fibrinous to a fibrous stage is rapid, and an "ovulation tag" is formed. The manual expression of a persistent corpus luteum in the cow sometimes is followed by severe hemorrhage. Organization of the blood clot can result in adhesions between the ovary and adjacent structures, such as fimbriae of the uterine tube or ovarian bursa, and cause infertility.

Atretic follicles are those that become arrested at any stage of development and then regress. Atretic follicles are, in most cases, normal. In any estrus cycle, only one or a small number of follicles is destined to mature, whereas the others undergo atresia at various stages of maturation. A similar process occurs in seasonal anestrus and in all domestic species during pregnancy, except for the mare. Follicular atresia is considered abnormal when it is a part of any disease process that interferes with the release of, or the pituitary response to, GnRH. Development of the follicle can be arrested at any stage, and after an undetermined amount of time, it degenerates. The ovum undergoes apoptosis first; then the granulosa cells become pyknotic, vacuolated, and desquamate. The follicle either persists as a cyst with a partial thin lining of granulosa cells or is infiltrated by macrophages, theca cells, and fibrous connective tissue, eventually becoming a small scar.

Cystic ovarian (Graafian) follicles, or follicular cysts, are important in cows and sows. The disease in cows is called cystic ovarian degeneration (COD). In dairy cows, the prolongation of the postpartum interval to first estrus (days-open) is the main consequence of cystic follicles. Ovulation does not occur. These cysts probably develop because of an abnormality of the hypothalamo-hypophyseal-ovarian axis that causes a deficiency of LH or of the LH receptor in the ovary, although the mechanism is not defined. Cystic ovarian degeneration is treated with GnRH (that causes release of LH in the pituitary) and with chorionic gonadotrophin (high in LH). Evidence is available that stress may be involved wherein adrenocorticotropic hormone (ACTH) or cortisol inhibits GnRH release from the hypothalamus and prevents up-regulation of LH receptors in the ovary. Higher concentrations of progesterone can have a similar effect. The end result is an inadequate LH surge and failure of ovulation. In a similar way, postpartum uterine infection can cause cystic ovaries in dairy cows.

Cystic ovaries have been linked with the recovery of *Escherichia coli* from the uterus and increased concentrations of serum $PGF_{2\alpha}$ metabolites and cortisol. Because of these findings, it has been proposed that bacterial endotoxins, or the prostaglandins produced because of damage caused by endotoxins, stimulate the adrenal cortical secretion of cortisol; cortisol excess suppresses the preovulatory release of LH, resulting in the development of cysts. Bovine cystic follicles are 2.5 cm or more in diameter (Fig. 18-11) and persist for 10 or more days without the formation of a corpus luteum. Cystic follicles were common lesions in a large slaughterhouse survey of beef heifers.

An anovulatory luteinized cyst is likely caused by delayed or insufficient release of LH and is therefore part of COD (Table 18-2). It occurs in cows and sows more often than in other species. Ovulation does not occur. The cystic cavity is lined by fibrous tissue, surrounded by an adjacent zone of luteinized theca cells. Cystic follicles and luteinized cysts can occur in the same ovary. The extent of luteinization that must occur in a cystic follicle to justify its designation as a luteal cyst has not been defined.

Cystic corpus luteum is of uncertain pathogenesis. In cows, it must be distinguished from anovulatory luteinized cyst and from the small central cyst that can occur normally in a corpus luteum. Ovulation occurs and a large irregular cyst develops (Fig. 18-12), but without interfering with the length of the estrous cycle.

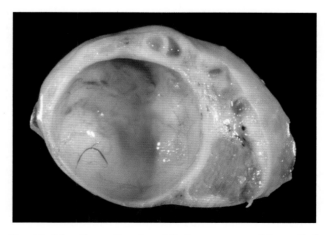

Fig. 18-11 **Cystic Graafian follicle, ovary, cow (also called follicular cysts).** Follicular cysts are larger than normal follicles and usually greater than 2.5 cm in diameter. They are the macroscopic lesions of cystic ovarian disease in the cow. They arise when ovulation of a normal follicle does not occur.
(Courtesy Dr. R.B. Miller, Ontario Veterinary College, University of Guelph.)

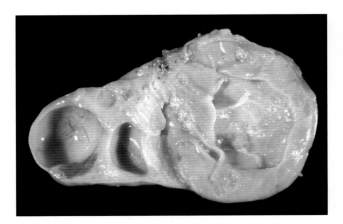

Fig. 18-12 **Cystic corpus luteum, ovary, cow.** A cystic corpus luteum is a normal corpus luteum complete with an ovulation papilla and a prominent cystic center. There is also a normal Graafian follicle *(left)* present. *(Courtesy Dr. R.B. Miller, Ontario Veterinary College, University of Guelph.)*

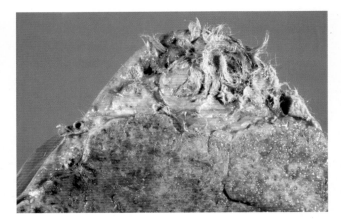

Fig. 18-13 **Ovarian teratoma, ovary, bitch.** These tumors have cells derived from all three germ cell lines: ectodermal (epithelium, including neuroepithelium), mesodermal (mesenchymal tissue), and endodermal (intestine and respiratory tissues). The most common tissues seen macroscopically include hair, cartilage, and bone. This teratoma was 30 cm in diameter and surrounded by a bursa, but residual ovarian tissue was not found. Hair and bone are the main structures visible. *(Courtesy Dr. R. A. Foster, Ontario Veterinary College, University of Guelph.)*

It has been suggested that at least in sows the cysts found in ovaries are different stages of the same aberration. The morphologic form, whether an ovulated or unovulated follicle or a corpus luteum, is determined by the stage at which the physiologic process became abnormal.

Supernumerary follicles are induced in bovine ovaries by chorionic gonadotropin or follicle-stimulating hormone used in doses to cause superovulation in preparation for embryo transfer. In these cows, it is not unusual for more than a dozen well-developed ovarian follicles or corpora lutea of the same age to be present.

NEOPLASMS

There are three main groups of primary ovarian neoplasia in domesticated animals: germ cell, sex-cord stromal, and epithelial neoplasms. These represent the major histogenic origins of the cells of the ovary. Little is known of ovarian carcinogenesis, although there is evidence in human beings that estrogen (and the lack of pregnancy) may be involved.

Germ cell neoplasms

It would be expected that neoplasms arising from germ cells could differentiate along either embryonic or extraembryonic lines and could be benign or malignant or undifferentiated. The great majority of neoplasms of germ cells are benign and undifferentiated (dysgerminoma) or benign with somatic differentiation (teratoma).

Dysgerminoma is a rare neoplasm of bitches, sows, cows, and mares and is composed of cells resembling primitive germ cells. The neoplasm is usually a solid lobulated mass with areas of hemorrhage and necrosis. It is analogous to seminoma in the male. Mitotic rate is high, but metastases are rare.

Ovarian teratomas are rare, usually well differentiated, and benign. They arise from totipotential primordial germ cells and have disorganized elements of at least two of the three embryonic germ layers. Skin is often a significant component (Fig. 18-13). Malignant teratomas occur less often, except in the bitch.

Gonadal stromal neoplasms

Granulosa cell neoplasms are the most common ovarian neoplasms in large animals. They are unilateral, smooth surfaced, and round and can be 20 to 30 cm in diameter. They can be solid, cystic, or polycystic (Fig. 18-14, *A* and *B*). The cysts can vary from microscopic size to several centimeters in diameter. Often the fluid within the cysts is red-brown. Microscopically the granulosa cells are not different from normal granulosa cells and often are arranged as they would be in normal Graafian follicles, that is, in single or multiple rows of round to columnar cells lining fluid-filled spaces (Fig. 18-14, *C*). In less differentiated areas, the neoplastic cells are arranged in sheets. Sometimes, especially in queens, Call-Exner bodies are present in the fluid. These bodies are rosettes of granulosa cells, some containing an eosinophilic body in the central space. The stroma can be sparse or plentiful; if the stroma predominates, the neoplasm is a thecoma. The cytoplasm of some thecoma cells contains lipid droplets. Areas of luteinization in granulosa-theca cell neoplasms are not uncommon, but luteomas, neoplasms with a uniform

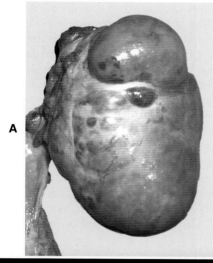

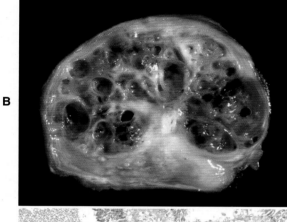

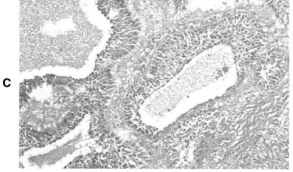

Fig. 18-14   Granulosa cell tumor, ovary, cow. A, This large, lobulated neoplasm has obliterated the normal structure of the ovary. They can be solid (as in this case) or multicystic. **B,** Multiple fluid-filled cysts and solid areas have caused the dramatic ovarian enlargement. Granulosa cell tumors are part of the group of neoplasms known as gonadal stromal tumors. **C,** This granulosa cell tumor has solid and cystic regions. The cysts are lined by cells that resemble granulosa cells of the follicle. H&E stain. (*A and C, Courtesy College of Veterinary Medicine, University of Illinois. B, Courtesy Dr. M.D. McGavin, College of Veterinary Medicine, University of Tennessee.*)

population of luteinized cells, are rare. Luteomas can probably develop from either granulosa or theca cells. Granulosa cell neoplasms are often malignant in the queen and sometimes in the bitch, but in the cow and mare, sex cord stromal neoplasms are usually benign. Many stromal neoplasms produce estrogens or androgens. The mare can have signs of anestrus, nymphomania, or stallion-like behavior; the bitch is likely to have prolonged estrus and may develop pyometra.

Epithelial neoplasms

The ovaries are covered by coelomic epithelium, the same layer of tissue that invaginates in early fetal life to form the lining of the reproductive tract. Neoplasms of the ovarian surface epithelium can thus resemble the several neoplastic types of the endometrium. The serous type is the only important one in animals. Serous papillary cystadenoma and cystadenocarcinoma occur commonly in the bitch (Fig. 18-15, *A*). The other main type is the cystadenoma and cyst adenocarcinoma. They originate from the surface epithelium or from subsurface rests within the ovary or from the rete ovarii. The neoplasms are frequently bilateral, with a shaggy surface and up to 10 cm in diameter. Malignant forms spread over the peritoneal surface by both lateral extension and seeding (Fig. 18-15, *C*). Ascites results either from obstruction of the diaphragmatic lymph vessels, which reabsorb peritoneal fluid, or from excess fluid secretion by the neoplasm.

UTERINE TUBES

Most lesions of the uterine tubes are either incidental or secondary to lesions elsewhere in the reproductive tract. In dogs and cats, commonly seen lesions of the uterine tubes are unlikely to affect reproductive performance. Lesions commonly encountered in dogs and cats are duct remnants in the mesosalpinx, more often of mesonephric ductal (simple tubular structures lined by low columnar to cuboidal cells) than paramesonephric ductal (lined by a folded mucosa similar to the uterine tube mucosa) origin.

Congenital or acquired hydrosalpinx, distention of the uterine tubes by clear fluid, is caused by mechanical or functional obstruction of the lumen. The obstruction can be at either end of the uterine tube. The distention can be uniform or irregular; the wall is thin, and the tube increases in length and tortuosity. Multiloculated cysts are numerous in the mucosa. The congenital type result from segmental aplasia of the uterine tube, as is present in freemartins, or more likely to segmental aplasia of the horn of the uterus. The acquired type is secondary to trauma or chronic inflammation; acute inflammation will cause pyosalpinx rather than hydrosalpinx. Trauma by manual interference with a corpus luteum in cows can cause an

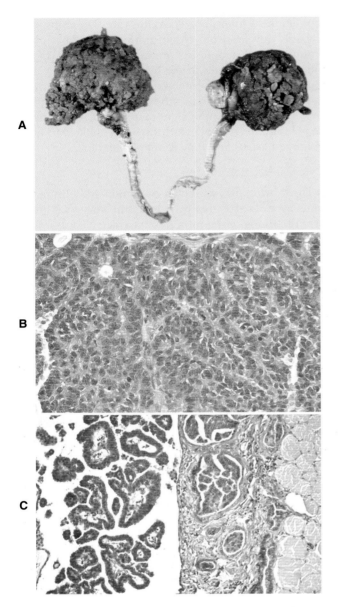

Fig. 18-15   Papillary ovarian carcinoma, ovary, bitch.
A, Both ovaries are enlarged by neoplastic epithelium that has formed papillary structures that give the masses a shaggy outer surface. These neoplasms are often malignant and bilateral, and they seed the abdomen, producing carcinomatosis.
B, Neoplastic epithelial cells are arranged in cords and papillae, are pleomorphic, and have many mitoses. H&E stain. **C,** This papillary carcinoma has seeded the abdominal cavity, implanted on the peritoneum, invaded into the muscle of the diaphragm, and is in subserosal lymphatics adjacent to the diaphragmatic skeletal muscle (*right*) H&E stain. (*A,* Courtesy Dr R.B. Miller, Ontario Veterinary College, University of Guelph. *B,* Courtesy Dr. M.D. McGavin, College of Veterinary Medicine, University of Tennesse. *C,* Courtesy Dr. K. McEntee, Reproductive Pathology Collection, University of Illinois.)

organizing hematoma about the uterine tube, resulting in obstruction by external pressure. This same manipulation can force inflammatory exudate from the uterus into the uterine tube, causing inflammation of tubular mucosa and obstruction of the lumen. Inflammatory exudate can be forced manually or under the pressure of therapeutic uterine infusion, not only into the uterine tube but also into the ovarian bursa, where the ensuing inflammation can result in fibrous bands that compress the uterine tube. Hydrosalpinx, or a bacteriologically sterile pyosalpinx, is one of the most common causes of sterility in pigs. It occurs almost exclusively in nulliparous animals and is almost always bilateral. The cause is unknown, but some evidence points to obstruction by embryonal rests of the mesonephric duct.

Salpingitis is uncommon in domestic species and results from spread of infection from the uterus to the uterine tubes; it is often bilateral. Generally, gross lesions are few, except perhaps for some hyperemia and thickening of the mucosa and small amounts of luminal exudate. Perioophoritis is a likely sequela and can cause infertility. Microscopically the inflammation ranges from mild to severe and from acute to chronic. Early mild lesions are loss of cilia and desquamation of epithelial cells at the tips of the mucosal folds. When severe, salpingitis involves other parts of the mucosa and sometimes the muscle layer. Exudate is present in the lumen. With time, adhesions form between the denuded areas and adjacent mucosa becomes cystic, reepithelializes, or is replaced by granulation tissue.

Pyosalpinx has similar pathogenetic events to salpingitis but is more severe, as suppurative exudate accumulates in the lumen. Obstruction of the lumen occurs, likely secondary to accumulation of exudate, or to scarring. Neutrophils predominate and form large lakes in the lumen or in mucosal cysts derived from the glands of the tube. The epithelium is damaged by the causative agent and by the products of neutrophilic granules that are released during phagocytosis and death, with the result that there is erosion and subsequent granulation, or the epithelium undergoes squamous metaplasia.

Ectopic pregnancy, as occurs in human beings, does not occur in domesticated mammals. Traumatic rupture of the pregnant uterus and release of the fetus into the abdomen is the usual cause of so-called ectopic pregnancy in dogs and cats.

UTERUS

INFLAMMATION

Uterine disease is a significant cause of infertility and, in some cases, mortality. Foremost of these are inflammatory diseases, usually the result of contamination of the uterus with bacteria.

Most uterine infections are the result of ascending infection that arises when the cervix is open—at estrus, parturition, or postpartum involution. Occasionally, infection can occur from a descending spread or via the hematogenous route, particularly in pregnancy when the uteroplacental interface is the site for preferential localization of organisms. It is assumed that the placenta is the target and the endometrium is secondarily affected, but the interface of the two systems is an area where a unique environment exists that is suitable for many infectious agents to multiply. Resistance of the uterus to infection is influenced by physical factors, the hormonal environment, and the humoral and cellular immune mechanisms as discussed previously.

Endometritis is inflammation limited to the endometrium, usually due to seminal fluid and bacterial infection in nonpregnant animals, and in cows, herpesviral infections are the usual causes. In pregnancy, organisms that cause placentitis, fetal infection, and abortion, in most cases, also spread and cause inflammation of the endometrium. Postpartum endometritis occurs to some extent even after a normal pregnancy and parturition, but endometritis is especially common and more severe following an abnormal parturition. Lochia, the fluid and debris that is discharged from the uterus for a short time after parturition, is an excellent nutrient medium for bacterial growth.

Mild cases of acute endometritis are not detected grossly. It can induce cystic endometrial hyperplasia in dogs and cats. In more severe cases of acute endometritis, the mucosa is swollen and has a rough surface, often with adherent shreds of fibrin and necrotic debris. At microscopic examination, a few to many neutrophils are found in the stroma and in the glands, with a range of surface changes from desquamation of a few surface epithelial cells to severe necrosis of the endometrium. Mild lesions resolve completely or incompletely with residual changes of cystic glands and periglandular fibrosis. Severe acute endometritis often becomes chronic, and the necrotic endometrium is replaced by granulation tissue devoid of glands, and ultimately this matures to form fibrous tissue. Acute endometritis can stimulate the synthesis of $PGF_{2\alpha}$ in large animals that have had 4 or 5 days of progesterone priming, causing premature regression of the corpus luteum and shortening of the estrous cycle. The loss of endometrium in chronic endometritis can result in reduced production of $PGF_{2\alpha}$, and this decrease in $PGF_{2\alpha}$, especially in the mare and the cow, results in a persistent corpus luteum.

In the mare, endometrial biopsy is used as a breeding management tool because the severity of endometritis is correlated directly with the inability of the uterus to carry a fetus to term. To give a prognosis based on the features of the endometrium, focal and diffuse inflammatory cell infiltration of the stroma, contents of the glands, and frequency and severity of periglandular fibrosis are scored (Fig. 18-16). The endometrium of individual mares is categorized as predicted high, reduced, or low likelihood of the animal completing pregnancy.

Persistent mating-induced endometritis is a problem in mares. Affected animals are unable to resolve the acute endometritis that usually follows mating. The inflammation that occurs at mating, presumably because of the local effects of seminal fluid, lasts 24 to 36 hours in normal mares. Those mares that fail to clear this inflammation accumulate fluid in the uterus, and edema also persists. This persistence is now believed to be an inability of some mares to adequately clear uterine contents (including seminal fluids) after mating because of a defect in uterine contractility. There appears to be an intrinsic dysfunction in myometrial contraction, and accumulation of nitric oxide and its absorption may interfere with uterine myoelectrical activity. Greater susceptibility is believed to occur with repeated pregnancies, loss of body condition, and genetics. The position of the uterus plays a role, and normal mares have a more horizontal uterus than the more drooped or vertical orientation of susceptible mares.

Metritis is inflammation of all layers of the uterine wall. It is a more severe and advanced form of endometritis. In the acute stage, in addition to endometritis, the serosa is dull, finely granular, and has

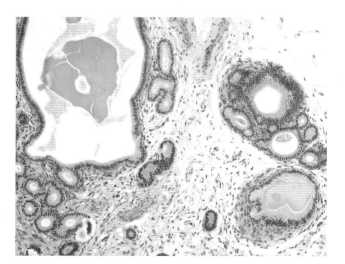

Fig. 18-16 Endometrial fibrosis, endometrial biopsy, mare. Fibrosis from endometrial inflammation and edema results in endometrial glands forming nests (*right*) and cysts (*left*). This fibrosis results in reduced fertility due to a lack of attachment of the conceptus, or a failure of formation of normal microcotyledons and a reduced placental area. H&E stain.
(Courtesy Dr. R. A. Foster, Ontario Veterinary College, University of Guelph.)

petechial hemorrhages and fine adhering strands of fibrin. Microscopically the subserosal tissue, muscle layers, and the endometrium are edematous and infiltrated by neutrophils.

Pyometra occurs as a sequela to endometritis or metritis. It is an acute or chronic infection of the uterus with accumulation of pus in the lumen (Fig. 18-17). The closure of the cervix is not always complete, and some discharge occurs. In some instances, the obstruction of the cervix is mechanical, but most cases are caused by a functional obstruction of the cervix, just as with diestrus, and is under the influence of progesterone produced by a retained corpus luteum. In the cow, the persistence of the corpus luteum is usually secondary to a pathologic process in the uterus. In the bitch and queen, most cases of pyometra follow endometritis (see the section on cystic endometrial hyperplasia later in this chapter) (Fig. 18-18, A and B). The color and consistency of the exudates vary with the infecting bacteria. Exudate is viscid and brown with *Escherichia coli* infection and creamy yellow with streptococcal infection. The uterus can be greatly distended, but not necessarily uniformly. Grossly, necrotic, ulcerated, and hemorrhagic areas are present in the uterine mucosa, along with dry, white, thickened, finely cystic areas. Microscopically the dry white areas have changes of hyperplasia and squamous metaplasia of surface epithelium, a common occurrence in chronic inflammation of

any mucous membrane. The cystic areas are caused by cystic endometrial hyperplasia (Fig. 18-19). Lesions outside the genital tract such as bone marrow depression, widespread extramedullary hematopoiesis, and immune complex glomerulopathy are common in the bitch.

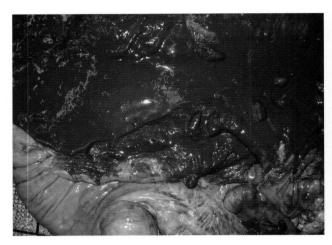

Fig. 18-17   Pyometra, uterus, cow. The uterus is distended and filled with foul-smelling dark brown fluid. The endometrium was red-black and dull, indicating an endometritis secondary to bacterial infection. This cow developed a severe pyometra immediately after calving. *(Courtesy Dr. R. A. Foster, Ontario Veterinary College, University of Guelph.)*

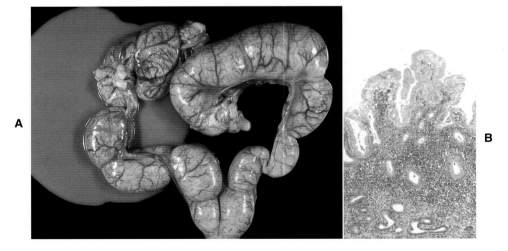

Fig. 18-18   Metritis-pyometra-endometrial hyperplasia, uterus, bitch. A, Pyometra occurs several weeks after estrus. Bacteria grow in the uterus and induce a suppurative response. The uterus fills with pus and is distended. **B,** Endometritis and pyometra. There are large numbers of lymphocytes and plasma cells in the endometrial stroma. The surface epithelium is hyperplastic and papillary. The luminal epithelial cells are highly vacuolated. Pus in the lumen of the uterus was removed during processing of the histologic section. H&E stain. (**A,** *Courtesy Dr. J. Wright, College of Veterinary Medicine, North Carolina State University; and Noah's Arkive, College of Veterinary Medicine, The University of Georgia.* **B,** *Courtesy Dr. R. A. Foster, Ontario Veterinary College, University of Guelph.)*

NONINFLAMMATORY DISEASES

Torsion of the uterus occurs in pregnant animals, mainly in the cow. To a lesser extent, it occurs in the pregnant bitch and queen (Fig. 18-20) and when the uterus is enlarged by pyometra (accumulation of pus in the uterine lumen) or mucometra (accumulation of mucus in the uterine lumen). The mesovarium is a fixed point in both the cow and the bitch, with the other fixed point influenced by the length of the horns and the presence and rigidity of the ligament between

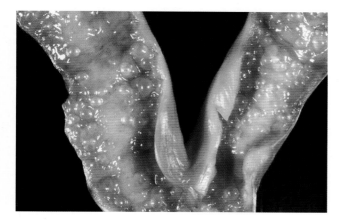

Fig. 18-19   Cystic endometrial hyperplasia, uterus, bitch. Note the cysts in the mucosa of the endometrium. This change occurs under the influence of progesterone after estrus. Cystic hyperplasia may provide a suitable environment for bacteria to grow and cause pyometra, or alternatively, cystic hyperplasia may be secondary to uterine infection and endometritis. *(Courtesy Dr. W. Crowell, College of Veterinary Medicine, The University of Georgia; and Noah's Arkive, College of Veterinary Medicine, The University of Georgia.)*

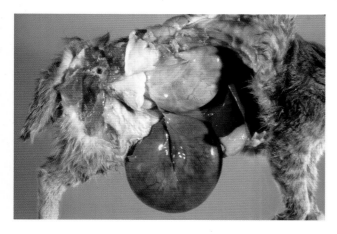

Fig. 18-20   Uterine torsion, cat. The dark red black structure (*bottom center*) is a twisted uterine horn that contains a fetus. Its color is the result of venous infarction. *(Courtesy Dr. R. A. Foster, Ontario Veterinary College, University of Guelph.)*

the horns. The rotation is around the mesometrium and tends to occur at the level of the cervix in the cow and the junction of the uterine horn and body in the bitch and queen. The result of torsion is circulatory compromise and venous infarction. The veins, being of a lower pressure and thinner walled, are compressed and occluded before the arteries. The uterine wall and placenta become congested and edematous. The fetus dies and mummifies or putrefies if the cervix is open enough to allow the entrance of bacteria or fungi to colonize the fetus. The uterine wall is friable and prone to rupture. Rupture of the uterus is also likely in severe dystocia and during treatment of uterine diseases by infusion of drugs and fluids. Rupture can be incomplete, involving just the mucosa, or complete. The torsion and dystocia-related ruptures are likely to be in the caudal part of the uterus and are often fatal because of hemorrhage or infection. The rupture that follows overvigorous infusion of medications into the uterus occurs at the lesser curvature of a horn, dissects beneath the serosa and into the mesometrium, and results in perimetritis.

Prolapse of the uterus is important in the ewe, cow, and sow after parturition. Factors that cause uterine inertia, such as prolonged dystocia, hypocalcemia, and ingestion of estrogenic plants, usually contribute to prolapse of the uterus. A flaccid uterus and excessive straining are predisposing conditions. The anatomic structures that are prolapsed can be restricted to the previously pregnant horn, cervix, or vagina or can include all of the uterus, the bladder, and sometimes some of the small intestine. As the structures prolapse, there is vascular compromise, and congestion and edema result (Fig. 18-21). Constriction by the vaginal and vulval tissues exacerbates this, and as edema develops, the tissues exposed to the outside environment continue to swell and hang down. They dry and become traumatized, further exacerbating the swelling. Continued straining and the effects of gravity on the prolapsed tissues continue to contribute to stretching of internal structures, such as ligaments and blood vessels. Hemorrhage and shock can cause death; even if the uterus is returned to its normal anatomic position in the abdominal cavity via palpation and the animal survives, the intervening drying, trauma, venous infarction, and infection that occur will prevent future fertility.

Subinvolution of placental sites is the longer than normal persistence of placental sites in the uterus after parturition in the bitch, beyond the normal 12 to 15 weeks. In the normal placenta, trophoblasts are found in the endometrium and around the small blood vessels of the myometrium, but they rapidly degenerate in the postpartum period. In the bitch, subinvolution of placental sites is characterized clinically by an excessive bloody vaginal discharge that lasts for weeks or months

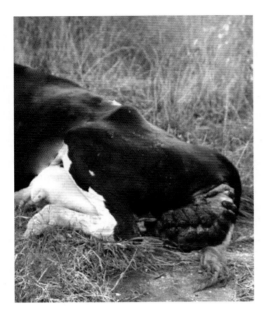

Fig. 18-21   Uterine prolapse, cow. Part of the uterus, and all of the cervix and vagina have prolapsed. The uterus has become swollen from dependent edema and from reduced venous outflow. The mucosae (e.g., caruncles) are exteriorized and exposed to the environment, and thus they have become dehydrated and traumatized. *(Courtesy Dr. C. Wallace, College of Veterinary Medicine, The University of Georgia; and Noah's Arkive, College of Veterinary Medicine, The University of Georgia.)*

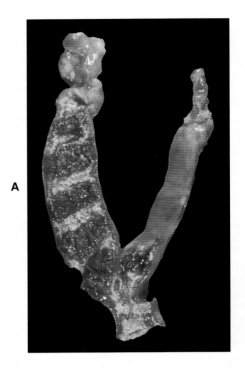

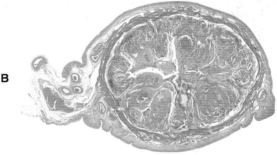

Fig. 18-22   Subinvolution of placental sites, uterus, bitch. A, Incompletely involuted placental sites. The red transverse stripes are placental sites with hemorrhage, fibrin, and necrotic debris. They are larger than normal sites for the same stage after parturition and remain long after normal sites would have disappeared (12 to 15 weeks postpartum). **B,** Transverse section of the uterus at a subinvoluted placental site. The two pink outer layers are normal myometrium and underlying endometrial stroma. Most of the distended lumen is filled with large irregularly sized clots of blood, fibrin, and necrotic debris around which are endometrial epithelium and trophoblastic cells. H&E stain. *(A and B, Courtesy Dr. M.D. McGavin, College of Veterinary Medicine, University of Tennessee.)*

after delivery instead of the normal 1 to 6 weeks. Grossly, subinvoluted placental sites are about twice the size of normal sites for the same time after parturition, but their appearance is identical to normal except that fibrin adherent to the site is more prominent (Fig. 18-22). As such, multiple segmental thickenings of the walls of the uterine horns are identifiable from the serosal surface. The luminal surface of each site is a raised, rough, ragged, gray-to-brown plaque of hemorrhage and fibrin. Microscopically the superficial part of the plaque near the lumen consists of cell debris, hematoma, thrombus, and regenerating endometrium. In the deeper part of the site, the changes are collagen deposition, hemorrhage, distention, and decreased density of endometrial glands. Trophoblast-like cells are more numerous in subinvolution sites than in normal placental sites and are abundant at the base of the deposited collagen; these cells can invade the myometrium and penetrate the full thickness of the wall and perforate the uterus. Because affected animals have a bloody discharge, anemia can result, and those dogs with coagulation disorders, such as von Willebrand's disease, can exsanguinate. The uterus is prone to develop postpartum infection and endometritis, and open pyometra can occur or worsen.

Pseudopregnancy is an exaggerated form of a normal physiologic process. Every entire female dog has a prolonged luteal phase of estrus, and this has been referred to as covert pseudopregnancy or physiologic pseudopregnancy. Some dogs, especially of the toy breeds, develop this exaggerated reaction, and prolactin or its receptors play a role, but it is poorly understood. The presence of progesterone is permissive of the changes that occur. Overtly pseudopregnant dogs either have an increased concentration of prolactin, or they have increased sensitivity to prolactin. This can occur with a more rapid than usual decline in progesterone when dogs are spayed during diestrus. Hyperprolactinemia that occurs in response to visual stimuli of the presence of surrogate neonates results in the mammary development, lactation, maternal behavior, and other clinically apparent changes of pseudopregnancy. Uterine changes in pseudopregnancy can include the formation of placental sites and mucometra in the absence of fetuses.

Endometrial atrophy is usually due to loss of ovarian function secondary to hypopituitarism, and the endometrial atrophy of old age is not seen in domestic species. In the mare, diffuse endometrial atrophy occurs in anestrus and also occurs, but much less commonly, because of the ovarian inactivity of debility and chromosomal aberrations. Focal endometrial atrophy of unknown cause sometimes occurs in the mare. Atrophic endometrium is thin and flat. In the mare, the longitudinal folds are indistinct in atrophic areas, and in the cow, the caruncles are flattened. The uterus of the mare has been most studied microscopically because data from uterine biopsies are frequently used for the management of breeding. The endometrium of the uterus of the anestrous mare has cuboidal luminal and glandular epithelium, with short, straight glands.

Endometrial polyps are common lesions in older bitches and queens. They are localized increases in endometrial stroma and glands. Their cause is not known and may be an age-associated change. They are localized swellings or nodules, and some have a narrow base (Fig. 18-23). They can cause obstruction and mucometra.

Endometrial hyperplasia can be localized or generalized, is an important lesion in the ewe, bitch, and queen, and is rare in the mare. In farm animals, it is caused by prolonged hyperestrogenism. Ingested estrogenic clover such as subterranean (*Trifolium subterraneum*) and red (*Trifolium pratense*) clover is the most likely source of estrogen in the ewe. Cystic follicles, granulosa cell tumors, and estrogens from plants are causes of endometrial hyperplasia in the cow. The mycotoxin zearalenone obtained from moldy feed is a cause in the sow. In ewes, endometrial hyperplasia results in reduced fertility, dystocia, and uterine prolapse because of uterine hypotonicity. Glands of the endometrial type can develop in the cervical mucosa. Even when nonpregnant, ewes have mammary gland enlargement. Endometrial cysts, about 1 cm in diameter in the ewe, are filled with clear fluid. The cysts are both beside and beneath the caruncles. Endometrial hyperplasia is not

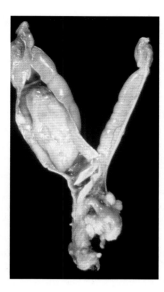

Fig. 18-23 **Endometrial polyp, cat.** The uterine horn on the left is distended by a solid cylindrical polyp that is connected to the endometrium by a narrow stalk. *(Courtesy Dr. G. Foley, Pfizer Inc.)*

precancerous in domestic animals, as it can be in women.

In the bitch, and presumably the queen, cystic endometrial hyperplasia (CEH) is a common response of the uterus (Fig. 18-19). It occurs mostly in diestrus. The disease can be reproduced by estrogen priming of dogs followed by progesterone administration, but this may not be the physiologic mechanism. Bacteria are almost always present in the uterus of dogs with CEH. Increased concentration of progesterone in late estrus or early diestrus and aberrant hormonal function may alter hormonal receptor expression. This may prime the uterus so that inflammation or irritation by bacteria (or other substances, such as suture material and oil) stimulates the uterus to undergo hyperplasia and the type of change seen in early pregnancy—the so called decidual reaction.

Simple endometrial hyperplasia can be overlooked or be recognizable grossly when mild and patchy or diffuse thickening involves the endometrium. When it progresses to the stage of cystic endometrial hyperplasia, the lesion is readily recognized at necropsy. Microscopically the main component of endometrial hyperplasia is an increase in the size and number of glands with no change in the stroma except for edema. The glandular epithelium is progestational in appearance, (i.e., the cells are columnar, hypertrophic, and hyperplastic, and have clear cytoplasm) (Fig. 18-18, *B*). As the glands become cystic, the pressure of retained secretion is increased, and the epithelium of the glands becomes flattened. Bitches and queens are likely to progress to pyometra. In all species, the cystic lesions are probably irreversible.

Mucometra and hydrometra are the accumulation of mucus and clear fluid, respectively, in the uterine lumen (Fig. 18-24, A and B). The cause is congenital or acquired obstruction of the outflow of mucus initially produced in normal amounts. However, mucometra can be due to the production of excessive amounts of mucus in cases of hyperestrogenism. Mucometra occurs in pseudopregnancy, where it resolves spontaneously. Mucometra or hydrometra from obstructive lesions will contribute to infertility.

Adenomyosis is occasionally encountered in domestic animals, notably the bitch, queen, and cow. Adenomyosis is the presence of nests of endometrium within the myometrium, and the effect generally is negligible in domestic animals, which do not menstruate. Sometimes the uterus undergoes diffuse symmetric or focal asymmetric enlargement (Fig. 18-25). Microscopically, endometrial glands or stroma or both have extended from the basal endometrium beyond the junction between endometrium and myometrium. Endometriosis is a lesion of importance only in primates, in which the endometrium goes through the proliferative, secretory, and menses (shedding) phases. Endometriosis is the presence of endometrial glands or stroma in locations outside the uterus, such as the ovary, the mesometrium, the peritoneum, and peritoneal surgical scars. The phases of the menstrual cycle result in a buildup of the products of menses in the extrauterine sites that cause inflammation, fibrosis, and pain.

NEOPLASMS

Uterine neoplasms are not common in domestic animals. The primary ones that do occur with any significant frequency are carcinoma in the cow and leiomyoma in the bitch. Lymphosarcoma in the cow is the most often encountered metastatic neoplasm.

Leiomyomas in the bitch are often multiple neoplasms, not only in the uterus, but also in the cervix and vagina (Fig. 18-26, A and B). Estrogens likely have a role

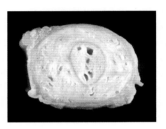

Fig. 18-25   Adenomyosis, uterine body, bitch. Formalin fixed specimen. The myometrium (*outer portion*) is infiltrated and expanded by multiple cysts of endometrial stroma and glands. Many of these glands are filled with pus, and the endometrium is expanded as a result of inflammation secondary to bacterial infection. *(Courtesy Dr. R.B. Miller, Ontario Veterinary College, University of Guelph.)*

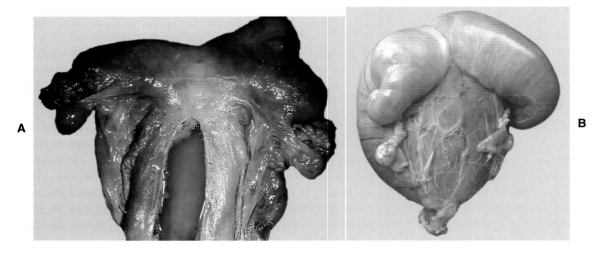

Fig. 18-24   Mucometra and hydrometra, uterus. A, Mucometra, mare. Note the accumulation of mucus within the opened body of the distended uterus. **B,** Hydrometra, goat. The uterine horns and body are filled with clear watery fluid. *(**A,** Courtesy Dr. K. McEntee, Reproductive Pathology Collection, University of Illinois; and Dr. J. King, College of Veterinary Medicine, Cornell University. **B,** Courtesy Dr. P. W. Ladds, James Cook University of North Queensland.)*

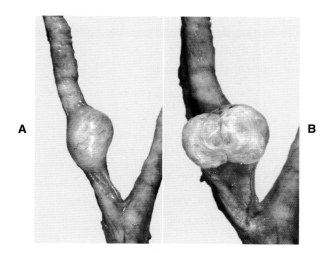

Fig. 18-26   Leiomyoma, uterus, bitch. A, Note the well-circumscribed, firm mass in the left uterine horn. **B,** The cut section of the leiomyoma reveals gelatinous content with bands of smooth muscle and connective tissue. This mass is within and arising from the myometrium. *(A and B, Courtesy Dr. D. D. Harrington, College of Veterinary Medicine, Purdue University; and Noah's Arkive, College of Veterinary Medicine, The University of Georgia.)*

of the uterine wall. Microscopically the neoplasm is readily distinguished from normal endometrium by the increased size, pleomorphism, and disarray of the glandular epithelial cells and the accompanying scirrhous reaction. Metastases occur to the regional lymph nodes (iliosacral) and lungs, and they seed the serosal surfaces of the abdomen.

Lymphosarcoma in the cow in the enzootic form is caused by the bovine leukemia retrovirus and commonly affects a tetrad of organs, namely the heart, abomasum, lymph nodes, and uterus. In the uterus, as in other locations, infiltration of neoplastic cells can be focal, multifocal, or multifocally coalescing and up to 3 cm thick (Fig. 18-27). Affected areas are light yellow, slightly friable, and sometimes centrally necrotic and thicken or replace any or all layers of the uterine wall. It is not uncommon for the cervix, vagina, and uterus to have lesions. In such cows, the vaginal lesions are multiple, small, often hemorrhagic, but nonulcerated nodules. An extensively involved uterus can support pregnancy even to an advanced stage.

in provoking and maintaining these neoplasms in the bitch. In other species, however, these neoplasms are rare, tend to be single, and have no unusual hormonal background. The neoplasms are well demarcated but not encapsulated, are usually spherical, and vary greatly in size. Depending on size, they can be confined within the wall of the vagina, cervix, or uterus or can protrude into the lumen or project to the serosal surface or into the pelvic canal. Some luminal neoplasms, especially those in the vagina, are pedunculated, making them liable to trauma or torsion. They are usually firm, pink or white, and occasionally calcified or edematous. The color is related to the amount of fibrous tissue present along with the whorled smooth muscle cells; in the grossly white neoplasms, fibrous tissue is the predominant component.

Carcinoma of the endometrium is rare in domestic animals as a clinical problem, but it is well known as a lesion of the bovine uterus found at the time of meat inspection. In the cow, the early carcinoma is found most often in the depths of the endometrial glands of the horns and less often in the body of the uterus. As it increases in size, the neoplasm thickens the uterine wall without any distortion of the overlying endometrium. A scirrhous response, the deposition of large amounts of fibrous tissue, is a characteristic lesion and makes the neoplasm firm and causes localized constriction bands on the external surface. The neoplasms can be small and annular or involve a large area

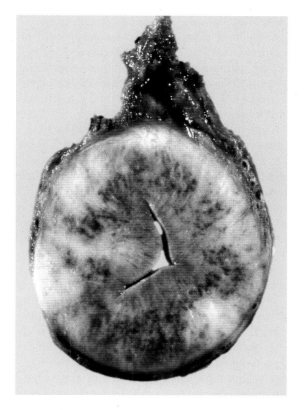

Fig. 18-27   Lymphoma (lymphosarcoma), uterus, cross section, cow. The mucosa, lamina propria, and myometrium are all heavily infiltrated by neoplastic lymphocytes. The dark-red to brown regions are areas of necrosis and hemorrhage. *(Courtesy Dr. R. A. Foster, Ontario Veterinary College, University of Guelph.)*

PLACENTA AND FETUS
FAILURE OF PREGNANCY

Maintenance of pregnancy is one of those miraculous events that often defy logic, and there is probably more that is not known than is known about pregnancy and embryonic and fetal development. The fetus is allogenic and therefore foreign to the mother. Yet it survives, even though both fetus and mother could mount an immune response to each other. Tolerance or suppression of the maternal immune system is required, but the mechanisms are incompletely understood, and there is little agreement about how this actually occurs. Theories, particularly in those species in which the fetal tissues invade the maternal system, involve the role of several potential processes, including an active role of systems like the Fas/Fas ligand system in which active immune cells undergo apoptosis when in contact with cells (trophoblasts) expressing the Fas ligand. Another system involving the suppression of material immunity in the uterus is indolamine 2,3 dioxygenase (IDO), which inhibits tryptophan, an amino acid necessary in the growth and development of T lymphocytes. Combined with the relative lack of MHC expression on trophoblasts, alteration of T helper lymphocyte balance and suppressor lymphocytes combine to partially explain the paradox that is pregnancy.

Immunologic considerations are only a part of the pregnancy equation. There are hormonal influences, especially maintenance of progesterone concentration. Stressors and systemic cytokines, such as prostaglandin, can cause luteolysis of the corpus luteum (where appropriate) and terminate pregnancy.

It is generally believed that fetuses initiate their own parturition. In conditions of fetal stress—such as maternal or fetal illness, hyperthermia, and hypoxia—they initiate the cascade of events that results in parturition. Initiation of birth by this process should result in a fresh (nonautolyzed) fetus, whereas rapid fetal death is believed to result in loss of pregnancy by other mechanisms, and the fetus, having spent additional time at body temperature, will be autolyzed.

The conceptus is the product of conception, and it is composed of the embryo, that part of the conceptus that gives rise to the adult, and the membranes. Embryos become fetuses at the time they develop features that allow their species and sex to be determined phenotypically. This occurs at about 35 to 45 days of age in large animals. Movement of the fetus occurs at this time. Loss of pregnancy is divided into stages based on the fetus's development and potential viability. Early embryonic mortality occurs at the embryonic stage, and abortion occurs during fetal development but when the fetus is not independently viable. Stillbirth occurs when the fetus is potentially viable. Fetal death later in development will lead to

Table 18-3   Failure of Pregnancy

GUIDE TO FETAL AUTOLYSIS*

Time Since Death	Change
12 hr	Cornea cloudy, amnionic fluid blood tinged
24 hr	Fluid in body cavities
36 hr	Gelatinous fluid in subcutis
72 hr	Eyes dehydrated
144 hr	Carcass dehydrated, no abomasal contents

COMMON CAUSES OF FETAL MUMMIFICATION

Horse	Twinning
Cattle	BVD virus infection, trichomoniasis
Dog	Canine herpesvirus
Cat	Torsion of a uterine horn
Sow	Parvoviral infection

ABORTOGENIC AGENTS COMMON TO ALL SPECIES

Brucella sp.
Campylobacter sp.
Chlamydophila abortus
Coxiella burnetii
Herpesviruses
Leptospira interrogans
Listeria monocytogenes
Mycoplasma and Ureaplasma
Neospora caninum
Salmonella sp.
Toxoplasma gondii

BVD, Bovine viral diarrhea.
*Data from Dillman RC, Dennis SM: Am J Vet Res 37: 403-407, 1976.

abortion, mummification, or maceration (Table 18-3). Mummified fetuses may be retained indefinitely if there is only one fetus. *Maceration* means to become soft and liquefy and requires bacterial infection of the fetus.

Embryonic and fetal death deprive the fetomaternal unit of whatever contribution the conceptus makes to the continuation of pregnancy. Parturition and (presumably) abortion in most animal species is initiated by the fetal adrenal gland. A signal, perhaps a stressful event, causes the fetal pituitary to secrete ACTH that in turn results in glucocorticoid production by the adrenal gland. Corticosteroids increase the synthesis of estrogens in the placenta, which in turn causes the synthesis and release of $PGF_{2\alpha}$ from the endometrium and myometrium. This causes luteolysis and a decreased progesterone production. In large animals, the loss of very small embryos does not influence the time of return to estrus. If embryonic loss occurs later, the interval to the next estrus will be somewhat increased because the corpus luteum will have been programmed for prolongation of its life. The importance of the fetal component and the necessity of the presence of a corpus luteum for the entire pregnancy vary with species. For instance, the corpus luteum of the sow is necessary throughout pregnancy because progesterone production by the placenta is small, but in the mare, the corpus luteum regresses halfway through pregnancy and placental progesterone maintains pregnancy. Regardless of the source of hormones responsible for maintaining pregnancy in large animals, embryonic or fetal death permits the release of $PGF_{2\alpha}$ and expulsion of the embryo or fetus. The exact outcome is unpredictable and is influenced, among other things, by species, stage of gestation, and number of fetuses. In the bitch and queen, the life span of the corpus luteum is not very different between pregnant and nonpregnant animals. When embryonic or fetal death occurs in domestic carnivores, the demise of the corpus luteum is definite and dead products of conception may be retained until approximately the normal time of parturition. Fetal autolysis is therefore common.

Mummification is one of the possible outcomes of fetal death. Rather than being expelled soon after death, the fetus is retained and progressively dehydrates to become a firm, dry mass, which is discolored by degraded hemoglobin to brown or black, and consists of leathery skin enclosing the harder parts of the fetus (Fig. 18-28). The cause of death can be infectious or noninfectious, but requisites for mummification are organisms that promote lysis of dead tissue be absent and that the cervix be closed to prevent the entry of putrefactive organisms. The situations in which mummification most commonly occurs are listed in Table 18-3. In twin pregnancy in the mare, the mummified fetus and the longer surviving fetus are aborted together before term. In parvovirus infection in the sow, mummified fetuses are retained and born at term

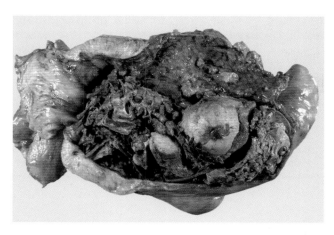

Fig. 18-29   Failure of pregnancy, macerated fetus, lamb. Fetal bones, hair, and brown pasty material fill the uterus. The ewe was infertile. *(Courtesy Dr. R. A. Foster, Ontario Veterinary College, University of Guelph.)*

along with live fetuses. In any species with a single fetus pregnancy, the mummified fetus can be expelled at any time or retained indefinitely.

Maceration of a dead fetus requires the presence of bacterial organisms in the uterus. These bacteria could be the ones that caused the fetal death in the first place or could be putrefactive organisms that entered the uterus via the cervix after the death of the fetus. In addition to disintegration of the fetus (Fig. 18-29), the uterus has lesions also. Endometritis or pyometra is present; the type of lesion depends on whether the cervix is open or closed. Endometritis and pyometra tend to become severe and chronic, with voluminous pus in the case of pyometra. Emphysema occurs with the invasion of the fetus by clostridial organisms. Maternal toxemia and death are likely. Fetal bones resist maceration, and if the uterus eventually regains some muscular tone, the bones can cause perforation.

The general diagnostic rate for determination of the cause of failure of pregnancy is low and with few exceptions is less than 40%, although success is usually much greater in outbreaks (Table 18-4). Many of the recognized causes are infectious because infections are usually easy to diagnose (Table 18-3). This has led to the general approach of determining if the loss of pregnancy is infectious or not.

Examination of fetus and membranes

Early embryonic mortality or death of the embryo or loss of pregnancy at this early stage of gestation is thought to result in dissolution, but it is also valid that the conceptus is so small that it is not found. The absence of material for diagnostic purposes often hampers the identification of the cause. There are recognized infectious causes of infertility, and the infection

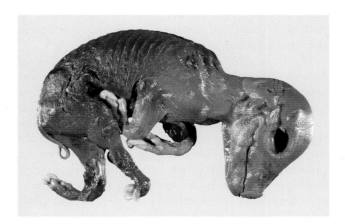

Fig. 18-28   Failure of pregnancy, mummified fetus, pig. This fetus died in utero, and the fluids were resorbed. Dehydration of a fetus in utero usually takes longer than 1 week to occur. *(Courtesy Ontario Veterinary College, University of Guelph.)*

Table **18-4**   Occurrence of Causes of Sporadic Failure of Pregnancy in Various Domesticated Species

Cause	Equine (%)	Bovine	Ovine	Caprine	Porcine
No diagnosis	40	60	60	52	53
Noninfectious	26*	3	5	10	1
Infectious	34	36	35	38	46
Placentitis	12	5	9	3	7
Viral	9	3	0	0	20
Bacterial	10	16	25	31	32
Protozoal	0	16	10	7	0

*See Box 18-5.

Table **18-5**   Specific or Regionally Important Diseases That Cause Failure of Pregnancy

Species	Cause
Equine	Insufficient serum progesterone
	Equine herpesvirus 1
	Fescue toxicosis (*Neotyphodium coenophialum*)
	Thyroid hyperplasia/musculoskeletal syndrome
Bovine	*Brucella abortus*
	Foothills abortion
	Ponderosa pine abortion
	Campylobacter fetus
	Tritrichomonas foetus
Ovine	*Listeria monocytogenes*
	Brucella ovis
	Wesselsbron
	Rift Valley fever
	Cache Valley virus
	Salmonella sp.
	Iodine deficiency
Caprine	*Brucella melitensis*
	Iodine deficiency
Porcine	Leptospirosis

These are not the most common in all areas. Common causes are listed in Table 18-4.

often occurs at or near the time of coitus or conception. Agents such as *Campylobacter*, *Tritrichomonas*, and *Ureaplasma* and nonspecific endometrial infections are among the common examples.

It appears that chromosomal abnormalities account for the majority of noninfectious causes. Regardless of which species is involved, investigation of abortion or stillbirth requires a keen sense of what can be achieved. Depending on the situation, the investigation may have an economic impact, a zoonotic impact, or it may appeal to your scientific curiosity. Maternal, fetal, and placental factors should be considered. There are causes that are common across all species that are listed in Table 18-3 and causes that are species specific or are regionally important causes of abortion that are listed in Table 18-5.

Examination of the fetus and membranes, and sampling of tissue primarily answers the question: Are there any fetal or placental abnormalities to explain the abortion or stillbirth? Some of the lack of success in determining the cause is the failure to submit the appropriate specimens. Where feasible, send the whole fetus and membranes to the laboratory. When this is not feasible, success in ruling out fetal factors depends on submission of the correct specimens, and this in part depends on knowing what specimens to send. Each diagnostic laboratory has a recommended list of samples that are suggested to maximize diagnostic success in their particular locale.

Each species and breed of animal has an expected rate of development and an average size at birth. Variance of this normal development indicates an abnormality that needs to be explained. Fetal and placenta weight, fetal size, including crown-rump length, and degree of development for gestation length are basic parameters that may indicate increased or inadequate maternal nutrition, concurrent disease, or placental sufficiency.

The degree of fetal autolysis and evidence of fetal distress will provide an indication of the fetal state just before the loss. When distressed and hypoxic, a fetus will gasp and aspirate amniotic contents, and meconium will be released into the amniotic fluid. Meconium staining of the skin can be seen grossly (Fig. 18-30). Keratin squames and meconium from the amniotic fluid will be found in the lungs when histologic assessment is done. A fetus that is caught in the birth canal for a sufficient period of time will develop localized swellings, such as a swollen tongue and face (Fig. 18-30). Fetal autolysis was studied in sheep and gives an approximation of the time of fetal death before expulsion. It is generally believed that an autolyzed fetus dies too quickly for it to initiate its own

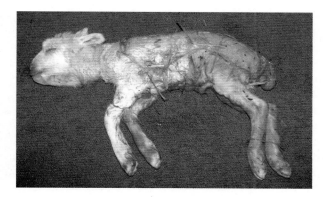

Fig. 18-30   Dystocia, lamb. This large lamb died during parturition. It was trapped in the birth canal by the shoulders and right foreleg, which has flexed (folded back). The lamb became hypoxic and defecated meconium, visible as a yellow deposit on the skin of the body caudal to the shoulder. The head and left foreleg became swollen and the skin dry. The skin of the rest of the body is moist from amniotic fluid (and meconium), indicating that this portion of the body was in the vagina and uterus. *(Courtesy Dr. R. A. Foster, Ontario Veterinary College, University of Guelph.)*

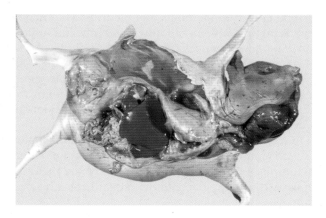

Fig. 18-31   Iodine deficiency, goiter, goat fetus. This fetus has bilaterally extremely enlarged thyroid glands, alopecia, and myxedema evident subcutaneously over the thorax and abdomen, the classic lesions of severe hypothyroidism. *(Courtesy Dr. R. A. Foster, Ontario Veterinary College, University of Guelph.)*

parturition, as would occur with fetal sepsis or viremia. A fresh fetus initiates its own parturition.

Fetal mummification occurs periodically in animals and has a common cause for each species, which is listed in Table 18-3.

The fetus is similar to an adult in the general response to diseases (Fig. 18-31), particularly near parturition, but many of the responses will be rudimentary, depending on the stage of gestation. To our knowledge, the fetus is in a sterile environment, and has no flora or fauna. Exposure to environmental or pathogenic agents

occurs from contact with the external environment or with maternal infection. Many of the pathogens have an affinity for the reproductive tract and may infect and/or initiate failure of pregnancy in many species. Agents common to all species are listed in Table 18-3. Some of them are discussed next.

Species-specific failure of pregnancy

Each species has its known causes and profile of lesions and conditions that result in the failure of the pregnancy. Table 18-4 lists the likely diagnostic success and the types of diseases and conditions to expect. Some of the conditions are specifically discussed in the following sections. Horses are unique in having a large number of noninfectious causes of abortion (Box 18-5), related in many instances to the apparent lack of placental reserve and microcotyledonary placentation. Examination of the placenta for lesions requires knowledge of normal anatomy, and there are many features and structures that are normal but have the appearance of being a lesion (Box 18-6). It is important to assess the equine

---

Box 18-5

Noninfectious Causes of Failure of Equine Pregnancy

Twinning
Umbilical cord anomalies
- Excessive length
- Torsion
- Too short

Inadequate villous development
- Endometrial fibrosis

Thyroid hyperplasia and musculoskeletal disease
Premature placental separation
Body pregnancy

Box 18-6

Normal Structures of the Equine Placenta Confused with Lesions

Amniotic plaques
Avillous regions of:
- Chorioallantoic pouches
- Large vessels
- Insertion of cord
- Location of uterine tube
- Cervical star

Hippomane
Allantoic pouches
Yolk sac remnant

Box 18-7

Lesions of Chronic Placentitis in Ruminants

Placental edema
Intercotyledonary opacity
Intercotyledonary fibrosis
Cupping of cotyledon
Cotyledonary necrosis
Exudates

placenta for anything that reduces placental area, such as avillous areas, involvement of the cervical star (Fig. 18-35), examination of the umbilical cord for excessive length (normal is 36 to 84 cm) and torsion (Fig. 18-40), and lesions of the amnion.

The placentation of ruminants is cotyledonary, and as such there is a large potential space between the placentomes for exudates and agents to accumulate. As such, chronic placentitis centered on the pericotyledonary area and the intercotyledonary portion of the chorion is more common (Box 18-7). Porcine, feline, and canine placentas rarely have lesions.

INFECTIOUS DISEASES

The most common diseases of the fetus and placenta across the species are infectious, except perhaps in the mare. Bacterial, viral, and protozoal agents and combinations all occur. With each agent, however, the significance of the infection should be determined by association with lesions or the known pathogenetic mechanisms.

Bacterial diseases

Bacterial species causing inflammation of the placenta and fetus are numerous. Almost any organism that causes septicemia can infect the pregnant uterus, but the following discussion concerns those organisms that target the placenta or fetus, or both. The route of invasion of the uterus and fetus for many animal species and many bacteria (such as salmonellae and brucellae) is hematogenous, after the organisms have entered the dam either through the digestive or genital tract. For some diseases, the method of spread is venereal (*Campylobacter* sp., *Ureaplasma* sp.). In the mare, most placental pathogens enter the pregnant uterus through the cervix.

Brucellosis is now a rare or sporadic disease of all species, but there are many similarities in the lesions and pathogenesis among the domesticated species. *Brucella abortus* infection in cattle is now eradicated from many states and provinces. It is, however, a much studied and classic cause of abortion. The placental

lesions are stereotypical and are shared by other agents. *Brucella abortus* is ingested with feed contaminated by an infected aborted fetus or placenta. The initial lesion is a persistent nasopharyngeal lymphadenitis. Bacteria are released into the blood in waves, causing bacteremia and bacteria to colonize the spleen, lymph nodes, mammary glands, testes, male accessory genital glands, and joint capsules, bursae, and tendon sheaths. *Brucella* organisms are removed from most organs, but a small nidus of infection usually persists in some organ. The pregnant uterus is particularly susceptible to infection, and the uterine disease process becomes chronic, eventually resolving after abortion or parturition.

Gross lesions in the placenta are edema of the intercotyledonary chorioallantois that is opaque with a leathery texture, light brown exudate on the chorionic surface, and various extents of necrosis of the cotyledons. A placenta with such lesions is grossly indistinguishable from the placenta of cases of mycotic abortion (Fig. 18-32) or the rare case of campylobacteriosis with a late-term abortion. The fetal lesions are nonspecific and consist of edema and fluid accumulation in body cavities; often more specific lesions include bronchopneumonia and pleuritis. Microscopic lesions include inflammation with edema and infiltration of mononuclear cells and a few neutrophils of both the intercotyledonary chorion and the chorionic villi. A striking feature is the presence of numerous gram-negative coccobacilli within trophoblasts, many of which are desquamated and form the considerable debris between maternal and fetal tissues.

In ruminants, *Brucella abortus* moves from the maternal circulation into the hemophagic organ where erythrophagocytosis occurs at the tips of the maternal septa within the placentome. Organisms are then

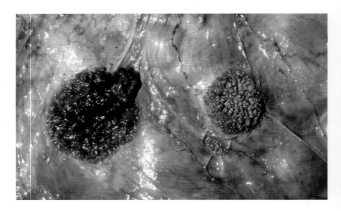

Fig. 18-32   Mycotic intercotyledonary placentitis, cow. Marked edema, fibrosis, and thickening of the intercotyledonary placenta has caused it to be opaque. The cotyledon on the right is necrotic. *(Courtesy Dr. R. A. Foster, Ontario Veterinary College, University of Guelph.)*

phagocytosed by the erythrophagocytic trophoblasts at the nearby base of the chorionic villi. Replication occurs in adjacent periplacentomal chorioallantoic trophoblasts. Replication is followed by trophoblast necrosis and chorioallantoic ulceration. Organisms enter the uterine lumen and chorionic villi to finally disseminate hematogenously to fetal viscera. *Brucella abortus* appears to be taken up by endocytosis through erythrophagocytic trophoblasts and replicates in the rough endoplasmic reticulum of the periplacentomal and interplacentomal trophoblasts, a unique mechanism of intracellular parasitism. Vasculitis occurs in both maternal and fetal tissues and the lesion could be a response to endotoxin released from the *Brucella* organisms. Most fetuses have pneumonia that ranges from minimal to severe. Microscopically the pneumonia is either a chronic bronchopneumonia with an exudate of numerous mononuclear cells and some neutrophils or a fibrinous pneumonia. Microscopic granulomas that include multinucleate giant cells occur in various organs, such as the lung, liver, spleen, and lymph nodes.

Brucella canis is acquired by the dog either through ingestion or venereally. Both sexes have lymphadenitis, especially of the nodes of the head and neck, and bacteremia. Epididymitis and testicular degeneration are the lesions in male dogs, and females have placentitis and fetal endocarditis, pneumonia, and hepatitis. Microscopically, trophoblasts are packed with *Brucella* organisms. Other fetal lesions include renal hemorrhage, subacute inflammation of the pelvic connective tissue, and lymphadenitis.

Brucella ovis in sheep is probably transmitted venereally from a ram with epididymitis shedding large numbers of organisms in the semen. Gross placental lesions are essentially similar to those produced by *Brucella abortus* in cattle. Fetal lesions at necropsy are nonspecific (e.g., edema and fluid accumulation in the body cavities). Calcified plaques on the hooves have been noted but are not specific for this agent. Microscopically, as with *Brucella* sp. infections in other species, large numbers of coccobacilli are found in trophoblasts and are free in the chorionic mesenchyme. Vasculitis involves the larger chorionic vessels. Lesions in the fetus are pneumonia, lymphadenitis, interstitial nephritis, and pericholangitis. In younger fetuses, infiltrates of monocytes and macrophages are present, whereas older fetuses have well-formed nodules of lymphocytes and plasma cells. *Brucella melitensis* infection in sheep and goats occurs mainly in Mediterranean countries. The infection has a septicemic phase, but inflammation is localized to the mammary gland and pregnant uterus. Goats have more severe febrile disease and more severe mastitis than do sheep.

Brucella suis causes a disease in pigs that differs in several respects from brucellosis in ruminants. The lesions are more widespread and have a predilection for bones and joints. Necrosis with caseation occurs in many lesions. Pregnancy is not a prerequisite for endometritis in porcine brucellosis. Miliary granulomas in the endometrium are mixed with multiple hyperplastic lymphoid nodules. Endometrial glands become distended with mucus and leukocytes, and the surface epithelium is partly desquamated and focally has squamous metaplasia. Between placentas of the pregnant uterus, the lumen has a mucopurulent exudate in which intracellular and free organisms are plentiful. The chorioallantoic membranes have nonspecific lesions of edema and congestion.

Campylobacteriosis is a sporadic disease in most species, but is particularly seen in ruminants. *Campylobacter fetus* var. *venerealis* can be a long-term inhabitant of the preputial cavity of bulls. It is transmitted venereally and can survive for some time on the vaginal mucosa, but the cow must become pregnant for it to establish itself in the uterus. Early embryonic death is the most likely manifestation of campylobacteriosis and often the only clinical abnormalities are irregular estrus cycles or the return to estrus of an animal thought to be pregnant. Much less frequently abortion occurs at a later stage of pregnancy. Cows become resistant to subsequent infections by the bacterium. Gross and microscopic lesions in placentas are similar to those described in brucellosis (edema of the intercotyledonary chorioallantois and necrosis of cotyledons with microscopic inflammation of both) but are less severe and with fewer organisms in the desquamated trophoblasts. Fetal lesions are nonspecific.

Campylobacter fetus ssp. *fetus* and *Campylobacter jejuni* are primarily intestinal inhabitants and cause similar lesions in sheep. The organisms are transmitted by ingestion, and abortions occur in outbreaks. Infection of the pregnant uterus results in late-term abortion or the birth of live, but sick lambs. Immunity is gained after the first infection. The placentitis is characterized by an edematous intercotyledonary chorioallantois and friable, yellow cotyledons. Grossly, about 25% of the fetuses have multiple yellow areas of hepatic necrosis from 10 to 20 mm in diameter with red, depressed centers. Microscopically the chorioallantois is infiltrated by a mixture of cells, mostly neutrophils, but many cells are necrotic and cannot be identified. Inflammation is especially severe in the chorionic villi. *Campylobacter* organisms are abundant among the inflammatory cells. A diagnostically useful lesion in campylobacterial infection is the presence of large, dense emboli of bacteria in the capillaries of the chorionic villi. The fetal lesions are those of a severe multifocal necrotizing hepatitis with abundant organisms. *Flexispira rappini* causes similar lesions in the ovine placenta and fetus, but infections are sporadic.

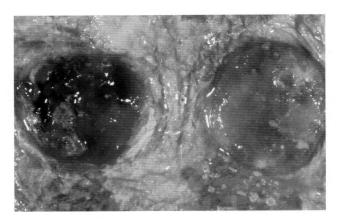

Fig. 18-33   Intercotyledonary placentitis (Coxiella burnetii), goat. Note the opacity of the intercotyledonary placenta caused by thickening from inflammation and fibrosis. The cotyledons have variable areas of gray discoloration, indicating necrosis and inflammatory exudates. The gross appearance of the lesions of placentitis tends to be similar, regardless of the etiologic agent identified by microbiological examination. *(Courtesy Dr. R.A. Foster, Ontario Veterinary College, University of Guelph.)*

Coxiella burnettii, the cause of Q fever in human beings, is responsible for abortion or the birth of dead or weak lambs or kids. Abortion occurs in newly exposed animals and repeat infection with abortion is possible. Infection of goats is more common. Transmission of the organism is either by ingestion or by inhalation. The organism is shed in vaginal discharges at parturition and in the milk. This organism is readily transmitted to human beings by the same ways. In affected goats, the intercotyledonary chorioallantois is thick, leathery, yellow, and covered with surface exudate (Fig. 18-33). Gross fetal lesions are nonspecific. Microscopically the placental lesions of acute inflammatory infiltration are most severe in the intercotyledonary areas. Hypertrophic trophoblasts are filled with *Coxiella* organisms. Fetal lesions, if present, consist of peribronchiolar, renal medullary, and hepatic portal lymphoid accumulations.

Enzootic abortion of ewes is caused by *Chlamydophila abortus* and is one of the most common abortifacient agents in sheep. It occurs in outbreaks when newly introduced into flocks, or as an enzootic condition of ewe lambs. It occurs in all sheep-producing countries, producing late-term abortion in ewes. Transmission is generally oral and ewes seem to be immune to reinfection after the first abortion, but they may remain as carriers. Ewes infected before 5 or 6 weeks of gestation abort in late gestation, but ewes infected after 5 or 6 weeks of gestation abort the subsequent pregnancy. The placenta in affected ewes grossly is similar to the placenta in *Coxiella* infection and in ovine brucellosis. Microscopically the chorioallantois is infiltrated by neutrophils. Cotyledons have more severe inflammation than the intercotyledonary areas. The organisms distend the trophoblasts but are difficult to visualize without special stains, such as modified Ziehl-Neelsen or Gimenez stains. In the fetus, subacute inflammatory foci may be present in several organs, especially the liver, lungs, and muscle.

Epizootic bovine abortion, also known as foothills abortion, occurs in California and adjacent states. The causative agent is unknown, with *Chlamydophila*, *Borrelia*, a spirochete, and viruses having been suggested and excluded. Abortion or the birth of weak calves occurs only in cows newly introduced into the territory of the tick *Ornithodorus coriaceus*. The fetal disease is chronic with notable microscopic lesions 50 days after tick exposure of the dam. The lesions are of sufficient specificity for a diagnosis in fetuses whose gestational age is greater than 100 days. Gross lesions include petechial hemorrhages of the conjunctiva and oral cavity, an enlarged nodular liver and ascites (presumably from heart failure secondary to myocarditis), and enlarged lymph nodes and spleen. Lymphoid follicles are hyperplastic and have large numbers of histiocytes. The thymus is atrophic because of the loss of cortical lymphocytes. The thymic parenchyma and interstitium are infiltrated by histiocytes. Foci of acute necrosis are present in several organs, especially the lymph nodes and spleen. These foci frequently develop into pyogranulomas. Vasculitis, acute or subacute, occurs in several organs. Deposits of IgG and IgM are present in the vascular lesions.

Leptospirosis is another possible cause of abortion. Results of serologic studies indicate that a large percentage of cattle and pigs are infected, but most animals do not have clinical signs. Several different serovars are associated with abortion, especially *Leptospira interrogans* serovar *hardjo* in cattle and serovar *pomona* in pigs. In adult animals, the organisms localize in the kidneys after the septicemic phase. Pregnant sows or cows abort weeks after the septicemic phase, usually in the last trimester. Placental lesions are usually limited to edema. Fetal lesions often are mild and obscured by autolysis. Some dead fetuses expelled near term without extensive autolysis have gross lesions of ascites and fibrinous peritonitis. Microscopic lesions include subacute interstitial nephritis and subacute necrotizing hepatitis. With or without morphologic changes in the fetal kidneys, leptospiral organisms may be demonstrated in peritoneal or pleural cavity fluid by dark field microscopy and in renal tubular lumens by silver stains or by immunohistochemical techniques. Measurement of the leptospiral antibody in fetal fluids (serum, cavity fluids) is a major method for diagnosis.

Listeriosis caused by *Listeria monocytogenes* is a cause of sporadic abortions in cattle, sheep, and goats and of outbreaks of abortion in sheep. Although both nervous disease and reproductive disease occur in the same flock or herd, this is rare. Listerial abortions occur in the last trimester of pregnancy. Some aborting dams are septicemic and have endometritis. The placental lesions include severe diffuse necrotizing and suppurative inflammation of both the cotyledons and the intercotyledonary areas. Fetal lesions are an enlarged liver with numerous 1-mm yellow foci. These yellow foci are areas of acute multifocal necrotizing hepatitis in which the necrotic cells are also filled with gram-positive *Listeria* organisms. Other fetal organs have similar microscopic lesions. Microscopically, severe inflammation involves the mesenchyme of the villi and the upper intercotyledonary chorion, with some of the cells degenerated beyond recognition. Trophoblasts, especially in the areas between the villi, are filled with gram-positive listerial bacilli.

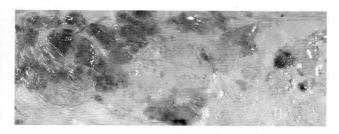

Fig. 18-34   **Amnionitis,** *Ureaplasma diversum* **infection, cow.** The amnion has large, opaque, red and white areas of granulation tissue and fibrous tissue, respectively. Amnionitis without placentitis in cattle is a good indicator of *Ureaplasma* sp. infection. *(Courtesy Dr. R.B. Miller, Ontario Veterinary College, University of Guelph.)*

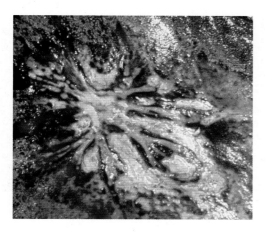

Fig. 18-35   **Bacterial placentitis, cervical star, mare.** The chorion at the cervical star is thickened by edema, and there is fibrin, necrotic debris, and suppurative exudate on the surface. *(Courtesy Dr. K. McEntee, Reproductive Pathology Collection, University of Illinois.)*

Organisms that cause bacteremia in adult animals are capable of causing lesions in the placenta and fetus. Thus in cattle, bacteria such as *Salmonella, Mannheimia,* and *Pasteurella* spp. and *Histophilus somni* are potential causes of placentitis, fetal inflammatory lesions, and abortion. In pigs, various *Streptococcus* spp. can cause similar lesions. *Ureaplasma diversum* can cause abortion in cattle. The placental lesions include focal or diffuse reddening of the amnion and chorioallantois, accompanied by thickening and yellow discoloration of the amnion (Fig. 18-34). Fibrosis, edema, inflammation, and necrosis of the amnion occur together with focal inflammation and necrosis of the cotyledons and the intercotyledonary chorioallantois.

Because ascending infection is the most common route of infection of the placenta in the mare (Fig. 18-35), various bacterial organisms are involved. Hemolytic streptococci (especially *Streptococcus zooepidemicus*) are the most frequently recovered from fetal organs, placentas, and uterine discharges. Other commonly encountered organisms are *Escherichia coli* and *Pseudomonas, Klebsiella,* and *Staphylococcus* spp. Although some infections are hematogenous, the ascending route of infection, through the cervix, is the rule. Inflammation of the chorioallantois is most severe opposite the cervix, and the area involved usually extends further ventrally than dorsally because of gravitational spread. Affected parts of the placenta are edematous and brown and covered by small amounts of fibrinonecrotic exudate. Gross fetal lesions are enlarged liver and increased abdominal and thoracic fluid. Microscopically the lesions are severe subacute inflammation of the stroma of the chorionic microcotyledons and desquamation of chorionic epithelium. Microscopic fetal lesions are rare, despite the ease with which bacteria can be recovered from many fetal organs. The prelude to abortion is either fetal death from septicemia or placental insufficiency.

Fungal diseases

Aspergillus and the zygomycetes (*Absidia, Mortierella, Rhizopus, Mucor*) cause sporadic abortions in cows and mares. In cows, the organisms spread to the placenta hematogenously, as indicated by the fact that the placentomes are involved first and there is random involvement of the placentomes. In the mare, as with bacterial placentitis, the fungi enter through the cervix because the lesions in the chorioallantois are most severe in or even confined to the cervical area. In the affected bovine placenta, the cotyledons become enlarged, brown, and friable and the intercotyledonary chorioallantois becomes leathery and covered with a brown exudate (Fig. 18-32 and Fig. 18-36, *A* and *B*). Thus the gross appearance of the placenta is similar to the classic descriptions of the placenta in bovine brucellosis.

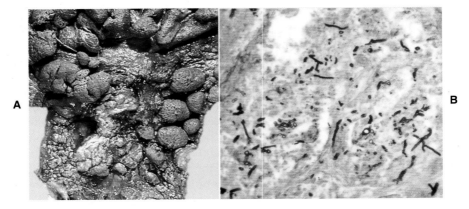

Fig. 18-36   **Mycotic endometritis, postpartum uterus, cow. A,** The endometrial surface of the middle and lower portion of this uterus is irregularly thickened and corrugated. Caruncles are small or missing. **B,** The placenta is necrotic, and the numerous fungal hyphae (*black*) are irregular in diameter, do not have regular septation, and branch at odd angles, all features typical of *Mucor* spp. Gomori's methenamine silver stain. (**A,** *Courtesy Dr. J. King, College of Veterinary Medicine, Cornell University.* **B,** *Courtesy Dr. K. McEntee, Reproductive Pathology Collection, University of Illinois.*)

Affected areas of the equine chorioallantois are brown, initially thickened, and later shrunken and friable. In both bovine and equine species, the amnion has thick, white or yellow, leathery areas. Small, white, raised plaques are present on the skin of the bovine fetus and sometimes on the equine fetus. Microscopically the lesions include inflammatory cell infiltration of amniotic and chorioallantoic mesenchyme and desquamation of trophoblasts. In the bovine species, the lesions of vasculitis and fungal vascular invasion involve the larger vessels at the base of the cotyledons. Lesions in the fetus are confined to the skin and include subacute dermatitis and hyperkeratosis. Fungal hyphae, septate in the case of *Aspergillus* and nonseptate in the case of the mucorales and hyphomycetes, are abundant in the lesions of the placenta and the skin of the fetus. Fungi can be recovered from the fetal stomach, presumably from swallowed amniotic fluid.

Viral diseases

Herpesviruses are well established as causes of outbreaks of abortion in cows, mares, and sows and are described in goats and dogs. Generally, the gross lesions in affected fetuses are multiple randomly distributed pale gray to white foci in affected organs characteristic of acute necrosis (Fig. 18-37, *A*). Lymphoid necrosis occurs in the spleen, thymus, and lymph nodes, whereas multiple small foci of necrosis, mild acute inflammation, and intranuclear inclusion bodies occur in parenchymal cells in a wide range of organs, especially the liver, lungs, and adrenal glands. Often the fetal liver is enlarged, and the necrotic foci are large enough to be visible as 1- to 2-mm white areas (Fig. 18-37, *B*). Pulmonary lesions usually include hyperplasia, focal necrosis, and desquamation of bronchiolar epithelium.

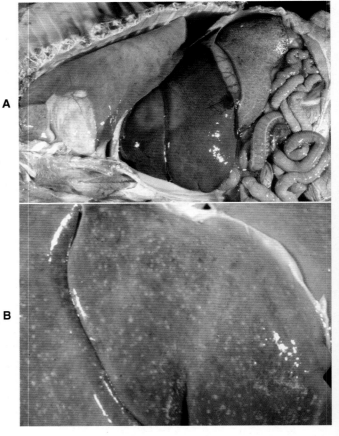

Fig. 18-37   **Equine herpesvirus 1 infection, aborted equine fetus. A,** The changes typical of herpesviral abortion include solid rubbery lungs, multiple foci of necrosis in the liver, and splenomegaly. **B,** Randomly distributed multiple 1-mm white foci in the liver are characteristic of necrosis caused by herpesviral infection. This case is more florid than most. (**A,** *Courtesy Dr. R.B. Miller, Ontario Veterinary College, University of Guelph.* **B,** *Courtesy Dr. J. King, College of Veterinary Medicine, Cornell University.*)

Fibrinous bronchiolitis, grossly visible, is present in some fetuses, especially equine. The placenta can be edematous, but only in the sow are inflammation and inclusion bodies readily observed in the chorion.

Equine herpesvirus 1 (EHV-1) could be the most economically significant abortigenic animal herpesvirus. Viral infection of maternal uterine endothelial cells has a major role in the pathogenesis of abortion. Damage to these endothelial cells results in thromboses accompanied by perivascular infiltration of lymphocytes, neutrophils, and monocytes and perivascular edema and subsequent infarction of the endometrium. The fluid that escapes through the damaged endometrium causes separation of the maternal and fetal layers of the placenta, and this separation could allow virus from maternal leukocytes and lysed endothelial cells to enter the fetus. Fetal endothelial cells and the cells of a wide range of organs are targets for the virus. The classic lesions are focal hepatic necrosis, pneumonia with fibrin casts in the trachea, and prominent lymphoid follicles in the spleen.

BHV-1 is a sporadic cause of bovine abortion. In addition, infectious bovine rhinotracheitis virus produces an acute necrotizing endometritis in the uterine body or caudal parts of the uterine horns of the cow, particularly in the postpartum period. Microscopically the lesions range from mild focal lymphocytic endometritis to severe diffuse necrotizing metritis.

Pestiviruses in cattle (bovine viral diarrhea [BVD] virus), sheep (border disease virus), and pigs (classical swine fever virus) can cause fetal death or malformation, depending on viral strain, fetal age, and stage of development of the fetal immune system. Placental and fetal lesions are either absent or are restricted to microscopic lymphocytic infiltrates in the heart and brain. Fetal malformations caused by these are discussed elsewhere.

Porcine parvovirus is an important cause of embryonic and fetal loss and causes death and mummification of a proportion of affected litters (SMEDI) (Fig. 18-38). Pig fetuses infected before immunocompetence have widespread necrotizing lesions, together with inflammation and inclusion bodies, especially in the liver, lungs, kidneys, and cerebellum. Damage to the fetal circulatory system results in edema, hemorrhage, and the accumulation of serosanguinous fluid in body cavities.

Arteriviruses are important in causing failure of pregnancy in animals. Transplacental infection of pig fetuses with porcine reproductive and respiratory syndrome (PRRS) virus causes segmental or diffuse hemorrhage in the umbilical cords as a result of necrotizing arteritis. Few stillborn fetuses have specific microscopic lesions; lesions are more common in live littermates. Gross lesions include ascites, hydrothorax, and edema of perirenal tissue, splenic ligament, and mesentery. Microscopically, mild to moderate segmental arteritis occurs in the lungs, heart, and kidneys. Alveolar septa in the lungs are thickened by mononuclear cell accumulation and proliferation of type 2 pneumocytes. Aggregates of lymphocytes, plasma cells, and macrophages are present in blood vessels in the heart, portal tracts, and cerebellar white matter. Various degrees of endometritis and myometritis also occur with lymphohistiocytic perivascular cuffs and edema.

Equine viral arteritis virus (an arterivirus) in the mare causes abortion, but in the majority of cases no lesions are in the fetus. In this species, the mechanism is probably fetal anoxia due to compression of uterine blood vessels by virus-induced myometritis, although a few cases of arteritis in the chorion and myocardium of aborted fetuses have been described.

Bunyaviruses, such as Akabane virus and Cache Valley virus, cause fetal infection and abortion in sheep and other ruminants. The virus produces a range of lesions in the developing fetal central nervous system, including hydranencephaly, microencephaly, cerebellar hypoplasia, and loss of spinal cord ventral horn neurons. The loss of ventral horn neurons causes denervation muscle atrophy. The atrophy and myositis are responsible for arthrogryposis (fixation of limb joints) and skeletal deformities, such as torticollis and scoliosis.

Bluetongue virus (Orbivirus) is an important viral infection of the ovine fetus in those areas where the bluetongue occurs. Fetal lambs with this infection develop hydranencephaly as a result of infection with bluetongue virus. They have viral antigen in immature neural cells in areas of necrosis in the periventricular

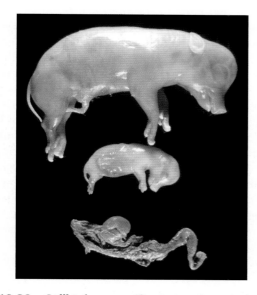

Fig. 18-38   Stillbirth, mummification, embryonic death and infertility (SMEDI), abortion, pig fetus. Viruses such as porcine parvovirus and porcine enteroviruses induce SMEDI. These viruses affect the fetuses to differing degrees and at different stages of gestation. Those fetuses that die early in gestation are usually mummified (*bottom fetus*) or resorbed. *(Courtesy College of Veterinary Medicine, University of Illinois.)*

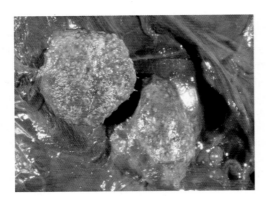

Fig. 18-39   Ovine protozoal placentitis, toxoplasmosis, abortion, placenta, sheep. The cotyledons have hundreds of white foci of necrosis, a lesion that is characteristic of *Toxoplasma gondii*-induced abortion in sheep and goats. (*Courtesy Ontario Veterinary College, University of Guelph.*)

zone of the cerebral hemispheres. Bluetongue is discussed elsewhere.

Protozoal diseases

Toxoplasma gondii is an important cause of abortion in ewes. The organism has a cat-sheep life cycle, with contamination of sheep feed by cat feces. Gross lesions in the fetal membranes include edema of the intercotyledonary chorioallantois and white 1- to 2-mm foci in the cotyledons (Fig. 18-39). A small percentage of fetuses with toxoplasmosis have leukoencephalomalacia that is likely a nonspecific effect of fetal anoxia secondary to placentitis. Microscopically the cotyledonary lesions are distinctive and consist of multiple foci of necrosis with rare groups of toxoplasma organisms within trophoblasts. Immunohistochemistry is particularly useful to detect organisms.

Neospora caninum is now recognized as a major cause of abortion in cows. Fetuses are 3 to 9 months' gestational age and have no gross lesions. In the fetal brain, multiple foci of necrosis or proliferated microglial cells are often adjacent to capillaries with hyperplastic endothelium. Groups of *Neospora caninum* in or around these foci are either extracellular or occur in neural cells or endothelial cells. In the heart, the lesions include subacute multifocal epicarditis, myocarditis, endocarditis, and protozoal organisms either in myofibers or endothelial cells. Mononuclear portal hepatitis, multifocal hepatocellular necrosis, and fibrin thrombi in sinusoids are also seen. Foci of mononuclear inflammatory cells are present in additional organs, including the placenta.

Tritrichomonas foetus in cattle is another protozoal organism that can cause abortion, although it usually causes early embryonic mortality. Mild placentitis, with no fetal lesion, is present. The standard method of diagnosis is the demonstration of protozoa in the contents

of the fetal abomasum. Endometritis can be severe, and pyometra is a possible sequela. Infiltration of the endometrium with mononuclear cells is moderate to severe. Lymphoid nodules and secondary follicles develop; these are likely sites of local production of IgA.

NONINFECTIOUS DISEASES AND CONDITIONS

Twinning is a common noninfectious cause of abortion in mares. Normally, chorionic villi develop where contact is made between the endometrium and the chorion. In other areas, such as the contact area between chorion and endocervix and the contact area between the placentas of twins, chorionic villi do not develop and the chorionic surface is smooth. Thus the combined functional area of the chorions of both twins is only slightly larger than that for a normal nontwin foal. Twin fetuses often have growth retardation. Aborted twin equine fetuses often appear to have died at different times. Death is thought to be because of placental insufficiency. When the available space in the uterus is divided evenly, which is approximately 80% of cases, both twins usually die and are aborted in midgestation. In cases in which great disparity exists in the apportioning of space, the favored twin has a chance of survival, whereas the other dies and mummifies.

In the mare, endometrial fibrosis, often the result of a previous endometritis, reduces the area of the endometrium available for formation of a diffuse placenta (Figs. 18-16 and 18-35). Chorionic villi do not develop where there is no endometrium with glands for the formation of interdigitations between fetal and maternal parts of the placenta. In large areas of endometrial fibrosis, the chorion does not develop microcotyledons and their villi. Clearly demarcated and smooth areas of chorionic surface mirror the affected areas of the endometrium. Severely affected mares become pregnant but do not carry the fetus to term because the functional area of the placenta is too small.

Premature placental separation in the mare has been described in two forms. One form occurs around the time of parturition, causing the chorioallantois to appear at the vulva with the cervical star intact. Although the caudal part of the chorioallantois is detached from the uterus, the cranial part remains in place, and there is tearing of the chorioallantois across its body. The other form occurs some time before parturition. Prematurely detached areas become brown and dehydrated.

Another equine disease, albeit a rare one, in which fetal death and abortion occur as a result of placental insufficiency and fetal malnutrition is uterine body pregnancy. The fetus occupies the uterine body rather than the body and horns, and the placenta is underdeveloped in the horns.

There are several abnormalities of the equine umbilical cord, including excessive length (or inadequate

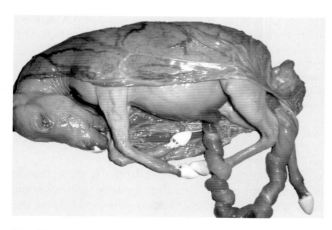

Fig. 18-40 Umbilical cord torsion, equine fetus. This aborted fetus, wrapped in its amnion, has a very long and twisted umbilical cord. Twisted cords are often longer than 83 cm, a risk factor for torsion of the cord. *(Courtesy College of Veterinary Medicine, University of Illinois.)*

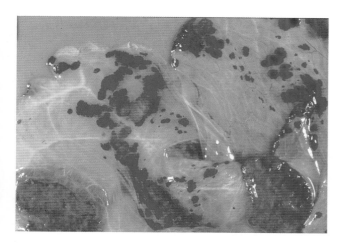

Fig. 18-41   Adventitial placentation, placenta, chorion cow. Additional sites of placentation are visible in the intercotyledonary chorion. They appear as red plaques, sometimes with villi, that extend from cotyledons. There is a corresponding change on the endometrium. *(Courtesy Drs. W. Crowell and Tyler, College of Veterinary Medicine, University of Georgia; and Noah's Arkive, College of Veterinary Medicine, University of Georgia.)*

length) and torsion. In torsion of the umbilical cord, the cord is long, excessively twisted, and the twists are difficult to undo. For a twisted cord to qualify as pathologic, lesions caused by compromise of the umbilical vessels must be present. The cord is edematous and hemorrhagic, and congested distended segments alternate with constricted twisted segments (Fig. 18-40). Fibrin is often present on the surface of affected areas of the cord. Lesser degrees of torsion occur without seriously affecting the umbilical blood vessels and killing

the fetus. The urachus is thinner and more pliable than the umbilical arteries or vein and is more easily constricted. Local distentions of the urachus can occur anywhere along its course in the cord from the umbilicus to the allantoic cavity. They are useful in confirming the obstructive effects of torsion of the cord.

Adventitial placentation in ruminants is the formation of additional placentomas (Fig. 18-41). It is thought to be an age-associated change because more are seen in cows with a higher parity. It is also considered a hyperplastic response to inadequacy of the placentomal surface area. A reduction in the area of placentomes due to loss of caruncles can occur as a result of endometritis, removal of cotyledons during aggressive manipulations, removal of retained placental membranes, and chronic placentitis. Adventitial placentation is also seen in hydroallantois and when fetuses are the result of cloning. Compensation for a reduced placentomal area can be achieved by enlargement of the existing functional maternal caruncles and the establishment of additional areas of contact by simple villous interdigitation. These adventitious areas form initially adjacent to the placentomes but can expand to involve much of the surface.

Just as adventitial placentation may be a "normal" or age-associated change in many situations, so there are structures in the placenta of most species that may be confused with lesions. These are particularly numerous in the mare and are listed in Box 18-6. It is important to know the normal or incidental findings before describing lesions. All species have amniotic plaques (Fig. 18-42, A). They are small raised plaques of epidermal tissue, and some may have hair growing from them. In ruminants they are up to 2 cm in diameter and only on the amnion on the same side as the fetus. Ruminants in particular have mineralization of the placenta, which appears as a white lacy change especially to the chorion. The equine placenta has many others, including normal avillus areas, allantoic pouches, and chorioallantoic pouches. Two structures that often cause confusion are the hippomane and the yolk sac remnant. Almost all equine placentas have a hippomane in the allantoic cavity. These are rubbery concrements of allantoic precipitates that vary in color from white to tan to red (Fig. 18-42, B). Also confused with a lesion or anomaly is the yolk sac remnant. This is a circular cystic structure found in the allantoic portion of the umbilical cord, from the junction of the amnion and the cord to the junction with the chorioallantois. It may be surrounded by the umbilical vessels or extend from the tissue of the cord from a stalk (Fig. 18-42, C). This remnant is often mineralized and, when opened, has a fluid-filled center and an ossified wall. The outer surface is smooth, but the inner surface has a pattern that resembles the inner surface of the calvarium. It is sometimes mistaken for the skull of a twin or an amorphous globosus (see later; Fig. 18-44).

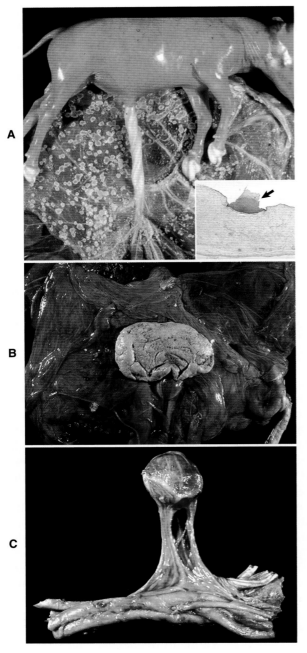

Fig. 18-42, cont'd   containing blood vessels and is located at the junction of the umbilical cord and the allantois. (**A,** *Courtesy Department of Veterinary Biosciences, The Ohio State University; and Noah's Arkive, College of Veterinary Medicine, The University of Georgia.* **Inset,** *Courtesy Dr. M.D. McGavin, College of Veterinary Medicine, University of Tennessee.* **B,** *Courtesy Dr. M. McCracken, College of Veterinary Medicine, University of Tennessee; and Noah's Arkive, College of Veterinary Medicine, The University of Georgia.* **C,** *Courtesy Dr. J. King, College of Veterinary Medicine, Cornell University.*)

Hydramnios and hydrallantois refer to the excessive accumulation of fluid in the amniotic and allantoic sacs, respectively. These lesions occur mostly in the cow, are rare, and usually do not occur together. Accumulation of excessive amniotic fluid occurs in association with some fetal facial muscle and skeletal

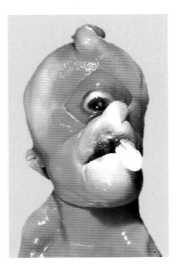

Fig. 18-43   Cyclopia, porcine fetus. A defect of ocular and cranial development has resulted in fusion of the eyes (cyclops) and a proboscis above the eye. Cyclopia can occur in the lambs of ewes that ingest the plant *Veratrum californicum* on the fourteenth day of gestation. *(Courtesy Dr. J. King, College of Veterinary Medicine, Cornell University.)*

Fig. 18-42   Incidental structures, placentas. A, Amniotic plaques, bovine fetus and placenta. Multiple white, raised circular plaques up to 1.5 cm in diameter are present on the fetal side of the amnion. They are normal incidental structures composed of stratified squamous keratinizing epithelium. *Inset:* An amniotic plaque (*arrow*). H&E stain. **B,** Hippomane, allantois, equine placenta. These rubbery flattened discs up to 10 cm in diameter are the end result of aggregation of sediments of allantoic fluid in the horse and other equids. They are incidental findings. **C,** Mineralized yolk sac remnant, umbilical cord, equine fetus. Yolk sac remnants seen on the allantoic portion of the umbilical cord are incidental structures. Note that in this case the yolk sac is connected by a stalk

(Continued)

abnormalities. The implication is that serious nervous abnormalities impair the muscles responsible for the fetal drinking reflex. An association has been found between fetal adrenal insufficiency and hydramnios. Allantoic fluid is formed in part from fetal urine received through the urachus. In the cow, hydrallantois occurs in conjunction with adventitial placentation and in some twin pregnancies. Abortion or dystocia follow, with a dead and sometimes small anasarcous and ascitic fetus. The allantoic fluid composition changes from normal to that closely resembling maternal or fetal extracellular fluid. When these membranes are retained after delivery of a fetus, fluid sometimes continues to accumulate.

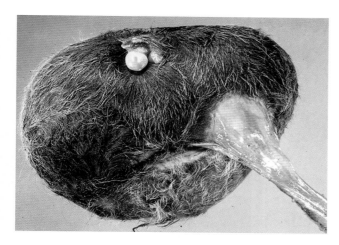

Fig. 18-44   Acardiac monster (bovine amorphous globosus). This structure, covered with hair, is the remnant of a twin fetus and is attached to the placenta of the normal twin by a stalk. It is a rare finding in cattle and is usually of little consequence. *(Courtesy Dr. J. Edwards, College of Veterinary Medicine, Texas A&M University; and Dr. J. King, College of Veterinary Medicine, Cornell University.)*

Fetal anomalies can take innumerable forms. Some of those that directly influence the reproductive process are mentioned here. First, certain anomalies cause prolonged gestation because a fetal adrenal gland does not make the necessary hormonal contribution to the birth process. Alteration of the pituitary-adrenal axis, such as aplasia or hypoplasia of the adrenal glands or anomalies of the anterior pituitary, will prolong gestation. One classic example is prolonged gestation in ewes that ingest the plant *Veratrum californicum* on the fourteenth day of gestation. Along with the cyclopia (Fig. 18-43) and holoprosencephaly that occurs, the pituitary may be absent. Absence of the pituitary gland also occurs, probably as an inherited disease, in Guernsey and Jersey cattle. Absence of the pituitary gland can occur alone or as part of hydranencephaly or anencephaly.

The second large group of fetal anomalies interferes with the reproductive process by causing mechanical problems at parturition (dystocia). Examples are hydrocephalus, hydrops fetus, and arthrogryposis.

Amorphous globosus is a rare and incidental finding in bovine placentas especially. It is a type of acardiac monster, and it is a severely anomalous second fetus. It is usually spherical, covered in hair, and attached to the placenta by a cord (Fig. 18-44). Histologically, various organs can be identified within the structure.

Retention of fetal membranes for longer than normal after parturition is common, especially in the cow. In cows, membranes are considered retained if not expelled by 12 hours postpartum. During normal pregnancy, there is a turnover of maternal epithelial cells of the caruncle. As parturition approaches, there

is a gradual loss and flattening of the cells. Trophoblasts compensate by hyperplasia. Normal separation of cotyledon from caruncle involves reduced cell proliferation and increased apoptosis of placental tissue. Parturition before there is complete "maturation" of the epithelium is believed to result in retention of placental membranes; thus retention is common in cases where caesarian section is necessary because there may be insufficient time for complete maturation to occur. Infectious, nutritional, hormonal, circulatory, hereditary, and weather factors may inhibit the "maturation" process. Retained membranes can act as a nutrient medium for growth of contaminant bacteria and for the development of severe endometritis from the transient mild postparturient endometritis. The endometritis can even cause systemic disease, such as septicemia or disseminated intravascular coagulation.

CERVIX

Disease of the cervix is rare in domestic mammals and is usually part of more generalized disease. There is considerable variation in the anatomy of the cervix, and this has an impact on uterine health because of the function of the cervix.

ANOMALIES

Two entire cervices or a single bifurcated cervix, along with a divided vagina and two uteri, can result from failure of proper fusion of the paired paramesonephric ducts. In cows, some developmental abnormalities are restricted to the cervix. These include hypertrophy or hypoplasia of the whole structure, aplasia of one or more of the usual five rugae, tortuosity, and dilation or diverticulum formation of the cervical canal.

DEGENERATIVE DISEASE

Ewes exposed to estrogenic substances in subterranean and red clover develop a permanent infertility because of alteration of the cervix. Affected animals have a cervix that has fused cervical folds and uterine-like glands that produce a less viscous mucus. Alteration of cervical mucus affects spermatozoal migration and results in reduced fertility.

INFECTIOUS DISEASES

Cervicitis usually occurs as a minor lesion concurrently with more severe endometritis or vaginitis. This distribution is observed in specific infectious diseases, such as contagious equine metritis caused by *Taylorella equigenitalis*, and in nonspecific postparturient metritis, cervicitis, and vaginitis. As a single lesion, inflammation of the cervix can result from poorly performed traumatic artificial insemination. In cows with acute cervicitis, the caudal rugae are edematous and prolapse into the vagina. Inflammatory exudate covers the cervical mucosa and collects in the vagina. The cervical mucosa is relatively thin, and the underlying fibromuscular tissue is relatively impervious to infection; thus most cases of cervicitis resolve readily. Those infections that follow traumatic dystocia are likely to involve the muscle layer from the onset and have the potential to produce severe lesions. These lesions include paracervical abscesses, local peritonitis with granulating tracts into the connective tissue of the pelvic canal, stenosis with adhesions across the lumen of the cervix in areas denuded of epithelium, or cysts filled with mucus in the lining.

NEOPLASMS

Neoplastic disease of the cervix of domestic animals is very rare.

VULVA AND VAGINA

The two main categories of disease of the vagina and vulva are similar to those of other parts of the female reproductive tract, being (1) infectious and inflammatory disease and (2) noninfectious conditions, including neoplasia, anomalies, and hyperplasia.

INFLAMMATORY DISEASE

Postparturient vulvitis and vaginitis occur when these organs are lacerated during dystocia and become infected. Trauma unrelated to parturition also can progress similarly. Inflammation of the cervix and proximal vagina following dystocia can have a more serious outcome because of the possible local spread of infection into and through the vaginal wall into the peritoneal cavity.

Granular vulvitis describes the clinical appearance of the vulva and vagina in inflammatory diseases. Inflammation causes the red coloration (hyperemia) and exudates, and the granular appearance is to a large extent the result of enlargement of the lymphoid follicles of the region (Fig. 18-45). Thus any infectious agent can be a cause. In bitches, this appearance is relatively common in so-called nonspecific vaginitis or vulvitis. Granular vulvitis in cattle occurs with *Ureaplasma diversum* infection. In the acute stage, there is a profuse purulent vulvular discharge and a hyperemic vulvular mucosa with 2-mm raised granules. The disease can become chronic, and lesions resolve within 3 months. In about 10% of affected cows, discrete, raised, white epithelial inclusion cysts, 2 to 5 mm in diameter, occur in rows or clusters on the dorsolateral wall of the vulva. Infection of cows is usually self-limiting, but herds can have a persistent infection. Bulls and semen can remain infected and spread the infection during mating or artificial insemination. Reduced fertility with return to service or abortion is seen with pathogenic strains of the organism as a sequela to infection and inflammation of the embryo or fetal membranes.

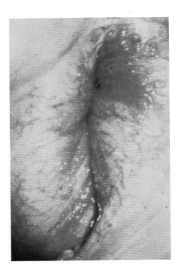

Fig. 18-45 **Granular vulvitis, vulva, cow.** Granular vulvitis is a nonspecific condition resulting from development and hyperplasia of subepithelial lymphoid follicles of the vulva and vestibule. Inflammation of the vulva, in the initial stages, causes hyperemia. There is subsequent hyperplasia of lymphoid tissue, visible as 1 to 2 mm raised white nodules on the vulval mucosa (*upper portion*). It is commonly seen in cows with infection of the vulva or vagina with *Ureaplasma diversum* and results in a granular appearance of the mucosa. (*Courtesy Dr. R.B. Miller, Ontario Veterinary College, University of Guelph.*)

Infectious pustular vulvovaginitis of cattle is caused by BHV-1, which is similar to the BHV-1 that is the cause of infectious bovine rhinotracheitis (IBR). The two diseases behave as separate entities, but their occurrence can overlap in a herd or in an individual. Vulvovaginitis is transmitted by coitus, artificial insemination, and possibly nose-to-vulva contact. The first evidence of the disease includes hyperemia and edema of the vagina and vulva; these lesions are followed by petechial hemorrhages and slight nodularity of the mucosal surfaces. A rapidly coalescing multifocal erosion and ulceration of the mucosa follows, beginning over the lymphoid nodules (Fig. 18-46). Microscopically, changes can be detected in the epithelium, the lamina propria, and the lymphoid nodules. The epithelium with eosinophilic intranuclear inclusions undergoes ballooning degeneration followed by necrosis, neutrophil infiltration, and desquamation, but without discrete stages of vesicle or pustule formation. The lamina propria is hyperemic, edematous, and infiltrated by inflammatory cells, mostly lymphocytes and plasma cells. The subepithelial lymphoid nodules are hyperplastic. Resolution of the disease is rapid, and the lesions that remain are slightly thickened epithelium and hyperplastic lymphoid nodules. Lesions are similar in the penis of affected bulls.

Caprine herpesvirus 1 causes lesions in goats similar to those of bovine vulvovaginitis (Fig. 18-47). In the

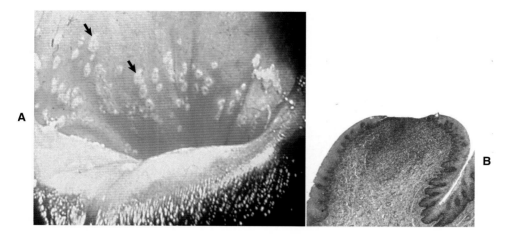

Fig. 18-46   **Infectious pustular vulvovaginitis, bovine herpesvirus 1 infection, cow.** **A,** Focal ulceration of mucosa of the vestibule. The multiple white regions (*arrows*) are areas of necrotic epithelium and ulceration. **B,** Ulceration of mucosa of the vestibile. Note the ulcer with loss of the epithelium over an aggregate of lymphocytes. H&E stain. (*A* and **B,** *Courtesy Dr. K. McEntee, Reproductive Pathology Collection, University of Illinois.*)

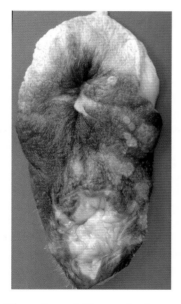

Fig. 18-47   **Ulcerative vulvitis, caprine herpesviral infection, goat.** The vulva (*lower*) has numerous vesicles on the mucosa. The skin of the perineal region around the anus (*upper*) and vulva has multiple circular regions of epithelial necrosis and erosion. Herpesviral infection of the genital tract has the classic lesions of vesicles that rupture to form ulcers, which are irregularly distributed on the affected areas. (*Courtesy Dr. P.W. Ladds, James Cook University of North Queensland.*)

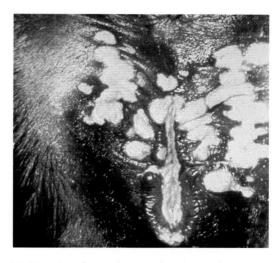

Fig. 18-48   **Coital exanthema, ulcerative vulvitis, mare.** **Large full-thickness ulcers around the perineum and on the vulvular skin heal with depigmented regions.** (*Courtesy Dr. K. McEntee, Reproductive Pathology Collection, University of Illinois.*)

NONINFLAMMATORY DISEASE

Tumefaction of the vulva is normal during estrus. Overly large or persistent swelling is abnormal. Abnormal tumefaction occurs in hyperestrogenism, such as with estrogen-producing ovarian neoplasms and exposure to estrogenic substances (Fig. 18-49). The vaginal mucosa becomes swollen with edema and protrudes through the vulva, exposing the mucosa. Toxicosis of pigs by the mycotoxin zearalenone found in moldy corn is a cause. Other effects of the mycotoxin are precocious mammary development, tenesmus leading to rectal prolapse, and the luteotrophic activities that induce anestrus or pseudopregnancy.

equine species, equine herpesvirus 3 (as distinct from EHV-1, and responsible for respiratory disease, nervous disease, and abortion) is the cause of coital exanthema characterized by transient vesicles and erosions morphologically similar to those observed in IBR on the external genitalia of both mares and stallions (Fig. 18-48).

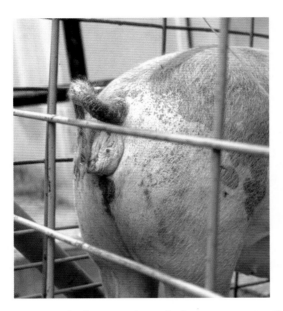

Fig. 18-49   Vulva hypertrophy and edema, estrogenic effect, sow. The vulva of this sow is swollen with edema. This swelling is typical of hyperestrogenism secondary to mycotoxicosis. (*Courtesy Dr. J. Simon, College of Veterinary Medicine, University of Illinois.*)

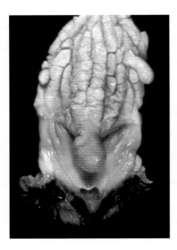

Fig. 18-50   Polyps, vulva, bitch. There are several vaginal polyps arising from the wall of the vagina. The larger caudal polyp adjacent to the urethra protrudes caudally through the labia of the vulva and is ulcerated. (*Courtesy Dr. K. McEntee, Reproductive Pathology Collection, University of Illinois.*)

Vaginal hyperplasia, hypertrophy, and/or prolapse of bitches is a common disease seen during the follicular stage (proestrus) of the first to third estrus periods in young animals, particularly of the brachiocephalic breeds. These animals are assumed to have an increased sensitivity to estrogen and develop excessive edema. The vaginal mucosa swells and interferes with coitus. Dramatic swelling can, if severe, result in the tissue protruding from the vulval labia to produce a prolapse that

becomes excoriated and ulcerated. Spontaneous regression during diestrus is the norm.

Vaginal polyps are relatively common in older bitches (Fig. 18-50). They are usually solitary, up to several centimeters in diameter, and have a thin stalk of attachment to the vaginal wall. Excision is usually curative.

Cysts in the vaginal wall of the cow arise from mesonephric duct remnants (Gartner's ducts) or major vestibular (Bartholin's) glands. Causes of cyst formation include inflammation of the lining of the duct or gland, and hyperestrogenism, in which edema caused by estrogen stimulation is prolonged. Gartner's ducts normally do not open into the vagina. When they become cystic, they form single or multiple cysts or a tortuous channel in the floor of the vagina somewhere between the cervix and near the urethral opening. Major vestibular glands are found on the ventral and lateral walls of the vestibule and become cystic when edema, inflammation, or scar tissue obstructs their openings. Other anomalies include persistent hymen, vaginal septum (double vagina), and stricture or stenosis of the vagina or vestibule that follow traumatic injury at parturition.

NEOPLASMS

Transmissible venereal tumor (TVT) of the dog is transmitted by coitus and the transfer of intact neoplastic cells. TVT cells have 59 chromosomes compared with the normal canine number of 78. Immunohistochemical evaluation with tumor markers suggests that these tumors may have a histiocytic origin, although a complete characterization is not reported. Both sexes are affected. The neoplasm begins as a nodule beneath the genital mucosa and when enlarged breaks through the overlying mucosa. In the bitch, the lesion often begins in the dorsal wall of the vagina at the junction with the vestibule. It proliferates into the lumen of the vagina and can protrude through the vulva as an ulcerated, friable mass (Fig. 18-51, A). Microscopically the neoplastic cells are large, round or oval, and uniform in size (Fig. 18-51, B) but with occasional large, bizarre nuclei. Cytoplasm is poorly defined, is lightly staining, and may have peripheral vacuoles. This neoplasm can spontaneously regress and have multifocal necrosis, infiltration of lymphocytes, likely cell-mediated neoplastic cell lysis, and deposition of collagen. This neoplasm is exquisitely sensitive to vincristine. A few dogs have metastases in other sites, although in countries with stray dogs and dogs in poor health, neoplasms with metastases are relatively common.

Squamous cell carcinoma of the vulva occurs in the mature cow, ewe, and mare (Fig. 18-52). Solar radiation has been established as an etiologic factor. Ewes subjected to the Mules operation (surgery of the perineum and inguinal areas intended to redirect the tip of the vulva to prevent urine wetting the wool) and

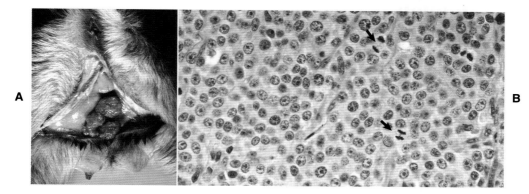

Fig. 18-51   Transmissible venereal tumor (TVT), vulva and vagina, bitch. A, The multinodular tumors markedly distend the vagina and vestibule and are grossly characteristic of TVT. **B,** Neoplastic cells are round and often divided into packets by a fine fibrous stroma. Mitoses are frequent (*arrows*). H&E stain. (**A,** *Courtesy Dr. J. King, College of Veterinary Medicine, Cornell University.* **B,** *Courtesy Dr. M. J. Abdy, College of Veterinary Medicine, The University of Georgia; and Noah's Arkive, College of Veterinary Medicine, The University of Georgia.*)

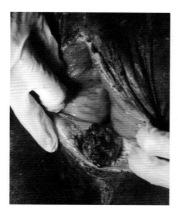

Fig. 18-52   Squamous cell carcinoma, vulva, mare. The clitoris has been replaced by a multinodular and ulcerated tumor. *(Courtesy Dr. J. King, College of Veterinary Medicine, Cornell University.)*

to short tail docking have a greater exposure of the vulva and greater incidence of squamous cell carcinoma of the vulva. Correlation can be made of incidence with exposure to sunlight and, at least in the cow, with the lack of pigmentation of the vulva. The squamous cell carcinoma originates on the hairless and less pigmented skin of the vulva and has the appearance and biologic behavior of squamous cell carcinomas in other sites. The neoplasm metastasizes late in the course of the disease to the iliosacral lymph nodes.

Carcinoma of the vulva or vagina in bitches is uncommon. Involvement of the urethra with transitional cell carcinoma and the development of a polypoid neoplasms and masses that extend from the urethral orifice, however, is a recognized entity in bitches and other domestic species.

Bitches develop multiple leiomyomas of the vagina. These only occur in entire bitches, so a hormonal link is proposed. Ovariohysterectomy may be curative, further indicating hormonal dependence. The common differential diagnoses of leiomyoma are vaginal polyps (see previous discussion). These have a similar appearance, and histologic examination is usually required to differentiate them because each has well-circumscribed nodules up to several centimeters in diameter that arise from the vaginal wall (Fig. 18-50).

MAMMARY GLAND
INTRODUCTION

Mastitis and mammary neoplasia are the major diseases of the mammary gland; most of the others represent aberrations or extreme manifestations of physiologic states.

Mastitis is inflammation of the mammary gland. Galactophoritis is inflammation of the mammary ducts. Most cases of mastitis begin with galactophoritis. Mastitis is the most economically important disease of the mammary glands, and although it occurs in all species, it is a particular problem in animals used for milk production.

Galactostasis is a condition in which the glands become engorged, hot, and painful. It occurs after weaning or in pseudopregnancy. Clinical signs are associated with milk retention, and there is no systemic illness. It is presumed to be the result of inadequate oxytocin release because of fear, stress, or lack of mammary stimulation.

Agalactia is a rare condition, and the cause is unknown. In goats there may be an association with the caprine arthritis and encephalitis virus (CAEV). The udders are hard, but no milk is produced. It is called "hard udder," and there is usually microscopic interstitial inflammation present.

Galactorrhea (also called inappropriate lactation and precocious lactation) is also unusual and, in bitches, occurs at the termination of diestrus when there is a prolactin surge in response to a reduction in progesterone concentration. It occasionally occurs following ovariohysterectomy during diestrus. Galactorrhea is seen in male goats of high milk production lines.

Inappropriate mammary development and lactation is relatively common in bitches as part of pseudopregnancy and was discussed previously.

MAMMARY DISEASE OF DOGS

Neoplasia of the mammary glands is common in the dog, and it has the highest incidence of all domesticated species (Fig. 18-53). Most canine mammary tumors are benign. There has been much interest in canine mammary neoplasia both from the view-point of prognosis and treatment, from a logical pathogenetic viewpoint, and as a tool in comparative oncology. Although the phenomenon of mammary neoplasia is well recognized, the cause is not. There are obvious risk factors, especially desexing at a young age. Ovariohysterectomy after the second estrus dramatically increases the prevalence of this disease. The window of susceptibility is up to 2 years of age. A high-protein diet decreases susceptibility, whereas treatment with medroxyprogesterone acetate and being a purebred increases it.

Mammary neoplasms are a diverse group that are dominated by epithelial (and myoepithelial) tumors.

Stromal tumors, such as fibrosarcoma and osteosarcoma, are much less common but are particularly aggressive and metastatic. The embryology of the mammary gland involves a close association between the epithelium and mesenchyme, so it is not surprising that tumors are often combinations of stroma and epithelium with the so called complex adenomas having a mixture of epithelial and myoepithelial components, and the mixed mammary tumor having those elements plus cartilage and bone.

The development of mammary epithelial neoplasia can proceed from ductal or lobular hyperplasia to dysplasia and on to neoplasia and progression from the benign adenomas and papillomas to carcinoma in situ and to invasive forms (Fig. 18-54). Once progression begins, an individual will often continue to develop neoplasia, and the development of multiple mammary masses is likely. The prognosis for each subsequent mass is not dependent on the previous one, so that many different types of neoplasia can be found in one animal.

Predicting behavior of mammary neoplasms is an inexact science. From a pragmatic and simplistic view, invasion is an indicator of a poor prognosis. It is the reason that excisional biopsy is the best procedure for diagnosis in dogs; cytology can be of use in identifying inflammation and malignant stromal neoplasms but can give a false impression of malignancy. The neoplasms that arise are pleomorphic in their characteristics, and, as such, there are many different classification schemes.

General principles of neoplasia apply, and, in dogs, those that are locally invasive are more likely to be life threatening. The threat increases with the lack of

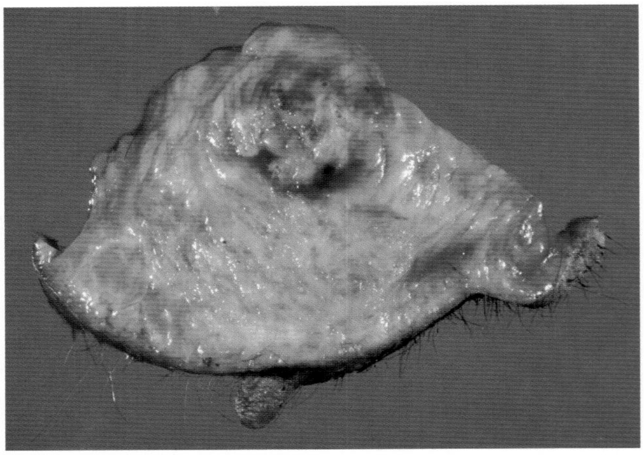

Fig. 18-53   Mammary carcinoma, mammary gland, bitch. This mammary carcinoma has infiltrated and replaced normal mammary gland and contiguous soft tissue. The upper nodule is the neoplasm, and the lower and surrounding white tissues are composed of infiltrating neoplastic cells and fibrous tissue, the result of a desmoplastic response. *(Courtesy Dr. R. A. Foster, Ontario Veterinary College, University of Guelph.)*

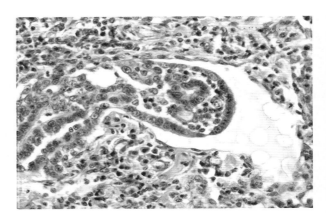

Fig. 18-54   Adenocarcinoma, invasion into lymphatic vessels, bitch. Note the neoplastic cells infiltrating through the wall of the lymphatic (*above left*). Microscopic invasion by mammary carcinoma into a lymphatic, as depicted here, is an indicator of a poor prognosis. In this case, there are lymphocytes and plasma cells in the perilymphatic tissues. H&E stain. *(Courtesy Dr. M. Domingo, Autonomous University of Barcelona; and Noah's Arkive, College of Veterinary Medicine, The University of Georgia.)*

differentiation, and there is an increasing risk of metastasis with tubulopapillary, solid, and anaplastic carcinomas, respectively. Those with metastasis to the local lymph node have an especially poor prognosis. Because there is a potential for progression from benign to malignant, neoplasms (either because of rapid growth or having additional time to develop) larger than 5 cm in diameter have a poorer prognosis.

In dogs, mastitis caused by bacteria or *Mycoplasma* occurs early in lactation or pseudopregnancy. Staphylococci, streptococci, and *Escherichia coli* are major isolates. It is assumed that the pathogenetic pathways of mastitis in dogs is the same as for dairy animals and will be discussed in detail later. Infection of fissures in nipples and adjacent skin spreads via the ducts and lymphatics into the gland and results in suppurative inflammation and/or abscesses. The glands become swollen, large, firm, and edematous because the toxins and tissue destruction by the agents, or the cytokine and contents of inflammatory cell granules, cause acute inflammation. It may be superimposed on mammary hyperplasia or mammary neoplasia, especially on tumors of ducts. Systemic illness is often seen. The effect of mastitic milk on puppies is not known.

MAMMARY DISEASE OF CATS

Fibroadenomatous hyperplasia (mammary hypertrophy) occurs in young intact female cats. Those less than 2 years old are most likely to develop mammary enlargement, which usually occurs in the spring and with the first several estrus cycles. Much of what is known about this disease is based on its coinciding with the luteal phase of estrus, early in pregnancy or after progestin therapy. High concentrations of progesterone or progesterone-like substances is the common link. As expected, megestrol acetate treatment of an old neutered male or female can induce this also. What is difficult to explain is that not only can all glands be affected, but only one gland, or parts of one gland, may be as well. Occasionally, only nodules may arise. The lesion is the result of notable proliferation of mammary ducts and adjacent stroma (Fig. 18-55). This overstimulation of an otherwise normal process is likely to be the result of a local dysregulation of tissue growth with the stimulation of receptors by progesterone. Some have theorized an exaggerated response to prolactin as well. Hemorrhages, coagulative necrosis, and/or ulceration of affected areas can occur. In young females, resolution is spontaneous or ovariohysterectomy is effective. Older neutered animals on progestin require drug withdrawal and sometimes mastectomy.

Mammary neoplasia in cats is relatively uncommon, so studies of causal factors have been limited. There does not appear to be the same relationship with early desexing as there is with dogs. Progression from focal hyperplasia to adenoma to carcinoma is recognized, but this progression is presumably rapid, as many of the carcinomas are small.

The majority of neoplasms in cats are carcinomas. They are usually single and occur in the subcutaneous tissue adjacent to the nipple; 75% to 96% are adenocarcinomas and show rapid growth (Fig. 18-56). They metastasize to regional lymph nodes, either the axillary or superficial inguinal nodes, lungs, or other mammae. The average age of affected animals is 10.7 years, and there is a 7- to 9-year-old risk plateau. Intact animals

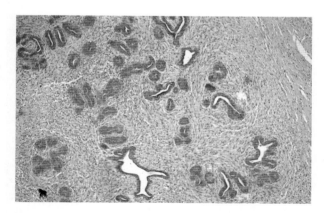

Fig. 18-55   Mammary hypertrophy (fibroadenomatous hyperplasia), mammary gland, cat. Mammary ducts have proliferated and are surrounded by abundant loosely arranged stromal tissues. Typically, cats with mammary hypertrophy are young and develop enlargement of one or several mammary glands, in the spring. H&E stain. *(Courtesy Dr. W. Crowell, College of Veterinary Medicine, The University of Georgia; and Noah's Arkive, College of Veterinary Medicine, The University of Georgia.)*

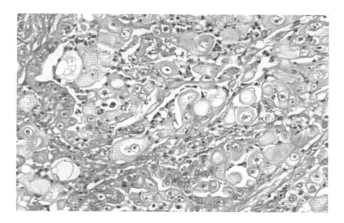

Fig. 18-56   Mammary carcinoma, mammary gland, cat. The cells of this anaplastic neoplasm do not resemble those of normal epithelium but are large and round. They are arranged either in clusters or as individual cells within a fibrous stroma. Inflammatory cells, including neutrophils and lymphocytes, are also present. H&E stain. *(Courtesy College of Veterinary Medicine, University of Illinois.)*

are at a slightly greater risk, but there is no beneficial effect of early spaying. The poorest prognosis is in older cats with neoplasms that are greater than 3 cm in diameter, with the presence of regional lymph node involvement, with increased number of mitoses, and with the presence of necrosis. Well-differentiated tumors have a better prognosis. The interval between diagnosis and death is often short, less than 1 year, but the range is wide. There is no or only a weak correlation between histologic features, including proliferation indices and prognosis, except perhaps size.

MAMMARY DISEASE OF COWS

Mastitis in dairy cattle is an extremely important disease. Most of the organisms responsible for mastitis are bacteria. The number of bacterial pathogens of the mammary gland are staggering in their number and range of lesions they cause. The majority of cases are caused by *Staphylococcus aureus* and are of the subclinical or moderate clinical forms.

Mammary pathogens can be divided into groups based on the source of infection for other cows. In one group are those organisms such as *Streptococcus agalactiae*, *Staphylococcus aureus*, and *Mycoplasma* sp., for which the mammary gland is the principal site of persistence or reservoir. Coliform organisms are in the group that is acquired from the external environment, such as fecal matter, soil, water, or bedding. An overlap group has members, such as *Streptococcus uberis* and *Streptococcus dysgalactiae*, capable of persisting in either location. Cow-to-cow transmission is important for the mammary reservoir group, whereas contamination of the teat end is important for disease caused by the environmental group. The rates of new mammary gland infections in dairy cows caused by environmental pathogens are greatest during the first and the last 2 weeks of a 60-day non-lactating period. Coliform and streptococcal infections that are established during the nonlactating period with organisms from the environment are present at the time of parturition and cause clinical mastitis soon afterward.

Another way to group the pathogenic organisms is by the disease they cause. The three main groups, based on their virulence and effects including systemic disease, are the gram-negative pathogens, gram-positive pathogens that cause acute severe necrotizing disease, and gram-positive pathogens that cause chronic suppurative mastitis. Gram-negative organisms, particularly *Escherichia coli*, can cause severe mastitis and systemic effects because of endotoxin release. Gram-positive pathogens cause disease that ranges from subclinical mastitis to gangrenous mastitis. Many induce a chronic suppurative disease.

Gram-negative bacteria gain access to the glands and release endotoxins, and the cytokine release they invoke results in necrosis and severe vascular leakage (Fig. 18-57). A systemic acute phase reaction induced by

the endotoxins and cytokines results in fever, anorexia, leukopenia, hyperfibrinogenemia, and hypocalcemia. This latter feature can be mistaken for primary milk fever. Edema of the mammary gland and surrounding areas is often prominent. Local changes include necrosis and sequestration of glandular tissue, wherein regions of the gland become dry, friable, and surrounded by a red border of hyperemia and hemorrhage (Fig. 18-58). The massive outpouring of edema fluid causes the gland to be dramatically swollen and hard and the "milk" to be watery and/or contain fibrin that can obstruct the ducts and sinuses. Not only is this type of mastitis potentially

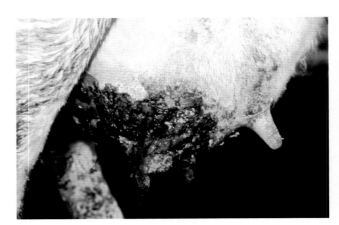

Fig. 18-57   Severe necrotic mastitis, coliform mastitis, mammary gland, cow. Serum oozes through the dead skin of the affected right rear quarter. *(Courtesy Dr. M.D. McGavin, College of Veterinary Medicine, University of Tennessee.)*

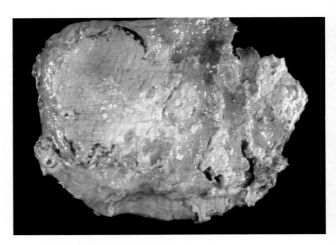

Fig. 18-58   Necrotizing mastitis, coliform mastitis, mammary gland, transverse section of quarter, cow. Note the dry and pale area, typical of coagulative necrosis, to the left of center. The necrotic tissue is partially surrounded by a zone of edema and by a thin light-gray band of fibrous tissue. Encapsulated necrotic tissue is designated a "sequestrum." *(Courtesy College of Veterinary Medicine, University of Illinois.)*

life threatening because of endotoxemia, the severe effects on the gland often lead to reduced defenses to other pathogens so that secondary, pus-forming pathogens also proliferate.

Severe acute mastitis is caused when necrotizing gram-positive bacteria, including virulent *Staphylococcus aureus* and streptococci, gain entry to the glands. With severe staphylococcal mastitis, there is neutrophilic infiltration within minutes to hours of introduction, and the products of neutrophils contribute to the necrosis of the glandular tissue. Cell surface–associated (adhesions, protein A, and capsular polysaccharides) and extracellular secretory products (leukotoxins, extracellular enzymes, and coagulase) of these organisms contribute to the damaging effect of these bacteria. The combined result is hemorrhage and necrosis of the gland, with the result that the gland or part of the gland becomes gangrenous, hard, dry, and red-black. When severe, systemic effects of the acute phase response caused by systemic cytokines induce fever, anorexia, weight loss, leukopenia, and hyperfibrinogenemia.

The pus-forming bacteria tend not to produce or induce the degree of necrosis, vascular effects, or systemic effects of the first two groups. These bacteria invoke a neutrophilic response that dominates the lesion and results in the build up of the characteristic necrotic leukocytic debris that typifies the suppurative response. The lesions they induce are often centered on the lactiferous ducts and sinus, and result in the filling of these tubes with suppurative exudate (Fig. 18-59). *Arcanobacterium pyogenes, Mycoplasma bovis, Streptococcus dysgalactiae* and various aerobes and anaerobes are prime candidates. Nocardial mastitis can be included in this group as well. Infection with these organisms, especially *Arcanobacterium pyogenes*, can occur with long-acting intramammary preparations used in the nonlactating or dry cow period. The occurrence in dry cows, initially recognized in the summer months, led to the name "summer mastitis." Careful culture of these cases will reveal a mixed culture of organisms and often up to five or six different species of the *Arcanobacterium, Streptococcus, Bacteroides, Peptostreptococcus,* and *Fusobacterium* genera. Because these are found in other pyogenic infections, it can be assumed that they are environmental contaminates. Dry cows are often not examined closely, so the mastitis is typically chronic, with thick intramammary exudates and fibrosis. Mycoplasma mastitis is similar in type, but infection can be from a systemic infection. Spread of the organism to calves and resultant otitis, arthritis, and pneumonia can occur.

Streptococcus agalactiae was the most important pathogen of the bovine mammary gland in the era before adequate mammary gland hygiene and efficient antibacterial drugs. Resistance of cows to mastitis

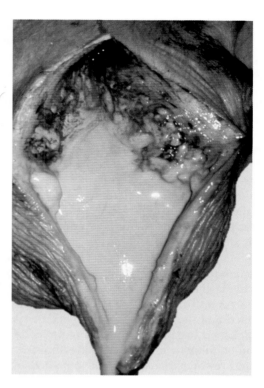

Fig. 18-59   Suppurative mastitis, mammary quarter, cow. The lactiferous sinus and ducts are filled with viscous yellow pus. *(Courtesy College of Veterinary Medicine, University of Illinois.)*

caused by this organism is subject to great individual variation; in general, resistance decreases with age. The mammary gland is the only organ affected by this organism. *Streptococcus agalactiae* does not persist long in the environment. Once a cow is infected, however, the organism persists in the lactiferous sinus, with periodic waves of multiplication, increase in virulence, and tissue invasion. The initial response to invasion of *Streptococcus agalactiae* is interstitial edema and an influx of neutrophils into the interstitium and alveoli. The alveolar epithelium undergoes either brief hyperplasia or vacuolation and then is desquamated. Macrophages quickly become a component of the cell population of infected alveoli, and fibrosis rapidly obliterates the lumen of these alveoli. Edema, cellular infiltration, and fibrosis are lesions found in infected and adjacent alveoli, so that pressure is increased within the lobule and within adjacent lobules. The increased pressure causes stagnation of milk flow, thereby initiating premature involution of a portion of the gland. After the acute phase, periductal fibrosis occurs and granulation tissue replaces part of the normal cuboidal to columnar epithelium of smaller ducts. Fibrous polyps can completely obstruct milk flow. Restoration of ductal epithelium can occur after the granulation tissue has matured and contracted. The lactiferous ducts and sinuses, with their normally two-layered columnar epithelium, are similarly but less severely affected, often going through a phase of squamous metaplasia of the epithelium.

The gross appearance of a mammary gland with mastitis caused by *Streptococcus agalactiae* depends on the stage of the disease; different stages are to be expected in different areas of a gland. Usually more than one quarter of the gland is involved. In the acute stage, hyperemia involves the mucosa of the lactiferous sinus. Milk quality is altered, and strands or clumps of debris are present in the milk, or the milk is transformed into pus. The areas of parenchymal edema and cellular infiltration are gray and turgid. Groups of alveoli, in which the secretion is retained because of obstruction of the duct by granulation tissue, resemble small abscesses. Involuting parenchyma and fibrotic parenchyma appear similar to one another and can be difficult to differentiate grossly. The mucosa of the lactiferous sinus becomes granular and thickened because of underlying projecting areas of granulation tissue and surrounding fibrosis.

Isolates of *Staphylococcus aureus* obtained from the bovine mammary gland range from nonpathogenic to highly pathogenic. The severest form of staphylococcal mastitis is the gangrenous form (Fig. 18-60), usually seen shortly after parturition and involving a variable proportion of the udder. Severe acute inflammation, with classic heat, redness, swelling, and pain, progresses to necrosis with its coldness of the affected area, blue-black color, and fluid exudation.

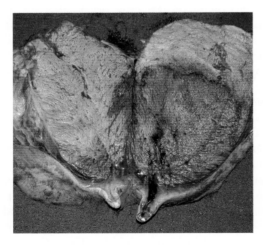

Fig. 18-60   Gangrenous mastitis (*Clostridium* sp.), mammary gland, transverse section of udder, cow. Most of the right quarter and some of the adjacent left quarter are dark red with hemorrhage. A well-demarcated hyperemic border has formed at its junction with the adjacent normal gland (*right udder*). There is also marked subcutaneous edema between the gland and the skin. (*Courtesy Dr. R. A. Foster, Ontario Veterinary College, University of Guelph.*)

Microscopically, during the first 48 hours after infection with toxigenic *Staphylococcus aureus*, the infected tissue has severe interstitial edema that increases the interalveolar stromal area and reduces the alveolar luminal area. Progressive swelling, vacuolar degeneration, and focal erosion and ulceration occur throughout the duct system and are most prominent near the junction of stratified squamous epithelium and columnar epithelium in the area of the papillary duct. The organism attaches to epithelial cells, causing focal damage, and later can be seen on, within, and below ductal and alveolar epithelium. Inflammatory cellular response is rapid, with neutrophils initially in the subepithelial tissues of the distal parts of the duct system, then within the epithelium, and later in the interstitial and epithelial tissue of alveoli.

Staphylococcal mastitis in the less acute form follows a course similar to that of streptococcal mastitis. Initially, damage occurs to the epithelium of the lactiferous sinus and larger lactiferous ducts. Organisms extend rapidly along the ducts and produce acute inflammation in groups of adjacent terminal alveoli. In chronically infected quarters, macrophages are the principal inflammatory cell type in epithelial lining, in lumens, and especially in the glandular interstitium. Lymphocytes also increase in number, but some investigators have reported a lack of increase in plasma cells. These observations suggest that mammary gland lymphocytes could become hyporesponsive to antigenic stimulation in quarters chronically infected with *Staphylococcus aureus*. Some data indicate that mammary gland lymphocyte function is compromised; blastogenesis is depressed in lymphocytes recovered from quarters infected with *Staphylococcus aureus*. Studies have documented that plasma cells are prevalent in the stroma of mammary glands with chronic *Staphylococcus aureus* mastitis; more cells produce IgA than IgG antibodies, and IgA-containing cells increase in number as the disease progresses. The extent of regeneration is uncertain; it is unclear whether damaged alveoli redevelop secretory tissue or remaining healthy tissue undergoes compensatory hypertrophy, or whether both processes occur.

Staphylococcus aureus has a greater propensity than *Streptococcus agalactiae* to invade the interstitial tissue between alveoli. The initial inflammatory reaction is necrotizing; abscess formation can follow. Abscesses, scattered and often coalescing, vary in size from those that are microscopic to those grossly visible. Sometimes the staphylococcal organisms are surrounded by rosettes of club-shaped material. (The obsolete term *botryomycosis* was applied to such lesions.) An equally important and parallel set of events occurring in the lobules not invaded by bacteria is the obstruction of milk flow by granulation tissue and pressure from surrounding fibrosis, resulting in involution of those uninvaded lobules. Multiple, small, soft cream to pink nodules, some containing pus, are separated by bands of fibrous tissue. Disease caused by less pathogenic strains of staphylococci, such as nonhemolytic coagulase-negative strains, progresses less dramatically and not necessarily with obvious abscess formation. However, the same components of granulation tissue and fibrosis are present, causing obstruction and pressure, which in turn cause atrophy of adjacent lobules.

Coliform mastitis is caused after organisms from the environment contaminate the opening of the papillary duct at the distal end of the teat and ascend the duct. The most common organisms are *Escherichia coli*, *Enterobacter aerogenes*, and *Klebsiella pneumoniae*. The coliform organisms probably exert their damaging effect via endotoxin acting on the vasculature. In the acute form of the disease, the lesions are hyperemia, hemorrhages, and edema of the affected areas centered around the lactiferous ducts. The secretion in the lactiferous sinus is cloudy and blood stained and has clumps of fibrin (Fig. 18-61). Microscopically, interlobular septa are edematous and fibrin thrombi are in lymph vessels. Epithelium of ducts and alveoli is necrotic, and very few inflammatory cells are present in the alveoli. Coliform organisms are numerous in the alveoli. Large numbers of organisms are phagocytosed by the secretory epithelium. The severity of the disease in postparturient cows is attributed to a delay in the influx of neutrophils. The cow's response to endotoxin is influenced by the stage of the reproductive cycle. The nonlactating mammary gland is much less sensitive to the effects of endotoxin than the lactating gland.

If the cow survives endotoxemia, the necrotic mammary tissue, which can be a large portion of a quarter, becomes separated from the viable tissue and is sequestered or eventually sloughs (Fig. 18-62). Cows in early lactation with less severe coliform mastitis often develop chronic mastitis that has alterations of hyperplasia, disorganization, and filiform processes of the epithelial lining of the papillary duct and lactiferous sinus.

Arcanobacterium pyogenes causes a mastitis in lactating, nonlactating, and even immature bovine mammary glands that is characterized by abscesses in the tissue of the small and large lactiferous ducts. Abscesses range from those microscopic in size to those grossly visible. Fistulas from the abscesses can form at the base of the teat. Fibrosis of the abscess walls can result in loss of small unaffected ducts and involution and fibrosis of the parenchyma they drain. The wall of large abscesses is thickened by granulation tissue.

Mycoplasma mastitis in cows occurs as individual sporadic cases or in outbreaks. Several mycoplasmas are capable of causing bovine mastitis, but *Mycoplasma*

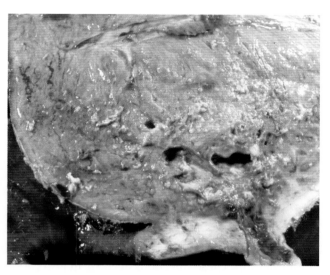

Fig. 18-61   Coliform mastitis, mammary gland, cow. There is marked thickening of the walls of the lactiferous ducts. White to yellow fibrin and pus have collected in the lactiferous ducts and the upper portion of the lactiferous sinus. *(Courtesy College of Veterinary Medicine, University of Illinois.)*

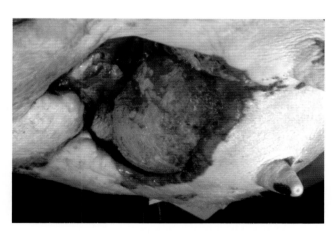

Fig. 18-62   Sloughed quarter, mammary gland, necrotizing mastitis, cow. The necrotic right rear quarter has recently sloughed, leaving a large ulcerated area covered by a thin gray layer of exudate. The surface is finely granular, indicating the formation of granulation tissue. *(Courtesy College of Veterinary Medicine, University of Illinois.)*

bovis is by far the most prevalent. The disease caused by *Mycoplasma bovis* can affect one quarter or involve the whole gland. Experimental inoculation of one quarter will often spread to all quarters. Hematogenous spread and contamination of the teat are therefore routes by which the gland becomes infected. Affected quarters initially are enlarged, firm, and light brown and have a nodular parenchyma. The nodules are abscesses that can be up to 10 cm in diameter. Exudation of neutrophils into the lobular interstitium and alveoli is intense in the early stages. The exudate changes with chronicity to include mononuclear cells. Early vacuolation and degeneration of alveolar epithelium is followed by hyperplasia of alveolar and ductular epithelium, and then by metaplasia to a relatively undifferentiated multilayered epithelial lining. Focal erosions of duct epithelium are filled in by granulation tissue. Aggregates of lymphocytes occur in the lobular interstitium and around ducts. Interstitial fibrosis and lobular atrophy are found in the late stages.

Granulomatous mastitis in the cow generally occurs when drugs for the treatment or prevention of mastitis are introduced through the teat and are contaminated with *Nocardia asteroides*, *Cryptococcus neoformans*, atypical *Mycobacterium* sp. (other than *Mycobacterium bovis*), or *Candida* spp. These infectious agents can also cause spontaneous mammary gland disease from organisms normally existing in the environment. Nocardial mastitis is the best known of these diseases because it occurs in outbreaks. Severely affected cows develop pyrexia that may last for several weeks. They become lethargic and lose weight, as would be expected with cytokine release. The glands are hot and swollen and may have multiple abscesses or granulomas. Small white particles may be found in the exudate. Lesions in the glands are centered on the lactiferous ducts and sinuses, as galactophoritis (inflammation of these structures) is the prominent finding. Because the infection is chronic and ascending, lobules are affected to a varying degree. Granulomas and pyogranulomas predominate microscopically. These are usually surrounded by fibrous tissue, and extensive involvement results in the gland being replaced by a framework of fibrous tissue surrounding pockets of inflammatory cells and central necrotic debris (Fig. 18-63). An udder affected with cryptococcal mastitis has the same yellow gelatinous material that is typical of cryptococcal lesions elsewhere.

MAMMARY DISEASE OF SHEEP AND GOATS

There are two main agents recovered from the mammary gland of sheep: *Mannheimia hemolytica* and *Staphylococcus aureus*. In many sheep flocks, the main manifestation of infection with these agents is unexpected death, because these bacteria are responsible for an acute necrotizing or gangrenous mastitis. It is difficult to be certain, but the morbidity can be about 5% and mortality 20%. Mastitis in goats is similar, and as with the disease in sheep, is assumed to have a similar pathogenesis as the disease in cattle. *Mycoplasma agalactiae* or *Mycoplasma mycoides* ssp. *mycoides* are usually the causative agents.

Goats develop a manifestation of infection with CAEV that causes "hard udder." This disease is seen in herds with CAEV infection, and affects does in the first

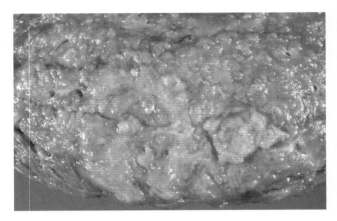

Fig. 18-63 **Chronic mastitis and galactophoritis (*Nocarida* spp.), mammary gland, transverse section, cow.** Chronic inflammation of the lactiferous ducts and adjacent mammary gland has resulted in the replacement of most of this gland by pyogranulomas and abscesses containing yellow pus. The adjacent normal glandular tissue has involuted. This cow was infected when the dry cow medication was contaminated by *Nocardia* spp. *(Courtesy Dr. R. A. Foster, Ontario Veterinary College, University of Guelph.)*

few days of lactation. The udder is hard, and little milk can be expressed from the teat. Recovery occurs, but milk production is reduced. The pathology of this disease is not fully described, but histologically there are large numbers of lymphocytes and lymphoid follicles in the interstitium between the glands. The virus grows in mammary epithelium and is present in milk. The newborn is infected through infected milk. A similar disease is seen with infection with the ovine lentivirus of the maedi-visna virus complex that is responsible for the diseases of ovine progressive pneumonia and the neurologic disease ovine lentiviral encephalitis or visna. This chronic lymphoproliferative disorder affects many organs, the mammary gland being one.

SUGGESTED READINGS

Alves D, McEwen B, Hazlett M et al: Trends in bovine abortions submitted to the Ontario Ministry of Agriculture, Food and Rural Affairs, 1993-1995 *Can Vet J* 37:287-288, 1996.

Boos A, Janssen V, Mulling C: Proliferation and apoptosis in bovine placentomes during pregnancy and around induced and spontaneous parturition as well as in cows retaining the fetal membranes, *Reproduction* 126:469-480, 2003.

Corbeil LB, BonDurant RH: Immunity to bovine reproductive infections, *Vet Clin North Am Food Anim Pract* 17:567-583, 2001.

Dillman RC, Dennis SM: Sequential sterile autolysis in the ovine fetus: macroscopic changes, *Am J Vet Res* 37:403-407, 1976.

Dunne HW. Abortion, stillbirth, fetal death and infectious infertility. In Leman AD, editor: *Diseases of swine*, ed 4, Ames, 1975, Iowa State University Press.

Feldman EC, Nelson RW: *Canine female reproduction in canine and feline endocrinology and reproduction,* ed 3, St Louis, 2004, Saunders.

Giles RC, Donahue, Hong CB et al: Causes of abortion, stillbirth and perinatal death in horses: 3527 cases (1986-1991) *J Am Vet Med Assoc* 203(8):1170-1175, 1993.

Gobello C, Concannon PQ, Verstegen J: Canine pseudopregnancy: a review. In Concannon PW, England G, Verstegen J, editors: *Recent advances in small animal reproduction,* Ithaca, NY, 2001, International Veterinary Information Service (*www.ivis.org*).

Hall MR, Hanks D, Kvasnicka W et al: Diagnosis of epizootic bovine abortion in Nevada and identification of the vector, *J Vet Diagn Invest* 14:205-210, 2002.

Jamakluddin AA, Case JT, Hird DW et al: Dairy cattle abortion in California: evaluation of diagnostic laboratory data, *J Vet Diagn Invest* 8:210-218, 1996.

Kawate N: Studies on the regulation of expression of luteinizing hormone receptor in the ovary and the mechanism of follicular cyst formation in ruminants, *J Reprod Develop* 50:1-8, 2004.

Kerr K, Entrican G, McKeever D et al: Immunopathology of *Chlamydophila abortus* infection in sheep and mice, *Res Vet Sci* 78:1-7, 2005.

Kirkbride CA: Etiologic agents detected in a 10 year study of bovine abortions and stillbirths, *J Vet Diagn Invest* 4:175-180, 1992.

Kirkbride CA: Diagnoses in 1,784 ovine abortions and stillbirths, *J Vet Diagn Invest* 5:398-402, 1993.

Leblanc MM: Persistent mating induced endometritis in the mare: pathogenesis, diagnosis, and treatment. In BA Ball, editor: *Recent advances in equine reproduction,* Ithaca, NY, 2003, International Veterinary Information Service (*www.ivis.org*).

McEntee K: *Reproductive pathology of domestic mammals,* New York, 1990, Academic Press.

Noakes DE, Dhaliwal GK, England GCW: Cystic endometrial hyperplasia/pyometra in dogs: a review of the causes and pathogenesis, *J Reprod Fert Suppl* 57:395-406, 2001.

Peter AT: An update on cystic ovarian degeneration in cattle, *Reprod Dom Anim* 39:1-7, 2004.

Quayle AJ: The innate and early immune response to pathogen challenge in the female genital tract and the pivotal role of epithelial cells, *J Reprod Immunol* 57:61-79, 2002.

Ramadan AA, Johnson III GL, Lewis GS: Regulation of uterine immune function during the estrus cycle and in response to infectious bacteria in sheep, *J Anim Sci* 75:1621-1632, 1997.

Robertson SA: Control of the immunological environment of the uterus, *Rev Reprod* 54:164-174, 2000.

Sordillo LM, Nickerson SC: Morphologic changes in the bovine mammary gland during involution and lactogenesis, *Am J Vet Res* 49:1112-1120, 1988.

Sordillo LM, Streicher KL: Mammary gland immunity and mastitis susceptibility, *J Mammary Gland Biol Neoplasia* 7:135-146, 2002.

Tengelsen LA, Yamini B, Mullany TP et al: A 12-year retrospective study of equine abortion in Michigan, *J Vet Diagn Invest* 9:303-306, 1997.

Thatcher WW, Guiszeloglu A, Mattos et al: Uterine-conceptus interactions and reproductive the failure in cattle, *Theriogenology* 56(9):1435-1450, 2001.

Whitwell KE: Morphology and pathology of the equine umbilical cord, *J Reprod Fert Suppl* 23:599-603, 1975.

Whitwell KE, Jeffcott LB: Morphological studies on the fetal membranes of the normal singleton foal at term, *Res Vet Sci* 19:44-55, 1975.

19

Male Reproductive System*

ROBERT A. FOSTER

The reproductive system is arguably the most important in terms of survival of a species. In production animals, reproduction is essential for the continued supply of product, be it meat, fiber, milk, or any of the many other by-products. Most production animals rely on a small number of males as breeding stock, so in addition to being 50% of the reproductive team, an infertile male or one carrying an undesirable trait can have a major impact.

The male reproductive system usually receives little attention and time; with some exceptions, replacement of a breeding male is often more effective than diagnosis and treatment. Fertility in the male is difficult to reverse unless the cause can be readily found and then corrected. This is where knowledge of the processes, responses to injury, and prognosis are so important.

Companion animals have not been given the same amount of study as production animals, especially the bull and ram. The aim here is to emphasize the diseases of all species and highlight the mechanisms and reactions of the male reproductive tract by examining the diseases of each anatomic location.

INTRODUCTION

ORGANIZATION OF THE MALE REPRODUCTIVE SYSTEM

The male reproductive tract can be separated into three major areas based not only on anatomic location but also on functional characteristics and on important disease processes. The three main areas are the scrotum and its contents, the accessory genital glands, and the penis and prepuce.

---

*Chapters on this subject in earlier editions were written or partially written by Dr. H. Acland of the Pennsylvania Veterinary Laboratory, Harrisburg, Pennsylvania.

THE SCROTUM AND CONTENTS

The purpose of the scrotum and its contents is to supply spermatozoa for transportation to the female. Although the general focus is on the testis and its germinal epithelium contained in the seminiferous tubules, other parts have important functional characteristics that allow this to happen. Testicular development is quiescent until puberty when spermatogenesis begins. The testes therefore are small until puberty, when they increase to their adult size. The testes are covered by a tunica albuginea, which is relatively nonexpansile and usually maintains the testicular contents under slight pressure. Within the testis are the interstitial and intratubular regions. Within the interstitium are the interstitial endocrine cells, blood vessels, lymphatics, and occasional macrophages. Each seminiferous tubule has a lining of myoid cells and a limiting membrane. There is a basement membrane between these structures. The arrangement of the seminiferous tubules varies from species to species, but the end result is the formation of spermatozoa. After spermatogenesis, spermatozoa are transported through rete tubules into the efferent ductules and then into the epididymis, a single and extremely long duct. In doing so, the spermatozoa mature and are concentrated. The pathway out of the scrotal area is through the ductus deferens.

The purpose of the scrotum, tunica vaginalis, and the spermatic cord (ductus deferens, pampiniform plexus, and cremaster muscle) is to protect and maintain spermatogenesis at a temperature slightly lower than body temperature. The testes are raised or lowered, according to ambient temperature, by the cremaster muscle. There is a counter current vascular system that allows the testes to be at a lower temperature than body temperature; the pampiniform plexus assists this process. The pulsatile nature of arterial blood flow is altered in this process to form a continuous but lower pressure system. In addition, the scrotal skin, which is thin, often hairless, and in most species has abundant apocrine sweat glands, helps to maintain a lower testicular and epididymal temperature. The tunica vaginalis, being an outpouching of the peritoneum, allows for free movement of the testes within the scrotal sac. The scrotum is composed of skin, tunica dartos, and scrotal fascia. It is fused with the parietal layer of the tunica vaginalis. The skin has a thin dermis, few hairs, and many apocrine sweat glands.

THE ACCESSORY GENITAL GLANDS

The purpose of the accessory glands is to provide nutrition and a transport medium for spermatozoa. There are four main accessory glands: the ampullae, vesicular glands, prostate, and bulbourethral glands. There is considerable species variation in the size, type, and number of these accessory glands. Ruminants and horses have all four glands, although the prostate of ruminants is either very small (bull) or is disbursed within the pelvic urethra (ram and buck). Pigs lack ampullae, dogs have only a prostate, and cats have a small prostate and bulbourethral glands. The secretion of the vesicular gland and prostate is serous, but the bulbourethral gland typically has a viscous mucoid product.

THE PENIS AND PREPUCE

There is considerable structural difference between the penis and prepuce of the various species. In prepubertal animals, the prepuce is attached to the penis, but they become separated at sexual maturity. The penis of the horse is erectile and is located within a prepuce that produces a thick, waxy material called smegma. Ruminants and pigs have a long fibrous penis that has some erectile tissue. To accommodate a penis of sufficient length, there is a series of bends called the sigmoid flexure, and there is retractor muscle to hold the penis in the prepuce. There is an extension of the urethra in small ruminants that is called the vermiform appendage or the urethral process. This, during ejaculation, spins and sprays semen onto the cervix. The glans of the penis of the boar has a corkscrew shape that allows it to insert into the cervix. The penis of dogs and to a lesser extent cats is erectile and has an os penis. The cat has projections of penile epithelium called spines or barbs on its penis, and they are testosterone dependent.

CELLS OF THE MALE REPRODUCTIVE SYSTEM

The function of the male reproductive system revolves around the production and transportation of spermatozoa. Spermatozoa are formed from germ (stem) cells by a process of spermatogenesis. Spermatogenesis occurs in three stages, the proliferative, meiotic, and spermatogenic stages. The proliferative phase involves the mitotically active spermatogonia. They are present at

the periphery of the seminiferous tubules on the basement membrane. The second phase is the meiotic phase, in which spermatocytes are formed. In the spermatogenic phase, spermatids and finally spermatozoa are formed. Spermatozoa have a head, body, and tail. The head contains the nucleus and an acrosome, which contains enzymes required for the penetration of the zona pellucida. The body or midpiece contains mitochondria and the tail is a flagellum.

Sertoli cells provide support, nutrients, and other environmental factors to allow spermatogenesis to happen. During spermatogenesis, the cells pass into a region that is separated from and external to the immune system of the body. The barrier is called the blood-testis barrier, and it is maintained by the Sertoli cells (Fig. 19-1). Control of spermatogenesis is achieved through a combination of both central (luteinizing hormone [LH] on the interstitial endocrine cells and follicle-stimulating hormone [FSH] of Sertoli cells) and local (paracrine factors, including testosterone) factors, and there is considerable crosstalk between germ cells, Sertoli cells, and

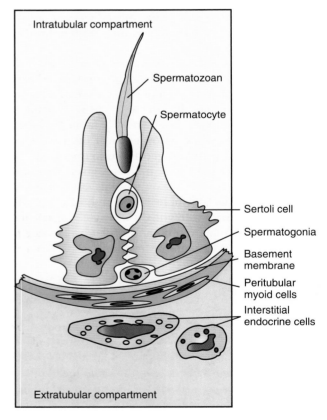

Fig. 19-1   Schematic diagram of the normal components of the testis. The Sertoli cells, germ cells, and interstitial endocrine cells are closely integrated, and considerable messaging occurs between them. The blood-testis barrier is at the level of the Sertoli cells, with contributions from the myoid cells and basement membrane. Spermatogonia are on the interstitial side of the blood-testis barrier.

interstitial endocrine cells. Local modification to spermatogenesis is achieved through apoptosis at any stage of development. Many of the diseases and conditions that affect spermatogenesis increase or decrease the apoptotic rate.

The cells lining the various ducts, including the rete tubules, efferent ductules, and epididymides, are epithelial cells that have a variety of functions in addition to being a barrier. Absorption, phagocytosis, and secretion are all part of their physiologic role. Movement of spermatozoa along these ducts and tubules is achieved through smooth muscle contraction and the cilia.

In the accessory genital glands, storage of spermatozoa (particularly in the ampulla, where present) and secretion of various substances are the major roles for the epithelium of these glands. From the pelvic urethra and through the penile urethra, the lining cells are urothelial in type.

RESPONSES OF THE MALE REPRODUCTIVE SYSTEM TO INJURY

Injury to the male reproductive system comes in many different forms, and there are many potential targets, including the pituitary and endocrine control, interstitial endocrine cells, Sertoli cells, spermatogenic epithelium, and the various ducts. Apart from the obvious redundancy of having bilateral systems, the male reproductive tract has very little functional reserve and cannot undergo compensatory change to any significant degree. Some testicular compensatory hypertrophy is possible and will be discussed later in this chapter.

The formation of spermatic granulomas (Fig. 19-2) is one of the most dramatic and important responses of the male reproductive system to injury. Spermatic granulomas occur with rupture of a duct; spermiostasis and spermatocele are the usual preliminary stages. Spermatozoa are "foreign" to the body. Immunity to spermatozoa with the formation of antisperm antibody is a well-recognized phenomenon. Exposure of tissue to spermatozoa results in a dramatic local inflammatory response. The cell wall constituents and the high chromatin content make them very difficult to degrade. Any injury that exposes spermatozoa to the tissue of the body results in severe inflammation, mostly of a granulomatous type. This can be a foreign body type response, an immunologic response, or both. The inflammation produced is usually chronic and results in severe scarring, which further obstructs tubules and ducts, leading to even more inflammation so that it becomes self-perpetuating. It is therefore critical to prevent such injury.

Injury to the testis can be the result of a primary attack on a target cell or may be secondary to interruption of hormonal regulation, be it systemic or local. The end point of an injury can therefore be far reaching. Regardless of the primary target, most injurious events result in germ cell degeneration and depletion. Germ cells are sensitive, but Sertoli cells are relatively resistant

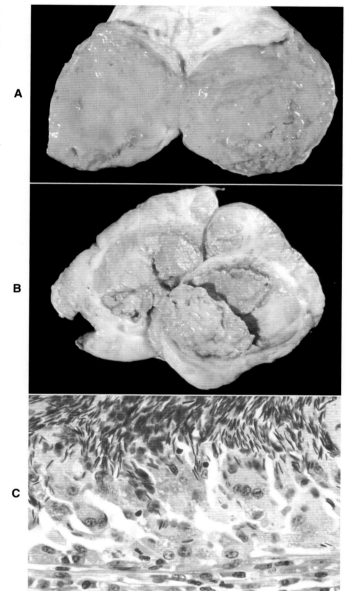

Fig. 19-2   Spermatic granulomas, tail of the epididymis, ram. A, The parenchyma has been replaced by a white-tan, semiliquid spermatic granuloma. These granulomas may be any color from white to red. They are frequently and incorrectly called abscesses. **B,** Multiple encapsulated (chronic) spermatic granulomas with white caseous centers. **C,** A mass of spermatozoa free in the interstitium (*upper*) is surrounded by epithelioid macrophages and multinucleated giant cells, some of which have phagocytosed spermatozoa. Lymphocytes, plasma cells, and fibrous connective tissue surround these granulomas (*lower*). H&E stain. (*A* and *B*, *Courtesy Drs. P. W. Ladds and R. A. Foster, James Cook University of North Queensland.* **C,** *Courtesy Dr. R. A. Foster Ontario Veterinary College, University of Guelph.*)

to injury. As a result, severe injury will often result in seminiferous tubules containing only spermatogonia and Sertoli cells. As Sertoli cells degenerate, they become vacuolated and swollen. Exfoliation of normal germ cells can also occur. The spermatogenic epithelium responds to injury by increasing or decreasing apoptosis, resulting in spermatogenic arrest or a complete failure of spermatogenesis. As long as spermatogonia remain, spermatogenesis can restart. Failure of release of spermatozoa is an early indication of degeneration. The formation of multinucleated spermatid giant cells and phagocytosis of spermatozoa by Sertoli cells occur.

A major effect of injury to interstitial endocrine cells is the failure of the release of testosterone. This can effectively stop spermatogenesis by increasing apoptosis and by inhibiting maturation of spermatids. Direct damage to spermatozoa can affect motility and fertilizing capability. Recovery from injury, while taking time, is achieved by restarting spermatogenesis from the relatively resistant spermatogonia.

The testis is a specialized immunologic environment and has a reduced immune responsiveness, no doubt because of the importance of not developing an immunologic response to germ cells. Unfortunately, if an inflammatory response does occur within the testis, it is likely to be sustained.

Injury to the epididymis can have permanent and devastating effects. Not only can injury affect the functions of the epididymides—including maturation and storage of spermatozoa, resorption of fluid, and secretion of materials—but also severe injury will result in inflammation. Any constriction of the epididymal duct will result in spermiostasis, potential rupture, and the formation of spermatic granulomas. Because the epididymis is very limited in its responses, alteration to the structure and function of the epididymis is often permanent and affects fertility in a dramatic fashion.

Injury to the accessory genital glands it is not common, and they can recover, often with a reduced function. Functional reserve is often sufficient to maintain fertility.

The peritesticular tissues, in particular the tunica vaginalis, is also prone to injury from peritoneal reactions secondary to epididymal disease or from a direct penetrating injury. The reaction of these tissues is identical to that of the peritoneum, and as such, fibrosis and adhesion are a common response. Adhesion can limit the movement of the testes and alter its ability to thermoregulate.

PORTALS OF ENTRY INTO THE MALE REPRODUCTIVE SYSTEM

There are three main portals of entry of infectious and injurious agents to the male reproductive tract (Box 19-1). They include direct penetration and injury, ascending infection, and hematogenous localization.

The external location of the penis, prepuce, and scrotum makes them prone to direct penetrating injury. Surprisingly, this is a relatively rare occurrence.

Box 19-1

Portals of Entry to the Male Reproductive System

Direct penetration
Ascending infection
Hematogenous localization
Peritoneal spread

Ascending infection is relatively common. It occurs sporadically in adults but curiously is particularly a problem in pubertal animals when hormonal changes make the system more prone to infection from bacteria (such as *Actinobacillus seminis* and *Histophilus somni*) that are resident flora of the prepuce of sheep. The accessory genital glands in particular are targets, but there can be further ascension to the epididymis. It is exceedingly rare, because of the long length of the epididymis, for the testis to be involved in ascending infection. The male reproductive tract is also a target of pathogens that are spread by sexual activity. Spread from females or in some circumstances from other males is recognized.

Hematogenous localization is a recognized portal of entry by specific pathogens, such as the various brucellae. The epididymis and the accessory genital glands are particular targets.

The tunica vaginalis is an extension of the peritoneum, being an outpouching of the peritoneal cavity. Any process affecting the peritoneum, be it infectious or neoplastic, will affect the peritesticular tissues.

DEFENSE MECHANISMS OF THE MALE REPRODUCTIVE SYSTEM

The male reproductive tract, and in particular the internal genitalia, is so exquisitely sensitive to injury that it is extremely important to prevent rather than respond to injury. The combined effect of the high antigenicity of spermatozoa and the exceedingly long and very narrow duct system means that there is little tolerance for inflammation, necrosis, or other injurious situations. Much of the reproductive system relies on isolation for protection and the prevention of infection or injury.

INNATE IMMUNITY

There are multiple factors that prevent infection and injury to the vulnerable tissues. The testes and epididymides are hidden from the external environment by their intrascrotal location and by the extremely long and narrow tube that connects them to the outside world. The thin luminal diameter and extreme length of the ductus deferens makes ascending infection unlikely. There is almost continuous flow of fluid along the ductus deferens and the epididymis, and so the flushing action is protective. Even the accessory genital glands are protected by the flushing action of urine and by the extremely long length of the urethra in species such as ruminants and the pig.

Testicular and epididymal fluid has antibacterial properties. The high chlorine content may be partially responsible. Antimicrobial proteins in seminal plasma are numerous and include bovine seminalplasmin, lactoferrin, and β-defensins. Most of these are acquired in the epididymis, where they are bound to spermatozoa. There are also numerous cytokines normally produced in the tract. Epithelial cells of the reproductive tract have physical barrier proteins, including mucin, that prevent infection.

Nonspecific cellular defenses are relatively few. Neutrophils are not normally present in seminal plasma but can infiltrate rapidly if required. Macrophages are present within tissue and particularly within the testes, where they are recruited and maintained by the interstitial endocrine cells. Their presence inhibits immune response (by producing tolerance). Little is known of the presence of natural killer cells in the male reproductive tract.

ADAPTIVE IMMUNITY

Much of the reproductive tract can produce an adaptive immune response if called upon to do so. Where it is important is in the more distal portions of the tract, particularly the accessory genital glands and the prepuce. Unfortunately, development of an adaptive response in the testis and the epididymis is often "too little, too late." Also, development of adaptive responses in the testis is inhibited by local immunosuppressive factors. This does not, however, prevent adaptive immunity from developing in the testis. The epididymis and ductus deferens do not have a developed mucosal immune system, but there is evidence that such a system exists in the accessory genital glands, particularly the ampulla and bulbourethral glands. When infection occurs, local immunity and transfer of serum immunoglobulin is present. Preputial immunity is also mediated by local humoral and cellular mechanisms. Immunoglobulin G (IgG)- and IgA-based systems are present. Little is known of cell-mediated immune mechanisms in the male reproductive tract.

Using local immunity to protect against infectious disease, particularly those important sexually transmitted diseases, has had little success. Response to vaccination has been variable with some individuals having protective immunity, particularly with *Campylobacter fetus* infection in bulls. Systemic immunity to reproductive disease has also been of variable effectiveness. Although protecting against systemic infection, challenge to the reproductive tract has in some instances increased the response to the infection and caused more damage than would normally occur.

INFLAMMATION OF THE MALE REPRODUCTIVE SYSTEM

In general terms, inflammation of the male reproductive tract is similar to that of other systems. What is unique about the male genital tract is inflammation to spermatozoa. Spermatozoa and germ cells outside the blood-testis barrier are antigenic. There are also antigenic components within seminal fluid. Spermatozoa have antigens that attract immune cells, and they also nonspecifically bind immunoglobulin. These reactions can have a minimal effect on the tissues directly and act by agglutinating spermatozoa or by opsonization. In some instances, the effect is much more dramatic and immunization against spermatozoa can result in a severe inflammatory response. This inflammation can be local or spermatozoa can be "attacked" in those areas where the tissue-spermatozoal barrier is the weakest. In many species, this is the region of the efferent ductule and the epididymis. This so-called autoimmune reaction to spermatozoa can be experimentally created, but a clinical correlate is infrequent. Local effects, however, are much more recognized. Direct damage to testicular parenchyma can result in granulomatous inflammation centered on the seminiferous tubules, the so-called intratubular orchitis. Where spermatozoa are exposed to the tissues of the body, the reaction is that of granulomatous inflammation. Macrophages and multinucleate giant cells are found adjacent to spermatozoa (Fig. 19-2, C). Initially at least, CD4+ T cells are abundant. Immunoglobulin-producing cells, particularly IgG-containing cells, are found. Granulomas are formed with the characteristic appearance of layers of epithelioid macrophages with multinucleate giant cells and then lymphocytes and plasma cells with a surrounding layer of fibrous tissue. In advanced cases, inspissated spermatozoa are found within a fibrous capsule. The production of a fibrous capsule and resultant contraction leads to further obstruction of the various ducts and tubules, with the result that additional spermiostasis, spermatocele, and spermatic granuloma formation continues. This inflammation therefore has devastating affects on fertility. Further complications occur if spermatozoa are released into the cavity of the tunica vaginalis because a severe periorchitis develops and results in fibrosis and the lack of ability to adequately thermoregulate the testes.

DISEASES OF THE MALE REPRODUCTIVE SYSTEM

There are many different ways to approach diseases of the male reproductive system (see Appendix 19-1). Each approach has its own advantages and disadvantages. Some of the diseases affect more than one region, yet there are many diseases that have a primary manifestation in one or more areas. Approaching diseases from a pathogenetic viewpoint is logical; however, it does not always account for clinical relevance or assist in the correlation between clinical signs and prognosis. We will approach diseases based on their anatomic location, that being scrotal contents, accessory genital glands, and the penis and prepuce, because this is more clinically relevant. Before doing so, it is prudent to examine ambiguous sexual development because this forms a distinct category.

ANOMALIES, INTERSEX, AND AMBIGUOUS DEVELOPMENT

There are a large number of anomalies of the male reproductive system (Box 19-2). Some have clinical relevance and others do not. Differentiating between these is very important. Some of the anomalies represent the most common disease of a particular species. Where this is the case, the disease will be handled under diseases of a particular anatomic location because this is the most clinically relevant place. We have attempted to divide the various anomalies into those that are major and minor based on effects on fertility and on the future breeding potential of the animal. Some anomalies have a genetic basis and such individuals should not be used as a stud animal, even though the animal may still be fertile.

Box **19-2**

Selected Congenital Anomalies

MAJOR ANOMALIES

Cryptorchidism
Testicular hypoplasia
Spermatic granuloma of the epididymal head
Ambiguous genitalia
- Tricolor cat (chimera)
- Persistent Müllerian duct syndrome
- Testicular feminization syndrome

Immotile cilia syndrome
Segmental aplasia of mesonephric duct

MINOR ANOMALIES

Inclusion cysts
Remnants of mesonephric ducts
- Paradidymis interna and externa

Remnants of paramesonephric (Müllerian) ducts
- Appendix testis
- Cystic uterus masculinus

Hypospadias
Retained preputial band

MALE EMBRYOLOGY

In males, the differentiation of a gonad to a testis is dependent on the presence of a sex-determining region of the Y chromosome (SRY) that codes for a testis-determining factor and on other genes that cause the germ cells to go into mitotic arrest. Supporting cells become the Sertoli cells, the steroid-producing cells become the interstitial endocrine cells of Leydig, and the mesenchyme develops the appearance of a testis. Further development requires the activation of many other genes that are not on the Y chromosome. The expression of SRY occurs briefly in the somatic cells of the indifferent gonads (or genital ridges). Because expression ceases shortly before Sertoli cells can be recognized, it is proposed that the functional gene product of SRY influences other genes, such as Sox9, that ensure the differentiation and maintenance of Sertoli cells. Sox9 is up-regulated in XY individuals just before gonadal differentiation. Sertoli cells signal the other supporting cell precursor lines to differentiate along the male pathway. Early in sex differentiation, the embryo has a double set of ducts. The paramesonephric (Müllerian) ducts are female precursors, arising by invagination of the celomic cavity. The mesonephric (Wolffian) tubules and ducts are male precursors, arising from the primitive kidney, the mesonephros. The rete testis and efferent ductules are derived from mesonephric tubules. There are about 20 efferent ductules, although the number varies with species. The epididymis is derived from the part of the mesonephric duct within the mesonephros. The ductus deferens, ampulla, and vesicular gland are derived from the distal part of the mesonephric duct, outside the mesonephros (Fig. 19-3).

After germ cells migrate from the yolk sac and the testes develop in the tissue of the genital ridge, the testes produce two hormones. Sertoli cells secrete the polypeptide hormone Müllerian-inhibiting substance (MIS) during embryonic development and at lower concentrations postnatally. MIS causes regression of the ipsilateral paramesonephric duct, indirectly through action on mesenchymal tissue. Sertoli cells stimulate differentiation of interstitial endocrine cells from the cells of the interstitium. Interstitial endocrine cells secrete the steroid hormone testosterone, which causes persistence and differentiation of the mesonephric ducts. Testosterone is likely transported down the mesonephric ducts rather than moving by simple diffusion. A third hormone, dihydrotestosterone, which is a metabolite of testosterone, is required for formation of the prostate gland, the closing of the urethral folds, and the formation of the penis and scrotum. The enzyme steroid 5α-reductase is produced by cells in the urogenital sinus, genital tubercle, and genital swellings and reduces testosterone to dihydrotestosterone. Functional androgen

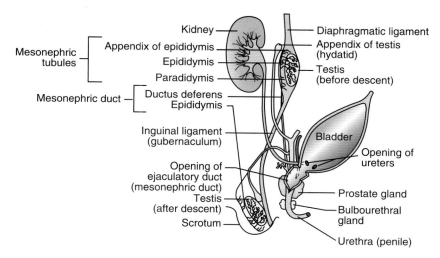

Fig. 19-3   Schematic diagram of the normal components of the male reproductive system and the embryonic structures, especially the mesonephric (Wolffian) duct and urogenital sinus and tubercle, from which they were derived. The rete tubules and efferent ductules are formed from the mesonephric ductules; the epididymis, ductus deferens, ampullae, and vesicular glands form from the mesonephric duct; the prostate and bulbourethral glands form from the urogenital sinus; and the penis, prepuce, and scrotum form from the genital tubercle and swellings.

receptors on target tissues are necessary for androgen-dependent differentiation and growth. Species differences exist in whether the production of testosterone by interstitial endocrine cells is under the control of gonadotropin produced by the fetal pituitary gland or the placenta. Fetal interstitial cells are replaced by postnatal interstitial cells, which are relatively quiescent until puberty. The production of testosterone is regulated by LH, which is under the control of LH-releasing hormone (LHRH) from the hypothalamus. Also under the control of LHRH is FSH, which is produced by the anterior pituitary gland. FSH regulates the activity of Sertoli cells and can thus influence MIS production. Sertoli cells stimulated by FSH produce a glycoprotein, androgen-binding protein, which fosters high testosterone concentration around the germ cells for the progression of spermatogenesis.

The external genitalia form when the genital tubercle is masculinized by the presence of androgens. Elongation of the tubercle forms the phallus; opposing urethral folds form the penile urethra; and the genital swellings fuse to form the scrotum.

TESTICULAR DESCENT

The testes and epididymides undergo descent from their original location to the scrotum. There are two main phases in testicular descent: the intraabdominal and the inguinal-scrotal phases. The developing gonads are held in place by cranial and caudal ligaments. The caudal ligament, the primitive gubernaculum testis, attaches the developing testis to the site of the inguinal canal. It develops into an intraabdominal and extraabdominal part that protrudes into the scrotum. Evagination of the peritoneum forms the inguinal canal and the tunica vaginalis.

With the intraabdominal phase particularly, stimulation of gubernaculum mesenchymal cells may be controlled by a low molecular weight factor that resembles the insulin-like peptide hormone INSL3. The receptor for INSL appears to be LGR8. Other molecules are also involved. Exposure to estrogen-like compounds will inhibit testicular descent. The exact mechanisms are yet to be elucidated, but they will no doubt be complex and involve an interrelationship of systemic and local factors.

The inguinoscrotal phase of testicular descent is mediated by the hypothalamopituitary-induced production of gonadal androgens. Having said this, domestic animals with failure of testicular descent into the scrotum seldom have hypogonadotropic hypogonadism. Other factors, such as a balance between androgen receptors and estrogen receptors, affect the genitofemoral nerve, and calcitonin gene–related proteins or binding sites might be involved.

MAJOR ANOMALIES

The most common and important major anomaly of the male reproductive system is failure of testicular descent, or cryptorchidism. Testicular hypoplasia and segmental aplasia of the epididymis are a close second.

These diseases and conditions will be discussed further under diseases of the testis. Much less common, but nevertheless important, are other diseases of sexual ambiguity and intersex.

SEXUAL AMBIGUITY AND INTERSEX

Errors of chromosomal, gonadal, or phenotypic sex are usually manifested by abnormalities in sexual dimorphism. Many of the abnormalities result in a female phenotype and are mentioned in more detail in Chapter 18. We will deal with those diseases that involve genotypic males, animals that have male gonads, or predominantly phenotypic males. One cannot always tell the underlying cause of sexual ambiguity by examining phenotype or even identifying the gonadal type. Complete definition of an anomaly requires knowledge of all three components: chromosomal, gonadal, and phenotypic types.

Sex chromosomes can be abnormal in structure or number. Two examples of abnormal structure of the Y chromosome are deletion of the short arm and isochromosome formation (duplication of one arm and loss of the other). Affected individuals have a female phenotype and extremely hypoplastic gonads. A few cattle have been identified with an isochromosome Y. With duplication of one of the sex chromosomes in an individual with a Y chromosome (XYY or XXY), or a mosaic (as occurs with the calico or tricolor male cats), the external genitalia are male in character. Klinefelter's syndrome (XXY) is discussed under testicular hypoplasia. Chimeras, such as XX/XY, are phenotypically sexually ambiguous, and the degree depends on the relative amounts of each chromosome.

Animals with an XY genotype may have an abnormality of gonadal sex. Hermaphrodites have abnormal gonads, and the gonads possess both testicular and ovarian tissue. There can be a separate testis and ovary, or one or both gonads can be mixed. The mixed organ is termed an ovotestis. Some ovotestes have an end-to-end arrangement of ovarian and testicular tissue, with clear demarcation between the two. Others have central testicular tissue with a periphery of ovarian structures. Bilateral hermaphrodites have an ovotestis on each side; unilateral hermaphrodites have an ovotestis on one side; and lateral hermaphrodites have a testis on one side and an ovary on the other. The genital tract in hermaphrodites is ambiguous. Hermaphrodites occur in canine, porcine, and caprine XX sex reversals and bovine freemartin XX/XY chimeras. In many other cases, the basic mechanism for the production of hermaphrodites is unknown.

Sex reversal is the term used when the gonad is not the type corresponding to the XX or XY chromosomal makeup of the individual. XX males have been identified in several species, and they have a testis-determining region on another chromosome. They are discussed under the female system. XY females are rare, but they have been identified in mice, horses, and human beings and have a deletion or mutation of the testis-determining region of the Y chromosome. XY females have hypogonadotropic hypogonadism with no secondary sexual characteristics. The gonad is a streak of ovarian stroma.

Male pseudohermaphrodites have abnormalities of phenotypic sex. Individuals that are clearly male with respect to their chromosomes (XY) and gonads (testes), but whose reproductive tract's phenotypic appearance is ambiguous, are termed male pseudohermaphrodites (Figs. 19-4 and 19-5). The differentiation of the tract can be slightly or greatly abnormal. In many cases, the mechanism for the abnormal differentiation is unknown. Ample scope exists for deficiencies in enzymes, hormones, or receptors to cause imperfect differentiation of the tract to match the gonads.

Three such syndromes in which the pathogenesis is understood are persistent Müllerian duct syndrome (PMDS), androgen insensitivity, and steroid 5α-reductase deficiency.

PMDS is a rare disorder of Müllerian inhibitory substance (MIS) production or function. MIS can be absent or present in affected human beings, with the syndrome being a result of either a mutation in the MIS gene or the MIS gene receptor. In animals, the syndrome

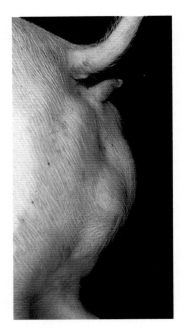

Fig. 19-4   Male pseudohermaphrodite, external genitalia, boar. This pig has a scrotum and intrascrotal testes, but the penis is small and clitoris-like and has a terminal urethral opening (ventral to the tail). *(Courtesy Dr. D. Dodd; and Noah's Arkive, College of Veterinary Medicine, The University of Georgia.)*

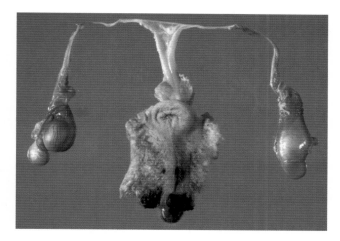

Fig. 19-5   Male pseudohermaphrodite (male feminization syndrome), reproductive tract, ram. This sheep has testes, ductus deferentes, and accessory genital glands but also a vulva and a prominent clitoris. An androgen receptor defect would explain these anomalies. *(Courtesy Ontario Veterinary College, University of Guelph.)*

is described in miniature schnauzer dogs with an autosomal recessive mode of inheritance, and in a goat with unknown mode of inheritance. Affected dogs have XY (or XXY) chromosomes and externally are normal males with the common exception of unilateral or bilateral cryptorchidism. The testes, however, are attached to the cranial ends of uterine horns. When a testis has descended into the scrotum, the uterine horn passes through the inguinal ring. Ductus deferentes can be found microscopically within the myometrium. The cranial vagina and the prostate gland are often present. MIS is present in the testes of normal male dogs up to 143 days of age. MIS is present in the testes of young affected dogs also and is bioactive. A mutation in the structural gene for the MIS receptor results in MIS resistance in PMDS-affected dogs. Dogs with unilateral or bilateral scrotal testes can be fertile. Sertoli cell tumor, hydrometra, and pyometra are diseases to which PMDS-affected dogs are subject. Testicular abnormalities in PMDS, such as reduced spermatogenesis and tubular sclerosis, could be attributable to cryptorchidism. Cryptorchidism could be due to interference with the MIS-controlled first phase of the function of the gubernaculums, the phase in which the testis migrates to the inguinal area.

Deficiency of 5α-reductase type 2, inherited as an autosomal recessive trait in human beings, has not yet been documented in animals, but in all likelihood exists. The enzyme converts testosterone to dihydrotestosterone, which is required for the masculinization of the urogenital sinus, tubercle, and genital swellings. Without dihydrotestosterone, these structures become caudal vagina, vestibule, clitoris, and vulva. Internally,

mesonephric structures (ductus deferens, epididymis) develop. The testes are likely to be retained.

Androgen receptor disorders are becoming increasingly recognized as causes of male pseudohermaphroditism. Most cases are due to a mutation in the androgen receptor gene, which is located on the X chromosome and thus in a single copy. Hundreds of mutations have been identified, and the effects range from complete androgen insensitivity with female external genitalia (testicular feminization) (Fig. 19-5) to mild male pseudohermaphroditism. Affected individuals are chromosomally male and have testes. The testes produce testosterone, but the stimulation of the mesonephric system is not normal because of defective androgen receptors. The normal androgen receptor has a hormone-binding and a DNA-binding domain; once activated by androgen, the domain changes shape and is able to bind to specific DNA sequences and regulate the transcription of other specific genes, leading to normal male differentiation. In human beings with androgen insensitivity, the gene is rarely deleted, but numerous point mutations in the receptor gene have been identified, mostly in the hormone-binding and DNA-binding domains. Whether the result is partial or complete androgen insensitivity depends on the location of the mutation and the change in function of the receptor. Dihydrotestosterone binds to the androgen receptor with greater affinity than that of testosterone, and the receptor, when it acts as a transcriptional factor, might interact with different genes other than the testosterone-bound receptor. In domestic animals, complete androgen insensitivity has been described in the equine, bovine, and feline species. The testes are often cryptorchid and are in the inguinal area. The first phase of testicular migration is normal. The inguinoscrotal second phase, which is under the control of androgens, does not occur. MIS produced by the testes causes regression of the paramesonephric ducts. External genitalia are female in complete androgen insensitivity, with a cranial blind end to the vagina, and neither the paramesonephric nor mesonephric ductal system is present.

SEGMENTAL APLASIA OF MESONEPHRIC DUCT DERIVATIVES

Segmental aplasia of the structures of mesonephric ductal origin (epididymis, ductus deferens, ampulla, or vesicular gland) can involve any of the structures but most commonly involves the epididymis alone (Fig. 19-6), and less commonly other structures. Segmental aplasia is reported mainly in the bull and most commonly involves the body and tail of the epididymis and is unilateral. Its inheritance is thought to be autosomal recessive. Spermatozoa become impacted because the epididymal duct is blind ending; local dilation or rupture occurs secondarily, allowing escape of spermatozoa and formation of spermatic granulomas.

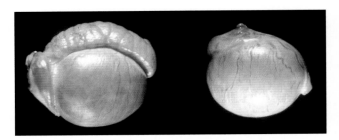

Fig. 19-6   Segmental aplasia, epididymis, dog. There is no tail of the epididymis of the right testis. This portion of the mesonephric duct did not develop. The left testis is normal. *(Courtesy College of Veterinary Medicine, University of Illinois.)*

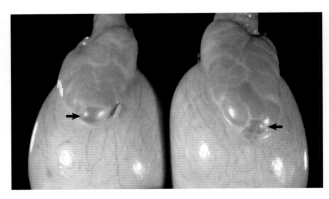

Fig. 19-7   Congenital inclusion cysts, testis and epididymis, ram. These 7-mm cysts *(arrows)* in the tissue between the head of the epididymis and testis are incidental findings and are not significant. *(Courtesy Drs. P. W. Ladds and R. A. Foster, James Cook University of North Queensland.)*

IMMOTILE CILIA SYNDROME

One or more of several defects in the axoneme of cilia throughout the body and of the flagellum of spermatozoa causes immotile cilia syndrome, a rare disease identified in human beings, dogs, pigs, mice, and rats. An autosomal recessive mode of inheritance is proposed. In dogs, heterogeneity of ultrastructural abnormalities of microtubule doublets and their dynein arms or central microtubules is reported. The effect on the reproductive system is immotile or hypomotile spermatozoa caused by flagellar lesions or to oligospermia (a subnormal concentration of spermatozoa) or azoospermia (no spermatozoa), presumably because of defective cilia in the epididymis and ductus deferens. Because of defective cilia in the nasal mucosa, bronchial and bronchiolar mucosa, and ependyma, commonly associated lesions are rhinitis, bronchopneumonia, bronchiectasis, and hydrocephalus. Also associated is situs inversus, but the pathogenesis of the reversal of the normal left and right orientation of organs is unclear. Female infertility is related to defective function of cilia of the uterine tube.

MINOR ANOMALIES

There are a myriad of minor of anomalies and they are of little consequence except when they are confused with other conditions that do affect fertility. Foremost of the minor anomalies are the various cysts that occur as a result of duplication or failure of regression of embryonic ducts and tubules.

CYSTS OF THE MALE TRACT

It is often difficult to identify the origin of an individual cyst or group of cysts. In many instances, anatomic location is the determining factor. Many of the cysts are simply called "inclusion cysts" (Fig. 19-7). These have a wall of compressed collagen, a thin lining of flattened cells, and a clear fluid content. They are found where mesothelial cells are trapped adjacent to a serosal surface. Inclusion cysts attached to the head of the epididymis are good examples.

The testis is derived from gonadal cords that form between the gonadal ridge on the medial side of the mesonephros and remnants of mesonephric tubules. The rete testis and efferent ductules are derived from mesonephric tubules. Within the mesonephros, many mesonephric tubules enter the single mesonephric duct. It is from the within the mesonephric part of the duct that the epididymis is derived. The ductus deferens, ampulla, and vesicular gland are derived from the more caudal part of the mesonephric duct, outside the mesonephros. In the developed testis, about 20 efferent ductules are found, but the number varies with the species. Efferent ductules normally link in the head of the epididymis. Blind efferent ductules result when there is no connection to the epididymis and can be resorbed or persist and enlarge to form cysts or rupture. Blind-ending efferent ductules can be present in sufficient numbers to cause spermiostasis, spermatocele, and spermatic granulomas. The condition known as spermatic granuloma of the epididymal head (SGEH; see later discussion) is thus formed.

Unconnected with the lumen of the epididymal duct and efferent ductules, remnants of tubules of the mesonephros can form cysts adjacent to the head of the epididymis (paradidymis externus) or within the head of the epididymis (paradidymis internus). Cysts, both connected and unconnected with the ductular system, are lined by ciliated columnar epithelium. They are clinically significant if they become large enough to cause stasis of spermatozoa in adjacent structures, or if they rupture and liberate spermatozoa into the surrounding tissue. Of no clinical significance is the remnant of the paramesonephric duct, called the appendix testis, located on the cranial or cranioventral surface (depending on the species orientation of the testes) of the testis near the head of the epididymis. Sometimes this small nodule of tissue can appear cystic. A similar

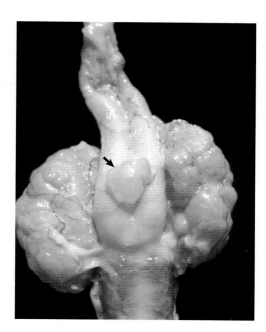

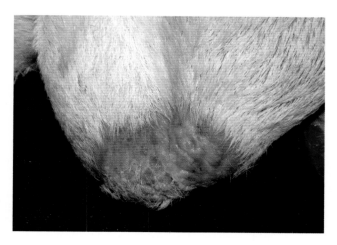

Fig. 19-9   Frostbite, scrotum, ram. The skin of the lower portion of the scrotal sac has sloughed. The ventral scrotal skin is alopecic, or covered by crusts from previous frostbite. *(Courtesy Dr. R. A. Foster, Ontario Veterinary College, University of Guelph.)*

Fig. 19-8   Cystic uterus masculinus, accessory genital glands, ram. This sheep has a 1-cm thin-walled cyst in the tissue between the ampullae of the ductus deferentes *(arrow)*. *(Courtesy Drs. P. W. Ladds and R. A. Foster, James Cook University of North Queensland.)*

cystic structure is found in the band of tissue between the ampullae. It is called the cystic uterus masculinus (Fig. 19-8). Some prostatic cysts of dogs have a similar origin.

DISEASES OF THE SCROTUM AND CONTENTS

The approach to the diseases of the scrotal contents is based on a clinical approach where the scrotal skin, then the vaginal tunics are examined before the testis and epididymis. The most important diseases, though, are those that affect the testis and epididymis. We should not forget the importance of diseases of the scrotal skin and tunics, if not for their direct effects on thermoregulation, but also because they can be confused with disease of the testis, epididymis, or spermatic cord.

THE SCROTUM

The fusion of the paired primordia of scrotal skin depends on hormones produced by cells of the gonad after it has differentiated into a testis. Disturbances in the formative stages can lead to various defects in the scrotum, such as failure of fusion, cleft formation, or bifurcation of the scrotum. Defects can be local, confined to the scrotum and penis, or part of a wider range of defects in an intersex animal. Hypospadias, where the urethra opens on the ventral side of the penis, can be part of these anomalies.

Dermatitis of the scrotal skin is common. Often it is nonspecific or involved in generalized dermatopathies. Dermatitis restricted to the scrotum can be the result of trauma, frostbite (Fig. 19-9), or exposure to environmental irritants, such as cement dust. Some pathogens have the scrotum as a predilection site. These include *Dermatophilus congolensis* and *Besnoitia besnoiti* in the bull, and *Chorioptes bovis* in the ram (Fig. 19-10). The heat generated in scrotal dermatitis can interfere with the thermoregulatory function of the scrotum, leading to testicular degeneration.

Neoplasms of any of the types that occur in the skin can occur in the scrotum, but are much less common in the scrotal skin. Neoplasms occasionally encountered are mast cell tumors, melanomas, and hemangiomas in

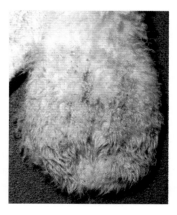

Fig. 19-10   Scrotal dermatitis (*Chorioptes bovis*), scrotum, ram. There is extensive crusting and exudation of the skin in response to the chronic irritation and inflammation caused by the mites. *(Courtesy Dr. R. A. Foster Ontario Veterinary College, University of Guelph.)*

the dog and papillomas in the boar. Testicular tumors occur in the scrotum of previously castrated males, presumably from cells inadvertently transplanted at surgery. Vascular abnormalities, which are probably hamartomas, occur on the scrotum of the boar and dog. The scrotal veins of bulls sometimes become varicose.

TUNICA VAGINALIS

The tunica vaginalis is the extension of the peritoneum that lines the scrotal sac as the parietal layer and covers the testis, epididymis, and spermatic cord as the visceral layer. The cavity between the two layers is continuous with the peritoneal cavity. The tunics and the cavity thus are subject to all the diseases of the peritoneum and peritoneal cavity. Neoplastic lesions are uncommon; mesothelioma is the most frequently encountered. Parasitic disease, especially the cysts of *Cysticercus tenuicollis* in rams occurs periodically and can be confused with cysts or spermatic granulomas.

Inflammation of the tunica vaginalis as part of a systemic disease, such as feline infectious peritonitis, will have the characteristics of that disease. Inflammation of the tunica vaginalis without initial inflammation of the abdominal peritoneum can be the result of trauma or infection. The latter is likely to be an extension from epididymitis. Especially well-known causes are *Brucella ovis* and *Actinobacillus seminis* in rams, and trypanosomes in bulls, rams, and male goats. In general, traumatic inflammation of the tunica vaginalis is mild and focal, and inflammation with an infectious cause is severe and diffuse. Adhesions between the parietal and visceral tunica vaginalis, also called periorchitis, are fibrinous at first and later fibrous.

TESTIS AND EPIDIDYMIS

The testis and epididymis are inseparable, and disease of one usually results in disease of the other. Scrotal palpation is the main clinical method for identification of abnormalities of this region, and the changes in size are usually the most obvious. We will therefore approach disease from a size approach, beginning with those that cause small scrotal contents, then with those that result in enlargement of one or more of the intrascrotal structures (Box 19-3).

Missing or aplastic components are rare. Segmental aplasia of the mesonephric duct, usually aplasia of the epididymal tail (Fig. 19-6), is one example. It is described earlier under major anomalies. If one side of the scrotal contents is missing, unilateral castration may have been performed or the affected animal may have been a unilateral cryptorchid. The maldescended testis and epididymis subsequently descended, or the castration operator may have missed a testis and epididymis. Affected sheep, for example, often have had the scrotum removed and the testis is located beneath the

---

Box **19-3**

Intrascrotal Disease-Based Differences in Size

DECREASED SIZE

Cryptorchidism
Hypoplasia
Testicular degeneration
Segmental aplasia

INCREASED SIZE (INCLUDING MASSES)

Spermatic granuloma of epididymal head
Epididymitis
Orchitis
Periorchitis
Testicular neoplasia
- Seminoma, teratoma
- Sertoli cell tumor
- Interstitial cell tumor
Congenital cysts
Varicocele
Torsion
Inguinal hernia
Scrotal lymphadenopathy

---

underlying skin. A lack of both sides of the scrotal contents can represent castration or bilateral cryptorchidism and requires additional investigation, including measurements of hormonal concentrations, especially after treatment with gonadotrophin-releasing hormone, or surgical exploration. Searching for secondary characteristics that are testosterone dependent, such as the barbs on the penis of the cat, and the presence of a prostate in dogs, can be of assistance in separating behavioral characteristics from similar behaviors in incompletely castrated males.

CRYPTORCHIDISM

A small testicular size is of great importance, especially to production animals, as daily sperm output is correlated to testicular volume and weight. A small size indicates hypoplasia or atrophy. It can be extremely difficult to differentiate these unless there is a history of size change. Hypoplasia is a congenital condition in which the testis does not increase to its full size at puberty. It is often seen as part of other syndromes, most commonly cryptorchidism. Cryptorchidism is incomplete descent of the testis (normal testicular descent is discussed earlier). In most mammalian species, the testis normally has descended into the scrotum by the time of birth. Cryptorchidism is more often unilateral than bilateral, with the side being somewhat species dependent. Many maldescended testes are on the right side. In the horse, the distribution of maldescent is equally distributed left to right, and in the bull, cryptorchidism

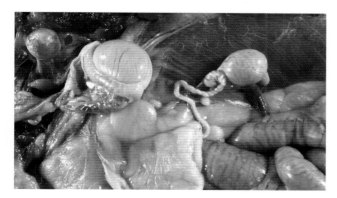

Fig. 19-11   Cryptorchid testis, intraabdominal, dog. The retained testis and epididymis (*right*) are hypoplastic (small). The other descended testis (*left*) is normal. Intestines are below the right testis. *(Courtesy Dr. Y. Niyo, College of Veterinary Medicine, Iowa State University; and Noah's Arkive, College of Veterinary Medicine, The University of Georgia.)*

epididymal differentiation is slowed in many cases of cryptorchidism.

Cryptorchidism is the most common disorder of sexual development in the dog and cat; it occurs in as many as 13% of male dogs. It may have a genetic basis and a reasonable working hypothesis is a sex-limited autosomal recessive mode of inheritance. It has been suggested that one gene might control internal testicular descent, and placement of the epididymis and ductus deferens and another gene might control external testicular descent.

In the horse, left and right testicular retention are almost equal in occurrence and the left retained testis is more likely to be abdominal than inguinal in location. Three breeds (Percheron, American saddle horse, and American quarter horse), ponies, and crossbred horses were significantly overrepresented in a large hospital-based study of cryptorchidism.

Abnormalities in the gubernaculum could cause cryptorchidism by its failure to develop, improper positioning, excessive growth, or failure to regress. Some other possible predisposing or contributing factors for cryptorchidism include testicular hypoplasia, estrogen exposure in pregnancy, breech labor compromising blood supply to the testes, and late closing of the umbilicus, delaying the ability to increase abdominal pressure.

usually affects the left side. The undescended testis can be anywhere along its path from caudal to the kidney (Figs. 19-11 and 19-12, *A*) to the scrotum, including just inside the inguinal ring and just outside the inguinal ring, but not in the scrotal sac. Epididymal differentiation is coordinated with testicular descent, and consequently,

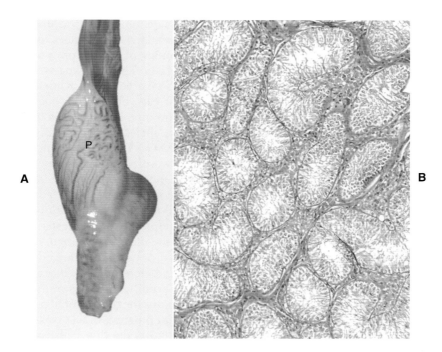

Fig. 19-12   Cryptorchid testis. A, Cryptorchild testis and epididymis, bull calf. The testis and epididymis are hypoplastic and are barely larger than the pampiniform plexus above (*P*). There are no attachments to the tunica vaginalis. **B,** Cryptorchid testis, dog. There is complete absence of spermatogenesis; however, the Sertoli cells are normal. H&E stain. (*A, Courtesy Dr. R.A. Foster, Ontario Veterinary College, University of Guelph. B, Courtesy Dr. J.A. Ramos-Vara, College of Veterinary Medicine, Michigan State University; and Noah's Arkive, College of Veterinary Medicine, The University of Georgia.)*

Atrophy occurs in the cryptorchid testis after puberty. The testis is small and fibrotic and has interstitial collagen deposition, hyaline thickening of the tubular basement membranes, and degeneration of germinal epithelium so that only a few spermatogonia remain along with the normal complement of Sertoli cells (Fig. 19-12, B). Spermatogenesis is dependent on the relatively cool scrotal temperature. Apoptosis (programmed cell death) of germ cells in the higher temperature environment of the abdomen is probably mediated by the regulatory protein p53. Interstitial endocrine cells appear relatively more numerous than in descended testes.

Cryptorchid testes are much more prone to neoplasia than scrotally placed ones. In the dog, Sertoli cell tumors are more likely to occur in the testes present in the abdomen (Fig. 19-13), whereas seminomas tend to develop more commonly in inguinally placed testes. The contralateral testis is also at increased risk for developing a neoplasm, even if the testis is located in the scrotum. A retained testis, especially if enlarged by a neoplasm, is prone to torsion.

Sexually ambiguous or intersex individuals (both hermaphrodites and pseudohermaphrodites) commonly have cryptorchid testes. The greater the ratio of testicular to ovarian tissue, the more likely an ovotestis will have descended into the scrotum. A testis most often lies in the scrotum, and an ovary is in its normal position. The ovary or ovarian portion of an ovotestis is histologically normal, but the seminiferous tubules of a testis or ovotestis are abnormal because of a combination of

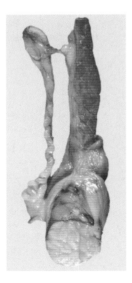

Fig. 19-13   Sertoli cell tumor, cryptorchid testis, dog. The testicular parenchyma has been replaced by a white multilobular neoplasm. The texture is firm, indicating fibrosis. This dog had bilaterally retained testes and epididymides and bilateral Sertoli cell tumors. *(Courtesy Dr. R. A. Foster, Ontario Veterinary College, University of Guelph.)*

cryptorchidism and the effects of estrogen produced by the ovarian tissue. Except for a few cases of scrotal testes, the tubules of testis or ovotestis are lined by Sertoli cells with only rare spermatogonia.

HYPOPLASIA

Hypoplasia of the testes is a very common condition, and it is often present in anomalies such as cryptorchidism and sexual ambiguity. We will deal specifically with the condition of hypoplasia of the testis and epididymis in an otherwise normal male.

It is difficult to distinguish hypoplasia from testicular atrophy by using morphologic features. Both testicular hypoplasia and atrophy can occur alone, with no apparent contributing or influencing factors; either can also be associated with, secondary to, or part of some other lesion. Testicular and epididymal hypoplasia (Fig. 19-14, A and B) has been causally related to poor general nutrition, zinc deficiency, specific genes in the Swedish red and white breed of cattle, and endocrine and cytogenetic abnormalities. Endocrine disturbances causing testicular hypoplasia are those related to reduced production of either luteinizing hormone by the pituitary gland, which in turn influences testosterone production by the interstitial endocrine cells, or follicle-stimulating hormone by the pituitary gland, which stimulates the nurturing function of the Sertoli cells.

A wide range of cytogenetic abnormalities, from translocations and mosaics to nondisjunctions causing polysomies of sex chromosomes, result in testicular hypoplasia. The best known example of polysomy is the XXY karyotype of Klinefelter's syndrome seen in tricolor cats, bulls, dogs, boars, and stallions. In cats, the syndrome is recognized in males with the tricolor, tortoise shell, or calico coat types. These cats can be XXY, XX/XXY, or more complex chimeras or mosaics with two or more X chromosomes and one or more Y chromosomes. The gene for black and the gene for orange are carried one per X chromosome, and so a normal male cat should not have hair of both colors.

Hypoplasia of the testis can theoretically occur when the number or length of seminiferous tubules is reduced, or when there are no or insufficient germ cells. Usually before puberty, the seminiferous tubules have only Sertoli cells and spermatogonia (Fig. 19-14, B). At puberty, the tubules of hypoplastic testes undergo an irregular progressive sclerosis and become collagenous. Interstital endocrine cells appear to be hyperplastic and clumped.

Hypoplasia of the testes is not apparent until after puberty. Unilateral hypoplasia is more common than bilateral hypoplasia, but this difference in prevalence could be a reflection of the relative ease of recognizing a size abnormality when the normal is available for

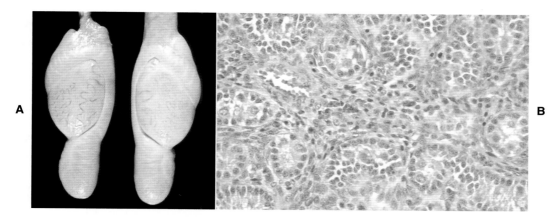

Fig. 19-14   Bilateral hypoplasia, testes, yearling ram. A, Both testes and epididymides from this yearling ram are very small compared with normal age-matched controls. **B,** The seminiferous tubules are lined only by Sertoli cells, and there is no spermatogenesis. H&E stain. (*A and **B**, Courtesy Dr. R. A. Foster, Ontario Veterinary College, University of Guelph.*)

ready comparison. Unilateral hypoplasia is difficult to explain because most of the causes seem to act systemically and therefore should produce a bilateral effect.

The size range of a hypoplastic testis generally is from a prepubertal size (Fig. 19-14, *A*) to almost normal. The consistency of a hypoplastic testis is near to normal. The severity of the hypoplasia can be graded histologically by the proportion of hypoplastic tubules scattered through the organ. Hypoplastic tubules have a small diameter, are lined by Sertoli cells and a few stem cells and spermatogonia, have a thickened basement membrane, and are surrounded by collagen. Interstitial endocrine cells appear proportionally more numerous, but this is only because the tubular area is reduced and the relative amount of interstitium is increased. In severe testicular hypoplasia, most or all of the tubules are abnormal; the tubules have a small diameter and a uniform microscopic appearance with only infrequent vacuolation of Sertoli cells and without a thickened basement membrane. In moderate hypoplasia, fewer tubules are small, those of normal size have some differentiation of the seminiferous epithelium, and a few tubules reach an advanced stage of development. In most tubules, however, when the stage of spermatocyte formation is reached, the spermatocytes undergo degeneration, leaving tubules lined by Sertoli cells with a vacuolated cytoplasm. The lumen of such tubules can contain cellular debris and multinucleate cells that are formed when dividing cells fail to separate. When hypoplasia is mild, only a few small tubules are lined mostly by Sertoli cells, whereas most of the tubules are active, many producing spermatozoa. Multinucleate spermatid giant cells can be present in the tubular lumens of some of these testes. Mild hypoplasia is difficult to distinguish from testicular degeneration.

The number of hypoplastic tubules would not be expected to increase with age because hypoplastic tubules do not arise after puberty.

TESTICULAR ATROPHY

Testes that reduce in size after puberty are atrophic, and the microscopic charge is degeneration of the seminiferous tubules. Testicular atrophy is a relatively common lesion. Mild testicular degeneration can be detected only microscopically, but when it is severe and chronic, the testis is small and firm (Fig. 19-15). The causes are many, and in a particular individual, the specific cause is often unknown. Degeneration can be unilateral or bilateral, depending on whether the cause is local or systemic. In young growing males, the distinction between testicular degeneration and hypoplasia is often difficult to make using morphologic features. Both lesions are often present together because hypoplastic testes are prone to degeneration. Inflammation also can be superimposed on degeneration when there is obstruction, leading to back pressure, rupture of seminiferous tubules, and spermatic granuloma formation. Recovery of a testis with degeneration back to a normal testis is possible if the injurious agent is eliminated and damage is not too severe.

Specific causes of testicular degeneration are numerous (Box 19-4), and accumulating data indicate that many agents act via apoptosis of germ cells. Fever or local heat from inflammation of the scrotal skin is a classic cause of degeneration. Obstruction of flow of spermatozoa causes testicular degeneration. Obstruction can be due to developmental anomalies such as segmental aplasia of mesonephric duct derivatives, local injury, or inflammation of the epididymis. Vascular events, such as impairment of aging, torsion, or severe crushing

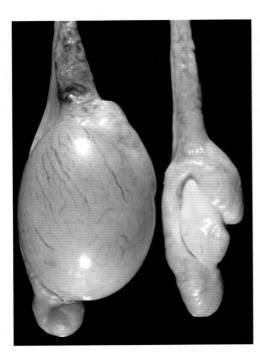

Fig. 19-15   Unilateral testicular atrophy and epididymitis, testis and epididymis, ram. The affected testis *(right)* is small, and testicular veins are not visible on the tunica albuginea due to fibrosis and contraction of the connective tissue. The other testis *(left)* is bulbous, indicating hypertrophy. *(Courtesy Drs. P. W. Ladds and R. A. Foster, James Cook University of North Queensland.)*

Box **19-4**

Some of the Known Causes of Testicular Degeneration in Mammals, Including Rodents

Advancing age
Chlorinated naphthalenes
Epididymitis
Chemicals
- Chemotherapy
- Halogenated compounds, including hexachlorophene
- Nitrogen-containing compounds, including benzimidazoles and nitrofurans

Heat
Hormones
- Dexamethasone
- Estrogen
- Testosterone
- Zeranolone

Metal compound toxicosis
Neoplasia
- Pituitary tumors
- Sertoli cell tumors

Nutritional disorders
- Negative energy balance
- Fatty acid deficiency
- Hypovitaminosis A
- Hypervitaminosis A
- Hypovitaminosis B
- Hypovitaminosis E
- Hypovitaminosis C
- Protein and amino acid deficiency
- Zinc deficiency

Plants
- Locoweed (*Astragalus*)
- Lysine seeds

Radiation
Stress/Corticosteroid therapy
Trauma
Ultrasound
Viral infection
- PRRS virus

PRRS, Porcine reproductive and respiratory syndrome.

of the spermatic cord, will cause degeneration. Systemic injurious factors include nutritional deficiency, hormonal aberrations, toxins, and irradiation. Hypovitaminosis A and zinc deficiency are specific nutritional deficiencies; general malnutrition also causes testicular degeneration. Interference with gonadotropin-releasing hormones, or luteinizing hormone and its control of androgen production by interstital endocrine cells, or follicle-stimulating hormone and its effect on the production of androgen-binding protein by Sertoli cells can have a deleterious effect on the seminiferous epithelium. Such interference could happen, for instance, when a neoplasm of the pituitary gland causes local compression of the pituitary gland, the hypothalamus, or both. Estrogen produced by Sertoli cell tumors induces testicular degeneration. Some therapeutic drugs, such as amphotericin B, gentamycin, and chemotherapeutic compounds, cause testicular degeneration.

Of the many toxins capable of causing testicular degeneration, most damage the spermatogonia and dividing primary spermatocytes, but some damage later stages, spermatocytes and spermatids, or injure Sertoli cells. Degeneration of seminiferous epithelium can occur secondary to injury of Sertoli cells.

A testis undergoing degeneration initially is softer than normal, and as the degeneration progresses, the testis becomes smaller. The cut surface of the normal testis and the acutely degenerated testis bulges slightly. After the acute phase, the testis becomes firmer and has small flecks or large areas of mineralization, especially in ruminants. Degeneration can be either generalized or regional, occurring in the dorsal part of the testis (near the head of the epididymis) in rams or in the ventrum of bulls. If the degeneration is due to ischemia after a vascular accident in the spermatic cord, small islands of parenchyma can survive the infarction because of diffusion of oxygen from vessels of the epididymis and tunica albuginea. Degeneration can occur locally around a lesion, such as a neoplasm, that expands and causes compression.

Microscopically, testicular degeneration has similar features to testicular hypoplasia; small seminiferous tubules with a thickened basement membrane, decreased numbers of germinal cells, vacuolated Sertoli cells, intratubular giant cells, and interstitial fibrosis (Fig. 19-16, A and B). The vacuolation of the Sertoli cells is likely to be more severe in the testis undergoing degeneration than in testicular hypoplasia because of the degeneration of Sertoli cells and the loss of germinal cells. A key lesion in the differentiation of testicular degeneration from testicular hypoplasia is the wavy basement membrane found in testicular degeneration because affected tubules had at some stage reached

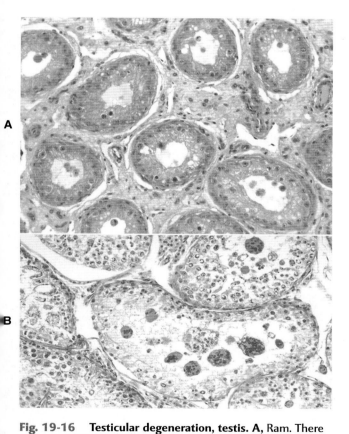

Fig. 19-16   Testicular degeneration, testis. A, Ram. There is interstitial fibrosis that separates the seminiferous tubules. Spermatogenic arrest at the spermatocyte stage, vacuolation of Sertoli cells, and a wavy basement membrane due to a reduction in tubular diameter are present. H&E stain. **B,** Dog. In addition to reduced spermatogenesis, there is formation of multinucleated spermatids (*centrally*) as a result of failure of spermatids to separate. This is a common change in testicular degeneration. (*A* and *B,* Courtesy Dr. R. A. Foster, Ontario *Veterinary College, University of Guelph.*)

full size and then subsequently collapsed. Because the basement membranes are thickened, they can be seen without special staining. At the end stage of testicular degeneration, Sertoli cells are the only lining cells remaining, but with time, these also disappear, leaving only the basement membranes. Mineralization can involve intratubular cellular debris, tubular basement membranes, or the interstitium.

Degeneration of the epididymis is less well studied but does occur. In degenerative conditions, the epididymis is much less likely to be reduced in size. This lack of reduction in size can be helpful in differentiating testicular atrophy from hypoplasia. In the former the epididymis will approximate adult size, whereas in hypoplasia the epididymis is also small in size.

EPIDIDYMITIS AND SPERMATIC GRANULOMAS

There are several diseases that result in testicular and epididymal enlargement. Foremost is inflammation, especially epididymitis, and testicular neoplasia.

Spermatic granuloma of the epididymal head is a unique disease of most species that is congenital in origin. It is not an infectious condition, but inflammation predominates as a response to extravasated spermatozoa. It affects the efferent ductule region first, and then spreads to involve the head of the epididymis (Fig. 19-17, A). All efferent ductules should link in the head of the epididymis, but blind-ended efferent ductules result when there is no connection with the single epididymal duct. At puberty, the blind-ending ductules fill with spermatozoa and the resultant spermiostasis can proceed to formation of a spermatocele, and spermatic granulomas (Fig. 19-17, B). These progress over time and result in infertility because of obstruction. The back pressure produced by the spermatic granulomas causes dilation of the mediastinum of the testis and testicular atrophy.

Epididymitis is very important in rams (Fig. 19-18) and dogs (Fig. 19-19) and is rare in other species. The tail of the epididymis is almost always affected, allowing the majority of cases to be differentiated from spermatic granuloma of the epididymal head. Because the epididymis is only a single coiled tube, any lesion along its length has potential for causing obstruction of spermatozoal flow and for the formation of spermatic granulomas. Thus epididymitis is frequently accompanied by spermatic granulomas and periorchitis. Epididymitis can be focal or multifocal or diffuse, unilateral, or bilateral. It is most frequently encountered in unilateral, chronic, focal, or multifocal form and thus can be recognized by comparing the size and shape of the abnormal organ with the normal one. In acute inflammation, the epididymis is soft and swollen; in chronic inflammation, it is firm and enlarged because of the deposition of fibrous tissue and likely to be nodular

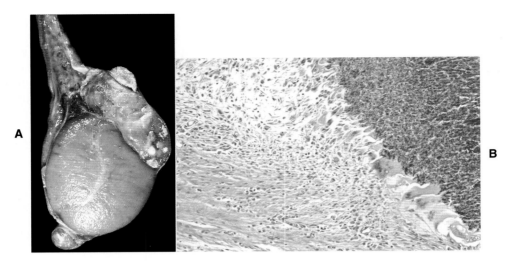

Fig. 19-17   Spermatic granuloma, head of the epididymis, dog. A, The head of the epididymis is tremendously enlarged because of spermatic granulomas *(white-yellow masses).* The body and tail of the epididymis *(ventral)* are small, as the spermatic granulomas have obstructed the flow of spermatozoa from the testis to the epididymis. **B,** The mass of spermatozoa *(right)* in the interstitial connective tissue of the epididymis is surrounded by macrophages and multinucleated giant cells. H&E stain. **(A,** *Courtesy College of Veterinary Medicine, University of Illinois.* **B,** *Courtesy Dr. K. McEntee, Reproductive Pathology Collection, University of Illinois; and Dr. J. King, College of Veterinary Medicine, Cornell University.)*

because of the distention of segments of the duct and the presence of spermatic granulomas. Epididymitis is one of the causes of testicular degeneration. The testis on gross appearance is atrophic. Focal fibrinous or fibrous adhesions occur between the visceral tunica vaginalis over the epididymis and the parietal tunica vaginalis lining the scrotal sac (Fig. 19-18). If a spermatic granuloma ruptures into the cavity of the tunica vaginalis, diffuse inflammation of the tunics can result, followed by adhesions across the cavity (Fig. 19-20). In some cases, fistulas discharge through the scrotum .

Infectious epididymitis occurs in two main ways: hematogenously by *Brucella* sp., and by ascending infection with bacteria such as *Actinobacillus seminis, Histophilus somni,* and *Escherichia coli.* Regardless of the causative agent, the lesion is similar and is dominated grossly and microscopically by the formation of

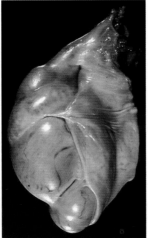

Fig. 19-18   Epididymitis (*Brucella ovis*), tunic adhesions, epididymis, ram. Note the dramatic enlargement of the epididymis and the adhesion of the parietal tunica vaginalis to the visceral tunica vaginalis around the affected epididymis. *(Courtesy Dr. K. McEntee, Reproductive Pathology Collection, University of Illinois; and Dr. J. King, College of Veterinary Medicine, Cornell University.)*

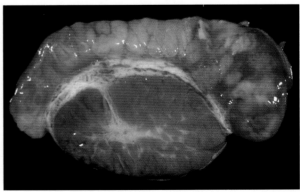

Fig. 19-19   Acute epididymitis, epididymis, dog. The head *(left)* and tail *(right)* of the epididymis are grossly hyperemic and contain pale foci of suppurative exudate and spermatozoa. *(Courtesy Dr. K. McEntee, Reproductive Pathology Collection, University of Illinois; and Dr. J. King, College of Veterinary Medicine, Cornell University.)*

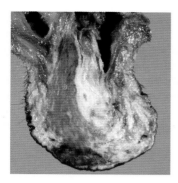

Fig. 19-20   Scrotal cellulitis and periorchitis, scrotum (testis has been removed), dog. The tunica vaginalis is thickened by inflammatory exudate, granulation tissue, and fibrous connective tissue. The inflammation extends into the skin. There is an ulcer ventrally from self-mutilation. *(Courtesy Dr. R. A. Foster, Ontario Veterinary College, University of Guelph.)*

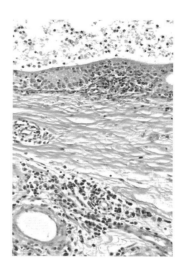

Fig. 19-21   Chronic epididymitis, epididymis, ram. Note the intertubular fibrosis and large numbers of lymphocytes and plasma cells in the interstitium. The epithelium of the duct *(top)* is hyperplastic, and the lumen contains neutrophils and spermatozoa. H&E stain. *(Courtesy Dr. R. A. Foster, Ontario Veterinary College, University of Guelph.)*

spermatic granulomas. Microscopically, in epididymitis, the lumen has a mixture of inflammatory cells, in which neutrophils are present and macrophages are prominent, together with desquamated epithelial cells, intact and fragmented spermatozoa, and spermatozoa within multinucleate foreign-body type giant cells. If the wall of the tubule is breached, inflammation spreads to the interstitium, and macrophages become more numerous in the inflammatory exudate and collagen is deposited. Hyperplasia of the luminal epithelium of the epididymis occurs. The epithelial cells proliferate irregularly, so that thick areas of epithelium appear to enclose thin areas, leading to "intraepithelial lumen" formation. Squamous metaplasia of the epithelium is another possible outcome in chronic epididymitis. The interstitial cellular reaction is usually dominated by lymphocytes and plasma cells, and with edema and fibrosis.

In rams, *Brucella ovis*, *Actinobacillus seminis*, or *Histophilus somni* infections produce a suppurative inflammatory response, with subsequent ductal epithelial hyperplasia and intraepithelial lumen formation as lesions of the early infection (Fig. 19-21) and spermatic granulomas in more chronic cases. Testicular atrophy occurs secondarily. *Brucella ovis* affects animals of breeding age, and they are often exposed during the breeding season or from other rams when not breeding. *Actinobacillus seminis* or *Histophilus somni* infect rams at puberty mostly, when hormonal alterations allow bacteria resident in the prepuce to ascend the reproductive tract, affecting the accessory genital glands first and then the epididymis.

Brucella abortus infection in bulls is the main infectious agent of the testis and epididymis. The disease is similar to *Brucella ovis* infection in rams, but orchitis predominates (see later discussion). The epididymis is also affected.

Epididymitis occurs most commonly in mature dogs. Gram-negative organisms, such as *Escherichia coli*, and presumably an ascending infection cause most cases. In acute disease, dogs suffer the effects of endotoxemia and the systemic response to infection with lethargy, fever, and a large painful and doughy scrotum. The epididymis and tunica vaginalis are usually affected, but in some cases a severe orchitis also is seen. Dogs will lick and chew at the affected scrotum and create a fistula to the scrotal contents (Fig. 19-20). Testicular degeneration is an invariable consequence of epididymitis. *Brucella canis* infection causes epididymitis also, followed by testicular degeneration and atrophy. The lesions are often unilateral and occur together with scrotal hyperemia, dermatitis, and prostatitis. The epididymis can become greatly enlarged, especially the tail, as a result of interstitial inflammation, fibrosis, and spermatic granulomas (Fig. 19-18).

Noninfectious causes of epididymitis are exceedingly rare, and often cases that have no recoverable agent are dominated by spermatic granulomas that remain after a previous infection has been otherwise controlled.

ORCHITIS

True orchitis is much less common than epididymitis, probably because the testis is much further "upstream" than the epididymis and possibly because of the altered immunologic environment, which is antiinflammatory. Orchitis is, unfortunately, the common clinical term for inflammation of the scrotal contents. Most cases are epididymitis. Orchitis is usually accompanied by epididymitis and may be an extension of epididymitis. Primary orchitis is usually hematogenous, with examples including *Brucella abortus* in bulls, *Brucella suis* in boars, and *Corynebacterium pseudotuberculosis* in rams. It happens in several forms. Intratubular orchitis is centered on the seminiferous tubules, so it is assumed the agent and the inflammatory reaction begins there. Intratubular orchitis appears grossly as poorly defined, up to 1-cm yellow foci that become firm and white as the lesions become chronic. Initially the affected tubules have acute inflammatory debris. The lining of the tubules is lost, but the tubular outlines are present for some time. Spermatic granulomas can form any time spermatozoa make contact with extratubular tissue. In the center of these granulomas, spermatozoa can be seen free and within macrophages. Macrophages and lymphocytes infiltrate around the core of spermatozoa and macrophages and, with time, collagen is deposited at the edge of the lesion. When the lesion is predominantly in the interstitium, it is called interstitial orchitis (Fig. 19-22).

Necrotizing orchitis, such as is caused by *Brucella abortus* and *Brucella suis*, is the most severe form of orchitis. It is a more severe form of intratubular or interstitial orchitis, but in some cases the affected areas are so severely inflamed and the necrosis is so extensive that the original structures have formed a caseous mass. Gray-brown, initially soft and later firm, necrotic debris replaces an irregular, but large, portion of the testis. In a few extremely severe cases, a fistula develops through the scrotum. One manifestation of feline infectious peritonitis is a fibrinous and necrotic orchitis (Fig. 19-23).

Granulomatous orchitis, especially tuberculous orchitis, is now very rare as countries move toward being free of *Mycobacterium bovis*. Mycotic orchitis caused by *Blastomyces dermatitidis*, for example, occurs sporadically in endemic areas.

Inflammation of the tunica vaginalis or the epididymis can be secondary to intratubular, necrotizing, or granulomatous orchitis.

NEOPLASIA

Testicular neoplasms are common in older dogs, much less frequent in horses, and rare in other species. They usually arise from germ cells, Sertoli cells, or interstitial endocrine cells. Occasionally, neoplasms of testicular mesenchymal structures or metastatic neoplasms are found. The three common primary testicular neoplasms are seminoma, interstitial cell tumor, and Sertoli cell tumor; they occur singly or in combination. These primary neoplasms are almost always benign, and there are no features that indicate the likelihood of metastasis. Metastasis, when it does occur, is identified by nodules in the spermatic cord, scrotal lymph node, or beyond.

Germ cell neoplasms are seminoma, teratoma, and other less common types such as embryonal carcinoma. Seminomas are the second most common canine testicular neoplasm (Fig. 19-24, A) and the most common testicular neoplasm in the aged stallion. They are more prevalent in cryptorchid testes than in descended testes. Multicentric origin within the testis and local invasiveness are characteristic, but metastasis

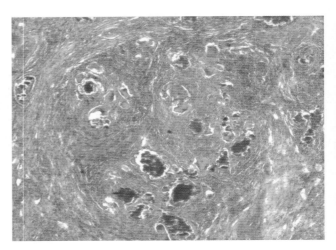

Fig. 19-22   Granulomatous interstitial orchitis, testis, ram. There is granulomatous inflammation surrounding aggregates of spermatozoa and mineral that replaced the seminiferous tubules after they were destroyed. Lymphocytes and plasma cells predominate in the surrounding interstitium. H&E stain. *(Courtesy Dr. R. A. Foster, Ontario Veterinary College, University of Guelph.)*

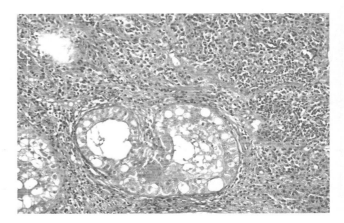

Fig. 19-23   Severe fibrinous interstitial orchitis, feline infectious peritonitis (FIP), testis, cat. Note the severe orchitis with a mixture of fibrin and plasma cells in the interstitium. The tubules are degenerate and not directly involved. The testicular lesion was the first manifestation of FIP in this cat. H&E stain. *(Courtesy Dr. R. A. Foster, Ontario Veterinary College, University of Guelph.)*

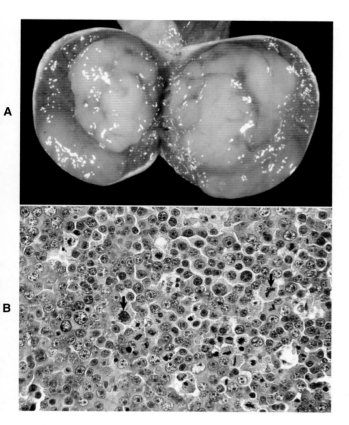

Fig. 19-24   Seminoma, testis, dog. A, Note the pale pink to beige circumscribed homogenous mass. The cut surface has a gelatinous texture and has bulged slightly on incision. The contralateral testis was atrophic. **B,** Seminomas consist of round germinal cells with a high nuclear-to-cytoplasmic ratio and frequent mitoses (*arrows*). Despite this "malignant" appearance, most are behaviorally benign. H&E stain. (**A,** *Courtesy Dr. K. Read, College of Veterinary Medicine, Texas A&M University; and Noah's Arkive, College of Veterinary Medicine, The University of Georgia.* **B,** *Courtesy Dr. R. A. Foster, Ontario Veterinary College, University of Guelph.*)

is rare. The neoplasm is homogenous, white or pink-gray, and firm; bulges when cut; and has fine fibrous trabeculae. Seminomas are either intratubular or diffuse, and the neoplastic cells are large, polyhedral, discretely demarcated round cells with a large nucleus, variable nuclear size, and very little cytoplasm. The mitotic rate is usually high. Giant cells, with either a single nucleus or multiple nuclei, are sometimes present (Fig. 19-24, *B*). Lymphoid aggregates are often present around blood vessels in seminomas and are a useful diagnostic feature.

Teratomas arise from totipotential primordial germ cells. They are uncommon but are best known in the young horse, especially in a cryptorchid testis. The neoplasms can be large, cystic, or polycystic and can contain recognizable hair, mucus, bone, or even teeth. Histologically, at least derivatives of two of the three embryonic germ layers (ectoderm, mesoderm, and endoderm) are present. Most teratomas have well-differentiated tissue and are benign.

Interstitial cell tumors are the most common testicular neoplasms of the dog, cat, and bull. They are readily identifiable grossly by their tan to orange color, often with hemorrhage. The neoplasm is spherical and well demarcated (Fig. 19-25, *A*). These neoplasms are almost always benign. They likely begin as regions of nodular hyperplasia. Some cases produce hormones, including estrogenic substances. Microscopically the cells of the bovine neoplasms vary little, but in the dog the cells can be large, round, polyhedral, or spindle shaped. The cells have abundant cytoplasm that is often finely vacuolated and often has brown pigment. The cells are arranged in solid sheets or packeted into small groups by a fine fibrovascular stroma (Fig. 19-25, *B*). Although hemorrhage, necrosis, and cyst formation are common, interstitial cell tumors are noninvasive and finely encapsulated.

Sertoli cell tumor is the third most common testicular neoplasm of the dog. It is rare in other species. In the dog, more than 50% of Sertoli cell tumors are located in undescended testes. The neoplasm is firm, white, and lobulated by fibrous bands and can cause enlargement of the affected testis (Fig. 19-26, *A*). The neoplasm can invade the spermatic cord and occasionally metastasize to the regional lymph node. Metastases beyond the regional lymph node have been reported but are rare. The neoplastic Sertoli cells either resemble normal Sertoli cells or are more pleomorphic. They can have an intratubular or a diffuse arrangement. The abundant fibrous connective tissue in Sertoli cell tumors distinguishes them from the other two common types of testicular neoplasm. Neoplastic cells tend to palisade along the fibrous stroma or form tubular structures (Fig. 19-26, *B*). In addition to the effects of pressure and local invasion, the other important consequence of the presence of Sertoli cell tumors is that about a third of them produce a feminizing effect, causing gynecomastia (enlargement of the mammary glands). Although some may produce estrogen, excessive inhibin secretion altering the balance between estrogen and testosterone production is thought to be responsible. A possibly life-threatening effect of hyperestrogenism is myelotoxicity, resulting in a poorly regenerative anemia, granulocytopenia, and thrombocytopenia. Other effects include alopecia, hyperplasia or squamous metaplasia of the acini of the prostate gland (Fig. 19-26, *C*), and adenomyosis of the epididymis. The amount of hormone produced is generally proportional to the size of the neoplasm.

Mixed germ cell–stromal neoplasms have been described in old dogs. The neoplasm-bearing testis is large and often cryptorchid. The testis is partially or

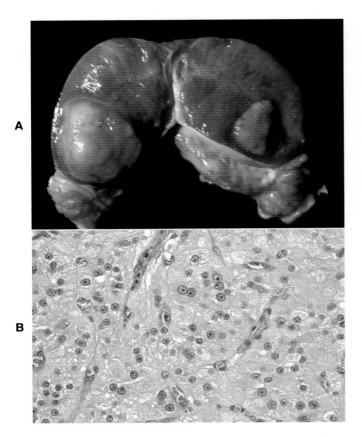

Fig. 19-25 **Interstitial cell tumor, testis, dog. A,** Note the well-demarcated, yellow-tan mass, which has bulged on incision. Such masses become hemorrhagic when they are large. Atrophy of an affected testis due to pressure is common when the tumor is large. **B,** Cells are arranged in packets surrounded by a fine fibrovascular stroma typical of endocrine cells. Their cytoplasm is pale, eosinophilic, and abundant and often has fine vacuoles. Mitoses are rare. H&E stain. *(A, Courtesy Dr. M.D. McGavin, College of Veterinary Medicine, University of Tennessee. B, Courtesy Dr. W. Crowell, College of Veterinary Medicine, The University of Georgia; and Noah's Arkive, College of Veterinary Medicine, The University of Georgia.)*

completely replaced by a firm, gray-white to tan, single multilobed mass. Intimate intermingling of germ cells and Sertoli cells occurs in tubular structures of various sizes. The germ cell component extends into the surrounding tissue.

DISEASES OF THE SPERMATIC CORD

The spermatic cord and associated structures comprise the ductus deferens, pampiniform plexus, and cremaster muscle. The scrotal lymph node and the inguinal canal are related structures.

Varicocele is the local dilation of the spermatic vein in the pampiniform plexus. Older rams are most commonly affected, and the thrombosed and dilated vessels are so large that they interfere with the ability of

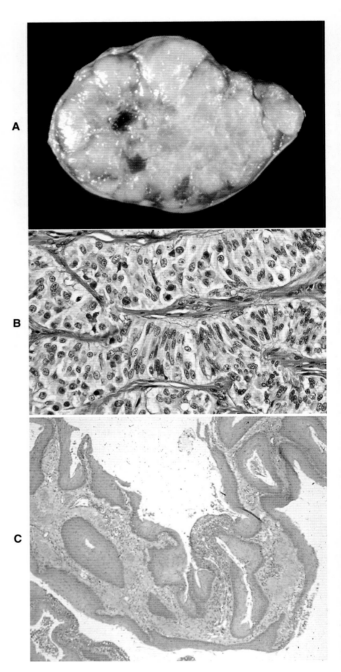

Fig. 19-26 **Sertoli cell tumor, testis, dog. A,** Sertoli cell tumors are firm, white, and often lobulated, and the lobules are surrounded by fibrous bands. **B,** Histologically, Sertoli cell tumors have tubular structures lined by cells that resemble Sertoli cells and are surrounded by septa of fibrous tissue. H&E stain. **C,** Prostate, squamous metaplasia. Functional Sertoli cell tumors that secrete estrogen can induce hyperplasia and/or squamous metaplasia of the prostate gland. Normal epithelium of the prostatic ducts (transitional) and glandular acini (columnar) is replaced by stratified squamous keratinizing epithelium. H&E stain. *(A, Courtesy Dr. K. McEntee, Reproductive Pathology Collection, University of Illinois. B, Courtesy Dr. R. A. Foster, Ontario Veterinary College, University of Guelph. C, Courtesy Dr. W. Crowell, College of Veterinary Medicine, The University of Georgia; and Noah's Arkive, College of Veterinary Medicine, The University of Georgia.)*

the testis to be raised or to thermoregulate normally. This is thought to lower fertility by creating poor spermatozoal motility, immature spermatozoa in the semen, and testicular degeneration. The dilation in the venous plexus is located near the inguinal ring and does not involve the complex distal part of the pampiniform plexus (Fig. 19-27). About half the cases are bilateral, and the unilateral cases are evenly divided between the left and right side. Thrombosis of affected vessels is common.

Torsion of the spermatic cord is seen in undescended testes, especially when there is a testicular neoplasm present. Torsion also occurs periodically in the stallion and is a cause of colic. Torsion causes venous occlusion with a resultant venous infarction of the testis especially and also of the epididymis.

Inflammation of the spermatic cord (funisitis, scirrhous cord) occurs after the contamination of a castration wound. Sometimes the lesion is acute and necrotizing, but more often it is chronic and a scirrhous cord is encountered. Great enlargement of the distal part of the cord is due to exuberant granulation tissue in which numerous small pockets of pus are scattered. Staphylococci are the organisms frequently recovered from the pus in the horse. The term "botryomycosis" has been used for these staphylococcal pyogranulomas. Radiating club-shaped eosinophilic deposits (Splendore-Hoeppli reaction) are present around the central clusters of bacteria.

Inguinal hernia and lymphadenopathy of the scrotal lymph nodes are a differential diagnosis for masses or swellings in the region of the spermatic cords. Older rams and stallions are particularly prone to inguinal hernia, which is a cause of scrotal enlargement and colic in stallions. Caseous lymphadenitis in rams and lymphoma in dogs are a cause of scrotal lymphadenopathy.

DISEASES OF THE ACCESSORY GENITAL GLANDS

The accessory genital glands include the ampullae, vesicular glands, prostate, and bulbourethral glands. The ampullae and vesicular glands are derived from the mesonephric duct, and the prostate and bulbourethral glands are derived from the urogenital sinus. Their hidden location within the pelvic canal means that they are often neglected in examination of the reproductive tract.

AMPULLAE

There are very few diseases of the ampullae, and the majority are microscopic. Bulls have variation in the patterns of insertion of ampullae at the seminal colliculus. They can be above and below the vesicular glands. The membrane between the ampullae is the location for the remnants of the paramesonephric duct—the cystic uterus masculinus—in rams and bulls. Hyperestrogenism can cause these to become greatly enlarged.

Ampullitis is a feature of infection with agents that cause epididymitis and vesicular adenitis, including but not restricted to *Brucella abortus, Brucella ovis, Actinobacillus seminis, Histophilus somni,* and many other agents. It may precede epididymitis as part of an ascending infection or occur when organisms and inflammatory products descend into the ductus from an inflamed epididymis.

VESICULAR GLANDS

The major disease of the vesicular glands (seminal vesicles) is inflammation of the gland, and often it is clinically silent, except in the bull. Vesicular adenitis (seminal vesiculitis) is a significant disease in the bull because it reduces fertility, particularly in young bulls. Inflammation in the vesicular glands contributes inflammatory cells and mediators to the semen, thus reducing the ability of spermatozoan to survive freezing. Young bulls, in their first breeding season, are especially affected. The cause is most likely infectious; various organisms including viruses, protozoa, *Chlamydophila, Ureaplasma, Mycoplasma, Brucella abortus,* and other bacteria having been investigated over the years. The pathogenesis is uncertain, but hypotheses include ascending infection, descending infection, hematogenous spread, congenital malformation preventing excretion of fluid and spermatozoa, and reflux of spermatozoa or urine into the glands.

The common form of vesicular adenitis is a chronic interstitial inflammation (Fig. 19-28, *A* and *B*). In some

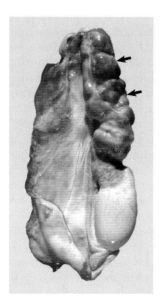

Fig. 19-27   Varicocele, pampiniform plexus, ram. This extremely large varicocele (*arrows*) is larger than the testis. It is multinodular from large thromboses filling the dilated veins. (*Courtesy Dr. P. W. Ladds, James Cook University of North Queensland.*)

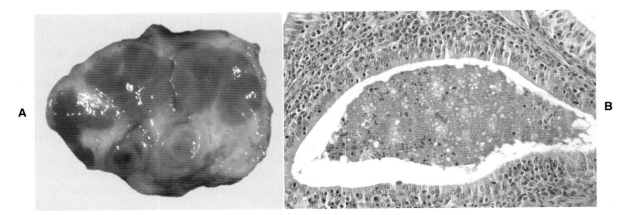

Fig. 19-28   Chronic vesicular adenitis, vesicular gland, cut surface, ram. A, The normal lobulation of the vesicular gland is distorted by fibrous tissue that surrounds the glandular tissue. **B,** Chronic vesicular adenitis (*Brucella ovis*) (different than Fig. 19-28, A). Glandular acini are filled with degenerating neutrophils and debris, and neutrophils are migrating through the acinar epithelium. The interstitium is heavily infiltrated by plasma cells and lymphocytes. H&E stain. (**A** and **B,** *Courtesy Dr. R. A. Foster, Ontario Veterinary College, University of Guelph.*)

cases, the glands are enlarged and firm and have loss of lobulation. Collagen is deposited between the acini. Lymphocytes, plasma cells, macrophages, and a few neutrophils and eosinophils are present in the interstitium. The lumens have neutrophils, desquamated epithelial cells, and debris (Fig. 19-28, B). Metaplasia of glandular epithelium to a stratified squamous type is common. In some bulls, much disorganization and denuding involve the epithelium of inflamed vesicular glands.

Vesicular adenitis can be part of the range of lesions caused by *Burkholderia pseudomallei* in boars and the many *Brucella* species, especially *Brucella ovis* in sheep. Vesicular adenitis is occasionally seen in stallions.

PROSTATE GLAND

The prostate gland is derived from the urogenital sinus. Both estrogens and androgens have trophic action on the prostate gland.

The only animal with any frequency of prostatic disease is the dog. There are three main diseases and their prevalence is, in order, hyperplasia, neoplasia, and prostatitis.

Prostatic hyperplasia is a common age- and testosterone-dependent condition. The dog is the only domestic animal species that spontaneously develops prostatic hyperplasia with age (Fig. 19-29, A and B). Clinical consequences of prostatic hypertrophy include constipation from the "ball valve" effect of a large prostate forced into the pelvis during attempted defecation. Although obstruction of the urethra is a feature of prostatic hyperplasia in humans, stenosis of the urethra only occasionally occurs in the canine disease. Enlargement of the prostate is hormone related, but the precise mechanisms are unknown. Hypertrophy of

the gland does not occur in castrated dogs, and removal of androgens by castration of affected dogs is therapeutic. Administration of estrogens causes enlargement of the gland. Acinar hyperplasia possibly is caused by androgen excess (Fig. 19-29, C), and fibromuscular hyperplasia is caused by estrogen excess, but the contribution of these two elements to the enlargement of the gland can overlap considerably. Enlargement of the gland is usually uniform. On occasion the hyperplasia is cystic, and in extreme cases, a large single cyst or multiple small cysts are found. Microscopically, there is hyperplasia of the acinar epithelium and hyperplasia of the interlobular and to a lesser extent the intralobular fibromuscular stroma. Some acini are distended with fluid and have a flattened epithelium.

Estrogen-induced hypertrophy of the canine prostate gland, most often because of the presence of Sertoli cell tumor, has the added feature of squamous metaplasia of acinar epithelium, ducts, prostatic urethra, and uterus masculinus (Fig. 19-26, C). Flattened keratinized epithelial cells are desquamated into the acini, and neutrophils and other inflammatory cells are present. Squamous metaplasia of the prostate gland in dogs is not preneoplastic.

Prostatic and paraprostatic cysts occur periodically in dogs, and their origin has been debated for years. Some may be an enlarged cystic uterus masculinus (see Cysts of the Reproductive Tract), but many are likely to be hyperplastic cysts formed when cystic acini extrude through the incomplete muscular layer of the prostatic capsule, in a manner similar to adenomyosis of the uterus. Paraprostatic cysts can attain giant proportions, as large as 30 cm in diameter. Some become infected and abscessed.

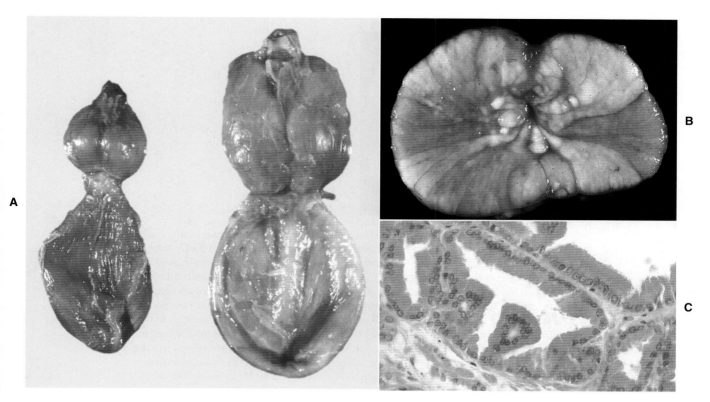

Fig. 19-29   **Prostatic hyperplasia, prostate, dog. A,** Prostates of two dogs of different ages *(oldest on the right).* Both prostates are bilaterally and symmetrically larger than normal pubertal prostates. **B,** The lighter white tissues that in some areas bulge from the cut surface are areas of hyperplasia. A hyperplastic prostate is symmetrically enlarged and detectable on rectal palpation, ultrasonography, or by gross examination at necropsy. **C,** The prostatic acini are larger than normal, as the epithelium is hyperplastic and the cells enlarged (hypertrophy). Note the abundant granular apical cytoplasm and the uniform size and shape of the cells. Mitotic activity is very low. H&E stain. (**A,** *Courtesy Dr. R. A. Foster, Ontario Veterinary College, University of Guelph.* **B,** *Courtesy Department of Veterinary Biosciences, The Ohio State University; and Noah's Arkive, College of Veterinary Medicine, The University of Georgia.* **C,** *Courtesy Dr. R.K. Myers, College of Veterinary Medicine, Iowa State University.*)

Carcinoma of the prostate in the dog is the only prostatic neoplasm of any importance in domestic animals (Fig. 19-30, *A*). A similar disease is exceedingly rare in the cat. The cause, possibly related to an abnormal hormonal environment, has not been well defined. Prostatic hyperplasia appears not to precede neoplasia, although the two lesions are found together in intact dogs. Some of the clinical signs of carcinoma of the prostate are similar to those of prostatic hyperplasia because of the enlargement of the organ. Carcinoma and its metastases cause cachexia and locomotor abnormalities through pressure and invasion of nearby structures, including bones. Grossly, there are two general appearances. The most obvious is the type that causes increased firmness, asymmetric enlargement (Fig. 19-30, *B*), partial or complete loss of the median raphe, and cystic cavities in the prostate gland. The prostate gland becomes large and attached to other pelvic structures. The second type is mostly periurethral, with a necrotic and cystic cavity within the prostatic capsule. It causes minimal enlargement of the gland, but urinary obstruction and metastatic disease are present. Castrated dogs are usually affected.

Much has been written and said about the prevalence of different types of neoplasia of the prostate. Some authors have divided them into adenocarcinoma and transitional cell carcinoma; the latter presumably arise from the pelvic urethra or from prostatic ducts. This is perhaps too simplistic, as there is also an intermediate category of mixed glandular and transitional types. A detailed study of the cellular origins of carcinomas was unsuccessful as there are no specific markers to separate those derived from acinar or urothelial tissue. This is possibly because of a common origin of prostatic ducts and glands, and for urothelium in general. Because of this, we choose to use the term "carcinoma of the prostate" as a general term and to

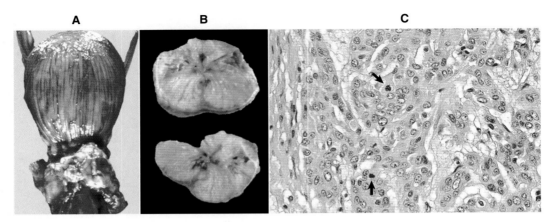

Fig. 19-30   Carcinoma, prostate, dog. A, The pelvic tissues of this dog contain many coalescing nodules of metastatic carcinoma that have spread from the prostate, which is barely recognizable beneath the bladder (*opened, upper*). Prostatic carcinomas are usually asymmetric and lobulated white-to-gray masses that expand the size of the gland and may compress the urethra (dysuria) and the colon (difficulty defecating, ribbon stools). **B,** Cross section. Note the asymmetric enlargement. The focal white areas are regions of necrosis within a gland that is enlarged by neoplastic epithelial cells that induce the abundant fibrous tissue that is also present. **C,** Note the anaplastic prostatic epithelial cells arranged in acini and solid lobules. Mitotic figures are common (*arrows*). There also may be stromal or lymphatic invasion and desmoplasia (scirrhous response). H&E stain. (*A,* Courtesy Dr. M. Howard, College of Veterinary Medicine, Iowa State University; and Noah's Arkive, College of Veterinary Medicine, The University of Georgia. *B,* Courtesy Dr. J. A. Ramos-Vara, College of Veterinary Medicine, Michigan State University; and Noah's Arkive, College of Veterinary Medicine, The University of Georgia. *C,* Courtesy Dr. L. Borst, College of Veterinary Medicine, University of Illinois.)

refer to adenocarcinoma, mixed carcinoma, squamous cell carcinoma, and transitional cell carcinoma when the histologic type is purely glandular, mixed squamous, or urothelial.

Microscopically, prostatic intraepithelial neoplasia, described as a precursor of human prostatic cancer, has been recognized in the dog, but only in conjunction with concurrent carcinoma of the prostate. The features are disruption of basal cell layer, increased mitotic index, and increased density of small blood vessels. The appearance of a carcinoma reflects attempted differentiation toward glandular, urothelial, or epidermal tissues, or mixtures of two or more (Fig. 19-30, C). There are varying degrees of stroma between the neoplastic epithelial cells. Some mixed neoplasms also contain sarcomatous tissue. In dogs, no specific regions of the prostate have a predilection for the development of hyperplasia or neoplasia.

The prognosis for carcinoma of the prostate is generally poor. About 40% are in sexually intact dogs, 80% of affected dogs have metastases to a lymph node and/or lung at the time of diagnosis, and 20% of these have metastasized to bone.

Prostatitis is seen periodically and can be clinically significant if toxemia accompanies the infection or if the gland becomes large enough to cause urinary obstruction. In the dog, prostatitis can be found in old animals, often together with hyperplasia, or in young animals without hyperplasia. Although increased concentrations of zinc in prostatic fluid are associated with antimicrobial properties in men and dogs, resistance to infection and resolution of infection are not correlated with zinc concentrations in prostatic tissue in the dog. Prostatitis can usefully be divided into acute, chronic, abscess formation, and specific (*Brucella canis*) forms. Organisms such as *Escherichia coli, Proteus vulgaris,* and others invade from the urethra. The affected organ can be diffusely or focally involved, swollen, congested, and edematous (Fig. 19-31, A). The early microscopic lesion is catarrhal to purulent inflammation of the acini, expanding later to involve the interstitium, with abscess formation (Fig. 19-31, B). The abscesses can persist or be replaced by fibrous tissue. Prostatitis is part of the spectrum of lesions caused by *Brucella canis* in the dog, and the prostate can be the site of persistence of the organism. A subacute interstitial inflammation causes enlargement and fibrosis of some lobules (Fig. 19-31, C). Dogs have a common, clinically insignificant, chronic prostatitis of unknown cause.

BULBOURETHRAL GLANDS

The bulbourethral gland, as with the prostate, is derived from the urogenital sinus. There are few lesions of the bulbourethral glands, no doubt because of their dense structure and lack of lumina to allow bacterial growth and persistence. The major disease of this gland is seen

A   B   C

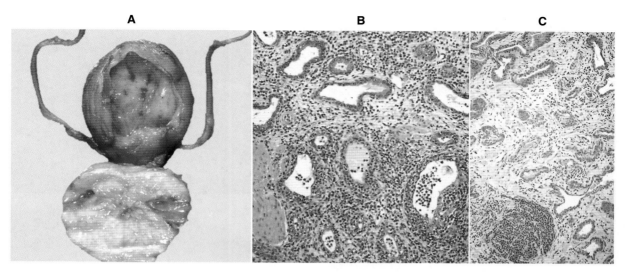

Fig. 19-31   Prostatitis, prostate, dog. A, Acute prostatitis, cut surface. The prostate is enlarged with edema, and there are myriad white foci of inflammatory cells instead of the usually smooth red surface. Clinically, this condition is usually painful. **B,** Acute prostatitis. Note that the glands and interstitium contain large numbers of neutrophils. Most of these infections are of bacterial origin and develop after bacteria ascend the urethra. H&E stain. **C,** Chronic prostatitis. Note that the glands and interstitium contain large numbers of lymphocytes and macrophages and a large lymphoid nodule (*bottom*). Follicular lymphoid hyperplasia is a common finding in chronically infected tissue. The abundant interstitial stromal is from fibroplasia and chronic inflammation. Most cases of chronic prostatitis have a bacterial origin. H&E stain. (*A, B, and* **C,** *Courtesy Dr. W. Crowell, College of Veterinary Medicine, The University of Georgia; and Noah's Arkive, College of Veterinary Medicine, The University of Georgia.*)

in castrated male sheep grazing clover pasture with a high estrogen content. The glands of these wethers have hypertrophy, squamous metaplasia, and cyst formation that can be massive and cause perineal swellings.

DISEASES OF THE PENIS AND PREPUCE

Disease of the penis and prepuce is relatively rare, yet infection is common and extremely important for food-producing animals. Many of the venereally transmitted diseases, such as trichomoniasis, campylobacteriosis, herpesviruses, and papillomaviruses, are present in the prepuce and do not cause severe disease or have a mild and self-limiting course. The penis is protected from trauma and drying by the prepuce, and this very environment is permissive of many infectious diseases. Some induce an immune reaction and or inflammation.

Phimosis is the inability to extrude the penis, and paraphimosis is the inability to retract the penis into the prepuce.

DEVELOPMENTAL ABNORMALITIES

Persistent frenulum is a relatively common and minor anatomic abnormality rather than a serious defect, but it can have an important deleterious effect in limiting the extent to which the penis can be protruded from the sheath and in causing the erect penis to be curved instead of straight (Fig. 19-32). Persistent frenulum is of importance in bulls and boars. Judging by the frequent occurrence of large flaps and tags of tissue on the ventral raphe of the penis, transitory persistence of the frenulum is quite common. The raphe of the penis and prepuce are remnants of the frenulum, a thin membrane ventral to the penis that normally ruptures at puberty, probably as the result of simple mechanical forces. Persistent segments of frenulum are well vascularized, usually occur at the distal end of the penis, and can connect the penis to the prepuce or the penis to itself.

The penis is subject to many abnormalities of size and form, such as congenital absence, hypoplasia, duplication, directional deviations, and, in ruminants, absence of the sigmoid flexure and abnormal locations of the insertions of the retractor muscles. None of these lesions is common.

Hypospadias and epispadias are malformations of the urethral canal that create abnormal openings of the urethra on the ventral surface of the penis (hypospadias) or on the dorsal surface (epispadias). In hypospadias, the urinary opening is anywhere from the glans to the penile shaft, penoscrotal junction, or the perineum. Their importance is in the potential for causing urinary obstruction and in interference with normal insemination.

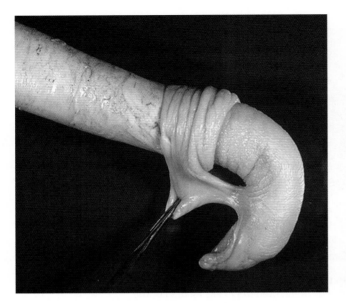

Fig. 19-32   Persistent frenulum, penis, bull. A tag of tissue *(forceps)* connecting the penis and prepuce has caused the penis to be curved ventrally, thus making intromission impossible. *(Courtesy Dr. W. Crowell, College of Veterinary Medicine, The University of Georgia; and Noah's Arkive, College of Veterinary Medicine, The University of Georgia.)*

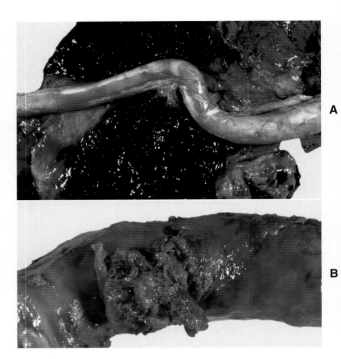

Fig. 19-33   Penile hematoma, penis, bull. A, The large hemorrhage around the penis at the sigmoid flexure is a hematoma from rupture of the penis during forced deviation. **B,** Illustrated is the site of rupture of the penis with a blood clot filling the rupture site. (**A** and **B,** *Courtesy Dr. M.D. McGavin, College of Veterinary Medicine, University of Tennessee.)*

HEMORRHAGE AND PENILE HEMATOMA

The penis is a highly vascular structure, and the presence of erectile tissue and high pressures during erection and coitus make the potential for severe or even fatal hemorrhage high. Trauma to the penis is usually responsible; cuts, lacerations, and surgical incisions bleed profusely. This is particularly evident with penile hematoma (penile deviation; broken penis) in bulls. A similar disease in the ram is reported. During mating, the penis of the bull probes for the vulva, and when appropriate, the copulatory thrust and ejaculation is done with great force. If the penis deviates from its intended target, tremendous pressure is applied to the region of the sigmoid flexure and insertion of the retractor penis muscles, resulting in rupture and hemorrhage (Fig. 19-33). Hematomas develop just cranial to the scrotum. Small hematomas heal without complications, but depending on the extent of the injury and hematoma, granulation and scar tissue is formed and prevents extension (phimosis) of the penis. In severe cases, hemorrhagic shock can occur. Some hematomas become infected and result in a penile abscess.

INFLAMMATION

Inflammation of the penis is phallitis, of the glans penis is balanitis, and of the prepuce is posthitis. Inflammation of the penis and prepuce (phaloposthitis or balanoposthitis) occurs mostly in castrated animals. This could be the result of alterations to structure because of a lack of testosterone and/or normal development and the tendency of these animals to urinate within their prepuce. Retention of urine in the preputial cavity creates an environment for the overgrowth of bacteria. Those that produce urease split urea to ammonia, a toxic molecule that damages the preputial epithelium, causing erosion and ulceration.

Ovine posthitis (pizzle rot) is a disease of wethers mostly and is caused by urease-producing *Corynebacterium renale.* When the urine has a high concentration of urea, *Corynebacterium renale* produces ulceration of the prepuce near the orifice. A high-protein diet predisposes to the disease. Lack of testosterone is also involved because the disease can be prevented by administration of androgens to wethers. If the preputial orifice becomes blocked by swelling, the disease becomes much more severe, spreading beyond the initial small ulcer on the hairless skin of the prepuce to diffusely involve the mucosa, with ulceration of the glans penis and loss of the urethral process. Scarring and phimosis can result.

In severe cases, the preputial orifice becomes blocked and the animals die from urinary retention.

Nonspecific posthitis occurs in all species and, in the gelding, is believed to occur because of a lack of extrusion of the penis with a resultant buildup of the waxy smegma and bacterial overgrowth. A foul-smelling prepuce and posthitis is the result. Dogs commonly develop a nonspecific and purulent discharge of the prepuce. Foreign material sometimes is found in the prepuce; bulls, rams, and bucks can have matted hair around their penis to form a constricting ring (colloquially called "hair ring"). This can cause a posthitis or even avascular penile necrosis. It is assumed the deposition of hair in this location is because of homosexual activity, and the rubbing of the penis on the posterior of other animals. Dogs, especially those of the chondrodystrophic breeds with short legs, will impact the prepuce with sand.

All species can have traumatic wounds of a variety of types and severity, resulting from mating injuries. Mating or attempting to mate through fences can cause lacerations of varying severities. Owners attempting to "untie" mating dogs can cause degloving injuries to the penis. Horses with penile laceration can develop exuberant granulation tissue ("proud flesh") of the penis.

Trauma is part of the pathogenesis of preputial prolapse in bulls. Bulls of Bos indicus type have a pendulous sheath that is easily lacerated by sticks or other sharp objects. Temporary eversion of the prepuce is common in these and other bulls and is related to inadequate muscular control. The everted preputial mucosa is subject to injury and to edema and inflammation. The prepuce remains everted (prolapsed), swells, dries, and is further lacerated, leading to a cycle of injury and inflammation that are permanent.

Preputial diverticulitis in boars is unique to this species because they are the only domesticated animal to have this anatomic structure normally. The pathogenesis is not completely known, but deflection of the penis into the normal preputial diverticulum of the boar because of malformation or masturbation will predispose this diverticulum to local infection. The diverticulum is also a location for papillomas to develop.

Herpesviruses can cause a multifocal phaloposthitis in several species. Bovine herpesvirus 1 causes a phaloposthitis in the bull, progressing over the course of a few days from hyperemia and swelling to vesicles and pustules and then 1- to 2-mm ulcers, especially of the glans penis (Fig. 19-34). In the vesiculopustular stage, intranuclear inclusion bodies are present briefly in epithelial cells of the penis and prepuce. Ulcerative balanoposthitis with acidophilic intranuclear inclusions has been observed in goats and is considered a result of caprine herpesvirus infection. Equine herpesvirus 3 is the cause of equine coital exanthema, a

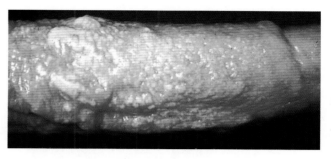

Fig. 19-34 **Phaloposthitis, bovine herpesvirus 1, penis (free part), bull.** Note the vesicles and pustules. Bovine herpesvirus 1 causes hyperemia, swelling, vesicles, pustules, and 1- to 2-mm ulcers, especially of the glans penis. Intranuclear inclusion bodies are present microscopically, briefly in epithelial cells of the penis and prepuce during the vesiculopustular stage. *(Courtesy Dr. K. McEntee, Reproductive Pathology Collection, University of Illinois; and Dr. J. King, College of Veterinary Medicine,*

disease of stallions and mares with a similarly short clinical course, but with larger (15 mm) ulcers with a predilection for the body rather than the glans of the penis. Canine herpesvirus reportedly causes inflammation at the base of the penis and the reflection of the prepuce but does not cause the formation of pustules or ulcers. Resolution of these lesions in the affected species is rapid, leaving only hyperplastic mucosal lymphoid nodules and small areas of depigmented mucosa. Bovine herpesvirus 1, suid herpesvirus 1 (pseudorabies virus) in pigs, caprine herpesvirus 1, and canine herpesvirus can persist in a latent state, capable of becoming reactivated by stress or treatment with corticosteroids.

Papillomaviruses affect the penis of many species. Typical "warts" are produced in the dog, sarcoids are seen in horses, and the bull develops fibropapilloma (Fig. 19-35, *A* and *B*). The bovine disease is discussed in the section on penile neoplasia.

Other organisms are capable of causing phaloposthitis. These include *Strongyloides papillosus* in the bull and the larvae of *Habronema* spp. in the horse. In equine habronemiasis, the gross lesion has the same elevated nodular bleeding surface as granulation tissue or a sarcoid. Microscopically, however, the lesions are distinct tracks of larval migration filled with debris and surrounded by fibrovascular tissue rich in eosinophils. The well-known bovine venereally transmitted diseases of campylobacteriosis and trichomoniasis cause no lesions or minimal nonspecific lesions of the penis and prepuce, even though they reside there.

Obstruction of the penile urethra, especially the urethral process of small ruminants, is common with urolithiasis. The narrowest part of the urethra is the

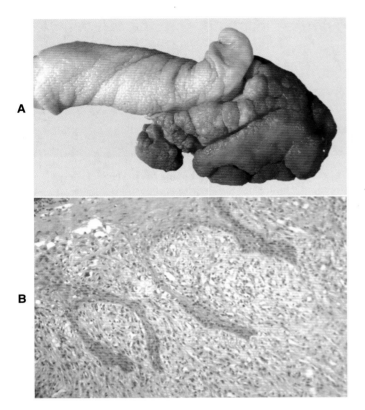

Fig. 19-35   Penile fibropapilloma, glans penis, bull.
A, There is a large exophytic papillary mass protruding from the penile epithelium. This large proliferative lesion on the penis is typical of a fibropapilloma. **B,** Note the abundant connective tissue covered by hyperplastic stratified squamous epithelium that is thickened and has elongated epidermal-dermal interdigitations that penetrate deeply into the connective tissue. H&E stain. (**A,** Courtesy Dr. R. A. Foster, Ontario Veterinary College, University of Guelph. **B,** Courtesy Dr. J. Simon, College of Veterinary Medicine, University of Illinois.)

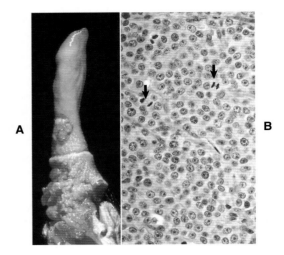

Fig. 19-36   Transmissible venereal tumor, penis, dog.
A, There is a large multinodular mass involving the penis and the prepuce at its reflection from the penis. **B,** Neoplastic cells are round, uniform in size, and often divided into packets by a fine fibrous stroma. Mitoses are frequent (*arrows*). H&E stain. (**A,** Courtesy Dr. M.D. McGavin, College of Veterinary Medicine, University of Tennessee. **B,** Courtesy Dr. M. J. Abdy, College of Veterinary Medicine, The University of Georgia; and Noah's Arkive, College of Veterinary Medicine, The University of Georgia.)

urethral process, and small uroliths that pass through the rest of the urethra become lodged near the tip. Depending on the degree of obstruction, necrosis, and rupture, penile and preputial necrosis can occur. Many animals die of bladder rupture before necrosis of the urethral process or penis occurs.

NEOPLASMS

Primary neoplasms of the penis and prepuce are mostly restricted to a limited number of types and species. Metastatic or multicentric neoplasms affect these tissues rarely.

Transmissible venereal tumor (TVT) of the dog is the only naturally transmitted neoplasm of any species, as it is a type of xenotransplantation. TVT is a round cell neoplasm. The primary neoplasm is usually on the external genitalia, but extragenital primaries and metastatic neoplasms also occur. In the male dog, the neoplasm is found on the penis, more often on the proximal parts, and not often on the prepuce (Fig. 19-36, *A*). The neoplasm can be single or multiple, a few millimeters to 10 cm in diameter, with an inflamed, ulcerated, cauliflower-like surface. Microscopically the neoplasm is the same as it is in the bitch, composed of sheets of round cells and minimal stroma. The neoplastic cells are large and uniform, with a large nucleus and nucleolus, distinct cell outline, and numerous mitotic figures (Fig. 19-36, *B*). Regression and recovery are the rule. The cells express major histocompatibility complex class II antigen, and there is infiltration of inflammatory cells, including increased numbers of T lymphocytes during the regression of the neoplasm. Based on data obtained from immunologic, cytogenetic, and nucleotide sequence studies, the neoplasm is thought to arise from a specific genetic alteration of canine histiocytes, followed by the transmission of abnormal cells from dog to dog.

Squamous cell carcinoma of the penis is of importance in the horse and to a lesser extent in the dog. In the horse, both stallions and geldings have neoplasms, and the common site is the glans penis (Fig. 19-37, *A*). Although proliferative masses do occur, the usual growth habit is one of infiltration with sclerosis, which results in an enlarged penis that is focally necrotic and ulcerated. Microscopically the neoplasm is well differentiated, with well-developed keratin pearls (Fig. 19-37, *B*).

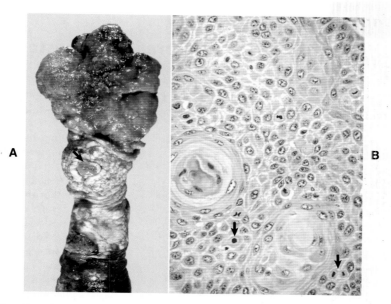

Fig. 19-37   **Squamous cell carcinoma, penis, horse (gelding). A,** A very large ulcerated mass protrudes from the glans penis. The urethral opening is visible (*arrow*). **B,** Neoplastic squamous epithelial cells are often arranged around "keratin pearls." Mitoses are frequent (*arrows*). H&E stain. (*A, Courtesy Dr. R. A. Foster, Ontario Veterinary College, University of Guelph. B, Courtesy Dr. M. J. Abdy, College of Veterinary Medicine, The University of Georgia; and Noah's Arkive, College of Veterinary Medicine, The University of Georgia.*)

Metastasis to the superficial inguinal (scrotal), deep inguinal, and medial iliac lymph nodes can occur. The sheath becomes edematous because of lymphatic obstruction, and the preputial cavity becomes distended by retained smegma, inflammatory debris, and urine.

Papilloma (or fibropapilloma) occurs on the glans penis of young bulls (Fig. 19-35, *A* and *B*). It is attributable to bovine papillomavirus type 1 infection, but the exact pathogenesis has not been elucidated. The papillomaviral origin is expected, as affected animals are young, usually in their first breeding season, and the lesions are self-limiting. They are histologically typical of fibropapillomas elsewhere, including the occasional observation of intranuclear inclusion bodies. The single or multiple warty growths have a significant fibrous core and a papilliferous epithelial covering. The proportions of epithelial and fibrous tissue vary greatly from case to case. Surface ulceration is often extensive following spontaneous necrosis or trauma. Larger neoplasms can interfere with breeding by causing pain or by their physical size. Affected bulls can develop an aversion to mating. The disease is usually self-limiting.

SUGGESTED READINGS

Cornell KK, Bostock DG, Cooley DM et al: Clinical and pathologic aspects of spontaneous canine prostate carcinoma: retrospective analysis of 76 cases, *Prostate* 45:173-183, 2000.

Hall SH, Hamil KG, French FS: Host defense proteins of the male reproductive tract, *J Androl* 23:585-597, 2002.

Heindel JJ, Treinen KA: Physiology of the male reproductive system: endocrine, paracrine and autocrine regulation, *Toxicol Pathol* 17:411-445, 1989.

Klonisch T, Fowler PA, Hombach-Klonisch S: Molecular and genetic regulation of testis descent and external genitalia development, *Develop Biol* 270:1-18, 2004.

Ladds PW: The male genital system. In Jubb KV, Kennedy PC, Palmer N, editors: *Pathology of domestic animals*, San Diego, 1993, Academic Press.

McEntee K: *Reproductive pathology of domestic mammals*, New York, 1990, Academic Press.

Russell LD, Ettlin RA, Sinha Hikim AP et al: *Histological and histopathological evaluation of the testis*, Clearwater, Fla, 1990, Cache River Press.

APPENDIX 19-1

Common Diseases of the Male Reproductive System Based on Species

Species	Common Diseases
Bull	Scrotum and contents
	Cryptorchidism
	Testicular hypoplasia
	Testicular degeneration
	Accessory genital glands
	Vesicular adenitis
	Penis and prepuce
	Preputial prolapse
	Fibropapilloma
	Penile hematoma
Stallion	Scrotum and contents
	Cryptorchidism
	Seminoma and teratoma
	Torsion
	Inguinal hernia
	Penis and prepuce
	Squamous cell carcinoma
Dog	Scrotum and contents
	Cryptorchidism
	Epididymitis
	Testicular neoplasia
	Sertoli cell tumor
	Interstitial cell tumor
	Seminoma
	Accessory genital glands
	Prostatic hyperplasia
	Carcinoma of prostate
	Prostatitis
	Paraprostatic cysts
	Penis and prepuce
	Nonspecific posthitis
	Transmissible venereal tumor
	Papilloma

Species	Common Diseases
Cat	Scrotum and contents
	Cryptorchidism
	Penis and prepuce
	Urolithiasis
Ram	Scrotum and contents
	Testicular hypoplasia
	Testicular degeneration
	Epididymitis
	Varicocele
	Accessory genital glands
	Vesicular adenitis
	Penis and prepuce
	Ovine posthitis
	Urolithiasis
Buck	Scrotum and contents
	Testicular degeneration
	Penis and prepuce
	Hair ring
	Caprine herpesvirus
Boar	Scrotum and contents
	Scrotal hemangiomas
	Cryptorchidism
	Testicular degeneration
	Penis and prepuce
	Preputial diverticulitis

20

Eye, Eyelids, Conjunctiva, and Orbit*

BRIAN P. WILCOCK

INTRODUCTION

Because of its superficial anatomic location and the transparency of its anterior pole, the globe is the only organ that can be directly examined in great detail by the clinician. As a result, the evaluation of the gross lesions of the eye is really the realm of the clinical practitioner and especially the clinical ophthalmologist. The terminology of ophthalmic pathology is identical to the terminology of clinical ophthalmology, which unfortunately is complex and seemingly designed to intimidate anyone other than the most determined.

Examining a globe is really a miniature postmortem in itself. The embryologic development, general reactions to injury, and specific diseases are as different among the cornea, uvea, and retina as they are among the lung, liver, and kidney. Therefore it is traditional to consider the diseases of the eye as a series of relatively separate topics defined by the anatomic portion of the eye under consideration. There are certainly some diseases affecting the eye as a whole, but they are actually in the minority.

All adult mammalian globes have similar general anatomy, depicted in Fig. 20-1. The globe is a spherical biologic camera with an elaborate autofocus lens derived from surface ectoderm and a light-absorbing film plate (retina) created by an outgrowth of specialized neurons from the brain. All other structures within and surrounding the globe are simply there to ensure the optimal function of the cornea, lens, and retina.

The eye develops as a tentacle of brain tissue that reaches out to just under the skin surface of the developing embryo. The eye's purpose is to gather sensory information in the form of photons of light, which are absorbed by neurons specifically adapted to convert light into electrical energy. To facilitate access by those photons to the light-sensitive neurons of the retina, the surface ectoderm, which would normally form ordinary skin, undergoes specialized differentiation into the cornea and lens as the tentacle of the brain comes into proximity with it. Details of embryogenesis will be discussed in later sections of this chapter.

The details of ocular anatomy can be found in any histology text, but there are some specific features that are particularly relevant to ocular pathology. A few of the most important features are emphasized here:

1. The globe is a sealed, fluid-filled sphere, which is protected from noxious influences by a bony orbit, mobile eyelids, a thick fibrous outer shell of cornea and sclera, and a series of vascular and epithelial tight junctions within the uvea and retina referred to as the blood-eye barrier.

2. Although the anatomy and physiology of the globe serve to protect it from many injuries affecting other parts of the body, the same unique features make it extremely susceptible to the propagation of injury once those defenses have been overcome. The fluid media within the globe allows diffusion of infectious agents and chemical mediators of inflammation throughout the globe. The same defenses that prevent entry of various types of chemical or biologic agents also prevent drainage of dangerous by-products of tissue injury and inflammation.

3. Proper visual function requires that very precise anatomic relationships be maintained among the constituent parts of the globe. Minor changes in those relationships that would be insignificant in most other tissues can have devastating results

*Chapters on this subject in earlier editions were written or partially written by Dr. W.W. Carlton, College of Veterinary Medicine, Purdue University; and Dr. J.A. Render, Pfizer Global Research and Development.

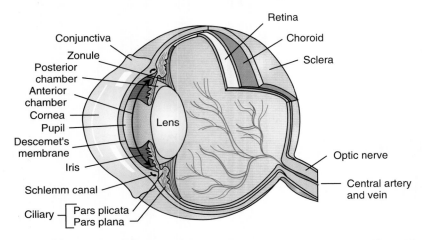

Fig. 20-1   Schematic diagram of the anatomy of the eye. *(Modified from Kumar V, Abbas AK, Fausto N: Robbins & Cotran pathologic basis of disease, ed 7, Philadelphia, 2005, Saunders; and Slatter D: Fundamentals of veterinary ophthalmology, ed 3, Philadelphia, 2001, Saunders.)*

within the globe. Common examples include blindness resulting from minor accumulations of serous exudate behind the retina (serous retinal detachment), or accumulation of edema fluid within the cornea that significantly alters corneal clarity even to the point of blindness. Many of the critical tissues within the globe are unforgiving even of minor changes associated with inflammation or wound healing that, in most other tissue, would be regarded as insignificant.

4. Most of the visually critical tissues within the globe have negligible regenerative capacity. Some, like the adult retina, are essentially postmitotic and cannot regenerate at all. Others, such as the lens and cornea, are capable of limited regeneration, but the regeneration never recreates a perfect structural or functional replica of the original tissue. Many of the most significant intraocular lesions are related to events of wound healing (epithelial proliferation, angiogenesis, and fibrosis), which are desirable events in most tissue but cause serious functional impairments in the globe.

5. Unlike most other tissue, the eye has essentially no reserve capacity. In many tissues we struggle to determine whether a lesion is or is not "functionally significant." There is probably no such thing as a functionally insignificant lesion within the globe. Every single focus of necrosis, inflammation, or scarring probably has a visual consequence even if the degree of impairment is not easily measured.

6. Vision requires that the cornea, lens, and fluid media within the globe remain optically clear. This means that accumulation of exudates, or changes in refractive properties related to conditions such as edema and fibrosis, are extremely damaging even

though these reactions to injury may be beneficial to the survival of the globe itself. There is not much point in having a globe that has survived, but has forfeited vision.

7. Ocular bystander injury occurs when injury to one component of the globe "spills over" and affects other parts of the globe. Examples include the following:
   - Inflammatory effusion from choroiditis, which can cause retinal detachment
   - Alteration in aqueous composition and flow, which can lead to cataracts
   - Organization of intraocular exudates, which can cause tractional retinal detachment or glaucoma secondary to pupillary block or peripheral anterior synechia
   - Chemical mediators of wound healing in chronic uveitis that stimulate preiridal fibrovascular membranes and corneal stromal vascularization

STRUCTURE AND FUNCTION
CORNEA

The cornea is the anterior third of the fibrous tunic that provides structural support for the retinal and uvea. It is a three-layered sandwich about 1 mm thick. It has a thick center of densely compacted collagen fibrils covered on its anterior surface by stratified squamous epithelium derived from fetal surface ectoderm. On its inner (posterior) surface, it is covered by a single layer of cuboidal epithelial cells, known as the corneal endothelium, which is derived from periocular mesenchyme (Fig. 20-2). The corneal epithelium is 6 to 10 cells thick and has a turnover time of 5 to 7 days. The adult corneal endothelium of most domestic mammals does not replicate.

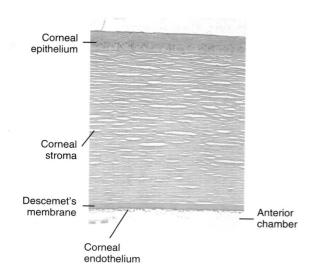

Corneal epithelium

Corneal stroma

Descemet's membrane

Corneal endothelium

Anterior chamber

Fig. 20-2   Normal cornea, dog. H&E stain. *(Courtesy Dr. B. Wilcock, Ontario Veterinary College.)*

The cornea is an adaptation of skin. These adaptations to the epidermis are designed specifically to render it transparent. The surface epithelium differs from that of skin in that there is no keratinization, pigmentation, hair follicles, or adnexal glands. The corneal stroma resembles dermis, except that it lacks blood vessels, hair follicles, and leukocytes. It has relatively few fibroblast-like cells (keratocytes) and a highly regimented organization of its collagen fibrils. These fibrils are arranged in compact lamellae with a space between them that matches the wavelength of visible light. Thus the cornea allows the passage of light without any scattering. To further facilitate the unimpaired passage of light, the corneal stroma is maintained in a dehydrated state compared with that of most other tissue. That dehydrated state is maintained passively by intercellular junctions within the corneal epithelium and endothelium, which exclude water from the tear film and anterior chamber, respectively. It is further maintained by the active removal of electrolytes (and thus water) by energy-dependent membrane pumps within the corneal endothelium and to a much lesser degree the overlying epithelium. The avascular cornea is permitted to exist in this highly privileged anatomic and physiologic state only as long as its "support system" is working properly. It must be protected from desiccation and irritation by properly functioning eyelids and lacrimal secretion, nourished by a tear film that is biochemically normal and delivered in adequate amounts, and replenished by germinal cells resident in the adjacent conjunctiva and sclera. The failure of any of these support systems results in corneal decompensation, seen clinically either as necrosis or as reversion of the cornea to a skinlike state, which although much more durable is unfortunately also opaque.

UVEA

The uvea is the nourishing vascular tunic of the globe. It is made up of the iris, ciliary body, and choroid. It includes the pigmented stroma and muscles of the iris and ciliary body, and the light-reflecting mirror known as the tapetum, which is buried within the dorsal choroid of all domestic species except the pig. It borders the fluid-filled cavities of the globe: the anterior chamber, posterior chamber, and vitreous. The uvea is surrounded exteriorly by the sclera.

The uvea is formed in part by neurectoderm from the primary optic vesicle, and in part by periocular mesenchyme. Its primary function is to provide nutrients to the avascular lens and to the outer half of the retina. In its general structure, it is similar to the lamina propria of the various tubular organs, such as the intestine or reproductive tract. It is rich in fibrous tissue, nerves, blood vessels, and melanocytes. In contrast to the lamina propria of other tissue, however, it contains virtually no resident lymphocytes or plasma cells. Although the vasculature of the uvea is in free communication with systemic vasculature, access by infectious agents or tumor cells from the blood into the globe via the uvea is normally prevented by a series of strategically located tight junctions, which are collectively referred to as the blood-eye barrier (see later discussion under Defense Mechanisms).

LENS

The lens is a biconvex, avascular, transparent accumulation of elongated epithelial cells, suspended within the pupillary aperture. Its shape and elasticity vary greatly by species and with age. It is surrounded by the lens capsule, which is a thick basement membrane (predominantly type IV collagen) produced throughout life by the lens epithelium. That germinal epithelium forms a single layer of cuboidal epithelial cells just below the capsule along the anterior surface of the lens. The epithelium is absent from the posterior surface of the lens. Near the equator of the lens, these epithelial cells migrate inwardly and elongate to become lens fibers. As they elongate, the cells also lose most of their cytoplasmic organelles and eventually lose their nuclei. They develop complex "ball and socket" interdigitations of their plasma membranes and many gap junctions that allow each lens fiber to adhere tightly to all of its adjacent fibers.

New lens fibers are recruited from the germinal cells of the lens epithelium throughout life, so the lens continues to grow. Its net growth is partially counterbalanced by a progressive increase in the density of the center of the lens (the lens nucleus), which is formed by the oldest lens fibers. Gradually the increasing number of aged fibers within the progressively expanding lens nucleus makes the lens less transparent (so-called nuclear sclerosis) and less flexible, so that at least in some species, there is a loss of focusing ability (accommodation) with age.

The purpose of the lens is to further refract light that has passed through the cornea and to focus that light onto the retina. To accomplish this, the lens obviously must remain transparent and in its proper location within the pupillary aperture. Its transparency depends on its highly regimented structure, the paucity of cytoplasmic organelles, the very precise molecular character of its intracellular crystalline proteins, and on its maintenance of a critical state of dehydration. That dehydration is maintained primarily by excretion of electrolytes through an active sodium-potassium–dependent adenosinetriphosphatase pump, located mostly in the anterior lens epithelium.

The location of the lens within the pupillary aperture (with the iris resting on its anterior surface and its posterior surface embedded in a depression in the anterior surface of the vitreous) is maintained by a ring of transparent elastin-like fibers (the lens zonules or zonular fibers) stretching from the lens capsule to the nonpigmented ciliary epithelium. The exact arrangement of these fibers varies greatly by species. Contraction and relaxation of the ciliary muscles alters tension on these fibers and allows the lens to change shape or position, and thus to focus.

The health of the lens is almost totally dependent on the aqueous humor delivering nutrients and removing its waste products. Lens metabolism is primarily via anaerobic glycolysis. Glucose is delivered via the aqueous humor and is absorbed across the lens capsule, which is impermeable to most other substances. This metabolic peculiarity of the lens is vital in the understanding the development of diabetic cataracts (see later discussion).

RETINA AND VITREOUS

The retina is the raison d'etre for the entire globe. The cornea, lens, uveal tract, and sclera are simply a "supporting cast" to allow the retina to do its job of converting photons of visible light into electrical impulses, which are transmitted to the visual cortex of the brain. It is the most fascinating of the ocular tissues, yet at the same time the one that we can influence the least. It is one of the sad realities of ocular disease that we are often powerless spectators, able to view the evidence of active or previous retinal disease, yet with virtually no ability to influence it. Most frequently, at the time of clinical examination, the eye is already blind from retinal detachment, inherited photoreceptor disease, or the devastating effects of glaucoma.

The retina is, quite literally, an outpouching of brain tissue. It is formed from the neurectoderm of the anterior half of the primitive optic vesicle. As that optic vesicle invaginates to form the optic cup, the presumptive retinal neurectoderm is pushed into apposition with the neurectoderm from the posterior half of that optic vesicle, which will form the retinal pigment epithelium (RPE). The proper development of the retina requires that proximity to the retinal pigment epithelium. This dependence of retina on the retinal pigment epithelium continues throughout life. It is impossible to review all significant features of the very complex retinal structure and function here, but those features that are most important in understanding the retinal diseases are as follows:

1. Macroscopically the retina resembles a slightly opaque vascularized membrane, resembling tissue paper, held against the RPE, choroid, and sclera by the gel-like vitreous. It is not actually attached to that RPE and/or choroid except at the optic disc and at its very periphery, where it becomes continuous with the epithelium of the pars plana of the ciliary body (the site of transition is known as the ora ciliaris retinae).

2. The retina consists of three layers of neurons (ganglion cells, inner nuclear layer, and outer nuclear layer) separated by cell-free layers created by the intermingling of the axons and dendrites of those neurons. The innermost layer, adjacent to the vitreous, is the nerve fiber layer. It is made up of the ganglion cell axons that, as they exit the globe, become the optic nerve. The RPE is usually listed as the outermost layer of the retina, but it is derived from the posterior half of the optic vesicle and is not directly involved in vision. The RPE, anatomically and functionally, is more appropriately considered a part of the choroid. The combination of retina, RPE, choroid, and tapetum that is responsible for the ophthalmoscopic appearance of the posterior pole of the globe is known as the ocular fundus (Fig. 20-3).

3. The outer nuclear layer is formed by the cell bodies of the photoreceptors, which are specialized cilia containing photoactivated pigments, which are responsible for converting light into electrical impulses. These photoreceptors are embedded into crevices within the surface of the adjacent RPE, but there are no actual cellular junctions. This intimate contact is essential to allow the RPE to deliver nutrients to, and to remove waste products from, the metabolically demanding photoreceptors. The potential space between the photoreceptors and the RPE is the remnant of the lumen of the primary optic vesicle. It is in this space that hemorrhage, edema fluid, and inflammatory exudate accumulate, resulting in exudative retinal detachment.

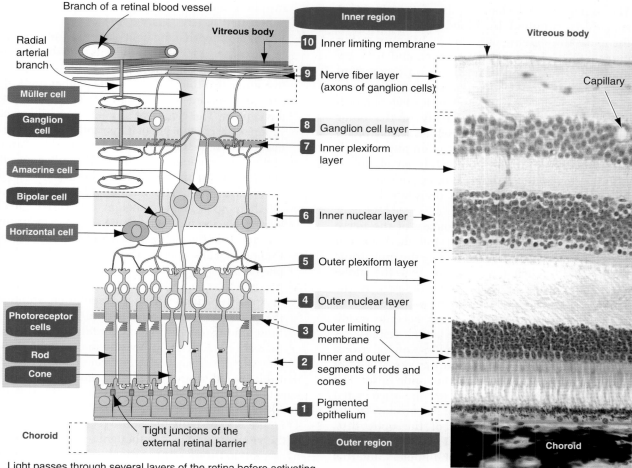

Light passes through several layers of the retina before activating the rod and cone photoreceptor cells. The layers of the retina observed in the photomicrograph are represented in the adjacent diagram. The synapses between the cells of each layer of the retina are also illustrated.

Radial branches from blood vessels (arteries and veins)—located on the retinal surface—are interconnected by capillary beds present in the inner layers of the retina. Retinal capillary beds are lined by endothelial cells linked by tight junctions creating an internal blood-retinal barrier. An external retinal barrier is formed by tight junctions linking the cells of the pigmented epithelium.

Note that:

The nuclei of rods and cones are present in the outer nuclear layer.

The axons of the cones and rods project into the outer plexiform layer and synapse with dendrites of the bipolar cells.

Nuclei of the bipolar cells contribute to the inner nuclear layer.

Axons of the bipolar cells synapse with dendrites of the ganglion cells in the inner plexiform layer.

Axons of the ganglion cells become part of the optic nerve.

Müller cells span most of the retina. The inner limiting membrane represents their basal lamina. Their nuclei form part of the inner nuclear layer.

The outer limiting membrane corresponds to junctional complexes (zonula adherens) between rods, cones, and Müller cells.

Horizontal cells synapse with several rods and cones.

Amacrine cells synapse with axons of bipolar cells and dendrites of ganglion cells.

Fig. 20-3 **Normal mammalian retina.** *(From Kierszenbaum AL: Histology and cell biology: an introduction to pathology, St Louis, 2002, Mosby.)*

4. The inner (vitreal) half of the retina in most species is supplied by blood vessels entering the globe through the optic nerve. In contrast, the outer nuclear layer, photoreceptors, and RPE are totally dependent on diffusion of nutrients from the adjacent choroid. Separation of the retina from the RPE results in rapid ischemic degeneration of photoreceptors, and eventually of the outer nuclear layer. In the horse, in which retinal blood vessels are almost absent, the assumption is that the retina relies almost completely on choroidal diffusion to obtain nutrients, and the consequences of retinal detachment should therefore be even more devastating.

5. The optic nerve is the continuation of the nerve fiber layer of ganglion cell axons into the brain and uses the preexistent tube formed by the embryonic optic stalk. Ganglion cell axons exit the globe through a series of perforations, known as the lamina cribrosa, in the sclera at the posterior pole of the globe. In most species, axons become myelinated at about the level of the lamina cribrosa, as the leave the globe. The combination of axons, myelin, and supporting glia on the vitreal side of that lamina cribrosa forms the optic disc. The amount of myelin and how far the myelinated fibers extend into the retina are responsible for the ophthalmoscopic appearance of the optic disc, which varies among species (Fig. 20-4). In dogs, the myelin extends several millimeters internal (anterior) to the lamina cribrosa and this is responsible for the prominence of the optic disc in that species. Because the optic nerve is a tract of the brain rather than a true peripheral nerve, the myelin is laid down by oligodendrocytes instead of Schwann cells (see Chapter 14).

6. Vision requires that the light gathered and refracted by the cornea is focused by the lens onto the photoreceptors. Light passes through the minimally absorptive inner two thirds of the retina so that most of it can be absorbed by the pigments within the photoreceptors. The electrical signal generated by activation of the photopigment is transmitted in a stepwise fashion from the outer nuclear layer to the neurons of the inner nuclear layer, then to the ganglion cells, and finally via the nerve fiber layer to the optic nerve and brain. The number of photoreceptors "feeding" to a single ganglion cell varies greatly among species and is one of the variables determining visual acuity and the efficacy of dim-light vision. Photons not absorbed on the initial pass through the photoreceptors will, in all domestic animals except the pig, then be reflected back by the cytoplasmic crystals embedded within the tapetum to stimulate the photoreceptors a second time. The tapetum is therefore assumed to be a choroidal adaptation to increase the efficiency of vision in dim light.

The vitreous is an optically clear, gelatinous mass that fills the interior of the globe from the back of the lens to the retina. It is about 99% water, with collagen and hyaluronic acid making up most of the remaining 1%. Little is known about the production and turnover of the vitreous humor. It is thought to be made mostly by secretion from nonneuronal cells of the retina and the nonpigmented epithelium of the ciliary body. The vitreous contains only a scattering of histiocyte-like cells, known as hyalocytes, and a few fibroblasts. Along the anterior surface of the vitreous is a shallow depression known as the hyaloid fossa, in which lies the posterior surface of the lens. The anterior surface of the vitreous undergoes condensation to form the anterior hyaloid membrane, which separates the vitreous from the aqueous humor. The vitreous seems to function mainly to maintain the shape of the globe and to help support the retina in its normal position against the RPE and choroid.

EYELIDS, CONJUNCTIVA, AND ORBIT

The central theme in ophthalmology is the degree to which proper ocular function rests on the ability of the critical visual tissues, such as the retina and lens, to function thanks to a carefully controlled, protected environment. The eye is thus entirely dependent on a long list of factors in a "supporting cast" to protect the sensitive visual tissues against the external environment. The first line of defense is the eyelids, conjunctiva, and bones of the orbit that create a wall around the globe. That protective wall is designed to let in light and nutrients, but to exclude the many elements

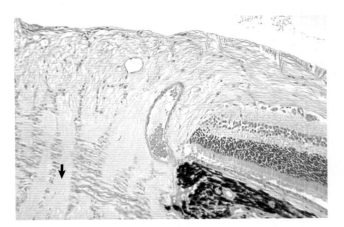

Fig. 20-4   Normal optic disc, dog. The dense fibrous tunic of the sclera becomes fenestrated to permit the exit of the nerve, creating the lamina cribrosa (*arrow*). H&E stain.
(*Courtesy Dr. B. Wilcock, Ontario Veterinary College.*)

of the external environment that might injure this very sensitive organ.

From the perspective of a pathologist, the diseases of the eyelids, conjunctiva, and orbit are much less intriguing than those of the globe itself. From a clinical perspective, however, the diseases of the eyelid and conjunctiva form a major part of what the primary care veterinarian is likely to diagnose and treat.

EYELIDS

The epithelium of the eyelids develops from the surface ectoderm adjacent to the cornea. After separation of the lens vesicle, the surface ectoderm regains continuity to form the cornea. Ectoderm at the periphery of the cornea then migrates over the surface of the embryonic cornea, accompanied by some underlying periocular mesenchyme to form the eyelids. The ectoderm will form the surface epithelium and glands; the accompanying periocular mesenchyme will form the deeper dermis and the eyelid muscles. These ingrowing lid buds fuse with each other over the central cornea. How long this fusion persists varies with the species. In dogs and cats, it persists until about 2 weeks after birth and provides the immature cornea with a secure, sterile environment in which to complete its embryologic development.

The mature eyelids are moveable folds of skin that slide across the surface of the cornea on a film of mucus and fluid known as the tear film. This blinking movement serves to help distribute the protective tear film across the corneal surface and to remove unwanted particulate debris from the corneal surface. Each eyelid has an anterior surface of haired skin, with all of the adnexal glands as seen in skin anywhere else. The dermis is modified by the addition of striated muscle (orbicularis oculi and levator muscles). The inner surface of the eyelid, which rests against the cornea, is covered by a mucus membrane known as the palpebral conjunctiva (see conjunctiva section). The site of transformation from eyelid skin to palpebral conjunctiva at the eyelid margin is characterized by the presence of a row of very large modified sebaceous glands known as Meibomian glands and by the emergence of several rows of large modified hairs that are the eyelid cilia (eyelashes). The Meibomian glands contribute a lipid component to the tear film, which aids in the dispersal of the aqueous component of the tear film and helps prevent evaporation. The cilia are largest and most numerous along the margin of the upper eyelid; they may be infrequent or absent along the lower eyelid.

CONJUNCTIVA

The conjunctiva is a mucous membrane extending from the palpebral margin of the eyelid to the periphery of the cornea. That portion of conjunctiva that covers the posterior surface of the eyelid is the palpebral conjunctiva. That portion attached to the surface of the globe, and continuous with the peripheral cornea at the limbus, is the bulbar conjunctiva.

The palpebral conjunctiva consists of stratified squamous nonkeratinized epithelium near its origin at the eyelid margin but quickly becomes stratified columnar epithelium with numerous goblet cells. At the base of the eyelid, it is reflected back onto the surface of the sclera. Now named the bulbar conjunctiva, it extends over the eyeball as far as the periphery of the cornea. The epithelium of the bulbar conjunctiva lacks goblet cells. It becomes continuous with the corneal epithelium at the limbus. At that junction between bulbar conjunctiva and corneal epithelium, there is a population of germinal cells that are the permanent replicative cells of the corneal epithelium. They are the source of replacement corneal epithelial cells in cases of persistent corneal ulceration.

The space between the palpebral and bulbar conjunctiva is the conjunctival sac. The space between the upper and lower eyelid is known as the palpebral fissure. The medial (nasal) limit of the palpebral fissure (where the upper and lower eyelids join) is the medial canthus. The lateral (temporal) margin of the palpebral fissure is known as the lateral canthus. It is the palpebral fissure that determines what most people would regard as the "shape of the eye," which has considerable importance in the breeding of purebred dogs. It is the careless genetic manipulation of the shape of the palpebral fissure that is responsible for the frequency of some of the most common eyelid diseases (see later discussion under Entropion and Ectropion).

The lamina propria of both the palpebral and bulbar conjunctiva resembles the lamina propria of any other mucus membrane. It has an abundance of blood vessels, loose connective tissue, variable numbers of lymphocytes, plasma cells, and diffuse lymphoid tissue and lymphoid nodules (MALT). The MALT responds immunologically to the microbial flora within the conjunctival sac. In patients with chronic conjunctivitis, the lymphoid nodules are often grossly visible, indicating the intensity and duration of the response of the MALT to antigenic stimuli.

The ventral conjunctiva, as it transforms from palpebral to bulbar conjunctiva, undergoes an additional specialization in the form of the third eyelid or nictitating membrane. This large fold of conjunctiva protrudes from the ventral-medial canthus over the anterior surface of the cornea, and contains a central supporting plate of cartilage and a stroma of dense fibrous tissue, containing an accessory lacrimal gland. Both its anterior and posterior surfaces are covered by stratified squamous nonkeratinized epithelium. In most domestic species, its movement is passive, serving to cover the globe and provide an extra level of protection when the globe is retracted into the orbit by the retractor bulbi muscle.

ORBIT

The orbit is the bony fossa that surrounds most of the globe, except the cornea, and separates the globe from the brain. Along its posterior border are numerous foramina through which blood vessels and nerves reach or leave the globe. The orbit is formed by the fusion of five to seven bones, depending on the species. It is a complete bony shell, except in dogs, cats, and pigs, in which the dorsal roof of the orbit is formed only by the supraorbital ligament that extends from the frontal bone to the zygomatic bone, leaving the dorsal orbit incomplete. The orbit contains not only the globe itself but also the extraocular muscles, abundant fat, lacrimal gland, zygomatic salivary gland, and all the muscles and nerves that support these structures.

The lacrimal gland is a specialized serous salivary gland located in the orbit, dorsolateral to the eyeball. Along with the histologically similar gland of the third eyelid, it is responsible for the production of the serous component of tears. It empties through 15 to 20 small excretory ducts at the lateral part of the fornix of the superior conjunctival sac.

It is unclear how much interdependence there is between the ocular and orbital embryologic development. On one hand, animals with severe microphthalmia often have a relatively normal orbit, but usually there is some reduction in size and distortion of shape. It may be that the critical issue is the stage of embryogenesis at which the developing globe is injured and subsequently atrophies (remember that most microphthalmia in domestic animals is "secondary" and is due to in utero atrophy rather than true hypoplasia).

PORTALS OF ENTRY

CORNEA

Portals of entry into the cornea are listed in Box 20-1. Injury to the cornea may arise from altered homeostasis of the corneal surface, by penetrating injury through the surface epithelium, secondary to injury to corneal endothelium, or rarely by migration into the cornea from the blood vessels at the limbus. Regardless of the route of entry, virtually all significant corneal diseases reflect stromal injury, whether this stromal injury was the primary lesion or simply a consequence of injury to the surface epithelium or to the endothelium of the cornea.

UVEA

Portals of entry into the uvea are listed in Box 20-2. Microbes and other injurious agents enter the uvea via the blood stream (hematogenous), penetrating injury,

---

Box 20-1

Portals of Entry for Corneal Injury

DESTRUCTION OF CORNEAL EPITHELIUM

Desiccation
Trauma
Chemical injury

PENETRATION OF THE CORNEAL STROMA
DIFFUSION INTO STROMA FROM LIMBAL BLOOD VESSELS
INJURY TO CORNEAL ENDOTHELIUM

Glaucoma
Lens luxation
Leukocyte-mediated injury

Box 20-2

Portals of Entry for Uveal Injury

HEMATOGENOUS

Toxins
Infectious agents
Neoplastic emboli

PENETRATING INJURY INTO ONE OR MORE OF THE OCULAR CHAMBERS
VIA AQUEOUS OR VITREOUS

Diffusion of chemical mediators of inflammation

---

or aqueous or vitreous. Hematogenous entry is used by toxins, infectious agents, and metastatic neoplasia. Injury to the blood vessels themselves (thrombosis, occlusion by neoplastic emboli) may cause ischemic damage. Penetrating injury provides infectious agents entry into one or more of the ocular chambers, causing either uveal injury either by production of toxins or (more often) by stimulating a uveal inflammatory response. Injury that causes lens rupture can initiate a phacoclastic uveitis (see later discussion). Chemical mediators of inflammation released from an injured cornea, lens, or retina diffuse into and throughout the aqueous or vitreous, thus providing the opportunity for additional injury in contiguous tissues.

LENS

Portals of entry into the lens are listed in Box 20-3. Although the lens is occasionally injured by a direct perforating injury (see later discussion under Phacoclastic Uveitis) or becomes displaced by blunt trauma (lens luxation), the vast majority of injuries to the lens are

Box **20-3**

Portals of Entry into the Lens

RADIATION

Light
Therapy (x-rays, cancer treatment)
Incidental or accidental exposure

PERFORATION

Through the cornea
Through the sclera
By lens-adapted organisms

BLUNT TRAUMA

Rupture of lens capsule
Dislocation of lens

VIA AQUEOUS HUMOR

Altered chemical composition
Altered volume and/or flow
Toxins
- Inflammatory mediators
- Chemicals
- Biotoxins

related to defective lens nutrition. This involves either inadequate delivery of nutrients because of defective flow of aqueous humor or chemically abnormal aqueous humor. That aqueous humor may contain by-products of intraocular necrosis or inflammation, or excessive/deficient levels of specific chemicals. Common examples include cataracts caused by excessive glucose levels in animals with diabetes mellitus and cataracts associated with systemic hypocalcemia. Degenerative changes in the lens are also seen in dogs with inherited photoreceptor disorders (so-called progressive retinal atrophy), probably caused by diffusion of toxic by-products of photoreceptor degeneration. Inherited cataracts in dogs are the single most frequent type of cataract seen in veterinary practice, but virtually nothing is known about the specific biochemical pathogenesis.

Among the more exotic causes of lens injury are injury from therapeutic radiation; electrical shock, including lightning strike; and penetrating intralenticular metallic foreign bodies. Dietary imbalances, excessive sunlight exposure, and parasitic migration are common causes of cataracts in some nonmammalian species (especially fish) but have rarely been reported in domestic mammals. Cataracts have been reported in puppies and wolf cubs fed a commercial milk replacer, and in kittens fed feline milk replacer. Cataract development was attributed to a dietary deficiency of arginine, although the precise nature of the dietary deficiency was not identified in every instance.

Because the lens is avascular and surrounded by a dense collagenous capsule, it is relatively impervious to the entry of infectious agents from elsewhere in the globe. The one rare exception in domestic mammals is the seemingly specific targeting of the lens capsule by systemic aspergillosis and presumably by other species of hyphal fungi occurring as a sequelae to mycotic abomasitis in calves or opportunistic mycoses in dogs immunosuppressed by cancer chemotherapy. These fungi exhibit a tropism for basement membranes throughout the body, including the lens capsule. In rabbits, the lens capsule is frequently penetrated by the protozoon *Encephalitozoon cuniculi*, which causes spontaneous lens rupture. In fish, cataracts induced by the selective intralenticular penetration by fluke larvae are exceedingly prevalent. Several viral diseases, notably bovine viral diarrhea, are occasionally associated with congenital cataracts as a consequence of generalized systemic infection in utero before the establishment of the blood-eye barrier.

RETINA AND VITREOUS

It has been said that anything in notable excess or deficiency is harmful. That statement is particularly applicable to the retina, which, despite its sheltered intraocular niche, probably is injured by a wider range of noxious stimuli arriving by a wider variety of routes than any other tissue in the body.

Portals of entry into the retina are listed in Box 20-4. The retina can be injured by light and other types of radiation arriving through the cornea and lens, by hematogenous dissemination of chemical or infectious agents, by objects penetrating through the cornea or through the sclera, and by microorganisms arriving via the optic nerve. Because the retina is part of the brain, it is susceptible to most of the infectious, degenerative, and metabolic diseases of the brain, including the storage diseases. Exactly how frequently the retina is involved in diseases affecting primarily the brain is unknown, but the risk appears to be quite low.

The retina is sensitive to injury from chemical mediators of inflammation and toxic products of infectious agents within the vitreous and is particularly sensitive to increased intraocular pressure. Especially in purebred dogs, there is also a huge list of inherited defects in photoreceptor metabolism, which result in progressive destruction of photoreceptors and their nuclei.

The most important and most frequent causes of injury are those related to retinal detachment (see later discussion), increased intraocular pressure, vascular hypertension, and genetically determined photoreceptor diseases. It is important to view this list in perspective. Despite the long list of potentially injurious stimuli and the innumerable routes by which such stimuli can impact the retina, retinal disease is actually quite infrequent.

Box 20-4

Portals of Entry into the Retina

HEMATOGENOUS

Infectious
Toxic
Vascular hypertension
Thrombosis/Thromboembolism
Metastasis

TRAUMATIC

Perforation
Blunt trauma

TRANSCORNEAL

Light
Therapeutic radiation

VITREOUS

By-products of endophthalmitis
Traction detachment
Liquefaction
Glaucoma

CHOROID

Exudative detachment

RETINAL PIGMENT EPITHELIUM (RPE)

RPE disease (Vogt-Koyanagi-Harada syndrome, central progressive retinal atrophy)

OPTIC NERVE

Dieback retinopathy
Retrograde infection
Retrograde malignancy

GENETIC

Canine progressive retinal atrophy syndromes
  • Primary retinal dysplasia

EYELIDS, CONJUNCTIVA, AND ORBIT

EYELIDS

The outer surface of the eyelid is skin and therefore is susceptible to the same diseases as the skin elsewhere on the body. For palpebral skin, the portals of entry are the same as for skin at other sites:

1. Through the skin's surface or through adnexal glands by colonization of niche-adapted infectious agents
2. Penetrating injury
3. Hematogenous localization

CONJUNCTIVA

The conjunctiva is a mucous membrane similar in structure to other mucous membranes and is therefore susceptible to injury from the same range of physical and chemical injuries affecting any other mucous membrane. The routes of entry are predictable:

1. Colonization of the epithelial surface by niche-adapted infectious agents
2. Absorption of injurious antigenic stimuli across an intact epithelium
3. Implantation via penetrating injury
4. Direct physical or chemical injury to the epithelial surface, allowing opportunistic infection
5. Hematogenous localization

ORBIT

Portals of entry into the orbit are as follows:

1. Orbital fractures from external trauma
2. Extension of inflammatory or neoplastic disease originating within the gingiva or the nasal cavity
3. Extension of intraocular inflammatory or neoplastic disease through the sclera
4. Direct extension of inflammatory or neoplastic foci from the conjunctiva or eyelid
5. Penetrating injuries through the skin or upwardly through the mouth, or migrating foreign bodies implanting infectious agents
6. Hematogenous localization of microorganisms, neoplasms, and influx of antibodies in immune-mediated diseases (muscle, lacrimal gland)
7. Extension from the cranial vault via the optic nerve or through one of the other foramina; this is rare

Of these portals of entry, infectious orbital cellulitis resulting from penetrating foreign body or migration from tooth root cellulitis is the most common. In dogs and cats, spread of osteolytic nasal carcinoma, oral squamous cell carcinoma, or malignant melanoma into the orbit is relatively frequent. In cattle, the orbit is a frequent location for metastatic malignant lymphoma in those animals that survive long enough with the disease.

DEFENSE MECHANISMS

CORNEA

The cornea is defended against injury by its protected anatomic location, by several reflexes, and by the tear film (Box 20-5). Passive (anatomic) protection is provided by the eyelids, the eyelashes, and the bony orbit. Various reflexes are activated by mechanical stimulation of eyelids, eyelashes, or the cornea itself. The blink reflex causes the eyelids to close when the eyelids or eyelashes are stimulated by contact with any solid material or even strong air currents. The menace reflex causes the eyelids to blink when there is visual perception of a threat to the globe. The corneal reflex causes the eyelids to close when the cornea itself is

Box **20-5**

Corneal Defenses against Infection

Intact corneal epithelium
Constant washing of the corneal surface
- Tears rich in antimicrobial substances (e.g., immunoglobulin A, lysozyme, and lactoferrin)
- Surface mucus inhibits bacterial colonization
Leukocytes
- Present in small numbers within the tear film
- Rapid recruitment from the capillaries at the limbus

irritated by external stimuli. Reflex retraction of the globe into the orbit, with subsequent passive sliding of the third eyelid to cover the cornea, occurs in response to corneal trauma.

The tear film is a serous secretion produced by the lacrimal gland and by the gland of the third eyelid, with contributions from goblet cells in the conjunctiva and several accessory glands within the conjunctival lamina propria. It not only provides the majority of the nourishment for the avascular cornea, but also provides a mucus coat to prevent evaporation of the protective fluid, soluble antibacterial chemicals, and a flushing action to protect the cornea against colonization by bacteria and fungi that live in the conjunctival sac.

UVEA

The uveal tract, like any other lamina propria, is in free communication with the peripheral blood and is therefore not protected against any noxious agents in circulation. It is protected from physical injury (as are most other parts of the globe) by the thick fibrous tunic of the sclera and by the bony orbit.

Direct uveal injury, however, seems to be less important to the globe than the spread of the uveal disease to other parts of the eye that are less able to resist an insult or regenerate (particularly the lens and retina). The protection of other portions of the globe from inflammation in the uvea rests on two main mechanisms: the blood-ocular barrier, and the unique immunologic phenomenon known as anterior chamber immune deviation.

The blood-ocular barrier is created by tight junctions between endothelial cells of the iris and retinal blood vessels, and tight junctions between adjacent epithelial cells of the inner nonpigmented ciliary epithelium and the retinal pigment epithelium. Unless the damage to the uvea itself is so severe as to disrupt these tight junctions, they prevent most chemical and infectious agents from gaining access to vulnerable intraocular tissues, such as the lens and retina.

The location of this barrier is important in understanding the different reactions to injury by different parts of the uveal tract. For example, the presence of tight junctions between the RPE cells is extremely important in preventing exudate from within the choroid gaining access to the subretinal space. Subretinal fluid accumulation can cause vision-threatening retinal detachment, so the blood-eye barrier at that site provides important protection.

In the anterior chamber, however, the situation is quite different. Here the barrier is at the level of the endothelial cells of the iris. During any substantial inflammation, this barrier is broken as part of the increased vascular permeability inherent in any acute inflammation. This allows infectious agents, inflammatory mediators, and leukocytes to flood into the stroma of the iris. Because the iris has no "barrier" along its anterior surface, these agents, cells, and chemicals then quickly diffuse into aqueous humor of the anterior chamber. From here, they may disperse throughout the globe and damage the lens or even the retina.

Anterior chamber-associated immune deviation (ACAID) is a specialized immune response by which infectious agents and many other antigens introduced into the anterior chamber cause only a highly controlled immune response that effectively eliminates the provoking antigen, while producing minimal bystander tissue injury that would threaten nearby ocular tissue. ACAID protects the eye from antigen-specific, immune-mediated injury from delayed-type hypersensitivity (DTH). The eye contains no lymphoid tissue. To initiate an immune response, antigens within the anterior chamber must first be captured by intraocular antigen presenting cells, exit the globe through the normal aqueous outflow pathways, and reach the marginal zones of the spleen. Here antigen-specific T cells are activated to differentiate into regulatory cells that interfere with the induction of DTH, thus muting DTH and sparing the eye from inflammation induced by DTH.

LENS

The defenses of the lens against injury are almost purely passive. They are the fibrous tunic of the cornea and sclera, the bony orbit, the eyelids, and a thick collagenous resilient lens capsule.

RETINA AND VITREOUS

The retina and vitreous, like the lens, rely mostly on their protected intraocular niche, and like the lens, its active defense mechanisms are negligible. They are protected from most physical and chemical injury by the bony orbit, the fibrous shell of cornea and sclera, and by the uvea and from infectious (and, to some extent, from toxic and metabolic) diseases by the blood-eye barrier created by tight junctions between RPE cells and by the tight junctions of the retinal vascular endothelium. The retina has essentially no defense against infectious agents, radiation, or noxious chemicals arriving through the vitreous. Ischemic injury is a major threat to retinal viability. It is protected by having an autoregulated vascular system that allows retinal perfusion to remain relatively normal despite wide fluctuations in systemic blood pressure. The injured retina also produces angiogenic growth factors and has a powerful system of scavengers to counteract the damaging effects of excitatory neurotoxins, nitric oxide, and other potentially damaging by-products of ischemia. The retina and vitreous have no resident phagocytes or other cellular components of the immune system.

EYELIDS, CONJUNCTIVA, AND ORBIT
EYELIDS

Like skin anywhere else, the defenses of eyelid against injury include both structural and cellular defenses, including hair, keratin, epithelial tight junctions, and a potent intraepithelial and superficial dermal immune system (see discussion on skin). Like skin, it becomes susceptible to infectious disease when those defenses are compromised by excessive moisture, metabolic disease, or mechanical injury. The eyelid is susceptible to all of the same infectious, nutritional, and immune diseases as skin in any other location.

CONJUNCTIVA

The conjunctiva is protected from most physical and chemical injuries by the eyelids and by the tear film. It has tight junctions between the epithelial cells to prevent easy access by infectious or chemical agents into the underlying lamina propria. It is capable of rapid replication in the event of injury, and readily undergoes squamous metaplasia as an adaptive survival mechanism in response to chronic low grade irritation of any type. The resident mucosal immune system (MALT) functions similarly to immune systems in other mucosal sites, such as the upper respiratory tract, lungs (BALT), and gastrointestinal tract (GALT) (see Chapter 13).

RESPONSE TO INJURY
CORNEA

Injury to the corneal epithelium occurs from chemical or physical injury, from deficiency in the quantity or quality of the tear film, or by colonization of the corneal epithelium by infectious agents specifically adapted to that environmental niche. Common examples of such damage include abrasion from misdirected eyelashes or improperly structured eyelids, irritating plant or other foreign bodies within the conjunctival sac, or lacerations inflicted in the course of fighting or running through heavy brush. The cornea is also very susceptible to changes in the quality or quantity of the tear film that may result from primary disease of the lacrimal gland or from desiccation caused by enlargement of the globe or impaired closure of the eyelids.

The corneal endothelium may be injured by increased intraocular pressure (glaucoma), mechanical damage from an anteriorly displaced lens, or from injury mediated by leukocytes (so-called corneal endothelialitis).

The corneal stroma is most frequently injured as a sequela to epithelial damage. It may also be directly injured by lacerations and penetrating injury, implantation of infectious agents subsequent to penetrating injury, or (rarely) by percolation of chemical or infectious agents into the corneal stroma from the blood vessels at the limbus. Injury to the corneal endothelium will also affect the stroma, allowing the dehydrated but strongly hydrophilic stroma to absorb fluid from the aqueous humor. This results in corneal edema and substantial visual impairment (Box 20-6).

The great majority of corneal lesions encountered in clinical practice result from epithelial injury as a result of trauma or desiccation. Almost all corneal diseases listed in clinical textbooks reflect one or more of only three pathologic processes: adaptive cutaneous metaplasia in response to mild irritation, epithelial and/or stromal necrosis, and repair (wound healing) (Box 20-7). The varied clinical manifestations of these three fundamental processes are often given specific clinical names that serve to confuse rather than clarify.

ADAPTIVE CUTANEOUS METAPLASIA TO MILD PERSISTENT IRRITATION

The usual response of the cornea to persistent mild irritation is cutaneous metaplasia, which is a combination of keratinization, epithelial hyperplasia, epithelial pigmentation, subepithelial fibrosis, and

---

Box 20-6

Causes of Corneal Edema

Injury to corneal epithelium
- Resulting in osmotic absorption of water from the tear film

Injury to corneal endothelium from:
- Anterior lens luxation
- Increased intraocular pressure (glaucoma)
- Primary corneal endothelial dystrophy
- Immune-mediated inflammatory destruction

Inflammation of the cornea
- Corneal stromal ingrowth of new, leaky blood vessels

Box **20-7**

Corneal Responses to Surface Injury

ADAPTIVE METAPLASIA

Keratinization
Rete ridge formation
Epithelial and stromal pigmentation
Superficial stromal fibrosis and vascularization from the
limbus

SHALLOW ULCERATION

Edema
Return to normal via epithelial regeneration

DEEP ULCERATION

Edema
Inflammation (primarily neutrophilic)
Neutrophil-mediated stromal lysis
Stromal repair via ingrowth of fibroblasts and blood
vessels from the limbus
Return to nearly normal via epithelial regeneration
following stromal rebuilding

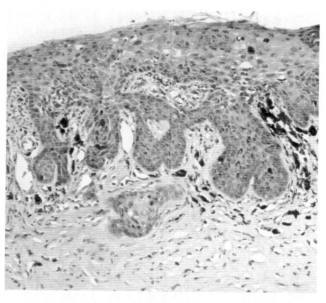

Fig. 20-6   Corneal cutaneous metaplasia, keratoconjunctivitis sicca, cornea, dog. Chronic desiccation has caused adaptive epithelial hyperplasia, epithelial and stromal pigmentation, and stromal scarring. H&E stain. *(Courtesy Dr. B. Wilcock, Ontario Veterinary College.)*

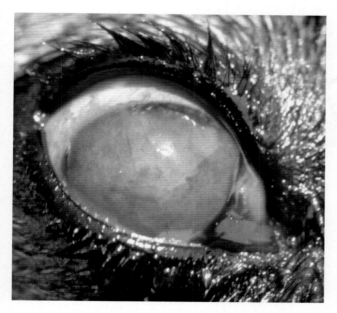

Fig. 20-5   Corneal cutaneous metaplasia, keratoconjunctivitis sicca, cornea, dog. The diffuse corneal opacity is caused by a combination of epithelial hyperplasia and keratinization, as well as stromal scarring and vascularization. *(Courtesy Dr. B. Wilcock, Ontario Veterinary College.)*

vascularization (Figs. 20-5 and 20-6). In short, a cornea that is challenged to adapt to mild persistent irritation does so by recalling its genetic heritage as skin, and comes to resemble skin in every way except for the acquisition of hair follicles. Not all examples of cutaneous metaplasia involve the entire range of adaptive changes; it is possible, for example, to have keratinization without pigmentation, or epidermal metaplasia without accompanying stromal fibrosis and vascularization. It depends on the nature of the irritation. The most common causes for such adaptation include chronic desiccation and mechanical irritation from eyelid diseases, such as entropion or anomalous placement or direction of eyelashes. Desiccation may result from defective production of tears as in keratoconjunctivitis sicca, from improper distribution of tears because of improper eyelid structure or function, or because of ocular enlargement that prevents the lids from closing. Because the cornea is permitted to exist in its privileged state only because it is constantly bathed in a protective and nourishing tear film, the partial or complete removal of that tear film represents a significant challenge to corneal homeostasis. If the change occurs slowly, the cornea will successfully adapt by undergoing cutaneous metaplasia. If, on the other hand, the desiccation occurs very rapidly, then the cornea will likely ulcerate.

Cutaneous metaplasia is a complex event that probably reflects the failure of conjunctival epithelial cells and stroma to acquire corneal phenotypes as they grow toward the center of the cornea to replace injured corneal tissue. The corneal epithelium has a finite number of replicative cycles. Persistent injury that exceeds the replicative ability of the corneal epithelium itself will require ingrowth of germinal cells that reside in the bulbar conjunctiva at the limbus. Similarly, injured corneal stroma will often need to recruit fibroblasts from the adjacent conjunctival lamina propria or sclera. What chemical signals are required to induce conjunctival or scleral tissue to undergo maturation into more appropriate "corneal" structure remain unknown.

Some of the lesions of cutaneous metaplasia are reversible, albeit only very slowly. Stromal fibrosis, however, is a permanent change and the corneal stroma will never again recover complete transparency (see discussion on corneal wound healing). It is easy to think of corneal cutaneous metaplasia as an undesirable pathologic event, but in fact it is an eye-saving response to a pathologic change in the corneal environment. Failure to undergo cutaneous metaplasia would lead to corneal disintegration and subsequent destruction of all of the intraocular tissues.

Clinical entities characterized by corneal cutaneous metaplasia include pigmentary keratitis (corneal desiccation in brachycephalic dogs), keratoconjunctivitis sicca, band keratopathy secondary to eyelid closure defects, chronic keratitis secondary to irritation from eyelids or eyelashes, and chronic corneal desiccation as a consequence of chronic glaucoma.

Epithelial and/or stromal necrosis

Injuries to the cornea that occur too quickly or with too much severity to permit cutaneous metaplasia result in corneal necrosis. Because most of the injuries are from external insults, it is the corneal epithelium that is most commonly affected. The usual result is corneal ulceration. The causes are numerous, including rapidly progressing desiccation, severe mechanical injury, injury from exogenous chemicals, and a few niche-adapted infectious diseases such as herpesvirus infection in cats and *Moraxella bovis* infection in cattle.

Following full-thickness epithelial loss, there is immediate osmotic absorption of water from the tear film into the anterior stroma, resulting in focal superficial stromal edema that is the clinical hallmark of corneal ulceration. The absorption of water increases the spacing between the stromal collagen fibers and results in increased scattering of light, which clinically appears as corneal opacity. Coloring the tear film with water-soluble dyes like fluorescein is a very common clinical diagnostic technique to accentuate the edema within the stroma. Within hours, neutrophils from that tear film are also absorbed into the cornea (Fig. 20-7). In small "physiologic" numbers, they aid in defending the denuded cornea against opportunistic infection, provide growth factors for subsequent wound healing, and help with a small amount of corneal stromal

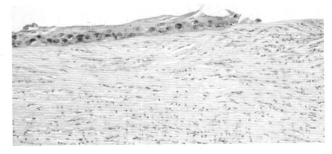

Fig. 20-7 Early healing, shallow ulcer, cornea, dog. The corneal epithelium is sliding along the surface of the denuded intact stroma that now has substantial staining pallor and separation of collagen fibers typical of edema. Numerous neutrophils have migrated into the stroma from the tear film. The neutrophils, although necessary in moderation, have the potential to cause enzymatic digestion of the stroma (keratomalacia) and are sources of fibroblastic and angioblastic growth factors. H&E stain. *(Courtesy Dr. B. Wilcock, Ontario Veterinary College.)*

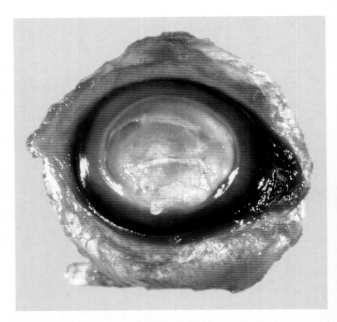

Fig. 20-8 Suppurative keratomalacia, enucleated globe, horse. An initial corneal laceration became infected with *Pseudomonas* spp. The infection has resulted in proteolytic destruction of the stoma caused mostly by the release of digestive enzymes from neutrophils in the inflammatory exudate. Healing will result in a large amount of stromal scarring. *(Courtesy Dr. B. Wilcock, Ontario Veterinary College.)*

débridement necessary for wound healing. If the wound becomes infected and the neutrophils migrate from the tear film and limbus in large numbers, their lytic enzymes create enough bystander injury to result in stromal destruction, known as suppurative keratomalacia (Fig. 20-8).

Corneal injuries of greater magnitude result in deep ulcers with substantial stromal loss, even to the point of disappearance of the entire stroma exterior to Descemet's membrane. This is most commonly seen in rapidly progressing ulcers contaminated with bacteria, resulting in neutrophil-induced keratomalacia. These ulcers, known as "melting ulcers," may progress over just a day or two to full-thickness stromal dissolution. Descemet's membrane is the last barrier. It will bulge anteriorly into the defect created by the loss of the overlying stroma and epithelium to create a descemetocele (Fig. 20-9). In most instances, this fragile membrane (Descemet's membrane) ruptures, resulting in a perforating ulcer, which leads to the loss of anterior chamber fluid and the strong probability of iris prolapse. Iris prolapse may also result from corneal perforation from trauma.

Keratitis is a common clinical term indicating inflammation of the cornea. Because the normal cornea is avascular, true inflammation cannot occur until later in the disease process, after the injured cornea has been vascularized as part of wound healing (see later discussion). Nonetheless, corneal ulcers are very susceptible to opportunistic infection from normal conjunctival flora or organisms from the environment. This is probably particularly true of mycotic keratitis in horses, particularly when the fungal infection is given an unfair advantage because of inappropriate use of antibiotics and/or corticosteroids in the management of minor corneal lacerations. The presence of such organisms within the cornea results in a marked acceleration of leukocyte immigration from the tear film and blood vessels of the limbus. Although these leukocytes may be effective in neutralizing the infectious agent, they usually create substantial bystander injury to the stroma or the epithelium, resulting in a delay in wound healing and an increase in scarring.

REPAIR (WOUND HEALING)

Those injuries limited to just a portion of the epithelial thickness will be rapidly repaired by epithelial sliding and eventual mitotic regeneration. Such injuries are unlikely to ever receive veterinary attention. Deeper defects that involve the full thickness of the epithelium and varying depths of stroma initiate a stereotypic series of events that are clinically significant, easily observed in clinical practice, and amenable to both medical and surgical intervention. Because the cornea is optically clear and readily accessible for continuous observation following injury, it is a favorite model for the in vivo study of the basic events of wound healing in mammalian tissue. From a pragmatic clinical perspective, the vast majority of corneal lesions encountered in clinical practice are already past the stage of initial injury and are at the stage of corneal wound healing. If healing is less than optimal, an array of antimicrobial agents, surgical procedures, and chemical agents to modify the wound healing response is commonly used.

Most models of corneal wound healing use a mild, controlled nonseptic epithelial injury. The sequence of events and the biochemical signaling involved in such injury are not necessarily the same as those in naturally occurring massive corneal injuries and subsequent infections seen in veterinary practice, but nonetheless these carefully controlled models provide the only information available.

Following full-thickness destruction of a portion of the corneal epithelium, the sequence of events is depicted in Fig. 20-10. Briefly, the injured epithelial cells release cytokines, such as interleukin-1 and platelet-derived growth factor (PDGF). Within minutes of lethal epithelial injury, these chemical mediators cause necrosis and/or apoptosis of stromal cells within the very superficial corneal stroma. At the same time, injured epithelial cells at the margin of the ulcer release epidermal growth factor (EGF), keratocyte growth factor (KGF), and hepatocyte growth factor (HGF) to stimulate epithelial migration and proliferation. Additionally, the production of these growth factors is up-regulated in the tear film. The increase in EGF and other growth factors results in flattening and sliding of viable suprabasilar epithelial cells from the adjacent intact epithelium. These cells dissolve their intercellular

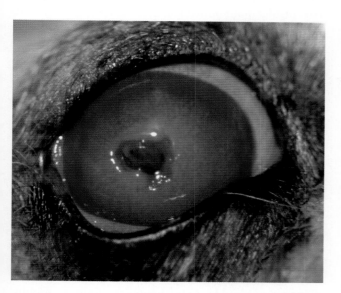

Fig. 20-9 **Deep central corneal ulcer (with descemetocele and early iris prolapse), dog.** Note the diffuse corneal edema (diffuse gray appearance) caused mostly by imbibition of tear fluid, with some contribution from the blood vessels which are growing (angiogenesis) into the injured cornea as part of wound healing (the circumferential red "brush border" from the limbus). *(Courtesy Dr. J. Wolfer, Islington Animal Clinic.)*

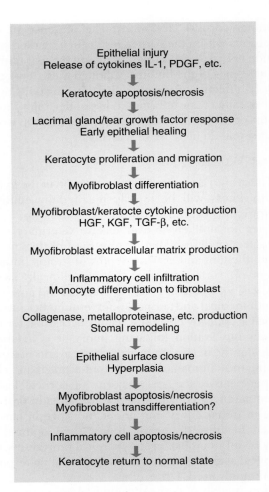

Epithelial injury
Release of cytokines IL-1, PDGF, etc.

↓

Keratocyte apoptosis/necrosis

↓

Lacrimal gland/tear growth factor response
Early epithelial healing

↓

Keratocyte proliferation and migration

↓

Myofibroblast differentiation

↓

Myofibroblast/keratocte cytokine production
HGF, KGF, TGF-β, etc.

↓

Myofibroblast extracellular matrix production

↓

Inflammatory cell infiltration
Monocyte differentiation to fibroblast

↓

Collagenase, metalloproteinase, etc. production
Stomal remodeling

↓

Epithelial surface closure
Hyperplasia

↓

Myofibroblast apoptosis/necrosis
Myofibroblast transdifferentiation?

↓

Inflammatory cell apoptosis/necrosis

↓

Keratocyte return to normal state

Fig. 20-10   Schematic diagram of the corneal wound healing cascade. *HGF,* Hepatocyte growth factor; *IL-1,* interleukin-1; *KGF,* keratocyte growth factor; *PDGF,* platelet-derived growth factor; *TGF-β,* transforming growth factor-β. *(Redrawn from Klenkler B, Sheardown H: Exp Eye Res 79:677-688, 2004.)*

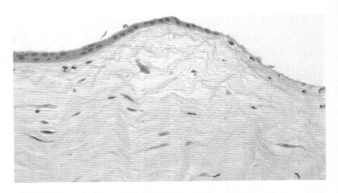

Fig. 20-11   Corneal epithelial cell migration (epithelial sliding), early wound healing, cornea, dog. Corneal epithelial cells are migrating (sliding) to cover the corneal ulcer (*right*). The stroma is edematous and contains a few neutrophils derived from the tear film. H&E stain. *(Courtesy Dr. B. Wilcock, Ontario Veterinary College.)*

junctions and migrate across the exposed stromal surface, adhering to a temporary scaffold of fibronectin and other adhesion molecules (Fig. 20-11). As long as the underlying stroma is healthy enough to support epithelial migration, excessive numbers of neutrophils are not present, and if the event that caused the original corneal injury is no longer active, those epithelial cells will slide with remarkable speed (as much as 1 mm per day) across the denuded surface in an attempt to close the defect. There are many other cytokines and adhesion molecules involved in corneal epithelial sliding and regeneration, suggesting that rapid sealing of the defect must be exceedingly important. Closure of the defect by even a thin layer of epithelium halts the continued recruitment of neutrophils, which are responsible for the keratomalacia, vision-impairing stromal fibroplasia, and vascularization from the limbus. Closure of the corneal defect also prevents further

edema and limits access by potentially injurious infectious agents.

Lagging behind the epithelial activation and sliding, which occur within minutes to hours of injury, is rebuilding of the injured stroma, which starts within a few days. It is not clear how the cornea recognizes the need for stromal rebuilding. There are some cases in which even a deep stromal defect does not initiate ingrowth of fibroblasts and blood vessels to rebuild the stroma. Instead the epithelium simply slides across whatever small amount of normal stroma remains. This results in an optically clear, but precariously thin, healed cornea (Fig. 20-12). Migration of neutrophils from the tear film and from the limbus into the corneal wound is a powerful stimulus for the recruitment of both blood vessels and fibroblasts from the limbus. Neutrophil immigration begins about 12 hours after mild injury in response to chemotactic factors released by injured epithelium and stroma. This delay in neutrophil recruitment presumably allows the epithelium to slide and seal small defects, and thus prevents excessive immigration of neutrophils (and its negative consequences as outlined later). Additional stimulation of stromal fibroplasia and angiogenesis comes from release of growth factors, such as PDGF, vascular endothelial growth factor (VEGF), and transforming growth factor-β (TGF-β) from the injured epithelium, migrating neutrophils, and the injured stromal keratocytes. Not only does injury stimulate activation and migration of fibroblasts and angioblasts from the limbus, but it also changes the morphology and activity of the resident stromal fibroblasts (keratocytes). These cells undergo myofibroblastic metaplasia, become mobile and contractile, and produce increased amounts of various matrix proteins, growth factors, and metalloproteinases essential for stromal remodeling.

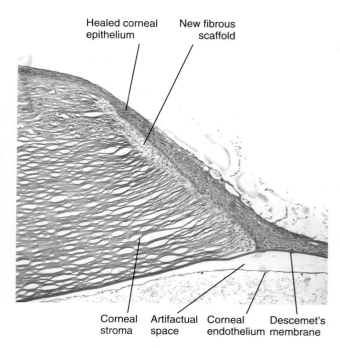

Healed corneal epithelium   New fibrous scaffold

Corneal stroma   Artifactual space   Corneal endothelium   Descemet's membrane

Fig. 20-12   Chronic descemetocele, cornea, dog. On the right, at the site of a former deep corneal ulcer, the epithelium has healed by corneal epithelial cell migration (sliding) into the ulcer, with subsequent epithelial hyperplasia and return of the corneal epithelium to normal or even increased thickness. However, because there has been no replacement or remodeling of the stroma (*right*), the epithelium is positioned directly on the surface of Descemet's membrane instead of on a reconstituted fibrous stroma. This process is "unsuccessful" wound healing, because the "healed" cornea, lacking stroma, is too fragile to survive. Masson trichrome stain. (*Courtesy Dr. B. Wilcock, Ontario Veterinary College.*)

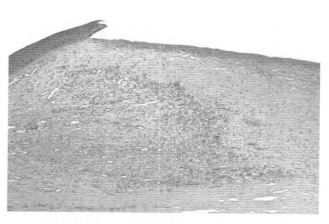

Fig. 20-13   Normal wound healing, cornea, dog. Following shallow ulceration that had damaged both the epithelium and the superficial stroma, the stroma is repaired and returned to near normal function by ingrowth of blood vessels and fibroblasts (wound healing) from the limbus. Such repair of the stroma is usually a prerequisite for epithelial regeneration following any large corneal ulceration. H&E stain. (*Courtesy Dr. B. Wilcock, Ontario Veterinary College.*)

The histologic events of stromal rebuilding following significant injury are less complicated than are the innumerable biochemical signaling interactions involved. Mild stromal injuries are repaired by in situ enlargement and sluggish proliferation of resident keratocytes, which undergo fibroblastic metaplasia. Following significant stromal injury, however, repair using just local keratocytes/monocytes is not adequate. Such repair must await the arrival of reinforcements in the form of fibroblasts and blood vessels from the limbus. Histologically, enlargement and hyperchromasia of limbal fibroblasts and angioblasts is visible within a day or two of injury, but detectable migration is not evident until about 4 days. Fibroblasts and blood vessels, preceded by a halo of edema and stromal proteolysis, migrate with a maximum speed of 1 mm per day until they reach the site of injury (Fig. 20-13). Here, they rebuild the injured stroma to provide a scaffold suitable for the migration, adhesion, and eventual normalization of the epithelium. Over time, this fibroblastic-angioblastic matrix of granulation tissue matures to histologically resemble normal stroma. However, it is never able to replicate the very specific lamellar structure of normal stroma and even with optimal stromal wound healing, corneal clarity is permanently impaired.

It is worth mentioning here that a lamellar ingrowth of blood vessels from the limbus into the middle third of a perfectly normal corneal stroma occurs as a bystander effect of chronic uveitis (see section on uveitis: Delayed Responses to Injury).

To summarize, the epithelial and stromal events of wound healing are stimulated by a complex interaction of dozens of growth factors, adhesion molecules, and other chemical signals. It is far from understood exactly how these interact. It is clear that the cellular responses are greatly influenced not only by what chemicals are present but also by the context into which they are introduced. The action triggered by any of these mediators is influenced by other mediators in the environment, when the mediators are generated in relation to the wound healing process, and by what cells are targeted (Fig. 20-14).

UVEA
UVEAL INFLAMMATION

The nomenclature of uveal inflammation is the same as that is used in clinical ophthalmology (Box 20-8). Hypopyon is the accumulation of neutrophils and fibrin that settles ventrally within the anterior chamber (Fig. 20-15). Inflammation within the iris and ciliary

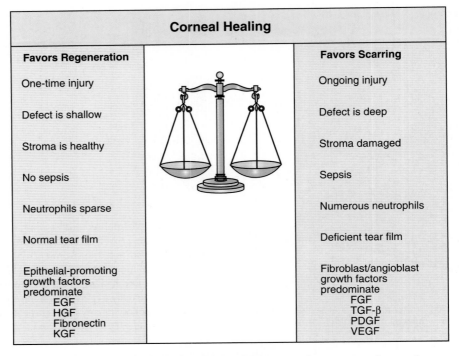

Corneal Healing

Favors Regeneration	Favors Scarring
One-time injury	Ongoing injury
Defect is shallow	Defect is deep
Stroma is healthy	Stroma damaged
No sepsis	Sepsis
Neutrophils sparse	Numerous neutrophils
Normal tear film	Deficient tear film
Epithelial-promoting growth factors predominate EGF HGF Fibronectin KGF	Fibroblast/angioblast growth factors predominate FGF TGF-β PDGF VEGF

Fig. 20-14   Schematic diagram of corneal wound healing. The outcome of corneal wound healing depends in part on the balance among growth factors coming from the tear film, injured epithelium and stroma, and immigrating leukocytes. *EGF,* Epidermal growth factor; *FGF,* fibroblast growth factor; *HGF,* hepatocyte growth factor; *KGF,* keratocyte growth factor; *PDGF,* platelet-derived growth factor; *TGF-β,* transforming growth factor-β; *VEGF,* vascular endothelial growth factor.

Box 20-8

Histologic-Clinical Correlation in Uveitis

The uveal tract responds to inflammatory stimuli as do other tissues. The macroscopic manifestations detectable by clinical examination are as follows:

- Aqueous flare: an increase in protein content within the aqueous humor increases light scattering
- Iris swelling and color change: iris stromal hyperemia, edema, and leukocyte accumulation
- Conjunctival reddening: hyperemia of the superficial and deep conjunctival blood vessels in response to vasoactive chemicals generated by the nearby uveitis
- Hypopyon: the accumulation of neutrophils and fibrin that settles ventrally within the anterior chamber
- Keratic precipitates: small clusters of macrophages and/or neutrophils adherent to the corneal endothelium
- Peripheral corneal midstromal vascularization: persistent inflammation results in the generation of enough angiogenic growth factors to stimulate "accidental" migration of limbal blood vessels into the peripheral cornea

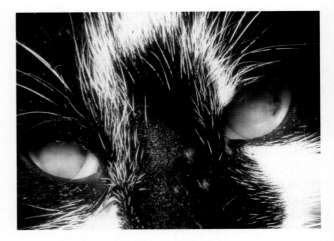

Fig. 20-15   Hypopyon (bilateral), feline infectious peritonitis, cat. A mixture of fibrin and neutrophils is present within the anterior chamber of the eyes. *(Courtesy Dr. B. Wilcock, Ontario Veterinary College.)*

body is usually referred to as anterior uveitis, although iridocyclitis is equally accurate. Inflammation limited to the choroid is choroiditis; inflammation limited to the vitreous is hyalitis; inflammation throughout the uveal tract is panuveitis; and inflammation involving the uveal tract and the adjacent ocular cavities (anterior chamber, posterior chamber, and vitreous) is endophthalmitis. Inflammation that spreads to involve sclera is known as panophthalmitis. Although these terms are widely used in clinical ophthalmology, in reality the vascular tunic within the globe is a unified structure and virtually all examples of clinically significant uveal inflammation involve all portions of the uvea at least to some degree and have at least a little bit of effusion into the ocular chambers. Furthermore, the globe is a sealed sphere filled with fluid, so that inflammatory mediators or toxic products of infectious agents are likely to be widely disseminated within the globe. Thus from a purely histologic perspective, virtually all cases of uveitis can be correctly classified as endophthalmitis.

A further source of confusion between histopathologic and clinical terminology is a consequence of identification of the predominant leukocyte in the exudate. As is true of lesions in many other tissues, histopathologic examination underestimates the number of rapidly migrating granulocytes and is misled by the gradual accumulation of nonemigrating mononuclear leukocytes. Neutrophils rapidly accumulate within the aqueous or vitreous humors where they can be detected by clinical or cytologic examination. Unless bound up in fibrin, those leukocytes are washed away during histologic processing, leaving only the predominantly mononuclear population within the uveal stroma. This is not unique to the globe: An identical opportunity for confusion exists in correlating cytologic and histologic lesions in immune-mediated joint disease, chronic rhinitis, and pyometra (among others).

CAUSES OF UVEITIS

Uveitis can be initiated by a wide array of infections, immune responses, and trauma. Tissues of the globe usually act as an integrated unit, so injury to one part almost always has at least some influence on the health of other parts of the globe. The globe is filled with fluid, thereby allowing chemical messengers generated in one part of the globe to be absorbed by distant intraocular tissue. The iris stroma, in particular, is highly reactive because there is free communication between it and the aqueous humor. Any toxins, chemical mediators of inflammation, or growth factors secreted into the aqueous will be absorbed by the iris, causing that portion of the uveal tract to react. (See later discussion under Preiridal Fibrovascular Membrane).

Most of the infectious causes of uveitis are ocular responses to systemic viral, bacterial, or parasitic diseases in which the uveal tract is only one of many tissues affected. Endophthalmitis as the sole manifestation of infectious disease is usually seen only as a sequela to penetrating injuries or perforating ulcers that allow the entry of environmental organisms into the globe. There are no viral causes of endophthalmitis, although there are a few systemic viral infections that cause vasculitis or retinitis that result in a uveal inflammatory response. Aberrant migration of nematode or trematode larvae will occasionally cause endophthalmitis, as will ocular colonization by a variety of protozoal parasites that cause systemic disease (toxoplasmosis and encephalitozoon in particular). Uveal involvement in systemic mycoses and prototheocosis is particularly common in animals in certain geographic regions.

Immune-mediated uveitis is a particularly frequent finding. In only a few types is there a reasonable understanding of the pathogenesis, as in uveodermatologic syndrome and phacoclastic uveitis (see later discussion). In the great majority, there is a chronic lymphocytic-plasmacytic endophthalmitis with no demonstrable infectious agent, and a moderately successful clinical response to immunosuppressive therapy (see Idiopathic Lymphonodular Uveitis later). The lesion is clearly the result of an immunologic response, but it is not known whether such a lesion reflects primary immune-mediated disease, or simply a response to an elusive infectious agent that has long since disappeared.

Ocular trauma is a frequent cause of transient endophthalmitis. The uvea will also respond to afferent neural signals and chemical factors released from an injured cornea, so that with any significant corneal ulceration or keratitis one can expect to have at least a mild anterior uveitis.

IMMEDIATE RESPONSE TO INJURY: UVEITIS

Because the uveal tract has a fibrovascular stroma similar to the lamina propria of intestine or the dermis of skin, it undergoes all of the usual inflammatory reactions. There is nothing at all unique about these reactions. What is unique, however, is the importance of the consequences of that inflammation for other parts of the globe.

DELAYED RESPONSES TO INJURY

What is most distinctive about uveitis is not the macroscopic or microscopic character of the inflammatory reaction itself, but the consequences of that inflammation for adjacent portions of the globe. These bystander effects, which include anterior and posterior synechiae, retinal detachment, cataract, corneal vascularization, preiridal fibrovascular membrane, and glaucoma, are clinically significant and are frequently the targets of therapeutic intervention.

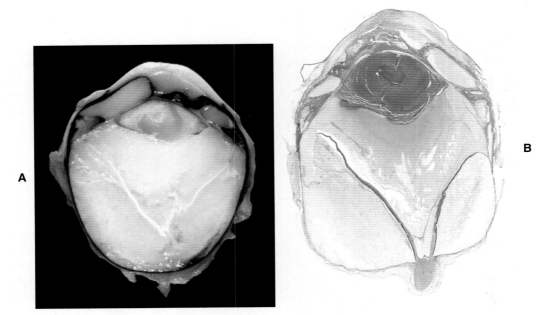

Fig. 20-16   Posterior synechia, pupillary block and iris bombé, eye, sagittal section, dog.
A, The iris has adhered to the lens, creating a pupillary block and subsequent iris bombé. Cloudy exudate fills the vitreous, and its accumulation in the subretinal space has caused complete retinal detachment. These changes occurred as a consequence of corneal perforation and secondary septic endophthalmitis. **B,** Same globe as Fig. 20-16, A. The serous effusion from the choroid has caused retinal detachment, which has serious implications for retinal survival. Additional lesions include posterior synechia, iris bombé, ciliary-lenticular adhesions, and circumferential cortical cataract. The combination of posterior synechia, pupillary block, iris bombé, and secondary peripheral anterior synechia is an exceedingly common sequence in the pathogenesis of glaucoma secondary to uveitis. H&E stain. (**A** and **B,** Courtesy Dr. B. Wilcock, Ontario Veterinary College.)

Synechiae are adhesions between the inflamed, sticky iris and either the lens or cornea. Adhesion to the anterior capsular surface of the lens (in the normal globe, the iris lies against the lens capsule) is known as posterior synechia. The adhesion is initially fibrinous but, if allowed to persist, will become a firm fibrous adhesion. If that adhesion is sufficiently extensive around the pupillary margin (i.e., approaching the full circumference of the pupil), there will be significant impairment of aqueous outflow from the posterior chamber to the anterior chamber (pupillary block) and inevitable secondary glaucoma. Increased pressure within the posterior chamber in the presence of a circumferential posterior synechia results in anterior bowing of the iris known as iris bombé (Fig. 20-16, A).

Anterior synechia is a focal-to-diffuse iridocorneal adhesion. Because the iris is not normally in proximity to the cornea, anterior synechia is much less prevalent than posterior synechia. It is most commonly seen as a sequela to iris prolapse, in which the flexible iris is literally "sucked up" into the corneal defect, where it then becomes anchored by fibrin and later by fibrosis. Peripheral anterior synechia commonly accompanies iris bombé and preiridal fibrovascular membranes (see later discussion).

Retinal detachment is a common sequela to uveitis and/or endophthalmitis by one of two mechanisms. Increased vascular permeability within the choroid results in effusion of fluid and cells into the subretinal space, resulting in so-called exudative detachment (Fig. 20-16, B). The normal retina is not actually adhered to the RPE. Fluid leaving the choroid during inflammation will preferentially accumulate in the potential space between the retina and RPE because its only alternative would be to try to escape through the dense fibrous shell of the sclera. Alternatively, replacement of fibrinous exudates by fibrous tissue within the vitreous may result in tractional detachment. The immediate and delayed visual consequences of retinal detachment are discussed later (see discussion on diseases of the retina). If there is a lot of fibrovascular ingrowth as a consequence of organization of vitreal exudate, the maturing fibrovascular tissue routinely creates a dense membrane across the anterior surface of the vitreous (just posterior to the lens). This cyclitic membrane is anchored into the

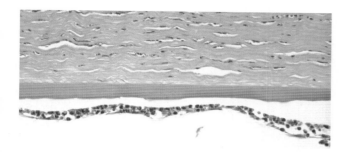

Fig. 20-17 Corneal endothelialitis, cornea, cat. Neutrophils adhere to and have accumulated on and in the corneal endothelium. When numerous, they separate the corneal endothelial cells from the adjacent Descemet's membrane. This is a relatively frequent complication of anterior uveitis in cats and especially cats with feline infectious peritonitis. The leukocytes may be predominantly neutrophils or lymphocytes, depending on the pathogenesis and the duration of the uveitis. H&E stain. *(Courtesy Dr. B. Wilcock, Ontario Veterinary College.)*

ciliary epithelium, and often incorporates remnants of the detached retina.

Cataracts are frequent sequela to uveitis, but the exact mechanisms are poorly understood. We do know that the avascular lens is entirely dependent on the aqueous humor for the delivery of nutrients and the removal of metabolic waste products. In eyes with uveitis, there is a notable drop in the production of aqueous humor (ocular hypotension is one of the clinical features of uveitis), resulting in lens "malnutrition." It is assumed that the lens is also susceptible to injury by mediators of inflammation and other toxic products in the aqueous humor of inflamed globes.

Corneal endothelialitis is characterized by an infiltration of neutrophils and/or lymphocytes into the corneal endothelium (Fig. 20-17). It usually is seen in globes with other lesions of chronic uveitis, but sometimes it is the most obvious histologic lesion of a uveitis that has almost disappeared (at least histologically) from other parts of the globe. It is much more prevalent in feline globes with feline infectious peritonitis (FIP) and idiopathic lymphonodular uveitis than in any others. Its pathogenesis is unknown. It was once a common lesion as a delayed sequela to vaccination with modified live vaccines containing canine adenovirus 1, and occasionally to canine adenoviral hepatitis. Complement-fixing antibodies against the virus were present within the endothelium as a result of a previous viral infection, resulting in attraction of neutrophils and subsequent bystander injury to the endothelium. If the endothelial damage was of sufficient magnitude, the result was the development of severe and sometimes permanent corneal edema, commonly referred to as "blue eye."

Preiridal fibrovascular membrane refers to a layer of granulation tissue on the anterior surface of the iris. It is created by budding and migration of capillaries

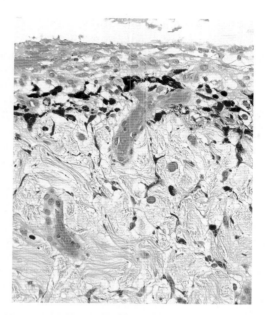

Fig. 20-18 Preiridal fibrovascular membrane, iris, dog. A membrane formed by proliferating fibroblasts and capillaries has grown out from the iris stroma and has adhered to the anterior surface of the iris (represented here by the thin layer of pigmented melanocytes). These membranes form in response to growth factors within the aqueous humor, originating from such varied sources as intraocular neoplasms, or follow retinal detachment or chronic uveitis. H&E stain. *(Courtesy Dr. B. Wilcock, Ontario Veterinary College.)*

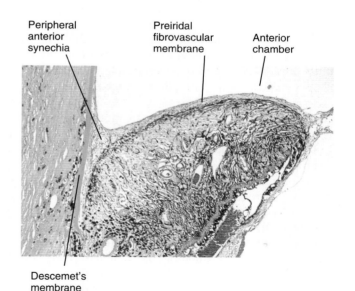

Fig. 20-19 Mature preiridal fibrovascular membrane, iris, dog. A layer of mature granulation tissue has adhered to the anterior surface of the iris. Contraction of the maturing membrane has distorted the shape of the iris and has caused it to adhere to the posterior surface of the cornea (peripheral anterior synechia). If extensive, the anterior synechia will result in secondary glaucoma. H&E stain. *(Courtesy Dr. B. Wilcock, Ontario Veterinary College.)*

from the iris stroma and recruitment of fibroblasts as a routine response to cytokine mediators of wound healing (Fig. 20-18). It is no different from granulation tissue anywhere else in the body, but in typical ocular fashion, it achieves special significance within the globe. If the granulation tissue migrates across the anterior face of the lens, it creates a pupillary block resulting in secondary glaucoma. Alternatively, this granulation tissue can also migrate across the anterior face of the filtration angle to create a peripheral anterior synechia and once again cause secondary glaucoma (Fig. 20-19). Like any immature granulation tissue, it is also susceptible to hemorrhage and is a frequent cause of anterior chamber hemorrhage, known as hyphema. Wound healing following uveitis is only one of several mechanisms for the development of preiridal fibrovascular membranes, which are described in greater detail in the section on glaucoma.

Midstromal corneal vascularization is an extremely common and clinically useful clue pointing to the presence of chronic uveitis. The vessels grow inwardly from the limbus. It has no known functional significance and appears to be a purely accidental lesion because the blood vessels of the limbus respond to angiogenic growth factors being produced within the globe as part of the ongoing inflammation and repair.

Phthisis bulbi refers to a shrunken, disorganized endstage globe. It is not a sequela only to uveitis, but severe uveitis is the most common cause.

LENS

The stereotypic histologic response of the lens to injury is hydropic swelling of the injured lens fibers, fiber disintegration resulting in cortical liquefaction, and abortive efforts at regeneration. This combination of changes is essentially identical, regardless of pathogenesis. They all result in opacification of the lens, referred to by the generic term "cataract."

In clinical ophthalmology, cataracts are extensively subclassified by location within the lens, by age of onset, by the macroscopic appearance, or by the state of progression. This gives rise to an exceedingly complicated list of purely descriptive adjectives that are not at all reflective of the pathogenesis. Such classification is used mostly when dealing with inherited cataracts in dogs to ensure that the data being collected about the frequency or behavior of a cataract in a specific breed are indeed referring to the same disease.

The stereotypic microscopic changes of cataracts (Figs. 20-20 and 20-21) are various combinations of the following, listed in order of overall frequency:

1. Fragmentation and liquefaction of cortical fibers, creating spherical globules of denatured lens protein known as Morgagnian globules.
2. Hydropic swelling of cells, known as bladder cells, attempting but failing to regenerate

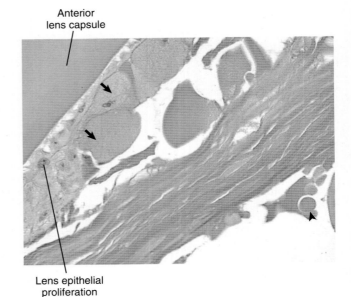

Anterior lens capsule

Lens epithelial proliferation

Fig. 20-20   Cataract, lens, dog. There is epithelial hyperplasia of the lens with fibroblastic metaplasia, formation of bladder cells (*arrows*), and a Morgagnian globule (*arrowhead*). H&E stain. (*Courtesy Dr. B. Wilcock, Ontario Veterinary College.*)

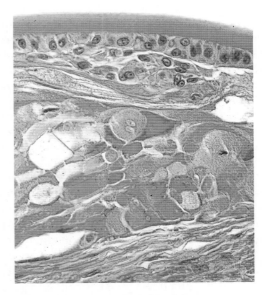

Fig. 20-21   Anterior cortical cataract, lens, fish. Note the lens epithelial proliferation, fibroblastic metaplasia, and prominent bladder cells. (*Courtesy Dr. B. Wilcock, Ontario Veterinary College.*)

3. Hyperplasia and fibrous metaplasia of lens epithelium; the epithelial hyperplasia may create plaquelike thickening with or without fibroblastic metaplasia
4. Posterior lens epithelial migration; the lens epithelium migrates from the equator to lie under the posterior lens capsule; the normal adult lens has no epithelium posterior to the equator

5. More variable changes include lens swelling in acute cataracts, lens shrinking with wrinkling of the lens capsule in advanced ("hypermature") cataracts, and intralenticular mineralization

The lens is capable of additional responses to injury other than those associated with cataracts, but these are much less frequent. As discussed in the section on phacoclastic uveitis, rupture of the lens capsule allows regenerative lens epithelium to escape from the lens, undergo fibroblastic metaplasia, and migrate within the anterior and posterior chambers, sometimes with devastating consequences. The same type of proliferation complicates cataract surgery, producing thick plaques of fibroblast-like epithelial cells that are aesthetically displeasing and reduce visual acuity.

RETINA AND VITREOUS

The general pathology of the retina resembles that of the brain. The neuronal elements of the adult retina of higher mammals do not regenerate; the outer segments of the photoreceptors, however, have a rapid turnover and have among the highest metabolic activity in the body. As long as the cell body within the outer nuclear layer remains viable, photoreceptors can be quickly regenerated.

The RPE remains mitotically active throughout life. Like other epithelia, it repairs itself, first by sliding viable cells into the area where cells have been lost and then by mitosis. Fibroblastic metaplasia is common (see later discussion).

The glial elements of the retina, particularly the astrocytes that reside within the inner nuclear layer (Müller cells), are exceedingly hardy and capable of proliferation. Repair of most cases of retinal necrosis

occurs primarily by proliferation of Müller cells, which eventually form a dense glial scar, sometimes with a contribution from migrating RPE cells that can also undergo fibroblastic metaplasia (Fig. 20-22). Occasionally the astrocytes proliferate along the vitreal face of the retina, forming a preretinal fibroglial membrane. Subretinal membranes (between the photoreceptors and the RPE) of a similar microscopic appearance are seen with chronic detachments and originate from migrating Müller cells or from retinal pigment epithelium that has undergone fibroblastic metaplasia.

The vast majority of retinal lesions fall into three categories:

1. Inflammation as a result of extension from endophthalmitis or encephalitis. Inflammation targeting the retina specifically is exceedingly uncommon. The character of the inflammation within the retina is exactly the same as it is within the brain: neuronal necrosis, perivascular cuffing, and gliosis. What is different about the retina, however, is its susceptibility to exudative retinal detachment. Fluid and cells escaping from inflamed retinal vessels are most likely to accumulate in the subretinal space and result in the separation of the photoreceptors from the RPE and the choroidal vasculature (Fig. 20-23). The photoreceptors are therefore likely to become necrotic, not only from the by-products of inflammation, but from ischemia and other forms of malnutrition resulting from their anatomic dislocation from the RPE (remember that the photoreceptors are entirely dependent on their intimate contact with the RPE and their proximity to the choroid for their nutrition). Serious photoreceptor damage will occur within days.
2. Noninflammatory photoreceptor degeneration from inherited metabolic disease, retinal detachment, or toxicity. Histologically, almost all of these

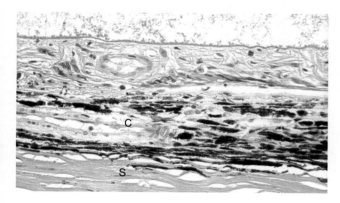

Fig. 20-22   Retinal atrophy (advanced), retina, dog. There is virtually complete loss of all retinal layers, including photoreceptors, leaving only a few surviving blood vessels and glial cells. The impression of retinal fibrosis is mostly the result of fibrous astrocytosis originating within the inner nuclear layer. This lesion could be the end stage of almost any severe retinitis or retinal necrosis (including retinal detachment, retinal hypertension, glaucoma, or trauma). C, Choroid; S, sclera. H&E stain. *(Courtesy Dr. B. Wilcock, Ontario Veterinary College.)*

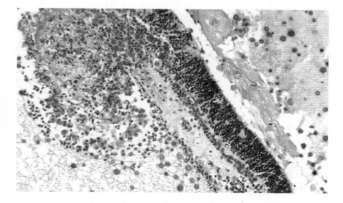

Fig. 20-23   Retinitis, retinal necrosis (with exudative retinal detachment), cryptococcosis, retina, dog. *Cryptococcus neoformans* organisms are numerous within the subretinal exudate. A mixture of fibrin, leukocytes, and organisms has replaced a portion of retina and created a focal preretinal exudate. Periodic acid-Schiff reaction. *(Courtesy Dr. B. Wilcock, Ontario Veterinary College.)*

photoreceptor diseases are indistinguishable from one another. The changes are the same regardless of whether the damage is from inborn metabolic errors (especially the innumerable inherited photoreceptor dysplasias of purebred dogs), excessive exposure to light or other radiation, or to toxic chemicals.

3. Destruction of the neural elements of the inner retina (nerve fiber layer, ganglion cells, and inner nuclear layer) as a result of glaucoma. The pathogenesis of the inner retinal destruction, and destruction of the optic nerve, remains a source of great controversy and probably varies among species and with the type of glaucoma. Some of the damage is probably from pressure-induced collapse of retinal and even choroidal blood vessels, and some is probably the result of pressure-induced interference with the axoplasmic flow of nutrients within the optic nerve and nerve fiber layer (see Glaucoma section).

RETINAL DETACHMENT

The neurosensory retina (not including the RPE) is physically anchored only at the ora ciliaris and at the optic disc. It is held in apposition to the RPE partly by the physical presence of the gel-like vitreous and partially by the membrane forces related to the intricate interdigitations between photoreceptors and surface crevices in the RPE. The potential space between the photoreceptors and the RPE is the remnant of the lumen of the primary optic vesicle, and it persists throughout life. Retinal detachment (sometimes referred to as retinal separation by those who correctly point out that the retina is never really attached at all) is a frequent and serious complication of many different ocular diseases. It may be focal or more diffuse. The distance of separation between the photoreceptors and the RPE may only be slight (so-called flat detachments) or the entire retina may be separated and suspended in the vitreous (Fig. 20-24) supported only by its durable attachments to the ciliary body and optic nerve (so-called morning glory detachment because of its resemblance to a tubular flower when viewed by clinical examination through the pupil).

The most frequent types of retinal detachment are as follows:

1. Exudative retinal detachment: accumulation of serous, fibrinous, or cellular exudates (or hemorrhage) within the subretinal space as a consequence of choroiditis, retinitis, or retinal vascular hypertension (Fig. 20-25; also Figs. 20-34 and 20-36).

2. Rhegmatogenous retinal detachment: leakage of liquefied vitreous into the subretinal space through traumatic or degenerative breaks in the peripheral retina. This may occur secondary to trauma or to a very frequent aging lesion known as microcystoid peripheral retinal degeneration.

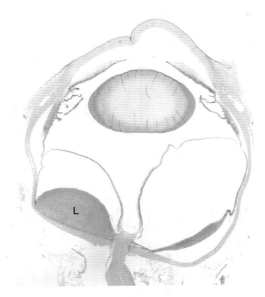

Fig. 20-24 **Retinal detachment (complete), globe, sagittal section, dog.** Serous effusion from the growth of metastatic lymphoma (L) within the choroid and subretinal space has caused a complete retinal detachment. H&E stain. *(Courtesy Dr. B. Wilcock, Ontario Veterinary College.)*

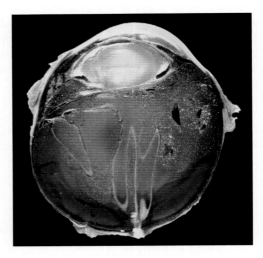

Fig. 20-25 **Retinal detachment (traumatic), globe, sagittal section, dog.** The detachment has been caused by accumulation of subretinal hemorrhage. The retina remains attached only at the sites of true anatomic attachment: the optic disc and its junction with the pars plana of the ciliary body. *(Courtesy Dr. B. Wilcock, Ontario Veterinary College.)*

3. Tractional retinal detachment: maturation of hemorrhage or fibrin within the vitreous, which pulls the retina away from the choroid. As it matures, the combination of fibrous tissue, fibrin, and detached retina lies as a membrane stretching from ciliary body to ciliary body across the posterior surface of the lens, a lesion known as a cyclitic membrane.

Retinal detachment is immediately significant because the image on the retina is out of focus, but more serious is the rapidity with which the photoreceptors are damaged. The outer segments of the photoreceptors, responsible for light absorption and electrical signal generation, are lost within 2 weeks following experimental saline-induced flat detachment (Fig. 20-26). Histologic and clinical evidence in natural disease suggests that this degeneration occurs much more rapidly (a few days at most) in the presence of toxic by-products of inflammation, or when the distance between the retina and the RPE is great. The inner segments of the photoreceptors and the cell bodies within the outer nuclear layer are much more resistant to injury and may remain viable for months (Fig. 20-27).

The retinal consequences of detachment probably vary by species, depending on how much intrinsic retinal vasculature is present. There is virtually no published information, but the almost avascular retina of horses should be much more susceptible to full-thickness ischemic injury than the well-vascularized retinas of dogs or cats (in which the inner half of the retina remains unaffected by detachment).

The detached retina in every species produces a variety of angiogenic growth factors presumably intended to increase its own blood supply. In species other than primates, however, there is a little evidence of stimulation of retinal angiogenesis. Instead, these growth factors percolate through the vitreous and are absorbed into the iris stroma where they stimulate the production of a preiridal fibrovascular membrane. The result is a substantial risk of secondary glaucoma from either pupillary block or occlusion of the filtration angle (see under Glaucoma).

EYELIDS, CONJUNCTIVA, AND ORBIT
EYELIDS

The responses of the eyelids to injury, the spectrum of potentially injurious agents, and the susceptibility to neoplasia are exactly the same as for skin and will not be discussed further.

Although the responses of the eyelid itself to injury may be identical to those of skin elsewhere, there may be unique consequences for other parts of the globe, particularly the nearby conjunctiva and cornea. There may be direct spread of inflammation or neoplasia from the eyelid to the nearby conjunctiva or even to the cornea. Physical distortion of the eyelid from inflammation, scarring, or neoplasia may interfere with the ability of the eyelid to distribute the tear film, or to properly protect the cornea from injury. The abnormal eyelid may even cause mechanical injury by scraping the cornea that it was designed to protect.

There are only a few inflammatory diseases and neoplasms with a predilection for the eyelids, and

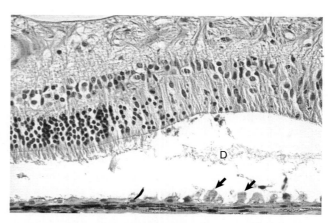

Fig. 20-26   Retinal detachment (serous), retina, dog. Floccular eosinophilic debris (*D*), the histologic counterpart of a serous exudate, has pushed the retina away from the retinal pigment epithelium (RPE). There is hypertrophy (*arrows*) of the RPE, degeneration of the photoreceptors, and focal loss of neurons from the outer nuclear layer. RPE hypertrophy occurs after just a few hours of detachment. The rapidity of progression of the photoreceptor degeneration depends on the magnitude of the detachment and the toxicity of the fluid within the subretinal space. H&E stain. (*Courtesy Dr. B. Wilcock, Ontario Veterinary College.*)

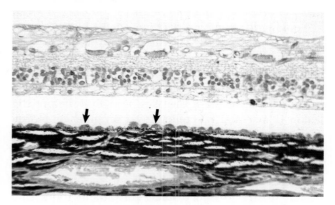

Fig. 20-27   Retinal detachment (chronic), retina, dog. There is hypertrophy of the retinal pigment epithelium (*arrows*), with loss of nuclei from the outer nuclear layer as well as disintegration of the photoreceptors. At this stage, the loss of vision from this portion of retina is irreversible. H&E stain. (*Courtesy Dr. B. Wilcock, Ontario Veterinary College.*)

these are discussed later under specific diseases. It is appropriate to be skeptical when attempting to prove an infectious cause for blepharitis in any species. There is a tendency to assume that whatever infectious agents are isolated from swabs of the eyelid margin or from expressed Meibomian secretion must be the cause of the blepharitis. This is flawed logic because ordinarily those same organisms are readily isolated from the conjunctival sac, or the eyelid margin, of perfectly healthy animals.

Cᴏɴᴊᴜɴᴄᴛɪᴠᴀ

The reaction of conjunctiva to injury is the same as that of any other mucous membrane. It has a narrow spectrum of responses to injury and only seldom can an etiologic diagnosis be made by histologic examination of a conjunctival biopsy. The epithelium responds to acute injury with ulceration. With chronic mild injury, there is squamous metaplasia. In animals with pigmented conjunctivae, chronic irritation also stimulates hyperpigmentation, just as it often does in skin. If there is desiccation, the areas of squamous metaplasia will often be keratinized.

The underlying lamina propria usually responds with a stereotypic lymphocytic-plasmacytic accumulation, with the development of hyperplastic lymphoid nodules if the stimulation is persistent. Neutrophils are seldom numerous within the tissue; if present at all, they are usually found migrating through the epithelium en route to the conjunctival sac where they will do battle with the infectious agents that might be present as opportunistic pathogens. Eosinophils are occasionally present in poorly defined allergic conjunctivitis in dogs, cats, and horses. They are present in greater numbers in the more discrete collagenolytic granulomas in horses with habronemiasis.

Looking for specific infectious agents in sections of conjunctiva is usually a waste of time. It is true that some of the viral diseases and chlamydial infections can leave specific footprints in the form of inclusion bodies, but these are usually present only very early in the course of these diseases, at a time before the lesion is assessed by conjunctival scraping or biopsy examination.

Oʀʙɪᴛ

There is nothing specific about the reaction of orbital tissues to injury. Each constituent (bone, fat, and muscle) reacts to injury in an identical fashion to that in the same type of tissue elsewhere. As has been a recurring the theme in discussions of diseases in other parts of the globe and ocular adnexa, an event at one site almost always causes significant consequences for other parts of the globe, such as the following:

1. Accumulation of fluid, cellular exudates, or tumor cells in the orbit, resulting in protrusion of the globe (exophthalmus) with the resulting risk of corneal ulceration secondary to desiccation
2. Destruction of orbital tissue and loss of fat from emaciation having the opposite effect; the globe sinks into the orbit, creating the risk of secondary entropion and resultant corneal irritation
3. Injury to extraocular muscles, resulting in abnormal positioning of the globe, thus predisposing the cornea to ulceration from eyelid trauma or desiccation
4. Significant damage to the function of the lacrimal gland, resulting in injury to the cornea via desiccation
5. Space-occupying orbital lesions, particularly neoplasms, which may cause injury to the optic nerve and result in blindness

DISEASES OF THE EYE, EYELID, CONJUNCTIVA, AND ORBIT

ANOMALIES OF THE GLOBE AS A WHOLE

The globe has a complex embryogenesis involving carefully orchestrated interactions of neurectoderm, surface ectoderm, and periocular mesenchyme throughout embryogenesis and in carnivores into the fifth or sixth the week after birth. The opportunity for developmental error is thus substantial. This also means that, especially in carnivores, all developmental errors are not necessarily congenital. Because the globe is not essential for postnatal survival, even severe anomalies are encountered with considerable frequency. Selective breeding practices have increased the frequency of ocular anomalies. Those that are important or prevalent will be discussed in sections dealing with diseases of the specific ocular segment affected.

As a general framework for understanding ocular anomalies, they are most conveniently divided into failures of initial induction, failures in remodeling, and late failures in atrophy. Included in this section are only those anomalies in very early induction that affect the eye as a whole. Those lesser anomalies that result from later defects in remodeling or atrophy are discussed in the sections devoted to diseases of the most severely affected components of the eye.

The eye begins very early in gestation as an outgrowth from the primitive forebrain. This primary optic vesicle grows outwardly from the brain toward the overlying surface ectoderm, remaining connected to the brain by the optic stalk. As the primary optic vesicle approaches the overlying ectoderm, it induces a focal thickening in that ectoderm, known as the lens placode. That placode thickens, separates from the surface ectoderm, and migrates inwardly to indent the spherical optic vesicle. As the lens pushes into that optic vesicle, the vesicle collapses upon itself to form a bilayer optic cup (Fig. 20-28). When the lens vesicle separates from the surface ectoderm, that ectoderm re-forms over the lens and forms the presumptive corneal epithelium. The presence of the epithelium seems to act as a magnet to attract one or more waves of periocular mesenchyme that will form the primitive corneal stroma and endothelium. This periocular mesenchyme is derived from the neural crest, and eventually will also form the sclera, uveal stroma, and a well-developed but transient intraocular network of blood vessels (hyaloid artery and tunica vasculosa lentis) that nourish the developing retina and lens (Fig. 20-29). The eyelids, extraocular muscles, lacrimal

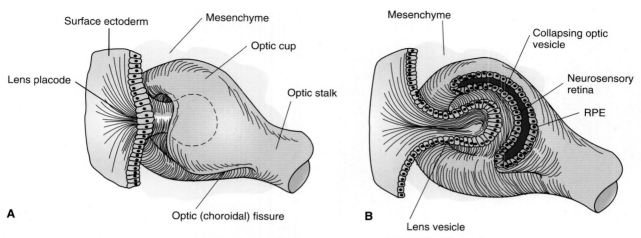

Fig. 20-28 **Schematic diagram of the formation of the primary optic vesicle and optic cup.** Note that the optic fissure is present because the optic cup is not yet fused inferiorly. **A,** Formation of lens vesicle and optic cup with inferior choroidal or optic fissure. Mesenchyme surrounds the invaginating lens vesicle. **B,** Surface ectoderm forms the lens vesicle with a hollow interior. Note that the optic cup and optic stalk are of surface ectoderm origin. *RPE,* Retinal pigment epithelium. (*A* and *B,* *From Cook CS, Sulik K, Wright K: Embryology. In Wright KW, ed:* Pediatric ophthalmology and strabismus, *St Louis, 1995, Mosby.*)

gland, and orbit are formed more or less independent of the globe and are generally not affected by those diseases that impair development of the eye itself.

Anophthalmia is a very rare condition in which there is no detectable development even of the primary optic vesicle. It is usually bilateral. The vast majority of the cases clinically diagnosed as "anophthalmia" are in fact severe microphthalmia, and some vestige of a globe is found somewhere within the orbit.

Microphthalmia is the presence of a miniature, disorganized globe in an orbit of relatively normal size. In the great majority of cases, the anomaly does not reflect a primary maldevelopment but rather involution following some type of exogenous injury to a globe that up to that stage was normal in its development. This includes in utero trauma, ischemic injury, and infection. Such globes can be remarkably small; usually it is a tiny pigmented nodule somewhere within the abundant fat and muscle still present within the orbit (Fig. 20-30). Microscopically the most durable and therefore the most recognizable remnants of the previously normal globe are the pigmented ciliary processes. If they are present, then one can be sure that the globe had reached a reasonably advanced state of embryologic development before undergoing regression.

Congenital cystic eye results from the failure of the primary optic vesicle to invaginate under the influence of the developing lens.

Cyclopia and synophthalmia are perceived clinically as a single midline globe, and virtually always occur in animals with other major developmental anomalies. They reflect failure of division of the very

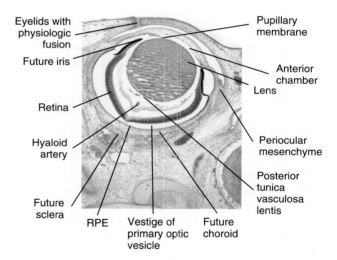

Fig. 20-29 **Fetal globe, gestational age day 34, dog.** The periocular mesenchyme is organizing to form the choroid and sclera. The anterior chamber has been formed, but the anterior lip of the optic cup has not yet folded inwardly to induce the formation of the iris and ciliary body. The relatively large lens is surrounded by a rich vascular tunic derived from the hyaloid artery and pupillary membrane. *RPE,* Retinal pigment epithelium. H&E stain. (*Courtesy Dr. B. Wilcock, Ontario Veterinary College.*)

primitive optic primordium into paired symmetric optic stalks and vesicles (or perhaps subsequent fusion), which therefore results in a single midline globe. Most examples have some degree of duplication of intraocular structures, such as the retina or lens, and are properly termed synophthalmia (Fig. 20-31).

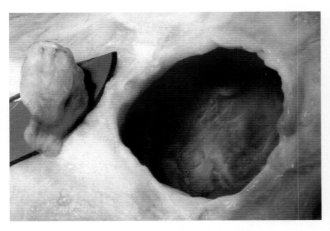

Fig. 20-30   Microphthalmia, globe and orbit, calf.
Note that the orbit *(right)* remains relatively normal, probably indicating that the initial development of the globe was normal and that its current small size *(on the scalpel blade, left)* is a result of in utero injury and subsequent atrophy (indicating so-called secondary microphthalmia rather than a primary failure of ocular development). *(Courtesy Dr. B. Wilcock, Ontario Veterinary College.)*

As naturally occurring developmental anomalies, cyclopia and/or synophthalmia are exceedingly rare. However, ewes grazing pastures of the alpine legume *Veratrum californicum* on day 15 of gestation will give birth to lambs with this malformation. Ingestion of the plant before day 15 results in fetal death but no anomalies. Ingestion after day 15 results in various skeletal anomalies and cleft palate, but the globes are apparently normal. Similar ocular lesions have been experimentally induced in goats and cattle.

Coloboma is the least severe of the developmental abnormalities affecting the globe as a whole. When used in this context, the word refers to a defect in the closure of the optic fissure, which is a normal channel in the floor of the optic cup that remains open long enough to allow the entry of the blood vessels that form the hyaloid artery and the perilenticular vascular tunic. This fissure normally closes in the last third of gestation, persisting longest near the posterior pole of the globe just ventral to the optic disc. If it persists for too long, there is the possibility that the developing retina will accidentally grow outwardly through this defect (i.e., coloboma) to cause a retrobulbar cyst lined by retinal neurectoderm (Fig. 20-32). This is a lesion made famous by its occurrence as one of the hallmarks of collie eye anomaly. The same defect occurs sporadically in other breeds of dogs and in horses, cattle, and cats. In Charolais cattle, colobomas at or near the optic disc are inherited as an autosomal dominant trait with incomplete penetrance.

The stepwise closure of the optic fissure appears to be orchestrated by soluble factors released from the retinal pigmented epithelium, which is developing

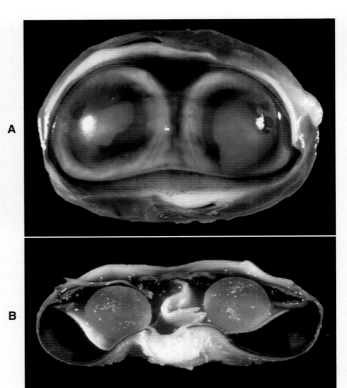

A

B

Fig. 20-31   Synophthalmia, globe, calf. A, This fused globe has two lenses, two corneas, and partial duplication of the retina. **B,** Horizontial section of the fused globe revealing two lenses but a shared fused midline retina. *(A and B, Courtesy Dr. B. Wilcock, Ontario Veterinary College.)*

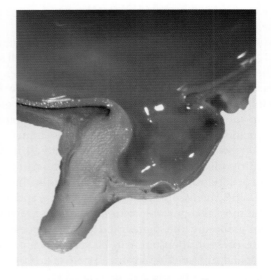

Fig. 20-32   Posterior polar coloboma, collie eye anomaly, globe, sagittal section, dog. Failure of closure of the most posterior portion of the optic fissure has allowed outpouching of the developing retina, adjacent fo the optic nerve. The protruding retina is covered by sclera. This result has prevented proper local formation of choroid and sclera, resulting in so-called scleral ectasia. Such globes always have choroidal hypoplasia. *(Courtesy Dr. B. Wilcock, Ontario Veterinary College.)*

from the neurectoderm of the posterior layer of the primitive optic cup. Because such colobomas are most commonly found in color-dilute animals, we assume that the proper chemical signaling is somehow related to the proper acquisition of pigment (or pigment-producing capability) by this neurectoderm (see later under Choroidal Hypoplasia).

DISEASES OF THE GLOBE AS A WHOLE
GLAUCOMA

Glaucoma is not a single disease but a group of diseases sharing specific physiologic and structural characteristics. It is a clinical syndrome characterized by a sustained increase in intraocular fluid pressure that is detrimental to the health of the optic nerve and the retina, resulting in loss of vision and eventual blindness. Glaucoma causes changes in virtually every tissue within the globe, but changes in the retina and optic nerve are the most important. The syndrome is most prevalent in dogs, followed by cats and horses. It is rarely documented in other species but undoubtedly exists in all. Glaucoma is extremely prevalent as a cause for ocular pain and blindness in dogs, and it is by far the leading reason for surgical removal of the globe (enucleation). It is relatively less common in cats, yet it is still the leading cause for enucleation in that species. Its frequency in horses may be greatly underestimated because of its variable clinical presentation in that species and because ocular pressure is not routinely measured in horses.

Theoretically, glaucoma may result from an increase in the production of aqueous humor or a decrease in its removal. In practical terms, however, all examples of glaucoma in domestic animals result from impairment of aqueous outflow. Glaucoma is usually divided into primary and secondary glaucoma. *Primary glaucoma* refers to those examples occurring without any known acquired intraocular disease to explain the increase in pressure. The great majority of these result from developmental errors in the structure and function of the aqueous drainage pathways. Secondary glaucoma refers to those examples in which there are changes such as lens luxation, pupillary block, or intraocular neoplasia to explain the impairment of aqueous humor outflow.

The aqueous humor that fills the anterior and posterior chambers is a low-protein transparent fluid just slightly denser than water. It is formed continuously by a combination of plasma filtration and active secretion by ciliary epithelium. Its chemical composition varies somewhat among species, but it always has a very low total protein concentration (about 5% of total plasma protein) but an amino acid concentration 50% higher than that of plasma. It contains glucose and electrolytes in concentrations roughly equivalent to those in plasma. The aqueous humor produced within the ciliary body circulates past the lens to provide nutrients to it and remove waste products, enters the anterior chamber through the pupil, circulates within the anterior chamber to nourish corneal endothelium and stroma, and then exits through slitlike spaces at the junction between peripheral cornea and iris. This iridocorneal angle extends circumferentially around the globe and normally has tremendous reserve capacity to accommodate fluctuations in aqueous production and to provide a substantial margin of safety against the development of glaucoma secondary to partial blockage of the aqueous outflow by accumulations of blood or inflammatory debris.

The maintenance of intraocular fluid pressure is a balance between aqueous production and outflow and in domestic animals is influenced primarily by resistance to outflow. The rate of production varies from 2.5 µl per minute in dogs to 15 µl per minute in cats. The outflow pathway is through the iridocorneal angle and more specifically through a series of perforations in the connective tissue of the peripheral cornea, sclera, and iris stroma that makes up the trabecular meshwork. The microscopic anatomy of this outflow pathway varies by species, but all examples are quite similar in general design.

The trabecular meshwork is a series of mesenchymal sieves that occupies the iridocorneal angle and extends circumferentially around the globe. Embryologically the trabecular meshwork is formed by rarefaction of the same mesenchyme that forms iris stroma. In carnivores this remodeling continues for several weeks after birth (Fig. 20-33). This area of perforated mesenchyme is referred to as the ciliary cleft. It is bordered externally by sclera, posteriorly by the muscles of

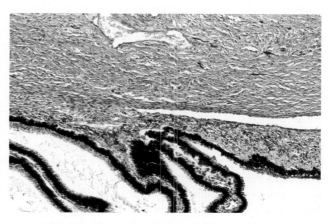

Fig. 20-33 **Normal neonatal globe, immature ciliary cleft, trabecular meshwork and iris stroma, dog.** The trabecular meshwork will develop by rarefaction and remodeling of this ciliary cleft over a period of a few weeks during normal maturation. H&E stain. *(Courtesy Dr. B. Wilcock, Ontario Veterinary College.)*

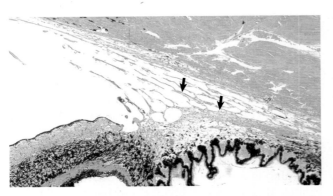

Fig. 20-34 **Normal adult ciliary cleft, trabecular meshwork and other portions of the drainage pathway, cat.** The arrows indicate the predominant pathway for aqueous outflow in carnivores. H&E stain. (*Courtesy Dr. B. Wilcock, Ontario Veterinary College.*)

Box **20-9**

The Most Frequent Histologic Lesions in Glaucoma

Atrophy of the nerve fiber layer and ganglion cell layer
   of the retina
Loss of neurons from the inner nuclear layer
Collapse of the trabecular meshwork
Corneal edema
Cataracts
Optic nerve atrophy
Optic disc cupping
Atrophy of ciliary processes
Corneal striae

---

the ciliary body, and internally by the iris stroma. Its anterior border, separating it from the anterior chamber, is formed by the pectinate ligament. With proper instrumentation (gonioscopy), the pectinate ligament is visible through the cornea as a series of cobweb-like branching cords (carnivores) or a fenestrated sheet (ungulates), stretching from the termination of Descemet's membrane to the anterior portion of the iris root (Fig. 20-34).

Ultrastructurally the trabecular meshwork is a series of connective tissue beams covered (completely or incompletely, depending on the species) by a single layer of trabecular endothelial cells connected to each other by delicate cytoplasmic tendrils. The cells are phagocytic and are probably important in regulating the outflow of aqueous humor. Most of that flow is probably by transcellular movement of pinocytotic vesicles across the cytoplasm of the trabecular endothelium.

In most species, the most functionally significant portion of the trabecular meshwork exists in the deep peripheral corneal stroma and inner sclera, and is known as the corneoscleral meshwork. Aqueous humor passing through this portion of the meshwork then enters a network of large veins, known as the scleral venous plexus, which is embedded in the peripheral sclera. The aqueous humor entering these veins will then be returned to the systemic circulation. A small percentage of the aqueous humor entering the filtration angle will exit via a more posterior route known as the uveoscleral meshwork, percolating into the veins of the ciliary body and choroid rather than into the scleral venous plexus (Fig. 20-34). The proportion of aqueous humor leaving the globe by this more posterior route varies by species: 3% in cats, 15% in dogs, and a larger (but undetermined) percentage in horses. Differences in the proportion of fluid leaving the globe by different routes might explain differing

susceptibilities to different types of glaucoma among the domestic animals, and it also creates at least the potential for different types of therapeutic interventions.

These outflow pathways are not just passive conduits through which the aqueous humor can flow. There is an important physiologic resistance to outflow responsible for the maintenance of normal intraocular pressure. The exact anatomic and physiologic constituents of this outflow resistance remain incompletely defined but include important contributions from the endothelial cells lining the collagen beams within the trabecular meshwork, the glycosaminoglycans embedded in the matrix supporting those endothelial cells, and blood pressure within the scleral venous plexus.

The clinical (macroscopic) lesions of glaucoma are related to the secondary effects of increased pressure on various components of the globe. Although the increase in pressure is the result of obstruction of outflow in the anterior chamber, the pressure elevation is distributed throughout the fluid medium of the globe, and the effects are thus felt by all parts of the globe. These effects are the same, regardless of the pathogenesis of the glaucoma, and they vary with the rapidity of onset, the magnitude of the pressure elevation, and the duration of the elevation. They are also influenced by the age of the patient and by the species. The most obvious of the macroscopic changes include ocular enlargement, corneal cloudiness because of edema, pupillary dilation, and excavation of the optic disc. The most frequent microscopic changes in glaucoma are listed in Box 20-9.

MORPHOLOGIC CHANGES SECONDARY TO GLAUCOMA

Buphthalmos (megaloglobus) is stretching of the globe secondary to increased intraocular pressure. It is most obvious in dogs and least obvious in horses (Fig. 20-35). Histologically the sclera becomes thin, and the anterior chamber increases in its anterior-posterior dimension.

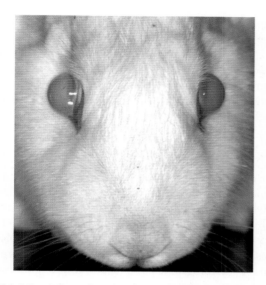

Fig. 20-35   Bilateral primary glaucoma (inherited), eye, rabbit. The eyes are protruding and have diffuse gray corneal opacity typical of edema. Distinguishing ocular enlargement caused by glaucoma from exophthalmos caused by a retrobulbar mass is based on clinical assessment of intraocular pressure, the ability to push the globe more deeply into the orbit (retropulsion), and the presence or absence of an orbital mass as detected by radiography or other imaging techniques. *(Courtesy Dr. B. Wilcock, Ontario Veterinary College.)*

The enlargement is significant because it probably causes pain, and it prevents the eyelids from closing over the cornea, thus resulting in corneal desiccation, which can lead to either corneal cutaneous metaplasia or ulceration (depending on the speed of onset and the severity of the desiccation).

Corneal edema develops when the aqueous pressure exceeds the ability of the sodium pump within the corneal endothelium (in dogs, at about 40 mm Hg). More severe corneal edema then develops as a result of pressure-induced injury to that endothelium, and that injury may become permanent if the endothelial injury is so extensive that it exceeds the capacity of the corneal endothelium to repair itself by sliding, usually when there is a loss of more than 50% of corneal endothelial cells. Corneal edema secondary to glaucoma is much more frequent in dogs than in cats for reasons that remain unclear.

Corneal striae are breaks in Descemet's membrane occurring secondary to corneal stretching. They are visible on clinical examination as serpentine tracts of deep corneal stromal opacity.

Atrophy of the iris and ciliary processes occurs late in the course of glaucoma, probably as a consequence of chronic pressure-induced ischemia. Atrophy of the iris causes the initial physiologic pupillary dilation typical of glaucoma to become permanent. Atrophy of the ciliary processes eventually leads to normalization

of intraocular pressure and even eventual hypotony, seen as part of very endstage glaucoma.

Cataracts are common in glaucoma, presumably as result of the stagnation of aqueous flow that results in inadequate delivery of nutrients to, and impaired removal of, metabolic waste products from the lens.

Lens luxation probably results from stretching of the zonules secondary to ocular enlargement. Pressure-induced degenerative change in the zonules is another possibility. The luxation may be into the anterior chamber or into the posterior chamber. Luxation into the posterior chamber requires that the vitreous has already liquefied. Such vitreal liquefaction is a common sequela to inflammation that may have preceded the glaucoma, and it also occurs as a sequela to the glaucoma itself. In globes with vitreal liquefaction, whether the dislocated lens moves anteriorly or posteriorly seems to be just a matter of chance.

Retinal degeneration is the most important secondary change in glaucoma and is the one against which most therapeutic efforts are directed. It is very important because it causes blindness as a result of damage to the ganglion cells, which cannot regenerate, even if the glaucoma is eventually brought under control. The exact pathogenesis for the characteristic retinal and optic nerve changes probably varies among species and among different types of glaucoma. At least some of the contributing factors include the following:

1. Pressure-induced ischemic damage following collapse of blood vessels in the retina, optic nerve, or choroid in response to increased pressure in the vitreous
2. Interference with ganglion cell nutrition by impairment of axoplasmic flow caused by pressure-induced compression of the axons passing through the lamina cribrosa
3. Direct damage to ganglion cells by elevated local production of excitatory amino acids, notably glutamate, from injured optic nerve and retina

The degeneration characteristically causes atrophy of the nerve fiber layer and ganglion cells, and later loss of neurons from the inner nuclear layer. The hardy astrocytes within the inner nuclear layer (Müller cells) remain intact. In classic glaucomatous retinal atrophy, the outer nuclear layer and photoreceptors remain unaffected for years (Fig. 20-36). This pattern of "inner retinal atrophy" with sparing of the outer nuclear layer and photoreceptors is virtually unique to glaucoma (remembering that inherited, nutritional and toxic retinopathies all target photoreceptors). In dogs with high-pressure glaucoma, however, it is common to also see destruction even of outer portions of the retina. Such destruction sometimes occurs quite quickly, presumably in response to pressure-induced collapse of the superficial choroidal blood vessels (choriocapillaris) responsible for the nutrition of the photoreceptors

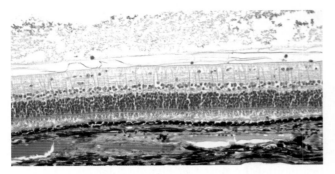

Fig. 20-36   Retinal atrophy, glaucoma, retina, horse. There is loss of density in the nerve fiber layer and loss of virtually all the ganglion cells (*top*), but excellent preservation of the outer nuclear layer and photoreceptors. Retinal microscopic changes in glaucoma vary with its severity and duration and with the species affected. H&E stain. (*Courtesy Dr. B. Wilcock, Ontario Veterinary College.*)

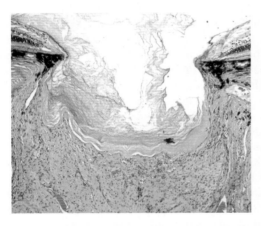

Fig. 20-37   Cupping of the optic disc, galucoma, eye, dog. The exact pathogenesis for the cupping in response to increased intraocular pressure probably involves many mechanisms and varies from species to species and among the different types of glaucoma. H&E stain. (*Courtesy Dr. B. Wilcock, Ontario Veterinary College.*)

and outer nuclear layer. In such cases, there is also necrosis of RPE.

Optic nerve changes are among the most controversial lesions seen in glaucoma. Much of the controversy centers around whether the optic nerve changes are just a consequence of glaucoma, or whether they can occur independently of the pressure changes. The answer probably varies with the species and with the type of glaucoma under consideration. The situation is greatly confused by incautious extrapolation of the results from human glaucoma research. Glaucoma in human beings is substantially different from that seen in most of our domestic animals. Microscopic changes in the optic nerve include degeneration of axons (Wallerian degeneration) and astrogliosis secondary

to the loss of the ganglion cells, and pressure-induced posterior displacement of the lamina cribrosa. Optic disc cupping is almost pathognomonic for glaucoma. It may occur very quickly as a result of pressure-induced posterior displacement of the lamina cribrosa, or more slowly as a result of atrophy of the optic nerve itself from the loss of axons (Fig. 20-37).

THE CLASSIFICATION OF GLAUCOMA
Primary glaucoma

Primary glaucomas are those glaucomas occurring without any significant contribution from disease elsewhere within the globe. Primary glaucomas are subdivided into those cases where there is detectable maldevelopment of the trabecular meshwork (goniodysgenesis), and those cases in which there are no primary histologic lesions (open-angle glaucoma). A very small proportion of these are truly congenital glaucomas in which clinical signs of glaucoma are evident in the first few weeks of life. The vast majority, however, have no clinically detectable increase in pressure or clinical signs related to glaucoma until middle-age or even older. The reasons for this delay in clinical onset are unknown.

Goniodysgenesis. Goniodysgenesis is a general term denoting imperfect development of the trabecular meshwork. It reflects incomplete remodeling of the solid mass of anterior chamber mesenchyme that gives rise to the stroma of the cornea and anterior uvea. In carnivores, most of this remodeling occurs in the first few weeks of life and involves rarefaction of what was previously a solid mesenchymal mass. In truly congenital glaucoma, there may be virtually no rarefaction (so-called trabecular hypoplasia), but in the great majority of cases there is reasonably complete development of the trabecular meshwork and other portions of the drainage system. The most common histologic anomaly is failure of the most anterior portion of the trabecular meshwork to be adequately remodeled, resulting in what looks like an abnormal solid or imperforate pectinate ligament (Figs. 20-38 and 20-39). The great majority occur as inherited disease in purebred dogs, with at least 20 different breeds known to be affected. The correlation between the severity of the goniodysgenesis and the frequency of glaucoma varies among breeds. It is sometimes quite poor, suggesting that there are other factors, perhaps functional rather than morphologic, involved in the pathogenesis of glaucoma.

The reasons for the delay in the onset of clinical signs of glaucoma, often for 5 years or more, are poorly understood. There may be age-related changes in the composition of trabecular meshwork matrix components or in lens position that result in a small decrease in aqueous outflow. Such minor decreases would

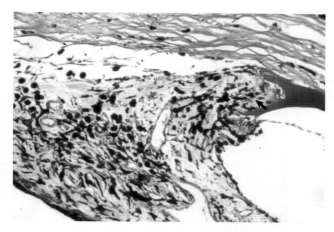

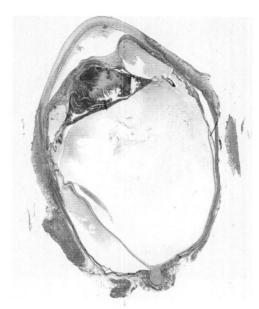

Fig. 20-38   Goniodysgenesis, primary glaucoma, dog.
Note the absence of a normal pectinate ligament. Descemet's membrane (*right*) inserts directly into a broad band of stroma (*arrow*) continuous with the iris stroma. The rest of the trabecular meshwork is microscopically normal. Periodic acid-Schiff reaction. *(Courtesy Dr. B. Wilcock, Ontario Veterinary College.)*

Fig. 20-40   Secondary glaucoma (from posterior synechia), iris bombé and peripheral anterior synechia, globe, sagittal section, dog. The original injury was a penetrating wound of the cornea that caused phacoclastic uveitis. The inflamed iris adhered to the ruptured lens, causing a pupillary block and then iris bombé. The anterior displacement of the iris resulted in narrowing of the iridocorneal angle, in this case with adhesion of the base of the iris to the peripheral cornea (peripheral anterior synechia). Note the retinal detachment and the abnormal shape of the lens (the latter resulting from loss of lens material at the time of perforation). Masson trichrome stain. *(Courtesy Dr. B. Wilcock, Ontario Veterinary College.)*

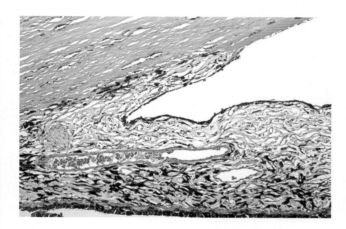

Fig. 20-39   Goniodysgenesis, primary glaucoma, dog.
Note the almost complete hypoplasia of the trabecular meshwork, the result of a profound arrest in remodeling of the mesenchyme within the ciliary cleft. H&E stain. *(Courtesy Dr. B. Wilcock, Ontario Veterinary College.)*

normally be insignificant, but they may be critical to a dog that already has impaired aqueous drainage. Alternatively, acquired changes, such as preiridal fibrovascular membrane or minor cellular infiltrates associated with a normally insignificant uveitis, might provide the "final straw" that triggers glaucoma in these predisposed individuals. There is no reason to presume that the triggering events are the same in each individual.

Primary open-angle glaucoma.   Some examples of primary glaucoma in dogs, cats, and horses occur in globes in which there is no visible abnormality in the structure of the trabecular meshwork or other portions of the aqueous outflow pathways. The best known is open-angle glaucoma in beagles. It has been widely used as a laboratory model, but its frequency outside of the laboratory appears to be very low. These dogs develop increased intraocular pressure by about a year of age, but usually do not have clinical signs of glaucoma (such as conjunctival congestion, corneal edema, and pupillary dilation) until they are between 2 and 4 years of age. In the early stages of glaucoma, all portions of the aqueous outflow pathways are histologically and ultrastructurally normal.

Secondary glaucoma

Anything capable of obstructing the flow of aqueous through the pupil or its exit through the trabecular meshwork can cause secondary glaucoma. The most common are listed next more or less in the order of frequency in dogs, the species in which glaucoma is by far the most prevalent. These mechanisms are not mutually exclusive, and frequently several different mechanisms act together to produce glaucoma. It is also undoubtedly true that dogs with goniodysgenesis

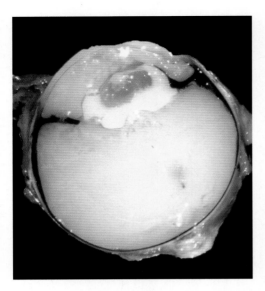

Fig. 20-41   Secondary glaucoma (from intumescent cataract), globe, sagittal section, dog. Hydropic swelling of the lens (intumescent cataract) secondary to diabetes mellitus has caused the iris to be compressed against the peripheral cornea, resulting in a functional peripheral anterior synechia and a secondary glaucoma. The lens has subsequently ruptured, triggering a phacoclastic uveitis that explains the coagulated protein visible within the lens and ocular chambers. *(Courtesy Dr. B. Wilcock, Ontario Veterinary College.)*

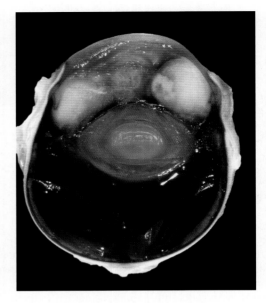

Fig. 20-42   Secondary glaucoma (from metastatic lymphoma), globe, sagittal section, dog. The trabecular meshwork has been occluded by metastatic lymphoma within the anterior uvea and anterior chamber. *(Courtesy Dr. B. Wilcock, Ontario Veterinary College.)*

are particularly prone to the development of secondary glaucoma, even when the degree of pupillary or trabecular occlusion is less than would be required to produce glaucoma in normal dogs.

Pupillary block.   The passage of aqueous through the pupil may be blocked by the anterior movement of the vitreous following primary anterior lens luxation by posterior synechiae as a sequela to fibrinous iridocorneal adhesions or by extension of a preiridal fibrovascular membrane (Fig. 20-40). Blockage may also occur from migration and fibroblastic metaplasia of lens epithelium that has been freed by rupture of the lens capsule or by massive swelling of the lens in what is known as intumescent cataract (Fig. 20-41). Displacement of the lens into the posterior chamber (posterior lens luxation) does not result in prolapse of the vitreous or in glaucoma.

Trabecular occlusion.   The trabecular meshwork extends the full circumference around the iridocorneal angle, and no one is sure how much occlusion is required to produce glaucoma. The general consensus among ophthalmologists is that it must be at least 80%. The most common causes for this type of diffuse occlusion are infiltration by neoplastic cells (Fig. 20-42 and Box 20-10), peripheral iridocorneal adhesions by preiridal fibrovascular membranes (Fig. 20-43), or

---

Box 20-10

How Intraocular Neoplasms Cause Glaucoma

Direct infiltration of the trabecular meshwork
- Feline diffuse iris melanoma
- Canine anterior uveal melanocytoma

Production of angiogenic growth factors that cause a preiridal fibrovascular membrane leading to pupillary block and/or trabecular occlusion
- Iridociliary adenoma/adenocarcinoma

Triggering of intraocular inflammation with posterior synechia and pupillary block or serous choroidal effusion with retinal detachment and preiridal fibrovascular membrane
- Metastatic carcinomas
- Malignant lymphoma

Primary intraocular neoplasms, with the exception of feline ocular sarcoma, have little metastatic risk and usually become medically significant by causing glaucoma.

---

mechanical compression of the base of the iris by intumescent cataract or by large posterior chamber neoplasms. The tumors that most frequently cause glaucoma by infiltration of the trabecular meshwork are anterior uveal melanocytoma and metastatic lymphoma in dogs, and diffuse iris melanoma and metastatic lymphoma in cats. Glaucoma caused by compression of the base of the iris is less frequent because it requires

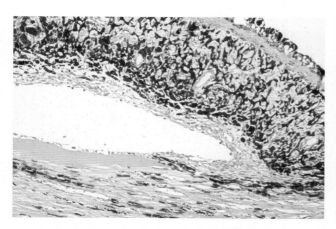

Fig. 20-43   Secondary glaucoma (from preiridal fibrovascular membrane), globe, sagittal section, dog. The mature membrane has grown across the anterior surface of the pectinate ligament, creating peripheral anterior synechia. The trigger for the formation of the preiridal fibrovascular membrane was a small, otherwise insignificant iridociliary adenoma (not visible here). H&E stain. *(Courtesy Dr. B. Wilcock, Ontario Veterinary College.)*

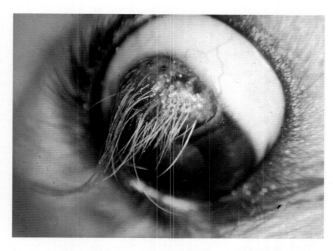

Fig. 20-44   Dermoid, cornea, dog. A plaque of haired skin exists in place of the normal peripheral cornea. What triggers the failure of normal corneal maturation from pluripotential fetal ectoderm is unknown. Its clinical significance depends on how much corneal irritation is caused by the hair. Such dermoids may arise in cornea or, more commonly, bulbar conjunctiva. *(Courtesy Dr. B. Wilcock, Ontario Veterinary College.)*

a very large tumor to cause the nearly circumferential occlusion. Only anterior uveal melanocytomas in dogs are likely to fulfill this requirement.

Very occasionally glaucoma is caused by the occlusion of the trabecular meshwork by particulate material, such as erythrocytes or leukocytes. It might seem that such occlusion would be prevalent, but such material usually settles by gravity and temporarily occludes only the ventral portion of the filtration angle.

DISEASES OF THE CORNEA
CORNEAL ANOMALIES
DERMOID

Dermoid is the only corneal anomaly that is reasonably prevalent. It reflects the failure of the fetal ectoderm to undergo complete corneal "metaplasia," with the result that a portion of the cornea remains as skin. Clinically, it is visible as a focus of corneal opacity in which there is hair, and histologically as a segment of cornea that is more or less identical to normal skin (Fig. 20-44). The degree of skinlike change varies from complete development of skin and hair follicles to a less extreme version in which only vestigial hair follicles are present.

ACQUIRED CORNEAL DISEASES
SUPERFICIAL STROMAL SEQUESTRATION/CANINE PERSISTENT ULCER

In dogs, cats, and horses (and probably in other species), there is a syndrome in which injury to the

corneal epithelium is followed by an increased amount of superficial stromal apoptosis above the small amount that normally follows any corneal epithelial injury. In dogs and horses, this results in an inability of the sliding corneal epithelium to properly adhere to the underlying stroma, which is a prerequisite for full epithelial regeneration. Initially, adhesion of the sliding epithelium is to fibronectin and other transient adhesion molecules, but permanent adhesion requires the reformation of basement membrane, hemidesmosomes, and hemidesmosomal anchoring filaments, which extend through the basement membrane to anchor into the superficial stroma. If that stroma is abnormal, these filaments cannot grip, and the regenerating epithelium is easily swept away with even the mildest trauma (Fig. 20-45). The cause for the excessive amount and/or persistence of the superficial stromal degeneration is not known. The most effective therapy is to surgically remove the superficial stroma (i.e., superficial keratectomy) to permit the epithelium to anchor into the normal deeper stroma.

In cats, the magnitude of the stromal devitalization is much greater, and there is imbibition of brown-colored pigment (thought to be derived from porphyrins in the tear film) into the dead stroma. This results in a very characteristic central corneal dark brown pigmentation that is the predominant and essentially pathognomonic feature of this disease (Figs. 20-46 and 20-47). The overlying epithelium may be ulcerated as it is in dogs or horses, but in many

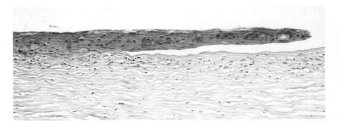

Fig. 20-45   Persistent ulcer, cornea, dog. The epithelium is thickened and disorganized and has failed to adhere to the adjacent corneal stroma. This failure of adhesion results in ineffective wound healing, seen clinically as either persistent or repeated ulceration. The failure of epithelial adhesion probably occurs because the hemidesmosomal anchoring filaments are unable to "anchor" in the injured stroma. H&E stain. *(Courtesy Dr. B. Wilcock, Ontario Veterinary College.)*

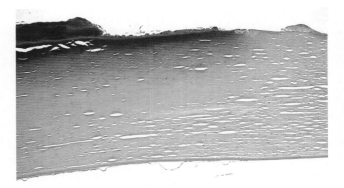

Fig. 20-47   Corneal sequestrum, cornea, cat. Note the complete loss of epithelium on the right two thirds of the cornea (ulcer) and the necrosis of the remaining epithelium (*left third*). The stroma under the ulcer is necrotic (deeper eosinophilic) to a depth of approximately half the thickness of the cornea. The necrotic epithelium, the thickened basement membrane, and some of the necrotic stroma are accentuated by brown porphyrin pigment from the tears. Corneal sequestra also occur in the dog and horse, but they do not become pigmented. H&E stain. *(Courtesy Dr. B. Wilcock, Ontario Veterinary College.)*

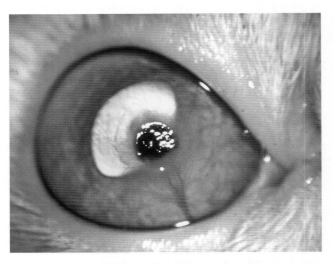

Fig. 20-46   Corneal sequestrum, cornea, cat. The axial corneal ulcer has been accentuated by the absorption of a brown pigment, probably derived from porphyrins in the tear film. The gray halo of corneal edema and the prominent vascular ingrowth from the limbus to the edge of the ulcer are frequent but inconsistent features. *(Courtesy Dr. M. Zigler, Mississuaga-Oakville Veterinary Emergency Clinic.)*

cases it re-forms over the surface of the dead stroma. The frequency of this disease is much higher in those breeds with flat faces and prominent eyes, such as Persians and Himalayans, presumably because these eyes are predisposed to desiccation and other types of mechanical corneal injury. In non-Persian breeds with normal facial configuration, there is some evidence that ulceration caused by the herpesvirus is the most common predisposing cause.

Suppurative keratomalacia ("melting ulcer")

Ulcers that become contaminated with bacteria or fungi are prone to suppurative destructive keratomalacia.

Most of the stromal dissolution is probably the result of bystander injury from neutrophils recruited because of infection, but part of the damage may be associated with proteases of bacterial or fungal origin. Pseudomonas and streptococcus are the bacteria most likely to cause suppurative keratomalacia, which sometimes rapidly progress to descemetocele and corneal perforation (Fig. 20-51). Contamination by opportunistic hyphal fungi (especially *Aspergillus* spp.) is a particularly frequent cause of keratomalacia in horses (see Equine Keratomycosis).

INFECTIOUS BOVINE KERATOCONJUNCTIVITIS

Infectious bovine keratoconjunctivitis (commonly known as "pink-eye") is a worldwide contagious disease of considerable economic importance that has been recognized for more than 100 years. It is caused by specific strains of the gram-negative bacillus *Moraxella bovis*, which is part of the normal conjunctival and nasal flora of cattle. Virulent strains have capsular pili, which facilitate corneal colonization, and most of the virulent strains are also hemolytic. In contrast, most of the strains recovered from the conjunctiva of healthy animals are nonhemolytic and nonpiliated. It is not clear exactly what is responsible for emergence of the virulent strains. *Moraxella bovis* is transmitted from animal to animal by mechanical vectors such as flies, by direct contact, and by fomites. In natural outbreaks, face flies (*Musca autumnalis*) appear to be the most important vectors. The concurrent presence of other infectious agents, such as *Mycoplasma* or infectious rhinotracheitis virus, often increases the severity of the disease.

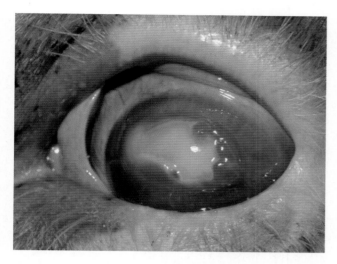

Fig. 20-48   Infectious bovine keratoconjunctivitis ("pink-eye"), cow. The axial half of the ulcerated cornea is filled with neutrophils (supperative keratomalacia) and surrounded by a border of red fleshy granulation tissue. The initial lesions are shallow corneal ulcers and foci of suppurative superficial stromal keratitis with conjunctival hyperemia, followed by circumferential superficial vascular ingrowth from bulbar conjunctiva toward the central ulcers. *(Courtesy Dr. M.D. McGavin, College of Veterinary Medicine, University of Tennessee.)*

The initial lesions are shallow corneal ulcers, which are probably the direct result of epithelial cytotoxin produced by adherent *Moraxella*. The organisms then gain access to the stroma, which results in attraction of large numbers of neutrophils from the limbus and from conjunctival blood vessels via the tear film. Inevitably, there is bystander injury from the degranulating neutrophils, but *Moraxella* also produces a potent cytotoxin, which accelerates neutrophil destruction. Lesions are initially unilateral but eventually become bilateral. Progression of a lesion is rapid during the initial 48 to 72 hours following infection, and usually results in a shallow painful corneal ulcer and foci of suppurative superficial stromal keratitis that gradually heal over the next few weeks. There is usually severe conjunctival hyperemia, followed by circumferential superficial vascular ingrowth from bulbar conjunctiva toward the central ulcers (Fig. 20-48). Healing involves the usual events of fibrovascular ingrowth from the limbus, resulting in permanent central corneal scarring, which is usually not functionally significant. In severe cases, the ulcer may progress to descemetocele, iris prolapse, and destruction of the globe.

Similar clinical and histologic entities exist in sheep, goats, and pigs associated with corneal colonization by *Chlamydia* spp. and *Mycoplasma* spp.

FELINE HERPETIC KERATITIS

Feline herpesvirus 1 (FHV-1) is an exceedingly common cause of acute-to-chronic keratitis in cats.

Viral infection of the corneal epithelial cells results in shallow intraepithelial branching tracts of necrosis, known as "dendritic" ulcers. FHV-1 can also cause a more severe delayed, deeper stromal accumulation of lymphocytes and plasma cells that appears to be a syndrome separate from the dendritic ulcers. In cats with deeper stromal keratitis, there is concurrent non-dendritic regional epithelial ulceration, necrosis of superficial stroma, and an intense accumulation of lymphocytes and plasma cells that presumably have migrated from the limbus. The histologic pattern is nonspecific, and a more definitive etiologic diagnosis requires the demonstration of viral antigen within the injured epithelium or in the deep stromal lesion. Most cases of herpetic stromal keratitis probably result from activation of latent infections precipitated by concurrent disease or the topical application of corticosteroids. The specific etiologic diagnosis can be problematic because viral antigen can be difficult to demonstrate in chronic lesions laden with a lot of neutralizing antibody. In addition, many cats are asymptomatic carriers and so the mere demonstration of the FHV-1 (by immunohistochemistry or polymerase chain reaction [PCR] done on diseased corneas) is not sufficient to establish causation.

EOSINOPHILIC KERATITIS

Eosinophilic keratitis is a unique disease that occurs predominantly in cats but has been seen occasionally in horses. The macroscopic appearance is characteristic: a granular white proliferative lesion extending inwardly along what seems to be the corneal surface from the medial or lateral limbus. Many cases have similar lesions in the adjacent conjunctiva, and in a few cases the lesions are exclusively conjunctival. Most begin as a unilateral disease, but soon both eyes are involved. The histologic lesion is a nonulcerative superficial stromal infiltration of a mixture of eosinophils, plasma cells, mast cells, and macrophages. The percentage of each cell type within the lesion varies with the duration of the disease and is significantly influenced by therapy, but eosinophils are always present and are a requirement for the diagnosis. The granular appearance of the macroscopic lesion is created by the degranulation of eosinophils, which create a thick refractile eosinophilic coagulum along the surface of the lesion (Fig. 20-49). The diagnosis is usually made on the basis of clinical appearance and the presence of eosinophils in a superficial corneal scraping. Even a few eosinophils in a superficial stromal keratitis with compatible clinical signs should be diagnosed as chronic eosinophilic keratitis, even though the majority of the leukocytes are plasma cells or other mononuclear leukocytes.

The cause and pathogenesis are unknown. Affected cats do not have concurrent skin lesions of eosinophilic granuloma complex or any other concurrent disease.

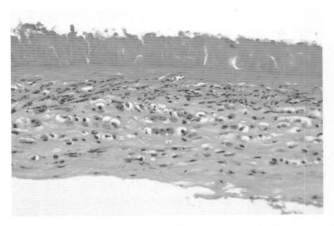

Fig. 20-49   Feline eosinophilic keratitis, cornea (keratectomy sample), cat. The corneal epithelium and superficial stroma have been replaced by a coagulum of eosinophil granules. A mixture of leukocytes, predominantly eosinophils, has infiltrated the underlying stroma. The histologic changes are highly variable depending on the stage of the disease, but eosinophils are always present. H&E stain. *(Courtesy Dr. B. Wilcock, Ontario Veterinary College.)*

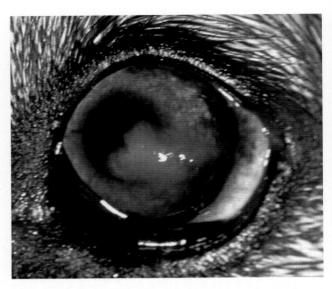

Fig. 20-50   Pannus keratitis, cornea, German shepherd dog. Note the fleshy gray-pink superficial stromal ingrowth from the lateral limbus *(right)* into the anterior stroma of the cornea. This appearance is classic for pannus. *(Courtesy Dr. B. Wilcock, Ontario Veterinary College.)*

Between 70% and 80% of lesions contain the DNA of FHV-1; the problem is that ocular herpesviruses infection is so common in cats that a definitive causal link is difficult to establish.

CANINE PANNUS KERATITIS (CHRONIC SUPERFICIAL KERATITIS, UBERREITER'S SYNDROME)

Pannus is a clinically and histologically distinctive superficial stromal keratitis seen primarily, but not exclusively, in German shepherd dogs. The disease usually begins at the lateral limbus as red conjunctival thickening. The lesion spreads toward the axial cornea as a superficial, fleshy, vascularized stromal infiltrate, involving both eyes (Fig. 20-50). Older lesions become intensely pigmented, and eventually the entire superficial stroma may be vascularized, scarred, and pigmented. The frequency and the severity of the disease increase proportionately as altitude increases, suggesting that sunlight exposure is important either in the initiation or the progression of the disease.

The histologic changes are almost identical to those seen in cutaneous discoid lupus, another disease with a predilection for German shepherds and related breeds. Discoid lupus is also exacerbated by sunlight. The early lesion is characterized by infiltration of plasma cells and smaller numbers of lymphocytes into the basilar half of the epithelium and the adjacent superficial corneal stroma near the limbus. There is vacuolation and then patchy loss of basal cells, followed by the dispersal of pigment from the injured epithelial cells. This is phagocytosed by macrophages, which

accumulate within the superficial stroma. As the disease progresses, cellular infiltration is accompanied by corneal vascularization and fibrosis.

The disease is successfully treated (but never cured) by immunosuppressive therapy identical to that used to treat cutaneous discoid lupus. The inability to identify an infectious agent and the response to immunosuppressive therapy suggests that the disease has an immunologic pathogenesis, but the exact mechanism remains elusive.

EQUINE KERATOMYCOSIS

Equine keratomycosis (mycotic keratitis) is probably always a manifestation of opportunistic contamination of corneal wounds by fungi that are common within the environment around horses. *Aspergillus* spp. is by far the most common agent isolated. Similar infection occurs, much less frequently, in dogs, cats, and other species. Alteration of the corneal defenses or the normal microbial environment by the prolonged use of antibiotics or corticosteroids in the management of corneal wounds is a strong predisposing factor in all species. In all species there are two different syndromes: opportunistic infection of dead superficial stroma by huge numbers of fungal hyphae in the almost complete absence of inflammation, or deep stromal infection that evokes an intense suppurative keratomalacia that, if untreated, often progresses to corneal perforation and iris prolapse. The deep stromal keratitis in cases in which the stroma and epithelium have healed over the top of a deep stromal infection is referred to as a

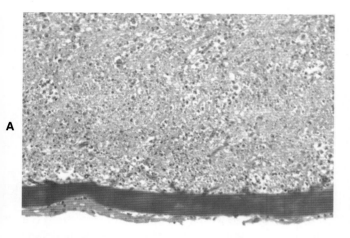

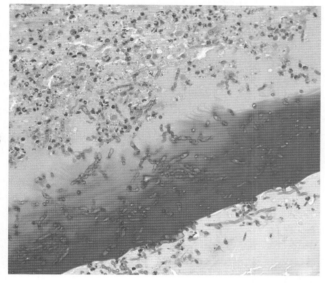

Fig. 20-51   **Suppurative keratomalacia (deep stromal), posterior cornea, keratomycosis, horse. A,** The deep portion of the corneal stroma contains numerous neutrophils, resulting in stromal destruction (keratomalacia). Descemet's membrane *(red)* is thickened and irregular and contains fungal hyphae. This is the most common histologic form of the disease. H&E stain. **B,** Higher magnification to show fungal hyphae within and adjacent to Descemet's membrane. Note the loss of the normal appearance of the stroma and the infiltration by neutrophils and edema fluid. H&E stain. (*A* and *B,* Courtesy Dr. B. Wilcock, Ontario Veterinary College.)

"stromal abscess." The fungi exhibit strong tropism for Descemet's membrane (as they do for basement membranes in other tissues), and may be absent from the stroma of the superficial (anterior) half of the cornea (Fig. 20-51). This explains why confirmation of infection by means of corneal scrapings is often unsuccessful. It also explains why topical application of antifungal medication alone is rarely successful. In many cases, successful management of the disease requires surgical débridement of the cornea to remove

most of the infected tissue and the damaging leukocytes. One peculiarity of this disease is that there is virtually never spread of the infection into the globe itself, even though the fungi can be seen dangling within the anterior chamber. There must be something unique to the corneal environment that is essential for fungal virulence or survival.

CORNEAL DYSTROPHIES AND DEPOSITIONS

Macroscopic examination of the cornea often reveals various types of colored or refractile stromal deposits. Some of these have already been discussed (superficial stromal pigmentation as part of cutaneous metaplasia or accumulation of leukocytes as part of stromal inflammation). Most other corneal deposits are composed of lipid and/or mineral. Among the domestic animals, they are most often seen in dogs. These deposits generally have characteristic clinical features (breed, age, exact anatomic location, and macroscopic appearance) that allow a diagnosis to be made without the need for histopathologic examination. They fall into two broad categories: inborn errors of metabolism known as corneal dystrophies, and acquired corneal deposits resulting from previous corneal disease or as incidental manifestations of systemic metabolic abnormalities that have "overflowed" into the cornea.

Genetically conditioned canine corneal stromal dystrophies include a seemingly endless array of lipid or mineral deposits somewhere within the corneal stroma. By definition, the defect is bilateral and congenital, even though the clinical or histologic manifestation of the abnormality may not be visible until later in life. The list of affected breeds grows daily. In each breed, the location, clinical character, and progression of the lesion is characteristic. In many, the exact nature of the deposit has not been characterized, but cholesterol, phospholipid, or lipid-calcium complexes, either alone or in combination, have been identified in some.

Corneal endothelial dystrophy is seen in several breeds of dogs as bilateral, diffuse corneal edema secondary to the progressive destruction of corneal endothelial cells. The edema is not accompanied by any evidence of inflammation or stromal fibrosis (Fig. 20-52) and usually begins at the lateral peripheral cornea and progresses over months-to-years to create diffuse edema. The microscopic lesion is extremely difficult to see because the corneal endothelial cells are generally not well preserved in histologic sections. Scanning electron microscopy and other specialized techniques demonstrate a progressive decrease in the number of corneal endothelial cells over time. The exact pathogenesis remains unknown.

Acquired corneal lipidosis (lipid keratopathy) results in milky or crystallin stromal deposits of serum lipids within the corneal stroma. The location depends

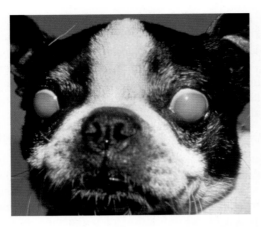

Fig. 20-52   Corneal endothelial dystrophy (inherited), cornea, Boston terrier, dog. The gray appearance of the corneas is due to severe diffuse corneal edema. The edema is secondary to progressive loss of corneal endothelial cells. The pathogenesis of this loss is unknown, but because these cells are critical in regulating the movement of water and electrocytes from the aqueous humor into the corneal stroma, their loss results in passive absorption of water into the cornea from the aqueous humor. *(Courtesy Dr. M. Nasisse, Carolina Veterinary Specialists.)*

on the pathogenesis. Any animal with an excessively high serum lipid concentration is predisposed to the deposition of neutral fat and cholesterol within the peripheral corneal stroma, reflecting an overflow from the limbal blood vessels. The lipid deposits become greatly accentuated if there is corneal inflammation because vascularization is increased and immature blood vessels are notoriously leaky.

The microscopic changes associated with corneal lipid deposition include the presence of the lipid material and variable degrees of reaction to those deposits. Stromal keratocytes may accumulate small lipid vacuoles, and clefts of cholesterol will usually be found among the stromal fibers. In some cases there is virtually no inflammatory reaction, whereas in other dogs there is a well-developed granulomatous inflammatory reaction.

DISEASES OF THE UVEA
UVEAL ANOMALIES

The epithelium on the posterior surface of the iris, the inner surface of the ciliary body, and the retinal pigment epithelium on the inner surface of the choroid are all derived from portions of the original optic vesicle. The bulk of the uvea is fibrovascular stroma derived from the periocular mesenchyme that originates from the neural crest (Fig. 20-29). Following outgrowth and later invagination of the primary optic vesicle to form the optic cup, the intraocular migration

Table 20-1   Uveal Anomalies

Failure of Formation	Failure of Remodeling
Iris hypoplasia	Goniodysgenesis
Choroidal hypoplasia and sequelae	Persistent pupillary membrane
	Persistent hyaloid/primary vitreous
	Anterior segment dysgenesis

Lists are arranged from most prevalent to least prevalent.

of this mesenchyme and its subsequent remodeling seem to be guided by soluble factors released from the neurectoderm; failures of proper induction, remodeling, and eventual atrophy of portions of this mesenchyme are among the most prevalent of ocular anomalies.

The anomalies of the uveal tract can be divided into those resulting from a failure of initial induction or migration, a failure of later remodeling, or a failure of eventual atrophy (Table 20-1). During early embryogenesis there is a persistent gap between the anterior lip of the optic cup and the overlying corneal epithelium. Through that gap will migrate several waves of periocular mesenchyme to form the corneal stroma and endothelium, the stroma of the anterior uvea, and the anterior portion of the perilenticular vascular tunic. The ingrowth of mesenchyme to form the iris stroma is guided by the infolding of the most anterior margin of the optic cup, which will form the two layers of the future iris epithelium. Later, papillary proliferation of that iris epithelium gives rise to the epithelium of the ciliary processes. Proper inward migration of the neurectoderm at the anterior lip of the optic cup seems to be a prerequisite for the subsequent migration of the mesenchyme to form the stroma of the iris and ciliary body (Fig. 20-53). Similarly, proper maturation of the future retinal pigment epithelium from the posterior neurectoderm of the optic cup is required for the proper maturation of the retina, choroid, and overlying sclera.

IRIS HYPOPLASIA

Failure of ingrowth of the future iris epithelium results in the relatively rare anomaly of extreme iris hypoplasia, clinically referred to as aniridia (Fig. 20-54). This is relatively more frequent in horses than in other species. At least in some cases (and probably in most), it is inherited.

CHOROIDAL HYPOPLASIA

Choroidal hypoplasia is a common anomaly in the eyes of dogs and cats and is often associated with inadequate pigmentation of the retinal pigment epithelium and choroid. There are many examples in which lack of pigmentation and thinning of the

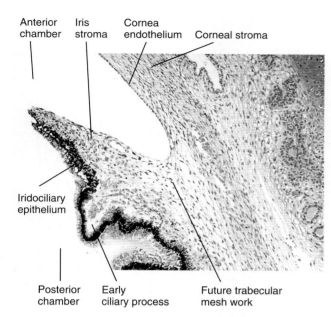

Fig. 20-53   Normal anterior uvea, 1-day-old puppy. The iris is just beginning to be formed by ingrowth of neurectoderm and associated mesenchyme from the anterior lip of the optic cup. Formation of the ciliary processes and trabecular meshwork will follow. H&E stain. *(Courtesy Dr. B. Wilcock, Ontario Veterinary College.)*

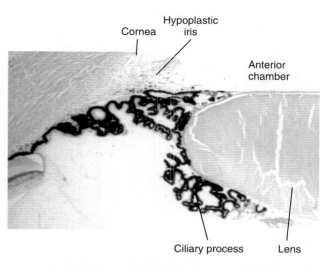

Fig. 20-54   Iris hypoplasia, piglet. There is no ingrowth of iris epithelium, and the periocular mesenchyme has therefore not migrated inward to form the iris stroma. Unexpectedly, the ciliary processes have formed normally but have arrested maturation in that they have not retracted from the lens capsule. H&E stain. *(Courtesy Dr. B. Wilcock, Ontario Veterinary College.)*

choroid seems to have no effect on vision or any other aspect of ocular health (the so-called subalbinotic fundus). There is often an association between choroidal hypopigmentation, choroidal hyperplasia, and color dilution within the hair coat. Some are accepted as "normal for the breed" by genetic screening registries, although perhaps unwisely.

There are other instances in which choroidal hypoplasia is part of a significant developmental anomaly involving the choroids, retina, optic nerve, and sclera. By far the most important example is collie eye anomaly. There are very similar anomalies in phenotypically related breeds, such as the Shetland sheepdog and Australian shepherd dog.

Collie eye anomaly was first described in 1953 as a widespread disease in smooth and rough collies in North America, Europe, and England. During the 1970s, it was found in more than 70% of collies within United States, often with devastating consequences for vision. The multitude of anomalies can all be explained by a single fundamental defect in the proper induction of the retinal pigment epithelium. The most basic and most prevalent of those inductive failures is hypoplasia and hypopigmentation of the choroid, which is why the disease is included here.

The fundamental defect in this anomaly appears to be improper inductive chemical signaling from the developing RPE. Choroidal development (in dogs and many other species) is in some way linked to the acquisition of melanin pigmentation. As a result of this defective signaling, the periocular mesenchyme destined to form the choroid and the sclera receives insufficient stimulation. In the choroid, this outcome is manifest as hypopigmentation and hypoplasia, including hypoplasia of the tapetum (Fig. 20-55). Within the fibrous tunic of the sclera, the most common manifestation is arrested growth, which results in delayed closure of the optic fissure along the ventral floor of the optic cup. That delay in closure allows the growing retina to bulge outwardly through the most posterior portion of this optic fissure. This outward protrusion of retina, usually just ventral to the optic disc, permanently prevents the proper closure of the embryonic fissure and sclera. The combined defect is referred to as posterior polar (or optic disc) coloboma, which produces a bulging of the sclera known as scleral ectasia (Fig. 20-56).

Other common defects in collie eye anomaly include mild microphthalmia, congenital retinal folding, tapetal hypoplasia, and retinal detachment. Detachment is usually delayed until the puppy is a few months of age and is not present at birth. Both the microphthalmia (which is usually just mild) and the retinal folding (see later under Retinal Dysplasia) probably represent improper coordination of the rates of retinal and scleral growth and are probably another manifestation of improper signaling from the RPE. A retinal growth rate that exceeds that of the scleral shell will inevitably result in folding of the redundant retina (interestingly, these retinal folds will usually disappear as retinal and

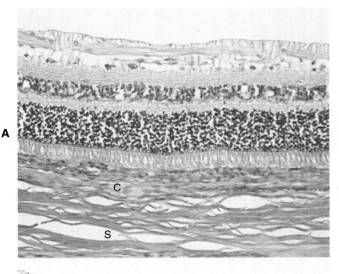

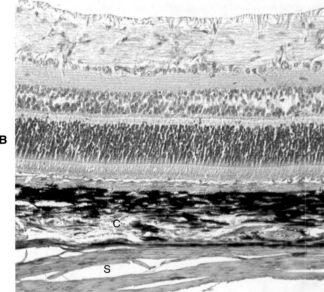

Fig. 20-55   Choroidal hypoplasia, collie eye anomaly, choroid, dog. A, The choroid is only about half normal thickness and has no pigment. These lesions are the most consistent of those described for collie eye anomaly, but the molecular basis remains unknown. H&E stain. **B,** Normal canine retina and choroid, age-matched control. **C,** Choroid; **S,** sclera. H&E stain. (**A** and **B,** Courtesy Dr. B. Wilcock, Ontario Veterinary College.)

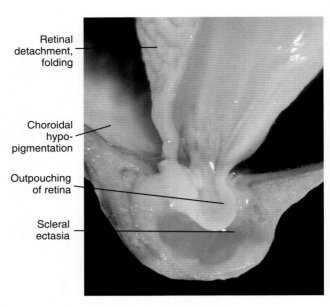

Fig. 20-56   Posterior polar scleral ectasia (at a site of coloboma), collie eye anomaly, eye, posterior pole, sagittal section, dog. The retina protrudes through a defect in the posterior pole of the globe, a sequel to the delayed closure of the posterior margin of the embryonic fissure. The protruding retina is covered by sclera that also bulges posteriorly to accommodate the retinal protrusion. The lack of synchronization between the retinal and scleral growth rate that is part of collie eye anomaly causes retinal folding and, later, retinal detachment. (Courtesy Dr. B. Wilcock, Ontario Veterinary College.)

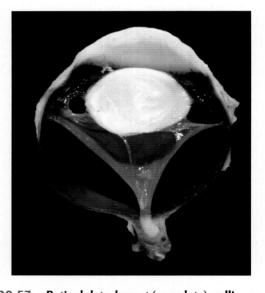

Fig. 20-57   Retinal detachment (complete), collie eye anomaly, globe, sagittal section, dog. The retina remains attached only at the sites of its true anatomic attachment: the optic disc and its junction with the pars plana of the ciliary body. (Courtesy Dr. B. Wilcock, Ontario Veterinary College.)

scleral growth eventually normalize). Conversely, normal growth of the scleral shell, accompanied by deficient retinal growth, will stretch the retina and eventually result in complete retinal detachment (Fig. 20-57).

OTHER UVEAL ABNORMALITIES

Goniodysgenesis is maldevelopment of the filtration angle and is exceedingly common as a cause of primary glaucoma in dogs, but it is much less frequent

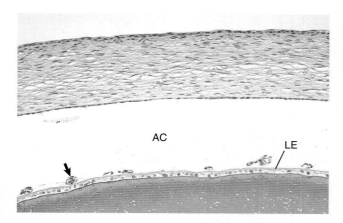

Fig. 20-58   Tunica vasculosa lentis (anterior portion [*arrow*]), 1-day-old kitten. The vessels on the anterior surface of the lens will gradually disappear during the first few weeks of postnatal life. *AC,* Anterior chamber; *LE,* lens epithelium. H&E stain. *(Courtesy Dr. B. Wilcock, Ontario Veterinary College.)*

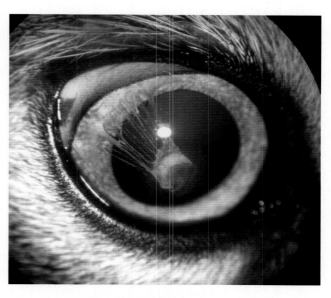

Fig. 20-59   Persistent pupillary membrane, 6-month-old dog. These persisting portions of the tunica vasculosa lentis have adhered to the anterior surface of the lens, causing anterior polar lens opacity. *(Courtesy pathology archives, Ontario Veterinary College.)*

in other species. It results from incomplete atrophy of the mesenchyme at the base of the iris. Most of this remodeling occurs in the first few weeks of life. For reasons that are poorly understood, clinical manifestations of glaucoma attributed to this developmental anomaly are not usually detected until middle-age or even later. Goniodysgenesis is described in more detail in the section under Glaucoma.

Persistent pupillary membranes and *persistent primary vitreous* refer to abnormal persistence of portions of the perilenticular vascular tunic or the vascular network within the developing vitreous. Such anomalies are common in dogs. The embryonic lens is encased in a network of blood vessels known as the tunica vasculosa lentis (Fig. 20-58). That network is created by contributions from the same mesenchyme that forms the iris stroma and from vasogenic mesenchyme growing into the developing vitreous through the posterior portion of the slowly closing optic fissure. The latter vessels, growing in from near the optic disc, are the hyaloid artery system (Fig. 20-29). Together with other nonangiogenic mesenchymal elements, these vessels form the primary vitreous. This embryonic hyaloid artery system creates a temporary vascular network along the surface of the developing retina and also joins with the anterior chamber vessels to complete the tunica vasculosa lentis. All portions of this elaborate vascular system undergo atrophy before maturation of the globe. Persistence of one or more portions is common. The most common is persistence of the anterior portion of the tunica vasculosa lentis. This is usually referred to as persistent pupillary membrane. Macroscopically, these are seen as fine threads originating from the minor arterial circle of the iris. They are usually

bloodless but are often pigmented. They may be inserted into the anterior stroma of the iris, or they may contact the surface of the lens (Fig. 20-59). Occasionally, in what is probably a more significant anomaly, they insert into the cornea. These membranes become clinically significant if they contact the lens or cornea, where they interfere with proper development of corneal or lens epithelium, or their associated basement membranes (Descemet's membrane and lens capsule, respectively). Histologically, persistent pupillary membranes are thin endothelial tubes accompanied by varying amounts of mesenchymal stroma. At sites of corneal contact, they may cause fibrous metaplasia of the corneal endothelium. Where they contact the lens, there will usually be epithelial proliferation and dysplasia of the lens capsule, resulting in a permanent focal cataract (Fig. 20-60). Those cases in which the pupillary membranes contact the cornea are probably more correctly classified as a minor expression of anterior segment dysgenesis (see later discussion).

Persistence of various portions of the hyaloid artery system, with or without other portions of the primary vitreous, include much less common anomalies known as persistent hyaloid artery, and persistent (hyperplastic) primary vitreous (Fig. 20-61). When persistent blood vessels are accompanied by hyperplastic nonangiogenic mesenchymal spindle cells, the resulting anomaly is known as persistent hyperplastic primary vitreous. It has been described as a prevalent familial lesion in several breeds of dogs, particularly Doberman

Persistent pupillary membrane   Anterior polar cataract   Pupillary margin of Iris

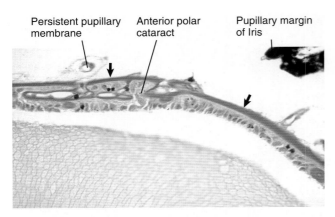

Fig. 20-60 Persistent pupillary membrane, dog. These membranes (*arrows*) have adhered to the anterior lens capsule, resulting in disorganized proliferation of lens epithelium and lens capsule. The result is an anterior polar cataract. Periodic acid–Schiff reaction. (*Courtesy Dr. B. Wilcock, Ontario Veterinary College.*)

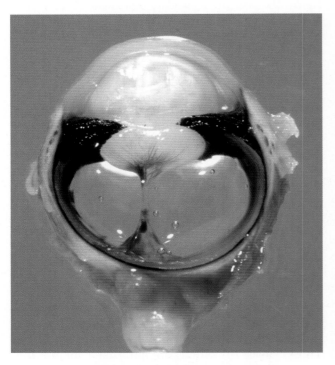

Fig. 20-61 Persistent hyaloid artery and posterior portions of the tunica vasculosa lentis, globe, sagittal section, dog. A stalk of fibrovascular tissue (the fetal hyaloid artery and associated mesenchyme) extends from the optic disc to ramify over the posterior surface of the lens. Opacity and deformity of the posterior pole of the lens are frequent complications. (*Courtesy Dr. B. Wilcock, Ontario Veterinary College.*)

pinschers. The nonangiogenic mesenchyme undergoes notable fibroblastic proliferation, sometimes with cartilaginous metaplasia. Most affected dogs have concurrent anomalies, such as persistent pupillary membrane, microphthalmia, congenital cataract, and abnormal

lenticular shape. Many of the described cases do not have the full range of lesions required for the diagnosis of persistent hyperplastic primary vitreous. Most would be better classified as persistent posterior tunica vasculosa lentis because the "hyperplastic" lesions of vitreal mesenchymal proliferation are absent.

Anterior segment dysgenesis is a blanket term for a variety of rare anomalies in which there is a failure of remodeling of the periocular mesenchyme destined to create the corneal stroma, corneal endothelium, iris stroma, and the anterior portion of the tunica vasculosa lentis. The usual clinical observation is absence of anterior chamber and the apparent fusion of the iris stroma to the corneal stroma, and no corneal endothelium or Descemet's membrane. The vast majority of these cases are not primary developmental anomalies but the result of perinatal corneal perforation. The loss of the anterior chamber is thus the result of a diffuse anterior synechia, usually secondary to traumatic corneal perforation or perforating ulcers that result in subsequent iris prolapse.

ACQUIRED UVEAL DISEASES

There are in excess of 50 different etiologic types of uveitis in dogs alone, but in most of these the uveitis is only an incidental part of a systemic disease. The macroscopic or microscopic lesions within the globe are usually not distinctive, and diagnosis of the disease is rarely made on the basis of ocular lesions. Even when uveitis is the only clinical sign of disease, rarely is an etiologic diagnosis made. Many of the specific examples of uveitis listed in clinical textbooks are syndromes made distinctive by clinical features or by identification of a causal agent, rather than by distinctive histologic lesions. Listed next and in Table 20-2 are the most common and most important examples of uveitis that do have distinctive histologic features.

IDIOPATHIC LYMPHONODULAR UVEITIS

Although not really a specific disease, this is by far the most common histologic pattern seen in uveitis. This may reflect in part a genuinely high frequency of immune-mediated uveitis. More likely, however, it is simply an indication of the chronicity of the uveitis because microscopic evaluation of globes with uveitis is usually done only in the chronic stages of disease, after all attempts at therapy have failed. Lymphonodular uveitis may therefore imply nothing more than a stereotypic endstage of uveitis that initially had a more distinctive and more variable histologic appearance. Lymphonodular uveitis was made famous by recurrent uveitis in horses. It is the only example of lymphonodular uveitis for which we have some insight into the actual cause, and for that reason it serves as the archetype for this group.

Equine recurrent uveitis (periodic ophthalmia, moon blindness) (ERU) is a frequent cause of blindness

Table **20-2**   **Frequent Causes of Uveitis**

Dog	Cat	Horse
Idiopathic causes	Idiopathic causes	Recurrent uveitis
Phacolytic uveitis	Cryptococcosis	
Trauma	Feline infectious	
Foreign body	peritonitis	
Blastomycosis		
Phacoclastic uveitis		

Lists are arranged from most prevalent to least prevalent.

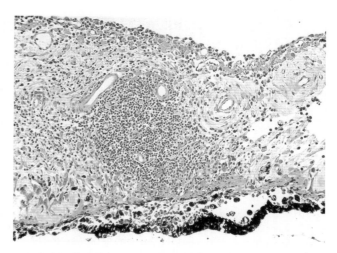

Fig. 20-62   Equine recurrent uveitis, iris, horse. Perivascular lymphocytic-plasmacytic aggregates within the iris stroma are typical of equine recurrent uveitis, but the same lesion is commonly seen in idiopathic uveitis in various species. H&E stain. *(Courtesy Dr. B. Wilcock, Ontario Veterinary College.)*

in horses. It is characterized by unpredictable episodes of severe uveitis with a tendency to become increasingly frequent and increasingly severe over time. It is likely that several different diseases are included under this diagnostic umbrella, but at least one of the causes is an immunologic reaction against intraocular leptospiral antigens. It is thought to be a delayed reaction to a systemic infection with *Leptospira interrogans* (most often serovar *pomona*). The evidence supporting a role for leptospirosis in the pathogenesis of equine recurrent uveitis is substantial even if not absolutely conclusive:

1. Horses with high serum titers to *Leptospira interrogans* are 13 times more likely to have uveitis than horses with no such titers.
2. Antileptospiral antibodies rise during episodes of uveitis and decrease during quiescent phases.
3. The disease can be reproduced by infection of naive horses with *Leptospira interrogans* serovar *pomona*. Not all infected horses developed uveitis, and the onset of ocular signs is usually delayed for a year or more after infection. In the original study, 22 of 36 of the eyes of Shetland ponies inoculated subcutaneously with small numbers of *Leptospira interrogans* serovar *pomona* eventually developed classic recurrent uveitis. All ponies developed leptospiremia soon after inoculation, but none developed ocular disease until at least 50 weeks later.
4. There is cross reaction between leptospiral antigens and various intraocular antigens, particularly those of the corneal endothelium and lens. This creates the possibility that the ongoing immune-mediated inflammation is not necessarily in response to persisting leptospiral antigens. Leptospirosis may cause the initial uveitis, but may not be responsible for its perpetuation.

The most common alternative agent implicated in a syndrome clinically indistinguishable from leptospira-associated recurrent uveitis is *Onchocerca cervicalis*. Intraocular dead or dying microfilaria have been proposed as sources of antigen responsible for the disease.

The microscopic lesions depend on the stage of the disease and represent a continuum from anterior uveitis to endophthalmitis with retinal scarring, or even phthisis bulbi. The earliest lesion is an anterior uveal inflammation that is transiently neutrophilic but rapidly becomes predominantly lymphocytic. Even during intervals in which the clinical disease is quiescent, the histologic lesions of perivascular lymphocytic anterior uveitis persist (Fig. 20-62). Peripheral corneal vascularization becomes increasingly prominent, eventually extending across the entire diameter of the corneal stroma. Choroidal inflammation is usually most obvious near the optic disc and may cause exudative retinal detachment. Even if the retina reattaches, there will be residual lesions of photoreceptor loss, or even full thickness retinal scarring as a result of ischemic injury during periods of detachment. This peripapillary retinal scarring is sometimes the only lesion seen in horses with a clinical history suggesting chronic, episodic ERU.

A characteristic lesion of chronic ERU is an eosinophilic hyaline membrane that seems to cover the ciliary epithelium. This material, in fact, lies within the apical cytoplasm of the nonpigmented ciliary epithelium and resembles amyloid. Its pathogenesis is unknown, but it serves as a useful marker for the disease.

Feline idiopathic lymphonodular uveitis is by far the most frequent histologic pattern of the uveitis in cats. It is important as a cause of the clinical signs of uveitis itself, but it is even more important as a very common cause of glaucoma in cats. The mechanism by which the uveitis causes the glaucoma is unknown; it is not by

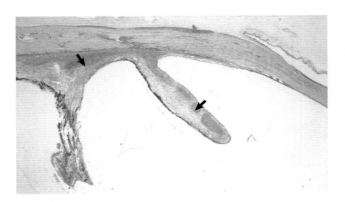

Fig. 20-63   Idiopathic lymphonodular uveitis, anterior uvea, cat. The iris and ciliary body contain numerous coalescing perivascular lymphocytic-plasmacytic nodules *(arrows)*. This lesion is the most common cause of glaucoma in cats (vying with diffuse iris melanoma for that distinction), but the mechanism by which it causes glaucoma is unknown. H&E stain. *(Courtesy Dr. B. Wilcock, Ontario Veterinary College.)*

the usual mechanisms of posterior synechia or preiridal membrane formation. At the initial clinical presentation, the lesion may be unilateral, but in most cases the uveitis eventually becomes bilateral.

The microscopic lesions are essentially identical to those seen in equine recurrent uveitis: perivascular accumulations of lymphocytes and plasma cells throughout the anterior uvea, and with less regularity, within the choroid and around small vessels in the retina. The iris tends to have the greatest accumulation, and here the lymphocytic-plasmacytic perivascular aggregates may become so large as to be clinically visible (Fig. 20-63). The degree of iris thickening and pallor may be sufficient to make this lesion macroscopically indistinguishable from that of lymphoma (lymphosarcoma).

The cause remains a complete mystery despite considerable investigation. The syndrome is presumed to be immune mediated, but the identity of the antigen or antigens is unknown. Affected cats are no more likely to be seropositive or PCR-positive for the various feline systemic infectious agents (FIV, FIP, leukemia virus, etc.) than are healthy cats, but no credible cause has been demonstrated by immunohistochemical or PCR investigation of affected globes. Some believe strongly that a previous infection with *Toxoplasma* is somehow involved, but the evidence remains inconclusive.

Canine lymphocytic uveitis has the most frequent histologic pattern of uveitis seen in dogs (as it is in cats and horses), a lymphocytic-plasmacytic panuveitis that tends to be more severe in the anterior uvea than in the choroid. It should not really be considered a specific disease but rather a histologic pattern that is probably shared by many different diseases. As in the other species, the disease may be unilateral or bilateral and tends to occur in multiple episodes interrupted by periods of quiescence. The cause remains unknown, and it is likely that there are multiple different agents capable of inducing this identical histologic change. In contrast to the situation in cats, it does not cause glaucoma. The main differential diagnosis is phacolytic uveitis, and indeed in some cases the histologic distinction is impossible.

UVEODERMATOLOGIC SYNDROME IN DOGS (VOGT-KOYANAGI-HARADA SYNDROME)

Despite the exotic-sounding name, this disease is relatively frequent in the most susceptible breeds (Akitas, Siberian huskies, Samoyeds). The clinical syndrome of facial dermal depigmentation and severe bilateral uveitis is distinctive, although many dogs with the uveitis do not have skin lesions. The canine syndrome closely parallels that of the human disease, except that the encephalitis, which is the least frequent part of the human syndrome, has not been confirmed in dogs. The histologic lesion is a destructive granulomatous endophthalmitis with abundant dispersal of melanin, a consequence of T-lymphocyte–mediated destruction of melanin-producing cells of the RPE and uvea. The disease is slowly progressive and is always eventually bilateral even though initially it may not affect both eyes.

SYSTEMIC MYCOSES

Systemic mycoses such as blastomycosis, cryptococcosis, histoplasmosis, and coccidioidomycosis are frequent causes of severe uveitis in those geographic areas where the organisms are common environmental contaminants. Immunodeficient animals may develop endophthalmitis as part of generalized disease caused by saprophytic fungi such as *Aspergillus* spp. or *Candida* spp., but these cases are rare; these same agents will occasionally cause endophthalmitis when introduced by penetrating plant foreign bodies.

The frequency with which endophthalmitis accompanies systemic mycosis is unknown. The majority of cases are found in dogs, except for the inexplicable predilection of cryptococcosis for cats. Ocular involvement is part of systemic disease, but fairly frequently ocular disease is the only obvious clinical sign. Blastomycosis is by far the most prevalent example of an endophthalmitis caused by systemic mycosis, and it will serve here as the prototype for this group.

Blastomycosis is the most frequently reported intraocular mycosis in dogs, but it is rare in cats. It is estimated that about 25% of dogs with the systemic disease have clinically obvious ocular disease: unilateral or bilateral endophthalmitis with a very high frequency of exudative retinal detachment. The microscopic lesion is severe diffuse pyogranulomatous endophthalmitis, which tends to be more severe in the choroid and subretinal space than in the anterior uvea. The greatest accumulation of both leukocytes and organisms is usually in the subretinal space. The disease is pyogranulomatous and very destructive. The organisms may be numerous or extremely sparse, probably depending on the duration of the disease and on therapy. They are either free or within the cytoplasm of macrophages and have the typical features of *Blastomyces* spp.: thick-walled yeast 4 to 20 µm in diameter, with occasional broad-based budding. The diagnosis can often been made by cytologic evaluation of subretinal exudates in eyes that are already blind because of retinal detachment (one would probably not dare to attempt aspiration of the subretinal space in a globe that still had vision). Other lesions in affected globes are those seen in any severe uveitis: intraocular hemorrhage, posterior synechia, preiridal fibrovascular membrane, and cataract. Spread into the optic nerve and even orbit is an infrequent complication.

Cryptococcosis is similar to blastomycosis in that the lesions are predominantly within the retina, choroid, and optic nerve. As mentioned earlier, ocular cryptococcosis is immeasurably more prevalent in cats than in dogs or any other domestic animal. As is typical of cryptococcosis in other feline tissue, the granulomatous inflammatory response is often minimal. Large collections of poorly stained pleomorphic yeasts, surrounded by wide capsular halos, impart a typical "soap-bubble" appearance in hematoxylin and eosin (H&E) stained sections. The organisms are usually numerous and vary greatly in size and shape. In a few cases, the granulomatous reaction is much more severe and mimics that seen in blastomycosis. In such lesions, organisms are typically scarce.

The ocular disease caused by *Coccidioides immitis* resembles blastomycosis but is more suppurative, more destructive, and more prone to progress to outright panophthalmitis. Involvement of the anterior uvea is perhaps more common than in the other systemic mycoses. The disease is seen only in animals that live in (or have visited) the very restricted geographic regions in which the organism is common. The great majority of cases are seen in dogs from the desert regions of the American Southwest (Fig. 20-64).

The lesions caused by ocular infection with *Histoplasma capsulatum* are distinctive and quite different from those of the other systemic mycoses. There is usually a diffuse granulomatous and lymphocytic choroiditis with little suppuration and without much of the destruction that characterizes blastomycosis and coccidioidomycosis. Organisms are usually very numerous and visible as small spherical bodies within the cytoplasm of macrophages.

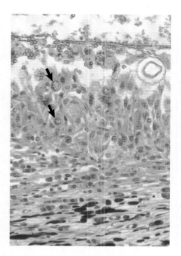

Fig. 20-64 **Granulomatous choroiditis (destructive), coccidioidomycosis, choroid, dog.** The retina is absent because inflammatory exudate has caused retinal detachment. Organisms are usually difficult to find, but two spherules (*arrows*) are amid the macrophages. H&E stain. *(Courtesy Dr. B. Wilcock, Ontario Veterinary College.)*

Protothecosis is included here because the organisms can easily be mistaken for yeast and because the clinical and histologic features closely resemble those of the systemic mycoses described earlier. Prototheca are colorless saprophytic algae capable of causing enteric, cutaneous, or generalized granulomatous disease in a variety of mammalian species. Ocular lesions have been described only in dogs with the disseminated form of the disease. The lesions are essentially identical to those seen with blastomycosis and are distinguishable only by the detection of the pleomorphic algae (which usually are very numerous). In histologic section, the algae are free or within macrophages. The organisms are spherical to oval, from 2 to 20 µm in diameter, and have a refractile cell wall that stains with periodic acid–Schiff (PAS) reaction or Gomori's methenamine silver stain. Prototheca reproduces by asexual multiple fission, so that multiple daughter cells form enclosed within a single cell wall. There is no budding as with blastomyces and cryptococcus.

FELINE INFECTIOUS PERITONITIS–ASSOCIATED UVEITIS

The coronavirus of feline infectious peritonitis causes a diffuse uveitis that is probably immune-mediated. The frequency of ocular lesions is unknown because the eyes are not regularly examined in cats with the disease. The histologic lesions in the globe are always bilateral and are similar to those seen in any other organ affected with the disease. As elsewhere, the lesions vary in the relative proportions of the different leukocyte types, the amount of fibrin, and the

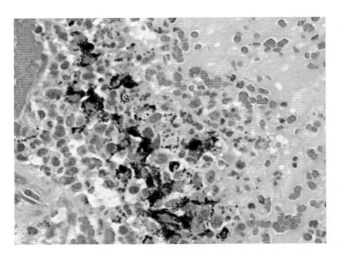

Fig. 20-65   Lymphocytic, granulomatous, and neutrophilic iridocyclitis (destructive), feline infectious peritonitis, ciliary body, cat. Lymphocytes and plasma cells tend to predominate within the uveal stroma (*left*), whereas neutrophils, fibrin, and macrophages predominate within the adjacent aqueous humor of the posterior chamber (*right*). These lesions are typical of feline infectious peritonitis. H&E stain. *(Courtesy Dr. B. Wilcock, Ontario Veterinary College.)*

amount of necrosis. In most cases the disease is primarily an anterior uveitis with a mixture of lymphocytes, plasma cells, neutrophils, and macrophages. Especially within the globe, the often-repeated statement that FIP causes "pyogranulomatous" inflammation is greatly exaggerated. The exudate within the anterior chamber is usually predominantly neutrophilic, yet in the choroid the inflammation is usually lymphocytic-plasmacytic. Formation of keratic precipitates and a neutrophilic corneal endothelialitis are strong indicators of an FIP-associated uveitis (Fig. 20-65). In many cases, there are also typical histologic lesions in the orbital soft tissue adjacent to the sclera and in the meninges of the optic nerve. There is no other cause of uveitis in cats that is also routinely involved in orbital cellulitis. Classic necrotizing vasculitis is seen only rarely, and if present, it is likely to be in the retina. Sequelae such as pupillary block and secondary glaucoma are rarely seen, simply because cats with ocular lesions of FIP are usually in the advanced stages of the systemic disease and do not survive long enough for those potential sequelae to develop.

Bovine Malignant Catarrhal Fever–Associated Uveitis

The majority of cattle with malignant catarrhal fever have prominent ocular lesions in the form of peripheral midstromal corneal vascularization and obvious anterior uveitis. These lesions help to clinically distinguish this disease from mucosal disease and acute severe bovine viral diarrhea (BVD). The histologic lesions

within the eye resemble those elsewhere in the body: arterial necrosis with perivascular and intramural accumulation of lymphoblasts, among which are a few with mitotic figures. The vasculitis is most often identified within the iris, but it can be found anywhere within the uveal tract or retina. The accompanying uveitis is predominantly lymphocytic right from the start. Of great diagnostic significance from a clinical perspective is a ring of peripheral corneal stromal vascularization extending into the cornea from the limbus. The vascular ingrowth is accompanied by notable corneal edema. Although this is a routine lesion seen in any chronic severe uveitis, it is not seen in keratoconjunctivitis associated with several other bovine infectious diseases. There may be a concurrent lymphocytic corneal endothelialitis contributing to the corneal edema.

The pathogenesis of the disease remains controversial. The appearance of the vasculitis suggests that it should be an immune-mediated vasculitis, yet intramural deposition of immunoglobulin or complement is not a significant feature of the vascular lesion. A T-lymphocyte dependent, type IV immune pathogenesis has been suggested.

Lens-Induced Uveitis

Phacolytic uveitis is an extremely common, mild lymphocytic-plasmacytic anterior uveitis that occurs in a large proportion of animals with cataracts in which the lens protein is beginning to disintegrate and leak through the intact lens capsule. Although seldom significant as the cause of clinical signs, it significantly reduces the success of cataract surgery, unless the surgery is preceded by a course of antiinflammatory drugs.

Phacoclastic uveitis is predominantly an immune-mediated disease in response to the release of large amounts of intact lens protein through a traumatically ruptured lens capsule. The severity and character of the reaction seem to be influenced by the amount of lens material lost, the speed of the loss, the age of the animal, and the species. The disease is most commonly seen in dogs because of their habit of running into sharp objects or having unpleasant encounters with the neighborhood cat. Lens rupture may also occur following blunt trauma, in which case the rupture is usually of the thin posterior capsule. Phacoclastic uveitis will also occur following spontaneous lens rupture, not associated with trauma. This occurs in rabbits as a result of penetration of the lens by *Encephalitozoon cuniculi* and in dogs with rapidly progressing diabetic cataracts.

The clinical syndrome is quite distinctive: The initial clinical signs are related to corneal perforation and uveitis as direct consequences of the penetrating injury and/or subsequent sepsis. Those are often managed successfully with antiinflammatory and antibiotic therapy, and everything seems to be healing very well until the development of a severe and therapeutically refractory anterior uveitis that most commonly occurs about 2 weeks after the initial injury. Once the phacoclastic uveitis is initiated, the prognosis for saving the globe becomes poor.

The lesions of phacoclastic uveitis are of two different types, usually occurring concurrently. The typical lesions in acute disease include rupture of the lens capsule, accumulation of intralenticular neutrophils, and a perilenticular inflammatory reaction that is initially neutrophilic. With time it becomes progressively more granulomatous but remains distinctly perilenticular (Fig. 20-66). After a few days, the inflammatory reaction is accompanied by proliferation, fibroblastic metaplasia, and perilenticular migration of lens epithelial cells that have escaped through the site of perforation (Fig. 20-67). Because the perforating injuries causing phacoclastic uveitis may also implant bacteria or foreign material into the globe, it is not always possible to determine what part of the posttraumatic lesion is phacoclastic uveitis and what part is in response to a foreign body or infection. True phacoclastic uveitis is distinctly perilenticular, with minimal reaction in more distant portions of the uvea, such as the choroid.

The pathogenesis of the inflammatory component of phacoclastic uveitis is probably an immunologic response to the release of large amounts of strongly antigenic lens protein into the aqueous humor.

Although lens protein is not truly "foreign," the body has tolerance for only small amounts of lens protein. The sudden release of large amounts following capsular rupture overwhelms this immune tolerance, resulting in a suppurative-to-pyogranulomatous reaction centered on the lens. This immune pathogenesis explains the lag between lens rupture and development of the phacoclastic uveitis. It also explains why small perforations might not cause the disease and why removal of the injured lens shortly after perforating injury prevents the development of the disease.

The fibrous metaplasia and migration of lens epithelium are critical prognostic events. This epithelium, once out of the lens, recognizes no barriers to its proliferation and will cause pupillary block, occlusion of the filtration angle, and secondary glaucoma. In cats, probably it is this same epithelium that undergoes malignant transformation to the clinically significant and uniquely feline entity of posttraumatic primary ocular sarcoma (see discussion on neoplasia).

Phacoclastic uveitis can be a serious complication of cataract surgery in which too much lens material is left behind within the lens capsular bag. In most instances, complications arise primarily from the migration and fibroblastic metaplasia of this residual lens epithelium. This can result in opacification of the pupil (and of any artificial lens implant) and possibly pupillary block, causing secondary glaucoma.

NEOPLASMS OF THE UVEA

Primary uveal neoplasms are common only in dogs and cats, but they are exceedingly important in both

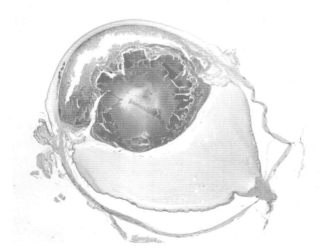

Fig. 20-66 **Phacoclastic uveitis, encephalitozoonosis, eye, sagittal section, rabbit.** The anterior lens capsule has disintegrated, with substantial loss of lens material from the anterior cortex. The scalloped remnant of lens is now covered by a mixture of fibrin and leukocytes that fills the anterior chamber. In all species, the sudden release of intact lens protein triggers massive suppurative and granulomatous perilenticular inflammation that is typically delayed until 10 to 14 days after lens rupture. H&E stain. *(Courtesy Dr. B. Wilcock, Ontario Veterinary College.)*

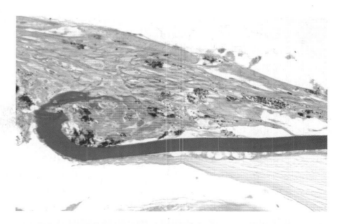

Fig. 20-67 **Chronic phacoclastic uveitis, eye, horse.** The predominant lesion is now a plaque of fibroblast-like cells on the anterior surface of the lens adjacent to the site of capsular rupture *(lower left)*. This plaque is created by metaplasia of lens epithelium that has escaped through the capsular defect. These proliferating cells frequently cause pupillary blockage and secondary glaucoma. H&E stain. *(Courtesy Dr. B. Wilcock, Ontario Veterinary College.)*

Table **20-3**   **Common Primary Intraocular Neoplasms**

Dog	Cat	Horse
Anterior uveal melanocytoma	Diffuse iris melanoma	Medulloepithelioma
Iridociliary adenoma	Iridociliary adenoma	
	Primary ocular sarcoma	

Lists are arranged from most prevalent to least prevalent.

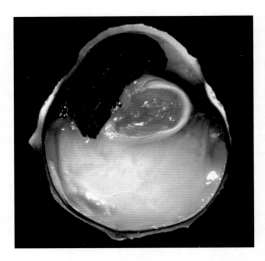

Fig. 20-68 **Anterior uveal melanocytoma, eye, sagittal section, dog.** A large black tumor has replaced the anterior half of the uvea and filled much of the anterior chamber. *(Courtesy Dr. B. Wilcock, Ontario Veterinary College.)*

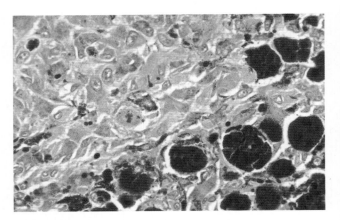

Fig. 20-69 **Anterior uveal melanocytoma, iris, dog.** Large, heavily pigmented polygonal "plump cells" predominate. The smaller number of lightly pigmented spindle cells are germinal cells. The paucity of mitotic figures is a predictor that the tumor is benign. H&E stain. *(Courtesy Dr. B. Wilcock, Ontario Veterinary College.)*

species and vie with glaucoma as the most common reason for enucleation (Table 20-3). Primary tumors (melanocytic tumors and iridociliary epithelial tumors) are considerably more prevalent than metastatic tumors in the globe, with the possible exception of metastatic uveal lymphoma in cats.

In all species, melanocytic tumors are by far the most common of all ocular tumors. Those tumors predicted to be behaviorally benign are referred to as melanocytomas; those predicted to be malignant are classified as melanomas. As with melanocytomas and melanomas elsewhere, there is substantial variation in biologic behavior depending on species and location. These site and species variables are more important in establishing the prognosis than are many of the histologic and cytologic features.

Canine anterior uveal melanocytoma is by far the most common primary intraocular tumor of dogs, arising from the melanocytes within the stroma of the iris or ciliary body. They ordinarily form a solid, deeply pigmented mass that protrudes into the anterior or posterior chamber. Growth is expansive rather than invasive (Fig. 20-68). The typical tumor has an inconspicuous germinal population of cytologically bland and poorly pigmented spindle cells, and a much larger proportion of huge ballooned "plump cells" distended with pigment (Fig. 20-69), which are assumed to be postmitotic endstage neoplastic melanocytes. These tumors have very little metastatic potential, and the few that are likely to metastasize can be identified by a notable increase in the numbers of mitotic figures. All of these tumors, sooner or later, grow large enough to cause obstruction of aqueous outflow and secondary glaucoma.

Histologically identical melanocytoma will very occasionally arise within the choroid as a slowly expanding subretinal mass. They are significant because they cause retinal detachment.

Feline diffuse iris melanoma has a distinctive clinical presentation: unilateral coalescing hyperpigmentation of the iris that slowly (often over many years) progresses to diffuse iris thickening and secondary glaucoma (Fig. 20-70). This is a uniquely feline disease. The tumor originates from the layer of melanocytes that forms the anterior border layer of the normal iris. The transformed cells have enlarged nuclei and hyperchromasia and proliferate slowly to replace the normal iris architecture. The fully developed tumor, as the name implies, results in a diffuse iridal infiltration by pleomorphic round-to-epithelioid melanocytes. Their appearance in cytologic preparations is extremely variable. Tumors vary from amelanotic to heavily pigmented, and from round cell to epithelioid to spindle cell (and mixtures of all of the above), but none of these variables has any prognostic significance. Mononuclear gigantism is frequently seen (Fig. 20-71). None of these variables has any prognostic significance.

The prognosis has been the subject of great debate over the past 10 years. Retrospective studies that have attempted to establish histologic predictors of behavior have been thwarted by poor overall follow-up data (cats lost to follow-up, very few necropsies). Nonetheless, emerging from these studies is the general consensus that although these tumors are substantially more likely to eventually metastasize than are canine uveal melanomas, the overall risk of an affected cat developing clinical signs related to metastatic disease seems to be low. The probability that the affected eye will eventually develop glaucoma secondary to tumor infiltration of the trabecular meshwork is exceedingly high, although it may take years.

Rarely, cats will develop caninelike nodular uveal melanocytomas (and dogs will occasionally develop felinelike diffuse melanomas).

Iridociliary tumors vary from well-differentiated papillary adenomas to solid carcinomas. They all arise from the neurectoderm of the posterior iris or ciliary body. The histologic distinctions have no apparent relevance to biologic behavior, because all of these tumors are benign. These are relatively common intraocular tumors in dogs (second in frequency only to melanocytoma), are occasionally seen in cats, and infrequently seen in other species. They usually grow as discrete, expansile nodules that protrude into the posterior chamber and are thus visible through the pupil. They are populated by cuboidal and columnar epithelial cells resembling normal iridociliary epithelium and usually form cords and papillary structures reminiscent of disorganized ciliary processes (Fig. 20-72). Some have a more primitive cytologic and histologic appearance, but extraocular metastasis is so rare as to be nonexistent. Even small tumors may become clinically significant because they habitually produce fibroblastic and angiogenic growth factors that stimulate the development of preiridal fibrovascular membranes, causing secondary glaucoma or intractable hyphema.

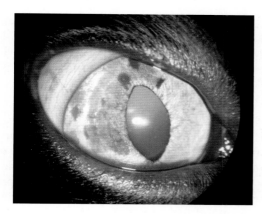

Fig. 20-70   Diffuse iris melanoma, eye, cat. Coalescing areas of brown pigmentation have caused thickening of the iris. In many cats, the extent of the pigmentation and thickening progresses over many years, and eventually the tumor may cause glaucoma secondary to trabecular occlusion. Enucleation may then be necessary. *(Courtesy pathology archives, Ontario Veterinary College.)*

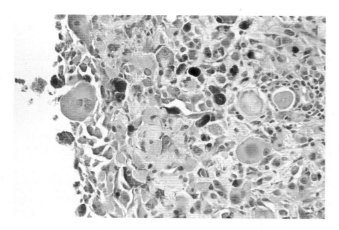

Fig. 20-71   Diffuse iris melanoma, iris, cat. Note the extreme variation in cellular morphology: threefold variation in cellular size, nuclear gigantism, and variation in cell shape from round to spindle. The marked variation in the histologic and cytologic appearance of this tumor from case to case has no proven prognostic significance. H&E stain. *(Courtesy Dr. B. Wilcock, Ontario Veterinary College.)*

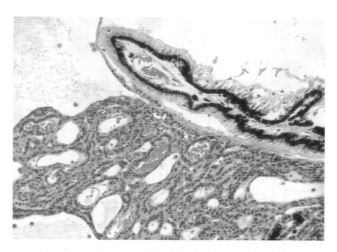

Fig. 20-72   Iridociliary adenoma, well-differentiated, posterior chamber, dog. Although almost always benign, even small tumors of this type may induce the formation of a preiridal fibrovascular membrane that leads to secondary glaucoma. H&E stain. *(Courtesy Dr. B. Wilcock, Ontario Veterinary College.)*

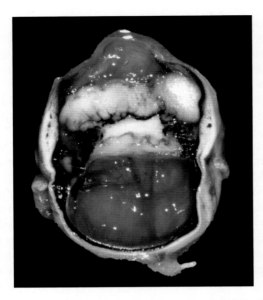

Fig. 20-73   Primary ocular sarcoma, eye, saggital section, cat. A solid white stromal sarcoma surrounds remnants of a ruptured lens. Wrinkled remnants of the lens capsule are still visible near the posterior margin of the tumor. *(Courtesy Dr. B. Wilcock, Ontario Veterinary College.)*

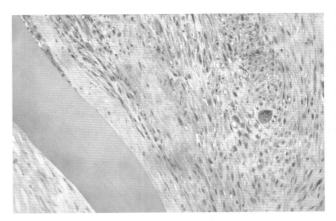

Fig. 20-74   Primary ocular sarcoma, eye, cat. Pleomorphic fibroblast-like cells, thought to be derived from lens epithelium, lie adjacent to remnants of lens capsule (*left*). Virtually all cases are preceded by rupture of the lens capsule. H&E stain. *(Courtesy Dr. B. Wilcock, Ontario Veterinary College.)*

Medulloepithelioma is a relatively rare congenital counterpart of iridociliary adenoma. It has the distinction of being the most common primary intraocular tumor of horses. The histologic appearance reflects its embryonic origin from primitive neurectoderm still capable of both iridociliary and retinal differentiation. The tumor is populated by hyperchromatic cuboidal cells that make structures reminiscent of ciliary processes and sometimes tubular structures resembling the rosettes seen in retinal dysplasia. In horses, they often incorporate foci of cartilage, bone, and even brain tissue; these are known as teratoid medulloepitheliomas. Although they are by definition congenital tumors, their growth is slow and they may not be diagnosed until many years later.

Feline primary ocular sarcoma (posttraumatic sarcoma) is a high-grade spindle cell neoplasm that probably arises from lens epithelial cells that have escaped through ruptures in the lens capsule. These cells routinely undergo fibroblastic metaplasia as part of ineffective wound healing (see discussion on phacoclastic uveitis), but only in cats does the metaplasia progress to outright sarcoma. The tumor begins as a distinctly perilenticular mass and then grows to fill the globe (Fig. 20-73). As with histologically similar postvaccinal sarcomas, these tumors may have fibroblastic, osteoblastic, or cartilaginous areas in the same tumor (Fig. 20-74). The interval between trauma and detection of tumor can be many years, but the key word here is "detection." It is very common for cats with this tumor to be presented for veterinary attention only after the tumor has filled the globe. We do not know the rapidity of microscopic tumor development following injury. These tumors frequently invade the optic nerve and then extend into the brain. They are also capable of distant metastasis.

Neoplasms metastatic into the globe are much less frequent than tumors originating within the globe. Virtually any metastatic neoplasm can localize within the uveal tract and spread from there into other portions of the globe. Their histologic appearance is the same as that of the primary tumor. By far the most prevalent is lymphoma (lymphosarcoma), seen in many species but particularly prevalent in cats. It causes diffuse thickening and pallor of the iris and less frequently the choroid. It is clinically almost indistinguishable from severe idiopathic uveitis, and the distinction is usually made on the basis of additional clinical evidence.

DISEASES OF THE LENS
ANOMALIES OF LENS

The lens is derived from the thickening of the ectoderm induced by contact with the primary optic vesicle. This lens placode then migrates inwardly to cause the optic vesicle to invaginate upon itself to form the primary optic cup. As it does so, the lens placode grows to become a lens vesicle and separates from the overlying ectoderm, which will become corneal epithelium (Fig. 20-29). This vesicle initially is just a single layer of cuboidal epithelial cells surrounded by a very thin capsule. The epithelial cells along its posterior surface elongate to obliterate the lumen of this primitive vesicle, creating the primary lens fibers that will persist throughout life as the lens nucleus. The subsequent development of the cortical fibers of the postnatal lens depends entirely on mitotic activity from the anterior lens epithelium. No epithelium remains along the posterior half of the lens any time after the stage of the primary lens vesicle.

Anomalies of the lens are of minor importance when contrasted with anomalies of other portions of the globe. The lens has a central inductive role in ocular development, so significant anomalies of the lens are almost always accompanied by multiple ocular anomalies, such as microphthalmia. It is likely that many of the lens anomalies reflect acquired degenerative changes (even if occurring in utero), resulting in regression of what was a normally developing lens. Such changes include an abnormally small lens (microphakia), an abnormally shaped lens (lenticonus and lentiglobus), and a congenital lens luxation, which is presumably secondary to some congenital abnormality in the zonules.

LENS LUXATION

Dislocation of the lens may be partial (subluxation) or complete (luxation). It may fall forward into the anterior chamber, or it may remain trapped in the posterior chamber. A completely dislocated lens is likely to develop a diffuse cataract, presumably because of its inadequate access to aqueous humor. Anterior lens luxation (Fig. 20-75) is much more significant

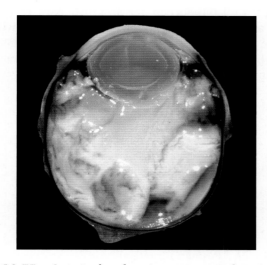

Fig. 20-75   Anterior lens luxation, eye, saggital section, dog. The dislocated, swollen lens has moved anteriorly to lie against the posterior surface of the cornea and has compressed the iris, creating pupillary blockage and secondary glaucoma. There is coagulation and opacification of the aqueous humor and the vitreous because of increased protein from inflammation. *(Courtesy Dr. B. Wilcock, Ontario Veterinary College.)*

because it predisposes to glaucoma (see under Glaucoma). Lens luxation may be primary or secondary.

Primary lens luxation refers to that occurring without any known trauma or other ocular disease. It may be congenital or it may be seen later in life. Congenital luxation is usually the result of a developmental error that causes abnormal or insufficient zonules. Much more prevalent are spontaneous luxations that occur in young adult dogs of specific breeds (notably terriers). The luxation is almost always bilateral, even if not simultaneous in onset. The ultrastructural and biochemical defect within the lens zonules have not been defined.

Secondary lens luxation is almost always a manifestation of blunt trauma, that causes avulsion of the zonules, or excessive stretching of zonules within a globe that has become greatly enlarged secondary to glaucoma. It may also occur as a result of lysis of zonules by neutrophil enzymes or perhaps bacterial proteases in septic endophthalmitis.

The potential consequences of lens luxation are numerous, but the most significant is glaucoma. This is particularly frequent with anterior lens luxation. The pathogenesis may involve several factors including anterior dislocation of the vitreous causing pupillary block and accumulation of degenerate zonular material within the trabecular meshwork. It is sometimes impossible to decide whether the luxation caused the glaucoma, or the glaucoma caused the luxation.

DIABETIC CATARACT

Rapidly progressing bilateral cataracts develop in at least 70% of spontaneously diabetic dogs (but not in cats). Progression to complete cortical opacity usually occurs within a few weeks. The swelling may be so rapid that the lens actually ruptures. The pathogenesis of the cataract has traditionally been ascribed to the excessively high level of glucose within the aqueous. Glucose is normally the major energy source for lens fibers via anaerobic glycolysis. When the rate-limiting enzyme of this pathway, hexokinase, is overloaded with glucose, most of the excess glucose absorbed by the lens is shunted to the sorbitol pathway where it is transformed into the polyalcohol sorbitol, which is then slowly reduced to a ketose. Sorbitol may accumulate to very high concentrations within the lens where it osmotically attracts water, resulting in rapid swelling of the lens and disruption of its critical architecture. Sorbitol-induced osmotic disruption alone is not sufficient to explain all of the structural and metabolic changes in sugar-induced cataracts. The efficacy of antioxidants in slowing the progression of such cataracts, the nature of intralenticular biochemical alterations, and detection of increased intralenticular oxidants all point to some kind of oxidative damage as an additional promoter of cataracts.

DISEASES OF THE RETINA

RETINAL ANOMALIES
RETINAL DYSPLASIA

Retinal dysplasia is a general term denoting an abnormal retinal differentiation characterized by jumbling of retinal layers. In the past, the term has been used rather loosely to include not only the rare genuine primary developmental anomalies, but also postnecrotic and/or postinflammatory retinal scarring within the developing retina, and retinal folding without any true disorganization. They should be considered as separate entities.

Primary retinal dysplasia is a rare anomaly that probably results from improper induction of retinal maturation by the RPE. Whether the failure relates to delayed and/or inadequate apposition between the two layers or a failure in the production of appropriate signaling molecules by the RPE is not known. The result is a retina with patchy-to-diffuse jumbling of the retinal layers (Fig. 20-76). Primary retinal dysplasia as the sole anomaly is seen as an inherited disease in a few breeds of dogs, but most examples are a part of multiple ocular anomalies. The significance of the lesion varies with the extent of dysplasia. Such retinas are prone to detachment (and in severe cases, the retina may never have been attached at all).

Postnecrotic retinal dysplasia is a much more frequent phenomenon, seen as a sequel to acquired retinal necrosis of the developing retina. In dogs and cats, the period of susceptibility extends for at least 6 weeks after birth, during which time the retina continues to develop. Most of the documented examples are sequelae to viral infection, but in theory virtually any kind of retinal injury during its development could result in postnecrotic retinal "dysplasia." In contrast to the adult retina, which retains no mitotic capability within the neurons of its various layers, the developing retina can still react with at least some neuronal regeneration. Such regeneration is usually mixed with glial scarring and does not restore perfect retinal architecture (Fig. 20-77).

The viruses most often implicated in causing retinal dysplasia in domestic animals are bovine virus diarrhea virus in cattle, bluetongue virus in sheep, herpesvirus in dogs, and both parvovirus and choroid virus in cats. The histologic lesions can be quite variable, but usually there is a combination of very subtle residual inflammation along with postnecrotic scarring in the retina, optic nerve, and perhaps the choroids. Only if these viral infections damage the retina while its neurons still have proliferative capacity, will there be additional findings of disorganized neuronal proliferations with blending of nuclear layers. Proliferation also occurs in the RPE, which may be stimulated to migrate into the overlying scarred retina or to proliferate in situ as plaques of fibroblast-like cells. The pathogenesis of the "dysplasia" is the same as for lesions caused by these agents in the brain—infection, and subsequent destruction of neurons (and possibly other cell types). The dysplasia is not specific to the mechanism of the cellular injury; it reflects only the unsuccessful attempts at postnecrotic healing in a retina still capable of at least some neuronal replication.

The window of susceptibility for the development of retinal dysplasia depends on the species (simply because the timetable for retinal development varies with the species). Infection of calves with bovine virus diarrhea virus between 79 and 150 days gestation regularly results in postnecrotic retinal dysplasia, which is the most frequent and certainly the most studied of the virally induced retinal dysplasias. The initial ocular lesion is necrotizing lymphocytic endophthalmitis with

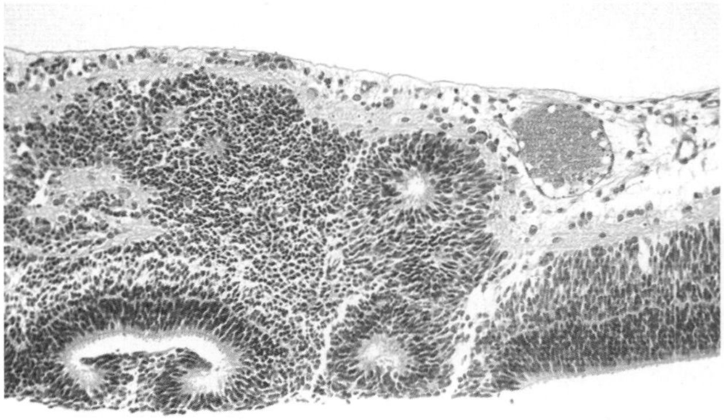

Fig. 20-76 **Primary retinal dysplasia, retina, puppy.** The cells of the retinal layers are poorly organized and arranged haphazardly, sometimes creating acinar-like structures known as retinal rosettes. H&E stain. (*Courtesy Dr. B. Wilcock, Ontario Veterinary College.*)

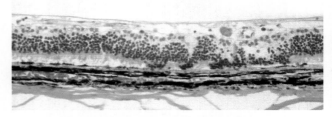

Fig. 20-77 **Postnecrotic retinal dysplasia (so-called), in utero bovine viral diarrhea (BVD) virus infection, retina, calf.** There is loss of nuclei from all retinal layers as a sequela to the in utero destruction of retinal neurons by BVD virus. In some instances, this loss is followed by efforts at retinal regeneration, resulting in disorganization that may be considered as a retinal dysplasia. H&E stain. (*Courtesy Dr. B. Wilcock, Ontario Veterinary College.*)

random retinal necrosis. The inflammation gradually subsides, so there is scant evidence of inflammation in fetuses aborted later or in dead neonatal calves. Those ocular structures (cornea, uvea, optic nerve) that are already well differentiated at the time of the endophthalmitis may remain normal or exhibit some postnecrotic scarring; only the retina will exhibit abortive efforts at regeneration. Because the peripheral retina remains mitotically active for several weeks after the central retina has matured, dysplastic lesions may be found only in the peripheral retina. It is said that all calves with BVD-associated retinal dysplasia will also have cerebellar hypoplasia. The same is probably true of cats with retinal dysplasia caused by in utero or perinatal infection with panleukopenia virus.

Retinal folding is by far the most common type of so-called retinal dysplasia. The great majority of such lesions are seen in juvenile purebred dogs. Most examples are inherited as autosomal recessive traits (sadly, so common in some breeds that they are now accepted as "normal variants"). The ophthalmoscopic findings and effect on vision vary from breed to breed. The histologic lesion is different from true retinal dysplasia and postnecrotic retinal dysplasia in that there is no jumbling of retinal layers, and there is no scarring. The exact pathogenesis for these retinal folds has not been determined, and it may not be the same among all breeds. What seems logical, however, is that the retinal folds represent nothing more than buckling of excessive retina within a globe because growth of the retina has been greater than that of the surrounding choroidal/scleral shell (Fig. 20-78). Supporting this speculation is the observation that such retinal folds are often transient and disappear as the puppy ages (implying that the growth rate of the scleral shell finally

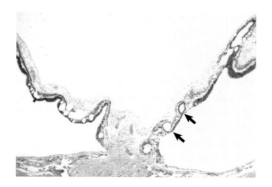

Fig. 20-78   Inherited retinal folds and retinal detachment, eye, posterior chamber, dog. The acinar-like structures *(arrows)* within the detached retina are transverse sections through retinal folds. These folds probably arise because the growth rate of the retina temporarily exceeds that of the sclera, forcing the retina to fold on itself. H&E stain. *(Courtesy Dr. B. Wilcock, Ontario Veterinary College.)*

"catches up" to that of the retina). The most severe examples occur in dogs with developmental retinal nonattachment. These have extensively folded retinas because the distance from optic disc to ora ciliaris in a straight line is shorter than the convex route taken by a normally attached retina.

Optic Nerve Hypoplasia

The true frequency of optic nerve hypoplasia is unknown. Most examples are seen in toy breeds of dogs, with the diagnosis being made by clinical examination. Because there is no apparent visual defect, these eyes are almost never available for histologic assessment and the exact nature of the defect (true hypoplasia versus atrophy) remains unknown. Genuine hypoplasia of the optic nerve is the expected result of prenatal or neonatal destruction of ganglion cells from any intraocular disease (including congenital glaucoma, viral infection, and neonatal septicemia with embolic endophthalmitis). The lesion should therefore be correctly classified as atrophy rather than hypoplasia, although the distinction becomes muddy when talking about injuries in the prenatal and perinatal periods.

A distinctly different pathogenesis explains optic nerve hypoplasia in calves born from cows with vitamin A deficiency or in young calves with persistent perinatal dietary deficiency. Atrophy of the nerve results from compression as it passes through an abnormally flattened foramen. The reason for the flattening is improper regulation of osteoblastic activity around the periphery of the developing foramen. Optic nerve damage is not seen if the deficiency in vitamin A occurs after 2 years of age.

ACQUIRED RETINAL DISEASE (TABLES 20-4 AND 20-5)
Canine Progressive Retinal Atrophy

Progressive retinal atrophy is the traditional designation for a large group of inherited bilateral degenerative retinopathies of dogs. These have become widespread because of deliberate restrictions of genetic diversity imposed by current line-breeding practices in purebred dogs. Innumerable breeds are affected, and the list grows daily. They all have a similar clinical and microscopic appearance, but that is where the uniformity ends. In reality, this group of diseases includes a genetically and biochemically diverse collection of photoreceptor dysplasias and degenerations that looked similar only when our methods of detection were limited to ophthalmoscopic evaluation and histopathologic examination. Its inclusion here as an acquired retinal disease rather than as a developmental disease is in deference to its clinical presentation and because at least some of this group are indeed true degenerations.

Table **20-4** **Acquired Retinal Diseases (Classified by Lesion)**

Photoreceptor Atrophy	Ganglion Cell Atrophy	Full-Thickness Necrosis	Retinitis	Other
PRA	Glaucoma	High pressure glaucoma (dogs only)	Localization of systemic infections	Storage diseases
Retinal detachment	Optic nerve injury (dieback)	Ischemic injury	Bystander reaction to endophthalmitis	Anomalies
Light-induced retinopathy		Vascular hypertension		
Drug toxicity		Vascular occlusion (thromboemboli, tumor)		
Nutritional deficiency				
Choroidal ischemia				

PRA, Progressive retinal atrophy.

Table **20-5** **Acquired Retinal Diseases (Classified by Pathogenesis)**

Ischemia	Inflammation	Trauma	Toxic/Metabolic	Developmental Error
Glaucoma*	Hematogenous infection	Detachment	Inherited photoreceptor dysplasias/degenerations	Retinal dysplasia
Detachment	Infection via penetrating injury	Hemorrhage/Infarction	Nutritional deficiency	
Hypertension	Bystander injury from endophthalmitis	Optic nerve trauma/ dieback neuropathy	Light-induced retinopathy	
Thromboembolism/ metastasis			Neuronal storage diseases	

*The role of ischemia in glaucomatous retinal atrophy is controversial and probably varies by type of glaucoma and by species.

The stereotypic features seen by light microscopy are loss of photoreceptor outer segments followed by progressive loss of inner segments and eventually loss of neurons from the outer nuclear layer. The result is collapse and thinning of the retina. Other portions of the retina remain normal, and there is no inflammation.

Currently, these bilateral noninflammatory photoreceptor dysfunctions are divided into developmental photoreceptor dysplasias and later-onset purely degenerative diseases. The classification of these various syndromes is under continuous review because in some cases what was once thought to be a degenerative disease affecting previously normal photoreceptors has been discovered to be an inborn biochemical error with a delayed phenotypic manifestation. The list of breeds in which photoreceptor dysplasia or degeneration has been described grows daily, so this brief discussion is not intended to be inclusive.

PHOTORECEPTOR DYSPLASIAS

The majority of the photoreceptor dysplasias cause clinical signs of bilateral, progressive blindness in juvenile dogs. The fundamental defect varies by breed; the defect may specifically target rods or cones, or affect both. Most examples have a simple, autosomal recessive inheritance pattern. The most thoroughly studied is the combined rod-cone dysplasia of Irish setter dogs. It is beyond the scope of this text to discuss all of the various photoreceptor dysplasias, so this one example will serve to illustrate the general model.

Rod-cone dysplasia of Irish setters is inherited as a simple autosomal recessive trait. Dogs homozygous for the defect have arrested differentiation and then deterioration of the rod external segments, with cones being much less affected. The defect is detected ultrastructurally as early as 16 days after birth, at which time the outer rod segments adjacent to the retinal pigment epithelium should be developing. There is essentially diffuse loss of all rod photoreceptors by 12 weeks of age. This is followed by loss of cones and cells of the outer nuclear layer. The central retina is affected earlier and more severely than is the peripheral retina. Biochemical abnormalities are detected as early as 1 week of age. There is a severe deficiency of the activity of the phosphodiesterase responsible for the continuous hydrolysis of cyclic guanine monophosphate (cGMP) within outer segments. This results in a tenfold excess of cGMP, which has been shown to be toxic to photoreceptors in vitro, and also inhibits photoreceptor development. The basic defect is defective messenger RNA in the gene encoding the outer segment-specific phosphodiesterase.

PHOTORECEPTOR DEGENERATIONS

Photoreceptor degeneration refers to an equally diverse group of diseases in which early development is (as far as we can currently detect) normal, and degeneration occurs later in life. Prototype for this group is a rod-cone degeneration in toy and miniature poodles (with virtually identical diseases seen in English and American cocker spaniels, Labrador retrievers, and Portuguese water dogs). This disease is classified as a true degeneration in that photoreceptor differentiation seems to be normal until 6 to 9 weeks of age. After this time, and progressing at an unpredictable rate, photoreceptor outer segments degenerate. Rods are affected earlier and with greater severity than are cones. The disease progresses at an unpredictable rate; affected dogs may not have clinical or ophthalmoscopic evidence of disease until 3 to 5 years of age (which, in breeding dogs, means that they will already have passed on the genetic defect). The macroscopic and histologic lesions begin centrally, around the optic disc, but eventually (by 6 to 7 years of age) the entire retina is affected and the dog is blind. The biochemical basis for the degeneration remains unknown.

INHERITED RETINAL DEGENERATION AND DYSPLASIA IN OTHER SPECIES

Inherited retinal dysplasias and degenerations have been reported as sporadic occurrences in a variety of cat breeds, but only in the Abyssinian breed has the syndrome been adequately studied. In this breed, there are two different diseases: early onset rod-cone dysplasia and late onset retinal degeneration affecting rods much sooner than cones. The early onset dysplasia is inherited as an autosomal dominant trait and is almost identical to the rod-cone dysplasia of Irish setter dogs. Retinal function deteriorates rapidly, with virtually all affected cats being blind before 1 year of age. In contrast, the late onset retinal degeneration is inherited as an autosomal recessive, and affected cats usually show no clinical signs until about 2 years of age; they may retain at least some useful vision throughout life. The earliest structural changes are loss of neurons from the outer nuclear layer and disintegration of rod outer segments.

Congenital stationary night blindness in horses (nyctalopia) is a poorly documented disease affecting the Appaloosa breed (occasionally others). At least in Appaloosas, it seems to be inherited. The visual defects and associated behavioral abnormalities are seen in foals in dim light. In most cases, it does not progress sufficiently to cause obviously defective vision in daytime. Retinal histology is normal.

OTHER (NONINHERITED) PHOTORECEPTOR DISEASES

Sudden acquired retinal degeneration (SARD) is an enigmatic, rapidly progressing, photoreceptor degeneration that is histologically identical to those of the inherited progressive retinal atrophies. Blindness occurs very rapidly (over a period of a few days to a few weeks). Affected dogs are adult or even elderly, and the disease can affect any breed or crossbreed. The funduscopic lesion is bilaterally symmetric and diffuse across the retina. Histologic studies of the early lesions are very few because there is no ethical justification for the surgical removal of these globes as the dogs are otherwise healthy. The disease has not been experimentally reproduced. The cause is unknown, but its occurrence is sometimes associated with polyuria, polydipsia, elevated serum cholesterol concentration, and increased serum alkaline phosphatase activity. Some, but not even the majority, of the affected dogs have adrenal cortical hyperfunction. How this malfunction causes the irreversible retinopathy, if indeed it does, is unknown. One small study demonstrated circulating, complement-fixing antibody to retinal S-antigen and interphotoreceptor retinoid-binding protein, raising the possibility that the disease is a cytotoxic autoimmune phenomenon.

Light-induced retinopathy is an important cause of blindness in animals maintained under inappropriate lighting conditions. The intensity and especially the duration of the light are important. Those species which, in their natural habitat, are preferentially nocturnal are particularly susceptible. The most susceptible group of all are deep-water fish maintained in aquariums with continuous artificial lighting or in shallow outdoor tanks without protection from sunlight. Outbreaks of blindness in different species of laboratory animals (especially albino rats) housed under continuous fluorescent lighting were the first to focus attention on this phenomenon.

The initial lesion is disruption of rod outer segment disks, followed by destruction of all photoreceptors and then their nuclei. At higher light intensities, but still within the range for "normal" room lighting, there may also be damage to neurons of the inner nuclear layer, and to astrocytes and Müller cells. The histologic changes are the same as those for most other photoreceptor diseases, so this specific etiologic diagnosis is made based on the circumstantial evidence of abnormally bright light or an inappropriate balance between high-light and low-light intervals. The mechanism by which "ordinary" light damages the retina is still incompletely understood. Even normal vision is a "destructive" event, with light activation of photopigments generating a lot of free radicals and requiring physiologic replacement of photopigments and photoreceptor membrane discs during periods of sleep. The most popular theory is that of light-induced excessive oxidation of the very abundant polyunsaturated long-chain fatty acids of the rod discs, with the generation of free radicals. These cause cell membrane damage, and without adequate dark intervals there is reduced opportunity for regeneration.

Taurine deficiency as a cause for photoreceptor degeneration is seen only in cats. It is now largely a historical disease because all commercial feline diets are supplemented with taurine. Cats are unable to synthesize taurine from cysteine in amounts adequate for retinal function. Cats eating inappropriate diets (most often, stealing dog food) develop focal retinal atrophy in a horizontal streak dorsal to the optic disc. The disease, at least in some cases, progresses slowly to generalized retinal atrophy and blindness. The clinical features are identical to those of a historical disease known as feline central retinal degeneration. It is now assumed that the two diseases are the same, but that may not be true in every single case. The histologic lesion is photoreceptor degeneration, initially involving cone outer segments, but eventually affecting rods as well. The rods of the peripheral retina are the last to degenerate.

Hypovitaminosis A as a cause for retinopathy is occasionally seen in groups of cattle or pigs receiving a ration deficient in vitamin A over a prolonged interval. Because most pastures have more than adequate vitamin A, deficiencies in cattle are likely to be seen only in animals raised in confinement and fed a poor quality ration (especially hay or grain that has been stored for a very long time). In adult animals, the effects of hypovitaminosis A first involve photoreceptor outer segments, slowly progressing to diffuse photoreceptor atrophy, loss of the outer nuclear layer, and eventually to complete retinal atrophy. These lesions have been reproduced in all domestic animals by feeding them specially formulated diets, but naturally occurring retinal lesions are seen almost exclusively in cattle. The deficiency of vitamin A results in a deficiency of rhodopsin within the photoreceptors. The initial ultrastructural lesion is swelling, followed by disintegration and fragmentation of the outer segments. Initially this can be reversed with vitamin A therapy until inner segments have also been affected.

Ischemic retinopathy may occur as a sequela to vascular occlusion within the retina itself or within the choroidal vasculature by tumor metastases or thromboemboli, as a sequela to retinal detachment, or as one of the mechanisms for retinal atrophy in glaucoma. Retinal ischemic injury may also occur subsequent to retinal or choroidal vasculitis associated with immune disease or a few infectious diseases, such as thrombotic meningoencephalitis of cattle or Rocky Mountain spotted fever or ehrlichiosis in dogs (Fig. 20-79). The microvascular disease associated with diabetes mellitus is an exceedingly important cause of ischemic retinopathy in human beings, but examples in domestic animals with spontaneous diabetes are rare.

Vascular hypertension is an additional and relatively common cause for devastating retinal ischemic

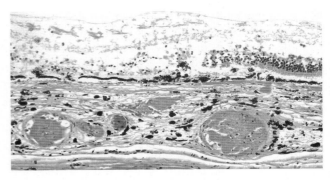

Fig. 20-79 **Choroidal vasculitis with thrombosis, choroid and retina, horse.** Dilated choroidal blood vessels contain fibrin thrombi and are surrounded by edema and some hemorrhage. There is ischemic necrosis of the overlying retina. The horse retina, with its very limited intrinsic vasculature, should theoretically be more susceptible to infarction secondary to choroidal vascular disease than the retina of any other domestic mammal. Such lesions are occasionally seen with disseminated intravascular coagulation regardless of the pathogenesis, as well as with idiopathic coagulopathies. H&E stain. *(Courtesy Dr. B. Wilcock, Ontario Veterinary College.)*

damage in dogs and cats. It is usually secondary to chronic renal failure. At least 60% of dogs with chronic renal failure are hypertensive.

The clinical disease is characterized by hemorrhage within the retina or from the retina into the posterior vitreous and retinal detachment secondary to serous effusion from injured retinal and choroidal blood vessels. The histologic lesions are primarily in retinal and choroidal vessels, but they may be found throughout the uvea. Characteristic changes are most easily found in the small retinal muscular arteries and larger arterioles. The vessel lesions include mural edema that may progress to fibrinoid necrosis of the tunica media and perivascular fibrosis. Muscular hypertrophy may occur in larger vessels, particularly those of the choroid. Changes occurring as a consequence of the vascular damage include localized retinal necrosis, serous retinal separation with resultant atrophy of photoreceptors and hypertrophy of retinal pigmented epithelium, and intraretinal hemorrhage (Fig. 20-80). There may be necrosis and/or repair of cells of the RPE, and sclerosis within the choroid. The severity of the retinal necrosis varies from focal infarcts in the inner retina to (more commonly) extensive full-thickness hemorrhagic infarcts in large segments of retina. The larger lesions probably reflect the effects of widespread choroidal and retinal vascular degeneration. At least some of the retinal lesions are not the direct result of vascular necrosis, but are the result of exaggerated autoregulatory vasoconstriction of precapillary sphincters attempting to protect the retinal capillary bed from the systemic hypertension.

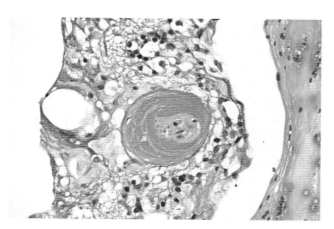

Fig. 20-80   Retinal hypertensive vasculopathy, retina, dog. There is fibrinoid necrosis of the retinal arteriole and nonselective ischemic necrosis of the surrounding retina. The dog had end-stage retinal disease. H&E stain. *(Courtesy Dr. B. Wilcock, Ontario Veterinary College.)*

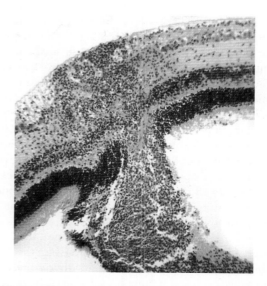

Fig. 20-81   Suppurative embolic retinitis, retina, steer. There is focal obliteration of the retina by a combination of necrosis and inflammation. The leukocytes extend through the outer nuclear layer into subretinal space. This lesion is common in bovine thrombotic meningoencephalitis but is occasionally seen in other bacteremic or septicemic diseases. H&E stain. *(Courtesy Dr. B. Wilcock, Ontario Veterinary College.)*

Sustained vasoconstriction leads to ischemic necrosis of the deprived retina, RPE or choroid, and necrosis of vascular endothelium distal to the constricted precapillary sphincters. Any blood that does manage to pass through the constricted sphincters into the capillaries enters blood vessels already damaged by a drop in perfusion pressure, so there is inevitable transmural leakage of serum and even blood.

RETINITIS

Retinitis as the sole ocular lesion is rare. When it does occur, however, it is almost always in the course of neurotropic virus infections, such as canine distemper, rabies, and pseudorabies. Additional diseases that frequently cause prominent retinal lesions (albeit virtually never retinal lesions alone) include toxoplasmosis, canine ehrlichiosis and Rocky Mountain spotted fever, and thrombotic meningoencephalitis of cattle (Fig. 20-81). The lesions in the retina are the same as those in any the other tissue affected by these systemic diseases. Retinal lesions also occur in the course of visceral larval migrans caused by the migration of the larvae of *Toxocara canis* and *Baylisascaris procyonis*.

DISEASES OF THE EYELIDS
DEVELOPMENTAL ANOMALIES

Anomalies in the formation of eyelids, including the shape of the palpebral fissure, are exceedingly common in dogs because "eye shape" has been so extensively manipulated during the evolution of the various breeds. In some instances, the "anomaly" is even a required feature for the breed (as with ectropion in Bloodhounds and Saint Bernards, for example). Most of these anomalies

are not examined microscopically because they are macroscopically obvious. They are important in clinical ophthalmology, and so they are considered in much greater detail in clinical textbooks than they are here.

EYELID AGENESIS AND COLOBOMA

Particularly in cats, there may be partial or complete absence of an eyelid. The most common by far is a partial defect (i.e., coloboma) involving only the upper eyelid. The notchlike defect results in localized corneal desiccation followed by cutaneous metaplasia.

PREMATURE EYELID SEPARATION

The normal fusion of eyelids (known as physiologic ankyloblepharon) in carnivores is essential to protect the immature cornea from infection and desiccation. Premature eyelid separation (technically a "maldevelopment" because it occurs before the maturation of the globe) seriously predisposes the eye to infectious keratitis, desiccation, and even corneal rupture.

ENTROPION AND ECTROPION

Entropion is the inward rolling of the eyelid margin because of inadequate overall length. The usual result is irritation of the cornea by the eyelid skin, cilia, and/or hair. It is a very common anomaly in purebred dogs because they have been selected for breeding based partly on the shape of the palpebral fissure, which is a factor in determining facial "expression."

The extent and magnitude of the defect varies greatly among individual animals, but tends to be relatively uniform within an affected breed. Clinical textbooks have extensive accounts of the manifestations of entropion and ectropion in different breeds and the innumerable techniques for their repair. The outcome for the cornea varies from corneal cutaneous metaplasia to outright ulceration, depending on the severity of the irritation. Entropion may also be acquired as the result of inflammation and subsequent contracture of a scar in the eyelid.

Ectropion is created by undue laxity of an excessively long eyelid, resulting in an outward gaping of the eyelid margin. As with entropion, its extent and severity vary greatly among individual animals and among breeds. The lower eyelid is more frequently affected to a clinically significant degree than the upper, presumably because the effect of gravity on the upper eyelid makes ectropion there less obvious. The anomaly has less significance than entropion because there is no direct corneal irritation. The protruding conjunctiva may entrap debris and become chronically inflamed and because of the failure of the lids to close properly, there may be some chronic exposure keratitis.

ANOMALIES OF EYELASHES: TRICHIASIS, DISTICHIASIS, AND ECTOPIC CILIA

These are prevalent in dogs and may or may not cause clinical signs, depending on whether they irritate the cornea or not. They are mentioned here only for the sake of completeness because these are almost never evaluated histologically. Distichiasis is the presence of an ectopic row of cilia originating from the ducts of the Meibomian glands. The defect is usually bilateral. It may be clinically silent or cause corneal irritation. Trichiasis is misdirection of the normal cilia, so that they contact the cornea. Ectopic cilia are abnormally placed cilia within the lamina propria of the conjunctiva. Their emergence through the palpebral conjunctiva may result in profound corneal irritation.

ACQUIRED DISEASES

Chalazion is sterile granulomatous inflammation in response to the leakage of Meibomian secretion into the surrounding dermis. It is much more common in dogs than in any other species. Although it can theoretically occur in response to any type of injury to the Meibomian gland, in almost all cases, the inflammation is found adjacent to Meibomian adenomas. Histologically the inflammation is an accumulation of large foamy macrophages and multinucleated cells around the abnormal Meibomian gland. Some of the lipid may occur in the form of extracellular lakes of unstained free lipid, especially in cats. The macrophages contain distinctive slender, birefringent, intracellular crystals, which are readily visible under polarized light.

Idiopathic granulomatous marginal blepharitis is seen only in dogs as a series of coalescing nodules that eventually create a diffuse thickening of one or both eyelid margins. The histologic lesion is a coalescence of suppurating granulomas in the subconjunctival tissue of the eyelid margin, without any proven association with any particular adnexal structure, such as a Meibomian gland or hair follicle. The lesion is very similar to those of cutaneous sterile pyogranuloma syndrome and other idiopathic granulomatous panniculitides, for all of which the pathogeneses are unknown. No infectious agent has ever been identified.

NEOPLASMS OF THE EYELIDS

Meibomian adenoma is by far the most common tumor of the canine eyelid, accounting for in excess of 80% of all eyelid tumors in that species. Eyelid tumors in any other species are infrequent to rare. The tumor is an exact counterpart of sebaceous adenomas seen elsewhere in skin: a smooth expansile growth populated by intermingled basal cells and mature sebaceous cells. The tumor usually retains well-developed lobular architecture and in some cases differs from a normal gland only by its much greater overall size (Fig. 20-82). Many are populated almost exclusively by basal cells with just a few foci of sebaceous differentiation. Many contain substantial amounts of melanin pigment. Behaviorally, they are benign and are easily cured by excision.

Melanocytoma is the second most common tumor of the canine eyelid. It is identical in all respects to superficial dermal melanocytomas found elsewhere in the skin, and it is universally benign (Fig. 20-83).

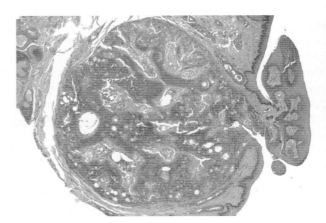

Fig. 20-82 **Meibomian adenoma, eyelid, dog.** The tumor is a well-demarcated, encapsulated, expansile nodule consisting of intermingled basal and sebaceous cells. The accompanying papillary hyperplasia of the overlying epidermis is a common secondary reactive change. H&E stain. *(Courtesy Dr. B. Wilcock, Ontario Veterinary College.)*

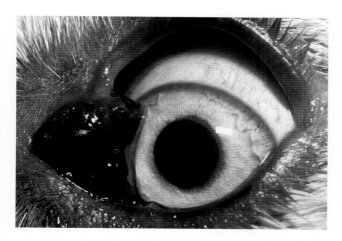

Fig. 20-83   Cutaneous melanocytoma, eyelid skin, dog.
A nodule of firm black tissue has replaced a wedge of the eyelid skin at its margin. Determining the exact location of the mass is clinically critical because a similar tumor arising even a few millimeters away on the palpebral conjunctiva would probably be behaviorally malignant. (*Courtesy Dr. R. Peiffer, University of North Carolina.*)

Other neoplasms affecting the eyelid with greater-than-usual frequency include nerve sheath tumors in dogs and cats, squamous cell carcinoma and mast cell tumors in cats, and sarcoids in horses. They are identical in histologic appearance and behavior to those tumors occurring anywhere else in skin.

DISEASES OF THE CONJUNCTIVA
DEVELOPMENTAL ANOMALIES
CONJUNCTIVAL DERMOID

As with corneal dermoid, this is the presence of ectopic hair follicles and adnexal glands within the conjunctiva. Ordinarily, it is the bulbar conjunctiva that is affected. The ectopic tissue ranges from just a few scattered sebaceous glands to mature hair follicles with a full complement of adnexa.

ACQUIRED CONJUNCTIVAL DISEASES
INFECTIOUS DISEASES

Infectious bovine rhinotracheitis (bovine herpesvirus 1) is usually accompanied by serous to purulent conjunctivitis, which can be confused clinically with infectious bovine keratoconjunctivitis caused by *Moraxella bovis*. However, corneal involvement with rhinotracheitis is uncommon, and it is never the major presenting complaint and never reaches the severity seen in infectious bovine keratoconjunctivitis. Following the acute serous conjunctivitis, hyperplasia of the resident conjunctival lymphoid nodules (follicular lymphoid hyperplasia) frequently occurs. Macroscopically, this is evident as a series of glistening gray-white protruding nodules a few millimeters in diameter, visible through the epithelium of the bulbar and palpebral conjunctiva.

Feline infectious conjunctivitis is caused by mycoplasma, chlamydia, or herpesvirus. The microscopic lesions are not specific except for the presence of inclusion bodies characteristic of the specific infectious agent. Unfortunately, inclusion bodies are present only during the first few days of disease and are almost never present by the time cytologic or histologic samples are obtained. Thus the presumptive diagnosis is usually based on the clinical characteristics of the conjunctival disease, and especially on the presence of other clinical signs. Because these agents are all quite widely distributed in the healthy feline population, one must use great caution in interpreting a positive result of a serologic or PCR test as indicating a causal role for that organism in the disease in that patient.

Feline herpesvirus 1 causes a combination of conjunctivitis, keratitis, and upper respiratory disease when it first affects young cats, but it may cause conjunctivitis alone as a recurring infection in older cats that have recovered from the initial, more widespread disease. Herpesvirus is a more significant cause of keratitis in cats.

Mycoplasma felis and *Mycoplasma gatae* have been reported to cause suppurative, erosive conjunctivitis. However, a review of the available evidence suggests that it is more likely that these mycoplasmas, which are members of the normal feline conjunctival flora, act only as significant opportunists in disease initiated by herpesvirus or chlamydia.

Chlamydia psittaci usually causes unilateral conjunctivitis in cats of any age, without any other associated disease. The conjunctivitis is initially neutrophilic but rapidly becomes a subepithelial mixture of neutrophils, macrophages, lymphocytes, and plasma cells. Early in the disease (between days 7 and 14), typical intracytoplasmic inclusion bodies can be seen, and their detection is improved by immunofluorescent staining. Because the clinical signs are characteristic and disease is easily treated, histologic assessment is rarely required. By the time histologic assessment is required in the few cases not responding to therapy, it is too late: The lesions have become completely nonspecific lymphonodular conjunctivitis with no visible inclusion bodies.

Thelazia are thin, rapidly motile nematodes 7 to 20mm in length that inhabit the conjunctival sac and lacrimal duct of a variety of wild and domestic mammals. They are perhaps not exactly "normal" in the conjunctival sac, but only a small proportion of animals infected with the parasite have clinical disease. They are transmitted from animal to animal by face flies, which ingest larvae in lacrimal secretions. In North America, they are of minor significance as parasites of horses, and cause only a mild lymphonodular conjunctivitis.

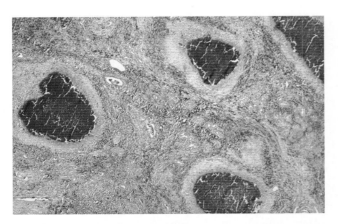

Fig. 20-84   Granulomatous conjunctivitis with eosinophils (focal), habronemiasis, conjunctiva, horse. Note the multiple coalescing eosinophil-rich granulomas within the conjunctival lamina propria. These granulomas are old larval migration tracts, but habronema larvae are rarely visible in them by the time such lesions are sampled for histological examination (usually to rule out neoplasia). H&E stain. *(Courtesy Dr. B. Wilcock, Ontario Veterinary College.)*

Habronemiasis is a far more significant disease in horses. It causes oozing eosinophilic granulomas, up to one centimeter in diameter, in the palpebral and bulbar conjunctivae. The macroscopic lesion is a firm nodule with yellow, caseous gritty debris in the center. The lesion is in response to nematode larvae deposited by a fly intermediate host, usually *Musca domestica* or *Stomoxys calcitrans*. They are attracted to this location by the moisture collecting in the medial canthus. Larvae of *Habronema muscae*, *Habronema microstoma* or *Draschia (Habronema) megastoma* are also capable of causing the same histologic lesion that is identical to cutaneous habronemiasis, a chronic eosinophilic and granulomatous inflammation surrounding live or dead larvae that are difficult to find in histologic sections (Fig. 20-84).

IDIOPATHIC AND IMMUNE DISEASES

Idiopathic eosinophilic conjunctivitis is probably the conjunctival counterpart of the eosinophilic keratitis syndrome seen in cats and occasionally in horses. Rarely the conjunctival lesion exists without any obvious corneal involvement. Lesions may be unilateral or bilateral. The microscopic lesions are greatly influenced by age and the previous antiinflammatory therapy, so it is hard to know what the "real" lesions are. In biopsy samples, the usual changes include ulceration, epithelial hyperplasia, squamous metaplasia, and a notable lymphocytic infiltration with a large number of eosinophils. The presence of eosinophils is a requirement for the diagnosis. They are not present as part of a granulomatous disease as in habronemiasis, nor are they associated with collagenolysis as seen in insect bite reactions.

Protrusion and/or prolapse of the gland of the third eyelid is quite common in dogs and is thought to be the result of laxity in the connective tissue anchoring the gland to the cartilage of the third eyelid. Because the prolapsed mass is unsightly and resembles a neoplasm, it is sometimes excised and submitted for histologic examination, which reveals that the gland is usually completely normal or has mild nonspecific changes in response to desiccation or chronic edema.

Nodular granulomatous episcleritis (NGE) is a prevalent nodular lesion of the conjunctival lamina propria of dogs. It has been known by many names over the years, reflecting confusion about its exact status as an immune-mediated proliferative disease or a histiocytic neoplasm. Some of the synonyms include ocular nodular fasciitis, fibrous histiocytoma, or collie granuloma. It is not known whether this is one disease or several different diseases with the same histologic appearance. The disease is defined by its histopathologic changes: a discrete nodular accumulation of macrophages, fibroblasts, lymphocytes, and plasma cells anywhere in the conjunctival lamina propria. These cells are uniformly intermingled, without the formation of discrete granulomas. There is no collagenolysis, and usually there is not a significant number of granulocytes. The lateral limbus is the most frequent site, but the third eyelid is also frequently affected. In most instances, the lesion is unilateral and solitary, but bilateral involvement is not uncommon.

Necrotic scleritis is another canine idiopathic "immune-mediated" disease that may be mistaken for NGE. It often begins as a nodular thickening of the bulbar conjunctiva or underlying sclera just posterior to the limbus. Microscopically, however, it is a more destructive lesion with collagenolysis and (at least in the early disease) numerous eosinophils in addition to the macrophages, fibroblasts, and lymphocytes, which are also seen in NGE. It is a rapidly progressive and destructive lesion, capable of spreading rapidly to involve large areas of the sclera. Late in the disease it may spread into the globe, causing destructive coalescing granulomas throughout the uvea.

NEOPLASMS OF THE CONJUNCTIVA

Squamous cell carcinoma is an exceedingly prevalent and economically significant neoplasm affecting the sunlight-exposed, nonpigmented epithelium of the eyelids, bulbar conjunctiva, usually at the lateral limbus and third eyelid of cattle living outdoors in sunny environments. The frequency is highest in areas in which livestock are likely to be exposed to ultraviolet radiation: areas with high altitude and lots of sunshine. Animals with poor pigmentation of eyelids and conjunctiva are particularly susceptible because this increases the risk of chronic cellular injury from solar radiation. Viruses such as bovine papillomavirus and bovine herpesvirus 5 have been detected within bovine ocular squamous cell carcinomas, but their causal role has not been proven. An identical tumor occurs in horses living in the same environments.

As occurs with sunlight-induced squamous cell carcinoma in other cutaneous locations, the ocular tumor goes through a series of precancerous changes in response to actinic injury. The sequence of lesions is squamous plaque (acanthosis), keratoses (localized foci of hyperkeratosis), squamous papilloma, dysplasia, squamous carcinoma in situ, and eventually invasive squamous cell carcinoma (Fig. 20-85). Keratoses can sometimes develop into cutaneous horns. These are usually conical, can reach a length of a few centimeters, and consist of compacted laminated keratin (Fig. 20-86). Occasionally, they are on the surface of a papilloma. Like actinic keratoses they are considered

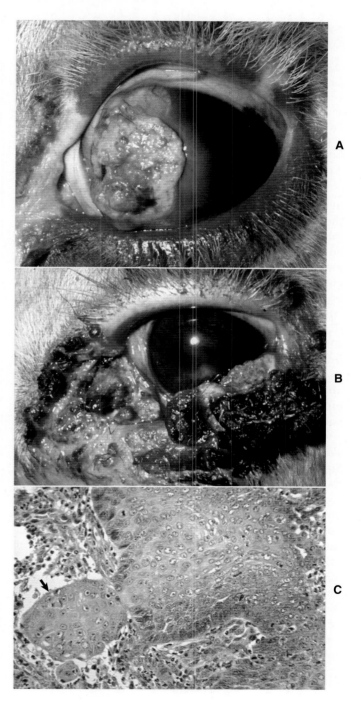

Fig. 20-85   Squamous cell carcinoma, eye and eyelids, Hereford cow. A, Medial limbus. The carcinoma has spread over the cornea as an exophytic growth from its original site on the medial limbus. Note the corneal edema (*gray area*) adjacent to the margin of the carcinoma. Pigmentation of the eyelids, as shown here, does not protect the conjunctiva or the limbus from developing an actinic (exposure to sunlight) squamous cell carcinoma. **B,** Third and lower eyelids. Note the early exophytic squamous cell carcinoma on the third eyelid, nodules of acanthosis on the lateral half of the lower lid conjuctiva and on the skin of the medial canthus, and keratoses on the lower lid. **C,** Early infiltrative squamous cell carcinoma, lower lid. A small group (*arrow*) of epithelial cells has infiltrated through the basement membrance of the mucosal squamous epithelium. Note that these cells are atypical. The basal cells have lost their polarity and now lie horizontal to the edge of the infiltrating mass instead of vertically, as do normal basal cells (perpendicular to the basement membrane). H&E stain. (*A, B,* and *C, Courtesy Dr. M.D. McGavin, College of Veterinary Medicine, University of Tennessee.*)

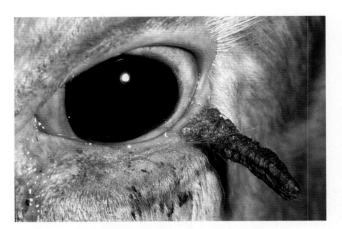

Fig. 20-86   Cutaneous horn, lower eyelid, mucocutaneous junction. The cutaneous horn on the lower lid is an exaggerated form of a keratosis. The unpigmented skin of the lower lid and medial canthus is erythematous, and the surface of the medial aspect of the lower lid is slightly roughed by white foci of acanthosis. *(Courtesy Dr. M.D. McGavin, College of Veterinary Medicine, University of Tennessee.)*

to be premalignant. The stepwise transition from acanthosis to eventual carcinoma in situ is characterized by increasing nuclear pleomorphism, hyperchromasia, and loss of polarity of the cells and maturational jumbling of cells within the stratum spinosum. The only absolutely unequivocal proof of malignant transformation is invasion by cords of malignant cells through the basement membrane into the underlying lamina propria (Fig. 20-85, C). The mass of invading cells is usually surrounded by an intense lymphocytic-plasmacytic inflammatory reaction, a reaction which is interpreted as an immune response to the developing tumor. Not all precursor lesions develop into carcinomas. The efficacy of the immune response in destroying precursor lesions and early carcinomas is unknown.

In cats, squamous cell carcinoma usually affects the skin of the eyelid itself rather than conjunctiva. Squamous cell carcinoma is inexplicably rare in either the eyelids or the conjunctiva of dogs.

Benign squamous papillomas with no inclination for malignant progression are frequent tumors of the bulbar conjunctiva of dogs. They are formed by multiple slender fronds consisting of conjunctival lamina propria covered by hyperplastic, but otherwise orderly and mature stratified squamous nonkeratinized epithelium. There is often substantial melanin pigment within the basal cells and lamina propria, so these tumors can be mistaken on clinical examination for conjunctival melanomas. There is no evidence that these papillomas are caused by a viral infection.

Primary conjunctival melanomas arise within the epithelium of the bulbar conjunctiva of dogs and cats.

In dramatic contrast to the benign melanotic tumors of the haired skin of the eyelid or those arising deeper within the stroma of the limbus (see later discussion), these are aggressively invasive with a high risk of metastasis. They resemble oral melanomas in histologic and cytologic appearance, and in the frequency of being amelanotic. Microscopically, they form solid endocrine-like packets of 20 to 30 cells supported by a delicate fibrous stroma. Intraepithelial clusters (junctional activity) are often present. The cells generally are pleomorphic epithelioid cells with frequent nuclear gigantism and hyperchromasia. They are markedly invasive, a feature often visible in histologic sections. Postoperative recurrence is extremely frequent. Pigment, when present, is most frequently found in tumor cells within or near the epithelium.

Limbal melanocytomas are relatively common tumors in dogs. They are infrequent but not rare in cats. They arise from the pigmented cells within the limbus, which is the junction of the corneal stroma and sclera. They form a slowly expanding, heavily pigmented discrete nodule populated by heavily pigmented large plump cells identical to those seen in the more common anterior uveal melanocytoma. They have no metastatic potential, and surgical excision is curative. They may bulge outwardly to distend the overlying conjunctiva, but histologic examination reveals that they do not infiltrate the epithelium and they are therefore easily distinguished from the more dangerous primary conjunctival malignant melanoma.

Hemangioma and hemangiosarcoma are vascular endothelial neoplasms arising within the conjunctival lamina propria at the lateral edge of the third eyelid, and in the lateral bulbar conjunctiva of dogs, cats, and (occasionally) horses. About 30% of canine cases are bilateral. The sites of predilection and the increased risk of disease in outdoor dogs in sunny climates and high altitudes suggest that this disease is probably triggered by chronic actinic radiation injury (as is true for at least some examples of cutaneous hemangioma and hemangiosarcoma in dogs). Those tumors that are well circumscribed and consist of bland endothelium are classified as hemangiomas, and those formed by hyperchromatic endothelium with at least moderate anisokaryosis and peripheral invasion are classified as hemangiosarcomas. However, there is a continuum in the histologic appearance from hemangioma to hemangiosarcoma. Many are intermediate, or even show a continuum of lesions from benign to malignant within the same tumor. Distinguishing benign from malignant is based primarily on the degree of peripheral invasion. At least in dogs (the species most often affected), this distinction appears to have no behavioral significance, as almost all are benign and surgically curable.

In horses, some (but not all) of the vascular tumors involving the third eyelid are solid primitive hemangiosarcomas. Some of these tumors are very invasive and have a high risk of metastasis to the regional lymph node.

Adenocarcinoma of the gland of the third eyelid is a tumor of very old dogs (rarely cats), which is usually seen as a well-differentiated, slowly expanding tubular adenocarcinoma at the dorsal margin of the third eyelid. It replaces the normal gland of the third eyelid but only slowly invades adjacent tissue. The risk of metastasis is very low.

Lymphoma (lymphosarcoma) occasionally arises within the lamina propria of the third eyelid in animals (most often in cats) that do not have any evidence of disseminated lymphosarcoma. The cells are similar in histologic appearance to those of lymphomas elsewhere, but it takes courage to make this diagnosis when the tumor appears to be present in only a single, unlikely location, such as the third eyelid.

DISEASES OF THE ORBIT

Orbital cellulitis is not a specific disease but inflammation of soft tissue in response to infectious agents introduced via a penetrating wound, a migrating foreign body, or an inflammatory focus from some adjacent tissue (often, a tooth root abscess). Only rarely does panophthalmitis extend into the orbit to cause orbital cellulitis because the sclera seems to be an effective barrier to the migration of leukocytes and infectious agents.

Lymphocytic interstitial dacryoadenitis is a progressive idiopathic lymphocytic inflammation of the lacrimal gland and/or gland of the third eyelid of dogs. It is present as a histologic lesion in most cases of spontaneous keratoconjunctivitis sicca. The initial lesion is an interstitial lymphocytic infiltration with epithelial necrosis, followed by glandular atrophy and extensive interstitial fibrosis with residual nests of lymphocytes. Because no infectious agent can be found and because the disease can be successfully managed with immunosuppressive therapy (particularly cyclosporin), it is assumed to represent a T-lymphocyte–dependent autoimmune disease.

Orbital extraocular myositis affects all the extraocular muscles except the retractor bulbi. It is a rare disease of dogs. Histologically, there is a lymphocytic myositis that results in myonecrosis, followed by attempts at regeneration and eventually muscle atrophy and fibrosis. The acute disease causes enough swelling to result in pain and exophthalmos. In the chronic disease, there is a notable enophthalmos (retraction of the globe into the orbit). An immune-mediated attack directed specifically against the extraocular muscles is suspected to be the cause of this disorder. Because the extraocular muscles are a difficult site from which to obtain a biopsy, diagnosis is generally based on the typical clinical findings. Corticosteroid therapy is effective, but episodes can recur.

Orbital neoplasms are surprisingly frequent in dogs. They are rare in other domestic animals with the exception of cattle, in which malignant lymphoma occurs. Most orbital tumors are not discovered until they are large enough to cause exophthalmos or blindness, by which time the majority of cases are no longer amenable to surgical cure. Many different tumors in the orbit have been reported, but the only ones that are relatively frequent are optic nerve meningioma and multilobular osteochondroma in dogs, nasal carcinoma and gingival squamous cell carcinoma in dogs and cats, and malignant lymphoma in cattle. These tumors are all histologically identical to those in other locations.

SUGGESTED READINGS

Brown MH et al: Infectious bovine keratoconjunctivitis—a review, *J Vet Intern Med* 12:259-266, 1996.

Cook CS: Ocular embryology and congenital malformations. In Gelatt KN, editor: *Veterinary ophthalmology*, ed 3, Baltimore, 1999, Lippincott Williams & Wilkins.

Dubielzig RR et al: Morphologic features of feline ocular sarcomas in 10 cats: light microscopy, ultrastructure, and immunohistochemistry, *Prog Vet Comp Ophthalmol* 4:7-12, 1994.

Dubielzig RR et al: Iridociliary epithelial tumors in 100 dogs and 17 cats: a morphological study, *Vet Ophthalmol* 1:223-231, 1998.

Gelatt KN, Brooks DE: The canine glaucomas. In Gelatt KN, editor: *Veterinary ophthalmology*, ed 3, Baltimore, 1999, Lippincott Williams & Wilkins.

Grahn B et al: Equine keratomycosis: clinical and laboratory findings in 23 cases, *Prog Vet Comp Ophthalmol* 3:2-7, 1993.

Klenkler B, Sheardown H: Growth factors in the anterior segment: role in tissue maintenance, wound healing and ocular pathology, *Exp Eye Res* 79:677-688, 2004.

McKenna KC, Kapp JA: Ocular immune privilege and CTL tolerance, *Immunol Res* 29:103-112, 2004.

Paulsen ME et al: Feline eosinophilic keratitis: a review of 15 clinical cases, *J Am Anim Hosp Assoc* 23:63-68, 1987.

Peiffer RL Jr, Wilcock BP: Histopathologic study of uveitis in cats: 139 cases (1978-1988), *J Am Vet Med Assoc* 198:135-138, 1991.

Peiffer RL, Wilcock BP, Yin H: The pathogenesis and significance of pre-iridal fibrovascular membrane in domestic animals, *Vet Pathol* 27:41-45, 1990.

Van der Woerdt A: Lens-induced uveitis, *Vet Ophthalmol* 3:227-234, 2000.

Whiteley HE: Dysplastic canine retinal morphogenesis, *Invest Ophthalmol Vis Sci* 32:1492-1498, 1991.

Wilcock BP, Dubielzig RR, Render JA: *Histological classification of ocular and otic tumors of domestic animals*, WHO international histologic classification of tumors of domestic animals, second series, Washington, 2002, AFIP.

Wilcock BP, Peiffer RL Jr: Morphology and behavior of primary ocular melanomas in 91 dogs, *Vet Pathol* 23:418-424, 1986.

Wilcock BP, Peiffer RL Jr: The pathology of lens-induced uveitis in dogs, *Vet Pathol* 24:549-553, 1987.

Index